Advances and Innovations in Heart Failure (AIHF)

A Textbook of Cardiology

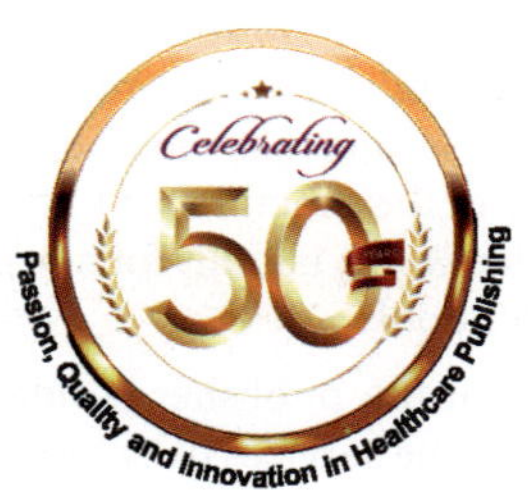

DISCLAIMER

The views and opinions expressed in this book are solely those of the original contributor (s)/author (s) and do not necessarily represent those of editor (s) of the book.

All brand names and product names used in this book are trade names, service marks, trademarks or registered trademarks of their respective owners. The publisher is not associated with an product or vendor mentioned in this book.

Medical knowledge and practice change constantly. This book is designed to provide accurate, authoritative information about the subject matter in question. However, readers are advised to check the most current information available on procedures included and check information from the manufacturer of each product to be administered, to verify the recommended dose, formula, method and duration of administration, adverse effects and contraindications. It is the responsibility of the practitioner to take all appropriate safety precaution. Neither the publisher nor the author (s)/ editor (s) assume any liability for any injury and /or damage to persons or property arising from or related to use of material in this book.

This book is sold on the understanding that the publisher is not engaged in providing professional medical services. If such advice or services are required, the services of a competent medical professional should be sought.

Every effort has been made, where necessary, to contact holders of copyright to obtain permission to reproduce copyright material. If any has been inadvertently overlooked, the publisher will be pleased to make the necessary arrangements at the first opportunity.

Advances and Innovations in Heart Failure (AIHF)

A Textbook of Cardiology

Editors-in-Chief

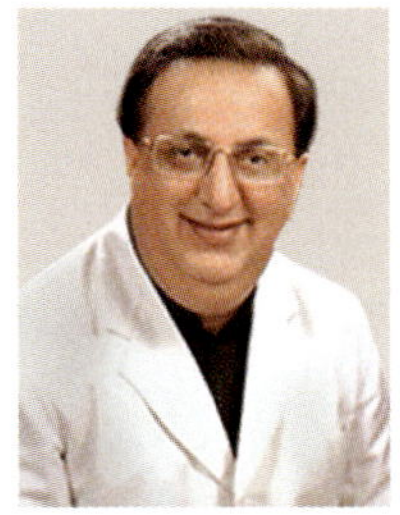

HK Chopra
National President, IAE- 2017
National President, CSI -2015
Chairman, World Wellness Foundation
Country Head, American Heart Association
Chief Cardiologist, Moolchand Medcity
New Delhi, India

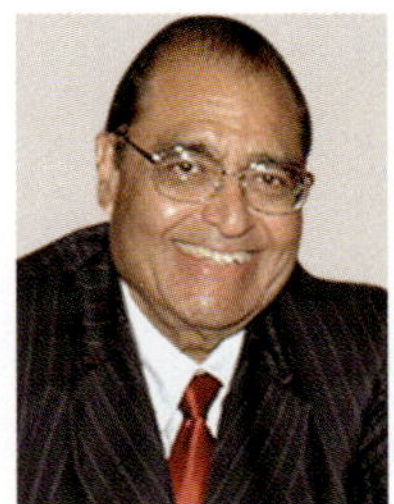

Navin C Nanda
Distinguished Professor of Medicine and
Cardiovascular Disease
University of Alabama at Birmingham
Birmingham Alabama, USA
Editor-in-Chief, Echocardiography A Journal of
Cardiovascular Ultrasound and Allied Techniques

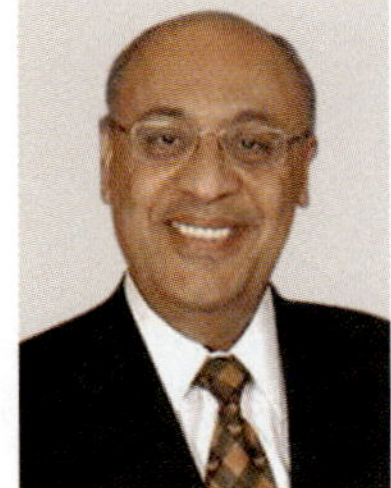

Jagat Narula
Trustee, American College of Cardiology
Director, Cardiovascular Imaging Program
Mount Sinai Cardiovascular Institute
Editor-in-Chief, JACC: CV Imaging
New York, USA

Principal Editors

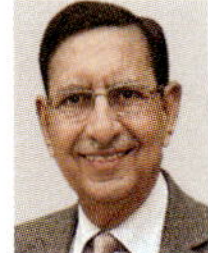

KK Sethi
Director of Cardiology
Chairman and Managing Director
Delhi Heart and Lung Institute
New Delhi, India
Past President, CSI

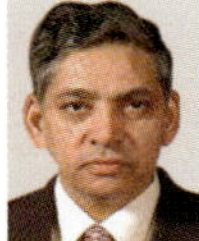

KK Talwar
Chairman, Department of Cardiology
Max Super Specialty Hospital
New Delhi, India
Formerly Director, PGIMER
Chandigarh, India

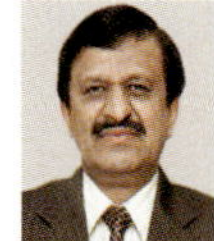

CN Manjunath
Professor of Cardiology
Director, Sri Jayadeva Institute of
Cardiovascular Sciences and Research
Bengaluru, Karnataka, India

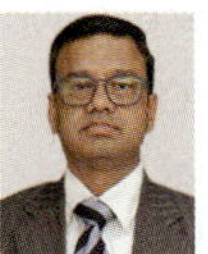

Viveka Kumar
Director, Cath Lab
Senior Consultant Interventional
Cardiologist, Max Super Specialty Hospital
New Delhi, India

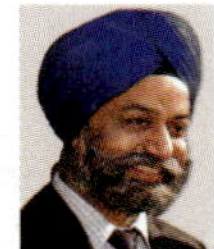

GS Wander
Professor and Head of Cardiology
Hero DMC Heart Institute
Dayanand Medical College and Hospital
Ludhiana, Punjab, India
Past President, API

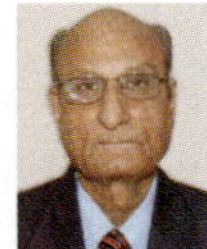

SK Parashar
Director, Non-Invasive Cardiac Laboratory
Metro Hospitals and Heart Institute
Past president, National CSI & IAE
New Delhi, India

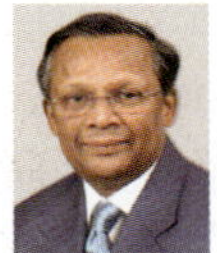

G Vijayaraghavan
Dean, Postgraduate Medical Studies
Vice Chairman, Kerala Institute
of Medical Sciences
Thiruvananthapuram, Kerala, India
Past President, IAE

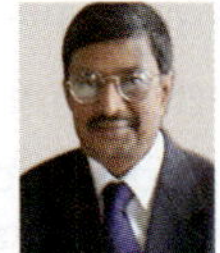

P Krishnam Raju
Senior Consultant Cardiologist
Department of Cardiology
CARE Hospitals
Hyderabad, Telangana, India
Past President, IAE

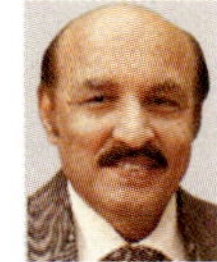

AK Pancholia
Head of Department
Clinical Cardiology
Arihant Hospital & Research center
Indore, Madhya Pradesh, India

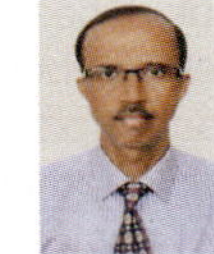

CK Ponde
Consultant Cardiologist
PD Hinduja National Hospital and
Medical Research Center
Mumbai, Maharashtra, India

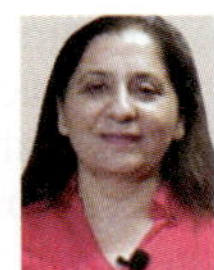

Poonam Malhotra Kapoor
Professor, Department of Cardiac Anesthesia
Cardio-Neuro Center (CNC)
All India Institute of Medical Sciences
New Delhi, India

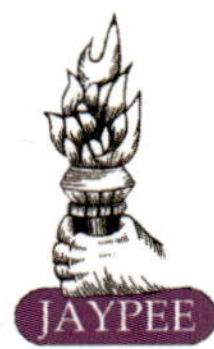

JAYPEE BROTHERS MEDICAL PUBLISHERS

The Health Sciences Publisher

New Delhi | London

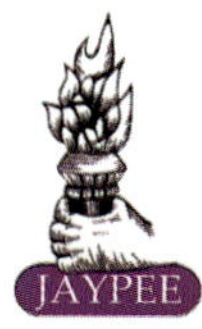

Jaypee Brothers Medical Publishers (P) Ltd

Headquarters
Jaypee Brothers Medical Publishers (P) Ltd
4838/24, Ansari Road, Daryaganj
New Delhi 110 002, India
Phone: +91-11-43574357
Fax: +91-11-43574314
Email: jaypee@jaypeebrothers.com

Overseas Offices
J.P. Medical Ltd
83 Victoria Street, London
SW1H 0HW (UK)
Phone: +44 20 3170 8910
Fax: +44 (0)20 3008 6180
Email: info@jpmedpub.com

Website: www.jaypeebrothers.com
Website: www.jaypeedigital.com

Advances and Innovations in Heart Failure (AIHF): A Textbook of Cardiology

First Edition: **2020**

ISBN: 978-93-89587-89-0

Printed at Sanat Printers

Dedicated to

Cardiological Society of India
Our parents, our teachers
All the members of CSI
Our colleagues
patients, students and our families

Contributors

A George Koshy
Professor
Department of Cardiology
Government Medical College
Thiruvananthapuram, Kerala, India

Aarya Naik
NHL Municipal Medical College and VS Hospital
Ahmedabad, Gujarat, India

Abhijit Biswas
Visiting Cardiologist
Department of Non-invasive Cardiology
Vivekananda Institute of Medical Sciences
Kolkata, West Bengal, India

Abhimanyu Bhatia
Moolchand Medcity
New Delhi, India

Aditya Kapoor
Professor
Department of Cardiology
Sanjay Gandhi Postgraduate Institute of Medical Sciences
Lucknow, Uttar Pradesh, India

Adrian Chong
Department of Cardiology
Princess Alexandra Hospital
University of Queensland
Brisbane, Australia

Ahmed Khurshid Pasha
Mayo Clinic Health System Mankato
Minnesota, USA

Ahmed M Dohain
Department of Pediatrics
Division of Pediatric Cardiology
Cairo University
Cairo, Egypt

Ahmed Y Salama
Division of Cardiovascular Disease
University of Alabama at Birmingham
Birmingham, Alabama, USA

Ajay Kumar Sinha
Ex-Director- Cardiology
Consultant, Cardiology
Paras HMRI Hospital
Patna, Bihar, India

Ajay Naik
Cardiac Electrophysiologist
CIMS Hospital
Ahmedabad, Gujarat, India

Ajmer Singh
Director, Cardiac Anesthesia
Institute of Critical Care and Anesthesiology
Medanta–The Medicity
Gurugram, Haryana, India

AK Pancholia
Head, Department of Clinical and Preventive Cardiology
Arihant Hospital and Research Center
Indore, Madhya Pradesh, India

Akshaya Kumar Samal
Professor and Head
Department of Cardiology
Hi-Tech Medical College
Bhubaneswar, Odisha, India

Amit Garg
Consultant, Department of Radiodiagnosis and Imaging
Fortis Escorts Heart Institute
New Delhi, India

Amit K Gupta
Fortis Escorts Heart Institute
New Delhi, India

Amit Nanda
Division of Cardiovascular Disease
University of Tennessee
Memphis, Tennessee, USA

Amitabh Poonia
Consultant Interventional Cardiologist
National Heart Institute
New Delhi, India

Amrish Agrawal
Senior Consultant
Department of Cardiology
Fujairah Hospital, MOHAP
Fujairah, UAE

Andrew Thai Nguyen
Harvard Medical School
Boston, USA

Anil Bharani
Former Professor and Head
Department of Medicine and Division of Cardiology
Mahatma Gandhi Memorial Medical College and
Maharaja Yashwant Rao Hospital
Indore, Madhya Pradesh, India

Anil Dhall
Consultant Cardiologist
Delhi Heart and Lung Institute
New Delhi, India

Anil Pareek
President, Medical Affairs and Clinical Research
Ipca Laboratories Limited
Mumbai, Maharashtra, India

Aniruddha De
Department of Non-invasive Cardiology
Apollo Gleneagles Hospital
Kolkata, West Bengal, India

Anjan Lal Dutta
Clinical Director
Senior Consultant and Head
Department of Cardiology
Peerless Hospital and BK Roy Research Center
Kolkata, West Bengal, India

Anju Nohria
Cardiovascular Division
Brigham and Women's Hospital
Boston, MA

Anuj Sangal
Department of Cardiothoracic Surgery
Max Healthcare
New Delhi, India

Anuradha Sridhar
Senior Consultant Interventional Cardiologist
Ashwin Clinic, Dr Mehta's Hospital
Apollo Group of Hospitals
Chennai, Tamil Nadu, India

Anurag Garg
Professor and Head
Cardiothoracic Vascular Surgery
Dr DY Patil Medical College, Hospital and Research Center
Pune, Maharashtra, India

Aparna Jaswal
Additional Director
Cardiac Pacing and Electrophysiology
Fortis Escorts Heart Institute
New Delhi, India

Arnab Banerjee
Rabindranath Tagore International
Institute of Cardiac Sciences
Kolkata, West Bengal, India

Arti Shah
Cardiovascular and Arrhythmia Consultants
Mount Sinai Health System
New York, USA

Arun Chutani
Cardiovascular and Arrhythmia Consultants
Mount Sinai Health System
New York, USA

Arvind Balaji
Department of Cardiology
All India Institute of Medical Sciences
New Delhi, India

Asha Moorthy
Senior Consultant Cardiologist
SRM Institutes for Medical Science
Chennai, Tamil Nadu, India

Ashish Jaikishan
Associate consultant
Fortis Escorts Heart Institute
New Delhi, India

Ashish Kumar Jain
Dharma Vira Heart Center
Sir Ganga Ram Hospital
New Delhi, India

Ashok H Punjabi
Medical Director
Krishna Cardiac Care Centre
Honorary Cardiologist
Lilavati Hospital and Research Center
Mumbai, Maharashtra, India

Ashok Seth
Fortis Escorts Heart Institute
New Delhi, India

Aslaniff Roslan
Institute Jantung Negara
Kuala Lumpur, Malaysia

Avishek Bagchi
Department of Cardiology
Max Super Speciality Hospital
New Delhi, India

Avneesh Prasad
National Heart Institute
East of Kailash, New Delhi, India

Bagirath Raghuraman
Senior Consultant
Heart Transplant, Cardiology - Adult
Narayana Institute of Cardiac Sciences
Bengaluru, Karnataka, India

Bantwal Vivek Baliga
Baliga Diagnostics
Bengaluru, Karnataka, India

Bhanu Mishra
Nephrology and Transplant Services
BLK Super Speciality Hospital
New Delhi, India

Bharat Kantharia
Cardiovascular and Arrhythmia Consultants
Mount Sinai Health System
New York, USA

Bhavik Dhirawani
Department of Cardiology
Holy Family Hospital and
Research Center
Mumbai, Maharashtra, India

Bhupinder Singh
Associate Professor of Cardiology
Hero DMC Heart Institute
Dayanand Medical College and Hospital
Ludhiana, Punjab, India

Bicky Vettichira
Stony Brook University Medical Center
Stony Brook, New York

Binoy John
Chief Consultant Interventional Cardiologist
Department of Cardiology
Interventional Cardiology
Advanced Heart Diseases
Heart-Failure and Cardiac Transplant Medicine
Dr Rela Institute and Medical Center
Chennai, Tamil Nadu, India

Biswaranjan Mishra
Chief Consultant Cardiologist
Max Diagnostic Center
Cuttack, Odisha, India

Biswarup Sarkar
Assistant Professor
ICVS, RG Kar Medical College and Hospital
Kolkata, West Bengal, India

Brian Pinto
Chief Cardiologist
Holy Family Hospital and
Research Center
Mumbai, Maharashtra, India

C Venkata S Ram
Director
Apollo Institute for Blood Pressure Management
and Apollo Blood Pressure Clinics, Apollo Hospitals
Hyderabad, Telangana, India
Director, World Hypertension League/WHO (South Asia)
Editor-in-Chief, Hypertension Journal

Chandramukhi Sunehra
Department of Cardiac Imaging
Care Hospital
Banjara Hills, Hyderabad, Telangana, India

Chandrashekhar K Ponde
Consultant Interventional Cardiologist and
Electrophysiologist
Head, Department of Cardiology
PD Hinduja National Hospital and
Medical Research Center
Mumbai, Maharashtra, India

Chandril Chugh
Head, Interventional Neurology
Max Super Specialty Hospital
Saket, New Delhi, India

Charan Reddy KV
Department of Cardiology
Lilavati Hospital and Research Center
Mumbai, Maharashtra, India

Chetan P Shah
Department of Cardiology
Lilavati Hospital and Research Center
Mumbai, Maharashtra, India

Christopher M Bianco
Division of Cardiology
West Virginia University Heart and Vascular Institute
Morgantown, WV

Clive Goulbourne
Stony Brook University Medical Center
Stony Brook Heart Institute
New York, USA

Danish H Kazmi
Consultant Cardiologist
Era Medical College and Hospital
Lucknow, Uttar Pradesh, India

Dayasagar Rao V
Department of Cardiology
Krishna Institute of Medical Sciences
Secunderabad, Telangana, India

Debabrata Roy
Senior Interventional Cardiologist and
Academic Co-Coordinator
Rabindranath Tagore International Institute
Kolkata, West Bengal, India

Dinkar Bhasin
Assistant Professor
Department of Cardiology
Vardhman Mahavir Medical College and Safdarjung Hospital and
New Delhi, India

Dipak Ranjan Das
Assistant Professor, Department of Cardiology
SCB Medical College and Hospital
Cuttack, Odisha, India

G Justin Paul
Professor, Institute of Cardiology
Madras Medical College
Chennai, Tamil Nadu, India

GN Mahapatra
Senior Consultant and Head
Department of Nuclear Medicine
Seven Hills Hospital, Mumbai
Director, West Coast Medical Center
Maharashtra Housing and Area Development Authority (MHADA)
Mumbai, Maharashtra, India

G Vijayaraghavan
Vice Chairman and Director
Kerala Institute of Medical Sciences
Thiruvananthapuram, Kerala, India

Gaser A Abdelmohsen
Department of Pediatrics
Division of Pediatric Cardiology
Cairo University
Cairo, Egypt

Gautam Rege
Department of Cardiology
Jupiter Hospital
Mumbai, Maharashtra, India

Geetha Subramaniam
Professor
Department of Cardiology
Institute of Medical Sciences
Banaras Hindu University
Varanasi, Uttar Pradesh, India
Emeritus Professor
Department of Cardiology
The Tamil Nadu DR MGR Medical University
Chennai, Tamil Nadu, India

Girish MP
Professor
Department of Cardiology
Govind Ballabh Pant Institute of Postgraduate
Medical Education and Research
New Delhi, India

GR Kane
Senior Consultant Interventional Cardiology
Hiranandani Hospital
A Fortis Network Hospital
Vashi, Mumbai, Maharashtra, India

Gunjan Garg
Director General of Health Services (Addl)
Professor and Chief Cardiologist
Vardhman Mahavir Medical College
and Safdarjung Hospital
New Delhi, India

Gurpreet S Wander
Professor and Head of Cardiology
Unit Hero DMC Heart Institute
Dayanand Medical College and Hospital
Ludhiana, Punjab, India

HK Chopra
Chief Cardiologist
Moolchand Medcity
New Delhi, India

Hala ElMarsafawy
Professor of Pediatrics and Pediatric Cardiology
Director Cardiac Catheterization Laboratory
Children Hospital
Mansoura University, Egypt

Hanumanth K Reddy
Adjunct Professor of Clinical Medicine
St Louis University Medical School
St Louis, USA

Harikrishnan S
Professor
Department of Cardiology
Sree Chitra Tirunal Institute for
Medical Sciences and Technology
Thiruvananthapuram, Kerala, India

Harmeet Singh
Head, Critical Care
Department of Emergency
and Urgent Care
Moolchand Medcity
New Delhi, India

Harsh Wardhan
Professor and Head
Department of Cardiology
Mahatma Gandhi Medical College and Hospital
Jaipur, Rajasthan, India

Harshita Singh
Department of Cardiology
All India Institute of Medical Science
New Delhi, India

Himanshu Agarwal
Consultant Interventional Neurology
Max Super Speciality Hospital
Saket, New Delhi, India

Hosam Rashwan
C/o Dr Hala ElMarsafawy
Professor of Pediatrics and Pediatric Cardiology
Director Cardiac Catheterization Laboratory
Children Hospital
Mansoura University
Mansoura City, Egypt

I Sathyamurthy
Consultant and Interventional Cardiologist
Apollo Main Hospitals
Chennai, Tamil Nadu, India

IB Vijayalakshmi
Professor Emeritus (RGUHS)
Professor of Pediatric Cardiology (PMSSY)
Bengaluru Medical College and Research Institute
Bengaluru, Karnataka, India

Ira Gupta
C/o Dr KK Aggarwal
Padma Shri Awardee
Senior Consultant Cardiologist
President, Heart Care Foundation of India
New Delhi, India

J Cecily Mary Majella
Assistant Professor
Institute of Cardiology
Madras Medical College
Chennai, Tamil Nadu, India

Jabir A
Senior Consultant Cardiologist
Lisie Hospital
Kochi, Kerala, India

Jain T Kallarakkal
Senior Interventional Cardiologist
St Mary's Hospital
Thodupuzha, Kerala, India

Jamshed J Dalal
Director, Cardiac Sciences
Kokilaben Dhirubhai Ambani Hospital and Medical Research Institute
Mumbai, Maharashtra, India

Jayakhanthan Kolathaivelu
Indraprastha Apollo Hospital
Delhi, India

Jayanta Sharma
C/o Mrinal Kanti Das
Senior Consultant and Interventional Cardiologist
CK Birla Hospital
Kolkata, West Bengal, India
President Elect National CSI and
Chairman Scientific Committee, CSICON-2019

Jeemon P
Sree Chitra Tirunal Institute for
Medical Sciences and Technology
Thiruvananthapuram, Kerala, India

Jimmy George
Consultant Cardiologist
Lisie Hospital, Kochi
Kochi, Kerala, India

John Gorcsan
Division of Cardiology
Washington University
St Louis, MO, USA

Jostol Pinto
Assistant Professor
Department of Cardiology
Government Medical College
Thiruvananthapuram, Kerala, India

JPS Sawhney
Chairperson, Department of Cardiology
Dharma Vira Heart Center
Sir Ganga Ram Hospital
New Delhi, India

Jui Shah
Cardiovascular and Arrhythmia Consultants
Mount Sinai Health System
New York, USA

K Venugopal
Professor and Head
Department of Cardiology
Pushpagiri Institute of Medical Sciences
Tiruvalla, Kerala, India

Kamal K Sethi
Director of Cardiology
Chairman and Managing Director
Delhi Heart and Lung Institute
New Delhi, India

Karishma Landge
Department of Cardiology
All India Institute of Medical Sciences
New Delhi, India

Karishma Walia
Moolchand Medcity
New Delhi, India

Kavita Tyagi
Consultant
Sir Ganga Ram Hospital
New Delhi, India

Kayan Siodia
C/o Dr GR Kane
Senior Consultant Interventional Cardiology
Hiranandani Hospital
A Fortis Network Hospital
Vashi, Mumbai, Maharashtra, India

Keval D Patel
Division of Cardiology
Washington University
St Louis, MO, USA

Kewal C Goswami
Professor
Department of Cardiology
All India Institute of Medical Sciences
New Delhi, India

KK Aggarwal
Padma Shri Awardee
Senior Consultant Cardiologist
President, Heart Care Foundation of India
New Delhi, India

KK Kapur
Chief Consultant Non-invasive Lab
Indraprastha Apollo Hospital
New Delhi, India

KK Shalia
Sir HN Medical Research Society
Sir HN Reliance Foundation Hospital
and Research Center
Mumbai, Maharashtra, India

KN Srinivasan
Consultant and Interventional Cardiologist
Apollo Hospitals
Chennai, Tamil Nadu, India

Kriti Mittal
C/o Sanjay Mittal
Director Clinical Cardiology and Research
Medanta-The Medicity
Gurugram, Haryana, India

Kumar Hrishikesh
C/o Dr Simmi Manocha
Associate Director Cardiology
Head, Non-invasive Cardiology
Asian Institute of Medical Sciences
Faridabad, Haryana, India

Kush Kumar Bhagat
Department of Interventional Cardiology
Eternal Heart Care Centre and Research Institute
Mount Sinai New York Affiliate
Jaipur, Rajasthan, India

Kushal Madan
Cardiac Rehabilitation Consultant
Dharma Vira Heart Center
Sir Ganga Ram Hospital
New Delhi, India

Lokesh Khandelwal
Govind Ballabh Pant Institute of Postgraduate
Medical Education and Research
Maulana Azad Medical College
New Delhi, India

Madhu Mary Minz
Senior Consultant Cardiology
Medanta–The Medicity
Gurugram, Haryana, India

Manish Bansal
Associate Director Cardiology
Medanta–The Medicity
Gurugram, Haryana, India

Manish Gaba
Moolchand Medcity
New Delhi, India

Manish Kumar Sharma
Dharma Vira Heart Center
Sir Ganga Ram Hospital
New Delhi, India

Masood Ahmad
Medical Director
Echocardiography Laboratory
Division of Cardiology
Department of Internal Medicine
301 University Blvd. JSA 5.106
Galveston, TX, USA

Mayank Jain
Consultant Interventional Cardiologist
Choithram Hospital and Research Center
Indore, Madhya Pradesh, India

Md Talha Khan Abid
Lokmanya Tilak Municipal Medical College and General Hospital
Mumbai, Maharashtra, India

Mehul Oswal
PD Hinduja National Hospital
Mumbai, Maharashtra, India

Milind Phadke
Associate Professor
Department of Cardiology
Lokmanya Tilak Municipal Medical College
and General Hospital
Interventional Cardiologist
Global Hospital
Mumbai, Maharashtra, India

Mohamed K Ahmed
Division of Cardiovascular Disease
University of Alabama at Birmingham
Birmingham, Alabama, USA

Mohammed Sadiq Azam
Department of Cardiology
Krishna Institute of Medical Sciences
Secunderabad, Telangana, India

Mohan Bhargava
Associate Director
Interventional Cardiology
Max Super Speciality Hospital
Saket, New Delhi, India

Mohit D Gupta
Professor
Department of Cardiology
Govind Ballabh Pant Institute of Postgraduate
Medical Education and Research
New Delhi, India

Mohit M Bhagwati
Max Super Speciality Hospital
Saket, New Delhi, India

Mona Bhatia
Director and Head
Department of Radiodiagnosis and Imaging
Fortis Escorts Heart Institute
New Delhi, India

Mrinal Kanti Das
Senior Consultant and Interventional Cardiologist
CK Birla Hospital
Kolkata, West Bengal, India
President Elect National CSI and
Chairman Scientific Committee, CSICON-2019

Musna PJ
Department of Cardiology
Lisie Hospital
Kochi, Kerala, India

Nandini Nair
Division of Cardiology
Department of Medicine
Texas Tech University Health Sciences Center
Lubbock, TX, USA

Naveen Garg
Clinical Cardiologist
BK Hospital
Faridabad, Haryana, India

Navin C Nanda
Division of Cardiovascular Disease
University of Alabama at Birmingham
Birmingham, Alabama, USA

Neeraj Kumar
Consultant Neurologist
Moolchand Medcity
New Delhi, India

Neeraj A Desai
Department of Cardiology
Holy Family Hospital and
Research Centre
Mumbai, Maharashtra, India

Niraj Pandey
Cardiac Radiology
All India Institute of Medical Sciences
New Delhi, India

Nirmal Ghati
Department of Cardiology
All India Institute of Medical Sciences
New Delhi, India

Nisarg Patel
Moolchand Medcity
New Delhi, India

Nitin Aggarwal
Senior Consultant Interventional Cardiology
Sri Balaji Action Medical Institute and
Rajiv Gandhi Cancer Institute and Research Center
New Delhi, India

Nitin Burkule
Consultant Cardiologist
Jupiter Hospital
Mumbai, Maharashtra, India

Nitish Naik
Professor
Department of Cardiology
All India Institute of Medical Sciences
New Delhi, India

NN Khanna
Senior Consultant Interventional
Cardiology and Vascular Interventions
Advisor-Apollo Group of Hospitals
Coordinator-Cardiology, Cath Lab
and Vascular Services
Indraprastha Apollo Hospitals
New Delhi, India

OP Yadava
CEO and Chief Cardiac Surgeon
National Heart Institute
New Delhi, India

P Krishnam Raju
Consultant Cardiologist
CARE Hospital
Hyderabad, Telangana, India

Parneesh Arora
Principal Consultant Cardiology
Fortis Hospital
Noida, Uttar Pradesh, India

Partho P Sengupta
Division of Cardiology
West Virginia University Heart and Vascular Institute
Morgantown, WV

Parveen Batra
Department of Radiodiagnosis and Imaging
Fortis Escorts Heart Institute
New Delhi, India

Pawan K Sharma
Assistant Professor of Medicine
Division of Cardiology
Adjunct Assistant Professor of Radiology
University of Utah School of Medicine
Salt Lake City, Utah, USA

PB Jayagopal
Director and Interventional Cardiologist
Lakshmi Hospital
Palakkad, Kerala, India

Peter D Farjo
Division of Cardiology
West Virginia University Heart and Vascular Institute
Morgantown, WV

Poonam Malhotra Kapoor
Professor, Cardiac Anesthesia
Cardio-Thoracic Center
All India Institute of Medical Sciences
New Delhi, India

PP Mohanan
Director and Head
Department of Cardiology
Westfort Hi-tech Hospital Ltd
Thrissur, Kerala, India

Prabhakar Dorairaj
Senior Consultant Interventional Cardiologist
Ashwin Clinic, Dr Mehta's Hospital
Apollo Group of Hospitals
Chennai, Tamil Nadu, India

Prateek Bajaj
C/o Dr Simmi Manocha
Associate Director Cardiology
Head, Non-invasive Cardiology
Asian Institute of Medical Sciences
Faridabad, Haryana, India

Praveen Chandra
Chairman, Interventional Cardiology
Heart Institute, Medanta Super Speciality Hospital
Gurugram, Haryana, India

Priyanka Gussain
Moolchand Medcity
New Delhi, India

Priya Jagia
Professor
Cardiovascular Radiology
and Endovascular Interventions
All India Institute of Medical Sciences
New Delhi, India

Qiangjun Cai
Division of Cardiology
University of Texas Medical Branch
Galveston, Texas, USA

Raghuveer Kura
Assistant Professor of Clinical Medicine
St Louis University Medical School
USA

Rahul Mehrotra
Director and Head
Department of Non-invasive Cardiology
Max Super Specialty Hospital
New Delhi, India

Raj Kumar
Senior Consultant
Non-invasive Cardiology
Max Super Specialty Hospital
New Delhi, India

Raja Vijendra Reddy Janke
C/o Dr D Prabhakar
Senior Consultant Interventional Cardiologist
Ashwin Clinic, Dr Mehta's Hospital
Apollo Group of Hospitals
Chennai, Tamil Nadu, India

Rajeev Gupta
Preventive Cardiology
Eternal Heart Care Center and Research Institute
Mount Sinai New York Affiliate
Jaipur, Rajasthan, India

Rajendra Kumar Agarwal
Consultant Cardiology
Max Super Specialty Hospital
Saket, New Delhi, India

Rajesh Janardhanan
Sarver Heart Center
Division of Cardiology
Department of Medicine
Banner-University Medical Center
Tucson, Arizona, USA

Rajneesh Malhotra
Senior Director–CTVS
Max Super Specialty Hospital
New Delhi, India

Rajni Saijpaul
Department of Biochemistry
Vardhman Mahavir Medical College
and Safdarjung Hospital
New Delhi, India

Rakesh Varma
Director, General of Health Services (Addl)
Professor and Chief
Department of Cardiologist
Vardhman Mahavir Medical College and
Safdarjung Hospital
New Delhi, India

Rami N Khouzam
Division of Cardiovascular Disease
University of Tennessee,
Memphis, Tennessee, USA

Ravi Komatireddy
Assistant Clinical Professor
University of California
San Diego, USA

Ravi Prakash
Senior Consultant
Moolchand Medcity
New Delhi, India

Ravi R Kasliwal
Chairman
Clinical and Preventive Cardiology
Medanta–The Medicity
Gurugram, Haryana, Haryana

Raziye E Akdogan
Division of Cardiovascular Disease
University of Alabama at Birmingham
Birmingham, Alabama, USA

Rekha Mishra
Consultant Cardiologist
National Heart Institute
New Delhi, India

Ritesh Sanguri
Consultant Cardiologist
Venkateshwar Hospital
Dwarka, New Delhi, India

RJ Manjuran
Emeritus Professor of Cardiology
Pushpagiri Medical College
Tiruvalla, Kerala, India

Rohit Tandon
Senior Consultant Physician
Dayanand Medical College and Hospital
Unit Hero DMC Heart Institute
Ludhiana, Punjab, India

Rudrani Sharma
Consultant Cardiology
Delhi Heart and Lung Institute
New Delhi, India

RVA Ananth
Consultant Cardiologist
Jeyalakshmi Heart Center
Madurai, Tamil Nadu, India

S Sivasankaran
Sree Chitra Tirunal Institute for
Medical Sciences and Technology
Thiruvananthapuram, Kerala, India

S Shanmugasundaram
Emeritus Professor of Cardiology
The Tamil Nadu Dr MGR Medical University
Chennai, Tamil Nadu, India

Sadanand Shetty
Emeritus Professor
Dr D Y Patil University School of Medicine
Head, Department of Cardiology
Somaiya Superspeciality Institute
CMD - Sadanand Healthy Living Center Ltd
Mumbai, Maharashtra, India

Sameer Srivastava
Director, Non-Invasive Cardiology
Fortis Escorts Heart Institute
New Delhi, India

Samuel Kim
Stony Brook University Medical Center
Stony Brook, New York, USA

Sanchit Sharma
C/o Dr KK Aggarwal
Padma Shri Awardee
Senior Consultant Cardiologist
President
Heart Care Foundation of India
New Delhi, India

Sandeep Seth
Professor
Department of Cardiology
All India Institute of Medical Sciences
New Delhi, India

Sanjay G
Sree Chitra Tirunal Institute for
Medical Sciences and Technology
Thiruvananthapuram, Kerala, India

Sanjay Mittal
Director, Clinical Cardiology and Research
Medanta-The Medicity
Gurugram, Haryana, India

Sanjeev Kumar
Associate Professor
Department of CTVS
All India Institute of Medical Sciences
Patna, Bihar, India

Sanket Garg
Head of Cardiac Sciences and
Chief Cardiovascular Surgeon
Cardiac Sciences
Manipal Hospital
New Delhi, India

Santhosh KG Koshy
Division of Cardiology
Department of Medicine
Texas Tech University Health Sciences Center
Lubbock, TX, USA

Satender Yadav
Nephrology and Transplant Services
BLK Super Speciality Hospital
New Delhi, India

Satish C Govind
Narayana Institute of Cardiac Sciences
Narayana Health City
Bengaluru, Karnataka, India

Satish K Parashar
Director, Senior Consultant Cardiologist
Non-invasive Cardiac Laboratory
Metro Hospital and Heart Institute
New Delhi, India

Satyanarayan Routray
Professor and Head
Department of Cardiology
SCB Medical College
Cuttack, Odisha, India

Saumitra Ray
Professor, Vivekananda Institute of Medical Sciences
Director of Invasive Cardiology
AMRI(S) Hospital
Kolkata, West Bengal, India

Saurabh Bhardwaj
National Heart Institute
East of Kailash, New Delhi, India

Saurabh Mehrotra
Additional Professor of Cardiology
Postgraduate Institute of Medical Education and Research
Chandigarh, India

SC Manchanda
Senior Consultant
Department of Cardiology
Dharma Vira Heart Center
Sir Ganga Ram Hospital
New Delhi, India

SG Prasad
Department of Telemedicine
CARE Foundation
Hyderabad, Telangana, India

Shariq Hoda
Manipal Hospital
New Delhi, India

Shashank Jain
Department of Radiodiagnosis and Imaging
Fortis Escorts Heart Institute
New Delhi, India

Shishu Shankar Mishra
Professor and Director
Department of Cardiology
Hi-Tech Medical College, Bhubaneswar, Odisha
Director and Senior Consultant Cardiologist
Med 'N' Heart Clinic
Cuttack, Odisha, India

Shraddha Ranjan
Department of Cardiology
Medanta–The Medicity
Gurugram, Haryana, India

Siddharthan Deepti
Assistant Professor
Department of Cardiology
All India Institute of Medical Sciences
New Delhi, India

Simardeep K Khangura
Government Medical College
Amritsar, Punjab, India

Simmi Manocha
Associate Director, Cardiology
Head of Department
Non-invasive Cardiology
Asian Institute of Medical Sciences
Faridabad, Haryana, India

Sivasubramanian Ramakrishnan
Professor
Department of Cardiology
All India Institute of Medical Sciences
New Delhi, India

SKM Sarjun Basha
Cardiologist, Taj Cardiac and Diabetic Clinic, Arakkonam
Peacock Hospital
Tiruttani, Tamil Nadu, India

Smadar Kort
Stony Brook University Medical Center
Stony Brook, New York, USA

Smita Mishra
Consultant and Head
Department of Pediatric Cardiology
Manipal Hospital
New Delhi, India

SN Narasingan
Vice Chairman, Lipid Association of India
Dean, Prof. M Viswanathan Diabetes Research Center
Formerly Adjunct Professor
The Tamil Nadu Dr MGR Medical University
Managing Director, SNN Specialties Clinic
Chennai, Tamil Nadu, India

SN Pathak
Consultant Interventional Cardiology
Pushpawati Singhania Research Institute and Hospital
New Delhi, India

Sonia A El-Saiedi
Department of Pediatrics, Division of Pediatric Cardiology
Cairo University
Cairo, Egypt

Soumik Chaudhuri
Consultant Cardiologist
Peerless Hospital and BK Roy Research Center
Kolkata, West Bengal, India

Soumitra Kumar
Professor and Head
Department of Cardiology
Vivekananda Institute of Medical Sciences
Kolkata, West Bengal, India

Sravan Kumar V
Department of Cardiology
Govind Ballabh Pant Institute of Postgraduate
Medical Education and Research
Maulana Azad Medical College
New Delhi, India

Srikant Sharma
Senior Consultant Physician
Moolchand Medcity
New Delhi, India

SS Iyengar
Manipal Hospital
Bengaluru, Karnataka, India

Sudhir Wahi
Associate Professor, Department of Cardiology
Princess Alexandra Hospital
University of Queensland
Brisbane, Australia

Sundeep Mishra
Professor of Cardiology
All India Institute of Medical Sciences
New Delhi, India

Sunil Prakash
Director and Head
Nephrology and Transplant Services
BLK Super Speciality Hospital
New Delhi, India

Surabhi Awasthi
Head of Department, Critical Care
Moolchand Medcity
New Delhi, India

Surendra K Chutani
Cardiovascular and Arrhythmia Consultants
Mount Sinai Health System
New York, USA

SV Shah
Southern Railway HQ Hospital
Ayanavaram/Perambur
Chennai, Tamil Nadu, India

Tapan Sinha
Consultant Cardiologist
Kothari Medical Centre
Kolkata, West Bengal, India

Thair Al Jumaily
Specialist Interventional Cardiology
Fujairah Hospital, MOHAP
Fujairah, UAE

Thirupathi K Reddy
C/o Dr Hanumanth K Reddy
Adjunct Professor of Clinical Medicine
St Louis University Medical School
USA

Uday M Jadhav
Cardiology and Cardiovascular Imaging
MGM New Bombay Hospital
Mumbai, Maharashtra, India

Uday S Yadav
Associate Consultant Cardiologist
National Heart Institute
New Delhi, India

Upendra Kaul
Chairman and Dean Academics and Research
Batra Heart Center and Batra Hospital
and Medical Research Center
New Delhi, India

V Amuthan
Emeritus Professor of Cardiology
The Tamil Nadu Dr MGR Medical University
Formerly, Professor and Head
Department of Cardiology
Madurai Medial College
Madurai, Tamil Nadu, India

Vasanthakumar Venugopal
Head, Medical Imaging Research
Centre for Advanced Research in Imaging
Neuroscience and Genomics
Mahajan Imaging
New Delhi, India

Vidur Mahajan
Head of Research and Development
Centre for Advanced Research in Imaging
Neuroscience and Genomics
Mahajan Imaging
New Delhi, India

Vidyut Jain
Cosultant Cardiologist
Choithram Hospital and Research Center
Indore, Madhya Pradesh, India

Vijay Bang
Professor and Senior Cardiologist
Lilavati Hospital and Research Center
Mumbai, Maharashtra, India

Vijay Kumar Trehan
Director Professor
Department of Cardiology
Govind Ballabh Pant Institute of Postgraduate
Medical Education and Research
Maulana Azad Medical College
New Delhi, India

Vijay Kumar
Fortis Escorts Heart Institute
New Delhi, India

Vikas Singh
Consultant
Intervention Cardiologist
Daksh Heart Care and 4A Heart Hospital
Patna, Bihar, India

Vineet Bhatia
Senior Consultant Cardiology
Fortis Hospital
Noida, Uttar Pradesh, India

Vinod Mittal
Senior Consultant Diabetologist
Delhi Heart and Lung Institute
Director, Delhi Diabetes Care Centre
New Delhi, India

Vinod Sharma
Senior Consultant Cardiologist
National Heart Institute
East of Kailash, New Delhi, India

Vishal Agrawal
Department of Accident and Emergency
Royal Albert Edward Infirmary
Wigan, UK

Vishal Batra
Assistant Professor
Department of Cardiology
Govind Ballabh Pant Institute of Postgraduate
Medical Education and Research
Maulana Azad Medical College
New Delhi, India

Vishal Rastogi
Fortis Escorts Heart Institute
New Delhi, India

Vivek Chaturvedi
Senior Consultant Cardiology and
Director Cardiac Electrophysiology
Narayana Superspeciality Hospital
Gurugram, Haryana, India.

Vivek Kumar
Consultant
Interventional Cardiology
Max Super Specialty Hospital
New Delhi, India

Viveka Kumar
Director, Cath Lab
Senior Consultant Interventional
Cardiologist and Electrophysiologist
Max Super Specialty Hospital
New Delhi, India

Vivudh P Singh
Fortis Escorts Heart Institute
New Delhi, India

VK Shah
Sir HN Reliance Foundation Hospital
and Research Centre
Mumbai, Maharashtra, India

Wasim Rashid
Associate Consultant
Cardiac Pacing and Electrophysiology
Fortis Escorts Heart Institute
New Delhi, India

Yatin Mehta
Chairman–Medanta Institute of
Critical Care and Anesthesiology
Medanta–The Medicity
Gurugram, Haryana, India

Yugal K Mishra
Head of Cardiac Sciences and
Chief Cardiovascular Surgeon
Cardiac Sciences
Manipal Hospital
New Delhi, India

Foreword

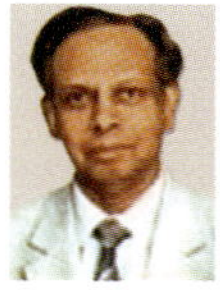 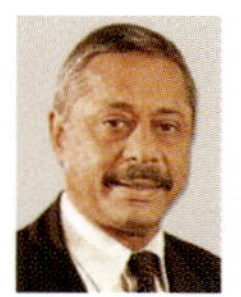 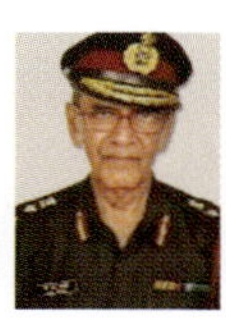 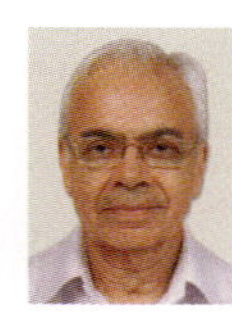 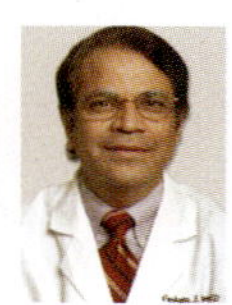 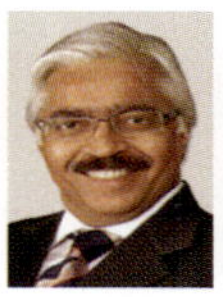 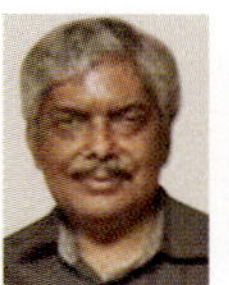 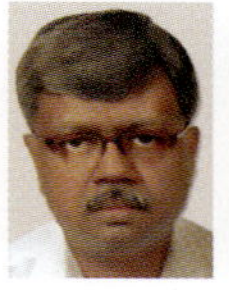 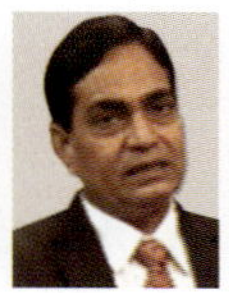 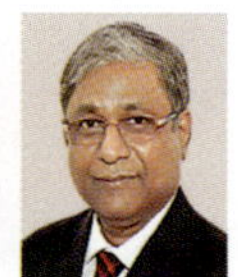

We are honored and have a great pleasure to write the Foreword for the state-of-art book *Advances and Innovations in Heart Failure: A Textbook of Cardiology* being released on the occasion of Dr BC Roy Oration Function of 71st Annual Conference of CSI at Delhi, India. The textbook on AIHF was long due considering the wealth of data, new strategies which are diagnostically, prognostically and therapeutically imaging and biomarker-based in the clinical practice. It is one of the most needed, comprehensive, illustrative, well-structured books, published with enormous information about advances in clinical, imaging including echocardiography and interventions for better cardiovasular disease management with morbidity and mortality reduction in various clinical situations.

This book is an excellent and outstanding educational initiative by the joint efforts of 3 Editors-in-Chief, 11 Principal Editors, 18 International Editors, 50 National Editors and over 250 Contributing Authors. This book comprises 128 chapters across, 15 sections, including Clinical, Echo, Imaging, Coronary Artery Disease, Stroke, Arrhythmia, Hypertension, Valvular, Congenital Heart Disease, Metabolic, Nutritional, Cardio-oncology, Inflammatory Disorders and Heart Failure including Rehabilitation, Legal and Ethical Issues and Future Directions.

The chapters are well outlined, organized and well written with authentic references. The writing style of every chapter is vivid, concise and practical. There are excellent graphics, tables and figures that present the relevant information. The printing and binding is of excellent quality. This book will represent a milestone for Advances and Innovations in Heart Failure management strategies in the world.

We congratulate the Editors-in-Chief HK Chopra, Navin C Nanda, Jagat Narula, Principal Editors, International, National Editors and the contributors for accomplishing this prodigious achievement of great clinical relevance in cardiology practice today for meticulous heart failure management.

M Khalilullah
Director and Senior Consultant Cardiologist
The Heart Centre
New Delhi, India
Past President, National CSI

Naresh Trehan
Chairman and Managing Director
Medanta—The Medicity
Gurugram, Haryana, India

GS Sainani
Emeritus Director
Department of Medicine
Jaslok Hospital and Research Centre
Mumbai, Maharashtra, India
Past President, National CSI

SC Manchanda
Senior Consultant Cardiologist
Dharma Vira Heart Centre
Sir Ganga Ram Hospital
New Delhi, India

C Venkata S Ram
Director, Apollo Institute for Blood Pressure Management
World Hypertension League/ South Asia Office
Apollo Hospitals
Hyderabad, Telangana, India
Texas Blood Pressure Institute
Dallas, Texas, USA

Ashok Seth
Chairman
Fortis Escorts Heart Institute
New Delhi, India
President, APSIC
Past President, National CSI

PK Deb
Formerly Chief Cardiologist
ESI PG Institute of Medical Sciences
Kolkata, West Bengal, India
Chairman, Academic National CSI
Past President, National CSI

Santanu Guha
Professor and Head
Department of Cardiology
Medical College
Kolkata, West Bengal, India
Past President, National CSI

KC Goswami
Professor
Department of Cardiology
All India Institute of Medical Science
New Delhi, India
President, National CSI

MK Das
Senior Consultant and Interventional Cardiologist
CK Birla Hospital
Kolkata, West Bengal, India
President, Elect-National CSI
Chairman, Scientific Committee, CSICON 2019

Preface

The Emerging War and Consensus in Heart Failure Management

Heart failure is a complex clinical syndrome resulting from impairment of ventricular filling or ejection of blood associated with symptoms of dyspnea, fatigue and peripheral and/or pulmonary edema. Although there have been dramatic innovations in medical and device treatments for heart failure in recent decades, the incidence of heart failure is still rising and is the menace in the globe. The heart failure syndrome affects more than 38 million patients worldwide, a number that is increasing with the aging population. It is the most common diagnosis in patients aged 65 years or older admitted to hospital and in all income nations. The prevalence of HFpEF is rising with uncontrolled resistant hypertension, obesity, diabetes, dyslipidemia and CKD in India. Despite significant progress, the prognosis of heart failure is still worse than that of most cancers. Because of the seriousness of the condition, a declaration of emerging war and consensus in the heart failure management a need of the hour. The heart failure epidemic has a staggering impact on quality of life, functioning, and longevity, while imposing heavy costs on the health care system. The identification of the syndrome of advanced heart failure requires an iterative clinical assessment integrating routinely available clinical risk markers. Pharmacotherapy and nonpharmacological interventions are the mainstay in the heart failure management today. Device therapy long-term ventricular assistance devices are now used increasingly as a destination therapy in patients with advanced heart failure. In selected patients, left ventricular assistance can lead to myocardial recovery and explanation of the device. The approaches to the treatment of heart failure described, when used alone or in combination, could become important weapons in the Emerging War and Consensus in Heart Failure Management.

The results of the management of heart failure, as described in practice guidelines, are mixed. In patients with chronic heart failure with reduced ejection fraction, both the survival and quality of life have improved with the use of β-adrenoreceptor blockers, with drugs that block the renin-angiotensin-aldosterone system, and, according to a recent report, with an angiotensin receptor-neprilysin inhibitor and with devices, including pacemakers, which enhance cardiac synchronization and implanted cardiac defibrillators. However, we are unable to do much more than reduce congestion with diuretics in patients with chronic heart failure with preserved ejection fraction, which occurs in almost half of the population with heart failure. The outlook for patients with acute decompensated heart failure, irrespective of ejection fraction, is also grave. In patients older than 65 years in the USA, the 30-day hospital mortality rate for patients admitted to the hospital with heart failure is fairly constant at about 11%, and the 30-day hospital readmission rate is around 30%. Similar outcomes have been reported in England and Wales and in Europe. The 5-year survival rate for heart failure is worse than it is for most cancers and the annual cost of care for heart failure in the USA has been estimated to exceed US $30 billion, most of it spent on hospital care. Although the increased application of clinical practice guidelines in high-income countries, especially in patients with heart failure with reduced ejection fraction, has resulted in some improvement in outcome, many patients now experience a more prolonged course, resulting in increases in the prevalence of the disorder, and in the economic burden on the health-care system. Heart failure is a particular threat in middle-income and low-income countries where the adjusted hazard ratios for case fatality were 2.61 and 3.72, with high-income countries as the referent.

For centuries, drugs that increase the power of contraction of the failing heart have been used for the treatment of congestive heart failure (dropsy). The cardiac effect is due to the content of cardiac glycosides. *Digitalis purpurea,* is mentioned in writings as early as 1250; a Welsh family, known as the Physicians of Myddvai, collected different herbs and digitalis was included in their prescriptions. However, the drug was used erratically until the 18th century, when William Withering, an English physician and botanist, published a monograph describing the clinical effects of an extract of the foxglove plant. Later, in 1785, the indication and the toxicity of digitalis were reported in his book, "An account of the foxglove and some of its medical uses with practical remarks on dropsy, and other diseases". *Digitalis* is used to strengthen contractions of the heart muscle. Belonging to a group of drugs called cardiac glycosides, digitalis is most commonly used to restore adequate circulation in patients with congestive heart failure, particularly as caused by atherosclerosis or hypertension. The drug is also used to slow the rate of ventricular contraction in patients with atrial fibrillation or flutter. Digitalis directly increases the contractile power of the heart muscle, enabling a disease-weakened heart to keep up with the body's demand for heart action.

Prior to 1980, during the "*Non-pharmacologic Era*," treatments focused on lifestyle changes or limitations such as bed rest, inactivity, and fluid restrictions. Hemodynamic agents, digitalis, and diuretics comprised the mainstay of treatment at this time. The 1980s marked the beginning of the "*Pharmacologic Era*," which was heralded by the first Vasodilator-Heart Failure Trial (V-HeFT). During this time, digitalis and diuretics continued to be mainstays, but vasodilators particularly the combination of nitrates and hydralazine, played a prominent role, with some or limited benefits. The use of positive inotropes also became prevalent.

The "*Pharmacologic Era*" continued into the 1990s, but the decade brought neurohormonal interventions to the forefront. Angiotensin-converting enzyme (ACE) inhibitors, beta-blockers, and spironolactone (for the treatment of advanced heart failure) were shown to alter the natural history of disease progression. The goals of treatment of Congestive heart failure (CHF) today are the reduction of symptoms, minimization of the number of hospitalizations and prevention of premature death. *The mainstay of treatment is lifestyle modifications and pharmacologic therapy. Implantable devices and surgery may be needed in selective patients*. Angiotensin-converting enzyme inhibitors (ACEIs) or angiotensin receptor blockers (ARBs), beta-blockers (BBs) and mineralocorticoid receptor antagonists (MRAs) have been shown to improve clinical condition and survival of patients with CHF with reduced ejection fraction (HFrEF). Diuretic therapy helps to reduce cardiac load with improvement in left ventricular (LV) function. Mortality and morbidity after symptomatic CHF have remained high although variable which could be due to differences in severity of disease and appropriate use of evidence-based treatment.

Since 1960s, when beta-blockers were first introduced for the management of angina, their use has increased substantially across a wide range of cardiac diseases. This has been driven by the results of several large, randomized controlled trials (RCTs) conducted mostly in the 1980s and 1990s that demonstrated reductions in mortality and morbidity with the use of β-blockers following myocardial infarction (MI) and in those with HFrEF. *Within the last 40 years beta-blocker therapy status in chronic heart failure has changed from being the most hazardous drug to the most effective therapy.* Beta-blockers are classified as non-selective beta-blockers or selective beta-blockers according to their selectivity for one of the three subtypes of beta-receptors. Beta-blockers may be administered both intravenously and orally.

The ACC/AHA as well as the European Society of Cardiology guidelines specifically recommend Bisoprolol, Metoprolol Succinate, or Carvedilol for treatment of heart failure.

It was not until the 20th century that diuretics were developed. The early, mercurial agents, however, were associated with substantial toxicity, unlike the thiazide diuretics, which were introduced in the 1950s.

Recent robust Diuretics review has suggested that diuretics are of tremendous clinical applications in Heart Failures to reduce congestion based on echo variables. While they relieve symptoms associated with HF, they are generally regarded as not affecting the underlying disease pathophysiology. In clinical practice, careful management of a patient's fluid status with diuretics can prevent or delay admission to hospital with acute decompensated HF. This finding is echoed in a meta-analysis of diuretic use in congestive HF, *suggesting a mortality benefit with their use and a reduction of admission.* Amongst the diuretic *chlorthalidone (CTD)* gives more "*Bang for the Buck*" and has been found to be superior to HCTZ. It has been documented in *23 years follow-up Cohort data CTD is a "Gift that keeps on giving*" and can be combined with loop diuretics and MRA.

In the mid-1960s, experimental work on molecules under screening as coronary dilators allowed the discovery of the mechanism of calcium entry blockade by drugs later named calcium channel blockers. Studies on pharmacology of calcium function were initiated in the mid-1960s and their therapeutic applications globally occurred in the 1980s. In studies, it was also shown that *Calcium channel blockers were less beneficial than diuretics, β-blockers, or ACE inhibitors in the prevention of heart failure.*

The discovery of the ACE inhibitors and the creation of captopril was one of the really great advances in cardiovascular medicine, alongside beta-blockers, calcium channel blockers and statins. Angiotensin-converting enzyme (ACE) inhibitors reduce morbidity and mortality in HFrEF. Randomized controlled trials (RCTs) clearly establish the benefits of ACE inhibition in patients with mild, moderate, or severe symptoms of HF and in patients with or without coronary artery disease. *ACE inhibitors can produce angioedema and should be given with caution to patients with low systemic blood pressures, renal insufficiency or elevated serum potassium. ACE inhibitors also inhibit kininase and increase levels of bradykinin, which can induce cough but also may contribute to their beneficial effect through vasodilation.*

Angiotensin receptor blockers (ARBs) were developed with the rationale that angiotensin II production continues in the presence of ACE inhibition, driven through alternative enzyme pathways. *ARBs do not inhibit kininase and are associated with a much lower incidence of cough and angioedema than ACE inhibitors*; but like ACE inhibitors, ARBs should be given with caution to patients with low systemic blood pressure, renal insufficiency, or elevated serum potassium. Long-term therapy with ARBs produces hemodynamic, neurohormonal, and clinical effects consistent with those expected after interference with the renin-angiotensin system and have been shown in RCTs to reduce morbidity and mortality, especially in ACE inhibitor–intolerant patients.

In ARNI, an ARB is combined with an inhibitor of neprilysin, an enzyme that degrades natriuretic peptides, bradykinin, adrenomedullin, and other vasoactive peptides. In a trial that compared the first approved ARNI, valsartan/sacubitril, with enalapril in symptomatic patients with HFrEF tolerating an adequate dose of either ACE inhibitor or ARB, the ARNI reduced the composite endpoint of cardiovascular death or HF hospitalization significantly, by 20%. The benefit was seen to a similar extent for both death and HF hospitalization and was consistent across subgroups. The use of ARNI is associated with the risk of hypotension and renal insufficiency and may lead to angioedema, as well.

Mineralocorticoid receptor antagonists are the latest in the addition. *They exhibit pleiotropic effects, but their renal effects consist of modulating the expression/activity of sodium and potassium channels in the distal nephron. MRAs have a class I recommendation as a disease-modifying therapeutic agent in symptomatic chronic HFrEF, counteracting the aldosterone escape generated by neurohormonal overactivation.*

Heart rate (HR) reduction with drugs is known to improve the outcomes in patients with Heart Failure, partly by reducing and even reversing the progression of left ventricular remodeling. Advantages of HR reduction are decreased myocardial oxygen consumption, prolonging the duration of diastole and thereby supports diastolic filling and coronary blood flow and lastly the force-frequency relationship is inverted. Besides highly selective beta-blockers such as Bisoprolol, *Ivabradine* I(f) inhibitor is appealing with respect to its ability to reduce hospitalizations in patients with HF as well as its ease of dosing and monitoring in a clinical setting. Combined therapy with beta-blockers is effective and well tolerated and results in significant benefits including improved quality of life among patients with chronic HF. According to the 2017 focused update of the ACC/AHA and the Heart Failure Society of America guideline for the management of HF, Ivabradine can be useful for reducing hospitalization due to HF in patients with symptomatic stable chronic HF with reduced ejection fraction (i.e. LVEF of 35% or less) and mortality reduction has been documented only by beta-blockers. Ivabradine also help in reducing vascular stiffness E/e' and NT Pro BNP level.

Sodium-glucose cotransporter 2 inhibitors (SGLT-2i) are a novel class of anti-diabetic agents which act by inhibiting glucose reabsorption in proximal convoluted tubules of kidney. Apart from maintaining glucose homeostasis they exert a number of positive effects on the cardiovascular system like weight loss, decreasing blood pressure, preserving renal function, reducing triglycerides, natriuresis and improving endothelial dysfunction. In large clinical trials, all the three prototype agents including Canagliflozin, Empagliflozin, and dapagliflozin have shown reductions in major adverse cardiovascular events including cardiovascular deaths, nonfatal MI, stroke and heart failure (HF) hospitalizations. The reduction in heart failure hospitalization is a surprising finding and trials of these drugs are now underway for HF also. More surprising is the fact that the benefits are comparable or even better that achieved by recently approved novel drugs for HF.

Renal artery denervation (RDN) moderates the SNS to improve physiological parameters in resistant hypertension with or without heart failure. Despite the recent failure of SYMPLICITY HTN-3 to reach its primary endpoint, burgeoning evidence in many alternative areas suggests the potential to overcome current therapeutic hurdles. Preliminary data continue to support the use of RDN to regulate SNS-derived pathology, with suggestions for benefit outside of strictly antihypertensive effects. SPYRAL HTN-OFF MED support the usefulness in resistant hypertension with heart failure.

Device therapy including LVAD (left ventricular assist device), ICD (implantable cardioverter-defibrillator), CRT (cardiac resynchronization therapy) are cornerstone in modern treatment of heart failure and help reducing the morbidity and mortality. Device therapies for HFpEF including InterAtrial Shunt by left atrial (LA) decompression, V wave device, IASD, atrial flow regulator, LV expanders including LVAD, Corrola, ImCardia and electrical therapies including Intra-atrial Dyssynchrony, LA permanent pacing trials are in progress.

Echocardiography is most practical besides other modalities of imaging and is the cornerstone of diagnosis and prognostication in HFpEF and HFrEF including 2D echocardiography, conventional Doppler, tissue Doppler, 3D echocardiography and transesophageal echocardiography. Various echo variables which are of tremendous clinical relevance are left atrial diameter, left atrial volume index, filling pressures evaluation including left atrial pressure, pulmonary capillary wedge pressure and left ventricular end-diastolic pressure by most specific and sensitive tissue Doppler variable E/e', left ventricular hypertrophy, left ventricular mass index, right atrial and right ventricular function evaluation including pulmonary artery pressure, LV, LA, RV, RA, strain and strain rate including LA stiffness index are also of great clinical relevance to diagnose, prognosticate and assess effect of therapeutic intervention. Periodic echocardiographic navigation is a must in all patients of heart failure for appropriate timely therapeutic intervention. One can have echo, NT pro BNP, screening evaluation correlation for diagnostic, prognostic and therapeutic assessment.

There remains a large unmet need for new therapies in the treatment of HFrEF and heart failure with preserved ejection fration (HFpEF). In the early drug development phase, the therapeutic potential of a drug is not yet fully understood and trial endpoints other than mortality are needed to guide drug development decisions. Managing patients with heart failure remains a clinical challenge and current therapies have impacts on short-term morbidity and mortality benefits and data is yet awaited on long-term mortality and morbidity benefits.

Gene therapy for patients with heart failure is on the edge of being successfully translated from the experimental to clinical arena. It is no longer a hypothetical vision but realistic opportunity for the future treatment in patients with HFrEF. This attributed to the understanding of optimization of the various AAV serotypes. The identification of new HFrEF—causing mutations in large-scale genomic studies may enhance appropriate genotype therapeutic intervention.

However, prevention of heart failure will include the cooperation of individuals, institutions, cardiology organizations and governments. There is a tremendous need of continuing medical education, and continuing public health education by print, electronic such as TV, radio and digital media on enhancing awareness and preventive strategies about heart failure as such as salt restriction, weight reduction, no alcohol, no smoking, guarded exercises, control of hypertension and control of diabetes, etc. Several ethical, regulatory, legal and financial issues also need to be addressed. Managing with patient with heart failure still remains a clinical challenge and current therapies need to be developed for a long-term morbidity and mortality benefits. Early echo guided therapeutic intervention especially in hypertensive, diabetics and obese individuals may help reducing the rising menace of heart failure.

Bringing up Advances and Innovations in Heart Failure was a phenomenal task and requires well-structured team efforts with immense dedication, devotion and coordination. We have made every possible effort to maintain the quality and standard of *Advances and Innovations in Heart Failure*. We are sure this book will serve as an important reference guide for postgraduate students, fellows, internists, cardiologists, neurologists, critical care providers, pulmonologists, pediatricians, pediatric surgeons, cardiovascular surgeons, imaging experts and nutritionists, etc.

We express our gratitude to all the eminent cardiologists including M Khalilullah, Naresh Trehan, GS Sainani, SC Manchanda, C Venkata S Ram, Ashok Seth, PK Deb, Santanu Guha, KC Goswami, MK Das for writing the Foreword of this book.

We also express our thanks to each and every member of CSI, manuscript contributors, industry and our Principal Editors KK Sethi, KK Talwar, CN Manjunath, Viveka Kumar, GS Wander, SK Parashar, G Vijayaraghavan, P Krishnam Raju, AK Pancholia, CK Ponde, Poonam Malhotra Kapoor and all the editors for their constant support.

We dedicate this state-of-the-art book to Cardiological Society of India, our teachers, all the members of CSI, our parents, our colleagues, patients, students and our family for being supportive and encouraging throughout in bringing out this Book.

We also express our thanks to M/s Jaypee Brothers Medical Publishers (P) Ltd, New Delhi, India, for publishing this book so well. We also thank Shri Jitendar P Vij (Group Chairman), Mr Ankit Vij (Managing Director), Mr MS Mani (Group President), Ms Chetna Malhotra Vohra (Associate Director-Content Strategy), Ms Pooja Bhandari (Production Head), Ms Nikita Chauhan (Senior Development Editor), Ms Seema Dogra (Cover Visualizer), Mr Binay Kumar (Proofreader), Mr Dinesh Bhardwaj (DTP Operator), and Mr Gopal Singh Kirola (Graphic Designer) for their help, guidance and timely active intervention in composing, designing and editing of the book.

Our sincere thanks to Soban Singh, who worked really hard to keep the record of every minor and finer communication.

Albert Einstein once said:

"Learn from yesterday, live for today, hope for tomorrow. The important thing is not to stop questioning".

HK Chopra, Navin C Nanda, Jagat Narula

Preface

Advances and Innovations in Echocardiography for HF Evaluation

Heart failure which represents failure of the heart to deliver enough blood to adequately meet the demands of the body, is one of the most common disorders encountered in day-to-day clinical cardiology practice. This serious condition affects millions of persons throughout the world. It is estimated that 1 out of every 15 individuals all over the world will develop heart failure some time during their life span. In USA alone more than 6 million individuals have been diagnosed to have heart failure. Broadly, patients with heart failure can be divided into two categories, those with reduced left ventricular ejection fraction (≤40%) and those with normal (≥50%) or near normal (41–49%) ejection fraction. The former typically present with a dilated left ventricle with reduced contractility and the latter with a normally contracting but stiff, often hypertrophied ventricle which is unable to accommodate flow coming in from the left atrium. Several disorders can result in heart failure. A major cause is coronary artery/ischemic heart disease but other causes are also important. These include, to name a few, systemic hypertension (an important cause of heart failure with normal or near normal ejection fraction specially in older, obese females), type two diabetes mellitus, valvular heart disease, cardiomyopathies, myocarditis, rhythm disorders such as atrial fibrillation, pulmonary hypertension, obstructive sleep apnea, endocrine disorders and congenital heart problems. The literature is replete with several scholarly articles on heart failure and updated guidelines have been published by prestigious cardiology societies and associations in USA, Europe and other countries. However, there is still a need for a compact compendium which would condense the vast knowledge available on heart failure with emphasis on recent advances and innovations into a succinct monograph. We hope this book with chapters written by an array of well-recognized national and international experts with masterly proficiency in various aspects of heart failure will go a long way to fulfil this important need.

This book consists of 15 sections. The Section 1 is large and comprehensively covers clinical aspects of heart failure including diagnosis, management and therapeutic strategies with emphasis on recent advances and innovations. Prevention, pathophysiology, endothelial dysfunction, lipids and heart failure, clinical guidelines, heart failure registry, biomarkers, anticoagulants, ACE inhibitors, ARBs, mineralocorticoid antagonists, ARNI, stem cells and gene therapy, other advances in drug therapy, cardiogenic shock, cardiac devices, sleep apnea, critical care, etc. are extensively described. The Section 2 deals with the role of various imaging modalities in the assessment of heart failure. These include two- and three-dimensional echocardiography, nuclear medicine, magnetic resonance imaging and cardiac computed tomography. Telemedicine and the impact of artificial intelligence in the management of heart failure are also described in this section. Sections 3 to 5 respectively cover heart failure and coronary artery disease, stroke and arrhythmia. Hypertension, valvular heart disease, congenital heart disease, and metabolic and nutritional aspects are dealt with in sections 6 to 10. Cardio-oncology, inflammatory release syndrome with multiorgan failure and cardiogenic shock and cardiac rehabilitation are well covered in Sections 11 to 13. Section 14 represents an important section dealing with legal and ethical issues. Finally, future directions are well described in the last section.

Navin C Nanda, HK Chopra, Jagat Narula

Preface

Advances & Innovations in Heart Failure

It is indeed a pleasure for three of us to be coming out with our second annual presentation—Advances and Innovations in Heart Failure. One of the most common cardiovascular disease globally, heart failure contributes more than 10% of deaths in high-income and up to 30% of cardiovascular deaths in low- and middle-income countries. The highest prevalence of heart failure is reported from North America (2%) and lowest prevalence in Africa (0.25%); less symptomatic cases in the developing world go unreported. The greatest 10-year growth in prevalent cases is expected to be nearly 40% in Latin America, Caribbean and Asia-Pacific region, and the lowest just over 20% in Europe. The burden is likely to increase because of the aging population (https://doi.org/10.1093/eurheartj/ehx502.P2452).

The last five years have demonstrated renewed interest in heart failure, especially due to novel pharmacological interventions. While ARNI invigorated the neurohumoral axis, SGLT2 inhibitors opened the alternative pathways of intervention. It seems that such approaches may eventually find use in heart failure with preserved ejection fraction. Novel drugs have become available for the treatment of amyloidosis and select small molecules are being experimented for molecular intervention of genetic cardiomyopathies. Remote continuous implantable hemodynamic monitoring solution has become available with end in view to restricting readmissions in frequent flyers. New devices have been developed to release heightened pressure in the left atrium in patients with high left atrial pressures and noncompliant left ventricles. New intermediary phenotypes of heart failure are being described including heart failure with mid-range ejection fraction (be it worsening or recovery), hypokinetic-nondilated cardiomyopathy, heart failure with non-obstructive artery disease, arrhythmogenic cardiomyopathies and more. Genetic characterization and new MOGES classification of cardiomyopathies is gaining popularity. Phenotypic assessment by echocardiographic and magnetic resonance imaging has matured with strain imaging, vortex velocity imaging, native T1 and T2 mapping, etc. The success of other established drugs, resynchronization and defibrillator therapy has stood the test of time.

Consolidation of the effective therapy in heart failure and burgeoning advances necessitate a compendium for ready reference. We embarked upon this task last year during the annual scientific sessions of the Cardiology Society of India. We invited 128 chapters, classified into 15 major section headings to tackle the latest in the field for an easy read. We hope you will enjoy the collection. We promise you with another one in the series that will be on stands next year, at the same time, on the same occasion of the annual scientific sessions. Happy reading folks.

Jagat Narula, HK Chopra, Navin C Nanda

International Editors

National Editors

The Scientific committee of Advances and Innovations in Heart Failure. A Textbook of Cardiology Express their gratitude and thanks to the following Academic Partners.

Platinum Academic Partners

USV Private Limited

IPCA Laboratories Limited

Gold Academic Partners

Merck Limited

Novartis Healthcare Private Limited

Silver Academic Partners

Sun Pharmaceutical Industries Limited

Emcure Pharmaceutical Limited

Bronze Academic Partners

Eris Lifesciences Private Limited
Zepsilon Healthcare Private Limited
Nutrabuff Nutraceuticals

Zydus Cadila Healthcare Limited
J B Chemical & Pharmaceuticals Ltd

For rendering unrestricted education support which made this book possible in its current enhanced form as "Global Education Initiative".

Contents

SECTION 1: CLINICAL

SECTION 2: ECHO, IMAGING AND HEART FAILURE

SECTION 3: CORONARY ARTERY DISEASE AND HEART FAILURE

SECTION 4: STROKE AND HEART FAILURE

SECTION 5: ARRHYTHMIA AND HEART FAILURE

SECTION 9: METABOLIC

SECTION 10: NUTRITIONAL

SECTION 11: HEART FAILURE AND CARDIO-ONCOLOGY

SECTION 12: SYSTEMATICS INFLAMMATORY RELEASE SYNDROME WITH MULTIORGAN FAILURE AND CARDIOGENIC SHOCK

SECTION 13: REHABILITATION

SECTION 14: LEGAL AND ETHICAL ISSUES

SECTION 15: FUTURE DIRECTIONS

SECTION 1

Clinical

1

CHAPTER

Heart Failure in Indian Scenarios: Issues and Challenges in 2019 and Beyond

Simardeep K Khangura, Bhupinder Singh, Gurpreet S Wander

INTRODUCTION

Heart failure is a global pandemic affecting an estimated 26 million people worldwide and resulting in more than 1 million hospitalizations annually in both the United States and Europe.[1] It is a clinical syndrome that results when abnormalities in the structure and function of the myocardium impair cardiac output or decrease filling of the ventricles. The incidence and prevalence estimates of heart failure in India are rather difficult to predict as there are no adequate surveillance systems to capture this data. The estimated prevalence of heart failure in India due to coronary heart disease, hypertension, obesity, diabetes, and rheumatic heart disease is estimated to range from 1.3 million to 4.6 million with an annual incidence of 491,600–1.8 million. This does not include a few other important causes of heart failure such as alcohol abuse, cardiomyopathies, congenital heart diseases, pericardial diseases, etc.[2] In contrast to the Western world, untreated congenital heart disease and rheumatic heart disease still contribute significantly to the burden of heart failure in the South Asia region (Table 1).[3]

Patients admitted with heart failure in the South Asia region are relatively younger as compared to their western counterparts (Fig. 1).[3]

Heart failure is one of the leading causes of hospitalizations and readmissions. Moreover heart failure is associated with a postadmission mortality rate of 20–30%. There are differences in the in-hospital mortality of heart failure patients in India and the rest of the world (Fig. 2).[4,5]

TABLE 1: Comparison of etiologies of heart failure in India and western countries.[4,5]

	Western world	*India*
Ischemic etiology	63%	71%
DCM	17%	13%
RHD	-	8%
Valvular heart disease (non-RHD)	5%	2.5%
Hypertension	4%	2%

(DCM: dilated cardiomyopathy; RHD: rheumatic heart disease)

Medication adherence for Indian heart failure patients ranges from 25% to 30% and medication tolerance for guideline-based treatment is also low for Indian patients.[6] Despite all the advances in treatment, prognosis of patients with heart failure is poor. While a number of studies have documented a higher mortality in patients with heart failure with reduced ejection fraction (HFrEF), a few others have reported the mortality in both HFrEF and heart failure with preserved ejection fraction (HFpEF) to be the same. In a study, the 1-year, 3-year, 5-year, and 10-year survival rates in the congestive heart failure patients were found to be 78.5%, 59.8%, 50.4%, and 14.7%, respectively.[7]

Key differences of heart failure scenario in India and the Western countries: [3,5]

- More prevalence in younger age group
- Male predominance
- Higher prevalence of coronary artery disease
- Longer length of hospital stay with higher in-hospital mortality
- Higher mortality in heart failure patients.

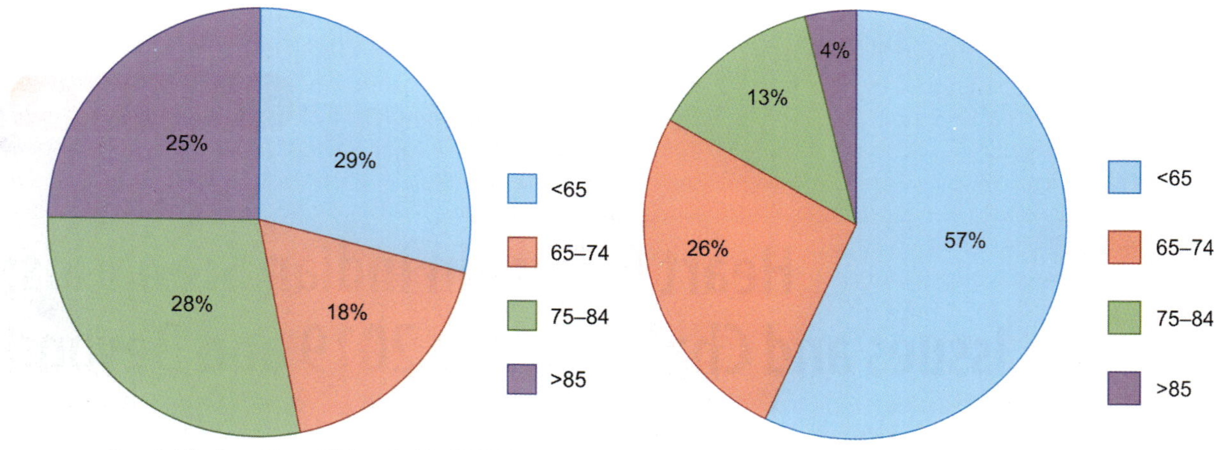

Fig. 1: Comparison of age distribution of heart failure patients in India and US.[4,5]
(ADHERE: Acute Decompensated Heart Failure National Registry)

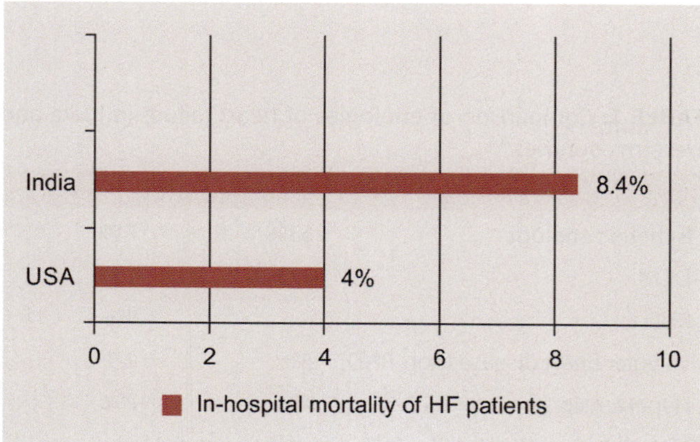

Fig. 2: Comparison of in-hospital mortality in heart failure patients.[4,5]
(HF: heart failure)

PRESENT ISSUES AND CHALLENGES

Increasing Risk Factors of Heart Failure

There is a trend of rapid urbanization throughout the country. According to 2011 Census, urban population grew to 377 million showing a growth rate of 2.76% per annum during 2001–2011.[8] The urban population in developing countries is projected to double between 2000 and 2030.[9] This demographic transition has increased the magnitude of lifestyle associated disorders and diseases.

- *Diabetes*: About 425 million people have diabetes in the world with 82 million in the Southeast Asian region and from which around 72,946,400 cases of diabetes were present in India in 2017 with a prevalence of 8.8% in adults.[10] Patients with diabetes and heart failure both have a higher risk of mortality compared with patients without diabetes or heart failure.[11] Furthermore antidiabetic medications increase the mortality and hospitalization for heart failure in patients with and without pre-existing heart failure.[12] So it is important to focus attention on controlling diabetes in order to address the increasing prevalence of heart failure and decreasing hospitalization in diabetic heart failure patients.
- *Hypertension*: About 33% urban and 25% rural Indians are hypertensive of which only one-tenth of rural and one-fifth of urban Indian hypertensive population have their blood pressure under control.[13] The number of adults with hypertension has nearly doubled from 442 million to 874 million worldwide in the past 25 years.[14] Longstanding hypertension is one of the leading risk factors of heart failure. The lowering of blood pressure over a 3–5 years period of time is effective in preventing severe disease, left ventricular (LV) hypertrophy, and congestive heart failure.[15]
- *Coronary artery disease (CAD)*: CAD is a major contributor to the progression of LV systolic dysfunction and heart failure. Most of the risk factors for CAD and heart failure are the same. Moreover data suggests that in patients with heart failure, CAD is associated with an increased mortality.[16] Despite the acknowledged role of CAD in the development of heart failure, the role of coronary revascularization in reducing heart failure associated morbidity and mortality remains controversial.[17]
- *Obesity and sedentary lifestyle*: Obesity worldwide has nearly tripled since 1975. In 2016, more than 1.9 billion adults, 18 years and older, were overweight. Out of

these, over 650 million were obese.[18] 1.6 million deaths annually can be attributed to insufficient physical activity.[19] There is convincing evidence supporting the adverse impact of obesity on the structure and function of heart affecting hemodynamics and cardiac performance leading to heart failure.[20] The role of weight reduction in improving the prognosis of obese heart failure patients is yet to be established.

- *Salt and water intake*: Excess salt and/or sodium intake has been attributed to 4.1 million annual deaths.[19] Almost all heart failure guidelines recommend low sodium and salt intake. WHO recommends <2,000 mg of sodium or <5 g of salt per day.[21] Although exact amount of salt consumption per day in Indian diet is not exactly known, but population salt consumption usually far exceeds the daily recommended salt intake. This problem could only be addressed by patient education which reinforces various behavioral strategies to ensure adequate compliance with low sodium and low salt diet.

Inadequate Access to Healthcare

Access to healthcare in India is mostly urban biased. So people living in the rural areas are at a disadvantage. Although there are a number of government funded centers at all levels in India, but the facilities provided in such institutions is not adequate for proper management of heart failure and decreasing mortality. Moreover there is also a lack of government-funded programs for the poor. There is also a lack of understanding and lack of recognition of the initial symptomatology of heart failure so that the patients only present to the hospital at an advanced stage which places a higher burden on healthcare as a number of interventions are needed at that stage in order to decrease morbidity and mortality. This increases the burden on already overburdened Indian health system. Moreover high incidences of poverty and low levels of literacy are also the contributing factors to this inadequate access. Primary prevention is one of the most neglected components of health in India. As people do not go in for routine checkups, there is very limited scope to tackle the risk factors of heart failure in order to halt the progression of patients to heart failure. Medication adherence along with dietary and lifestyle modifications constitute a very crucial part in the management of heart failure. This can only be achieved with patient education and patient compliance. Management of heart failure requires a number of pharmacologic, nonpharmacologic, and invasive strategies. Although newer devices such as an implantable cardioverter defibrillator (ICD), left ventricular assist device (LVAD), cardiac resynchronization therapy (CRT), etc. are now available in India, these devices in addition to being expensive are not so widely available so as to be readily available to all sectors. Only 19% of patients with left ventricular systolic dysfunction (LVSD) during hospital admission received guideline-based treatment (beta-blockers + angiotensin converting enzyme inhibitors/angiotensin II receptor blockers + aldosterone receptor blocker) while only 25% received guideline-based treatment on discharge.[5]

All these problems could only be addressed by public education and improving access to quality healthcare to all strata of society. Physicians can also play a pivotal role in patient education, which consequently will improve compliance and improve morbidity and mortality of heart failure. Moreover, a number of studies have proven that the early detection of asymptomatic patients with an LV ejection fraction ≤40% is important because effective therapy delays the onset of heart failure and prolongs life, further emphasizing the need of public education and timely intervention.[22,23]

Increase in the Aged Population

The share of population over the age of 60 years is projected to increase from 8% in 2015 to 19% in 2050. According to the United Nations Fund for Population Activities (UNFPA) estimates, by the end of the century, the elderly will constitute nearly 34% of the total population in the country.[24] This superimposed by improved and better survival after cardiac insults due to a number of advances in medical field has contributed to the increased prevalence of heart failure as risk of heart failure increases with advancing age with a high rate of early rehospitalization for heart failure. This age group is also prone to polypharmacy, multiple comorbidities, and differences in medication tolerance. So, due consideration has to be given to frame policies that ensure easy and affordable access to healthcare for this population.

Quality of Life Issues

A study has found that the number of physical symptoms, depression scores, and spiritual well-being in heart failure patients is similar to that of cancer patients. In fact, severe heart failure patients with worse health status had a greater number of physical symptoms, higher depression scores, and lower spiritual well-being than patients with advanced cancer.[25] So considering that, severe heart failure patients do need a great deal of palliative care and access to mental health. This emphasizes the importance of having a multidisciplinary approach for managing the symptoms and complications of heart failure in patients.

CONCLUSION

As the risk factors leading to heart failure are on the rise, so is the incidence and prevalence of heart failure. The three main factors that are important in the management of heart failure are medications, dietary, and lifestyle modifications. Patient education and compliance along with access to quality healthcare are the only things which can assure this. In order to prevent heart failure incidence from rising, early detection and treatment of high-risk candidates by general practitioners and physicians at all levels is required. Initiation of effective therapy at a stage where the patient is not symptomatic and there is only evidence of decreased LV ejection fraction is very important as it will help decrease the progression of heart failure to later stages. If this is done, not only will it lead to better long-term outcomes for the patient, it will also lessen the financial burden on the system, as early preventative interventions usually tend to be more cost effective, versus more advanced stage disease interventions.

REFERENCES

1. Ambrosy AP, Fonarow GC, Butler J, et al. The global health and economic burden of hospitalizations for heart failure: lessons learned from hospitalized heart failure registries. J Am Coll Cardiol. 2014;63(12):1123-33.
2. Huffman MD, Prabhakaran D. Heart failure: epidemiology and prevention in India. Natl Med J India. 2010;23(5):283-8.
3. Pillai HS, Ganapathi S. Heart failure in South Asia. Curr Cardiol Rev. 2013;9(2):102-11.
4. Fonarow GC, Yancy CW, Heywood JT, et al. Adherence to heart failure quality-of-care indicators in US hospitals: analysis of the ADHERE Registry. Arch Intern Med. 2005;165(13):1469-77.
5. Harikrishnan S, Sanjay G, Anees T, et al. Clinical presentation, Management, in-hospital and 90-day outcomes of heart failure patients in Trivandrum, Kerela, India: the Trivandrum Heart Failure Registry. Eur J Heart Fail. 2015;17(8):794-800.
6. Seth S, Ramakrishnan S, Parekh N, et al. Heart failure guidelines for India: Update 2017. J Pract Cardiovasc Sci. 2017;3:133-8.
7. Matoba M, Matsui S, Hirakawa T, et al. Long term prognosis of patients with congestive heart failure. Jpn Circ J. 1990;54(1):57-61.
8. Bhagat RB. Urbanisation in India: Trend, Pattern and Policy Issues. Working Paper No. 17. Mumbai: International Institute for Population Sciences; 2018.
9. Wild S, Roglic G, Green A, et al. Global prevalence of diabetes: estimates for the year 2000 and projections for 2030. Diabetes Care. 2004;27(5):1047-53.
10. International Diabetes Federation. (2019). IDF SEA members. [online] Available from https://www.idf.org/our-network/regions-members/south-east-asia/members/94-india.html [Last accessed November, 2019].
11. Metra M, Zacà V, Parati G, et al. Cardiovascular and noncardiovascular comorbidities in patients with chronic heart failure. J Cardiovasc Med (Hagerstown). 2011;12(2):76-84.
12. Rosano GM, Vitale C, Seferovic P. Heart failure in Patients with Diabetes Mellitus. Card Fail Rev. 2017;3(1):52-5.
13. Anchala R, Kannuri NK, Pant H, et al. Hypertension in India: a systematic review and meta-analysis of prevalence, awareness, and control of hypertension. J Hypertens. 2014;32(6):1170-7.
14. Forouzanfar MH, Liu P, Roth GA, et al. Global Burden of Hypertension and Systolic Blood Pressure of at Least 110 to 115 mm Hg, 1990-2015. JAMA. 2017;317(2):165-82.
15. Moser M, Herbert PR. Prevention of disease progression, left ventricular hypertrophy and congestive heart failure in hypertension treatment trials. J Am Coll Cardiol. 1996;27(5):1214-8.
16. Gheorghiade M, Flaherty JD, Fonarow GC, et al. Coronary artery disease, coronary revascularization, and outcomes in chronic advanced systolic heart failure. Int J Cardiol. 2011;151(1):69-75.
17. Lala A, Desai AS. The role of coronary artery disease in heart failure. Heart Fail Clin. 2014;10(2):353-65.
18. WHO. (2018). Obesity and Overweight. [online] Available from http://www.who.int/mediacentre/factsheets/fs311/en/index.html [Last accessed November, 2019].
19. WHO. (2014). Global status report on noncommunicable diseases 2014. [online] Available from http://www.who.int/nmh/publications/ncd-status-report-2014/en/ [Last accessed November, 2019].
20. Hamzeh N, Ghadimi F, Farzaneh R, et al. Obesity, Heart failure, and Obesity Paradox. J the Univ Heart Ctr. 2017;12(1):1-5.
21. WHO. (2013). WHO issues new guidance on dietary salt and potassium. [online] Available from https://www.who.int/mediacentre/news/notes/2013/salt_potassium_20130131/en/ [Last accessed November, 2019].
22. Yusuf S, Pitt B, Davis CE, et al. Effect of enalapril on mortality and the development of heart failure in asymptomatic patients with reduced left ventricular ejection fractions. N Engl J Med. 1992;327(10):685-91.
23. Garg R, Yusuf S. Overview of randomized trials of angiotensin-converting enzyme inhibitors on mortality and morbidity in patients with heart failure. Collaborative Group on ACE Inhibitor Trials. JAMA. 1995;273(18):1450-6.
24. UNFPA India. (2017). Caring for Our Elders: Early Responses India Ageing Report 2017. [online] Available from https://india.unfpa.org/en/publications/caring-our-elders-early-responses-india-ageing-report-2017 [Last accessed November, 2019].
25. Bekelman DB, Rumsfeld JS, Havranek EP. et al. Symptom burden, depression, and spiritual well being: a comparison of heart failure and advanced cancer patients. J Gen Intern Med. 2009;24(5):592-8.

CHAPTER 2

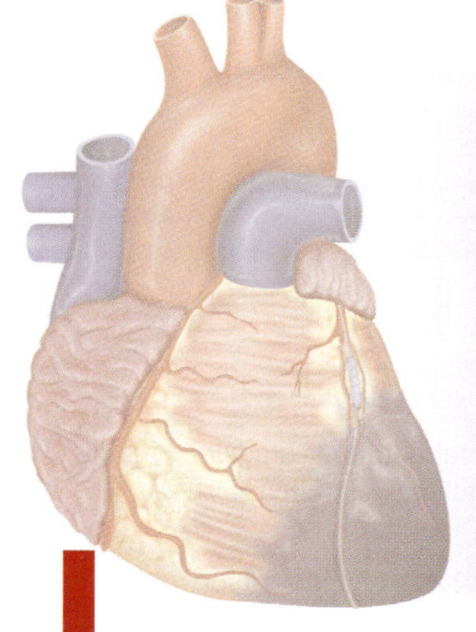

Pathophysiology and Prevention of LV Diastolic Heart Failure

Hanumanth K Reddy, Ravi Komatireddy, Raghuveer Kura, Thirupathi K Reddy

INTRODUCTION

The prevalence of diastolic heart failure is increasing exponentially with rising age of the population, obesity, and inactivity. Left ventricular (LV) diastolic dysfunction and diastolic heart failure with preserved ejection fraction (HFpEF) are usually associated with hypertension, coronary artery disease (CAD), valvular heart disease, hypertrophic and restrictive cardiomyopathies, tachycardia, and atrial fibrillation. Close to 50% of heart failure patients have preserved LV ejection fraction along with diastolic dysfunction.[1] High morbidity and mortality are associated with this condition. Although, left ventricular end-diastolic pressure (LVEDP) has shown to be elevated in these patients on a consistent basis.[2,3] Impaired cardiac reserve, especially during exercise, plays a major role. This is due to a complex interplay of subtle systolic dysfunction (altered strain, twisting, and suction) and impaired diastolic function. Impaired LV diastolic relaxation with stiffness has many causes. Interstitial fibrosis, alteration of structural, architectural, and biochemical properties of actin-myosin complex and reduced SERC-ATPase required for active relaxation. Furthermore, atrioventricular synchrony and coupling, ventricular interaction, ventricular geometry, pericardial restraint as well as ventriculovascular coupling play critical roles in diastolic dysfunction. Although multiple factors are involved, elevated LVEDP and decreased cardiac reserve constitute the clinical substrate for diastolic heart failure. Increased LVEDP causes pulmonary congestion, pulmonary hypertension, and right-sided congestion and dyspnea. Decreased cardiac reserve leads to effort intolerance, fatigue, and dyspnea. Increased heart rate, atrial fibrillation, uncontrolled hypertension, and renal dysfunction may complicate the patient's clinical course. The goals of management include adequate diuresis, control of heart rate and blood pressure, possible cardioversion, and promotion of physical exercise.

PATHOPHYSIOLOGY OF DIASTOLIC HEART FAILURE

Left ventricular diastolic heart failure is multifactorial in origin. A wide variety of risk factors are involved in this type of heart failure. However, all individuals with similar risk factors do not develop diastolic heart failure indicating the fact that some individuals have genetic predisposition to this condition. In fact, there are some reports suggesting genetic predisposition to ventricular stiffness, diastolic dysfunction, and diastolic heart failure.

GENETIC BASIS OF LEFT VENTRICULAR DIASTOLIC HEART FAILURE

Genetic basis for LV diastolic dysfunction (LVDD) has not been well-worked out. Multiple authors have reported a role of micro-ribonucleic acids (miRNAs) in diastolic heart failure. miRNAs work as regulators of gene expression by controlling messenger RNAs (mRNAs). In vitro experiments, either knockdown or overexpression of miRNAs in cultured cardiomyocytes was shown to influence cardiomyocyte hypertrophy.[4] Van Rooij et al. reported that overexpression of miRNA-195 in rodent hypertrophic hearts resulted in dilated cardiomyopathy and heart failure.[5] There is continuous flow of new information about the seminal role of miRNAs in the pathophysiology of diastolic heart failure and cardiomyopathies. In the near future, miRNAs are going to be new therapeutic targets in the management of heart failure.

GROSS STRUCTURAL AND SUBCELLULAR SUBSTRATES OF LV DIASTOLIC DYSFUNCTION

Left Ventricular Relaxation

Left ventricular relaxation during diastole is a highly energy dependent process. Any impairment of the energy utilization during diastole is associated with LVDD. This impairment is more evident in late diastole since atrial contribution plays an important role at this stage. Certain individuals have structural predisposition to LVDD based on the type of titin isoform.

Role of Titin in Left Ventricular Diastolic Dysfunction

Titin or elastin is a giant elastic protein noted in human myocardial cells. It is the third most commonly available protein in the human myocardium after myosin and actin. Because of its large size, it is named after the Greek mythological giant *Titan*. Titin molecules link thick filaments to Z-disk and the M-line thus networking sarcomeres and playing an important role in their normal stretching and stretch recovery. It is composed of immunoglobulin and fibronectin like domains. Its kinase domain provides signaling and elasticity properties to the cardiomyocyte. In other words, it works as a molecular spring needed for the normal LV diastolic function. Furthermore, it plays a critical role in myocyte postcontraction recovery and prevention of overstretching of the myocyte. Titin mutations cause dilated cardiomyopathy. Human myocardium has two types of titin isoforms. N2B is the stiffer titin isoform commonly found in patients with LVDD and increased LV stiffness may be attributed to this type of titin (Fig. 1). Borbely et al. showed in heart failure patients that hypophosphorylation of the stiff N2B isoform may contribute to increased myocardial stiffness.[6] N2BA is relatively softer titin isoform and is predominantly present in patients with dilated cardiomyopathy. Alternatively, ventricular relaxation may be related to changes in troponin I protein kinase A (PKA) phosphorylation. This PKA mediated troponin I phosphorylation is energy dependent and leads to reduced myofibrillar calcium sensitivity, increased calcium dissociation from troponin C, and

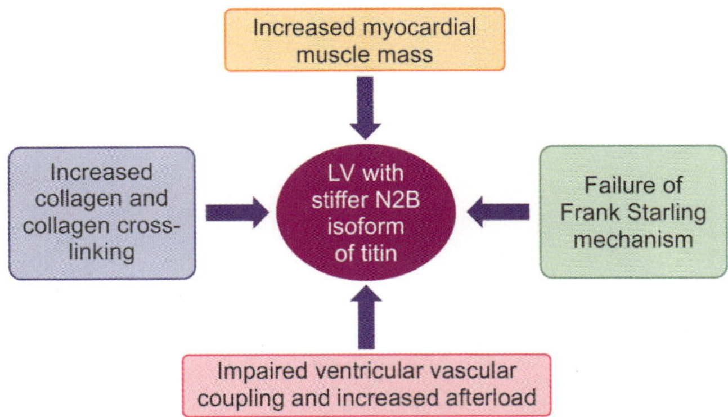

Fig. 1: Interaction of structural and physiological variables in left ventricular diastolic dysfunction (LVDD).

enhanced myocardial relaxation. Decreased reserves of energy at rest mediate impaired LV relaxation at rest and also cause limited contractile reserve (during exercise with decreased phosphocreatine/adenosine triphosphate ratio). The causes of this decrease in resting myocardial energy include aging, insulin resistance, neuroendocrine activation, mitochondrial dysfunction, and impaired substrate metabolism. A phenotype for this pathophysiology is hypertrophic cardiomyopathy where decreased creatine phosphate (PCr)/ATP correlated with fibrous area of the LV myocardium.

Influence of Cellular and Biochemical Homeostasis on Cardiomyocytes and Fibroblasts in LVDD

There is a delicate interplay of cellular and biochemical elements in patients with LVDD. There is an active signal mediated crosstalk among coronary microvascular endothelial cells, cardiomyocytes, and fibroblasts via a myriad of mediators including nitric oxide (NO), cyclic guanosine monophosphate (CGM), and protein kinase G (PKG) (Fig. 2). Normally, these molecules maintain the active relaxed state of the left ventricle and depletion of these elements with inflammation and oxidative stress leads to cardiomyocyte hypertrophy, fibroblast proliferation, and LV stiffness (Figs. 1 and 2).

Hemodynamic Basis and Clinical Presentation

Normal left ventricle has a finite range of elastic properties beyond which LV diastolic pressure rises steeply with an increase in volume. Impaired ventricular elasticity or increased stiffness may be secondary to altered actin-myosin calcium and titin complex associated with genetic abnormality and may be an acquired process related to

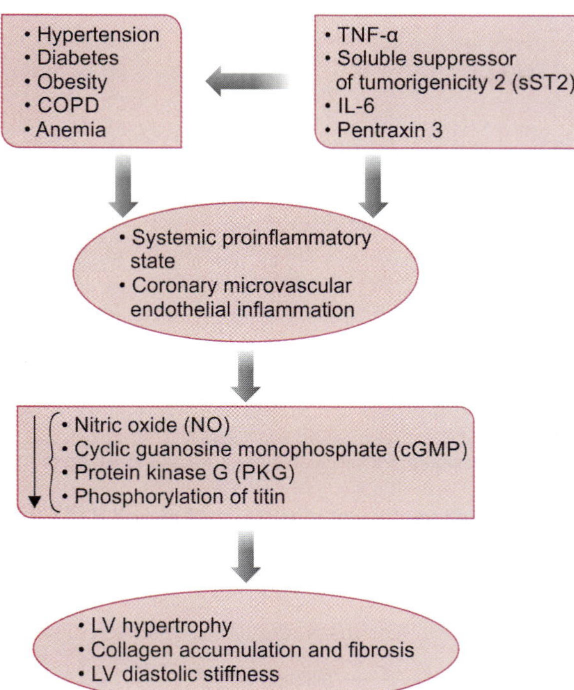

Fig. 2: Proposed mechanisms linking risk factors to LV diastolic dysfunction.

(COPD: chronic obstructive pulmonary disease; IL-6: Interleukin 6; LV: left ventricular; TNF-α: tumor necrosis factor-α)

Source: Paulus WJ, Tschöpe C. A novel paradigm for heart failure with preserved ejection fraction: comorbidities drive myocardial dysfunction and remodeling through coronary microvascular endothelial inflammation. J Am Coll Cardiol. 2013;62(4):263-71.

A 52-year man with STEMI with improving LVDD post intervention.

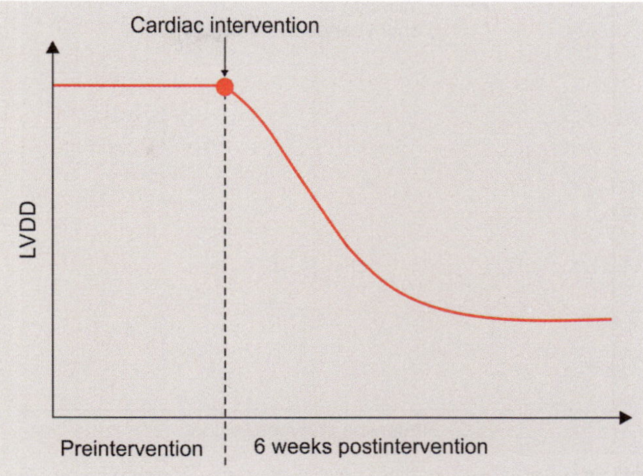

Fig. 3: Impact of ST-elevation myocardial infarction (STEMI) and intervention on left ventricular diastolic dysfunction (LVDD).

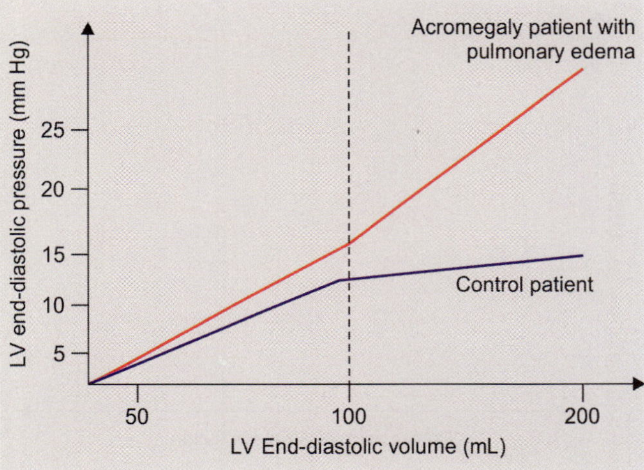

Fig. 4: Interaction between LVDD with severe LVH, pulmonary edema undergoing diuresis in a 57-year-old man with acromegaly.

(LV: left ventricular; LVDD: left ventricular diastolic dysfunction; LVH: left ventricular hypertrophy)

ventricular hypertrophy, dilatation, and scarring. LVDD may be due to dynamic pathophysiological processes such as volume or pressure overload associated with congenital heart disease with shunts, valvular heart disease, obesity/hypoventilation, hypertrophic cardiomyopathy, dilated cardiomyopathy, atrial fibrillation, sleep apnea, anemia, uncontrolled hypertension, and active myocardial ischemia/myocardial infarction (MI) with CAD (Figs. 3 to 10). Dynamic LVDD may be partially or totally normalized with effective management of the causative factors. The time course of LVDD recovery may be short or prolonged based on the severity and duration of the underlying process. In some cases of advanced structural and congenital myocardial abnormalities, LVDD may become severe and irreversible.

Increased Left Ventricular End-diastolic Pressure in Diastolic Heart Failure

The hemodynamic end product of various pathophysiological mechanisms of LVDD is elevated LVEDP which translates into fluid congestion and congestive heart failure (CHF). LVDD is an early partner of LV systolic dysfunction often clinically manifesting as pulmonary edema in situations such as acute MI, papillary muscle rupture, and acute onset of atrial fibrillation with rapid ventricular rate, especially in hypertrophic obstructive cardiomyopathy (HOCM), valvular aortic stenosis, and uncontrolled hypertension patients. With prompt therapy, LVDD mostly improves to a variable degree in these patients (Figs. 3 to 6 and Fig. 10). Chronic LVDD is a slow and an incremental process occurring over a period of decades. Initially subtle in its clinical presentation, LVDD finally manifests itself as LV

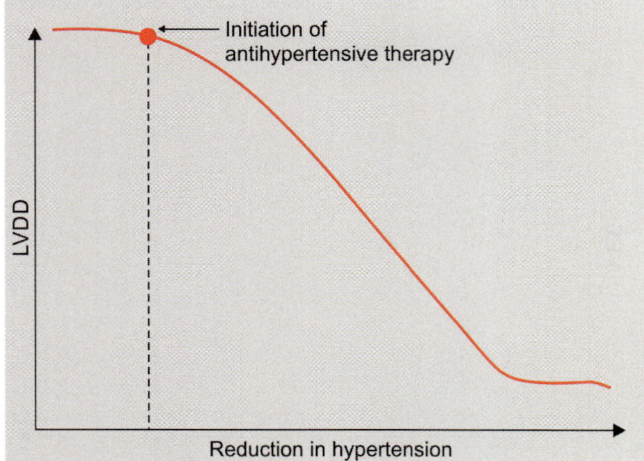

Fig. 5: Left ventricular diastolic dysfunction (LVDD) changes in a 67-year-old man with uncontrolled hypertension, before and after control of hypertension.

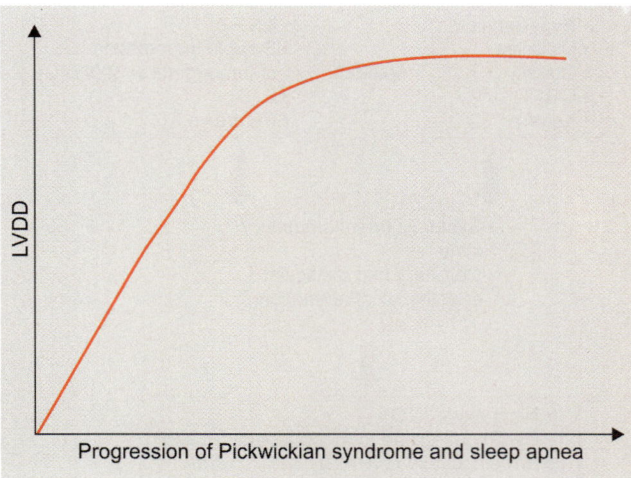

Fig. 7: Left ventricular diastolic dysfunction (LVDD) associated with Pickwickian syndrome and sleep apnea.

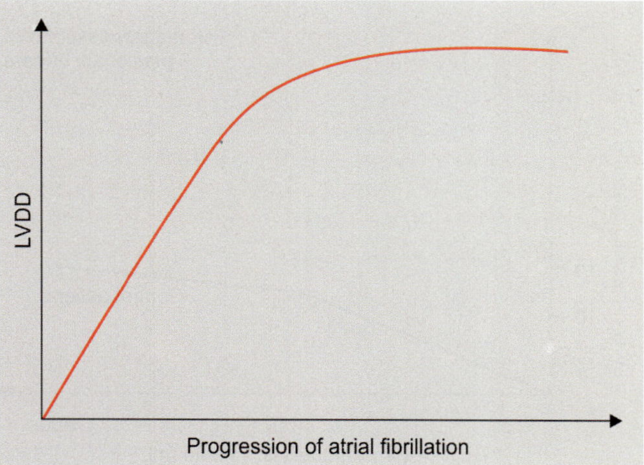

Fig. 6: Left ventricular diastolic dysfunction (LVDD) and atrial fibrillation.

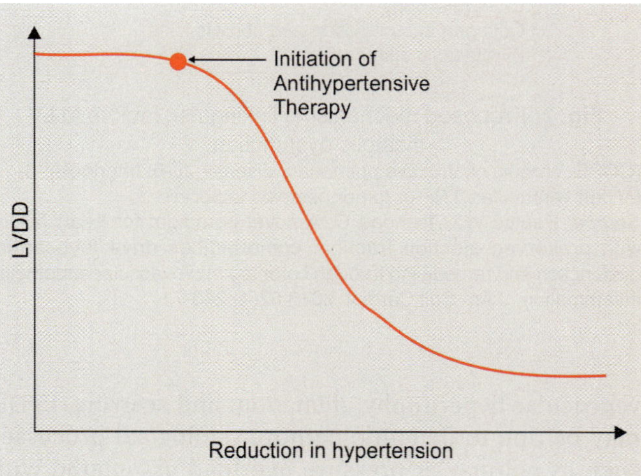

Fig. 8: Left ventricular diastolic dysfunction (LVDD) related to obesity—deconditioning and small vessel disease with hypertensive treatment.

diastolic heart failure often in later stages of life. LVDD becomes an integral part of various clinical conditions as shown in Figures 3 to 10. Chronic elevation in LVEDP is gradually compensated by pulmonary vasculature, both the atria, right ventricle (RV), peripheral veins, lymphatics, and the third space. Structural and electrical remodeling of the atria occurs. Atria are dilated and become dysfunctional, loosing their booster pump function. Cardiac output decreases and the frequently associated atrial fibrillation which makes diastolic heart failure worse. The right-sided compensatory mechanisms with RV dilatation, pulmonary hypertension, and peripheral fluid congestion prevent pulmonary vascular congestion and pulmonary edema thus avoiding a lethal outcome to the patient.

Impaired Cardiac Output and Vasodilator Reserve with Altered Ventricular-arterial Coupling

In patients with diastolic heart failure, increased stiffness is seen both in the left ventricle and the large peripheral arteries.[7] This combined ventricular-vascular stiffness associated with reduced LV diastolic filling leads to decreased cardiac output at rest and during exercise. Furthermore, in these patients, left bundle branch block (LBBB) and atrial fibrillation may cause ventricular-arterial decoupling and further compromise in cardiac output. In fact, peak exercise cardiac output and maximal oxygen uptake ($VOmax_2$) have been reported to be limited in these patients.

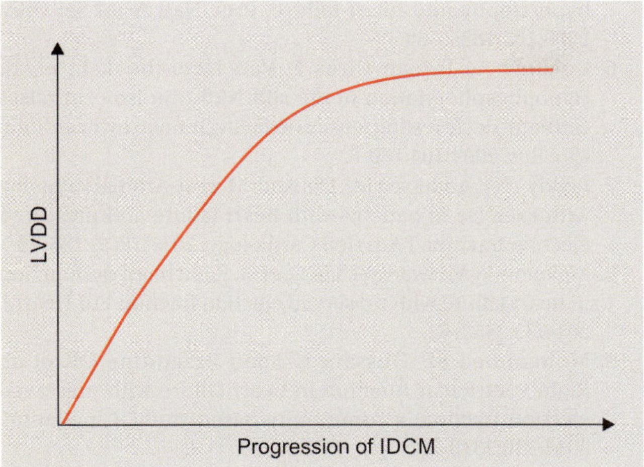

Fig. 9: Left ventricular diastolic dysfunction (LVDD) in patients with idiopathic dilated cardiomyopathy (IDCM).

LVDD

Progression of HOCM

Fig. 10: Left ventricular diastolic dysfunction (LVDD) associated with hypertrophic obstructive cardiomyopathy (HOCM).

Atrial Dysfunction

Left atrial (LA) volume progressively increases leading to LA myopathy and an eventual loss of booster pump function in patients with diastolic heart failure. Furthermore, LA strain decreases, LA stiffness increases, and LA diastolic dysfunction ensues.

Right Ventricle Dysfunction and Pulmonary Hypertension

While the focus has been on the LVDD in diastolic heart failure, the roles of peripheral circulation, vasodilator reserve, atrial and RV dysfunction, and pulmonary hypertension cannot be overestimated. A significant number of diastolic heart failure patients have peripheral circulatory dysfunction, right ventricular dilatation and dysfunction (RVD), pulmonary hypertension, and right heart failure.[8,9] This is an advanced stage of diastolic heart failure and is often irreversible.

Risk Factors for Left Ventricular Diastolic Hear Failure

Diastolic heart failure is more commonly associated with aging, female sex, obesity, metabolic syndrome, hypertension, chronic obstructive pulmonary disease, anemia, and chronic kidney disease.

Primary Prevention

With an alarming rise in childhood and adult obesity and metabolic syndrome, there has been an epidemic of LVDD and diastolic heart failure in the industrialized countries. Outcomes are poor in diastolic heart failure patients and there is no proven and effective therapy. Therefore, the best way to prevent the most common type of LVDD is to prevent metabolic syndrome from childhood. Promotion of the culture of physical activity at home, gymnastic, and sports activities at school and work place should be the fashionable modus operandi of each community. Excessive consumption of calories in the absence of physical activity should be strongly discouraged.

Aerobic Exercise in Patients with LVDD and Diastolic Heart Failure

Aerobic exercise has been shown to prevent and improve diastolic heart failure in patients with LVDD.[10,11] In patients with regular aerobic exercise, it is easier to modify the coexisting risk factors such as obesity, hypertension, and diabetes. Randomized controlled and single center studies as well as meta-analysis of several studies have shown improvement in aerobic capacity and quality of life in diastolic heart failure patients.[12]

Control of Hypertension and Diabetes

Adequate control of blood pressure preferably with angiotensin-converting enzyme (ACE) inhibitors, angiotensin receptor blockers (ARBs), and beta-blockers will prevent and mitigate LVDD and eventual diastolic heart failure. Diuretics are often needed in these patients. Optimal diabetic therapy with sodium-glucose cotransporter-2 (SGLT2) inhibitors has been shown to prevent CHF hospitalizations.

Secondary Prevention

In patients with diastolic heart failure due to advanced LVDD, optimal medical therapy is unavailable at the present time. In addition to aerobic exercise, drugs including diuretics, ACE inhibitors, ARBs, beta-blockers and vasodilators, aggressive therapies with atrial fibrillation ablation, and biventricular pacing may be needed. However, prognosis in these patients is quite poor.

REFERENCES

1. Owan TE, Hodge DO, Herges RM, et al. Trends in prevalence and outcome of heart failure with preserved ejection fraction. N Engl J Med. 2006;355:251-9.
2. Grossman W. Diastolic dysfunction in congestive heart failure. N Engl J Med. 1991;325:1557-64.
3. Bonow RO, Udelson JE. Left ventricular diastolic dysfunction as a cause of congestive heart failure. Mechanisms and management. An Intern Med. 1992;117:502-10.
4. Sayed D, Hong C, Chen IY, MicroRNAs play an essential role in the development of cardiac hypertrophy. Circ Res. 2007;100:416-24.
5. van Rooij E, Sutherland LB, Liu N, et al. A signature pattern of stress-responsive microRNAs that can evoke cardiac hypertrophy and heart failure. Proc Natl Acad Sci USA. 2006;103:18255-60.
6. Borbely A, Talcao-Pires I, Van Heerebeek L, et al. Hypophosphorylation of the stiff N2B titin isoform raises cardiomyocyte resting tension in failing human myocardium. Circ Res. 2009;104:780-6.
7. Reddy YNV, Andersen MJ, Obokata M, et al. Arterial stiffening with exercise in patients with heart failure and preserved ejection fraction. J Am Coll Cardiology. 2017;70(2):136-48.
8. Melenovsky V, Hwang SJ, Lin G, et al. Right heart dysfunction in heart failure with preserved ejection fraction Eur Heart J. 2014;35:3452-62.
9. Mohammed SF, Hussain I, Abou Ezzeddine OF, et al. Right ventricular function in heart failure with preserved ejection fraction: a community-based study. Circulation. 2014;130:2310-20.
10. Howden EJ, Sarma S, Lawley JS, et al. Reversing the cardiac effects of sedentary aging in middle age-a randomized controlled trial. Circulation. 2018;137:1549-60.
11. Edemann F, Gelbrich G, Dungen HD, et al. Exercise training improves exercise capacity and diastolic function in patients with heart failure with preserved ejection fraction: results of the Ex-DHF (Exercise training in Diastolic Heart Failure) pilot study. J Am Coll Cardiol. 2011;58, 1780-91.
12. Ponikowski P, Voors AA, Anker SD, et al. 2016 ESC guidelines for the diagnosis and treatment of acute and chronic heart failure. Rev Esp Cardiol (Engl Ed). 2016;69(12):1167.

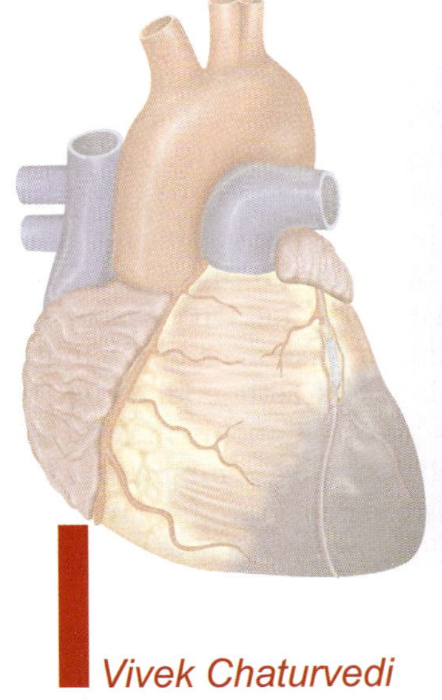

Heart Failure: From India to the Globe

Vivek Chaturvedi

INTRODUCTION

Heart failure (HF) is the modern plague of our times and is likely to remain so in the foreseeable future. While the etiologies may be different, there is no doubt that the burden of HF is increasing worldwide. And while tremendous progress has been achieved in its treatment, increasing age at presentation, comorbidities and better survival from acute episodes have meant that the outcomes are still dismal and not very different than 3 decades ago. This chapter attempts to briefly outline the current epidemiology of HF in India, and worldwide.

BURDEN OF HEART FAILURE

While lower income countries have HF burden primarily due to infectious, nutritional, and hypertension-related heart disease, in lower middle-income countries like India there is a double burden of rheumatic heart disease (RHD) as well as hypertension and atherosclerotic heart disease. Most of the HF in developed nations emanates from ischemic heart disease (IHD) and multicausal diastolic HF. Further, congenital heart disease and cardiomyopathies (region specific as well as worldwide) also contribute to this burden. It is estimated that in 2012, 26 million people worldwide were living with HF.[1] To put this in perspective, similar number are living worldwide with cancer (32 million). This was responsible for more than 10% of total health expenditure in USA and probably similar proportion in other countries with managed healthcare.[2] In USA approximately 5.8 million people are living with HF while China had about 4.2 million people with HF in 2010 and 500,000 new cases were diagnosed each year.[3] In Japan approximately 1 million people have HF while almost 9 million people suffer from HF in Southeast Asian countries.

In general, the overall prevalence of HF in adults worldwide is about 1–2%,[1] but this varies a lot depending on the age group with dramatic increases seen above age of 80 years. In terms of lifetime risk, it has been estimated that at the age of 40 years, one out of every five adults is likely to develop HF in his lifetime.[4] In developed countries, with better treatment of coronary artery disease (CAD) and hypertension, the rates of heart failure with reduced ejection fraction (HFrEF) is decreasing while prevalence of heart failure with preserved ejection fraction (HFpEF) is increasing. Contemporary magnitude of HF in UK was provided by Conrad et al. in 2018[5] amongst a representative community based sample of 4 million individuals. They showed that between 2002 and 2014, the incidence of HF decreased by 7% from 358 to 332 per 100,000 population. While a decline in new onset HF in the 60–85 years age group was responsible for this decrease, the same period saw a rising incidence in the older people. Thus, the absolute number of newly diagnosed HF increased by 12%. New onset HF cases were more in number than newly reported cases of breast, lung, bowel, and prostate cancers put together! The prevalence in population was about 1.6%, an increase of 23% during this period, due to rising age and better survival after myocardial infarction (MI). Socioeconomically disadvantaged were more likely to develop HF and at an earlier age as well. The age at diagnosis also increased significantly and so did the associated comorbid conditions (from mean 3.4 to 5.4). Approximately two-thirds had hypertension, half had IHD, and 245 had kidney dysfunction or failure.

As a primary diagnosis, HF accounts for 1–4% of all hospital admissions in developed nations.[1] The number is likely to rise further if HF as a secondary diagnosis or misclassification is accounted for. In India, in one tertiary hospital in North India, it accounted for 20% of all admissions to medical cardiology services.[6] The hospital burden for HF is enormous because the average hospital stay for HF patients is 5–10 days and uptil a quarter are readmitted in a month and two-thirds within a year.[1] Quality of life suffers tremendously in chronic HF. Data from Sweden has shown that premature life years lost due to HF (66,318 in men and 59,535 in women) in Sweden are more than that from cancer (55,364 and 64,533, respectively).[7]

BURDEN OF HEART FAILURE IN INDIA

In India, there is no large representative population or cohort data to reliably inform the incidence and prevalence of HF. However of concern, the main cardiovascular diseases (CVDs) contributing to HF, IHD, hypertensive heart disease (HHD) and RHD have seen a rise in their burden. Total deaths attributable to CVD increased from 15% to 28% from 1990 to 2016.[8] Similarly the proportion of total disability adjusted life years (DALYs) attributable to CVD increased from 7% to 14%. In 2016, this meant that the chief causes of HF (IHD, HHD, and RHD) were responsible for 20% of total mortality and 10% of DALYs. Approximate estimated prevalence of IHD in India in 2016 was 24 million. During the same period, the prevalence of high blood pressure, high blood glucose, and high total cholesterol increased across the entire nation. While not a direct proof, these data do indicate that the incidence and prevalence of HF is set to rise dramatically in India. We[6] estimated the prevalence of HF burden in India, using projections made by both age-specific extrapolations from developed countries (assuming similar prevalence of CAD and HHD) and data regarding development of HF in the presence of risk factors. The estimated prevalence of HF is about 1% of the total population or about 8–10 million individuals in India. The estimated mortality attributable to HF is about 0.1–0.16 million individuals per year. Other has estimated this prevalence to be between 1.3 million and 4.6 million, which is probably an underestimate.

The causes and type of HF are heterogeneous across world populations. In the high-income countries, while significant control of traditional risk factors for HF has taken place, there have been neutral or even declining, trends in prevalence of HFrEF which in these countries, is driven more by increasing survival after MI. On the other hand, HFpEF is on the rise because of increasing age, obesity, hypertension, atrial fibrillation, kidney disease, etc. In low- and middle-income countries there is still a large legacy of unique infectious causes of HF like Chagas disease, human immunodeficiency virus (HIV) and RHD. In Latin America, Chagas disease is responsible for more than half of all HFs.[9,10] In Sub-Saharan Africa, the most common cause of HF is HHD (39%) and IHD is relatively uncommon (7%) as compared to Western nations.[11] India, and South Asia in general, has variable etiology of HF owing to different regions and strata being in different states of transition. While RHD is still a common cause of HF in socioeconomically disadvantaged groups, HHD and CAD as an etiology for HF are present across the entire socioeconomic spectrum. In the Indian centers of the International Congestive Heart Failure (INTER-CHF) study, IHD was the etiology in 46%, while the Trivandrum Heart Failure Registry had 72% patients with IHD.[13]

While in developed nations, 80% of patients are above the age of 65 years, more than half of HF patients in Sub-Saharan Africa are younger than 50 years.[14] The average age of HF patients in Indian studies has been 55–60 years. While HFpEF accounts for more than half of HF patients in developed nations, in Trivandrum Registry only 25% patients were admitted with HFpEF, possibly because of decreased survival after acute coronary events and shorter life expectancy.

OUTCOMES OF HEART FAILURE

Across the globe, 17–45% of patients admitted to a hospital with HF die within 1 year of admission and the majority die within 5 years of admission.[1] Disappointingly, this has stayed true over last 3–4 decades despite significant advances in medical and interventional management of HF. Table 1 shows the short- and long-term outcomes of patients admitted with acute decompensated HF in India and across the world.

European Society of Cardiology Long-Term heart Failure Study[19] is an important long-term prospective observational registry from 21 European countries with data collected on 12,440 acute heart failure (AHF) and chronic heart failure patients between 2011 and 2013. The study aimed to describe the clinical characteristics and 1 year outcomes of HF patients across varied European health systems. The mean age was 65–70 years and 40% presented with AHF. IHD was present in half and almost 40% had left ventricular ejection fraction (LVEF) more than 40%. Almost a quarter (23.6%) of those admitted initially with AHF died over a period of 1 year while

TABLE 1: Contemporary studies on short- and long-term outcomes of acute heart failure patients.

Study	*Number*	*Mean age*	*Common causes*	*In-hospital mortality*	*Intermediate mortality*	*Long-term mortality*	*Hospitalization*
Trivandrum Heart Failure Registry 2013[13,15]	1,205 31% women	61 years	IHD (72%) 25% HFpEF	HFrEF 10% HFpEF 5%	1 year mortality 31%	45% At 3 year	30% 1 year
Trivandrum 2018[16]	287 33% women	65 years	IHD 63%			425 IHD 30% NIHD	90 days IHD 56%, NIHD 33%
Delhi 2015[17]	90 37% women	53 years	IHD 54%	31%			
ADHERE International-Asia Pacific Registry[18]	10,171 57% men	67 years		5%			
ESC Long-term HF Registry[19]	5,038			5%	1 year morality 24%		19% at 1 year
OPTIMIZE-HF Registry, USA, 2007[20]	>41,000 patients	HFrEF 70 years HFpEF 75 years	Roughly half each with HFrEF and HFpEF	HFrEF-3.9% HFpEF 2.9%	60–90 day mortality: HFrEF 9.8 HFpEF 9.5%		60–90 days hospitalization HFpEF 29% HFrEF 30%
Get with the Guidelines-HF and Medicare data, 2014[21–23]	>40,000 patients		47% had HFpEF, 14% had HF with borderline EF (HFbEF) and 39% had HFrEF			Median survival 2 years 5 years mortality in all groups 75%	
Latin America meta-analysis[24]		Mean age ~60 years	Chagas (highest mortality) Ischemic Dilated CM Hypertensive	12%	1 year 25%	5 year 47%	1 year hospitalization rate 31%

(ADHERE: Acute Decompensated Heart Failure National Registry; CM: cardiomyopathy; ESC: European Society of Cardiology; HFpEF: heart failure with preserved ejection fraction; HFrEF: heart failure with reduced ejection fraction; IHD: ischemic heart disease; NIHD: nonischemic heart failure; OPTIMIZE-HF: Organized Program to Initiate Lifesaving Treatment in Hospitalized Patients with Heart Failure)

almost a third died or were hospitalized within 1 year. The 1 year mortality and mortality or hospitalization rates for patients with congestive heart failure (CHF) were 6% and 15%, respectively. Among the CHF patients, outcomes were further stratified according to the baseline LVEF, with EF <40% as HFrEF, EF 40–50% as HF with mid-range EF (HFmrEF), and EF> 50% as HFpEF. Mortality among the three groups was 8.8%, 7.6%, and 6.3%. Combined incidence of death and hospitalization at 1 year was 21.2%, 15%, and 14.6%, respectively.

An important landmark in HF research has been the INTER-CHF study.[12] The study aimed to measure HF mortality at 1 year and its prognostic factors in patients with HF in Africa, China, India, the Middle East, Southeast Asia and South America. It enrolled 2,105 in-hospital admissions for HF and 3,695 HF patients presenting in outpatients from 108 centers worldwide in 6 geographical regions. They were followed up at 6 months and 1 year to record symptoms, medications, and outcomes. Mean age of the group was 59 years (56 in India) and 61% were males. The combined 1 year mortality was 16.5%, highest in Africa (34%) and India (23%), intermediate in Southeast Asia (15%) and lowest in China, South America, and Middle East (7–9%). The population characteristics of the patients enrolled and the outcomes in India are presented in Table 2. Despite the younger age, mortality for both AHF and CHF was significantly higher among Indians as compared to high-income countries.

The Asian Sudden Cardiac Death in Heart Failure (ASIAN-HF) is a contemporary outpatient based prospective registry of HF with reduced EF <40% across 46 centers and 11 Asian regions (India, Southeast Asia, China, and East Asia).[24] The mean age of the cohort (n = 5,276) was only 59 years with more than three-fourths being men. About 80%

TABLE 2: Population characteristics of patient enrolled in India in the INTER-CHF study (n = 858).

Mean age (years)	56
% women	38
Hospital inpatient (%)	45
Ischemic/hypertensive/valvular heart disease (%)	46/14/12
Idiopathic dilated cardiomyopathy	11
Others (hypertrophic, congenital, metabolic, and alcohol)	7
Reduced LV ejection fraction (<40%)	53
NYHA III or IV (%)	50%
History of diabetes (%)	26
Illiterate/rural residence (%)	29/48
Health insurance (%)	19
All cause mortality at 1 year (%)	23
Mortality by admission status at baseline inpatient/outpatient (%)	35–40/10–15

(INTER-CHF: International Congestive Heart Failure; NYHA: New York Heart Association)

were in New York Heart Association (NYHA) class II/III and approximately half of HF was due to IHD. The mortality rate among 4,052 patients completing 6 month follow-up was 6.9%. A recent paper that compared outcomes in HFrEF globally by combining data from ASIAN-HF and comparing to regions of Western Europe (reference region), Eastern Europe, North, and Latin America.[25] The all-cause death rate per 100 patient-years was 7.1 in Western Europe, 8.8 in Eastern Europe, 8.2 in North America, 10.9 in South America, 8.8 in China, 4.6 in Japan, and 9.0 in India.

CONCLUSION

Heart failure continues to be a significant cause of mortality and morbidity worldwide, with incidence and prognosis similar to those of cancer. The overall prevalence of HF is about 1–2% worldwide, but this rises dramatically with increasing age, which has sinister implications in an aging human population. While the high-income countries now encounter more HF from survivors of acute coronary events and sicker older patients with multiple comorbidities, the low- and middle-income countries are facing a double whammy of residual infectious causes for HF as well as a rising burden of CAD, diabetes, and hypertension in a younger population. This coupled to inadequate healthcare facilities and poorly penetrating preventive policies makes a compelling case for urgently considering HF as a truly ominous epidemic by all the stakeholders alike.

REFERENCES

1. Ponikowski P, Anker SD, AlHabib KF, et al. Heart failure: preventing disease and death worldwide. ESC Heart Fail. 2014;1:4-25.
2. Lund LH, Savarese G. Global Public Health Burden of Heart Failure. Card Fail Rev. 2017;3:7-11.
3. Hu SS, Kong LZ, Gao RL, et al. Outline of the report on cardiovascular disease in China, 2010. Biomed Environ Sci. 2012;25:251-6.
4. Mozaffarian D, Benjamin EJ, Go AS, et al. Heart Disease and Stroke Statistics-2016 Update: A report from the American Heart Association. Circulation. 2016;133:e38-360.
5. Conrad N, Judge A, Tran J, et al. Temporal trends and patterns in heart failure incidence: a population-based study of 4 million individuals. Lancet. 2018;391:572-80.
6. Chaturvedi V, Parakh N, Seth S, et al. Heart failure in India: The INDUS (INDia Ukieri Study) study. J Pract Cardiovasc Sci. 2016;2:28-35.
7. Stewart S, Ekman I, Ekman T, et al. Population impact of heart failure and the most common forms of cancer: a study of 1 162 309 hospital cases in Sweden (1988 to 2004). Circ Cardiovasc Qual Outcomes. 2010;3:573-80.
8. India State-Level Disease Burden Initiative CVD Collaborators. The changing patterns of cardiovascular diseases and their risk factors in the states of India: the Global Burden of Disease Study 1990-2016. Lancet Glob Health. 2018;6:e1339-e1351.
9. Huffman MD, Prabhakaran D. Heart failure: epidemiology and prevention in India. Natl Med J India. 2010;23:283-8.
10. Bocchi EA, Marcondes-Braga FG, Bacal F, et al. Updating of the Brazilian guideline for chronic heart failure—2012. Arq Bras Cardiol. 2012;98:1-33.
11. Agbor VN, Essouma M, Ntusi NAB, et al. Heart failure in sub-Saharan Africa: A contemporaneous systematic review and meta-analysis. Int J Cardiol. 2018;257:207-15.
12. Dokainish H, Teo K, Zhu J, et al. Global mortality variations in patients with heart failure: results from the International Congestive Heart Failure (INTER-CHF) prospective cohort study. Lancet Glob Health. 2017;5:e665-e672.
13. Harikrishnan S, Sanjay G, Anees T, et al. Clinical presentation, management, in-hospital and 90-day outcomes of heart failure patients in Trivandrum, Kerala, India: the Trivandrum Heart Failure Registry. Eur J Heart Fail. 2015;17:794-800.
14. Damasceno A, Mayosi BM, Sani M, et al. The causes, treatment, and outcome of acute heart failure in 1006 Africans from 9 countries. Arch Intern Med. 2012;172:1386-94.
15. Sanjay G, Jeemon P, Agarwal A, et al. In-Hospital and Three-Year Outcomes of Heart Failure Patients in South India: The Trivandrum Heart Failure Registry. J Card Fail. 2018;24:842-8.
16. OSS, GV, ARM, et al. Long-term outcomes of patients admitted with heart failure in a tertiary care center in India. Indian Heart J. 2018;70(Suppl 1):S85-S89.
17. Seth S, Khanal S, Ramakrishnan S, et al. Epidemiology of acute decompensated heart failure in India: The AFAR study (Acute failure registry study). J Pract Cardiovasc Sci. 2015;1:35-8.

18. Atherton JJ, Hayward CS, Wan Ahmad WA, et al. Patient characteristics from a regional multicenter database of acute decompensated heart failure in Asia Pacific (ADHERE International-Asia Pacific). J Card Fail. 2012;18: 82-8.
19. Crespo-Leiro MG, Anker SD, Maggioni AP, et al. European Society of Cardiology Heart Failure Long-Term Registry (ESC-HF-LT): 1-year follow-up outcomes and differences across regions. Eur J Heart Fail. 2016;18:613-25.
20. Cheng RK, Cox M, Neely ML, et al. Outcomes in patients with heart failure with preserved, borderline, and reduced ejection fraction in the Medicare population. Am Heart J. 2014;168:721-30.
21. Shah KS, Xu H, Matsouaka RA, et al. Heart failure with preserved, borderline, and reduced ejection fraction: 5-year outcomes. J Am Coll Cardiol. 2017;70:2476-86.
22. Ciapponi A, Alcaraz A, Calderon M, et al. Burden of heart failure in Latin America: a systematic review and meta-analysis. Rev Esp Cardiol. 2016;69:1051-60.
23. Chioncel O, Lainscak M, Seferovic PM, et al. Epidemiology and one-year outcomes in patients with chronic heart failure and preserved, mid-range and reduced ejection fraction: an analysis of the ESC Heart Failure Long-Term Registry. Eur J Heart Fail. 2017;19:1574-85.
24. Lam CS, Teng TK, Tay WT, et al. Regional and ethnic differences among patients with heart failure in Asia: the Asian sudden cardiac death in heart failure registry. Eur Heart J. 2016;37:3141-53.
25. Dewan P, Jhund PS, Shen L, et al. Heart failure with reduced ejection fraction: comparison of patient characteristics and clinical outcomes within Asia and between Asia, Europe and the Americas. Eur J Heart Fail. 2019;21:577-87.

CHAPTER

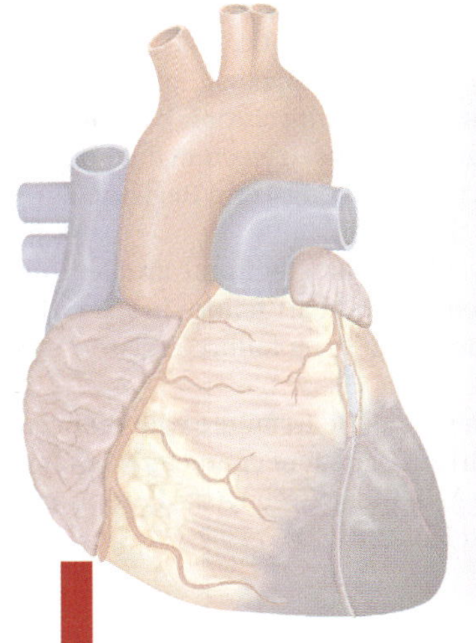

Trivandrum Heart Failure Registry

Harikrishnan S, Sanjay G, Jeemon P

INTRODUCTION

Cardiovascular disease (CVD) is the leading cause of mortality and morbidity globally. The rapid epidemiological transition in the last 2–3 decades in the low-income and middle-income country (LMIC) settings resulted in disproportionately higher burden of noncommunicable diseases as compared to communicable diseases or conditions related to maternal and child health. Consequent to the epidemiological transition, CVD emerged as the leading cause of death and disability even in the LMIC settings.[1]

Heart failure (HF), one of the prominent chronic conditions in surviving individuals with CVD, is currently a major public health problem in LMIC. It accounts for a huge health care spending and to the tune of 1–2% of total healthcare expenditure in the west. HF is also the leading cause of hospitalization, accounting for 1–2% of total hospital admissions.[2]

Heart failure is a disease with high morbidity and mortality. With 1-year mortality of 30% and 5-year reported mortality of 50%, it is worse than the estimates for common cancers of breast and the colon.

Even though HF is a major health issue, epidemiological data from the LMIC are scarce.[3] There is only a small study on the prevalence[4] of HF from India and the rest of the data are from a few registries.[3,5-7] There are also a few estimates and projections of burden of HF based on risk factor data.[4,8,9]

The prevalence of HF increases with age. Hence, the number of people with HF is likely to increase as the population is ageing in India.[8] The second reason for increasing prevalence of HF is the rising prevalence of atherosclerotic vascular diseases and their risk factors.[10] The third is the persisting burden of conditions like rheumatic heart disease (RHD), chronic obstructive pulmonary disease, and untreated congenital heart diseases which add to the HF burden. Based on all the available data, we can predict that the burden of HF is likely to increase in India in the next few decades.

THE TRIVANDRUM HEART FAILURE REGISTRY

The Trivandrum Heart Failure Registry (THFR) is a prospective HF registry setup in 2013 in Trivandrum district, the southernmost district of Kerala. The THFR was initiated with financial support from Indian Council of Medical Research (ICMR). The study was conducted in two areas in Trivandrum district, the Trivandrum city area (urban) and in a suburban rural area, about 25 kilometers from the city. The Trivandrum city urban area had a population of 957,000 (area 215 sq km). The selected rural area, the Athiyannoor block panchayat had a population of 166,549 and an area of 60 sq km.[3]

We invited all the hospitals in the region where HF patients are likely to get admitted and requested the concerned physicians to participate in the registry. All the 12 hospitals in the urban area and the 5 of 5 eligible hospitals in the rural area joined the registry. The key objectives of THFR were: (1) to describe the demographic and clinical characteristics of patients admitted with HF in the hospitals in the region, (2) to describe the diagnostics and therapeutic approaches routinely followed by the treating physicians and the hospitals and (3) to assess the in-hospital and short- and long-term mortality outcomes in patients with HF and the factors associated with mortality.

All the participating hospitals enrolled consecutive patients who were admitted with HF satisfying the European Society of Cardiology (ESC) 2012 criteria.[11] However, septicemia-related HF and those patients who were unwilling to participate or not willing to provide the informed consent were excluded from the registry. The patients enrolled were classified into one of the following categories: (1) acute de novo HF (defined as those patients who were admitted with HF for the first time and (2) acute on chronic HF (defined as acute decompensation needing admission in a patient already known to have HF). The registry enrolled patients for a period of 1 year from January to December 2013. Optimal treatment was defined as a combination of beta-blockers, angiotensin-converting enzyme inhibitors (ACEIs) or angiotensin receptor blockers (ARBs), and aldosterone receptor blockers in HF patients with reduced ejection fraction (HFrEF).[12] The THFR registry was subsequently converted to a cohort and now being followed-up at regular intervals. 5-year follow-up has been just concluded. The cohort is being supported by ICMR.

WHAT DID WE FIND IN TRIVANDRUM HEART FAILURE REGISTRY?

The THFR recruited 1,205 patients in 1 year. Males formed 70% of the cohort, while in the west the sex ratio is almost equal. Mean age of the patients in THFR was 61.2 [standard deviation (SD) = 13.7] years. Indian patients with HF in the THFR were younger by 10 years compared to the western data from US and Europe. The proportion of patients below 65 years was 57% in TFHR, whereas it was 29% in the US population (Fig. 1).

Additionally, the proportion of patients above 85 years was 25% in Acute Decompensated Heart Failure National Registry (ADHERE) while it was 4% in THFR. Hence in India, HF affects a much younger, predominantly male population. With respect to the risk factor profile, prevalence of diabetes and smoking was much higher in THFR compared to the western data (Table 1). The high prevalence of diabetes mellitus (DM) is in concordance with its high prevalence in the general population in India, and especially Kerala, where the registry was conducted. There were no significant differences between men and women with regard to risk factors like hypertension and diabetes. However, women reported more atrial arrhythmias–atrial fibrillation/flutter at baseline (18.3%) compared to men (13.1%). The most common etiology of HF in THFR was ischemic heart disease (IHD) (71%) (Table 2). ADHERE data also shows predominance of IHD, but the proportion was slightly less (63% vs. 71%). While RHD contributed 8% of the HF burden in THFR, it was negligible in the US patients with HF. This shows that even now in India, old-age diseases like RHD are contributing to the burden of HF. The most common etiology of HF in both men and women was IHD (74.3% and 66.3%, respectively). Women reported a higher prevalence of RHD (11.6%) compared to men (6.2%).

The patients were classified into different groups based on ejection fraction (EF).[13] HF with preserved ejection fraction (HFpEF: defined as EF >50%) constituted 236 patients (19.6%) of the population. HF with mid-range ejection fraction

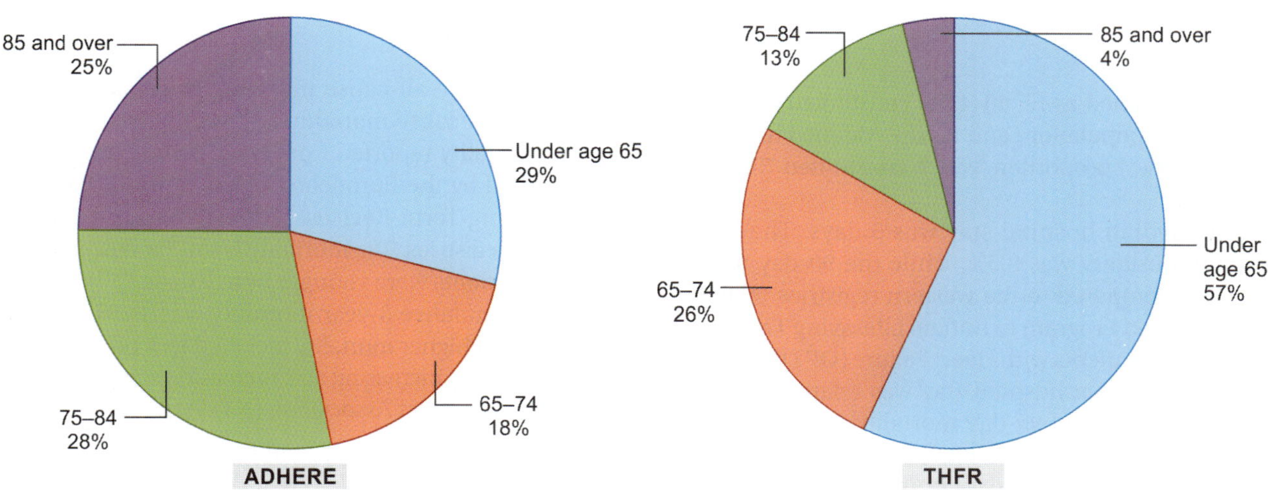

Fig. 1: Age distribution—comparison of Trivandrum Heart Failure Registry (THFR) (right) with the Acute Decompensated Heart Failure National Registry (ADHERE) of US (left).

TABLE 1: Baseline characteristics of patients in the Trivandrum Heart Failure Registry.

Variables	*Total (N = 1,205)*
Age in years, mean (SD)	61.23 (13.68)
Women, n (%)	371 (30.79)
Etiology, n (%)	
Coronary heart disease	866 (71.87)
Dilated cardiomyopathy	156 (12.95)
Hypertrophic cardiomyopathy	27 (2.24)
Rheumatic heart disease	95 (7.88)
Diastolic heart failure	11 (0.91)
Miscellaneous	50 (4.15)
Tobacco use, n (%)	
Current use	188 (15.60)
Past use	301 (24.98)
Alcohol use, n (%)	
Current use	234 (19.42)
Past use	21 (1.74)
History of hypertension, n (%)	696 (57.76)
History of diabetes, n (%)	662 (54.94)
Atrial arrhythmia, n (%)	177 (14.69)
History of stroke, n (%)	75 (6.22)
History of COPD, n (%)	186 (15.44)
History of CKD, n (%)	216 (17.93)
Heart rate >100 beats/minute, n (%)	720 (60.05)
NYHA Class 4, n (%)	382 (32.87)
LV ejection fraction <35, n (%)	544 (45.15)

(CKD: chronic kidney disease; COPD: chronic obstructive pulmonary disease; LV: left ventricular; NYHA: New York Heart Association; SD: standard deviation)

(HFmrEF: defined as EF 40–49%) constituted 217 patients (18%) of the population, and HFrEF (defined as EF <40%) was the highest proportion, which constituted 752 patients (62.4%).

The median hospital stay was 6 days. The total in-hospital mortality was 8.5%, while the 90-day mortality was 18%. Compared to the western registries, ADHERE[14] and Organized Program to Initiate Lifesaving Treatment in Hospitalized Patients with Heart Failure (OPTIMISE-HF),[15] THFR showed that hospital stay was relatively long, and both in-hospital and 90-day mortality rates were higher. Despite being younger patients, the HF mortality was higher in THFR as compared to data from US. This could be due to the relatively higher prevalence of comorbidities and comparatively lower EF in THFR cohort.

TABLE 2: Etiology of heart failure in the Trivandrum Heart Failure Registry.

Etiology	*Percentage*
CAD	71%
Ischemic cardiomyopathy	36%
Acute coronary syndrome (ACS)	35%
Dilated cardiomyopathy	13%
Rheumatic heart disease	8%
HFpEF (>45%)	25%
Miscellaneous	5%
Non-RHD valve diseases	2.50%
Isolated right heart failure	1.50%
Congenital heart disease	1.30%
Peripartum cardiomyopathy	0.25%

(CAD: coronary artery disease; HFpEF: heart failure with preserved ejection fraction; RHD: rheumatic heart disease)

"Guideline-based" medical treatment was defined as the combination of beta-blockers, ACEIs or ARBs, and aldosterone receptor blockers in patients with HFrEF. Only a fourth (25%) of the patients with left ventricular (LV) systolic dysfunction received optimal treatment at discharge. There were no gender differences in prescription of guideline-directed medical treatment status at discharge (25.3% in men compared with 22.9% in women).

Patients who did not receive guideline-based therapy experienced higher mortality than those who received guideline-based therapy ($p < 0.001$).[3] Only one-fourth of the total study population received guideline-based medical treatment, which indicates gross underutilization of evidence-based therapies.

ONE-YEAR AND THREE-YEAR OUTCOMES

The cumulative all-cause mortality at 1-year was 30.8% (n = 371). All-cause mortality at 1-year of 30.8% is similar to the mortality reported from US and the European data as reported by the European Society of Cardiology Heart Failure Long-Term Registry (ESC-HF-LT) and American ADHERE registries. The mortality is similar despite the fact that the patients were younger by a decade.[16,17]

The cumulative 3-year mortality was 44.8% (Table 3). Predictors of higher mortality included lack of goal directed therapy (GDT), increasing age, increasing serum creatinine, and New York Heart Association (NYHA) functional class IV.

Readmissions and Outcomes

The 1-year hospital readmission was 30.2% (n = 333) among the 1,103 participants discharged from the index

TABLE 3: Cumulative all-cause mortality in the Trivandrum Heart Failure Registry cohort.

Variable	*Number (percentage) Total N = 1,205*
In-hospital mortality	102 (8.5)
Cumulative 30-day mortality	151 (12.5)
Cumulative 90-day mortality	218 (18.1)
Cumulative 1-year mortality	371 (30.8)
Cumulative 2-year mortality	492 (40.8)
Cumulative 3-year mortality	540 (44.8)

BOX 1: Key points from the 3-year follow-up of the Trivandrum Heart Failure Registry.

- Higher 1 and 3-year mortality than the western population for patients with both reduced and preserved left ventricular ejection fraction.
- Continuing survival benefit for patients who were initiated on guideline-directed therapy.
- Rehospitalizations are associated with higher long-term mortality.

(Reproduced from reference 8, published with permission of Elsevier)

hospitalization. There was no gender difference in readmissions, men (30.3%) and women (30.9%). Those patients who had readmissions had higher mortality at 1-year. Of the 30.2% patients readmitted after the index hospitalization, 24.3% were readmitted specifically for HF exacerbation. The predictors of readmission were two—NYHA functional class IV symptom at index hospitalization and not receiving optimal guideline-directed medical therapy.

The impact of readmissions on outcomes was evident at the 3-year follow-up. At 3 years, readmissions were a predictor of mortality (Box 1). The impact of readmission on long-term mortality rates as illustrated in Figure 2.[6]

CONCLUSION

In summary, the data from THFR shows that patients hospitalized with HF were younger by a decade, more likely to be men and had a higher prevalence of coronary artery disease. The patients reported longer length of hospital stay and higher in-hospital mortality compared with published data from other registries from the West. Guideline-based therapy was found to improve outcomes, but remained dismally suboptimal (25%). The readmission ratio at 1 year was 30%. Majority of readmissions were for HF exacerbation. Lack of GDT predisposed to readmissions and readmission was a predictor of mortality. Given the suboptimal rates of utilization of guideline-directed therapy on the prognosis,

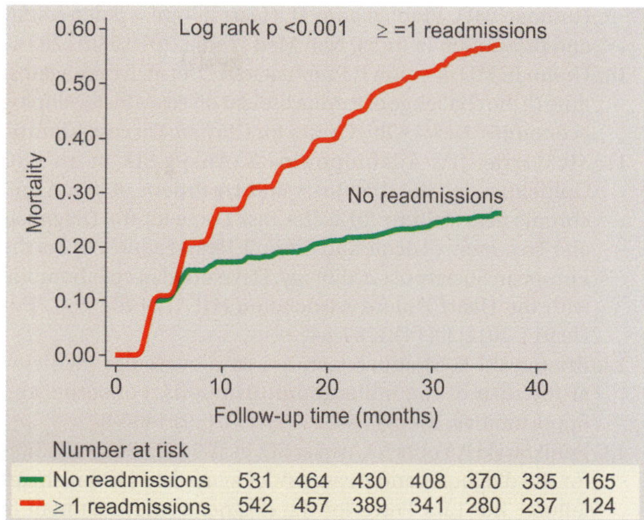

Fig. 2: Long-term readmission and mortality rates in the Trivandrum Heart Failure Registry.

physicians and healthcare administrators should initiate hospital-based quality improvement measures aimed at focused care which can improve the outcomes of patients with HF in the developing world.

REFERENCES

1. Mozaffarian D, Benjamin EJ, et al. Heart Disease and Stroke Statistics-2016 Update: A Report from the American Heart Association. Circulation. 2016;133:e38-360.
2. Ambrosy AP, Fonarow GC, Butler J, et al. The Global health and economic burden of hospitalizations for heart failure lessons learned from hospitalized heart failure registries. J Am Coll Cardiol. 2014;63(12):1123-33.
3. Harikrishnan S, Sanjay G, Anees T, et al. Clinical presentation, management, in-hospital and 90-day outcomes of heart failure patients in Trivandrum, Kerala, India: the Trivandrum Heart Failure Registry. Eur J Heart Fail. 2015;17(8):794-800.
4. Chaturvedi V, Parakh N, Seth S, et al. Heart failure in India: The INDUS (INDia Ukieri Study) Study. J Pract Cardiovasc Sci. 2016;2:28-35.
5. Harikrishnan S, Sanjay G, Agarwal A, et al. One-year mortality outcomes and hospital readmissions of patients admitted with acute heart failure: Data from the Trivandrum Heart Failure Registry in Kerala, India. Am Heart J. 2017;189:193-9.
6. Sanjay G, Jeemon P, Agarwal A, et al. In-Hospital and Three-Year Outcomes of Heart Failure Patients in South India: The Trivandrum Heart Failure Registry. J Card Fail. 2018;24(12):842-8.
7. Dokainish H, Teo K, Zhu J, et al. Heart Failure in Africa, Asia, the Middle East and South America: The INTER-CHF study. Int J Cardiol. 2016;204:133-41.
8. Pillai HS, Ganapathi S. Heart failure in South Asia. Curr Cardiol Rev. 2013;9(2):102-11.

9. Huffman MD, Prabhakaran D. Heart failure: epidemiology and prevention in India. Natl Med J India. 2010;23(5):283-8.
10. Huffman MD, Jeemon P, Prabhakaran D, et al. A race against time II: the challenge of cardiovascular diseases in developing economies. New Delhi: Centre for Chronic Disease Control.
11. McMurray JJV, Adamopoulos S, Anker SD, et al. ESC Guidelines for the diagnosis and treatment of acute and chronic heart failure 2012: The Task Force for the Diagnosis and Treatment of Acute and Chronic Heart Failure 2012 of the European Society of Cardiology. Developed in collaboration with the Heart Failure Association (HFA) of the ESC. Eur Heart J. 2012;33(14):1787-847.
12. Braunwald E. Shattuck lecture—cardiovascular medicine at the turn of the millennium: triumphs, concerns, and opportunities. N Engl J Med. 1997;337(19):1360-9.
13. Ponikowski P, Voors AA, Anker SD, et al. 2016 ESC Guidelines for the diagnosis and treatment of acute and chronic heart failure: The Task Force for the diagnosis and treatment of acute and chronic heart failure of the European Society of Cardiology (ESC) Developed with the special contribution of the Heart Failure Association (HFA) of the ESC. Eur Heart J. 2016;37(27):2129-200.
14. Adams KF, Fonarow GC, Emerman CL, et al. Characteristics and outcomes of patients hospitalized for heart failure in the United States: rationale, design, and preliminary observations from the first 100,000 cases in the Acute Decompensated Heart Failure National Registry (ADHERE). Am Heart J. 2005;149(2):209-16.
15. Abraham WT, Fonarow GC, Albert NM, et al. Predictors of in-hospital mortality in patients hospitalized for heart failure: insights from the Organized Program to Initiate Lifesaving Treatment in Hospitalized Patients with Heart Failure (OPTIMIZE-HF). J Am Coll Cardiol. 2008;52(5):347-56.
16. Callender T, Woodward M, Roth G, et al. Heart failure care in low- and middle-income countries: a systematic review and meta-analysis. PLoS Med. 2014;11(8):e1001699.
17. Kociol RD, Hammill BG, Fonarow GC, et al. Associations between use of the hospitalist model and quality of care and outcomes of older patients hospitalized for heart failure. JACC Heart Fail. 2013;1(5):445-53.

The Importance of Physical Examination in Patients with Heart Failure

Anil Bharani

INTRODUCTION

Early diagnosis of heart failure is crucial for initiating appropriate management. The physical examination (history and clinical examination) is considered to have a central role for the diagnosis and follow-up of heart failure patients. Regrettably the art of physical examination has been facing a threat by the declining emphasis on it and by increasing reliance on the imaging and biomarkers.[1] Diagnostic value of physical examination has been questioned.[2,3] Kelder, et al. in a large cohort of patients with suspected heart failure demonstrated that focused history and physical examination can accurately predict the presence or absence of heart failure.[4] Physical examination by trained clinicians has been demonstrated to be accurate for cardiac diagnosis compared to echo imaging.[5] Among heart failure patients about half of them have left ventricular ejection fraction (LVEF) ≥50% called heart failure with preserved ejection fraction (HFpEF) and majority of remaining patients have heart failure with reduced (LVEF ≤ 40%) (HFrEF), prevalence of HFpEF increases with age and is more common in elderly and women. Identifying these syndromes early is essential for planning further management. The vast array of symptoms of heart failure are not specific to HFpEF versus HFrEF, however, physical examination should help in differentiating them.[6-8]

HISTORY

Evaluation of the patients with known or suspected cardiac failure begins with a focused history and targeted physical examination. The common signs and symptoms include dyspnea, orthopnea, bendopnea, paroxysmal nocturnal dyspnea, angina, fatigue, palpitations, edema, right upper quadrant abdominal pain, and ascites.

Worsening dyspnea is a cardinal symptom of heart failure but its absence does not exclude the diagnosis. Severe and sudden onset dyspnea indicates acute pulmonary edema that should be differentiated from acute pulmonary embolism and pneumothorax. *Orthopnea* is not specific for heart failure and can occur in patients with asthma, ascites or esophageal reflux. *Paroxysmal nocturnal dyspnea* is one of the most reliable indicators of heart failure. The *Cheyne-Stokes periodic breathing* may be apparent when the patient is awake and is common in advanced heart failure. The prevalence of central sleep apnea or *Cheyne-Stokes breathing* is reported in 20–62% of patients with heart failure in various studies with associated high mortality risk.[9]

Clinically evident *edema* or weight gain over days indicates fluid retention. *Tender hepatomegaly and ascites* indicate advanced right heart failure. Gastrointestinal (GI) symptoms such as nausea, vomiting, and early satiety are common in right heart failure and indicate decreased GI blood flow and bowel edema. *Fatigue* is a cardinal symptom of heart failure indicative of reduced cardiac output and abnormal skeletal muscle metabolic responses to exercise.[10] Unintended weight loss, often leading to cachexia suggest poor prognosis.[11] Information about patient's past and current medical problems, family history, alcohol and drug abuse should be obtained. Cancer chemotherapy, certain diabetes drugs, NSAID, etc. are associated with incident heart failure.

The predictive value of various signs and symptoms of heart failure have been explored. In a systematic review orthopnea only modestly predicted heart failure.[12] Dyspnea and edema were more predictive when combined with other physical findings such as *S3, raised jugular venous pressure (JVP), abdominojugular reflux,* and *rales.* A total of three or more signs predicted over 90% likelihood of increased filling pressures. The Framingham criteria for diagnosis of heart failure in patients with HFrEF have only modest specificity (63%) and sensitivity (63%).[11]

Wang et al. reviewed 22 studies on adults presenting to emergency department (ED) with dyspnea, the probability of heart failure was predicted by a past history of heart failure [likelihood ratio (LR) 5.8; 95% confidence interval (CI), 4.1–8.0], paroxysmal nocturnal dyspnea (LR 2.6; 95% CI, 1.5–4.5), or a third heart sound (LR 11; 95% CI, 4.9–25).[13] Physicians initial clinical impression of heart failure was strong predictor of this diagnosis (LR 4.4; 95% CI, 1.8–10). The addition of testing for N-terminal pro b-type natriuretic peptide (NTproBNP) increased diagnosis accuracy only modestly (C-statistic, 0.83 versus 0.13).

PHYSICAL EXAMINATION

Physical examination findings and medical history complement each other in defining the presence and severity of heart failure. No physical finding in heart failure is pathognomonic for HFpEF versus HFrEF.[4] Presence and severity of heart failure should be assessed from patient's general appearance, examination of heart and pulses, assessment of other organs for evidence of congestion, hypoperfusion or indications of comorbid conditions. The most definitive method for assessing patient's volume status is by measurement of JVP. An elevated JVP has good sensitivity (70%) and specificity (79%) for elevated left-sided filling pressures.[4] The sensitivity and specificity of the JVP in detecting congestion can be improved by eliciting hepatojugular reflux. Changes in JVP with therapy usually parallel changes in left-sided filling pressures. Pulmonary congestion is associated with pleural effusion, rales and rhonchi. Pulmonary rales due to heart failure are fine in nature and extend from base upwards. Rales and rhonchi may be absent in congested patients with advanced heart failure. Dependent edema is a common sign in volume overloaded heart failure patients but may occur in venous insufficiency or as side effect of certain medication (calcium channel blockers).

Detecting reduced cardiac output and systemic hypoperfusion are key components of examination. Poor systemic perfusion is indicated by weak pulses accompanied by low systolic and narrow pulse pressure. However, many patients with systolic pressure of 80 mm Hg may have adequate perfusion. Reduced cardiac output is suggested by decreased urine output, cool extremities, and poor mentation. Thus, assessment for systemic congestion taken together with evaluation for reduced cardiac output may be useful to categorize patients into "dry-warm" (no congestion with normal perfusion) "wet-warm" (congested with normal perfusion), "dry-cold" (no congestion but hypoperfused) and "wet-cold" (congestion with hypoperfused). A patient with heart failure is considered "wet" if the estimated pulmonary capillary wedge pressure (PCWP) is ≥ 22 mm Hg. If the estimated cardiac index is ≤2.2 L/min/m^2 the patient is considered "cold". It has been found that physicians have superior ability to assess congestion rather than adequacy of perfusion.[14] These categories are prognostic and useful in making treatment decisions.[9] Patients discharged with "wet" or "cold" profile experience worse outcomes [hazard ratio (HR), 1.5; 95% CI, 1.1-12.1; p = 0.017] compared with those discharged "warm and dry" (HR, 0.9; 95% CI, 0.7–2.1; p = 0.5).[8,9]

By observing or palpating the apical impulse, clinician can determine heart size in majority and know about volume or pressure overload on left ventricle depending on whether the apex is hyperdynamic or heaving in nature. In severe heart failure, a palpable third heart sound may be present. Auscultation may reveal mitral or tricuspid regurgitation murmurs that become softer as volume overload is treated with resultant reduction in ventricular cavity size and annular diameters.

A third heart sound is highly specific for heart failure and suggest increased ventricular filling volume. A fourth heart sound usually indicates reduced ventricular compliance.[15] In heart failure patients an S3 is equally prevalent in those with or without left ventricular systolic dysfunction. Marcus et al. reported that presence of third heart sound predicted elevated left ventricular end-diastolic pressures (>15 mm Hg) and BNP (>100 pg/mL) and depressed left ventricular systolic functions (LVEF < 50%) with low sensitivities (32–52%). A fourth heart sound had low sensitivity and moderate specificity (72–80%) compared to third heart sound.[12] Diagnostic value of physical examination for predicting presence of heart failure was tested using a multivariate model in a cohort of 721 patients. The history and physical examination accurately predicted presence or absence of heart failure that was added by a single additional test, the NTproBNP levels (C-statistic 0.83). Displaced apex beat [odds ratio (OR) 5.37, 95% CI, 2.75–10.5], irregularly irregular pulse (OR 4.08, 95% CI, 2.17–7.62) basal rales (OR 2.12, 95% CI, 1.31–3.75) tachycardia (per 10 bpm) (OR 1.27, 95% CI, 1.11-1.45), mitral regurgitation (OR 2.45, 95% C1, 1.34–4.49) and elevated JVP (OR 2.78, 95% CI, 1.35–5.7) predicted presence of heart failure.[4] Table 1 gives sensitivity, specificity, and predictive value of various signs and symptoms of heart failure.

TABLE 1: Utility of physical examination in detecting elevated left ventricular filling pressures (LVFP).

Physical sign	Sensitivity (%)	Specificity (%)	Predictive value		Author	Ref. No.
			Positive (%)	Negative (%)		
Elevated jugular venour pressure	65	64	75	52	Drazner MH, et al.	1
	58	100	-	-	Stevenson LW, et al	16
	10	97	3	-	Watson RD, et al.	2
Hepatojugular reflux	83	27	65	49	Drazner MH, et al	1
Hepatomegaly	15	93	78	39	Drazner MH, et al	1
Edema	41	66	67	40	Drazner MH, et al	1
	10	93	3	-	Watson RD, et al.	2
S3	62	32	61	33	Drazner MH, et al	1
	41	92	81	65	Marcus GM, et al.	15
	31	95	61	-	Watson RD, et al.	2
Rales	15	89	69	38	Drazner MH, et al	1
	13	91	27	-	Watson RD, et al.	2
Orthopnea	86	25	66	51	Drazner MH, et al	1
	21	81	2	-	Watson RD, et al.	2
S4	21	81	2	-	Watson RD, et al.	2
	46	80	66	64	Marcus GM, et al.	15
Cardiomegaly	62	67	-	-	Watson RD, et al.	2

Proportional Pulse Pressure

Pulse pressure in normotensive individuals is determined by the stroke volume and peripheral resistance and can be used to assess cardiac output. Proportional pulse pressure (systolic – diastolic/systolic) correlated well with cardiac index ($r = 0.82$) and when less than 25%, it had 97% sensitivity and 83% specificity for predicting a cardiac index below 2.2 L/min/m^2.[1,16]

Bendopnea is a symptom of dyspnea, which develops within 30 seconds on bending forward at the waist in an attempt to touch the toes. It is associated with increased filling pressures particularly in the setting of low cardiac output and have prognostic utility in heart failure. In a study of 250 patients with decompensated heart failure, bendopnea was associated with increased 6 months mortality. However, it can occur in other conditions such as morbid obesity allergic bronchopulmonary aspergillosis, etc.[17]

Valsalva Maneuver

The blood pressure response to Valsalva maneuver allows estimation of the PCWP noninvasively. Physiologically, the blood pressure drops during the strain phase due to decrease in pulmonary venous return. However, patients with elevated left ventricular filling pressures (LVFP) show a "square wave" pattern of response. The blood pressure rises with strain and remains stably elevated throughout the strain, returning to baseline after strain release. There is no decrease in blood pressure during strain despite decreased pulmonary venous return, because the left ventricle remains adequately filled given the prestrain elevated left ventricular filling pressure. The "square-root" response to the Valsalva maneuver was associated with the invasively measured PCWP.[18-20]

Limitations of Physical Examination in Assessing Hemodynamics in Heart Failure

Although pulmonary rales, dependent edema, and pleural effusion can be seen in decompensated heart failure, these signs have limitations. Patients with advanced chronic heart failure with elevated LVFP may not have rales because of body's adaptation by increasing the lymphatic drainage. Similarly patient with heart failure may have clear lung fields in chest X-rays despite having elevated filling pressures.

Dependent edema may be common but it represents extravascular rather than intravascular volume. Other conditions such as venous insufficiency, obesity, nephrotic syndrome or chronic liver diseases may be associated with peripheral edema. Its specificity as a sign of heart failure is increased in the presence of elevated JVP.[16,21]

CONCLUSION

Despite technological advances, the physical examination (history and clinical examination) remain fundamental in the management of patients with heart failure. It provides information regarding diagnosis, hemodynamic status, and prognosis in patients with heart failure. The physical examination is more accurate in the assessment of elevated ventricular filling pressures rather than in the detection of a low cardiac index. Currently, elevated LVFP are inferred from findings of elevated right atrial pressures. For prognosticating and choosing optimal therapy in patients with heart failure, judging the volume and perfusion status of heart failure patients clinically and categorizing them as "warm-dry", "warm-wet", "cold-dry", and "cold-wet" is useful. Determination of "wet" is based on detection of elevated jugular venous pressure, hepatojugular reflux, orthopnea, bendopnea and a "square wave" response in blood pressure during Valsalva maneuver. The adequacy of perfusion can be judged by narrow pulse pressure, cool extremities, low blood pressure, low urine output, and the global assessment of "cool" made by the clinician.

REFERENCES

1. Drazner MH, Hellkamp AS, Leier CV, et al. Value of clinician assessment of hemodynamics in advanced heart failure: The ESCAPE trial. Circ Heart Fail. 2008;7:170-7.
2. Watson RD, Gibbs CR, Lip GY. ABC of heart failure. Clinical features and complications. BMJ. 2000;320:236-9.
3. Khunti K, Baker R, Grimshaw G. Diagnosis of patients with chronic heart failure in primary care: usefulness of history, examination, and investigation. Br J Gen Pract. 2000;50:50-4.
4. Kelder JC, Cramer MJ, van Wijngaarden J, et al. The diagnostic value of physical examination and additional testing in primary care patients with suspected heart failure. Circulation. 2011;124:2865-73.
5. Patel A, Tomar NS, Bharani A. Utility of physical examination and comparison to echocardiography for cardiac diagnosis. Indian Heart J. 2017;69:141-5.
6. Mozaffarian D, Benjamin EJ, Go AS, et al. Executive summary: heart disease and stroke statistics-2016 update: a report from the American Heart Association. Circulation. 2016;133: 447-54.
7. Roger VL. Epidemiology of heart failure. Circ Res. 2013;113:646-59.
8. Thibodeau JT, Drazner MH. The role of the clinical examination in patients with heart failure. JACC Heart Fail. 2018;6:543-51.
9. Brack T, Theur I, Clarenbach CF, et al. Day time Cheyne-Stokes respiration in ambulatory patients with severe congestive heart failure is associated with increased mortality. Chest. 2007;132:1463-71.
10. Yu DS, Chan HY, Leung DY, et al. Symptom clusters and quality of life among patients with advanced heart failure. J Geriatr Cardiol. 2016;13:408-14.
11. Rahman A, Jabry S, Jeejeebhoy K, et al. Malnutrition and cachexia in heart failure. JPEN J Parenter Entera Nutr. 2016;40:475-86.
12. Drazner MH. Hemodynamic assessment in heart failure and cardiomyopathy. ACCSAP. 2016.
13. Wang CS, FitzGerald JM, SchulzerM, et al. Does this dyspneic patient in the emergency department have congestive heart failure? JAMA. 2005;294:1944-56.
14. Nohria A, Tsang SW, Fang JC, et al. Clinical assessment indentifies hemodynamic profiles that predict outcomes in patients admitted with heart failure. J Am Coll Cardiol. 2003;41:1797-804.
15. Marcus GM, Gerber IL, Mckeown BH, et al. Association between phonocardiographic third and fourth heart sounds and objective measures of left ventricular functions. JAMA. 2005;293:2238-44.
16. Stevenson LW, Perloff JK. The limited reliability of physical signs for estimating hemodynamics in chronic heart failure. JAMA. 1989;261:884-8.
17. Thibodeau JT, Turer AT, Gualano SK, et al. Characterization of a novel symptom of advanced heart failure: bendopnea. JACC Heart Fail. 2014;2:24-31.
18. McIntyre KM, Vita JA, Lambrew CT, et al. A noninvasive method of predicting pulmonary capillary wedge pressure. N Engl J Med. 1992;327:1715-20.
19. Zema MJ, Masters AP, Margouleff D. Dyspnoea: the heart or the lungs? Differentiation at bedside by use of the simple Valsalva maneuver. Chest. 1984;85:59-64.
20. Zema MJ. Diagnosing heart failure by the Valsalva maneuver. Isn't it finally time? Chest. 1999;116:851-3.
21. Butman SM, Ewy GA, Standen JR, et al. Bedside cardiovascular examination in patients with severe chronic heart failure: importance of rest or inducible jugular venous distention. J Am Coll Cardiol. 1993;22:968-74.

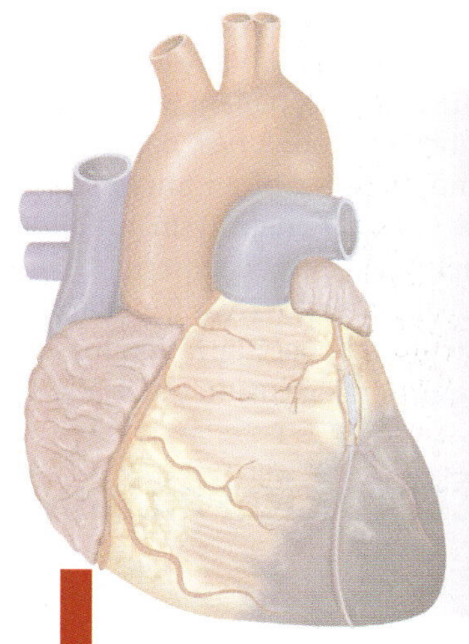

Heart Failure: Bench to Bedside

Harsh Wardhan, Nitin Aggarwal

INTRODUCTION

Heart failure (HF) is a debilitating disease in which abnormal function of the heart leads to inadequate supply of blood to tissues and organs to meet their metabolic demands. Various factors can contribute to HF pathogenesis, such as myocardial infarction, ischemia, hypertension or cardiomyopathies. Heart failure is a significant global health problem which is becoming worse as the population ages.[1,2] Despite significant advances in cardiovascular medicine and management, mortality rates remain high, with almost 50% of HF patients dying within 5 years of diagnosis.[3] Further, conventional pharmacological treatments largely delay disease progression and death due to HF, but they do not cure HF.[4] As a multifactorial clinical syndrome, HF still represents an epidemic threat, highlighting the need for deeper insights into disease mechanisms and the development of innovative therapeutic strategies.

Our understanding of pathophysiological processes in HF has increased tremendously over the last several decades, yet the pace at which these discoveries have translated into new therapies for patients has been frustratingly slow. In this review of heart failure "From Bench to Bedside", we will highlight how our current understanding of pathophysiology has translated into development of new pharmacologic agents which have been tested in clinical trials in recent years and many more which are still being investigated in clinical trials.

CONVENTIONAL PHARMACOLOGICAL THERAPIES

A host of clinical trials have demonstrated that careful pharmacologic management can reduce symptoms, slow progression of the disease, and improve survival in majority of HF patients. Conventional pharmacological therapies include beta-blockers, a number of agents that inhibit the deleterious effects of the renin–angiotensin–aldosterone system (RAAS), and diuretics.

Inhibition of the Renin–angiotensin–aldosterone System

Vasoconstriction, sodium and water retention, aldosterone release, ventricular remodeling, and myocardial hypertrophy are well-known detrimental consequences of excessive circulating angiotensin II. A number of current medications target different points of the RAAS to attenuate these effects, including angiotensin-converting enzyme inhibitors (ACE inhibitors), angiotensin II receptor antagonists (ARBs), and mineralocorticoid receptor antagonists (MRAs).[5-7] The beneficial effects of ACE inhibitors have been studied in thousands of patients with varying etiologies and stages of HF.[8] Angiotensin-converting enzyme inhibition has repeatedly been shown to attenuate cardiac remodeling and improve heart function in patients with HF and after myocardial infarction. Angiotensin II receptor antagonists are an appealing option in patients who are intolerant to ACE inhibitors. Several clinical trials have illustrated a reduction in morbidity and mortality in patients with left ventricular dysfunction.[5,8] Mineralocorticoid receptor antagonists, spironolactone, and eplerenone have shown reduction in hospitalization and total mortality in patients with severe HF.[9]

Beta-blockers

Beta-blockers are administered to control HF symptoms (such as shortness of breath, high blood pressure or weakness), which occur due to the release of excess catecholamines. Beta-blockers have produced almost uniformly beneficial effects in patients with HF from various causes and in all stages. This is due in large part to their inhibition of the harmful effects of chronic activation of the sympathetic nervous system, which is a hallmark of HF. Significant effects have included improvement in survival, morbidity, ejection fraction, quality of life, remodeling, hospitalization, and incidence of sudden death.[6,10]

Diuretics

Diuretics remain a major component of drug therapy in both hypertension and HF and are combined with an ACE inhibitor, beta-blocker or MRA. They are often necessary to combat the water and sodium retention elicited by angiotensin II and aldosterone. Diuretics allow for a rapid improvement in signs and symptoms of HF but their effect on morbidity and mortality remains somewhat unclear.[7]

HYDRALAZINE AND ISOSORBIDE DINITRATE

There is no clear evidence to suggest the use of this fixed-dose combination therapy in all patients with heart failure with reduced ejection fraction (HFrEF). The combination of hydralazine and isosorbide dinitrate may be considered in symptomatic patients with HFrEF who can tolerate neither ACEI nor ARB (or they are contraindicated) to reduce mortality. However, this recommendation is based on the results of the Veterans Administration Cooperative Study, which recruited symptomatic HFrEF patients who received only digoxin and diuretics.[11]

New Pharmacological Agents Targeting Pathophysiological Features of the Failing Heart

Next generation HF therapeutics are required that can improve clinical outcome. Potential pharmacological agents have been identified that target pathophysiological features of the failing heart. Neurohormonal antagonists have been shown to improve survival in patients with HFrEF and are recommended for the treatment of every patient with HFrEF, unless contraindicated or not tolerated. A new compound (LCZ696) that combines the moieties of an angiotensin receptor blocker (ARB; valsartan) and a neprilysin inhibitor (sacubitril) has recently been shown to be superior to an angiotensin-converting enzyme inhibitor (ACEI; enalapril) in reducing the risk of death and of hospitalization for HF in a single trial with strict inclusion/exclusion criteria.[12]

ANGIOTENSIN RECEPTOR NEPRILYSIN INHIBITOR

Background

Currently, blockade of the RAAS is the cornerstone of the treatment of HF. However, the combination of RAAS blockade with inhibition of neprilysin, an enzyme that degrades natriuretic peptides (NPs), has recently emerged as a potentially superior treatment strategy.[12] In July 2015, the Food and Drug Administration (FDA) approved sacubitril/valsartan (previously known as LCZ696) for use in patients who have chronic and stable but symptomatic HF and who have an left ventricular ejection fraction (LVEF) of less than 40%. The drug should be used in conjunction with other HF therapies but in place of ACE inhibitors or ARBs, and is contraindicated in patients with a history of ACE inhibitor or ARB-induced angioedema.

Mechanism of Action

The first-in-class is LCZ696, which is a molecule that combines a neprilysin inhibitor (sacubitril) and an ARB (valsartan) in a single substance. Neprilysin is a zinc-dependent neutral endopeptidase that is responsible for the degradation of several vasoactive peptides such as NPs, bradykinin, and adrenomedullin and contributes to the breakdown of angiotensin II.[13] High circulating A-type natriuretic peptide (ANP) and B-type natriuretic peptide (BNP) exert physiologic effects through binding to NP receptors and the augmented generation of cyclic guanosine monophosphate (cGMP), thereby enhancing diuresis, natriuresis and myocardial relaxation, and anti-remodeling.[14]

PARADIGM Trial

The PARADIGM-HF trial was conducted in 8,399 patients who had New York Heart Association (NYHA) Class II-IV

HF and an LVEF of not more than 40% (this was changed to ≤35% during the study) and who were randomly assigned to LCZ696 or enalapril.[12] The trial was stopped early because of an overwhelming benefit with LCZ696 therapy. LCZ696 was also associated with significant reductions in all-cause mortality, cardiovascular mortality, and hospitalization for worsening HF as compared to enalapril [hazard ratio (HR) 0.80, 95% confidence interval (CI): 0.73–0.87, $p < 0.001$]. Furthermore, those patients who received LCZ696 had lower levels of the biomarkers NT-proBNP and troponin compared with those receiving enalapril. Interestingly, levels of BNP actually increased: this is consistent with the mechanisms of action of neprilysin inhibition.[15] This trial provided strong evidence for superiority of the angiotensin receptor neprilysin inhibitor (ARNI) in patients with HFrEF.[12]

IF-CHANNEL INHIBITOR

Background

One novel potential therapeutic option for HF is heart rate (HR) control. An elevated HR, probably reflecting activation of the sympathetic nervous system, is associated with worse cardiovascular outcomes. Although beta-blockers are used mainly for reducing HR in HF treatment, uptitration of beta-blockers can be associated with an increased risk of adverse reactions.[16] Ivabradine, which acts by directly and selectively inhibiting the I_f current in the sinoatrial node and therefore should only be used for patients in sinus rhythm. It has potential benefits of pharmacologic modification of HR in HF. The European Medicines Agency (EMA)[17] approved ivabradine for use in Europe in patients with HFrEF with LVEF ≤ 35% and in sinus rhythm with a resting HR ≥ 75 bpm.

SHIFT Trial

The SHIFT trial was an randomized controlled trial (RCT) in 6,558 patients with stable symptomatic HF and an LVEF of not more than 35% in sinus rhythm with an HR of at least 70 bpm.[18] In this trial, ivabradine significantly reduced the primary endpoint of a composite of cardiovascular death or hospital admission for worsening HF and deaths due to HF. The effect was consistent across all prespecified subgroups, including the elderly. Further analyses proved that high HR as a risk factor in HF and lowering HR improve outcomes. Other analyses showed that ivabradine reduces the risk of rehospitalization for HF and is associated with an improvement in quality of life. Given its promising therapeutic value, ivabradine is clearly desirable in patients with symptomatic LV systolic dysfunction, elevated HR, and intolerance to beta-blockers.

NEWER AGENTS TO PREVENT HYPERKALEMIA DURING RAAS INHIBITION

Background

As the use of RAAS inhibitors and MRA in patients with HF increases, hyperkalemia has become a more common electrolyte disturbance in clinical practice, especially in patients with chronic kidney disease (CKD). Moreover, hyperkalemia is a major limiting factor to titrate these drugs fully in these patients who are most likely to benefit from treatment. Currently, noninvasive treatment of hyperkalemia is limited by a lack of safety, efficacy, and tolerability. Thus, agents to control reliably the plasma concentration of potassium while maintaining the use of RAAS inhibitors or MRA are needed. Now, there are two novel potassium absorbents, *(1) patiromer calcium and (2) sodium zirconium cyclosilicate (ZS-9)*, that are designed to increase potassium loss via the gastrointestinal tract. Although they have not yet been approved by the FDA, both have demonstrated efficacy and safety in recent trials.

Mechanism of Action

Patiromer

Patiromer is a nonabsorbable polymer that binds potassium in exchange for calcium throughout the gastrointestinal tract. This agent, which is an orally administered drug, increases fecal excretion of potassium and consequently decreases plasma potassium levels. Prior patiromer clinical trials have also demonstrated the drug's utility in treating hyperkalemia in at-risk populations for periods ranging from a few days to up to 12 weeks.[19]

Sodium Zirconium Cyclosilicate

Sodium zirconium cyclosilicate is a high-specificity inorganic crystal that entraps potassium in the intestinal tract. Instead of exchanging calcium, ZS-9 exchanges sodium and hydrogen ions for potassium. Dose-dependent excretion of potassium occurs in the feces, whereas urinary excretion decreases with dose.

Clinical Trial

HARMONIZE Study

The HARMONIZE study was an RCT evaluating the long-term efficacy and safety of ZS-9 in 258 patients with hyperkalemia.[20] Patients achieving normokalemia were randomly assigned to different doses of ZS-9 (5, 10, or 15 g) or placebo for 28 days in the maintenance phase.

Mean baseline potassium was 5.6 mEq/L and declined to 4.5 mEq/L after 48 hours of 10 g ZS-9 treatment in the acute phase. A significant reduction in potassium was observed within 1 hour of ZS-9 administration, and 84% of patients achieved normokalemia at 24 hours, and 98% at 48 hours.[21] Furthermore, studies assessing the long-term efficacy and safety profile of this novel drug are ongoing.

NEWER VASODILATORS

Relaxin

Serelaxin is a recombinant form of the human hormone relaxin, which is a naturally occurring hormone that is produced by the corpus luteum and placenta in pregnancy. Recent studies have shown that relaxin is also produced by the vasculature and failing myocardium. Relaxin interacts with a G protein-coupled receptor, leading to increased cyclic adenosine monophosphate (cAMP). As a result, nitric oxide production is increased. Additionally, relaxin upregulates the activity of vascular matrix metalloproteinase-2 (MMP-2), which can activate endothelin-1 leading to endothelin-B receptor activation and subsequent nitric oxide production. Activation of the endothelin-B receptor is probably involved in the relaxin-mediated increase in renal blood flow.[22] Thus, relaxin increases cardiac output, arterial compliance, and renal blood flow, supporting important physiological changes during pregnancy. Given its potent vasodilator properties as well as its ability to increase renal perfusion, relaxin became of interest as a potential therapy for acute HF.

Ularitide

Decongestion is an important part of managing both acute and chronic HF, and retention of fluid and sodium metabolism play a fundamental role in this. Natriuretic peptides are activated in HF and exert compensatory effects by inhibiting the RAAS and inducing vasodilatation and natriuresis. Therefore, NPs have received much interest as a potential therapy in acute decompensated heart failure (ADHF). Natriuretic peptides consist of ANP, BNP, C-type NP (CNP), D-type NP (DNP), and urodilatin. Urodilatin was first isolated from human urine in 1988 as a modified version of pro-ANP. It is produced mainly by distal renal tubule cells and is secreted into urine and is involved in renal sodium handling.[23] When it is administered to patients with ADHF, a rapid reduction of pulmonary capillary pressure and consequent relief of dyspnea often result because of natriuresis, diuresis, and venous and arterial dilation.

THERAPIES THAT TARGET IMPAIRED CARDIAC CONTRACTILITY

Activation of SERCA2a using Viral Vectors

Abnormal handling of calcium ions by cardiomyocyte is a key pathophysiological mechanism in HF. The SERCA2a pump is responsible for calcium reuptake during excitation–contraction coupling.[24] The importance of SERCA2a has been reflected in numerous studies that demonstrate reduced SERCA2a activity and expression in animal models of HF and in the human failing myocardium. Preclinical studies in small and large HF animal models have convincingly shown significant improvement in cardiac function and remodeling as a consequence of overexpression of SERCA2a using adenoviral vectors (Fig. 1).[25] Following successful preclinical studies, clinical trials were conducted and SERCA2a was delivered to the myocardium of patients with HF using an adeno-associated viral (AAV) vector approach. These studies demonstrated that AAV-*SERCA2a* gene therapy increased SERCA2a protein levels, was safe and improved cardiac function in HF patients.[20] Further, after a 12-month follow-up, patients with advanced HF displayed improved signs and symptoms of HF and cardiac function.[26] However, results from a recent international clinical trial (CUPID-2) suggested that AAV-SERCA2a was no different to the placebo when added to a maximal, optimized HF drug and device regimen.[27] Several factors may have contributed to the primary endpoint not being achieved in this study. These include dose, less uptake of the vector, patient population, delivery method, and the distribution of AAV1 neutralizing antibodies is greater in European than USA populations, which can limit effective gene transfer.[28] Second- or third-generation AAV vectors designed using mosaics are being developed, and the therapeutic formulation can be optimized which will be important for future studies.[27]

A schematic representing gene-based or small-molecule based therapies that manipulate SERCA2a activity by directly targeting SERCA2a or by SUMOylation. Cardiac myosin activators such as omecamtiv mecarbil targets contractile apparatus of the heart increasing the contracting of the left ventricle of the heart.

Cardiac Myosin Activators

Decreased cardiac contractility is a central feature of systolic HF. Omecamtiv mecarbil is a small molecule, cardiac-specific myosin activator. It speeds up the transition of myosin from a weak actin-binding to a strong actin-binding force generating state, thereby increasing the contraction of the left ventricle[29] (Fig. 1). In preclinical studies, cardiac

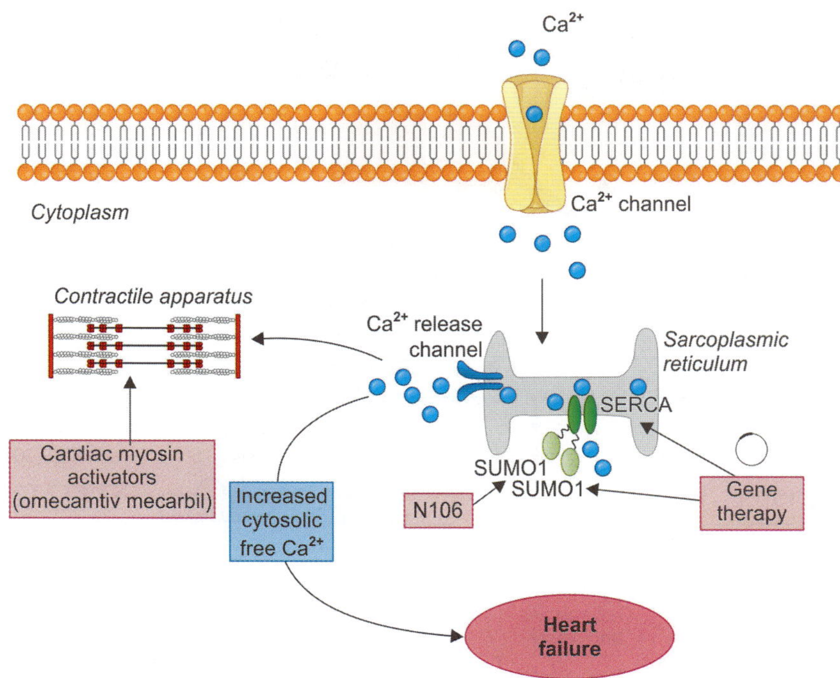

Fig. 1: Promising therapies targeting impaired cardiac contractility.

myosin activators increased systolic function, stroke volume and cardiac output without desensitization or increasing myocardial oxygen consumption.[30,31] However, Omecamtiv mecarbil failed to improve symptoms of ADHF in a second phase II trial ATOMIC-AHF (Acute Treatment with Omecamtiv Mecarbil to Increase Contractility in Acute Heart Failure),[32] raising some concern for future studies, including possible effects of a myosin activator on diastolic function. Combined data from ATOMIC-HF and from the ongoing COSMIC-HF (Chronic Oral Study of Myosin Activation to Increase Contractility in Heart Failure)[33] will be utilized to determine whether the phase II clinical trials assessing the effect of omecamtiv mecarbil in patients with acute or chronic HF will be pursued.

TARGETING NON-CODING RIBONUCLEIC ACIDS FOR THE TREATMENT OF HEART FAILURE

MicroRNAs

The multifaceted pathophysiology of HF limits the effectiveness of current therapeutics. Thus, fine-tuning gene expression using microRNA-based drugs may represent a novel therapeutic approach for the treatment of HF. MicroRNAs (miRNAs) are small, noncoding RNA (ncRNA) molecules that regulate gene expression by directing their target mRNAs for degradation or translational repression.[34] These tiny RNA molecules, once thought of as “genomic junk”, play crucial roles in health and disease, including the development of cardiac hypertrophy and HF.[35] The actions of disease-causing miRNAs can be blocked by synthetic oligonucleotides, some of which have been shown to improve cardiac function and pathology in preclinical rodent models. Studies have targeted miRNAs involved in calcium homeostasis, contractility, adaptive heart growth (i.e. cardiac protection) or myocyte proliferation as potential therapies for HF (Fig. 2). SERCA2a is an important regulator of calcium reuptake in the sarcoplasmic reticulum and is inhibited by miR-25. Blocking miR-25 in a mouse model of HF was associated with improved contractility, survival and restoration of SERCA2a activity (Fig. 2).[36] Other studies have investigated the therapeutic potential of miR-208a. miR-208a is encoded by the α-myosin heavy chain gene and regulates the cardiac stress response and contractility. In a rodent model of salt-induced hypertension, inhibition of miR-208a was able to ameliorate hypertrophy, attenuate fibrosis and improve cardiac function.[37]

MicroRNAs implicated in calcium homeostasis, cardiac contractility, adaptive heart growth or myocyte proliferation are dysregulated in the diseased heart. Administration of miRNA inhibitors or mimics in preclinical models of cardiac stress reduced pathology and improved heart function. This demonstrates the therapeutic potential of miRNAs for the treatment of HF.

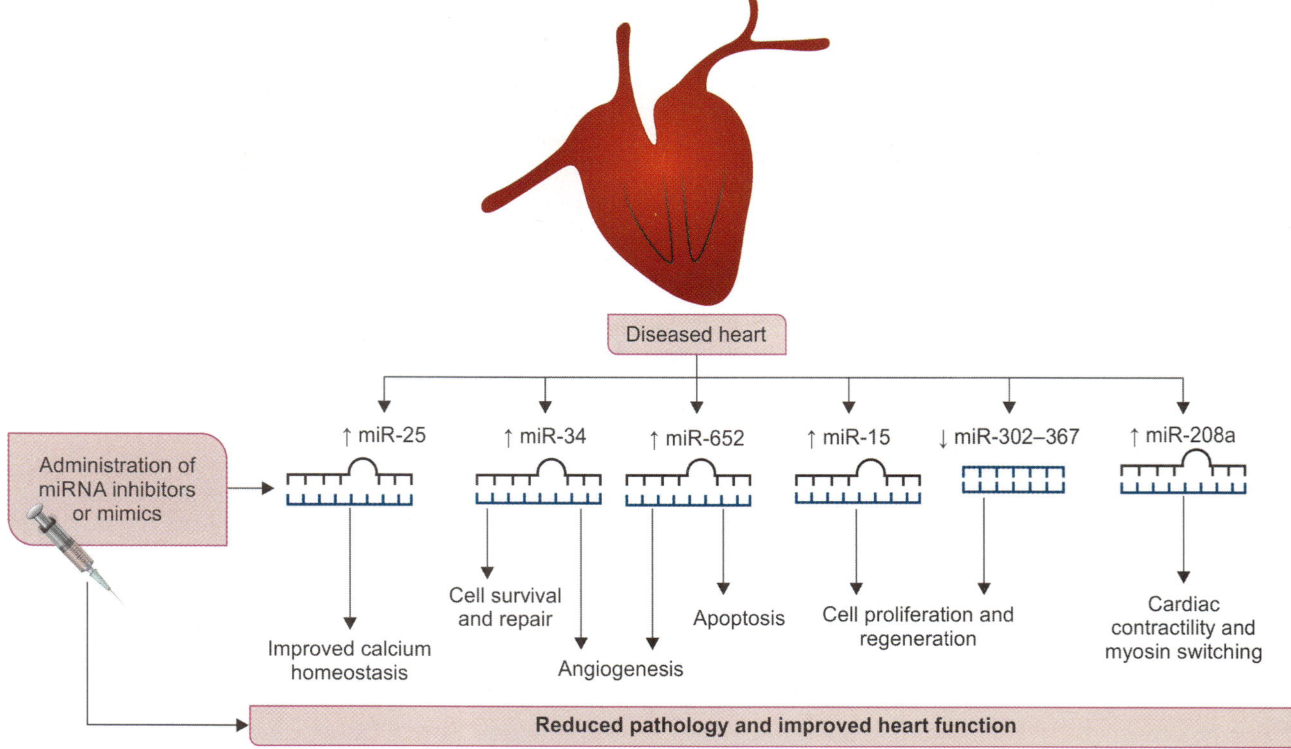

Fig. 2: MicroRNA (miRNA)-based therapies for the treatment of heart failure.

The adult mammalian heart has a limited capacity to regenerate following injury. The loss of cardiomyocyte in adult hearts is a key component of most HF pathogenesis. Thus the potential of applying miRNAs to restore lost cardiomyocyte in the damaged heart would be of considerable therapeutic value. The miR-15 family plays an important role in the cardiac regenerative response by regulating a number of cell-cycle genes including checkpoint kinase 1. Prolonged inhibition of the miR-15 family was able to promote cardiomyocyte proliferation in the infarct region of the heart.[38] The miR-17-92 cluster is among the best-studied miRNA clusters. Expression of this cluster has been shown to promote cell proliferation and suppress apoptosis in cancer cells.[39,40] Cardiac-specific overexpression of the miR-17-92 cluster has been shown to be sufficient to induce cardiomyocyte proliferation in adult hearts and in response to cardiac injury and this was associated with improved cardiac function. More recently, the miR-302-367 cluster has been shown to be crucial for cardiomyocyte proliferation during development, and functions in part, through repression of Hippo signaling, a pathway that governs cell proliferation and organ size.[39] Inhibition of miR-34, miR-34a, or miR-652 with miRNA inhibitors was associated with reduced pathology and improved cardiac function in mouse models of cardiac disease via mechanisms that are associated with preserved angiogenesis, decreased fibrosis, and a more favorable cardiac molecular profile (e.g. attenuation of ANP, BNP gene expression).[41-43] Thus, targeting miRNAs appear to be a promising approach for the development of a novel miRNA-based therapy for the failing heart (Fig. 2).

Although these preclinical studies are encouraging, a major obstacle in translating miRNA-based therapeutics into a therapy for HF patients is how to deliver miRNA inhibitor oligonucleotides to the sites where their actions are needed. Dosing, specificity and side effects should be carefully assessed when developing miRNA-based therapies. However, the translational efficacy and safety of miRNA-based therapeutics to patients has been shown in phase IIa clinical trials for the treatment of hepatitis C virus, where results indicate that the treatment was well tolerated in patients.[44]

Long Noncoding Ribonucleic Acids

In addition to small noncoding RNAs (ncRNAs), high-throughput analyses of the transcriptome have identified other functional classes of transcripts, which are larger than 200 nucleotides, collectively known as long noncoding RNAs (lncRNAs). There is increasing evidence that lncRNAs have a role in numerous cellular processes, however our understanding of lncRNAs is limited.[45] In the heart, several studies have characterized the expression of lncRNAs involved in cardiac development and disease.[46-48] Chemically modified antisense oligonucleotides called "gapmeRs" can be used to downregulate the expression of lncRNAs. As individual lncRNAs have distinct biological functions and target a specific molecular process (e.g. apoptosis, hypertrophy, angiogenesis), inhibition of their function might lead to novel treatments for HF. One of the first pharmacological inhibition studies using gapmeRs for cardiac or vascular disease was performed in an animal model of hind limb ischemia to inhibit *Malat1*.[49] Inhibition of *Malat1* decreased vascularization, suggesting *Malat1* as a potential target for angiogenic processes.[49] Further understanding of the involvement of lncRNAs in cardiac development and disease will aid in the development of new therapeutic strategies for the failing heart.

CONCLUSION

Heart failure is the end result of a variety of disease states, including coronary artery disease and hypertension. Heart failure remains a challenge to treat, and the incidence continues to rise with an aging population. The treatment of HF has evolved rapidly over the past few years and many aspects of this evolution have been discussed in this article. Patients are often complex, with multiple comorbidities, and being under specialist care has been shown to be associated with greater use of evidence-based therapies and improved survival. With current HF drugs largely delaying HF progression, some of the new therapeutic approaches discussed in this review may show potential in improving heart function and reversing adverse cardiac remodeling. Future clinical trials with adequately powered, more appropriate study designs, optimal clinical endpoints, and proper patient selection are mandatory to assess the true efficacy of these treatments.

REFERENCES

1. Braunwald E. The war against heart failure: the Lancet lecture. Lancet. 2015;385:812-24.
2. Mozaffarian D, Benjamin EJ, Go AS, et al. Heart Disease and Stroke Statistics—2015 Update: A Report from the American Heart Association. Circulation. 2015;131:e29-e322.
3. Liu L, Eisen HJ. Epidemiology of Heart Failure and Scope of the Problem. Cardiol Clin. 2014;32:1-8.
4. Braunwald E. Research Advances in Heart Failure: A Compendium. Circ Res. 2013;113:633-45.
5. Tham YK, Bernardo BC, Ooi JY, et al. Pathophysiology of cardiac hypertrophy and heart failure: signaling pathways and novel therapeutic targets. Arch Toxicol. 2015;89:1401-38.
6. Falvey J, Blaxall BC. Pharmacologic therapy. In: Bisognano JD, Baker ML, Earley MB (Eds). Manual of Heart Failure Management. Springer Dordrecht Heidelberg London New York: Springer; 2009. pp. 85-96.
7. Yancy CW, Jessup M, Bozkurt B, et al. 2013 ACCF/AHA Guideline for the Management of Heart Failure: A Report of the American College of Cardiology Foundation/American Heart Association Task Force on Practice Guidelines. Circulation. 2013;128:1810-52.
8. Lang CC, Struthers AD. Targeting the renin-angiotensin-aldosterone system in heart failure. Nat Rev Cardiol. 2013;10:125-34.
9. Pitt B, Zannad F, Remme WJ, et al. The effect of spironolactone on morbidity and mortality in patients with severe heart failure. Randomized Aldactone Evaluation Study Investigators. N Engl J Med. 1999;341:709-17.
10. Frishman WH. Beta-adrenergic blockers. Circulation. 2003;107:e117-e9. 23.
11. Cohn JN, Archibald DG, Ziesche S, et al. Effect of vasodilator therapy on mortality in chronic congestive heart failure. Results of a Veterans Administration Cooperative Study. N Engl J Med. 1986;314:1547-52.
12. McMurray JJ, Packer M, Desai AS, et al. Angiotensin-neprilysin inhibition versus enalapril in heart failure. N Engl J Med. 2014;371:993-1004.
13. Daniels LB, Maisel AS. Natriuretic peptides. J Am Coll Cardiol. 2007;50:2357-68.
14. Mangiafico S, Costello-Boerrigter LC, Andersen IA, et al. Neutral endopeptidase inhibition and the natriuretic peptide system: an evolving strategy in cardiovascular therapeutics. Eur Heart J. 2013;34:886-893c.
15. Packer M, McMurray JJ, Desai AS, et al. Angiotensin receptor neprilysin inhibition compared with enalapril on the risk of clinical progression in surviving patients with heart failure. Circulation. 2015;131:54-61.
16. de Groote P, Isnard R, Assyag P, et al. Is the gap between guidelines and clinical practice in heart failure treatment being filled? Insights from the IMPACT RECO survey. Eur J Heart Fail. 2007;9:1205-11.
17. Böhm M, Borer J, Ford I, et al. Heart rate at baseline influences the effect of ivabradine on cardiovascular outcomes in chronic heart failure: analysis from the SHIFT study. Clin Res Cardiol. 2013;102:11-22.
18. Böhm M, Swedberg K, Komajda M, et al. Heart rate as a risk factor in chronic heart failure (SHIFT): the association between heart rate and outcomes in a randomised placebo-controlled trial. Lancet. 2010;376:886-94.
19. Weir MR, Bakris GL, Bushinsky DA, et al. Patiromer in patients with kidney disease and hyperkalemia receiving RAAS inhibitors. N Engl J Med. 2015;372:211-21.
20. Jaski BE, Jessup ML, Mancini DM, et al. Calcium upregulation by percutaneous administration of gene therapy in cardiac disease (CUPID Trial), a first-in-human phase 1/2 clinical trial. J Card Fail. 2009;15:171-81.
21. Anker SD, Kosiborod M, Zannad F, et al. Maintenance of serum potassium with sodium zirconium cyclosilicate (ZS-9) in heart failure patients: results from a phase 3 randomized,

double-blind, placebo-controlled trial. Eur J Heart Fail. 2015;17:1050-6.
22. Jeyabalan A, Novak J, Danielson LA, et al. Essential role for vascular gelatinase activity in relaxin-induced renal vasodilation, hyperfiltration, and reduced myogenic reactivity of small arteries. Circ Res. 2003;93:1249-57.
23. Mitrovic V, Seferovic PM, Simeunovic D, et al. Haemodynamic and clinical effects of ularitide in decompensated heart failure. Eur Heart J. 2006;27:2823-3.
24. Lou Q, Janardhan A, Efimov IR. Remodeling of calcium handling in human heart failure. Adv Exp Med Biol. 2012;740:1145-74.
25. Byrne MJ, Power JM, Preovolos A, et al. Recirculating cardiac delivery of AAV2/1SERCA2a improves myocardial function in an experimental model of heart failure in large animals. Gene Ther. 2008;15:1550-7.
26. Jessup M, Greenberg B, Mancini D, et al. Calcium Upregulation by Percutaneous Administration of Gene Therapy in Cardiac Disease (CUPID): a phase 2 trial of intracoronary gene therapy of sarcoplasmic reticulum Ca^{2+}-ATPase in patients with advanced heart failure. Circulation. 2011;124:304-13.
27. Ratner M. Heart failure gene therapy disappoints but experts keep the faith. Nat Biotech. 2015;33:573-4.
28. Calcedo R, Vandenberghe LH, Gao G, et al. Worldwide Epidemiology of Neutralizing Antibodies to Adeno-Associated Viruses. J Infect Dis. 2009;199:381-90.
29. Malik FI, Morgan BP. Cardiac myosin activation part 1: From concept to clinic. J Mol Cell Cardiol. 2011;51:454-61.
30. Shen YT, Malik FI, Zhao X, et al. Improvement of cardiac function by a cardiac Myosin activator in conscious dogs with systolic heart failure. Circ Heart Fail. 2010;3:522-7.
31. Malik FI, Hartman JJ, Elias KA, et al. Cardiac myosin activation: a potential therapeutic approach for systolic heart failure. Science. 2011;331:1439-43.
32. Teerlink JR, Clarke CP, Saikali KG, et al. Dose-dependent augmentation of cardiac systolic function with the selective cardiac myosin activator, omecamtiv mecarbil: a first-in-man study. Lancet. 2011;378:667-75.
33. Cleland JG, Teerlink JR, Senior R, et al. The effects of the cardiac myosin activator, omecamtiv mecarbil, on cardiac function in systolic heart failure: a double-blind, placebo-controlled, crossover, dose-ranging phase 2 trial. Lancet. 2011;378:676-83.
34. Bernardo BC, Ooi JY, Lin RC, et al. miRNA therapeutics: a new class of drugs with potential therapeutic applications in the heart. Future Med Chem. 2015;7:1751-69.
35. Hata A. Functions of microRNAs in cardiovascular biology and disease. Annu Rev Physiol. 2013;75:69-93.
36. Wahlquist C, Jeong D, Rojas-Munoz A, et al. Inhibition of miR-25 improves cardiac contractility in the failing heart. Nature. 2014;508:531-5.
37. Montgomery RL, Hullinger TG, Semus HM, et al. Therapeutic inhibition of miR-208a improves cardiac function and survival during heart failure/clinical perspective. Circulation. 2011;124:1537-47.
38. Porrello ER, Mahmoud AI, Simpson E, et al. Regulation of neonatal and adult mammalian heart regeneration by the miR-15 family. Proc Natl Acad Sci U S A. 2013;110:187-92.
39. Tian Y, Liu Y, Wang T, et al. A microRNA-Hippo pathway that promotes cardiomyocyte proliferation and cardiac regeneration in mice. Sci Transl Med. 2015;7:279ra38.
40. Mogilyansky E, Rigoutsos I. The miR-17/92 cluster: a comprehensive update on its genomics, genetics, functions and increasingly important and numerous roles in health and disease. Cell Death Differ. 2013;20:1603-14.
41. Bernardo BC, Gao XM, Tham YK, et al. Silencing of miR-34a attenuates cardiac dysfunction in a setting of moderate, but not severe, hypertrophic cardiomyopathy. PLoS One. 2014;9:e90337.
42. Bernardo BC, Gao XM, Winbanks CE, et al. Therapeutic inhibition of the miR-34 family attenuates pathological cardiac remodeling and improves heart function. Proc Natl Acad Sci U S A. 2012;109:17615-20.
43. Bernardo BC, Nguyen SS, Winbanks CE, et al. Therapeutic silencing of miR-652 restores heart function and attenuates adverse remodeling in a setting of established pathological hypertrophy. FASEB J. 2014;28:5097-110.
44. Janssen HL, Reesink HW, Lawitz EJ, et al. Treatment of HCV infection by targeting microRNA. N Engl J Med. 2013;368:1685-94.
45. Jiang X, Ning Q. The emerging roles of long noncoding RNAs in common cardiovascular diseases. Hypertens Res. 2015;38:375-9.
46. Thum T, Condorelli G. Long noncoding RNAs and microRNAs in cardiovascular pathophysiology. Circ Res. 2015;116:751-62.
47. Uchida S, Dimmeler S. Long Noncoding RNAs in Cardiovascular Diseases. Circ Res. 2015;116:737-50.
48. Devaux Y, Zangrando J, Schroen B, et al. Long noncoding RNAs in cardiac development and ageing. Nat Rev Cardiol. 2015;12:415-25.
49. Michalik KM, You X, Manavski Y, et al. Long noncoding RNA MALAT1 regulates endothelial cell function and vessel growth. Circ Res. 2014;114:1389-97.

7

CHAPTER

Myocarditis and Heart Failure

Ahmed Khurshid Pasha, Rajesh Janardhanan

INTRODUCTION

Myocarditis is an old term first coined in the 19th century by Corvisart.[1] Myocarditis is an inflammation of myocardium which is diagnosed by accepted histological, immunological, and immunohistochemical criteria (Table 1).[2] Acute myocarditis remains a challenging diagnosis due to the heterogeneity in clinical presentation, despite the position statement by European Society of Cardiology Working Group on Myocardial and Pericardial Diseases.[2] The purpose of this review is to summarize the evidence available for clinical presentation, diagnosis and management.

ETIOLOGY AND PATHOGENESIS

Myocarditis is caused by a variety of different causes: infectious agents (viruses, bacteria, fungi), systemic diseases, drugs, toxins or physical agents (Box 1).[3] Myocarditis has diverse clinical presentation and progression.[4]

CLINICAL PRESENTATION

The exact prevalence and incidence of myocarditis is unknown. A study stated 0.5% of cardiovascular-related admissions were due to myocarditis.[5] Myocarditis presents in a multitude of ways ranging from asymptomatic presentation to life-threatening cardiogenic shock and fatal arrhythmias affecting individuals of all ages. Due to its varied presentation, the diagnosis requires a high level of suspicion early in the course of the disease.

Asymptomatic acute myocarditis: Transient elevation of troponins after an acute viral illness or vaccination has been reported.[6] Acute dilated cardiomyopathy (DCM) is a syndrome characterized by dyspnea, fatigue, edema, and paroxysmal nocturnal dyspnea is the most dramatic presentation after a recent (upper respiratory or gastrointestinal) infection signifying viral myocarditis. Majority of these patients improve with guideline-directed medical therapy for heart failure (HF).[7] Chronic dilated cardiomyopathy/chronic HF: these patients have heart failure symptoms of more than 3 months duration with periodic exacerbations. These patients develop chronic ventricular dysfunction and periodically manifest signs and symptoms of dyspnea, fatigue, atypical chest pain or arrhythmia. These patients have persistent symptoms of HF despite guideline-directed medical therapy. 25% of patients will progress to transplantation or death and another 25% will have improvement in their symptoms.[8] Myocarditis resembling acute coronary syndrome (ACS): these patients present with acute chest pain, elevated troponin, electrocardiographic (EKG) changes

TABLE 1: Defining myocarditis per criteria.[2,27]

Histologic Dallas criteria	*Immunohistochemical criteria*
Presence of inflammatory infiltrates within the myocardium along with associated myocyte degeneration and necrosis which is nonischemic in origin.	Abnormal inflammatory infiltrate to be defined as ≥14 leukocytes/mm^2 including up to 4 monocytes/mm^2 with the presence of CD 3 positive T-lymphocytes ≥7cells/mm^2

BOX 1: Etiology of myocarditis (some examples in each section are provided below).[2,23]

Infectious:
- *Bacterial*: *Staphylococcus, Streptococcus, Pneumococcus, Salmonella, Mycoplasma pneumoniae*
- *Spirochaetal*: *Borrelia, Leptospira*
- *Fungal*: *Aspergillus, Actinomyces, Blastomyces, Candida*
- *Protozoal*: *Trypanosoma cruzi, Toxoplasma gondii*
- *Parasitic*: *Trichinella spiralis, Taenia solium*
- *Rickettsial*: *Coxiella burnetii* (Q fever), Rickettsia rickettsii
- *Viral*: Coxsackievirus A and B, echoviruses, polioviruses, influenza A and B, adenovirus, parvovirus B19, cytomegalovirus, Epstein-Barr virus

Immune-mediated myocarditis:
- *Allergens*: Tetanus toxoid, vaccines, serum sickness
- *Drugs*: Penicillin, furosemide, isoniazid, tetracycline, amitriptyline
- *Alloantigens*: Heart transplant rejection
- *Autoantigens*: Systemic lupus erythematosus, rheumatoid arthritis, Churg–Strauss syndrome, Kawasaki disease, scleroderma, polymyositis, myasthenia gravis

Toxic myocarditis:
- *Drugs*: Amphetamines, anthracyclines, cocaine, cyclophosphamide, lithium, clozapine, trastuzumab, ethanol, fluorouracil, catecholamines, hemetine
- *Heavy metals*: Copper, iron, lead
- *Miscellaneous*: Scorpion sting, snake, bee and wasp stings
- *Hormones*: Pheochromocytoma, vitamins: beriberi
- *Physical* agents: Radiation, electric shock

consistent with myocardial ischemia, segmental or global echocardiographic wall motion abnormalities but a normal coronary angiogram.[9] Cardiac conduction abnormalities: myocarditis can affect cardiac conduction system which can infrequently cause sudden cardiac death.[10]

DIAGNOSTIC EVALUATION

Before diagnosis of myocarditis is made, common cardiovascular diseases (CVDs), such as atherosclerotic and valvular CVD should be ruled out as per various guidelines.[11,12]

Electrocardiography

Electrocardiography (EKG) is the initial screening tool despite having low sensitivity.[13] ST-T segment elevation which is concave in nature, in contrast to convex in myocardial ischemia, and diffuse changes without reciprocal changes are more suggestive of myocarditis.

Cardiac Biomarkers

Cardiac troponins are sensitive markers of myocyte injury when compared to creatine kinase levels, but a normal troponin level does not exclude myocarditis.[14] Increased troponin I can be detected in one-third of the patients with myocarditis[15] but it does not have same prognostic value in myocarditis as it has in ACS.[16]

Inflammatory Biomarkers

Erythrocyte sedimentation rate (ESR) and C-reactive protein (CRP) are usually elevated in myocarditis, but again, they are nonspecific.[17]

Echocardiography

Echocardiography is a useful imaging modality for suspected myocarditis as it helps to rule out valvular heart disease and monitor various echocardiographic parameters for HF: cardiac chamber size, systolic and diastolic functions, wall thickness, wall motion abnormalities, and pericardial effusion. It does not provide direct evidence of myocarditis but provides important information about the cardiomyopathy, which can be followed longitudinally to document improvement/resolution of HF.[18]

Cardiovascular Magnetic Resonance

Cardiovascular magnetic resonance (CMR) imaging provides valuable information about the tissue characterization noninvasively. T2-weighted (T2W) images (noncontrast) are indicative of tissue free water (edema) and an increased T2 signal is seen during an inflammatory process like myocarditis (Fig. 1). Contrast-enhanced (CE) CMR has a high sensitivity for detecting areas of myocardial damage in acute myocarditis because of signal intensity between myocardial regions with and

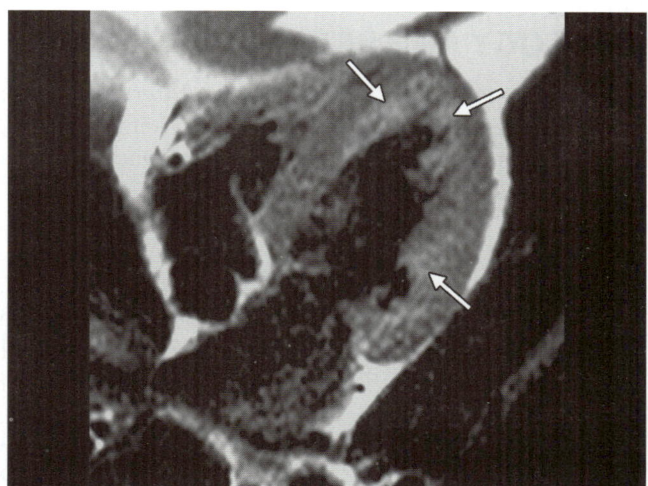

Fig.1: A4C T2 image: Arrows showing increased T2 signal in myocarditis.

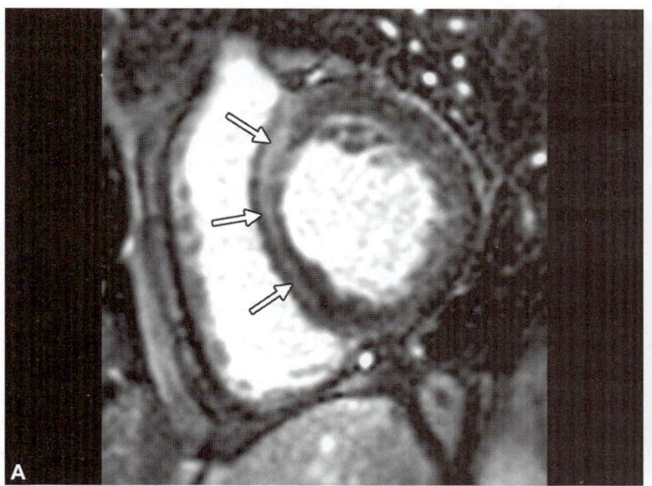

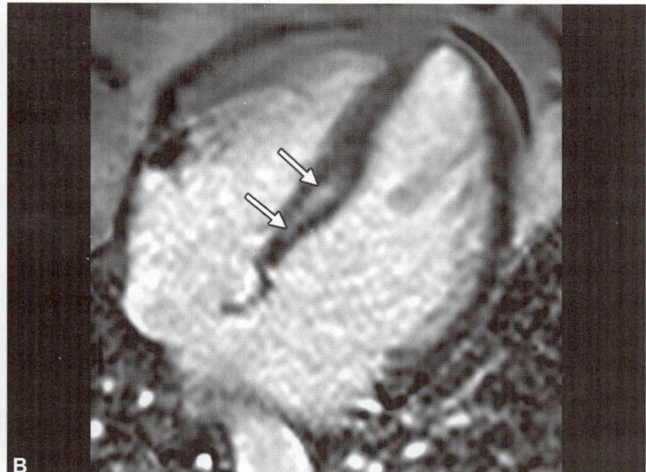

Figs. 2A and B: Midwall delayed enhancement in the septum. (A) Short axis with midwall stripe (arrows); (B) A4C delayed (arrows).

without gadolinium due to its uptake in disease and healthy heart tissue.[19] Severe inflammation, due to inflammatory mediators, can lead to myocytes necrosis, fibrosis and scarring. This provides enhanced volume for the contrast (gadolinium) to be distributed including the myocyte intracellular space.[20] Late gadolinium enhancement (LGE) imaging has two common patterns of enhancement: (1) mid-wall delayed enhancement, often seen in the septum (Figs. 2A and B) and (2) subepicardial in the left ventricle lateral free wall. The sensitivity and specificity of CE-CMR is high when compared to endomyocardial biopsy (EMB).[21]

Contrast-enhanced-CMR is usually performed in clinically stable patients usually before EMB. CE-CMR can identify the area of inflammation, and hence can provide a road map for EMB sampling when necessary. The International Consensus Group on CMR Diagnosis of Myocarditis has published recommendations for use of CMR in myocarditis (Lake Louise Criteria).[20,22]

Endomyocardial Biopsy

The gold standard for diagnosis of myocarditis is EMB. It not only helps in the diagnosis but also aids in the underlying etiology and type of inflammation which has implications in treatment and prognosis.[23] Criteria of acute myocarditis is defined by Dallas Criteria (Table 1). Immunohistochemistry is gaining importance as EMB is susceptible to sample bias and expertise of observer while reviewing the histopathological specimens. European Society of Cardiology recommends early institution of EMB for histology, immunohistochemistry and viral polymerase chain reaction (PCR) analysis.[7] Number of biopsies revealing myocarditis has substantially increased with use of immunohistochemistry methods.[24]

Endomyocardial biopsy could sometimes be repeated to monitor the response. Depending upon the clinical scenario or imaging finding (noted on CMR) decision should be made to biopsy both ventricles or a single ventricle. When performed in experienced hands, right and left heart biopsies are safe with complication rate of <1%.[25]

MANAGEMENT

In general, patients with myocarditis have decreased ventricular function. These should be managed according to the guideline-directed therapy for HF utilizing beta-blockers, angiotensin-converting enzyme (ACE) inhibitors or angiotensin receptor blockers (ARBs), aldosterone antagonists and diuretics. Avoidance of physical therapy is recommended until complete resolution of disease. Specific/specialized care includes antiviral therapy, high dose intravenous immunoglobulin (IVIG), and immunosuppression depending upon the etiology.

PROGNOSIS

Prognosis in myocarditis depends upon the clinical presentation, hemodynamic stability and EMB findings. Patient with myocarditis who have preserved systolic function generally have a favorable prognosis.[26,27]

CONCLUSION

Myocarditis is a complex condition, which is under diagnosed and has a broad spectrum of clinical presentations. It also has numerous etiologies. Some patients demonstrate complete recovery of ventricular function, while others might progress to heart failure. A high index of suspicion is required so that patients could be selected for further extensive molecular testing to confirm or refute the diagnosis, but this should be undertaken once the common cardiovascular diseases have been ruled out.

REFERENCES

1. Mattingly TW. Changing Concepts of Myocardial Diseases. JAMA. 1965;191:33-7.
2. Caforio AL, Pankuweit S, Arbustini E, et al. Current state of knowledge on aetiology, diagnosis, management, and therapy of myocarditis: a position statement of the European Society of Cardiology Working Group on Myocardial and Pericardial Diseases. Eur Heart J. 2013;34:2636-48, 48a-48d.
3. Sagar S, Liu PP, Cooper LT Jr. Myocarditis. Lancet 2012; 379:738-47.
4. Mason JW, O'Connell JB, Herskowitz A, et al. A clinical trial of immunosuppressive therapy for myocarditis. The Myocarditis Treatment Trial Investigators. N Engl J Med. 1995;333:269-75.
5. Felker GM, Thompson RE, Hare JM, et al. Underlying causes and long-term survival in patients with initially unexplained cardiomyopathy. N Engl J Med. 2000;342:1077-84.
6. Engler RJ, Nelson MR, Collins LC Jr, et al. A prospective study of the incidence of myocarditis/pericarditis and new onset cardiac symptoms following smallpox and influenza vaccination. PLoS One. 2015;10:e0118283.
7. Fung G, Luo H, Qiu Y, et al. Myocarditis. Circ Res. 2016;118: 496-514.
8. Magnani JW, Dec GW. Myocarditis: current trends in diagnosis and treatment. Circulation. 2006;113:876-90.
9. Dec GW Jr, Waldman H, Southern J, et al. Viral myocarditis mimicking acute myocardial infarction. J Am Coll Cardiol. 1992;20:85-9.
10. Drory Y, Turetz Y, Hiss Y, et al. Sudden unexpected death in persons less than 40 years of age. Am J Cardiol. 1991;68: 1388-92.
11. Heart Failure Society of America, Lindenfeld J, Albert NM, et al. HFSA 2010 Comprehensive Heart Failure Practice Guideline. J Card Fail. 2010;16:e1-194.
12. Dickstein K, Cohen-Solal A, Filippatos G, et al. ESC guidelines for the diagnosis and treatment of acute and chronic heart failure 2008: the Task Force for the diagnosis and treatment of acute and chronic heart failure 2008 of the European Society of Cardiology. Developed in collaboration with the Heart Failure Association of the ESC (HFA) and endorsed by the European Society of Intensive Care Medicine (ESICM). Eur J Heart Fail. 2008;10:933-89.
13. Morgera T, Di Lenarda A, Dreas L, et al. Electrocardiography of myocarditis revisited: clinical and prognostic significance of electrocardiographic changes. Am Heart J. 1992;124: 455-67.
14. Heymans S. Myocarditis and heart failure: need for better diagnostic, predictive, and therapeutic tools. Eur Heart J. 2007;28:1279-80.
15. Smith SC, Ladenson JH, Mason JW, et al. Elevations of cardiac troponin I associated with myocarditis. Experimental and clinical correlates. Circulation. 1997;95:163-8.
16. Kobayashi D, Aggarwal S, Kheiwa A, et al. Myopericarditis in children: elevated troponin I level does not predict outcome. Pediatr Cardiol. 2012;33:1040-5.
17. Caforio AL, Brucato A, Doria A, et al. Anti-heart and anti-intercalated disk autoantibodies: evidence for autoimmunity in idiopathic recurrent acute pericarditis. Heart. 2010;96: 779-84.
18. Pinamonti B, Alberti E, Cigalotto A, et al. Echocardiographic findings in myocarditis. Am J Cardiol. 1988;62:285-91.
19. Simonetti OP, Kim RJ, Fieno DS, et al. An improved MR imaging technique for the visualization of myocardial infarction. Radiology. 2001;218:215-23.
20. Ferreira VM, Schulz-Menger J, Holmvang G, et al. Cardiovascular Magnetic Resonance in Nonischemic Myocardial Inflammation: Expert Recommendations. J Am Coll Cardiol. 2018;72:3158-76.
21. Mahrholdt H, Goedecke C, Wagner A, et al. Cardiovascular magnetic resonance assessment of human myocarditis: a comparison to histology and molecular pathology. Circulation. 2004;109:1250-8.
22. Friedrich MG, Sechtem U, Schulz-Menger J, et al. Cardiovascular magnetic resonance in myocarditis: A JACC White Paper. J Am Coll Cardiol. 2009;53:1475-87.
23. Dennert R, Crijns HJ, Heymans S. Acute viral myocarditis. Eur Heart J. 2008;29:2073-82.
24. Schultheiss HP. [Dilated cardiomyopathy—a chronic myocarditis? New aspects on diagnosis and therapy]. Z Kardiol. 1993;82 (Suppl 4):25-32.
25. Kindermann I, Kindermann M, Kandolf R, et al. Predictors of outcome in patients with suspected myocarditis. Circulation. 2008;118:639-48.
26. Blauwet LA, Cooper LT. Myocarditis. Prog Cardiovasc Dis. 2010;52:274-88.
27. Sinagra G, Anzini M, Pereira NL, et al. Myocarditis in Clinical Practice. Mayo Clin Proc. 2016;91:1256-66.

8

CHAPTER

Biomarkers of Heart Failure: Diagnostic, Prognostic and Therapeutic Implications

Srikant Sharma, HK Chopra, Harmeet Singh, Nisarg Patel

INTRODUCTION

Heart failure (HF) is a common condition, with over 5.7 million affected and over 1 million hospitalizations annually.[1] HF represents an increasing problem worldwide and has an advancing trend, predominantly in elderly patients. The prevalence rate in general population is 0.4–2.0% and rapidly increases with age.[2] At the age of 50, the prevalence rate is about 1%, whilst at the age of 80 and above, it is 10%.[3] After establishing a HF diagnosis, nearly 60% of men and 45% of women will die within 5 years.[4] HF is a clinical diagnosis but often times presents with nonspecific symptoms, and delays in accurate diagnosis and treatment, thereby associated with worse clinical outcomes. Biomarkers provide a low cost, low risk, and quick turnaround method to confirm or exclude a HF diagnosis, help to establish prognosis and optimize treatment.

BIOMARKERS

National Institutes of Health Biomarkers Definitions Working Group defined a biomarker as a characteristic that is objectively measured and evaluated as an indicator of normal biological processes, pathogenic processes or pharmacological responses to a therapeutic intervention.[5] The World Health Organization has defined a biomarker as any substance, structure or process that can be measured in the body or its products and influence or predict the incidence of outcome or disease.

Proposed Biomarkers in Heart Failure

Proposed biomarkers in heart failure has been described in Figure 1.

Natriuretic Peptides

B-type natriuretic peptide (BNP) is a protein hormone one among the nine natriuretic peptides (seven are atrial in

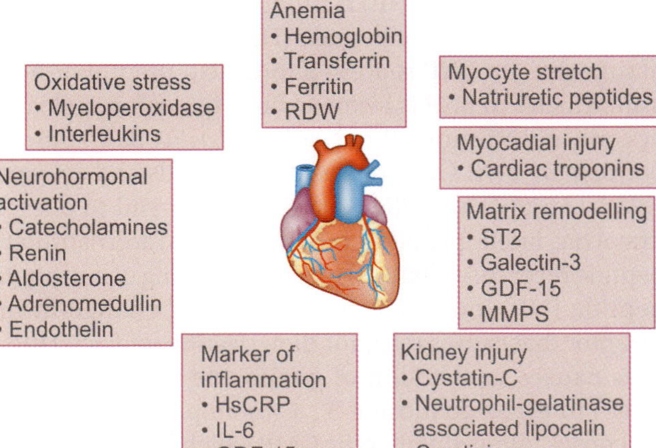

Fig. 1: Proposed biomarkers in heart failure.
(ADM: adrenomedullin; GDF-15: growth differentiating factor-15; MMPS: matrix metalloproteinases; RDW: red cell distribution width)

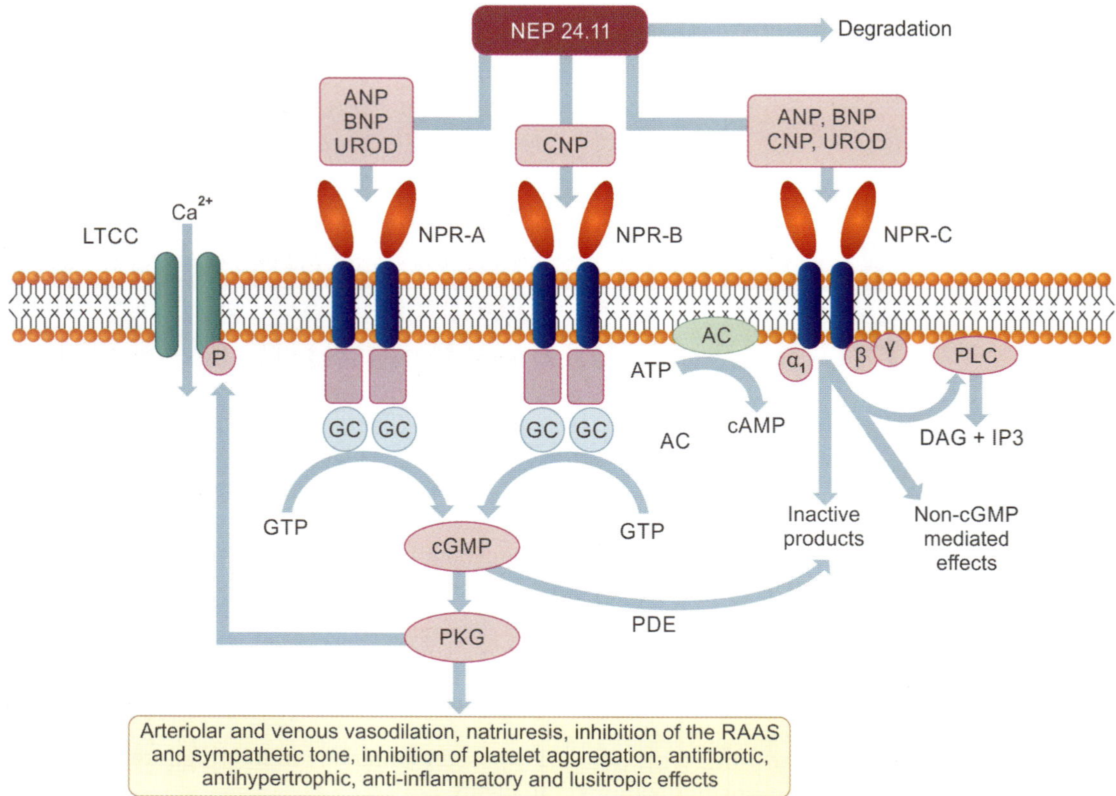

Fig. 2: Function of natriuretic peptides.

(ANP: atrial natriuretic peptide; BNP: B-fype natriuretic peptiae; CNP: C-type natriuretic peptide; cGMP: cyclic guanosine monophospate; DAG: diaciglicerol; GC: guanylyl cyclase-A; GMP: guanosine monophosphate; GTP: guanosine triphosphate; IP3: inosital 1,4,5'trifosfato; LTCC: L-type calcium channel; NEP - nepritysin (neutral endopeptidase); NPR: natriuretic peptide receptor, PDE: phosphodiesterase; PKG: protein kinase G; PLC: phosphadypase C; RAAS: renin-angiotensin-aldosterone system; UROD: urodilatin).

origin). Atrial natriuretic peptide (ANP) is produced from muscle cells of atria, BNP is produced from ventricles, C-type natriuretic peptide (CNP) is produced from blood vessels and D-type natriuretic peptide (DNP) is formed in blood plasma. Prepro BNP is a 134 amino acid preprohormone from which Pro BNP is formed which thereafter is cleaved by corin into NT-proBNP and *biological active 32 amino acid polypeptide BNP.* Once released, BNP binds and activates NPRA (Atrial Natriuretic Factor receptor) and to a lesser extent natriuretic peptide receptor-B (NPRB) and natriuretic peptide receptor-C (NPRC) receptor. Binding of natriuretic peptide (NP) induces a conformational change in the receptor that causes receptor dimerization and activation. This causes conversion of guanosine 5′-triphosphate (GTP) to cyclic guanosine 3′, 5′-monophosphate (GMP) and raises intracellular cyclic GMP which *activates a cyclic GMP dependent kinase (PKG).* This leads to actions like *natriuresis, vasodilatation, increased glomerular filtration rate, increased renal blood flow, enhancement of ventricular relaxation, antifibroblastic, antithrombotic, suppression of renin angiotensin aldosterone system and sympathetic nervous system.*[6]

Neutral endopeptidase (NEP) also known as neprilysin is the enzyme that metabolizes natriuretic peptide, less than 5% is excreted via the kidney (Fig. 2). NT-proBNP rely solely on kidney for excretion.

There are *3 volume regulating systems,* two salt saving systems, the renin angiotensin aldosterone system (RAAS), renal sympathetic system (RSS); and the third salt excreting natriuretic peptide (NP) a hormone system. When the vascular space contracts, the RASS and RSS are turned on when the atria expands natriuretic peptide are turned on.

BNP may increase with increasing atrial dimensions[7] rather than atrial pressure. Hence NP is also increased in atrial fibrillation, supraventricular tachycardia and after pericardiocentesis.

DIAGNOSTIC IMPLICATION

B-type natriuretic peptide is an effective method for detecting HF with or without systolic dysfunction. BNP monitoring in HF also correlates with pulmonary capillary wedge pressure.[8] Original studies by Troughton et al.,[9]

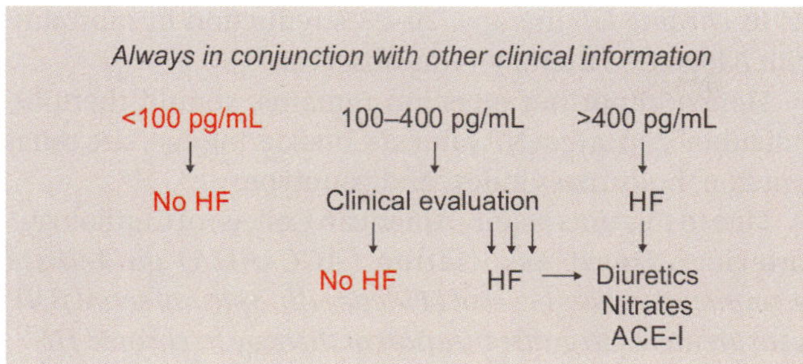

Fig. 3: Interpretation of BNP levels in patients with acute dyspnea.

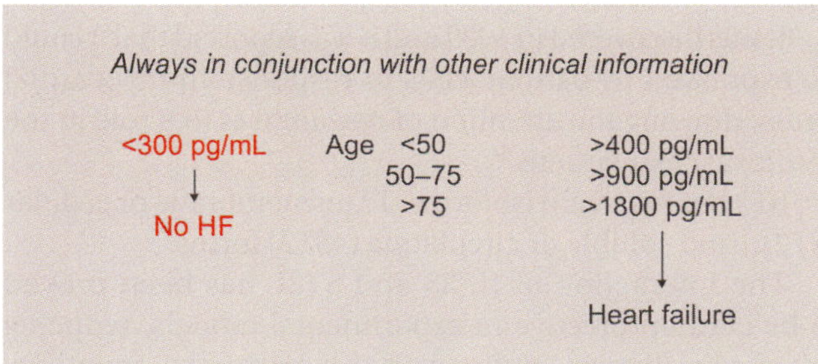

Fig. 4: Interpretation of NT-proBNP levels in patients with acute dyspnea.

Maisel et al.,[10] Januzzi et al.,[11] and others demonstrated that NP are extremely useful in diagnosis of HF. Normal BNP excludes HF by 98%. Between normal and HF zone is the grey zone.

In patients with kidney disease with *glomerular filtration rate of less than 60 mL/minute, BNP of 200-225 pg/mL* is the appropriate cutoff value to rule out HF.[12,13] In patients with severe *obesity (with BMI more than 35), BNP cutoff value of 60 pg/mL* to rule out, and 200 pg/mL to rule in HF, as the cause of dyspnea.[14,15] In *Intensive Care Unit (ICU), BNP lower cutoff of 150 pg/mL* to rule out HF as the cause of respiratory failure, and 600 pg/mL as a reasonable higher cutoff value to rule in HF (Figs. 3 and 4).[16-18]

BNP increased levels in noncardiac cases are, increased age and female gender. A single nucleotide polymorphism in the promoter region of the *BNP gene* (rs 198389; also referred to as T-381C) *was associated with 30% higher BNP* levels per C-allele.[19-24] BNP also increases in lung disease, advanced liver disease, overactive thyroid, cortisol excess, brain hemorrhage, certain tumors, chronic hypoxia, renal failure,[25] pulmonary embolism and pulmonary hypertension.[26-28]

BNP increased levels in cardiac cases are acute coronary syndrome, valvular heart disease (aortic stenosis, mitral regurgitation), high blood pressure with left ventricular hypertrophy. Atrial fibrillation also causes high BNP. BNP are also high in diastolic dysfunction, hypertrophic cardiomyopathy or associated systolic dysfunction. A study "breathing not properly" trial, and PRIDE (ProBNP investigation of dyspnea) study support the accuracy for diagnosis in heart failure.

B Type Natriuretic Peptide in Risk Population

Wang et al. showed in the Framingham offspring study that in *asymptomatic individuals with mild elevation in* BNP (after adjustment for cardiovascular risk factors)[29] was associated with increased risk of death, first cardiovascular event, HF, atrial fibrillation and stroke or transient ischemic attack. There is an increasing interest in using BNP measurement to target at *risk populations*, without HF, for preventing strategy. Two randomized clinical trials, PONTIAC (NT ProBNP guide of primary prevention of cardiovascular events in Diabetic patients)[30] and STOP-HF (screening to prevent HF)[31] have demonstrated improvement in clinical outcome; with a strategy of using BNP to identify high-risk patients for more aggressive HF prevention strategy.

McKie et al. confirm in a *general population* of Olmsted County, MN, that higher BNP and NT-proBNP levels are associated with increased mortality.[32]

PROGNOSTIC IMPLICATIONS

The BNP are among the most powerful prognostic markers in all forms of clinical HF, including HF with reduced ejection fraction[33] with preserved ejection fraction,[34] and acute HF.[35] In the acute setting, both elevations of the initial value at the time of presentation[35] and changes with therapy (value at hospital discharge) are strong predictors of short[36] and long-term outcomes.[37] Persistence of higher than 5000 pg/mL NT-proBnp levels long after decongestion portends poor outcomes, as per PROTECT (proBNP outpatient Tailored chronic HF trial).[38] For chronic cases, data from Val-HeFT, where both baseline values changes and over 3 months in BNP and NT-proBNP have been shown to be among the most powerful predictors of future outcomes.[39]

A change from normal to elevated BNP indicates an increase in risk, but, once elevated, this increased risk persisted regardless of subsequent changes. BNP reduction more than 80% was associated with risk reduction, while an increase from below to above 500 pg/mL was associated with an increased risk. *BNP increase of 100 pg/mL causes a 35% increase in risk of death.* Also, BNP is potentially more useful than traditional predictors of mortality [e.g. age, etiology, ischemic, left ventricular ejection fraction (LVEF), New York Heart Association (NYHA) class, s-creatinine level].[40]

We should try to achieve *predischarge BNP* levels below 350–400 pg/mL[41,42] with up titration of drugs. Patients of acute HF with a predischarge BNP levels of 350–700 pg/mL had a five times increased mortality or readmission for HF risk as compared to patients with predischarge BNP below 350 pg/mL. Once the predischarge BNP was above 700 pg/mL, mortality or readmission for HF risk increased by a factor 15 and reached a rate of 90%. Similar results were reported for NT-proBNP.[36]

Admission BNP is an independent powerful marker of early and late cardiac mortality in patients with *acute chest pain* without ST-segment elevation. BNP correlated with *severity of hepatic cirrhosis*[43] and with heart dysfunction.[44]

TREATMENT IMPLICATIONS

BNP correlates well with *pulmonary capillary wedge pressure,*[8] hence maybe a tool for monitoring treatment response.

The prognostic importance of NP levels and their modulation with treatment have created interest in the use of serial NP measurements to guide HF therapy. Patients with high biomarker levels should receive more intensive disease modifying therapy. The overall *results* of NP guided treatment *are mixed*[45-53] with the largest studies showing no clear evidence of benefit.

There is little evidence that the benefit of HF therapy varies according to HF severity or NP levels. Excessive reliance on NP levels to assess volume status, rather than HF symptoms, might prompt inappropriate dose of drugs among patients without significant congestion; and hence increase the rate of hypotension, renal dysfunction, and other adverse events. Troughton et al. in patients with symptomatic chronic HF with low ejection fraction (<40%)[54] French multicenter study (STARS -BNP),[55] and Berger et al. (64 B) favored NP guided therapy.

Treatment which proved benefit in HF patients with reduced EF, include angiotensin-converting-enzyme (ACE) inhibitors,[56] angiotensin II receptor blockers (ARB),[57] spironolactone,[58] beta-blockers,[59] and cardiac resynchronization therapy,[60] appear to decrease BNP levels in parallel with improvements in cardiac remodeling and clinical outcomes.

The TIME-CHF (Trial of intensified BNP guided) suggested, mortality was reduced with BNP guidance in the younger group, but not in the older group. Reason may be that the older patient group was associated with worse renal function, and more comorbidities.

In *chronic HF* therapy, 20–25% reduction in mortality with NP guided therapy[61] was observed.

Hence important question remains, should there be individualized target NP values? Considering age, sex, renal function, body mass index, and genotype.

Due to this uncertainty American College of Cardiology/American Heart Association (*ACC/AHA) guidelines recommend (Class-Level of Evidence IIb-B) use of serial BNP measurements to guide titration of therapy in chronic HF.*

sST2

ST2 that stands for "suppression of tumorigenicity 2", is the member of the interleukin 1 receptor family.[62,63]

It was discovered in 1989 and it was reported that it could be expressed by cardiac cells in response to myocardial stress, drawing the attention of researchers to a role in the cardiovascular system.[64]

ST2 has two main isoforms: Transmembrane or cellular (ST2L) and soluble or circulating (sST2) forms.[62]

The interaction of IL-33 and ST2L has been proved to be cardioprotective in experimental models, reducing myocardial fibrosis, cardiomyocyte hypertrophy, apoptosis, and improving myocardial function.

This cardioprotective action occurs exclusively through the ST2L receptor and not through the soluble receptor. The IL-33/ST2 system is up regulated in cardiomyocytes and fibroblasts in response to cardiac injury. sST2 avidly binds to IL-33 competing with ST2L. The interaction of this soluble receptor with IL-33 blocks the IL-33/ST2L system and, as a result, eliminates the cardioprotective effects described above. Therefore, sST2 is considered a decoy receptor.[65]

In outpatient, with prior high sST2 levels, showed high 1 year mortality, even among nonHF cases.[66]

In patients with acutely decompensated heart failure (ADHF), In PRIDE (Pro-Brain Natriuretic Peptide Investigation of Dyspnea in the Emergency Department) sST2 was measured. Levels of sST2 were significantly higher in patients with ADHF than nonHF patients. Patients who died at 1 year had higher values than survivors and sST2 levels were significantly correlated with mortality rates; with greater concentrations predicting the highest risk. Hence sST2 was a powerful predictor of mortality.[67]

GREAT (Global Research on Acute Conditions Team) study with 5,306 ADHF patients were carried out with great number of biomarkers (measured at admission), among them ST2 emerged as the strongest biomarker for death risk. ST2 was the best predictor of both 30-day and 1-year mortality.[68]

In chronic HF, ST2 has been shown to predict myocardial remodeling. The association of this biomarker with the remodeling process raises the possibility of identifying those most likely to respond to antiremodeling therapies. For example, in the setting of ADHF, patients with high sST2 levels benefit most from beta-blocker and antiremodeling therapies [mineral corticoid receptor antagonist, ARB and angiotensin receptor neprilysin inhibitor (ARNI)]. Hence can be used also to guide therapy in remodeling in HF.[69]

Serial measurements of SST 2 was carried out in patients admitted with ADHF and demonstrated that patients whose values decrease rapidly after admission had a good short-term outcome, and in contrast those with an increase in sST2 values had a high probability of dying at 6 months (Boisot et al.).[70]

The performance of sST2 was not influenced by renal function (Barcelona study), age, gender, body mass index, as observed with Natriuretic peptides.[71]

sST2 and galectin-3 are both associated with fibrosis and cardiac remodeling. Head-to-head comparison of these two biomarkers revealed that sST2 was superior to galectin-3 in risk stratification.[72]

sST2 is also associated with inflammatory and immune processes, especially regarding the regulation of mast cells and type 2 CD4 T- helper cells and production of Th2 associated cytokines. Thus, a role for IL-33/ST2 system has been demonstrated in diseases associated with a predominant Th2 response such as asthma, pulmonary fibrosis, rheumatoid arthritis, collagen vascular disease, sepsis, trauma, malignancy, fibroproliferative diseases, helminthic infections and ulcerative colitis.

Galectin-3

Galectin 3 (Gal-3) is a macrophage lectin product that plays a role in a cascade of events leading to tissue fibrosis. In animal models of heart failure, galectin-3 highly expressed in failing vs. functionally compensated hearts.[73] Intrapericardial administration of galectin-3 significantly increases left ventricular (LV) collagen content and reduces LV ejection fraction.

Cardiac remodeling is an essential feature of heart failure, and it is linked to disease progression. Recently, a role for Gal-3 in cardiac remodeling and heart failure has been suggested. Fibrosis is a pivotal process in maladaptive cardiac response. Fibroblasts and macrophages are responsible for the initiation and progression of tissue fibrosis.

The first clinical data for galectin-3 in HF came from the PRIDE study where in patients with ADHF, galectin-3 concentrations were strongly predictive of 60-day mortality or the combination of death/recurrent HF within 60 days; the combination of NT- proBNP with galectin-3 was a better predictor of mortality than either biomarker alone.[74]

An elevated level of Gal-3 was the best independent predictor of 60-days mortality or recurrent HF within 60 days. Higher circulating Gal-3 concentrations are associated with a high risk of new onset HF and all-cause mortality in apparently healthy subjects.

In chronic HF, the prognostic ability of gal-3 is more variable, with other biomarkers such as sST2 or nitropeptides frequently showing superiority for prognostication.

This marker is not specific to heart, since it is found in spleen, lung, stomach, colon, adrenal gland, uterus and ovary. Gal-3 is also a biomarker associated with atherosclerosis, stroke, diabetes mellitus, vasculitis and connective tissue disease.

sST2, galectin-3 testing received a class II recommendation in the American College of Cardiology/American Heart Association/Heart Failure Society of America HF guidelines for risk prediction in HF.[75]

High Sensitivity Troponin

The troponin complex regulates myocyte contraction and consists of 3 subunits: C, I, and T.[76] The isoforms of troponin T and I are unique to the heart, allowing targeted assays to these proteins.

The AHA/ACC Foundation guidelines endorse measuring troponin in acute HF to assess for acute coronary syndrome and risk stratification. Elevated concentrations of high sensitivity troponin (hsTn) are seen in patients with both ADHF and chronic HF even in the absence of ischemic heart disease. Mechanism for this being subendocardial stress, myocyte degeneration, and toxic effects of noncardiovascular disorders (such as renal failure).

It has been unequivocally shown that an elevated troponin measured with conventional assays is associated with an increased in hospital mortality in acute heart failure.[77]

Conventional troponin (CTn) with an elevated level, in AHF have found to increase risk of adverse events. In the EFFECT (enhanced feedback for effective cardiac treatment) study a peak cTn >0.5 Ug/L measured in the first 48 hours of hospitalization was an independent predictor of all-cause mortality at 1 year; regardless of with or without ischemia.[78]A persistently elevated CTn level on repeated admissions, especially if >0.04 ng/mL is associated with increased long-term mortality rates.[78]

Serial measurements of hsTn during a hospitalization for acute heart failure can risk-stratify patients, for 90-day mortality and readmission. Patients whose discharge troponin value rose compared with admission or was above a certain cutoff had the greatest risk.[79]

As with NPs in outpatients with chronic heart failure, hsTn is prognostic for mortality and disease severity.[80]

High sensitivity troponin is especially valuable in identifying patients at high risk for developing heart failure. hsTn can predict which individuals are at increased risk for developing heart failure or experiencing a cardiovascular death.[81]

This prognostic ability is enhanced when hsTn is combined with NPs.[82]

A potential use for hsTn is assessing response to therapy. In the RELAX studies, an elevated hsTn as well as 20% increase in hsTn was associated with increased mortality.[83]

Similarly, therapy with LCZ696 can significantly reduce hsTn values.[84] Targeting either a value of hsTn or a delta change of hsTn to institute therapies for heart failure (e.g. nitrates, ranolazine) may have beneficial effects in patients with subendocardial ischemia.

The Heart Type of Fatty Acid Binding Protein

The heart type of fatty acid binding protein (hFABP) is normally essential for the long-chain fatty acids reuptake, regulation of calcium homeostasis in cardiomyocytes and mediating inflammatory reaction.[85] Because hFABP is tissue-specific biomarker of myocardial injury and necrosis, it is reserved as predictor of myocardial infarction at the early hours of development of the disease. Recent studies have shown that circulating levels of hFABP are elevated in cardiac dysfunction and closely predicted cardiovascular (CV) outcomes and HF-related events in in-patients especially in those who had fluid retention and lung congestion.[85-87] Although elevated serum level of hFABP exhibited better prognostic information on survival in individuals with acute and advanced HF when compared to NPs, cardiac troponins and even galectin-3 taken alone.

Procalcitonin

Procalcitonin is determined a propeptide of calcitonin, which is normally produced by the parafollicular C cells of the thyroid gland.[88] Recent preclinical and clinical studies have shown that extrathyroidal production of procalcitonin markedly increases in cases of systemic inflammatory reaction, severe infections (viral, bacterial, fungal and parasitic), and shock.[89,90] Large clinical trials are required regarding a predicted role of procalcitonin in exacerbated heart failure individuals.

Mid-regional Pro-adrenomedullin

Mid-regional Pro-adrenomedullin (MR-proADM) was associated with mortality with a prognostic value beyond natriuretic peptides as evidenced by BACH (Biomarkers in Acute Heart Failure) study,[91] and Australia-New Zealand heart failure[92] study. Although MR-proADM is rather prognostic, but the marker lacks specificity for HF because of its expression in multiple tissues. More studies are needed to determine the utility and prognostic value of MR-proADM in HF.

Copeptin

Copeptin is C-terminal derivate of the arginine vasopressin that normally acts as regulator of water and electrolyte homeostasis. Direct arginine vasopressin measurement is difficult as the peptide is unstable; copeptin, the C-terminal segment of provasopressin has been reported to be a suitable surrogate, predictive marker of adverse outcomes in patients with ADHF.[93]

Although plasma levels of copeptin are very variable and tightly related to blood/urine osmolality, copeptin appears to be in higher concentrations in sever hypertension, stroke, acute and chronic HF, myocardial infarction, diabetes mellitus, advanced kidney diseases, and in critical conditions.[94] As quantitative biomarker of endogenous biomechanical stress, elevated level of copeptin was found in close positive association with increased CV mortality and CV disease, in out-patients and all-cause mortality in critical ill patients.[95] The serial measurements of copeptin levels may provide an important information for discrimination of a risk for all-cause mortality, HF-related outcomes and CV events.[96-98]

Cystatin C

Increased cystatin C is a predictor of CV death and HF related complications, in reduced ejection fraction heart failure patients, rather than preserved ejection fraction heart failure patients.[99-101] Cystatin C was found as an endogenous inhibitor of cysteine proteases. Despite cystatin C has validated a predictor of kidney injury, the discriminative ability of this biomarker in chronic HF patients is lower to hs-CRP and NPs.[101]

Serum Uric Acid

As strong oxidative factor uric acid triggers inflammation and may impair vascular function.[102] In contrast, uric acid in peripheral tissues could act as scavenger of free radicals and protects against an oxidative stress.[103,104]

TABLE 1: American College of Cardiology Recommendation

Biomarker	*Indication for use*	*Recommendation*	*Level of evidence*
BNP/NT-proBNP	Prognosis at hospital admission Diagnosis Prognosis after discharge Prevention To guide therapy	I I IIa IIa IIb	A A B B B
Troponin T or I	Hospital admission prognosis	I	A
sST2 , Galectin-3	Prognosis	IIb	B

(BNP: B-type natriuretic peptide)

Moreover, serial measures of serum uric acid (SUA) levels are accurate predictor of clinical outcomes in acute HF than in chronic HF,[100,105,106] while SUA undoubtedly remains a risk factor of poor outcomes in HF independently of LVEF.[100,101]

Recent studies have revealed the elevated level of SUA could be common feature for patients with HF, hypertension, atherosclerosis, obesity, diabetes mellitus and chronic renal disease.[107,108]

In the OPT-CHF (Oxypurinol Therapy in Congestive Heart Failure) study,[109] oxypurinol, a xanthine oxidase inhibitor, reduced uric acid levels, but failed to show improvement in the hospitalization or cardiovascular death.

Myeloperoxidase

Myeloperoxidase (MPO) is oxidative stress biomarker, released from activated neutrophils and monocytes during periods of inflammation.

Plasma MPO levels increased in parallel with increasing NYHA class of heart failure and were also correlated with plasma BNP concentrations.[110]

In ADHF patients, MPO concentration >99 pmol/L were associated with significant increase in 1 year mortality.[111] Plasma MPO levels in chronic HF were significantly elevated compared with those of healthy control.[110]

Matrix Metalloproteinase

Development of HF strongly associates with CV remodeling, biomechanical and oxidative myocardial stress, neurohormonal and inflammatory activation that are modulated by MMPs. It has demonstrated that MMPs determine extracellular accumulation of collagen and mediate pro-fibrotic processes.[112] Excessive collagen cross-linking is associated with hospitalization for HF in hypertensive patients.[113]

Matrix metalloproteinase (MMP)-2 concentrations were an independent predictor of mortality in patients with HF.[114] Subsequently, Buralli et al.[115] demonstrated that MMP-3 and MMP-9 were univariate predictors of all-cause mortality in patients with HF reduced ejection fraction (rEF).

AMERICAN COLLEGE OF CARDIOLOGY RECOMMENDATION

American College of Cardiology Recommendations have been specified in Table 1.

PRACTICAL USE OF NOVEL BIOMARKER

Practical use of novel biomarkers is described in Flowchart 1.

CONCLUSION

The biomarkers evaluation in acute HF has diagnostic, prognostic and therapeutic implications. In acute HF, screen the patients at admission may be subjected to evaluation with NT-proBNP, hsTn, sST2/Galectin-3 etc. If hsTn >99%le and 3 hours after repeat hsTn is increased, then treat as myocardial infarction. If sST2 >35, BNP >400 and NT-proBNP is significantly raised; treat acute HF and check biomarkers prior to discharge. If NT-proBNP is elevated, i.e. <30% decline than prior estimated or BNP >250 mg/mL; hsTn, sST2/galectin-3 elevated then early titration of optimal HF therapy and early follow-up is needed. If hsTn, sST2/Galectin-3 improved than prior estimated, then follow-up as outpatient with repeat NT-proBNP, SST2, hsTn levels. If there is rising trends, then timely optimization of HF therapy is necessary to enhance morbidity and mortality benefits.

Flowchart 1: Choosing of biomarkers in acute heart failure.

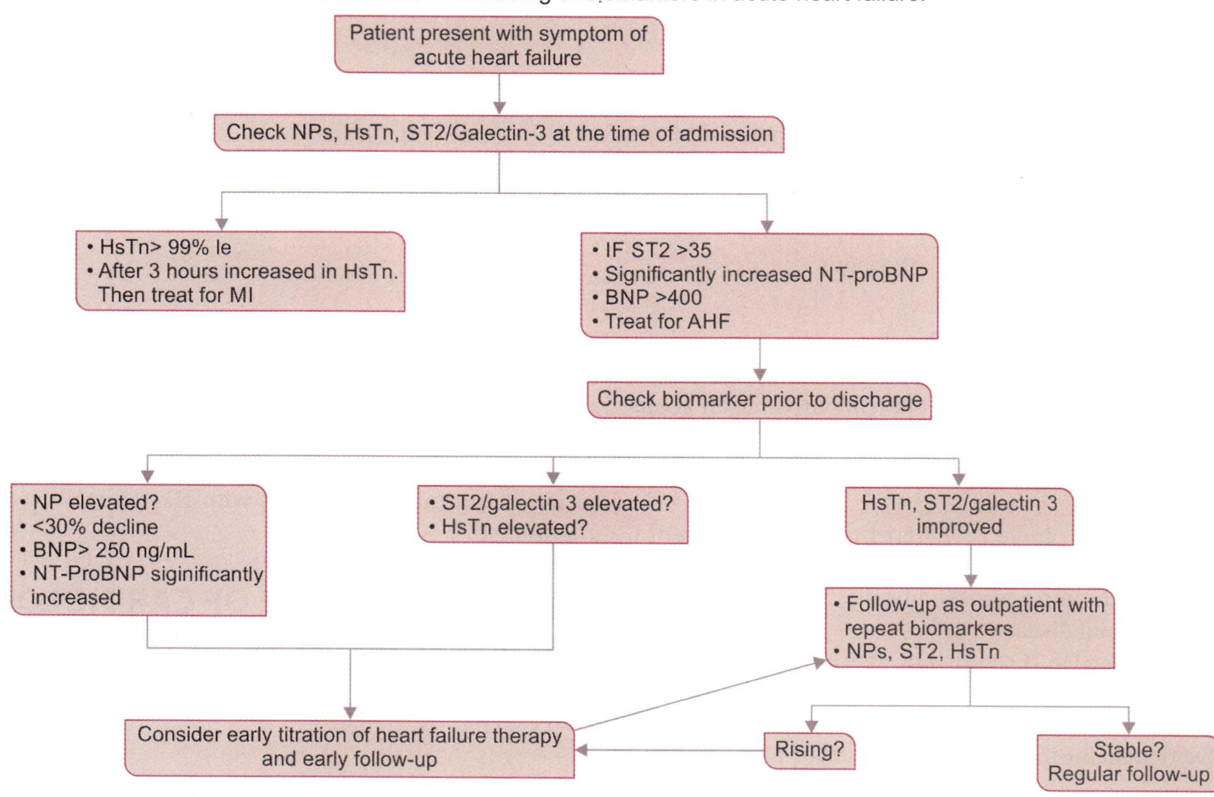

REFERENCES

1. Mozaffarian D, Benjamin EJ, Go AS, et al. Heart disease and stroke statistics—2015 update: a report from the American Heart Association. Circulation. 2015;131(4):e29-e322.
2. McKee PA, Castelli WP, McNamara PM, et al. The natural history of congestive heart failure: the Framingham study. N Engl J Med. 1971;285(26):1441-6.
3. Eriksson H. Heart failure: a growing public health problem. J Inter Med. 1995;237(2):135-41.
4. Writing Group Members, Lloyd-Jones D, Adams RJ, et al. Heart disease and stroke statistics-2010 update: a report from the American Heart Association. Circulation. 2010;121(7):e46-e215.
5. Atkinson A, Colburn W, DeGruttola V, et al. Biomarkers and surrogate endpoints: preferred definitions and conceptual framework. Clin Pharmacol Ther. 2001;69(3):89-95.
6. Sharma S, Chhabra S. ARNI in heart failure with cardiodiabetes: The way forward. In: Kasliwal RR, Chopra HK, Wander GS, Kumar V, Pancholia AK, Joshi SR (Eds). Cardiodiabetes Update: A Textbook of Cardiology. New Delhi: Jaypee Brothers Medical Publishers (P) Ltd; 2018. pp. 505-13.
7. Agnoletti G, Rodella A, Ferrari R, et al. Release of atrial natriuretic peptide-like immunoreactive material during stretching of the rat atrium in vitro. J Mol Cell Cardiol. 1987;19(3):217-20.
8. Kazanegra R, Cheng V, Garcia A, et al. A rapid test for B-type natriuretic peptide correlates with falling wedge pressures in patients treated for decompensated heart failure: a pilot study. J Card Fail. 2001;7(1):21-9.
9. Sharma S, Chopra HK, Babu M, Awasthi S, Patel N. Biomarker B-type natriuretic peptide imaging in heart failure. In: Advances in clinical cardiovascular imaging echocardiography & intervention. New Delhi: Jaypee Brothers Medical Publishers (P) Ltd; pp. 1115-25.
10. Maisel AS, Krishnaswamy P, Nowak RM, et al. Rapid measurement of B-type natriuretic peptide in the emergency diagnosis of heart failure. N Engl J Med. 2002;347(3):161-7.
11. Januzzi JL Jr, Camargo CA, Anwaruddin S, et al. The N-terminal Pro-BNP investigation of dyspnea in the emergency department (PRIDE) study. Am J Cardiol. 2005;95(8):948-54.
12. McCullough PA, Duc P, Omland T, et al. B-type natriuretic peptide and renal function in the diagnosis of heart failure: An Analysis from the breathing not properly multinational study. Am J Kidney Dis. 2003;41(3):571-5.
13. Mueller C, Laule Kilian K, Scholer A, et al. B-type natriuretic peptide for acute dyspnea in patients with kidney disease: insights from a randomized comparison. Kidney Int. 2005;67(1):278-84.
14. Wang TJ, Larson MG, Levy D, et al. Impact of obesity on plasma natriuretic peptide levels. Circulation. 2004;109(5):594-600.

15. McCord J, Mundy BJ, Hudson MP, et al. Relationship between obesity and B-type natriuretic peptide levels. Arch Intern Med. 2004;164(20):2247-52.
16. McLean AS, Tang B, Nalos M, et al. Increased B-type natriuretic peptide (BNP) level is a strong predictor for cardiac dysfunction in intensive care unit patients. Anaesth Intensive Care. 2003;31(1):21-7.
17. McLean AS, Huang SJ, Nalos M, Tang B, et al. The confounding effects of age, gender, serum creatinine, and electrolyte concentrations on plasma B-type natriuretic peptide concentrations in critically ill patients. Crit Care Med. 2003;31(11):2611-8.
18. Silver MA, Maisel A, Yancy CW, et al. BNP consensus panel 2004: a clinical approach for the diagnostic, prognostic, screening, treatment monitoring, and therapeutic roles of natriuretic peptides in cardiovascular diseases. Congest Heart Fail. 2004;10(3):10-11.
19. Wang TJ, Larson MG, Levy D, et al. Heritability and genetic linkage of plasma natriuretic peptide levels. Circulation. 2003;108(1):13-6.
20. Meirhaeghe A, Sandhu MS, McCarthy MI, et al. Association between the T-381C polymorphism of the brain natriuretic peptide gene and risk of type 2 diabetes in human populations. Hum Mol Genet. 2007;16(11):1343-50.
21. Lanfear DE, Stolker JM, Marsh S, et al. Genetic variation in the B-type natriuretic peptide pathway affects BNP levels. Cardiovasc Drugs Ther. 2007;21(1):55-62.
22. Costello-Boerrigter LC, Boerrigter G, Ameenuddin S, et al. The B-type natriuretic peptide T-381C polymorphism is associated with increased BNP plasma immunoreactivity and higher prevalence of type 2 diabetes mellitus and atrial fibrillation. Eur Heart J. 2008;29:766.
23. Redfield MM, Rodeheffer RJ, Jacobsen SJ, et al. Plasma brain natriuretic peptide concentration: impact of age and gender. J Am Coll Cardiol. 2002;40(5):976-82.
24. Costello-Boerrigter LC, Boerrigter G, Redfield MM, et al. Amino-terminal pro-B-type natriuretic peptide and B-type natriuretic peptide in the general community: determinants and detection of left ventricular dysfunction. J Am Coll Cardiol. 2006;47(2):345-53.
25. Siebenhofer A, Ng LL, Plank J, et al. Plasma N-terminal pro-brain natriuretic peptide in type 1 diabetic patients with and without diabetic nephropathy. Diabet Med. 2003;20(7):535-9.
26. Kucher N, Goldhaber SZ. Cardiac biomarkers for risk stratification of patients with acute pulmonary embolism. Circulation. 2003;108(18):2191-4.
27. Pruszczyk P, Kostrubiec M, Bochowicz A, et al. N-terminal pro-brain natriuretic peptide in patients with acute pulmonary embolism. Eur Respir J. 2003;22(4):649-53.
28. Burke MA, Cotts WG. Interpretation of B-type natriuretic peptide in cardiac disease and other comorbid conditions. Heart Fail Rev. 2007;12(1):23-36.
29. Wang TJ, Larson MG, Levy D, et al. Plasma natriuretic peptide levels and the risk of cardiovascular events and death. N Engl J Med. 2004;350(7):655-63.
30. Huelsmann M, Neuhold S, Resl M, et al. PONTIAC (NT-proBNP Selected Prevention of cardiac events in a population of diabetic patients without A history of Cardiac disease): a prospective randomized controlled trial. J Am Coll Cardiol. 2013;62(15):1365-72.
31. Ledwidge M, Gallagher J, Conlon C, et al. Natriuretic peptide-based screening and collaborative care for heart failure: the STOP-HF randomized trial. JAMA. 2013;310(1):66-74.
32. McKie PM, Rodeheffer RJ, Cataliotti A, et al. Amino-terminal pro-B-type natriuretic peptide and B-type natriuretic peptide: biomarkers for mortality in a large community-based cohort free of heart failure. Hypertension. 2006;47(5):874-80.
33. Anand IS, Fisher LD, Chiang YT, et al. The Val-HeFT Investigators Changes in brain natriuretic peptide and norepinephrine over time and mortality and morbidity in the Valsartan Heart Failure Trial (Val-HeFT) Circulation. 2003;107(9):1278-83.
34. Anand IS, Rector TS, Cleland JG, et al. Prognostic value of baseline plasma amino-terminal pro-brain natriuretic peptide and its interactions with irbesartan treatment effects in patients with heart failure and preserved ejection fraction: findings from the I-PRESERVE trial. Circ Heart Fail. 2011;4(5):569-77.
35. Fonarow GC, Peacock WF, Phillips CO, et al. The ADHERE Scientific Advisory Committee and Investigators Admission B-type natriuretic peptide levels and in-hospital mortality in acute decompensated heart failure. J Am Coll Cardiol. 2007;49(19):1943-50.
36. Bettencourt P, Azevedo A, Pimenta J, et al. N-terminal-pro-brain natriuretic peptide predicts outcome after hospital discharge in heart failure patients. Circulation. 2004;110(15):2168-74.
37. Kociol RD, Horton JR, Fonarow GC, et al. Admission, discharge, or change in B-type natriuretic peptide and long-term outcomes: data from Organized Program to Initiate Lifesaving Treatment in Hospitalized Patients with Heart Failure (OPTIMIZE-HF) linked to Medicare claims. Circ Heart Fail. 2011;4(5):628-36.
38. Gaggin HK, Truong QA, Rehman SU, et al. Characterization and prediction of natriuretic peptide "nonresponse" during heart failure management: results from the ProBNP Outpatient Tailored Chronic Heart Failure (PROTECT) and the NT-proBNP-Assisted Treatment to Lessen Serial Cardiac Readmissions and Death (BATTLESCARRED) study. Congest Heart Fail. 2013;19(3):135-42.
39. Masson S, Latini R, Anand IS, et al. The Val-HeFT Investigators Prognostic value of changes in N-terminal pro-brain natriuretic peptide in Val-HeFT (Valsartan Heart Failure Trial) J Am Coll Cardiol. 2008;52(12):997-1003.
40. Doust JA, Pietrzak E, Dobson A, et al. How well does B-type natriuretic peptide predict death and cardiac events in patients with heart failure: systematic review. BMJ. 2005;330(7492):625.
41. Logeart D, Thabut G, Jourdain P, et al. Predischarge B-type natriuretic peptide assay for identifying patients at high risk of readmission after decompensated heart failure. J Am Coll Cardiol. 2004;43(4):635-41.
42. Verdiani V, Nozzoli C, Bacci F, et al. Pre-discharge B-type natriuretic peptide predicts early recurrence of

decompensated heart failure in patients admitted to a general medical unit. Eur J Heart Fail. 2005;7(4):566-71.

43. Henriksen JH, Goetze JP, Fuglsang S, et al. Increased circulating probrain natriuretic peptide (proBNP) and brain natriuretic peptide (BNP) in patients with cirrhosis: relation to cardiovascular dysfunction and severity of disease. Gut. 2003;52(10):1511-7.
44. Kneiseler G, Herzer K, Marggraf G. The interaction between liner and heart. Heart-Thorax-Vascular-Surgery. 2010;24(6):334-40.
45. Troughton RW, Frampton CM, Yandle TG, et al. Treatment of heart failure guided by plasma aminoterminal brain natriuretic peptide (N-BNP) concentrations. Lancet. 2000;355(9210):1126-30.
46. Jourdain P, Jondeau G, Funck F, et al. Plasma brain natriuretic peptide-guided therapy to improve outcome in heart failure: the STARS-BNP Multicenter Study. J Am Coll Cardiol. 2007;49(16):1733-9.
47. Shah MR, Califf RM, Nohria A, et al. The STARBRITE trial: a randomized, pilot study of B-type natriuretic peptide-guided therapy in patients with advanced heart failure. J Card Fail. 2011;17(8):613-21.
48. Pfisterer M, Buser P, Rickli H, et al. BNP-guided vs symptom-guided heart failure therapy: the Trial of Intensified vs Standard Medical Therapy in Elderly Patients With Congestive Heart Failure (TIME-CHF) randomized trial. JAMA. 2009;301(4):383-92.
49. Lainchbury JG, Troughton RW, Strangman KM, et al. N-terminal pro-B-type natriuretic peptide-guided treatment for chronic heart failure: results from the BATTLESCARRED (NT-proBNP-Assisted Treatment to Lessen Serial Cardiac Readmissions and Death) trial. J Am Coll Cardiol. 2009;55(1):53-60.
50. Eurlings LW, van Pol PE, Kok WE, et al. Management of chronic heart failure guided by individual N-terminal pro-B-type natriuretic peptide targets: results of the PRIMA (Can PRo-brain-natriuretic peptide guided therapy of chronic heart failure Improve heart failure morbidity and mortality?) study. J Am Coll Cardiol. 2010;56(25):2090-100.
51. Januzzi JL, Rehman SU, Mohammed AA, et al. Use of amino-terminal pro-B-type natriuretic peptide to guide outpatient therapy of patients with chronic left ventricular systolic dysfunction. J Am Coll Cardiol. 2011;58(18):1881-9.
52. Berger R, Moertl D, Peter S, et al. N-terminal pro-B-type natriuretic peptide-guided, intensive patient management in addition to multidisciplinary care in chronic heart failure a 3-arm, prospective, randomized pilot study. J Am Coll Cardiol. 2010;55(7):645-53.
53. Persson H, Erntell H, Eriksson B, et al. Improved pharmacological therapy of chronic heart failure in primary care: a randomized Study of NT-proBNP Guided Management of Heart Failure–SIGNAL-HF (Swedish Intervention study–Guidelines and NT-proBNP Analysis in Heart Failure). Eur J Heart Fail. 2011;12(12):1300-8.
54. Troughton RW, Frampton CM, Yandle TG, et al. Treatment of heart failure guided by plasma aminoterminal brain natriuretic-peptide (N-BNP) concentrations. Lancet. 2000;355(9210):1126-30.
55. Jourdain P, Funck F, Gueffet P, et al. Benefit of BNP plasma levels for optimising therapy: the systolic heart failure treatment supported by BNP multicenter trial (STARS-BNP). J Am Coll Cardiol. 2005;45(16):1001-151.
56. Motwani JG, McAlpine H, Kennedy N, et al. Plasma brain natriuretic peptide as an indicator for angiotensin-converting-enzyme inhibition after myocardial infarction. Lancet. 1993;341(8853):1109-13.
57. Latini R, Masson S, Anand I, et al. Effects of valsartan on circulating brain natriuretic peptide and norepinephrine in symptomatic chronic heart failure: the Valsartan Heart Failure Trial (Val-HeFT). Circulation. 2002;106(19):2454-8.
58. Tsutamoto T, Wada A, Maeda K, et al. Effect of spironolactone on plasma brain natriuretic peptide and left ventricular remodeling in patients with congestive heart failure. J Am Coll Cardiol. 2001;37(5):1228-33.
59. Stanek B, Frey B, Hülsmann M, et al. Prognostic evaluation of neurohumoral plasma levels before and during beta-blocker therapy in advanced left ventricular dysfunction. J Am Coll Cardiol. 2001;38(2):436-42.
60. Cleland JG, Daubert JC, Erdmann E, et al. The effect of cardiac resynchronization on morbidity and mortality in heart failure. N Engl J Med. 2005;352(15):1539-49.
61. Troughton R, Felker GM, Januzzi JL. Natriuretic peptide-guided heart failure management. Eur Heart J. 2014;35(1):16-24.
62. Pascual-Figal DA, Januzzi JL. The biology of ST2: The international ST2 consensus panel. Am J Cardiol. 2015;115:3B-7B.
63. Tominaga S. A putative protein of a growth specific cDNA from BALB/c-3T3 cells is highly similar to the extracellular portion of mouse interleukin 1 receptor. FEBS Lett. 1989;258(2):301-4.
64. Weinberg EO, Shimpo M, De Keulenaer GW, et al. Expression and regulation of ST2, an interleukin-1 receptor family member, in cardiomyocytes and myocardial infarction. Circulation. 2002;106(23):2961-6.
65. Schmitz J, Owyang A, Oldham E, et al. IL-33, an interleukin-1-like cytokine that signals via the IL-1 receptor-related protein ST2 and induces T helper type 2-associated cytokines. Immunity. 2005;23(5):479-90.
66. Gagging HK, Szymonifka J, Bhardwaj A, et al. Head-to-head comparison of serial soluble ST2, growth differentiation factor-15, and highly-sensitivity troponin T measurements in patients with chronic heart failure. JACC Heart Fail. 2014;2(1):65-72.
67. Januzzi JL, Peacock WF, Maisel AS, et al. Measurement of the interleukin family member ST2 in patients with acute dyspnea: results from the PRIDE (Pro-Brain Natriuretic Peptide Investigation of Dyspnea in the Emergency Department) Study. J Am Coll Cardiol. 2007;50(7):607-13.
68. Lassus J, Gayat E, Mueller C, et al. Incremental value of biomarkers to clinical variables for mortality prediction in acutely decompensated heart failure: the Multinational

Observational Cohort on acute heart failure (MOCA) Study. Int J Cardiol. 2013;168(3):2186-94.

69. Manzano-Fernández S, Januzzi JL, Pastor-Pérez FJ, et al. Serial monitoring of soluble interleukin family member ST2 in patients with acutely decompensated heart failure. Cardiology. 2012;122(3):158-66.
70. Boisot S, Beed J, Isakson S, et al. Serial sampling of ST2 predicts 90-day mortality following destabilized Heart failure. J Card Fail. 2008;14(9):732-8.
71. Bayes-Genis A, Zamora E, De Antonio M, et al. Soluble ST2 serum concentration and renal function in heart failure. J Card Fail. 2013;19(11):768-75.
72. Bayes-Genis A, De Antonio M, Villa J, et al. Head-to-head comparison of 2 myocardial fibrosis biomarkers for long-term heart failure risk stratification: ST2 versus galectine-3. J Am Coll Cardiol. 2014:63(2):158-66.
73. Sharma UC, Pokharel S, van Brakel TJ, et al. Galectin-3 marks activated macrophages in failure-prone hypertrophied hearts and contributes to cardiac dysfunction. Circulation. 2004;110(19):3121-8.
74. van Kimmenade RR, Januzzi JL, Ellinor PT, et al. Utility of amino-terminal pro-brain natriuretic peptide, galectin-3, and apelin for the evaluation of patients with acute heart failure. J Am Coll Cardiol. 2006;48(6):1217-24.
75. Yancy CW, Jessup M, Bozkurt B, et al. 2017 ACC/AHA/HFSA Focused Update of the 2013 ACCF/AHA guideline for the management of heart failure: a report of the American College of Cardiology/American Heart Association Task Force on Clinical Practice Guidelines and the Heart Failure Society of America. Circulation. 2017;136(6):e147-e239.
76. Parmacek MS, Solaro RJ. Biology of the troponin complex in cardiac myocytes. Prog Cardiovasc Dis. 2004;47(3):159-176.
77. Peacock WF, De Marco T, Fonarow GC, et al. Cardiac troponin and outcome in acute heart failure. N Engl J Med. 2008;358(20):2117-26.
78. Tu JV, Donovan LR, Lee DS, et al. Effectiveness of public report cards for improving the quality of cardiac care. The EFFECT study: a randomized trial. JAMA. 2009.
79. Xue Y, Clopton P, Peacock WF, et al. Serial changes in high sensitive troponin I predict outcome in patients with decompensated heart failure. Eur J Heart Fail. 2011;13(1):37-42.
80. Latini R, Masson S, Anand IS, et al. Prognostic value of very low plasma concentrations of troponin T in patients with stable chronic heart failure. Circulation. 2007;116(11):1242-9.
81. Saunders JT, Nambi V, de Lemos JA, et al. Cardiac troponin T measured by a highly sensitive assay predicts coronary heart disease, heart failure, and mortality in the Atherosclerosis Risk in Communities Study. Circulation. 2011;123(13):1367-6.
82. Nambi V, Liu X, Chambless LE, et al. Troponin T and N-terminal pro- B-type natriuretic peptide: a biomarker approach to predict heart failure risk-the atherosclerosis risk in communities study. Clin Chem. 2013;59(12):1802-10.
83. Felker GM, Mentz RJ, Teerlink JR, et al. Serial high sensitivity cardiac troponin T measurement in acute heart failure: insights from the RELAX-AHF study. Eur J Heart Fail. 2015;17(12):1262-70.
84. Packer M, McMurray JJ, Desai AS, et al. Angiotensin receptor neprilysin inhibition compared with enalapril on the risk of clinical progression in surviving patients with heart failure. Circulation. 2015;131(1):54-61.
85. Kitai T, Kim YH, Kiefer K, et al. Circulating intestinal fatty acid-binding protein (I-FABP) levels in acute decompensated heart failure. Clin Biochem. 2017;50(9):491-5.
86. Chmurzyńska A. The multigene family of fatty acid binding proteins (FABPs): function, structure, and polymorphism. J Appl Genet. 2006;47(1):39-48.
87. Qian HY, Huang J, Yang YJ, et al. Heart-type Fatty Acid Binding Protein in the Assessment of Acute Pulmonary Embolism. Am J Med Sci. 2016;352(6):557-62.
88. Ryu JA, Yang JH, Lee D, et al. Clinical Usefulness of Procalcitonin and C-Reactive Protein as Outcome Predictors in Critically Ill Patients with Severe Sepsis and Septic Shock. PloS One. 2015;10(9):e0138150.
89. Hayashida K, Kondo Y, Hara Y, et al. Head-to-head comparison of procalcitonin and presepsin for the diagnosis of sepsis in critically ill adult patients: a protocol for a systematic review and meta-analysis. BMJ Open. 2017;7(3):e014305.
90. Simon L, Gauvin F, Amre DK, et al. Serum procalcitonin and C-reactive protein levels as markers of bacterial infection: a systematic review and meta-analysis. Clin Infect Dis. 2004;39(2):206-17.
91. Maisel A, Mueller C, Nowak R, et al. Mid-region pro-hormone markers for diagnosis and prognosis in acute dyspnea: results from the BACH (Biomarkers in Acute Heart Failure) trial. J Am Coll Cardiol. 2010;55(19):2062-76.
92. Zairis MN, Tsiaousis GZ, Georgilas AT, et al. Multimarker strategy for the prediction of 31 days cardiac death in patients with acutely decompensated chronic heart failure. Int J Cardiol. 2010;141(3):284-90.
93. Morgenthaler NG. Assay for the measurement of copeptin, a stable peptide derived from the precursor of vasopressin. Clin Chem. 2006;52(1):112-9.
94. Moayedi Y, Ross HJ. Advances in heart failure: a review of biomarkers, emerging pharmacological therapies, durable mechanical support and telemonitoring. Clin Sci (Lond). 2017;131(7):553-66.
95. Remde H, Dietz A, Emeny R, et al. The cardiovascular markers copeptin and high-sensitive C-reactive protein decrease following specific therapy for primary aldosteronism. J Hypertens. 2016;34(10):2066-73.
96. Berezin AE. Biological markers of cardiovascular diseases. Part 4. Diagnostic and prognostic value of biological markers at risk stratification among patients with heart failure. Moskow: LAMBERT Academic Publishing GmbH; 2015. p. 329.
97. Herrero-Puente P, Prieto-García B, García-García M, et al. Predictive capacity of a multimarker strategy to determine short-term mortality in patients attending a hospital emergency Department for acute heart failure. BIO-EAHFE study. Clin Chim Acta. 2017;466:22-30.
98. Yan JJ, Lu Y, Kuai ZP, et al. Predictive value of plasma copeptin level for the risk and mortality of heart failure: a meta-analysis. J Cell Mol Med. 2017;21(9):1815-25.

99. Otaki Y, Watanabe T, Kinoshita D, et al. Association of plasma xanthine oxidoreductase activity with severity and clinical outcome in patients with chronic heart failure. Int J Cardiol. 2017;228:151-7.
100. Berezin A. Does serum uric acid play a protective role against tissue damage in cardiovascular and metabolic diseases? Ann Clin Hypertens. 2017;1:39-41.
101. Berezin A. Biomarkers in heart failure. J Blood Lymph. 2017;7:172-9.
102. Berezin AE, Kremzer AA. Serum uric acid as a marker of coronary calcification in patients with asymptomatic coronary artery disease with preserved left ventricular pump function. Cardiol Res Pract. 2013;2013:129369.
103. Berezin AE. Serum uric acid as a metabolic regulator of endothelial reparative processes in heart failure patients. Stem Cell and Translational Investigation 2014;3(1):e432.
104. Berezin AE, Kremzer AA, Martovitskaya YV, et al. Serum Uric Acid Predicts Declining of Circulating Proangiogenic Mononuclear Progenitor Cells in Chronic Heart Failure Patients. J Cardiovasc Thorac Res. 2014;6(3):153-62.
105. Huerta A, López B, Ravassa S, et al. Association of cystatin C with heart failure with preserved ejection fraction in elderly hypertensive patients: potential role of altered collagen metabolism. J Hypertens. 2016;34(1):130-8.
106. Kim H, Yoon HJ, Park HS, et al. Potentials of cystatin C and uric acid for predicting prognosis of heart failure. Congest Heart Fail. 2013;19:123-9.
107. Grassi D, Ferri L, Desideri G, et al. Chronic hyperuricemia, uric acid deposit and cardiovascular risk. Curr Pharm Des. 2013;19(13):2432-8.
108. Borghi C, Rosei EA, Bardin T, et al. Serum uric acid and the risk of cardiovascular and renal disease. J Hypertens 2015;33(9):1729-41.
109. Krishnan E. Hyperuricemia and incident heart failure. Circ Heart Fail. 2009;2(6):556-62.
110. Tang WH, Brennan ML, Philip K, et al. Plasma myeloperoxidase levels in patients with chronic heart failure. Am J Cardiol. 2006;98(6):796-9.
111. Reichlin T, Socrates T, Egli P, et al. Use of myeloperoxidase for risk stratification in acute heart failure. Clin Chem. 2010;56(6):944-51.
112. van Kimmenade RR, Januzzi JL. Emerging biomarkers in heart failure. Clin Chem. 2012;58(1):127-38.
113. López B, Ravassa S, González A, et al. Myocardial collagen cross-linking is associated with heart failure hospitalization in patients with hypertensive heart failure. J Am Coll Cardiol. 2016;67(3):251-60.
114. George J, Patal S, Wexler D, et al. Circulating matrix metalloproteinase-2 but not matrix metalloproteinase-3, matrix metalloproteinase-9, or tissue inhibitor of metalloproteinase-1 predicts outcome in patients with congestive heart failure. Am Heart J. 2005;150(3):484-7.
115. Buralli S, Dini FL, Ballo P, et al. Circulating matrix metalloproteinase-3 and metalloproteinase-9 and tissue Doppler measures of diastolic dysfunction to risk stratify patients with systolic heart failure. Am J Cardiol. 2010;105(6):853-6.

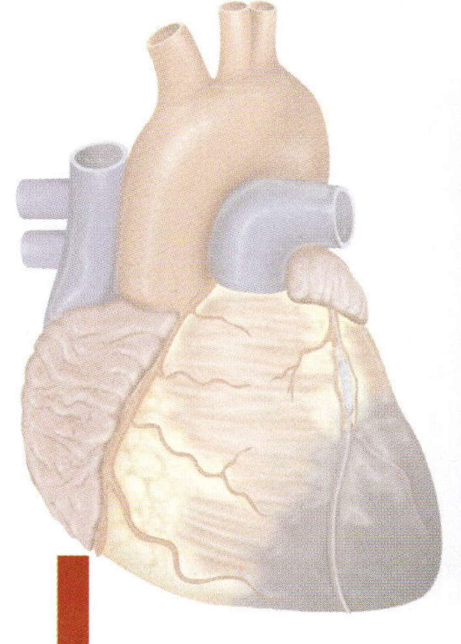

Heart Failure and End Organ Damage

Ajay Kumar Sinha, Vikas Singh, Sanjeev Kumar

PREAMBLE AND BACKGROUND

> **New breakthrough treatments for heart failure offer hope for millions**
>
> **PUBLISHED FRI, MAR 2, 2018**
>
> Roni Jacobson, special to CNBC.com

- From hype to hope, heart disease continues to be the leading causing of death in the United States, responsible for 1 in 4 deaths every year, reports the Centre of Disease Control (CDC).
- Almost 6 million Americans currently have heart failure, a figure that is expected to increase 46 percent, to 8 million, by 2030.
- About half of people with heart failure (HF) die within 5 years of diagnosis.
- With recent dramatic leaps in sensor and soft robotics technology, scientists are turning to innovative medical devices to prolong the life of patients with heart failure.
- Unlike western countries where heart failure is predominantly a disease of the elderly, in India it affects a younger age group. The actual burden of the problem is unknown but as per projections there are at least 8–10 million patients with HF in India with a prevalence of about 1% adult population with a high in-hospital mortality rate of 30.8% and with high post-discharge 6 months rehospitalization and mortality rates of 40% and 26%, respectively.[1-3]. Many patients remain symptomatic despite guideline-directed medical therapy (GDMT) (Fig.1).

INTRODUCTION

Heart failure has assumed the status of modern day epidemic; contributing considerably to morbidity, mortality and financial burden in both developed and developing countries. Heart failure syndrome (HFS) is the currently accepted term describing the heart's inability to supply oxygenated blood, including metabolites, to end organs and peripheral tissues, and in turn affecting several organs.

Organ involvement, ranging from subtle injury to gross impairment are commonly observed in patients with heart failure. Congestion is an essential pathophysiological mechanism mediating the same in a large number of these patients; a smaller proportion presents with peripheral hypoperfusion or cardiogenic shock.[1,2] The injury and dysfunction of target organs in the setting of HF are associated with increased risk for mortality and hence their prevention and correction represents a therapeutic target of interest in HF.[3]

> In the past five years the direction has been to decrease readmission, by developing some sort of technology that we can monitor the patient before the symptoms actually start. Because the data shows that if the patient comes to us and they are short of breath and having symptoms, it is already too late.
>
> **Rami Kahwash, Ohio State University Wexner Medical Center**

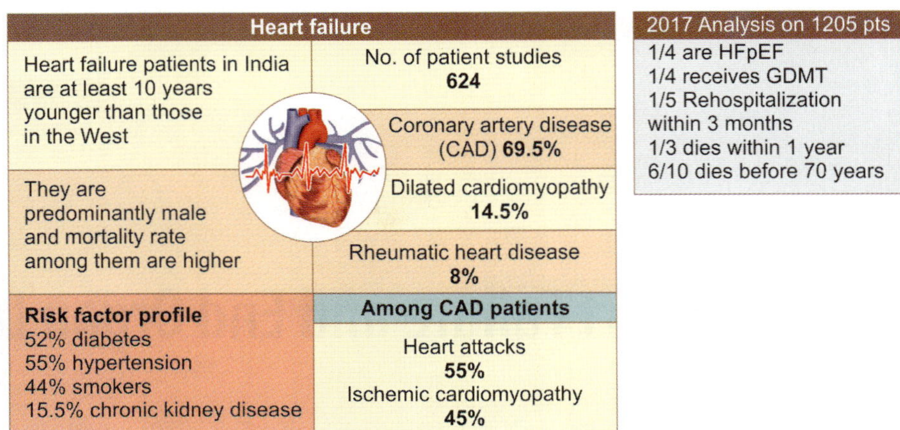

Fig. 1: Guidelines directed medical therapy.

Source: Harikrishnan S, Sanjay G, Agarwal A, et al. One-year mortality outcomes and hospital readmissions of patients admitted with acute heart failure: Data from the Trivandrum Heart Failure Registry in Kerala, India. Am Heart J. 2017;189:193-9.

In the continuum from asymptomatic to symptomatic stages of heart failure, several counterregulatory mechanisms are activated. Inadequate stroke volume induces sympathetic nervous system activation (Fig. 2), which increases cardiac output. The positive effect of this adaptation is halted and at times reversed after tachycardia reaches a threshold of 140–150 beats/ min. Augmentation of intravascular volume simultaneously occurs via neurohormonal system activation, which results in increasing intravascular volume, enlarging ventricular chambers, and improvement in myocardial fiber tension.[4] The inotropic effect via the Frank-Starling mechanism increases myocardial contraction power, but this positive effect reverses after the sarcomere length reaches the upper limit of 2.2 μm. At this stage, no physiologic mechanism can improve the contractility, stroke volume, and cardiac decompensation, and the left ventricle (LV) undergoes progressive alterations from reversible cellular to irreversible myocardial remodeling.

Neurohormonal alterations act as a complex and combined compensatory mechanism to support and maintain tissue perfusion during the HFS. However, after a certain point, these neurohormonal responses become maladaptive, in large part because of uncontrollable activation and promote progression of heart failure.

Congestion and to a lesser extent, hypoperfusion are primarily responsible for organ injury, impairment and, ultimately, the failure of target organs (i.e. heart,

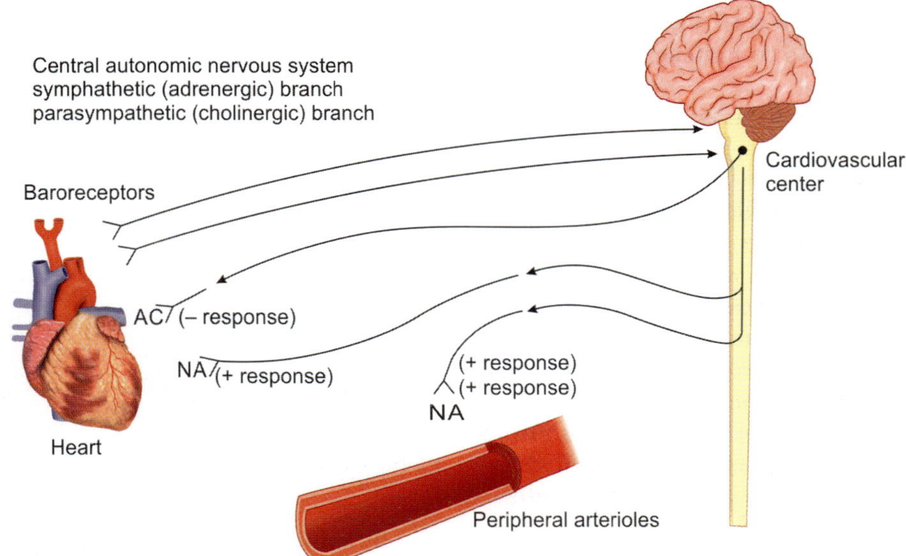

Fig. 2: Autonomic nervous system function.

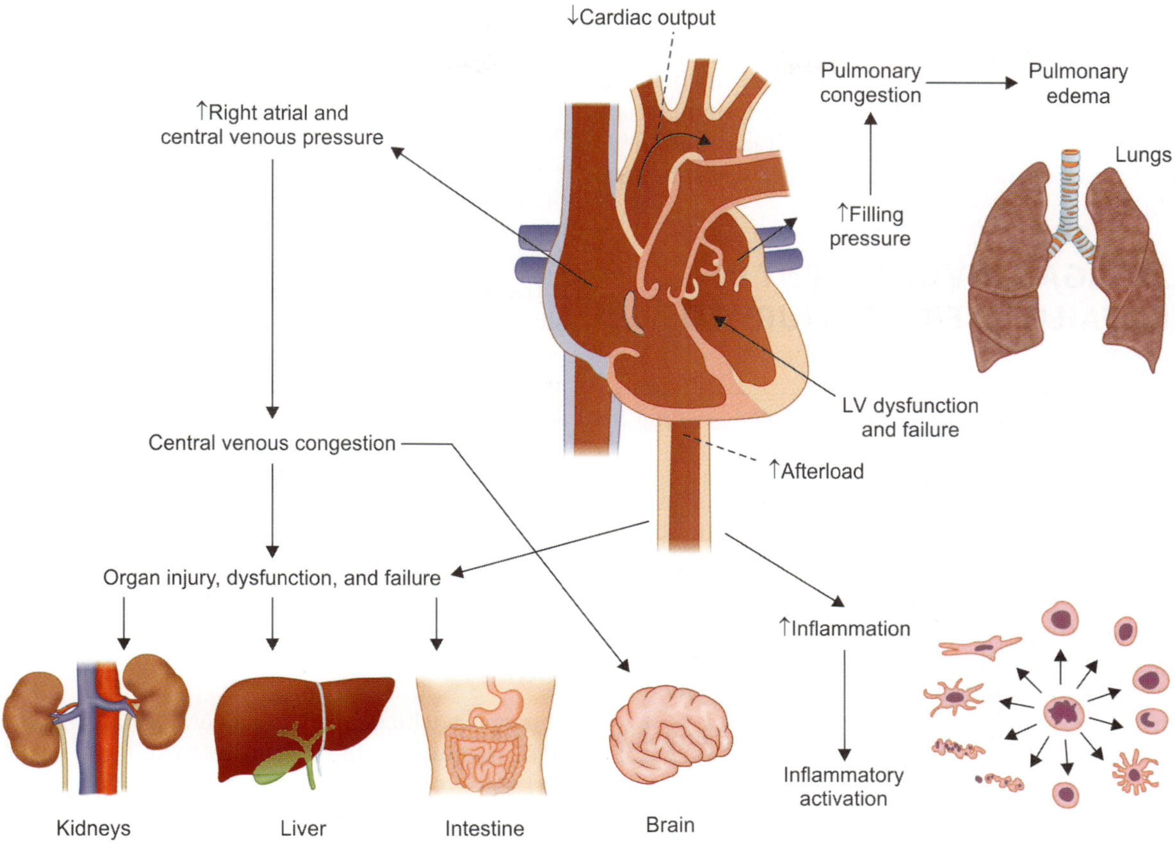

Fig. 3: Relationship between congestion and end organs.
Source: Harijola et al. 2017, European Journal of Heart Failure.

lungs, kidneys, liver, intestine, and brain). There are in addition many other factors which also play a role in the pathophysiology. Elderly patients with comorbidities are in particular predisposed to organ injury.

Congestion: Increased left atrial pressure causes the blood to remain upstream of the left ventricle leading to pulmonary congestion and pulmonary edema, whereas congestion of organs in the abdominal cavity ensues when blood remains upstream of the right ventricle (Fig. 3).[5,6] Both pulmonary and organ congestion may occur separately or simultaneously, and one part may dominate. Raised intra-abdominal pressure due to organ congestion and/or ascites may further contribute to injury or impairment of the end-organs. Cardiac filling pressure, however, may not be a true reflection of volume overload. In one study, 54% of patients hospitalized for acute heart failure (AHF) gained ≤0.9 kg during the 30 days prior to admission,[7] suggesting that volume overload incompletely characterizes the pathophysiology of AHF. Similarly, weight loss during hospitalization is not necessarily always associated with improved in-hospital or post-discharge morbidity or mortality.[8] It appears more near to accurate that redistribution (from venous capacitance beds to the central venous system) rather than absolute volume overload may be a frequent cause of increased cardiac filling pressures.

Organ hypoperfusion: A clinical profile of low cardiac output and subsequent organ hypoperfusion (cold-dry or cold-wet) is much less common than a profile of congestion with normal perfusion. It is usually associated with low systolic blood pressure (<90 mm Hg) and mean arterial pressure (<65 mm Hg) (i.e. cardiogenic shock). Due to inadequate tissue perfusion, aerobic metabolism suffers and leads to the sequence of cell death, tissue injury and organ failure. One has to be cautious while using diuretics in this group of patients as it may reduce cardiac preload, thereby diminishing stroke volume and contributing to the shock state iatrogenically.[9] The neurohormonal and inflammatory response to systemic congestion and/or peripheral hypoperfusion, if present, may further contribute to organ injury.[9-11] In heart failure, neurohormonal alterations disrupt glycosaminoglycan (GAG) structure, leading to loss of the interstitial buffer capacity and disproportionate interstitial fluid accumulation.

Nowadays, in clinical practice, well-validated and inexpensive biomarkers are available to quantify injury or impairment of the heart, kidneys or liver and can be used routinely (e.g. natriuretic peptides, cardiac troponin, serum creatinine, cystatin C, albuminuria, blood urea nitrogen, transaminases, coagulation factors, alkaline phosphatase, bilirubin).[12]

MULTIORGAN INVOLVEMENT IN HEART FAILURE: FROM INJURY TO FAILURE

> ***The Heart, Kidneys and Brain: Three Pieces of the Same Puzzle?***
>
> Heart failure, diabetes, kidney disease and atrial fibrillation are separate diseases, but in reality these conditions are seldom seen in isolation. The interactions between these conditions, the impact on patient treatment and outcomes, will define future of cardiology. HF specialists see patients with comorbidities every day, so they know the importance of holistic management.
>
> **Professor Martin Cowie (London).**

Heart

Venous congestion increases preload, which leads to increased ventricular wall stress, valvular regurgitation, myocardial stretch, remodeling, ventricular myocyte necrosis and a progressive decline in cardiac function.[13] In response to these changes of wall stress, the atria or ventricle releases natriuretic peptides to counter the wall stress and decrease preload. With the use of high-sensitivity assays,[14] it is common to find raised cardiac troponins in a large proportion of patients with HF in the absence of ischemia, suggesting nonischemic myocyte injury or necrosis.

In the Relaxin in Acute Heart Failure (RELAX-AHF) study, 90% of patients had high-sensitivity troponin T (TnT) levels above the 99th upper reference limit, with a median value of 0.033 μg/L.[15]

In emergency room, when the cause of dyspnea is not clear and HF is suspected, natriuretic peptides are recommended to establish the diagnosis. Obesity and some other conditions may lead to falsely low natriuretic peptide levels, and sepsis, renal dysfunction and many other conditions may be the cause of false positive which should be kept in mind. Procalcitonin levels may aid in the differential diagnosis of pneumonia in patients with HF and suspected concomitant infection.

Lungs

Raised left atrial pressure and mitral regurgitation are transmitted backward as increased pressure to the pulmonary capillaries, creating an imbalance in capillary Starling forces. These changes cause fluid accumulation in the interstitium and may cause dyspnea. When interstitial pressure exceeds pleural pressure and surpasses drainage capacity of the lymphatics, fluid moves to pleural and intra-alveolar spaces, causing pleural effusion and alveolar edema.[16] An inflammation-triggered increase in permeability of the pulmonary vasculature may play a role in patients who develop pulmonary edema despite relatively low hydrostatic pressures.[17]

Repetitive decompensations of this sort may result in cardiopulmonary remodeling (i.e. endothelial dysfunction, proliferation of myofibroblasts, fibrosis and thickening of the extracellular matrix) with an impairment in alveolar gas diffusion properties,[18] pulmonary vasoconstriction and, finally, pulmonary hypertension.[19]

Kidneys

The reported incidence of worsening renal function during AHF hospitalization is 20–30%, the large variation in incidence to a large part because of the different definitions of renal dysfunction used in different studies.[20] Cardiorenal syndrome describes the entire extent of interaction between the heart and the kidneys. Elevated central venous pressure may worsen renal function through several different mechanisms, including pressure-induced reduction in renal blood flow, renal hypoxia, increased interstitial pressure and interstitial fibrosis.[21] In a study, systemic congestion was a stronger predictor of worsening renal function than cardiac output or mean arterial pressure.

Impaired baseline renal function is the strongest risk factor for acute kidney injury,[22] suggesting that underlying intrinsic kidney disease is an important determinant of kidney reserve and the renal response to HF and aggressive diuretic treatment.

Transient worsening of renal function in conjunction with clinical heart failure improvement, also referred as "pseudo worsening renal function" may not always be detrimentaland.[23] It is mostly the result of changing intraglomerular hemodynamics rather than renal injury. It is worth noting that some degree of "worsening renal function" is acceptable while effective decongestion is ongoing. Very few patients with cardiac improvement will have renal tubular injury and experience an irreversible decline in GFR that is prognostically important.

Kidney injury can be detected and quantified using a combination of urine output and blood biomarkers of renal function [e.g. cystatin C, serum creatinine to calculate estimated glomerular filtration rate (GFR), albuminuria, blood urea nitrogen],[23] or blood and/or urine markers of tubular injury [e.g. neutrophil gelatinase-associated lipocalin (NGAL), pen-enkephalin and KIM-1], although these may not be widely available in clinical practice.

The therapeutic goal is to achieve the lowest venous filling pressures without deteriorating cardiac output. Ultrafiltration may be considered in patients in whom decongestion goals are not met with vasodilators or loop diuretics. Inotropes may be considered in patients with deteriorating cardiac output and renal perfusion in the setting of decongestion. Nephrotoxic agents and procedures should be avoided, if feasible during the AHF presentation.

Liver

Hepatic dysfunction is present in 20–30% of patients with AHF.[24,25] Hepatic dysfunction is also closely related to renal dysfunction in AHF (i.e. cardio-renal-hepatic syndrome). When venous congestion is marked, increased levels of alkaline phosphatase, bilirubin and Gamma-Glutamyl Transferase (GGT) is often seen because of cholestatsis.[26,27]

Hypoxic liver injury is the most common cause of massively raised aminotransferase levels in hospital,[28] signaling liver cell necrosis and is a strong risk factor for mortality in the intensive care unit (ICU). Coagulation factors reflect hepatic synthetic function in acute organ failure, whereas albumin represents hepatic synthetic capacity in chronic stable conditions.

Liver impairment can impact the pharmacokinetics of some drugs commonly used in heart failure, potentially leading to adverse effects or toxicity caused by elevated serum concentrations of some drugs (e.g. warfarin).

Intestine

Intestinal morphology, permeability and absorption are altered in heart failure,[29,30] leading to a state of chronic inflammation and malnutrition. Systemic/venous congestion, sympathetic vasoconstriction and low cardiac output contribute to decreased flow in the splanchnic microcirculation and increase the risk for bowel ischemia. Ischemia causes epithelial cell dysfunction and loss of the barrier function of the intestine, which allows lipopolysaccharide or endotoxin produced by gram-negative gut bacteria to enter the circulatory system. These effects trigger systemic inflammation and cytokine generation, leading to several abnormalities of cardiomyocyte function and energetics.

Brain

Depression, cognitive dysfunction, and delirium are not uncommon in patients with heart failure. Prevalence of cognitive impairment in AHF of 54–75% has been reported.[31] Delirium is an acute disorder of inattention and global cognitive dysfunction and is a poor predictor in HF. Hypoxemia is the primary cause of cerebral dysfunction in AHF, but other factors (e.g. inflammation, stress and neurohormonal dysregulation) may also play significant roles.

Silent cerebral infarctions, hypotension, disturbances of cerebral metabolism, cardiac embolism, frailty and low adherence to medications may also contribute to cognitive dysfunction and depression in AHF.[32]

GAPS IN UNDERSTANDING: FUTURE DIRECTIONS

Real clinical challenge is defining adequate endpoints of decongestion in patients with HF. Change in body weight is often used as a guide, but this approach is frequently inadequate as body weight is not increased in all patients and does not reflect congestion caused by vascular type fluid redistribution. Evidence based clinical and biochemical indicators of adequate decongestion are lacking. Vasodilator or diuretic dose adjustments are largely empirical.

Novel, effective and safe pharmacological or mechanical methods to achieve decongestion are needed.

The patterns of congestion in AHF with preserved ejection fraction are not well characterized and warrant investigation, although the available evidence suggests that patients with heart failure from reduced or preserved ejection fraction have similar characteristics of congestion at presentation.

Organ-specific injury markers suitable for clinical practice are lacking for many organs (e.g. brain, lung, intestine, endothelium, vasculature). Injury markers for these organs would be valuable, along with evidence based recommendations for monitoring, leading to possible intervention strategies. Even where organ specific injury markers exist (e.g. cardiac troponin, markers of renal or hepatic injury), research is needed to guide their interpretation.

The clinical progression of organ injury to dysfunction and ultimately failure is not well characterized and the extent to which injury and dysfunction are reversible or irreversible in the setting of AHF is not known. The clinical importance of low levels of detectable troponin is not well understood and whether or not treatments that target troponins alter risk is unknown. The same is true for novel prognostic markers such as mid-region adrenomedullin and soluble ST2. It remains uncertain whether decongestion-targeting reduction in traditional markers of heart failure (i.e. natriuretic peptides) is more beneficial than clinical guidance. More research is needed to establish the appropriate pathway (i.e. discharge or further evaluation) in otherwise stable patients with persistently elevated biomarkers.

Furthermore, no therapy has shown simultaneous benefits in symptomatic relief, hemodynamic improvement, and increased survival and end organ protection.

New methods such as thoracic impedance monitoring have been used to detect pulmonary edema in the research setting.

The concept that treatment of congestion can reduce or prevent organ injury needs to be tested in randomized trials, and the effects of preventing organ injury on morbidity; survival and health economics require validation.

CONCLUSION

Heart failure is responsible for substantial morbidity and mortality worldwide. Its prevalence is increasing because of aging of the population and improved treatment of acute cardiovascular events, despite the efficacy of many therapies for patients with heart failure with reduced ejection fraction, such as angiotensin converting enzyme (ACE) inhibitors, angiotensin receptor blockers (ARBs), β-blockers, and mineralocorticoid receptor antagonists, and advanced device therapies. Combined angiotensin receptor blocker neprilysin inhibitors (ARNIs) have been associated with improvements in hospital admissions and mortality from heart failure compared with enalapril, and guidelines now recommend substitution of ACE inhibitors or ARBs with ARNIs in appropriate patients. Improved safety of left ventricular assist devices means that these are becoming more commonly used in patients with severe symptoms. Antidiabetic therapies might further improve outcomes in patients with heart failure. New drugs with novel mechanisms of action, such as cardiac myosin activators, are under investigation for patients with heart failure with reduced left ventricular ejection fraction. Heart failure with preserved ejection fraction is a heterogeneous disorder that remains incompletely understood and will continue to increase in prevalence with the aging population. Managing patients with HF has improved a lot over time, particularly in the domain of chronic heart failure. The use of therapies that prevent or reverse organ injury may represent a strategy that would prove more successful in times to come. Understanding the pathophysiology of organ dysfunction is the essential first step in that direction. A lot has been learned over the years, but many missing links need to be established still.

"It's gonna take a lot more research and a lot more development before we have a 3-D printed heart that we can put into a patient". it is estimated that they are at least 15 to 20 years out from this point. Getting there will also take a lot of capital investment. "We are still at the proof-of-concept stage, but we believe that at some point it is going to be the future".

— By Roni Jacobson, special to CNBC.com

REFERENCES

1. Ponikowski P, Voors AA, Anker SD, et al. 2016 ESC Guidelines for the diagnosis and treatment of acute and chronic heart failure: the Task Force for the diagnosis and treatment of acute and chronic heart failure of the European Society of Cardiology (ESC). Eur J Heart Fail. 2016;18(8):891-975.
2. Nieminen MS, Brutsaert D, Dickstein K, et al. Euro Heart Failure SurveyII (EHFSII): a survey on hospitalized acute heart failure patients: description of population. Eur Heart J. 2006;27(22):2725-36.
3. Mebazaa A, Longrois D, Metra M, et al. Agents with vasodilator properties in acute heart failure: how to design successful trials. Eur J Heart Fail. 2015;17(7):652-64.
4. Gaggin HG, Januzzi JL Jr. Biomarkers and diagnostics in heart failure. Biochim Biophys Acta. 2013;1832(12):2442-50.
5. Nikolaou M, Parissis J, Yilmaz MB, et al. Liver function abnormalities, clinical profile, and outcome in acute decompensated heart failure. Eur Heart J. 2013;34(10):742-9.
6. Ronco C, Haapio M, House AA, et al. Cardiorenal syndrome. J Am Coll Cardiol. 2008;52(19):1527-39.
7. Chaudhry SI, Wang Y, Concato J, et al. Patterns of weight change preceding hospitalization for heart failure. Circulation. 2007;116(14):1549-54.
8. Mehta RH, Rogers JG, Hasselblad V, et al. Association of weight change with subsequent outcomes in patients hospitalized with acute decompensated heart failure. Am J Cardiol. 2009;103(1):76-81.
9. Rudiger A. Understanding cardiogenic shock. Eur J Heart Fail. 2015;17(5):466-7.
10. Calfee CS, Matthay MA. Clinical immunology: culprits with evolutionary ties. Nature. 2010;464(7285):41-2.
11. Hochman JS. Cardiogenic shock complicating acute myocardial infarction: expanding the paradigm. Circulation. 2003;107(24):2998-3002.
12. Metra M, Cotter G, Davison BA, et al. Effect of serelaxin on cardiac, renal, and hepatic biomarkers in the Relaxin in Acute Heart Failure (RELAX-AHF) development program: correlation with outcomes. J Am Coll Cardiol. 2013;61(2): 196-206.
13. Parrinello G, Greene SJ, Torres D, et al. Water and sodium in heart failure: a spotlight on congestion. Heart Fail Rev. 2015;20(1):13-24.
14. Januzzi JL Jr, Filippatos G, Nieminen M, et al. Troponin elevation in patients with heart failure: on behalf of the

third Universal Definition of Myocardial Infarction Global Task Force: Heart Failure Section. Eur Heart J. 2012;33(18): 2265-71.

15. Felker GM, Mentz RJ, Teerlink JR, et al. Serial high sensitivity cardiac troponin T measurement in acute heart failure: insights from the RELAX-AHF study. Eur J Heart Fail. 2015;17(12):1262-70.
16. Ware LB, Matthay MA. Clinical practice. Acute pulmonary edema. N Engl J Med. 2005;353(26):2788-96.
17. Ritter S, Rudiger A, Maggiorini M. Transpulmonary thermodilution-derived cardiac function index identifies cardiac dysfunction in acute heart failure and septic patients: an observational study. Crit Care. 2009;13(6):R133.
18. Guazzi M, Phillips SA, Arena R, et al. Endothelial dysfunction and lung capillary injury in cardiovascular diseases. Prog Cardiovasc Dis. 2015;57(5):454-62.
19. Guglin M, Khan H. Pulmonary hypertension in heart failure. J Card Fail. 2010;16(6):461-74.
20. Damman K, Valente MA, Voors AA, et al. Renal impairment, worsening renal function, and outcome in patients with heart failure: an updated meta-analysis. Eur Heart J. 2014;35(7):455-69
21. Legrand M, Mebazaa A, Ronco C, et al. When cardiac failure, kidney dysfunction, and kidney injury intersect in acute conditions: the case of cardiorenal syndrome. Crit Care Med. 2014;42(9):2109-17.
22. Hsu CY, Ordonez JD, Chertow GM, et al. The risk of acute renal failure in patients with chronic kidney disease. Kidney Int. 2008;74(1):101-7.
23. Damman K, Testani JM. The kidney in heart failure: an update. Eur Heart J. 2015;36(23):1437-44.
24. Auer J. What does the liver tell us about the failing heart? Eur Heart J .2013;34(10):711-4.
25. Biegus J, Hillege HL, PostmusD, et al. Abnormal liver function tests in acute heart failure: relationship with clinical characteristics and outcome in the PROTECT study. Eur J Heart Fail. 2016;18(7):830-9.
26. Moller S, Bernardi M. Interactions of the heart and the liver. Eur Heart J. 2013;34(36):2804-11.
27. Samsky MD, Patel CB, DeWald TA, et al. Cardiohepatic interactions in heart failure: an overview and clinical implications. J Am Coll Cardiol. 2013;61(24):2397-405.
28. Whitehead MW, Hawkes ND, Hainsworth I, et al. A prospective study of the causes of notably raised aspartate aminotransferase of liver origin. Gut. 1999;45(1):129-33.
29. Rogler G, Rosano G. The heart and the gut. Eur Heart J. 2014;35:426-30.
30. Sandek A, Bauditz J, Swidsinski A, et al. Altered intestinal function in patients with chronic heart failure. J Am Coll Cardiol. 2007;50(16):1561-9.
31. Sokoreli I, de Vries JJ, Pauws SC, et al. Depression and anxiety as predictors of mortality among heart failure patients: systematic review and meta-analysis. Heart Fail Rev. 2016;21(1):49-63.
32. Kindermann I, Fischer D, Karbach J, et al. Cognitive function in patients with decompensated heart failure: the Cognitive Impairment in Heart Failure (CogImpair-HF) study. Eur J Heart Fail. 2012;14(4):404-13.

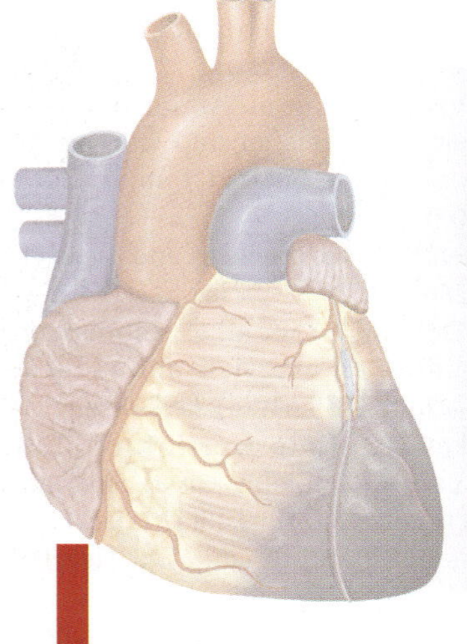

Natural History and Prognostic Factors in Alcoholic Cardiomyopathy with Heart Failure

GR Kane, Kayan Siodia

INTRODUCTION

For more than 3,000 years, alcoholic beverages have been consumed in heterogeneous societies through the centuries and cultures. Pulverized antimony was used as eye shadow by Egyptian women and named al-Kol. Over the centuries, "the good and the bad" of alcohol was evaluated clinically and scientifically. As early as 1855, Wood incriminated alcohol as a cause of heart failure. In 1861, Friedrich reported idiopathic hypertrophy as associated with alcoholism. In his 1972 review article, Bridgen was the first to introduce the term alcoholic cardiomyopathy (ACM). ACM is a disease associated with chronic long-term use of alcohol leading to heart failure (HF). It customarily manifests in the form of dilated cardiomyopathy (DCM). Multitude of causative factors and pathogenic features of alcohol and the byproducts produced thereof are responsible for the genesis of cardiomyopathy. Excessive alcohol intake is a sizable health issue in developed countries. Notwithstanding light-to-moderate alcohol intake has been historically related to reduction in coronary artery disease (CAD) and HF; heavy consumption is associated with development of left ventricular (LV) dysfunction.[1] Excess alcohol consumption has been implicated in 40%[2] cases of DCM. ACM shares similar features to other causes of DCM, but diagnosis is one of exclusion in a patient with long history of alcohol consumption.

OVERVIEW

Long duration of excess alcohol intake remains the sine qua non of ACM. The duration and the amount vary with race, ethnicity, and sex. The most accepted definition of heavy alcohol consumption being defined as alcohol intake of 80 g/day (eight standard drinks) over a period of 5 years. Corollary to diagnosis of ACM being that alcohol abuse must have been maintained until at least 3 months prior to diagnosis of DCM.[3]

Proposed mechanisms of injury in ACM include the following:

- Inhibition of protein synthesis
- Inhibition of oxidative phosphorylation
- Fatty acid ester accumulation
- Free radical damage
- Inhibition of calcium-myofilament interaction
- Inflammatory and immunologic factors
- Receptor abnormalities
- Disruption of cell membrane structure
- Coronary vasospasm
- Synergy with concomitant conditions
- Activation of the renin-angiotensin system.

NATURAL HISTORY

Quantity of alcohol is the chief decisive factor for evolution of ACM.

- An inverse relationship between total lifetime intake and ejection fraction and fractional shortening.
- A direct relationship between total lifetime intake and LV mass. In persons who consumed 70 g of ethanol [or the equivalent of 7 oz of whiskey, 20 oz of wine, or 72 oz of beer (i.e. six 12-oz cans)] per day for 20 years, 36% had an abnormal ejection fraction.
- Age and nutritional status appeared to play little or no role.[4]

Continuous, rather than episodic, drinking was a major risk factor for the development of HF and this effect was unrelated to the hypertensive effect of alcohol.

Binge drinking induces a systemic inflammatory reaction, which may lead to alcohol-induced myocardial inflammation. One study indicated that patients who repeatedly expose themselves to excessive amounts of alcohol may demonstrate evidence on magnetic resonance imaging (MRI) scans of alcohol-induced myocardial inflammation, but not show deterioration in indices of LV performance.

In general, approximately one-third of patients with ACM died or underwent heart transplant, a third remained clinically stable without improvement in cardiac function, and a third experienced substantial left ventricular ejection fraction (LVEF) recovery.

Figure 1 outlines the above findings.[5]

The difference in presentation and outcomes has been greatly attributed to genetic factors.

After the advent of angiotensin-converting enzyme (ACE) inhibitors, beta-blockers, and aldosterone antagonists, the overall transplant-free survival has improved.

Flurry of data are available for the progression of ACM, but remain riddled with controversies. Many have proven that abstinence may cause a reversibility of the ACM, however contradictory trials are present. However, it has been proven beyond any reasonable doubt that the prognosis is far better in ACM as compared to idiopathic dilated cardiomyopathy (IDCM).[6]

It has also been noted from previous studies that alcohol abusers tend to be men smokers with a higher body mass index (BMI).

The natural history of patients with ACM depends greatly on each patient's ability to cease alcohol consumption completely. Multiple case reports and small retrospective and prospective studies have clearly documented marked improvement in, or in some patients, normalization of cardiac function with abstinence.

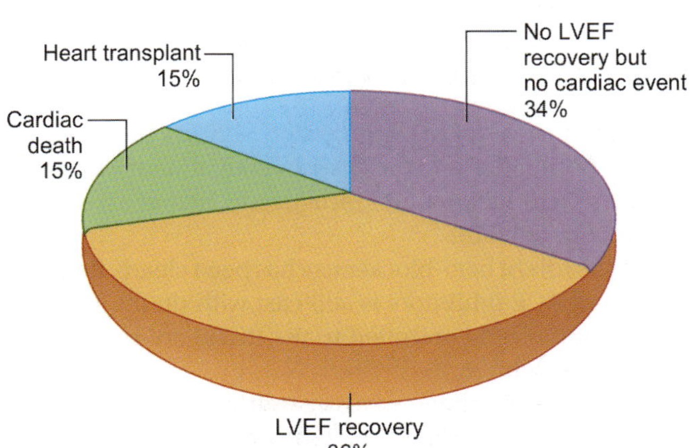

Fig. 1: Long-term cardiovascular evolution of ACM.[5]
(ACM: alcoholic cardiomyopathy; LVEF: left ventricular ejection fraction)

Complete abstinence from ethanol is advocated in all ACM patients. However, the need for complete alcohol abstinence in advanced ACM is a controversial issue. Although it is suggested that the clinical outcome of ACM could be improved if patients abstain from alcohol, other studies have shown that complete alcohol abstinence may not be necessary to improve LVEF.

Moreover, some of the previous ACM studies that advocated complete abstinence included light-to-moderate drinkers in the abstainers' group or reported good improvement in moderate drinkers.

Demakis and colleagues found that, overall, the two factors that were associated with a better prognosis in ACM were abstinence and a shorter duration of symptoms before the initiation of therapy. In their study, perhaps the largest evaluation of the natural history of ACM, the investigators prospectively followed 57 patients with ACM and divided them into three groups: 15 patients who improved clinically, 12 patients who remained stable, and 30 patients whose conditions deteriorated. Of the 39 patients who continued to drink, only four patients improved. 11 of the 18 patients who abstained improved; however, the condition of three patients who abstained continued to deteriorate.[7]

Complete abstinence from ethanol is advocated in all ACM patients. It is found that ACM patients who decreased their alcohol intake to moderate levels had better outcomes than IDCM patients and outcomes similar to those of ACM patients who abandoned alcohol completely. Moreover, LVEF during follow-up increased significantly to a similar extent as in abstainers among ACM patients who reduced their alcohol intake to moderate levels. Of note, although all patients who reduced alcohol intake to <80 g/day were classified as moderate drinkers, the vast majority of these patients reduced alcohol intake to <20–30 g/day (two to three standard drinks). This amount of alcohol is similar to the amount described in studies which reported that low-to-moderate alcohol consumption is associated with lower mortality and incidence of nonischemic heart failure (Table 1).[8-10]

Finally, the type of beverage has no difference in any of the endpoints studied.

PROGNOSIS

Variables have the maximal effect on the outcomes in ACM.

- Abstinence
- QRS duration (more than 120 ms)
- Presence of atrial fibrillation
- Lack of use of beta-blockers

TABLE 1: Published studies on alcoholic cardiomyopathy (ACM).

	Demakis, 1974[7]	*Prazak, 1996*[6]	*Fauchier, 2000*[2]	*Gavazzi, 2000*[3]	*ACC, 2015*
Number of patients with ACM	57	23	50	79	94
Mean age (years)	40.5	47 ± 8	49 ± 11	45 ± 10	49.6 ± 10
Duration of HF symptoms (months)	10.5	20 ± 22	20 ± 28	20 ± 27	32 ± 5
NYHA III–IV (%)	Not available	52	44	35	67
AF (%)	Not available	22	Not available	15	35
LVEF (%)	Not available	30 ± 12	35 ± 12	28 ± 9	26 ± 9
MPAP (mm Hg)	Not available	23 ± 10	18 ± 8	22 ± 11	33 ± 13
PCW (mm Hg)	Not available	17 ± 8	13 ± 8	18 ± 11	23 ± 12
CI (L/min/m^2)	Not available	Not available	3.06 ± 0.9	3.01 ± 0.95	2.2 ± 0.5
ACEI/ARB (%)	0	Not available	78	81	90
Beta-blockers (%)	0	0	3	9	60
Aldosterone antagonists (%)	0	Not available	Not available	Not available	49
Abstainers (%)	31.6	Not available	45	74.6	62.7
Nonabstainers (%)	68.4	Not available	55	25.4	37.3
Persistent heavy drinkers (%)	Not available	Not available	30	Not available	5
Transplant-free survival (%)	Overall: 58% (3 years)	Overall: 81% (10 years)	Overall: Not available Abstainers: ≈50% (10 years) Nonabstainers: 32% (10 years)	Overall: 41% (7 years) Abstainers: 45% (7 years) Nonabstainers: 27% (7 years)	Overall: 67% (10 years) Abstainers: 66% Moderate drinkers: 77% (10 years) Persistent heavy drinkers: 20% (10 years)

(ACC: American College of Cardiology; ACEI: angiotensin-converting enzyme inhibitor; AF: atrial fibrillation; ARB: angiotensin receptor blocker; CI: cardiac index; HF: heart failure; LVEF: left ventricular ejection fraction; MPAP: mean pulmonary artery pressure; NYHA: New York Heart Association; PCW: pulmonary capillary wedge)

- Systolic blood pressure
- The New York Heart Association (NYHA) class on admission.

Other variables affecting the outcome albeit minutely were:

- Positive hepatojugular reflux
- Use of diuretics
- Left ventricular end-systolic diameter.

QRS prolongation is well known to occur in the general population, with an incidence that increases sharply with age. Patients with organic heart disease often have wide QRS complexes due to bundle branch blocks, and the presence of wide QRS complexes on electrocardiogram (ECG) has been accepted as a traditional prognostic clinical marker in varied clinical settings.

Several studies have indicated that QRS prolongation is a significant predictor of mortality and arrhythmias in HF and DCM. QRS duration of <118 ms was an independent protective factor for sudden cardiac death in patients with DCM.[11]

Absence of treatment with beta-blockers, the presence of atrial fibrillation, a QRS duration >120 ms, a shorter distance in the 6-minute walking test, and the use of digoxin were factors associated with the occurrence of major cardiac events (cardiovascular death or heart transplantation) in ACM patients.

Stated further that a QRS duration >120 ms, the presence of atrial fibrillation, and the absence of treatment with beta-blockers were independent prognostic factors associated with a poor outcome.

As the role of beta-blocker use has been clearly defined, the use of ACE inhibitors is still cast with doubt. Further, large randomized controlled trials (RCTs) are required to preclude its role.

Many studies have investigated whether excessive alcohol consumption contributes to a higher baseline blood pressure (both systolic and diastolic).

Contrary to popular beliefs, hypotension was a recognized predictor of poor prognosis in patients with

HF, and patients with HF and a low systolic blood pressure (SBP) had a much higher incidence of in-hospital and postdischarge mortality.

There is an association between higher NYHA functional classes and poorer outcomes in HF patients were widely recognized. In recent years, it is argued that the NYHA class assessment demonstrated prognostic value among individuals with acute HF and emerged as a significant independent predictor of all-cause mortality in patients with DCM.

Last but certainly not the least, the role of abstinence is clearly defined and is beyond any reasonable doubt the most important factor which has been discussed earlier herein with.

CONCLUSION

Various variables in ACM with HF have prognostic implications including abstinence, QRS duration (more than 120 ms), presence of atrial fibrillation, lack of use of beta-blockers, SBP, the NYHA class on admission, positive hepatojugular reflux, use of diuretics, and LV end-systolic diameter to stratify the prognosis in ACM with HF, thereby helping early and timely therapeutic intervention to reduce the morbidity and mortality.

REFERENCES

1. Elliott P, Andersson B, Arbustini E, et al. Classification of the cardiomyopathies: a position statement from the European Society of Cardiology Working Group on Myocardial and Pericardial Diseases. Eur Heart J. 2008;29:270-6.
2. Fauchier L, Babuty D, Poret P, et al. Comparison of long-term outcome of alcoholic and idiopathic dilated cardiomyopathy. Eur Heart J. 2000;21:306-14.
3. Gavazzi A, De Maria R, Parolini M, et al. Alcohol abuse and dilated cardiomyopathy in men. Am J Cardiol. 2000;85: 1114-8.
4. Urbano-Marquez A, Estruch R, Navarro-Lopez F, et al. The effects of alcoholism on skeletal and cardiac muscle. N Engl J Med. 1989;320:409-15.
5. Guzzo-Merello G, Segovia J, Dominguez F, et al. Natural history and prognostic factors in alcoholic cardiomyopathy. JACC Heart Fail. 2015;3:78-86.
6. Prazak P, Pfisterer M, Osswald S, et al. Differences of disease progression in congestive heart failure due to alcoholic as compared to idiopathic dilated cardiomyopathy. Eur Heart J. 1996;17:251-7.
7. Demakis JG, Proskey A, Rahimtoola SH, et al. The natural course of alcoholic cardiomyopathy. Ann Intern Med. 1974;80:293-7.
8. Abramson JL, Williams SA, Krumholz HM, et al. Moderate alcohol consumption and risk of heart failure among older persons. JAMA. 2001;285:1971-7.
9. Walsh CR, Larson MG, Evans JC, et al. Alcohol consumption and risk for congestive heart failure in the Framingham Heart Study. Ann Intern Med. 2002;136:181-91.
10. Djousse L, Gaziano JM. Alcohol consumption and risk of heart failure in the Physicians' Health Study I. Circulation. 2007;115:34-9.
11. Lelakowski J, Piekarz J, Rydlewska A, et al. Determinants of patient survival rate after implantation of a cardioverter-defibrillator without resynchronisation capability. Kardiol Pol. 2012;70:1099-110.

CHAPTER

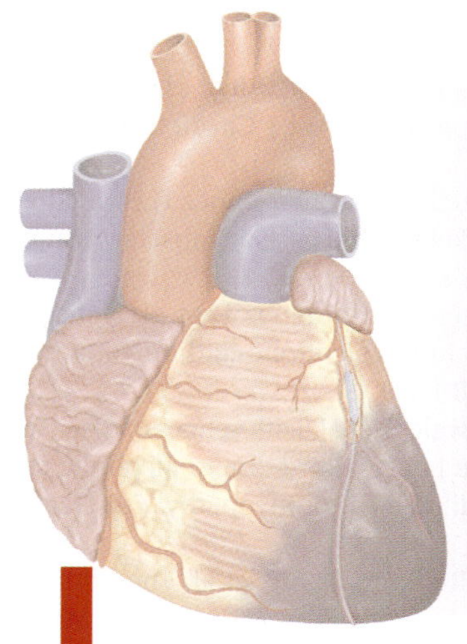

Treatment Priorities in Heart Failure

Nirmal Ghati, Siddharthan Deepti, Nitish Naik

INTRODUCTION

Heart failure remains the leading cardiovascular cause of hospitalization. Treatment priorities in heart failure include improvement in symptoms, reduction in need for hospitalization, prevention of progression of disease, and prolongation of survival. This review will elaborate on optimizing medical therapy and devices for treatment of heart failure.

PHARMACOLOGIC THERAPY

Contemporary pharmacologic therapy for heart failure with reduced ejection fraction (HFrEF) includes a three-pronged strategy including inhibition of renin-angiotensin-aldosterone axis via angiotensin-converting enzyme inhibitors (ACEIs) or angiotensin receptor blockers (ARBs), counteracting sympathetic activation via beta (β)-adrenergic receptor blockers, and a mineralocorticoid/aldosterone receptor antagonist (MRA). The latest kid on the block is the angiotensin receptor neprilysin inhibitor (ARNI) which has proven beneficial in a selected group of patients. All these agents have been shown in multiple landmark trials to have significant mortality benefit.

Preventing of Progression of Disease

Angiotensin-converting Enzyme Inhibitors in Heart Failure with Reduced Ejection Fraction

Angiotensin-converting enzyme inhibitors are the cornerstone of pharmacotherapy in patients with current or prior heart failure with left ventricular (LV) systolic dysfunction. In contrast to other vasodilators used in heart failure, ACEI reduce symptoms, hospitalization, and mortality not only by a reduction in preload and afterload but also by inhibiting deleterious effect of renin-angiotensin-aldosterone system (RAAS) on heart, blood vessels, and kidney. ACEI not only antagonizes circulating angiotensin and aldosterone, but also inhibits their tissue counterparts resulting in the prevention of cardiac remodeling like hypertrophy and fibrosis.[1] The other possible beneficial effects of ACEI are reduction in central sympathetic tone, improvement in the compliance of the central arteries, improvement in the endothelial functions, and increase in the blood kinin levels.[2-4]

The benefit of ACEI in HFrEF is a class effect. Among the ACEIs, enalapril has been tested in most of the landmark clinical trials (Table 1). Additional evidence for short-term and long-term benefit of ACEIs on LV systolic dysfunction due to myocardial infarction can be observed in few clinical trials that used other ACEIs like trandolapril, lisinopril, captopril, and ramipril.[5] The list of evidence is still growing up not only for patients with HFrEF, but also for those with heart failure with preserved ejection fraction (HFpEF) and asymptomatic LV dysfunction.

Angiotensin-converting enzyme inhibitors are usually administered in combination with optimum dose of β-blockers and mineralocorticoid receptor blockers for the purpose of disease modulation in heart failure patients. Although current evidence supports ARNI in those who tolerate ACEI for further mortality benefit, ACEI is still the treatment of choice in patients who cannot tolerate or afford

TABLE 1: Landmark RCTs evaluating benefit of ACEI in heart failure patients.

Study names	*Number of patients recruited*	*Agents tested*	*Mortality reduction in 1 year (relative risk reduction)*	*P value*
CONSENSUS-1[16]	253	Enalapril versus placebo	31%	0.01
SOLVED-Rx[17]	2,569	Enalapril versus placebo	21%	0.02
SAVE[18]	2,231	Captopril versus placebo	18%	0.11
AIRE[19]	1,986	Ramipril versus placebo	22%	0.01
TRACE[20]	1,749	Trandolapril versus placebo	16%	0.04

(ACEI: angiotensin-converting enzyme inhibitor; RCTs: randomized controlled trials)

ARNI. Ideally, ACEIs are started before initiating β-blockers and mineralocorticoid receptor blockers. Initially starting with a low dose, ACEI should be first titrated up to a moderate dose and the β-blocker should be initiated. After achieving an optimum dose of β-blocker, ACEI should also be titrated up to the highest dose showing benefit in randomized controlled trials (RCTs) which is 10 mg twice daily for enalapril, 50 mg three times daily for captopril, and 40 mg daily for lisinopril.[6]

Angiotensin-converting enzyme inhibitors are usually well tolerated. Renal parameters like estimated glomerular filtration rate (eGFR), serum creatinine levels, and serum potassium levels should be adequately monitored, especially during the initiation of therapy and during dose uptitration. ACEI-induced nonproductive cough usually manifests within 1–2 weeks of initiating therapy. In case it interferes with the quality of life, ACEI should be replaced with ARBs. Another serious side effect is angioedema which usually occurs within first week to 3 months of therapy. In such cases, ACEI should be stopped. ARB can be started, but the patient should be kept in close observation as angioedema has been reported rarely with ARBs also. Symptomatic or asymptomatic hypotension can occur during the initiation and uptitration of ACEI. Though it usually improves with time, sometime a reduction in the dose or even stoppage of ACEI may be required if hypotension persists even after taking care of other possible causes like excessive diuretic and inappropriate calcium channel blockers usage.[7]

Angiotensin Receptor Blockers

Both ARBs and ACEIs result in inhibition in angiotensin II (AT) receptor activity but through different mechanisms. ACEIs reduce production of the angiotensin II enzymes whereas ARBs directly inhibit the action of AT type 1 receptors. Furthermore, ACEIs also result in an increase in the blood kinin levels by inhibiting their degradation by ACEs (kininase activity). Although the exact mechanism is still a topic of investigation, these differences of action may be the basis of superiority of ACEI in comparison to ARBs in the domain of heart failure therapy.[8]

The therapeutic benefits of ARBs have been tested in several trials. In the CHARM-Alternative trial, a total 2,028 heart failure patients with LV systolic dysfunction [left ventricular ejection fraction (LVEF) < 40%] were randomized to either Candesartan or placebo.[9] All these patients were intolerant to ACEI. The trial showed a significant reduction in the composite of cardiovascular death and heart failure hospitalization [hazard ratio (HR) 0.70; 95% confidence interval (CI) 0.60–0.81] at a median 33.8 months of follow-up. A later meta-analysis of nine RCTs also showed a significant benefit of ARBs in comparison to placebo in patients with intolerance to ACEI.[10] However, the benefit was borderline in comparison to the encouraging results of ACEI in heart failure patients. As a result, the major heart failure guidelines recommend ACEI therapy as the first choice to achieve a greater mortality and symptomatic benefit.[7,11] ARBs should be advised in case of ACEI-induced troublesome nonproductive cough and angioedema. However, angioedema can occur rarely with ARBs, the risk of which should be properly counseled to the patients. The risk of hypotension, hyperkalemia, and renal impairment by ARBs are same as ACEI therapy requiring a regular monitoring.

The effect of addition of ARBs to the ACEI therapy was tested in the Val-HeFT, CHARM-Added, and VALIANT trials.[12-14] All these RCTs and one large meta-analysis which included the Val-HeFT and CHARM-Added trials have shown no significant difference in total mortality, cardiovascular mortality, and heart failure hospitalization with combination therapy instead of ACEI alone.[10] Although, the adverse events were more common with the combination therapy resulting in more numbers of drug withdrawal. As a result, the current guidelines do not recommend combination of ARBs and ACEIs in heart failure management.[7,11]

Although, ARBs have class effect in heart failure patients, the strongest evidence is for valsartan (starting dose—20–40 mg twice daily, target dose—160 mg twice daily) and candesartan (starting dose—4–8 mg daily, target dose—32 mg daily).[12,13] For losartan, a higher dose

150 mg is considered effective although the evidence is low. ARBs are contraindicated in pregnant and breastfeeding mothers.[15] A close watch on serum potassium and renal parameters is also a prerequisite for starting ARBs in heart failure patients.[16-20]

Beta-adrenergic Receptor Blockers

In HFrEF, chronic inhibition of beta (β)-adrenergic receptors especially β1 receptors has been shown to reverse ventricular remodeling, improve symptoms, reduce hospitalization, and prolong life. Three β-blockers have been shown to have mortality benefit in patients with chronic HFrEF. These include bisoprolol and sustained-release metoprolol succinate both of which competitively inhibit the β1-adrenergic receptor, and carvedilol which blocks the α1-, β1-, and β2-adrenergic receptors. All three agents have been rigorously tested in well-controlled trials and shown to have mortality benefit. A brief summary of these studies is presented in Table 2.[21-25]

Initiation and/or uptitration of dosing of these agents may lead to worsening of fluid retention because of the abrupt withdrawal of adrenergic support to the heart and the circulation. Therefore, the dose of diuretic agent needs to be optimized before initiation of β-blockers and uptitration of dose should be cautious and should proceed no sooner than at 2-week intervals.

In patients hospitalized for acute decompensated heart failure, β-blockers can be safely initiated before discharge, provided that the patient is stable and does not require intravenous therapy. Though the majority of patients tolerate β-blockers eventually, a subset (10–15%) remains intolerant due to worsening of fluid retention or symptomatic hypotension.

TABLE 2: Landmark RCTs evaluating benefit of β-blockers in heart failure (HF) patients.

β-blockers	*Study*	*N*	*Study patients*	*Results*
Metoprolol SR	MERIT-HF[21]	3,991	Patients with chronic HF in the NYHA functional class II–IV and with ejection fraction (EF) of 40% or less, stabilized with optimum standard therapy (primarily ACE inhibitors and diuretics)	Significant reduction in all-cause mortality by 34% (7.2% vs 11%) compared with placebo. Reduction in mortality from both sudden cardiac death and progressive pump failure. Prevention of one death for treatment of every 27 patients with metoprolol CR/XL for 1 year
Bisoprolol	CIBIS-II[22]	2,647	Patients with chronic heart failure in the NYHA functional class III–IV and with EF of 35% or less receiving standard therapy with diuretics and ACE inhibitors Clinical stability was a prerequisite for inclusion during the preceding 6 weeks for HF or 3 months for acute myocardial infarction or unstable angina	Significant reduction in all-cause mortality by 34% (11.8% vs 17.3%) compared with placebo Significant reduction in sudden deaths by 44% (3.6% vs. 6.3% deaths), HF hospitalizations by 30% (11.9% vs 17.6%), and all-cause hospitalizations by 15% (33.6% vs 39.6%)
Carvedilol	COPERNICUS[23]	2,289	This trial included patients with more advanced HF. Clinically euvolemic patients with symptoms at rest or on minimal exertion for at least 2 months and an EF of 0.25 or less, receiving standard therapy with diuretics and ACE inhibitors for at least 2 months	Significant reduction in 12-month mortality by 38% and in relative risk of death or HF hospitalization by 31%
Carvedilol	CAPRICORN[24]	1,959	Patients with acute myocardial infarction (MI) and a left ventricular EF of ≤40%	Significant reduction in relative risk of total mortality by 23%, cardiovascular mortality by 25%, and nonfatal MI by 41%. The trial, however, failed to show a reduction in the prespecified primary endpoint of mortality plus cardiovascular hospitalization
Carvedilol	COMET[25]	1,511	This trial compared carvedilol with immediate release of metoprolol in chronic HF (NYHA II–IV), previous cardiovascular hospitalization, and an EF of less than 0.35 receiving diuretics and ACE inhibitors	Significant 33% reduction in all-cause mortality

(ACE: angiotensin-converting enzyme; NYHA: New York Heart Association; RCTs: randomized controlled trials)

TABLE 3: Studies of ARNI in acute decompensated heart failure.

Name of trials	Study population	Intervention	Control arm	Primary endpoint	Result
TRANSITION-HF[27]	Patients admitted with acute decompensated heart failure with reduced ejection fraction (HFrEF)	Pre- versus postdischarge initiation of sacubitril/valsartan	Nil	Proportion of patients achieving 200 mg BD dose at 10 weeks	Target doses achieved in 62% and 68% in pre- and postdischarge groups, respectively
PIONEER-HF	Patients with HFrEF admitted for acute decompensation	Sacubitril/valsartan (target dose 200 mg BD)	Enalapril (target dose 10 mg BD)	Time averaged proportional change in NT-proBNP at 4 and 8 weeks	Significant reduction in NT-proBNP of the sacubitril/valsartan arm

(ARNI: angiotensin receptor neprilysin inhibitor; NT-proBNP: N-terminal pro B-type natriuretic peptide)

Angiotensin Receptor Neprilysin Inhibitor

Neprilysin is a neutral endopeptidase responsible for degradation of endogenous natriuretic peptides. In addition to degrading natriuretic peptides, neprilysin also inhibits a host of vasodilator and vasoconstrictor peptides. Initial efforts of supplementing exogenous natriuretic peptides resulted in short-term hemodynamic improvement. However, on long-term, there was no significant benefit. Subsequently, omapatrilat, a combination of ACE inhibition and neprilysin inhibition, led to modest benefits. However, there was a higher incidence of angioedema. Neprilysin also hydrolyzes angiotensin I and angiotensin (1–7), an inhibitor of angiotensin II. Hence, neprilysin inhibition alone leads to increase in angiotensin II activity neutralizing the beneficial effects of neprilysin inhibition.

LCZ696 was the first in class ARNI having 1:1 combination of valsartan and sacubitril. The PARADIGM-HF was a double-blind, RCT comparing sacubitril/valsartan with enalapril in patients with HFrEF and ejection fraction less than 40%, who were in the New York Heart Association (NYHA) class II–IV and having B-type natriuretic peptide (BNP) or N-terminal pro B-type natriuretic peptide (NT-proBNP) levels at least 150 pg/mL or 600 pg/mL, respectively.[26] The primary outcome was a composite of cardiovascular death and heart failure hospitalization. The primary composite outcome was significantly lower in the ARNI group [21.8% vs. 26.5%; HR 0.80, 95% CI (0.73–0.87)]. The number needed to treat one occurrence of primary outcome was only 21. There were significantly higher symptomatic hypotension episodes in ARNI group. However, there was no difference in drug discontinuation attributed to hypotension. There were no significant differences in other adverse effects. Currently, heart failure guidelines of various professional bodies recommend sacubitril/valsartan, as class I indication in patients with HFrEF whose are symptomatic despite maximum tolerable doses of β-blockers, ACEI/ARB, and mineralocorticoid receptor blockers.

Subsequently, two trials have shown safety and efficacy of initiating ARNI in acute decompensated heart failure (Table 3).[27] Various trials are ongoing looking into utility of ARNI in HFpEF and postmyocardial infarction LV dysfunction (Table 4).

DEVICE THERAPY IN HEART FAILURE

Despite remarkable advancement in pharmacologic therapy, the high rate of mortality and morbidity is still a concern in management of HFrEF. Sudden cardiac death (SCD) and progressive pump failure remain the leading causes of mortality in patients with HFrEF.[28] Almost 40% of cases of SCD in HFrEF are due to cardiac arrhythmias, most commonly ventricular tachycardia (VT) degenerating into ventricular fibrillation (VF).[29] Other major reasons for SCD are pump failure and mechanical complications of myocardial infarction. Though SCD is a major cause of mortality in heart failure patients, its contribution to the total deaths is not uniform in all the NYHA functional classes. The proportion of SCD to total death is higher in the NYHA class II and III than in the NYHA class IV or resistant heart failure cases where progressive pump failure contributes to a significant number of deaths.[21] The main necessity of implantable device therapy in heart failure treatment armamentarium is for prevention of SCD by terminating life-threatening arrhythmias and prevention of pump failure by the establishment of synchronicity during cardiac contraction. Other newer indications are hemodynamic monitoring, remote monitoring, and acute hemodynamic support, but the evidence behind these newer technologies are not very robust till now.

Implantable Cardioverter Defibrillator

Implantable Cardioverter Defibrillator for Secondary Prevention of Sudden Cardiac Death

Medical management to correct the reversible factors is the main goal of therapy in cardiac arrest survivors with

TABLE 4: Ongoing trials on sacubitril/valsartan.

Name of trials	Study population	Intervention	Control arm	Primary endpoint	Duration
PARAGON-HF	HFpEF with elevated NT-proBNP	Sacubitril/valsartan	Valsartan	Composite of CV death and heart failure hospitalizations	57 months
PARALLEL-HF	Same as PARADIGM-HF in Japanese population	Sacubitril/valsartan	Enalapril	Composite of CV death and heart failure hospitalizations	40 months
PARABLE	Elevated NT-proBNP, LAVI > 28 mL/m^2, and CV risk factors	Sacubitril/valsartan	Valsartan	Change in LAVI at 18 months	18 months
PARADISE-AMI	Postmyocardial infarction with LVEF < 40%	Sacubitril/valsartan	Ramipril	Composite of CV death and heart failure hospitalization or outpatient heart failure	32 months
PARTHENON	Canadian population taking sacubitril/valsartan	Sacubitril/valsartan	None	Change in NT-proBNP	36 months
PARALLAX	HFpEF, NYHA class II–IV	Sacubitril/valsartan	Enalapril, valsartan, or placebo	Change in NT-proBNP	24 weeks
PERSPECTIVE	HFpEF, NYHA class II–IV	Sacubitril/valsartan	Valsartan	Change in cognitive state and global cognitive composite score	156 weeks

(CV: cardiovascular; HFpEF: heart failure with preserved ejection fraction; LAVI: left atrial volume index; LVEF: left ventricular ejection fraction; NT-proBNP: N-terminal pro B-type natriuretic peptide; NYHA: New York Heart Association)

a transient or reversible cause. Implantable cardioverter defibrillator (ICD) is indicated for secondary prevention in patients with history of sustained VT or VF without any reversible cause. Multiple trials have shown a reduction in the incidence of SCD and total mortality with ICD implantation when compared to antiarrhythmic drugs in patients with sustained life-threatening VT/VF with or without LV dysfunction.[30] Among them, three landmark trials and one meta-analysis are worth mentioning. The AVID trial was the first and the largest of the landmark trials which included a total of 1,016 patients with history of hemodynamically unstable VF or VT with syncope and LV dysfunction (LVEF < 40%).[31] Most of the patients had severe LV dysfunction (ejection fraction ~31%) with history of coronary artery disease. In the RCT, ICD therapy was compared with antiarrhythmic therapy (mainly amiodarone and sotalol). There was 39%, 24%, and 31% relative risk reduction of mortality with ICD therapy at 1, 2, and 3 years of follow-up, respectively. The reduction in mortality was more significant in patients with severe LV dysfunction (LVEF ≤ 35%). β-blockers were administered less frequently in the antiarrhythmic arm because of increased risk of bradycardia in this trial, but the significant mortality benefit of ICD therapy persisted even after adjusting for β-blocker therapy.

Another landmark trial, the CASH study[32] recruited 288 patients with a history of hemodynamically unstable VT/VF and LV dysfunction. The mean ejection fraction was 45% and coronary artery disease was the cause of LV dysfunction in most patients. The study patients were randomized to receive either ICD or antiarrhythmic drugs (metoprolol, propafenone, and amiodarone). The mean follow-up period was 57 months. The propafenone arm was stopped after 11 months of study due to significant incidence of mortality in comparison to the ICD arm. There was no statistically significant reduction in all-cause mortality with ICD therapy compared to amiodarone/metoprolol in the trial (36.4% vs 44%). In comparison to the AVID trial, the negative result in this trial might be due to lack of study power as well as lesser severity of LV dysfunction in the study population (46% vs 31%). The secondary endpoint of SCD was significantly reduced by the ICD therapy than amiodarone/metoprolol in this trial.

Another landmark trial, the Canadian Implantable Defibrillator Study (CIDS) randomized 659 patients with history of unstable VF, VT, and unmonitored syncope to either ICD arm or amiodarone arm.[33] Most of these patients had severe LV dysfunction (mean ejection fraction ~34%) with coronary artery disease. It was also a negative study with no significant reduction in all-cause mortality with ICD therapy in comparison to amiodarone after 5 years of follow-up.

Except AVID, both CIDS and CASH trials did not show any significant survival benefit of ICD implantation in heart failure patients with history of cardiac arrest resuscitation.

This discrepancy may be because of smaller sample size, lack of power, and referral bias where patients with highest risk of recurrence of cardiac arrest were referred for ICD implantation instead of recruitment in the trials.[34] To clarify the dispute, one meta-analysis included all the three landmark trials and one smaller RCT that evaluated the secondary prevention of ICD in patients with LV dysfunction.[35] In this study, there was 7% absolute risk reduction of all-cause mortality (to prevent one death, 15 patients need ICD therapy) and 25% relative risk reduction of arrhythmic death with ICD in comparison to medical therapy. Furthermore, patients with LVEF ≤ 35% had more benefit than those with LVEF > 35%.

On the basis of the above evidence, ICD is the treatment of choice to prevent SCD in cardiac arrest survivor heart failure patients. However, two points need to be kept in mind before advising the ICD therapy. First, all the major trials of ICD for secondary prevention were conducted almost 2 decades back when the benefits of optimum medical therapy of heart failure with ACEI, ARB, MRAs, ARNI, and β-blockers were not well-recognized. Although ICD is essential for SCD prevention, additional optimum medical therapy can further reduce the risk of mortality by decreasing progression of pump failure and sympathetic nervous system activation. Second, at the terminal phase of heart failure, ventricular arrhythmias may become resistant to ICD shocks and even after ICD implantation. SCD can occur due to resistant terminal VT/VF, pulseless electrical activity, pulmonary embolism, and mechanical complications of myocardial infarction.

Implantable Cardioverter Defibrillator for Primary Prevention of Sudden Cardiac Death

Sudden cardiac arrest may be the first manifestation of cardiac arrhythmias in heart failure patients underscoring the need for ICD implantation for primary prevention of SCD. Several large trials evaluated the extent of benefit of ICD therapy for this intent. Among them, the first study was the Multicenter Automatic Defibrillator Implantation Trial (MADIT) which recruited selected high-risk patients with history of severe LV dysfunction (LVEF < 35%), past history of myocardial infarction (MI), recurrent spontaneous nonsustained VT, and inducible nonsuppressible ventricular tachyarrhythmias with programmed electrical stimulation.[36] 196 subjects were randomized to receive either ICD or antiarrhythmic medication predominantly amiodarone. In this trial, ICD therapy resulted in 54% relative risk reduction of all-cause mortality and SCD in comparison to antiarrhythmic medications. This encouraging result was mainly due to significant mortality benefit in patients with LVEF < 26%, clinical heart failure, and intraventricular conduction defect. The next major trial was Multicenter Unsustained Tachycardia Trial (MUSTT) which enrolled 704 post-MI patients with LVEF less than 40%, asymptomatic spontaneous nonsustained VT, and inducible-sustained VT by programmed electrical stimulation.[37] The patients were randomized to receive antiarrhythmic drug therapy decided by programmed electrical stimulation or ICD. There was 76% relative risk reduction of mortality due to cardiac arrhythmia with ICD therapy in comparison to the antiarrhythmic therapy in this trial.

The MADIT II included patients with coronary artery disease and LVEF of less than 30%, prior MI at least 30 days before the enrolment or history of coronary artery bypass grafting (CABG) at least 90 days before recruitment for randomization to either ICD or conventional medical therapy alone arm.[38] This was the first study to remove the electrical inducibility criteria for patient recruitment unlike the previous MADIT and MUSTT trials. There was a 31% relative risk reduction of mortality predominantly due to reduction in SCD with ICD implantation in comparison to the conventional medical therapy alone. Two findings were unique to this trial. First, there was an increased incidence of heart failure hospitalization in the ICD arm in spite of survival benefit. Second, the mortality benefit was achieved primarily after 9 months of ICD implantation which was later in comparison to the previous studies. The allotment of sicker patients in the previous trials and better usage of conventional medical therapy in this trial may be the reason behind these results.

The Defibrillators in Nonischemic Cardiomyopathy Treatment Evaluation (DEFINITE) study was the first major RCT which randomized 458 patients with nonischemic cardiomyopathy patients with LVEF less than 36%, nonsustained VT, and ventricular premature complexes to either conventional medical therapy or single chamber ICD arm.[39] The mean LVEF of the study population was ~21% which was much lower than previous trials. ICD implantations over and above conventional medical therapy resulted in significant reduction in mortality due to cardiac arrhythmia, but there was nonsignificant reduction in all-cause mortality in this trial. The Sudden Cardiac Death in Heart Failure Trial (SCD-HeFT) was the largest primary prevention trial which recruited 2,521 patients with both ischemic and nonischemic cardiomyopathy patients with LVEF ≤ 35%, the NYHA class II/III for at least 3 months duration to receive either amiodarone or placebo or ICD in addition to conventional medical therapy.[40] There was a net survival benefit with ICD therapy in comparison to amiodarone or placebo with a 23% relative risk reduction of mortality. Moreover, there was no significant difference between ischemic and nonischemic cardiomyopathy patients in terms of survival benefit with ICD therapy in the trial.

The most recent Danish Study to Assess the Efficacy of ICDs in Patients with Non-ischemic Systolic Heart Failure on Mortality (DANISH) trial was designed to improve the evidence base for ICD implantation for primary prevention in nonischemic cardiomyopathy.[41] The study enrolled 1,116 patients with nonischemic cardiomyopathy (LVEF ≤ 35%) and symptomatic heart failure to either ICD implantation with medical therapy or conventional medical therapy alone. Approximately, 58% of patients received cardiac resynchronization therapy (CRT) in both the study groups, if eligible. The study showed 50% relative risk reduction of SCD, although there was no significant reduction in all-cause mortality by the ICD implantation in addition to standard medical treatment.

The benefit of ICD in the prevention of life-threatening cardiac arrhythmias and SCD in the early post-MI or revascularization phase was assessed in several trials. Among them, the DINAMIT and IRIS trials recruited patients with LV dysfunction 5–6 days after and within 40 days of MI.[42,43] Whereas in the CABG patch trial, heart failure patients with abnormal signal-averaged electrocardiogram were randomized to CABG and intraoperative ICD implantation or CABG alone.[44] None of the above trials showed any significant survival benefit of ICD in the early post-MI or revascularization patients mainly due to increased non-SCD deaths in the ICD arm. As a result, current guidelines do not recommend ICD implantation in the immediate post-MI or revascularization phase as a measure of primary prevention of SCD.

Although the major guidelines recommend ICD implantation in certain high-risk subsets of heart failure patients (Table 5), there are several caveats in the current risk stratification methods. A significant number of patients never experience any ICD shocks in spite of poor LV function and functional class. Moreover, the DANISH trial has shown that the survival benefit of ICD therapy in nonischemic cardiomyopathy may not be as robust as its ischemic counterpart. This may be partly because of a very low rate of mortality in the DANISH trial due to optimum usage of conventional medical therapy and high rate of CRT implantation in both the study arms which is impractical in most of the resource-limited scenarios. Further larger trials are needed to reanalyze the utility of ICD therapy for primary prevention in both ischemic and nonischemic cardiomyopathy in the era of highly effective drugs like ARNI.

Although ICD is primarily implanted to gain survival benefit, recent trials have shown poor survival with appropriate or inappropriate ICD shocks partly because of advanced stage of heart failure and partly due to suboptimal programming of device.[45] Multiple trials have shown that increasing the tachycardia detection time, threshold rate for VT detection, and programming two to three bursts of adenosine triphosphate (ATP) therapy, while the ICD is getting charged, result in significant decrease in ICD shocks without compromising its lifesaving effect during unstable VT/VF.[46] Finally, the MADIT-RIT trial has shown a significant survival benefit with appropriate ICD programming as described above.[47] On the basis of these evidence, proper programming of the ICD devices depending upon the patient's need is strongly recommended.

Cardiac Resynchronization Therapy

Cardiac resynchronization therapy prevents the progression of ventricular remodeling and improves the quality of life in heart failure patients with LVEF ≤ 35%. The benefit is highest in patients with left bundle branch block (LBBB) and QRS duration ≥150 ms (Table 6). It has also shown survival benefit in selected group of patients in addition to conventional medical therapy.

TABLE 5: Indications for ICD implantation.

Class I indications	• Cardiac arrest due to hemodynamically unstable VT or VF in the absence of reversible causes • Spontaneous sustained VT • LVEF ≤ 35% due to past MI, at least 40 days post-MI, or >90 days postrevascularization with the NYHA class II/III • LVEF ≤ 30% due to prior MI, at least 40 days post-MI, or >90 days postrevascularization with the NYHA class I • Nonsustained VT with past history of MI, LVEF ≤ 40%, and inducible VF or sustained VT on EP testing • Syncope of undetermined origin in ischemic heart disease with inducible sustained VT on EP testing.
Class II indications	• Sustained VT and normal or near-normal left ventricular function • Nonhospitalized but are candidates for heart transplantation or left ventricular assist device implantation.
Class III indications	• Do not have a reasonable expectation of survival with an acceptable functional status for at least 1 year • Incessant VT or VF • The NYHA class IV and refractory heart failure who are not candidate for cardiac transplantation, left ventricular assist device, or CRT.

(CRT: cardiac resynchronization therapy; EP: electrophysiology; ICD: implantable cardioverter defibrillator; LVEF: left ventricular ejection fraction; MI: myocardial infarction; NYHA: New York Heart Association; VF: ventricular fibrillation; VT: ventricular tachycardia)

TABLE 6: Indications for CRT implantations (major guidelines).

Recommendations for patients with LBBB						
	QRS ≥ 150 ms		*QRS 130–149 ms*		*QRS 120–129 ms*	
Guidelines (year)	*NYHA class III/IV*	*NYHA class II*	*NYHA class III/IV*	*NYHA class II*	*NYHA class III/IV*	*NYHA class II*
ESC HFA (2016)	IA	IA	IB	IB	IIIA	IIIA
ESC EHRA (2013)	IA	IA	IB	IB	IB	IB
ACC/AHA/HRS (2013)	IA	IB	IIa B	IIa B	IIa B	IIa B
Recommendations for patients without LBBB						
	QRS ≥ 150 ms		*QRS 130–149 ms*		*QRS 120–129 ms*	
Guidelines (year)	*NYHA class III/IV*	*NYHA class II*	*NYHA class III/IV*	*NYHA class II*	*NYHA class III/IV*	*NYHA class II*
ESC HFA (2016)	IIa B	IIa B	IIb B	IIb B	IIIA	IIIA
ESC EHRA (2013)	IIa B	IIa B	IIb B	IIb B	IIb B	IIb B
ACC/AHA/HRS (2013)	IIa A	IIb B	IIb B	IIIB	IIb B	IIIB
Other indications for CRT						
Guidelines (year)	*Atrial fibrillation and heart failure (HF)*			*LV dysfunction with symptomatic HF and requirement of ventricular pacing (high %)*		
ESC HFA (2016)	IIa B			IA		
ESC EHRA (2013)	IIa B			IIa B		
ACC/AHA/HRS (2013)	IIa B			IIa C		

(ACC: American College of Cardiology; AHA: American Heart Association; CRT: cardiac resynchronization therapy; EHRA: European Heart Rhythm Association; ESC: European Society of Cardiology; HFA: Heart Failure Association; HRS: Heart Rhythm Society; ICD: implantable cardioverter defibrillator; LBBB: left bundle branch block; LV: left ventricular; NYHA: New York Heart Association)

The first major landmark trial, the Multisite Stimulation in Cardiomyopathy (MUSTIC) study, recruited heart failure patients with LVEF < 35%, the NYHA class III, and QRS duration >150 ms.[48] In this study, CRT implantation resulted in significant improvement in the quality of life and exercise tolerance. Similarly, the Multicenter InSync Randomized Clinical Evaluation (MIRACLE) trial also evaluated CRT pacing in the NYHA class III or IV heart failure patients (LVEF < 35%) with QRS width >130 ms and showed a significant symptomatic benefit.[49]

The survival benefit of CRT was first described in the Comparison of Medical Therapy, Pacing and Defibrillation in Heart Failure (COMPANION) trial which randomized total 1,520 patients with heart failure, LVEF < 35%, QRS width >120 ms, and the NYHA class III or IV to receive either medical therapy with CRT-P or CRT-D or medical therapy alone.[50] The primary endpoints were time to death or time to first hospitalization for any cause. Both CRT-D and CRT-P significantly reduced the primary outcome with HR of 0.80 and 0.81, respectively. The relative risk of all-cause death was reduced by 24% in the CRT-P arm and by 36% in the CRT-D arm.

The survival benefit in the NYHA class III and IV heart failure patients with LVEF < 35%, LV end-diastolic diameter >30 mm indexed to height, and QRS duration >150 ms was further tested in the Cardiac Resynchronization-Heart Failure (CARE-HF) trial where 813 patients were randomized to receive medical therapy with CRT-P implantation or medical therapy alone.[51] Additional echocardiographic dyssynchrony criteria like aortic preejection delay and interventricular mechanical delay were used first time in this trial for enrolment of patients with QRS width 120–149 ms. The trial's primary endpoints, time to death due to any cause and time to first hospitalization due to major cardiovascular event, were reached in 39% patients in the CRT group and 55% in the medical therapy alone group. The risk of all-cause death was also reduced significantly by CRT implantation (20%) in comparison to the medical therapy alone (10%). The other benefits of CRT implantations were improvement in the quality of life, intraventricular conduction delay, and reduction in secondary mitral insufficiency.

The efficacy of CRT in the NYHA class I and II heart failure patients with LVEF ≤ 30% and QRS duration ≥130 ms was first evaluated in the MADIT-CRT trial.[52] In this study, total 1,820 patients were randomized to either CRT-D or ICD alone arm. The primary outcome was all-cause mortality or heart failure hospitalization whichever comes first. Although there was no significant reduction in the all-cause mortality, the primary endpoint reduced significantly in the CRT-D arm than in the ICD arm (17.2% vs 25.3%, respectively) predominantly due to effect on heart failure hospitalization. The RAFT trial was the first randomized trial to show a survival benefit of CRT-D in comparison to ICD alone in patients with mild-to-moderate heart failure symptoms.[53] The trial enrolled 1,798 heart failure patients with the NYHA class II and III symptoms, LVEF ≤ 30%, and QRS duration ≥120 ms. The primary study outcomes were all-cause mortality or heart failure-related hospitalization. There was a 25% relative risk reduction in all-cause mortality and 32% relative risk reduction in heart failure hospitalization by CRT-D in comparison to ICD implantation alone.

In spite of the frequent use of CRT devices in the eligible heart failure patients with electrical dyssynchrony, a significant number of cases do not respond to CRT due to inadequate risk stratification criteria. The role of echocardiographic signs of mechanical dyssynchrony for guiding CRT implantation in patients with narrow QRS was tested in the Echocardiography-Guided Cardiac Resynchronization Therapy (ECHO-CART) trial.[54] 809 patients with LVEF ≤ 35%, the NYHA class III/IV functional class, QRS width <130 ms, and echocardiographic evidence of mechanical dyssynchrony were enrolled to undergo CRT implantation. The patients were then randomized to either of the CRT on or off groups for a follow-up. The primary endpoint of all-cause mortality was significantly higher in the CRT pacing arm underscoring the greater importance of electrical dyssynchrony rather than mechanical dyssynchrony for patient selection. This result was further supported by the RethinQ trial which showed no benefit of CRT pacing in the heart failure patients with narrow QRS in improving peak oxygen consumption with exertion.[55] Another subset of eligible patients who may benefit with CRT pacing are those with mild-to-moderate LV dysfunction, but with wide QRS duration (>150 ms) and complete LBBB. The indication becomes much stronger if the patient requires frequent pacing (>40% of the time). The benefit of CRT pacing in reducing morbidity, mortality, and ventricular remodeling in patients with mild LV dysfunction (LVEF < 50%) and atrioventricular (AV) block requiring high pacing burden were evaluated in the BLOCK-HF trial.[56] CRT pacing significantly reduced mortality and heart failure hospitalization resulting in the recommendation of CRT implantation instead of pacemaker in patients with LVEF < 50%, AV block, and expected pacing burden >40%.

Apart from the appropriate patient selection, proper LV lead positioning is also very important to achieve the maximum benefit of CRT pacing. The posterolateral segment of the left ventricle is the last part to contract in cases of LBBB. Targeting this segment is very important during LV lead positioning as the MADIT-CRT trial has shown a significant risk of suboptimal response with an apical position of the LV lead. Another important reason behind the nonresponse to CRT is the inadvertent placement of the LV lead on the myocardial scars.[57] Preprocedure speckle tracking echocardiography or gadolinium-enhanced MRI may be helpful to place LV lead at the site of late mechanical activation away from the myocardial scar tissue. Recently, multisite pacing with the quadripolar leads has gain popularity because of flexibility to change the LV pacing vector to avoid diaphragmatic pacing and achieve adequate synchronicity. Although, these newer concepts need further evaluation before gaining a strong recommendation for routine use.

CONCLUSION

Pharmacologic therapy for heart failure with reduced ejection fraction (HFrEF) includes ACEIs, ARBs, β-blockers, MRA, ARNI,which has proven beneficial in a selected group of patients. All these agents have been shown in multiple landmarks trials to have significant mortality benefit. Besides this Device Therapy and CRT have also shown morbidity and mortality benefits in selected group of patients.

REFERENCES

1. Dzau VJ. Tissue renin-angiotensin system in myocardial hypertrophy and failure. Arch Intern Med. 1993;153(8): 937-42.
2. Giannattasio C, Achilli F, Failla M, et al. Radial, carotid and aortic distensibility in congestive heart failure: effects of high-dose angiotensin-converting enzyme inhibitor or low-dose association with angiotensin type 1 receptor blockade. J Am Coll Cardiol. 2002;39(8):1275-82.
3. Witherow FN, Helmy A, Webb DJ, et al. Bradykinin contributes to the vasodilator effects of chronic angiotensin-converting enzyme inhibition in patients with heart failure. Circulation. 2001;104(18):2177-81.
4. Varin R, Mulder P, Tamion F, et al. Improvement of endothelial function by chronic angiotensin-converting enzyme inhibition in heart failure: role of nitric oxide, prostanoids, oxidant stress, and bradykinin. Circulation. 2000;102(3):351-6.
5. Flather MD, Yusuf S, Køber L, et al. Long-term ACE-inhibitor therapy in patients with heart failure or left-ventricular dysfunction: a systematic overview of data from individual patients. ACE-Inhibitor Myocardial Infarction Collaborative Group. Lancet. 2000;355(9215):1575-81.
6. Yancy CW, Jessup M, Bozkurt B, et al. ACCF/AHA guideline for the management of heart failure: a report of the American College of Cardiology Foundation/American Heart Association Task Force on Practice Guidelines. J Am Coll Cardiol. 2013;62(16):e147-239.
7. Ponikowski P, Voors AA, Anker SD, et al. ESC Guidelines for the diagnosis and treatment of acute and chronic heart

failure: The Task Force for the diagnosis and treatment of acute and chronic heart failure of the European Society of Cardiology (ESC) Developed with the special contribution of the Heart Failure Association (HFA) of the ESC. Eur Heart J. 2016;37(27):2129-200.
8. Goldsmith DJ. Angiotensin receptor antagonists. Lancet. 1997;349(9060):1255.
9. Granger CB, McMurray JJ, Yusuf S, et al. Effects of candesartan in patients with chronic heart failure and reduced left-ventricular systolic function intolerant to angiotensin-converting-enzyme inhibitors: the CHARM-Alternative trial. Lancet. 2003;362(9386):772-6.
10. Heran BS, Musini VM, Bassett K, et al. Angiotensin receptor blockers for heart failure. Cochrane Database Syst Rev. 2012;(4):CD003040.
11. Yancy CW, Jessup M, Bozkurt B, et al. ACC/AHA/HFSA Focused Update on New Pharmacological Therapy for Heart Failure: An Update of the 2013 ACCF/AHA Guideline for the Management of Heart Failure: A Report of the American College of Cardiology/American Heart Association Task Force on Clinical Practice Guidelines and the Heart Failure Society of America. Circulation. 2016;134(13):e282-93.
12. Cohn JN, Tognoni G. A Randomized Trial of the Angiotensin-Receptor Blocker Valsartan in Chronic Heart Failure. N Engl J Med. 2001;345(23):1667-75.
13. McMurray JJ, Ostergren J, Swedberg K, et al. Effects of candesartan in patients with chronic heart failure and reduced left-ventricular systolic function taking angiotensin-converting-enzyme inhibitors: the CHARM-Added trial. Lancet. 2003;362(9386):767-71.
14. McMurray J, Solomon S, Pieper K, et al. The effect of valsartan, captopril, or both on atherosclerotic events after acute myocardial infarction: an analysis of the Valsartan in Acute Myocardial Infarction Trial (VALIANT). J Am Coll Cardiol. 2006;47(4):726-33.
15. Konstam MA, Neaton JD, Dickstein K, et al. Effects of high-dose versus low-dose losartan on clinical outcomes in patients with heart failure (HEAAL study): a randomised, double-blind trial. Lancet. 2009;374(9704):1840-8.
16. CONSENSUS Trial Study Group. Effects of enalapril on mortality in severe congestive heart failure. Results of the Cooperative North Scandinavian Enalapril Survival Study (CONSENSUS). N Engl J Med. 1987;316(23):1429-35.
17. Yusuf S, Pitt B, Davis CE, et al. Effect of enalapril on survival in patients with reduced left ventricular ejection fractions and congestive heart failure. N Engl J Med. 1991;325(5):293-302.
18. Pfeffer MA, Braunwald E, Moye LA, et al. Effect of captopril on mortality and morbidity in patients with left ventricular dysfunction after myocardial infarction. Results of the survival and ventricular enlargement trial. The SAVE Investigators. N Engl J Med. 1992;327(10):669-77.
19. Effect of ramipril on mortality and morbidity of survivors of acute myocardial infarction with clinical evidence of heart failure. The Acute Infarction Ramipril Efficacy (AIRE) Study Investigators. Lancet. 1993;342(8875):821-8.
20. Køber L, Torp-Pedersen C, Carlsen JE, et al. A clinical trial of the angiotensin-converting-enzyme inhibitor trandolapril in patients with left ventricular dysfunction after myocardial infarction. Trandolapril Cardiac Evaluation (TRACE) Study Group. N Engl J Med. 1995;333(25):1670-6.
21. Effect of metoprolol CR/XL in chronic heart failure: Metoprolol CR/XL Randomised Intervention Trial in Congestive Heart Failure (MERIT-HF). Lancet. 1999;353(9169):2001-7.
22. The Cardiac Insufficiency Bisoprolol Study II (CIBIS-II): a randomised trial. Lancet. 1999;353(9146):9-13.
23. Packer M, Fowler MB, Roecker EB, et al. Effect of carvedilol on the morbidity of patients with severe chronic heart failure: results of the carvedilol prospective randomized cumulative survival (COPERNICUS) study. Circulation. 2002;106(17):2194-9.
24. Dargie HJ. Effect of carvedilol on outcome after myocardial infarction in patients with left-ventricular dysfunction: the CAPRICORN randomised trial. Lancet. 2001;357(9266):1385-90.
25. Poole-Wilson PA, Swedberg K, Cleland JG, et al. Comparison of carvedilol and metoprolol on clinical outcomes in patients with chronic heart failure in the Carvedilol or Metoprolol European Trial (COMET): randomised controlled trial. Lancet. 2003;362(9377):7-13.
26. Jhund PS, Fu M, Bayram E, et al. Efficacy and safety of LCZ696 (sacubitril-valsartan) according to age: insights from PARADIGM-HF. Eur Heart J. 2015;36(38):2576-84.
27. Wachter R, Senni M, Belohlavek J, et al. Sacubitril/valsartan initiated in hospitalized patients with heart failure with reduced ejection fraction after hemodynamic stabilization: primary results of the TRANSITION study. J Cardiac Fail. 2018;24(8):S15.
28. Narang R, Cleland JG, Erhardt L, et al. Mode of death in chronic heart failure. A request and proposition for more accurate classification. Eur Heart J. 1996;17(9):1390-403.
29. Cleland JG, Erhardt L, Murray G, et al. Effect of ramipril on morbidity and mode of death among survivors of acute myocardial infarction with clinical evidence of heart failure. A report from the AIRE Study Investigators. Eur Heart J. 1997;18(1):41-51.
30. Antiarrhythmics versus Implantable Defibrillators (AVID) Investigators. A comparison of antiarrhythmic-drug therapy with implantable defibrillators in patients resuscitated from near-fatal ventricular arrhythmias. N Engl J Med. 1997;337(22):1576-83.
31. Domanski MJ, Sakseena S, Epstein AE, et al. Relative effectiveness of the implantable cardioverter-defibrillator and antiarrhythmic drugs in patients with varying degrees of left ventricular dysfunction who have survived malignant ventricular arrhythmias. AVID Investigators. Antiarrhythmics versus Implantable Defibrillators. J Am Coll Cardiol. 1999;34(4):1090-5.
32. Kuck KH, Cappato R, Siebels J, et al. Randomized comparison of antiarrhythmic drug therapy with implantable defibrillators in patients resuscitated from cardiac arrest: the Cardiac Arrest Study Hamburg (CASH). Circulation. 2000;102(7):748-54.
33. Connolly SJ, Gent M, Roberts RS, et al. Canadian implantable defibrillator study (CIDS): a randomized trial of the

implantable cardioverter defibrillator against amiodarone. Circulation. 2000;101(11):1297-302.
34. Hussein AA, Wilkoff BL. Cardiac Implantable Electronic Device Therapy in Heart Failure. Circ Res. 2019;124(11):1584-97.
35. Lee DS, Green LD, Liu PP, et al. Effectiveness of implantable defibrillators for preventing arrhythmic events and death: a meta-analysis. J Am Coll Cardiol. 2003;41(9):1573-82.
36. Moss AJ, Hall WJ, Cannom DS, et al. Improved survival with an implanted defibrillator in patients with coronary disease at high risk for ventricular arrhythmia. Multicenter Automatic Defibrillator Implantation Trial Investigators. N Engl J Med. 1996;335(26):1933-40.
37. Buxton AE, Lee KL, Fisher JD, et al. A randomized study of the prevention of sudden death in patients with coronary artery disease. Multicenter Unsustained Tachycardia Trial Investigators. N Engl J Med. 1999;341(25):1882-90.
38. Moss AJ, Zareba W, Hall WJ, et al. Prophylactic implantation of a defibrillator in patients with myocardial infarction and reduced ejection fraction. N Engl J Med. 2002;346(12):877-83.
39. Kadish A, Dyer A, Daubert JP, et al. Prophylactic defibrillator implantation in patients with nonischemic dilated cardiomyopathy. N Engl J Med. 2004;350(21):2151-8.
40. Bardy GH, Lee KL, Mark DB, et al. Amiodarone or an implantable cardioverter-defibrillator for congestive heart failure. N Engl J Med. 2005;352(3):225-37.
41. Kober L, Thune JJ, Nielsen JC, et al. Defibrillator Implantation in Patients with Nonischemic Systolic Heart Failure. N Engl J Med. 2016;375(13):1221-30.
42. Hohnloser SH, Kuck KH, Dorian P, et al. Prophylactic use of an implantable cardioverter-defibrillator after acute myocardial infarction. N Engl J Med. 2004;351(24):2481-8.
43. Steinbeck G, Andresen D, Seidl K, et al. Defibrillator implantation early after myocardial infarction. N Engl J Med. 2009;361(15):1427-36.
44. Bigger JT. Prophylactic use of implanted cardiac defibrillators in patients at high risk for ventricular arrhythmias after coronary-artery bypass graft surgery. Coronary Artery Bypass Graft (CABG) Patch Trial Investigators. N Engl J Med. 1997;337(22):1569-75.
45. Poole JE, Johnson GW, Hellkamp AS, et al. Prognostic importance of defibrillator shocks in patients with heart failure. N Engl J Med. 2008;359(10):1009-17.
46. Wilkoff BL, Fauchier L, Stiles MK, et al. 2015 HRS/EHRA/APHRS/SOLAECE expert consensus statement on optimal implantable cardioverter-defibrillator programming and testing. Heart Rhythm. 2016;13(2):e50-86.
47. Ruwald MH, Okumura K, Kimura T, et al. Syncope in high-risk cardiomyopathy patients with implantable defibrillators: frequency, risk factors, mechanisms, and association with mortality: results from the Multicenter Automatic Defibrillator Implantation Trial–Reduce Inappropriate Therapy (MADIT-RIT) study. Circulation. 2014;129(5):545-52.
48. Cazeau S, Leclercq C, Lavergne T, et al. Effects of multisite biventricular pacing in patients with heart failure and intraventricular conduction delay. N Engl J Med. 2001;344(12):873-80.
49. Abraham WT, Fisher WG, Smith AL, et al. Cardiac resynchronization in chronic heart failure. N Engl J Med. 2002;346(24):1845-53.
50. Bristow MR, Saxon LA, Boehmer J, et al. Cardiac-resynchronization therapy with or without an implantable defibrillator in advanced chronic heart failure. N Engl J Med. 2004;350(21):2140-50.
51. Cleland JG, Daubert JC, Erdmann E, et al. The effect of cardiac resynchronization on morbidity and mortality in heart failure. N Engl J Med. 2005;352(15):1539-49.
52. Moss AJ, Hall WJ, Cannom DS, et al. Cardiac-resynchronization therapy for the prevention of heart-failure events. N Engl J Med. 2009;361(14):1329-38.
53. Tang AS, Wells GA, Talajic M, et al. Cardiac-resynchronization therapy for mild-to-moderate heart failure. N Engl J Med. 2010;363(25):2385-95.
54. Ruschitzka F, Abraham WT, Singh JP, et al. Cardiac-resynchronization therapy in heart failure with a narrow QRS complex. N Engl J Med. 2013;369(15):1395-405.
55. Beshai JF, Grimm RA, Nagueh SF, et al. Cardiac-resynchronization therapy in heart failure with narrow QRS complexes. N Engl J Med. 2007;357(24):2461-71.
56. Curtis AB, Worley SJ, Adamson PB, et al. Biventricular pacing for atrioventricular block and systolic dysfunction. N Engl J Med. 2013;368(17):1585-93.
57. Ypenburg C, Schalij MJ, Bleeker GB, et al. Impact of viability and scar tissue on response to cardiac resynchronization therapy in ischaemic heart failure patients. Eur Heart J. 2007;28(1):33-41.

12 CHAPTER

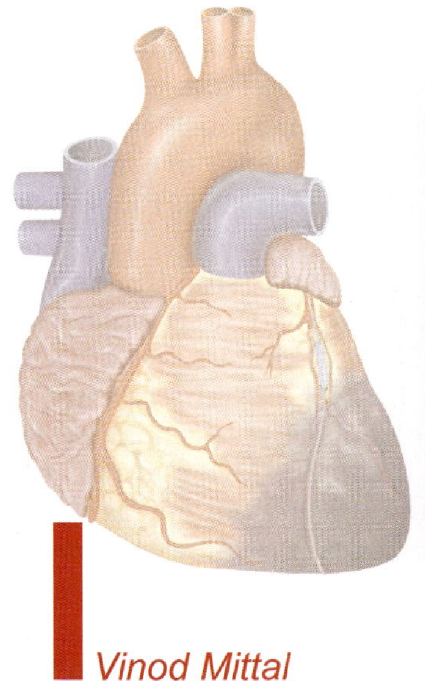

Optimizing Treatment in Heart Failure

Vinod Mittal

INTRODUCTION

The correct use of approved medications is the single most important tool for the management of chronic heart failure (HF). The evidence supporting pharmacologic recommendations for heart failure with reduced ejection fraction (HFrEF) is substantially stronger than supporting recommendations for heart failure with preserved ejection fraction (HFpEF). The classes of pharmacologic agents available for HF treatment are shown in Box 1.

ANGIOTENSIN-CONVERTING ENZYME INHIBITORS, ANGIOTENSIN-RECEPTOR BLOCKERS, AND VALSARTAN-SACUBITRIL

Angiotensin-converting enzyme inhibitors (ACEi) interfere with the upstream conversion of angiotensin I (Ang I) to angiotensin II (Ang II). In contrast, angiotensin receptor blockers (ARBs) competitively inhibit the downstream binding of Ang II to angiotensin (AT)[1] receptors in heart, kidney, and vascular tissue. Because of these differences in mechanism of action, the two classes of drugs are not equivalent.[1]

Angiotensin-converting Enzyme Inhibitors

Evidence and experience with ACEi agents in severe HF now span almost three decades, dating from the CONSENSUS trial[2] and the SOLVD trial.[3] ACEis act more proximally in the renin–angiotensin–aldosterone system (RAAS) than ARBs and have distinctly different pharmacology. In addition to suppression of angiotensin II (Ang II) formation, some of the effects of ACE inhibitors may be related to the accumulation of kinins, particularly bradykinin, due to ACE inhibition.[4]

Clinical trial data in HFrEF patients show that ACEi treatment is associated with reduction in both mortality and hospitalizations across the spectrum of severity and in both ischemic and nonischemic patients. As a consequence, ACE inhibition remains the recommended first step in constructing a pharmacologic approach to HFrEF in both the American College of Cardiology/American Heart Association (ACC/AHA)[5] and European Society of Cardiology (ESC) 2016 guidelines[6] updates. On the other hand, ACE inhibition is associated with a more significant burden of adverse effects (Table 1).

BOX 1: Classes of pharmacologic agents available for heart failure treatment.

ACEi/ARB and sacubitril/valsartan:
- β-blockers and ivabradine
- Mineralocorticoid receptor antagonists
- Hydralazine-nitrates
- Loop-blocking diuretics
- Digitalis glycosides
- Antithrombotic agents: Antiplatelet agents, warfarin, and novel anticoagulants
- Agents specifically targeting pulmonary hypertension

(ACEi: angiotensin-converting enzyme inhibitors; ARB: angiotensin receptor blocker)

TABLE 1: Adverse effects of ACEis and ARBs.

	ACE Inhibitors	*ARBs*
Hypotension	✓	✓
Azotemia	✓	✓
Hyperkalemia Angioedema	✓	✓
Cough	✓	✓
Taste disorder		✓

(ACEi: angiotensin-converting enzyme inhibitors; ARB: angiotensin receptor blocker)

Angiotensin Receptor Blockers

As a class of therapeutic agents, the ARBs are remarkably well tolerated, however there is limited data directly comparing the safety and efficacy of an ACEi vs an ARB. The ONTARGET trial[7] involved more than 25,000 subjects in a three-way comparison of ramipril, telmisartan, or the combination in patients with vascular disease or high-risk diabetes. The primary composite outcome was death from cardiovascular (CV) causes, myocardial infarction (MI), stroke, or hospitalization for HF. The median follow-up was 56 months. The primary outcome occurred in 1,412 patients in the ramipril group (16.5%) compared with 1,423 patients in the telmisartan group [16.7%; relative risk (RR), 1.01; 95% confidence interval (CI), 0.94 to 1.09].

Compared with subjects in the ramipril group, those receiving telmisartan had less cough (1.1% vs 4.2%, P < 0.001) and angioedema (0.1% vs 0.3%, P = 0.01) and more hypotensive symptoms (2.6% vs 1.7%, P < 0.001); the occurrence of syncope was 0.2% in both groups (0.2%). Combination therapy with both active agents had no additional benefit and was associated with more adverse events and a greater number of total study discontinuations, including discontinuations due to hypotension and syncope.

With regard to treatment of HFpEF, in a meta-analysis of 30 studies that included 53,878 HFpEF patients, treatment with standard agents for HFpEF including ACEis and ARBs improved exercise tolerance but did not have the dramatic impact on mortality that is seen in HFrEF.[8] Since hypertension often plays a major role in the development of HFpEF, careful control of blood pressure in HFpEF with the use of ACEi or ARB agents as primary antihypertensives, may offer benefits.

Sacubitril/Valsartan (Angiotensin Receptor Blocker-neprilysin Inhibitor)

Natriuretic peptides (NPs), especially B-type natriuretic peptide (BNP), have primarily been regarded as biomarkers in heart failure (HF). However, they are also possible therapeutic agents due to their potentially beneficial physiological effects. The combination of sacubitril, a neprilysin inhibitor, and valsartan, an ARB, is a unique chemical entity, since the combination actually crystallizes in a fixed ratio. This agent represents a first of a new drug class, the combined angiotensin receptor blocker-neprilysin inhibitor or ARNI.[9]

The ARNI, sacubitril/valsartan, simultaneously augments the natriuretic peptide system (NPS) by inhibiting the enzyme neprilysin (NEP) and inhibits the RAAS by blocking the angiotensin II receptor.[9] The two major human NPs, atrial NP (ANP) and BNP, play an important counterregulatory role to the RAAS. ANP and BNP are cleared from the circulation by different mechanisms. BNP is largely cleared by cell surface clearance receptors. However, ANP is predominantly cleared by a circulating enzyme called neprilysin.

Sacubitril, an orally effective neprilysin inhibitor (NEPi), was described in 1995. Neprilysin inhibition with sacubitril is associated with increases in circulating ANP and the typical effects of ANP on CV physiology.[10] However, sacubitril also inhibits the degradation of angiotensin II and when administered as a single agent, it showed limited efficacy in the treatment of HF or high blood pressure.

In the large, randomized, double-blind PARADIGM-HF trial, replacement of an ACEi (enalapril) with sacubitril/valsartan resulted in a significant improvement in morbidity and mortality in patients with HFrEF. Sacubitril/valsartan was superior to enalapril in reducing the risk of CV death or HF hospitalization (composite primary endpoint) and all-cause death, and in limiting progression of HF. Sacubitril/valsartan was generally well tolerated, with a comparable safety profile to enalapril; symptomatic hypotension was more common with sacubitril/valsartan, whereas renal dysfunction, hyperkalemia, and cough were less common compared with enalapril. Sacubitril/valsartan was therefore found to be a superior alternative to ACE inhibitors/ARBs in the treatment of HFrEF, a recommendation that is reflected in many HF guidelines. It has recently been approved in the EU and the USA for the treatment of chronic HFrEF [New York Heart Association (NYHA) class II-IV].[11]

BETA-BLOCKERS AND IV ABRADINE

Beta (β)-adrenergic blocking agents have become widely accepted as first-line therapy for HFrEF over the last decade. The available β-blockers are B1 selective β-blockers and metabolic friendly bisoprolol, others are not selective B1 such as carvedilol, metoprolol succinate, which differ in their selectivity for adrenergic receptors and their effects on the peripheral circulation. In the absence of robust head-to-head trials, the potential differences in β-blockers for HFrEF were assessed using meta-analysis approaches. The network meta-analysis by Chatterjee et al. included 23,122 patients and showed, "no obvious differences when comparing the different β-blockers head-to-head for the risk of death, sudden cardiac death, death due to pump failure, or drug discontinuation". In addition, "improvements in left ventricular ejection fraction (LVEF) were also similar, irrespective of the individual study drug".[12]

Another meta-analysis of the impact of β-blockers on mortality and morbidity in HFpEF patients included 15 observational studies and two randomized control trials involving a total of 27,099 patients. In the observational studies, β-blockers were associated with lower all-cause mortality [RR 0.81 (0.72–0.90), P < 0.001] but not with reductions in HF hospitalization [RR 0.79 (0.57–1.10), P < 0.001]. Most importantly, in the randomized controlled trails (RCTs), β-blockers were not associated with improvement in all-cause mortality [RR 0.94 (0.67–1.32), P = 0.72] or rates of HF hospitalization [0.90 (0.54–1.49), P = 0.68].[13]

An elevated heart rate (HR), probably reflecting activation of the sympathetic nervous system, has been associated with worse CV outcomes. Although β-blockers reduce HR in HF treatment, uptitration of β-blockers can be associated with an increased risk of adverse reactions.[14,15] Ivabradine lowers HR by inhibiting the specific sinus node pacemaker. If current and does not adversely affect echocardiographic indices of LV function in patients with LV dysfunction.[16,17]

The SHIFT (Systolic HF Treatment with If Inhibitor Ivabradine) trial was an RCT with 6,558 patients with HFrEF (LVEF ≤ 35%) in sinus rhythm with HR ≥ 70 bpm.[18] In SHIFT, ivabradine significantly reduced the primary efficacy end-point, the composite of CV death or hospital admission for worsening HF and deaths due to HF.

MINERALOCORTICOID RECEPTOR ANTAGONISTS

In addition to Ang II, aldosterone is the other potent effector hormone of the RAAS. Aldosterone is a steroid hormone released primarily from the adrenal cortex in response to increased Ang II and increased plasma [K^+]. Aldosterone binds to a mineralocorticoid receptor (MR), and activation of the receptor is associated with increased salt and water reabsorption, increased blood volume, and alterations in ion-channel expression. The currently approved receptor antagonists, spironolactone and eplerenone, competitively inhibit aldosterone binding to MRs in the heart, kidney, and peripheral vasculature.

Mineralocorticoid Receptor Antagonists in HFrEF

The current ACC/AHA guidelines give MRAs a class 1 recommendation, level of evidence A for, "NYHA class II–IV HF and who have LVEF of 35% or less, unless contraindicated, to reduce morbidity and mortality. Patients with NYHA class II HF should have a history of prior CV hospitalization or elevated plasma natriuretic peptide levels to be considered for aldosterone receptor antagonists."[5] However, perhaps more than for any other pharmacologic approach to HF, the decision to employ an MRA for management of chronic HFrEF is complicated by comorbidities and polypharmacy, since treatment-related hyperkalemia is a significant concern.

All HF patients should have regular, frequent monitoring of electrolytes and renal function; however, this is particularly important in those receiving MRAs. In addition, patients should discontinue MRA therapy, if they experience diarrhea or dehydration, or while loop diuretic therapy is interrupted.

The major clinical differentiation between eplerenone and spironolactone is in their selectivity of aldosterone receptor antagonism, not their receptor blocking activity. The Randomized Aldactone Evaluation Study (RALES) trial randomized 822 HFrEF patients to receive 25 mg of spironolactone daily, and 841 to receive placebo (27% of both groups were female). There was a 32% reduction in the risk of the composite end-point of death from cardiac causes or hospitalization for cardiac causes in the spironolactone group compared with the placebo group (RR, 0.68; 95% CI, 0.59 to 0.78; P < 0.001). Serious hyperkalemia occurred in 14 spironolactone patients vs 10 patients in the placebo group. However, gynecomastia or breast pain was reported by 10% of the men in the spironolactone group vs 1% of the men in the placebo group (P < 0.001), with the result that more men in the spironolactone group discontinued treatment (10 vs 1, P = 0.006).[19]

In the Eplerenone Post-Acute Myocardial Infarction Heart Failure Efficacy and Survival Study (EPHESUS), 6,642 patients were randomized to eplerenone (25 mg per day) or matching placebo for 4 weeks, then the eplerenone dose was increased to a maximum of 50 mg per day. 885 patients in the eplerenone group (26.7%) and 993 patients in the placebo group (30.0%) had an end-point event, death from CV causes or hospitalization for CV events (RR, 0.87; P = 0.002). The incidence of gynecomastia in males was 0.5% and 0.6% for eplerenone and control patients, respectively.[20]

A systematic review and meta-analysis of eight trials involving 3,929 patients concluded that MRAs were superior to the control for reduction of all-cause mortality (RR 0.79, 95% CI 0.66, 0.95) and in reduction of rehospitalization for cardiac causes (RR 0.62, 95% CI 0.52, 0.74, P = 0.52).[21] In a detailed review of the literature aimed at integrating evidence into clinical practice, a group of expert trialists concluded that "The morbidity and mortality benefits of MRAs may be mediated by several proposed actions, including antifibrotic mechanisms that slow HF progression, prevent or reverse cardiac remodeling, or reduce arrhythmogenesis. Both eplerenone and spironolactone have demonstrated survival benefits in individual clinical trials. Pharmacologic differences exist between the drugs, which may be relevant for therapeutic decision making in individual patients. Although serious hyperkalemia events were reported in the major MRA clinical trials, these risks can be mitigated through appropriate patient selection, dose selection, patient education, monitoring, and follow-up. When used appropriately, MRAs significantly improve outcomes across the spectrum of patients with HFrEF."[22]

Mineralocorticoid Receptor Antagonists in HFpEF

A meta-analysis that included 11 randomized controlled trials with 942 participants (weighted mean follow-up of 9.1 ± 3.0 months) assessed the impact of MRA therapy on echocardiographic parameters, surrogate measures for myocardial fibrosis [markers of collagen turnover such as carboxy-terminal peptide of procollagen type I (PICP) and amino-terminal peptide of procollagen type II (PIIINP)], and surrogate clinical outcomes (exercise capacity and serum potassium levels) in patients with HFpEF or asymptomatic left ventricular diastolic dysfunction (LVDD). Six trials included patients with symptomatic HFpEF and five included patients with asymptomatic LVDD and/or LVH. Eight of the trials used spironolactone; two used eplerenone and one used canrenone. The principal findings were that MRA therapy was associated with improved diastolic function, blood pressure, and markers of myocardial fibrosis without significant changes in indexed LV mass or LV cavity size.[23]

These positive findings with surrogate end-points in HFpEF provided the rationale for the Treatment of Preserved Cardiac Function Heart Failure With an Aldosterone Antagonist (TOPCAT) trial. TOPCAT randomized 3,445 patients to spironolactone or placebo: 1,767 in North and South America (United States, Canada, Brazil, and Argentina) and 1,678 in Russia and the Republic of Georgia. The primary efficacy outcome was the composite of CV death aborted cardiac arrest, or hospitalization for HF. In the patients randomized from North and South America, this end-point occurred in 11.5 of 100 patients per year, while in patients from Russia and Georgia, it was only 2.4 of 100 patients per year.[24]

HYDRALAZINE/NITRATES

Hydralazine (H) and nitrates (Ns), when combined, have been shown to reduce morbidity and mortality in some trials of chronic heart failure (CHF). A systematic review of randomized trials assessing the effects of H and N in CHF, with end-points of all-cause mortality and cardiovascular mortality considered was published recently. [25]

In seven trials evaluating H and N in 2,626 patients, combination therapy reduced all-cause mortality (OR 0.72; 95% CI 0.55–0.95; P = 0.02), and cardiovascular mortality (OR 0.75; 95% CI 0.57–0.99; P = 0.04) compared to placebo. However, when compared to ACEis, combination therapy was associated with higher all-cause mortality (OR 1.35; 95% CI 1.03–1.76; P = 0.03), and cardiovascular mortality (OR 1.37; 95% CI 1.04–1.81; P = 0.03). For N alone, ten trials including 375 patients reported all-cause mortality and showed a trend to harm (13 deaths in those assigned to nitrates and 7 to placebo; OR 2.13; 95% CI 0.88–5.13; P = 0.09). For H alone, three trials showed no difference in all-cause mortality compared to placebo (OR 0.96; 95% CI 0.37–2.47; P = 0.93), and two trials suggested inferiority to ACEI (OR 2.28; 95% CI 1.03–5.04; P = 0.04). In conclusion, "compared to placebo, H and N reduces mortality in patients with CHF. Whether race or background therapy influences benefit is uncertain, but on direct comparison H and N appears inferior to ACEi. There is little evidence to support the use of either drug alone in CHF, according to the authors.

DIURETICS

Thiazide diuretics are a cornerstone of antihypertensive treatment, and thus in the management of Stage A and B HF, both HFrEF and HFpEF. Among the thiazide diuretics, hydrochlorothiazide and chlorthalidone, recent evidence may suggest that chlorthalidone is a more effective agent. In the antihypertensive and Lipid-lowering Treatment to Prevent Heart Attack Trial (ALLHAT),[26] a randomized, double-blind, active-controlled clinical trial, a total of 33,357 participants aged 55 years or older with hypertension and at least one other CHD risk factor were randomized to treatment with chlorthalidone, 12.5–25 mg/day (n = 15,255); amlodipine, 2.5–10 mg/day (n = 9048); or lisinopril, 10–40 mg/ day (n = 9054) for planned follow-up of approximately 4–8 years. The primary outcome was combined fatal CHD or nonfatal MI, analyzed by intent-to-treat. Systolic blood pressure was lower with chlorthalidone, and the primary outcome occurred in 2,956 participants, with no difference between treatments.

In a network analysis of nine randomized, controlled comparisons (n = 78,350) in which either hydrochlorothiazide or chlorthalidone was used as the base diuretic, chlorthalidone was associated with a 21% highly significant ($P < 0.0001$) reduction in CV events.[27]

DIGOXIN

Digoxin is one of the oldest compounds used in cardiovascular medicine. Positive inotropic and neurohormonal modulation properties are attributed to digoxin, and it was the mainstay of heart failure therapeutics for decades. However, since the institution of β-blockers and aldosterone antagonists as part of modern heart failure medical therapy, digoxin prescription rates have reduced. The fact that digoxin is still listed as a valid therapeutic option in both American and European Heart Failure guidelines has not altered clinicians' attitude toward the drug. Since the publication of original Digitalis Investigation Group trial data, a series of reports based predominately on observational studies and post hoc analyses have raised concerns about the clinical efficacy and long-term safety of digoxin. [28]

The most recent results from the Polish part of ESC Heart Failure Long-term Registry showed that digoxin is associated with increased risk of death in HFrEF patients without AF history receiving the guideline-directed treatment. However, the authors indicate that digoxin seems to be employed in patients with worse clinical status, which may at least partial explain its association with increased risk of death.[29]

CONCLUSION

Heart failure is one of the most common causes of hospitalization, hospital readmission, and death. Patients with HF have many complications, with multiple coexisting diagnoses, which result in polypharmacy. Improved self-management will increase compliance, promote patient quality-of-life, advance clinical outcomes, reduce hospital readmission, and will decrease hospitalization costs.

REFERENCES

1. Ferrari R, Rosano GM. Not just numbers, but years of science: putting the ACE inhibitor-ARB meta-analyses into context. Int J Cardiol. 2013;166(2):286-8.
2. The CONSENSUS Trial Study Group. Effects of enalapril on mortality in severe congestive heart failure. Results of the Cooperative North Scandinavian Enalapril Survival Study. N Engl J Med. 1987;316:1429-35.
3. The SOLVD Investigators. Effect of enalapril on survival in patients with reduced left ventricular ejection fractions and congestive heart failure. N Engl J Med. 1991;325:293-302.
4. Dezsi CA. Differences in the clinical effects of angiotensin converting enzyme inhibitors and angiotensin receptor blockers: a critical review of the evidence. Am J Cardiovasc Drugs. 2014;14:167-73.
5. Yancy CW, Jessup M, Bozkurt B, et al. 2017 ACC/AHA/HFSA Focused Update of the 2013 ACCF/AHA Guideline for the Management of Heart Failure: A Report of the American College of Cardiology/American Heart Association Task Force on Clinical Practice Guidelines and the Heart Failure Society of America. Circulation. 2017;136(6):e137-61.
6. Ponikowski P, Voors AA, Anker SD, et al. Authors/Task Force members; Document Reviewers. 2016 ESC Guidelines for the diagnosis and treatment of acute and chronic heart failure. The Task Force for the diagnosis and treatment of acute and chronic heart failure of the European Society of Cardiology (ESC). Developed with the special contribution of the Heart Failure Association (HFA) of the ESC. Eur J Heart Fail. 2016;18(8):891-975.
7. Yusuf S, Teo KK, Pogue J, et al. Telmisartan, ramipril, or both in patients at high risk for vascular events. N Engl J Med. 2008;358(15):1547-59.
8. Holland DJ, Kumbhani DJ, Ahmed SH, et al. Effects of treatment on exercise tolerance, cardiac function, and mortality in heart failure with preserved ejection fraction. J Am Coll Cardiol. 2011;57:1676-86.
9. Singh JSS, Burrell LM, Cherif M, et al. Sacubitril/valsartan: beyond natriuretic peptides. Heart. 2017;103(20):1569-77.
10. Ksander GM, Ghai RD, deJesus R, et al. Dicarboxylic acid dipeptide neutral endopeptidase inhibitors. J Med Chem. 1995;38:1689-1700.
11. Marques da Silva P, Aguiar C. Sacubitril/valsartan: An important piece in the therapeutic puzzle of heart failure. Rev Port Cardiol. 2017;36(9):655-668.
12. Chatterjee S, Biondi-Zoccai G, Abbate A, et al. Benefits of β-blockers in patients with heart failure and reduced ejection fraction: network meta-analysis. BMJ. 2013;346:55.
13. Bavishi C, Chatterjee S, Ather S, et al. Beta-blockers in heart failure with preserved ejection fraction: a meta-analysis. Heart Fail Rev. 2015;20(2):193-201.
14. Böhm M, Swedberg K, Komajda M, et al. Heart rate as a risk factor in chronic heart failure (SHIFT): the association between heart rate and outcomes in a randomised placebo-controlled trial. Lancet. 2010;376(9744):886-94.
15. Butler J, Arbogast PG, BeLue R, et al. Outpatient adherence to beta-blocker therapy after acute myocardial infarction. J Am Coll Cardiol. 2002;40(9):1589-95.
16. Borer JS, Fox K, Jaillon P, et al. Antianginal and anti-ischemic effects of ivabradine, an I (f) inhibitor, in stable angina: a randomized, double-blind, multicentered, placebo-controlled trial. Circulation. 2003;107(6):817-23.
17. Manz M, Reuter M, Lauck G, et al. A single intravenous dose of ivabradine, a novel I(f) inhibitor, lowers heart rate but does not depress left ventricular function in patients with left ventricular dysfunction. Cardiology. 2003;100(3):149-55.
18. Swedberg K, Komajda M, Böhm M, et al. Ivabradine and outcomes in chronic heart failure (SHIFT): a randomized placebo-controlled study. Lancet. 2010;376(9744):875-85.
19. Pitt B, Zannad F, Remme WJ, et al. Randomized Aldactone Evaluation Study Investigators. The effect of spironolactone

on morbidity and mortality in patients with severe heart failure. N Engl J Med. 1999;341:709-17.
20. Pitt B, Remme W, Zannad F, et al. Eplerenone Post-acute Myocardial Infarction Heart Failure Efficacy and Survival Study Investigators. Eplerenone, a selective aldosterone blocker, in patients with left ventricular dysfunction after myocardial infarction. N Engl J Med. 2003;348(14):1309-21.
21. Hu L, Chen Y, Deng S, et al. Additional use of an aldosterone antagonist in patients with mild to moderate chronic heart failure: a systematic review and meta-analysis. Br J Clin Pharmacol. 2012;75:1202-12.
22. Zannad F, Gattis Stough W, Rossignol P, et al. Mineralocorticoid receptor antagonists for heart failure with reduced ejection fraction: integrating evidence into clinical practice. Eur Heart J. 2012;33:2782-95.
23. Pandey A, Garg S, Matulevicius SA, et al. Effect of mineralocorticoid receptor antagonists on cardiac structure and function in patients with diastolic dysfunction and heart failure with preserved ejection fraction: a meta-Analysis and systematic review. J Am Heart Assoc. 2015;4:e002137.
24. Pitt B, Pfeffer MA, Assmann SF, et al. TOPCAT Investigators. Spironolactone for heart failure with preserved ejection fraction. N Engl J Med. 2014;370(15):1383-92.
25. Farag M, Mabote T, Shoaib A, et al. Hydralazine and nitrates alone or combined for the management of chronic heart failure: A systematic review. Int J Cardiol. 2015;196: 61-9.
26. ALLHAT Officers and Coordinators for the ALLHAT Collaborative Research Group. The Antihypertensive and Lipid-lowering Treatment to Prevent Heart Attack Trial. Major outcomes in high-risk hypertensive patients randomized to angiotensin-converting enzyme inhibitor or calcium channel blocker vs diuretic: The Antihypertensive and Lipid-lowering Treatment to Prevent Heart Attack Trial (ALLHAT). JAMA. 2002;288(23):2981-97.
27. Roush GC, Holford TR, Guddati AK. Chlorthalidone compared with hydrochlorothiazide in reducing cardiovascular events: systematic review and network meta-analyses. Hypertension. 2012; 59:1110-7.
28. Konstantinou DM, Karvounis H, Giannakoulas G. Digoxin in Heart Failure with a Reduced Ejection Fraction: A Risk Factor or a Risk Marker. Cardiology. 2016;134(3):311-9.
29. Migaj J, Kałużna-Oleksy M, Nessler J, et al. Impact of digoxin on risk of death in heart failure patients treated with β-blockers. Results from Polish part of ESC Heart Failure Long-Term Registry. Kardiol Pol. 2018;76(7):1064-72.

Nonpharmacologic Therapies in Heart Failure

Girish MP, Mohit D Gupta, Rajni Saijpaul

INTRODUCTION

The prevalence of heart failure is increasing worldwide, particularly in patients <50 years of age.[1,2] The prevalence of heart failure with preserved ejection fraction (HFpEF) is rising faster than the heart failure with reduced ejection fraction (HFrEF).[3] Heart Failure in younger patients has been largely attributed to an increase burden of risk factors, mainly obesity and its comorbidities and in India rheumatic heart disease.[2,4] Modern lifestyle includes unhealthy food choices (poor-quality diet and increased caloric intake), sedentary lifestyle, and high levels of mental stress. These are probably contributing to the rapidly changing epidemiology of heart failure.[5] The evidence for prevention of development of heart failure is stronger than for treatment of established heart failure. Despite this, lifestyle changes can be effective through the different stages of heart failure. The evidence for lifestyle changes is limited.

NONPHARMACOLOGICAL STRATEGIES

The lifestyle disorders at risk for development of heart failure include hypertension, diabetes mellitus and coronary artery disease.

Diet in Heart Failure Prevention

Diets containing larger amounts of plant-based foods like fruits, vegetables, nuts, seeds, legumes are beneficial for both coronary artery disease as well as heart failure prevention.[6-9] Men who consumed more vegetables and fruits were at a lower risk of developing heart failure in the Physician's Health Study.[10] At the other end, animal products like red meat, cheese, and eggs appear to increase the risk for myocardial infarction, stroke, heart failure and death.[11] In randomized controlled trials, high vegetable and fruit intake have been linked to improved cardiovascular outcomes.[12] DASH (Dietary Approaches to Stop Hypertension) diet is associated with reduction in blood pressure and reduced incidence of heart failure in men and women in two large prospective Swedish cohorts.[13] In women who had greater adherence to Mediterranean style diet (more vegetables, fruits, nuts, whole grains, legumes, fish, and low in red meat) is associated with lower heart failure risk.[14] Dietary approaches with healthy eating patterns like plant-based diet, whole grains, Mediterranean diet, and DASH diets may offer protection from development of heart failure. The evidence is only modest.

Sodium Restriction

Adherence to the DASH diet, which advocates salt reduction, was inversely proportional to heart failure incidence.[13] Meta-analysis and trials provide strong scientific support for salt restriction to prevent hypertension, stroke and cardiovascular disease but whether sodium restriction specifically reduces the incidence of heart failure are lacking.[13,15,16] However, population-based studies have demonstrated an association between higher salt intake and an increased incidence of heart failure.[17] The American Heart Association (AHA) recommends limiting dietary sodium intake to <1,500 mg/day.[18] In patients with known heart failure, the Heart failure Society of America guidelines recommend dietary sodium restriction to 2–3 g/day.[19] In the 2013 AHA/American College of Cardiology guidelines for the management of heart failure, sodium restriction is considered reasonable (Class IIa recommendation) for patients with symptomatic heart failure to reduce congestive symptoms.[20] However, adherence to dietary sodium restriction is poor. In one analysis, only 34% of patients consumed <2,000 mg/day of salt.[21] Evidence is adequate to support sodium restriction to prevent hypertension, stroke and cardiovascular disease. Also, there is strong link between hypertension and heart failure and hence it is reasonable to recommend limitation of salt intake.

Dietary Antioxidants and Nutritional Supplements

Deficiencies of micronutrients like selenium and zinc have been shown in patients with heart failure.[22,23] The use of antioxidant supplements has not been effective in prevention of coronary artery disease and has not been well studied for heart failure. Some of the supplements which have been studied are coenzyme Q10, L-carnitine, taurine, thiamine, and other B vitamins. Amongst these, coenzyme Q10 has a stronger evidence for use than for other supplements and is one of the dietary therapies, which has been directly studied in stage C to D heart failure. Coenzyme Q is present in food, but the quantity in which it is present is insufficient to affect heart failure incidence or progression. Meta-analysis of RCTs with coenzyme Q10 in heart failure have indicated a positive effect on ejection fraction with or without associated improvement in New York Heart Association (NYHA) functional class. These studies were small, heterogeneous, and lacked information on clinically relevant endpoints like mortality.[24-26] The Q-SYMBIO RCT that included 420 patients with NYHA class III or IV heart failure, coenzyme Q10 supplementation over 2 years was associated with significantly lower major adverse cardiovascular events, cardiovascular death, urgent cardiac transplantation, mechanical support, total mortality, heart failure-related hospitalizations and improvement in functional class.[27] Genetic causes of carnitine deficiency are associated with cardiomyopathy and reduced L-carnitine content has been documented in the failing heart.[28] Studies of L-carnitine supplementation in the doses ranging from 1.5 g/day to 6 g/day and with a follow-up periods lasting from 7 days to 3 years showed benefits on cardiac remodeling after myocardial infarction, increase in exercise capacity, improvement in ejection fraction, and improved clinical outcomes in patients with heart failure.[29-31] However, these studies are small and heterogeneous in nature and there is little to no evidence for the use of L-carnitine supplements in the prevention of heart failure.

Prolonged treatment of heart failure with diuretics, especially in large doses may be associated with thiamine deficiency.[32] Repletion of thiamine in such patients has been associated with improvement in left ventricular (LV) function in one study[33] but other studies have shown mixed results.[34,35] There is lack of studies on the effects of routing vitamin B supplementation in patients with heart failure or at risk for heart failure. Deficient vitamin D levels have been in reported in heart failure patients and have been correlated with the severity of heart failure.[36,37] Studies of vitamin D supplementation involving a small number of vitamin D-deficient patients have shown to improve left ventricular ejection fraction in the elderly, decrease serum aldosterone levels and improve NYHA functional capacity.[38,39]

Exercise Training and Physical Rehabilitation

The beneficial effects on health due to physical activity are multifactorial in nature.[40] The "2013 AHA/ACC Guideline on Lifestyle Management to Reduce Cardiovascular Risk" recommends 40 minutes of moderate-to-vigorous activity 3–4 days/week to help control BP and to improve blood cholesterol levels.[41] Exercise training has been proven to be efficacious in HFrEF as well as in HFpEF. In the randomized trial (HF-ACTION), exercise (consisting of 36 supervised sessions followed by home-based training) did not significantly affect all-cause mortality or all-cause hospitalization; however, there was a reduction in mortality seen after adjustment for covariates. In subanalysis, exercise training in women with heart failure was associated with a larger reduction in rate of the combined endpoint of all-cause mortality and hospital stay than in men.[42,43] In HFpEF, the data is not so encouraging for physical training. However, recent evidence suggests that HFpEF patients had greater peak VO2 improvement in response to 16-week supervised moderate intensity endurance training compared with those with HFrEF.[44] Exercise training is strongly associated with reduced incident heart failure in HFrEF and HFpEF. However, survival benefit is seen only with HFrEF.

Yoga and Meditation

Yoga mediates its beneficial effects by increasing the parasympathetic and reducing the sympathetic activities.[45] In a meta-analysis, there was a 22% improvement in VO2 in the intervention group. The quality of life indices also improved by 24% in the yoga group.[46] Yoga should be offered to all patients with heart failure. A pooled analysis from two studies in patients with hypertension, meditation was associated with 30% relative risk reduction in cardiovascular mortality and 23% relative risk reduction in all-cause mortality.[47] In HFrEF, meditation improved 6 minutes' walk test, depression scores, and quality of life indices but there was no effect on death or hospitalization at 1 year.[48]

Weight Management in Obese Patients

There is a dose-dependent relationship between increasing weight and risk of heart failure.[49] Aiming for a body weight < 30.0 kg/m^2 over an average period of 21.5 years in older adults was associated with an adjusted hazard ratio of 0.70 for heart failure development[50] making it one of the most important goal in the prevention of heart failure. A minimum of 10% reduction in body weight is necessary to achieve a favorable effect in reducing the risk of developing heart failure or reducing hospitalizations.[51] A significant amount of sustained weight loss is achieved through bariatric surgery. This has been associated with reduction in LV mass as well as in reduction in new cases of heart failure.[52] Hence we can safely conclude that maintaining a normal body weight is strongly protective against development of heart failure.

Vaccination in Heart Failure

Vaccination per se does fit in the pharmacological management of heart failure. However, it is yet find its place as a standard of care. Looking into the importance of vaccination which might be a low-cost treatment, it is discussed in this section on heart failure. Influenza is a serious health hazard for a patient with heart failure, however very little is known about the association between vaccination against influenza and outcomes in patients with heart failure. In their editorial, Adam D DeVore and Ankeet S Bhatt mentioned that >50% of heart failure decompensation is triggered by a respiratory infection.[53] Influenza vaccination is grossly underutilized as reported in a Cohort study Daniel Modin et al.[54] The vaccine coverage in the study ranged from 16% to 54% during the study period. Annual vaccination, vaccination early in the year (September to October) and greater cumulative number of vaccinations were associated with larger reductions in the risk of death compared to intermittent vaccination. The post hoc analysis of the PARADIGM-HF trial demonstrated that influenza vaccination was associated with a lower risk for all-cause mortality, whereas in propensity adjusted models, the composite outcome of cardiovascular death and heart failure hospitalization did not reach statistical significance.[55] With regard to the clinical outcomes of pneumococcal vaccination in heart failure patients, there is a paucity of high level of evidence that requires further research.

Nonpharmacologic Therapies in Acute Heart Failure

Acute heart failure (AHF) constitutes a heterogeneous syndrome of signs and symptoms of new onset or gradual/rapidly worsening heart failure. AHF has a complex pathophysiology.[56] Despite recent advances in pharmacological management, its morbidity and mortality remain high. As a result, in addition to pharmacologic therapies, nonpharmacologic therapies are being developed and increasingly used. Some of the non-pharmacologic therapies are:

- *Positive airway pressure (both invasive and noninvasive)*: One of the valuable nonpharmacological tools in the management of AHF is positive airway pressure (PAP). PAP has effects on both circulatory system (reduces systemic venous system and right ventricular unloading by increase in intrathoracic pressure, changes in total systemic vascular resistance)[57,58] and respiratory system (prevention of alveolar collapse, shift of fluid back from interstitial and alveolar space to pulmonary circulation and reduction in respiratory muscle load).[59]

  One of the most often used PAP method is by noninvasive ventilation. Noninvasive positive pressure ventilation (NPPV) should be encouraged to alleviate signs and symptoms of respiratory distress due to cardiogenic pulmonary edema. NPPV is achieved either through continuous PAP (CPAP) or bilevel PAP. Evidences suggest that noninvasive ventilation improves symptoms and physiological variables, reducing rates of invasive ventilation and mortality in selected patients.[60,61] Currently, there is still uncertainty regarding the real prognostic impact of noninvasive ventilation. European guidelines generally recommend the use of NPPV therapy in AHF patients with a respiratory rate >20 breaths/min and signs of pulmonary edema without shock (recommendation IIa B).[62]
- *Ultrafiltration*: Congestion and fluid retention is the hallmark of heart failure and is a primary cause of hospital admissions in about 90% of the patients. These patients have higher neurohumoral activation, cellular dysregulation, and increase in oxidative stress.[63] The optimum method for achieving successful decongestion is an area of intensive research. Also successful treatment of congestion cannot simply be translated into clinical improvement. Peripheral venovenous ultrafiltration, a mechanical strategy to remove fluid has emerged as an adjunctive/alternative modality to diuretic therapy in patients with AHF. It allows for an effective removal of sodium and water across a semi-permeable membrane in response to a transmembrane gradient driven by the hydrostatic pressure difference. Ultrafiltration removes more sodium (than potassium) than diuretics for an equivalent volume loss.[64] The mechanism underlying the long-term positive effect of ultrafiltration remains unclear. There is a scarcity of vigorous clinical trials in the field of ultrafiltration therapy for AHF. Most of the studies are retrospective involving small study population without controls and with a short follow-up.

The RAPID-CHF trial was the first randomized control trial with only 48 patients. For the primary endpoint of weight loss at 24 hours, there was no significant difference between groups. However, fluid removal after 24 hours and dyspnea and heart failure symptoms at 48 hours, were significantly improved with ultrafiltration.[65] The UNLOAD trial is the largest trial that randomized 200 patients with AHF to either ultrafiltration or loop diuretic therapy within 24 hours of admission. The UNLOAD trial showed a decrease in rehospitalization for heart failure with ultrafiltration compared with diuretic therapy. However, there was a trend toward worsening renal function in the ultrafiltration group.[66]

The safety and efficacy of ultrafiltration depend upon the ability to remove fluid without causing hemodynamic instability and worsening renal function. To achieve this goal, the amount and rate of fluid removal must be clearly established. A safe way of doing this is ultrafiltration should be initiated at low ultrafiltration rates, i.e. 100–200 mL/hr.

- *Mechanical circulatory support*: The rationale in using mechanical circulatory support (MCS) in patients with cardiogenic shock is to restore adequate systemic perfusion, systemic pressure, and gaining time to ventricular recovery (as acute myocardial infarction is the single largest cause of cardiogenic shock). The roles of MCS can be the following:
  - Bridge to transplantation
  - Destination therapy: An alternative for patients contraindicated for a heart transplantation
  - Bridge to recovery
  - Bridge to bridge: For those patients who present with severe shock or following cardiac arrest and are supported with a temporary device to evaluate, if they could become candidates for long-term support
  - Bridge to decision: Used when the best option for a given patient is unclear at the time of device implantation.

An ideal device is the one which would provide both hemodynamic support and myocardial protection. At present the available devices for MCS are—intra-aortic balloon pump (IABP), extracorporeal life support (ECLS) and ventricular assist devices (VADs). Current European guidelines recommend the use of percutaneous assist device to provide for a quick and easy initiation, with no preference for device selection (recommendation IIa C).[67]

The major determinants of success are timing of device implantation and patient selection. IABP is the most commonly used and less expensive form of MCS. It helps in improving peak diastolic pressure and coronary blood flow while reducing afterload and myocardial oxygen consumption.[68] The venoarterial configuration of ECLS can completely replace cardiopulmonary function and is indicated in the severe form of cardiogenic shock and refractory cardiac arrest. Blood is withdrawn via the venous system (femoral vein or right atrium) and pumped through an oxygenator, where gas exchange takes place. It is then returned to the arterial system (femoral artery or ascending aorta).[69] VADs are flow pumps connected to the patient's circulation that replace the function of either left heart, right heart or both. The 2014 European Society of Cardiology and the European Association for CardioThoracic Surgery guidelines on myocardial revascularization recommend left VAD implantation in younger patients with no contraindication for cardiac transplantation as a bridge to transplantation and in patients not eligible for transplantation as a bridge to recovery or with the goal of destination therapy.[70]

CONCLUSION

Heart failure incidence is rising by the day due the increasing prevalence of lifestyle disorders like hypertension, diabetes and coronary artery disease. Nonpharmacological management of these lifestyle disorders especially weight management, salt restriction, and exercise training have shown to prevent the development of heart failure in stage A heart failure. Evidence for routine antioxidant supplement is limited and is seen with only coenzyme Q10. Vaccination (against influenza) though underutilized if used annually and regularly is associated with reduced risk of both all cause mortality and cardiovascular mortality. Non-pharmacological management of AHF is being used increasingly to complement the established pharmacological management that includes IV diuretics and the other drugs in the treatment of AHF.

REFERENCES

1. Christiansen MN, Kober L, Jeppensen J, et al. Age specific trends in incidence, mortality and comorbidities of heart failure in Denmark, 1995 to 2012. Circulation. 2017;135: 1214-23.
2. Seth S, Khanal S, Ramakrishnan S, et al. Epidemiology of acute decompensated heart failure in India: The AFAR study (Acute Failure Registry Study). J Pract Cardiovasc Sci. 2015;1:35.
3. Oktay AA, Rich JD, Shah SJ. The emerging epidemic of heart failure with preserved ejection fraction. Curr Heart Fail Rep. 2013;10:401-10.
4. Rosamond WD, Johnson A. Trends in heart failure incidence in the community: a gathering storm. Circulation. 2017;135:1224-6.
5. Andersson C, Vasan RS. Epidemiology of cardiovascular disease in young individuals. Nat Rev Cardiol. 2018;15: 230-40.

6. Micha R, Penalvo JL, Cudhea F, et al. Association between dietary factors and mortality from heart disease, stroke and type 2 diabetes in the United States. JAMA. 2017;317:912-24.
7. Barnard ND, Levin SM, Yokoyama Y. A systematic review and meta-analysis of changes in body weight in clinical trials of vegetarian diets. J Acad Nutr Diet. 2015;115:954-69.
8. Wang F, Zheng J, Yan B, et al. Effects of vegetarian diets on blood lipids. A systematic review and meta-analysis of randomized controlled trials. J Am Heart Assoc. 2015;4:e002408.
9. Yokoyama Y, Nishimura K, Barnard ND, et al. Vegetarian diets and blood pressure: a meta analysis. JAMA Intern Med. 2014;174:577-87.
10. Djousse L, Driver JA, Gaziano JM. Relation between modifiable lifestyle factors and lifetime risk of heart failure. JAMA. 2009;302:394-400.
11. Tang WH, Hazen SL. The contributory role of gut microbiota in cardiovascular disease. J Clin Invest. 2014;124:4204-11.
12. Miller V, Mente A, Dehghan M, et al. Fruit, vegetable, and legume intake and cardiovascular disease and deaths in 18 countries (PURE): a prospective cohort study. Lancet. 2017;100:320S-8S.
13. Levitan EB, Wolk A, Mittleman MA. Consistency with DASH diet and incidence of heart failure. Arch Intern Med. 2009;169:851-7.
14. Tektonidis TG, Akesson A, Gigante B, et al. A Mediterranean diet and risk of myocardial infarction, heart failure and stroke: a population based cohort study. Atherosclerosis. 2015;243:93-8.
15. He FJ, MacGregor GA. Salt reduction lowers cardiovascular risk: meta-analysis of outcome trials. Lancet. 2011;378:380-2.
16. Cook NR, Appel LJ, Whelton PK. Lower levels of sodium intake and reduced cardiovascular risk. Circulation. 2014;129:981-9.
17. He J, Ogden LG, Bazzano LA, et al. Dietary sodium intake and incidence of congestive heart failure in overweight US men and women. First National Health and Nutrition Examination Survey epidemiologic follow up. Arch Intern Med. 2002;162:1619-24.
18. Whelton PK, Appel LJ, Sacco RL, et al. Sodium, Blood pressure, and cardiovascular disease: further evidence supporting the American Heart Association sodium reduction recommendations. Circulation. 2012;126:2880-9.
19. Lindenfeld J, Albert NM, Boehmer JP, et al. for the Heart Failure Society of America. HFSA 2010 comprehensive heart failure practice guideline. J Card Fail. 2010;16:e1-194.
20. Yancy CW, Jessup M, Bozkurt B, et al. 2013 ACC/AHA guidelines for the management of heart failure: a report of the American College of Cardiology Foundation/American Heart Association Task Force on practice guidelines. J Am Coll Cardiol. 2013;62:e147-239.
21. Lemon SC, Olendzki B, Magner R, et al. The dietary quality of persons with, heart failure in NHANES 1999-2006. J Gen Intern Med. 2010;25:135-40.
22. Saliba W, Fakih RE, Shaheen W. Heart failure secondary to selenium deficiency, reversible after supplementation. Int J Cardiol. 2010;141:26-7.
23. Ripa S, Ripa R, Giustiniani S. Are failure cardiomyopathies a zinc deficit related disease? A study on Zn and Cu in patients with chronic failure dilated and hypertrophic cardiomyopathies. Minerva Med. 1998;89:397-403.
24. Fotino AD, Thompson Paul AM, Bazzano LA. Effect of coenzyme Q10 supplementation on heart failure: A meta-analysis. Am J Clin Nutr. 2013;97:268-75.
25. Sharma A, Fonarow GC, Butler J, et al. Coenzyme q10 for heart failure. Cochrane Database Syst Rev. 2014;6:e002639.
26. Madmani ME, Yusuf Solaiman A, et al. Coenzyme q10 for heart failure. Cochrane Database Syst Rev. 2014:CD008684.
27. Mortensen SA, Rosenfeldt F, Kumar A, et al. The effect of coenzyme q10 on morbidity and mortality in chronic heart failure: results from Q-SYMBIO: a randomized double blind trial. J Am Coll Cardiol HF. 2014;2:641-9.
28. Soukoulis V, Dihu JB, Sole M, et al. Micronutrient deficiencies an unmet need in heart failure. J Am Coll Cardiol. 2009;54:1660-73.
29. Iliceto S, Scrutinio D, Bruzzi P, et al. Effects of L-Carnitine Administration on Left Ventricular Remodeling After Acute Anterior Myocardial Infarction: The L-Carnitine Ecocardiografia Digitalizzata Infarto Miocardico (CEDIM) Trial. J Am Coll Cardiol. 1995;26(2):380-7.
30. Anand I, Chandrashekhan Y, De Giuli F, et al. Acute and chronic effects of propionyl l carnitine on the hemodynamics, exercise capacity and hormones in patients with congestive heart failure. Cardiovasc Drugs Ther. 1998;12:291-9.
31. Rizos I. Three-year survival of patients with heart failure caused by dilated cardiomyopathy and l-carnitine administration. Am Heart J. 2000;139(2 Pt 3):S120-3.
32. Hanninen SA, Darling PB, Sole MJ, et al. The prevalence of thiamine deficiency in hospitalized patients with congestive heart failure. J Am Coll Cardiol. 2006;47:354-61.
33. Shimon I, Almog S, Vered Z, et al. Improved Left ventricular function after thiamine supplementation in patients with congestive heart failure receiving long term furosemide therapy. Am J Med. 1995;98:485-90.
34. Pfitzenmeyer P, Guilland JC, d'Athis P, et al. Thiamine status of elderly patients with cardiac failure including the effects of supplementation. Int J Vitam Nutr Res. 1994;64:113-8.
35. Smithline H. Thiamine for the treatment of acute decompensated heart failure. Am J Emerg Med. 2007;25:124-6.
36. Zittermann A, Schleithoff SS, Tenderich G, et al. Low Vitamin D status: a contributing factor in the pathogenesis of congestive heart failure? J Am Coll Cardiol. 2003;41:105-12.
37. Belen E, Tipi FF, Aykan AC, et al. Clinical staging in chronic heart failure associate with low vitamin D and elevated parathormone levels. Acta Cardiol. 2014; 69:665-71.
38. Dalbeni ASG, Degan M, Minuz P, et al. Effects of six months of vitamin D supplementation in patients with heart failure: a randomized double-blind controlled trial. Nutr Metab Cardiovasc Dis. 2014;24:861-8.
39. Boxer RS, Hoit BD, Schmotzer BJ, et al. The effect of vitamin D on aldosterone and health status in patients with heart failure. J Card Fail. 2014;20:334-42.
40. Agha G, Loucks EB, Tinker LF, et al. Healthy lifestyle and decreasing risk of heart failure in women: The Women's

Health Initiative observational study. J Am Coll Cardiol. 2014;64:1777-85.
41. Eckel RH, Jakicic JM, Ard JD, et al. 2013 AHA/ACC guideline on lifestyle management to reduce cardiovascular risk: a report of the American College of Cardiology/American Heart Association Task Force on Practice Guidelines [published corrections appear in Circulation. 2014;129[suppl 2]:S100-S101 and Circulation. 2015;131:e326]. Circulation. 2014;129(suppl 2):S76–99.
42. O'Connor CM, Whellan DJ, Lee KL, et al. Efficacy and safety of exercise training in patients with chronic heart failure: HF-ACTION randomized controlled trial. JAMA. 2009;301:1439-50.
43. Pina IL, Bittner V, Clare RM, et al. Effects of exercise training on outcomes in women with heart failure: Analysis of HF-ACTION (Heart Failure-A Congrolled Trial Investigating Outcomes of Exercise Training) by sex. J Am Coll Cardiol HF. 2014;2:180-6.
44. Pandey A, Berry JD. Physical activity in heart failure with preserved ejection fraction: Moving toward a newer treatment paradigm. Circulation. 2017;136:993-5.
45. Krishna BH, Pal P, Pal G, et al. Effect of yoga therapy on heart rate, blood pressure and cardiac autonomic function in heart failure. J Clin Diagn Res. 2014;8:14-6.
46. Gomes-Neto M, Rodrigues ES Jr, Silva WM Jr, et al. Effects of yoga in patients with chronic heart failure: a meta-analysis. Arq Bras Cardiol. 2014;103:433-9.
47. Schneider RH, Alexander CN, Staggers F, et al. Long term effects of stress reduction on mortality in persons ≥ 55 years of age with systemic hypertension. Am J Cardiol. 2005;95:1060-4.
48. Sullivan MJ, Wood L, Terry J, et al. The support, education, and research in chronic heart failure study (search): a mindfulness based psychoeducational intervention improves depression and clinical symptoms in patients with chronic heart failure. Am Heart J. 2009;157:84-90.
49. Pandey A, LaMonte M, Klein L, et al. Relationship between physical activity, body mass index and risk of heart failure. J Am Coll Cardiol. 2017;69:1129-42.
50. Del Gobbo LC, Kalntarian S, Imamura F, et al. Contribution of major lifestyle risk factors for incident heart failure in older adults: The Cardiovascular Health Study. J Am Coll Cardiol HF. 2015:3:520-8.
51. Wing RR, Bolin P, Brancati FL, et al. Look AHEAD Research Group. Cardiovascular effects of intensive lifestyle intervention in type 2 diabetes. N Engl J Med. 2013;369(2):145-54.
52. Benotti PN, Wood GC, Carey DJ, et al. Gastric bypass surgery produces a durable reduction in cardiovascular disease risk factors and reduces the long term risks of congestive heart failure. J Am Heart Assoc. 2017;6:e005126.
53. DeVore AD, Bhatt AS. Influenza vaccination in patients with Heart Failure. Circulation. 2019;139:587-9.
54. Modin D, Jorgensen E, Gislason G, et al. Influenza vaccine in Heart Failure. Circulation. 2019;139:575-86.
55. Vardeny O, Claggett R, Udell JA, et al.; PARADIGM-HF Investigators. Influenza Vaccination in patients with Chronic Heart Failure: the PARADIGM-HF trial. JACC Heart Fail. 2016;4(2):152-8.
56. Ponikowski P, Jankowska E. Pathogenesis and clinical presentation of acute heart failure. Rev Esp Cardiol. 2015;68:331-7.
57. Guyton AC, Lindsey AW, Abernathy B, et al. Venous return at various right atrial pressures and the normal venous return curve. Am J Physiol. 1957;189:609-15.
58. Whittenberger JL, Mcgregor M, Beglund E, et al. Influence of state of inflation of the lung on pulmonary vascular resistance. J Appl Physiol. 1960;15:878-82.
59. Tobin MJ. Mechanical Ventilation. N Engl J Med. 1994;330:1056-61.
60. Masip J, Begtbese AJ, Paez J, et al. Noninvasive pressure support ventilation versus conventional oxygen theapy in acute cardiogenic pulmonary oedema: a randomised trial. Lancet. 2000;356:2126-32.
61. Nava S, Carbone G, DiBattista N, et al. Noninvasive ventilation in cardiogenic pulmonary edema: a multicentre randomized trial. Am J Respir Crit Care Med. 2003;168:1432-7.
62. McMurray JJ, Adamopoulos S, Anker SD, et al. The ESC guidelines for the diagnosis and treatment of acute and chronic heart failure 2012. Eur Heart J. 2012;33:1787-847.
63. Adams Jr KF, Fonarow GC, Emerman CL, et al. Characteristics and outcomes of patients hospitalized for heart failure in the United States: rationale, design and preliminary observations from the first 100000 cases in the Acute Decompensated Heart Failure National Registry (ADHERE). Am Heart J. 2005;294;1625-33.
64. Giglioli C, Landi D, Cecchi E, et al. Effects of ULTRAfiltration vs Diuretics on clinical, biohumoral and haemodynamic variables in patients with decompensated heart failure: the ULTRADISCO study. Eur J Heart Fail. 2011;13:337e46.
65. Bart BA, Boyle A, Bank AJ, et al. Ultrafiltration versus usual care for hospitalized patients with heart failure: the Relief for Acutely Fluid Overloaded patients with decompensated heart failure (RAPID-CHF) trial. J Am Coll Cardiol. 2005;46:2043-6.
66. Costanzo MR, Guglin ME, Saltzberg MT, et al. UNLOAD Trial investigators. Ultrafilitration versus intravenous diuretics for patients hospitalized for acute decomenpsated heart failure. J Am Coll Cardiol. 2007;49:675-83.
67. Steg PG, James SK, Atar D, et al. ESC guidelines for the management of acute myocardial infarction in patients presenting with ST segment elevation. Eur Heart J. 2012;33:2569-619.
68. Thiele H, Zeymer U, Neumann FJ, et al. IABP-SHOCK II Trial Investigators. Intraaortic balloon support for myocardial infarction with cardiogenic shock. N Engl J Med. 2012;367:1287-96.
69. Combes A, LePrince P, Luyt CE, et al. Extracorporeal membrane oxygenation (ECMO) for cardiopulmonary support. Reanimation. 2009;18:420-7.
70. Authors/Task Force members; Windecker S, Kolh P, Alfonso F, et al. 2014 ESC/EACTS Guidelines on myocardial revascularization: the Task Force on Myocardial Revascularization of the European Society of Cardiology (ESC) and the European Association for Cardio-Thoracic Surgery (EACTS) developed with special contribution of the European Association of Percutaneous Cardiovascular Interventions (EAPCI). Eur Heart J. 2014;35:2541-619.

Self-care in Heart Failure: Patient Empowerment for Better Management

Kush Kumar Bhagat, Rajeev Gupta

INTRODUCTION

Heart failure (HF) is a rapidly fatal condition and is an important clinical problem globally as well as in India.[1,2] The massive burden of heart failure in India behoove that all the participants in chain of management are properly empowered. It has been shown that strong health systems, hospital-based clinical pathways, physician level algorithms, and nursing and paramedic support can increase patient compliance to therapies and reduce heart failure mortality.[3,4] Prescription of evidence-based therapies (lifestyle, drugs, etc.) at the level of physicians and adherence to these therapies at the patient level has led to better outcomes.[3,4] Our studies over the last three decades have shown that 3-year survival from heart failure due to reduced ejection fraction (HFrEF) has increased from 10% to 20% in 1980s to more than 50% in the current era.[5,6] However, long-term survival following an acute heart failure syndrome still remains dismal as reported in a number of studies from India.[6-9] It is now abundantly clear that adherence to healthy lifestyles—walking and physical activity, healthy diet, fluid restriction, smoking,/tobacco, and alcohol cessation—is crucial in management of HF.[10,11] Lifestyle changes must be accompanied with adherence to evidence-based medications—beta adrenergic blockers, angiotensin converting enzyme (ACE) inhibitors or angiotensin receptor blockers (ARB) or angiotensin receptor neprilysin inhibitors (ARNI), mineralocorticoid receptor antagonists (MRA)—all of which improve survival in HF.[3,4,11] However, adherence to such therapies is low.[11] Survival is significantly lower in patients not adherent to these therapies as reported in multiple global studies[11] and also in a study from Kerala.[12] In this brief review, we summarize HF management components and approaches to promote patient empowerment for self-care.

PATIENT EMPOWERMENT: HEART FAILURE MANAGEMENT

Basic management strategies in HF include general management, management of comorbidities, lifestyle therapies, and drug therapies as outlines in American and European guidelines.[3,4] Advanced therapies including cardiac rhythm control devices, ventricular assist devices, and cardiac transplantation are beyond the scope of this article. Every patient should be empowered with knowledge about basic heart failure management, drug therapy, healthy lifestyles, and other nitty-gritties of the disease. Clinicians should aim to screen for and inform the patient regarding comorbidities such as hypertension, ischemic heart disease, diabetes mellitus, anemia and sleep-disordered breathing as these conditions tend to exacerbate HF.[10] Certain drugs are known to make HF worse and should be avoided, for example, nonsteroidal anti-inflammatory drugs, including cyclooxygenase 2 inhibitors, are not recommended in patients with chronic HF because the risk of renal failure and fluid retention is markedly increased in the presence of reduced renal function. Patients should receive immunization with influenza and pneumococcal vaccines to prevent respiratory infections and must be informed of its importance.[3,4] It is important to educate the patient and family about HF, the importance of proper diet, as well the importance of compliance with the medical regimen. Supervision of outpatient care by a specially trained nurse or physician assistant and/or in specialized HF clinics have all been found to be helpful, particularly in patients with advanced disease.[4]

A number of strategies exist to increase adherence to therapies among HF patients. These can occur at multiple levels of healthcare such as healthcare systems, healthcare providers, and patients (Table 1).[10] The patient is the most important part of the survival chain and should be the focus of all attempts to improve survival. Also, there are a number of specific strategies for improving patient participation (patient empowerment) in HF care. These are—understanding rationale and importance of commitment; development of communication skills; using reminder systems (verbal, telephonic or smartphone based); use of self-monitoring skills, development of problem-solving skills and use of social-support networks; defining own needs on basis of experience; and continuous validation of rationale to follow recommendations.[10,11]

TABLE 1: Strategies to improve adherence to evidence-based therapies in heart failure (HF).

Level of healthcare	*Strategy*
Healthcare organization	• Provide tracking and reporting systems • Provide education and training for providers • Provide adequate reimbursement for allocation of time for all healthcare professionals • Rapid translation of knowledge into practice • Technology training and creating technology-friendly environment for physician-patient interactions
Providers	• Foster effective communication with patients • Provide clear direct messages about importance of lifestyle and therapies in HF management • Include patients in decision-making process about prevention and treatment goals • Incorporate behavioral modification strategies at counseling • Document the patients' progress toward goals • Create an evidence-based practice • Assess patients' compliance at each visit • Develop reminder systems to ensure identification and follow-up • Technology enabled physicians for many of the above strategies • All patients must engage in prevention and treatment behaviors
Patients	• Decide to control risk factors • Negotiate goals with providers • Develop skills for adopting and maintaining recommended behaviors • Monitor progress towards goals • Resolve problems that block the achievement of goals • Communicate with physicians regularly • Technology enabled patients

COMPONENTS OF SELF-MANAGEMENT

The American Heart Association (AHA) and American Association of Cardiovascular and Pulmonary Rehabilitation (AACVPR) have defined the core components of clinic-based cardiac rehabilitation as optimization of cardiovascular risk reduction, to enhance healthy behaviors, and to reduce cardiovascular morbidity and mortality. Medication adherence has been added to the core components for home based rehabiliation.[13] Self-monitoring in HF patients should follow the same protocol (Table 2). A number of home-based activities are important in HF patients and summarized below.

Healthy Lifestyle

An important component of patient self-empowerment and self-care is adherence to healthy lifestyles. All patients must be informed of various aspects of lifestyles—graded exercise, dietary restrictions, salt and fluid restrictions, and alcohol and tobacco avoidance as cornerstone of HF management.[3,4]

Exercise

Although heavy physical labor is not recommended in HF, routine modest exercise has been shown to be beneficial in selected patients with HF. HF-ACTION trial, which was a controlled trial investigating outcomes of exercise training, showed that there was a trend toward decreased cardiovascular mortality or HF hospitalizations and quality of life was significantly improved in the exercise group.[14] For euvolemic patients, regular isotonic exercise such as walking or riding a stationary bicycle with an ergometer may be useful as an adjunctive therapy to improve clinical status after patients have undergone exercise testing to determine suitability for exercise training.[3,4] Exercise training is not

TABLE 2: Process and outcomes for cardiac rehabilitation and self-monitoring.

Interventions	*Target behaviors*	*Intermediate outcomes*	*Secondary prevention goals*
Exercise training	Physical activity	Exercise capacity Cardiovascular symptoms	Improved • Physical fitness • Functional capacity • Quality of life
Dietary education	Healthy eating	Body mass index Waist circumference	
Medication management	Medication adherence	Blood pressure, glycemic control Lipid levels	Reduced • Cardiovascular events • Hospitalizations • Mortality • Adverse events • Cost and resource use
Tabacco counseling	Smoking cessation	Tobacco use	
Psychosocial assessment	Stress management	Anxiety Depression	

recommended, however, for HFrEF patients who have had a major cardiovascular event or procedure within the last 6 weeks, patients with cardiac devices that limit the ability to achieve target heart rates, and patients with significant arrhythmia or ischemia during baseline cardiopulmonary exercise testing.

Diet

Dietary restriction of sodium (2–3 g daily) is recommended in all patients with HF and preserved or depressed EF. Further restriction (<2 g daily) may be harmful. Fluid restriction is generally unnecessary unless the patient develops hyponatremia (<130 mEq/L), which may develop because of activation of the renin-angiotensin system, excessive secretion of antidiuretic hormone, or loss of salt in excess amount of water from diuretic use. Fluid restriction (<1.5 L/day) should be considered in hyponatremic patients or for those whose fluid retention is difficult to control despite high doses of diuretics and sodium restriction.[3,4] Caloric supplementation is recommended for patients with advanced HF and unintentional weight loss or muscle wasting (cardiac cachexia); however, anabolic steroids are not recommended for these patients because of the potential problems with volume retention.

Smoking and Alcohol

Heart failure patients should be advised to stop smoking and to limit daily alcohol consumption to zero. Each puff of nicotine from tobacco smoke temporarily increases heart rate and blood pressure and also increases risk of atherosclerosis. People who quit smoking are more likely to have their heart failure symptoms improve.

Drugs and Devices

A number of drugs are available for chronic reduced ejection fraction heart failure management (Table 3).[3,4,15] The drugs are divided into three broad groups: (1) palliative therapies, (2) evidence-based long-term therapies and (3) supportive therapies and vaccines. An empowered patient should be aware of indications, contraindications and side-effects of these drugs. Self-titration of these drugs, especially diuretics, is important and part of patient education.

Diuretics

Many of the clinical manifestations of moderate to severe HF result from excessive water and sodium retention that leads to volume expansion and congestive symptoms. Diuretics are the only pharmacologic agents that can adequately control fluid retention in advanced HF [both HFrEF and heart failure due to preserved ejection fraction (HFpEF)] and they should be used to restore and maintain normal volume status in patients with congestive symptoms (dyspnea, orthopnea, and edema) or signs of elevated filling pressures (rales, jugular venous distention or peripheral edema).[3,4]

Beta-adrenergic Receptor Blockers

Beta blocker therapy represents a major advance in the treatment of patients with a HFrEF. These drugs interfere with the harmful effects of sustained activation of the adrenergic nervous system. When given in concert with ACE inhibitors, these drugs reverse the process of left ventricular remodeling, improve patient symptoms, prevent hospitalization, and prolong life.[3,4] Therefore beta blockers are indicated for patients with symptomatic or asymptomatic HF with EF <40%.

Angiotensin-converting Enzyme Inhibitors

There is an overwhelming evidence that ACE inhibitors should be used in symptomatic and asymptomatic patients with HFrEF (EF<40%) and to control hypertension in HFpEF.[3,4] ACE inhibitors should be initiated in low doses,

TABLE 3: Drugs used in heart failure management[15] important for self-management and identification of target doses. Class I or IIa recommendation in guidelines.[3,4]

Group	*Drug class*	*Examples (India)*	*Initiating dose (mg)*	*Target dose (mg)*
Symptom-limiting drugs	Diuretics (loop)	Furosemide	10 od	As required
		Torsemide	10 od	As required
	Diuretics (distal tubule)	Hydrochlorothiazide	25 od	As required
		Metolazone	2.5 od	As required
		Chlorthalidone	12.5 od	As required
	Digitalis	Digoxin	0.125 od	0.25 od (serum levels)
	If receptor inhibitors	Ivabradine	5 bid	15 od
Evidence-based beneficial therapies	Angiotensin converting enzyme inhibitors	Enalapril	2.5–5 bid	10 bid
		Lisinopril	2.5–5 od	20 od
		Ramipril	1.25–2.5 bid	5 bid
	Angiotensin receptor blockers	Losartan	12.5–25 od	50 od
		Valsartan	80 od	160 od
		Candesartan	16 od	32 od
	Angiotensin receptor neprilysin inhibitors	Sacubitril-Valsartan	24/26 bid	97/103 bid
	Beta-blockers	Metoprolol XL	25 od	150–200 od
		Carvedilol	10 od	40 od
		Bisoprolol	1.25 od	8.6 od
		Nebivolol	1.25 od	10 od
	Mineralocorticoid inhibitors	Spironolactone	12.5–25 od	25–50 od
		Eplerenone	25 od	50 od
	Direct vasodilators	Hydralazine-ISDN	25/37.5 tid	50/75 tid
		Hydralazine	25 qid	50–75 qid
		Isosorbide dinitrate	10–20 tid	20–80 tid
Supportive therapies	Anticoagulants	Heparin, low molecular weight heparins	aPTT response	aPTT response
	Direct oral anticoagulants	Dabigatran	110–150 bid	110–150 bid
		Rivaroxaban	10–20 od	10–20 od
		Apixaban	2.5–5 bid	5 bid
	Antiarrhythmic	Amiodarone	Loading	100–200 od
Vaccines	Polyvalent vaccines	Influenza A/B	Once a year	--
		Pneumococcal spp.	Once in 5 years	--
Note: Dosages and efficacy is different in heart failure with preserved ejection fraction.				

[aPTT: activated partial thromboplastin time; ISDN: Integrated Services Digital Network; od: once daily; bid: bis in die (twice daily); tid: ter in die (thrice daily); qid: quater in die (four times a day)]

followed by gradual increments and the doses should be increased until they are similar to those that have been shown to be effective in clinical trials (Table 3). Higher doses are more effective than lower doses in improving lifespan and preventing hospitalizations.

Angiotensin Receptor Blockers

These drugs are indicated in patients who are intolerant to ACE inhibitors because of cough, skin rash, and angioedema.[3,4,16] Although ACE inhibitors and ARBs inhibit the renin-angiotensin system, they do so by different mechanisms. When given in concert with beta-blockers in HFrEF, ARBs reverse the process of left ventricular remodeling, improve patient symptoms, prevent hospitalization, and prolong life.

Angiotensin Receptor Neprilysin Inhibitors

In ARNI, an ARB is combined with an inhibitor of neprilysin, an enzyme that degrades natriuretic peptides, bradykinin, adrenomedullin, and other vasoactive peptides. In an randomized controlled trial (RCT), that compared an ARNI— valsartan/sacubitril—with enalapril in symptomatic patients with HFrEF tolerating an adequate dose of either ACE inhibitor or ARB, this drug reduced composite endpoint of cardiovascular death or HF hospitalization significantly.[17] The use of ARNI is associated with the risk of hypotension and renal insufficiency and may lead to angioedema, as well. In patients with chronic symptomatic HFrEF, New York Heart Association (NYHA) class II or III who tolerate an ACE inhibitor or ARB, replacement by an ARNI is recommended to further reduce morbidity and mortality. ARNIs, however, should not be used with an ACE inhibitor and should not be used by patients with a history of angioedema.

Ivabradine

Ivabradine selectively inhibits the *If* current in the sinoatrial node, providing heart rate reduction. Ivabradine may be beneficial in reducing heart failure hospitalizations in patients with symptomatic stable heart failure with HFrEF who are receiving guideline-directed evaluation and management, including a beta blocker at a maximum tolerated dose, and who are in sinus rhythm with a heart rate ≥70/min at rest.[18]

Aldosterone Antagonists

Although classified as potassium-sparing diuretics, drugs that block the effects of aldosterone (spironolactone or eplerenone) have beneficial effects that are independent of the effects of these agents on sodium balance. Accordingly, the administration of an aldosterone antagonist is recommended for patients with class III-IV HF with HFrEF and who are receiving standard therapy, including diuretics, ACE inhibitors, and beta blockers.[3,4]

Device Therapy

Three types of devices could be used in HF patients: (1) implantable cardiac defibrillators for primary and secondary prevention of malignant arrhythmias and treatment; (2) cardiac resynchronization therapy for synchronizing and improving cardiac contractility depressed EF in suitable patients with intracardiac conduction abnormalities [left bundle branch block (LBBB)]; and (3) ventricular assist devices, left ventricular or biventricular, as a bridge to cardiac transplantation or destination therapy.[3] An empowered patient should be aware of these alternatives, indications and contraindications, and outcomes.

SELF-MONITORING AND ADHERENCE

Self-care in HF is described as a naturalistic decision-making process enabling engagement with healthy behaviors such as daily monitoring and adherence to the plan of care (self-care maintenance) and adequate management of symptoms and evaluation of applied treatment actions (self-care management). Important components of self-care in HF are self-monitoring of symptoms and adherence to therapies.[19] Use of technology is also important.[20,21] There are a number of barriers and facilitators of self-monitoring and adherence (Table 1). These should be overcome to promote self-care.[10]

Self-monitoring

Watching out for the warning signs that heart failure is getting worse will help to catch problems before they become too serious. At home, one should watch for changes in weight, pulse rate, and blood pressure. Various warning symptoms and signs are listed below. Patients must be encouraged to contact the healthcare provider immediately.

- Weight gain: if there is gain of ½ kg or more in a day or 2 kg or more in a week
- Swollen feet, ankles, legs, and abdomen
- Extreme fatigue
- New, more or worse dry coughing, increased difficulty in breathing not related to exercise, shortness of breath on lying down, or an hour or two after falling asleep
- Pulse gets very slow or very fast, or it is irregular
- Blood pressure is lower or higher than is normal.

Adherence

Medication adherence is the most important self-care behavior to prevent acute exacerbations of heart failure. Self-care behaviors help decrease all-cause hospital admission and readmission for heart failure exacerbations. Medication nonadherence is associated with more emergency department visits, frequent rehospitalizations, and higher medical cost.[4] Medication adherence rates have varied from 10% to 98% depending on the definition and measurement used to assess and analyze adherence.

Many factors contribute to medication nonadherence such as lack of support, finances, absent of symptoms, cognitive decline, adverse reactions, depression, poor attention span, poor knowledge about medication, multiple medications, difficulty swallowing large pills, and inconveniences of urinary frequency with diuretics. Researchers have explored various strategies such as the use of pharmacists, nurses, telemedicine, and interdisciplinary teams to provide interventions to improve medication adherence in heart failure.[4] Healthcare providers should continue to provide education, constantly reinforce the importance of taking medication as prescribed, and when feasible, utilize one of the successful evidence-based strategies to increase adherence (Table 1).[10]

Barriers and Facilitators to Self-care in Heart Failure

Despite the advantages of self-care, patients with heart failure, especially older people, face numerous difficulties in achieving optimal quality of self-care. Appreciating the factors that enable or inhibit self-care is critical in developing effective recommendations for self-care and effective health care interventions. Self-care is a complex and multi-faceted phenomenon that needs a comprehensive consideration of patients including their emotional situation, psychological characters, physical abilities, family support, living facilities, comorbidities and their ability for learning. Insufficient knowledge about heart failure, symptom recognition and ways of self-care along with hopelessness and psychological problems limited their abilities for an effective self-care. A supportive environment, motivation, and adequate care programs using effective educational methods that build self-care skills, should be recommended to healthcare providers and families.

TECHNOLOGY

Several studies have shown that home telemonitoring, including digital scales, blood pressure monitoring via smartphones, and pulse oximeters can reduce both hospital admissions and mortality. Guidelines recommendations also support technological interventions.[3,4] One meta-analysis of home telemonitoring, documented an insignificant 40–46% reduction in HF-related admissions, with a significant reduction in mortality (30–67%), and bed-days (53–62%).[20] A study from Italy, comparing home telemonitoring with usual care, demonstrated a highly significant reduction in the composite endpoint of mortality and rate of hospitalization.[21] Another meta-analysis including 21 studies (3,082 patients) reported that home telemonitoring reduced mortality [risk ratio = 0.64; 95% confidence interval (CI): 0.48–0.85] compared with usual care.[22] Several of the studies analyzed in the meta-analysis suggested reduction in hospitalizations. A 20% reduction in all-cause mortality and 21% reduction in rate of hospitalization were documented in a third meta-analysis.[23] However, another recent meta-analysis suggested that a decline mortality is short-lived; home telemonitoring reduced all-cause and heart failure-related mortality at 180 days, but not at 365 days.[24]

On the other hand in HF management, practice readiness is a more high-tech intervention than those discussed earlier, and requires coordination between primary care, cardiology and, often, home care telemonitoring staff; often nurses in a call center environment, must have shared protocols with contingency orders, as well as clear and open communication with providers managing the patient. When clinically meaningful changes are detected, the care team must act quickly to avoid unnecessary emergency room visits and hospitalizations. Technology use for symptom management is beneficial for both patients and physicians. Widespread acceptance of technology use in healthcare fuels continued development of technology with ever-increasing sophistication. New technologies are now being used to help manage and reduce hospital admissions for patients with HF.

CardioMEMS

The CardioMEMS HF System is the first and only Food and Drug Administration (FDA)—approved heart failure monitoring device that has been proven to significantly reduce hospital admissions when used by physicians to manage HF.[25] The system features a sensor that is implanted in the pulmonary artery during a nonsurgical procedure to directly measure artery pressure. Increased pressures appear before weight and blood pressure changes, which are often used as indirect measures that indicate worsening heart failure. The new system allows patients to transmit daily sensor readings from their homes to their healthcare providers, allowing for personalized and proactive management of the condition, and reduce complications and readmissions for care.

ZOLL HFAMS

This is an FDA-cleared patch-based, wireless system that employs novel radiofrequency technology to monitor pulmonary fluid levels, an early indicator for heart failure decompensation. The heart failure and arrhythmia management system (HFAMS) sensor is noninvasive and can be worn by patients 24 hours a day. It continuously records, stores, and transmits patient data, including thoracic fluid index, heart rate, respiration rate, activity, posture, and electrocardiogram (ECG) which eventually improve outcomes and reduce hospitalizations for heart failure patients with fluid management problems.[26]

Machine Learning and Artificial Intelligence

In the future, deep machine learning and artificial intelligence (AI) algorithms can be created to assess a broader array of clinical and patient-generated data to identify patients requiring more intensive intervention from a nurse or other clinician, improve outcomes, and further reduce the cost of care.[27,28] Furthermore, AI applications can analyze data in an electronic medical records (EMR crawlers) and suggest treatment optimizations.

HEART FAILURE ACTION PLAN

Every heart failure patient should have an action plan that includes daily monitoring and steps for getting emergency care quickly in the event of severe symptoms. According to the American Heart Association, a typical plan may fall into three zones:

1. Green = Stable. No noticeable changes in heart failure signs or symptoms. Weight is stable. No chest pain or shortness of breath. Continue daily weight checks and treatment plan as recommended.
2. Yellow = Warning. One should contact a doctor if there is new cough, shortness of breath with activity, increased swelling in legs or feet, or if sudden weight gain 2–5 pounds within a week. May not necessarily need an office visit but caution is needed. One may just need diet or medication changes.
3. Red = Danger. Immediately go to the emergency room if develop heart failure and have a weight gain of more than 5 pounds in a week, an inability to lie flat, shortness of breath at rest, increased swelling and discomfort in the lower body, or a constant, hacking cough.

Carefully following the action plan can help the physician more quickly treat any new health issues that develop and manage better. Sticking to action plans may result in fewer hospital admissions or shorter hospital stay. Clinical and upcoming technological interventions can ultimately lead to patient empowerment and an educated patient is the best resource for heart failure self-management.

CONCLUSION

Heart failure is an important clinical problem and is associated with high mortality with five-year survival rates of 15–50%. Two types of heart failure syndromes exist, reduced and preserved ejection fraction. Lifestyle modification along with evidence-based drug therapies can significantly reduce morbidity, prevent hospitalizations, and prolong life in heart failure with reduced ejection fraction. One of the important interventions in management of heart failure is self-care or patient empowerment. Self-care process involves understanding of the nature of the disease, symptom awareness, compliance to lifestyle changes, and adherence to drug therapies. Technological support using a variety of devices can augment process of self-care.

REFERENCES

1. Savarese G, Lund LH. Global public health burden of heart failure. Card Fail Rev. 2017;3:7-11.
2. Pillai HS, Ganapathi S. Heart failure in South Asia. Curr Cardiol Rev. 2013;9:102-11.
3. Yancy CW, Jessup M, Bozkurt B, et al. 2017 ACCF/ACC/HFSA focused update on new pharmacological therapy for heart failure: an update of the 2013 ACCF/AHA guidelines for the management of heart failure: a report of the American College of Cardiology Foundation/American Heart Association Task Force on Practice Guidelines and the Heart Failure Society of America. J Am Coll Cardiol. 2017;70:776-803.
4. Ponikowski P, Voors AA, Anker SD, et al. 2016 ESC guidelines for the diagnosis and treatment of acute and chronic heart failure. The Task Force for the diagnosis and treatment of acute and chronic heart failure of the European Society of Cardiology. Eur Heart J. 2016;37:2129-200.
5. Gupta R, Gupta KD. Prognostic significance of radiographic cardiomegaly in patients with coronary heart disease. J Assoc Physicians India. 1993;41:421-4.
6. Gupta R, Grover V, Roy S, et al. Heart failure etiologies, management and short-term outcomes in hospitalized and clinic-based patients in India. RUHS J Health Sciences. 2018;3:5-10.
7. Harikrishnan S, Sanjay G, Agarwal A, et al. One year mortality outcomes and hospital readmissions of patients admitted with acute heart failure: data from Trivandrum Heart Failure Registry in Kerala, India. Am Heart J. 2017;189:93-199.
8. Suman OS, Vijayaraghvan G, Muneer AR, et al. Long-term outcomes of patients admitted with heart failure in a tertiary care centre in India. Indian Heart J. 2018;70(Suppl 1): S85-9.
9. Teng TK, Tromp J, Tay WT, et al. Prescribing patterns of evidence based heart failure pharmacotherapy and outcomes in the ASIAN-HF registry: a cohort study. Lancet Glob Health. 2018;6:e1008-18.
10. Moser DK, Riegel B. Disease management in heart failure. In: Mann DL (Ed). Heart Failure: A Companion to Braunwald's Heart Disease, 2nd edition. St Louis, Missouri: Saunders; 2011. pp. 854-66.
11. Braunwald E. The war against heart failure: the Lancet lecture. Lancet. 2015;385:812-24.
12. Harikrishnan S, Sanjay G, Anees T, et al. Clinical presentation, management, in-hospital and 90-day outcomes of heart

failure patients in Trivandrum, Kerala: The Trivandrum Heart Failure Registry. Eur J Heart Fail. 2015;17:794-800.
13. Thomas RJ, Beatty AL, Beckie TM, et al. Home based cardiac rehabilitation: a scientific statement from the American Association of Cardiovascular and Pulmonary Rehabilitation, the American Heart Association and American College of Cardiology. J Am Coll Cardiol. 2019;74:133-53.
14. O'Connor CM, Whellan DJ, Lee KL, et al. Efficacy and safety of exercise training in patients with chronic heart failure: HF-ACTION randomized controlled trial. JAMA. 2009;301:1439-50.
15. Rosenthal JL, Tang WHW. Heart failure with systolic dysfunction. In: Griffin BP, Menon V, (Eds). Manual of Cardiovascular Medicine, 5th edition. New Delhi: Wolters Kluwer; 2019. pp. 98-119.
16. Granger CB, McMurray JJ, Yusuf S, et al. Effects of candesartan in patients with chronic heart failure and reduced left-ventricular systolic function intolerant to angiotensin-converting enzyme inhibitors: the CHARM-Alternative trial. Lancet. 2003;362:772-86.
17. McMurray JJ, Packer M, Desai AS, et al. Angiotensin-neprilysin inhibition versus enalapril in heart failure. N Engl J Med. 2014;371:993-1004.
18. Swedberg K, Komajda M, Bohm M, et al. Ivabradine and outcomes in chronic heart failure (SHIFT): a randomized placebo-controlled study. Lancet. 2010;376:875-85.
19. Gupta R. Patient empowerment: paradigm shift in health care. Electronic response. BMJ. 2003; 327:303.
20. Clark RA, Inglis SC, McAlister FA, et al. Telemonitoring or structured telephone support programs for patients with chronic heart failure: systematic review and meta-analysis. BMJ. 2007;334:942.
21. Antonicelli R, Testarmata P, Spazzafumo L, et al. Impact of telemonitoring at home on the management of elderly patients with congestive heart failure. J Telemed Telecare. 2008;14:3005.
22. Dang S, Dimmick S, Kelkar G. Evaluating the evidence base for the use of home telehealth remote monitoring in elderly with heart failure. Telemed J E Health. 2009;15:783-96.
23. Zhu Y, Gu X, Xu C. Effectiveness of telemedicine systems for adults with heart failure: a meta-analysis of randomized controlled trials. Heart Fail Rev. 2019; EPub.
24. Pekmezaris R, Torez L, Williams M, et al. Home telemonitoring in heart failure: a systematic review and meta-analysis. Health Affairs. 2018;37:1983-9.
25. Leung CC. Current role of the CardioMEMS device for management of patients with heart failure. Curr Cardiol Rep. 2019;21:98.
26. Abraham WT, Perl L. Implantable hemodynamic monitoring for heart failure patients. J Am Coll Cardiol. 2017;70:389-98.
27. Awan SE, Sohel F, Sanfilippo FM, et al. Machine learning in heart failure: ready for prime time. Curr Opin Cardiol. 2018;33:190-5.
28. Topol EJ. High performance medicine: the convergence of human and artificial intelligence. Nature Med. 2019;25: 44-56.

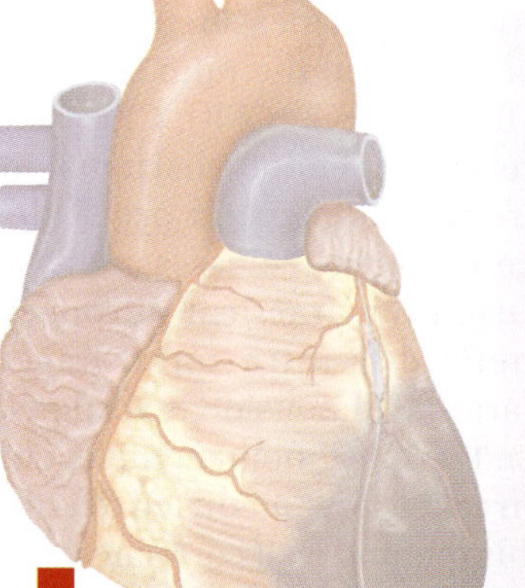

Endothelium in Heart Failure

Shishu Shankar Mishra, Biswaranjan Mishra, Satyanarayan Routray, Akshaya Kumar Samal

INTRODUCTION

The incidence of heart failure (HF) is gradually increasing. In spite of advancement in therapeutics, prognosis remains grim particularly in heart failure with preserved ejection fraction (HFpEF).[1] Of late significant improvement has occurred in medical management of heart failure with reduced ejection fraction (HFrEF). Drugs like beta-blockers, mineral corticoid antagonists, and renin-angiotensin blockers which influence outcome in HFrEF, do not have much influence in HFpEF.[2] Intense research in this field has generated interest in targeting endothelium in the therapeutics of HF.[3] HFpEF is now recognized as a distinct clinical entity which occurs in approximately half of the patients presenting with HF. Its association with hypertension, diabetes, old age, elderly females, other systemic and pulmonary diseases is well established.[4] Adaptation in different diseases involving neurohormonal activation, cytokine expression, and endothelial dysfunction (ED) are the different mechanisms thought to be involved in the genesis of HFpEF in various comorbidities.[5] Role of ED in the pathophysiology of HF particularly as an early marker remained a matter of research for the last several decades. Its role as an independent predictor of prognosis in various systemic diseases like diabetes and hypertension with or without HF has been well established.[6] Endothelial-dependent vasodilatation during exercise is the key to switching from aerobic to anaerobic metabolism and genesis of dyspnea, the cardinal symptom of HF. Several methods such as regular exercise have been seen to improve endothelial function in health and diseases including HF which is mediated through improvement in endothelial function.[7]

ENDOTHELIAL FUNCTION

Endothelium is no longer considered as a mere barrier in the vessel walls rather an active organ having endocrine, exocrine, and various regulatory function in health and disease. It plays an active role in maintaining blood flow and vascular tone that are essential to perfuse tissues.[8] The key molecule secreted by endothelial cells is nitric oxide (NO). In the endothelial cells, with appropriate stimuli such as inflammatory cytokines or mechanical shear stress, NO is formed from its precursor L-arginine with the help of the enzyme NO synthase. NO after its production from endothelial cells act as anti-inflammatory and antiproliferative agent with antiatherosclerotic properties. The mechanism of anti-inflammatory action includes inhibition of expression of leukocyte adhesion molecules apart from its property to diffuse from the endothelial cells into the adjacent smooth muscle cells and the circulatory platelets. It has inhibitory action on platelet aggregation by stimulation of the soluble guanylate cyclase (sGC), cyclic guanosine monophosphate (cGMP), protein kinase G (PKG) pathways. On the vascular smooth muscle NO acts as a strong stimulus for vascular relaxation, thereby acting as a potent vasodilator. In the heart NO released from coronary microvasculature and cardiac endocardial cells modulates cardiac function. NO has also the ability of mobilizing stem cells and other progenitor cells to the site of injury and plays an important role in vascular repair.[9] Studies have shown that risk factors for coronary artery such as diabetes, hypertension, smoking, and dyslipidemia mediate their adverse cardiovascular effects by means of ED.[10]

ENDOTHELIAL DYSFUNCTION

Deranged function of the endothelium refers to "endothelial dysfunction". In disease states ED is brought about by oxygen free radicals that combine with NO to form peroxynitrites. These are highly toxic. As NO level decreases, it disturbs physiological homeostasis, leading to inflammation, thrombosis, smooth cell proliferation, platelet aggregation, and progression of atherosclerotic cardiovascular disease (ASCVD). Endothelial NO release directly affects the arterial vasculature and heart. In ED raised levels of peroxynitrites increase diastolic calcium content impairing cardiomyocyte relaxation. Through its effects on sGC cardiomyocyte stiffness and hypertrophy are increased, NO also influences cGMP production causing increase in cellular PKG content. PKG causes reduced cardiomyocyte stiffness through phosphorylation of a giant protein called titin. Titin is responsible for passive myocardial stiffness. Downregulation of sGC-cGMP-PKG pathway in HF is one of the major factor in producing ED. NO has antifibrotic properties. It counteracts rennin–angiotensin–aldosterone system (RAAS) and also inhibits endothelin-1 receptors. Reduced NO levels will exacerbate these enzymes leading to smooth muscle proliferation and prothrombotic actions. Restoration of endothelial function is not achieved by proliferation of existing endothelial cells but by mobilization of bone marrow derived endothelial progenitor cells to the site of injury where they proliferate by means of secreting vascular growth factors, and finally integrate into the endothelial layer and later by differentiating into endothelial cells.[11]

Assessment of Endothelial Function

Endothelial dysfunction occurs earliest in the course of ASCVD, in the early stages, it is possible to reverse ED with appropriate measures thereby overt ASCVD can be prevented.[12] Therefore, assessing endothelial function before clinical ASCVD carries paramount importance. ED can be assessed by intra-arterial administration of acetylcholine or bradykinin which releases NO from endothelial cells causing vasodilatation and hyperemia. In the coronary arteries, coronary flow is measured at resting state and after vasodilator injection, the ratio of which is expressed as coronary flow reserve (CFR). CFR is an indicator of coronary microvascular endothelial function. However, invasive nature of this method precludes its clinical use. Therefore noninvasive assessment of endothelial function is used for practical purposes. The commonly used method is ultrasound based measurement of brachial arterial dimension in response to fore arm ischemia induced by sphygmomanometer cuff inflation and then deflation called flow-mediated dilation (FMD) (Figs. 1A and B). This method well correlates with gold standard invasive assessment of ED as well as with the severity and extent of atherosclerosis.[13] A reactive hyperemia index (RHI) can also be assessed by a finger tip probe EndoPAT™ (Itamar Medical, Israel) which also includes microvascular function unlike FMD which is a measure of a large conduit vessel.[14] The importance of micro- versus macrovascular ED has been highlighted by studies which found abnormal RHI in almost all studies involving patients of HFpEF but FMD in a large study did not have significant difference between patients with HFpEF and healthy control. RHI indicating microvascular ED has also been shown to be an important prognostic marker.[15]

Endothelial Dysfunction in Heart Failure

Bioavailability of NO is the principal factor responsible for structural and functional alteration of cardiomyocytes in HF. Muscle hypertrophy and interstitial fibrosis impairs ventricular relaxation and subsequently decreases ventricular compliance as the muscle become stiff. ED independent of atherosclerosis is seen in patients with HF. The causal role of ED in the development of HFpEF has been

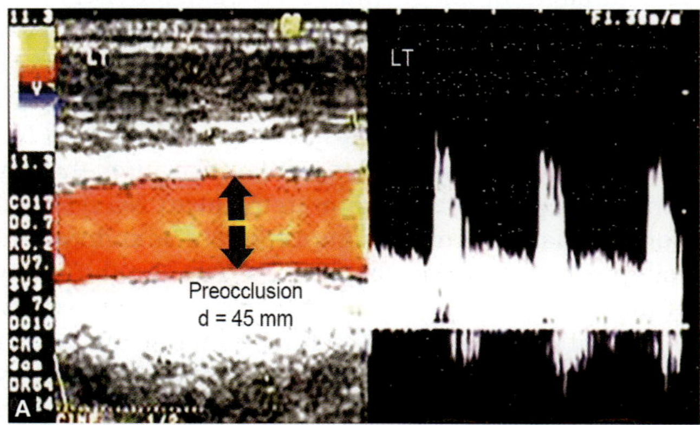

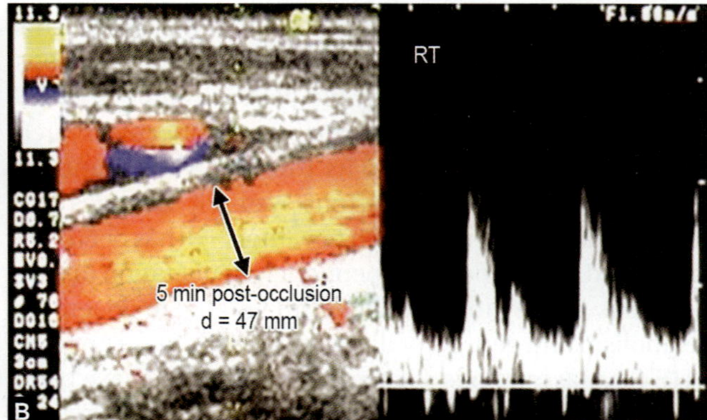

Figs. 1A and B: (A) Preocclusion brachial artery dimension 45 mm; (B) Post-occlusion dimension 47 mm, flow-mediated dilation = 47- 45/45 = 4. Percentage indicating severe endothelial dysfunction.

postulated.[16] Although the exact incidence and prevalence of ED in HF is not known, studies estimated the incidence of ED by use of FMD and RHI to be 42–50% in the population HF. By no means this appear to be an under estimation as they have taken different methodology and different parameters often in unmatched heterogeneous controls and with arbitrary cut-off values for FMD and RHI.[17]

The comorbid conditions associated in HF particularly HFpEF produce a state of systemic inflammation resulting in ED of the coronary circulation including the microvasculature of the heart. Markers of inflammation such as cytokine levels of are raised even before clinical development of HF, therefore highlighting role of these biomarker as predictors of future HF.[18] Circulating markers of inflammation such as cytokines produce a generalized state of endothelial inflammation and dysfunction which also includes the coronary microvasculature. This has been seen in animal models of HFpEF and in human cardiac biopsies.[19] Because of ED, NO signaling from dysfunctional endothelium decreases. It also affects the nearby cardiomyocytes and cardiac fibroblasts. Thus, ED leads to structural and functional changes in cardiomyocytes making them stiff, cardiomyocytes relax with difficulty because of interstitial fibrosis, they also become hypertrophied. All these lead to HFpEF.[20] HF by itself produce a state of inflammation and generates proinflammatory cytokines increasing production of reactive oxygen species resulting in neurohormonal activation, increased oxidative stress and increased collagen synthesis. Thus, ED promotes HF and HF aggravates ED setting a vicious cycle which spirals downward to worsens ED and cause progressive HF.[21]

Adequate endothelial function is crucial for delivering oxygen to the exercising muscles. Exercise tolerance and VO_2 peak is a measure that combines cardiovascular and skeletal muscle oxidative function. It also measures pulmonary ventilation and diffusion capacity. Assessment of VO_2 peak by cardiopulmonary exercise testing objectively determines endothelial function. VO_2 peak is considered a major prognostic marker in HF.[22] Exercise intolerance in HF is largely due to decrease in capillary blood flow and also decrease in peripheral O_2 extraction by decreased pO_2 driving gradient due to ED. These factors limiting VO_2 peak are proved by exercise hemodynamics and exercise echocardiography.[23] Decreased skeletal muscle mass, obesity associated decrease in lean leg mass, and mitochondrial dysfunction where O_2 is utilized intracellularly also contribute to exercise intolerance in HF. These skeletal muscle abnormalities are also shown to be linked to ED. In skeletal muscle, there occurs a switch from oxidative fiber to glycolytic fiber in HF increasing fatigability. There also occurs a reduced capillary density, decreased ratio of capillary to fiber, decreased diffusion of oxygen to muscle fibers, reduced vasodilatory capacity and increased skeletal muscle atrophy in these patients. Doppler studies of arterial flow also demonstrated decreased flow to exercising muscle compared to healthy subjects. In HFpEF, given the preserved heart rate and cardiac output, such decreased flow is attributed to ED.[24]

Pulmonary hypertension (PH) accompanies HF and is an indicator of worse prognosis. Generally raised pulmonary pressure is attributed to increased left ventricular end-diastolic pressure; it cannot be explained only as a passive transmission of pressure. It has been shown that ED and reduced NO bioavailability in pulmonary arterial bed is one of the major factor causing vascular remodeling, pulmonary vasoconstriction generating, and perpetuating PH. ED reduces pulmonary diffusion capacity involving the pulmonary microcirculation. It reduces lung function similar to skeletal muscles alterations occur in the diaphragmatic muscles which further reduces lung function.[25]

Renal dysfunction accompanies HF both as a cause and also effect. ED is impaired in patients with chronic kidney disease (CKD) as measured by RHI or FMD. It has been shown that ED cause decrease in glomerular filtration rate leading to renal vascular and glomerular injury, activation of sodium retention pathways, and impaired renal function.[26]

Correction of Endothelial Dysfunction

There are no specific treatment specially intended for correction of ED, however, one of the most promising therapeutic approach is to increase the bioavailability of NO. Several trials have used with positive outcomes with NO donor such as L-arginine which increases amounts of NO metabolites in subjects with ED. Studies have demonstrated improvement in FMD by L-arginine.[27]

Addressing the comorbidities is one of the major factors to improve outcome in HFpEF. Comorbidities frequently cluster in HFpEF patients and act as contributors to mortality and morbidity HFpEF. Therefore, correction of comorbidities such as diabetes, hypertension, obesity, sleep apnea, COPD, etc. are to be taken care of to prevent a HF.

Antioxidative therapy and anti-inflammatory drugs have shown to be beneficial effects in HF. Pleotropic effects of statins, RAAS blockers, and beta-blockers have also shown to improve diastolic function parameters.

The other easy way of improving ED is regular exercise training. Exercise has various beneficial effects in general and over the cardiovascular system in particular. Correction of endothelial function has been demonstrated objectively in those undergoing regular exercise.[28]

CONCLUSION

Endothelial dysfunction plays a key role in HF. Early identification and correction of ED is the most potential approach in the successful management of HF particularly HFpEF where prognosis and therapeutic approach is still gloomy. Research oriented to recognize factors producing ED and development of drugs particularly addressing endothelial function will definitely prevent and improve prognosis in HF whether reduced or preserved ejection fraction.

REFERENCES

1. Roger VL. Epidemiology of heart failure. Circ Res. 2013;113(6):646-60.
2. Pitt B, Pfeffer MA, Assmann SF, et al. Spironolactone for heart failure with preserved ejection fraction. N Eng J Med. 2014;370(15):1383-92.
3. De Keulenaer GW, Segers VFM, Zannad F, et al. The future of pleiotropic therapy in heart failure. Lessons from the benefits of exercise training on endothelial function. Eur J Heart Fail. 2017;19:603-14.
4. Bhatia RS, Tu JV, Lee DS, et al. Outcome of heart failure with preserved ejection fraction in a population-based study. N Eng J Med. 2006;355(3):260-9.
5. Borlaug BA. The pathophysiology of heart failure with preserved ejection fraction. Nat Rev Cardiol. 2014;11(10): 507-15.
6. Xu Y, Arora RC, Hiebert BM, et al. Non-invasive endothelial function testing and the risk of adverse outcomes: a systematic review and meta-analysis. Eur Heart J Cardiovasc Imaging. 2014;15(7):736-46.
7. Upadhya B, Haykowsky MJ, Eggebeen J, et al. Exercise intolerance in heart failure with preserved ejection fraction: more than a heart problem. J Geriatr Cardiol. 2015;12(3): 294-304.
8. Pacher P, Beckman JS, Liaudet L. Nitric oxide and peroxynitrite in health and disease. Physiol Rev. 2007;87(1):315-424.
9. Özüyaman B, Ebner P, Niesler U, et al. Nitric oxide differentially regulates proliferation and mobilization of endothelial progenitor cells but not of hematopoietic stem cells. Thromb Haemost. 2005;94(4):770-2.
10. Bruyndonckx L, Hoymans VY, Lemmens K, et al. Childhood obesity-related endothelial dysfunction: an update on pathophysiological mechanisms and diagnostic advancements. Pediatr Res. 2016;79(6):831-7.
11. Van Craenenbroeck EM, Van Craenenbroeck AH, Van Ierssel S, et al. Quantification of circulating CD34+/KDR+/CD45dim endothelial progenitor cells: analytical considerations. Int J Cardiol. 2013;167(5):1688-95.
12. Fischer D, Rossa S, Landmesser U, et al. Endothelial dysfunction in patients with chronic heart failure is independently associated with increased incidence of hospitalization, cardiac transplantation, or death. Eur Heart J. 2005;26(1):65-9.
13. Moens AL, Goovaerts I, Claeys MJ, et al. Flow-mediated vasodilation: a diagnostic instrument, or an experimental tool? Chest. 2005;127(6):2254-63.
14. Bruyndonckx L, Radtke T, Eser P, et al. Methodological considerations and practical recommendations for the application of peripheral arterial tonometry in children and adolescents. Int J Cardiol. 2013;168(4):3183-90.
15. Maréchaux S, Samson R, Van Belle E, et al. Vascular and microvascular endothelial function in heart failure with preserved ejection fraction. J Card Fail. 2016;22(1):3-11.
16. Paulus WJ, Tschöpe C. A novel paradigm for heart failure with preserved ejection fraction. J Am Coll Cardiol. 2013;62(4):263-71.
17. Borlaug BA, Olson TP, Lam CSP, et al. Global cardiovascular reserve dysfunction in heart failure with preserved ejection fraction. J Am Coll Cardiol. 2010;56(11):845-54.
18. Collier P, Watson CJ, Voon V, et al. Can emerging biomarkers of myocardial remodelling identify asymptomatic hypertensive patients at risk for diastolic dysfunction and diastolic heart failure? Eur J Heart Fail. 2011;13(10):1087-95.
19. Franssen C, Chen S, Unger A, et al. Myocardial microvascular inflammatory endothelial activation in heart failure with preserved ejection fraction. JACC Heart Fail. 2016;4(4): 312-24.
20. Van Heerebeek L, Hamdani N, Falcão-Pires I, et al. Low myocardial protein kinase G activity in heart failure with preserved ejection fraction. Circulation. 2012;126(7): 830-9.
21. Adams V, Alves M, Fischer T, et al. High-intensity interval training attenuates endothelial dysfunction in a dahl salt sensitive rat model of heart failure with preserved ejection fraction. J Appl Physiol. 2015;119(6):745-52.
22. Shafiq A, Brawner CA, Aldred HA, et al. Prognostic value of cardiopulmonary exercise testing in heart failure with preserved ejection fraction. The Henry ford HospITal CardioPulmonary EXercise testing (FIT-CPX) project. Am Heart J. 2016;174:167-72.
23. Dhakal BP, Malhotra R, Murphy RM, et al. Mechanisms of exercise intolerance in heart failure with preserved ejection fraction: the role of abnormal peripheral oxygen extraction. Circ Heart Fail. 2014;8(2):286-94.
24. Lee JF, Barrett-O'Keefe Z, Nelson AD, et al. Impaired skeletal muscle vasodilation during exercise in heart failure with preserved ejection fraction. Int J Cardiol. 2016;211:14-21.
25. Lam CSP, Brutsaert DL. Endothelial dysfunction: a pathophysiologic factor in heart failure with reserved ejection fraction. J Am Coll Cardiol. 2012;60(18):1787-9.
26. Ter Maaten JM, Damman K, Verhaar MC, et al. Connecting heart failure with preserved ejection fraction and renal dysfunction: the role of endothelial dysfunction and inflammation. Eur J Heart Fail. 2016;18(6):588-98.
27. Hambrecht R, Hilbrich L, Erbs S, et al. Correction of endothelial dysfunction in chronic heart failure: additional effects of exercise training and oral L-arginine supplementation. J Am Coll Cardiol. 2000;35(3):706-13.
28. Obokata M, Reddy YNV, Pislaru SV, et al. Evidence supporting the existence of a distinct obese phenotype of heart failure with preserved ejection fraction. Circulation. 2017;136(1): 6-19.

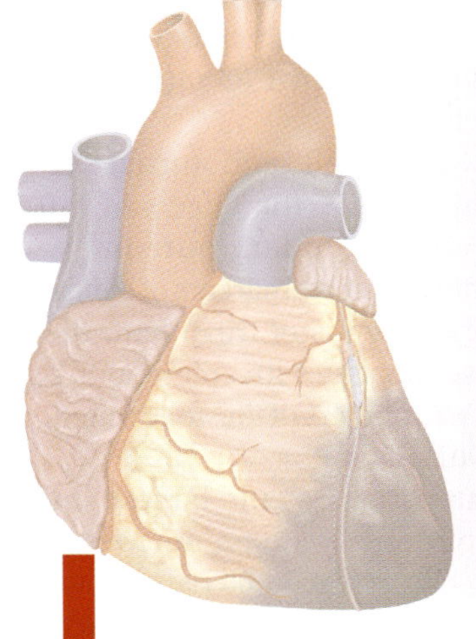

Therapies for HFpEF: Current Status and Future Directions

Kewal C Goswami, Dinkar Bhasin

INTRODUCTION

Nearly 50% of the patients admitted with decompensated heart failure (HF) have heart failure with preserved ejection fraction (HFpEF).[1] Outcomes of such patients in clinical trials have been better than those with heart failure with reduced ejection fraction (HFrEF) with many patients dying from noncardiovascular causes.[2]

APPROACH TO TREATMENT

No treatment modality has been shown to convincingly improve clinical outcomes in patients with HFpEF. Drugs such a beta-blockers, angiotensin-converting enzyme (ACE) inhibitors and angiotensin receptor blockers (ARBs) which have shown a survival benefit in patients with HFrEF have failed to do so in patients with HFpEF. The management of HFpEF is directed at treating volume overload with diuretics, treatment of comorbid conditions such as hypertension, improving exercise capacity, and interventions to decrease hospitalizations.[3,4]

TRIALS OF THERAPIES FOR HEART FAILURE WITH PRESERVED EJECTION FRACTION

Several trials have studied various interventions in patients with HFpEF. There has been significant intertrial variability in the inclusion criteria with respect to ejection fraction (range 35–50%) and primary outcomes which have varied from HF hospitalization to exercise capacity. The important trials are summarized below:

Angiotensin-converting Enzyme Inhibitors and Angiotensin Receptor Blockers

The CHARM-preserved randomized trial assessed the effects of angiotensin receptor inhibitor (ARB) candesartan on the primary outcome of cardiovascular death or hospitalization for chronic heart failure (CHF) in 3,023 patients with HFpEF [left-ventricular ejection fraction (LVEF) > 40%] who were in New York Heart Association (NYHA) class II–IV. After a median follow-up of 36.6 months, there was no difference in the primary outcome or cardiovascular deaths, but there was a significant reduction in hospitalization for CHF.[5] The PEP-CHF trial studied the effects of perindopril in patients ≥70 years of age with HFpEF. The primary end-point was a composite of all-cause death and unplanned hospitalizations for HF. The study had major limitations such as low event rates and patient withdrawal from medication by nearly 25% of the patients. Hence, the results were not definitive but a significant reduction was noted in the the primary end-point [hazard ratio (HR) 0.69: 95% CI 0.47–1.01; $P = 0.055$] and hospitalization for HF (HR 0.63: 95% CI 0.41–0.97; $P = 0.033$) at 1 year. There was an improvement in functional class ($P < 0.030$) and 6-minute walk distance ($P = 0.011$) in patients receiving perindopril.[6]

The I-PRESERVE trial assessed the utility of irbesartan in patients with HFpEF (EF > 45%) in 4,128 symptomatic patients with age ≥60 years. The primary end-point was all-cause death or hospitalization from a cardiovascular cause. The mean follow-up was for 49.5 months, and there was no difference in any of the outcomes.[7]

To summarize, there is insufficient evidence to support the routine use of ACE inhibitors or ARBs in patients with HFpEF. Patients with coexistent hypertension may derive benefit from the associated control of hypertension by these drugs.

Beta-blockers

The Japanese diastolic heart failure (J-DHF) trial was a small, randomized study with 245 patients with HFpEF (LVEF ≥ 40%) that was designed to investigate the effects of carvedilol on the composite outcome of death due to cardiovascular causes and unplanned HF hospitalization. There was no difference in the outcomes among patients receiving carvedilol or placebo after a median follow-up of 3.2 years. However, the median prescribed dose was 7.5 mg/day, which was much less than the target dose of 20 mg/day. In a subgroup analysis of patients treated with >7.5 mg/day of carvedilol, there was significant reduction in the composite outcome (HR 0.54, 95% CI 0.30–0.96; P = 0.034).[8]

The ELANDD trial included 116 symptomatic patients with HF and LVEF > 45% who were randomized to nebivolol or placebo to study the effect on clinical symptoms and exercise capacity. At the end of 6 months, there was no difference in peak oxygen uptake, 6-minute walk distance (6MWD), and functional class. A correlation was observed between the maximum exercise heart rate and peak oxygen uptake suggesting that the negative chronotropic effect of nebivolol may have counterbalanced any benefit from this drug on exercise capacity.[9] The SENIORS trial studied the effects of nebivolol on clinical outcomes in elderly patients with HF. Nebivolol is a beta-1 selective agent with vasodilatory properties mediated by the release of nitric oxide. The primary end-point was a composite of all-cause death or hospitalization due to cardiovascular causes. There was significant reduction in primary outcome in the entire population (31.1% vs 35.3%; HR = 0.86, 95% CI 0.74–0.99, P = 0.039). The benefit was similar in patients with LVEF < 35% and those with LVEF ≥ 35%. However, this trial did not truly study patients with EF ≥ 50%, and hence the utility of this drug in HFpEF remains unproven.[10,11]

Mineralocorticoid Receptor Antagonists

Mineralocorticoid receptor antagonists (MRAs) have been shown to improve outcomes in patients with HFrEF and have been studied in patients with HFpEF. The Aldo-DHF trial included 422 patients with NYHA class II or III HFpEF and randomized them to therapy with spironolactone or placebo. At the end of 6 months of treatment, there was a significant difference in the peak exercise capacity, symptom status, or quality of life parameters between the two groups. There was evidence of marginal improvement in diastolic dysfunction as assessed by E/e' ratio, but the implications of this are unclear.[12]

The RAAM-PEF trial was a small randomized study (n = 42 patients) designed to study the effects of MRA eplerenone on 6-MWD and secondary outcomes of diastolic dysfunction (E/e' ratio) and biomarkers of collagen metabolism. At the end of 6 months of treatment, there was no difference in exercise capacity with eplerenone but significant improvement in parameters of diastolic function and a decrease in collagen turnover.[13]

The TOPCAT multicenter trial was the largest study to evaluate the effect of spironolactone on outcomes in patients with HFpEF (EF ≥ 45%). Over 3,000 patients were randomized to receive either spironolactone or placebo and followed up over 3.3 years. The primary outcome was a composite of cardiovascular death, aborted cardiac arrest, or HF hospitalizations. There was no difference in primary outcome between the two groups (18.6% vs 20.4%; HR = 0.89, 95% CI = 0.77–1.94; P = 0.14). However, a significant reduction in HF hospitalizations (12.0% vs 14.2%; HR = 0.83; 95% CI 0.69–0.99; P = 0.04) was observed. There was no difference in the other components of the primary outcome. The incidence of hyperkalemia was nearly double (18.7% vs. 9.1%) and a more frequent increase in serum creatinine was observed. An important interaction was noted between the country of enrolment and outcomes in this study. The trial suffered from recruitment related issues in Russia and Georgia, where asymptomatic patients with HFpEF had also been included in the study and event rates were observed to be similar to controls.[14] A post-hoc analysis showed that after excluding patients from these countries, a significant reduction in the primary outcome was noted (HR = 0.82; 95% CI 0.69–0.98).[15]

Other Drugs

The RELAX trial was a small study designed to evaluate the effect of phosphodiesterase-5 inhibitor sildenafil in patients with HFpEF. Sildenafil failed to improve clinical status or exercise capacity at 24 weeks. A major criticism of this trial was lenient inclusion criteria with a large proportion of patients with mild diastolic dysfunction and many patients without pulmonary hypertension. Presence of comorbidities in patients with HFpEF may have confounded the use of exercise capacity as an outcome measure.[16] The NEAT-HFpEF study assessed the potential benefit with sustained release isosorbide mononitrate in patients with HFpEF. There was no improvement in patient activity or quality of life after 6 weeks of therapy.[17]

Digoxin

The DIG-PEF trial randomized 988 patients with HF and EF > 45% to receive digoxin or placebo. The primary outcome was a composite of death due to HF or HF Hospitalization. No benefit was observed with digoxin in either the primary outcome or any of its components. The group treated with digoxin showed a trend towards reduction in HF hospitalization which was counterbalanced by an increase in unstable angina-related hospitalizations. None of these differences were truly significant.[18]

Implantable Hemodynamic Monitors

Implantable hemodynamic monitors are devices implanted in the pulmonary artery which provide a or intermittent assessment of hemodynamic data, most importantly, the pulmonary artery pressure, and this data is used to guide patient management. The CHAMPION trial studied one such device—the wireless CardioMEMS™ heart sensor in 550 patients with HF. 119 patients had EF ≥ 40%, and 66 patients had EF ≥ 50%. After a median follow-up of 17.6 months, there was a significant reduction in HF hospitalization among patients with EF ≥ 40% randomized to management with the sensor (HR = 0.50; 95% CI 0.35–0.70; P < 0.0001). The benefit was consistent in patients with EF ≥ 50% (HR = 0.30; 95% CI 0.18–0.48; P < 0.0001). Patients with the sensor were prescribed more diuretics and vasodilators.[19,20]

REASON FOR FAILURE OF STANDARD HEART FAILURE THERAPIES IN HFpEF: DIFFERENCES IN ETIOPATHOGENESIS

Like HFrEF, patients with HFpEF present with signs and symptoms of HF, and a clinical distinction between the two entities is not possible. However, there are essential differences in etiopathogenesis of the two conditions which influence treatment and management. HFpEF constitutes a heterogeneous group of conditions with a broad spectrum of patient profiles with regard to etiology and comorbidities. Most trials have been unable to account for these differences. For instance, a patient with severe diastolic dysfunction secondary to hypertension and a patient with HFpEF because of hypertrophic cardiomyopathy may have similar clinical features; however, the management and outcomes may be greatly influenced by the underlying condition. Further, there is a fundamental difference in the pathophysiology of HFpEF. Presence of diastolic dysfunction results in restrictive left ventricular filling. Aggressive therapy with diuretics may improve the congestive symptoms but decrease preload resulting in symptoms of decreased cardiac output such as fatigue. Similarly, because cardiac output in such conditions is heart rate dependent, aggressive reduction in heart rate with beta-blockers may result in paradoxical decrease in cardiac output. This may be compounded by frequent coexistence of chronotropic incompetence in these patients. Also, unlike HFrEF, the activation of neurohormonal pathways may be only modest in HFpEF, probably explaining the failure of neurohormonal antagonists to improve outcomes.

TREATMENT OF CONGESTION

Most important limiting symptom in patients with HFpEF is dyspnea secondary to elevated filling pressures and pulmonary venous congestion. Diuretic therapy remains the cornerstone of symptomatic treatment. Basic principles are similar to HFrEF, but aggressive diuretic therapy can paradoxically decrease cardiac output and worsen fatigue while relieving dyspnea. Loop diuretics are the drugs of choice for initial therapy and should be combined with MRAs to avoid hypokalemia. Intermittent treatment with thiazide-like diuretics can provide additional diuresis but warrants careful electrolyte monitoring. Patients with diuretic resistance should be treated with intravenous diuretics.

MANAGEMENT OF COMORBIDITIES

The major comorbidities associated with HFpEF include hypertension, diabetes, obesity, sleep apnea, and chronic kidney disease. Hypertension is present in most patients with HFpEF, and appropriate management can decrease the risk of HF hospitalizations. The choice of drug therapy should be guided by coexistent conditions such as coronary artery disease, diabetes, and left ventricular hypertrophy. Most patients with hypertension and HF should be treated with diuretics. Patients with kidney disease may benefit from ACE inhibitors or ARBs. Vasodilatory beta-blockers are a viable treatment option, but these drugs should be avoided in patients with chronotropic incompetence. The presence of HFpEF does not modify the treatment pressure targets, but care should be taken to avoid orthostatic hypotension given the elderly age group, and concomitant therapy with diuretics. Diabetes is independently associated with diastolic dysfunction, and appropriate management of blood sugars is necessary.[21] A significant proportion of patients with HFpEF are obese. Obesity is associated with diastolic dysfunction, and weight loss strategies such as dietary modifications, exercise, and bariatric surgery should be considered.[22] Sleep apnea is independently associated with worse outcomes in patients with HF.[23] There should be a high suspicion in patients with HFpEF, and it should be managed with weight loss and continuous positive airway pressure therapy.

ATRIAL FIBRILLATION

Atrial fibrillation (AF) is commonly present in patients with HFpEF because of advanced age and coexistent condition such as hypertension. Because of diastolic dysfunction, patients with HFpEF are dependent on the atrial kick for maintaining cardiac output and are likely to deteriorate after the onset of AF. Management should be based on standard guidelines, but in patients with refractory HF, rhythm control should be preferred. Catheter ablation has emerged as an effective and safe alternative to pharmacological rhythm control, especially in patients with paroxysmal AF or early AF. Most of the patients are candidates for anticoagulation (elderly, HF and often hypertension) and direct-acting oral anticoagulants remain the drugs of first choice.

NONPHARMACOLOGICAL THERAPIES

Patients should be adequately educated about self-care such as monitoring of weight, dietary restrictions, adjustment of diuretic dose based on symptoms, regular exercise, and scheduled follow up. Dietary fluid and salt restriction (<2 g/day of sodium) is not necessary for all patients but may be useful for patients who are symptomatic despite a high dose of diuretics. Small studies have shown benefit with exercise training in symptom status, and quality of life.[24,25] Patients should be encouraged to engage in aerobic exercise daily for at least 30 minutes as dictated by their functional status and capacity. All patients should receive a pneumococcal vaccine and annual influenza vaccine.

PHENOTYPE-BASED APPROACH

As discussed, unlike HFrEF, patients with HFpEF represent a heterogeneous spectrum where generalizations to treatment cannot be made. Patients should be characterized into a phenotype to allow optimal management. For example, patients can be stratified based of presenting symptoms like congestive symptoms, features of decreased cardiac output such as fatigue or right HF. Patients can also be classified based on etiology such as hypertension, coronary artery disease (CAD), hypertrophic cardiomyopathy (HCM), or valvular heart disease. Such categorization allows better treatment decisions. For instance, a hypertensive patient presenting with predominantly congestive symptoms should be managed with diuretics and blood pressure control. While a similar patient presenting with symptoms of decreased cardiac output like fatigue, care must be taken to avoid aggressive diuresis and rate reduction with beta-blockers. A patient with CAD and HFpEF may benefit from revascularization and should be evaluated for the same.

FUTURE DIRECTIONS

Angiotensin Receptor Neprilysin Inhibitor

The combination of sacubitril-valsartan (LCZ696) has been shown to improve outcomes in patients with HFrEF. One small phase II randomized controlled trial (RCT) has shown benefit on biochemical and echocardiographic parameters in HFpEF. The PARAMOUNT study assessed the effect of angiotensin receptor neprilysin inhibitor (ARNI) on NT-proBNP in patients with HF and EF ≥45%. There was a significant reduction in NT-proBNP levels at 12 weeks in patients receiving LCZ696 compared to patients receiving only valsartan (ratio 0.77; 95% CI 0.64–0.92; p = 0.005) with no difference in serious adverse events.[26] There was a significant reduction in the global circumferential strain at 36 weeks in patients treated with ARNI compared with valsartan with no change in the global longitudinal strain.[27] A large study to assess the effect of this agent on clinical outcomes is underway (PARAGON-HF trial).[28]

Statins

Statins have been shown to have several pleomorphic effects such as membrane stabilization, improving endothelial function, and anti-inflammatory benefits. Most patients with HFpEF have an indication for statin use for either primary or secondary prevention. Evidence from observational studies suggests that treatment with statins may be associated with better outcomes in HFpEF patients. A meta-analysis of four observational studies with over 5,000 patients showed an association between statin therapy and decreased mortality.[29] However, the confounding effects of statin therapy on outcomes related to comorbidities of HFpEF cannot be adjusted completely in observational studies. A post-hoc analysis of TOPCAT trial after propensity score matching showed that among patients without CAD, treatment in statins resulted in a lower all-cause and cardiovascular mortality.[30] RCTs that systematically test this hypothesis are required.

Ivabradine

Ivabradine results in a slowing of heart rate and is recommended in patients with HFrEF who have fast rates and cannot tolerate beta-blockers. A small echocardiography based observational study showed improvement in parameters of diastolic dysfunction with ivabradine.[31] However, a crossover RCT showed that after 2 weeks of therapy, when compared with placebo, ivabradine resulted in a significant worsening of the peak oxygen consumption and reduction in the exercise capacity. No change was observed in plasma brain natriuretic peptide (BNP) or quality of life parameters.[32]

Interatrial Shunt Device

The interatrial shunt device (Corvia Medical, Massachusetts, the United States of America) has been designed to create and maintain a defect in the interatrial septum. It is a nitinol device with an external diameter of 18 mm deployed using a 16F delivery system. It produces an 8-mm atrial septal defect to allow a left to right shunt and decompress the left atrium, thereby decreasing the left atrial pressure and congestive symptoms. In a small phase II RCT, 44 patients with HFpEF with EF ≥ 40%, pulmonary capillary wedge pressure (PCWP) during exercise ≥ 25 mm Hg and PCWP right atrial pressure gradient ≥ 5 mm were randomized to undergo device implantation or a sham procedure. At 1 month follow-up, patients receiving the device experienced a significant reduction in PCWP during exercise with no significant periprocedural or 1 month major adverse events.[33] At 12-month follow-up, the device patency rates were 100% with no difference in cardiac or other adverse events.[34] A mid-term follow-up (median 792 days) of patients undergoing device implantation reported the mortality rates to be significantly lower than expected based on baseline characteristics of the cohort (3.4 per 100 patient years vs. 10.2 per 100 patient years; P = 0.02) suggesting that implantation of this device may be associated with better survival.[35] Another device, the V-Wave (V-Wave, Caesarea, Israel) is a nitinol implant shaped like an hourglass which is encapsulated by polytetrafluoroethylene (PTFE) and has porcine bioprosthetic valve allowing only one-way shunting to prevent paradoxical embolism. Initial observational data with the device suggest improvement in NYHA class and 6MWD at 3 months and 12 months of follow-up. All devices were patent at 3 months but the rates of shunt occlusion (14%) and shunt stenosis (36%) at 12 months were high suggesting a need for modifying the device.[36]

CONCLUSION

The burden of HFpEF is increasing; however, unlike HFrEF, there is little evidence to support the use of specific therapies to improve clinical outcomes. Management of such patients is centered around diuretic therapy for symptom control and management of comorbidities. There is some evidence to support the use of spironolactone to decrease hospitalizations with HF. Use of implantable hemodynamic monitors may be considered in refractory cases. Other nonpharmacologic therapies such as physical rehabilitation, dietary restrictions, vaccination, and self-care should be same as in HFrEF. In the future, evidence from RCTs may support the use of ARNI in HFpEF. With growing evidence, the interatrial shunt device may prove to be a viable option for patients who have refractory HF symptoms.

REFERENCES

1. Gladden JD, Linke WA, Redfield MM. Heart failure with preserved ejection fraction. Pflugers Arch. 2014;466(6):1037-53.
2. Campbell RT, Jhund PS, Castagno D, et al. What Have We Learned About Patients With Heart Failure and Preserved Ejection Fraction From DIG-PEF, CHARM-Preserved, and I-PRESERVE? J Am Coll Cardiol. 2012;60(23):2349-56.
3. Coats AJ, Shewan LG. The Management of Heart Failure with Preserved Ejection Fraction. Card Fail Rev. 2015;1(1):11-5.
4. Upadhya B, Kitzman DW. Heart Failure with Preserved Ejection Fraction in Older Adults. Heart Fail Clin. 2017;13(3):485-502.
5. Pfeffer MA, Swedberg K, Granger CB, et al. Effects of candesartan on mortality and morbidity in patients with chronic heart failure: the CHARM-Overall programme. Lancet Lond Engl. 2003;362(9386):759-66.
6. Cleland JGF, Tendera M, Adamus J, et al. The perindopril in elderly people with chronic heart failure (PEP-CHF) study. Eur Heart J. 2006;27(19):2338-45.
7. Massie BM, Carson PE, McMurray JJ, et al. Irbesartan in patients with heart failure and preserved ejection fraction. N Engl J Med. 2008;359(23):2456-67.
8. Yamamoto K, Origasa H, Hori M, et al. Effects of carvedilol on heart failure with preserved ejection fraction: the Japanese Diastolic Heart Failure Study (J-DHF). Eur J Heart Fail. 2013;15(1):110-8.
9. Conraads VM, Metra M, Kamp O, et al. Effects of the long-term administration of nebivolol on the clinical symptoms, exercise capacity, and left ventricular function of patients with diastolic dysfunction: results of the ELANDD study. Eur J Heart Fail. 2012;14(2):219-25.
10. Flather MD, Shibata MC, Coats AJS, et al. Randomized trial to determine the effect of nebivolol on mortality and cardiovascular hospital admission in elderly patients with heart failure (SENIORS). Eur Heart J. 2005;26(3):215-25.
11. van Veldhuisen DJ, Cohen-Solal A, Böhm M, et al. Beta-blockade with Nebivolol in Elderly Heart Failure Patients with Impaired and Preserved Left Ventricular Ejection Fraction: Data From SENIORS (Study of Effects of Nebivolol Intervention on Outcomes and Rehospitalization in Seniors With Heart Failure). J Am Coll Cardiol. 2009;53(23):2150-8.
12. Edelmann F, Wachter R, Schmidt AG, et al. Effect of Spironolactone on Diastolic Function and Exercise Capacity in Patients With Heart Failure With Preserved Ejection Fraction: The Aldo-DHF Randomized Controlled Trial. JAMA. 2013;309(8):781-91.
13. Deswal A, Richardson P, Bozkurt B, et al. Results of the Randomized Aldosterone Antagonism in Heart Failure with

Preserved Ejection Fraction trial (RAAM-PEF). J Card Fail. 2011;17(8):634-42.
14. Pitt B, Pfeffer MA, Assmann SF, et al. Spironolactone for heart failure with preserved ejection fraction. N Engl J Med. 2014;370(15):1383-92.
15. Pfeffer MA, Claggett B, Assmann SF, et al. Regional Variation in Patients and Outcomes in the Treatment of Preserved Cardiac Function Heart Failure With an Aldosterone Antagonist (TOPCAT) Trial. Circulation. 2015;131(1): 34-42.
16. Wang H, Anstrom K, Ilkayeva O, et al. Sildenafil Treatment in Heart Failure With Preserved Ejection Fraction: Targeted Metabolomic Profiling in the RELAX Trial. JAMA Cardiol. 2017;2(8):896-901.
17. Redfield MM, Anstrom KJ, Levine JA, et al. Isosorbide Mononitrate in Heart Failure with Preserved Ejection Fraction. N Engl J Med. 2015;373(24):2314-24.
18. Ahmed A, Rich MW, Fleg JL, et al. Effects of Digoxin on Morbidity and Mortality in Diastolic Heart Failure: The Ancillary Digitalis Investigation Group Trial. Circulation. 2006;114(5):397-403.
19. Abraham WT, Adamson PB, Bourge RC, et al. Wireless pulmonary artery haemodynamic monitoring in chronic heart failure: a randomised controlled trial. Lancet Lond Engl. 2011;377(9766):658-66.
20. Adamson PB, Abraham WT, Bourge RC, et al. Wireless pulmonary artery pressure monitoring guides management to reduce decompensation in heart failure with preserved ejection fraction. Circ Heart Fail. 2014;7(6):935-44.
21. Patil VC, Patil HV, Shah KB, et al. Diastolic dysfunction in asymptomatic type 2 diabetes mellitus with normal systolic function. J Cardiovasc Dis Res. 2011;2(4):213-22.
22. Tadic M, Cuspidi C. Obesity and heart failure with preserved ejection fraction: a paradox or something else? Heart Fail Rev. 2019;24(3):379-85.
23. Arikawa T, Toyoda S, Haruyama A, et al. Impact of Obstructive Sleep Apnoea on Heart Failure with Preserved Ejection Fraction. Heart Lung Circ. 2016;25(5):435-41.
24. Kitzman DW, Brubaker P, Morgan T, et al. Effect of Caloric Restriction or Aerobic Exercise Training on Peak Oxygen Consumption and Quality of Life in Obese Older Patients With Heart Failure With Preserved Ejection Fraction: A Randomized Clinical Trial. JAMA. 2016;315(1):36-46.
25. Pandey A, Parashar A, Kumbhani D, et al. Exercise training in patients with heart failure and preserved ejection fraction: meta-analysis of randomized control trials. Circ Heart Fail. 2015;8(1):33-40.
26. Solomon SD, Zile M, Pieske B, et al. The angiotensin receptor neprilysin inhibitor LCZ696 in heart failure with preserved ejection fraction: a phase 2 double-blind randomised controlled trial. Lancet Lond Engl. 2012;380(9851):1387-95.
27. Biering-Sorensen T, Shah A, Claggett B, et al. The Angiotensin Receptor Neprilysin Inhibitor (arni), Sacubitril/Valsartan, Improves Left Ventricular Myocardial Deformation in Heart Failure with Preserved Ejection Fraction (paramount Trial). J Am Coll Cardiol. 2019;71(11 Suppl):A2665.
28. Solomon SD, Rizkala AR, Gong J, et al. Angiotensin Receptor Neprilysin Inhibition in Heart Failure With Preserved Ejection Fraction: Rationale and Design of the PARAGON-HF Trial. JACC Heart Fail. 2017;5(7):471-82.
29. Fukuta H, Goto T, Wakami K, et al. The effect of statins on mortality in heart failure with preserved ejection fraction: a meta-analysis of propensity score analyses. Int J Cardiol. 2016;214:301-6.
30. Tsujimoto T, Kajio H. Favorable effects of statins in the treatment of heart failure with preserved ejection fraction in patients without ischemic heart disease. Int J Cardiol. 2018;255:111-7.
31. Cacciapuoti F, Magro VM, Caturano M, et al. The role of Ivabradine in Diastolic Heart Failure with preserved Ejection Fraction. A Doppler-Echocardiographic study. J Cardiovasc Echogr. 2017;27(4):126-31.
32. Pal N, Sivaswamy N, Mahmod M, et al. Effect of Selective Heart Rate Slowing in Heart Failure With Preserved Ejection Fraction. Circulation. 2015;132(18):1719-25.
33. Feldman Ted, Mauri Laura, Kahwash Rami, et al. Transcatheter Interatrial Shunt Device for the Treatment of Heart Failure With Preserved Ejection Fraction (REDUCE LAP-HF I [Reduce Elevated Left Atrial Pressure in Patients With Heart Failure]). Circulation. 2018;137(4):364-75.
34. Shah SJ, Feldman T, Ricciardi MJ, et al. One-Year Safety and Clinical Outcomes of a Transcatheter Interatrial Shunt Device for the Treatment of Heart Failure With Preserved Ejection Fraction in the Reduce Elevated Left Atrial Pressure in Patients With Heart Failure (REDUCE LAP-HF I) Trial: A Randomized Clinical Trial. JAMA Cardiol. 2018;3(10):968-77.
35. Kaye DM, Petrie MC, McKenzie S, et al. Impact of an interatrial shunt device on survival and heart failure hospitalization in patients with preserved ejection fraction. ESC Heart Fail. 2019;6(1):62-9.
36. Rodés-Cabau J, Bernier M, Amat-Santos IJ, et al. Interatrial Shunting for Heart Failure: Early and Late Results From the First-in-Human Experience With the V-Wave System. JACC Cardiovasc Interv. 2018;11(22):2300-10.

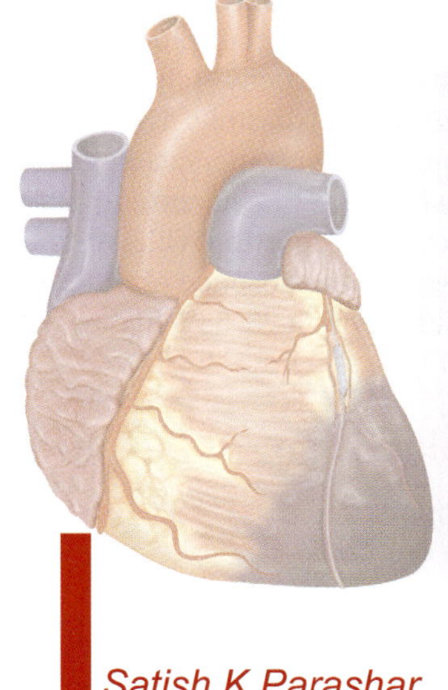

Heart Failure with Preserved Ejection Fraction: Few Newer Insights

Satish K Parashar

INTRODUCTION

Diastole is an important component of cardiac cycle and occupies most of it as compared to systole. It is an energy consuming process and is as active as systole. Moreover it is the first component to be affected in various disease processes. As this would be discussed later it is an important parameter for all clinical and subclinical heart failures. The heart failure (HF) is predominantly of three types: (1) HFrEF with left ventricular ejection fraction (LVEF) below 40%, (2) HFmrEF with LVEF from 41% to 49% and (3) HFrEF with LVEF > 50%. Diastolic dysfunction of the heart has assumed significant importance in last several years. This is because it can lead to isolated heart failure. It has now been recognized that almost 40–50% of all patients in western population with clinically diagnosed heart failure have a near normal ejection fraction. The incidence in overall population is 1–2%. This clinical entity, which occurs without significant valvular lesion or pericardial disease, is now referred as heart failure with preserved ejection fraction (HFpEF) which in the past was labeled as diastolic heart failure (DHF).

SIGNIFICANCE OF HEART FAILURE WITH PRESERVED EJECTION FRACTION

The clinical outcomes of HFpEF are similar to those with HFrEF, including in-hospital morbidity and hospital readmission rates. Although in-hospital mortality may be slightly higher in HFrEF, 30-day to 1-year mortality after discharge is similar between these groups. Patients with either HF syndrome have comparable functional limitations and poor quality of life. Health care costs are at par in both. Annual mortality in HFpEF ranges from 10% to 30%. Nearly two-third (60%) of HFpEF patients die from cardiovascular causes, mostly sudden death and heart failure related death. Key mortality risk factors include advance age, female gender, body mass index, comorbidity burden, renal impairment, hemodynamic instability ((hypotension and tachycardia) and coronary artery disease (CAD).

Clinical conditions/comorbidities usually responsible for it are older age, female gender hypertension, cardiomyopathy, CAD, diabetes mellitus, infiltrative disorders, obesity, sleep apnea, renal dysfunction, constrictive pericarditis, metabolic syndrome, etc. As such all vulnerable patients with dyspnea, either at rest or exertion, or heart failure should be evaluated for diastolic functions.

This syndrome has proven particularly challenging on many fronts: (a) consensus-based diagnostic criteria result in a heterogeneous population that has proven challenging for clinical studies and trials; (b) multiple mechanisms have been proposed but many remain hypothetical because of limited access to live human heart tissue; (c) good experimental models do not really exist, as many capture components of the human disease but do not reflect its integrative complexity; and (d) HFpEF patients are afflicted with multiple common comorbidities, as mentioned above that have a major impact on the syndrome and mortality. Given this, it is perhaps not surprising that we have yet to find an evidence-based HFpEF therapy beyond diuretics for fluid overload and conventional treatments for comorbidities.

METHODS TO ASSESS DIASTOLIC DYSFUNCTION

There are several methods to assess diastolic dysfunction as mentioned below:
- Invasive method like cardiac catheterization
- Echo-Doppler approach
- Nuclear approach
- cMRI/CT

Each technique has its own strengths and weaknesses. However considering the simplicity of technique and financial implications involved, echocardiography has emerged as the most practical approach because of its easy availability, portability, capability of performing repeated studies and giving immediate diagnosis. Moreover it has a fairly good correlation with invasively determined left ventricular filling pressure.

The diagnosis of HFpEF is primarily based on (a) presence of signs and symptoms of heart failure; (b) presence of normal or near normal left ventricular ejection fraction: ≥50%; (c) Normal left ventricular volume: LVEDVI < 97 mL/m^2, as >90% patients with HFpEF have normal LV chamber dimension, area, and volume; (d) signs of abnormal diastolic functions especially increased filling pressure with LVEDP > 15 mm Hg and mean LA Pressure: > 12 mm Hg; and (e) other helpful signs are left ventricular hypertrophy and/or left atrial enlargement.

Evaluation of diastolic parameters for assessing LV filling pressure are well known (Table 1 and Flowcharts 1 and 2) but are based on mainly four parameters: (1) Transmitral Doppler for recording mitral early filling velocity (E wave), late diastolic atrial velocity (A), E/A ratio, mitral deceleration slope; (2) Tissue Doppler (TDI) early diastolic annular velocity (e'), thereby calculating E/e' ratio-*importance*:. Mitral E depends on LA pressure, LV relaxation kinetics and age, e' depends on LV relaxation kinetics and age. E/e' eliminates two common factors, hence indicates LA pressure or LV filling pressure. So with increasing velocity of mitral 'E' wave and decreasing annular 'e; velocity, E/e' ratio progressively increases with increasing LV filling pressure; (3) Left atrial volume index; and (4) Tricuspid regurgitation jet velocity. Table 1 shows the various parameters for grading of diastolic dysfunction with increased LV filling pressure with increasing grade. *Concentric remodeling in which there* is increase in mass or thickness relative to (or out of proportion with) volume or dimension can occur even in the absence of frank LV hypertrophy. This is associated with a 25–35% higher risk of heart failure events.

Simple Diagnostic Algorithm

Step 1: Assess pretest likelihood
- Presence of dyspnea on exertion
- Assessment for presence of comorbidities
- N-terminal pro b-type natriuretic peptide (NT-pro BNP) if available
- Conventional echo for structural abnormalities like left ventricular hypertrophy (LVH), left atrial (LA) enlargement, etc.
- Electrocardiogram (ECG) and X-ray chest.

Step 2: Diastolic work-up
- N-terminal pro b-type natriuretic peptide if not already done
- Comprehensive work-up of diastolic functions as mentioned above.

Step 3: Advance work-up
- *Diastolic stress echo*: Many elderly patients of HT and LVH have symptoms mainly on exertion and may have normal resting echo, so more relevant to study with exercise, as it can unmask increased filling pressure on exercise
- Invasive studies in "gray zone or indeterminate patients" which can be as high as 30%.

Step 4: *Optional*: Etiology work-up
- cMRI
- Positron emission tomography (PET) scan
- Genetic testing.

TABLE 1: Diagnostic criteria of different grades of diastolic dysfunction.

LV relaxation, filling pressure and 2D and Doppler findings according to LV diastolic function				
	Normal	*Grade I*	*Grade II*	*Grade III*
LV relaxation	Normal	Impaired	Impaired	Impaired
LAP	Normal	Low or normal	Elevated	Elevated
Mitral E/A ratio	≥0.8	≤0.8	>0.8 to <2	>2
Average E/e' ratio	<10	<10	10–14	>14
Peak TR velocity (m/sec)	<2.8	<2.8	>2.8	>2.8
LA volume index	Normal	Normal or increased	Increased	Increased

Flowchart 1: 2016 American College of Cardiology/American Heart Association (ACC/AHA) criteria for diagnosis of heart failure with preserved ejection fraction (HFpEF)

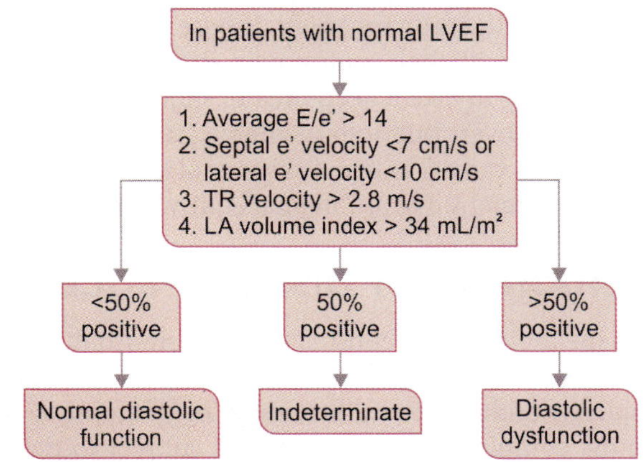

(LVEF: left ventricular ejection fraction)

HEART FAILURE WITH PRESERVED EJECTION FRACTION SCORING SYSTEM

Reddy et al. have proposed a scoring system from diagnosis and prognosis point of view. Points are given as follows:

- *Obesity > 30 kg/m²*: 2 points
- *Hypertension requiring more than two drugs*: 1 point
- *Atrial fibrillation, paroxysmal or persistent*: 3 points
- *Age*: >60 years: 1 point
- *LV filling pressure*: E/e' > 9—2 points.

More than 5 points indicates definite HFpEF. The higher the points the more adverse is the prognosis. This scoring also enables discrimination of HFpEF from noncardiac causes of dyspnea and can assist in determination of the need for further diagnostic testing in the evaluation of patients with unexplained exertional dyspnea.

Age related Differences in Patients with Heart Failure with Preserved Ejection Fraction (Tromp J et al.) (Table 2)

Caveats in diagnosis of HFpEF: (a) The availability of an objective parameter is essential to diagnosis of heart failure because it is a highly subjective condition. Indeed, it has been shown in a study that a majority of HF cases (90%) were undiagnosed and—equally alarmingly—that 76% of previous HF diagnoses were actually misdiagnosed. This illustrates the poor diagnostic reliability of the common signs and symptoms of HF. (b) Almost >30% may have normal diastolic function, which could also be related to fortuitous LV unloading because of prior administration of diuretics. (c) B-type natriuretic peptide (BNP) and N-t Pro BNP: BNP and N-terminal proBNP are elevated in patients

Flowchart 2: 2016 American College of Cardiology/American Heart Association (ACC/AHA) criteria for diagnosis of heart failure with preserved ejection fraction (HFpEF).

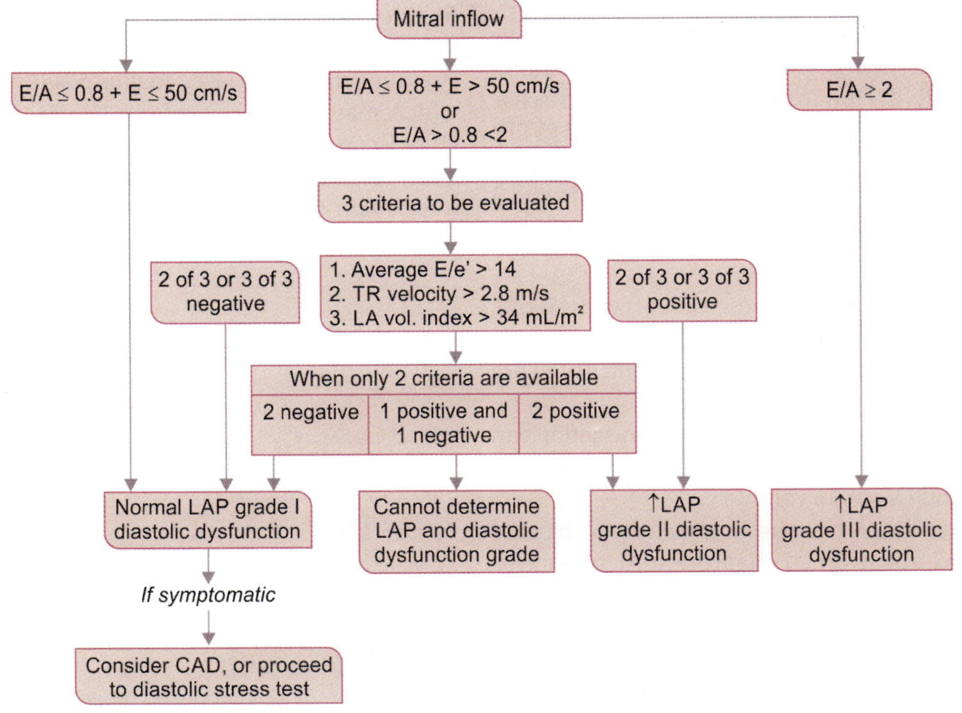

(CAD: coronary artery disease; LAP: left atrial pressure; LV: left ventricle; LVEF: left ventricular ejection fraction)

TABLE 2: Age related differences in patients with HFpEF.

	Young with HFpEF	*Elderly with HFpEF*
Clinical characteristics	Men	Women
	Increased obesity	Increased AF, HT, renal disease
Cardiac structure and function	Increased concentric LVH	Increased filling pressure
	Increased left atrial size	Increased LV volume
Clinical outcome	Increased CV death	Increased non-CV cause of death
	Increased SCD	

(AF: atrial fibrillation; CV: cardiovascular; HFpEF: heart failure with preserved ejection fraction; HT: hypertension; LVH: left ventricular hypertrophy; SCD: sudden cardiac death)

Source: Tromp J, Shen L, Jhund PS, et al. Age-related aspects of heart failure with preserved ejection fraction. J Am Coll Cardiol. 2019;74:601-12.

with HFpEF as compared with those persons without heart failure but are lower than in patients with HFrEF. Increased BNP is directly related to LV diastolic filling pressure and end-diastolic wall stress. Patients with HFpEF have a smaller LV cavity and thicker LV walls; hence, their end-diastolic wall stress is much lower than in HFrEF, even in the setting of high systolic and diastolic pressures, thus producing a lower stimulus for BNP production. On an average, patients with HFpEF presenting with acute decompensation have a BNP value of 100–500 pg/mL versus 500–1,500 pg/mL in patients with HFrEF. Elevation of BNP also indicates increased risk for subsequent events, even in asymptomatic persons. However, as almost a third of HFpEF patients have normal levels of BNP, then BNP cannot be used to exclude a diagnosis of HFpEF. (d) How to interpret diagnosis in a case of decreased global longitudinal strain with normal LVEF? Would such patients qualify for the diagnosis of HFpEF? and (e) many humans have abnormal diastolic function with a normal EF, and that this combination per se does not mean they have HF.

HFpEF and impaired response to stress: Patients with HFpEF have particular difficulty in tolerating certain hemodynamic stresses which thus need priority management. These are mentioned below:

- *Atrial fibrillation*, since the loss of atrial contraction can dramatically reduce left atrial emptying, left ventricular (LV) filling, and LV stroke volume.
- *Sinus tachycardia*, since the increase in heart rate shortens the duration of diastole and truncates relaxation, pressure decline, recoil, and diastolic filling.
- Elevations in systemic blood pressure, especially the abrupt, severe, or refractory elevations often seen with renovascular hypertension. It increases LV wall stress, which can worsen myocardial relaxation.
- *Myocardial ischemia*: The acute induction or worsening of diastolic dysfunction by ischemia raises left atrial and pulmonary venous pressure. This explains why many patients with coronary artery disease have respiratory symptoms with their anginal pain, including wheezing, an inability to take a deep breath, shortness of breath, and even overt pulmonary edema. These respiratory symptoms can occur in the absence of anginal pain and are often referred to as "anginal equivalents".

MECHANISMS OF DISEASE PROCESS

Given the multifaceted constellation of comorbidities that are almost invariably present in HFpEF patients and the complexity of the disease, its underlying pathophysiology remains complex, complicated, and subject to debate. Among the leading contenders are diastolic dysfunction, impaired systolic rest and/or reserve function, abnormal ventricular-arterial coupling, endothelial dysfunction, depressed heart rate response (chronotropic incompetence), altered myocardial energetic and peripheral skeletal muscle metabolism and perfusion, pulmonary hypertension (PH), and renal insufficiency. Several of these mechanisms are noncardiac. Ultimately there is LV structural and altered geometry and changes in LV and vascular compliance with alteration in LV relaxation and compliance. Some proposed mechanisms are shown in Figure 1.

ROLE OF INFLAMMATION

Results from LV endomyocardial biopsy, analyses of inflammatory cell markers suggest that increased oxidative stress and depressed NO signaling resulting in inflammation which may play a key role in HFpEF. The multitude of HFpEF comorbidities may contribute to a proinflammatory state; as such circulating inflammatory cytokines such as interleukin-6, tumor necrosis factor-α, soluble ST2, and pentraxin-3 are elevated in HFpEF.

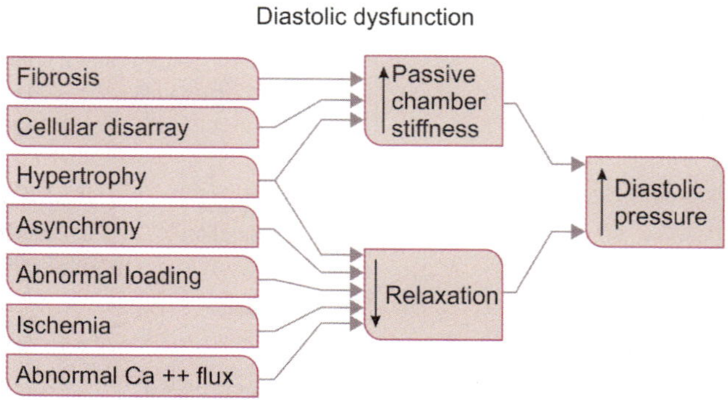

Fig. 1: Various proposed mechanisms for diastolic dysfunction.

TREATMENT

The treatment of HFpEF has traditionally been unsatisfactory with major stress on lifestyle management, and treating the comorbidities. Diuretics have been one of the mainstays to control sodium and water retention, and relieve breathlessness and edema. Targeting the RAAS and β-adrenergic stimulation pathways has long been considered reasonable for HFpEF, the former based on its link to hypertension, fibrosis, and fluid imbalance, and the latter to improve time for diastolic filling. Beta-blockers have been studied in various trials and results have been variable. Pooled data from few randomized controlled trials are suggestive of a positive impact on outcomes, with a trend toward a significant reduction in all-cause mortality, but not on recurrent hospitalization, hence the outcomes remain to be confirmed. In view of variable results, further randomized clinical trials are certainly warranted not only with beta-blockers but also other standard therapies in HFpEF. Yet, despite their clear success in HFrEF, no clinical trial of these standard therapies has revealed similar mortality benefits, and only a few trials have shown symptomatic improvement in HFpEF. Similar have been the results with endothelin antagonists, or metalloproteinase inhibitors in HFpEF. Most of the drugs that should be avoided in HFrEF should also be avoided in HFpEF; exceptions include verapamil and diltiazem, which are not recommended in HFrEF but can be used in HFpEF.

In 2013, the ALDO-DHF study tested the impact of an aldosterone antagonist in HFpEF with the primary endpoints being improved diastolic function and exercise capacity. Some measures of diastolic function improved, though maximal exercise capacity, clinical symptoms, and quality of life were not changed. One critique of the study was that patients had early-stage HFpEF without overt signs of volume overload. The larger 2014 TOPCAT (Treatment of Preserved Cardiac Function Heart Failure with an Aldosterone Antagonist trial) trial failed to demonstrate a benefit study and did not meet its primary composite endpoint (cardiovascular mortality, aborted cardiac arrest, or hospitalization for the management of HF).

FUTURISTIC TREATMENT

Some of the drugs are being studied but have still not found a foundation for treatment. Some of these include (a) one avenue for research concerns advanced glycation endproducts (AGEs), which have been surmised to play a role in HF and have therefore been considered as potential targets in HFpEF. It has resulted in improvements in LV mass and LV diastolic filling, along with improvements in quality of life on the Minnesota Living with Heart Failure score but will merit long-term study; (b) Another treatment which initially showed some promise is the angiotensin receptor–neprilysin inhibitor, which has been demonstrated to reduce NT-proBNP in a phase II trial in 300 patients with HFpEF (LVEF ≥ 45%). However phase III trial PARAGON-HF (Efficacy and Safety of LCZ696 compared to Valsartan on Morbidity and Mortality in Heart Failure Patients with Preserved Ejection Fraction study) it has not shown consistent benefit over Valsartan; (c) statins, ivabradine, and ronalazine are being explored in treatment. SGLT2 inhibitors have currently no significant role in established heart failure; and (d) Agents having antifibrotic, antihypertrophic and anti-inflammatory agents have shown positive results in HFpEF in registries.

Beyond formal treatment with pharmacological agents or other interventions, the effect of lifestyle changes in HFpEF, especially exercise programming, is also being explored.

EXERCISE THERAPY

Exercise intolerance is a major complaint of all HF patients. It is an independent predictor of morbidity and mortality and is increasingly a leading outcome in pharmacological trials of HFpEF. Exercise training has been used to improve outcomes in HFrEF, particularly in patients with ischemic disease, and is being viewed as a potential therapy for HFpEF. Kitzman et al. reported findings from the first randomized controlled study of exercise training in older patients with HFpEF during a 16-week period. The primary outcome of peak exercise oxygen uptake significantly improved in the exercise therapy group compared with controls. Improvements were also noted in exercise time, 6-minute walk distance, ventilatory anaerobic threshold, peak power output, and the physical component of the quality of life score. Some initial studies of exercise training are promising and suggest that exercise training should be considered part of the treatment algorithm, along with pharmacological agents, for the management of HFpEF.

CONCLUSION

Heart failure with preserved ejection fraction continues to be an intriguing disease, which is either over- or underdiagnosed. However considering its prognostic significance, every patient of unexplained dyspnea, either on rest or exertion should be evaluated for HFpEF. This is more so in presence of comorbidities which provoke HFpEF. Comprehensive echocardiography with 2D imaging, spectral Doppler, TDI, LA volume index and newer techniques like speckle strain echocardiography provide a complete assessment of diastolic function. Other ancillary methods like pulmonary venous Doppler, LV mass, LA strain, etc. are utilized in special situations. Various diagnostic algorithms are being proposed to aid in diagnosis. The management continues to be unsatisfactory and still relies on lifestyle management, exercise protocol, diuretics and strict control of comorbidities. However research is still being focused on developing newer management strategies.

BIBLIOGRAPHY

1. ACC/AHA/HFSA. Focused update of the 2013 ACCF/AHA Guideline for the Management of Heart failure. Circulation. 2017;136:e137-e161.
2. Bhatia RS, Tu JV, Lee DS, et al. Outcome of heart failure with preserved ejection fraction in a population-based study. N Engl J Med. 2006;355:260-9.
3. Bshiebish HAH, Al-Musawi AH, Khudeir SA. Role of global longitudinal strain in assessment of left ventricular systolic function in patients with heart failure and preserved ejection fraction. J Saudi Heart Assoc. 2019;31:100-5.
4. Cleland JGF, Bunting KV, Flather MD, et al. Beta-blockers for heart failure with reduced, mid-range, and preserved ejection fraction: an individual patient-level analysis of double-blind randomized trials. Eur Heart J. 2018;39:26-35.
5. Edelmann F, Wachter R, Schmidt AG, et al. Effect of Spironolactone on diastolic function and exercise capacity in patients with heart failure with preserved ejection fraction: the ALDO-DHF randomized controlled trial. JAMA. 2013;309:781-91.
6. Ferrari R, Bohm M, Cleland JG, et al. Heart Failure with Preserved Ejection Fraction: Uncertainties and Dilemmas. Eur J Heart Fail. 2015;15; 665-71.
7. Fonarow GC, Stough WG, Abraham WT, et al. Characteristics, treatments, and outcomes of patients with preserved systolic function hospitalized for heart failure: a report from the OPTIMIZE-HF Registry. J Am Coll Cardiol. 2007;50: 768-77.
8. Hoekstra T, Lesman-Leegte I, van Veldhuisen DJ, et al. Quality of life is impaired similarly in heart failure patients with preserved and reduced ejection fraction. Eur J Heart Fail. 2011;13:1013-8.
9. Kitzman DW, Brubaker PH, Morgan TM, et al. Exercise training in older patients with heart failure and preserved ejection fraction: a randomized, controlled, single-blind trial. Circ Heart Fail. 2010;3:659-67.
10. Lund LH, Claggett B, Liu J, et al. Heart failure with mid-range ejection fraction in CHARM: characteristics, outcomes and effect of candesartan across the entire ejection fraction spectrum. Eur J Heart Fail. 2018;123:1230-9.
11. Paulus WJ, Tschöpe C. A novel paradigm for heart failure with preserved ejection fraction: comorbidities drive myocardial dysfunction and remodeling through coronary microvascular endothelial inflammation. J Am Coll Cardiol. 2013;62:263-71.
12. Pitt B, Pfeffer MA, Assmann SF, et al. Spironolactone for heart failure with preserved ejection fraction. N Engl J Med. 2014;370:1383-92.
13. Reddy YNV, Carter RE, Obokata M, et al. A simple, evidence-based approach to help guide diagnosis of heart failure with preserved ejection fraction. Circulation. 2018;138(9): 861-70.
14. Seferovic PM, Ponikowski P, Anker SD, et al. Clinical practice update on heart failure 2019: pharmacotherapy, procedures, devices and patient management. An expert consensus meeting report of The Heart Failure Association of the European Society of Cardiology. Eur J Heart Fail. 2019;21:1169-86.
15. Solomon SD, Rizkala AR, Gong J, et al. Angiotensin Receptor Neprilysin Inhibition in Heart Failure with Preserved Ejection Fraction: Rationale and Design of the PARAGON-HF Trial. JACC Heart Fail. 2017 5:471-82.
16. Tromp J, Shen Li, Jhund PS, et al. Age-related aspects of heart failure with preserved ejection fraction. J Am Coll Cardiol. 2019;74:601-12.
17. Westermann D, Lindner D, Kasner M, et al. Cardiac inflammation contributes to changes in the extracellular matrix in patients with heart failure and normal ejection fraction. Circ Heart Fail. 2011;4:44-52.
18. Yancy CW, Lopatin M, Stevenson LW, et al. Clinical presentation, management, and in-hospital outcomes of patients admitted with acute decompensated heart failure with preserved systolic function: a report from the Acute Decompensated Heart Failure National Registry (ADHERE) Database. J Am Coll Cardiol. 2006;47:76-84.

Advanced Heart Failure: What is it? When to Refer?

Kriti Mittal, Sanjay Mittal

INTRODUCTION

The condition where the heart is unable to pump blood into the circulation in accordance to the requirements of the body without elevation of filling pressure (resulting in congestion) was simplistically described as heart failure. The definition however failed to emphasize that the defect has to lie in the heart to call it heart failure. The recent definition of heart failure in European guidelines[1] suggest that "Heart Failure is a clinical syndrome characterized by typical symptoms (like breathlessness, ankle swelling and fatigue) that may be accompanied by signs (like elevated jugular venous pressure, pulmonary crackles and peripheral edema) caused by a structural and/or functional cardiac abnormality, resulting in a reduced cardiac output and/or elevated intracardiac pressures at rest or during stress". The definition limits itself to describe symptomatic heart failure and fails to recognize that heart failure onset is usually much before the onset of symptoms. The staging of heart failure given by American College of Cardiology/American Heart Association (ACC/AHA)[2] is thus widely accepted world over. According to the staging of heart failure, the disease is understood to be a progressive one with advancement in only one direction, i.e. there is no moving backward to prior stages. Once symptoms develop, stage C heart failure is present and Stage B will never again be achieved.

Stage A heart failure: Includes patients at risk for heart failure who have not yet developed structural heart changes like those with diabetes, those with coronary disease without prior infarct.

Stage B heart failure: Includes yet asymptomatic patients with structural heart disease like reduced ejection fraction, left ventricular hypertrophy, and chamber enlargement.

Stage C heart failure: Includes patients who have developed symptoms of clinical heart failure.

Stage D heart failure: Includes patients with heart failure who remain symptomatic despite guideline directed medical therapy. These patients are also called as refractory heart failure or advanced heart failure as they require advanced intervention like biventricular pacemakers, left ventricular assist device, transplantation, etc.

Catching and managing patients in early stage of heart failure can reduce their progression to advanced heart failure. Though implementation of evidence-based therapies has improved outcomes in patients with heart failure, a large number still progress to an advanced stage of the disease. According to a rough estimate 1–10% of the overall heart failure population happen to be in advanced heart failure.[3] The prevalence of advanced heart failure is increasing due to the growing number of patients with heart failure and their better treatment and survival. Advanced heart failure, as the term implies, is associated with very high morbidity and mortality but is not unmanageable. Advanced therapies are possible in specialized heart failure setups for such patients if they are referred for the same in proper time. Thus, clinicians need to be appropriately equipped to identify patients that might be candidates for advanced heart failure therapies and to recognize the optimal time for referral. Of equal importance, physicians should be prepared to address the needs of patients who are clearly not eligible for advanced heart failure therapies, engage in discussions about changing goals of care, and optimize management strategies to lessen the symptomatic burden of advanced heart failure and improve quality of life.

In the following chapter we will describe the clinical characteristics to identify patients with advanced heart failure, markers of poor prognosis, optimal short-term management strategies to improve outcomes of advanced heart failure therapies, recognize the optimal time for referring patients to advanced heart failure centers and ensure collaboration between advanced heart failure, palliative or symptom-focused care including end-of-life care.

WHAT IS ADVANCED HEART FAILURE?

Common understanding is that stage D heart failure, where patients remain symptomatic despite goal-directed medical therapy, is advanced heart failure. A lot of questions still arise as to recognition of such patients. To try to answer this many definitions have been coined to describe advanced heart failure. A thorough definition of advanced heart failure is mandatory to facilitate appropriate application of treatment such as heart transplantation or long-term mechanical circulatory support (MCS) devices.

Advanced heart failure: Advanced heart failure was first defined in 1998 as a syndrome with a resting left ventricular ejection fraction <30% and the New York Heart Association (NYHA) class III to IV or a peak oxygen uptake (VO_2) below 14 mL/kg/min.[4] In 2004, a US consensus statement defined advanced heart failure as a "state in which patients have significant cardiac dysfunction with marked symptoms of dyspnea, fatigue, or symptoms relating to end-organ hypoperfusion at rest or with minimal exertion despite maximal medical therapy".. This definition did not include the criterion of a previous hospitalization and did not try objectively to assess the impairment of cardiac dysfunction and functional capacity. In 2007, the Heart Failure Association (HFA) of the European Society of Cardiology (ESC)[5] published a position statement in which the definition and clinical characteristics of advanced chronic heart failure were outlined. According to this definition, both symptoms of severe heart failure and objective evidence of severe cardiac dysfunction, impaired exercise capacity and an unstable clinical course must be present, despite optimal medical treatment. The definition was updated in 2018 by HFA as well as ESC to include additional clinical aspects, such as outpatient treatment of episodes of decompensation and the role of comorbidities, and an update of treatment, namely with the new mechanical circulatory support (MCS) devices.[2,6] The HFA criteria of the ESC were inserted into the American Heart Association/American College of Cardiology (AHA/ACC) Foundation criteria for destination therapy with cardiac devices.[2]

European Society of Cardiology Definition of Advanced Heart Failure[5]

- The New York Heart Association Class III–IV symptoms
- Episodes of volume overload and/or peripheral hypoperfusion
- Objective evidence of severe cardiac dysfunction [ejection fraction (EF) < 30%, Doppler pseudonormal or restrictive filling pattern, pulmonary capillary wedge pressure (PCWP) > 16 mm Hg or right atrial pressure (RAP) > 12 mm Hg]
- Severely impaired functional capacity (inability to exercise, 6-minute walking distance < 300 m, peak VO_2 < 12–14 mL/kg/min)
- Heart failure hospitalizations (>1 in past 6 months)
- Above occurring despite attempts to optimize diuretics, renin-angiotensin-aldosterone system (RAAS) antagonists, β-blockers (BB), cardiac resynchronization therapy (CRT) or in the setting of intolerance to optimal medical therapy (OMT).

Heart Failure Association Criteria—2018 Guidelines[6]

1. Severe and persistent symptoms of heart failure (NYHA Class II advanced or IV)
2. Severe cardiac dysfunction
   - Reduced left ventricular ejection fraction (LVEF) < 30%
   - Isolated right ventricular (RV) failure [e.g. arrhythmogenic right ventricular cardiomyopathy (ARVC)]
   - Nonoperable severe valve abnormalities
   - Congenital abnormalities.
3. Episodes of pulmonary or systemic congestion requiring high-dose intravenous diuretics (or diuretic combinations) or episodes of low output requiring inotropes or vasoactive drugs or malignant arrhythmias causing >1 unplanned visit or hospitalization in the past 12 months.
4. Severe impairment of exercise or low 6-minute walking test distance (<300 m) or peak VO_2 (<12–14 mL/kg/min) estimated to be of cardiac origin.

In addition to the above, extracardiac organ dysfunction resulting from heart failure (e.g. cardiac cachexia, or liver or kidney dysfunction) or type 2 pulmonary hypertension may be present, but are not required. Criteria 1 and 4 can be met in patients who have cardiac dysfunction (as described in criterion 2), but also have substantial limitation caused by other conditions (e.g. severe pulmonary disease, noncardiac cirrhosis or, most commonly, renal disease with mixed etiology). These patients have a limited quality of life and survival because of advanced disease and warrant the same intensity of evaluation as someone in whom the only disease is cardiac; however, the therapeutic options for these patients are usually more limited.

Comparison of various advanced heart failure definitions in different guidelines is shown in Table 1.

Sometimes terms like end-stage heart failure and refractory heart failure are used to describe advanced heart failure.

End-stage heart failure: Advanced heart failure should be kept distinct from end-stage heart failure. This term indicates an extremely advanced condition where no improvement with conventional heart failure treatment is possible and where palliative care, ventricular assist devices or heart transplantation are indicated. Indeed, there are remarkable differences between advanced and end-stage heart failure in terms of quality of life and outcomes. End-stage heart failure should be also distinguished from acute heart failure in which a certain degree of reversibility can be achieved.[3]

Refractory heart failure: Refractory heart failure is similar to end-stage heart failure and is observed in clinical practice when patients continue to be symptomatic at rest or develop recurrence of heart failure despite optimal contemporary pharmacotherapy proven to be of benefit in clinical trials. Physical examination, laboratory testing, multimodality imaging, and cardiopulmonary exercise testing are pivotal for the definition of refractory heart failure. These patients commonly have rapid clinical deterioration and may require inotropic agents to augment cardiac performance.[7,8]

TABLE 1: Comparison between guidelines.

		ACC/AHA	*HFSA*	*ESC*
Refractory symptoms	Severe symptoms	Yes	Yes	Yes
	Multiple hospitalizations	Yes	Yes	Yes
	Optimal therapy	Yes	Yes	Yes
	Inotropic support	…..	Yes	…..
	Fluid retention and/or peripheral hypoperfusion	…..	…..	Yes
Exercise intolerance	Severe functional capacity impairment	Yes	Yes	Yes
Objective evidence of severe cardiac dysfunction	Reduced ejection fraction	Yes	…..	Yes
	Doppler echocardiography	……	…..	Yes
	Hemodynamics	……	…..	Yes
	Elevated natriuretic peptides	…..	…..	Yes

(ACC: American College of Cardiology; AHA: American Heart Association; ESC: European Society of Cardiology; HFSA: Heart Failure Society of America)

Various reports describe advanced HF prevalence to be 6–25% of the overall HF population.[3,9,10] While the true overall and within HF prevalence of advanced HF remains uncertain, especially in India, the intense health care utilization and poor outcomes of advanced HF patients establish advanced HF as a major public health burden.

MANAGEMENT IN ADVANCED HEART FAILURE CENTERS: WHY REFER?

Advanced heart failure cannot be cured, but it can be treated. In fact, the increasing number of therapies and state-of-the-art technologies for advanced heart failure provide more choices than ever. Treatments can reduce your symptoms and help your heart pump as best it can. These treatments involve risks as well as benefits and can be delivered in specialized setups called heart failure centers.

Multidisciplinary care: It is often a general cardiologist who is responsible for directing patients to advanced heart failure resources and helping patients to navigate next steps in care. Thus, clinicians need to be appropriately equipped to identify patients that might be candidates for advanced heart failure therapies and to recognize the optimal time for referral. Of equal importance, physicians should be prepared to address the needs of patients who are clearly not eligible for advanced heart failure therapies, engage in discussions about changing goals of care, and optimize management strategies to lessen the symptomatic burden of advanced heart failure and improve quality of life.

Fundamental to the delivery of this complete package of care are multidisciplinary management programs designed to improve outcomes through structured follow-up with patient education, optimization of medical treatment, psychosocial support and improved access to care. Such strategies reduce HF hospitalization and mortality in patients discharged from the hospital. Key to the success of these programs is coordination of care along the continuum of HF and throughout the chain of care delivered by the various services within the health care system. This necessitates close collaboration between HF practitioners (primarily cardiologists, HF nurses and general practitioners).

When a patient with advanced heart failure presents to a multidisciplinary heart failure unit, a thorough assessment of the clinical status and risk factors determine the therapeutic strategy. There are three stages of management:

1. Assessment of precipitating causes of HF decompensation
2. Risk assessment
3. Short-term management and long-term management.

Assessment of Precipitating Causes

The risk factor assessment helps in identifying the urgency and the modality of therapy. For example, if a patient has a poor life expectancy of less than 1 year, that person is best suited for palliative long-term care. The identification of risk factors and risk scores are based on clinical, biochemical and imaging criteria. These are described later in the chapter.

Evaluation should also focus on identification of reversible precipitating factors for heart failure decompensation. Correcting these factors may obviate the need for advanced heart failure therapies. Precipitants for decompensated heart failure may include:[11]

- Nonadherence
  - Medication noncompliance
  - Dietary indiscretion
- Arrhythmias
  - Atrial fibrillation/atrial flutter
  - Ventricular tachycardia
- Infection
- Ischemia
- Valvular disease
  - Mitral regurgitation
  - Aortic stenosis
- Thyroid disease
- Renal failure
- Anemia

Risk Assessment

Despite improvements in treatment, heart failure (HF) continues to have a progressive clinical course characterized by worsening of cardiac function and clinical condition, leading to a stage of advanced chronic HF. At this stage, the clinical picture is characterized by severe symptoms, frequent episodes of decompensation, poor quality of life and poor survival. Evidence-based medical treatments and devices are no longer effective in controlling symptoms and improving the clinical course and, in the case of neurohormonal antagonists, may not frequently be tolerated. The rate of deterioration is faster once a patient has entered stage D or advanced heart failure stage. A relatively stable condition may deteriorate to unmanageable situation very fast. To confuse the issue even stage D heart failure patients have varied prognosis. There are patients who can be identified as worse prognosis even in the advanced heart failure settings. For identification of patients with worse prognosis various risk markers have been identified. These risk markers could be clinical, biochemical, imaging and functional. The problem with markers is that they present with various permutations of combination and is difficult to individualize the risk assessment. Various risk scores have thus been developed and validated to predict the high-risk group in patients with advanced heart failure.

- *Clinical markers of poor prognosis*: Clinical presentation of a patient with advanced heart failure may indicate adverse outcomes. These include increasing age, longer heart failure duration, higher NYHA class, poor quality of life, poor mobility, signs of congestion, lower BP, tachycardia and concomitant occurrence of cardiac and noncardiac comorbidities. The clinical biomarkers associated with adverse clinical outcomes in various studies have been listed below.[6]

Clinical Markers

- Presentation
  - Higher age
  - Male sex
  - Longer HF duration
  - Higher NYHA class
  - Poor quality of life
  - Recent/recurrent HF hospitalizations
  - Hemodynamic profiles
  - Reduced peripheral muscle strength
- Congestion—presence of:
  - S3
  - Rales
  - Edema, jugular venous distention (JVD), hepatomegaly, and ascites
- Cardiomegaly
- Electrocardiography
  - ↑ QRS duration
  - ↑ HR in sinus rhythm but not in atrial fibrillation
  - Reduced HR variability
- Blood pressure
  - Lower and labile SBP and lower DBP and MAP
  - Lower pulse pressure
- Cardiovascular comorbidity
  - Ischemic heart disease/prior myocardial infarction
  - Prior transient ischemic attack/stroke
  - Peripheral arterial disease atrial fibrillation
  - Ventricular arrhythmia, sudden cardiac death, ICD shocks
- Noncardiovascular comorbidity
  - Chronic kidney disease (CKD), liver dysfunction
  - Diabetes

- Chronic obstructive pulmonary disease (COPD)
- Anemia, iron deficiency
- Higher white blood cell count
- Sleep apnea and Cheyne-Stokes breathing
- Depression, cognitive dysfunction
- Frailty, cachexia
- Diuretic resistance.

- *Biochemical markers of adverse outcome*: There are several biomarkers that have been associated with cardiac injury, myocardial fibrosis, myocardial stretch and inflammation. Higher levels of these biomarkers indicate more severe and sometimes irreversible myocardial damage and are thus related to poor prognosis. The list of various poor prognostic biomarkers is given below.[6]

Biochemical Markers

- Copeptin
- Low sodium
- Cardiomyocyte injury
  - Troponin
- Cardiomyocyte stress
  - Higher B-type natriuretic peptide (BNP) and/or N-terminal pro B-type natriuretic peptide (NT-proBNP)
  - Increased NT-proBNP over time
  - Atrial natriuretic peptide (ANP)
  - Midregional pro-atrial natriuretic peptide (MR-pro ANP)
- Inflammation
  - C-reactive protein (CRP)
  - Erythrocyte sedimentation rate (ESR)
- Oxidative stress and fibrosis
  - ST2
  - Galectin-3
  - Growth differentiator 15 (GDF-15)
  - MR-pro ADM
  - Lower LDL
  - Uric acid
  - Low T3
  - Albuminuria.

The prognostic value of these markers is usually not quantifiable. However lot of work have been done on the value of various biochemical markers in predicting in-hospital, medium term and HF rehospitalization risk. Elevated serum creatinine has been associated with increased in-hospital mortality, 30-day mortality as well as heart failure rehospitalization. Similar observations have been reported for cystatin C, serum sodium levels, BNP levels and NT-pro-BNP levels. The comparative value of the biochemical markers is described in Table 2.

TABLE 2: Prognostic value of various biochemical markers of heart failure.

	In-hospital mortality	*Medium-term mortality*	*HF rehospitalization*
Creatinine	x	x	x
BUN	x	x	
Cystatin	x	x	x
Sodium	x	x	x
BNP	x	x	x
NT-proBNP	x	x	x
MR-proANP	x	x	x
MR-proADM		x	
Troponin	x	x	
CRP	x	x	
sST2	x	x	
Galectin-3		x	X

(BNP: b-type natriuretic peptide; BUN: blood urea nitrogen; CRP: C-reactive protein; HF: heart failure; MR-proADM: midregional proadrenomedullin; MR-proANP: midregional pro-A type natriuretic peptide; NT-proBNP: N-terminal pro b-type natriuretic peptide)

- *Imaging markers of poor prognosis*: Echocardiography is the most common tool to assess the extent of myocardial injury. Other imaging tools like MRI, CT scan, nuclear imaging and ultrasound, etc. could also help by identifying patients at higher risk. The most common imaging parameter associated with adverse outcome is LV ejection fraction. Lower the EF worse is the outcome. Many parameters obtained by imaging, mainly by Doppler echocardiography and cardiac magnetic resonance imaging, have greater prognostic value than LVEF. These include LV dilatation and hypertrophy, mitral regurgitation, left atrial function, valve abnormalities, right ventricular function, pulmonary arterial pressure estimates, and inferior vena cava diameter and dynamics. The accuracy of noninvasive measurements to estimate LV filling pressure is still controversial with the use of multiparametric approaches likely better than one single measurement such as the E/e' ratio.[12,13] Various imaging biomarkers implicated with poor prognosis have been listed below.[6]

Imaging Markers of Poor Prognosis

- Echocardiography
  - Lower LVEF
  - Large areas of hypo/akinesis
  - Left ventricular dilatation
  - Diastolic dysfunction
  - Mitral regurgitation
  - Aortic stenosis
  - Left ventricular hypertrophy

- Higher LV mass
- Left atrial enlargement
- Right ventricular function
- Pulmonary hypertension
- Resting dobutamine stress strain
- Other imaging
  - Pulmonary congestion by lung ultrasound
  - Inflammation and fibrosis on CMR
  - Poor viability on stress echo and CMR
  - Reduced miBG uptake.
- *Effort intolerance on cardiopulmonary exercise testing*: Cardiopulmonary exercise testing (CPET) provides objective information about the exercise capacity of ambulatory patients with HF. It is indicated for the selection of candidates for heart transplantation. Peak exercise oxygen consumption (VO_2) measured both as percent of maximal predicted values and as an absolute value, as well as minute ventilation/carbon dioxide production (VE/VCO_2) and an oscillatory pattern of ventilation during exercise have all been shown to have independent prognostic value.[14] Based on prognostic studies, heart transplantation is indicated when peak VO_2 is ≤14 mL/kg/min or ≤12 mL/kg/min in patients on beta-blockers. Achievement of a respiratory exchange rate >1.05 is important to define achievement of maximal aerobic capacity. Ventilatory response to exercise provides an objective assessment of exercise capacity, independently of patients' motivation and, along with the presence of an oscillatory pattern of ventilation, may further stratify the patients.[14] A low 6-minute walking test distance (6MWTD) may also be used in prognostic assessment.[15]

The various parameters studied have been described in the list below.[6]

- *Cardiopulmonary exercise test*:
  - pVO_2
  - 6-minute walking test
  - Minute ventilation/carbon dioxide production (VE/VCO_2) slope.
- *Development off risk scores*: Though numerous single risk markers have been identified but it is difficult to predict the life expectancy on the basis of concomitant multiple risk markers. For this very reason many risk scores have been developed and validated. These risk scores are important in identifying specific advanced heart failure therapies in a given individual. As these therapies are costly and also have associated morbidity and mortality of their own, they are reserved for situations where the predicted risk of action outweighs that of inaction. The problem is these studies are generally based on ambulatory patients or on those hospitalized for acute HF. Relatively little data specific to patients with advanced chronic HF is available. However, we have tried to describe below whatever risk scores were available for advanced heart failure risk stratification.[16]

Various composite scores have been given like:
- Interagency Registry for Mechanically Assisted Circulatory Support (INTERMACS)
- Meta-analysis Global Group in CHF (MAGGIC)
- BIOSTAT-CHF
- BCN Bio-HF
- Seattle heart failure Model (SHFM)
- Heart failure survival score (HFSS)
- UCLA score.

Short-term Management of Advanced Heart Failure

The purpose of short-term management is to stabilize acute decompensated heart failure till definitive therapy becomes a viable option. This helps in limiting the end-organ damage and helps to improve the outcome. The strategy may include:
- Intravenous vasoactive drugs
- Management of congestion
- Short-term circulatory support.
- *Intravenous vasoactive drugs*: Inotropes studied in randomized clinical trials have generally not been associated with improved outcomes, and have, in some studies, worsened prognosis, thus inotropes have no place in the routine treatment of advanced heart failure. However, there is expert opinion that inotropic support may be necessary in refractory heart failure in selected patients as a bridge to temporary mechanical circulatory support. Inotropes may also be used as short-term therapy in patients with low cardiac output and evidence of end-organ dysfunction, for instance during decongestion. Inotropes may improve hemodynamics and help reverse worsening end-organ function in advanced heart failure. Conversely continuous inotropes may be acceptable as a palliative measure for patients without other advanced treatment options. Some patients may respond to intermittent use of inodilators. Since levosimendan came in use long-term intermittent use of the drug has been reported to improve symptoms. The hemodynamic effects of levosimendan may last for >7 days after a 12–24 hours infusion because of the pharmacologically active metabolite with a long half-life.[17] While meta-analyses of several heterogeneous small trials of a repeated infusion strategy have suggested a positive effect on survival[18] and a reduction in hospitalizations,[19] such a survival

effect has not been demonstrated in a single, adequately sized, prospective study.

- *Management of congestion*: Most of the heart failure hospitalizations are due to signs and symptoms of fluid overload.[20] Recurrent congestion worsens patients' outcomes. Loop diuretics remain the cornerstone for the treatment of congestion in the patients with heart failure. Diuretic therapy is thoroughly described in the current guidelines for heart failure treatment and their further discussion goes beyond the aims of this article. The clinical course of patients with advanced heart failure is often characterized by kidney dysfunction (cardiorenal syndrome) and by diuretic resistance. The first may have multiple mechanisms including abnormal hemodynamics, neurohormonal activation, excessive tubular sodium reabsorption, inflammation, oxidative stress, and nephrotoxic drugs.[20] Loop diuretic resistance is generally due to a series of renal adaptations after diuretic use ("braking phenomenon") including hypertrophy and hyperfunction of other sites of the nephron and to increased renin secretion in the macula densa. Increased uremic anions and proteinuria also impair achievement of therapeutic concentrations at the diuretic's tubular site of action.[20] Concomitant administration of thiazide diuretics or metolazone with loop diuretics is used to overcome the braking phenomenon. However, no evidence from clinical trials exists to guide this practice.
- *Short-term mechanical circulatory support*: Advanced heart failure patients with cardiogenic shock have a very high mortality. Besides, the prolonged hypoperfusion may lead to multiorgan damage, thus complicating the issues. As previously discussed inotropes may increase arrhythmogenecity and mortality. Short-term MCS may be indicated in the setting of cardiogenic shock. Several percutaneous and paracorporeal devices are available which can be used for a few days, up to several weeks. The purpose of short-term mechanical circulatory assist devices is to allow cardiac recovery as well as recovery of other organs such as the kidneys, liver, and brain. Although insertion of most short-term devices is relatively simple and straightforward, the care of patients on short-term MCS requires specific expertise. Moreover there should also be continuous evaluation when not to expect any more chance of cardiac recovery thus a decision to go for long-term mechanical circulatory support device is taken. Short-term MCS can thus be used as a *bridge-to-decision* for long-term MCS or heart transplantation.[21] There are many devices as listed here. Each one has pros and cons and thus their use should be primarily guided by clinical judgment and local experience.[22]
- Intra-aortic balloon pump
- Extracorporeal membrane oxygenator
- Tandem heart percutaneous ventricular assist
- Impella ventricular support system
- Centrimag acute circulatory support system.

Long-term Management of Advanced Heart Failure

Advanced heart failure therapies are indicated when guideline-directed medical and device therapies have been implemented and optimized as appropriate in the individual patient but heart failure has progressed such that symptoms can no longer be adequately managed or end-organ function is compromised. Most of these procedures are surgical and require precision in diagnosis, patient selection, patient optimization, and management. The long-term therapies could be divided in four categories:

1. Conventional surgical procedures
2. Special interventional procedures
3. Heart transplant
4. Long-term mechanical ventricular assist devices.

- *Conventional surgeries: open-heart surgery:* Conventional surgeries are possible in certain patients with continued heart failure symptoms despite goal-directed medical management. In a specialized heart failure setup the risk of the procedure could be minimized and a good result can be obtained with decent improvement in outcomes. The various surgical therapies recommended for selected advanced heart failure patients could be:
  - *Coronary artery bypass graft:* The 10 years of follow-up in the Surgical Treatment for Ischemic Heart Failure (STICH) trial[23,24] clearly shows that in patients with LVEF ≤ 35% and CAD amenable to surgical revascularization, CABG in addition to medical therapy significantly improve all-cause mortality, cardiovascular mortality and cardiovascular hospitalization as compared to medical therapy alone. CABG surgery is recommended for patients with advanced heart failure having left main stenosis or left main equivalent.[25]
  - *Aortic valve replacement surgery:* In severe symptomatic aortic valve stenosis with mean gradient >40 mm Hg, aortic valve replacement (AVR) is recommended irrespective of the degree of left ventricular dysfunction. In "true" low-flow, low-gradient severe aortic stenosis[26] with a depressed LVEF, left ventricular function usually improves after AVR if left ventricular dysfunction is due to excessive afterload. In severe aortic regurgitation, AVR is recommended in all symptomatic patients as well as asymptomatic patients with LVEF ≤ 50%.[26]

- *Coronary artery bypass grafting (CABG) with mitral valve repair surgery:* In certain patients with LVEF <30% and severe functional mitral regurgitation due to coronary artery disease, but with evidence of myocardial viability, mitral valve surgery should be considered with revascularization.[26]
- *Specialized interventions:* Many interventional procedures are available in specialized heart failure setups for selected patients where conventional surgical options are considered to be at very high-risk. These may include:
  - *High-risk coronary interventions*: Patients with CAD especially significant left main disease, with unacceptably high surgical risk, coronary intervention is an option and may be facilitated under protection using an Impella device.[27]
  - *Transcutaneous aortic valve replacement:* In patients with severe aortic stenosis with prohibitive surgical risk due to comorbidities but with projected survival >1 year after aortic valve intervention, transcatheter aortic valve implantation should be considered. The growing experience and confidence is leading to fast expansion of indications.
  - *Percutaneous edge-to-edge mitral valve repair*: In selected patients with severe secondary MR and LVEF < 30% who remain symptomatic despite optimal medical management (including CRT if indicated) and who have no option for revascularization, percutaneous edge-to-edge procedure is a possibility. Using Mitraclip in such patients showed improved outcomes in COAPT trial.
- *Heart transplant*: Heart transplantation is the treatment of choice for carefully selected patients with advanced or end-stage heart failure. There is consensus within the cardiology community that heart transplantation significantly improves survival, exercise capacity, quality of life and return to work compared with conventional treatment, provided that proper selection criteria are applied.[1,28] The main limitation of heart transplantation is the limited supply of donor hearts, especially in our country. Heart transplantation requires a setup to monitor and maintain the patient with advanced heart failure till the time heart is available for transplant and even after the transplant for management of immunosuppressant therapy.
- *Indications of heart transplant:*[1,6]
  - End-stage HF with severe symptoms, a poor prognosis, and no remaining alternative treatment options
  - Motivated, well-informed, and emotionally stable
  - Capable of complying with the intensive treatment required postoperatively
- *Contraindications for heart transplant:*
  - Active infection
  - Severe peripheral arterial or cerebrovascular disease
  - Pharmacologic irreversible pulmonary hypertension (LVAD should be considered with subsequent re-evaluation to establish candidacy)
  - Cancer (a collaboration with oncology specialists should occur to stratify each patient as to their risk of tumor recurrence)
  - Irreversible renal dysfunction (e.g. creatinine clearance <30 mL/min)
  - Systemic disease with multiorgan involvement
  - Other serious comorbidity with poor prognosis
  - Pretransplant BMI > 35 kg/m^2 (weight loss is recommended to achieve a BMI < 35 kg/m^2)
  - Current alcohol or drug abuse
  - Any patient for whom social supports are deemed insufficient to achieve compliant care in the outpatient setting.
- *Long-term mechanical circulatory support*: In patients with advanced heart failure, long-term support with durable mechanical circulatory support (MCS) devices like LVAD have shown to improve survival and better quality of life as compared with conventional treatments in inotrope-dependent patients or in patients with contraindications for heart transplantation.[8] The Randomized Evaluation of Mechanical Assistance for the Treatment of Congestive Heart Failure (REMATCH) trial first showed improved 1-year survival in inotrope-dependent, transplant-ineligible patients with advanced heart failure treated with an LVAD, but 2-year survival was not statistically different.[29] Since then, technology of LVAD and conservative management have improved.[29,30] Managing patients with long-term MCS require a multidisciplinary Heart Team approach, and by gaining experience, centers may actually improve patient survival.[31] The classical indication for LVADs is as bridge to transplant but can be considered as a lifesaving therapy for patients who were ineligible for heart transplantation. The proportion of long-term MCS devices implanted for destination therapy (DT) to heart transplants is increasing.[32] Unfortunately the exorbitant prices of the devices limit the use of LVADs in a handful of patients. INTERMACS class 1 and 2 are usually too sick group of patients. Although MCS can be implanted in these patients, the risk of complications and poor outcomes is higher due to invariable co-occurrence of end-organ damage. These patients may require stabilization with short-term paracorporeal devices as described above, before definitive MCS use. INTERMACS 3 and 4 are best category of patients for long-term MCS.

ADVANCED HEART FAILURE: WHEN TO REFER?

The best time to refer is when intervention can be done so as to improve the outcome and alter the course of the disease in the patient. All heart failures are not safe or stable. On one hand, there are people who do very well with goal-directed therapy which can be handled by a general physician, i.e. ACEIs, ARBs, ARNIs, β-blockers, diuretics, CRT-Ds, etc. But, there is a crossroad, where these treatments cease to be beneficial. The treatment here on would be for advanced heart failure. At this point in time, where medical therapy has seized to work, there is a strategy which has to be made, that a person with heart failure may not have the best outcome in a general physician's hand and the patient has to be referred to a higher cardiac centers, where these kinds of therapies are available, that include—high-risk surgery for valvular surgeries like MVR, AV replacement, Mitraclip, TAVI, coronary artery bypass grafting, stem cell therapy, VADs, heart transplant surgery.

It is a tricky task and a huge responsibility to draw a line or define the level at which the physician realizes that the patient should be referred to a higher center. If the patient is referred too early, the patient's cost of the therapy and the outcome of that therapy may not match with the risk of continuing medical therapy. Hence, the staging is of paramount importance in making this decision. The guidelines are available in public domain.

Referring the patient too late leaves for very little or no room for an effective outcome and change in prognosis as compared to the toll it takes on them, and referring too early increases the financial cost to the patient which can easily be managed by a general physician.[6]

Role of INTERMACS Classification

The Interagency Registry for Mechanically Assisted Circulatory Support (INTERMACS) classification of identifying risk stages of patients with Stage D heart failure having NYHA class III or more symptoms is the most widely used model for the purpose of choosing patients with advanced heart failure for mechanical circulatory support devices. INTERMACS has created seven clinical profiles with increasing severity of symptoms and worsening of prognosis.[33,34] Profile 7 is the best and 1 is the worst. The clinical criteria and the action recommended are described in Table 3.

In a study of survival according to INTERMACS profile, estimated survival was modeled through 1 year using the Kaplan–Meier method with censoring at either ventricular assist device (VAD) or transplant. Survival was significantly different between INTERMMACS patient profile groups.

Whereas profile 7 and 6 had an annual survival of greater than 75%, the survival dropped below 60% in INTERMACS patient profile 4 or below. In INTERMACS class 1 and even 2 the outcomes of patients despite advanced heart failure therapies like LVAD, transplant, etc. are poor. Thus in these situations temporary mechanical support devices are of use till the time end-organ recovery happens. Thus INTERMACS 3–4 is when a patient should be considered for surgical management (VADs) so as to improve the outcome.[35,36]

Role of Multivariate Risk Scores

While INTERMACS classification is primarily focused on recommendations for mechanical circulatory devices, other heart failure scores like MAGGIC,[37] MECKI,[38] SHFM,[39] and HFSS[40] are prominent to overall assess the risk for ambulatory heart failure patients. The comparative description of these scores is given in Table 4. Most of the scores can be assessed online. Data points are fed in the required fields and predicted survival of the patient.

European Society of Cardiology Heart failure Association Guidelines[6]

In July 2018, heart failure association of European Society of Cardiology published the advanced heart failure position statement. According to the document there are recommendations on when to refer a patient of advanced heart failure to a specialized heart failure center. This tabulates clinical criteria, laboratory criteria, imaging criteria, and composite risk score criteria to consider a patient for referral. These recommendations have been described in Table 5.

This table reflects many clinically relevant but sometimes subjective and nonspecific criteria. With these criteria, sensitivity has been prioritized over specificity, i.e. many criteria may be present in patients who do not need referral, but by considering these criteria in a comprehensive assessment, there is a lower risk that high-risk patients may be missed or referred too late. While cut-offs exist for transplantation listing or left ventricular assist device implantation, there are no data to support specific cut-offs for referral to a HF center.

Heart Failure Association of European Society of Cardiology has also provided a flowchart of advanced heart failure patient management indicating the timing of referral.[6] The same is shown in Flowchart 1.

In nutshell, if a patient is having advanced heart failure, is aged less than 75 years, and has no comorbidity which shortens his survival to less than 1 year, such a person should be referred for advanced heart failure management to a heart failure setup. Bomwoul J has coined a mnemonic "I NEED HELP" to identify heart failure patients fit to be

TABLE 3: Prognostic value of various biomarkers.

INTERMACS profile	*Clinical description*	*Recommendation*
Profile 1: Critical cardiogenic shock "Crash and burn"	Cardiogenic shock with life-threatening hypotension despite rapidly escalating inotropic support, critical organ hypoperfusion	Definitive intervention needed within few hours
Profile 2: Progressive decline "Sliding on inotropes"	Patient with declining function despite intravenous inotropic support may be manifest by worsening renal function, nutritional depletion, and inability to restore volume balance. Also describes declining status in patients unable to tolerate inotropic therapy	Definitive intervention needed within few days
Profile 3: Stable but inotrope-dependent "Dependent stability"	Patient with stable blood pressure, organ function, nutrition, and symptoms on continuous intravenous inotropic support (or a temporary circulatory support device or both), but demonstrating repeated failure to wean from support due to recurrent symptomatic hypotension or renal dysfunction	Definitive intervention elective over a period of weeks to few months
Profile 4: Resting symptoms	Patient can be stabilized close to normal volume status but experiences daily symptoms of congestion at rest or during ADL. Doses of diuretics generally fluctuate at very high levels. More intensive management and surveillance strategies should be considered, which may in some cases reveal poor compliance that would compromise outcomes with any therapy. Some patients may shuttle between 4 and 5	Definitive intervention elective over a period of weeks to few months
Profile 5: Exertion intolerant	Comfortable at rest and with ADL but unable to engage in any other activity, living predominantly within the house. Patients are comfortable at rest without congestive symptoms, but may have underlying refractory elevated volume status, often with renal dysfunction. If underlying nutritional status and organ function are marginal, patients may be more at risk than INTERMACS 4, and require definitive intervention	Variable urgency depends upon maintenance of nutrition, organ function, and activity
Profile 6: Exertion limited "Walking wounded"	Patient without evidence of fluid overload is comfortable at rest and with ADL and minor activities outside the home but fatigues after the first few minutes of any meaningful activity. Attribution to cardiac limitation requires careful measurement of peak oxygen consumption, in some cases with hemodynamic monitoring to confirm severity of cardiac impairment	Variable, depends upon maintenance of nutrition, organ function, and activity level
Profile 7: Advanced NYHA class III	A placeholder for more precise specification in future, this level includes patients who are without current or recent episodes of unstable fluid balance, living comfortably with meaningful activity limited to mild physical exertion	Transplantation or circulatory support may not currently be indicated

(INTERMACS: Interagency Registry for Mechanically Assisted Circulatory Support; NYHA: New York Heart Association)

referred.[41] I—Inotropes (previous or ongoing), N—NYHA III/IV, E—End-organ damage (Kidney/Liver), E—Ejection fraction <20%, D—Defibrillator shocks (recurrent, appropriate), H - Hospitalizations (>1 over last 1 year), E—Edema (persisting despite increasing diuretics), L—Low BP (<90 mm Hg systolic), P—Prognostic medications (Inability to uptitrate). This is easy to remember and also clearly imparts the message to the patients and the primary physician to understand when not to delay and preferably refer the patient to advanced heart failure center.

CONCLUSION

Advanced heart failure remains a major clinical challenge. It is important to diagnose advanced heart failure early so that timely management could be beneficial to the patients. New biomarkers and imaging tools may allow better prognostic stratification and the assessment of mechanisms of disease progression. Once guideline-directed management therapy is insufficient, the patient may benefit from advanced heart failure therapies like short-term inotropes, long- and short-term mechanical assist devices and heart transplant besides high-risk conventional surgeries in selected patients. These procedures require multidisciplinary heart team approach, which is available at specialized heart failure centers. Timely recognition of refractory or advanced heart failure may empower the treating physician to refer the patient for advanced heart failure therapies to these heart failure centers. If the advanced failure therapies are offered too late, they do not improve outcomes. We as physicians

TABLE 4: Prognostic heart failure scores.

Score	Component	Comment
Heart failure survival score (HFSS)	• Presence/absence CAD • Resting heart rate • LVEF • MAP • Presence/absence IVCD • Serum sodium • Peak oxygen uptake	• Score is based on a sum of these variables multiplied by defined coefficients • Low-risk: HFSS ≥ 8.1, medium-risk: HFSS 7.20–8.09, high-risk: HFSS ≤ 7.1
Seattle heart failure model (SHFM)	• Demographics • Clinical characteristics • Medications • Laboratory data • Devices • www.seattleheartfailuremodel.org	Incorporates impact of interventions (medical and device) and provides estimates of 1, 2, and 5-year survival
Metabolic Exercise data with Cardiac and Kidney Indices (MECKI)	• Percent predicted peak VO_2 • VE/VCO_2 slope • Hemoglobin • Serum sodium • LVEF • eGFR by MDRD	Incorporates data from the CPET as well as kidney function
Meta-analysis Global group in CHF (MAGGIC)	• Age • Gender • LVEF • Systolic blood pressure • Body mass index • Serum creatinine • NYHA class • Smoking history • Comorbidities (e.g. diabetes, COPD) • Length of heart failure diagnosis • Medications • www.heartfailurerisk.org	Risk model converted into integer score generalizable to a broad spectrum of patients

(CAD: coronary artery disease; CPET: cardiopulmonary exercise testing; COPD: chronic obstructive pulmonary disease; eGFR: estimated glomerular filtration rate; IVCD: inferior vena cava dimension; LVEF: left ventricular ejection fraction; MAP: mean arterial pressure; MDRD: modification of diet in renal disease)

TABLE 5: Recommendations of clinical criteria, laboratory criteria, imaging criteria, and composite risk score criteria to consider a patient for referral.

Clinical	Laboratory	Imaging	Risk score data
• >1 HF hospitalization in last year • NYHA class III–IV • Intolerance of optimal dose of any GDMT HF drug • Increasing diuretic requirement • SBP < 90 mm Hg • Inability to perform CPET • 6MWT • CRT nonresponder clinically • Cachexia, unintentional weight loss • KCCQ • MLHFQ	• eGFR < 45 nL/min • SCr > 160 mmol/L • K > 5.2 or <3.5 mmol/L • Hyponatremia • Hb < 120 g/L • NT-proBNP > 1,000 pg/mL • Abnormal LFT • Low albumin	• LVEF < 30% • Large area of akinesis/ dyskinesis or aneurysm • Moderate–severe mitral regurgitation • RV dysfunction • PA pressure > 50 mm Hg • Moderate–severe tricuspid regurgitation • Difficult to grade aortic stenosis • IVC dilated or without respiratory variation	• MAGGIC predicted survival <80% at 1 year • SHFM predicted survival <80% at 1 year

(IVC: inferior vena cava; LVEF: left ventricular ejection fraction; MAGGIC: meta-analysis global group in CHF; NYHA: New York Heart Association; SHFM: Seattle heart failure model)

Flowchart 1: Referral of advanced heart failure patient.[6]

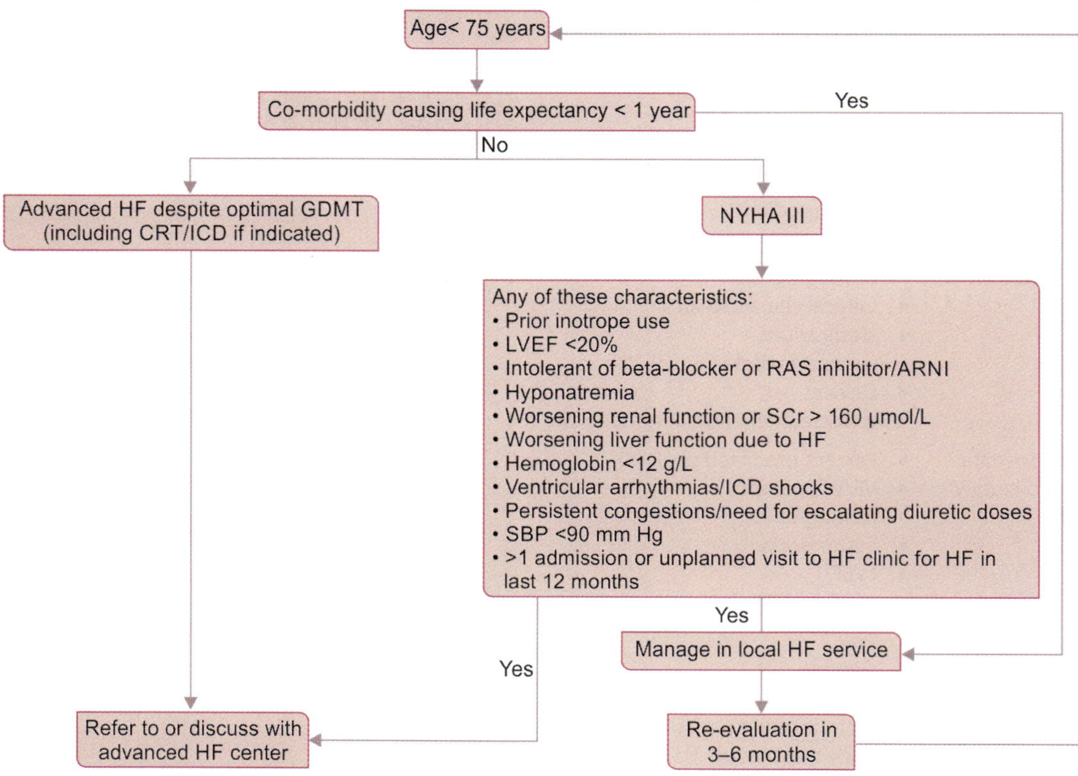

(CRT: cardiac resynchronization therapy; GDMT: guideline-directed medical therapy; HF: heart failure; ICD: implantable cardioverter-defibrillator; LVEF: left ventricular ejection fraction; NYHA: New York Heart Association; RAS: renin-angiotensin system)

should listen to the call of the patients with heart failure if the SOS is ***"I NEED HELP".*** Not too early and not too late is the mantra of ideal referral.

REFERENCES

1. Ponikowski P, Voors AA, Anker SD, et al. 2016 ESC guidelines for the diagnosis and treatment of acute and chronic heart failure: The Task Force for the diagnosis and treatment of acute and chronic heart failure of the European Society of Cardiology (ESC) Developed with the special contribution of the Heart Failure Association (HFA) of the ESC. Eur Heart J. 2016;37:2129-200.
2. Yancy CW, Jessup M, Bozkurt B, et al. 2013 ACCF/AHA Guideline for the Management of Heart Failure: A Report of the American College of Cardiology Foundation/American Heart Association Task Force on Practice - Guidelines. J Am Coll Cardiol. 2013;62:e147-239.
3. Bjork JB, Alton KK, Georgiopoulou VV, et al. Defining Advanced Heart Failure: A Systematic Review of Criteria Used in Clinical Trials. J Card Fail. 2016;22(7):569-77.
4. Adams KF Jr, Zannad F. Clinical definition and epidemiology of advanced heart failure. Am Heart J. 1998;135:S204-15.
5. Metra M, Ponikowski P, Dickstein K, et al. Advanced chronic heart failure: a position statement from the Study Group on Advanced Heart Failure of the Heart Failure Association of the European Society of Cardiology. Eur J Heart Fail. 2007;9:684-94.
6. Crespo-Leiro MG, Metra M, Lund LH, et al. Advanced heart failure: a position statement of the Heart Failure Association of the European Society of Cardiology. Eur J Heart Fail. 2018;20:1505-35.
7. Hunt SA, Abraham WT, Chin MH, et al. ACC/AHA 2005 guideline update for the diagnosis and management of chronic heart failure in the adult- summary article. A report of the American College of Cardiology/American Heart Association. Task Force on Practice Guidelines (Writing Committee to Update the 2001 Guidelines for the Evaluation and Management of Heart Failure). J Am Coll Cardiol. 2005;46:1116-43.
8. Ahmad T, Patel CB, Milano CA, et al. When the heart runs out of heartbeats: treatment options for refractory end-stage heart failure. Circulation. 2012;125:2948-55.
9. Xanthakis V, Enserro DM, Larson MG, et al. Prevalence, neurohormonal correlates, and prognosis of heart failure stages in the community. JACC Heart Fail. 2016;4:808-15.
10. Fang JC, Ewald GA, Allen LA, et al. Advanced (stage D) heart failure: a statement from the Heart Failure Society of America Guidelines Committee. J Card Fail. 2015;21:519-34.
11. Kittleson M, Kobashigawa J. Management of advanced heart failure: The Role of Heart Transplantation. Circulation. 2011;123:1569-74.

12. Nauta JF, Hummel YM, van der Meer P, et al. Correlation with invasive left ventricular filling pressures and prognostic relevance of the echocardiographic diastolic parameters used in the 2016 ESC heart failure guidelines and in the 2016 ASE/EACVI recommendations: a systematic review in patients with heart failure with preserved ejection fraction. Eur J Heart Fail. 2018;20:1303-11.
13. Nagueh SF. Non-invasive assessment of left ventricular filling pressure. Eur J Heart Fail. 2018;20:38-48.
14. Sakata Y, Shimokawa H. Epidemiology of heart failure in Asia. Circ J. 2013;77:2209-17.
15. Corra U, Agostoni PG, Anker SD, et al. Role of cardiopulmonary exercise testing in clinical stratification in heart failure. A position paper from the Committee on Exercise Physiology and Training of the Heart Failure Association of the European Society of Cardiology. Eur J Heart Fail. 2018;20:3-15.
16. Metra M, Dinatolo E, Dasseni N. The New Heart Failure Association Definition of Advanced Heart Failure. Card Fail Rev. 2019;5(1):5-8.
17. Thorvaldsen T, Benson L, Hagerman I, et al. Planned repetitive use of levosimendan for heart failure in cardiology and internal medicine in Sweden. Int J Cardiol. 2014;175:55-61.
18. Silvetti S, Nieminen MS. Repeated or intermittent levosimendan treatment in advanced heart failure: an updated meta-analysis. Int J Cardiol. 2016;202:138-43.
19. Silvetti S, Belletti A, Fontana A, et al. Rehospitalization after intermittent levosimendan treatment in advanced heart failure patients: a meta-analysis of randomized trials. ESC Heart Fail. 2017;4:595-604.
20. Costanzo MR, Ronco C, Abraham WT, et al. Extracorporeal ultrafiltration for fluid overload in heart failure: current status and prospects for further research. J Am Coll Cardiol. 2017;69:2428-45.
21. Barge-Caballero E, Almenar-Bonet L, Gonzalez-Vilchez F, et al. Clinical outcomes of temporary mechanical circulatory support as a direct bridge to heart transplantation: a nationwide Spanish registry. Eur J Heart Fail. 2018;20:178-86.
22. Rihal CS, Naidu SS, Givertz MM, et al. 2015 SCAI/ACC/HFSA/STS Clinical expert consensus statement on the use of percutaneous mechanical circulatory support devices in cardiovascular care: endorsed by the American Heart Assocation, the Cardiological Society of India, and Sociedad Latino Americana de Cardiologia Intervencion; Affirmation of Value by the Canadian Association of Interventional Cardiology-Association Canadienne de Cardiologied'Intervention. J Am Coll Cardiol. 2015;65:e7-e26.
23. Velazquez EJ, Lee KL, Deja MA, et al. Coronary-artery bypass surgery in patients with left ventricular dysfunction. N Engl J Med. 2011;364:1607-16.
24. Velazquez EJ, Lee KL, Jones RH, et al. Coronary-artery bypass surgery in patients with ischemic cardiomyopathy. N Engl J Med. 2016;374:1511-20.
25. Windecker S, Kolh P, Alfonso F, et al. 2014 ESC/EACTS Guidelines on myocardial revascularization: The Task Force on Myocardial Revascularization of the European Society of Cardiology (ESC) and the European Association for Cardio-Thoracic Surgery (EACTS). Developed with the special contribution of the European Association of Percutaneous Cardiovascular Interventions (EAPCI). Eur Heart J. 2014;35:2541-619.
26. Baumgartner H, Falk V, Bax J, et al. 2017 ESC/EACTS guidelines for the management of valvular heart disease. Eur Heart J. 2017;38:2739-91.
27. Baumann S, Werner N, Ibrahim K, et al. Indication and short-term clinical outcomes of high-risk percutaneous coronary intervention with microaxial Impella(R) pump: results from the German Impella® registry. Clin Res Cardiol. 2018;107:653-7.
28. Mehra MR, Canter CE, Hannan MM, et al. The 2016 International Society for Heart Lung Transplantation listing criteria for heart transplantation: a 10-year update. J Heart Lung Transplant. 2016;35:1-23.
29. Rose EA, Gelijns AC, Moskowitz AJ, et al. Long-term use of a left ventricular assist device for end-stage heart failure. N Engl J Med. 2001;345:1435-43.
30. Adlbrecht C, Hulsmann M, Wurm R, et al. Outcome of conservative management vs. assist device implantation in patients with advanced refractory heart failure. Eur J Clin Invest. 2016;46:34-41.
31. Lund LH, Matthews J, Aaronson K. Patient selection for left ventricular assist devices. Eur J Heart Fail. 2010;12:434-43.
32. Birks EJ. A changing trend toward destination therapy: are we treating the same patients differently? Tex Heart Inst J. 2011;38:552-4.
33. Stevenson LW, Pagani FD, Young JB, et al. INTERMACS profiles of advanced heart failure: the current picture. J Heart Lung Transplant. 2009;28:535-41.
34. Stevenson LW, Couper G. On the fledgling field of mechanical circulatory support. J Am Coll Cardiol. 2007;50:748-51.
35. Estep JD, Starling RC, Horstmanshof DA, et al. Risk assessment and comparative effectiveness of left ventricular assist device and medical management in ambulatory heart failure patients: results from the ROADMAP Study. J Am Coll Cardiol. 2015;66:1747-61.
36. Boyle AJ, Ascheim DD, Russo MJ, et al. Clinical outcomes for continuous-flow left ventricular assist device patients stratified by pre-operative INTERMACS classification. J Heart Lung Transplant. 2011;30:402-7.
37. Pocock SJ, Ariti CA, McMurray JJ, et al. Predicting survival in heart failure: a risk score based on 39372 patients from 30 studies. Eur Heart J. 2013;34:1404-13.
38. Agostoni P, Corra U, Cattadori G, et al. Metabolic exercise test data combined with cardiac and kidney indexes, the MECKI score: a multiparametric approach to heart failure prognosis. Int J Cardiol. 2013;167:2710-8.
39. Levy WC, Mozaffarian D, Linker DT, et al. The Seattle Heart Failure Model: prediction of survival in heart failure. Circulation. 2006;113:1424-33.
40. Aaronson KD, Schwartz JS, Chen TM, et al. Development and prospective validation of a clinical index to predict survival in ambulatory patients referred for cardiac transplant evaluation. Circulation. 1997;95:2660-7.
41. Baumwol J. "I Need Help"-A mnemonic to aid timely referral in advanced heart failure. J Heart Lung Transplant. 2017;36:593-4.

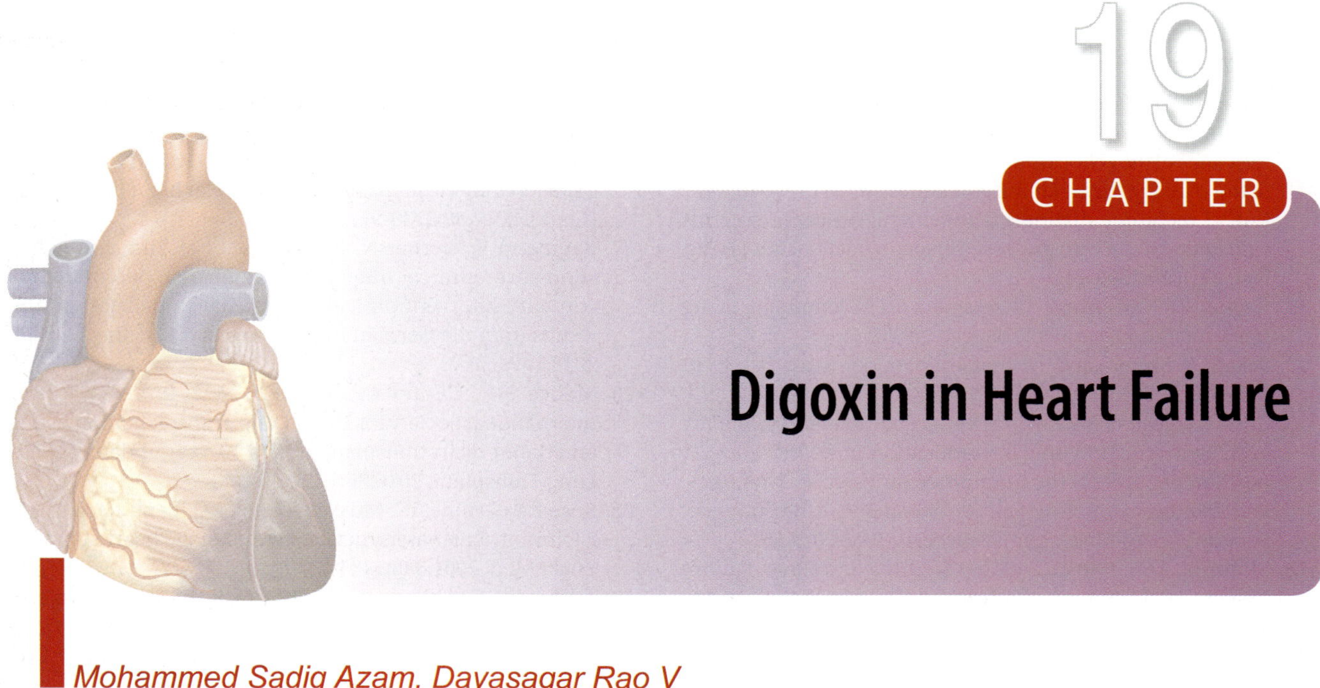

Digoxin in Heart Failure

Mohammed Sadiq Azam, Dayasagar Rao V

INTRODUCTION

"All that is gold does not glitter, not all those who wander are lost;
The old that is strong does not wither, deep roots are not reached by the frost."—JRR Tolkien

These few lines by the celebrated novelist JRR Tolkien probably are best to describe the prodigal son of the cardiologist's armamentarium, *digoxin*. From being a wonder drug in 1785 to being relegated to a last resort in 2018, digoxin is often said to be a "has-been", one whose time has come and gone, but is it so? Has this once celebrated molecule that gave a fresh lease of life to many a patient with debilitating heart failure truly run its course? This review hopes to answer these questions and address the use of digoxin in heart failure in today's day and age.

HISTORY

The discovery of digoxin is accredited to the Scottish doctor William Withering in the year 1775, who was then working as a physician in Staffordshire, and had a fascination for plants and botany. In 1775, one of his patients presented with what seemed to him like end-stage heart failure and he had little hope of his survival. However, a few months later he noticed the patient had dramatically improved, and on questioning discovered that he had taken a secret herbal therapy at a local gypsy and promptly improved! Excited by this, withering searched high and low for the gypsy and finally found her and demanded to know the secret. After much bargaining she finally revealed her secret, the remedy was made of a concoction of herbs but the active ingredient was the purple foxglove, *Digitalis purpurea*. After trying out various formulations of digitalis extracts on 163 patients, he found that if he used the dried, powdered leaf, he got amazingly successful results and introduced its use officially in 1785.

MECHANISM OF ACTION

Digoxin has a unique inotropic-bradycardic action when compared to the other sympathomimetic inotropic agents that all-cause tachycardia. In addition to being a weak positive inotrope, digoxin slows the ventricular rate, which leads to improved ventricular filling in heart failure (HF), especially in patients with atrial fibrillation (AF). It also decreases the sympathetic drive generated by the failing circulation which provided a rationale for its use in HF with sinus rhythm—a use that is now deemed controversial. Being a drug with an extremely narrow therapeutic window, its optimal use requires a thorough understanding of its various drug interactions and of the multiple factors governing its efficacy and toxicity. Since the effects of digoxin in an acutely ill patient often seen with electrolyte disturbances, hypoxia, altered homeostatic milieu, are difficult to predict and there is a dearth of concrete evidence of benefit in such a setting, its use is very seldom justified in acute heart failure. Nonetheless, it remains the only drug for chronic heart failure that inhibits the sodium pump.

Sodium Pump Inhibition

It is responsible for the myocardial cellular effect of digoxin. The sodium pump (Na/K-ATPase) inhibition leads to a transient increase in the intracellular sodium concentration close to the sarcolemma which promotes calcium influx by stimulating the sodium-calcium exchanger. The increase in intracellular calcium content leads to enhanced myocardial contractility, albeit with an increase in risk of arrhythmogenicity. This arrhythmogenic risk is greatly compounded in cases of digoxin toxicity where an increase in direct calcium entry into the cells via new transmembrane calcium channels is noted.[1]

Autonomic and Renin-angiotensin Effects

Sinus slowing and atrioventricular (AV) nodal inhibition with digoxin results from parasympathetic activation. Digoxin by increasing the vagal tone, slows AV nodal conduction and prolongs the AV refractory period. By inhibiting the sympathetic tone, digoxin exerts its beneficial effects in HF. Renin release is inhibited as a consequence of reduced activity of the sodium pump with consequent natriuresis which leads to vasodilation and offsetting of the direct vasoconstrictor effects of digoxin (Box 1).

TURNING POINT: THE DIG TRIAL

Digoxin was considered the cornerstone in the management of heart failure for almost two centuries until 1997 until the results of a large multicenter trial, the Digitalis Investigation Group (DIG) trial, shook the world. Twenty years since and the opponents of digoxin still quote this trial as evidence enough to say that digoxin is no longer a drug to be considered in the management of heart failure. The trial enrolled nearly 6,800 patients with symptomatic HF, an LVEF ≤45%, and normal sinus rhythm who were randomly assigned to digoxin or placebo and aimed at identifying the effect of digoxin on patient survival and hospitalization. Most patients enrolled in this trial had NYHA class II or III HF (84%), 70% had ischemic heart disease and 94% were treated with an ACE inhibitor. At the end of 3 years, digoxin failed to show a survival benefit compared to placebo. Digoxin had a statistically insignificant effect on reducing mortality secondary to worsening heart failure compared to placebo, however this benefit was offset by the increase in non-heart failure deaths, including arrhythmogenic deaths, in the digoxin treated group. Patients taking digoxin had a significant decrease in hospitalization, primarily due to decrease in hospitalization for HF. There was also a significant reduction in the combined end-point of death from HF and hospitalization for worsening HF which was independent of age.[2]

BOX 1: Pharmacokinetics of digoxin.

- Rapid absorption of 75% of oral dose
- Circulates in blood unbound to plasma proteins
- Blood $T_{1/2}$ approximately 36 hour
- Binds to tissue receptors in heart and skeletal muscle
- Lipid soluble; brain penetration +
- Mostly excreted unchanged in urine, 30% nonrenal clearance
- Reduced volume of distribution in chronic renal failure
- Reduced skeletal muscle binding with small lean body mass

Target Levels

Digoxin is a drug with a very narrow therapeutic window. Hence it is imperative to choose the appropriate dose so as to prevent its adverse effects and increased mortality. Many of the adverse effects and non-heart failure related deaths including arrhythmogenic deaths seen in the DIG trials can be ascribed to an increase in the serum digoxin levels beyond the desired range. Unfortunately, the only way to be sure of the correct dosing is to monitor the serum digoxin levels, which is a costly affair often out of reach of the majority of the population especially in the developing world where costs are prohibitory. For patients with HFrEF, the target serum digoxin level for maximum efficacy and minimal risk of toxicity is between 0.5 ng/mL and 0.8 ng/mL. Higher serum levels should be avoided as they are associated with an increased risk of toxicity without and evidence of enhanced efficacy. Clinical trials in patients with sinus rhythm that demonstrated benefit from digoxin therapy have targeted mean SDCs ranging from 0.5 ng/mL to 1.75 ng/mL.[2-4] The doses used to achieve these values ranged from 0.125 to 0.25 mg per day of digoxin. Post-hoc analyses of the DIG trial have shown that when patients were stratified according to the SDC, there was a correlation between the digoxin level and patient survival, such that mortality and hospitalizations were lesser in patients with a SDC between 0.5 ng/mL and 0.9 ng/mL regardless of the EF or gender compared to those with higher SDCs who consequently had an increased event rate.[5-7]

Only around 20% of participants (318 patients) enrolled in the DIG trial were women, a number that was too small to derive any meaningful statistical analysis of the effects of SDCs on event rate in this population. An initial retrospective subgroup analysis suggested that mortality may have been elevated in women taking digoxin,[8] subsequent analysis taking into account the SDCs found that only women with SDCs >1 ng/mL were at higher risk for mortality.[9] There was a significant 33% increase in mortality in women with SDCs between 1.2 ng/mL and 2 ng/mL (Fig. 1).

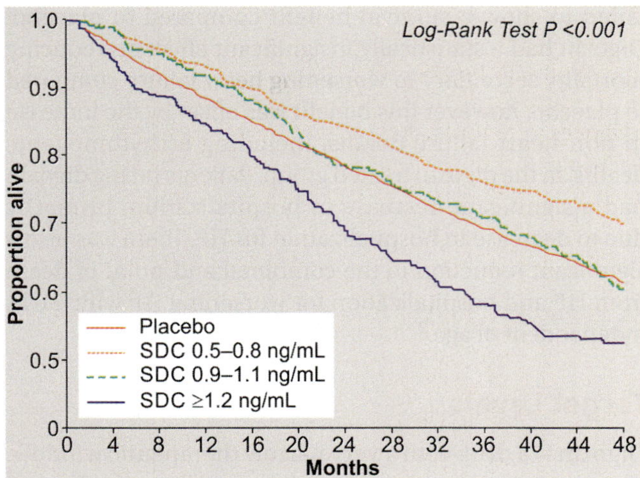

Fig 1: Kaplan-Meier survival analysis of all-cause mortality in association with serum digoxin levels

Source: Rathore SS, Curtis JP, Wang Y, et al. Association of serum digoxin concentrations and outcomes in patients with heart failure. JAMA. 2003;289:871-8.

USE OF DIGOXIN IN HEART FAILURE

Although there is a significant body of available data that has indicated that digoxin can provide clinical benefits in patients with HFrEF, its routine use in this setting is controversial and there has been a steady decline in its use over the last decade.[10] Since much of the controlled data on the use of digoxin in HF predates the advent and subsequent widespread use of contemporary guideline-directed medical therapies (GDMT), it is unclear whether and to what extent the observed benefits of digoxin apply to this population receiving GDMT. Though clinical benefits of digoxin were evident in controlled trials of digoxin in HFrEF, there was evidence to suggest an increase in adverse events when serum digoxin concentrations (SDC) exceeded 1.0 ng/mL. Hence, careful patient selection and drug dosing are important. The most frequently encountered clinical scenarios are:

- Chronic AF without overt HF is today the most widely accepted indication for the use of digoxin. However, even when used by experienced cardiologists in well-organized trials for AF, as in PALLAS, the mean levels were in the toxic range and could have contributed to the higher incidence of HF.[11] Digoxin may be combined with other rate control drugs like beta-blockers, diltiazem and verapamil, however, there is a significant interaction with verapamil which leads to a decreased non-renal clearance of digoxin.
- Chronic AF with HF has no good outcome data and its usage and dosage largely rests on clinical judgment. Use of digoxin in this setting with a beta blocker that not only controls ventricular rate but also improves exercise tolerance and ejection fraction.[12]
- Chronic HF with sinus rhythm—use of digoxin has shown very limited benefits in the DIG trial. A narrow therapeutic window and numerous drug interactions have largely restricted its use in this setting to an optional and potentially dangerous agent, if not carefully given in lower doses.[12]

MAJOR SOCIETY GUIDELINES

- The 2016 European Society of Cardiology (ESC) HF guidelines included a weak recommendation for use of digoxin in patients symptomatic despite GDMT.[13]
- *"Digoxin may be considered in symptomatic patients in sinus rhythm despite treatment with an ACE-I (or ARB), a beta-blocker and an MRA, to reduce the risk of hospitalization (both all-cause and HF-hospitalizations)."* (Class IIb, LOE: B)
- The 2013 American College of Cardiology/American Heart Association (ACC/AHA) HF guidelines included a more general statement that digoxin can be beneficial in patients with HFrEF to decrease hospitalizations for HF.[14] The guideline writing committee noted that digoxin may be added during initial therapy for HF with severe symptoms or may be used only in patients with persistent symptoms despite GDMT for HFrEF.
- *"Digoxin can be beneficial in patients with HFrEF, unless contraindicated, to decrease hospitalizations for HF."* (Class IIa, LOE: B)

Worsened Outcomes with Digoxin Withdrawal

Two randomized trials (PROVED and RADIANCE) examined the effects of digoxin withdrawal in stable HF patients treated with diuretics and digoxin (PROVED),[15] or diuretics, ACE inhibitors and digoxin (RADIANCE).[16] Both these studies showed that digoxin withdrawal was associated with a worsening of heart failure symptoms and an increased risk of clinical deterioration.

Digoxin in Ambulatory Patients

Based on data from the DIG trial, ambulatory patients with chronic HF and low SDC had lower mortality and hospitalizations. Low-dose digoxin (≤ 0.125 mg/day) was the strongest independent predictor of low SDC.[17] Studies on the effect of digoxin on exercise capacity have shown that exercise tolerance and peak V_{O2} improved with digoxin, an effect which was seen predominantly in patients in advanced degrees of HF.[18-22]

Digoxin not for Advanced Heart Failure

In patients awaiting transplant, otherwise optimally treated, digoxin was associated with a higher risk of death and there was a deterioration in major outcomes (combined death, urgent transplantation or insertion of LVAD) and increased hospitalization rates.

DIGOXIN CONTRAINDICATIONS

Hypertrophic obstructive cardiomyopathy, WPW syndrome with AF, significant AV block and diastolic dysfunction are contraindications for digoxin use. Relative contraindications are renal failure and older age where dosage reduction is strongly recommended to prevent dangerous toxicity.

Digoxin in Women and Older Adults

Only 22% of the participants in the DIG trial were women, in whom there was an unexplained increased 23% risk of all-cause mortality. The authors speculated that this could be a consequence of renal interaction with hormone replacement therapy which was concurrently used in a majority of the women participants in the study. In a post-hoc analysis of the data from the DIG trial, the authors found an absolute difference of 5.8% between men and women in the effect of digoxin on the rate of death from any cause. Specifically women randomly assigned to digoxin had a higher rate of death than women who were randomly assigned to placebo (33% vs. 28.9%), a difference that was not seen in men.[23] There has been sporadic data from two studies that showed an increased risk of breast cancer with digoxin use in women. While one study relates to use at any time, the other is related to increased risk of invasive cancer associated with continuous use for at least 2 years.[24,25] In older adults, decreased skeletal muscle mass, lean body mass and renal function increase digoxin levels. Digoxin half-life may be prolonged up to 73 hours, depending on renal function. Use of a digoxin dose <0.125 mg/day is recommended (such as 0.125 mg every alternate day).

DRUG INTERACTIONS

Verapamil reduces nonrenal clearance of digoxin leading to an increase of digoxin blood levels by as much as 50–75%. Amiodarone and propafenone also elevate serum digoxin levels. Loop diuretics, notably furosemide, may induce hypokalemia, which sensitizes the heart to digoxin toxicity, and shuts off tubular secretion of digoxin when the plasma potassium falls to <2–3 mEq/L.

CONCLUSION

Digoxin the once upon a time wonderkid has today turned into the prodigal son in the management of heart failure. With the advances in renin angiotensin system modulation therapies (ACE inhibitors, ARNI), beta blockers and mineralocorticoid receptor antagonists, digoxin has been relegated to the background. With monitoring of SDC, the patient can obtain benefits of digoxin while avoiding its dangerous adverse effects. The choice of digoxin in HF needs to be tailored to the individual patient, keeping in mind the gender, EF, NYHA class and associated comorbidities. Digoxin's role in HF today may be down but it is certainly not out. There remain clinical scenarios especially in the management of chronic HF with AF where digoxin has a place up, right and center.

REFERENCES

1. Arispe N, Diaz JC, Simakova O, et al. Digitoxin induces calcium uptake into cells by forming transmembrane calcium channels. Proc Nat Acad Sci USA. 2008;105:2610-5.
2. Digitalis Investigation Group. The effect of digoxin on mortality and morbidity in patients with heart failure. N Engl J Med. 1997; 336:525.
3. Guyatt GH, Sullivan MJ, Fallen EL, et al. A controlled trial of digoxin in congestive heart failure. Am J Cardiol. 1988; 61:371.
4. Comparative effects of therapy with captopril and digoxin in patients with mild to moderate heart failure. The Captopril-Digoxin Multicenter Research Group. JAMA. 1988;259:539.
5. Rathore SS, Curtis JP, Wang Y, et al. Association of serum digoxin concentration and outcomes in patients with heart failure. JAMA. 2003;289:871.
6. Goldberger ZD, Goldberger AL. Therapeutic ranges of serum digoxin concentrations in patients with heart failure. Am J Cardiol. 2012;109:1818.
7. Ahmed A, Rich MW, Love TE, et al. Digoxin and reduction in mortality and hospitalization in heart failure: a comprehensive post hoc analysis of the DIG trial. Eur Heart J. 2006;27:178.
8. Rathore SS, Wang Y, Krumholz HM. Sex-based differences in the effect of digoxin for the treatment of heart failure. N Engl J Med. 2002;347:1403.
9. Adams KF Jr, Patterson JH, Gattis WA, et al. Relationship of serum digoxin concentration to mortality and morbidity in women in the digitalis investigation group trial: a retrospective analysis. J Am Coll Cardiol. 2005;46:497.
10. Patel N, Ju C, Macon C, et al. Temporal trends of digoxin use in patients hospitalized with heart failure: analysis from the American Heart Association get with the Guidelines-Heart failure registry. JACC Heart Fail. 2016;4:348.
11. Connolly SJ, Camm AJ, Halperin JL, et al. Dronederone in high-risk permanent atrial fibrillation. New Engl J Med. 2012;366:1159.
12. Teerlink JR, Sliwa K, Opie LH. Heart Failure. In: Opie LH, Gersh BJ (Eds). Drugs for the Heart, 8th edition. New York: Elsevier; 2013. pp. 169-223.

13. Ponikowski P, Voors AA, Anker SD, et al. ESC Guidelines for the diagnosis and treatment of acute and chronic heart failure: the Task Force for the diagnosis and treatment of acute and chronic heart failure of the European Society of Cardiology (ESC) Developed with the special contribution of the Heart Failure Association (HFA) of the ESC. Eur Heart J. 2016;37:2129.
14. Yancy CW, Jessup M, Bozkurt B, et al. ACCF/AHA guideline for the management of heart failure: a report of the American College of Cardiology Foundation/American Heart Association Task Force on practice guidelines. Circulation. 2013;128:e240.
15. Uretsky BF, Young JB, Shahidi FE, et al. Randomized study assessing the effect of digoxin withdrawal in patients with mild to moderate chronic congestive heart failure: results of the PROVED trial. PROVED Investigative Group. J Am Coll Cardiol. 1993;22:955.
16. Packer M, Gheorghiade M, Young JB, et al. Withdrawal of digoxin from patients with chronic heart failure treated with angiotensin-converting-enzyme inhibitors. RADIANCE Study. N Engl J Med. 1993;329:1.
17. Ahmed A, Pitt B, Rahimtoola SH, et al. Effects of digoxin at low serum concentrations on mortality and hospitalization in heart failure: a propensity-matched study of the DIG trial. Int J Cardiol. 2008;123:138-46.
18. Guyatt GH, Sullivan MJ, Fallen EL, et al. A controlled trial of digoxin in congestive heart failure. Am J Cardiol. 1988;61:371.
19. DiBianco R, Shabetai R, Kostuk W, et al. A comparison of oral milrinone, digoxin, and their combination in the treatment of patients with chronic heart failure. N Engl J Med. 1989;320:677.
20. Uretsky BF, Young JB, Shahidi FE, et al. Randomized study assessing the effect of digoxin withdrawal in patients with mild to moderate chronic congestive heart failure: results of the PROVED trial. PROVED Investigative Group. J Am Coll Cardiol. 1993;22:955.
21. Fleg JL, Rothfeld B, Gottlieb SH. Effect of maintenance digoxin therapy on aerobic performance and exercise left ventricular function in mild to moderate heart failure due to coronary artery disease: a randomized, placebo-controlled, crossover trial. J Am Coll Cardiol. 1991;17:743.
22. Davies RF, Beanlands DS, Nadeau C, et al. Enalapril versus digoxin in patients with congestive heart failure: a multicenter study. Canadian Enalapril versus Digoxin Study Group. J Am Coll Cardiol. 1991;18:1602.
23. Rathore SS, Wang Y, Krumholz HM. Sex-based differences in the effect of digoxin for the treatment of heart failure. N Engl J Med. 2002;347:1403-11.
24. Biggar RJ, Wohlfahrt J, Oudin A, et al. Digoxin use and the risk of breast cancer in women. J Clin Oncol. 2011;29:2165-70.
25. Ahren TP, Lash TL, Sørensen HT, et al. Digoxin treatment is associated with an increased incidence of breast cancer: a population-based case-control study. Breast Cancer Res. 2008;10:R102.

20

CHAPTER

How to Choose Diuretics in Heart Failure

Lokesh Khandelwal, Girish MP, Mohit D Gupta

INTRODUCTION

Heart failure (HF) is a major public health problem having high morbidity and mortality. Incidence of heart failure hospitalizations has been on increasing trend. The main pathology is fluid overload and it is responsible both for acute decompensation and progression of HF. Mainstay of therapy is removal of excess extracellular fluid with diuretics to treat peripheral and/or pulmonary edema. Diuretics improve symptoms such as dyspnea and edema, however data supporting a mortality benefit or an alteration in disease progression is scarce. Determination of congestion and euvolemia, diuretic resistance and approach for choosing diuretics is discussed here.

DETECTION OF CONGESTION IN HEART FAILURE

The gold standard for determining congestion in HF is invasive measurement of right atrial pressure (RAP) and pulmonary capillary wedge pressure (PCWP). The important clinical signs of volume overload in HF patients are pulmonary edema, peripheral edema and elevated jugular venous pressure. Chest X-ray may show cardiomegaly, pulmonary venous congestion and pleural effusion. Lung ultrasound shows B-lines resulting from extravasated fluid into interstitium. Echocardiography measures RAP by estimation of inferior vena cava diameter and collapsibility with respiration. Doppler to estimate mitral inflow velocities and tissue Doppler can be used for left sided filling pressures. Measurement of natriuretic peptides should be done in all patients with acute HF. BNP <100 pg/mL and NT-proBNP <300 ng/mL indicates absence of congestion. Sensitivity and specificity of various clinical variables is shown in Table 1.[1]

DETERMINATION OF EUVOLEMIA IN HEART FAILURE

Evaluation of euvolemia before discharge is of prime importance because persistent volume overload at discharge is associated with higher morbidity and mortality. The role of diuretic therapy is to achieve and maintain euvolemia with the lowest dose. The best strategy to detect congestion at discharge is by using multi parameter based approach as shown in Figure 1.[1] When patient's dry weight is achieved, dose of diuretic should be adjusted to prevent dehydration which can result in hypotension and renal dysfunction.

Loop Diuretics

In treatment of ADHF loop diuretics play a major role and are utilized in over 90% of patients hospitalized for HF.[2] Loop diuretics include furosemide, torsemide and bumetanide, with furosemide most commonly used. On absorption, the majority of the drug becomes bound to plasma proteins and then secreted into tubular lumen by organic anion transporters. They inhibit $Na^+/K^+/2\ Cl$ cotransporter in ascending limb of loop of Henle. These agents induce renal prostaglandin synthesis resulting in vascular smooth muscle relaxation and venodilation. A threshold concentration of luminal diuretic is required to achieve increase in natriuresis. These drugs show a ceiling effect, in which there

TABLE 1: Sensitivity and specificity of different clinical and technical parameters to detect congestion.[1]

Clinical evaluation					
Right-sided			*Left-sided**		
Parameters	*Sensitivity*	*Specificity*	*Parameters*	*Sensitivity*	*Specificity*
JVP >8 cm	48%	78%	Dyspnea	50%	73%
Jugular venous reflux	50%	75%	Dyspnea on exertion	66%	52%
Hepatomegaly	51%	62%	Orthopnea	66%	47%
Bilateral leg edema	94%	10%	S3	73%	42%
			Rales	13%	90%
Echocardiographic evaluation					
Collapse (<50%) IVC	12%	27%	Mitral inflow E-wave velocity>50 (cm/s)	92%	28%
Inspiratory diameter IVC <12 mm	67%	91%	Lateral E/e' >12	66%	55%
			Deceleration time <130 ms	81%	80%
			Pulmonary vein S/D <1	83%	72%
			Diffuse B-lines on lung ultrasound[a]	85.7%	85.7%

*Sensitivity and specificity of right sided parameters as compared to RAP > 7 mm Hg and that of left-sided parameters compared with PCWP >18 mm Hg.
[a]More than three B-lines in more than two intercostal spaces bilaterally.
Source: Adapted from European Journal of Heart Failure.

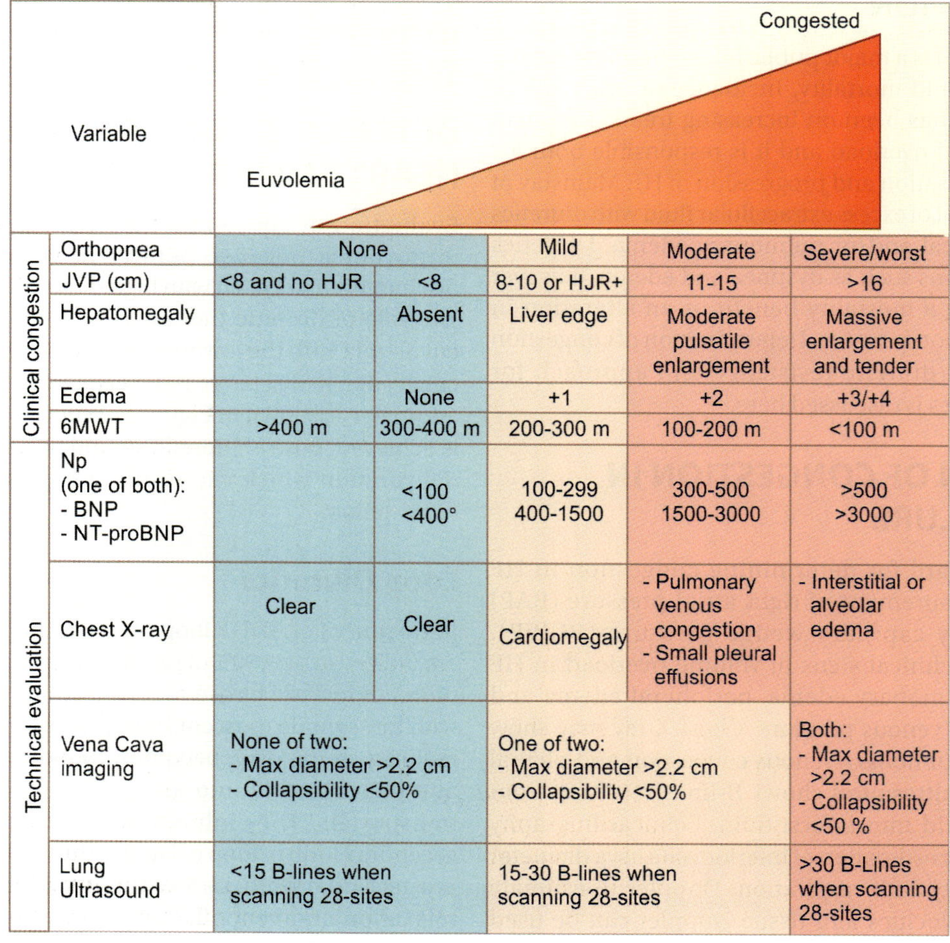

Fig. 1: Evaluation of euvolemia and congestion.
Source: Adapted from European Journal of Heart Failure.[1]

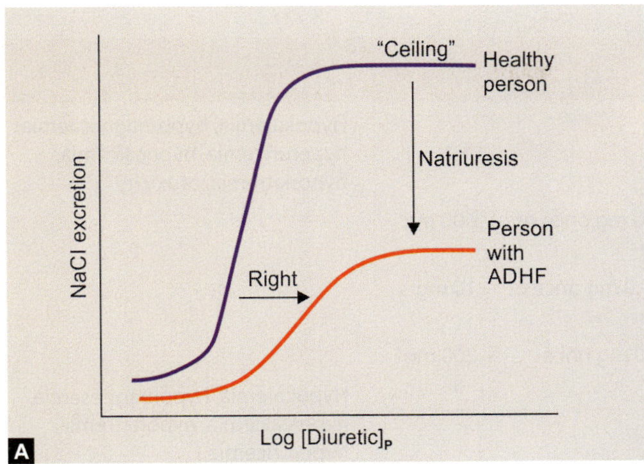

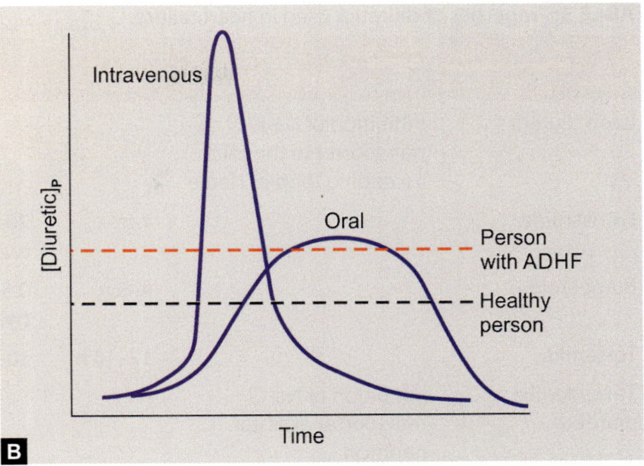

Figs. 2A and B: Properties of loop diuretics in person with ADHF versus healthy person:[3] (A) ADHF shifts the relation between the log of the plasma diuretic concentration ($[Diuretic]_P$) and sodium chloride excretion to the right and reduces the "ceiling" natriuresis; (B) The plasma concentration of loop diuretic $[Diuretic]_P$ as a function of time after an intravenous or oral dose. The natriuretic threshold (dashed lines) is increased in patients with ADHF than in healthy persons. Natriuresis is determined by, total time diuretic concentration is above natriuretic threshold.

is no increment in natriuresis when certain concentration of drug is achieved. In patients having reduced GFR, effect of loop diuretics is decreased as less drug is secreted into tubular lumen, therefore higher dose is required. In HF patients, efficacy of diuretics is decreased as compared to normal subjects as there is decreased absorption of oral diuretic due to gut wall edema and renal hypoperfusion,so less diuretic secreted into tubules with an increased sodium reabsorption due to activation of the RAAS (Fig. 2).

Furosemide has a variable bioavailability of 10–90% whereas torsemide and bumetanide have higher and consistent bioavailability of 80–100% (Table 2). Oral dose of furosemide is approximately twice the intravenous dose and food decreases its absorption. Twice daily dose is preferred for loop diuretics as they act for short time, to prevent post diuretic sodium retention. Properties of diuretics used in HF are given in Table 3.

TORsemide In Chronic heart failure (TORIC) was nonrandomized, post-marketing surveillance trial which showed the use of torsemide was associated with lower mortality than furosemide in patients with HF.[4]But there is not enough strong evidence to recommend torsemide and bumetanide over furosemide in HF and guidelines do not dictate which diuretic is to be preferred.

Braking phenomenon: When extracellular fluid volume drops there is activation of RAAS as well as sympathetic nervous system and hypertrophy of the distal nephron, therefore response to diuretic decreases. Long-term diuretic treatment can cause progressive contraction of ECF volume and breaking phenomenon is an adaptive response. But when it happens in patients having persistent congestion, it leads to diuretic resistance.

TABLE 2: Properties of loop diuretics.

	Furosemide	*Torsemide*	*Bumetanide*
Relative intravenous potency (mg)	40	20	1
Oral: Intravenous dosing	1:2	1:1	1:1
Bioavailability (%)	10–90	80–100	80–100

Urine output and post-diuretic spot urinary sodium content may be used for determining diuretic response. Volume overloaded patients having inadequate diuretic response can be detected by having a spot urine sodium <50–70 mEq/L after 2 hours and/or urine output <100–150 mL/hr. Approach for using diuretics in acute heart failure is shown in Flowchart 1.[1]

There are two approaches for choosing diuretic therapy in ADHF, continuous infusion and bolus injection. After a bolus dose there is sympathetic stimulation and post-diuretic sodium retention when diuretic concentration falls. Continuous infusion is advantageous as there are no rapid fluctuations in intravascular volume and persistent therapeutic dose of diuretic is maintained. Additionally continuous infusion may limit ototoxicity as there is overall lower dose requirement.

DOSE trial randomly assigned 308 patients to receive furosemide administered intravenously via either a bolus every 12 hours or continuous infusion and at either a low dose (equivalent to the patient's previous oral dose) or a high dose (2.5 times the previous oral dose).[5] There was no significant difference in patients' global assessment of symptoms or men change in creatinine level in bolus

TABLE 3: Properties of diuretics used in heart failure.

Drug	*Site of action*	*Duration of action*	*Starting dosage*	*Maximum dosage*	*Side effects*
Loop diuretics	Inhibition of Na-K-Cl co-transporter in the thick ascending loop of Henle				Hypokalemia, hypomagnesaemia, hyperuricemia, hypocalcemia, hyponatremia, otoxicity
Furosemide		7 h	20–40 mg once or twice	600 mg	
Bumetanide		4–6 h	0.5–1.0 mg once or twice	10 mg	
Torsemide		12–16 h	10–20 mg once	200 mg	
Thiazide-like diuretics	Inhibition of Na-Cl transporter at distal nephron				Hypokalemia, hypomagnesemia, hypercalcemia, hyponatremia, hyperuricemia
Chlorthalidone		24–72 h	12.5–25 mg once	100 mg	
Indapamide		36 h	2.5 mg once	20 mg	
HCTZ		12–24 h	25mg once	200 mg	
Metolazone		24 h	2.5 mg once	20 mg	
Potassium-sparing diuretics	Inhibition of mineralocorticoid receptor at distal nephron				Hyperkalemia
Amiloride		24 h	5 mg once	20 mg	
Spironolactone		24 h	12.5–25.0 mg once	50 mg	Gynecomastia
Eplerenone		12–24 h	25 mg once	50 mg	

versus continuous infusion. High-dose furosemide, compared with low-dose furosemide, produced greater net fluid loss, weight loss, and relief from dyspnea but also more frequent transient worsening of renal function. It suggested that intravenous continuous infusion and bolus loop diuretic therapy have similar efficacy in patients with ADHF.

Monitoring of blood urea and serum creatinine should be done as they often rise during HF treatment. BUN/serum creatinine ratio >20:1 suggests a prerenal kidney injury. If during therapy BUN increases and serum creatinine is stable it suggests preserved GFR. But when serum creatinine increases it reflects reduction in GFR and may suggest reduced perfusion to kidney and other organs. In patients with persistent congestion before achievement of euvolemic state, increase in serum creatinine portends worse prognosis. In these cases also fluid removal may be required to treat signs of congestion especially pulmonary edema. In contrast stable serum creatinine indicates maintained perfusion and if patient is volume overloaded diuresis can be continued.

If before achievement of euvolemia, hypotension or deteriorating renal function develops, diuresis should be slowed. In patients with asymptomatic mild to moderate decrease in blood pressure or renal function, diuresis should be continued if there is still hypervolemia. Persistently volume overload leads to decreased efficacy of diuretics and patients tend to have continued symptoms with increased mortality.

Loop Diuretic Resistance

It is the failure of diuretics to achieve decongestion, which is indicated by a low urine sodium concentration, despite the use of maximal recommended doses. There is decrease in diuretic efficiency, which is defined as net fluid loss per mg if diuretics. It is frequent and occurs in up to 25% of patients. Loop diuretics have failed to show any mortality benefit in heart failure but diuretic resistance has poor prognosis with increased hospitalizations for heart failure and higher mortality.[6]

Mechanisms

- In patients with HF there is gut wall edema, decreased splanchnic blood flow and decreased intestinal motility due to sympathetic stimulation.
- In patients with renal insufficiency, other organic acids such as blood urea nitrogen compete with loop diuretics for transport by the organic anion transporters.

- Post-diuretic effect: During periods of decreased drug levels between diuretic doses there is a rebound increase in sodium reabsorption.
- Braking phenomenon: After chronic diuretic use, hypertrophy of cells in the distal convoluted tubules leads to increased efficiency of sodium reabsorption.
- Use of NSAIDs.

Management

- Increase the diuretic dose.
- Change from one loop diuretic to another with better pharmacokinetics, e.g. from furosemide to torsemide which has more consistent bioavailability and the longer half-life which can counter the "post-diuretic" effect.
- Continuous intravenous infusion of a loop diuretic.

Flowcharts 1A and B: Diuretic use in acute heart failure. (A) Congestion with volume overload; (B) Treatment algorithm after 24 hours. Total loop diuretic dose can be administered either as continuous infusion or bolus infusion.

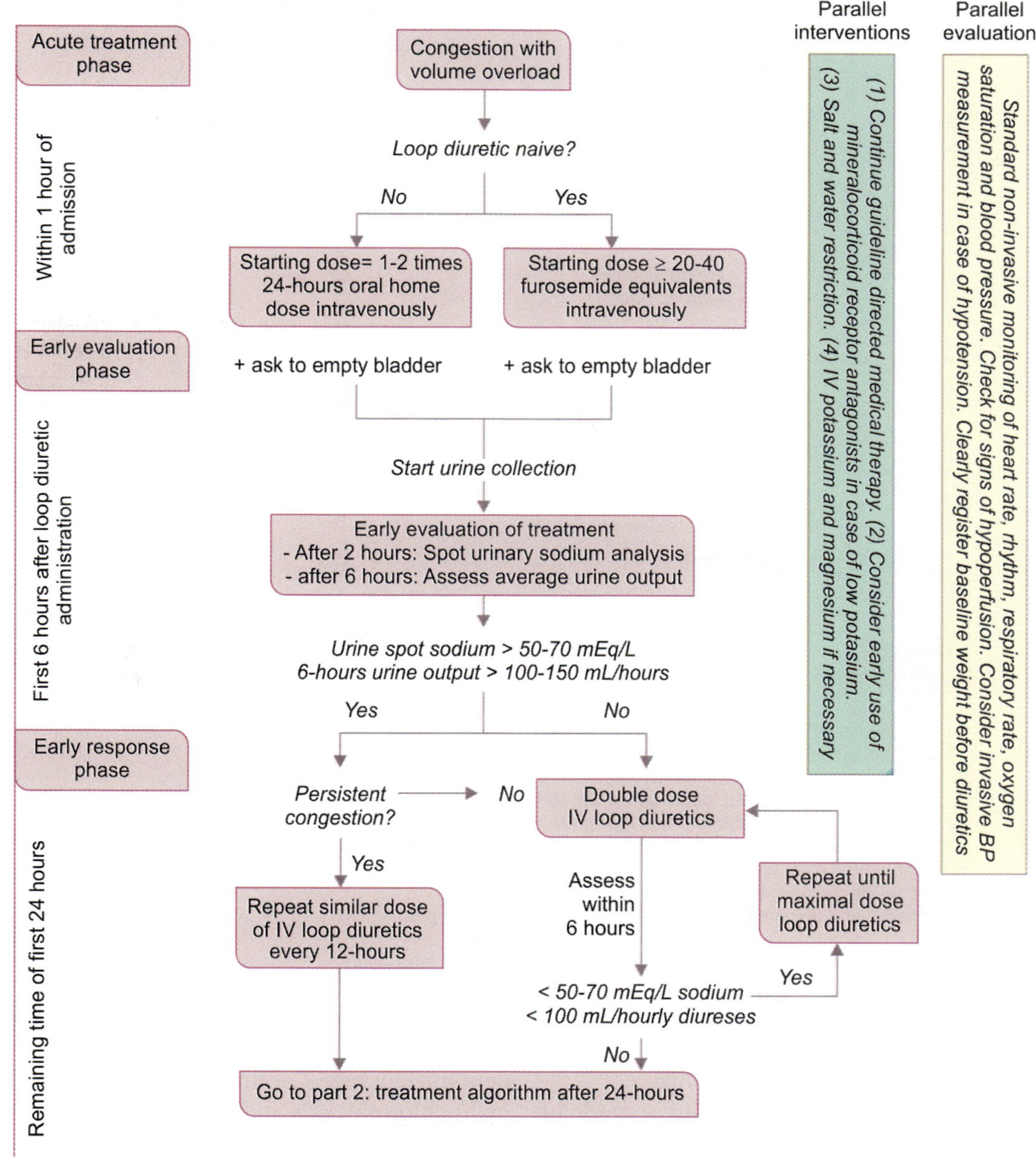

Contd...

Contd...

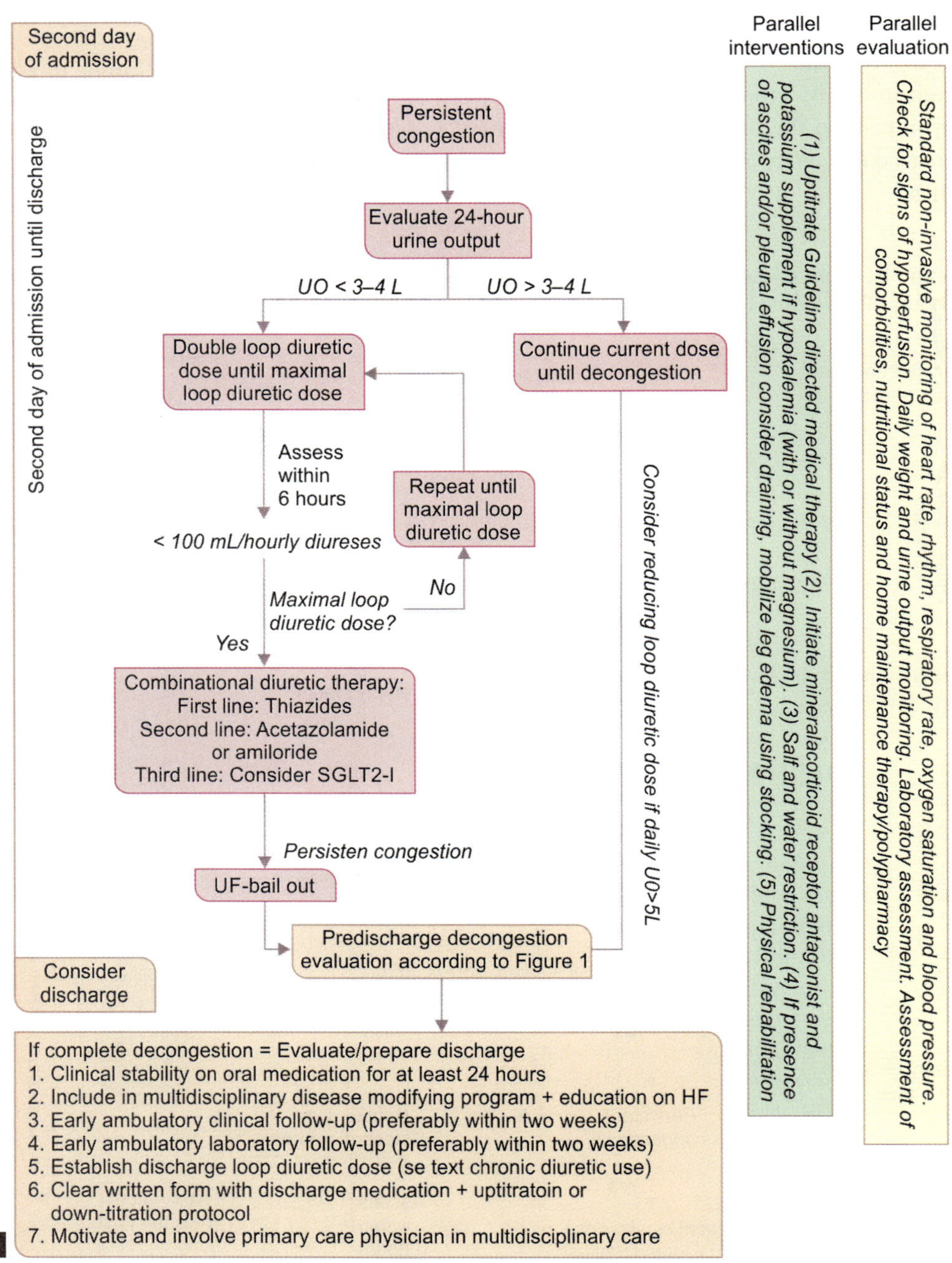

Source: Adapted from European Heart Journal.[1]

- Sequential nephron blockade by addition of a thiazide-type diuretic.
- Administration of an aldosterone antagonist.
- Ultrafiltration can be used in cases of volume overload refractory to diuretics.

Thiazide Diuretics

These have limited diuretic effect which is about 30-40% of loop diuretis.[7] They block Na^+-Cl^- cotransporter in the distal convoluted tubule and are frequently used with loop diuretics in resistant cases to achieve sequential nephron blockage. Common diuretics used are metolazone, hydrochlorothiazide and chlorthalidone.

They counter sodium reabsorption that occurs with the increased sodium load being delivered to the distal convoluted tubule after loop diuretic administration, as well as counter the increased sodium transport capacity or "braking phenomenon" that occurs with chronic loop diuretic use.

The increased delivery of sodium to the collecting ducts enhances the exchange of sodium with potassium and results in potassium depletion. Frequent monitoring of electrolytes and renal function is important when combination diuretic strategy is used because it can cause hypokalemia and less commonly, hyponatremia and hypochloremia. Metolazone is more potent than hydrochlorothiazide and retains its effectiveness even when there is severe reduction in GFR, so can be used in renal impairment.

Mineralocorticoid Receptor Antagonists

They inhibit actions of mineralocorticoids at cortical collecting duct. These are weak diuretics as only 3% of filtered sodium is reabsorbed at the collecting duct. In patients with HF aldosterone antagonists spironolactone and eplerenone have been shown to improve survival in RALES and EPHESUS trials.[8,9] At low doses studied, the primary effect of these drugs is due to inhibition of aldosterone rather than diuretic action. They give rise to hyperkalemia and may be beneficial in counteracting the hypokalemia from loop diuretics. They should be given prior to the addition of a thiazide diuretic in patients with a low or borderline serum potassium on loop diuretic therapy alone. They may also enhance diuresis in the resistant patient, but data to support the use of higher dose of aldosterone antagonist diuretics in heart failure is not available. Spironolactone is a non-selective aldosterone receptor antagonist so endocrine-related adverse effects, e.g. gynecomastia are relatively common. Eplerone has greater selectivity on the mineralocorticoid receptor so has lesser side effects.

These are recommended in patients who have New York Heart Association (NYHA) class II HF and left ventricular ejection fraction (LVEF) ≤30%; or NYHA class III to IV HF and an LVEF <35%; or are post-ST elevation myocardial infarction with an LVEF ≤40% and have either symptomatic HF or diabetes mellitus. An aldosterone antagonist (spironolactone or eplerenone) is preferred to a sodium channel blocker (amiloride or triamterene) because of evidence that aldosterone antagonist therapy improves outcomes in patients with HF.

Aldosterone Targeted Neurohormonal Combined with Natriuresis Therapy in Heart Failure (ATHENA-HF) trial evaluated high-dose MRA therapy in addition to standard loop diuretic therapy in acute heart failure. 100 mg of spironolactone per day versus 25 mg per day was not found superior in reducing NT-proBNP or increase urine output after 96 hours.[10] But, spironolactone is a pro-drug with onset of action only 48–72 hour after oral intake, which could count for the observed nil-effect. High-dose MRA was found to be safe, as it did not result in hyperkalemia or worsening of renal function.

Vasopressin Antagonists

Heart failure with concomitant severe hyponatremia is a poor prognostic indicator. Vasopressin antagonists increase in free water excretion by blocking aquaporin V2 receptor at the cortical collecting duct. They can also be helpful in cases with diuretic resistance.

Efficacy of Vasopressin Antagonism in Heart Failure Outcome Study with Tolvaptan (EVEREST) a multicenter, randomized, placebo-controlled trial in hospitalized chronic HF patients, evaluated the addition of tolvaptan 30 mg daily to standard therapy. There was no difference in the global clinical status in patients treated with tolvaptan or placebo, although the tolvaptan group had significantly decreased dyspnea on day 1 and decreased weight and edema after 7 days. Long-term primary outcome trial showed no significant difference in overall mortality.[11]

Tolvaptan is approved only for the treatment of clinically significant hypervolemic and euvolemic hyponatremia (serum Na^+<125 meq/L), which includes patients with HF and the syndrome of inappropriate antidiuretic hormone secretion.

OTHER APPROACHES

Ultrafiltration

Ultrafiltration (UF) moves water and small to medium weight solutes across a semipermeable membrane to reduce volume overload. Cardiorenal Rescue Study in Acute Decompensated Heart Failure (CARRESS-HF), which compared the effect of UF with that of stepped pharmacological therapy on renal function and weight loss in patients with HF who have worsening renal function and persistent congestion, patients in the UF group had a significantly greater increase in serum creatinine and more adverse events, including bleeding and vascular complications, as well as progressive renal dysfunction. Moreover, there was no significant difference in the outcome, including mortality and rehospitalization, at 60 days (Table 4).[12,13] According to guidelines, UF might be considered in patients having volume overload refractory to medical therapy.

CONCLUSION

Diuretics play a pivotal role in the management of heart failure by decreasing congestion and relieving symptoms. Loop diuretics are most commonly used, because

TABLE 4: ACC/AHA 2016 Update to 2013 heart failure clinical practice guidelines.[13]

Recommendation	*COR*	*LOE*
HF patients hospitalized with fluid overload should be treated with intravenous diuretics	I	B
HF patients receiving loop diuretic therapy, should receive an initial parenteral dose greater than or equal to their chronic oral daily dose, then doses should be serially adjusted	I	B
Serum electrolytes, urea nitrogen, and creatinine should be measured during the titration of HF medications, including diuretics	I	C
When diuresis is inadequate, it is reasonable to a) Give higher doses of intravenous loop diuretics; or b) Add a second diuretic (e.g. thiazide)	IIa	B
Low-dose dopamine infusion may be considered with loop diuretics to improve diuresis	IIb	B
Ultrafiltration may be considered for patients with obvious volume overload	IIb	B
Ultrafiltration may be considered for patients with refractory congestion	IIb	C
Intravenous nitroglycerin, nitroprusside or nesiritide may be considered an adjuvant to diuretic therapy for stable patients with HF	IIb	B
In patients hospitalized with volume overload and severe hyponatremia, vasopressin antagonists may be considered	IIb	B
Diuretics should be used for relief of symptoms due to volume overload in patients with HFpEF	I	C

they have the most potent natriuretic action. Diuretic resistance remains a clinical problem and it might not resolve with increased doses of diuretics or a change in the loop diuretic. A sequential nephron blockade where thiazide-like diuretics are administered in combination with loop diuretics is helpful in these cases. Despite having a weak diuretic effect, potassium sparing diuretics have been shown to improve the long-term outcomes in HF patients.

REFERENCES

1. Mullens W, Damman K, Harjola VP, et al. The use of diuretics in heart failure with congestion - a position statement from the Heart Failure Association of the European Society of Cardiology. Eur J Heart Fail. 2019;21(2):137-55.
2. Chioncel O, Mebazaa A, Harjola VP, et al. ESC Heart Failure Long-Term Registry Investigators. Clinical phenotypes and outcome of patients hospitalized for acute heart failure: the ESC Heart Failure Long-Term Registry. Eur J Heart Fail. 2017;19:1242-54.
3. Ellison DH, Felker GM. Diuretic Treatment in Heart Failure. N Engl J Med. 2017;377(20):1964-75.
4. Cosin J, Diez J. Torasemide in chronic heart failure: results of the TORIC study. Eur J Heart Fail. 2002;4:507-13.
5. Felker GM, Lee KL, Bull DA, et al. Diuretic strategies in patients with acute decompensated heart failure. N Engl J Med. 2011;364:797-805.
6. Aronson D, Burger AJ. Diuretic response: clinical and hemodynamic predictors and relation to clinical outcome. J Card Fail. 2016;22:193-200.
7. Knauf H, Mutschler E. Pharmacodynamic and kinetic considerations on diuretics as a basis for differential therapy. Klin Wochenschr. 1991;69:239-50.
8. Pitt B, Zannad F, Remme WJ, et al. The effect of spironolactone on morbidity and mortality in patients with severe heart failure. Randomized Aldactone Evaluation Study Investigators. N Engl J Med. 1999;341(10):709-17.
9. Pitt B, Remme W, Zannad F, et al. Eplerenone, a selective aldosterone blocker, in patients with leftventricular dysfunction after myocardial infarction. N Engl J Med. 2003;348(14):1309-21.
10. Butler J, Anstrom KJ, Felker GM, et al. Efficacy and safety of spironolactone in acute heart failure: the ATHENA-HF randomized clinical trial. JAMA Cardiol. 2017;9: 950-8.
11. Pang PS, Konstam MA, Krasa HB, et al. Effects of tolvaptan on dyspnea relief from the EVEREST trials. Eur Heart J. 2009;30:2233-40.
12. Bart BA, Goldsmith SR, Lee KL, et al. Ultrafiltration in decompensated HF with CRS. N Engl J Med. 2012;367:2296-304.
13. 2016 ACC/AHA/HFSA Focused Update on New Pharmacological Therapy for Heart Failure: An Update of the2013 ACCF/AHA Guideline for the Management of Heart Failure: A Report of theAmerican College of Cardiology/ American Heart Association Task Force on Clinical Practice Guidelines and the Heart Failure Society of America. J Card Fail. 2016;22(9):659-69.

21

CHAPTER

Chlorthalidone: A Diuretic of First Choice in Hypertension and Heart Failure

Anil Pareek, HK Chopra, C Venkata S Ram

INTRODUCTION

Heart failure (HF) is one of the major healthcare problems worldwide[1] and is a leading cause of morbidity, hospitalization, and mortality in older adults, placing a huge financial burden on the health care system.[2] Cardiovascular (CV) disease is the most common cause of death globally and HF represents the end phenotype of many CV disorders. Although advances in pharmacological and device-based therapies have reduced mortality rates in patients with HF, a recently published analysis of outcomes from a national primary care database in Scotland concluded that, HF remains as "malignant" as some of the common cancers in both men and women. In men, HF (5-year survival: 55.8%) had worse mortality outcomes than prostate cancer (5-year survival: 68.3%), and bladder cancer (5-year survival: 57.3%), while in women, HF (5-year survival: 49.5%) had worse mortality outcomes than breast cancer (5-year survival 77.7%).[3] Hypertension is a major risk factor for HF, preceding it in 75% of patients, and present in 60% to 89% of people with HF with preserved ejection fraction (HFpEF), perhaps representing the main causative factor.[4] Compared with those with an average systolic blood pressure (SBP) <120 mm Hg, the adjusted incidence of HF was increased 1.6, 2.2, and 2.6 times in those with average SBPs between 120 and 139 mm Hg, between 140 and 159 mm Hg, and ≥160 mm Hg, respectively.[5] In SPRINT, a more intensive intervention that targeted an SBP <120 mm Hg significantly reduced the incidence of HF, a component of the primary outcome, by 38% (HR: 0.62; 95% CI: 0.45–0.84).[6]

Despite this evidence, most of the clinical trials in past have evaluated HF as a "soft" endpoint, while major attention was being given to myocardial infarction and stroke.[7] A systematic review of recent hypertension trials to assess incidence of HF compared to coronary heart diseases and stroke revealed that incidence of HF is comparable with that of stroke and is more prevalent in "very high risk" individuals. Although achieving optimal BP control is important in HF prevention and control, the type of antihypertensive agent used also plays a role.[8] Increasing urinary sodium excretion is a logical and fundamental part of treatment of hypertension, as all monogenic forms of hypertension have sodium retention as the main mechanism of the increase in blood pressure.[9] Consistent with this understanding, thiazide diuretics are listed in hypertension guidelines as one of first-line antihypertensive options. Simultaneously, it is critical to understand that optimizing antihypertensive treatments aimed at preventing the progression to overt HF is essential.[8]

Antihypertensive agents like diuretics and angiotensin-converting enzyme inhibitors (ACE-I) have been shown to reduce incidence of HF in patients with hypertension.[10-13] A meta-analysis of 19 randomized controlled clinical trials involving 112,113 patients was conducted to evaluate whether thiazide diuretics, including thiazide-type and thiazide-like diuretics have additional cardioprotective effects. Treatment with thiazide diuretics was associated with reduction in the risks of HF [odds ratio (OR): 0.62; $p < 0.001$] and cardiac events (OR: 0.86; $p = 0.007$), but no difference was observed in stroke (OR: 0.92; $p = 0.438$)

or coronary heart diseases (CHDs) (OR: 0.95; p = 0.378) between thiazide diuretics and controls. Further analysis showed that thiazide-like diuretics have greater protective effects on cardiac events (OR: 0.78; p < 0.001), especially HF (OR: 0.57; p <0.001), than the thiazide-type diuretics; thus providing greater CV benefits in hypertensive patients.[14]

Antihypertensive Lipid-Lowering Treatment to Prevent Heart Attack Trial (ALLHAT) is the largest randomized hypertension outcomes trial (n = 42,418) designed to compare CV outcomes in high-risk hypertensive patients assigned to the ACE-I lisinopril, the calcium channel blocker (CCB) amlodipine, and the α-blocker doxazosin, in comparison to the thiazide-like diuretic chlorthalidone (CTD). The most intriguing finding of ALLHAT has been the lower rates of HF events observed in the CTD group compared to each of the three other treatment arms. HF was a secondary outcome, listed as a component of a major secondary outcome, combined CV disease.[15] The overall findings of the trial showed that CHD risk was not improved for any of the three newer agents compared with CTD. However, the doxazosin arm was discontinued prematurely as there was a significant 25% higher incidence of major CVD events in doxazosin group compared to the CTD group. Importantly, this included a doubled risk of CHF (RR, 2.04; 95% CI, 1.79–2.32). The event curves separated largely during the first year but continued to diverge thereafter.[16] Even for the other two arms, HF rates were significantly higher (p <0.001) (by 38% and 19% in the amlodipine and lisinopril groups, respectively) as compared to the CTD group. These results held true when examined by subgroups of age, race, sex, and diabetes status (Fig. 1).

Since, patients with a history of HF or known low ejection fraction were excluded, majority of the HF cases could be considered to be new-onset HF. Remarkably, the Kaplan–Meier event curves for patients hospitalized for HF or death due to HF begin to separate immediately after randomization, with relative risk (RR) of 2.22 [95% confidence interval (CI), 1.69–2.91; P < 0.001] versus CTD in the first year for hospitalized or fatal HF with amlodipine and of 2.08 (95% CI, 1.58–2.74; P < 0.001) with lisinopril versus CTD.[17] For lisinopril versus CTD, the curves converged between years 6 and 7, but for amlodipine versus CTD, they remain separated (Fig. 2).

Apart from ALLHAT, the significant effect of CTD in prevention of HF has been documented in other landmark trials too. The Systolic Hypertension in the Elderly Program (SHEP), a placebo-controlled, double-blind, randomized, multicenter clinical trial, demonstrated that in persons aged 60 years and older with isolated systolic hypertension, antihypertensive stepped care drug treatment with low-dose CTD as step 1 medication reduced the incidence of total stroke by 36% and of major CV events (including HF) by 32%. A sub-analysis focusing on the occurrence of HF in the active and placebo groups of SHEP among all patients as well as among those with a history of or ECG evidence of prior MI was carried out. It was seen that, during follow-up averaging 4.5 years, risk of fatal and nonfatal HF was reduced by almost 50% in the CTD arm (RR, 0.51; 95% CI, 0.37–0.71; P < 0.001). More importantly, risk reduction in the group with a history of or ECG evidence of MI at baseline ranged from 59% to 85% for the different HF endpoints examined.[18] The Treatment of Mild Hypertension Study (TOMHS) assessed the effect of five antihypertensive monotherapies (CTD, acebutolol, doxazosin, amlodipine and enalpril) on reduction of left ventricle mass (LVM) in 902 patients with "mild" (stage 1) hypertension. After 4 years of treatment,

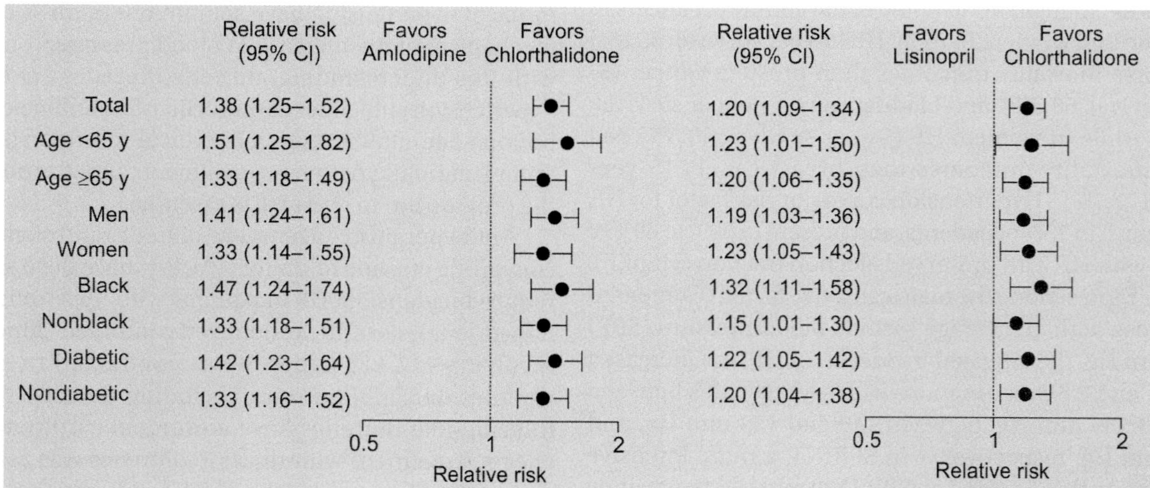

Fig. 1: Chlorthalidone is color-blind in effects—superior in preventing HF than amlodipine (left) and lisinopril (right) across different patient profiles.

Source: Adapted from ALLHAT, 2002.

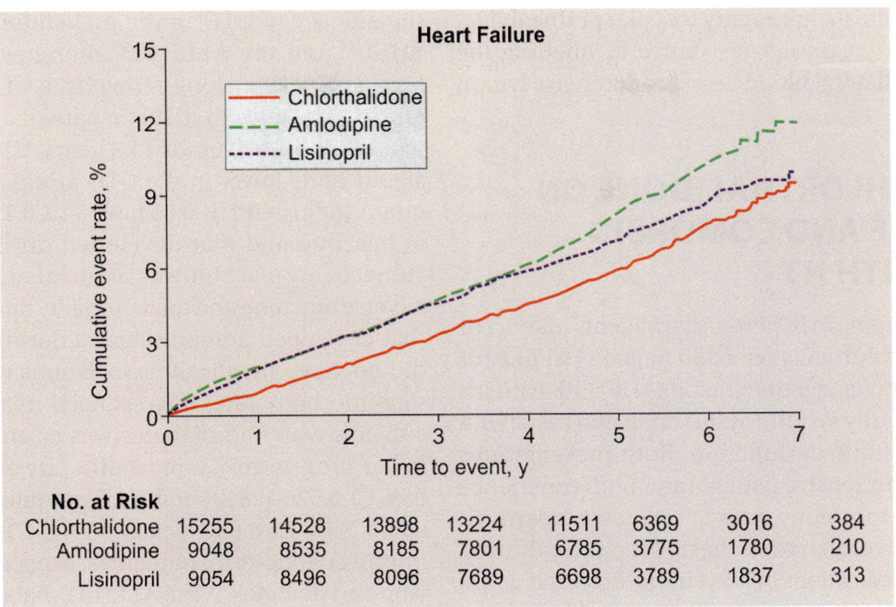

Fig. 2: Kaplan–Meier event curves for HF based on treatment.
Source: Adapted from ALLHAT, 2002.

all 5 therapies showed reduction in LVM from baseline; but only CTD declined LVM significantly more than placebo. Average decreases ranged from 34 g for participants given CTD to 23 g for participants given enalapril and 25 g with amlodipine (P = 0.05 for difference among the five drug-treatment groups). It was also observed that CTD caused a significantly larger decrease in LV internal dimension at end diastole compared to other drug treatments (P = 0.02).[19]

MECHANISMS OF HEART FAILURE PREVENTION WITH CHLORTHALIDONE

Although ALLHAT answered questions about the comparative effectiveness of antihypertensive treatments for HF prevention, the mechanisms behind this HF prevention remain incompletely understood. CCBs, particularly dihydropyridines, have been associated with higher rates of HF in several trials.[20] Surprisingly, ALLHAT showed that CTD was also superior in preventing HF compared to lisinopril, an ACE-I which has well-known protective effect in the prevention and treatment of HF. This was true in subgroups of black and nonblack persons.

Several reasons have been suggested for the superiority of CTD over the CCB amlodipine, the ACE-I lisinopril and the alpha-blocker doxazosin in preventing HF in ALLHAT; including the possibility that HF was misdiagnosed in patients with edema and fluid retention, which are known side effects of dihydropyridine CCBs and alpha-blockers.[21] However, results of an extensive validation study that excluded edema as adjudication criteria, confirmed the lower rates of HF events in the CTD group.[22] Another plausible explanation that has been discussed is that these findings may have been influenced by the antihypertensive medications taken by the ALLHAT participants prior to entry or its withdrawal at the time of study drug initiation. However, extensive analyses of the relation of HF events to patients' preceding antihypertensive therapy showed no significant evidence that pre-entry drug type explained observed hospitalized HF differences by ALLHAT treatment.[23] Perhaps the most interesting hypothesis has been recently tested and published. Johnson et al. aimed to quantify the extent to which the effects of lisinopril, amlodipine, and doxazosin (as compared with CTD) on incident HF are mediated by evolving left ventricular hypertrophy (LVH) and BP lowering. The causal mediation analysis of ALLHAT revealed that evolving ECG LVH and BP lowering explain up to 13% of the HF-preventive effect of CTD as compared to treatment with doxazosin, lisinopril, and amlodipine.[24] This clarifies that the mechanisms by which CTD prevents HF were not restricted to BP lowering and prevention of LVH; and in order to achieve the most effective HF prevention, BP lowering should not be the only criterion of hypertension treatment effectiveness. In addition to BP lowering, CTD has been shown to impart meaningful pleiotropic benefits including improving endothelial function and reducing inflammation and oxidative stress.[25] CTD has been shown to specifically diminish the expression of vascular endothelial growth factor-C (VEGF-C) and transforming growth factor-β3 (TGF-β3), as a result of which, it has also been postulated that CTD could diminish pulmonary vascular permeability, decrease pulmonary vascular resistance by abetting the development of collateral blood vessels or increase lymph flow.[26]

EFFECT OF CHLORTHALIDONE ON HFPEF, HFREF AND COMORBID DIABETES WITH HT

Heart failure developing in hypertensive patients may occur with preserved left ventricular ejection fraction (HFpEF) or reduced left ventricular ejection fraction (HFrEF). Patients with rEF have primarily systolic dysfunction and those with pEF, primarily diastolic dysfunction. Both presentations are common in hypertensive patients and both experience high mortality and morbidity rates.[27-29] Notably, not much is known about the comparative effects of commonly used antihypertensive medications in preventing these outcomes, because HFpEF patients are generally excluded from large clinical trials. In a subanalysis of the ALLHAT, effect of CTD, amlodipine, lisinopril or doxazosin were compared in high-risk hypertensive patients with regard to hospitalized HFpEF (defined as LVEF ≥50%) or HFrEF (LVEF <50%). Ejection fraction was available in 910 of 1,367 patients with hospitalized events, of whom, HFpEF was present in 404 (44%) cases and HFrEF was present in the remaining 506 (56%) cases. CTD significantly reduced the risk of HFpEF by 31%, 26% and 47% compared to amlodipine, lisinopril and doxazosin, respectively [corresponding HRs and 95% CIs were 0.69 (0.53-0.91; p = 0.009), 0.74 (0.56–0.97; p = 0.032), and 0.53 (0.38–0.73; p <0.001)]. The risk of HFrEF was also significantly reduced with CTD by 26% and 39% compared to amlodipine and doxazosin, respectively [HRs 0.74 (0.59–0.94; p = 0.013) and 0.61 (0.47–0.79; p <0.001)].[30]

The inability to identify therapies to improve clinical outcomes in patients with HFpEF has been particularly worrisome; more so considering that nearly half of all patients with HF symptoms have HFpEF.[31] Furthermore, HFpEF is emerging as a significant clinical problem for patients with diabetes, which is a common comorbid condition that is present in almost half of HFpEF patients and confers a nearly two-fold increase in morbidity and mortality in these patients.[32] Coexistence of hypertension and diabetes results in a negative synergistic effect on left ventricular (LV) diastolic mechanics and is associated with higher LV filling pressures than either condition alone.[33] In this context, it is noteworthy that patients with pEF may be more sensitive to fluid retention as a trigger for decompensation,[21] a likely explanation behind the higher HF rates with amlodipine.

Hyperglycemia is a known side-effect of thiazide diuretics including CTD; however this does not reduce the efficacy of CTD in the prevention of CV events. The SHEP[34] and the ALLHAT[35] diabetes extension studies have assessed the long-term effects of CTD-based therapy on CV outcomes in diabetic patients. In the SHEP study, at a mean follow-up of 14.3 years, CV mortality rate was significantly lower in the CTD group than in the placebo group (adjusted HR 0.854, 95% CI 0.751–0.972). Diabetes at baseline and that developed during the trial among subjects on placebo was associated with increased CV adverse outcome and total mortality rate. However, diabetes that developed among subjects during therapy with CTD did not have significant associations with CV mortality or total mortality rate. Interestingly, treatment with CTD in subjects who had diabetes was strongly associated with lower long-term CV mortality rate (adjusted HR 0.688, 95% CI 0.526–0.848) and total mortality rate (adjusted HR 0.805, 95% CI 0.680–0.952). Thus, CTD-based treatment improved long-term outcomes, especially among subjects who had diabetes.[34] The ALLHAT diabetes extension study assessed the cardiovascular disease (CVD) consequences of incident diuretic-associated diabetes compared to the effects of incident diabetes associated with CCBs and ACE inhibitor use. In this study, patients with baseline diabetes, incident diabetes (7.5% with CTD, 5.6% with amlodipine, and 4.3% with amlodipine), or no diabetes at 2 years of in-trial follow up were followed for a mean total of 6.9 years. The primary outcome was CV disease mortality that included death due to CHD, stroke, HF, or other CVD. Participants on CTD with incident diabetes versus no diabetes had consistently lower, non-significant risk for CVD mortality (HR 1.04, 95% CI 0.74–1.47), all-cause mortality (HR 1.04, 95% CI 0.82–1.30), and non-CVD mortality (HR 1.05, 95% CI 0.77–1.42) than participants with incident diabetes on amlodipine or lisinopril (HR's 1.22-1.53).[35] Considering the proven benefits of CTD in diabetic patients in these landmark studies, and amlodipine-associated fluid retention as a trigger for decompensation in pEF patients, it has been suggested that in diabetic hypertensive patients with diastolic dysfunction, thiazide-like diuretics should be preferred ahead of CCBs for blood pressure control.[36]

LIMITATIONS

Much of the current understanding about effects of antihypertensive therapies in preventing HF comes from the largest antihypertensive trial till date—ALLHAT. However, HF was not the primary outcome measure in ALLHAT, but a prespecified secondary outcome.[15] Although prior recognition of a primary end point assures statistical power to that end point, it does not mean that the other outcomes are less important. From a public health viewpoint and from the perspective of patients, all major clinical outcomes in ALLHAT are worthy of exploration because of its sheer size and large number of CV events including HF. Nonetheless, no study till date has assessed incidence of HF with different antihypertensive therapies as a primary outcome in hypertensive patients. Long-term follow-up studies with HF as a primary outcome are required.

CONCLUSION

Most longstanding hypertension, resistant hypertension ultimately leads to HF unless this sequence of events is otherwise interrupted by other outcome.[37] All antihypertensive agents reduce BP; however, literature reveals that all antihypertensives are not equal in terms of their ability to prevent HF. Although β-blockers remain cornerstone in the management of HF because of its mortality reduction potential in HF.[38] In a Cochrane meta-analysis, CCBs were associated with increased risk of HF events as compared with diuretics and ACE-I.[39] The HF preventive efficacy of diuretics as a group in 10 randomized controlled trials was clearly superior to other antihypertensives (RR: 0.84; 95% CI: 0.73–0.98).[40,41] Among diuretics, the thiazide-like diuretic CTD remains the treatment of choice for prevention of HF in hypertensive patients.

As described earlier, major clinical studies with long-term follow-up, that includes ALLHAT, SHEP and TOMHS, have demonstrated benefits of CTD in reducing LVM and preventing HF. In ALLHAT, CTD has been proven to be superior to doxazosin, lisinopril, and amlodipine in preventing HF. In diabetic patients too, CTD has been shown to exert beneficial effects in reducing CV events including HF. New-onset diabetes associated with CTD was also not associated with increased risk of CVD. Moreover, CTD is superior, metabolic friendly as it does not cause hyperglycemia, hyperuricemia or significant electrolyte imbalance, it has long half-life, morbidity and mortality reduction potential in hypertension, resistant hypertension and heart failure with preserved ejection fraction and reduce ejection fraction as evident by echo-guided management by reduction of E/E' and LAVI in heart failure with hypertension. CTD is therefore the diuretic molecule of first choice and has withstood the test of time of almost 60 years.

REFERENCES

1. Sciarretta S, Palano F, Tocci G, et al. Antihypertensive treatment and development of heart failure in hypertension: a Bayesian network meta-analysis of studies in patients with hypertension and high cardiovascular risk. Arch Intern Med. 2011;171(5):384-94.
2. Butrous H, Hummel SL. Heart Failure in Older Adults. Can J Cardiol. 2016;32(9):1140-7.
3. Mamas MA, Sperrin M, Watson MC, et al. Do patients have worse outcomes in heart failure than in cancer? A primary care-based cohort study with 10-year follow-up in Scotland. Eur J Heart Fail. 2017;19(9):1095-104.
4. Whelton PK, Carey RM, Aronow WS, et al. 2017 ACC/AHA/AAPA/ABC/ACPM/AGS/APhA/ASH/ASPC/NMA/PCNA guideline for the prevention, detection, evaluation, and management of high blood pressure in adults: a Report of the American College of Cardiology/American Heart Association Task Force on Clinical Practice Guidelines. Hypertension. 2018;71:e13-e115.
5. Butler J, Kalogeropoulos AP, Georgiopoulou VV, et al. Systolic blood pressure and incident heart failure in the elderly. The Cardiovascular Health Study and the Health, Ageing and Body Composition Study. Heart. 2011;97:1304-11.
6. Wright JT Jr, Williamson JD, Whelton PK, et al. A randomized trial of intensive versus standard blood-pressure control. SPRINT Research Group. N Engl J Med. 2015;373:2103-16.
7. Lewington S, Clarke R, Qizilbash N, et al. Prospective Studies Collaboration. Age-specific relevance of usual blood pressure to vascular mortality: a meta-analysis of individual data for one million adults in 61 prospective studies. Lancet. 2002;360(9349):1903-13.
8. Tocci G, Sciarretta S, Volpe M. Development of heart failure in recent hypertension trials. J Hypertens. 2008;26(7):1477-86.
9. Burnier M, Bakris G, Williams B. Redefining diuretics use in hypertension: why select a thiazide-like diuretic? J Hypertens. 2019;37(8):1574-86.
10. SHEP Cooperative Research Group. Prevention of stroke by antihypertensive drug treatment in older persons with isolated systolic hypertension: final results of the Systolic Hypertension in the Elderly Program (SHEP). JAMA. 1991;265:3255-64.
11. Staessen JA, Fagard R, Thijs L, et al. Randomised double-blind comparison of placebo and active treatment for older patients with isolated systolic hypertension. Lancet. 1997;350:757-64.
12. Yusuf S, Sleight P, Pogue J, et al. Effects of an angiotensin-converting-enzyme inhibitor, ramipril, on cardiovascular events in high-risk patients. N Engl J Med. 2000;342:145-53.
13. Turnbull F. Effects of different blood-pressure-lowering regimens on major cardiovascular events: results of prospectively-designed overviews of randomised trials. Lancet. 2003;362:1527-35.
14. Chen P, Chaugai S, Zhao F, et al. Cardioprotective Effect of Thiazide-Like Diuretics: a Meta-Analysis. Am J Hypertens. 2015;28(12):1453-63.
15. Davis BR, Cutler JA, Gordon DJ, et al; ALLHAT Research Group. Rationale and design for the Antihypertensive and Lipid Lowering Treatment to Prevent Heart Attack Trial (ALLHAT). Am J Hypertens. 1996;9:342-60.
16. Major cardiovascular events in hypertensive patients randomized to doxazosin vs chlorthalidone: the antihypertensive and lipid-lowering treatment to prevent heart attack trial (ALLHAT). ALLHAT Collaborative Research Group. JAMA. 2000;283(15):1967-75.

17. Davis BR, Piller LB, Cutler JA, et al. Role of diuretics in the prevention of heart failure: the Antihypertensive and Lipid-Lowering Treatment to Prevent Heart Attack Trial. Circulation. 2006;113(18):2201-10.
18. Kostis JB, Davis BR, Cutler J, et al. Prevention of heart failure by antihypertensive drug treatment in older persons with isolated systolic hypertension. SHEP Cooperative Research Group. JAMA. 1997;278(3):212-6.
19. Neaton JD, Grimm RH Jr, Prineas RJ, et al. Treatment of Mild Hypertension Study. Final results. Treatment of Mild Hypertension Study Research Group. JAMA. 1993;270(6):713-24.
20. Psaty BM, Lumley T, Furberg CD, et al. Health outcomes associated with various antihypertensive therapies used as first line agents: a network meta-analysis. JAMA. 2003;289:2534-44.
21. Massie BM. Prevention of heart failure with chlorthalidone in ALLHAT: placing the results into perspective. J Clin Hypertens (Greenwich). 2009;11(9):462-5.
22. Einhorn PT, Davis BR, Massie BM, et al. Antihypertensive and Lipid Lowering Treatment to Prevent Heart Attack Trial (ALLHAT) heart failure validation study: diagnosis and prognosis. Am Heart J. 2007;153:42-53.
23. Grimm RH, Davis BR, Piller LB, et al. ALLHAT Collaborative Research Group. Heart failure in ALLHAT: did blood pressure medication at study entry influence outcome? J Clin Hypertens (Greenwich). 2009;11(9):466-74.
24. Johnson K, Oparil S, Davis BR, et al. Prevention of Heart Failure in Hypertension-Disentangling the Role of Evolving Left Ventricular Hypertrophy and Blood Pressure Lowering: The ALLHAT Study. J Am Heart Assoc. 2019;8(8):e011961.
25. Roush GC, Buddharaju V, Ernst ME, et al. Chlorthalidone: mechanisms of action and effect on cardiovascular events. Curr Hypertens Rep. 2013;15(5):514-21.
26. Woodman R, Brown C, Lockette W. Chlorthalidone decreases platelet aggregation and vascular permeability and promotes angiogenesis. Hypertension. 2010;56(3):463-70.
27. Vasan RS, Larson MG, Benjamin EJ, et al. Congestive heart failure in subjects with normal versus reduced left ventricular ejection fraction: Prevalence and mortality in a population-based cohort. J Am Coll Cardiol. 1999;33:1948-55.
28. Mosterd A, Hoes AW, de Bruyne MC, et al. Prevalence of heart failure and left ventricular dysfunction in the general population; The Rotterdam Study. Eur Heart J. 1999;20:447-55.
29. Devereux RB, Roman MJ, Liu JE, et al. Congestive heart failure despite normal left ventricular systolic function in a population-based sample: The Strong Heart Study. Am J Cardiol. 2000;86:1090-6.
30. Davis BR, Kostis JB, Simpson LM, et al. Heart failure with preserved and reduced left ventricular ejection fraction in the antihypertensive and lipid-lowering treatment to prevent heart attack trial. Circulation. 2008;118(22):2259-67.
31. Sharma K, Kass DA. Heart failure with preserved ejection fraction: mechanisms, clinical features, and therapies. Circ Res. 2014;115:79-96.
32. Sandesara PB, O'Neal WT, Kelli HM, et al. The Prognostic Significance of Diabetes and Microvascular Complications in Patients with Heart Failure with Preserved Ejection Fraction. Diabetes Care. 2018;41(1):150-5.
33. Russo C, Jin Z, Homma S, et al. Effect of diabetes and hypertension on left ventricular diastolic function in a high-risk population without evidence of heart disease. Eur J Heart. Fail. 2010;12(5):454-61.
34. Kostis JB, Wilson AC, Freudenberger RS, et al. Long-term effect of diuretic-based therapy on fatal outcomes in subjects with isolated systolic hypertension with and without diabetes. Am J Cardiol. 2005;95(1):29-35.
35. Barzilay JI, Davis BR, Pressel SL, et al. Long-term effects of incident diabetes mellitus on cardiovascular outcomes in people treated for hypertension: the ALLHAT Diabetes Extension Study. Circ Cardiovasc Qual Outcomes. 2012;5(2):153-62.
36. Pareek AK, Mehta RT, Purkait I, et al. Diabetic Hypertensives and Diastolic Dysfunction: Use of Calcium Channel Blockers-A Clinical Concern. JACC Heart Fail. 2017;5(11):850-1.
37. Messerli FH, Rimoldi SF, Bangalore S. The Transition from Hypertension to Heart Failure: Contemporary Update. JACC Heart Fail. 2017;5(8):543-551.
38. Bangalore S, Wild D, Parkar S, et al. Beta-blockers for primary prevention of heart failure in patients with hypertension insights from a meta-analysis. J Am Coll Cardiol. 2008;52(13):1062-72.
39. Chen N, Zhou M, Yang M, et al. Calcium channel blockers versus other classes of drugs for hypertension. Cochrane Database Syst Rev. 2010;(8):CD003654.
40. Thomopoulos C, Parati G, Zanchetti A. Effects of blood pressure-lowering treatment: 6. Prevention of heart failure and new-onset heart failure–meta-analyses of randomized trials. J Hypertens. 2016;34:373-84.
41. Davis BR, Furberg CD, Wright JT Jr, et al. ALLHAT Collaborative Research Group. ALLHAT: setting the record straight. Ann Intern Med. 2004;141(1):39-46.

22 CHAPTER

Angiotensin Receptor Blockers and Heart Failure

Vijay Kumar Trehan, Vishal Batra, Sravan Kumar V

INTRODUCTION

Oral angiotensin receptor blockers (ARBs) were first approved for clinical use in 1995.[1] Since then many randomized control trials and meta-analyses were done to assess tolerability, safety, and efficacy in various clinical settings which include hypertension, chronic heart failure, diabetic nephropathy, heart failure, post-myocardial infarction (MI). This review focuses on the use of ARBs in heart failure.

MECHANISM OF ACTION

Renin-angiotensin system (RAS) is central to the pathogenesis of cardiovascular diseases through vasoconstriction, inflammatory response, an increase in reactive oxygen species, endothelial dysfunction, and atherosclerosis which leads to subsequent complications such as MI, LVH and LV dysfunction, congestive heart failure (CHF) and renal disease.[2] All these conditions are characterized by abnormal elevation and activity of angiotensin II (A-II), which represents the final effector of the RAS (Fig. 1).[3] Angiotensin II receptor blockers (ARBs) and angiotensin-converting enzyme (ACE) inhibitors reduce the stimulation of angiotensin II (AT) receptors via different mechanisms.[4] AT1 receptors predominate vasculature and nerve endings in myocardium whereas AT2 predominates in the myocardial interstitium. Initially, it was believed that ACE is the only enzyme that will catalyze the production of AII from AI. However, it is unclear how complete the blockade by ACE inhibitors is and if there is continuing angiotensin II formation during chronic treatment with ACE inhibitors. Numerous studies have now shown that some patients on long-term treatment with ACE inhibitors eventually have AII levels return to pretreatment levels, demonstrating that the blockade of the RAS by the ACE inhibitor is incomplete. This phenomenon is referred to as "ACE escape" and it may be the result of AII formation through non-ACE-dependent pathways. For example, chymase, a serine protease found in the human heart and other tissues, is able to form AII from AI and is not blocked by ACE inhibitors.[5] The physiological significance of these non-ACE-dependent pathways for AII formation is not known at the present time but patients who develop ACE escape have a poor prognosis. ARBs are believed to provide a more effective means of the blockade of the RAS than is possible with ACE inhibitors because this blockade at the receptor level is independent of the pathway for AII formation. Some differences between ACEI and ARBS are:[6]

- ACE inhibitors reduce the synthesis of Angiotensin II by the action of ACE while ARBs block the actions of Angiotensin II through AT1 receptors.
- Unlike ACE inhibitors, ARBs allow activation of AT2 receptors.
- ARBs cause an increase in circulating levels of Angiotensin II available to act on AT2 receptors. AT2 receptor activation is thought to have the opposite effect of those mediated by the AT1 receptor, which is beneficial to the cardiovascular system and helps protect target organs from damage.
- ACE inhibitors, but not ARBs, reduce the degradation of bradykinin.

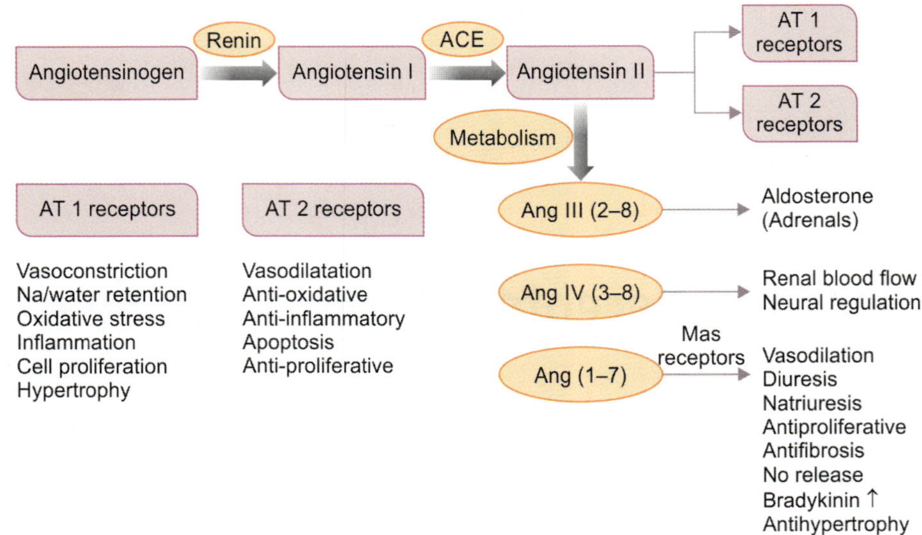

Fig. 1: Components of renin-angiotensin system (RAS). Angiotensin II produced at tissue level plays an important role in the pathophysiology of heart failure. Angiotensin II acts on both AT 1 and AT 2 receptors. Angiotensin II is metabolized into Angiotensin III, Angiotensin IV and Angiotensin 1-7 in which the latter mediates the physiological actions via Mas receptors.
(ACE: angiotensin-converting enzyme; AT1: angiotensin II receptor type 1; AT2: angiotensin II receptor type 2; Ang: angiotensin)

- Angiotensin (1-7) a metabolite of angiotensin II acts on Mas receptors mediating beneficial effects on the cardiovascular system.

GUIDELINES

The ACC/AHA 2016 guidelines suggested the use of ARBs:[7,8]

- The clinical strategy of inhibition of the renin-angiotensin system with ACEi or ARBs (Class I level of evidence A) or ARNI (Class I level of evidence B) in chronic heart failure with reduced ejection fraction.
- Use of ARBs might be considered to decrease hospitalizations in HFpEF (heart failure with preserved ejection fraction) (Class IIb level of evidence B).

The ESC guidelines 2016 recommend ARB in patients intolerant to ACEi to reduce heart failure hospitalization and cardiovascular mortality. (IB)

EVIDENCE

Several trials have shown a significant benefit of ACEI in terms of mortality and hospital admissions due to worsening heart failure. Not all the ARBs have been studied in heart failure. Losartan, Candesartan and Valsartan are the three ARBs which have been studied extensively in the heart failure population (Tables 1 and 2).

In Heart Failure with Reduced Ejection Fraction (HFrEF)

In the "Evaluation of Losartan in the Elderly (ELITE)" trial, the ARB losartan 50 mg once daily was compared with the ACE-I captopril 50 mg three times daily in 722 patients with heart failure. The primary endpoint was a measure of renal safety, a persisting increase in serum creatinine of 0.3 mg/dL or more, and the secondary endpoint was a composite of death and/or hospitalizations for heart failure. An unexpected 32% reduction in death and/or hospital admission for heart failure was found in patients treated with losartan. In addition, losartan was better tolerated than captopril and thus fewer patients discontinued losartan therapy due to adverse events.[9] These results prompted a large-scale follow-on study, the ELITE II trial, in which the effects on morbidity and

TABLE 1: Comparison of ARB trials in heart failure with reduced ejection fraction.

	ARB vs ACEI		*ARB vs Placebo*	*ARB + ACEI*		*ACEI*
Trial	ELITE	ELITE II	CHARM Alternative	CHARM-Added	Val-Heft	HEAAL
Patients	722	3,152	2,028	2,548	5,010	1,919
Intervention	Losartan		Candesartan	Candesartan + ACEI	Valsartan + ACEI	Losartan (150 mg or 50 mg)
Control	Captopril		Placebo	Placebo + ACEI	Placebo + ACEI	

TABLE 2: Results of major ARB trials in heart failure with reduced ejection fraction.

Trial	Result
ELITE	A 32% reduction in death and/or hospital admission for heart failure was found in patients treated with losartan
ELITE II	No differences in all-cause mortality, sudden death or resuscitated arrests between the two treatment groups
CHARM Alternative	Candesartan markedly reduced CV mortality and morbidity in patients who are intolerant to ACE-Is
CHARM-Added	Candesartan reduced CV death and hospital admission for CHF
VAL-HEFT	Valsartan modestly improved morbidity but not mortality in the entire group
HEAAL	Losartan 150 mg daily reduced the rate of death or admission for heart failure in patients with reduced left ventricular ejection fraction and intolerance to ACE-Is compared with losartan 50 mg daily

mortality in heart failure patients treated with losartan and captopril were evaluated. The results, however, did not confirm the initial finding of the ELITE study; there were no significant differences in all-cause mortality, sudden death or resuscitated arrests between the two treatment groups. The dose of losartan in this trial was 50 mg once daily which was lower than in other trials and also patients were naïve for ACEi at baseline so there was no ACE-escape.[10]

"Heart Failure Endpoint Evaluation of Angiotensin II Antagonist Losartan (HEAAL)" trial where 3,846 patients with heart failure were randomized to receive low-dose (50 mg) or high-dose (150 mg) losartan. The primary combined endpoint, admission for heart failure and mortality rate, significantly favored the high-dose group, mainly due to reduced hospital admissions, but no difference in mortality was observed.[11]

In the "Valsartan Heart Failure Trial (Val-Heft)"[12] a small morbidity benefit was demonstrated in 5,010 patients with heart failure of NYHA class II, III, or IV, 93% of whom were already pretreated with an ACE-I. However, in a post-hoc analysis of the small patient subgroup (7%) which was not being treated with an ACE-I, there was a 44.0% reduction in the combined endpoint of mortality and morbidity and a 33.1% reduction in mortality. Valsartan in Acute Myocardial infarction (VALIANT)[13] trial is the largest cohort of post-MI LV dysfunction in which valsartan was as effective as captopril. Valsartan dose in both the trials was up to 160 mg twice daily to attain maximum neurohormonal and hemodynamic benefit.

TABLE 3: Recommended dose of ARB in heart failure.

Drug	Initial daily dose	Maximum doses
Candesartan	4–8 mg QD	32 mg QD
Valsartan	20–40 mg BID	160 mg BID
Losartan	25–50 mg QD	50–150 mg QD

In the CHARM[14] program (Candesartan in Heart failure: Assessment of Reduction in Mortality and morbidity), a total of 7,601 patients with symptomatic CHF were allocated to either placebo or candesartan over three parallel component trials CHARM-alternative[15] (LVEF ≤40% and ACEI intolerant), CHARM-added[16] (LVEF ≤40% and already on ACEI) and CHARM preserved (LVEF >40%). The results showed that candesartan reduced the composite outcomes, cardiovascular mortality, hospital admissions for heart failure and all-cause mortality, particularly among patients with reduced left ventricular systolic function. Table 3 describes the dosage of ARBs in heart failure.

ACEi Combined with ARBs

A meta-analysis of outcomes of ARB plus ACE inhibitor therapy to ACE inhibitor therapy alone in patients with HF was dominated by the Val-HeFT and CHARM-Added results. There were no statistically significant differences in total mortality (RR 0.98, 0.90–1.06), cardiovascular mortality, or total mortality between combined ARB plus ACE inhibitor and ACE inhibitor monotherapy. Combination therapy with valsartan reduced hospitalization for HF (RR 0.81, 95% CI 074–0.89) and myocardial infarction (RR 0.64, 95% CI 0.44–0.92) compared with ACE inhibitor therapy alone but did not reduce total hospitalizations (RR 0.99, 95% CI 0.94–1.05). There were more withdrawals in the combination therapy group due to frequent adverse events.

There are many discrepancies between CHARM-added and the combination treatment arm of VALIANT. Firstly, the two studies recruited different patient populations and treatment was used in a different way. Importantly, many of the patients who were randomized into CHARM added were those who remained symptomatic despite treatment on the dose of an ACE inhibitor. These patients may have the most marked, chronic, neurohormonal activation and may have developed the phenomenon of ACE-escape. This might have led to reduced cardiovascular events as well as hospitalization for heart failure in CHARM-added trial.

ARBS IN HEART FAILURE WITH PRESERVED EJECTION FRACTION

There is no evidence from randomized clinical studies that ARB therapy directly improves overall morbidity or mortality in patients with heart failure with preserved ejection fraction (HFpEF). There is no evidence of improved diastolic function with ARB treatment as compared with other therapies in patients with asymptomatic LV diastolic dysfunction or overt HFpEF.[17]

Two large trials have investigated ARBs in patients with HFpEF:

1. In the CHARM-preserved[17] trial, 3,023 patients with symptomatic HF and an LVEF >40% and controlled blood pressure were randomly assigned to either candesartan or placebo. The mean LVEF was 54%. At a median follow-up of 37 months, there was a slight difference in the incidence of the primary endpoint of hospitalization for heart failure (22% vs 24%; adjusted HR 0.86, 95% CI 0.74–1.00) but no reduction in cardiovascular death. However, a significant number of patients discontinued candesartan because of renal dysfunction, hyperkalemia or hypotension.
2. In the I-PRESERVE trial,[18] 4,128 patients with symptomatic HF, controlled blood pressure, and an LVEF ≥45% were randomly assigned to either daily irbesartan 300 mg or placebo. The mean LVEF was 59%. At a mean follow-up of 49.5 months, there was no significant difference in the primary endpoint of death from any cause or hospitalization for a cardiovascular cause. There were also no significant differences in secondary outcomes, which included death or hospitalization for HF, death from any cause, hospitalization for a cardiovascular cause, and quality of life.

CONTRAINDICATIONS AND ADVERSE EFFECTS

- An ARB should not be administered during pregnancy given the potential risk of fetal harm based upon the observed fetal risk of ACE inhibitors. Given the lack of data, ARBs are not recommended in lactation.
- The most common adverse reactions of ARBs are hypotension, dizziness, worsening renal function, and hyperkalemia.
- In clinical HR trials, dizziness (17% with valsartan versus 9% with placebo) and hypotension (7% with valsartan versus 2% with placebo) were common adverse effects.
- In patients receiving any regimen including one or more inhibitors of the RAS system, precautions should be taken to avoid hyperkalemia, including careful screening of patients for baseline renal dysfunction or hyperkalemia and close periodic monitoring of renal function and serum potassium concentration, especially in patients with risk factors for hyperkalemia.[19]

CONCLUSION

Candesartan, valsartan and losartan are preferred ARBs in heart failure with reduced ejection fraction. Maximum tolerated target dose should be used to attain maximal neurohormonal and hemodynamic benefit. Routine use of the combination of an ACE inhibitor and an ARB is potentially harmful and should be avoided. ACE-Is and ARBs appear to be equally effective with respect to morbidity and mortality endpoints, but ARBs are better tolerated.

REFERENCES

1. Tomlinson B, Young RP, Chan JC, et al. Pharmacoepidemiology of ACE inhibitor-induced cough. Drug Saf. 1997;16(2):150-1.
2. Atlas SA. The renin-angiotensin-aldosterone system: Pathophysiological role and pharmacologic inhibition. J Manag Care Pharm. 2007;13(Suppl B):9-20.
3. Paul M, Poyan Mehr A, Kreutz R. Physiology of local renin-angiotensin systems. Physiol Rev. 2006;86:747-803.
4. Burneir M, Brunner HR. Angiotensin 11 receptor antagonists. Lancet. 2000;355:637-45.
5. Ennezat PV, Berlowitz M, Sonnenblick EH, et al. Therapeutic implications of escape from angiotensin-converting enzyme inhibition in patients with chronic heart failure. Curr Cardiol Rep. 2000;2(3):258-62.
6. Goldsmith DJ. Angiotensin receptor antagonists. Lancet. 1997;349:1255.
7. Yancy CW, Jessup M, Bozkurt B, et al. 2016 ACC/AHA/HFSA Focused Update on New Pharmacological Therapy for Heart Failure: An Update of the 2013 ACCF/AHA Guideline for the Management of Heart Failure: A Report of the American College of Cardiology/American Heart Association Task Force on Clinical Practice Guidelines and the Heart Failure Society of America. J Am Coll Cardiol. 2016;68:1476.
8. Ponikowski P, Voors AA, Anker SD, et al. 2016 ESC Guidelines for the diagnosis and treatment of acute and chronic heart failure: The Task Force for the diagnosis and treatment of acute and chronic heart failure of the European Society of Cardiology (ESC) Developed with the special contribution of the Heart Failure Association (HFA) of the ESC. Eur Heart J. 2016;37:2129.
9. Pitt B, Segal R, Martinez FA, et al. Randomised trial of losartan versus captopril in patients over 65 with heart failure. Lancet. 1997;349:747-52.
10. Pitt B, Poole-Wilson P, Segal R, et al. Effects of losartan versus captopril on mortality in patients with symptomatic heart failure rationale, design, and baseline characteristics of patients in the losartan heart failure survival study - ELITE II. J Cardiac Fail. 1999;5:146-54.
11. Konstam MA, Poole-Wilson PA, Dickstein K, et al. Design of the heart failure endpoint evaluation of AII-antagonist losartan (HEAAL) study in patients intolerant to ACE-inhibitor. Eur J Heart Fail. 2008;10(9):899-906.

12. Cohn JN, Tognoni G. Randomized Trial of the Angiotensin-Receptor Blocker Valsartan in Chronic Heart Failure. N Engl J Med. 2001;345:1667-75.
13. Pfeffer MA, McMurray JJ, Velazquez EJ, et al. Valsartan, captopril, or both in myocardial infarction complicated by heart failure, left ventricular dysfunction, or both. N Engl J Med. 2003;349:1893.
14. Pfeffer MA, Swedberg K, Granger CB, et al. Effects of candesartan on mortality and morbidity in patients with chronic heart failure: the CHARM-overall programme. Lancet. 2003;362(9386):759-66.
15. Granger CB, McMurray JJ, Yusuf S, et al. Effects of candesartan in patients with chronic heart failure and reduced left ventricular systolic function intolerant to angiotensin-converting-enzyme inhibitors: the CHARM-alternative trial. Lancet. 2003;362(9386):772-6.
16. McMurray JJ, Ostergren J, Swedberg K, et al. Effects of candesartan in patients with chronic heart failure and reduced left ventricular systolic function taking angiotensin-converting-enzyme inhibitors: the CHARM-added trial. Lancet. 2003;362(9386):767-71.
17. Yusuf S, Pfeffer MA, Swedberg K, et al. Effects of candesartan in patients with chronic heart failure and preserved left-ventricular ejection fraction: the CHARM-Preserved Trial. Lancet. 2003;362:777.
18. Massie BM, Carson PE, McMurray JJ, et al. Irbesartan in patients with heart failure and preserved ejection fraction. N Engl J Med. 2008;359:2456.
19. Palmer BF. Managing hyperkalemia caused by inhibitors of the renin-angiotensin-aldosterone system. N Engl J Med. 2004;351:585.

CHAPTER

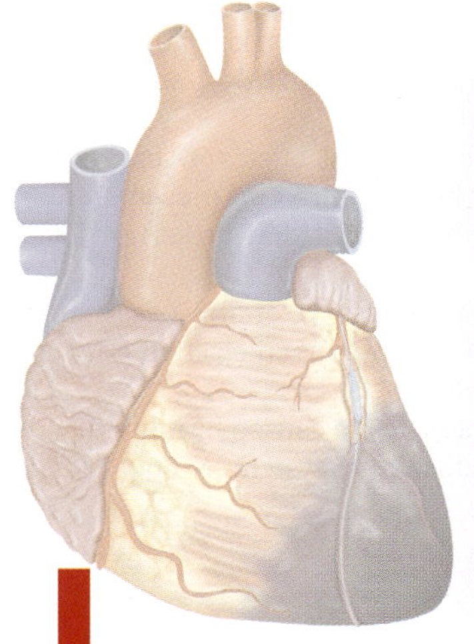

Angiotensin-converting Enzyme Inhibitor and Heart Failure

Satyanarayan Routray, Dipak Ranjan Das, Shishu Shankar Mishra

INTRODUCTION

Heart failure (HF) is best characterized as a progressive disease. Compensatory mechanisms like renin-angiotensin-aldosterone system (RAAS) are a hallmark of the bodily response in such circumstances. However, sometimes these responses may be either positively adaptive or maladaptive. Angiotensin-converting enzyme inhibitors (ACEIs) have been proven as instrumental in countering the maladaptive response of RAAS in HF with reduced ejection fraction (HFrEF). The long-term mortality and morbidity benefits derived from these agents have continuously placed them as a class-I treatment modality in all international heart failure guidelines.

PATHOPHYSIOLOGY

Changes in HFrEF that occur to the myocardial anatomy, specifically the left ventricle, are a result of myocyte death and neurohormonal activation. Compensatory mechanisms following myocardium injury lead to reconstruction of the heart's anatomy in a phenomenon known as remodeling, causing dilation of the ventricle, reduction in contractility, and decline in systolic function. The RAAS and sympathetic nervous system (SNS) are activated as the heart attempts to restore hemodynamic stability. Angiotensin II activates several cardiovascular and renal mechanisms through angiotensin I receptors, including systemic arterial vasoconstriction, renal arteriolar vasoconstriction, stimulation of renal tubular reabsorption of sodium and water, vascular smooth muscle contraction, cellular proliferation, oxidative stress and aldosterone release from the adrenal glands. Stimulation of the angiotensin I receptor by angiotensin II produces cellular and fibroblast hypertrophy and collagen deposition leading to myocardial fibrosis in the myocardium. Hypertrophy and fibrosis promote ventricular remodeling, a hallmark sign of HFrEF. Aldosterone stimulates collagen synthesis and increases the level of ACE in the heart, further increasing angiotensin II production. The activation of the RAAS and SNS is initially beneficial, but prolonged activation leads to cardiac and peripheral hemodynamic instability.[1] This leads to harmful effects not only on the heart, but also on blood vessels, kidneys, muscles, bone marrow, lungs and liver. Further damage continues in a positive feedback fashion leading to symptomatology and deficiency within the framework of the myocardium, including electrical abnormalities. As a result, a decreased quality of life, decrease in the functional capacity of the heart, decompensation, increase in hospitalizations and premature death from pump failure or ventricular arrhythmia occurs. ACE inhibitors are drugs that aim to halt the cycle created by this detrimental environment by working on RAAS.[2] As the name implies, ACE inhibitors (ACEIs) block the transformation of angiotensin I into angiotensin II by decreasing the production of the ACE enzyme. These agents also increase nitric oxide stimulation, causing positive outcomes on endothelial function by halting the breakdown of bradykinin. Additionally, cardiac hemodynamics and exercise capacity are improved by decreasing systemic vascular resistance. However, it is important to keep in mind that not all patients will tolerate these agents. Common side effects include hypotension,

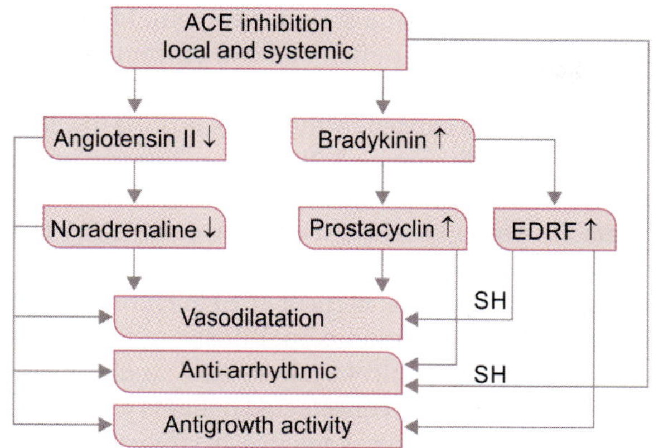

Fig. 1: The schematic diagram indicates the multidirectional benefits from ACEI.

dizziness and dry cough. Monitoring for severe adverse events, including angioedema and anaphylactic reactions, must also be taken into consideration (Fig. 1).[3]

ACEI AND LANDMARK TRIALS

There are several landmark trials that have demonstrated the impact of ACE inhibitors in HF patients starting with CONSENSUS. This study looked at patients with New York Heart Association (NYHA) class IV symptoms with a heart size greater than 550 mL/m^2 (women) and 600 mL/m^2 (men) receiving enalapril compared to placebo for a mean of 6.2 months. Patients were randomized to enalapril 5 mg twice daily and, as tolerated, were then increased to 10 mg twice daily after 1 week up to a goal (target) dose of 20 mg twice daily. Patients had to be on a diuretic and digoxin for at least 2 weeks. Other medications such as spironolactone, BB and vasodilators were allowed to help control symptoms. The primary endpoint was 6-month mortality. The secondary endpoint was 12-month and overall mortality. Originally planned to continue for several years, the Ethical Review Committee observed a consistent mortality difference in favor of enalapril after a year and a half, which ended the trial early. The mortality benefits observed were significantly different compared to placebo, showing a 40% relative risk reduction at 6 months ($p = 0.002$), 31% at 1 year ($p = 0.001$) and 27% reduction in total mortality over the entire study period ($p = 0.003$). Furthermore, cardiac death was significantly reduced compared to placebo ($p = 0.001$) as well as progression of congestive HF ($p = 0.001$). Additionally, heart size was significantly reduced in the enalapril group ($p = 0.02$). This investigation showed that enalapril in patients with severe HF can reduce mortality and improve symptoms. This was the first trial to demonstrate a mortality benefit of ACE inhibition in HF.[4] The SOLVD studies used echocardiography and radionuclide ventriculography to show that enalapril reduced ventricular volumes over 3–4 years. The radionuclide substudy of SOLVD showed, however, that the largest change in volume occurred in the first 4 months; thereafter there was no apparent difference in the rate of ventricular dilatation. The change in ventricular volumes did not seem to be solely due to an effect of enalapril on hemodynamics because, although ventricular volumes rose after withdrawal of enalapril for 2 weeks at the end of the study, they were still reduced compared with placebo. This group of studies proved conclusively that ACE inhibitors reduce both systolic and diastolic ventricular volumes in patients with heart failure, and this effect occurs within 6 weeks of starting treatment. Data from the SOLVD study suggest that long-term ACE inhibition reduces filling pressures to a lesser extent than ventricular diastolic volume: thus for a given ventricular volume, filling pressure tends to rise. This implies that ACE inhibitors reduce ventricular compliance towards normal.[5]

Survival and Ventricular Enlargement (SAVE) trial was designed to determine whether long-term ACE inhibition therapy would reduce morbidity and mortality among survivors of myocardial infarction. The SAVE study found the following risk reductions among captopril versus placebo recipients: death (all causes) 19% (95% confidence interval, 3–35%; $p = 0.019$); cardiovascular death 21% (95% confidence interval, 5–35%; $p = 0.014$); myocardial infarction 25% (95% confidence interval, 5–40%; $p = 0.012$). Myocardial infarction increases the risk of subsequent cardiovascular events (e.g. heart failure or another myocardial infarction) among survivors as compared with the general population. Left ventricular dysfunction is among the major risk factors for such adverse events. This trial outcome paved the way for mandatory inclusion of ACEI in secondary prevention in majority of patients of AMI for long-term benefits in reduction of heart failure related outcomes.[6]

In spite of the evidence for benefit of ACE inhibitors they are persistently used in lower doses in clinical practice than tested in the large-scale trials. This was so prevalent as to allow the conduct of a substantial study, the ATLAS trial, to compare high and low dose ACE inhibition. Its outcome clarified the concept that starting with a low dose is appropriate but the dose should be titrated then without undue delay to the maximum tolerable levels wherever possible. The evidence for benefit with these drugs had been obtained largely in patients with impaired systolic function.[7] However the AIRE study selected patients with clinical evidence of heart failure after myocardial infarction rather than with impaired systolic function. A substantial and long-term benefit was found from ACE inhibition.[8] A cohort of patients had ventricular function assessed and as anticipated almost one half had preserved systolic function. Whilst the absolute benefit in lives saved was greater in the higher risk/low ejection fraction group, the relative risk reduction was not significantly different between those with preserved or impaired systolic function.

The publication of the HOPE trial, although not a study of patients with heart failure, has clarified the situation considerably for those taking day to day care of patients. The HOPE study selected patients on the basis of high cardiovascular risk excluding those with known impaired systolic function. Although not an entry requirement for the study, ejection fraction was measured in a substantial majority and was above 40% indicating good number of patients with systolic dysfunction. The ACE inhibitor ramipril markedly reduced the combined end-point of cardiovascular death, stroke and myocardial infarction. Importantly there was a highly significant 20% risk reduction in the rate of myocardial infarction, a prospectively defined end-point, over the average four and a half-year follow-up.[9] Taken together with the retrospectively derived evidence from the heart failure trials there is now compelling evidence that the ACE inhibitors prevent myocardial infarction. The majority of patients with clinical heart failure have underlying ischemic heart disease. Prevention of myocardial infarction and control of blood pressure are two key factors in the management of these patients irrespective of systolic ventricular function. The ACE inhibitors like the beta-blockers therefore have a pivotal role in their management.

SIDE EFFECTS AND DOSE OF ACE INHIBITORS

Possible major ACE inhibitor side effects include—dry cough, hyperkalemia, fatigue, dizziness, headaches, loss of taste, etc. In rare cases—but more commonly in people of African heritage and in smokers—these can cause angioedema. If it occurs in the throat, the swelling can be life-threatening. Nonsteroidal anti-inflammatory drugs (NSAIDs), such as ibuprofen and naproxen sodium, decrease the effectiveness of ACE inhibitors. Taking an occasional dose of these medications should not change the effectiveness of your ACE inhibitor. Because ACE inhibitors can cause birth defects, they are absolutely contraindicated in any stage of pregnancy. The most common adverse reactions encountered in clinical practice are cough. There have never been any major studies to quantitate the incidence of this side effect among different agents of this class. It has also been observed that if patients manage this initial side effect for 2 weeks, subsequently the irritability of cough substantially comes down. Hyperkalemia is a relatively common occurrence. This should not be surprising in view of the effect of the ACE inhibitors on plasma aldosterone. When dietary potassium intake is regulated and sources of altered potassium excretion are identified, hyperkalemia is seldom a serious problem. Identification of sodium and water deficits allows corrections before the drugs are started, and the frequency of hypotension and hyperkalemia caused by the drugs is quite low if these factors are properly managed. The bottom line in countering the side effects to use ACEI in heart failure should be—when patients are properly selected and correctable risk factors are removed, serious side effects are uncommon.[1]

Majority of landmark RCTs of ACEI in HFrEF have used either maximal or supramaximal doses of these agents. Unlike randomized clinical trials, several studies included representative sample of unselected patients with CHF and reflecting real-world clinical practice. In large meta-analysis of such studies including more than 100,000 patients with CHF, approximately one-third were prescribed low doses of ACE inhibitors. Low-dose users had significantly greater all-cause mortality and CHF readmissions. It needs to be highlighted with greater emphasis that ACE inhibitors decreased mortality and the composite end point in a dose-dependent manner, with high-dose users having the best outcome. Availability of various ACEIs in different parts of the world like captopril, cilazapril, enalapril, fosinopril, lisinopril, benazepril, perindopril, quinapril, ramipril, and/or trandolapril has not been able to significantly alter the physician inertia in uptitrating the dose of this class of agents. Physicians should strive, whenever possible, to treat patients with CHF with high doses of ACE inhibitors to improve outcomes.[3]

THE STATUS OF ACEI IN HEART FAILURE BY CURRENT RECOMMENDATIONS FROM GUIDELINES

The recommendations from recent *European Heart Failure guidelines* suggest—"ACEIs have been shown to reduce mortality and morbidity in patients with HFrEF and are recommended unless contraindicated or not tolerated in all symptomatic patients. ACEIs should be uptitrated to the maximum tolerated dose in order to achieve adequate inhibition of the RAAS. ACE inhibitors remain initial treatment in all patients with LV systolic dysfunction and achieving the doses used in clinical trials is emphasized. ESC-CHF reminds that early intervention with ACE inhibitors reduces significantly the occurrence of heart failure in high cardiovascular risk populations such as patients with previous cardiovascular disease, diabetes, alone or with nephropathy and hypertension. ACEIs are also recommended in patients with asymptomatic left ventricular (LV) systolic dysfunction to reduce the risk of HF development, HF hospitalization and death." These statements have class I recommendation with level of evidence A.[10] The recommendations from ACC/AHA/HFSA guidelines mention—"ACE inhibitors have been shown in large RCTs to reduce morbidity and mortality in patients with HFrEF with mild, moderate, or severe symptoms of HF, with or without coronary artery disease. Data suggest that there are no differences among available ACE inhibitors in their effects on symptoms or survival. ACE inhibitors should be started at low doses and titrated upward to doses shown to reduce the risk of cardiovascular events in clinical trials. ACE inhibitors can produce angioedema and should be given with caution to patients with low systemic blood pressures, renal insufficiency or elevated serum potassium (>5.0 mEq/L). Angioedema occurs in <1% of patients who take an ACE inhibitor, but it occurs more frequently in blacks and women. Patients should not be given ACE inhibitors if they are pregnant or plan to become pregnant. ACE inhibitors also inhibit kininase and increase levels of bradykinin, which can induce cough in up to 20% of patients but also may contribute to beneficial vasodilation. If maximal doses are not tolerated, intermediate doses should be tried; abrupt withdrawal of ACE inhibition can lead to clinical deterioration and should be avoided.[11] Although the use of an ARNI in lieu of an ACE inhibitor for HFrEF has been found to be superior, *for those patients for whom ARNI is not appropriate, continued use of an ACE inhibitor for all classes of HFrEF remains strongly advised."*

CONCLUSION

Angiotensin-converting enzyme inhibitors have conclusively proven their safety and efficacy in treatment of heart failure with reduced ejection fraction. They have justified their status as the wonder drugs of 21st century which have ushered in a paradigm shift in therapy and outcome in suffering multitudes of HFrEF all across the globe. No clinical data exists as yet to validate its utility in HFpEF. A misplaced concern for the side effects among physicians is a significant hindrance to more appropriate and extensive utilization of this unique class of agents, which not only provide substantial morbidity benefits, but can also definitely bring in mortality benefits for patients of HFrEF.

REFERENCES

1. Demers C, Mody A, Teo KK, et al. ACEI and HF–what more do we need to know. Am J Cardiovasc Drug. 2005;5(6):351-9.
2. Konstam MA, Rousseau MF, Kronenberg MW, et al. Effects of the angiotensin converting enzyme inhibitor enalapril on the long-term progression of left ventricular dysfunction in patients with heart failure. Circulation. 1992;86:431-8.
3. De Sutter J, Mendes M, Franco OH. Cardioprotective drugs. In: Gielen S, De Backer G, Piepoli MF, Wood D (Eds). The ESC Textbook of Preventive Cardiology, 2nd edition. Oxford: Oxford University Press; 2016.
4. The CONSENSUS Trial Study Group. Effects of enalapril on mortality in severe congestive heart failure. Results of the Cooperative Scandinavian Enalapril Survival Study. N Engl J Med. 1987;316:1429-35.
5. SOLVD Investigators. Effect of enalapril on mortality and the North development of heart failure in asymptomatic patients with reduced left ventricular ejection fractions. N Engl J Med. 1992;327:685-91.
6. Pfeffer M, Braunwald E, Moye LA, et al. Effect of captopril on mortality and morbidity in patients with LV dysfunction after myocardial infarction. N Engl J Med. 1992;327: 669-77.
7. Parker M, Pole Wilson P, Armstrong PW, et al. ATLAS investigators. Comparative effects of low and high dose ACEI on chronic heart failure. Circulation. 1999;100:2312-8.
8. The Acute Infarction Ramipril Efficacy (AIRE) Study Investigators. Effect of ramipril on mortality and morbidity of survivors of acute myocardial infarction with clinical evidence of heart failure. Lancet. 1993;342(8884):1418-9.
9. Yusuf S, Sleight P, Pogue J, et al. Effects of an angiotensin-converting-enzyme inhibitor, ramipril, on cardiovascular events in high-risk patients. (HOPE). New Engl J Med. 2000;342(3):145-53.
10. Voors AA, Anker SD, Falk V, et al. 2016 ESC guidelines for the diagnosis and treatment of acute and chronic heart failure. Eur Heart J. 2016;37(27):2129-200.
11. Yancy WA, Jessup M, Butler J, et al. 2017 ACC/AHA/HFSA Focused update guideline on management of Heart failure. Circulation. 2017;136:e137-e161.

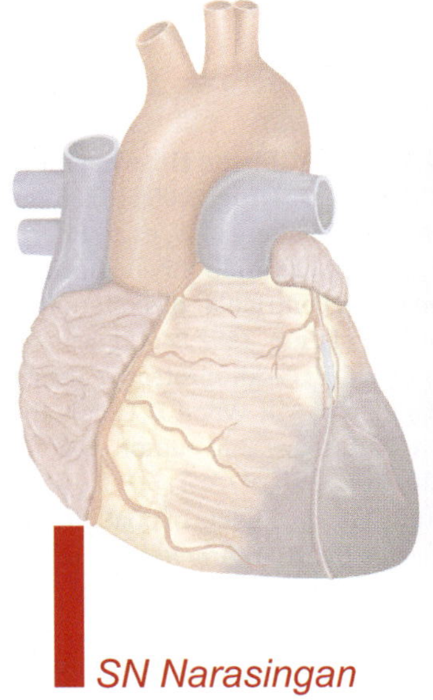

Lipid Management in Heart Failure

SN Narasingan

INTRODUCTION

We are now witnessing recent advances in the management of heart failure (HF) including medical and device therapies. HF is always a challenge facing clinicians. Incidence of HF is increasing in alarming proportions partly because of improved care of patients after acute myocardial infarction (AMI) who are left with damaged heart as well as an increase in aging population. Statins which are 3-hydroxy-3-methyl-glutaryl CoA reductase inhibitors are the cornerstone in the treatment of lipid disorders. Statin trials in primary and secondary prevention have shown huge benefit in reducing morbidity and mortality due to atherosclerotic cardiovascular disease (ASCVD). Incidence of MI in both settings decreased with lowering of low density lipoprotein cholesterol (LDL–C). Many cases of HF are due to myocardial infarction. By decreasing the incidence of MI, statins could prevent the development of HF probably through pleiotropic mechanisms. The use of statins with existing HF is always disputed. This chapter will focus on statins as lipid lowering therapy in HF-based on the available evidence with some newer concepts on triglycerides and ASCVD risk.

STATINS IN HEART FAILURE

- **Controlled Rosuvastatin Multinational Trial in Heart Failure (CORONA Trial):** The trial included 5,000 patients with CHF of ischemic etiology. Daily treatment with 10 mg of Rosuvastatin did not reduce the composite outcome of death from CV causes or nonfatal MI or stroke in elderly patients with ischemic, systolic heart failure. The patients had already received extensive treatment with other drugs. However, Rosuvastatin reduced the number of hospitalizations for cardiovascular causes. In addition, Rosuvastatin effectively reduced the levels of LDL-C and high-sensitivity C-reactive protein. *Comments on the trial:* Elderly persons (mean age: 73 years) constituted a large proportion of the recruited patients. Majority were in advanced CHF stages (NYHA functional class III and IV).[1] The study also revealed that patients with low plasma concentrations of galectin-3 may benefit from statin therapy, while high values of this indicator are associated with no response to statin. Perhaps galectin-3 will become a marker for identifying CHF patients in whom statin therapy can be successful.[2]
- **GISSI-HF study**: This included younger patients than those in the CORONA study; it also included fewer patients with ischemic CHF and advanced CHF (NYHA functional class III/IV). This study also failed to demonstrate a beneficial effect of Rosuvastatin therapy on reducing cardiovascular mortality.[3]
- These two studies did not support the usage of statins. Hence, protecting HF patients for further events and prolonging their survival by statin therapy is disappointing. Observational studies suggested benefits in subgroup of HF patients and positive results were seen in many smaller randomized and nonrandomized trials.[4]
- **Meta-analysis:** A recent large meta-analysis by Preiss and colleagues.[5] This was to determine whether statin therapy had an effect on major HF events through

examining comprehensive published and unpublished data from randomized trials. Mean follow-up of 4.3 years was seen. Thirteen of the 17 trials selected for overall analysis reported baseline HF amongst study participants. Main findings from the overall analysis of up to 132,568 pooled participants include a significant reduction in non-fatal MI and a significant but modest reduction in first non-fatal heart failure hospitalizations (HFH). The composite outcome of HF death and HFH was also significantly reduced in the statin treated groups. This was driven exclusively by a reduction in HFH. No significant effect on HF death was observed. In addition, another meta-analysis of trials in HF patients published in 2014, found that statin therapy reduced HF rehospitalizations by approximately 16%.[6] Meta-analysis raised more questions than answers for the usage of statins in HF.

Beneficial Actions of Statin

The mechanisms by which statin therapy reduced the risk of HFH is through their pleiotropic (i.e. non-LDL-C lowering) properties such as improving endothelial function, ameliorating inflammation, attenuating myocardial remodeling, and reducing cardiac arrhythmias in the setting of HF.[7,4] Statin appears to improve the autonomic cardiac control (heart rate variability, baroreflex sensitivity), to prevent post-infarction ventricular remodeling and reduce LV mass, as well as to improve renal function. Other important benefits included promotion of bone-marrow endothelial progenitor cells mobilization and re-endothelialization of injured arteries. In addition, antithrombotic action extends the list of beneficial effects of statins. Whether these effects are potent enough to improve mortality outcomes in patients with HF is unclear.

Does the Choice of a Particular Statin Really Matter?

A meta-analysis describes the particular statins used in each of the contributing trials. Recent evidence suggests that there is not a class effect for statin use in the setting of HF due to chemical differences between statin molecules. Statins can be classified as either hydrophilic or lipophilic. Lipophilic statins may be more readily taken up by cardiac muscles, thus leading to greater beneficial effects in the setting of HF.[4] Evidence from this meta-analysis showed a significant benefit of atorvastatin—a lipophilic statin—on all-cause mortality, left ventricular ejection fraction, and hospitalization due to HF, whereas similar effects were not observed in patients randomized to the hydrophilic rosuvastatin.[8] More recently, significant beneficial effect of lipophilic statins on left ventricular ejection fraction and plasma concentrations of multiple biomarkers including brain natriuretic peptide, high-sensitivity C-reactive protein, and interleukin-6 were observed in a separate analysis.[9] A meta-analysis of 7 clinical studies covering CHF patients demonstrated the efficacy of atorvastatin therapy in reducing the rates of all-cause mortality, cardiovascular mortality, and sudden cardiac death.[10] There was also a significant reduction in the frequency of hospitalization due to CHF. Another study also reported that including atorvastatin to CHF patients in the course of dilated cardiomyopathy may improve their prognosis.[11] In conclusion, lipophilic statins like atorvastatin is better than rosuvastatin in the setting of HF. The authors of the PEARL study (The study stands for a Pilot Randomized Clinical Trial of Early Coronary Angiography Versus No Early Coronary Angiography for Post-Cardiac Arrest Patients without ECG ST Segment Elevation) postulated a hypothesis that the type of the employed statin may significantly influence the benefits of treatment in CHF patients. It may be the case that pitavastatin used in the PEARL study is characterized by better bioavailability and lipophilicity in comparison with rosuvastatin, which may have been responsible for achieving treatment benefits with pitavastatin.

Effects of Statins to Reduce All–cause Mortality in Heart Failure Patients: Findings from the EPICAL2 Cohort Study[12]

An analysis data collected in the French Epidemilogie et Prognostic de I'Insuffisance Cardiaque Aigue en Lorraine (EPICAL2) cohort study, was questioned for the effects of statin use on 1 year survival after a HF related hospitalization. 2,254 patients hospitalized for HF complications for a follow up of 1 year were analyzed. Stain prescription at discharge was recorded in 45% of the patients versus 55% who were not prescribed statins and used as controls. After statistical analysis it was found that there were no survival benefits at the end of 1 year. *Conclusion:* Prescribing statins in a broad spectrum of patients hospitalized for HF complications (with preserved and reduced ejection fraction) statins use was not associated with improved 1 year survival. Potential benefits in specific subgroups of HF patients could not be dismissed. Insufficient statistical power was noted as another potential explanation for the lack of statin benefits in the EPICAL2 participants.

Limitations for the Use of Statins in Heart Failure

An inverse relationship between cholesterol and mortality in advanced HF and the elderly has raised concerns about statins use in elderly patients with HF. One of potential harms of statin use in HF is related to their lipid-lowering effects. Lipoproteins (LDL, HDL) downregulate inflammatory immune responses to bacterial lipopolysaccharides (the endotoxin-lipoprotein hypothesis). Statins may attenuate this protective role of lipoproteins in HF which may in turns lead to further activation of inflammatory cytokines (TNF-α). Another restriction on the use of statins in HF is related to their inhibitory effects on ubiquinone (CoQ10) synthesis, which may precipitate or aggravate myopathy or polyneuropathy. However, the absolute risk is small and the number of patients needed to treat to cause harm (NNTH) is approximately 5,000–10,000. Finally, interactions between statins and drugs used in HF treatment (e.g. digoxin, warfarin) may bring about undesirable effects.

TRIGLYCERIDE AND CV RISK: ROLE OF LIPID LOWERING DRUGS OTHER THAN STATIN

Recent evidence shows that triglycerides and triglyceride rich lipoprotein particles (TGRLP) such as VLDL, chylomicron and their remnants are involved in atherosclerosis. Elevated triglyceride levels are associated with increased cardiovascular risk which has been projected in many genetic and epidemiological studies. The residual risk seen in primary and secondary prevention trials using statin is attributed to increased triglycerides and TGRLP. There is no specific study which focused on heart failure management with drugs that lower triglycerides levels. Statins have shown modest effect in reducing triglycerides. Elevated triglycerides with low levels of HDL and higher levels of LDL particularly small dense LDL with increased apo-B concentration are considered under atherogenic dyslipidemia which is seen in people with metabolic syndrome and type 2 diabetes. The increased CV risk in these population is attributed to these lipid abnormalities. TGRLP are responsible for the conversion of LDL into small dense LDL cholesterol and lowering the levels of HDL cholesterol by deleting apo-A1. The drugs that are used other than statins do not have any role in the management of heart failure as per the evidence available. REDUCE-IT Trial has shown 25% reduction in primary endpoints by using icosapent ethyl ester which is an omega 3 fatty acid.[13] Future studies focusing on the role of omega 3 fatty acids and other drugs will give clear information on reducing triglycerides for a better cardiovascular outcome.

CONCLUSION

Heart failure is a clinical syndrome in which the key role is played by the stimulation of the renin-angiotensin-aldosterone and sympathetic nervous system, the release of proinflammatory cytokines, and impairments regarding nitric oxide synthesis, the use of statins for this disease should be pathophysiologically justified. It appears that treatment efficacy also depends on the stage of the disease. Introducing statins to the therapy at the late stage of advanced HF may be responsible for the lack of desired treatment effects. The mechanism of the potentially beneficial effect of statins on HF is not fully elucidated. It is worth noting that, apart from reducing lipid concentration, they exhibit pleiotropic activity. It is absolutely essential to conduct further multicenter randomized clinical studies using different statin agents in different HF patient populations, as the term chronic heart failure encompasses different stages of the disease, while adequate study conclusions may only be drawn on the basis of comparable populations.

REFERENCES

1. Kjekshus J, Apetrei E, Barrios V, et al. Rosuvastatin in older patients with systolic heart failure. N Engl J Med. 2007;357:2248-61.
2. Gullestad L, Ueland T, Kjekshus J, et al. Galectin-3 predicts response to statin therapy in the Controlled Rosuvastatin Multinational Trial in Heart Failure (CORONA). Eur Heart J. 2012;33:2290-96.
3. Tavazzi L, Maggioni AP, Marchioli R, et al. Effect of rosuvastatin in patients with chronic heart failure (the GISSI-HF trial): a randomised, double-blind, placebo-controlled trial. Lancet. 2008;372:1231-9.
4. Bonsu KO, Kadirvelu A, Reidpath DD. Statins in heart failure: do we need another trial? Vasc Health Risk Manag. 2013;9:303-19.
5. Preiss D, Campbell RT, Murray HM, et al. The effect of statin therapy on heart failure events: a collaborative meta-analysis of unpublished data from major randomized trials. Eur Heart J. 2015;36:1536-46.
6. Wang JQ, Wu GR, Wang Z, et al. Long-term clinical outcomes of statin use for chronic heart failure: a meta-analysis of 15 prospective studies. Heart Lung Circ. 2014;23:105-13.
7. Lipinski MJ, Abbate A, Fuster V, et al. Drug insight: statins for nonischemic heart failure—evidence and potential mechanisms. Nat Clin Pract Cardiovasc Med. 2007;4:196-205.
8. Lipinski MJ, Cauthen CA, Biondi-Zoccai GG, et al. Meta-analysis of randomized controlled trials of statins versus placebo in patients with heart failure. Am J Cardiol. 2009;104:1708-16.
9. Bonsu KO, Reidpath DD, Kadirvelu A. Effects of statin treatment on inflammation and cardiac function in heart failure: an adjusted indirect comparison meta-analysis of randomised trials. Cardiovasc Ther. 2015;33(6):338-46.
10. Xu M, Yuan G, Wei F. Effect of atorvastatin in patients with chronic heart failure insights from randomized clinical trials. Arch Med Sci. 2010;6:866-73.

11. Wojnicz R, Wilczek K, Nowalany-Kozielska E, et al. Usefulness of atorvastatin in patients with heart failure due to inflammatory dilated cardiomyopathy and elevated cholesterol levels. Am J Cardiol. 2006;97:899-904.
12. Al Gobari M, Agrinier N, Soudant M, et al. Effectiveness of drug interventions to prevent sudden cardiac death in patients with heart failure and reduced ejection fraction: an overview of systematic reviews. Am J Cardiovasc Drug. 2019;8(7):e021108.
13. Gabriel Steg P, Miller M, Brinton EA, et al. Cardiovascular Risk Reduction with Icosapent Ethyl for Hypertriglyceridemia. N Engl J Med. 2019;380:11-22.

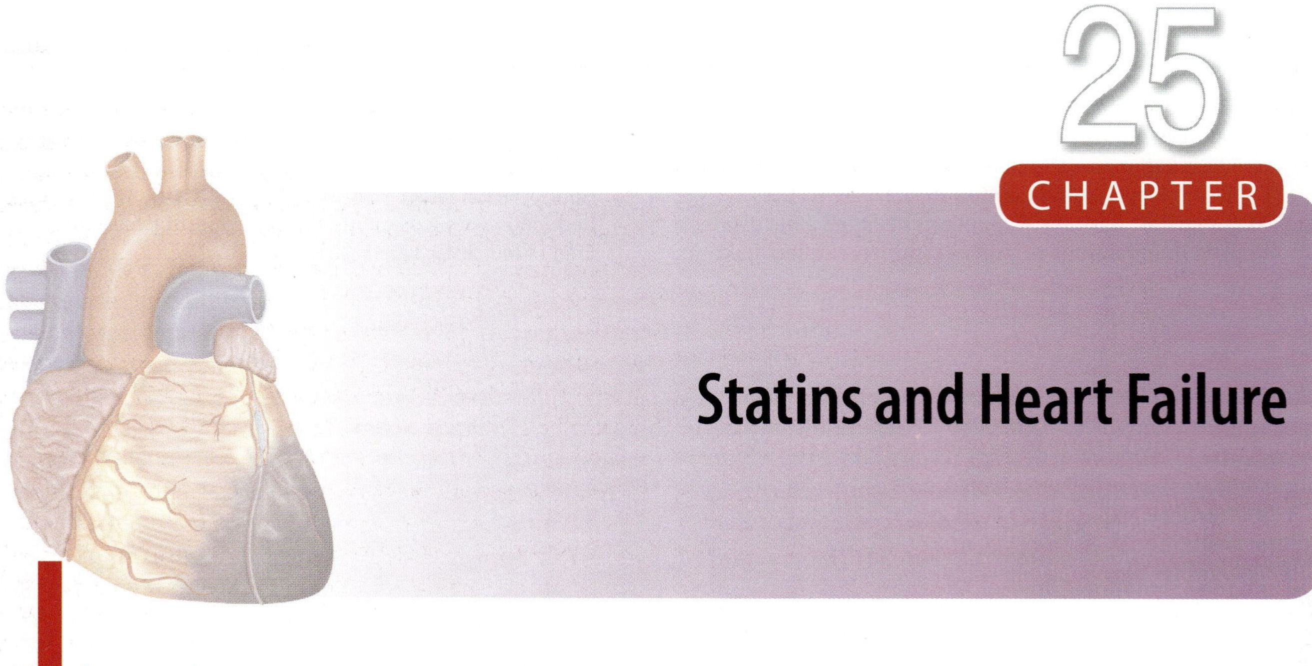

Statins and Heart Failure

Geetha Subramaniam, J Cecily Mary Majella

INTRODUCTION

Statins play a vital role in preventing atherosclerosis and thereby prevents cardiovascular events. They have consistently shown to retard and even at times reverse coronary and cerebral atherosclerotic events and to improve the outcomes in patients with ischemic heart disease (IHD) and preserved cardiac function.[1,2] Optimizing the dose of statins decrease major cardiovascular events by 20% for every 1 mmol/L decline in low-density lipoproteins (LDL).[3] The net benefit is entirely dose dependent, and intensive statin therapy may reduce further risk. Myocardial infarction presages cardiac failure, and the rapid reduction in the incidence of cardiac failure is partly accounted by more intensive lipid-lowering therapy. The exact correlation between acute coronary syndrome (ACS) and heart failure (HF) is not clear. The incidence of developing HF in the early period after an uncomplicated anterior wall infarct is primarily related to the infarct size and left ventricular dysfunction, and late-onset cardiac failure is related to the extent of coronary artery disease (CAD) and recurrent ischemic events.[4]

ROLE OF STATINS IN HEART FAILURE: OBSERVATIONS FROM VARIOUS STUDIES

The Scandinavian Simvastatin Survival Study (4S) revealed that patients with IHD without HF benefited from long-term simvastatin treatment by a reduction of 30% in all-cause mortality during 5.4 years follow-up.[5] Retrospective analysis also showed a 19% decline in new-onset HF.[6] Almost 50% of the patients who presents with new-onset HF would have a non-fatal myocardial infarct prior to heart failure. Incident of HF amplifies the risk for imminent cardiovascular events, and hence has significant clinical implications. Due to higher risk, absolute beneficial effect of treatment will be greater. More recent studies have added uncertainty to the preventive effects of statin therapy in incident HF.[7-9] The discrepancies are attributed to varying definitions of heart failure, with exclusion of early-onset HF after ACS because they are assumed to be one event, different statin regimens, and lack of high sensitive biomarkers of acute myocardial infarction and cardiac failure.

Hence it is commendable that Preiss and coworkers have evaluated the effects of statins and risk of HF hospitalizations and HF related mortality by reviewing all primary and secondary randomized controlled trials with statins between 1994 and 2014 in a standardized fashion.[10] Seventeen trials including 132,568 patients, virtually all without HF at baseline, were eligible. LDL was reduced by 0.97 mmol/L, resulting in 26% fewer non-fatal MIs on treatment. The authors observed reduced numbers of first HF hospitalizations [risk ratio (RR) 0.90, 95% confidence interval (CI) 0.84–0.97] and the composite of first non-fatal HF hospitalization or HF death (RR 0.92, 95% CI 0.85–0.99), but not HF death alone. The numbers needed to treat in the secondary prevention trials over 5 years was 200 to avoid one non-fatal HF hospitalization. Thus, the effect on HF hospitalization was modest. The efficacy of statins may have been underestimated because it could not account for repeated hospitalizations and the definition of HF differed between the involved trials. In the CORONA trial of patients with clinical HF, cumulated hospitalizations over a median follow-up of 33 months were reduced by rosuvastatin by approximately 15–20%.[11] The study did not show any varying effect of statins on HF outcomes related to an in-study MI or not. This is not surprising because it may take 6–12 months to identify the net outcome of statin therapy. It has been observed that early statin therapy for acute MI was associated with a significant decline in early complications including HF events. The results from the registry are difficult to interpret due to allocation bias. The interpretations are limited due to the fact that patients were not randomized for the occurrence or non-occurrence of acute MI.

The net result of statin therapy on the composite endpoint of non-fatal HF hospitalizations and HF death were exclusively driven by incident non-fatal HF hospitalization with no effect on HF mortality. Mortality due to HF is a terminal stage that follows severe left ventricular dysfunction. The mode and cause of death vary among patients with stable CAD without heart failure and patients with chronic decompensated HF. Patients without heart failure are likely to die from sudden onset of acute MI and arrhythmias especially ventricular fibrillation. In contrast, patients with HF die due to progressive HF and stroke.[4,12] It is therefore imperative that statins have no effect in preventing mortality due to heart failure. The same difference in statin effects on non-fatal HF hospitalization and HF deaths was observed in the CORONA and GISSI trials, where patients with documented HF were treated with rosuvastatin.[13,14] There was no effect of rosuvastatin treatment on HF death, but benefits for non-fatal HF hospitalization and atherosclerotic events were observed.[11]

Acute coronary events and incidence of HF are declining due to effective prevention of arteriosclerosis by statins, yet the prevalence of HF is increasing.[15] The improved survival among HF patients is caused by interventions that target downstream pathophysiological mechanisms by unloading the failing left ventricle and by blunting detrimental effects of neurohormonal activation (beta-blockers, renin-angiotensin-aldosterone inhibitors, and resynchronization devices), thereby reducing myocardial energy requirement and electrical instability. Conversely, beta-blockers and inhibitors of the renin-angiotensin-aldosterone system have small and insignificant effects in stable coronary disease without HF.[16]

Targets for statin therapy in stable CAD is prevention of coronary and cerebral arteriosclerosis,[1,2] but has minor impact in established HF[13] mainly because the events are due to the failing myocardium and less by progression of atherosclerosis. However, a retrospective analysis of CORONA, restricted to "atherothrombotic" events, defined as fatal and non-fatal MI and fatal and non-fatal non-ischemic strokes, showed a borderline significant difference favoring rosuvastatin (P = 0.05). Preiss et al. also suggest other explanations whereby statins may reduce the risk of developing HF by preventing ischemic events including pleiotropic anti-inflammatory effects unrelated to the LDL-lowering effect. This might be interesting especially because HF is a trigger for inflammation, but the lack of statin effects in established HF on major composite endpoints[13,14] and the recent positive results of the IMPROVE-IT with ezetimibe, a non-statin, cholesterol-lowering agent, probably brought this discussion to an end.[17]

The study by Preiss and coworkers is important because incident HF carries a dismal prognosis. It reminds us that prevention of new-onset HF can be achieved by statin treatment. This is different from prevention of HF death, which primarily is determined by mechanisms most probably dependent on left ventricular remodeling and myocardial dysfunction. The study therefore also suggests different etiologies for non-fatal HF events and fatal HF. For the same reason, the two endpoints should not be clumped together in clinical studies. Prevention of new-onset HF and HF hospitalization requires a treatment approach that is different from treatment of established HF and prevention of HF death.

Observations from CORONA and GISSI-Heart Failure Study

The observation that most patients with moderate-severe HFrEF die of progressive HF rather than ACS or other CV events led to the hypothesis that statins may not improve survival among this population. GISSI-HF studied this hypothesis among ischemic and non-ischemic HF patients, while CORONA investigated ischemic HF patients only.

The Controlled Rosuvastatin Multinational Trial in Heart Failure (CORONA) trial randomized 5,011 patients with ischemic heart failure, NYHA class II-IV symptoms and LVEF ≤40% (LVEF ≤35% with NYHA class II symptoms) to either rosuvastatin 10 mg daily or placebo. It found no significant difference in the primary composite outcome of cardiovascular death, nonfatal MI or nonfatal stroke (HR 0.92; 95% CI 0.83–1.02; P = 0.12). Notably, all-cause hospitalizations (a secondary outcome) were significantly reduced in the rosuvastatin group. Together, CORONA and GISSI-HF provide reasonably strong evidence against the routine initiation of statins for moderate-severe ischemic cardiomyopathy. Neither study supports the routine discontinuation of statins among heart failure patients; in particular, because hospitalizations for heart failure were reduced in CORONA's rosuvastatin group, routine discontinuation among ischemic patients may be associated with harm. A randomized controlled trial of statin discontinuation in heart failure is currently underway to help settle this issue.

Statins are indicated for the primary and secondary prevention of atherosclerotic cardiovascular events and demonstrably decrease the risk of myocardial infarction (MI) in both settings through lowering low-density lipoprotein cholesterol (LDL-C). Since many cases of HF are consequent to MI, statins could potentially prevent the development of HF by decreasing the incidence of MI or through other mechanisms. The use of statins in patients with existing HF, however, is disputed.

The controversy surrounding the use of statin therapy for HF patients stems mainly from the results of two large, randomized, prospective, placebo-controlled trials: (1) the CORONA trial and (2) the GISSI-HF trial. Both trials examined the effect of rosuvastatin on mortality and morbidity in HF patients. Although treatment was well tolerated, both trials failed to show a significant effect of the statin therapy on the predetermined endpoints, which contrasted with the positive results observed in many smaller randomized and non-randomized trials.

STATIN THERAPY AND MORTALITY IN PATIENTS WITH DIASTOLIC HEART FAILURE

In the last few years, numerous studies have also reported that statin therapy is associated with a decline of mortality in patients with HF and reduced LVEF. In a cohort of 551 patients with HF and LVEF <40%, Horowich et al. showed that statin therapy was associated with 55% reduction of the risk of death or need for urgent transplantation during 1-year follow-up.

PRAISE study reported beneficial effects of statins therapy in cause-specific cardiac mortality, where it was associated with 57% reduction of sudden death and a relative decrease in the risk of pump-failure death. Analysis in the ELITE II, CIBIS II and OPTIMAAL studies showed reduced mortality rates. There is little evidence about the possible effects of statin therapy in patients with DHF. The first study concerning this problem was recently published by Fukuta et al. In a small trial comprising only 137 patients with LVEF ≥50%, statin therapy significantly reduced long-term mortality [unadjusted hazard ratio (HR): 0.22; 95% confidence interval (CI): 0.07–0.64], and this was the only effective mortality-reducing treatment in this population.

Statin Therapy and Cardiovascular Hospitalizations in Patients with Diastolic Heart Failure

Safety of Statin Therapy in Chronic Heart Failure

Despite these encouraging results, there is still a lot of controversy about the possible use of statins in HF patients. It has been established that low levels of total and low-density lipoprotein (LDL) cholesterol are associated with higher mortality in this population. The similar phenomenon of "reverse epidemiology" in HF was also observed for body mass index (BMI) and blood pressure. Low cholesterol levels in patients with HF with reduced LVEF are commonly associated with the development of cardiac cachexia and systemic activation of the immune system, indicating depletion of metabolic reserve; however, in patients with DHF these conditions are infrequent. In the study conducted by Fukuta et al., 50% of patients with DHF had a lipid profile below that indicated as the target for treatment in the National Cholesterol Education Program Adult Treatment Panel III Guidelines.

Possible Explanations for the Beneficial Effects of Statins in Diastolic Heart Failure

Statins have been proved to have pleiotropic effects, which influence multiple mechanisms that underlie many cardiovascular diseases, including HF. The benefits from statin therapy in patients with HF may be related to both their lipid-dependent and lipid-independent effects. Zile and Brutsaert divide treatment of DHF into symptom-targeted, disease-targeted and mechanism-targeted treatment. The possible beneficial effects of statins in DHF may be also classified in this way.

The lipid-dependent effects of statins are thought to be mainly due to a decrease in vascular atherosclerosis, which results in a decrease in the prevalence of myocardial infarction, cerebral vascular accident or peripheral vascular accident, which are common in patients with HF with preserved LVEF. In epidemiological studies, CAD is present in more than half of patients with HF and preserved LVEF; we can anticipate that this group of patients will benefit the most from statin therapy. However, clinical studies have still not elucidated this association. Results of the recently published study CHARM-PRESERVED revealed that up to 30% of deaths in patients with HF and preserved LVEF were caused by myocardial infarction and cerebral accident. On the other hand, Ray et al. in a population-based retrospective cohort study with over 28,000 elderly patients with HF reported reduction in all-cause mortality in patients receiving statin therapy (adjusted HR: 0.67;

95% CI: 0.57–0.78), but they found a lack of effect of statin use on the prevalence of non-fatal myocardial infarction and non-fatal stroke. The second important group of possible beneficial effects of statins in patients with HF may be related to their lipid-independent properties. Both clinical studies and animal models have proved that statins lead to a decrease of LV mass and a decrease in LV fibrosis. Other important lipid-independent effects of statins in DHF are an increase in arterial compliance, a positive effect on myocardial cellular function, the induction of neoangiogenesis, downregulation of the AT1 receptor, restoration of autonomic function and inhibition of proinflammatory cytokines.

Observational studies suggest that adding statins to standard therapy may be a new therapeutic option to improve survival in patients with DHF. This is achieved through the multifactorial reflecting lipid-dependent and pleiotropic effects of statins. It is time to confirm these observations in large, randomized trials.

Figure 1 shows the different targets and treatment for first non-fatal heart failure and established heart failure, according to the mechanisms involved.

Statins and their effects on heart failure are given in Table 1.

TABLE 1: Statins and their effects on heart failure.

Possible beneficial mechanisms	*Potential deleterious effects*
• Slow progression of atherosclerosis (e.g., downregulation of AT1 receptor) • Reduce arterial and ventricular arrhythmias • Improve endothelial dysfunction • Reduce aortic stiffness • Reduce/inhibit proinflammatory cytokines • Antithrombotic effects • Reduce left ventricular hypertrophy • Prevent adverse left ventricular remodeling • Reduce neurohormonal activation	• Low cholesterol indicates poor prognosis in advanced heart failure • Cholesterol may limit lipopolysaccharide-induced production of cytokines, particularly during phases of clinical deterioration; thus, cholesterol lowering may increase risk • Statins decrease levels of ubiquinone (coenzyme Q10), which may impact ventricular function and exercise tolerance

CONCLUSION

Statin therapy is associated with improved outcomes in HF patients with borderline (LVEF 40–49%) or preserved (LVEF ≥50%) ejection fraction but not in those with reduced ejection fraction (LVEF <40%). Use of higher-intensity statins was not associated with improved outcomes in patients with LV dilation, cardiac hypertrophy, higher NYHA classes, or high BNP levels. These findings suggest that statin use was not associated with prognostic improvement in HF patients with advanced cardiac remodeling and symptoms. Second, the impact of both higher- and lower-intensity statins on

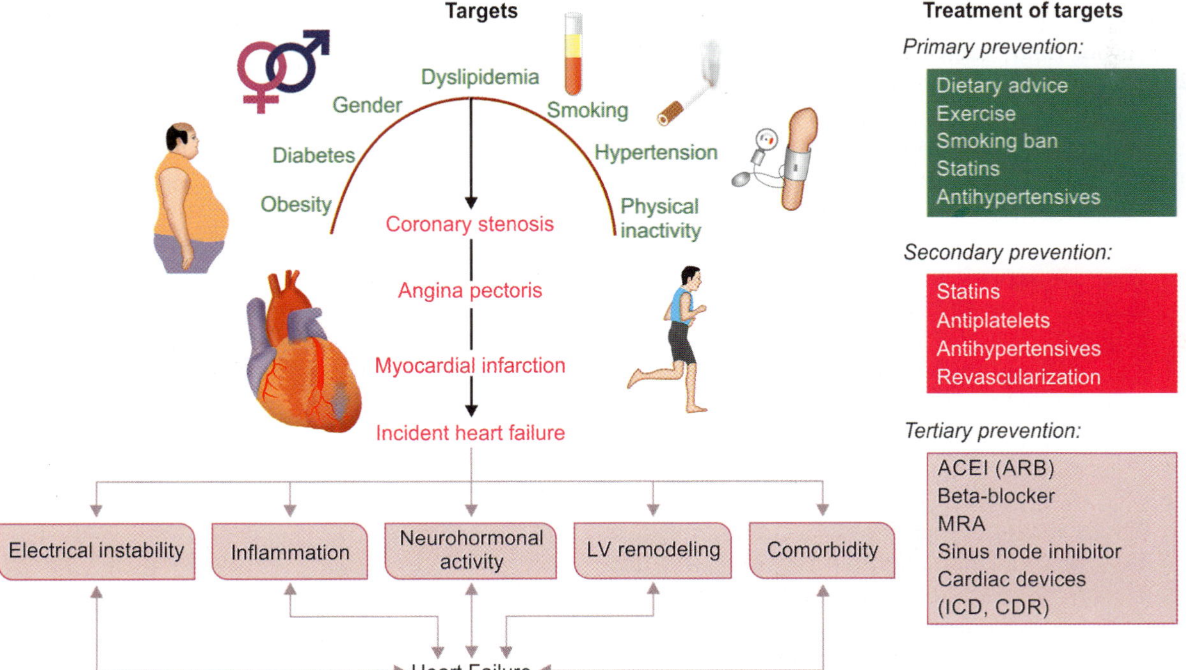

Fig. 1: Diagram showing different targets and treatment for first non-fatal heart failure and established heart failure, according to the mechanisms involved.

the incidence of the primary end point was more evident in patients with higher CRP levels. It is conceivable that pleiotropic effects of statins, including anti-inflammatory and antioxidant effects, may play more important roles in patients with higher CRP levels.

REFERENCES

1. Nissen SE, Nicholls SJ, Sipahi I, et al. Effect of very high-intensity statin therapy on regression of coronary atherosclerosis. The ASTEROID trial. JAMA. 2006;295:1556-65.
2. Hegland O, Kurz MW, Munk PS, et al. The effect of statin therapy on the progression of carotid artery stenosis in relation to stenosis severity. Acta Neurol Scand. 2010;121:11-5.
3. Cholesterol Treatment Trialists. The effects of lowering LDL cholesterol with statin therapy in people at low risk of vascular disease: meta-analysis of individual data from 27 randomized trials. Lancet. 2012;380:581-90.
4. Lystash JC, Gibson RS, Watson DD, et al. Early versus late congestive heart failure after initially uncomplicated anterior wall acute myocardial infarction. Am J Cardiol. 1995;75:653-8.
5. Randomised trial of cholesterol lowering in 4444 patients with coronary heart disease: the Scandinavian Simvastatin Survival Study (4S). Lancet. 1994;344:1383-9.
6. Kjekshus J, Pedersen TR, Olsson AG, et al. The effects of simvastatin on the incidence of heart failure in patients with coronary heart disease. J Card Fail. 1997;3:249-54.
7. ALLHAT Officers and Coordinators for the ALLHAT Collaborative Research Group. The Antihypertensive and Lipid-Lowering Treatment to Prevent Heart Attack Trial. Major outcomes in moderately hypercholesterolemic, hypertensive patients randomized to pravastatin vs usual care: the Antihypertensive and Lipid-Lowering Treatment to Prevent Heart Attack Trial (ALLHAT-LLT). JAMA. 2002;288:2998-3007.
8. LaRosa JC, Grundy SG, Waters DD, et al. Intensive lipid lowering with atorvastatin in patients with stable coronary disease. N Engl J Med. 2005;352:1425-35.
9. Shepherd J, Blauw GJ, Murphy MB, et al. Pravastatin in elderly individuals at risk of vascular disease (PROSPER): a randomised controlled trial. Lancet. 2002;360:1623-30.
10. Preiss D, Campbell RT, Murray HM, et al. The effect of statin therapy on heart failure events: a collaborative meta-analysis of unpublished data from major randomized trials. Eur Heart J. 2015;36:1536-46.
11. Rogers JK, Jhund PS, Perez AC, et al. Effect of rosuvastatin on repeat heart failure hospitalizations: the CORONA Trial (Controlled Rosuvastatin Multinational Trial in Heart Failure). JACC Heart Fail. 2014;2:289-97.
12. Ørn S, Dickstein K. How do heart failure patients die? Eur Heart J. 2002;4:D59-D65.
13. Kjekshus J, Apetrei E, Barrios V, et al. Rosuvastatin in older patients with systolic heart failure. N Engl J Med. 2007;357:2248-61.
14. Tavazzi L, Maggioni AP, Marchioli R, et al. Effect of rosuvastatin in patients with chronic heart failure (The GISSI-HF trial): a randomized, double-blind placebo-controlled trial. Lancet. 2008;372:1231-9.
15. Shafazand M, Rosengren A, Lappas G, et al. Decreasing trends in the incidence of heart failure after acute myocardial infarction from 1993–2004: a study of 175 216 patients with a first acute myocardial infarction in Sweden. Eur J Heart Fail. 2011;13:135-41.
16. Sorbets E, Labreuche J, Simon T, et al. Renin–angiotensin system antagonists and clinical outcomes in stable coronary artery disease without heart failure. Eur Heart J. 2014;35:1760-8.
17. American College of Cardiology. IMProved Reduction of Outcomes: Vytorin Efficacy International Trial (IMPROVE-IT). AHA Scientific Sessions November 2014. Washington, DC: ACC; 2014.

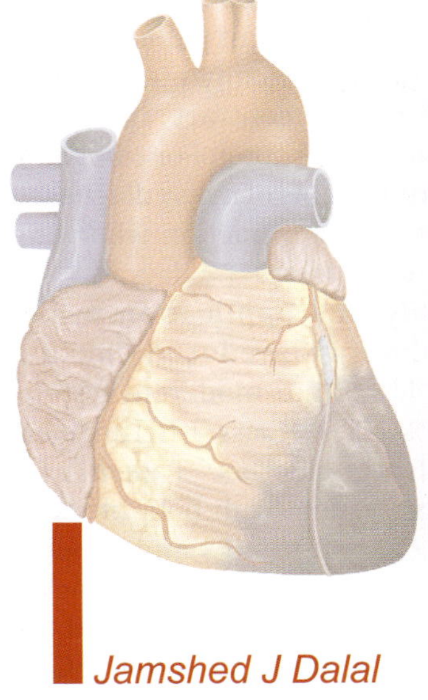

Beta-blockers in Heart Failure

Jamshed J Dalal

INTRODUCTION

With 26 million people worldwide affected by this disease, it has become a global pandemic.[1,2] The epidemiology of heart failure is evolving and it is estimated that up to one out of five people is expected to develop heart failure during their lifetime.[3] The prevalence of heart failure is reported to vary across different geographic locations. Even among similar ethnic population, the prevalence varies widely; for example, it is reported to range from less than 1% in India to 4.5% and 6.7% in Singapore and Malaysia, respectively.[4] Overall, the prevalence of heart failure in adults in developed countries is approximately 1–2%.[5] Though population-based studies for heart failure are lacking,[6] the epidemiological estimates of heart failure are derived from estimates reported due to coronary heart disease, hypertension, obesity, diabetes and rheumatic heart disease. The prevalence in India is estimated to range from 1.3 million to 4.6 million. These estimates are not precise as surveillance systems are lacking in our country. The estimated increasing prevalence rates may be due to the increase in aging population, rise in potential risk factors, epidemiological transitions, and changes in health status.[7] A prospective, observational, hospital-based heart failure registry (January 1, 2013 to December 31, 2013) showed that only one in six patients who received guideline-based in-hospital treatment for heart failure; and only this group had lower mortality. This registry unfurled the need for quality improvement in heart failure management.[8] Heart failure poses a huge burden. An average of 2.2% (range: 0.3–7.7%) hospital admissions in 31 low- and medium-income countries are reported to be due to heart failure.[8] Worldwide, about 15–45% patients hospitalized due to heart failure are reported to die within a year and the majority within 5 years of admission.[9-12] The economic burden of heart failure is reported to be due to drug and resource utilization.[13]

PHARMACOTHERAPY IN HEART FAILURE

Pharmacotherapy in heart failure aims to improve clinical status and quality of life, prevent hospitalization, and reduce mortality. Unless contraindicated neurohormonal antagonists, angiotensin-converting enzyme inhibitors, mineralocorticoid receptor antagonists, and beta-blockers are the mainstay of management in heart failure. Other pharmacotherapies include loop and thiazide diuretics, vasodilators, digoxin, metabolic modulators like trimetazidine and newer agents like the angiotensin receptor-neprilysin inhibitor (Sacubitril/valsartan) and the sinoatrial node modulator (Ivabradine)[14]. In patients with reduced ejection fraction, beta-blockers improve symptoms, reduce risk of hospitalization, and increase survival. The beta-blockers approved for use in heart failure include bisoprolol, carvedilol, and metoprolol.[5]

BETA-BLOCKERS IN HEART FAILURE

Benefits of beta-blockers in heart failure are explained by reductions in sympathetic neural activity, catecholamine levels, heart rate, and cardiotoxic effects of cyclic adenosine monophosphate-mediated calcium overload.[15]

Beta-blockers have been reported to reverse LVH in young/middle-aged hypertensives.[16] Along with ACEIs, beta-blockers are the cornerstone of management of systolic heart failure due to the inhibition of chronic beta-1 stimulation-induced myocardial apoptosis/necrosis/inflammation. Available evidence suggests that first-line treatment with bisoprolol is "non-inferior" to first-line enalapril in reducing all-cause death and is probably superior in reducing sudden death in heart failure.[17] The choice of beta-blocker is important and is not solely a class effect. Bisoprolol, metoprolol succinate, and carvedilol may be chosen for optimal efficacy.[16]

Pharmacology of Beta-blockers Used in Heart Failure

Carvedilol is an adrenoceptor antagonist, which inhibits beta-1-, beta-2-, and alpha-1-adrenergic receptors. Carvedilol has additional metabolic and antioxidant properties including inhibition of apoptosis, reduction in neutrophil infiltration and vascular smooth muscle migration and improvement of myocardial remodeling after acute myocardial infarction.[18] Bisoprolol is cardioselective for beta-1 receptors at low doses with little or no effect on beta-2 receptors at doses ≤20 mg. At therapeutic doses (5–10 mg/day), bisoprolol does not occupy the beta-2 receptors even at peak plasma concentrations.[19]Metoprolol is also a beta-1-selective adrenoceptor blocking drug.[20] In oral doses of less than 100 mg, metoprolol has minimal or no effects on beta-2 receptors.

The pharmacological properties of bisoprolol, metoprolol, and carvedilol are shown in Table 1. The half-life of bisoprolol with normal renal function is 10–12 hours and this is prolonged to 27–36 hours in renal compromise (<40 mL/min).[21] The long half-life offers a suitable once daily dosing option.[22] Metoprolol has a half-life of 3–4 hours, with high first pass metabolism.[23] Carvedilol has a half-life of 6 hours.[24] Metoprolol and carvedilol are available in immediate- and extended-release formulations.

Selecting Patients for Beta-blocker Therapy in Heart Failure

Patient characteristics are important determinants of approach to management in heart failure. Though beta-blockers are the standard therapy in heart failure with reduced ejection, their role in heart failure with preserved ejection is not clear.[5] In the latter class of patients, beta-blockers are not reported to improve any outcomes of hospitalization or death.[25] On the contrary, improved prognosis has been reported with bisoprolol or carvedilol in a prospective study in 2,704 patients of newly diagnosed heart failure and preserved ejection fraction who were followed up for a median duration of 1,877.4 days.[25]

Beta-blockers primarily find application in the management of heart failure with reduced ejection fraction. Patients with stable mild or moderate systolic heart failure with LVEF < 40% (NYHA Class II-III) are ideal candidates for treatment with beta-blockers.[26] Patients with severe heart failure may also benefit with beta-blockers depending upon patient characteristics and clinical decision making. In stabilized heart failure, beta-blocker therapy should be initiated as early as possible and these agents form the first-line of management along with ACE-I and mineralocorticoid receptor antagonists (MRA).[27] There is emerging evidence for use of beta-blockers in patients of heart failure with preserved ejection fraction. In the Medicare-linked Organized Program to Initiate Lifesaving Treatment in Hospitalized Patients with Heart Failure (OPTIMIZE-HF) registry, high dose beta-blockers (atenolol ≥ 100 mg/day, carvedilol ≥ 50 mg/day, metoprolol tartrate or succinate ≥ 200 mg/day, or bisoprolol ≥ 10 mg/day) was associated with a significantly lower risk of death in patients of heart failure with ejection fraction <50%. In patients who received high-dose (n = 730) and no beta-blockers (n = 1,740), all-cause mortality occurred in 63% and 68%, respectively during 6 years (median, 2.8) of follow-up (HR: 0.86; 95% CI: 0.75–0.98; P = 0.027) (Lam 2018).[28]

Dosing of Beta-blockers in Heart Failure

An ideal approach to beta-blocker therapy in heart failure is to begin with a low dose once patient is stabilized. The doses can then be titrated to achieve the target or highest tolerated dose. The doses can be doubled at intervals of not less than 2 weeks but may need step down of dose with worsening clinical signs and symptoms. The benefits are best evident in long-term treatment with beta-blockers. Upon initiation of treatment with beta-blockers, symptomatic improvement may develop slowly over 3–6 months or longer. Adherence

TABLE 1: Pharmacological properties of beta-blockers used in heart failure.

	Plasma half life	*Protein binding*	*Elimination*	*Intrinsic sympathomimetic activity*	*α-blocking activity*	*β1 selectivity*
Carvedilol	6 hours	95%	Liver	No	Yes	No
Bisoprolol	9–12 hours	30%	Kidney, liver	No	No	Yes
Metoprolol	3–7 hours	12%	Liver	No	No	yes

to the recommended approach to beta-blocker and other pharmacological therapy in heart failure has been reported to improve clinical outcomes. In QUALIFY, an international, prospective, observational, longitudinal survey (September 2013 to December 2014) in 6,669 outpatients with heart failure and reduced ejection, adherence to least 50% of recommended dosages was associated with better clinical outcomes during follow up at 6 months.[28]

Dosing is key for the use of beta-blockers in heart failure. The aim should be to attain the guideline recommended target doses.[5] Ouwerkerk et al. (2017) reported the characteristics and outcomes in 2,100 patients of heart failure with reduced ejection fraction across 11 European countries.[29] The recommended doses for beta-blocker therapy were achieved in only 12% patients. When compared to those achieving the target doses, patients treated with less than 50% of the dose of ACE-inhibitors/ARBs and beta-blockers seemed to have a greater risk of death and/or heart failure hospitalization. Chin et al. (2016) analyzed the prescribing patterns of common agents in heart failure.[30]In a systematic review (2000–2015) of 23 reports (n = 83,605 patients), beta-blockers were prescribed in 81.4% patients and 49% patients received ≥50 % of the guideline-recommended target doses. According to the authors, pharmacotherapy including beta-blockers was under prescribed in eligible patients of heart failure with reduced ejection fraction. In the recent Practice Innovation and Clinical Excellence (PINNACLE) study (2011–2015), quality of cardiovascular care was assessed in 11,965 patients with heart failure. When compared to men, women with ejection fraction ≤40% received significantly lower guideline-directed medical therapy with beta-blockers (30.8% vs 37.0%, $p \leq 0.001$) and beta-blockers/ACE-I or ARBs (24.6% vs 31.0%, $p \leq 0.001$). The gender disparities in treatment provide a cue for public health interventions to optimize the use of pharmacotherapy in HF.[31]

Appropriate dosing of beta-blockers is key to the management of heart failure. In a recent study,[32] effect of low and high dose (n = 36,168 each) of carvedilol and metoprolol was evaluated on mortality in patients with reduced ejection fraction heart failure. Independent of heart rate achieved, high dose was associated with lower overall mortality as compared to the low dose of beta-blockers (HR: 0.75, 95% CI: 0.73–0.77, $p < 0.01$). It is beneficial to achieve guideline recommended dose for beta-blockers. This is associated with survival benefits in heart failure. Once target doses are achieved, achievement of target heart rate (51–69 bpm) may additionally help to improve survival.[33]

The recommended starting dose of bisoprolol in heart failure is 1.25 mg daily, and target dose is 10 mg daily.[5] Adjustment of dose of bisoprolol is needed in moderately to severely decreased renal function. Patients with low body weight or low skeletal muscle index (SMI) are likely to have greater fluctuations and higher maximal plasma concentrations due to low volume of distribution.[34] Routine measuring of serum creatinine helps to determine the appropriate dosing of bisoprolol in patients on hemodialysis.[35] Additionally, the dose of bisoprolol should be optimized before any other concomitant medications are included in the treatment regimen, e.g. ivabradine to reduce heart rate. In heart failure, therapy with carvedilol can be titrated up to 25 mg twice daily as tolerated.[36] Abrupt cessation of therapy with beta-blockers should be discouraged as may lead to withdrawal syndrome including tachycardia, hypertension, angina, and myocardial infarction.[37]

Efficacy of Beta-blockers in Heart Failure

Beta-blockers can improve hemodynamics in chronic heart failure. The key clinical trials for bisoprolol, metoprolol, and carvedilol in heart failure are listed in Table 2.[38-42] Once daily metoprolol controlled release/extended release (CR/XL) when added to optimum standard therapy improves survival in patients with chronic heart failure (ejection fraction of ≤0.40) and New York Heart Association (NYHA) functional class II-IV (MERIT HF 1999). In the placebo-controlled Carvedilol Prospective Randomised Cumulative Survival (COPERNICUS) trial (n = 2,289), carvedilol significantly reduced all-cause mortality and the combined endpoint of death or hospitalization for any reason in severe chronic heart failure (Packer 2002).

The clinical efficacy of bisoprolol has been examined in stable chronic heart failure (NYHA class III or IV) in two major randomised, double-blind, placebo-controlled, multicentre trials: the Cardiac Insufficiency Bisoprolol Study CIBIS; (n = 641) and CIBIS II (n = 2,647). Bisoprolol was used concomitant with ACE inhibitors and diuretics in these trials. The results of these trials are summarized in Table 1. Regardless of dose, the all-cause mortality (primary endpoint) was significantly lower in bisoprolol than in placebo recipients in CIBIS II (11.8% vs 17.3%). All-cause mortality was also lower in CIBIS (16.6% vs 20.9%) although statistical significance was not achieved for the difference. In a meta-analysis of CIBIS and CIBIS II (n = 3,288), a relative reduction of 29% in the incidence of all-cause mortality was reported for bisoprolol when compared to placebo. Additionally, the analysis demonstrated reduction in mortality with bisoprolol in chronic heart failure regardless of etiology or severity.[43] Data from the CIBIS-II trial were analyzed to assess the effect of bisoprolol on perioperative outcomes in moderate to severe heart failure. Of the 2,647 patients randomized in the CIBIS-II study, 165 underwent surgery (87 patients receiving bisoprolol and 78 receiving placebo). When compared to placebo, the bisoprolol group did not demonstrate any significant reduction in mortality

(7.7% vs 5.8%, p = 0.76), postoperative hospital admission (24.4% vs 34.5%, p = 0.17), time to postoperative hospital admission (≤30 days/31–180 days/>180 days; placebo, n = 2/11/6; bisoprolol, n = 9/10/11; p = 0.14).[44]

Selecting Beta-blockers in Heart Failure

Differences in efficacy between beta-blockers have been studied in clinical trials and practice. From three registries in Norway, England, and Germany, Fröhlich et al. (2017) identified 6,010 outpatients with stable heart failure and reduced LVEF who were treated with either bisoprolol, carvedilol or metoprolol succinate and were individually matched with respect to both dose equivalents and the respective propensity scores for beta-blocker treatment. During a follow-up of 26,963 patient-years, death was reported in 302 (29.5%), 637 (37.0%), and 1,232 (37.7%) patients receiving bisoprolol, carvedilol, and metoprolol, respectively. When compared with metoprolol succinate, bisoprolol and carvedilol were both associated with lower mortality [HR: 0.80, 95% confidence interval (CI) 0.71–0.91, p < 0.01, and HR: 0.86, 95% CI 0.78–0.94, p < 0.01, respectively] in a univariate analysis. Similar mortality rates were reported for bisoprolol or carvedilol [HR: 0.94, 95% CI: 0.82–1.08, p = 0.37). In matched samples, all-cause mortality did not significantly differ for choice of beta-blocker (HR: 0.90; 95% CI: 0.76–1.06; p = 0.20; HR: 1.10, 95% CI: 0.93–1.31, p = 0.24; and HR: 1.08, 95% CI: 0.95–1.22, p = 0.26 for bisoprolol vs carvedilol, bisoprolol vs metoprolol succinate, and carvedilol vs metoprolol succinate, respectively).[45]

In a similar study, Perreault et al. (2017) reported no differential effect of beta-blockers on all-cause mortality in 3,197 patients with heart failure who were followed up for a median period of 2.8 years. The annual mortality rates (per 100 person-years) were 16, 14.9, and 17.7 for metoprolol tartrate, carvedilol, and bisoprolol, respectively. When compared to metoprolol, carvedilol, and bisoprolol showed no additional benefit for all-cause mortality after matching for propensity score.[46]

Bisoprolol is a preferred choice for treatment of heart failure with comorbidities. When compared to carvedilol and metoprolol, bisoprolol has shown a dose-response survival benefit in patients with coexisting heart failure and chronic obstructive pulmonary disease (COPD) in a nationwide population-based study in 11,558 patients who were followed up for a mean duration of 4.07 years. After adjustment for age, sex, comorbidities, and severity of HF and COPD, bisoprolol use showed a dose-response survival benefit [low dose: adjusted hazard ratio (HR) = 0.76, 95% CI = 0.59–0.97, P = 0.030; high dose: adjusted HR = 0.40,

TABLE 2: Clinical trials for beta-blocker therapy in heart failure.

Clinical trial and drug	*Mean follow-up*	*Key inclusion criteria*	*Key outcomes*
CIBIS: Bisoprolol (n = 320) vs placebo (n = 321).	1.9 years	LVEF ≤ 40%, NYHA III–IV	No significant difference in mortality: 67 patients died on placebo, 53 on bisoprolol (P = 0.22; RR, 0.80; 95% CI, 0.56 to 1.15). No significant difference in sudden death rate (17 on placebo, 15 on bisoprolol) or death related to documented ventricular tachycardia or fibrillation (7 on placebo and 4 on bisoprolol). Bisoprolol significantly improved the functional status of the patients: • Lesser hospitalization for cardiac decompensation (90 on placebo versus 61 on bisoprolol, P < 0.01) • More patients improved at least one NYHA functional class (48 on placebo versus 68 on bisoprolol, P = 0.04) at end of follow up.
CIBIS-II: Bisoprolol (n = 1,327) vs placebo (n = 1320)	1.3 years	LVEF ≤ 35%, NYHA III–IV	All-cause mortality reduced by 34% (12% vs 17%) (HR: 0.66; 95% CI: 0.54–0.81; P < 0.001). Significantly fewer sudden deaths with bisoprolol [48 (3.6%) vs 83 (6.3%) deaths] (HR: 0.56; 95% CI: 0.39–0.80, p = 0.0011). Reduction in combined cardiovascular mortality or cardiovascular hospitalization rate by 21% (P < 0.001).
MERIT-HF: Metoprolol CR/XL (n = 1991) vs placebo (n = 2001).	1.0 year	LVEF ≤ 40%, NYHA II–IV	All-cause mortality reduced by 34% (7% vs 11%) (P < 0.001). Reduction in the risk of cardiovascular death by 38% (P < 0.001), sudden death by 41% (P < 0.001) and death from aggravated HF by 49% (P = 0.002).
COPERNICUS: Carvedilol (n = 1,156) vs placebo (n = 1,133)	0.9 year	LVEF < 25%, NYHA IV	All-cause mortality reduced by 35% (11% vs 17%) (P < 0.001). Reduction in combined all-cause mortality and any hospitalization rate by 24% (P < 0.001).

(CI: confidence interval; CIBIS: the Cardiac Insufficiency Bisoprolol Study; CIBIS II: Cardiac Insufficiency Bisoprolol Study II; HF: heart failure; HR: hazard ratio; LVEF: left ventricular ejection fraction; MERIT-HF: Metoprolol CR/XL Randomised Intervention Trial in Congestive Heart Failure; NYHA: New York Heart Association; RR: relative risk)

95% CI = 0.26–0.63, P < 0.001] compared with nonusers. No survival difference was observed for carvedilol or metoprolol.[47]

The carvedilol or metoprolol European trial (COMET) compared loss of well-being with carvedilol (target dose of 25 mg twice daily) or metoprolol (target dose of 50 mg twice daily) in patients with stable heart failure. The total numbers of deaths in patients receiving carvedilol and metoprolol were 512 and 600, respectively (HR: 0.83; 95% CI: 0.74–0.93; P = 0.0017). Compared with metoprolol, carvedilol was associated with fewer days lost to death, with no increase in days lost due to impaired well-being or days in hospital. Carvedilol was shown to favorably impact patient journey over 4 years when compared to metoprolol.[48] This can be explained by the full adrenergic blockage and additional antioxidative properties of carvedilol which may result in better vascular protection.[49] However, there is contrary evidence reported for use of more beta-1 selective blockers when compared to carvedilol. Toyoda et al. (2017) compared the efficacy of bisoprolol (n = 38) and carvedilol (n = 29) in patients with chronic systolic heart failure (≤45% ejection fraction).[50] The two groups showed no differences in improvement of NYHA class, ejection fraction, or N-terminal pro-brain-type natriuretic peptide level. However, in the bisoprolol group, there was a decrease in troponin T [-4.1 ± 0.9 to -4.5 ± 0.8 log (ng/mL), P = 0.003] and an increase in forced expiratory volume in the first second [2.26 ± 0.70 to 2.40 ± 0.70 (L), P = 0.014]. These parameters did not show change in the carvedilol group, 4.4 ± 1.1 to -4.6 ± 0.8 log (ng/mL), P = 0.161 and 2.53 ± 0.71 to 2.59 ± 0.78 (L), P = 0.127, respectively. The authors concluded superior protection from myocardial injury and preserved pulmonary function in chronic systolic heart failure with bisoprolol.

Switching of Beta-blockers in Heart Failure

Switching of beta-blockers is a practical and safe approach to optimize treatment in patients with heart failure. The safety of switch has been explored in the COMET study wherein 1,321 out of 1,440 patients were transitioned to open-label treatment (76.8% to carvedilol) and followed up for 30 days. Serious adverse events in patients switching from carvedilol to metoprolol and metoprolol to carvedilol were 9.4% and 3.1% whereas CHF-related events were 4.7% and 1.5%, respectively. The switch from carvedilol to metoprolol was associated with highest mortality or hospitalization rate (12.3%) when compared to the switch from metoprolol to carvedilol (3.1%, p < 0.001) or no switch (carvedilol: 2.5%, p < 0.001; metoprolol: 4.2%, p = 0.04).[51]

Switch from metoprolol to bisoprolol in chronic stable heart failure has been reported to be safe. In 282 patients with NYHA class I–III heart failure and/or postinfarction reduced LVEF, bisoprolol was introduced after discontinuation of metoprolol tartarate. Of these, 28.5% patients reached the 10-mg target dose and 21.5%, 42.5%, 7.5%, received 7.5 mg, 5 mg, and 2.5 mg dose, respectively. Mean heart rate (84 bpm before the switch) dropped to 67 bpm with various doses of bisoprolol suggesting a more effective adrenergic blockage with bisoprolol.[52] The clinical, hemodynamic and neurohumoral effects of switching patients with chronic heart failure from nonrecommended adrenoblockers to bisoprolol were assessed in 35 patients in ambulatory practice. After 6 months of treatment with bisoprolol, there was significant improvement of clinical status with increase of 6 minutes walking distance, betterment of parameters of quality of life, and significant rise of LVEF combined with lowering of mean CHF functional class (all p < 0.01 compared with baseline). Irrespective of changes in heart rate, there was a lowering of initially elevated N-terminal fragment of pro-brain natriuretic peptide (NT pro-BNP) in blood serum.[53]

In a retrospective study in 23 patients with heart failure who could not increase dose of carvedilol due to dizziness or hypotension (systolic BP < 90 mm Hg), switch to bisoprolol resulted in relief from dizziness in all (100%) patients and from hypotension in 56% patients. At 6 months after bisoprolol therapy, LVEF improved significantly and there was increased exercise tolerance. The mean dose of carvedilol before switching was 5.60 ± 3.43 mg and that of bisoprolol immediately after and 6 months after switch was 1.84 ± 1.08 mg and 3.13 ± 1.74 mg, respectively.[54]

Safety and Tolerability of Beta-blockers in Heart Failure

Beta-blockers are generally well-tolerated in patients with heart failure. Common adverse events with beta-blocker therapy include bradycardia, heart block, fatigue, hypotension, cold extremities, dizziness, decreased libido, and depression. Glucose intolerance has been reported with metoprolol[37] though not with carvedilol.[55] Glucose tolerance and lipid profiles are minimally impacted by bisoprolol (Johns 1995).[56] Due to high beta-1 receptor selectivity, bisoprolol is devoid of metabolic disturbances, helps to improve vascular compliance, and does not adversely impact sexual functions.[57] Beta-blockers should be used with caution in patients with severe (NYHA Class IV) heart failure, recent (<4 weeks) or current exacerbation of heart failure, heart block, or falling heart rate (<50 bpm), signs of hypotension (<90 mm Hg) and congestion. Due to potential risk of bradycardia and atrioventricular block, beta-blocker therapy should be used with caution with concomitant digoxin, amiodarone, and ivabradine.

Concomitant therapy with verapamil and diltiazam should be discontinued. In CIBIS II, adverse events, regardless of causal association, reported more frequently for bisoprolol included dizziness, fatigue, bradycardia, and hypotension. Dyspnea or tachycardia was more frequently reported with placebo. In both the trials (CIBIS and CIBIS II) there was no significant difference in the incidence of permanent treatment withdrawal in the bisoprolol and placebo groups.[58,59]

The CIBIS II study has established superior safety of bisoprolol in comparison to placebo. Regardless of age, New York Heart Association (NYHA) functional class, and comorbidities, the all-cause mortality (11.8% vs 17.3%; $p < 0.0001$) and sudden death (3.6% vs 6.3%, $p < 0.002$) were reduced in patients treated with bisoprolol when compared with those on placebo. Further, the CIBIS III study (n = 1,010), patients receiving bisoprolol (target dose 10 mg QD; n = 505) or enalapril (target dose 10 mg BID; n = 505) for 6 months demonstrated comparable safety in the two groups.[17] Good tolerability of beta-blockers has been reported in a prospective observational study in 119 elderly (>70 years) with HF who were receiving bisoprolol or carvedilol in the last 1 month and were followed up for 6 months. Three deaths were reported during this period and none were related to use of beta-blockers. Treatment withdrawal was reported in 8.4% patients and the adverse reactions responsible for the withdrawal were symptomatic hypotension (2.5%); asymptomatic hypotension (0.8%); heart failure (1.7%); bradycardia (1.7%); bronchospasm (0.8%); and unknown cause (0.8%).[17] In a postmarketing surveillance for carvedilol, only 7% (164/2,226) of patients (83% of the total number received 25 mg daily for 12 weeks) withdrew from treatment because of adverse events, the most common ones being vertigo, headache, bronchospasm, fatigue, and skin reactions.[55]

Therapy with beta-blockers necessitates monitoring of blood glucose in patients with concomitant diabetes and should be administered with caution in patients with a history of asthma and reactive airway disease. Patients with heart failure should be monitored for signs of decompensation. Cardioselective beta-blockers are preferred agents in the treatment of heart failure in patients with diabetes and pulmonary obstructive diseases.[60]

Absolute contraindications to beta-blocker therapy include severe hypotension, severe bradycardia, AV block sick sinus syndrome, and severe decompensated heart failure requiring inotropic support.

CONCLUSION

Chronic heart failure represents a major health problem and is one of the leading causes of hospitalization, in particular in elderly patients. Benefits with beta-blockade in heart failure are not solely a class effect. Appropriate beta-blockers should be chosen and therapy should be tailored according to patient characteristics. Therapy and dose optimization is key in achieving a better outcome, especially in countries where less than one-fourth of patients receive guideline-based treatment for chronic heart failure. Data for reduction of all-cause mortality is available only with three beta-blockers, bisoprolol, metoprolol succinate and carvedilol. Cardioselective beta-blockers like bisoprolol and metoprolol are preferred agents in heart failure with obstructive pulmonary disease. When compared to carvedilol, bisoprolol offers superior protection from myocardial injury and preserved pulmonary function in chronic systolic heart failure. Carvedilol, however, has the advantage of vasodilatory properties which help to reduce after load. Beta-blockers when added to the standard treatment with ACEI and diuretics, improves survival, functional status, and reduces the need for hospitalization in patients with chronic stable heart failure.[61] They may be even combined with ivabradine if optimal heart rate is not obtained and hypotension prevents further increase in beta-blocker dose. Pharmacoeconomic studies in UK, France, and Germany have confirmed addition of bisoprolol to standard treatment as a cost-effective option when compared to standard treatment alone in chronic heart failure.[61] Newer formulations of beta-blockers are being investigated for better patient convenience and adherence with improved plasma concentration-time profiles. The efficacy and safety of switch from oral bisoprolol to once daily transdermal formulation was studied in a phase II trial in 40 patients with stable chronic heart failure. The dose conversion ratio of the oral to transdermal formulation was 5:8. The mean pre-switch left ventricular ejection fraction (50.13 ± 11.09%) was not significantly different from the post-switch value (50.87 ± 10.79%) after 16 weeks. There were no cardiovascular deaths, hospitalizations for worsening heart failure, or safety concerns during the 16-week period.[62] Efforts are also being made to individually tailor bisoprolol treatment according to genotype of the beta-1 adrenergic receptor gene (ADRB1) in heart failure.[63]

REFERENCES

1. Ambrosy AP, Fonarow GC, Butler J, et al. The global health and economic burden of hospitalizations for heart failure: lessons learned from hospitalized heart failure registries. J Am Coll Cardiol. 2014;63(12):1123-33.
2. Ponikowski P, Anker SD, AlHabib KF, et al. Heart failure: preventing disease and death worldwide. ESC Heart Failure. 2014;1:4-25.
3. Lloyd-Jones DM, Larson MG, Leip EP, et al. Lifetime risk for developing congestive heart failure: the Framingham Heart Study. Circulation. 2002;106:3068-72.

4. Savarese G, Lund LH. Global Public Health Burden of Heart Failure. Card Fail Rev. 2017;3(1):7-11.
5. Ponikowski P, Voors AA, Anker SD, et al. 2016 ESC Guidelines for the diagnosis and treatment of acute and chronic heart failure: The Task Force for the diagnosis and treatment of acute and chronic heart failure of the European Society of Cardiology (ESC) Developed with the special contribution of the Heart Failure Association (HFA) of the ESC. Eur Heart J. 2016;37(27):2129-200.
6. Callender T, Woodward M, Roth G, et al. Heart failure care in low- and middle-income countries: a systematic review and meta-analysis. PLoS Med. 2014;11(8):e1001699.
7. Huffman MD, Prabhakaran D. Heart failure: epidemiology and prevention in India. Natl Med J India. 2010;23(5):283-8.
8. Harikrishnan S, Sanjay G, Anees T, et al. Clinical presentation, management, in-hospital and 90-day outcomes of heart failure patients in Trivandrum, Kerala, India: the Trivandrum Heart Failure Registry. Eur J Heart Fail. 2015;17(8):794-800.
9. Barretto AC, Del Carlo CH, Cardoso JN, et al. Hospital readmissions and death from heart failure—rates still alarming. Arq Bras Cardiol. 2008;91:335-41.
10. Blair JE, Huffman M, Shah SJ. Heart failure in North America. Curr Cardiol Rev. 2013;9:128-46.
11. Bocchi EA, Arias A, Verdejo H, et al. The reality of heart failure in Latin America. J Am Coll Cardiol. 2013;62:949-58.
12. Maggioni AP, Dahlstrom U, Filippatos G, et al. EURObservational Research Programme: regional differences and 1-year follow-up results of the Heart Failure Pilot Survey (ESC-HF Pilot). Eur J Heart Fail. 2013;15:808-17.
13. Huang J, Yin H, Zhang M, et al. Understanding the economic burden of heart failure in China: impact on disease management and resource utilization. J Med Econ. 2017;20(5):549-53.
14. Shah A, Gandhi D, Srivastava S, et al. Heart Failure: A Class Review of Pharmacotherapy. P T. 2017;42(7):464-72.
15. Satwani S, Dec GW, Narula J. Beta adrenergic blockers in heart failure: review of mechanisms of action and clinical outcomes. J Cardiovasc Pharmacol Ther. 2004;9:243-55.
16. Cruickshank JM. Beta-blockers and heart failure. Indian Heart J. 2010;62(2):101-10.
17. Willenheimer R, van Veldhuisen DJ, Silke B, et al. Effect on survival and hospitalization of initiating treatment for chronic heart failure with bisoprolol followed by enalapril, as compared with the opposite sequence: results of the randomized Cardiac Insufficiency Bisoprolol Study (CIBIS) III. Circulation. 2005;112(16):2426-35.
18. Chen-Scarabelli C, Saravolatz L Jr, Murad Y, et al. A critical review of the use of carvedilol in ischemic heart disease. Am J Cardiovasc Drugs. 2012;12(6):391-401.
19. Wellstein A, Palm D, Belz GG, et al. Reduction of exercise tachycardia in man after propranolol, atenolol and bisoprolol in comparison to beta-adrenoceptor occupancy. Eur Heart J. 1987;8(Suppl M):3-8.
20. Brogden RN, Heel RC, Speight TM, et al. Metoprolol: a review of its pharmacological properties and therapeutic efficacy in hypertension and angina pectoris. Drugs. 1977;14(5):321-48.
21. Prichard BN. Bisoprolol: a new beta-adrenoceptor blocking drug. Eur Heart J. 1987;8 (Suppl M):121-9.
22. Leopold G, Ungethum W, Pabst J, et al. Pharmacodynamic profile of bisoprolol, a new beta-1-selective adrenoceptor antagonist. Br J Clin Pharmacol. 1986;22(3):293-300.
23. Morris J, Dunham A. Metoprolol. [Updated 2018 Dec 17]. In: StatPearls [Internet]. Treasure Island (FL): StatPearls Publishing; 2019 Jan. [online] Available from: https://www.ncbi.nlm.nih.gov/pubmed/30422518; https://www.ncbi.nlm.nih.gov/books/NBK532923/ [Last accessed Nov., 2019].
24. Stafylas PC, Sarafidis PA. Carvedilol in hypertension treatment. Vasc Health Risk Manag. 2008;4(1):23-30.
25. Ruiz G, Andrey JL, Puerto JL, et al. Prognosis of heart failure with preserved ejection fraction treated with β-blockers: A propensity matched study in the community. Int J Cardiol. 2016;222:594-602.
26. Chavey WE, Hogikyan RV, Van Harrison R, et al. Heart Failure Due to Reduced Ejection Fraction: Medical Management. Am Fam Phys. 2017;95(1):13-20.
27. Ponikowski P, Voors AA, Anker SD, et al. 2016 ESC Guidelines for the diagnosis and treatment of acute and chronic heart failure: The Task Force for the diagnosis and treatment of acute and chronic heart failure of the European Society of Cardiology (ESC). Developed with the special contribution of the Heart Failure Association (HFA) of the ESC. Eur J Heart Fail. 2016;18(8):891-975.
28. Komajda M, Cowie MR, Tavazzi L, et al. Physicians' guideline adherence is associated with better prognosis in outpatients with heart failure with reduced ejection fraction: the QUALIFY international registry. Eur J Heart Fail. 2017;19(11):1414-23.
29. Ouwerkerk W, Voors AA, Anker SD, et al. Determinants and clinical outcome of uptitration of ACE-inhibitors and beta-blockers in patients with heart failure: a prospective European study. Eur Heart J. 2017;38(24):1883-90.
30. Chin KL, Skiba M, Tonkin A, et al. The treatment gap in patients with chronic systolic heart failure: a systematic review of evidence-based prescribing in practice. Heart Fail Rev. 2016;21(6):675-97.
31. Kalra A, Pokharel Y, Glusenkamp N, et al. Gender disparities in cardiovascular care access and delivery in India: Insights from the American College of Cardiology's PINNACLE India Quality Improvement Program (PIQIP). Int J Cardiol. 2016;215:248-51.
32. Ajam T, Ajam S, Devaraj S, et al. Effect on Mortality of Higher Versus Lower β-Blocker (Metoprolol Succinate or Carvedilol) Dose in Patients With Heart Failure. Am J Cardiol. 2018;122(6):994-998.
33. Corletto A, Fröhlich H, Täger T, et al. Beta blockers and chronic heart failure patients: prognostic impact of a dose targeted beta blocker therapy vs. heart rate targeted strategy. Clin Res Cardiol. 2018;107(11):1040-1049.
34. CvanTrobec K, Grabnar I, Kerec Kos M, et al. Bisoprolol pharmacokinetics and body composition in patients with chronic heart failure: a longitudinal study. Eur J Clin Pharmacol. 2016;72(7):813-22.

35. Nikolic VN, Jankovic SM, Dimitrijevic ZM, et al. Population Pharmacokinetics of Bisoprolol in Hemodialysis Patients with Hypertension. Pharmacology. 2016;97(3-4):134-7.
36. Singh S, Preuss CV. Carvedilol. [Updated 2018 Dec 9]. In: StatPearls [Internet]. Treasure Island (FL): StatPearls Publishing; 2019 Jan. [online] Available from https://www.ncbi.nlm.nih.gov/books/NBK534868/ [Last accessed Nov., 2019].
37. Kukin ML, Mannino MM, Freudenberger RS, et al. Hemodynamic comparison of twice daily metoprolol tartrate with once daily metoprolol succinate in congestive heart failure. J Am Coll Cardiol. 2000;35(1):45-50.
38. A randomized trial of beta-blockade in heart failure. The Cardiac Insufficiency Bisoprolol Study (CIBIS). CIBIS Investigators and Committees. Circulation. 1994;90(4): 1765-73.
39. Effect of metoprolol CR/XL in chronic heart failure: Metoprolol CR/XL Randomised Intervention Trial in Congestive Heart Failure (MERIT-HF). Lancet. 1999;353(9169):2001-7.
40. The Cardiac Insufficiency Bisoprolol Study II (CIBIS-II): a randomised trial. Lancet. 1999;353(9146):9-13.
41. Flather MD, Shibata MC, Coats AJ, et al. Randomized trial to determine the effect of nebivolol on mortality and cardiovascular hospital admission in elderly patients with heart failure (SENIORS). Eur Heart J. 2005;26(3):215-25.
42. Packer M, Fowler MB, Roecker EB, et al. Effect of carvedilol on the morbidity of patients with severe chronic heart failure: results of the carvedilol prospective randomized cumulative survival (COPERNICUS) study. Circulation. 2002;106(17):2194-9.
43. McGavin JK, Keating GM. Bisoprolol: a review of its use in chronic heart failure. Drugs. 2002;62(18):2677-96.
44. Böhm M, Maack C, Wehrlen-Grandjean M, et al. Effect of bisoprolol on perioperative complications in chronic heart failure after surgery (Cardiac Insufficiency Bisoprolol Study II (CIBIS II)). Z Kardiol. 2003;92(8):668-76.
45. Fröhlich H, Torres L, Täger T, et al. Bisoprolol compared with carvedilol and metoprolol succinate in the treatment of patients with chronic heart failure. Clin Res Cardiol. 2017;106(9):711-21.
46. Perreault S, de Denus S, White M, et al. Older adults with heart failure treated with carvedilol, bisoprolol, or metoprolol tartrate: risk of mortality. Pharmacoepidemiol Drug Saf. 2017;26(1):81-90.
47. Su VY, Chang YS, Hu YW, et al. Carvedilol, Bisoprolol, and Metoprolol Use in Patients with Coexistent Heart Failure and Chronic Obstructive Pulmonary Disease. Medicine (Baltimore). 2016;95(5):e2427.
48. Cleland JG, Charlesworth A, Lubsen J, et al. A comparison of the effects of carvedilol and metoprolol on well-being, morbidity, and mortality (the "patient journey") in patients with heart failure: a report from the Carvedilol Or Metoprolol European Trial (COMET). J Am Coll Cardiol. 2006;47(8): 1603-11.
49. Remme WJ, Torp-Pedersen C, Cleland JG, et al. Carvedilol protects better against vascular events than metoprolol in heart failure: results from COMET. J Am Coll Cardiol. 2007;49(9):963-71.
50. Toyoda S, Haruyama A, Inami S, et al. Protective effects of bisoprolol against myocardial injury and pulmonary dysfunction in patients with chronic heart failure. Int J Cardiol. 2017;226:71-6.
51. Di Lenarda A, Remme WJ, Charlesworth A, et al. Exchange of beta-blockers in heart failure patients. Experiences from the poststudy phase of COMET (the Carvedilol or Metoprolol European Trial). Eur J Heart Fail. 2005;7(4):640-9.
52. Tomcsányi J, Wettstein A, Toldy-Schedel E, et al. Switching beta-blocker therapy in chronic heart failure. Int J Cardiol. 2008;130(3):497-9.
53. Ageev FT, Zhubrina ES, Ovchinnikov AG, et al. Clinical, hemodynamic and neurohumoral effects of switching patients with chronic heart failure from not recommended—adrenoblockers to bisoprolol in ambulatory practice. Kardiologiia. 2010;50(6):41-7.
54. Taniguchi T, Ohtani T, Mizote I, et al. Switching from carvedilol to bisoprolol ameliorates adverse effects in heart failure patients with dizziness or hypotension. J Cardiol. 2013;61(6):417-22.
55. McTavish D, Campoli-Richards D, Sorkin EM. Carvedilol. A review of its pharmacodynamic and pharmacokinetic properties, and therapeutic efficacy. Drugs. 1993;45(2): 232-58.
56. Johns TE, Lopez LM. Bisoprolol: is this just another beta-blocker for hypertension or angina? Ann Pharmacother. 1995;29(4):403-14.
57. Cruickshank JM. Are we misunderstanding beta-blockers? Int J Cardiol. 2007;120(1):10-27.
58. McGavin JK, Keating GM. Bisoprolol: a review of its use in chronic heart failure. Drugs. 2002;62(18):2677-96.
59. Böhm M, Maack C, Wehrlen-Grandjean M, et al. Effect of bisoprolol on perioperative complications in chronic heart failure after surgery (Cardiac Insufficiency Bisoprolol Study II (CIBIS II)). Z Kardiol. 2003;92(8):668-76.
60. Dézsi CA, Szentes V. The Real Role of β-Blockers in Daily Cardiovascular Therapy. Am J Cardiovasc Drugs. 2017;17(5):361-73.
61. McGavin JK, Keating GM. Bisoprolol: a review of its use in chronic heart failure. Drugs. 2002;62(18):2677-96.
62. Momomura SI, Saito Y, Yasumura Y, et al. Efficacy and Safety of Switching From Oral Bisoprolol to Transdermal Patch in Japanese Patients With Chronic Heart Failure. Circ J. 2017;82(1):141-7.
63. Lee HY, Chung WJ, Jeon HK, et al. Impact of the β-1 adrenergic receptor polymorphism on tolerability and efficacy of bisoprolol therapy in Korean heart failure patients: association between β adrenergic receptor polymorphism and bisoprolol therapy in heart failure (ABBA) study. Korean J Intern Med. 2016;31(2):277-87.

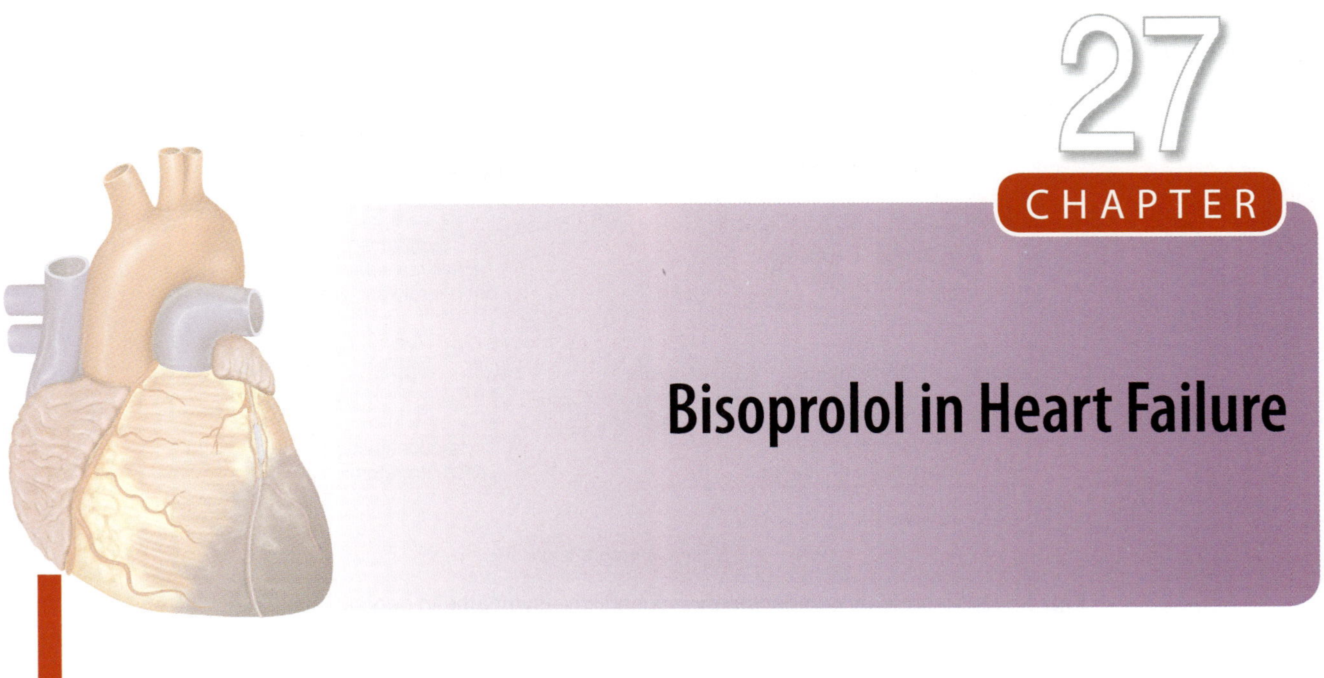

Bisoprolol in Heart Failure

Chandrashekhar K Ponde, Mehul Oswal, HK Chopra

INTRODUCTION

Heart failure (HF) is a global pandemic affecting at least 26 million people worldwide and is increasing in prevalence. Its prevalence ranges from 0.4% to 2%.[1-4] Despite the significant recent advances in therapies and prevention, mortality and morbidity are still high with poor quality of life. Initially, beta-blockers were contraindicated in the treatment of heart failure. The high catecholamine levels are useful in the early phase to maintain the cardiac output but become detrimental in long-term as they result in apoptosis, fibrosis, adverse remodeling and increased arrythmogenesis. Waagstein et al. were the first to report that a treatment with a beta-blocker may dramatically improve symptoms and ventricular function in patients with mild to severe heart failure due to idiopathic dilated cardiomyopathy.[5,6] Recently, multiple randomized control trials (RCTs) have clearly demonstrated the beneficial effects of beta-blocker therapy. Guidelines recommend only three beta-blockers for congestive heart failure (CHF): bisoprolol, metoprolol succinate and carvedilol (beta-1-beta-2 adrenoreceptor blocker with additional alpha-1 vasodilatory activity).[7] Bisoprolol is a highly selective β_1-adrenoceptor antagonist. Administration of bisoprolol to patients with chronic heart failure is associated with increase in left ventricular ejection fraction (LVEF), reduced hospitalization for heart failure and reduction in mortality even at low doses.

PATHOPHYSIOLOGICAL MECHANISMS IN HEART FAILURE

The introduction of beta-blockers in HF has been a major breakthrough in the interpretation and treatment of heart failure with reduced ejection fraction (HFrEF). In 1978, Prichard commented that patients with HFrEF or patients with incipient left ventricular insufficiency are critically dependent on sympathetic activity to the heart to maintain their cardiac output. However, later studies had shown the long-term deleterious effects of sympathetic activation on myocardial function patients with HFrEF. Increased cardiac sympathetic drive was shown to be associated with increased myocardial energy expenditure and possibly ischemia. It also causes secondary activation of renin-angiotensin-aldosterone system (RAAS), increased apoptosis, and increased arrhythmogenecity (Fig. 1).

Subsequently, beta-1 adrenergic receptors (ARs) stimulation was shown to be a powerful mechanism leading to accelerated cell death, through apoptosis,[8] and to major changes in the qualitative characteristics of myocardial cells with reduced contractility and abnormal intracellular calcium handling by the sarcoplasmic reticulum.[9] The role of sympathetic stimulation in all these quantitative and qualitative changes in myocardial characteristics was indirectly shown by their reversal with beta-blocker treatment.[10,11] The pharmacological basis for the beneficial effects of β-blockers in heart failure seems to be this reduction in catecholamine-driven detrimental changes.

BETA-BLOCKER THERAPY IN HEART FAILURE

Historical Notes

Small single-center trials showed the beneficial effects of beta-blockers on clinical symptoms and, to an even greater extent,

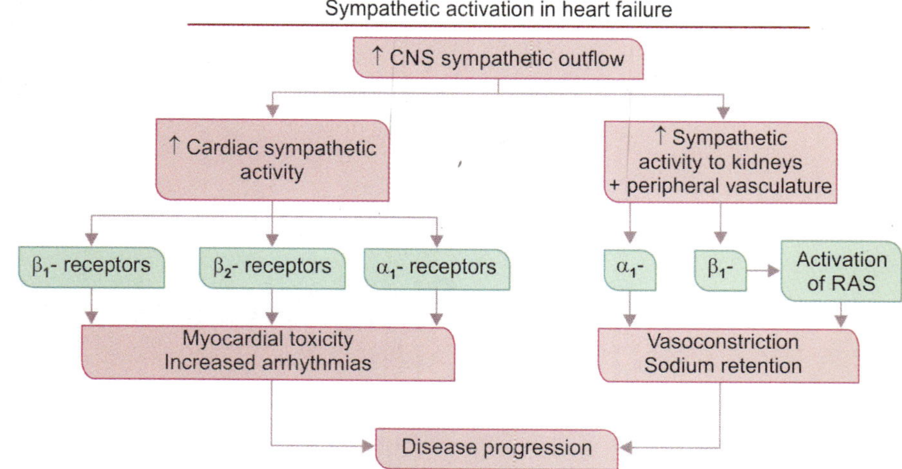

Fig. 1: Neurohormonal compensatory mechanism—sympathetic nervous system.
(CNS: central nervous system; RAS: renin-angiotensin system)
Source: Packer M. Beta-adrenergic blockade in chronic heart failure: principles, progress, and practice. Prog Cardiovasc Dis. 1998;41(Suppl 1):39-52.

on myocardial function. All the major changes associated with LV remodeling: LV dilatation, acquisition of a spherical shape, and mitral regurgitation, were reduced by the long-term administration of beta-blockers with a concomitant, highly significant, improvement in LVEF.[12-14] The magnitude of these changes is actually greater than that described with ACE inhibitors. Randomized controlled trials, having mortality as primary endpoint, showed the beneficial effects of beta-blockers on mortality and hospitalizations, with reductions in sudden cardiac deaths (SCD), HF deaths, cardiovascular hospitalizations, and HF hospitalizations.[15-16] This has led to the indication for beta-blocker therapy for all patients with chronic HF who do not have major contraindications.[4,7,17] Based on the results of early postinfarction trials as well as of the more recent Carvedilol Post-Infarct Survival Control in LV Dysfunction (CAPRICORN) trial,[18] beta-blockers are also recommended in patients with LV systolic dysfunction following myocardial infarction, regardless of whether they are symptomatic or not for HF.[4,7]

Bisoprolol has been extensively studied in the patients with chronic HF. In the following sections of this article we will describe its main pharmacokinetic and pharmacodynamics characteristics with respect to the treatment of HF.

ESSENTIAL CLINICAL PHARMACOLOGY

Beta-receptor Selectivity

Bisoprolol has high selectivity for beta-1 ARs with a beta-1 to beta-2 antagonist activity ratio of 75. Its selectivity for beta-1 ARs is higher compared with metoprolol, the other selective beta-blockers used in the treatment of HF

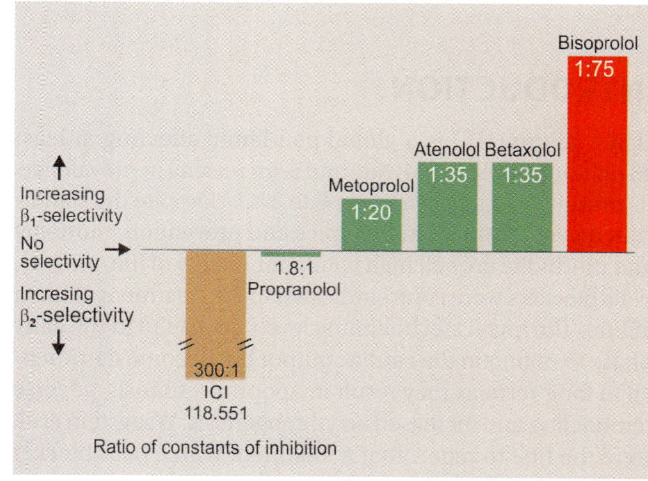

Fig. 2: Beta-1 to beta-2 selectivity ratios determined in ligand binding studies.

(beta-1 to beta-2 ratio, 20)[10] (Fig. 2). This high selectivity leads to better tolerability in patients with concomitant chronic obstructive pulmonary disease (COPD) as well as with peripheral vascular disease.[19-21]

Pharmacokinetics

Bisoprolol is almost completely absorbed in the enteric tract (90%) with very low liver first pass metabolism (10%). It has low plasma protein binding (30%) with a 1:1 ratio between hepatic metabolism and renal excretion (Fig. 3). In normal subjects, its half-life is long (10–11 hours) and is further prolonged in patients with HF (17 ± 5 hours) and/or with severe renal failure allowing once-daily administrations.[22] Bisoprolol does not interfere with the metabolism of other drugs.

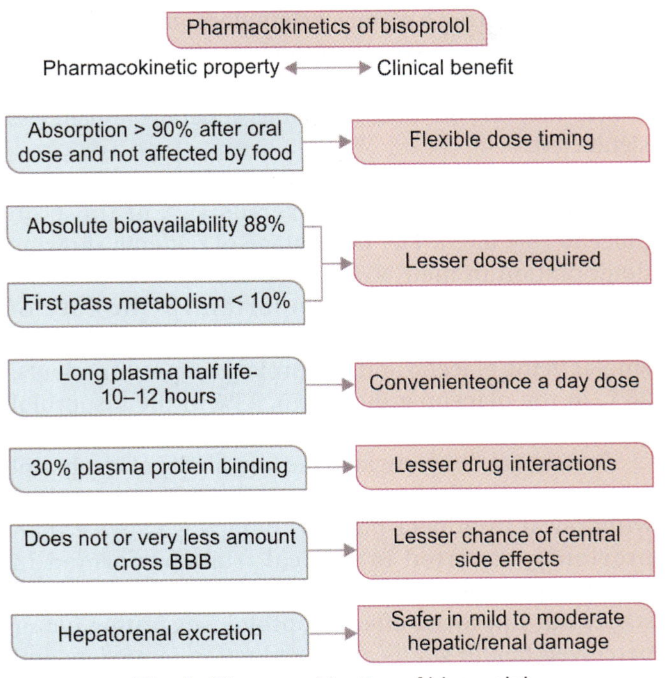

Fig. 3: Pharmacokinetics of bisoprolol.
(BBB: blood–brain barrier)
Source: Leopold G, Pabst J, Ungethüm W, Bühring KU. Basic pharmacokinetics of bisoprolol, a new highly beta-1 selective adrenoceptor antagonits. J Clin Pharmacol. 1986;26(8):616-21.

Modes of Administration

As with all beta-blockers in patients with HF, bisoprolol should be started with low doses with gradual (1- to 2-week intervals) uptitration to target doses. Treatment is generally started with 1.25 mg once daily with subsequent uptitration to 2.5 mg, 3.75 mg, 5 mg, 7.5 mg, and 10 mg/daily, if tolerated.[15] Interestingly, target dose of bisoprolol was 5 mg in the first Cardiac Insufficiency Bisoprolol Study (CIBIS) trial, in which bisoprolol did not significantly reduce mortality, while it was 10 mg in CIBIS-II, in which bisoprolol reduced mortality. Taking into account the differences in the initial as well as in the target doses (carvedilol, 3.125 mg bid to 25–50 mg bid, metoprolol succinate, 12–25 mg to 200 mg daily), similar protocols for initiation of therapy and uptitration must be used also for the other beta-blockers approved for HF treatment.[4,7,17]

The dose of the beta-blockers may be reduced in case of worsening HF or other adverse hemodynamic effects (hypotension and bradycardia). This may occur during the uptitration phase or, less often, while the patient is on stable maintenance doses. Bisoprolol, like any other beta-blocker indicated for HF treatment, should be completely withdrawn only in case of absolute intolerance. In addition to hemodynamic reasons (hypotension and bradycardia), the only absolute contraindication to beta-blocker treatment is asthma sensitive to the administration of beta-2 ARs agonists.[4,7,17,19] Patients with bronchial asthma may, however, show better tolerance to bisoprolol, compared with other beta-blockers, because of its greater beta-1 ARs selectivity.

Bisoprolol, like all other beta-blockers, should not be stopped abruptly as this may cause tachycardia, tachyarrhythmias, angina, and worsening HF. If the discontinuation is necessary, the dose should be decreased gradually.

EFFECTS IN THE PATIENTS WITH HEART FAILURE

Heart Rate

As expected with beta-blocker treatment, bisoprolol administration is associated with a reduction in HR. This has been consistently shown in CIBIS (–16.3 ± 15.3 vs –1.6 ± 13.4 bpm with bisoprolol and placebo, respectively; p < 0.001), as well as in CIBIS II (-9.8 ± 14.7 vs -0.2 ± 13.7 bpm with placebo).[23,24] In CIBIS, the changes in HR were predictive of survival, with a *longer survival in patients showing the greatest decrease in HR.*[23] Similarly, in CIBIS II, both baseline HR and its changes after 2 months of treatment were related to survival.[24] This analysis also showed that the beneficial effects of beta-blocker therapy (e.g. bisoprolol) were independent of the HR changes. *Patients on bisoprolol had a better survival, compared with those on placebo,* both in the subgroups of patients with lower or higher HR at baseline and in the patients with no change, a decrease or an increase in HR from baseline.

Blood Pressure

In CIBIS-II, bisoprolol reduced BP from baseline (–4.1 ± 16.4 vs –2.3 ± 16.4 mm Hg with placebo for systolic BP, and –2.6 ± 10.7 vs –0.9 ± 10.9 mm Hg with placebo, p < 0.0001 in both cases). There was no relation between changes in blood pressure and mortality in CIBIS.[23,24]

Left Ventricular Function

Bisoprolol is a beta-blocker with high selectivity for beta-1 ARs. It has no intrinsic sympathomimetic activity and no membrane stabilizing activity. Lacking of any ancillary property, it may probably be considered as "the purest" beta-1 AR blocker for the treatment of HF. Its hemodynamic effects in patients with HF were studied in single center trials[25-27] as well as in the two, large, randomized, placebo-controlled outcome trials.[15] In the study by Dubach et al.[26] the effects of bisoprolol on LV function were studied by nuclear magnetic resonance myocardial tagging in 28 patients with chronic HF randomized to bisoprolol or placebo. One-year treatment with bisoprolol was associated with an increase in LVEF (from 25 ± 7 to 36 ± 9%; $p < 0.05$) and a nonsignificant decline in LV end-diastolic and end-systolic volumes (–54 and –62 mL, respectively). No change occurred with placebo.

An improvement in LV function has been shown also with the other beta-blockers having beneficial effects on mortality in HF.[9,12,14] In a randomized comparison study, carvedilol has been associated with a greater improvement in LVEF, compared with metoprolol tartrate.[28] However, no comparison study with metoprolol succinate, as well as bisoprolol, has been concluded to our knowledge.

In a retrospective analysis of CIBIS, the changes in LV fractional shortening were related to subsequent prognosis both in the bisoprolol and the placebo groups. Patients who had a fractional shortening change >0.014 (median value) had a better survival than the others. The change in LV fractional shortening, the changes in HR, and bisoprolol administration were independent predictors of survival.[23]

These results were consistent with other studies showing that the changes in LVEF after beta-blocker therapy predict subsequent outcome.[29]

Neurohormonal Parameters and Inflammatory Markers

Pousset et al.[30] assessed HR variability (HRV) in 54 patients enrolled from CIBIS. Patients receiving bisoprolol showed an increase in HRV parameters related to parasympathetic activity [24-hour rMSSD (root mean square of successive RR interval differences), $p = 0.04$; 24-hour pNN50 (percentage of successive RR intervals that differ by more than 50 msec), $p = 0.04$; daytime SDNN (standard deviation of normal to normal intervals), $p = 0.05$ and daytime high-frequency power, $p = 0.03$]. These authors also analyzed scatterplots of R-R intervals consistently showing an increase in parameters related to parasympathetic tone with a decrease in parameters related to sympathetic tone.[31] All these changes are known to be associated with an improvement in prognosis.

Belenkov et al.[27] and colleagues showed that bisoprolol treatment can also decrease other neurohormonal parameters such as plasma rennin activity ($p < 0.05$), plasma levels of norepinephrine ($p < 0.05$), angiotensin II, and aldosterone ($p < 0.05$). Similarly to other beta-blockers, also the administration of bisoprolol has been associated with favorable effects on markers of inflammatory activity [tumor necrosis factor (TNF)-alpha, TNF-receptors, interleukins] both in animal models and clinical studies.[32-34]

Quality of Life

Beneficial effects on outcome are the main reason why beta-blocker therapy is now indicated for all the patients with HF who do not have major contraindications. However, an improvement in symptoms and quality of life remains the second important objective of treatment.[4,7] The effects of beta-blockers on these endpoints generally remain less significant.

In CIBIS, 21% of patients in the bisoprolol group improved their NYHA class versus 15% of those on placebo ($p < 0.03$). The percentage of patients showing deterioration in their NYHA class was similar between bisoprolol and placebo. Importantly, the rate of withdrawal of treatment caused by side-effects was similar in the placebo and bisoprolol groups (82 patients, 26%, in the placebo group vs 75, 23% in the bisoprolol group; nonsignificant).[35]

Baxter et al.[36] investigated the tolerability of bisoprolol treatment in elderly patients with CHF. The rate of withdrawal from beta-blocker therapy was twice than previously reported in clinical trials performed in younger patients. Quality of life, assessed through a score, was improved after bisoprolol, suggesting better perceived health status and a reduction in anxiety and depression.

EFFICACY STUDIES: CARDIAC INSUFFICIENCY BISOPROLOL STUDY TRIALS

Bisoprolol fumarate has the advantage to have been studied largely in three major mortality trials in stable CHF patients, demonstrating the important benefits of this beta-1 blocking agent and its good tolerability.

Cardiac Insufficiency Bisoprolol Study

Cardiac insufficiency bisoprolol study (CIBIS) was the *first randomized, double-blind, placebo-controlled study with the primary objective to evaluate the impact of bisoprolol on mortality in patients with heart failure.*[35]

Inclusion Criteria

- Ambulatory CHF patients in New York Heart Association (NYHA) class III–IV
- Left ventricular ejection fraction <40%, receiving diuretics and vasodilator therapy and not registered on a waiting list for heart transplantation.

Outcomes

- Primary endpoint was mortality
- Secondary endpoints were the tolerability of bisoprolol and analysis of all critical events.

An important prerequisite before inclusion was the need of a clinical phase of stability, without any episode

TABLE 1: Clinical characteristics of the different CIBIS[a] trials.

	CIBIS	*CIBIS-II*	*CIBIS-III*
n	641	2,647	1,010
Age, years (mean)	59	61	72
Female	17%	19%	32%
NYHA class III/IV	95%/5%	83%/17%	50%/0%
Ischemic heart failure	55%	50%	62%
Idiopathic dilated cardiomyopathy	36%	12%	10%
ACEI	90%	96%	-
Diuretics	100%	99%	90%
Heart rate, bpm	83 ± 1.5	81 ± 15	79 ± 13
Systolic blood pressure, mm Hg	126	130 ± 19	134 ± 17
Diastolic blood pressure, mm Hg	78	80 ± 11	80 ± 10
LVEF (%)	25 ± 0.9	27 ± 6	28.8 ± 5
Mean dose bisoprolol, mg	3.8 ± 0.2		

[a]for CIBIS, quantitative results are presented as mean ± SEM.

(ACEI: angiotensin converting enzyme inhibitor; CIBIS: Cardiac Insufficiency Bisoprolol Studies; LVEF: left ventricular ejection fraction)

of heart failure decompensation and the absence of major modification of heart failure therapy in the last 3 weeks before randomization.

The initial dose of bisoprolol was 1.25 mg once daily, which could be increased 48 hours later to 2.5 mg/day and 1 month after to the maximal dose of 5 mg/day. It was not a forced titration procedure and each investigator was free to give to their patient, according to their clinical status, one of the four doses: 1.25, 2.5, 3.75, or 5 mg/day.

Cardiac insufficiency bisoprolol study enrolled 641 patients with CHF with age between 18 years and 75 years, in NYHA class III in the vast majority (609, 95%). Clinical characteristics are summarized in Table 1.

Findings of the Study

- There were fewer deaths in the bisoprolol group (53 deaths, 16.6%) as compared to the placebo group (67 deaths, 20.9%) but this difference did not reach statistical significance (Fig. 4).
- Subgroup analyses showed additional benefits for certain patient groups:
  - Significant reduction in mortality ($p < 0.01$) in patients without history of myocardial infarction (MI) by 47% (Fig. 5).
  - Significant reduction in mortality ($p = 0.01$) in patients with dilated cardiomyopathy (DCM) by 53%.

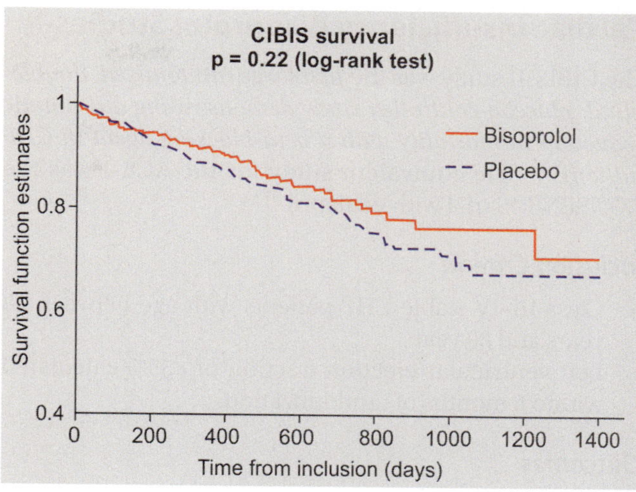

Fig. 4: Survival curves in cardiac insufficiency bisoprolol studies (CIBIS) patients.

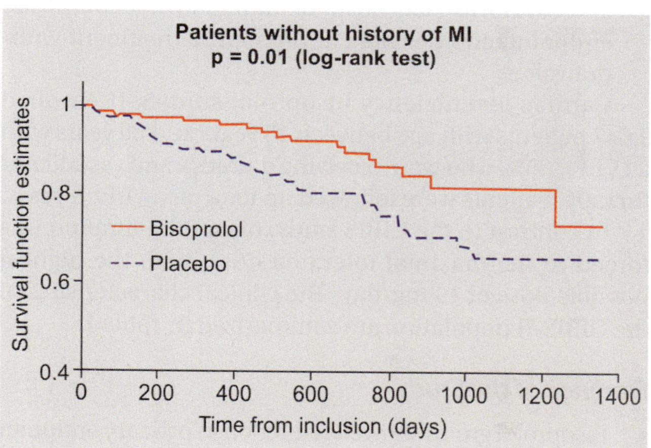

Fig. 5: Survival curves in cardiac insufficiency bisoprolol studies (CIBIS) patients without history of myocardial infarction (MI).

  - Significant reduction in mortality ($p = 0.05$) in patients with a ventricular rate >80 bpm by 42%.
  - No significant difference was seen in sudden death rate (17 on placebo, 15 on bisoprolol) or death related to documented ventricular tachycardia or fibrillation (7 on placebo, 4 on bisoprolol).
  - Bisoprolol group shown 21% improvement in one NYHA class as compared to 15% in the placebo group ($p = 0.04$).
  - Substantially fewer patients needed hospitalization for cardiac decompensation (61 on bisoprolol vs 90 on placebo, $p < 0.01$).

Despite this negative result, CIBIS was a very important study demonstrating the good tolerability of bisoprolol in a large CHF population, without evidence for any harmful effect of the beta-blocker therapy.

Cardiac Insufficiency Bisoprolol Studies-II

The CIBIS-II study was the *first large randomized, double-blind, placebo-controlled study demonstrating a dramatic reduction in mortality with a beta-blocking agent in CHF patients.*[15] The equivalent study for the ACE-I was the CONSENSUS trial with enalapril.[37]

Inclusion Criteria

- Class III–IV stable CHF patients with age between 18 years and 80 years.
- Left ventricular ejection fraction of <35% calculated within 6 months of randomization.

Outcomes

- Primary endpoint was all-cause mortality.
- Secondary endpoints were all-cause hospital admissions, cardiovascular mortality, cardiovascular mortality and cardiovascular hospital admissions, a composite endpoint, and permanent premature treatment withdrawals.

Cardiac insufficiency bisoprolol studies-II enrolled 2,647 patients with age between 18 years and 80 years with a LVEF < 35%, who were receiving diuretics and vasodilator therapy. Patients were followed up for a mean of 1.3 years.

In contrast to the CIBIS study, bisoprolol titration was forced to the maximal tolerated dose, with the highest possible dose of 10 mg/day. The clinical characteristics of the CIBIS-II population are summarized in Table 1.

Findings of the Study

- Bisoprolol group showed reduction in primary endpoint as compared to the placebo group [156 (11.8% vs 228 917.3%)] (p < 0.0001).
- Bisoprolol group showed lower annual mortality rate as compared to placebo group (8.8% vs 13.2%) hazard ratio 0.66 (95% CI: 0.54–0.81) (Fig. 6).
- Patients on bisoprolol showed significantly fewer cardiovascular deaths than placebo (p = 0.0049).
- Bisoprolol group showed significantly lesser admissions to hospital for all causes than placebo (p = 0.0006) as well as the combined endpoint of cardiovascular death and admission to hospital for cardiovascular events were lower in the bisoprolol group (p = 0.0004).
- Placebo group showed significantly higher number of sudden deaths as compared to bisoprolol group (83 vs 43) with a difference of 42% (p = 0.0011).
- 32% of difference in admissions to hospital for worsening heart failure was identified between the two groups.
- *Cardiac insufficiency bisoprolol studies-II is the only landmark trial which have analyzed the efficacy of BBs (Bisoprolol) in HF at low, moderate and high dose (Fig. 7).*

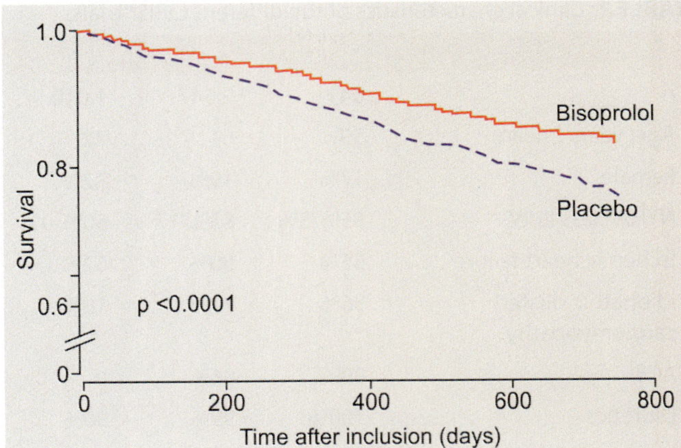

Fig. 6: Survival curves in cardiac insufficiency bisoprolol studies-II (CIBIS-II).

Bisoprolol induced a significant heart rate reduction (of 9.8 ± 14.7 beats/min), with a limited effect on blood pressure (systolic blood pressure reduction of 4.1 ± 16.4 mm Hg with bisoprolol but of 2.3 ± 16.4 mm Hg with placebo).[24]

The study was prematurely stopped because of the significant mortality benefit associated with bisoprolol.

The magnitude of the benefit was similar in NYHA subclasses, and independent of the etiology of heart failure. However, in patients with atrial fibrillation (n = 521, 20%), bisoprolol did not decrease total mortality when compared with placebo. This result must be taken with caution because of the limited number of patients with atrial fibrillation and the retrospective nature of the analysis.[24] Although heart rate at baseline and heart rate reduction were independently associated with survival, there was no interaction with bisoprolol, suggesting that the beneficial effect of bisoprolol was not influenced by these two parameters, and in particular by the extent of the heart rate reduction.[24]

In CIBIS, retrospective analysis suggested that patients with a LVEF ≤ 20% benefit more from bisoprolol than other patients.[38] However, this was not confirmed in CIBIS-II, where the beneficial effect of bisoprolol was independent of the level of left ventricular dysfunction.

Cardiac Insufficiency Bisoprolol Studies-III

The third important study with bisoprolol in CHF patients was *designed to determine what drug to initiate in a de novo, stable, CHF patient, either ACEI or beta-blocker.*[39] Because the beneficial effects of ACEI have been demonstrated first,[37] all the subsequent studies have studied the impact on mortality of a new drug or device on top of ACEI.[40] This question is of importance since the effects of beta-blockers in CHF patients are observed

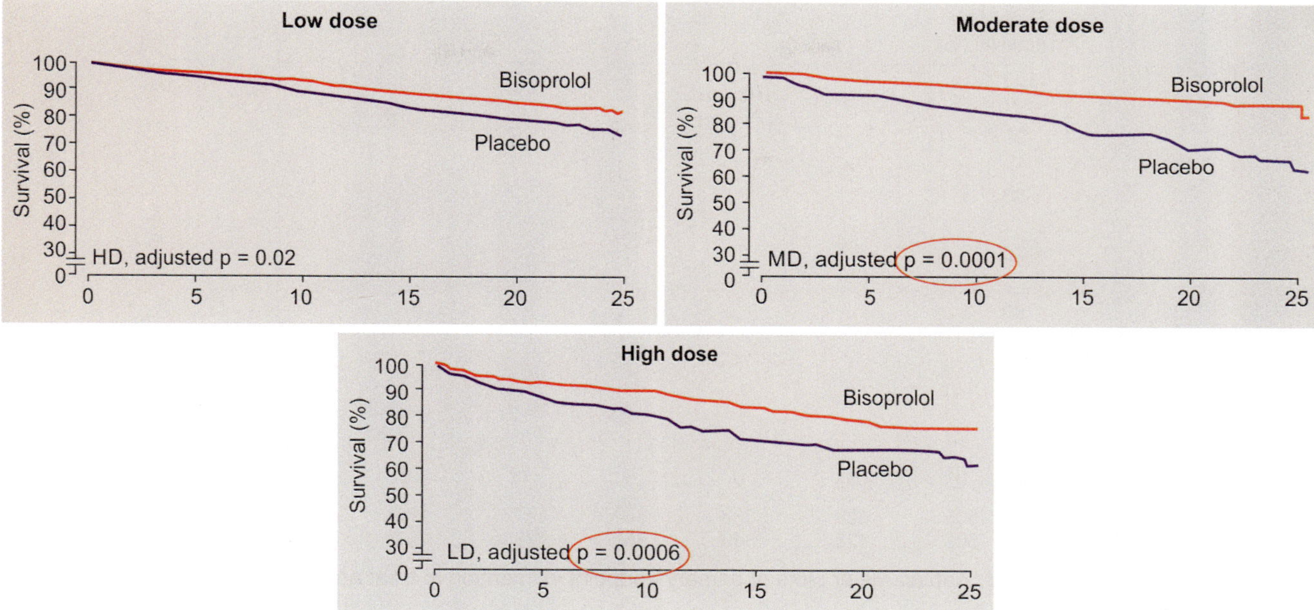

Fig. 7: Kaplan Meier survival curves in patients receiving placebo and bisoprolol at low dose, moderate dose and high dose.

quickly after their introduction, in particular with a reduction of sudden cardiac death, which is the most prevalent cause of death in this population. Moreover, instead of ACEI that blocks one system, beta-blockers effectively inhibit two systems, the sympathetic system and the renin angiotensin system.

Cardiac insufficiency bisoprolol studies-III was a multicenter, prospective, randomized, open label, blinded endpoint evaluation study, with two parallel groups.

Inclusion Criteria

- Patients older than 65 years in NYHA class II or III
- LVEF ≤ 35% and of course receiving neither ACEI nor beta-blocker.

All patients were clinically stable for at least 7 days before the inclusion. As in CIBIS-II, the titration was forced, depending on patient's tolerance, for both drugs with a target dose of 10 mg/day for bisoprolol and of 20 mg/day for enalapril.

There were two phases of treatment:

1. A monotherapy phase of 6 months, in which patients were randomized to receive either the β-blocker bisoprolol or the ACE inhibitor enalapril.
2. A combination therapy phase which varied in length as per the date of randomization, from 6 months (last included patient) to 1.5 years (all patients completed the study on the same day). Since the recruitment period was prolonged to 1.5 years, the combination therapy phase varied from 6 months to 2 years.

Outcomes

- The primary outcome was time-to-the-first-event of combined all-cause mortality or all-cause hospitalization throughout the study period.
- Secondary outcome was the combined endpoint at the end of the monotherapy phase and the individual components of the primary endpoint at the study end, as well as at the end of the monotherapy phase.

Cardiac insufficiency bisoprolol studies-III was designed as a noninferiority trial comparing the impact on the primary endpoint of the initiation of bisoprolol first compared with enalapril. CIBIS-III enrolled 1,010 patients who were followed during a mean period of 1.22 ± 0.42 years. Clinical characteristics of the study population are presented in Table 1. Because of the different inclusion criteria, some characteristics of CIBIS-III patients were different compared with those of patient enrolled in previous CIBIS studies. Patients in CIBIS-III were older, more often female, and less symptomatic (no NYHA class IV patients and half of the population was in NYHA class II). The results did not demonstrate any significant difference between the two strategies.

Findings of the Study

- The primary endpoint (all-cause mortality or all-cause hospitalizaton) occurred in 178 patients (35.2%) allocated to bisoprolol first versus 186 (36.8%) allocated to enalapril in the intention to treat (ITT) population: absolute difference—1.6%, 95% CI for absolute difference -7.6 to + 4.45; p = 0.019 (Fig. 8).

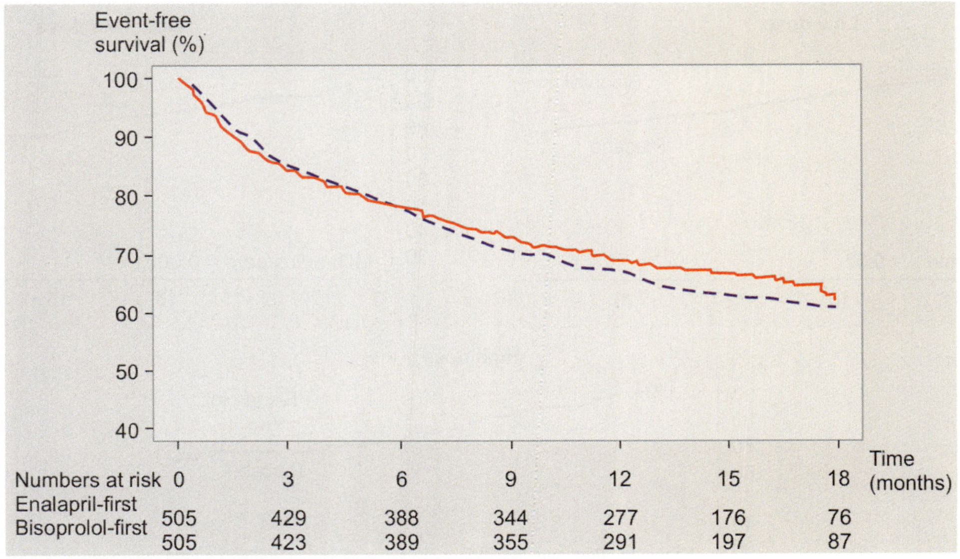

Fig. 8: Kaplan Meier plots of primary endpoint in intention to treat analysis.

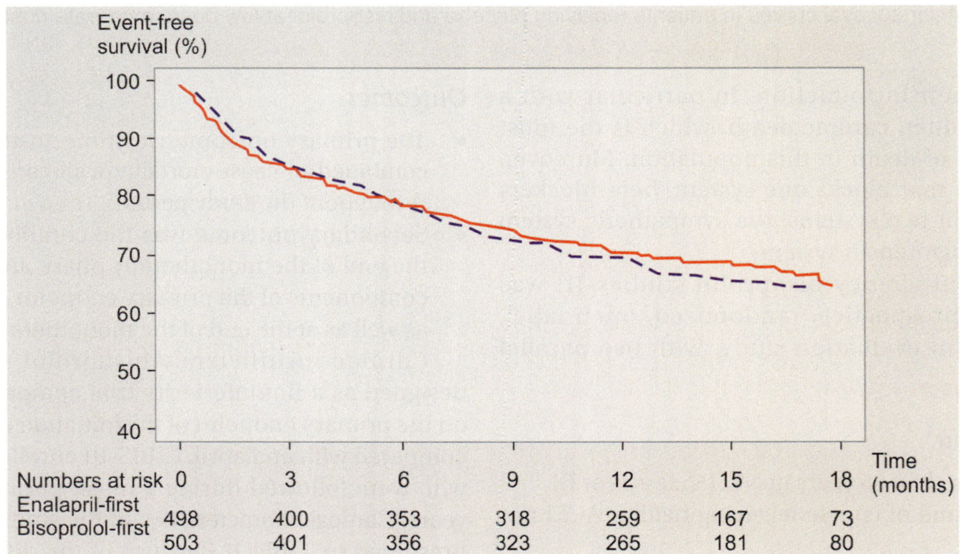

Fig. 9: Kaplan Meier plots of combined primary endpoints in per protocol populations.

- There were 163 events (32.4%) in the bisoprolol group versus 165 (33.1%) in the enalapril group in the per protocol (PP) population; the absolute difference for the primary endpoint was—0.7%, 95% CI, p = 0.04633. (Fig. 9).

There were fewer deaths in the bisoprolol-first group than in the enalapril first group, but the difference was not statistically significant [65 vs 73, HR: 0.88 (0.63–1.22), p = 0.44]. There was a nonsignificant increase in the number of patients having a hospitalization for worsening CHF in the bisoprolol first group compared with the enalapril-first group [63 vs 51 patients, respectively, HR = 1.25 (0.87–1.81), p = 0.23]. We can conclude, from the results of the CIBIS-III trial, that there was no difference in terms of efficacy and safety between the two strategies of treatment initiation in stable CHF patients.

Tolerability

Controlled trials have shown that treatment with bisoprolol is well tolerated. In CIBIS trials, withdrawal rates for lack of tolerance to bisoprolol were similar to placebo. Contraindications to bisoprolol initiation are the same as with all other beta-blockers and are clearly summarized in guidelines. They include sinus bradycardia, atrioventricular block, bronchial asthma sensitive to beta-agonist administration.[4,7,17,19] A recent episode of HF decompensation is a contraindication to the initiation of bisoprolol treatment, although recent data have shown that beta-blockers can be initiated during the same hospitalization caused by acute HF and this allows higher doses to be reached and better long-term outcome.[41]

Bisoprolol treatment as well as treatment with any other beta-blocker still needs implementation in clinical practice. Beta-blocker therapy is still underused and underdosed.[42]

Bisoprolol versus Carvedilol and Metoprolol in Heart Failure and Chronic Obstructive Pulmonary Disease

- In patients with coexisting HF and COPD, a study demonstrated a dose-response survival benefit of bisoprolol use, but not of carvedilol or metoprolol use.[43]
- The study included 11,558 subjects, with a mean follow-up period of 4.07 years.
- After adjustment for age, sex, comorbidities, and severity of HF and COPD, bisoprolol use showed a dose-response survival benefit [low dose: adjusted hazard ratio (HR) = 0.76, P = 0.030; high dose: adjusted HR = 0.40, P < 0.001] compared with nonusers, whereas no survival difference was observed for carvedilol or metoprolol.
- Compared with patients with HF alone, this special HF + COPD cohort received significantly fewer targeted β-blockers (P < 0.001) and bisoprolol (P < 0.001).

Role of Bisoprolol in Nephro Patients

Beta-blocker dialyzability and mortality in older patients receiving hemodialysis: Hemodialysis allows certain beta-blockers to be efficiently removed from the circulation (high dialyzability) whereas others are not removed (low dialyzability). This characteristic may impact the effectiveness of the beta-blockers among patients receiving long-term hemodialysis. Weir et al. conducted a propensity matched population-based retrospective cohort study using the linked healthcare databases of Ontario, Canada to determine whether new use of a high dialyzability beta-blocker compared with a low dialyzability beta-blocker associates with a higher rate of mortality in patients older than age 66 years receiving long-term hemodialysis.[44]

Patients were divided into:

- High dialyzability group (n = 3,294) (patients initiating atenolol, acebutolol, or metoprolol)
- Low dialyzability group (n = 3,294) (patients initiating bisoprolol or propanolol)

Results observed were:[44]

- In the hemodialysis cohort, a higher relative risk (RR) of death 40% was seen in patients prescribed a high dialyzability beta-blocker as compared to those prescribed a low dialyzability beta-blocker [RR: 1.4; 95% confidence interval (95%CI), 1.1–1.8; p < 0.01].
- The absolute risk increase was 1.4%, giving a number needed to harm of 71.
- The composite of death, myocardial infarction, or heart failure occurred more frequently in those prescribed a high dialyzability beta-blocker [RR: 1.2; (95% CI, 1.0–1.5; p = 0.03)].

GUIDELINES RECOMMENDING BETA-BLOCKERS

American College of Cardiology/American Heart Association 2017 Guidelines

Pharmacological Treatment for Stage C Heart Failure with Reduced Ejection Fraction Recommendations[45]

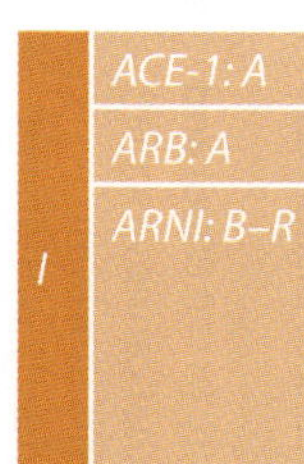

The clinical strategy of inhibition of the renin-angiotensin system with ACE inhibitors (*Level of Evidence: A*), *OR* ARBs (*Level of Evidence: A*), *OR* ARNI (Level of Evidence: B-R) in conjunction with evidence-based beta blockers, and aldosterone antagonists in selected patients, is recommended for patients with chronic HFrEF to reduce morbidity and mortality.

"Initial recommended dose of bisoprolol is 1.25 mg QD to maximum 10 mg QD".

European Society of Cardiology 2016 Guidelines

Pharmacological Treatments Indicated in Patients with Symptomatic (NYHA II-IV) Heart Failure with Reduced Ejection Fraction[46]

A beta-blocker is recommended, in addition an ACE-I, for patients with stable, symptomatic HFrEF to reduce the risk of HF hospitalization and death.

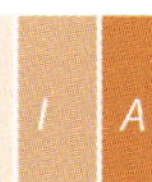

Recommendations to Prevent or Delay the Development of Overt Heart Failure or Prevent Death before the Onset of Symptoms

Beta-blocker is recommended in patients with asymptomatic LV systolic dysfunction and a history of myocardial infarction, in order to prevent or delay the onset of HF and prolong life.

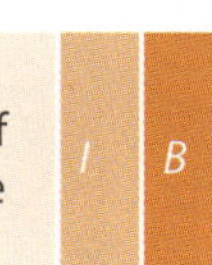

"Initial recommended dose of bisoprolol is 1.25 mg QD to maximum 10 mg QD".

INDIAN HEART FAILURE GUIDELINES 2017

Beta-blockers to be initiated only when the patient is:[47]

- Mobile
- Off IV diuretics and inotropes
- Having no systemic or pulmonary congestion
- Mobilized

"Start a very low dose of any approved beta-blocker (carvedilol, metoprolol succinate or bisoprolol) and build up the dose very gradually. Bisoprolol (1.25 mg QD->10 mg QD) is recommended".

Bisoprolol as in Various Studies (Table 2)

TABLE 2: Bisoprolol as in various studies.

Trial	*Medication dose/dosage*	*Target patient population*	*Clinical outcomes*	*Conclusion*
CIBIS-II investigators and committees, Lancet 1999	Bisoprolol 1.25 mg vs placebo	2,647 symptomatic patients in NYHA III or IV, with LVEF < 35% receiving standard therapy with diuretics and ACE inhibitors	• CIBIS-II was stopped early, after the second interim analysis, because bisoprolol showed a significant mortality benefit • All-cause mortality was significantly reduced with bisoprolol than with placebo • Significantly fewer sudden deaths among patients on bisoprolol than in those on placebo	Bisoprolol therapy reported to be beneficial for survival in stable heart failure patients
Funck Bretano C, et al. Am Heart J. 2001	Bisoprolol vs placebo	2,647 symptomatic patients in NYHA III or IV	• Withdrawal from bisoprolol therapy was more frequent in patients whose baseline heart rate was in the lower tertile of the distribution ($p = 0.0002$) but otherwise was not different between patients randomized to bisoprolol and placebo • Bisoprolol reduces mortality ($p = 0.0006$) and hospitalizations for nonlethal cardiovascular events ($p = 0.003$) in patients in whom treatment was not permanently withdrawn • Analysis of survival curves in patients who permanently discontinued treatment showed that bisoprolol did not reduce mortality compared with placebo in this population (RR: 1.03, 95% CI: 0.67; $p = 0.88$). Recurrent nonlethal events were reduced by bisoprolol.	In CIBIS-II, medical events were significantly influenced by treatment withdrawal. Patients who derive benefit from bisoprolol therapy are those in whom treatment is not permanently withdrawn
Simon T, et al. Circulation. 2001	Bisoprolol	2,647 patients with CHF	• Probability of all-cause mortality was significantly reduced by 36% in women compared to that in men • Bisoprolol shows 39% reduction in cardiovascular deaths among women and 70% reduction in deaths from pump failure compared with men • Bisoprolol shows significant reduction in all-cause mortality among women compared with men but not among women treated with placebo	In CIBIS-II, bisoprolol reduced the mortality rates for both men and women. Despite this beneficial effect, female sex is a significant independent predictor of survival in patients with severe heart failure

Contd...

Contd...

Trial	*Medication dose/dosage*	*Target patient population*	*Clinical outcomes*	*Conclusion*
Belenkov IuN, et al. Kardiologia, 2003	Bisoprolol 1.25 mg to 10 mg/day vs control	54 patients with NYHA III or IV and LVEF < 35%	• Bisoprolol shows improvement of heart failure functional class, lowering of heart rate (by 14%, $p < 0.01$), elevation of systolic blood pressure (by 7.2 ± 12.3 mm Hg, $p < 0.01$) and increase of walking distance (by 30.1 ± 29 m, $p < 0.01$) • No significant changes of these parameters occurred in control group. • Bisoprolol shows improvement in left ventricular end-diastolic and end-systolic volumes (by 85 ± 69.2 and 71 ± 51.5 mL, respectively, $p < 0.001$) and of LVEF (by 5.7+/7.3%, $p < 0.01$) after 12 months • These changes were significantly ($p < 0.0001$) higher than those in control group. • Bisoprolol reduces plasma renin activity (from 1.2 to 0.42 ng/mL/h), plasma concentrations of angiotensin II (from 17.1 to 13.1 pg/mL) and aldosterone (from 173 pg/mL to 148 pg/mL, $p < 0.05$)	Long-term use of bisoprolol was associated with improved clinical and hemodynamic status, increased systolic BP, blocked processes of pathological LV remodeling, lowered activity of not only sympathetic adrenal but also of main components of renin angiotensin system and improved heart rate variability
Jose R et al. Rev Esp Cardiol. 2003	Bisprolol 1.25 to 10 mg/day vs conventional treatment	334 patients with stable systolic heart failure	• 63% of the patients attained the maximum targeted dose; the mean dose at the end of follow up was 8.5 mg • Functional status, quality of life and ejection fraction improved significantly between the beginning and end of study	Bisoprolol can be used for therapy in a high percentage of outpatients with stable chronic heart failure, with acceptable tolerability at the maximum recommended dose
Simon T, et al. European Heart J. 2003	Bisoprolol vs placebo	2,647 patients with CHF	• Treatment withdrawal was associated with a significant increase in mortality in the bisoprolol group • Bisoprolol group shows significant reduction in all-cause mortality compared to placebo regardless of the dose level considered	Bisoprolol reduces mortality in CHF patients at all tolerated dose levels and its withdrawal increases the risk of mortality. Efforts should be made to maintain bisoprolol therapy based on individual patients tolerability
Groote P de, et al. Annals of Cardiology and Angiology, 2004	Bisoprolol (mean dose 8.8 ± 2.4 mg/d)	201 patients with stable CHF	• Bisoprolol shows significant improvement in NYHA classification • Bisoprolol shows significant reduction in HR at rest from 87 ± 17 to 66 ± 12 beats/min without any effect on ECG parameters • Bisoprolo shows significant improvement in LVEF from 31 ± 11 to 41 ± 13% ($p < 0.0001$), and significant decrease in end diastolic and end systolic LV diameters and volumes	Bisoprolol significantly improved LVEF with a reverse remodeling of the left ventricle, a decrease in hormonal activation and a modest improvement in exercise capacity

Contd...

Contd...

Trial	Medication dose/dosage	Target patient population	Clinical outcomes	Conclusion
			• Bisoprolol shows significant reduction in plasma levels of A type and of B type natriuretic peptides and of norepinephrines	
Dobre D, et al. Cardiovasc Drugs. 2008	1.25 mg QD Bisoprolol vs 2.5 mg BID enalapril	1,010 patients with mild to moderate HF and age >65 years	• Bisoprolol shows similar effect as enalapril on the combined endpoint of all-cause mortality or hospitalization (HR: 1.02; $p = 0.90$), as well as on each of the individual endpoints • More cases of worsening HF requiring hospitalization or occurring while in hospital were observed in the bisoprolol group (HR: 1.67; $p = 0.03$)	Bisoprolol and enalapril shows similar effect on the combined endpoint of mortality or hospitalization during 6 months monotherapy
Konishi M, et al. Circulation J. 2010	Bisoprolol vs carvedilol	655 patients with HF, categorized as NYHA class III or IV	• After 18 months of follow up, there were no significant differences in the survival and cardiac event free rates between the two groups • Bisoprolol group shows significantly improvement in heart rate and brain natriuretic peptide level than in the carvedilol group • Furthermore, more patients in the bisoprolol group were defibrillated from AF to sinus rhythm than those in the carvedilol group (48% vs 16%; $p = 0.03$)	Both beta-blockers are equally effective in the improvement of severe HF, but bisoprolol shows favorable effects in the patients with AF
Funck-Brentano, et al. Eur J Heart Fail. 2011	Uptitration of monotherapy with either bisoprolol (target dose 10 mg OD) or enalapril (target dose 10 mg BID) for 6 months, followed by their combination for 6–24 months	1,010 patients with stable CHF	• The study drug (ACEI or beta-blockers) was last prescribed at ≥50% of target dose to significantly more patients for the first initiated drug in both treatment groups (both $p < 0.001$) • 60% of endpoints were reached during the monotherapy phase and randomized treatment during monotherapy was not a predictor of the three assessed outcomes • Monotherapy phase was the strongest independent predictor of the outcome ($p < 0.0001$ for all endpoints)	The order of drug administration plays an important role in whether in CHF patients reached in target doses of bisoprolol or enalapril. For both study drugs, the dose level reached was associated with baseline charachteristics and adverse events
Fong Su, et al. Medicine. 2016	Defined daily doses (DDDs) of carvedilol 6.25 mg; bisoprolol 1.25 mg; metoprolol 25 mg	11,558 subjects with HF and concurrent COPD	Bisoprolol use showed a dose response survival benefit (low dose: adjusted HR = 0.76, 95% CI = 0.59–0.97, $p = 0.030$; high dose: adjusted HR = 0.40, 95% CI = 0.26–0.63, $p < 0.001$, compared with nonusers, whereas no survival difference was observed for carvedilol or metoprolol	This study demonstrated the suboptimal use of beta-blockers and revealed a dose-dependent benefit of bisoprolol in patients with coexisting COPD and H. There is no survival benefit of the other two beta-blockers recommended by the HF guidelines (carvedilol and metoprolol)

Contd...

Contd...

Trial	*Medication dose/dosage*	*Target patient population*	*Clinical outcomes*	*Conclusion*
Frohlich H, et al. Clin Res Cardiol. 2017	Bisoprolol 5 mg/day (2.5–10), carvedilol 25 mg/day (12.5–50) and metoprolol succinate 100 mg/day (50–150)	6,010 outpatients with stable CHF and a reduced LVEF	• In univariable analysis of the overall cohort, patients prescribed bisoprolol and carvedilol therapy both had lower mortality when compared with those prescribed metoprolol succinate (HR 0.80, 95% CI 0.71–0.91, $p < 0.01$, and HR 0.86, 95% CI 0.78–0.94, $p < 0.01$, respectively) • Patients prescribed bisoprolol or carvedilol had similar mortality (HR 0.94, 95% CI 0.82–1.08, $p = 0.37$) • However, there was no significant association between beta-blocker choice and all-cause mortality in any of the matched samples (HR 0.90; 95% CI 0.76–1.06; $p = 0.20$; HR 1.10, 95% CI 0.93–1.31, $p = 0.24$; and HR 1.08, 95% CI 0.95–1.22, $p = 0.26$ for bisoprolol vs carvedilol, bisoprolol vs metoprolol succinate and carvedilol vs metoprolol succinate, respectively)	In an international, real world cohort of CHF patients with reduced ejection fraction, no difference in all-cause mortality for patients treated with bisoprolol, carvedilol or metoprolol succinate was found. In accordance with current guidelines, this analysis suggests that bisoprolol, carvedilol, and metoprolol succinate may be used interchangeably in the treatment of patients with CHF
Tsutsui H, et al. Circ J. 2019	Bisoprolol 5 mg/day vs carvedilol 20 mg/day	217 patients with HFrEF	• The primary endpoint was achieved in 41.4% of patients with bisoprolol and 42.5% in carvedilol groups • The noninferiority of tolerability of bisoprolol compared with carvedilol was not supported, however, neither beta-blocker was superior with regard to tolerability • Heart rate decreased in both groups and its decrease from baseline was significantly greater in the bisoprolol group (20.3 vs 15.4 beats/min at 24 weeks, $p < 0.05$) • Plasma b-type natriuretic peptide (BNP) levels decreased in both groups and the decrease was significantly greater in the carvedilol group (12.4 vs 39% at 24 weeks, $p < 0.05$)	There were no significant differences between bisoprolol and carvedilol in the tolerability of target doses in Japanese HFrEF patients. The clinical efficacy and safety were also similar despite the greater reduction in HR by bisoprolol and plasma BNP by carvedilol

(AF: atrial fibrillation; CHF: congestive heart failure; CIBS: cardiac insufficiency bisoprolol; COPD: chronic obstructive pulmonary disease; HF: heart failure; HFrEF: heart failure with reduced ejection fraction; HR: heart rate; NYHA: New York Heart Association)

CONCLUSION

Bisoprolol fumarate is a potent, highly beta-1 selective adrenergic blocker. Large RCTs have clearly demonstrated the beneficial effects of bisoprolol on mortality and on morbidity in patients with HFrEF. These favorable effects are associated with a reverse remodeling of the left ventricle and a significant improvement in LVEF.

Advantages of bisoprolol include:

- Excellent safety particularly in elderly patients, patients with chronic obstructive pulmonary disease and patients with renal failure
- Improved patient compliance because of once a day dosing
- Very low rate of drug withdrawal in RCTs
- Mortality reduction occurs all range of dosages, a virtue which no other beta-blocker has demonstrated.

Therefore, bisoprolol should be considered as a beta-blocker of choice for treating patients of HFrEF.

REFERENCES

1. Cowie MR, Mosterd A, Wood DA, et al. The epidemiology of heart failure. Eur Heart J. 1997;18:208-25.
2. Cleland JG, Khand A, Clark A. The heart failure epidemic: exactly how big is it? Eur Heart J. 2001;22:623-6.
3. Stewart S, MacIntyre K, Hole DJ, et al. More 'malignant' than cancer? Five-year survival following a first admission for heart failure. Eur J Heart Fail. 2001;3:315-22.
4. Swedberg K, Cleland J, Dargie H, et al. Task Force for the Diagnosis and Treatment of Chronic Heart Failure of the European Society of Cardiology. Guidelines for the diagnosis and treatment of chronic heart failure: executive summary (update 2005). Eur Heart J. 2005;26:1115-40.
5. Swedberg K, Hjalmarson A, Waagstein F, et al. Prolongation of survival in congestive cardiomyopathy by beta-receptor blockade. Lancet. 1979;1:1374-6.
6. Waagstein F, Hjalmarson A, Varnauskas E, et al. Effect of chronic beta-adrenergic receptor blockade in congestive cardiomyopathy. Br Heart J. 1975;37:1022-36.
7. Hunt SA, Abraham WT, Chin MH, et al. ACC/AHA 2005 Guideline Update for the Diagnosis and Management of Chronic Heart Failure in the Adult: a report of the American College of Cardiology/American Heart Association Task Force on Practice Guidelines (Writing Committee to Update the 2001 Guidelines for the Evaluation and Management of Heart Failure): developed in collaboration with the American College of Chest Physicians and the International Society for Heart and Lung Transplantation: endorsed by the Heart Rhythm Society. Circulation. 2005;112:e154-235.
8. Communal C, Singh K, Pimentel DR, et al. Norepinephrine stimulates apoptosis in adult rat ventricular myocytes by activation of the beta adrenergic pathway. Circulation. 1998;98:1329-34.
9. Lowes BD, Gilbert EM, Abraham WT, et al. Myocardial gene expression in dilated cardiomyopathy treated with beta-blocking agents. N Engl J Med. 2002;346:1357-65.
10. Bristow MR. Beta-adrenergic receptor blockade in chronic heart failure. Circulation. 2000;101:558-69.
11. Metra M, Nodari S, D'Aloia A, et al. A rationale for the use of beta-blockers as standard treatment for heart failure. Am Heart J. 2000;139:511-21.
12. Metra M, Nardi M, Giubbini R, et al. Effects of short- and long-term carvedilol administration on rest and exercise hemodynamic variables, exercise capacity and clinical conditions in patients with idiopathic dilated cardiomyopathy. J Am Coll Cardiol. 1994;24:1678-87.
13. Metra M, Nodari S, Bordonali T, et al. Beta-blocker therapy of heart failure: an update. Expert Opin Pharmacother. 2007;8:289-98.
14. Lechat P, Packer M, Chalon S, et al. Clinical effects of beta adrenergic blockade in chronic heart failure: a meta-analysis of double-blind, placebo-controlled, randomized trials. Circulation. 1998;98:1184-91.
15. CIBIS-II Investigators and Committees. The Cardiac Insufficiency Bisoprolol Study: a randomised trial. Lancet. 1999;353:9-13.
16. MERIT-HF Study Group. Effect of metoprolol CR/XL in chronic heart failure: Metoprolol CR/XL Randomised Intervention Trial in Congestive heart failure (MERIT-HF). Lancet. 1999;353:2001-7.
17. McMurray J, Cohen-Solal A, Dietz R, et al. Practical recommendations for the use of ACE inhibitors, beta-blockers, aldosterone antagonists and angiotensin receptor blockers in heart failure: putting guidelines into practice. Eur J Heart Fail. 2005;7:710-21.
18. The CAPRICORN Investigators. Effect of carvedilol on outcome after myocardial infarction in patients with left-ventricular dysfunction: the CAPRICORN randomised trial. Lancet. 2001;357:1385-90.
19. Metra M, Nodari S, D'Aloia A, et al. Beta blockers in heart failure: issues in the management of individual patients. Heart Fail Rev. 1999;4:65-77.
20. Sirak TE, Jelic S, Le Jemtel TH. Therapeutic update: non-selective beta- and alpha-adrenergic blockade in patients with coexistent chronic obstructive pulmonary disease and chronic heart failure. J Am Coll Cardiol 2004;44:497-502.
21. Le Jemtel TH, Padeletti M, Jelic S. Diagnostic and therapeutic challenges in patients with coexistent chronic obstructive pulmonary disease and chronic heart failure. J Am Coll Cardiol. 2007;49:171-80.
22. Leopold G, Kutz K. Bisoprolol: pharmacokinetic profile. Rev Contemp Pharmacother. 1997;8:35-43.
23. Lechat P, Escolano S, Golmard JL, et al. Prognostic value of bisoprolol-induced hemodynamic effects in heart failure during the Cardiac Insufficiency BIsoprolol Study (CIBIS). Circulation. 1997;96:2197-205.
24. Lechat P, Hulot JS, Escolano S, et al. Heart rate and cardiac rhythm relationships with bisoprolol benefit in chronic heart failure in CIBIS II trial. Circulation. 2001;103:1428-33.

25. Nyolczas N, Dékàny M, Fiòk J, et al. Prediction of the effect of bisoprolol in dilated cardiomyopathy. Cardiovasc Drugs Ther. 2000;14:543-50.
26. Dubach P, Myers J, Bonetti P, et al. Effects of bisoprolol fumarate on left ventricular size, function, and exercise capacity in patients with heart failure: analysis with magnetic resonance myocardial tagging. Am Heart J. 2002;143:676-83.
27. Belenkov IuN, Skvortsov AA, Mareev VIu, et al. Clinical, hemodynamic and neuorohumoral effects of long-term therapy of patients with severe chronic heart failure with beta-adrenoblocker bisoprolol. Kardiologiia. 2003;43:10-2.
28. Metra M, Giubbini R, Nodari S, et al. Differential effects of β-blockers in patients with heart failure. A prospective, double-blind comparison of the long-term effects of metoprolol versus carvedilol. Circulation. 2000;102:546-51.
29. Metra M, Nodari S, Parrinello G, et al. Marked improvement in left ventricular ejection fraction during long-term beta-blockade in patients with chronic heart failure: clinical correlates and prognostic significance. Am Heart J. 2003;145:292-9.
30. Pousset F, Copie X, Lechat P, et al. Effects of bisoprolol on heart variability in heart failure. Am J Cardiol. 1996;7:612-7.
31. Copie X, Pousset F, Lechat P, et al. Effects of β-blockade with bisoprolol on heart rate variability in advanced heart failure: Analysis of scatterplots or R-R intervals at selected heart rates. Am Heart J. 1996;132:369-75.
32. Ohtsuka T, Hamada M, Hiasa G, et al. Effect of beta-blockers on circulating levels of inflammatory and anti-inflammatory cytokines in patients with dilated cardiomyopathy. J Am Coll Cardiol. 2001;37:412-7.
33. von Haehling S, Genth-Zotz S, Bolger AP, et al. Effect of noradrenaline and isoproterenol on lipopolysaccharide-induced tumor necrosis factor-alpha production in whole blood from patients with chronic heart failure and the role of beta-adrenergic receptors. Am J Cardiol. 2005;95:885-9.
34. Ichihara S, Yamada Y, Ichihara G, et al. Attenuation of oxidative stress and cardiac dysfunction by bisoprolol in an animal model of dilated cardiomyopathy. Biochem Biophys Res Commun. 2006;350:105-13.
35. CIBIS Investigators and Committees. A Randomized Trial of beta blockade in heart failure. The Cardiac Insufficiency Bisoprolol Study (CIBIS). Circulation. 1994;90:1765-73.
36. Baxter AJ, Spensley A, Hildreth, et al. Beta-blockers in older persons with HF: tolerability and impact on quality of life. Heart. 2002;88:611-4.
37. The CONSENSUS Trial Study Group. Effects of enalapril on mortality in severe congestive heart failure. Results of the Cooperative North Scandinavian Enalapril Survival Study (CONSENSUS). N Engl J Med. 1987;316:1429-35.
38. Funck-Brentano C, Lancar R, Le Heuzey JY, et al. Predictors of medical events in patients enrolled in the cardiac insufficiency bisoprolol study (CIBIS): a study of the interactions between beta-blocker therapy and occurrence of critical events using analysis of competitive risks. Am Heart J. 2000;139:262-71.
39. Willenheimer R, van Veldhuisen DJ, Silke B, et al. Effect on survival and hospitalization of initiating treatment for chronic heart failure with bisoprolol followed by enalapril, as compared with the opposite sequence: results of the randomized Cardiac Insufficiency Bisoprolol Study (CIBIS) III. Circulation. 2005;112:2426-35.
40. Pitt B, Zannad F, Remme WJ, et al. The effect of spironolactone on morbidity and mortality in patients with severe heart failure. N Engl J Med. 1999;341:709-17.
41. Gattis WA, O'Connor CM, Gallup DS, et al. IMPACT-HF Investigators and Coordinators. Predischarge initiation of carvedilol in patients hospitalized for decompensated heart failure: results of the Initiation Management Predischarge: Process for Assessment of Carvedilol Therapy in Heart Failure (IMPACT-HF) trial. J Am Coll Cardiol. 2004;43:1534-41.
42. Galatius S, Gustafsson F, Atar D, et al. Tolerability of beta-blocker initiation and titration with bisoprolol and carvedilol in congestive heart failure—a randomized comparison. Cardiology. 2004;102:160-5.
43. Su VY, Chang YS, Hu YW et al. Carvedilol, Bisoprolol, and Metoprolol Use in Patients with Coexistent Heart Failure and Chronic Obstructive Pulmonary Disease. Medicine (Baltimore). 2016;95(5):e2427.
44. Weir MA, Dixon SN, Fleet JL, et al. Beta blocker dialyzability and mortality in older patients receiving hemodialysis. J Am Soc Nephrol. 2015;26(4):987-96.
45. Yancy CW, Jessup N, Bozkurt B, et al. 2017 ACC/AHA/HFSA Focussed Update of the 2013 ACCF/AHA Guideline for the Management of Heart Failure: A Report of the American College of Cardiology/American Heart Association Task Force on Clinical Practice Guidelines and the Heart Failure Society of America. J Card Fail. 2017;23(8):628-51.
46. Ponikowski P, Voors AA, Anker SD, et al. 2016 ESC Guidelines for the diagnosis and treatment of Acute and Chronic Heart Failure: The Task Force for the diagnosis and treatment of acute and chronic heart failure of the European Society of Cardiology (ESC) Developed with the special contribution of the Heart Failure Association (HFA) of the ESC. Eur Heart J. 2016;37(27):2129-200.
47. Seth S, Ramakrishnan S, Parekh N, et al. Heart failure guidelines for India: Update 2017. J Pract Cardiovasc Sci. 2017;3:133-8.

NOAСs, Atrial Fibrillation and Heart Failure

PP Mohanan

ATRIAL FIBRILLATION AND HEART FAILURE

Heart failure (HF) and atrial fibrillation (AF) frequently coexist, sharing risk factors and pathophysiological mechanisms.[1,2] AF is prevalent up to 41% of heart failure patients. AF is the most common heart rhythm disorder in the elderly, and has important consequences in terms of morbidity, mortality and healthcare costs. As with HF, the prevalence of AF rises exponentially with age: 0.12–0.16% in subjects aged <49 years; 3.7–4.2% in those aged 60–70 years; and 10–17% in subjects aged >80 years.[3] As a consequence, AF and HF frequently coexist, and the burden of AF and HF is expected to increase with population aging. Indeed, both conditions share common risk factors: Older age, hypertension, diabetes mellitus, valvular heart disease and ischemic heart disease.[4] Moreover, from a pathophysiological point of view, it is also well-known that HF and AF beget one another: HF is associated with increased left ventricular filling pressures contributing to left atrial dilatation and AF. On the other hand, the loss of atrial systole associated or not with tachycardia impairs left ventricular filling and contributes to HF.[5]

The reported prevalence of AF in various HF series ranges from 13 to 27% and increases with rising severity of HF; thus, patients with New York Heart Association (NYHA) functional class I symptoms have an AF prevalence of ≤4% versus approximately 40% in patients with class IV symptoms. The Framingham study showed that patients with AF or HF who subsequently develop the other condition have a poor prognosis, regardless of which condition came first.[6] In this study, AF preceded HF about as often as HF preceded AF. In a French observational survey constituting a single day snapshot of all unplanned hospitalizations because of acute HF in 1,658 patients (72% with history of chronic HF), AF was one of the main precipitating factors (24%), along with infection (27%).[7]

HF increases the risk of stroke and systemic embolism in AF, and this appears to be largely independent of the type and severity of HF.[8] In a systematic literature review to assess the effect of HF in patients with AF, Agarwal et al.[9] recently reported that in studies in which HF was based on a clinical diagnosis, HF independently increased stroke/systemic embolism in five of 13 studies, conferring a 1.6-fold to 3.1-fold increase in risk. When HF was defined as impaired left ventricular function, the additive risk was evident in four of six studies, with a 1.7-fold to 2.6-fold increase in the risk of stroke/systemic embolism.

Before the development of persistent or permanent AF, multiple episodes of paroxysmal AF can occur in patients with HF. Often these AF episodes are asymptomatic, making detection of the arrhythmia unreliable via conventional detection methods. The interrogation of cardiac implanted devices has shown in several trials that more than 20–27% and up to 42% of patients with severe congestive HF thought to be persistently in sinus rhythm were having episodes of asymptomatic paroxysmal AF.[10] As paroxysmal AF is more prevalent than persistent AF in patients with acute stroke or transient ischemic attack, these results raise the question of the need for a more extensive diagnostic effort to detect these episodes in order to prevent the occurrence of ischemic stroke more efficiently. The AF burden threshold that confers an increased risk of thromboembolism is not precisely defined. In a pooled analysis of five prospective studies including >10,000 relatively unselected patients with an implanted cardiac device and no history of permanent AF, daily AF burden is associated with an increased risk of ischemic stroke and transient ischemic attack; among the evaluated thresholds, 1 hour was associated with the highest HR for ischemic stroke.[11] Although there was no information in this analysis on the proportion of patients with HF, patients with silent AF could merit consideration for anticoagulation.

PREVENTION OF THROMBOEMBOLISM IN PATIENTS WITH HF AND AF: ROLE OF NOACS

Most patients with AF and HF have a CHA2DS2-VASc score ≥2; for example, in a nation-wide prospective cohort study using Danish registries, 93.5% of patients with AF and HF had a CHA2DS2-VASc score ≥2.[12]

Vitamin K antagonists and antiplatelet agents have, until recently, been the only drugs used in the prevention of thrombosis and thromboembolism. However, the slow onset of action and the narrow therapeutic index of warfarin, along with its multiple drug and diet interactions, have negative effects on safety, compliance and efficacy.[13] It is often challenging to maintain the international normalized ratio within the therapeutic range, and this seems particularly true for patients with HF treated with vitamin K antagonists. Thus, from a subanalysis of the atrial fibrillation follow-up investigation of rhythm management (AFFIRM) trial, history of congestive HF and symptoms of HF were associated with less time in the therapeutic range [61% in history of congestive HF and 58% in symptomatic HF versus 65% in the absence of one of these factors (P <0.009 in the first case and P <0.004 in the second case)]. Also, during congestive HF episodes, HF patients are more sensitive to warfarin because of modification of the metabolism of vitamin K antagonists that can lead to increased hemorrhagic risk. Moreover, the risk of bleeding in the AF population is increased by 43% when associated with HF.[14]

In contrast to vitamin K antagonists, nonvitamin K antagonist oral anticoagulants (NOACs) target only one coagulation enzyme: Either thrombin (dabigatran) or factor Xa (rivaroxaban, apixaban and edoxaban). These new anticoagulant drugs have recently demonstrated effective and safe protection against stroke and systemic embolism in AF.[15-18] The pivotal studies for the four NOACs were included in a meta-analysis by Ruff et al., which included 42,411 patients who received a NOAC and 29,272 who received warfarin.[19] The rate of stroke or systemic embolic events in patients treated with NOACs was significantly reduced by 19% in comparison with warfarin (P <0.0001). This decrease was mainly related to a reduction in the rate of hemorrhagic strokes (relative risk: 0.49). The rates of all-cause mortality and intracranial hemorrhages were also reduced, but the rate of gastrointestinal bleeding was increased (Table 1).

TABLE 1: Meta-analysis of randomized trials: Comparison of the efficacy and safety of nonvitamin K antagonist oral anticoagulants with warfarin in patients with atrial fibrillation.

	Relative risk: NOAC versus warfarin	*P*
Stroke or embolic events		
RELY[16]	0.66	0.0001
ROCKET-AF[18]	0.88	0.12
ARISTOTLE[17]	0.80	0.012
ENGAGE-AF[15]	0.88	0.10
Combined	0.81	<0.0001
Efficacy		
Ischemic stroke	0.92	0.10
Hemorrhagic stroke	0.49	<0.0001
Myocardial infarction	0.97	0.77
All-cause mortality	0.90	0.0003
Safety		
Intracranial hemorrhage	0.48	<0.0001
Gastrointestinal bleeding	1.25	0.043

a. Dabigatran 150 mg twice daily.
b. Rivaroxaban 20 mg once daily.
c. Apixaban 5 mg twice daily.
d. Edoxaban 60 mg once daily.
(NOAC: nonvitamin K antagonist oral anticoagulant)

Renal insufficiency is frequently associated with HF,[20] and has been identified as a risk factor for major bleeding; it is included in the HAS-BLED risk score for bleeding.[21] As NOACs are predominantly excreted by the kidney, they are contraindicated in patients with severe renal impairment (estimated glomerular filtration rate <30 mL/min). This could be a concern in many patients with HF, as stated in the latest European guidelines for HF which recommend serial monitoring of renal function when using NOACs.[22]

Meta-analysis of HF patients enrolled in the four major trials on NOACs—55,011 patients by Gianluigi Savarese investigated the overall effects of these drugs on major efficacy and safety end-points. In these four trials, NOACs achieved efficacy and safety outcomes that were at least as good as warfarin in patients with HF.[23]

In the ARISTOTLE trial, apixaban significantly reduced the risk of SSE compared with warfarin, and the subgroup analysis comparing patients with HF with reduced ejection fraction to patients without HF demonstrated no significant interaction between treatments and subgroups. Risks of intracranial, major, and total bleeding were significantly reduced by apixaban compared with warfarin in the main trial and to a similar degree in subgroups stratified by HF, with no evidence of subgroup by treatment interaction for these safety end-points.

In RELY, no differences in treatment efficacy were reported between HF and no-HF subgroups. In both the patients with and those without HF, intracranial and any bleeding were significantly reduced by dabigatran, 150 mg twice daily, whereas no differences were observed between dabigatran and warfarin for major bleeding

In ROCKET AF, rivaroxaban compared with warfarin did not significantly reduce the risks of SSE, bleeding, CV death, or overall mortality in patients with or in patients without HF. In ENGAGE AF-TIMI 48, edoxaban, 60 mg was similar to warfarin for the prevention of thromboembolism, regardless of the presence or absence of prior HF. In addition, edoxaban significantly reduced CV death and CV hospitalization even in patients with severe HF. Regardless of HF severity, edoxaban significantly reduced the risk of major bleeding and intracranial hemorrhage compared with warfarin.

CONCLUSION

Patients with concomitant AF and HF are a high-risk group. Oral anticoagulation is well established and successful, and is recommended in evidenced based guidelines for patients with HF and AF. Similar outcomes for NOACs and warfarin were obtained in patient subgroups with both nonvalvular AF and HF in the pivotal studies of NOACs. The results of the recent meta-analysis of these four pivotal trials confirmed that NOACs in patients with HF and nonvalvular AF were more effective (less stroke/systemic embolism) and even safer (fewer cases of intracranial hemorrhage) than vitamin K antagonists. In the absence of evidence so far from specifically designed trials, there is no clinical argument for administering NOACs in patients with HF who are in sinus rhythm. Therefore, these recent analyses support the use of NOACs as an alternative to warfarin in patients with both nonvalvular AF and HF.

REFERENCES

1. Ferreira JP, Santos M. Heart failure and atrial fibrillation: from basic science to clinical practice. Int J Mol Sci. 2015;16:3133-47.
2. Benjamin EJ, Wolf PA, D'Agostino RB, et al. Impact of atrial fibrillation on the risk of death: the Framingham Heart Study. Circulation. 1998;98:946-52.
3. Zoni-Berisso M, Lercari F, Carazza T, et al. Epidemiology of atrial fibrillation: European perspective. Clin Epidemiol. 2014;6:213-20.
4. Benjamin EJ, Levy D, Vaziri SM, et al. Independent risk factors for atrial fibrillation in a population-based cohort. The Framingham Heart Study. JAMA. 1994;271:840-4.
5. Maisel WH, Stevenson LW. Atrial fibrillation in heart failure: epidemiology, pathophysiology, and rationale for therapy. Am J Cardiol. 2003;91:2D-8D.
6. Wang TJ, Larson MG, Levy D, et al. Temporal relations of atrial fibrillation and congestive heart failure and their joint influence on mortality: the Framingham Heart Study. Circulation. 2003;107:2920-5.
7. Logeart D, Isnard R, Resche-Rigon M, et al. Current aspects of the spectrum of acute heart failure syndromes in a real-life setting: the OFICA study. Eur J Heart Fail. 2013;15:465-76.
8. Boos CJ, Brown L. Anticoagulation in atrial fibrillation and chronic heart failure: the risk and drug of choice. Curr Opin Cardiol. 2016;31:229-34.
9. Agarwal M, Apostolakis S, Lane DA, et al. The impact of heart failure and left ventricular dysfunction in predicting stroke, thromboembolism, and mortality in atrial fibrillation patients: a systematic review. Clin Ther. 2014;36:1135-44.
10. Caldwell JC, Contractor H, Petkar S, et al. Atrial fibrillation is under-recognized in chronic heart failure: insights from a heart failure cohort treated with cardiac resynchronization therapy. Europace. 2009;11:1295-300.
11. Boriani G, Glotzer TV, Santini M, et al. Device-detected atrial fibrillation and risk for stroke: an analysis of >10,000 patients from the SOS AF project (Stroke preventiOn Strategies based on Atrial Fibrillation information from implanted devices). Eur Heart J. 2014;35:508-16.
12. Melgaard L, Gorst-Rasmussen A, Lane DA, et al. Assessment of the CHA2DS2-VASc Score in predicting ischemic stroke, thromboembolism, and death in patients with heart failure with and without atrial fibrillation. JAMA. 2015;314:1030-8.
13. Gonsalves WI, Pruthi RK, Patnaik MM. The new oral anticoagulants in clinical practice. Mayo Clin Proc. 2013;88:495-511.
14. DiMarco JP, Flaker G, Waldo AL, et al. Factors affecting bleeding risk during anticoagulant therapy in patients with atrial fibrillation: observations from the Atrial Fibrillation Follow-up Investigation of Rhythm Management (AFFIRM) study. Am Heart J. 2005;149:650-6.
15. Giugliano RP, Ruff CT, Braunwald E, et al. Edoxaban versus warfarin in patients with atrial fibrillation. N Engl J Med. 2013;369:2093-104.
16. Connolly SJ, Ezekowitz MD, Yusuf S, et al. Dabigatran versus warfarin in patients with atrial fibrillation. N Engl J Med. 2009;361:1139-51.
17. Granger CB, Alexander JH, McMurray JJ, et al. Apixaban versus warfarin in patients with atrial fibrillation. N Engl J Med. 2011;365:981-92.
18. Patel MR, Mahaffey KW, Garg J, et al. Rivaroxaban versus warfarin in nonvalvular atrial fibrillation. N Engl J Med. 2011;365:883-91.

19. Ruff CT, Giugliano RP, Braunwald E, et al. Comparison of the efficacy and safety of new oral anticoagulants with warfarin in patients with atrial fibrillation: a meta-analysis of randomised trials. Lancet. 2014;383:955-62.
20. Silverberg D, Wexler D, Blum M, et al. The association between congestive heart failure and chronic renal disease. Curr Opin Nephrol Hypertens. 2004;13:163-70.
21. Hart RG, Eikelboom JW, Ingram AJ, et al. Anticoagulants in atrial fibrillation patients with chronic kidney disease. Nat Rev Nephrol. 2012;8:569-78.
22. Ponikowski P, Voors AA, Anker SD, et al. 2016 ESC Guidelines for the diagnosis and treatment of acute and chronic heart failure. Eur J Heart Fail. 2016;37:2129-200.
23. Gianluigi S, Giugliano RP, Giuseppe MC. Rosano efficacy and safety of novel oral anticoagulants in patients with atrial fibrillation and heart failure: a meta-analysis. JACC: Heart Fail. 2016;4:11-5.

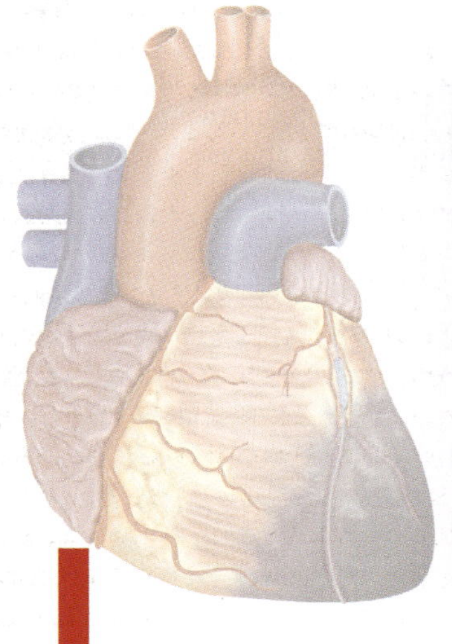

Ivabradine: A Therapeutic Agent in Heart Failure

I Sathyamurthy, KN Srinivasan

INTRODUCTION

Heart failure is a clinical syndrome identified by a combination of symptoms and signs of hypoperfusion and congestion in both systemic and pulmonary circulations. This could be secondary to abnormality of cardiac structure or function. The prevalence of heart failure (HF) increases with age. With early diagnosis and better treatment of coronary artery disease (CAD), there is significant reduction in CAD mortality and many patients are living longer with poor left ventricular (LV) function, who are the potential future candidates for HF. Despite better understanding and newer drugs for the treatment of HF, the overall prognosis remains poor. The commonly used, more relevant classification of HF is the one which categorizes HF into three groups according to LV ejection fraction (LVEF), namely HF with reduced EF (HFrEF) (EF <40%), HF with mid-range EF (HFmEF) (EF 41–49%) and HF with preserved EF (HFpEF) (EF>50%). The therapeutic goals of drug therapies in HF are to improve symptoms, prevent recurrent hospital admissions and to reduce mortality. Evidence based, guideline directed drug therapy (EGDT) for HFrEF includes angiotensin converting enzyme inhibitors (ACEI)/angiotensin receptor blockers (ARBS)/angiotensin receptor neprilysin inhibitor (ARNI), beta-blockers, and mineralocorticoid receptor antagonist (MRA). Elevated resting heart rate (HR) is an independent predictor of mortality and morbidity in chronic HF (with HFrEF or HFpEF). It creates an imbalance between the myocardial oxygen supply and demand. Hence Ivabradine is considered when the heart rate is more than 70/min, in spite of optimal medical therapy.

Various multicenter trials have shown that those with higher HR at admission are associated with poorer outcomes[1] and higher discharge heart rates are associated with increased mortality and hospital readmissions.[2] A meta-analysis of patients with HF has shown 18% reduction in all-cause mortality for every 5 beats/min reduction in heart rate.[3] Beta blockers and Ivabradine are the drugs which can be considered for reducing the HR in HF. If there are any contraindications for beta-blockers, or beta-blocker intolerance then Ivabradine will stand out as drug of choice.

PHARMACOKINETICS AND PHARMACODYNAMICS

Ivabradine selectively inhibits I_f (funny) channels in the sinoatrial node, thereby reduces the HR without having any effect on blood pressure, myocardial contractility and relaxation. Hyperpolarization-activated cyclic nucleotide-gated channel 4 (HCN4) isoform[4] is predominantly present in SA node. Ivabradine binds to this channel on their intracellular side, when the channel is open (active) which explains the use dependency effect of Ivabradine. Though, Ivabradine gets absorbed fully when taken orally, only 40% of the drug is bioavailable in the blood due to extensive first-pass metabolism by the gut and liver. It is predominantly excreted by liver (80%). It is metabolized by CYP450 3A4 enzyme and its active metabolite N-demethylated derivative is also metabolized by the same enzyme.

As Ivabradine is a weak inhibitor of CYP450 3A4, it does not influence the metabolism and plasma levels of other drugs that utilize the same enzyme. On the other hand, inducer of CYP450 3A4 (rifampicin, barbiturates, phenytoin) may decrease Ivabradine concentration and may require rise in dosing and strong inhibitors of CYP450 3A4 (azole antifungal, macrolides, HIV protease inhibitors, nefazodone) will increase Ivabradine concentration. Hence, their concomitant use with this agent is contraindicated. QT prolongation with Ivabradine may become significant especially when combined with QT prolonging agents.

Ivabradine is started with 5 mg twice daily and heart rate is monitored. After 2 weeks of initiation, dose can be up titrated to 7.5 mg twice daily if heart rate is high, or down titrated to 2.5 mg twice daily if heart rate is <60/min. It should also not be initiated in patients with a blood pressure <90/60 mm Hg. It should be stopped whenever heart rate is <50/min despite down titrating or when patient develops symptomatic bradycardia.

Adjustment of dose is not needed in mild to moderate hepatic impairment, mild to moderate renal impairment and no data available regarding usage in severe renal impairment. It is contraindicated in pacemaker dependent patients and in severe hepatic impairment (Child-Pugh C). The most common side effect of Ivabradine is phosphenes (a sensation of a ring or spot of light) (14.5%) which resolve spontaneously in 75% of patients during the treatment. The other common side effects are bradycardia (3.3%), headache and atrial fibrillation. It should not be used in patients with cardiogenic shock, high-grade AV block, sick sinus syndrome, pregnancy and during lactation.

EVIDENCE-BASED DATA

Beautiful trial (morbidity-mortality evaluation of the I_f inhibitor Ivabradine in patients with coronary disease and left-ventricular dysfunction trial[5]): This is the first multicenter, randomized, double-blinded, placebo-controlled trial in patients with CAD with LV dysfunction, wherein mortality and morbidity benefits of Ivabradine use was assessed. This trial included patients over the age of 55 years with stable CAD, in sinus rhythm with resting HR of at least 60 bpm, HFrEF with EF less than 40%, clinically stable for at least 3 months and on appropriate cardiovascular medication for 1 month. There was no difference in primary and secondary end-points noted in the overall population (Figs. 1A to D). There was no difference in any prespecified subgroups.

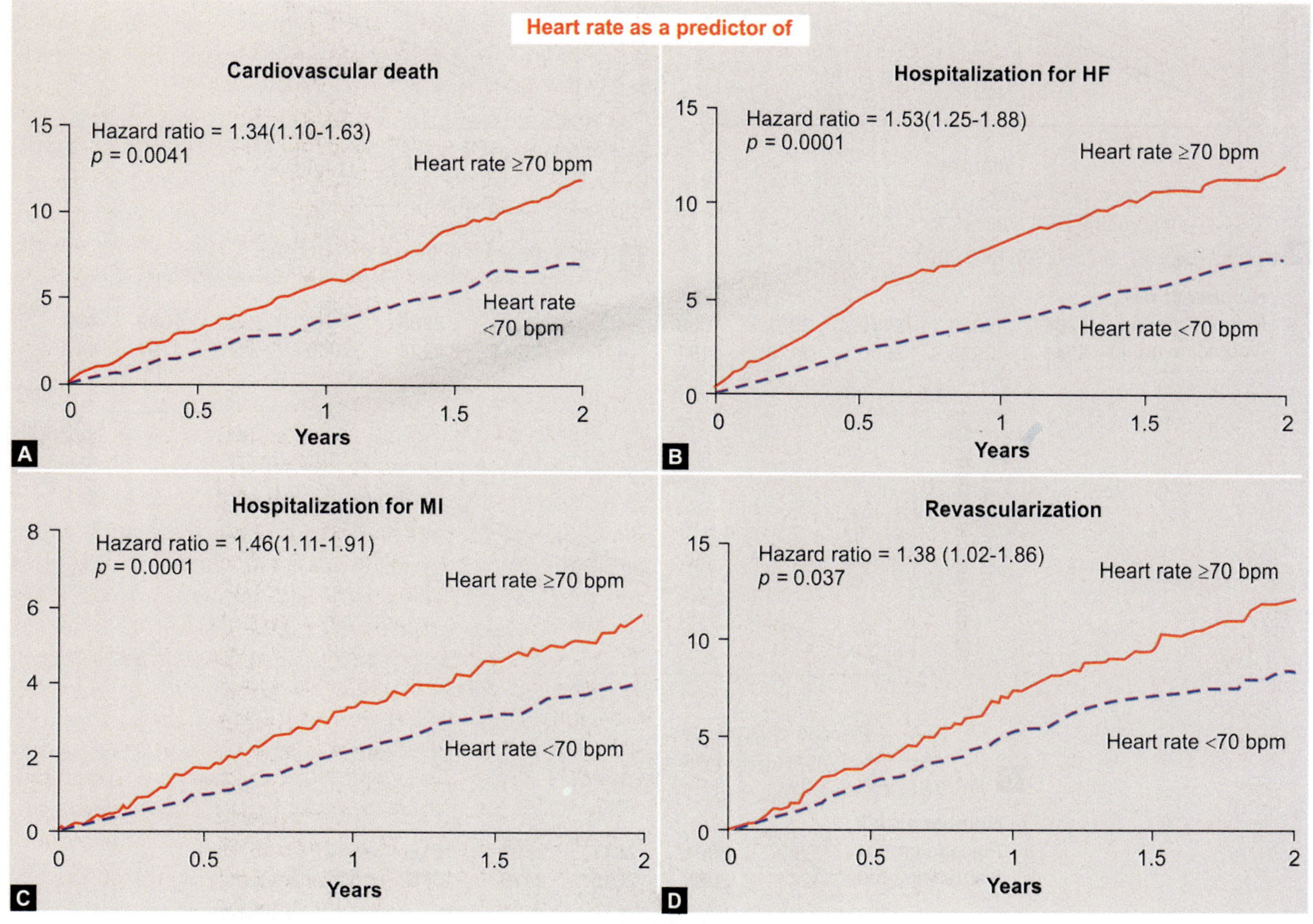

Figs. 1A to D: Beautiful trial results: Heart rate as a prognostic risk factor in patients with coronary artery disease with left ventricular dysfunction (Beautiful study): A subgroup analysis.[6]

However, Ivabradine appeared to reduce admissions for acute myocardial infarction (MI) by 36%, reduce composite admission for acute MI or unstable angina by 22% and additionally reduced coronary revascularization by 30% in a group of patients with HR at least 70 bpm.[6] As these end-points were prespecified in the overall population, should be interpreted with caution. The Systolic Heart Failure Treatment with the I_f Inhibitor Ivabradine *(SHIFT)* Trial[7] was a randomized, double-blind, multicenter, placebo-controlled trial of 6,558 patients with stable symptomatic chronic HF of NYHA class II-IV, with severe LV dysfunction (LVEF ≤35%) of both ischemic and nonischemic etiology. Patients were in sinus rhythm with resting HR 70/min or higher (mean 79.96/min). They were already on guideline directed medical therapy (GDMT) (beta-blocker 89%, ACE or ARB 91%, MRA 63%). Patients were randomized to receive either Ivabradine or placebo. Target HR was kept <70/min and the dose of Ivabradine was adjusted accordingly in the first month of study. The median follow-up was 22.9 months. The effect of Ivabradine over the GDMT for HF was assessed. There was a reduction in the primary end-points of cardiovascular death or hospitalization for worsening HF symptoms (HR 0.82, 95% CI 0.75–0.90, p <0.0001) (Figs. 2A to C). There was no difference in the secondary end-points (all cause or cardiovascular mortality) (HR 0.90, P = 0.092, and HR 0.91, P = 0.128, respectively). Ivabradine reduced all-cause hospitalizations (HR 0.89, P = 0.003). When the HR was more, Ivabradine offered more benefit with group having highest HR (HR >87/min), had maximum benefit in primary end points (HR 0.75, 95% CL 0.67–0.85).

Ivabradine did not significantly reduce the end-points in patients with baseline HR <75/min. Even

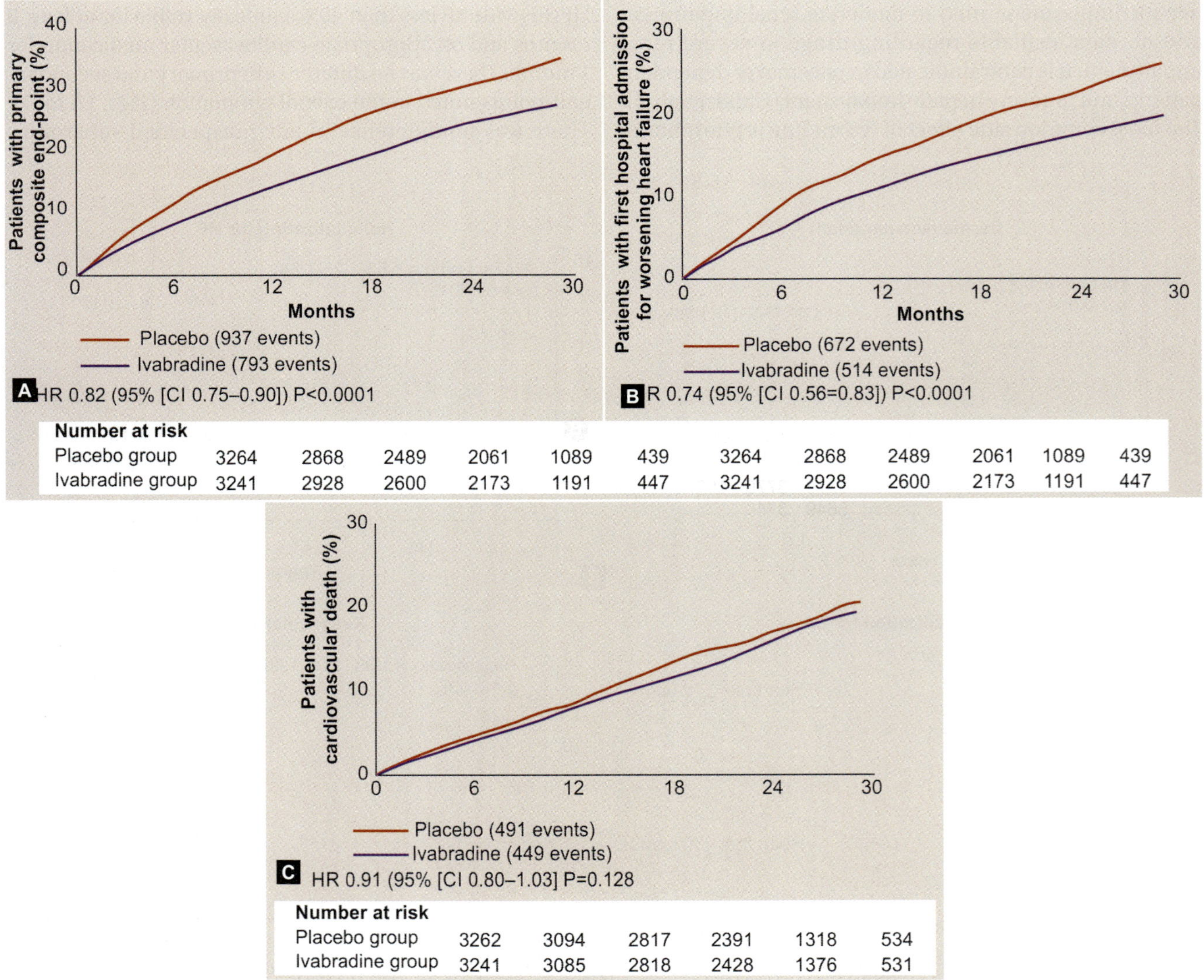

Number at risk												
Placebo group	3264	2868	2489	2061	1089	439	3264	2868	2489	2061	1089	439
Ivabradine group	3241	2928	2600	2173	1191	447	3241	2928	2600	2173	1191	447

Number at risk						
Placebo group	3262	3094	2817	2391	1318	534
Ivabradine group	3241	3085	2818	2428	1376	531

Figs. 2A to C: SHIFT trial results.[8]

though 90% of patients in the trial were on beta-blockers, only 26% were at target doses and it was found that Ivabradine reduced end-points significantly in patients taking less than 50% of target beta-blocker dose. Ivabradine is well tolerated in the SHIFT trial in combination with other HR-lowering agents with a lower rate of adverse effects seen in the placebo group (3,388 vs. 3,847 p = 0.025). Posthoc analysis of the SHIFT trial data showed that when the comorbidities were >3, there was maximum events in both the arms (Ivabradine and control arm), but the rate of hospitalization was lower in the Ivabradine group.[8]

Quality Scoring

From the Shift trial patient data, subgroup analysis was done and quality of life (QOL) scoring was analyzed using Kansas City Cardiomyopathy Questionnaire (KCCQ) at base line, 4 and 12 months. There was improvement in the QOL in the Ivabradine group as measured with the KCCQ by 1.8 for clinical summary scores (CSS), and 2.4 for overall summary score (OSS) (p ≤0.02, p <0.01 respectively). There was small flaw in the patient selection criteria in this study, as more patients with less severe symptoms (<class II NYHA) were included in this study.[9]

Similarly, an Italian trial with 60 patients analyzed QOL in patients with heart failure using Minnesota Living with Heart Failure Questionnaire scoring and found significant improvement in Ivabradine group at 3 months comparing to baseline (37.5 ± 1.9 P value <0.0001).[10]

Results of the *SIGNIFY study*[11] (Study assessInG the morbidity-mortality benefits of the I_f inhibitor Ivabradine in patients of CAD without heart failure), has shown lowering HR with Ivabradine in CAD patients without clinical HF does not reduce the risk of CV death or nonfatal MI (Fig. 3). In the subgroup of patients with angina (CCS class ≥II), there appeared to be an increase in CV deaths or nonfatal MIs. In the same subgroup, there appeared to be

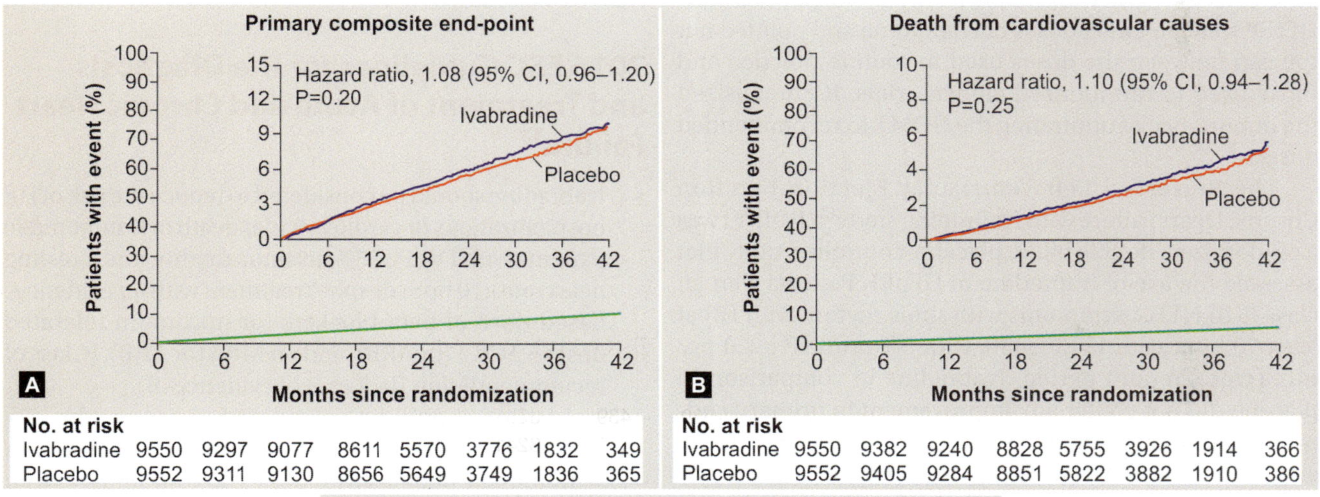

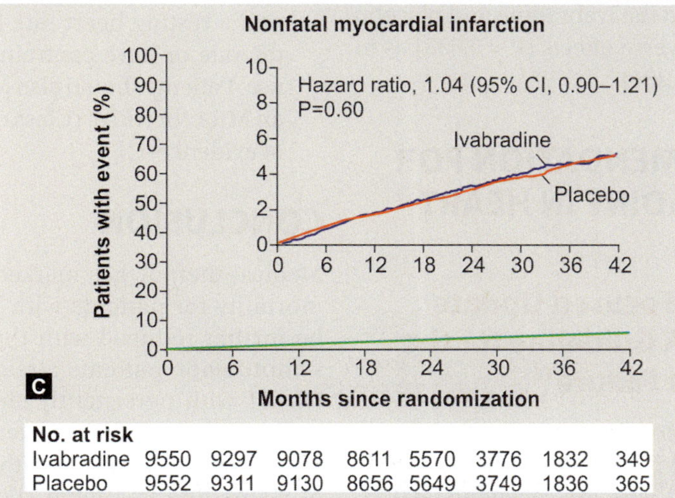

Figs. 3A to C. Signify trial results: Kaplan–Meier plots of the primary composite end point and its components.[12]

TABLE 1: Comparison of SHIFT and SIGNIFY trials.[13]

SHIFT: A study of patients with chronic HF	*SIGNIFY*: A study of patients with chronic stable CAD without HF
All patients with systolic HF	No patients with HF of any kind
LVEF ≤35%	LVEF >40%
All patients hospitalized for WHF within 12 months of randomization	No patients previously hospitalized with HF
All patients receiving guidelines suggested evidence-based background therapy for HF	All patients receiving nonprotocolized therapy for CAD; none for HF
Ivabradine given in doses not exceeding 7.5 mg BID (most received this dose throughout the trial)	Ivabradine titrated as high as 10 mg BID (not approved for clinical use) if HR target not achieved at lower doses

improvement in symptoms and need for elective coronary revascularization. This could be secondary to higher dose of Ivabradine used and the use of CYP450 3A4 inhibitor like diltiazem, verapamil. This trial results should not confuse the decision of using Ivabradine in patients with HFrEF secondary to CAD (Table 1).

QUALIFY registry[14] has shown only 30% of patients with HFrEF were on target doses of Ivabradine and pointed out the gap between the doses used in routine practice and those used in randomized clinical trials. It emphasized the importance of uptitrating the GDMT to recommended doses.

The Preserved Left Ventricular Ejection Fraction Chronic Heart Failure with Ivabradine study[15] (EDIFY) was a randomized, double blind, placebo-controlled study that assessed the use of Ivabradine in HFpEF. Patients were in class II-III NYHA symptoms with sinus rhythm with HR at least 70 bpm with LVEF ≤45% with NT-proBNP ≤220 pg/mL. Over 8 month period, Ivabradine in comparison to placebo did not confer any improvement in primary end-points [cardiac filling pressure (E/e'), exercise capacity and reduction in NT-proBNP]. There was no statistically significant difference between the Ivabradine and placebo group in the incidence of adverse effects (P = 0.633) as in rate of discontinuation (p = 0.261).

GUIDELINE RECOMMENDATION FOR THE USE OF IVABRADINE IN HEART FAILURE

2017 ACC/AHA/HFSA Focused Update of the 2013 ACCF/AHA Guideline for the Management of Heart Failure[16]

Ivabradine can be beneficial to reduce HF hospitalization for patients with symptomatic (NYHA class II-III), stable, chronic HF*r*EF (LVEF ≤35%) who are receiving GDEM, including beta-blockers at maximum tolerated dose, and who are in sinus rhythm with a heart rate of 70 bpm or greater at rest (Class of recommendation IIa, Level of evidence—B-R). The European Medicines Agency approved Ivabradine for use in Europe in patients with HFrEF with LVEF ≤35% and in sinus rhythm with a resting heart rate ≥75 bpm, because in this group Ivabradine conferred a survival benefit.

2016 ESC Guidelines for the Diagnosis and Treatment of Acute and Chronic Heart Failure[17]

- Ivabradine should be considered to reduce the risk of HF hospitalizations or cardiovascular death in symptomatic patients with LVEF ≤35%, in sinus rhythm and a resting heart rate ≥70 bpm despite treatment with an evidence-based dose of beta-blockers (or maximum tolerated doses), ACE-I (or ARB), and an MRA (or ARB). (Class of recommendation IIa, Level of evidence–B).
- Ivabradine should be considered to reduce the risk of HF hospitalization and cardiovascular death in symptomatic patients with LVEF ≤35%, in sinus rhythm and a resting heart rate ≥70 bpm who are unable to tolerate or have contraindications for a beta-blocker use. Patients should also receive an ACE-I (or ARB) and an MRA (or ARB). (Class of recommendation IIa, Level of evidence–C).

CONCLUSION

Medical therapy has markedly improved morbidity and mortality for patients with HFrEF. Hospitalization can be further reduced with the addition of Ivabradine to symptomatic patients already treated with maximized GDMT with persistently elevated HR and reduced EF. Ivabradine improves the exercise tolerance, quality of life and the overall prognosis in these sick patients. The benefits of Ivabradine treatment suggest the importance of HR reduction in the causal HF pathway.

REFERENCES

1. Bui AL, Grau-Sepulveda MV, HernandezAF, et al. Admission heart rate and in-hospital outcomes in patients hospitalized for heart failure in sinus rhythm and in atrial fibrillation. Am Heart J. 2013;165:567-74.
2. Laskey WK, Alomari I, Cox M, et al. AHA get with the guidelines®-heart failure program. Heart rate at hospital discharge in patients with heart failure is associated with mortality and rehospitalization. J Am Heart Assoc. 2015;22:e001626.
3. McAlister FA, Wiebe N, Ezekowitz JA, et al. Meta-analysis: beta-blocker dose, heart rate reduction, and death in patients with heart failure. Ann Intern Med. 2009;150: 784-94.
4. Thollon C, Bedut S, Villeneuve N, et al. Use-dependent inhibition of hHCN4 by Ivabradine and relationship with reduction in pacemaker activity. Br J Pharmacol. 2007;150(1):37-46.
5. Fox K, Ford I, Steg PG, et al. Ivabradine for patients with stable coronary artery disease and left ventricular systolic dysfunction (BEAUTIFUL): a randomised, double-blind, placebo-controlled trial. Lancet. 2008;372:807-16.
6. Fox K, Ford I, Steg PG, et al. Heart rate as a prognostic risk factor in patients with coronary artery disease and left-ventricular systolic dysfunction (BEAUTIFUL): a subgroup analysis of a randomised controlled trial. Lancet. 2008;372:817-21.
7. Swedberg K, Komajda M, Böhm M, et al. Effects on outcomes of heart rate reduction by Ivabradine in patients with congestive heart failure: is there an influence of beta-blocker dose?: findings from the SHIFT (Systolic Heart failure treatment with the I(f) inhibitor Ivabradine Trial) study. J Am Coll Cardiol. 2012;59:1938-45.
8. Böhm M, Robertson M, Ford I, et al. Influence of cardiovascular and noncardiovascular co-morbidities on outcomes and treatment effect of heart rate reduction with Ivabradine in stable heart failure (from the shift trial). Am J Cardiol. 2015;116:1890-7.
9. Ekman I, Chassany O, Komajda M, et al. Heart rate reduction with Ivabradine and health related quality of life in patients with chronic heart failure: results from the SHIFT study. Eur Heart J. 2011;32:2395-404.
10. Sarullo F, Fazio G, Puccio D, et al. Impact of "off-label" use of Ivabradine on exercise capacity, gas exchange, functional class, quality of life, and neurohormonal modulation in patients with ischemic chronic heart failure. J Cardiovasc Pharmacol Ther. 2010;15:349-55.
11. Fox K, Ford I, Gabriel P, et al. Rationale, design, and baseline characteristics of the Study assessInG the morbidity-mortality benefits of the If inhibitor Ivabradine in patients with coronary artery disease (SIGNIFY trial): A randomized, double-blind, placebo-controlled trial of Ivabradine in patients with stable coronary artery disease without clinical heart failure. Am Heart J. 2013;166:654-61.
12. Fox K, Ford I, Steg PG, et al. SIGNIFY Investigators. Ivabradine in stable coronary artery disease without clinical heart failure. N Engl J Med. 2014;371(12):1091-9.
13. Heart. Heart failure and recent heart rate trial data what does it signify? [online] Available from www.heart.org. [Last Accessed November, 2019].
14. Komajda M, Anker SD, Cowie MR, et al. Physicians' adherence to guideline recommended medications in heart failure with reduced ejection fraction: data from the QUALIFY global survey. Eur J Heart Fail. 2016;18:514-22.
15. Komajda M, Isnard R, Cohen-Solal A, et al. Effect of Ivabradine in patients with heart failure with preserved ejection fraction: the EDIFY. (prEserveD left ventricular ejectIon fraction chronic heart Failure with Ivabradine studY (EDIFY) Investigators)-randomized placebo-controlled trial. Eur J Heart Fail. 2017;19(11):1495-503.
16. 2017 ACC/AHA/HFSA Focused Update of the 2013 ACCF/AHA Guideline for the Management of Heart Failure. JACC. 2017;70:6.
17. 2016 ESC Guidelines for the diagnosis and treatment of acute and chronic heart failure The Task Force for the diagnosis and treatment of acute and chronic heart failure of the European Society of Cardiology (ESC). Eur Heart J. 2016;37:2129-200.

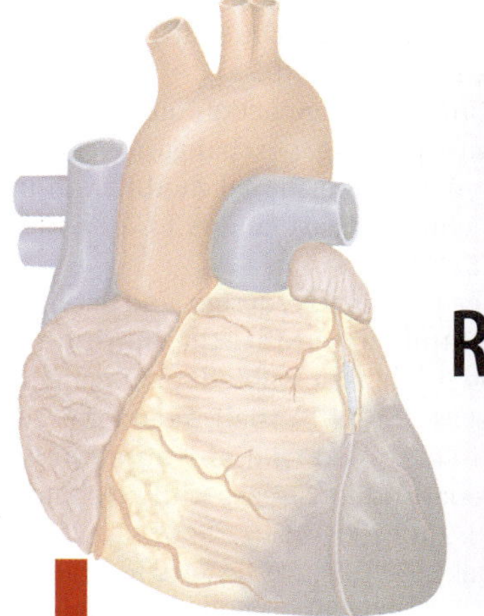

Real-world Data on Use of ARNI in HFrEF

Kamal K Sethi, Rudrani Sharma

INTRODUCTION

Heart failure is one of the leading causes of hospital admission and death across the globe. With a 5-year survival chance of only 50%, heart failure has a mortality rate similar to that of several cancer diagnoses.[1] Therefore, it is a serious and a costly disorder. Standard heart failure therapy is effective and refers to an angiotensin-converting enzyme (ACE) inhibitor or angiotensin receptor blocker (ARB), a beta-blocker, and a mineralocorticoid antagonist.[2] Even though standard treatment reduces the risk of death and heart failure hospitalization by up to 10–37%,[3-9] mortality is high, and many patients suffer from severe symptoms on a daily basis. New and more effective heart failure treatments are needed to improve standard of care.

Sacubitril–valsartan (LCZ696), an angiotensin receptor–neprilysin inhibitor (ARNI), is a new treatment option for heart failure. Sacubitril increases natriuretic peptides, causing vasodilation and diuresis. Valsartan blocks the angiotensin II receptor type 1, reducing vasoconstriction, sodium and water retention, and cardiac hypertrophy. Sacubitril–valsartan was approved by US Food and Drug Administration (FDA) and European Medicines Agency in 2015, based on the Phase III trial, Prospective Comparison of ARNI with ACE inhibitor to Determine Impact on Global Mortality and Morbidity in Heart Failure (PARADIGM-HF).[10] In PARADIGM-HF, 8,442 patients with stable heart failure and reduced ejection fraction (HFrEF) were randomized to either enalapril or sacubitril–valsartan. It was seen that sacubitril–valsartan reduced the primary endpoint cardiovascular death or hospitalizations for heart failure by 20%. The trial was stopped early, after a median follow-up of 27 months, owing to 16% risk reduction in death from any cause. Even though sacubitril–valsartan showed promising results in the PARADIGM-HF trial, it is unknown how applicable the results are to a real-world population.

Similar to most randomized controlled trials, PARADIGM-HF used strict enrollment criteria to minimize the risk of confounders, although this strategy reduces the eligibility.[11,12] For example, patients only qualified for randomization, if they had stable and symptomatic HFrEF, elevated natriuretic peptide plasma concentration, systolic blood pressure ≥ 95 mmHg, and plasma potassium level <5.4 mmol/L, and tolerated a run-in period of enalapril 20 mg daily and sacubitril–valsartan in target dose. The baseline characteristics in PARADIGM-HF were comparable with those of other landmark HFrEF trials.[13] However, these characteristics do not correspond to the real-world heart failure patients, who are generally older, about 50% being women, and have more comorbidities.[14-18] We therefore need to see if the PARADIGM-HF population is a fair representation of a real-world HFrEF population.

This article will try to address the following questions:

- What proportion of a real-world heart failure population is eligible for sacubitril–valsartan according to inclusion and exclusion criteria in the PARADIGM-HF trial?
- How comparable is the PARADIGM-HF population to a real-world heart failure population?

REAL-WORLD DATA FROM VARIOUS OTHER SMALL STUDIES IN HFREF AND USE OF ARNI

A community-based single-center study by Norberg et al.[19] selected patients eligible for sacubitril–valsartan treatment by applying the PARADIGM-HF enrollment criteria. Of the 401 HFrEF patients [left ventricular ejection fraction (LVEF) ≤ 35%], 155 patients (39%) were treated with ACE inhibitor/ARB in target dose and 95 patients were eligible for treatment with sacubitril–valsartan, which corresponds to 24% of the HFrEF population (n = 401) and 5% of the overall heart failure population (n = 1,924). As the entry criteria in PARADIGM-HF were first set to LVEF ≤ 40% and a pre-study dose of ACE inhibitor/ARB equivalent to enalapril 10 mg daily was used, which corresponds to half target dose, a second selection process with these criteria was done by Norberg et al. The latest echocardiography showed LVEF ≤40% in 622 patients, where of 414 patients (67%) were being treated with ACE inhibitor/ARB in at least half dose. After applying PARADIGM-HF exclusion criterion, 250 patients remained eligible for sacubitril–valsartan, corresponding to 40% of the HFrEF population (n = 622) and 13% of the overall heart failure population (n = 1924). Patients eligible for sacubitril–valsartan in the study population were more likely to be older (73.2 ± 10.3 vs 63.8 ± 11.5 years, P < 0.001), had higher systolic blood pressure (128 ± 17 vs 122 ± 15 mmHg, P < 0.001), and higher heart rate (77 ± 17 vs 72 ± 12 beats per minute , P < 0.001) than was the PARADIGM-HF population. Expanding the criteria to slightly higher ejection fraction and trying to titrate patients with only half dose ACE inhibitor/ARB, authors still ended up with only 250 patients. This study highlights the central problem of how valid clinical trials are to real-world patients. Clinical trials use strict inclusion and exclusion criteria to increase the chance of showing significant results with a smaller number of patients. Real-world patients may not fit into those tight frames, and we may have a substantial proportion of HFrEF patients who do not meet the entry criteria. Two more recent analyses from US HFrEF population, however, revealed fairly similar patient characteristics as reported in PARADIGM-HF trial.[20,21]

What are the patterns and factors associated with use and dose of medications for heart failure with reduced ejection fraction (HFrEF) in current practice?

Early adoption of sacubitril/valsartan for patients with heart failure with reduced ejection fraction using data from the AHA's Get With The Guidelines-Heart Failure (GWTG-HF) Registry, Luo et al. analyzed the prevalence and variation in ARNI prescription among a real-world HF population.[22] Patients discharged alive from 347 participating hospitals between July, 2015 and March, 2016 were assessed. Authors compared patient and hospital characteristics among HFrEF (EF ≤ 40%) patients with and without ARNI prescription at discharge. Of 13,831 HFrEF hospitalizations without documented contraindications, 221 (1.6%) were prescribed ARNI. Those prescribed ARNI were younger (median age 63 vs 70 years, P < 0.001), were less likely to have ischemic disease (35% vs 43%, P = 0.02), and had less renal dysfunction (14% vs 20%, P = 0.02) than those not prescribed ARNI. Patients prescribed ARNI had similarly high use of beta-blocker (90% vs 89%, P = 0.7) but higher use of aldosterone antagonist (42% vs 31%, P = 0.0004) at discharge compared to non-ARNI patients. At the 232 participating hospitals, 168 (72%) reported no discharge prescriptions of ARNI. Hospitals reporting no discharge prescriptions were not statistically different from those that prescribed ARNI. The authors concluded that less than 2% of HFrEF patients in a national registry were prescribed ARNI in the first 9 months following FDA approval.

The CHAMP-HF (Change the Management of Patients with Heart Failure) registry[23] cohort comprised of subjects from outpatients in the US cardiology plus general practice with chronic HFrEF receiving at least one oral medication for management of HF. The patients were characterized by baseline use and dose of guideline-directed medical therapy (GDMT) including angiotensin-converting enzyme inhibitor (ACEI)/angiotensin II receptor blocker (ARB), angiotensin receptor neprilysin inhibitor (ARNI), beta-blocker, and mineralocorticoid receptor antagonist (MRA). Among eligible patients, 27%, 33%, and 67% were not prescribed ACEI/ARB/ARNI, beta-blocker, and MRA therapy, respectively. When medications were prescribed, few patients were receiving target doses of ACEI/ARB (17%), ARNI (14%), and beta-blocker (28%), whereas most patients were receiving target doses of MRA therapy (77%). Among patients eligible for all classes of medication, only 1% were simultaneously receiving target doses of ACE/ARB/ARNI, beta-blocker and MRA. In adjusted models, older age, lower blood pressure, more severe functional class, renal insufficiency, and recent HF hospitalization generally favored lower medication utilization or dose. Patients receiving <50% target ARNI dose tended to have similar renal function, but lower blood pressure than those not receiving therapy. For ARNI therapy, multiple clinical factors were independently associated with lower likelihood of treatment, including older age, Hispanic ethnicity, chronic renal insufficiency, and higher EF (all p ≤ 0.009). The authors concluded that significant gaps in use and dose of GDMT remain. A 1-year follow-up of 2,588 patients in CHAMP-HF registry reported proportion of patients at baseline receiving target doses of GDMT to be as follows: mineralocorticoid receptor antagonist (25%), beta-blocker (20%), ACEI/ARB (11%), and ARNI (2%). After 1 year, the medicine initiation or dose increase was seen in

6% for MRA, 10% for beta-blockers, 7% for ACEI/ARB, and 10% for ARNI. Corresponding rates for reduction in dose or discontinuation in therapy were 4%, 7%, 11%, and 3% respectively.[24]

PARASAIL, a Canadian prospective, multicenter, open-label study, aimed at characterizing the real-life effectiveness and safety of sacubitril/valsartan in 302 patients with HFrEF treated for a 12-month period. The interim analysis results of the QoL (quality of life) and tolerability presented were those from patients who completed at least 12 weeks of treatment. The trial was designed to evaluate the real-life therapeutic effectiveness, tolerability, and safety of sacubitril/valsartan in HFrEF patients. Although the lack of a comparator group limits the interpretation, the results indicate a potential improvement in 2 of the 3 validated questionnaires in the first 12 weeks of treatment with ARNI.[25]

DISCUSSION

Given that hospitalization is a robust predictor of increased mortality in the HFrEF population, reduction of inpatient admissions is essential for improving patient morbidity and mortality outcomes. Sacubitril–valsartan (LCZ696) is a major breakthrough in heart failure treatment that should be used in patients who fulfill the inclusion criteria in the PARADIGM-HF study. There is a clear group within the heart failure population that should benefit from this treatment. However, only a quarter of the patients with HFrEF in a real-world setting clearly fulfill the inclusion criteria in the PARADIGM-HF trial. For the rest of the 75% of the HFrEF population, data are less clear. Previous studies have shown that between 10% and 66% of real-world patients managed to fulfill all enrollment criteria from heart failure RCTs. A recent study applying the strict PARADIGM-HF main criteria on a heart failure clinic showed that 21% of an HFrEF population was eligible for sacubitril–valsartan.[26] Studies highlight the central problem of how valid clinical trials are to real-world patients. Based on results of real world studies, the main validity issues of the PARADIGM-HF trial seem to be the LVEF level and ACE inhibitor/ARB doses. Some believe that LVEF ≤ 35% appears to be too strict, considering that the definition of HFrEF includes LVEF < 40%. Further, PARADIGM-HF only randomized patients who tolerated uptitration of enalapril and sacubitril–valsartan to target doses. Provided that results shown in PARADIGM-HF would persist, Norberg et al. suggested that using less strict criteria provides the opportunity to prescribe sacubitril–valsartan to a larger real-world HFrEF population. The TRANSITION study evaluated the ability to achieve target dose of ARNI at week 10 postrandomization in the pre- and postdischarge treatment initiation groups in patients with acute decompensated heart failure. About 24% patients were ARB/ACEI naive, and 29% had de novo heart failure. At 10 weeks, target dose could be achieved in 45–50% of patients.[27]

However, it is unclear how well a real-world population who has been under uptitration once but does not reach ACE inhibitor/ARB target doses tolerates a second attempt at uptitration. When the target ACE inhibitor/ARB dose criteria were strictly applied in the main selection process, a higher dropout was seen suggesting that reaching target doses is difficult in an unselected heart failure population. In clinical trials, however, the proportion of patients reaching the target dose is 49–84% for ACEI/ARB and 43–65% for beta-blockers. In the PARADIGM-HF trial, 12% of the patients withdrew during the run-in phase owing to adverse events of enalapril or sacubitril–valsartan. Hence, we cannot expect that ACE inhibitor/ARB target dose can be reached in all patients. In the 1-year follow-up of CHAMP HF registry, factors associated with initiation or dose increase were previous heart failure hospitalization, higher blood pressure, and lower ejection fraction. Similarly, HF hospitalization, impaired quality of life, and more severe functional class were also predictors for reduction in dose or discontinuation of therapy. Though medical reasons were more common for discontinuation or dose decrease, patient preference and economic reasons were also significant factors. If more emphasis is given on class III/IV patients and those with recent decompensation, we may be able to reduce rates of drug discontinuation or reduced dosing.[28] A bidirectional change in medication is seen in recent hospitalization with HF, involving both increase and decrease in doses, depending on physician's perception of clinical and patient's characteristics. Whereas, GDMT certainly needs to be augmented in such situations, withdrawal or decrease in therapy should be understood as an exceptionally high-risk situation for patients. It would be of great interest for additional studies to investigate why target doses cannot be reached in more heart failure patients.

Both FDA and European Medicines Agency have approved sacubitril–valsartan for a wider indication than the PARADIGM-HF trial inclusion criteria. This was shown in a real-world study where 149 of 210 (71%) hospitalized HFrEF patients met the FDA criteria for sacubitril–valsartan, but only 54 of 210 (26%) patients fulfilled the PARADIGM-HF criteria.[29] Apart from cost, an important factor that has contributed to slow adoption of ARNI is inclusion of only "stable outdoor patients". The PIONEER-HF trial[30] showed that ARNI can be initiated in a lower dose in acute decompensated heart failure with salutary effects, though its safety outcomes need more validation in real-world studies, as the confidence intervals for relative risk of each safety outcome (worsening renal function, hypotension, and hyperkalemia) were quite wide. To improve the external validity in RCTs, patients who represent the real-world population need to be included to a higher extent. Other study designs, such as registry-based randomized trials or observational studies on real-world patients, may be desirable to complement RCTs and increase eligibility. By using registry-based studies to a higher extent, it might be possible to increase the knowledge of novel drug's effect and safety in elderly patients before they are approved for an unselected and often more fragile population. In the sacubitril–valsartan case, it will be essential to perform real-life (Phase IV) studies to find out how the heart failure patients, we meet in clinical practice, actually respond.

CONCLUSION

While guidelines now recommend the use of ARNI in place of ACE inhibitors and angiotensin receptor blockers for select patients with heart failure and reduced ejection fraction, the utilization of ARNI among eligible patients in clinical practice remains low. Access, cost, tolerability, and physician's inertia are perceived barriers to use. Despite strong evidence of superior efficacy, adoption of ARNI in clinical practice after US market approval has been relatively slow, with reports ranging from 2% to 13% of patients with HFrEF. Only 24% of real-world HFrEF population was eligible for sacubitril–valsartan, and the real-world HFrEF patients were significantly older than the PARADIGM-HF population. The lack of data on a majority of the patients that we see in clinical practice is a real problem, and we are limited to extrapolation of results for a hitherto unstudied population. This is difficult to address, but perhaps registry-based studies will help to solve this issue. Although clinical or therapeutic inertia is influenced by clinicians and potential reluctance to implement novel therapies, if their patients are "doing fine", factors such as individual's reluctance to change therapy, nonadherence, comorbidities such as renal or pulmonary disease that prohibits concomitant use of certain GDMT, and cost also play a pivotal role in patients with heart failure with reduced ejection fraction taking GDMT. Can things get better? Looking at a ray of hope, if we can address the clinician, patient, and system factors that are modifiable, we may be able to improve the implementation of GDMT and in turn significantly reduce the morbidity and mortality associated with this deadly disease, viz. heart failure, while keeping the therapy affordable.

REFERENCES

1. Zarrinkoub R, Wettermark B, Wandell P, et al. The epidemiology of heart failure, based on data for 2.1 million inhabitants in Sweden. Eur J Heart Fail. 2013;15:995-1002.
2. Ponikowski P, Voors AA, Anker SD, et al. 2016 ESC Guidelines for the diagnosis and treatment of acute and chronic heart failure: The Task Force for the diagnosis and treatment of acute and chronic heart failure of the European Society of Cardiology (ESC). Developed with the special contribution of the Heart Failure Association (HFA) of the ESC. Eur Heart J. 2016;37:2129-200.
3. SOLVD Investigators, Yusuf S, Pitt B, et al. Effect of enalapril on survival in patients with reduced left ventricular ejection fractions and congestive heart failure. N Engl J Med. 1991;325:293-302.
4. Granger CB, McMurray JJ, Yusuf S, et al. Effects of candesartan in patients with chronic heart failure and reduced left-ventricular systolic function intolerant to angiotensin-converting-enzyme inhibitors: the CHARM-Alternative trial. Lancet. 2003;362:772-6.
5. Konstam MA, Neaton JD, Dickstein K, et al. Effects of high-dose versus low-dose losartan on clinical outcomes in patients with heart failure (HEAAL study): a randomised, double-blind trial. Lancet. 2009;374:1840-8.
6. Packer M, Fowler MB, Roecker EB, et al. Effect of carvedilol on the morbidity of patients with severe chronic heart failure: results of the carvedilol prospective randomized cumulative survival (COPERNICUS) study. Circulation. 2002;106:2194-9.
7. The Lancet. The Cardiac Insufficiency Bisoprolol Study II (CIBIS-II): a randomised trial. Lancet. 1999;353:9-13.
8. Pitt B, Zannad F, Remme WJ, et al. The effect of spironolactone on morbidity and mortality in patients with severe heart failure. Randomized Aldactone Evaluation Study Investigators. N Engl J Med. 1999;341:709-17.
9. Zannad F, McMurray JJ, Krum H, et al. Eplerenone in patients with systolic heart failure and mild symptoms. N Engl J Med. 2011;364:11-21.
10. McMurray JJ, Packer M, Desai AS, et al. Angiotensin–neprilysin inhibition versus enalapril in heart failure. N Engl J Med. 2014;371:993-1004.
11. Yandrapalli S, Aronow WS, Mondal P, et al. Limitations of sacubitril/valsartan in the management of heart failure. Am J Ther. 2017;24:e234-39.
12. Vaduganathan M, Desai AS. Angiotensin–neprilysin inhibition as a paradigm for all? Curr Cardiol Rep. 2016;18:115.
13. McMurray JJ, Packer M, Desai AS, et al. Baseline characteristics and treatment of patients in prospective comparison of ARNI with ACEI to determine impact on global mortality and morbidity in heart failure trial (PARADIGM-HF). Eur J Heart Fail. 2014;16:817-25.
14. Maggioni AP, Orso F, Calabria S, et al. The real-world evidence of heart failure: findings from 41413 patients of the ARNO database. Eur J Heart Fail. 2016;18:402-10.
15. Masoudi FA, Havranek EP, Wolfe P, et al. Most hospitalized older persons do not meet the enrollment criteria for clinical trials in heart failure. Am Heart J. 2003;146(2):250-7.
16. Hernandez AF, Mi X, Hammill BG, et al. Associations between aldosterone antagonist therapy and risks of mortality and readmission among patients with heart failure and reduced ejection fraction. JAMA. 2012;308:2097-107.

17. Kennedy-Martin T, Curtis S, Faries D, et al. A literature review on the representativeness of randomized controlled trial samples and implications for the external validity of trial results. Trials. 2015;16:495.
18. Lazzarini V, Mentz RJ, Fiuzat M, et al. Heart failure in elderly patients: distinctive features and unresolved issues. Eur J Heart Fail. 2013;15:717-23.
19. Norberg H, Bergdahl E, Lindmark K. Eligibility of sacubitril-valsartan in a real-world heart failure population: a community-based single-centre study. ESC Heart Fail. 2018;5(2):337-43.
20. Tahhan AS, Vaduganathan M, Greene SJ, et al. Enrollment of Older Patients, Women, and Racial and Ethnic Minorities in Contemporary Heart Failure Clinical Trials: A Systematic Review. JAMA Cardiol. 2018;3(10):1011-9.
21. DeVore AD, Mi X, Thomas L, et al. Characteristics and Treatments of Patients Enrolled in the CHAMP-HF Registry Compared with Patients Enrolled in the PARADIGM-HF Trial. J Am Heart Assoc. 2018;7(12):pii: e009237.
22. Luo N, Ballew NG, O'Brien EC, et al. Early impact of guideline publication on angiotensin-receptor neprilysin inhibitor use among patients hospitalized for heart failure. Am Heart J. 2018;200:134-40.
23. Greene SJ, Butler J, Albert NM, et al. Medical Therapy for Heart Failure with Reduced Ejection Fraction: The CHAMP-HF Registry. J Am Coll Cardiol. 2018;72(4):351-66.
24. Greene SJ, Fonarow G, DeVore AD, et al. Titration of Medical Therapy for Heart Failure with Reduced Ejection Fraction. JACC. 2019;73(19):2365-83.
25. Haddad BH, Bergeron S, Ignaszewski A, et al. The parasail study: patient reported outcomes from the Canadian real world experience use of sacubitril/valsartan in patients with heart failure and reduced ejection fraction. Canadian J Cardiol. 2017;33(10):S162-3.
26. Pellicori P, Urbinati A, Shah P, et al. What proportion of patients with chronic heart failure are eligible for sacubitril–valsartan? Eur J Heart Fail. 2017;19:768-78.
27. Pascual-Figal D, Wachter R, Senni M, et al. Rationale and design of TRANSITION: a randomized trial of pre-discharge vs. post-discharge initiation of sacubitril/valsartan. ESC Heart Fail. 2018;5(2):327-36.
28. Bhagat AA, Greene SJ, Vaduganathan M, et al. Initiation, Continuation, Switching, and Withdrawal of Heart Failure Medical Therapies During Hospitalization. JACC Heart Fail. 2019;7(1):1-12.
29. Perez AL, Kittipibul V, Tang WHW, et al. Patients not meeting PARADIGM-HF enrollment criteria are eligible for sacubitril/valsartan on the basis of FDA approval: the need to close the gap. J Am Coll Cardiol HF. 2017;5:460-3.
30. Velazquez EJ, Morrow DA, DeVore AD, et al. Angiotensin–Neprilysin Inhibition in Acute Decompensated Heart Failure for the PIONEER-HF Investigators February 7, 2019. N Engl J Med. 2019;380:539-48.

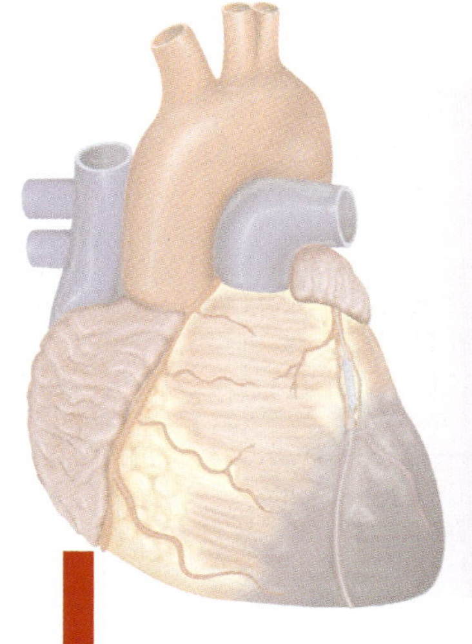

ARNI in NYHA Class II Heart Failure: What is the Evidence?

Vivek Kumar, Viveka Kumar

INTRODUCTION

Clinical instability is considered a potential criterion to determine which patients should be given angiotensin-converting enzyme inhibitors (ACEI)/angiotensin receptor blocker (ARB) and which ones should be considered for replacement therapy with sacubitril/valsartan. The results of PARADIGM-HF (Prospective comparison of ARNI with ACEI to Determine Impact on Global Mortality and morbidity in Heart Failure) established that clinically stable patients [defined as those with no prior heart failure (HF) hospitalization and New York Heart Association (NYHA) class II] at enrollment benefited as much from sacubitril/valsartan as less stable patients. This data suggested that stable patients on ACEI/ARBs might benefit from switching to sacubitril/valsartan for further reducing the mortality and hospitalization.[1]

Despite recent improvements in mortality rates among patients with HF, the 5-year survival rates remain at about 50%. Improvements in management are needed for a large number of patients with NYHA class II or III functional status.[1] Even patients with well-managed NYHA class II HF are at risk for poor outcomes, particularly sudden cardiac death (SCD). These patients are often perceived as "stable," however, sudden cardiac death remains the leading cause of mortality in these patients, and they account for the majority of HF-related hospitalizations and deaths. However, in multiple large clinical trials, the rates of SCD among patients with NYHA class II HF have been found to exceed those of patients with NYHA class III or IV HF. In an analysis of 10,538 HF patients enrolled in six randomized trials and several HF registries, rates of SCD as the cause of death among those with NYHA class II, III, and IV HF were 65%, 51%, and 45%, respectively.[2]

A study published in Desai et al.[3] aimed to understand the components of the mortality benefit of sacubitril/valsartan over enalapril based on the results of PARADIGM-HF trial. The effect of sacubitril/valsartan on mode of death was examined and ARNI was found to significantly reduce the number of sudden cardiac deaths by 20% compared with enalapril (Fig. 1) which does not differ amongst patients with or without an implantable cardioverter defibrillator (ICD). This antiarrhythmic effect was confirmed in a study in which ARNI decreased ventricular arrhythmias leading to a reduction of appropriate ICD shocks in a mainly ischemic HFrEF population with ICD under remote monitor.[4]

Patients with stable HF typically experience subtle disease progression that is often not clinically detectable. Even when patients are receiving guideline-directed medical treatment (GDMT), considerable cardiac damage and progression of HF can occur over time as a result of continued overactivation of RAAS and sympathetic nervous system pathways as well as inadequate effects of endogenous compensatory peptides such as natriuretic peptides.[5] Previous guideline recommendations focused on stacking newer therapies on older approved drugs and did not consider it appropriate to switch a patient's existing pharmacologic regimen. This is because all previous trials have compared the active drug against a placebo. However, the PARADIGM-HF trial tested sacubitril/valsartan against

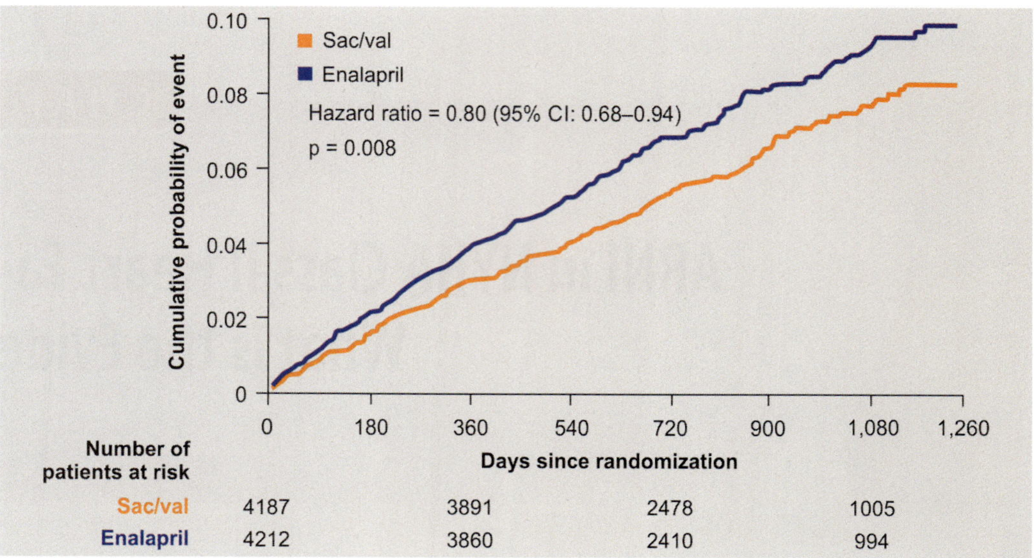

Fig. 1: A cumulative decrease of sudden cardiac death by sacubitril/valsartan as compared to enalapril.

the active comparator enalapril and found it to be superior. The 2016 ACC/AHA Guideline update specifically noted that patients with chronic, symptomatic HFrEF who have NYHA class II or III disease should be switched from an ACEI or ARB to the ARNI, sacubitril/valsartan, to further reduce morbidity and mortality.[5]

Cardiac remodeling is the center point of the pathophysiology of heart failure and it leads to changes in structure and functions of the heart in HFrEF patients.

Although patients with major remodeling demonstrate progressive worsening of cardiac function, slowing or reversing remodeling has recently become a goal of HF therapy. Sacubitril/valsartan was studied in PROVE HF study[6] to evaluate the correlation between changes in concentration of NT-proBNP and cardiac remodeling. This open label multicentric study enrolled 794 patients with HFrEF, NYHA class II and III. The results suggest that NT pro-BNP levels were reduced significantly from baseline to 12 months of ARNI initiation. Majority of the reduction in NT pro-BNP was observed in initial 2 weeks (Fig. 2).

In EVALUATE-HF (Effect of Sacubitril-Valsartan vs Enalapril on Aortic Stiffness in Patients with Heart Failure and Reduced Ejection Fraction), researchers randomized 464 patients with HFrEF to receive either sacubitril/valsartan or enalapril. After 12 weeks of therapy, the two groups did not differ significantly in changes in aortic characteristic impedance (an indirect measure of LV wall stress) or LVEF; however, sacubitril/valsartan recipients experienced significantly greater declines in LV and left-atrial (LA) volumes and in the mitral E/e' ratio, compared with enalapril recipients.[7]

The clinical implications from PROVE-HF (Prospective Study of Biomarkers, Symptom Improvement, and Ventricular Remodeling During Sacubitril/Valsartan Therapy for Heart Failure) and EVALUATE-HF suggests that guidelines recommend patients with new-onset HFrEF should have an ICD only after a trial of GDMT. Based on these two studies, it stands to reason that ARNI should be implemented before determining a patient's eligibility for an ICD and strongly suggest that ARNI therapy can promote cardiac reverse remodeling in patients with HFrEF.[8]

CONCLUSION

Several heart failure trials have proved the fact that the apparently stable patient with chronic HF remains at increased risk of asymptomatic progression of HF, death, and hospitalization. However, we now have new therapies that have been shown to be particularly beneficial for such patients. Patients with NYHA class II HF have mild symptoms that can be difficult to recognize for the clinician. Hence, this condition is typically underdiagnosed and undertreated, thereby complicating disease management. Clinicians are often hesitant to intensify therapies when patients appear to be stable and lack clinical evidence of progression, which makes it difficult to switch to a new therapy in stable patients. Additionally, suboptimal implementation of GDMT, including ACEI/ARB/ARNI therapy to prevent LV remodeling, contributes to disease progression. Thus, optimization of GDMT should reduce the risk of death in this patient population. The strong evidence of ARNI may help the clinicians to reach their main treatment goals for patients with NYHA class II HF by decreasing the risk for SCD, preventing disease progression and worsening symptoms, enhancing reverse remodeling, and improving the overall quality of life.

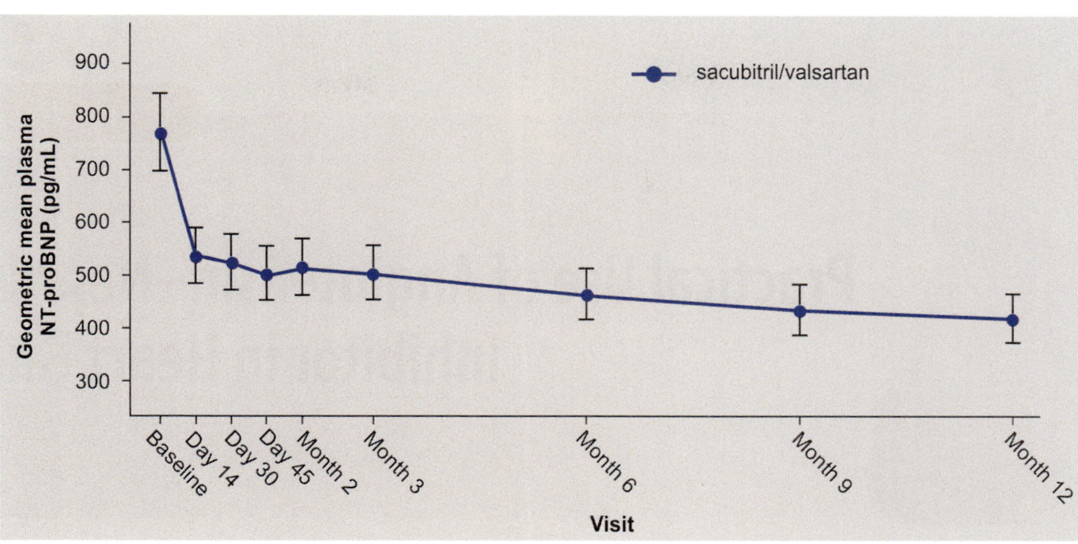

Fig. 2: Decrease in NT proBNP levels with the use of sacubitril/valsartan.

REFERENCES

1. Solomon, Scott D, et al. Benefit of sacubitril/valsartan therapy in clinically stable patients with heart failure and reduced ejection fraction. J Am Coll Cardiol. 2016;67(13):1349.
2. Gilbert EM, Xu WD. Rationales and choices for the treatment of patients with NYHA class II heart failure. Postgrad Med. 2017;129(6):619-31.
3. Desai AS, et al. Effect of the angiotensin-receptor-neprilysin inhibitor LCZ696 compared with enalapril on mode of death in heart failure patients. Eur Heart J. 2015;36(30):1990-7.
4. Anand I. Stable but progressive nature of heart failure: considerations for primary care physicians. Am J Cardiovasc Drugs. 2018;18(5):333-45.
5. De Diego C, González-Torres L, Núñez JM, et al. Effects of angiotensin-neprilysin inhibition compared to angiotensin inhibition on ventricular arrhythmias in reduced ejection fraction patients under continuous remote monitoring of implantable defibrillator devices. Heart Rhythm. 2018;15(3):395-402.
6. Januzzi J, Prescott MF, Butler J, et al. Association of change in N-Terminal Pro-B-Type natriuretic peptide following initiation of sacubitril-valsartan treatment with cardiac structure and function in patients with heart failure with reduced ejection fraction. JAMA. 2019:1-11.
7. Desai AS, Solomon SD, Shah AM, et al. Effect of sacubitril-valsartan versus enalapril on aortic stiffness in patients with heart failure and reduced ejection fraction: A randomized clinical trial. JAMA. 2019:1-10.
8. Drazner MH. Angiotensin receptor-neprilysin inhibition (ARNI) therapy and reverse remodeling in heart failure with reduced ejection fraction. JAMA. 2019:1-3.

CHAPTER

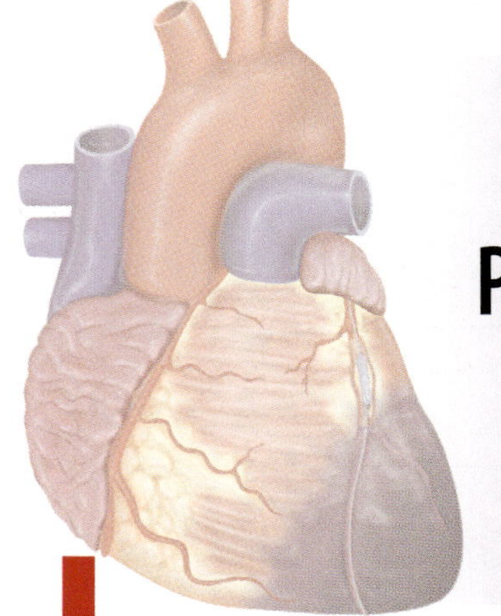

Practical Use of Angiotensin–Neprilysin Inhibitor in Heart Failure

Shraddha Ranjan, Manish Bansal, Ravi R Kasliwal, HK Chopra

INTRODUCTION

Years of experience and literature strongly suggest that blockade of the renin–angiotensin–aldosterone system (RAAS) is a key component in the treatment of patients with heart failure (HF) with reduced ejection fraction (HFrEF), i.e. the patients whose left ventricular ejection fraction (LVEF) is ≤40%. This strategy took care of one axis of neurohumoral system integral to HF pathophysiology by suppressing harmful effects of RAAS. However, the other axis of beneficial counter-regulatory systems like natriuretic peptides remained untouched. Inhibition of neprilysin enzyme augments levels of several beneficial endogenous vasoactive peptides, including natriuretic peptides, bradykinin, and adrenomedullin. The combination of neprilysin inhibitor plus angiotensin II receptor blocker (ARB) known as angiotensin receptor-neprilysin inhibitor (ARNI) therapy theoretically exploited both of the axes and when used practically in trials, also lived up to the expectations. The PARADIGM-HF (Prospective comparison of ARNi with ACEi to Determine Impact on Global Mortality and Morbidity in Heart Failure) trial demonstrated that ARNI was superior to an angiotensin-converting enzyme inhibitor (ACEi) in reducing mortality in patients with HFrEF.[1,2] As a result, ARNI has now become first-line therapy for the treatment of HFrEF.

EVOLUTION OF ARNI

PARADIGM-HF appears to represent a miraculous advance in the treatment of HFrEF but ARNI, prototype drug being LCZ696 (sacubitril–valsartan) did not arrive in the scene so easily. Its discovery is a result of series of preclinical and clinical trials over the years, which started with the discovery of renin more than 100 years back. Table 1 provides an overview of the journey of discovery of ARNI.

MECHANISM OF ARNI

To understand the mechanism of ARNI, we need to revisit the basics of pathophysiology of HF in brief.

Role of RAAS in HF

Neurohumoral activation of RAAS and the sympathetic nervous system (SNS) plays a major role in the development and progression of HF. RAAS exerts its actions through the hormones angiotensin II and aldosterone, and controls blood pressure (BP) and vascular tone by means of vasoconstriction and renal sodium and water retention. Any impairment of perfusion activates RAAS and SNS in order to maintain perfusion of vital organs. This is a compensatory protective mechanism in HF. However, prolonged activation of these systems leads to increased sodium and water retention as well as increased systemic vascular resistance. At the same time, these systems are also involved in regulating myocardial fibrosis and apoptosis at cellular level. Together, these actions lead to myocardial remodeling due to hypertrophy, fibrosis, and apoptosis, which accelerates the progression of HF and the end-result is a harmful sequence of events. This understanding about the role of RAAS in HF has led to the therapeutic use of RAAS inhibitors, which include ACEI/ARB/mineralocorticoid receptor antagonists (MRA) in the treatment of chronic HF.

TABLE 1: Evolution of angiotensin receptor neprilysin inhibitor (ARNI) therapy.

Year	*Event*
1900	Robert Tigerstedt and Per Bergman extracted renin from rabbit's renal cortex.[3]
1934	Goldblatt et al. demonstrated that constriction of the renal arteries of dogs caused persistent hypertension.[4]
1940–1950	Inactive decapeptide (angiotensin I) and the active pressor substance, the octapeptide (angiotensin II) were discovered. Role of ACE in inhibition of angiotensins and also the vasodilator peptide, bradykinin was studied.[5]
1965	Kininase/ACE inhibitor was isolated from venom of Bothrops Jararaca, the Brazilian pit viper, and work on developing synthetic analogs was started.[6]
1970	The earliest ACEI, teprotide was developed which required parenteral administration. It improved the disordered hemodynamics in patients with HF, demonstrating the important role of activation of the RAAS in HF.[7]
1970	Marshall et al. developed first ARB, which was an angiotensin II analog, Saralasin. It was also only parenterally active.[8]
1977	First orally active ACEI, Captopril was synthesized by Ondetti et al.[9]
1981	de Bold et al. found that infused crude extracts of rat atrium caused hypotension and a more than 30-fold increase of sodium excretion, whereas urine volume rose 10-fold and named this substance atrial natriuretic peptide.[10]
1988	Sudoh et al. identified a peptide in porcine brain, which is also found in heart ventricles and named it brain natriuretic peptide. C-type natriuretic peptide, was also extracted first from porcine brain, and then from endothelial cells.[11]
1993	Kitamura et al. isolated another novel, potent, hypotensive peptide adrenomedullin, which had similar vasorelaxant and natriuretic properties as natriuretic peptides.[12]
1995	Ksander et al. described Sacubitril, a neprilysin inhibitor which later became a component of LCZ696.[13]
2000	Omapatrilat, a dual inhibitor of ACE and neprilysin system, was used experimentally in trials but could not get approval due to increased incidences of angioedema.[14]
2003	Novartis Pharmaceutical Corporation applied for the patent of a drug comprising a combination of the ARB, valsartan, and a neprilysin inhibitor, sacubitril; LCZ696.
2014	The superiority of clinical outcomes in patients with HFrEF by the first ARNI over enalapril was established in the PARADIGM-HF trial.[2]

(ACE: angiotensin-converting enzyme; ACEI: angiotensin-converting enzyme inhibitor; ARB: angiotensin receptor blocker; ARNI: angiotensin receptor neprilysin inhibitor; HF: heart failure; HFrEF: heart failure with reduced ejection fraction; PARADIGM-HF: Prospective Comparison of ARNi with ACEi to Determine Impact on Global Mortality and Morbidity in Heart Failure; RAAS: renin–angiotensin–aldosterone system)

However, ACEI and ARB induce a reactive rise in plasma renin activity that may supersede their effect, and plasma aldosterone levels remain elevated in few patients despite therapy, a phenomenon known as aldosterone escape.[15-17]

Role of Natriuretic Peptides in HF

Although RAAS and SNS play an integral role in the pathophysiology of HF, other counter-regulatory pathways are also activated in HF. Most important of these is the role of natriuretic peptides. Natriuretic peptides inhibit many of the deleterious effects of RAAS/SNS and regulate BP and fluid status. There are primarily three natriuretic peptides—atrial natriuretic peptide (ANP), brain natriuretic peptide (BNP), and C-type natriuretic peptide (CNP). ANP is synthesized in atria, BNP is secreted from the ventricles in response to mechanical stretch due to raised intracardiac volume or pressure overload, and CNP is produced from endothelial and renal cells in response to endothelium-dependent agonists and proinflammatory cytokines. Natriuretic peptides activate three transmembrane receptors: natriuretic peptide receptor (NPR)-A, NPR-B, and NPR-C. The binding of natriuretic peptides to NPR-A and NPR-B activates guanylate cyclase and increases cyclic guanosine monophosphate (cGMP). This induces natriuresis, diuresis, vasodilation as well as inhibition of the RAAS and SNS. Given these beneficial effects of natriuretic peptides, augmentation of this pathway is a potential therapeutic target in HF. Neprilysin (neutral endopeptidase) is an enzyme, which catalyzes the degradation of ANP, BNP, and CNP as well as of other vasoactive peptides like bradykinin, adrenomedullin, endothelin-1, substance P, and angiotensin II. Neprilysin inhibition results in increase in their levels, but it also leads to activation of RAAS, which is undesirable (Fig. 1). Therefore, in order to be clinically beneficial, neprilysin inhibition requires concomitant inhibition of RAAS.[18,19]

Mechanism of Action of LCZ696

Combined RAAS/neprilysin inhibition was tried initially in the form of omapatrilat, which resulted in dual inhibition

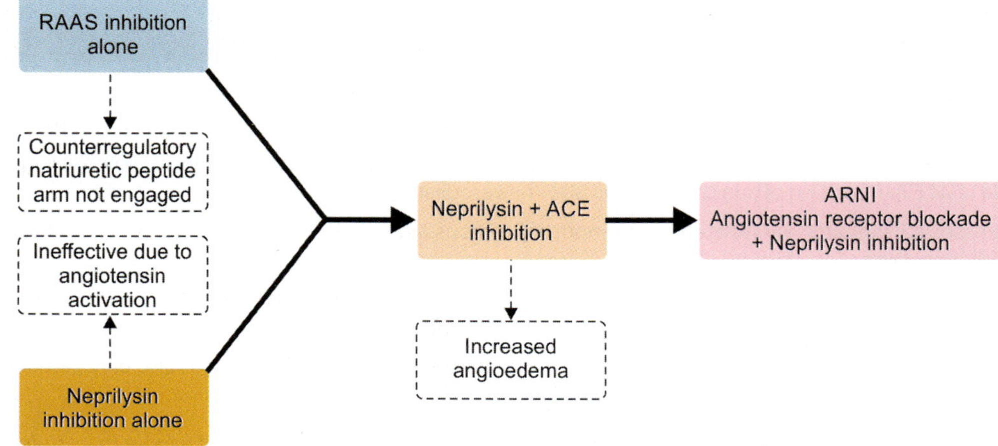

Fig. 1: The concept underlying angiotensin receptor neprilysin inhibitor.
(ACE: angiotensin-converting enzyme; ARNI: angiotensin receptor neprilysin inhibitor; RAAS: renin–angiotensin–aldosterone system)

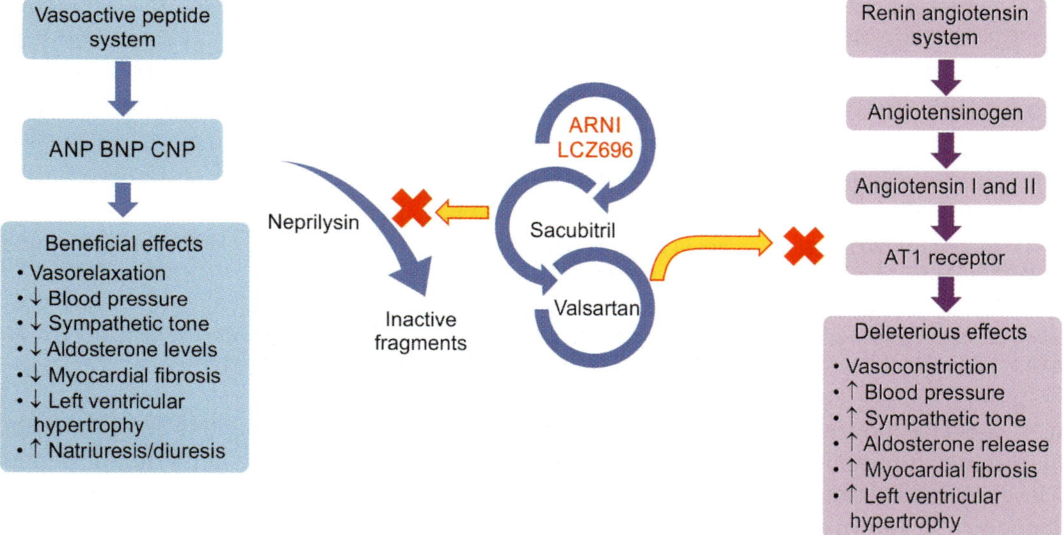

Fig. 2: Mechanism of action of sacubitril/valsartan.
(ANP: atrial natriuretic peptide; ARNI: angiotensin receptor neprilysin inhibitor; AT1: angiotensin II receptor type 1; BNP: brain natriuretic peptide; CNP: C-type natriuretic peptide)

of ACEI and neprilysin. However, it was unsuccessful due to increased instances of angioedema, perhaps due to increased bradykinin levels. Subsequently, the combination of neprilysin and an ARB, which has a lesser effect on bradykinin, was investigated. LCZ696 is the first drug in this category and is composed of two molecular moieties (in a 1:1 molar ratio) in a single crystalline complex comprising valsartan (an ARB) and sacubitril (a neprilysin inhibitor). It causes dose-dependent increase in ANP, plasma, and urinary cGMP as a result of neprilysin inhibition, and inhibition of vasoconstriction, Na^+ and water retention, aldosterone and vasopressin release by angiotensin II receptor type 1 (AT1) receptor blockade (Fig. 2).

However, the precise mechanism by which LCZ696 reduces cardiovascular mortality in HF patients is uncertain and is likely to be related to the incremental benefits of neprilysin inhibition, which may counteract the detrimental effects of RAAS and SNS activation. Reduction in ventricular wall stress, an improvement in ventricular function, decreased myocardial fibrosis and hypertrophy, attenuation of ventricular remodeling, and direct anti-arrhythmic properties are some of the actions that appear to be responsible for this drug's beneficial effects. Valsartan and sacubitril have similar pharmacokinetics, with rapid absorption, reaching maximum plasma concentrations within 1.5–4.5 hours, and a half-life of approximately

10–12 hours making the combination suitable for twice-daily dosing.[20]

EVIDENCE BASE WITH ARNI

Table 2 provides an overview of various clinical trials that have been completed or are underway to evaluate the role of ARNI in different clinical settings.

PRACTICAL USE OF ARNI IN HF

Sacubitril/valsartan resulted in 20% reduction in the incidence rate of death or HF hospitalization compared to enalapril in symptomatic HFrEF patients in the PARADIGM-HF trial and gained a place in guideline-directed medical therapy. However, translating the positive results of trials into true clinical benefit is often not so easy. HF is a polymorphic syndrome, often with multisystem involvement, in sick patients who are prone to decompensation, especially with a drug, which can be hemodynamically challenging to the already compromised hemodynamics. It is therefore imperative to discuss and familiarize clinicians with practical issues regarding the introduction and follow-up of sacubitril/valsartan.[2]

Indications for using ARNI

Chronic HFrEF is currently the primary indication for using ARNI. The latest European Society of Cardiology (ESC) guidelines for HF recommend sacubitril/valsartan as a replacement for an ACEI in ambulatory HFrEF patients, who remain symptomatic with New York Heart Association (NYHA) class II to IV symptoms despite optimal treatment with an ACEI, a beta-blocker and an MRA, to further reduce the risk of death and HF hospitalization.[21] The recently updated version of the American College of Cardiology (ACC)/American Heart Association (AHA) guidelines for HF recommend sacubitril/valsartan as a replacement for ACEI or ARB, for symptomatic chronic HFrEF patients with NYHA II or III symptoms who tolerate an ACEI or ARB, to further reduce morbidity and mortality.[22]

Following are the other potential clinical indications for which ARNI appears to be useful:

- *Acute decompensated heart failure*: TRANSITION (A Multicenter, Randomized, Open Label, Parallel Group Study Comparing Pre-discharge and posT-discharge tReatment Initiation With LCZ696 in heArt Failure patieNtS With Reduced ejectIon-fracTion hospItalized for an Acute decOmpensation eveNt) study analyzed the possibility of starting ARNI during hospital admission (pre-discharge) for acute decompensated heart failure (ADHF).[23] It was found to be safe and efficacious in these patients, similar to when prescribed in outpatient setting post-discharge. Additionally, its use in patients with de novo HF who were not already on any ACEI/ARB was also established. PIONEER-HF (Comparison of Sacubitril–Valsartan versus Enalapril on Effect on NT-proBNP in Patients Stabilized from an Acute Heart Failure Episode) trial which was published early this year (2109) reinforced these findings.[24] ARNI, when initiated during hospitalization for ADHF, was associated with reduction in N-terminal proBNP (NT-proBNP) levels and was generally well tolerated. However, as of now, the use of ARNI in ADHF has not been included in any of the guidelines.
- *Heart failure with preserved ejection fraction (HFpEF)*: After encouraging results of PARAMOUNT (Prospective comparison of ARNI with ARB on Management of heart failure with preserved ejection fraction), a phase II trial in HFpEF (LVEF ≥ 45%) which showed the safety and efficacy of ARNI,[25] another large trial PARAGON-HF (Prospective Comparison of ARNI with ARB Global Outcomes in HF With Preserved Ejection Fraction) is currently ongoing which has enrolled around 4,300 HFpEF patients with a primary objective to compare LCZ696 to valsartan.[26] The results are expected to be out soon.
- *Renal disease*: There is now good evidence that blockade of the RAAS by either ACEI or ARB slows progression in patients with chronic kidney disease, with and without diabetes. HF trials with ARNI have suggested that LCZ696 may be superior to other RAAS blockers with respect to renal function/dysfunction. This is being tested prospectively in the UKHARP (UK Heart and Renal Protection) III trial, which is comparing LCZ696 with irbesartan (an ARB) in patients with proteinuric renal disease.[27] Furthermore, because HF is a common, serious complication in patients with end-stage renal disease, LCZ696 might retard the development and/or progression of both conditions.

Initiating ARNI Therapy

It is usually prescribed along with other HF therapies like diuretics and beta-blockers, in place of an ACEI or an ARB. Accordingly, hemodynamic stability and ability to tolerate ACEI/ARB is a prerequisite for starting this drug. At present, the ideal guideline-recommended situation for sacubitril/valsartan is an ambulatory symptomatic chronic HFrEF patient on optimal treatment with an ACEI or ARB, a beta blocker, and a MRA, without hypotension (systolic BP ≥95 mmHg) or hyperkalemia (≤5.4 mmol/L) and with an estimated glomerular filtration rate ≥30 mL/min/1.73 m^2 and without a history of angioedema or other serious side effects associated with ACEI or ARB therapy.

TABLE 2: Clinical trial evidence with angiotensin receptor neprilysin inhibitor (ARNI).

Clinical setting	*Trial*	*Description of trial*	*Treatment*	*Primary end-point*	*Primary outcome*
Chronic heart failure with reduced ejection fraction	*PARADIGM-HF* (Prospective Comparison of Angiotensin Receptor-Neprilysin Inhibitor with Angiotensin-converting Enzyme Inhibitor to Determine Impact on Global Mortality and Morbidity in Heart Failure)[2]	Phase III trial 8,442 participants Mean age was 64 years, 21% were women, 60% had ischemic etiology, mean LVEF was 30%, and 35% had diabetes	LCZ696 (200 mg twice daily) OR enalapril (10 mg twice daily)	Composite of CV death or HF hospitalization	The trial was stopped prematurely due to overwhelming benefit in ARNI arm. After a median of 27 months, CV death or hospitalization for heart failure had occurred in 21.8% of the ARNI group vs 26.5% of the enalapril group ($p < 0.001$)
	PROVE-HF (Prospective Study of Biomarkers, Symptom Improvement, and Ventricular Remodeling during Sacubitril/Valsartan Therapy for Heart Failure)[28]	Phase IV-prospective study in 830 patients of HFrEF comparing biomarkers, symptom improvement, and ventricular remodeling	LCZ696 vs valsartan	Change from baseline in concentration of BNP, ANP, NT-proBNP and left ventricular indices at 1 year	Results are awaited. Study enrolment completed in 2018
Heart failure with preserved ejection fraction	*PARAMOUNT* (Prospective comparison of ARNi with ARB on Management Of heart failUre with preserved ejectioN fracTion)[25]	Phase II Double-blind randomized trial done with 301 patients test the safety and efficacy of ARNI in HFpEF	LCZ696 vs Valsartan	The primary end-point was to look for the decline in NT-proBNP at 12 weeks	Significant improvement in NT-proBNP levels, left ventricular indices and NYHA class in LCZ696 group than in the valsartan group
	PARAGON (Prospective Comparison of LCZ696 with ARB Global Outcome in HF with Preserved Ejection Fraction)[26]	Phase III trial: It has enrolled around 4,300 HFpEF patients with a primary objective to compare LCZ696 to valsartan	LCZ696 vs Valsartan	To compare the reduction of rate of the composite endpoint of CV death and HF hospitalization	Results are expected soon
Acute decompensated heart failure	*PIONEER-HF* (Comparison of Sacubitril–Valsartan versus Enalapril on Effect on NT-proBNP in Patients Stabilized from an Acute Heart Failure Episode)[24]	Biomarker-end-point trial that randomized 881 adults with ADHF	LCZ696 or enalapril	To find out whether initiation of ARNI in patients hospitalized with ADHF reduces NT-proBNP levels when compared to enalapril	LCZ696 was associated with a greater reduction in NT-proBNP than enalapril (-47% vs -25%) at 4 and 8 weeks without significant side effects

Contd...

Contd...

Clinical setting	*Trial*	*Description of trial*	*Treatment*	*Primary end-point*	*Primary outcome*
	TRANSITION (A Multicenter, Randomized, Open Label, Parallel Group Study Comparing Pre-discharge and posT-discharge tReatment Initiation With LCZ696 in heArt Failure patieNtS With Reduced ejectIon-fracTion hospItalized for an Acute decOmpensation event)[23]	Multicenter, randomized study evaluating feasibility, and safety of per-discharge initiation of sacubitril/valsartan therapy in patients with ADHF	Sacubitril–valsartan	To evaluate the proportion of patients achieving the target sacubitril/valsartan dose of 200 mg twice daily at the end of week 10	Up-titration of sacubitril/valsartan to target doses was achieved and maintained in about 62% of predischarge initiation, compared with 68% for postdischarge. The difference was not significant
Renal disease	*UKHARP* (UK Heart and Renal Protection) III trial[27]	Randomized study of ARNI vs Irbesartan in chronic kidney disease patients	LCZ696 vs ARB—irbesartan	Short-term safety and efficacy with respect to estimated glomerular filtration rate were compared	LCZ696 was equally effective at preserving renal function and reducing albuminuria
Hypertension	*PARAMETER* (Prospective comparison of Angiotensin Receptor neprilysin inhibitor with Angiotensin receptor blocker Measuring arterial stiffness in the Elderly)[29]	Multicenter, double blind randomized controlled trial done in 432 elderly hypertensive patients with a pulse pressure >60 mmHg.	LCZ696 (200 mg) vs olmesartan (20 mg)	Central aortic pressure, ambulatory blood pressure was assessed at 12 weeks	Results demonstrated superiority of LCZ696 vs olmesartan in reducing clinic and ambulatory peripheral BP and central aortic pressures in elderly population

(ADHF: acute decompensated heart failure; ANP: atrial natriuretic peptide; ARNI: angiotensin receptor neprilysin inhibitor; BNP: brain natriuretic peptide; CV: cardiovascular; HF: heart failure; HFpEF: heart failure with preserved ejection fraction; NT-proBNP: N-terminal pro-brain natriuretic peptide; NYHA: New York Heart Association)

When switching from an ACEI, a washout period of 36 hours is important to avoid the risk of angioedema. However, it is not so for ARB, which can be substituted with ARNI from the next dose itself. The recommended starting dose is 49/51 mg (sacubitril/valsartan) twice daily, to be increased after every 2–4 weeks to the target maintenance dose of 97/103 mg twice daily or as tolerated by the patient. A low starting dose of 24/26 mg twice daily for patients with borderline hemodynamics who are not currently taking an ACEI/ARB or those with renal dysfunction may be more suitable.[2,30]

Monitoring ARNI Therapy

Monitoring is essential when using ARNI. Important side effects that need to be watched out for are—symptomatic hypotension, rise in serum creatinine, hyperkalemia, and angioedema. The PARADIGM-HF study showed that sacubitril/valsartan was safer than enalapril in terms of hyperkalemia and renal function worsening. However, sacubitril/valsartan caused more episodes of hypotension, and though it did not lead to a higher treatment discontinuation, BP needs to be vigilantly followed. BP monitoring should be done preferably on a daily basis for the first few weeks after onset or up-titration of treatment, as well as on development of symptoms suggestive of hypotension.

In accordance to PARADIGM-HF, serum creatinine and potassium have to be checked within a week after treatment onset or uptitration, every 2–4 weeks thereafter during the first 4 months and every 4 months thereafter.

Treatment with sacubitril/valsartan initially (within 4 weeks of onset or uptitration) may cause a slight increase in BNP levels, which is due to neprilysin inhibition. In contrast, there is usually and a parallel small decline in NT-proBNP, which reflects the beneficial effect of the drug on cardiac wall stress. These aspects should be kept in consideration when interpreting the results of these biomarkers.[2,30]

Troubleshooting

- Correction of volume or salt depletion prior to administration is important to avoid hypotension. If hypotension occurs, dose adjustment of diuretics, concomitant antihypertensive drugs, and treatment of other causes of hypotension should be done, instead of immediately reducing or stopping ARNI (unless really necessary).
- If hyperkalemia (>5.5 mEq/L) occurs, reduction of dietary potassium or adjusting the dose of concomitant medications (e.g. potassium-sparing diuretics and potassium supplements) is usually enough to resolve the issue.
- In case of persistent hypotension (symptoms or systolic BP $\leq$95 mm Hg or both), hyperkalemia (serum potassium > 5.5 mmol/L), renal function worsening (eGFR < 30 mL/min/1.73 m^2 or eGFR decrease > 35%), or other adverse events, the dose of the drug may be halved or temporarily discontinued for a period of 2 weeks. Rechallenging with the previous dose may be considered, if adverse events are resolved. No starting dose adjustment is needed for mild or moderate renal impairment (i.e. indexed GFR >30 mL/min).
- No dose modification is required in mild hepatic impairment, whereas cautious use is recommended in moderate cases. The drug is contraindicated in severe hepatic insufficiency.[31]

Stopping ARNI Therapy

Permanent discontinuation of therapy is usually not required. However, if above measures are not helpful or in case of severe adverse events, drug discontinuation should be considered, and the patient should be monitored closely.

CONCLUSION

ARNI has emerged as a powerful therapy for patients with HFrEF. Initial clinical experience with this agent has matched the remarkable beneficial effects seen in PARADIGM-HF trial. This has resulted in an increasing uptake of this therapy in clinical practice. However, to be able to derive the maximum benefit with ARNI, clinicians need to familiarize themselves with appropriate indications and protocols for using this therapy.

REFERENCES

1. Braunwald E. The path to an angiotensin receptor antagonist-neprilysin inhibitor in the treatment of heart failure. J Am Coll Cardiol. 2015;65:1029-41.
2. McMurray JJ, Packer M, Desai AS, et al. Dual angiotensin receptor and neprilysin inhibition as an alternative to angiotensin-converting enzyme inhibition in patients with chronic systolic heart failure: rationale for and design of the Prospective comparison of ARNI with ACEI to Determine Impact on Global Mortality and morbidity in Heart Failure trial (PARADIGM-HF). Eur J Heart Fail. 2013;15:1062-73.
3. Marks LS, Maxwell MH. Tigerstedt and the discovery of renin. An historical note. Hypertension. 1979;1:384-8.
4. Goldblatt H, Lynch J, Hanzal RF, et al. Studies on experimental hypertension: I. The production of persistent elevation of systolic blood pressure by means of renal ischemia. J Exp Med. 1934;59:347-79.
5. Page IH, Helmer OM. Angiotonin-activator, renin- and angiotonin-inhibitor, and the mechanism of angiotonin tachyphylaxis in normal, hypertensive, and nephrectomized animals. J Exp Med. 1940;71:495-519.

6. Ferreira SH. A Bradykinin-potentiating factor (Bpf) present in the venom of Bothrops Jararca. Br J Pharmacol Chemother. 1965;24:163-9.
7. Blumberg AL, Denny SE, Marshall GR, et al. Blood vessel-hormone interactions: angiotensin, bradykinin, and prostaglandins. Am J Physiol. 1977;232:H305-10.
8. Marshall GR, Vine W, Needlemann P. A specific competitive inhibitor of angiotensin II. Proc Natl Acad Sci USA. 1970;67:1624-30.
9. Ondetti MA, Rubin B, Cushman DW. Design of specific inhibitors of angiotensin-converting enzyme: new class of orally active antihypertensive agents. Science. 1977;196:441-4.
10. De Bold AJ. Heart atria granularity effects of changes in water-electrolyte balance. Proc Soc Exp Biol Med. 1979;161:508-11.
11. Sudoh T, Kangawa K, Minamino N, et al. A new natriuretic peptide in porcine brain. Nature. 1988;332:78-81.
12. Kitamura K, Kangawa K, Kawamoto M, et al. Adrenomedullin: a novel hypotensive peptide isolated from human pheochromocytoma. Biochem Biophys Res Commun. 1993;192:553-60.
13. Ksander GM, Ghai RD, deJesus R, et al. Dicarboxylic acid dipeptide neutral endopeptidase inhibitors. J Med Chem. 1995;38:1689-700.
14. Robl JA, Sun CQ, Stevenson J, et al. Dual metalloprotease inhibitors: mercaptoacetyl-based fused heterocyclic dipeptide mimetics as inhibitors of angiotensin-converting enzyme and neutral endopeptidase. J Med Chem. 1997;40:1570-7.
15. von Lueder TG, Sangaralingham SJ, Wang BH, et al. Renin-angiotensin blockade combined with natriuretic peptide system augmentation: novel therapeutic concepts to combat heart failure. Circ Heart Fail. 2013;6:594-605.
16. Brewster UC, Setaro JF, Perazella MA. The renin-angiotensin-aldosterone system: cardiorenal effects and implications for renal and cardiovascular disease states. Am J Med Sci. 2003;326:15-24.
17. Radford MJ, Arnold JM, Bennett SJ, et al. ACC/AHA key data elements and definitions for measuring the clinical management and outcomes of patients with chronic heart failure: a report of the American College of Cardiology/American Heart Association Task Force on Clinical Data Standards (Writing Committee to Develop Heart Failure Clinical Data Standards): developed in collaboration with the American College of Chest Physicians and the International Society for Heart and Lung Transplantation: endorsed by the Heart Failure Society of America. Circulation. 2005;112:1888-916.
18. Mangiafico S, Costello-Boerrigter LC, Andersen IA, et al. Neutral endopeptidase inhibition and the natriuretic peptide system: an evolving strategy in cardiovascular therapeutics. Eur Heart J. 2013;34:886-893c.
19. Potter LR, Abbey-Hosch S, Dickey DM. Natriuretic peptides, their receptors, and cyclic guanosine monophosphate-dependent signaling functions. Endocr Rev. 2006;27:47-72.
20. Gu J, Noe A, Chandra P, et al. Pharmacokinetics and pharmacodynamics of LCZ696, a novel dual-acting angiotensin receptor-neprilysin inhibitor (ARNi). J Clin Pharmacol. 2010;50:401-14.
21. Ponikowski P, Voors AA, Anker SD, et al. 2016 ESC Guidelines for the diagnosis and treatment of acute and chronic heart failure: The Task Force for the diagnosis and treatment of acute and chronic heart failure of the European Society of Cardiology (ESC). Developed with the special contribution of the Heart Failure Association (HFA) of the ESC. Eur J Heart Fail. 2016;18:891-975.
22. Yancy CW, Jessup M, Bozkurt B, et al. 2017 ACC/AHA/HFSA Focused Update of the 2013 ACCF/AHA Guideline for the Management of Heart Failure: A Report of the American College of Cardiology/American Heart Association Task Force on Clinical Practice Guidelines and the Heart Failure Society of America. Circulation. 2017;136:e137-e161.
23. Wachter R, Senni M, Belohlavek J, et al. Initiation of sacubitril/valsartan in hospitalized patients with heart failure with reduced ejection fraction after hemodynamic stabilization: primary results of the TRANSITION study. Eur J Heart Fail. 2019;21:998-1008.
24. Velazquez EJ, Morrow DA, DeVore AD, et al. Angiotensin-neprilysin inhibition in acute decompensated heart failure. N Engl J Med. 2019;380:539-48.
25. Solomon SD, Zile M, Pieske B, et al. The angiotensin receptor neprilysin inhibitor LCZ696 in heart failure with preserved ejection fraction: a phase 2 double-blind randomised controlled trial. Lancet. 2012;380:1387-95.
26. Solomon SD, Rizkala AR, Gong J, et al. Angiotensin Receptor Neprilysin Inhibition in Heart Failure With Preserved Ejection Fraction: Rationale and Design of the PARAGON-HF Trial. JACC Heart Fail. 2017;5:471-82.
27. Haynes R, Judge PK, Staplin N, et al. Effects of sacubitril/valsartan versus irbesartan in patients with chronic kidney disease. Circulation. 2018;138:1505-14.
28. Januzzi JL, Butler J, Fombu E, et al. Rationale and methods of the Prospective Study of Biomarkers, Symptom Improvement, and Ventricular Remodeling During Sacubitril/Valsartan Therapy for Heart Failure (PROVE-HF). Am Heart J. 2018;199:130-6.
29. Williams B, Cockcroft JR, Kario K, et al. Effects of Sacubitril/Valsartan versus Olmesartan on Central Hemodynamics in the Elderly with Systolic Hypertension: The PARAMETER Study. Hypertension. 2017;69:411-20.
30. Farmakis D, Bistola V, Karavidas A, et al. Practical considerations on the introduction of sacubitril/valsartan in clinical practice: Current evidence and early experience. Int J Cardiol. 2016;223:781-4.
31. Jhund PS, McMurray JJ. The neprilysin pathway in heart failure: a review and guide on the use of sacubitril/valsartan. Heart. 2016;102:1342-7.

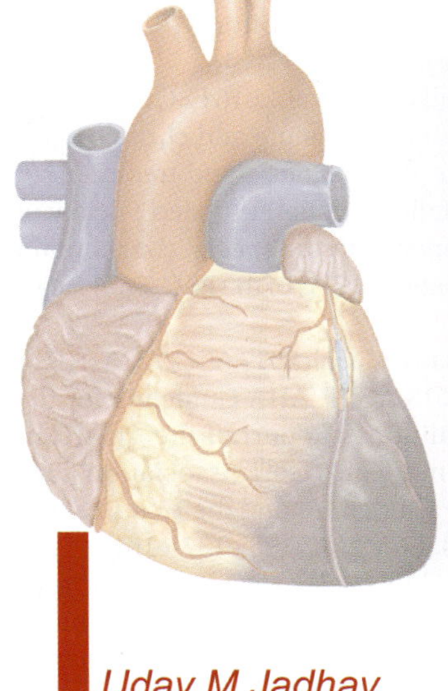

Sacubitril–Valsartan Initiation as In-hospital Therapy

Uday M Jadhav

INTRODUCTION

In the PARADIGM-HF (Prospective Comparison of ARNI with ACEI to Determine Impact on Global Mortality and Morbidity in Heart Failure) trial,[1,2] use of sacubitril–valsartan resulted in a 20% lower risk of death from cardiovascular causes or hospitalization for heart failure than the use of enalapril 10 mg daily, for a minimum of 4 weeks.[3] Acute heart failure (AHF) is the most common reason for hospitalization with substantial incidence ranging from 30% to 40% of patients getting rehospitalized within 12 months.[4] During the vulnerable 2-3 months postdischarge period, early rehospitalizations within 3 months have been reported to reach 25% during the first 30 days, and corresponding mortality figures of 10%.[5,6] Patients who were eligible for inclusion in the PARADIGM-HF trial included patients who were ambulatory outpatients. Patients with acute decompensated heart failure requiring intravenous therapy were excluded from the trial. Two recent studies PIONEER and TRANSITION highlighted the feasibility of initiation of sacubitril–valsartan during the in-hospitalization phase. These two studies have provided insights into the dosage, efficacy and safety of sacubitril–valsartan in in-hospital phase of acute heart failure.

PIONEER

PIONEER design included 881 patients who were randomly assigned to receive sacubitril–valsartan (n = 440, target dose, 97 mg of sacubitril with 103 mg of valsartan twice daily) or enalapril (n = 441, target dose, 10 mg twice daily).[7]

Key Inclusion Criteria

- Hospitalized for acute decompensated heart failure (ADHF)
- Left ventricular ejection fraction (LVEF) ≤40% within the last 6 months
- NT-proBNP ≥1,600 pg/mL or BNP ≥400 pg/mL
- Stabilized while hospitalized
  - Systolic blood pressure (SBP) ≥100 mm Hg in prior 6 hours; no symptomatic hypotension
  - No increase in IV diuretics in prior 6 hours
  - No IV vasodilators in prior 6 hours
  - No IV inotropes in prior 24 hours.

Primary Endpoint

Time-averaged proportional change in NT-proBNP from baseline at 4 and 8 weeks.

Safety

- Worsening renal function
- Hyperkalemia
- Symptomatic hypotension
- Angioedema.

Exploratory Clinical Outcomes

Serious clinical composite: Death, hospitalization for HF, LVAD, or listing for cardiac transplant.

Results

Reduction in the NT-proBNP concentration was significantly greater in the sacubitril-valsartan group than in the enalapril group [percent change –46.7% vs –25.3%; ratio of change with sacubitril-valsartan vs enalapril, 0.71; 95% confidence interval (CI), 0.63–0.81; P < 0.001].

- NT-proBNP concentration reduction with sacubitril-valsartan than with enalapril was evident as early as week 1 after therapy.
- Incidence of hyperkalemia (≥5.5 mmol/L) was similar for those assigned enalapril (9.3%) or sacubitril/valsartan (11.6%). This was a reassuring finding with consideration to patients receiving MRA in the PARADIGM-HF trial where sacubitril/valsartan reduced the risk of severe hyperkalemia (>6.0 mmol/L) as compared with enalapril (3.1 vs 2.2 per 100 patient-years; HR, 1.37; P = 0.02)
- Reduced re-hospitalization for HF
- Well tolerated with comparable rates of worsening renal function, hyperkalemia, symptomatic hypotension, and angioedema.

Conclusion

Investigators of PIONEER reported that among patients with heart failure with reduced ejection fraction who were hospitalized for acute decompensated heart failure, the initiation of sacubitril-valsartan therapy led to a greater reduction in the NT-proBNP concentration than enalapril therapy without any deleterious side effects and major safety concerns. It should be, however, noted that approximately 20% of the patients in each treatment group had discontinued treatment by 8 weeks mostly due to an adverse event. This will warrant caution and clinical status evaluation when initiating in-hospital. European Society of Heart Failure in a recent update highlights that the PIONEER trial provides limited evidence that it is safe to initiate sacubitril/valsartan in ACE-I naïve patients; more evidence would be very welcome.[8] PIONEER-HF was a randomized, double-blind trial of sacubitril/valsartan versus enalapril in hospitalized patients with ADHF following hemodynamic stabilization. Effects of circulating hsTnT, sST2, and urinary cGMP were assessed in 694 patients at baseline 1, 2, 4, and 8 weeks.[9] Sacubitril/valsartan led to a significantly greater decline in hsTnT and sST2 compared with enalapril. This effect was noted as early as 1 week for sST2 and was significant for hsTnT and sST2 at 4 weeks, 16% greater reduction in hsTnT (P < 0.001) and 9% greater reduction in sST2 (P = 0.0033). Serial urinary cGMP increased serially with sacubitril/valsartan compared with enalapril (P < 0.001, 1 week). The positive effect on biomarkers with sacubitril/valsartan reflects on reduction of myocardial injury and hemodynamic stress.

TRANSITION

TRANSITION was a multicenter, open-label study in which 1,000 adults hospitalized for ADHF with reduced ejection fraction were randomized to sacubitril/valsartan in a predischarge arm (initiated ≥ 24 hours after hemodynamic stabilization) or a postdischarge arm (initiated within 1–14 days after discharge).[10,11]

Aim of the Study

TRANSITION aimed to provide evidence on safety and tolerability of early initiation of sacubitril/valsartan in hospitalized HFrEF patients:

- Stabilized following an ADHF episode
- With pre-existing or newly diagnosed ("de novo") HF
- On any angiotensin-converting enzyme inhibitor (ACEI)/angiotensin receptor blocker (ARB) dose before admission or ACEI/ARB naïve.

Key Inclusion Criteria

- Male or female patients aged ≥ 18 years
- Hospitalized due to ADHF episode as primary diagnosis
- Diagnosis of HF New York Heart Association (NYHA) class II–IV and reduced ejection fraction at screening
- LVEF ≤ 40% at screening
- Patients who did not receive any IV vasodilators (except nitrates) and/or any IV inotropic therapy from the time of presentation for ADHF to randomization
- Stabilized (while in the hospital) for at least 24 hours leading to randomization defined as:
    - No need for IV diuretics in the past 24 hours prior to signing ICF
    - SBP ≥110 mm Hg for at least 6 hours prior to randomization.
- Meeting one of the following criteria:
    - Patients on any dose of ACEI or ARB before admission
    - ACEI/ARB naïve patients and patients not on ACEI or ARB for at least 4 weeks before admission.

Primary Objective

To evaluate the proportion of patients achieving the target dose of sacubitril/valsartan 200 mg BID at week 10 post-randomization in the pre- and postdischarge treatment initiation groups.

Results at 10 Weeks

- Comparable proportions of patients met the primary and secondary endpoints in the pre- and postdischarge initiation groups.
- About half of HFrEF patients stabilized after an ADHF event achieved the target dose of 200 mg sacubitril/valsartan BID within 10 weeks.
- At week 10, more than 86% of patients in both groups were receiving any dose for 2 weeks or longer without interruption.
- Incidence of AEs and sacubitril/valsartan discontinuations due to AEs was similar in in-hospital and ambulatory initiation groups.
- Initiation of sacubitril/valsartan in a wide range of HFrEF patients, early after ADHF event in hospital or shortly after discharge, was feasible and well tolerated.

What is known in heart failure therapy with angiotensin receptor–neprilysin inhibitor?

Sacubitril–valsartan is indicated for the treatment of stable patients with symptomatic heart failure with reduced ejection fraction.

Conclusion and Future Directions

Sacubitril–valsartan has tremendous morbidity and mortality reduction potentials with patients with heart failure. Some of the clinical situations are enumerated as follows in patients who are hospitalized for acute decompensated heart failure:

- Sacubitril–valsartan in patients who have new heart failure
- Sacubitril–valsartan in patients who have not been exposed to high doses of guideline-directed medications for heart failure
- Sacubitril–valsartan in patients who are not receiving conventional renin–angiotensin system inhibitors
- Sacubitril–valsartan low dose initiation (24 mg of sacubitril with 26 mg of valsartan)
- Sacubitril–valsartan initiation during the transition to home and throughout the subsequent out of hospital vulnerable period.

REFERENCES

1. McMurray JJ, Packer M, Desai AS, PARADIGM-HF Committees and Investigators, et al. Dual angiotensin receptor and neprilysin inhibition as an alternative to angiotensin-converting enzyme inhibition in patients with chronic systolic heart failure: rationale for and design of the Prospective comparison of ARNI with ACEI to Determine Impact on Global Mortality and morbidity in Heart Failure trial (PARADIGM-HF). Eur J Heart Fail. 2013;15:1062-73.
2. McMurray JJ, Packer M, Desai AS, PARADIGM-HF Investigators and Committees, et al. Angiotensin-neprilysin inhibition versus enalapril in heart failure. N Engl J Med. 2014;371:993-1004.
3. Packer M, McMurray JJ, Desai AS, PARADIGM-HF Investigators and Coordinators, et al. Angiotensin receptor neprilysin inhibition compared with enalapril on the risk of clinical progression in surviving patients with heart failure. Circulation. 2015;131:54-61.
4. Christ M, Stork S, Dorr M, et al. Heart failure epidemiology 2000–2013: insights from the German Federal Health Monitoring System. Eur J Heart Fail. 2016;18:1009-18.
5. Maggioni AP, Anker SD, Dahlstrom U, et al. Heart Failure Association of the ESC. Are hospitalized or ambulatory patients with heart failure treated in accordance with European Society of Cardiology guidelines? Evidence from 12,440 patients of the ESC Heart Failure Long-Term Registry. Eur J Heart Fail. 2013;15:1173-84.
6. Greene SJ, Fonarow GC, Vaduganathan M, et al. The vulnerable phase after hospitalisation for heart failure. Nat Rev Cardiol. 2015;12:220-9.
7. Velazque EJ, Morrow DA, DeVore AD, et al. Angiotensin–Neprilysin Inhibition in Acute Decompensated Heart Failure. N Engl J Med. 2019;380:539-48.
8. Seferovic PM, Ponikowski P, Anker SD, et al. Clinical practice update on heart failure 2019: pharmacotherapy, procedures, devices and patient management. An expert consensus meeting report of The Heart Failure Association of the European Society of Cardiology. Eur J Heart Fail. 2019;21:1169-86.
9. Morrow AD, Velazquez EJ, DeVore AD, et al. Cardiovascular biomarkers in patients with acute decompensated heart failure randomized to sacubitril-valsartan or enalapril in the PIONEER-HF trial. Eur Heart J. 2019;40:3345-52.
10. Pascual-Figal D, Wachter R, Senni M, et al. Rationale and design of TRANSITION: a randomized trial of pre-discharge vs. post-discharge initiation of sacubitril/valsartan. ESC Heart Fail. 2018;5:327-36.
11. Wachter R, Senni M, Belohlavek J, et al. Initiation of sacubitril/valsartan in haemodynamically stabilised heart failure patients in hospital or early after discharge: primary results of the randomized TRANSITION study. Eur J Heart Fail. 2019;21:998-1007.

CHAPTER

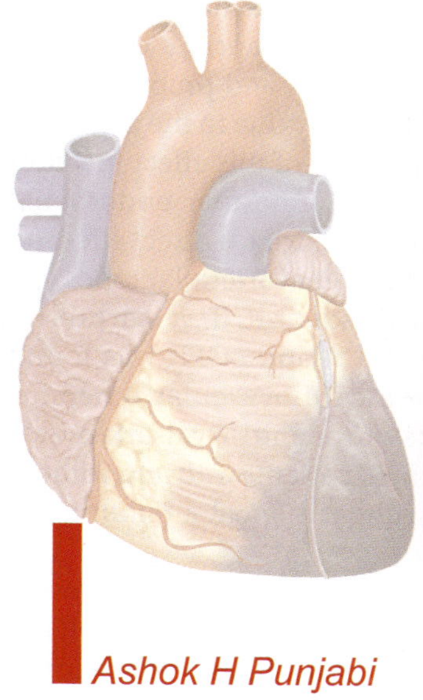

ARNI in HF with Comorbidities

Ashok H Punjabi

INTRODUCTION

Sacubitril/valsartan, the first-in-class angiotensin receptor-neprilysin inhibitors (ARNI), has been proved to significantly reduce the primary composite endpoint of cardiovascular death and heart failure hospitalization, sudden cardiac death, disease progression and improved quality of life, compared with enalapril, in patients of heart failure with reduced ejection fraction (HFrEF) on evidence-based background medical therapy.[1] This new pharmacological class of ARNI has encouraged a conceptual change in the treatment of HFrEF patients. This drug encouraged a paradigm shift in the treatment of HFrEF patients by moving from only the inhibition of the renin–angiotensin–aldosterone system (RAAS) and sympathetic nervous system (SNS) to a neurohormonal modulation strategy based on the concomitant pharmacological enhancement of endogenous natriuretic peptides.[2]

Natriuretic peptides (NPs) are structurally related signaling molecules namely atrial NP (ANP), B-type NP (BNP), and C-type NP (CNP) which play a variety of important physiological roles. In HF patients, the levels of ANP and BNP have long been known to significantly elevate in the heart subjected to stress. NPs are crucial for the homeostasis of blood pressure (BP) by exerting a direct vasodilator effect, through the suppression of the RAAS, the inhibition of endothelin-1, a vasoconstrictor, and the reduction of sympathetic tone. NPs are also important for the regulation of intravascular volume by their direct actions on endothelial permeability and their modulation in the kidneys of fluid and electrolyte balance. In addition, NPs enhance natriuresis and diuresis through effects on renal hemodynamics, mesangial cells, and glomerular filtration.[1]

HF WITH COMORBIDITIES: DIABETES AND CHRONIC KIDNEY DISEASE

The prevalence of HF increases with age and comorbidities, such as hypertension, obesity, and type 2 diabetes mellitus (T2DM). Diabetes and HF are called the "deadly duo" as both global epidemics add tremendous costs on society with increased rates of HF hospitalizations and worsened prognosis. HF and concomitant T2DM are a strong predictor for adverse outcomes and are associated with an approximately two-fold higher risk for CV or all-cause mortality.[3]

Chronic kidney disease (CKD) remains an insufficiently addressed complication of T2DM affecting nearly two of every five patients. Coexistence of CKD and T2DM represents a subset of patients who are at markedly increased risk of mortality. Patients with CKD are at increased risk of cardiovascular disease and this often manifests clinically like heart failure. Conversely, patients with heart failure frequently have reduced kidney function. The interconnectedness of these three chronic conditions—HF, T2DM, and CKD—is well known, while each condition acts as a prognostic risk factor for the other two.[3]

CLINICAL EVIDENCE OF ARNI IN HF AND CKD

The PARADIGM-HF trial conducted on sacubitril/valsartan provided a robust evidence that the combination of RAAS blockade and neprilysin inhibition is superior to RAAS blockade alone in reducing the mortality and hospitalization in HFrEF patients. One of the secondary endpoints of the trial was time to the first occurrence of a decline in renal function (defined as end-stage renal disease or as a decrease in the eGFR of at least 50% or a decrease of more than 30 mL/min/1.73 m^2 from randomization to less than 60 mL/minute/1.73 m^2).[4]

In PARADIGM-HF study, the researchers did not observe significant differences between sacubitril-valsartan and enalapril regarding decline in renal function (<50% eGFR from baseline). However, creatinine levels ≥2.5 mg/dL were less frequent in the sacubitril-valsartan group, with less episodes of renal impairment.[4]

To study the renal effects of sacubitril/valsartan further, a comprehensive analysis of the PARADIGM-HF was conducted to understand the comparative effects of sacubitril/valsartan and enalapril on eGFR and urine albumin-to-creatinine ratio (UACR) and the relationship between changes in eGFR and UACR in cardiovascular and renal outcomes. The results suggested that sacubitril/valsartan, compared to enalapril, slowed the rate of decrease in the eGFR and had favorable effects on cardiovascular and renal outcomes in HFrEF patients with and without CKD and in those with and without microalbuminuria or macroalbuminuria. These beneficial effects were observed even though sacubitril/valsartan increased the UACR compared with enalapril. The favorable effects of sacubitril/valsartan over enalapril on eGFR and other renal outcomes were similar in patients with baseline CKD, compared with those without CKD. These effects are therapeutically important because conventional RAAS blockers are often withdrawn in patients with heart failure and renal dysfunction.[5]

Voors et al. reanalyzed the data from PARAMOUNT trial to study the effect and impact of the sacubitril/valsartan in renal function. Their results showed that treatment with sacubitril/valsartan resulted in lower serum creatinine and higher eGFR after 36 weeks of treatment compared with valsartan. Additionally, the use of sacubitril/valsartan was accompanied by slightly higher albuminuria compared with valsartan (UACR = 2.4–2.9 vs 2.1–2.0 mg/mmol).[5]

In spite of the positive data on the renal impact of the drug, the studies performed in chronic HF patients treated with sacubitril/valsartan have reported a slight increase in urinary albumin excretion. The experts believe that even if albuminuria was slightly increased with sacubitril/valsartan, the overall impact of the drug could be beneficial if higher GFR or reduced CKD progression can be achieved. This is particularly relevant for nonproteinuric renal diseases where albuminuria reduction is not a therapeutic target.

Greater urinary albumin excretion has been associated with a more rapid worsening of renal function in patients with CKD (although it is not known whether this is also true in HFrEF). The investigators found that sacubitril/valsartan increased UACR compared with enalapril, a rapid and modest increase reflecting a distinct, and probably acute intrarenal hemodynamic effect likely due to the actions of natriuretic peptides. The possibility of this effect includes one or more of an increase in glomerular endothelial permeability and hydraulic conductivity, a direct effect on mesangial cells, or alterations in renal arteriolar tone.[6]

The effect observed with sacubitril/valsartan on renal outcomes including UACR and eGFR was found in addition to the effects on cardiovascular outcome. The cardiovascular benefits of sacubitril/valsartan over enalapril were also consistent in patients with and without CKD and in those with and without microalbuminuria and macroalbuminuria.[6]

Senni et al. conducted the TITRATION study to provide additional and complementary data to the PARADIGM-HF trial. The study compared two titration regimens of sacubitril/valsartan: Condensed (100 mg twice daily for 2 weeks followed by 200 mg twice daily) and conservative (50 mg twice daily for 2 weeks, 100 mg twice daily for 3 weeks, followed by 200 mg twice daily) in HF patients. The percentage of patients with increase in serum creatinine levels was negligible in both arms.[7]

The UK HARP-III trial was performed to study the role of sacubitril/valsartan in comparison to irbesartan in patients with CKD. The investigators assessed whether neprilysin inhibition improved kidney function in the short-to medium-term and its effects on cardiovascular biomarkers. No effect (compared to irbesartan control) was found on kidney function, however, the allocation to sacubitril/valsartan reduced the cardiac biomarkers more than irbesartan suggesting that this treatment might improve cardiovascular outcomes.[8,9]

CLINICAL EVIDENCE OF ARNI IN HF AND DIABETES

The pathophysiology for HF development in T2DM is complex and in addition to the general HF risk factors like advancing age, ethnicity, genetic predisposition, hypertension, and smoking, T2DM increases the risk of ischemic HF through increased risk of coronary artery disease, and affects the myocardium leading to structural and functional changes (diabetic cardiomyopathy). Hyperglycemia is a major contributor, and observational data suggest that with each 1%-point increase in HbA1c, there is an 8–16% increased risk of HF (Table 1).[10]

Of the 8,399 patients randomized in the PARADIGM-HF study, 8,274 had a measurement of HbA1c at baseline, a total of 2,907 patients (35%) had a known history of diabetes. Treatment with sacubitril/valsartan reduced the occurrence

TABLE 1: Clinical trials of sacubitril/valsartan and their results on tested renal parameters.

Study drug	*Dosage*	*Comparator*	*Trial name*	*Number of patients (n)*	*Results of renal parameters studies*
Sacubitril/valsartan	400 mg	Valsartan	HF (paramount)	301	Lower eGFR decline, lower incidence of worsening renal function, increased UACR from baseline vs valsartan
Sacubitril/valsartan	400 mg	Enalapril	HF (paradigm)	8442	Less patients with creatinine ≥2.5 mg/dL (3.3 vs 4.5%, p = 0.007), less patients with eGFR decline vs enalapril
Sacubitril/valsartan	400 mg	Different titration regimen	HF (titration)	498	0.6% patients with 200% increase of SCr from baseline; 0.2% patients with SCr >3.0 mg/dL
Sacubitril/valsartan	400 mg	Enalapril	HF (pioneer)	887	No significant difference between the rates of worsening renal function and hyperkalemia

of primary composite outcome as compared to enalapril across all the glycemic states (diabetes, prediabetes, and normoglycemic).[4]

In a posthoc analysis of PARADIGM-HF trial, the investigators studied the effect of sacubitril/valsartan versus enalapril on HbA1c in patients with diabetes and HFrEF enrolled in PARADIGM-HF, as well as the influence of these regimens on the initiation of oral antihyperglycemic and insulin therapy in patients with diabetes. The analysis showed that the level of HbA1c was consistently lower with sacubitril/valsartan as compared to enalapril over a follow-up period of 3 years (Fig. 1). The use of new insulin was reduced by 29% in the study arm taking sacubitril/valsartan as compared to the one taking enalapril in addition to the other background therapies.[10]

The above data suggest that in addition to the heart failure benefits established by PARADIGM-HF trial, sacubitril/valsartan might have favorable metabolic effects in patients with heart failure and diabetes.

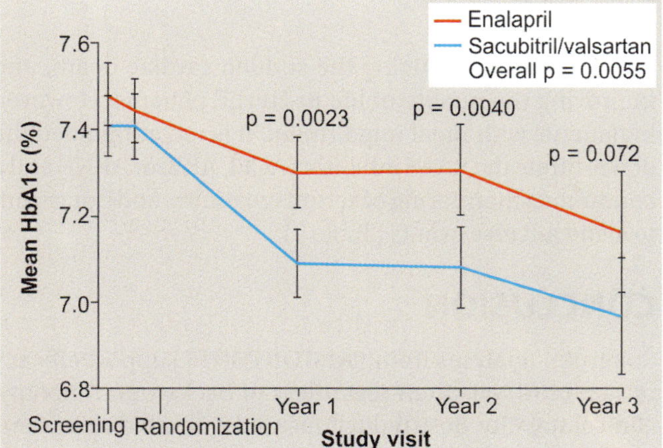

Fig. 1: Level of hemoglobin A1c (HbA1c) reduction with enalapril and sacubitril/valsartan therapy in heart failure with reduced ejection fraction (HFrEF) patients with type 2 diabetes mellitus (T2DM).[10]

Neprilysin, an enzyme which is inhibited by ARNI, is expressed in a wide variety of tissues (endothelial, epithelial and smooth muscle cells, cardiac myocytes, and adipocytes) and is responsible for the breakdown of a number of vasoactive peptides including natriuretic peptides, bradykinin, angiotensin I and II, and glucagon-like peptide 1 (GLP-1). Inhibition of neprilysin might lead to improvement in glycemic control through several possible mechanisms. Natriuretic peptides which are increased by neprilysin inhibition might have a crucial role in insulin sensitivity and metabolism. Neprilysin is known to promote lipid mobilization from adipose tissue, increase postprandial lipid oxidation, promote adiponectin release, enhance muscular oxidative capacity, and decrease blood glucose level (Fig. 2).[3]

Patients with HF and T2DM are associated with an accelerated decline in renal function and increased risk for chronic kidney disease which adversely influences risk for HF outcome. Neprilysin inhibition has been shown to have favorable effects in animal models of diabetic nephropathy, but its effects on renal function in patients with type 2 diabetes have not been evaluated in large-scale trials.[3]

A posthoc analysis of the PARADIGM-HF trial examined the effect of T2DM on the decline in renal function in patients with HFrEF, and evaluated the effects of sacubitril/valsartan versus enalapril on renal function in patients with and without diabetes (Fig. 3).[3]

A significantly greater decline in eGFR was observed in HFrEF patients with diabetes compared with those without diabetes. The benefit of sacubitril/valsartan on renal function in HFrEF patients with diabetes was twice as large as in HFrEF patients without diabetes.[3]

In addition, sacubitril/valsartan has shown to effectively reduce the risk of hyperkalemia in HFrEF patients. The

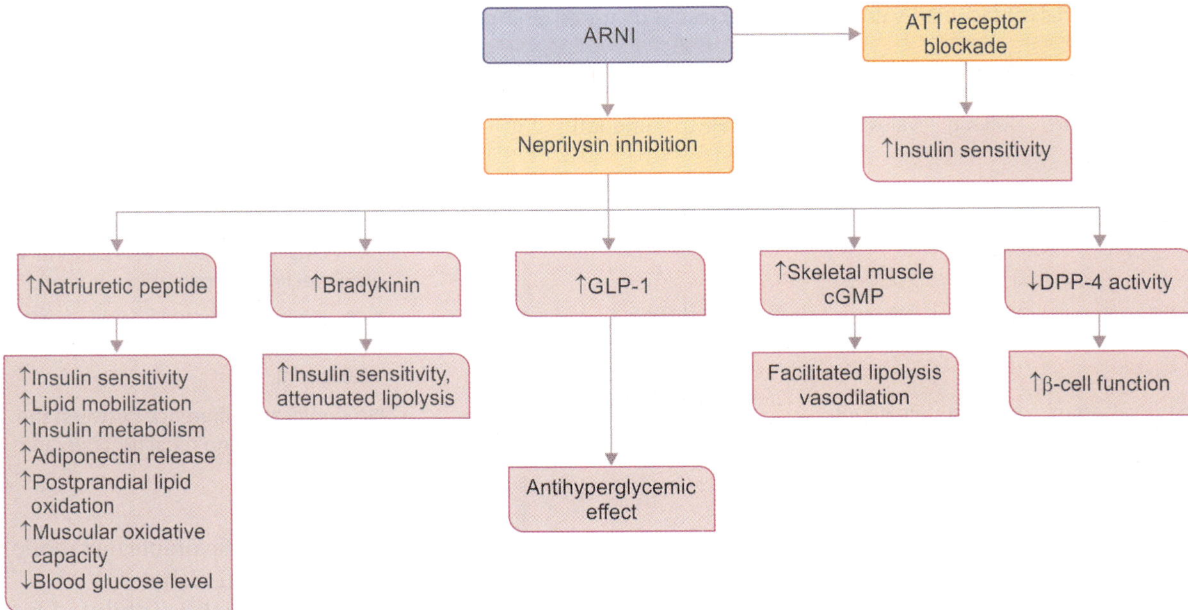

Fig. 2: Possible mechanisms of glycemic control by angiotensin receptor-neprilysin inhibitor (ARNI).[11]

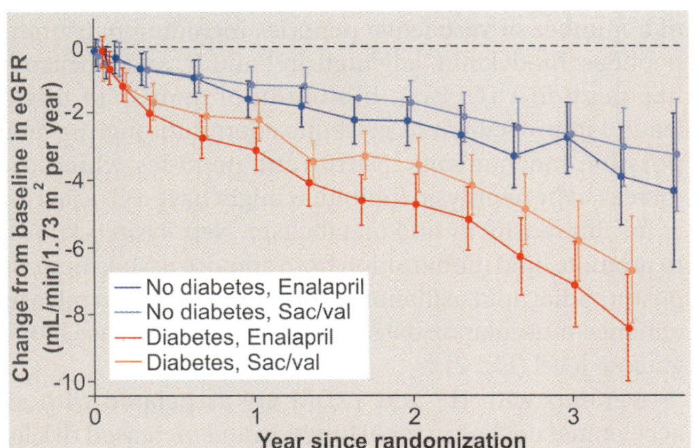

Fig. 3: The estimated glomerular filtration rate (eGFR) change from baseline in heart failure (HF) patients with and without diabetes on sacubitril/valsartan or enalapril.[3]

current ACC/AHA and ESC guideline recommends the addition of mineralocorticoid receptor antagonists (MRAs) for most HF patients who are symptomatic despite treating them with beta-blockers and RAAS inhibitors. Although MRAs are associated with reduction in risk of death or hospitalization in HFrEF, there is a heightened concern for the risk of hyperkalemia. A posthoc analysis of PARADIGM-HF proved that the incidence of severe hyperkalemia was less with sacubitril/valsartan as compared to enalapril in HFrEF patients.[12]

The robust data proves the superiority of sacubitril/valsartan over enalapril in reducing the CV mortality, HF hospitalization, reducing the sudden cardiac death, and improving the quality of life in HFrEF patients. However, in patients with renal impairment, it is recommended the down-titrate the RAAS inhibitor (ACEI, ARB, or ARNI) and a continuous monitoring of serum creatinine and potassium to avoid adverse events (Table 2).

TABLE 2: Dosing recommendation of sacubitril/valsartan as per the renal impairment.

Dosing	*Mild (eGFR ≥ 60 mL/min/1.73 m²)*	*Moderate (eGFR 59 – 30 mL/min/1.73 m²)*	*Severe (eGFR < 30 mL/min/1.73 m²)*
Starting	No dose adjustment required	No dose adjustment required	50 mg
Duration			2–4 weeks
Target maintenance dose			100 mg

(eGFR: estimated glomerular filtration rate)

Source: Adapted from the prescribing information of Vymada®.

CONCLUSION

Subgroup analyses from PARADIGM-HF support efficacy of sacubitril/valsartan regardless of background therapy, clinical stability, dose reductions, and comorbid conditions and reassure clinicians about the drug's effectiveness in broad patient populations.[2] According to ACC/AHA, ESC, and Canadian HF guidelines, it is beneficial to implement sacubitril/valsartan in eligible patients to provide further reductions in mortality and HF hospitalization. To conclude, an appropriate and timely use of sacubitril/valsartan has the potential to significantly improve global and public health.

REFERENCES

1. Yandrapalli S, Khan MH, Rochlani Y, et al. Sacubitril/valsartan in cardiovascular disease: evidence to date and place in therapy. Ther Adv Cardiovasc Dis. 2018;12(8):217-31.
2. Dargad RR, Prajapati MR, Dargad RR, et al. Sacubitril/valsartan: A novel angiotensin receptor-neprilysin inhibitor. Indian Heart J. 2018;70 Suppl 1:S102-S10.
3. Packer M, Claggett B, Lefkowitz MP, et al. Effect of neprilysin inhibition on renal function in patients with type 2 diabetes and chronic heart failure who are receiving target doses of inhibitors of the renin-angiotensin system: a secondary analysis of the PARADIGM-HF trial. Lancet Diabetes Endocrinol. 2018;6(7):547-54
4. McMurray JJV, Packer M, Desai AS, et al. Angiotensin–neprilysin inhibition versus enalapril in heart failure. N Engl J Med. 2014;371:993-1004.
5. Voors AA, Gori M, Liu LC, et al. Renal effects of the angiotensin receptor neprilysin inhibitor LCZ696 in patients with heart failure and preserved ejection fraction. Eur J Heart Fail. 2015;17:510-7.
6. Gervasini G, Robles NR. Potential beneficial effects of sacubitril-valsartan in renal disease: a new field for a new drug. Expert Opin Investig Drugs. 2017;26:651-9.
7. Senni M, McMurray JJ, Wachter R, et al. Initiating sacubitril/valsartan (LCZ696) in heart failure: results of TITRATION, a double-blind, randomized comparison of two uptitration regimens. Eur J Heart Fail. 2016;18(9):1193-202.
8. Haynes R, Judge PK, Staplin N, et al. Effects of Sacubitril/Valsartan versus Irbesartan in Patients with Chronic Kidney Disease. Circulation. 2018;138:1505-14.
9. Velazquez EJ, Morrow DA, DeVore AD, et al. Angiotensin-neprilysin inhibition in acute decompensated heart failure. N Engl J Med. 2019;380:539-48.
10. Seferovic JP, Claggett B, Seidelmann SB et al. Effect of sacubitril/valsartan versus enalapril on glycaemic control in patients with heart failure and diabetes: a post-hoc analysis from the PARADIGM-HF trial. Lancet Diabetes Endocrinol. 2017;5(5):333-40.
11. Giamouzis G, Butler J. Glycaemic control in heart failure: a PARADIGM shift for patients with concomitant diabetes? Lancet Diabetes Endocrinol. 2017;5(5):314-5.
12. Desai AS, Vardeny O, Claggett B, et al. Reduced risk of hyperkalemia during treatment of heart failure with mineralocorticoid receptor antagonists by use of sacubitril/valsartan compared with enalapril: a secondary analysis of the PARADIGM-HF trial. JAMA Cardiol. 2017;2:79-85.

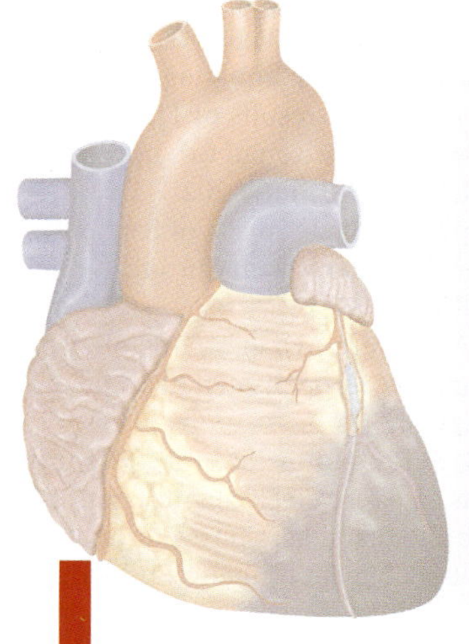

Ischemic Mitral Regurgitation

Anil Dhall, Anurag Garg, Ritesh Sanguri

INTRODUCTION

Ischemic mitral regurgitation (IMR) is a frequent complication after acute myocardial infarction (AMI) associated with a worse prognosis. IMR is highly dynamic, especially during the acute phase of ischemia over the course of emergency revascularization and may need surgical intervention beyond revascularization. The pathophysiological mechanisms of chronic IMR are not fully understood, but it is known that it is a complex process in which ventricular remodeling could be the main causal factor. Echocardiography has contributed significantly for clarifying the mechanisms that cause and progressively aggravate IMR. The role of surgical repair or catheter intervention for MR is still controversial with limited and conflicting data based on various surgical strategies.

ACUTE ISCHEMIC MITRAL REGURGITATION

About 3% of patients with an acute MI have severe mitral regurgitation with a 30-day mortality of 25% and a 1-year mortality of 50%.[1,2] A further 15% of patients have mild-to-moderate mitral regurgitation, which is often transient and usually has a good prognosis. In patients with cardiogenic shock, about 40% will have at least moderate and often severe mitral regurgitation; this doubles the mortality at 1 year compared with patients without mitral regurgitation. In patients with cardiogenic shock, acute ischemic mitral regurgitation was the underlying cause in 6.9%.[3,4]

Acute mitral regurgitation after MI can be due to:

- Papillary muscle dysfunction caused by fibrosis or ischemia of the papillary muscle
- Papillary muscle rupture (either partial or complete)
- Mitral annular dilatation associated with LV failure.

The blood supply to the posteromedial papillary muscle (derived only from the posterior descending artery) is more tenuous than that to the anterolateral papillary muscle (derived from both the LAD and the LCX). 90% of papillary muscle ruptures involve the posteromedial papillary muscle. This is fortuitous because the posteromedial papillary muscle usually has multiple heads (in contrast to the single head of the anterolateral papillary muscle), and rupture of an individual head is frequently survivable, at least in the short term. Complete transection of a LV papillary muscle is usually fatal because of massive sudden mitral regurgitation. Infarctions associated with papillary muscle rupture are usually small, and frequently there is only single-vessel coronary disease. Patients with papillary muscle rupture usually present up to 1 week after MI with acute pulmonary edema. The loudness of the mitral regurgitation murmur is variable and may not correlate with the degree of mitral regurgitation. The murmur may be completely absent in some patients with severe mitral regurgitation. A thrill is rarely present in acute mitral regurgitation. Large V waves are present in the pulmonary wedge tracing, and, more rarely, the regurgitant jet may be transmitted through the pulmonary vasculature to lead to increased oxygen saturation in the PA; this may suggest an erroneous diagnosis of ventricular septal rupture.

Echocardiography is the diagnostic imaging method of choice afterload reduction with sodium nitroprusside and placement of an intra-aortic balloon pump will temporarily improve patient hemodynamics by increasing forward cardiac output and decreasing the regurgitant fraction. Emergency cardiac surgery is generally indicated with an expected mortality of about 25%:[5,6] ideally the mitral valve should be repaired if there is no papillary muscle necrosis, but mitral valve replacement is often needed. Coronary artery bypass graft (CABG) at the time of mitral valve surgery improves outcome and in patient who survives surgery, long-term prognosis is often good. In acute ischemic mitral regurgitation, only papillary muscle rupture needs immediate repair. Other causes, such as left ventricular global or regional remodeling, or ischemic papillary muscle dysfunction, may resolve after revascularization and recovery of left ventricular function. Accordingly, only 46% of the patients in the SHOCK trial registry underwent mitral valve surgery. In contrast to VSD repair, surgery of papillary muscle rupture does not involve necrotic myocardium in suture lines. Therefore, mortality associated with this repair is lower, although is still high with an overall mortality of 55%. Nevertheless, the unpredictability and potential for rapid deterioration and death with papillary muscle rupture make early surgery necessary. There are few case reports with interventional edge-to-edge repair in acute ischemic mitral regurgitation; however, no larger series have been published.

CHRONIC ISCHEMIC MITRAL REGURGITATION

This may have components of:

- Regional wall motion abnormality with inadequate closure of MV leaflets (increased tethering forces)
- Mechanical damage to mitral valve apparatus
- Mitral valvular spatial disposition and geometry abnormality (the PM displacement that creates greater tension of the leaflets is posterolateral-apical, which explains why a located inferior AMI can produce a significant IMR, and why its incidence is much lower in the anterior AMI)
- *Functional mitral regurgitation due to LV and annular dilatation*: LV dilatation is more global, LV is more spherical, both papillary muscles are displaced, with a central regurgitant jet, contribution of annular dilatation is more important (anterior infarction):
  - Posterior infarction, local LV remodeling and distortion—apical, posterior, and lateral displacement of the posterior papillary muscle
  - More apical position of the leaflets, deformity of the anterior leaflet (seagull sign), reduced mobility of the posterior leaflet.
- Ruptured papillary muscle secondary to myocardial infarction is included as primary ischemic MR.
- True ischemic MR secondary to a transient active ischemic episode.
- Acute ischemic episodes linked to a severe stenosis of the left circumflex and/or the right coronary artery can induce "flash pulmonary edema".

Ischemic MR results from an imbalance between *increased tethering forces and reduced closing forces*, the latter including reduction in LV contractility, altered systolic annular contraction, reduced synchronicity between the two papillary muscles and global LV dyssynchrony, especially in basal. Inadequate closure of the mitral leaflets is the consequence of increased tethering forces. The most frequent pattern corresponds to a posterior infarction, usually transmural, leading to local LV pathological remodeling and distortion contributing to apical, posterior, and lateral displacement of the posterior papillary muscle. The papillary muscle contributes nonextensible chordae to both leaflets; its displacement results in a more apical position of the leaflets and their coaptation point, and a characteristic deformity of the anterior leaflet described as "*seagull sign*". The tethering process produces the shape of a tent between the annular plane and the displaced leaflets. The tenting volume relates closely to the regurgitant orifice area. In the case of posterior infarction and regional remodeling, the tenting area is asymmetric, predominates on the posterior leaflet close to the medial commissure, accompanied by reduced mobility of the posterior leaflet. In other patients, LV dilatation is more global; LV is more spherical; both papillary muscles are displaced; the tenting area is symmetric; the regurgitant jet is central; the contribution of annular dilatation and flattening is more important. This situation occurs in patients with previous anterior or both anterior and posterior infarctions.[7-9]

We can classify this as symmetric and asymmetric MR. Characteristics of symmetric and asymmetric ischemic MR are shown in Table 1.

The previously held notion that ischemic MR is caused by papillary muscle dysfunction is not true.

Pathophysiology of ischemic MR is much more complex than that of primary MR, since myocardial damage and LV dysfunction are the causes that precede MR (Figs. 1A and B). The consequences of MR depend on the severity of regurgitation, the driving force, and the acuteness of the lesion and in turn of LA compliance. Isolated papillary muscle infarction does not produce MR and may reduce the amount of MR. Fibrotic elongation of papillary muscle after myocardial infarction is an unusual lesion. In this situation, there is an association of some degree of leaflet tethering and leaflet prolapse. In the vast majority of patients in whom ischemic MR is chronic and complicates

TABLE 1: Characteristics of symmetric versus asymmetric CIMR tethering phenotypes.

	Symmetric CIMR	*Asymmetric CMR*
Major net tethering vectors	Apical	Posterior> apical
Tethered mitral leaflets	Anterior and posterior	Posterior
Associated myocardial infarct pattern (and vessels)	Anterior (left anterior descending/multiple coronary arteries)	Inferoposterior (right coronary > circumflex)
Archetype pattern of LV dysfunction	Global LV dilatation and wall motion abnormality	Inferoposterior wall motion abnormality and dilatation
Mitral valve coaptation zone displacement	Apically	Posteriorly; pseudoprolapse of anterior leaflet over posterior leaflet
Tethering angles	Anterior ≈ posterior	Posterior > anterior
Tenting volume	Higher	Lower
MR origin and direction	Central, non-eccentric	Posterior, posteriorly eccentric
Annular dilatation	Greater	Lesser
Annular height	Greater loss of non-planarity (flattened)	Less loss of height
MR relative severity	Less severe	More severe
Severity correlates best with	LV dilatation and sphericity	Degree of mitral valve deformation (greater tethering angles, more marked derangement of coaptation zone)

(CIMR: chronic ischemic mitral regurgitation)

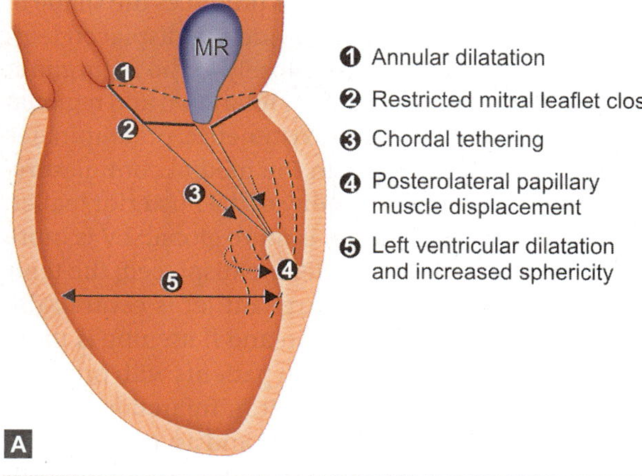

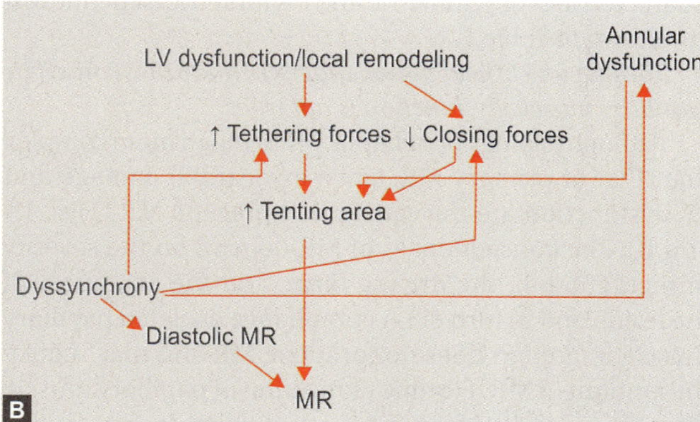

Figs. 1A and B: (A) Mechanism of ischemic MR; (B) Flowchart of mechanism of ischemic MR. (LV: left ventricular; MR: mitral regurgitation)

LV dysfunction and most often heart failure, LA is enlarged, more compliant, and the driving force is relatively low.[7-9] The volume overload due to MR contributes to a vicious circle: the more remodeled LV, the more severe MR, which begets further LV dilatation and thus, further MR. This cycle has important effects on LV geometry, leading to a rather spherical LV. The upstream consequences are high LA pressure and pulmonary arterial hypertension. An important characteristic of ischemic MR is its dynamic component. The effective regurgitant orifice (ERO) area can change during systole: it is less important in mid-systole when compared with early and late systole. These changes are determined by dynamic changes of transmitral pressure contributing to valve closure.[9,10] Echocardiographic and clinical characteristics of different subgroups of IMR are shown in Table 2.

Medical Management

Many patients with secondary MR will have a reduced left ventricular ejection fraction (LVEF). First-line medical treatment typically involves standard pharmacologic therapy for heart failure including beta-blockers, diuretics, and angiotensin-converting enzyme inhibitors or angiotensin receptor blockers. Another option in some patients is the use of cardiac resynchronization therapy (CRT), which has been shown to improve LV systolic and diastolic function and reduce MR. Numerous randomized controlled trials have demonstrated the benefit of CRT in heart failure with reduced EF.

TABLE 2: Echocardiographic and clinical characteristics of different subgroups of IMR.

	Asymmetric tethering	*Symmetric tethering*	*Prevalence of annular dilation/dysfunction*	*Ischemic prolapse*
Posterior leaflet tethering	+++	+	–	–
Apical leaflet tethering	+	+++	+	–
Eccentric jet	+++	+	–	+++
Central jet	+	+++	++	–
Coaptation depth	↑↑	↑↑↑	↔	–
Tenting area	↑↑	↑↑↑	↔	–
Annular dilation	↑↑	↑↑↑	↑↑↑	↑
Annular flattening	↑	↑↑↑	↑↑	–
Local remodeling	+++	+++	+	++
Global remodeling	+	+++	++	+
Anterior myocardial infarction	+	+++	+	–
Inferior-lateral myocardial infarction	+++	+	+	+++
Multiple myocardial infarction	+	+++	+	+
Single vessel disease	++	+	+	++
Multiple vessel disease	++	+++	+	+

Semiquantitative methods:

Color Doppler jet area
Maximum MR jet area/left atrium (LA) area (same frame)
<20%—mild MR, 20–40%—moderate MR, >40%—severe MR
Keep Nyquist limit between 40 cm/s and 50 cm/s. Optimize color gain. Add a grade, if MR jet eccentric or assess also laminar flow signals moving with turbulent MR jet. Check if MR pansystolic. Measure blood pressure.

Vena contracta width:
- <3 mm—mild MR
- 3–7 mm—moderate MR
- >7 mm—severe MR

Mitral inflow:
- Peak E velocity > 1.5 m/s—severe MR (in the absence of mitral stenosis)
- Pulsed Doppler mitral to aortic time velocity integral (TVI) ratio < 1m/s—mild MR, >1.4 m/s—severe MR

Pulmonary venous flow:
- Reverse systolic flow in pulmonary vein—severe MR. More accurate, if reverse flow in more than one pulmonary vein.
- Continuous wave Doppler MR jet intensity and morphology
- Dense MR signals with full envelope of equal intensity to antegrade flow—severe MR
- Blunting/notching of envelope—severe MR

Quantitative methods:

Flow convergence (PISA method):
- *Effective MR orifice area (EROA)*: <0.2 cm^2—mild MR, 0.2–0.29 cm^2—moderate MR, 0.30–0.39 cm^2—moderately severe MR, ≥0.40 cm^2—severe MR
- *MR volume*: <30 mL/beat—mild, 30–44 mL/beat—moderate MR, 45–59 mL/beat—moderately severe MR, >60 mL/beat—severe MR
- *MR fraction*: <30%—mild MR, 30–39%—moderate MR, 40–59%—moderately severe MR, >50%—severe MR
- *Three-dimensional assessment of vena contracta area*: <0.2 cm^2—mild MR, 0.2–0.4 cm^2—moderate, >0.4 cm^2—severe MR

(IMR: ischemic mitral regurgitation)

Guideline-directed medical therapy is important:

- Proportion of patients in mitral regurgitation (MR) grade 3+ or 4+ after CABG with/without MV repair are shown in Figure 2
- The benefits of individual drug classes are substantial
- Mortality benefits of drug classes are additive
- There is a reduction in secondary mitral regurgitation (SMR)
- Reducing filling pressures with diuretics also likely reduces SMR
- A reduction in SMR is strongly correlated with improved outcomes with GDMT and MitraClip®
- Congestion is a better predictor of outcomes than cardiac index
- Many patients with HFrEF and HFpEF are congested with high PA pressures
- Referred patients not in a HF clinic are rarely on *maximally tolerated* GDMT

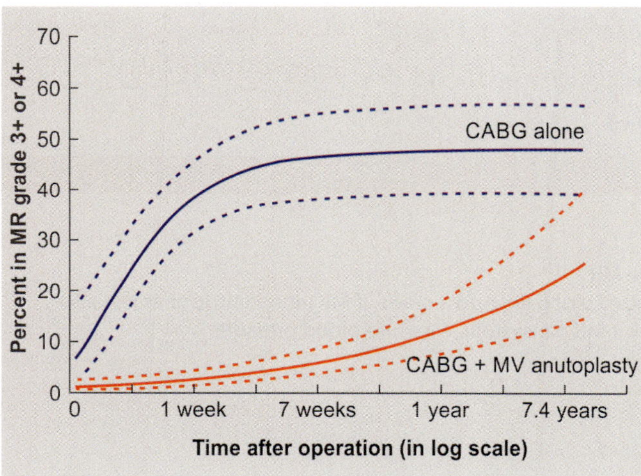

Fig. 2: Proportion of patients in mitral regurgitation (MR) grade 3+ or 4+.
(CABG: coronary artery bypass graft)

- Uptitrating GDMT after MitraClip® is likely to be important as it is after CRT.[10,11]

Surgical Options for IMR

Surgery is an established treatment for functional MR. *The gold standard of management remains an undersized mitral ring annuloplasty.* Mitral valve surgery is not currently recommended for isolated secondary regurgitation unless the patient is severely symptomatic and has class III/IV heart failure, but it is suggested (Class of Recommendation IIb, Level of evidence B) in those patients undergoing CABG or aortic valve replacement. However, recent studies have debated this recommendation as to whether there is benefit to any intervention on the MV for patients undergoing CABG as MV repair has a failure rate of 20–30% at 2 years (Fig. 2).

Mihaljevic and associates studied 390 patients who underwent CABG with or without MV annuloplasty. Although recurrent MR was reduced in patients who underwent annuloplasty, it did not appear to improve survival or functional status (Figs. 3 and 4).[10-13]

Mitral valve repair in moderate IMR remains a contentious issue with a number of very conflicting studies. However, some patients do benefit from MVA though this subset is yet to be definitively defined. It may be possible that these are patients with predominantly heart failure symptoms with raised BNP levels.

Recurrent MR was seen in the CSTN study and tethering/basal dyskinesia was the main mechanism as shown in Figure 5.[14-16]

A second question of whether to repair or replace the MV remains controversial as well. According to the Society of Thoracic Surgeons database (2008–2012), MV repair was favored in over 50% of patients undergoing MV surgery at the time of CABG.[14-16]

Reasons for this include reported lower perioperative morbidity and mortality thought to be due in part to

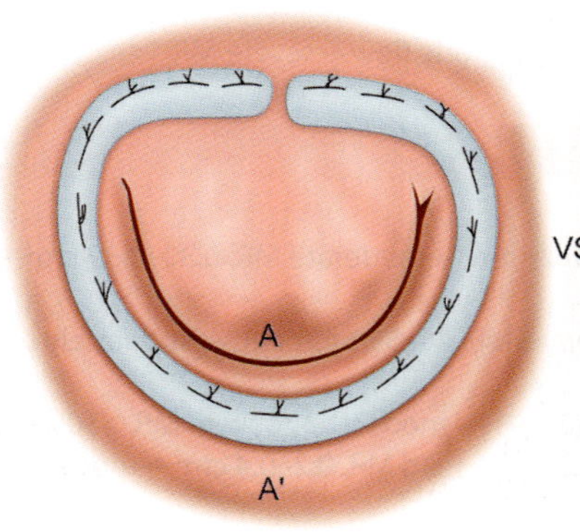

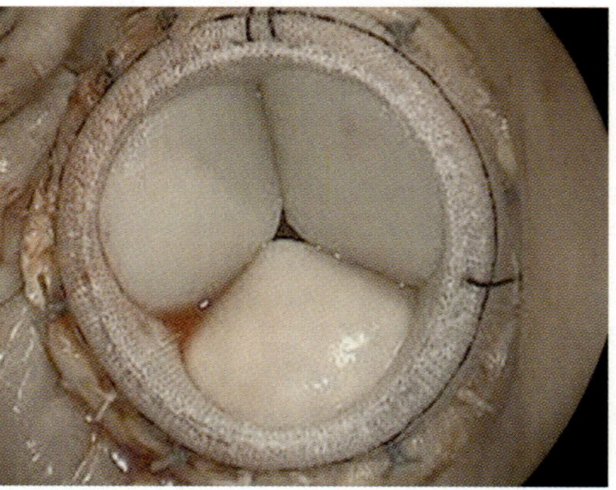

Fig. 3: Undersized ring annuloplasty and mitral valve replacement as treatment of IMR.

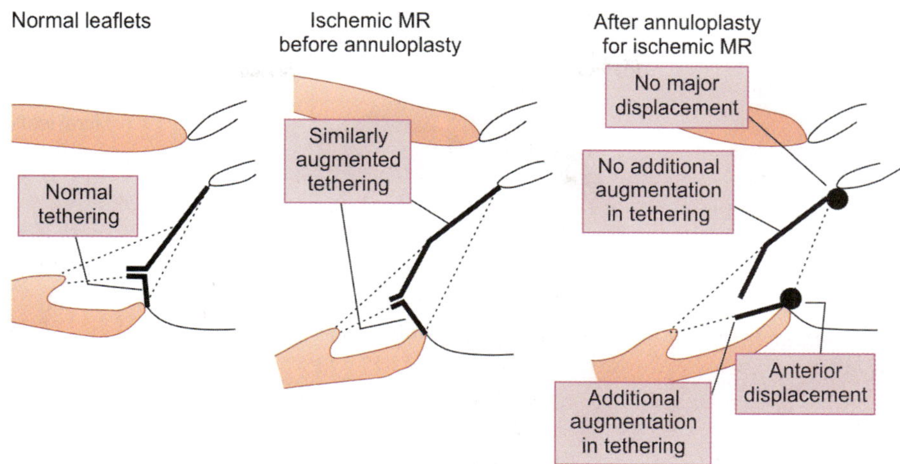

Fig. 4: Ischemic MR with and without annuloplasty.

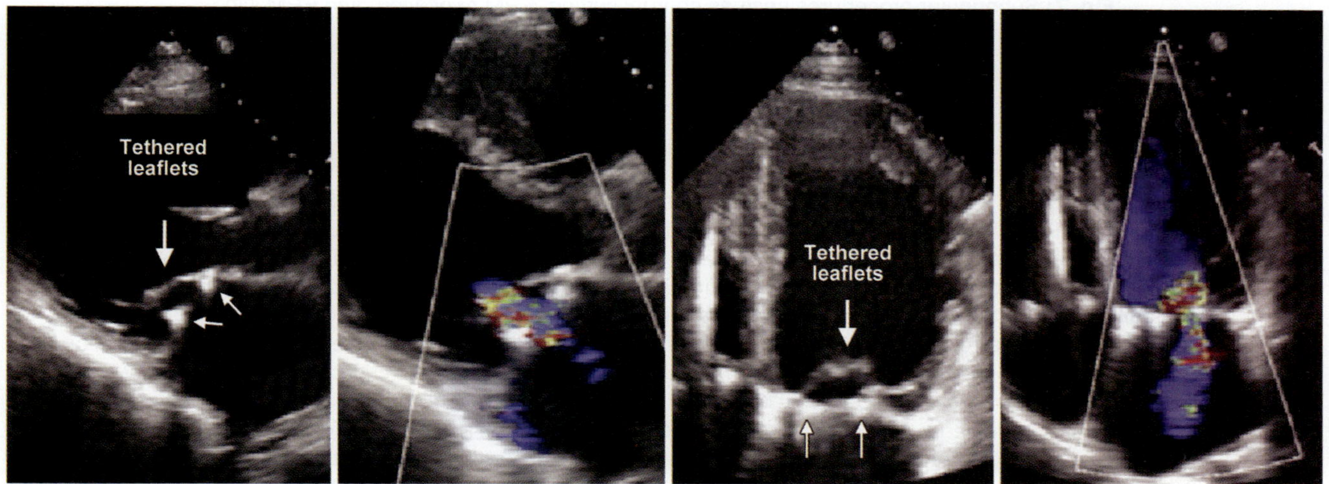

Fig. 5: Recurrent mitral regurgitation (MR) in CSTN trial.

Source: Kron IL, Hung J, Overbey JR, et al. Predicting recurrent mitral regurgitation after mitral valve repair for severe ischemic mitral regurgitation. J Thorac Cardiovasc Surg. 2015;149(3):752-61.e1.

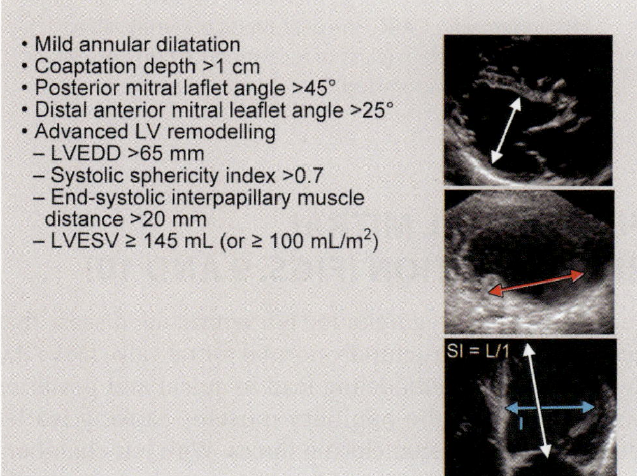

Fig. 6: Predictors of failure of undersized ring annuloplasty.

preservation of the subvalvular apparatus and lack of prosthetic valve complications such as endocarditis and bleeding among others. Several surgical options are available when considering MV repair for IMR. The primary approach is annular repair with a downsized ring annuloplasty (Fig. 6). Another option is leaflet repair using the edge-to-edge technique or posterior mitral leaflet augmentation. A repair of the subvalvular apparatus, which includes the papillary muscles and chordae tendineae, is sometimes performed as well. Secondary cords may be cut to alleviate restriction and papillary muscles may be relocated or approximated. All of the above may be combined with downsized ring annuloplasty. In an attempt to improve durability of MVR in FIMR, subannular procedures such as chordal cutting, PPM relocation, and PPM sling have been tried (Fig. 7).[16-20]

Secondary MR may demand different surgical approaches concomitant to restrictive annuloplasty (Fig. 8).

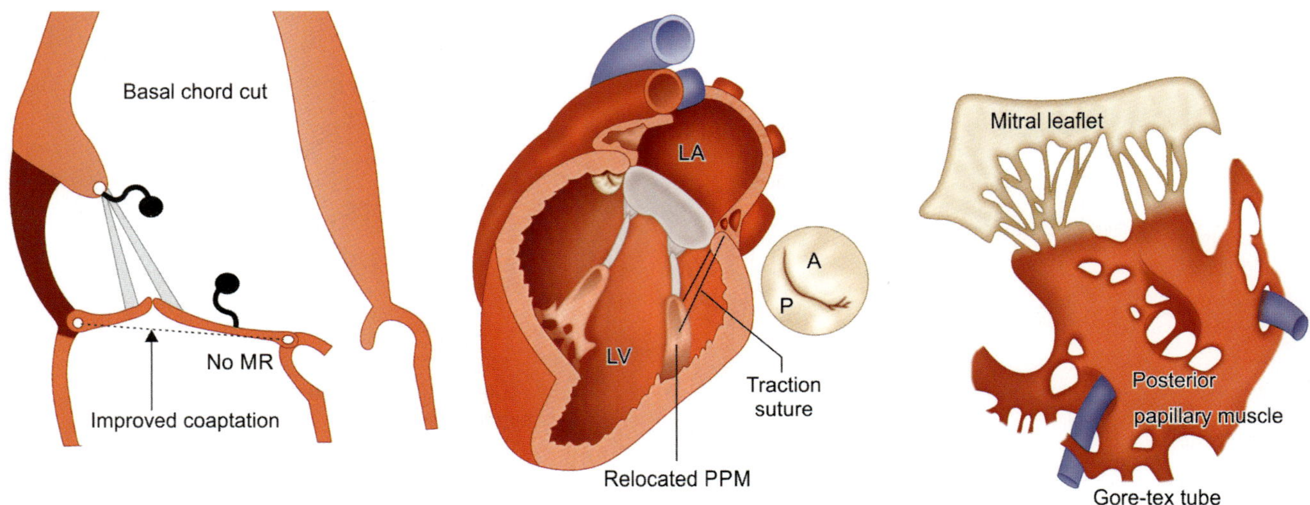

Fig. 7: Subannular procedures such as chordal cutting, PPM relocation, and PPM sling.

TABLE 3: Comparison of AATS and AHA/ACC guidelines.

	2016 AA TS Guideline	*2017 AHA/ACC Guideline*
Severe ischemic MR	"MV replacement is reasonable in patients with severe ischemic MR who remain symptomatic despite guideline-directed medical and cardiac device therapy (i.e. stage D), and who have a basal aneurysm/dyskinesis, significant leaflet tethering, and/or severe left ventricular dilatation (end-diastolic diameter > 6.5 cm) (class of recommendation IIa, level of evidence B)." "MV repair with an undersized complete rigid annuloplasty ring may be considered in patients with severe ischemic MR who remain symptomatic despite guideline-directed medical and cardiac device therapy (i.e. stage D) and who do not have a basal aneurysm/dyskinesis, significant leaflet tethering, or severe LV enlargement (end-diastolic dimension> 6.5 cm) (class of recommendation IIb, level of evidence B)."	"Mitral valve repair or replacement may be considered for severely symptomatic patients (New York Heart Association class III to IV) with chronic severe secondary MR (stage D) who have persistent symptoms despite optimal guideline-directed medical therapy for heart failure (class of recommendation IIb, level of evidence B)." "It is reasonable to choose chordal-sparing MV replacement over downsized annuloplasty repair if operation is considered for severely symptomatic patients (New York Heart Association class III to IV) with chronic severe ischemic MR (stage D) and persistent symptoms despite guideline-directed medical therapy for heart failure (class of recommendation IIa, level of evidence B-randomized)."
Moderate ischemic MR	"In patients with moderate ischemic MR undergoing CABG, mitral valve repair with an undersized complete rigid annuloplasty ring may be considered (class of recommendation IIb, level of evidence B)."	"In patients with chronic, moderate, ischemic MR (stage B) undergoing CABG, the usefulness of mitral valve repair is uncertain (class of recommendation IIb, level of evidence B-randomized)."

Isolated restrictive annuloplasty will be performed in Type I MR meanwhile subannular techniques are necessary for patients with Type IIIB. Subannular techniques are easy, safe, and reproducible and improve repair results. More follow-up data are necessary to investigate long-term results.[19,20]

Treating severe or even moderate MR surgically has been again a matter of varying opinion and the same is even reflected in the guidelines as shown in Table 3.

FUNCTIONAL MITRAL REGURGITATION (FIGS. 9 AND 10)

Functional mitral regurgitation is a ventricular disease that occurs despite a structurally normal mitral valve (MV). LV dysfunction and remodeling lead to apical and posterior displacement of the papillary muscles causing leaflet tethering and reduced closing forces. With left chambers enlargement, the mitral annulus dilates and loses its saddle

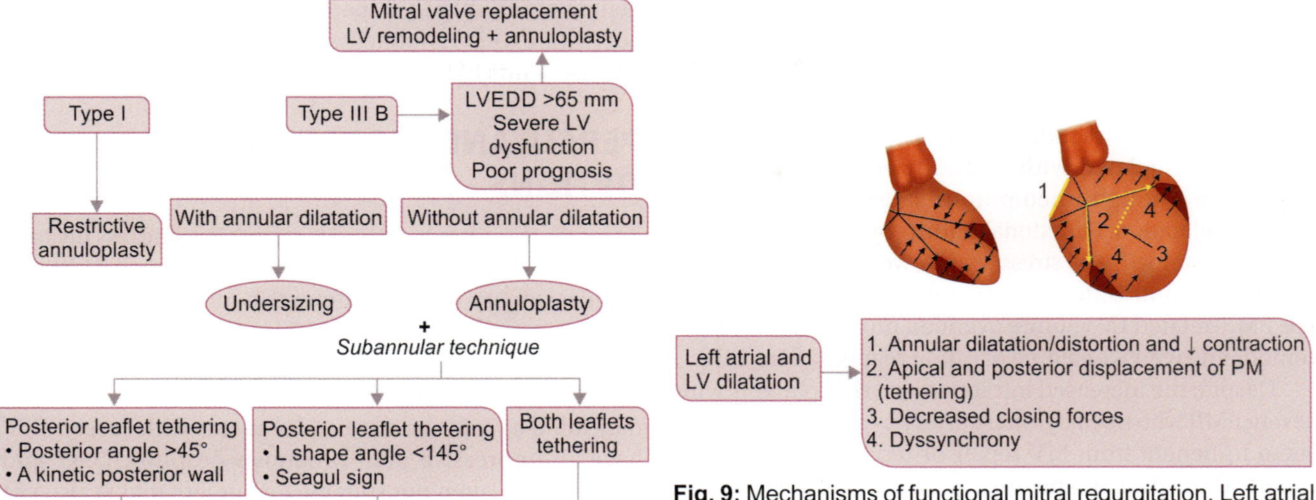

Fig. 8: Proposed algorithm for secondary mitral regurgitation.

Fig. 9: Mechanisms of functional mitral regurgitation. Left atrial and left ventricular (LV) dilatation lead to: annular dilatation/ distortion (1); apical and posterior displacement of papillary muscles (PM) causing leaflet tethering (2); reduced closing forces (3); and dyssynchrony (4).

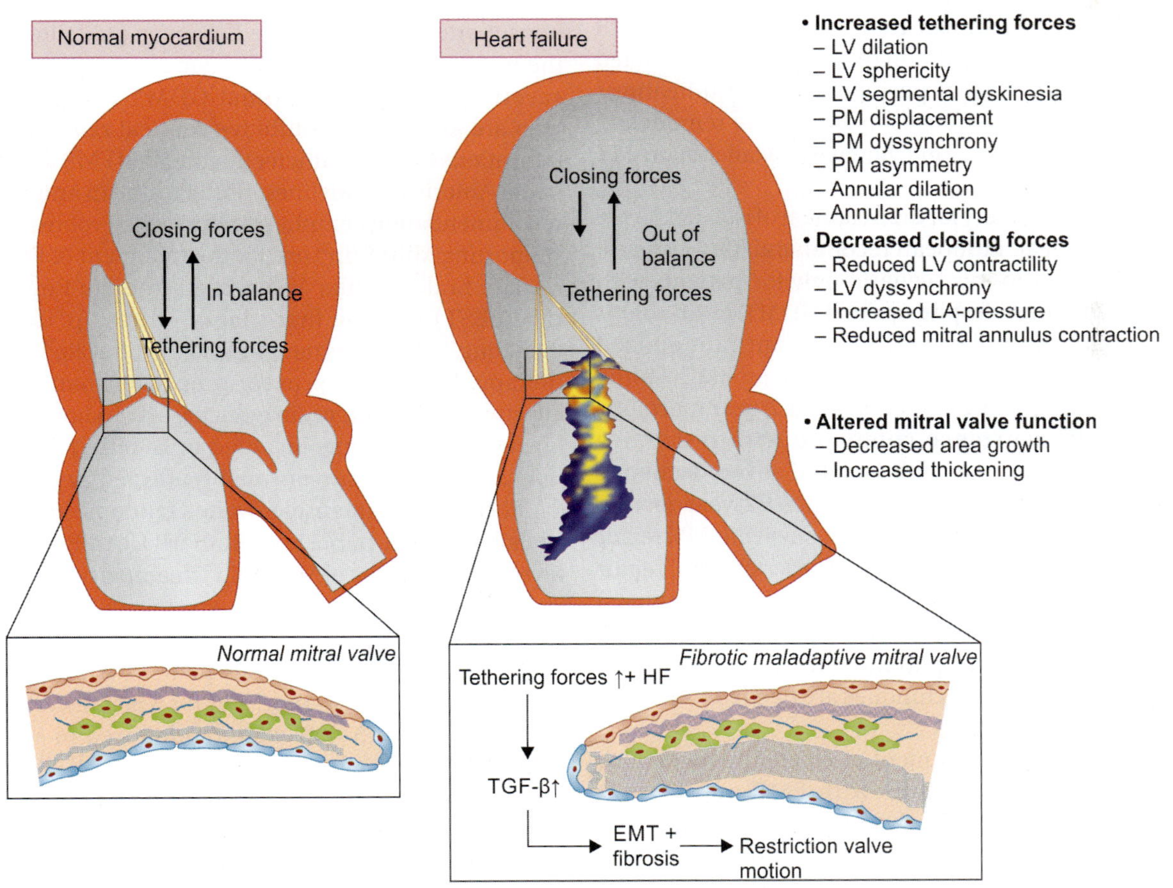

Fig. 10: Role of functional mitral regurgitation (FMR) in heart failure progression. Left ventricular (LV) remodeling leads to FMR. The latter induces LV volume overload promoting heart failure progression with further LV remodeling and worsening of mitral insufficiency.

shape, resulting in increased mitral leaflet stress and failure of coaptation. LV dyssynchrony may be an additional mechanism of FMR due to wall motion abnormalities involving the papillary muscles, with further leaflet dysfunction and retraction. Isolated left atrial enlargement, generally associated with atrial fibrillation, may be an additional, though uncommon, cause of FMR due to annulus dilatation. Functional mitral regurgitation leads to increased preload, wall stress, and LV workload, all of which negatively contribute, in a vicious circle, to progressive HF. FMR-related LV volume overload promotes further LV remodeling with worsening of mitral regurgitation (MR).

Despite the increased intraoperative risk, patients with severe FMR who need coronary artery bypass graft (CABG) seem to benefit from MV repair or replacement. As well stated in both the ESC and ACC/AHA guidelines even if with a low level of evidence (c), MV repair over-replacement is suggested in patients without basal aneurysm/dyskinesis, significant leaflet tethering, or severe LV dilatation. A much debated scenario regards patients with moderate FMR that are scheduled to undergo CABG, for whom the indication for MV surgery remains controversial. A recent randomized controlled trial has shown that in patients with FMR undergoing CABG, the addition of MV repair is associated with an increased rate of perioperative complications with no significant differences in LV reverse remodeling and mortality at 2 years. No evidence is available on MV replacement in this setting.

The role of MV surgery for the treatment of isolated severe FMR is also unclear. European recommendations suggest surgical treatment in this scenario only for patients with severe HF symptoms despite optimal GDMT, LVEF > 30%, and low comorbidity burden. In a recent randomized controlled trial, valve-sparing MV replacement resulted in similar LV remodeling and equivalent 2-year mortality, but lower MR recurrence compared with restrictive annuloplasty in patients with isolated severe ischemic FMR. However, in this study, the greatest 2-year reverse remodeling was obtained in patients receiving MV repair who had no MR recurrence. Thus, successful MV repair (probably not only annuloplasty but also other techniques) may have similar or better results than MV replacement. In this scenario, careful patient selection and further refinement of MV repair techniques are needed to achieve optimal and durable results.

At present, surgical treatment of isolated FMR remains uncommon because patients with FMR are often at high surgical risk due to LV dysfunction, older age, and comorbidities. In addition, evidence on the prognostic benefit of MV surgery in patients with severe FMR who do not require CABG is limited and mostly restricted to patients with ischemic FMR.

PERCUTANEOUS TREATMENT OPTIONS

Recently, there has been great interest in using less invasive approaches to minimize the morbidity associated with open cardiac surgery or as an alternative for high-risk patients that are not suitable candidates for MV replacement with functional MR lesions.

Transcatheter technologies for the treatment of FMR may fulfill a major unmet need. Patients with severe FMR have an impressive poor prognosis despite GDMT and CRT, and are often not suitable for surgery that is also not supported by sufficient evidence.

Although MitraClip® therapy has been deemed safe in select patients with degenerative MR, the outcomes in patients with functional MR remain unproven. In the ACCESS-EU trial and the GRASP Registry, 75% of the patients had functional MR but, MitraClip® therapy was shown to be nonsuperior to surgery. The European guidelines suggest the use of MitraClip® only for symptomatic patients with severe FMR despite optimal GDMT (including CRT) who are at high or prohibitive surgical risk, whereas no indications for transcatheter treatment of FMR are reported in the American guidelines. Both European and American recommendations emphasize the lack of robust evidence supporting MitraClip® use for the treatment of FMR.

The Endovascular Valve Edge-to-Edge Repair Study (EVEREST) II is the first trial of MitraClip® treatment, including 279 patients randomized to MitraClip® or surgical therapy. MitraClip® proved to be safer than but not as effective as open surgery in reducing MR. It should be noted, however, that patients included in EVEREST II were low-risk candidates for surgery mainly affected by primary MR.

Recently, two intensely awaited randomized controlled trials have been published. Both MITRA-FR and COAPT investigated the role of MitraClip® treatment in patients with ischemic or nonischemic FMR, who remained symptomatic (NYHA class II–IV) despite GDMT.

In the MITRA-FR trial, 304 patients with severe FMR (defined as EROA > 20 mm^2 and RV > 30 mL), NYHA class II–IV, and LVEF 15–40% were randomized to MitraClip® plus GDMT ($n = 152$) or GDMT alone ($n = 152$). The primary composite end-point (all-cause death and hospitalization for HF at 12 months) was similar between the two arms [54.6% in the device group vs 51.3% in the control group;

TABLE 4: Comparison of MITRA-FR and COAPT trials.

	MITRA-FR	*COAPT*
Centers	37	78
Duration, months	40	57
Funding	French Ministry of Health and Research National Program and Abbott Vascular	Abbott Vascular
Etiology	Ischemic and non-ischemic cardiomyopathy	Ischemic and non-ischemic cardiomyopathy
NYHA functional class	II-IV despite stable GDMT	II–IV despite stable GDMT
LVEF	15–40%	20–50%
LVESD	Not required	<70 mm
MR severity	EROA >20 mm^2 or RV >30 mL	EROA >30 mm^2 or RV >45 mL
Prior hospitalization and BNP	At least one HF hospitalization within 12 months BNP not required	At least one HF hospitalization within 12 months and/or BNP >300 pg/mL or NT-proBNP >1500 pg/mL
Right ventricular dysfunction and pulmonary hypertension	Included	Excluded SPAP > 70 mm Hg and moderate or severe right ventricular dysfunction
Primary end-point	Composite of all-cause death or unplanned hospitalization for HF at 12 months	Effectiveness: HF hospitalizations within 24 months of follow-up Safety: freedom from device-related complications at 12-month follow-up
Time to randomization	16 days	14 days
Eligibility committee	Local heart team assessment	Local heart team assessment and central eligibility committee
Crossover	Allowed	Not allowed

odds ratio 1.16, 95% confidence interval (CI) 0.73–1.84], and both single end-points did not significantly differ between groups. No significant differences were noted across specified subgroups.

In the COAPT trial, 614 patients with moderate-to-severe (3+) or severe (4+) FMR (EROA > 30 mm^2 and RV > 45 mL), NYHA class II–IV and LVEF 20–50% were randomized to MitraClip® plus GDMT (n = 302) or GDMT alone (n = 312). The primary effectiveness end-point (HF hospitalizations at 24 months) was significantly lower in the MitraClip® group compared to the GDMT group [35.8% vs 67.9% per patient-year; hazard ratio (HR) 0.53, 95% CI 0.40–0.70; P < 0.001] with a very favorable number needed to treat (NNT) of 3.1. Importantly, significant differences between groups were also observed in the composite of death and HF hospitalization at 1 year (45.7% in the device arm vs 67.9% in the control arm; HR 0.57, 95% CI 0.45–0.72; P < 0.001), all-cause mortality alone at 24 months (29.1% in the device arm vs 46.1% in the control arm; HR 0.62, 95% CI 0.46–0.82), and need for LV assist device at 1 year (3% in the device arm vs 7.1% in the control arm; HR 0.34, 95% CI 0.13–0.87; P = 0.02).

A favorable LV remodeling, improvement in symptoms, exercise capacity, and quality of life were observed. Finally, the primary safety end-point was significantly lower than expected. All results were consistent in the subgroup analysis.[21-23]

On 14 March 2019, FDA approved MitraClip® for treatment of select patients with severe secondary MR who remain symptomatic despite GDMT with a label. "The MitraClip™ NTR/XTR Clip Delivery System, when used with maximally tolerated guideline-directed medical therapy (GDMT), is indicated for the treatment of symptomatic, moderate-to-severe or severe secondary (or functional) mitral regurgitation (MR; MR ≥ Grade III per American Society of Echocardiography criteria) in patients with a left ventricular ejection fraction (LVEF) ≥ 20% and ≤ 50%, and a left ventricular end-systolic dimension (LVESD) ≤ 70 mm whose symptoms and MR severity persist despite maximally tolerated GDMT as determined by a multidisciplinary heart team experienced in the evaluation and treatment of heart failure and mitral valve disease."

CONCEPT OF PROPORTIONAL AND DISPROPORTIONATE MR (FIG. 11)

Paul Grayburn and Milton Packer[23] introduced a new concept to explain the differences in response to GDMT and mitral valve therapies. Patients with secondary MR represent a heterogeneous group, which can be usefully subdivided based on understanding that the effective regurgitant orifice area (EROA) is dependent on left ventricular end-diastolic volume (LVEDV). According to the Gorlin hydraulic orifice equation, patients with heart failure, an LV ejection fraction of 30%, an LVEDV of 220–250 mL, and a regurgitant fraction of 50% would be expected to have an EROA of 0.3 cm^2 independent of specific tethering abnormalities of the mitral valve leaflets. The MR in these patients is proportionate to the degree of LV dilatation and can respond to drugs and devices that reduce LVEDV. In contrast, patients with EROA of 0.3–0.4 cm^2 but with LVEDV of only 160–200 mL exhibit degrees of MR that are disproportionately higher than predicted by LVEDV. These patients appear to preferentially benefit from interventions directed at the mitral valve.

The LV dilatation causes papillary muscle displacement and in these cases, the degree of MR correlates to the LV volume. These can be called proportionate MR (Fig. 12).

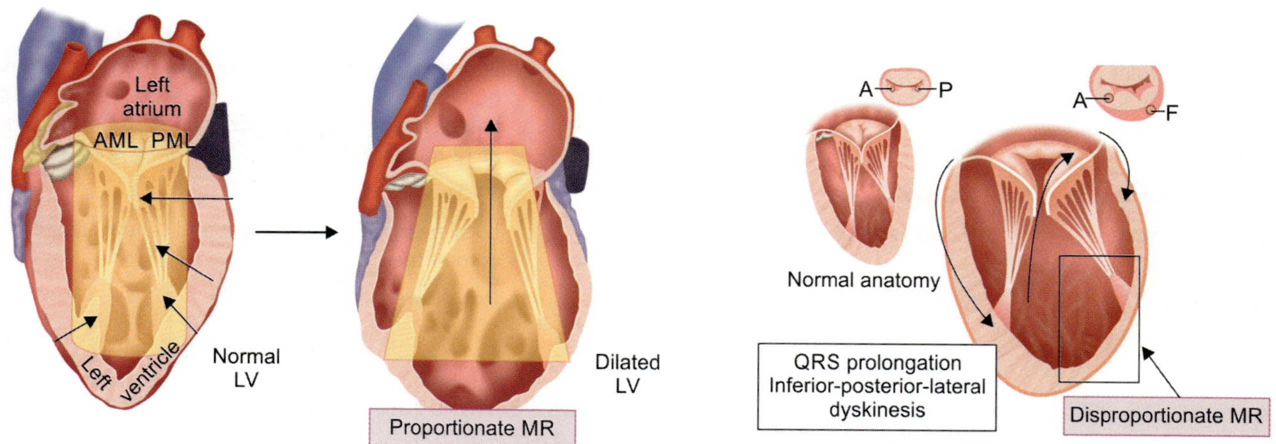

Fig. 11: Concept of proportionate and disproportionate mitral regurgitation.
(LV: left ventricular; MR: mitral regurgitation)

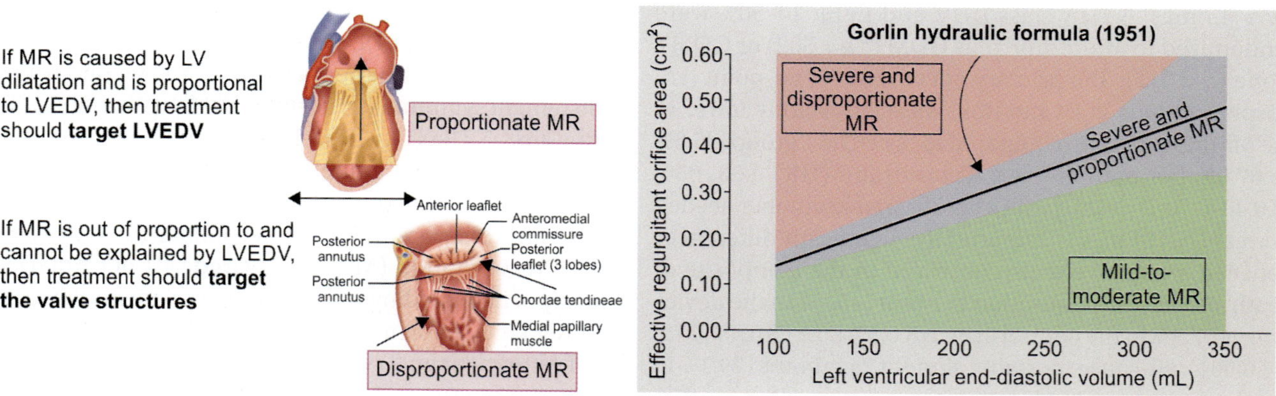

Fig. 12

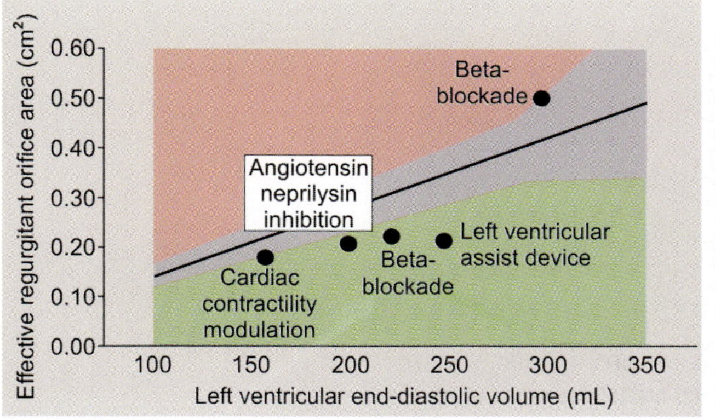

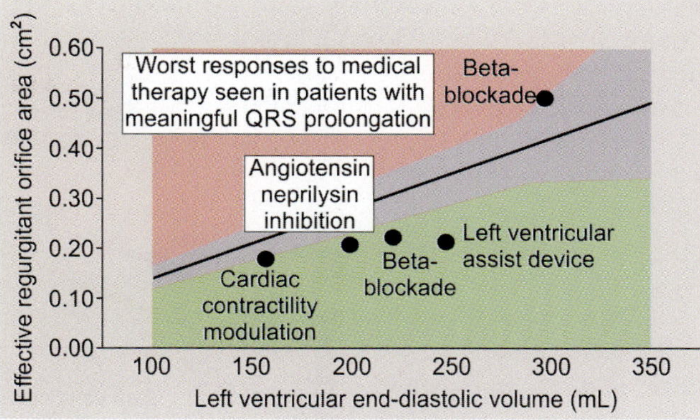

Fig. 13

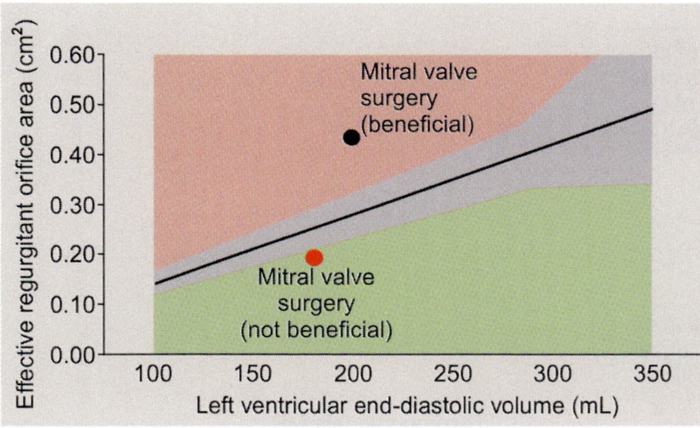

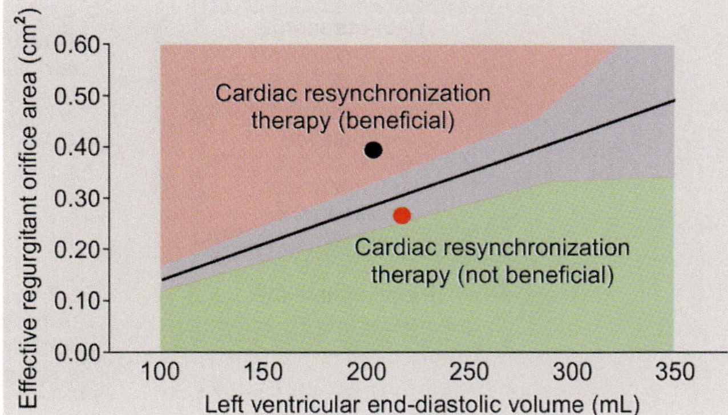

Fig. 14

On the other hand, intraventricular conduction delay or regional dyssynchrony causes MR that is disproportionate.

If we plot the MR against LV volumes, we get interesting relationship and this can be the basis of planning therapy for MR (Fig. 13).

In proportionate MR, LVEDV reduction will lead to substantial decrease in MR and can be achieved by pharmacotherapy.

The worst response to pharmacotherapy is in patients with significant QRS prolongation.

Treatments directed at the mitral valve yield benefit in disproportionate MR but not in proportionate MR. The response of MR to CRT may be explained by this concept (Fig. 14).

We can also use this concept to explain the differences between COAPT and MITRA-FR. We can see that MITRA-FR had more proportionate MR, which did not show benefit (Fig. 15).

What about sacubitril–valsartan?

The PRIME study recently randomly assigned 118 heart failure patients with chronic functional MR secondary to left ventricular (LV) dysfunction to receive either sacubitril/valsartan, in addition to standard medical therapy for heart failure.[24] The primary end-point was the change in effective regurgitant orifice area (EROA) of functional MR from baseline. Among patients with secondary functional MR, sacubitril/valsartan reduced MR to a greater extent than did valsartan suggesting that an ARNI might be considered for optimal medical therapy of patients with heart failure and functional MR. PRIME study was a small study with less MR and not analyzed for LVEDV and proportionate MR. It yet emphasizes the need for best-in-class GDMT.

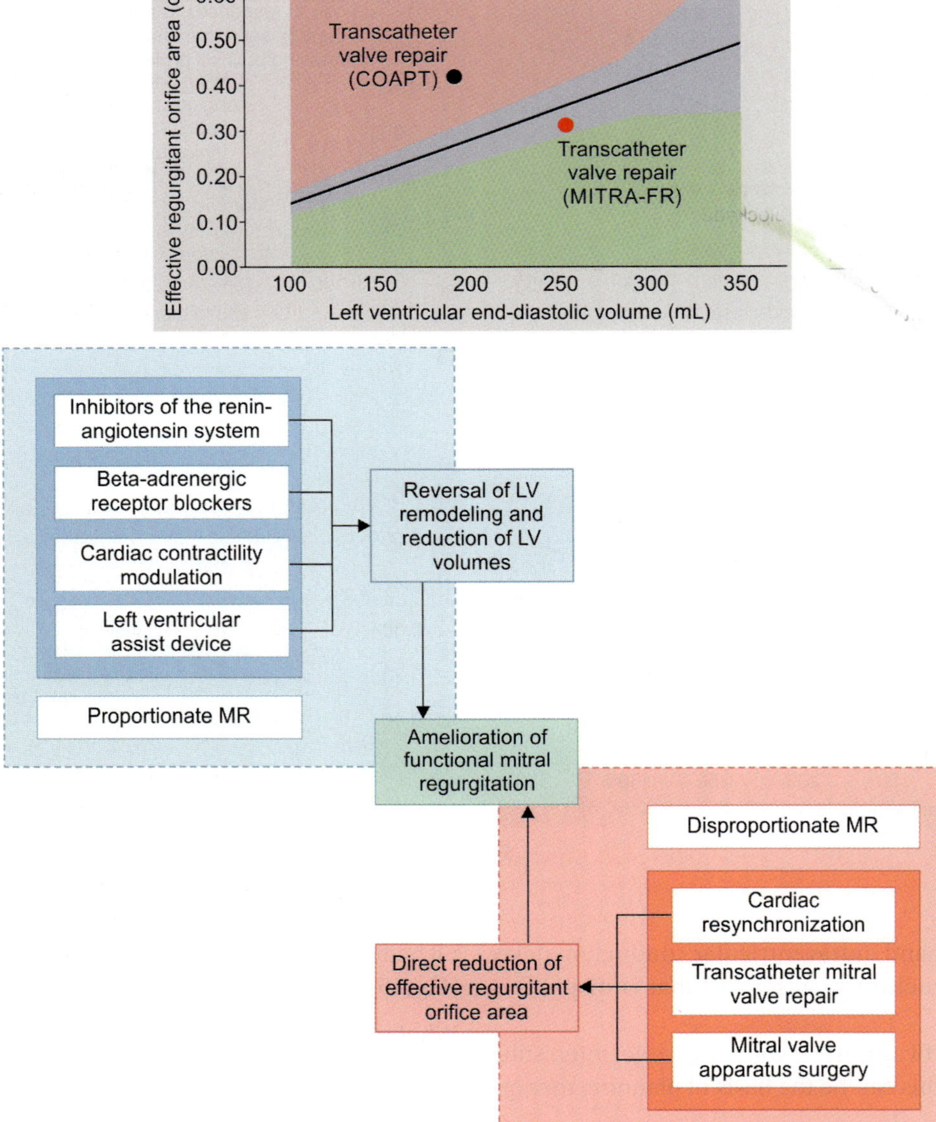

Fig. 15

REFERENCES

1. Tcheng JE, Jackman JD, Nelson CL, et al. Outcome of patients sustaining acute ischemic mitral regurgitation during myocardial infarction. Ann Intern Med. 1992;117: 18-24.
2. Thompson CR, Buller CE, Sleeper LA, et al. Cardiogenic shock due to acute severe mitral regurgitation complicating acute myocardial infarction: a report from the SHOCK Trial Registry. Should we use emergently revascularize occluded coronaries in cardiogenic shock? J Am Coll Cardiol. 2000;36 (3 suppl A):1104–9.
3. Reynold HR, Hochman JS. Cardiogenic shock: Current concepts and improving outcomes. Circulation. 2008;117:686-97.
4. Westabay S, Kharbanda R, Banning AP. Cardiogenic shock in ACS. Part 1: prediction, presentation and medical therapy. Nat Rev cardiol. 2011;9:158-71.
5. Gammie JS, Sheng S, Griffith BP, et al. Trends in mitral valve surgery in the united States: Results from the Society of Thoracic Surgeons Adult Cardiac Database. Ann Thorac Surg. 2009;87:1431-9.
6. Chatterjee S, Rankin JS, Gammie JS, et al. Isolated mitral valve surgery risk in 77,836 from the society of Thoracic Surgeons Database. Ann Thorac Surg. 2013;96:1587-94.

7. Castillo JG, Adams DH. Mitral valve repair and replacement. In: Otto CM, Bonow RO (Eds). Valvular Heart Disease: A Companion to Braunwald' s heart disease, 4th edn. Philadelphia: Saunders; 2013. pp. 326-40.
8. Agricola E, Oppizzi M, Maisano F, et al. Echocardiographic classification of chronic ischemic mitral regurgitation caused by restricted motion according to tethering pattern. Eur J Echocardiogr. 2004;5:326-34.
9. Helmcke F, Nanda NC, Hsuing MC, et al. Transthoracic and transesophageal echocardiographic assessment of mitral regurgitation severity: usefulness of qualitative and semiquantitative techniques. Echocardiography. 2005;22(9):748-69.
10. Enriquez-Sarano M, Avierinos JF, Messika-Zeitoun D, et al. Quantitative determinants of the outcome of asymptomatic mitral regurgitation. N Engl J Med. 2005;352(9):875-83.
11. Breithardt OA, Sinha AM, Schwammenthal E, et al. Acute effects of cardiac resynchronization therapy on functional mitral regurgitation in advanced systolic heart failure. J Am Coll Cardiol. 2003;41:765-70.
12. Mihaljevic T, Lam BK, Rajeswaran J, et al. Impact of mitral valve annuloplasty combined with revascularization in patients with functional ischemic mitral regurgitation. J Am Coll Cardiol. 2007;49(22):2191-201.
13. Chan KM, Punjabi PP, Flather M, et al. RIME Investigators. Coronary artery bypass surgery with or without mitral valve annuloplasty in moderate functional ischemic mitral regurgitation: final results of the Randomized Ischemic Mitral Evaluation (RIME) trial. Circulation. 2012;126(21):2502-10.
14. Smith PK, Puskas JD, Ascheim DD, et al. The Cardiothoracic Surgical trial networks. Surgical Treatment of Moderate Ischemic Mitral Regurgitation. N Engl J Med. 2014;371:2178-88.
15. Al-Radi OO, Austin PC, Tu JV, et al. Mitral repair versus replacement for ischemic mitral regurgitation. Ann Thorac Surg. 2005;79:1260-7.
16. McGee EC, Gillinov AM, Blackstone EH, et al. Recurrent mitral regurgitation after annuloplasty for functional ischemic mitral regurgitation. J Thorac Cardiovasc Surg. 2004;128:916-24.
17. Vassileva CM, Boley T, Markwell S, et al. Meta-analysis of short-term and long-term survival following repair versus replacement for ischemic mitral regurgitation. Eur J Cardiothorac Surg. 2011;39:295-303.
18. Acker MA, Parides MK, Perrault LP, et al. for the CTSN. Mitral-valve repair versus replacement for severe ischemic mitral regurgitation. N Engl J Med. 2014;370:23-32.
19. Magne J, Girerd N, Sénéchal M, et al. Mitral repair versus replacement for ischemic mitral regurgitation: comparison of short-term and long-term survival. Circulation. 2009;120(11 Suppl):S104-11.
20. Ciarka A, Braun J, Delgado V, et al. Predictors of mitral regurgitation recurrence in patients with heart failure undergoing mitral valve annuloplasty. Am J Cardiol. 2010;106(3):395-401.
21. Obadia JF, Messika-Zeitoun D, Leurent G, et al. for the MITRA-FR Investigators. Percutaneous Repair or Medical Treatment for Secondary Mitral Regurgitation. N Engl J Med. 2018;379:2297-306.
22. Stone GW, Lindenfeld JA, Abraham WT, et al. for the COAPT Investigators. Transcatheter Mitral-Valve Repair in Patients with Heart Failure. N Engl J Med. 2018;379:2307-18.
23. Packer M, Grayburn PA. Contrasting Effects of Pharmacological, Procedural, and Surgical Interventions on Proportionate and Disproportionate Functional Mitral Regurgitation in Chronic Heart Failure. Circulation. 2019;140:779-89.
24. Kang DH, Park SJ, Shin SH, et al. Angiotensin Receptor Neprilysin Inhibitor for Functional Mitral Regurgitation. Circulation. 2018;139:1354-65.

SGLT2 Inhibitor and HFrEF

PB Jayagopal, SKM Sarjun Basha

INTRODUCTION

Current standard of care for patients with heart failure with reduced ejection fraction (HFrEF) includes renin-angiotensin-aldosterone system (RAAS) inhibitor, angiotensin receptor neprilysin inhibitor (ARNI), diuretics, and digoxin to suppress neurohormones, reduce volume overload, and improve contractility. Despite current established therapy, heart failure (HF) remains a leading cause of hospitalization and mortality worldwide, highlighting the need for novel therapeutic targets to improve the prognosis of patients with HF. The EMPA-REG OUTCOME trial[1] (Empagliflozin Cardiovascular Outcome Event Trial in Type 2 diabetes mellitus patients) and the CANVAS Program[2] (Canagliflozin cardiovascular assessment study) demonstrated significant reduction in major adverse cardiovascular events (MACE) and HF hospitalization. The use of sodium glucose co-transporter 2 inhibitor (SGLT2i) results in favorable effects on biomarkers including glycemia, blood pressure, body weight, intrarenal hemodynamics, albuminuria, and may also reduce the risk of serious cardiovascular complications, kidney disease, and death.[3,4] We summarize the key effects of SGLT2i and the clinical evidence that support the rationale for the use of SGLT2i in patients with HFrEF who have type 2 diabetes mellitus (DM).

POTENTIAL MECHANISM OF CARDIOVASCULAR PROTECTION BY SGLT2i

High-capacity low-affinity SGLT2 is located in the renal proximal tubular epithelium and reabsorbs filtered glucose. Even in the presence of excess glucose, the proximal renal tubule continues to reabsorb more glucose. There is no negative feedback mechanism for resorption of glucose by the proximal renal tubule. SGLT2i are designed to prevent these uncontrolled glucose resorption by the kidney in patient with diabetes. The mechanism underlying cardiovascular and renal protection by SGLT2i type2 DM is multifactorial, complex, and discussed below.

Hemodynamic Effects

The cardiovascular benefits seen in EMPA-REG OUTCOME were related to reduction in blood pressure and intravascular volume. A decrease in systolic/diastolic blood pressure of 5/2 mm Hg was recorded during EMPA-REG OUTCOME[5] and was not associated with increased heart rate. This was due to decrease in preload due to natriuresis and osmotic diuresis, decrease in afterload due to decrease in arterial stiffness,[6] and effects on endothelial and vascular architecture namely vascular smooth muscle relaxation.[7]

Diuretic Effects

The natriuresis and diuresis are the main contributory mechanisms explaining the reduction in heart failure hospitalization observed during EMPA-REG OUTCOME.[8]

The SGLT2i differ from loop and thiazide diuretics in that:

- SGLT2i do not lead to reflex sympathetic nervous system activation (no observed increase in heart rate despite blood pressure lowering).
- Thiazide and loop diuretics are known to cause hyperglycemia and hyperuricemia whereas SGLT2i have positive effect on blood glucose and uric acid.
- Thiazide diuretics act on the distal tubule whereas SGLT2i act on the proximal tubule and cause increased urinary sodium and chloride delivery to the juxtaglomerular apparatus. It has been suggested that these effects of SGLT2 inhibition reinstate tubuloglomerular feedback resulting in afferent arteriolar vasoconstriction and decreased glomerular filtration by reducing intraglomerular pressure. Increased delivery of sodium and chloride to macula densa during SGLT2i treatment may influence other neurohormonal factor such as local RAAS inhibition, and this may result in reduced level of aldosterone and decreased sympathetic nerve activity, which could reduce the risk of cardiovascular death and heart failure.[9]

Hormonal Effects

Glucagon

As increase in glucagon levels in patients with SGLT2i may be due to increased glucosuria and reported direct effect on glucagon-secreting pancreatic α-cell.[10] Glucagon modulates cardiac function with positive inotropic and chronotropic effects. An increase in glucagon levels has been proposed as possible contributor for the reduced cardiovascular risk observed in EMPA-REG OUTCOME particularly when considering its inotropic effects in relation to heart failure. However, the impact of these changes in glucagon and cardiovascular risk remains to be clearly determined.

Insulin

SGLT2i-related glycosuria results is an insulin-independent HbA1c reduction of 0.7–1% in patient with type 2 DM and also body weight loss (2–3 kg) attributable to the induction of a negative caloric balance in patients with normal renal function.

RAAS

EMPA-REG OUTCOME trial found that RAAS activity was slightly increased, although within the normal range, which may be interpreted as a compensatory response to volume contraction. It has also been suggested that empagliflozin may act through the nonclassic RAAS pathways.[11] RAAS activation by empagliflozin could stimulate type 1 angiotensin II receptor, which is central in the pathogenesis of cardiovascular disease. However during EMPA-REG OUTCOME study, 81% of patients received angiotensin-converting enzyme inhibitor or type I angiotensin II receptor blockers. Empagliflozin could therefore have had additive cardioprotective effects through activation of type 2 angiotensin II receptor pathway and angiotensin 1–7 activation, which cause responses such as vasodilation, anti-inflammatory effects and positive inotropic effects.[11]

Erythropoietin

When SGLT2i dapagliflozin was administered to type 2 DM patients, the blood level of erythropoietin (EPO) increased after 1 week and peaked at 2 weeks, before returning to the pretreatment level after 2 months.[12] The reticulocyte count also increased along with increase in EPO, followed by elevation of both hemoglobin and hematocrit (hCT). Although hCT increased, the blood urea nitrogen (BUN) level and BUN/creatinine ratio usually showed no change. It has been proved in EMPA-REG OUTCOME trial that the change in HCT was most closely related to the decrease in cardiovascular death.

Metabolic Effects

Cardiac Fuel Energetics

In T2DM with heart failure, there is restricted fuel availability and low-energetic reserve. Hence, ketone bodies act as a "super fuel" by releasing energy more efficiently than fatty acid (or) glucose.[13] It has been demonstrated that SGLT2i can shift whole body metabolism from glucose to fatty acid oxidation,[14,15] and this could have beneficial effects for failing hearts.[16] In addition to being a circulating energy source, ketones have an important role in cellular and epigenetic signalling[17] and act as nongenomic antioxidants,[18] effects that could potentially contribute to reducing cardiovascular disease.

Plasma Lipid and Uric Acid

Small increases in both low-density lipoproteins (LDL) and high-density lipoproteins (HDL) and small reduction in plasma uric acid concentration when compared with placebo were observed in EMPA-REG OUTCOME. The significance of these changes in terms of cardiovascular risk is currently unclear.

INSIGHTS FROM CARDIOVASCULAR TRIALS WITH SGLT2i AND HEART FAILURE

The EMPA-REG OUTCOME trial[1] with empagliflozin demonstrated 35% reduction in the risk of hospitalization and 14% reduction in 3 point MACE (cardiovascular death, nonfatal myocardial infarction, and nonfatal stroke). Similarly in CANVAS program[2] with an overall HF prevalence of 14.4% where the primary endpoint 3-point MACE was significantly reduced and risk of hospitalization for HF was reduced by 33%. The progression of albuminuria was reduced by 27%. The majority of patients (90%) in the EMPA-REG OUTCOME and CANVAS program trial did not have HF at baseline suggesting the HF beneficial effects observed were attributable to a primary prevention effect. In Declare TIMI 58 trial[19] in patients with type 2 diabetes who had (or) were at risk for atherosclerotic cardiovascular disease (ASCVD) were randomized to receive dapagliflozin (or) placebo. Among 17,160 patients, 3,584 had history of myocardial infarction (MI). Dapagliflozin significantly reduced MACE by 16% in these patients with history of prior MI but not among those with no prior MI but with established ASCVD. In total, 671 patients (3.9%) were stratified as HFrEF although only 408 (24%) had a history of heart failure. Dapagliflozin led to significant reduction in cardiovascular death and hospitalization for heart failure when compared to placebo and there was greater reduction in patients with HFrEF compared to patients without HFrEF (HR 0.62 vs 0.88, P -0.046). However the awaited result of DAPA-HF, EMPEROR-REDUCED studies, which also considers NT-proBNP as inclusion criteria, will further add to the usefulness of SGLT2i in HFrEF.

SGLT2i VERSUS OTHER ORAL GLUCOSE LOWERING AGENTS FOR HEART FAILURE

In CVD Real 2 study[20]—a large multinational study, SGLT2i when compared with other glucose-lowering drugs was associated with lower rates of hospitalization for heart failure (HHF), death, and HHF (or) death with no significant heterogeneity by country. In CVD-Real Nordic[21]—a multinational observational analysis, SGLT2i when compared with other glucose-lowering drugs was associated with significantly decreased risk of cardiovascular mortality, MACE, and hospital events for heart failure.[21] Thus, large, international study across three major world region showed superiority of SGLT2i among other oral hypoglycemic agent for patient with cardiovascular risk.

SGLT2i: SAFETY AND COUNSELING

There is small increase in urinary tract infections, however, no increase in serious infections like pyelonephritis. Increase in genital infection was reported; hence, proper genital hygiene is to be maintained. Volume depletion may occur; hence, adequate hydration is to be advised. Renal adverse events occurred more frequently in dapagliflozin-treated patients, but they were mostly related to reversible small increase in serum creatinine. Amputation primarily at the level of the toe (or) metatarsal was documented with dapagliflozin.

CONCLUSION

Heart failure is the most disabling and deadly complication of diabetes. SGLT2i has emerged safe and effective adjunctive therapy for HF by significantly reducing hospitalization for heart failure. In real world practice, it is superior to other oral hypoglycemic agents in reducing HHF and death suggesting class effect applicable to a broad population of patients with type 2 DM.

REFERENCES

1. Zinman B, Wanner C, Lachin JM, et al. Empagliflozin, cardiovascular outcomes, and mortality in type 2 diabetes. N Engl J Med. 2015;373:2117-28.
2. Neal B, Perkovic V, Mahaffey KW, et al. Canagliflozin and Cardiovascular and Renal Events in Type 2 Diabetes. N Engl J Med. 2017;377:644-57.
3. Wanner C, Inzucchi SE, Lachin JM, et al. Empagliflozin and progression of kidney disease in type 2 diabetes. N Engl J Med. 2016;375:323-34.
4. Wu JH, Foote C, Blomster J, et al. Effects of sodium-glucose cotransporter-2 inhibitors on cardiovascular events, death, and major safety outcomes in adults with type 2 diabetes: a systematic review and meta-analysis. Lancet Diabetes Endocrinol. 2016;4:411-9.
5. Abdul-Ghani M, Del Prato S, Chilton R, et al. SGLT2 inhibitors and cardiovascular risk: lessons learned from the EMPAREG-OUTCOME study. Diabetes Care. 2016;39:717-25.
6. Chilton R, Tikkanen I, Cannon CP, et al. Effects of empagliflozin on blood pressure and markers of arterial stiffness and vascular resistance in patients with type 2 diabetes. Diabetes Obes Metab. 2015;17:1180-93.
7. Townsend RR, Machin I, Ren J, et al. Reductions in mean 24-hour ambulatory blood pressure after 6-week treatment with

canagliflozin in patients with type 2 diabetes mellitus and hypertension. J Clin Hypertens (Greenwich). 2016;18:43-52.

8. Scheen AJ. Reappraisal of the diuretic effect of empagliflozin in the EMPA-REG OUTCOME trial: comparison with classic diuretics. DiabetesMetab. 2016;42(4):224-33.
9. Marx N, McGuire DK. Sodium-glucose cotransporter-2 inhibition for the reduction of cardiovascular events in high-risk patients with diabetes mellitus. Eur Heart J. 2016;37(42):3192-200.
10. Bonner C, Kerr-Conte J, Gmyr V, et al. Inhibition of the glucose transporter SGLT2 with dapagliflozin in pancreatic alpha cells triggers glucagon secretion. Nat Med. 2015;21:512-7.
11. Muskiet MH, van Raalte DH, vanBommel EJ, et al. Understanding EMPA-REG OUTCOME. Lancet Diabetes Endocrinol. 2015;3:928-9.
12. Lambers Heerspink HJ, de Zeeuw D, Wie L, et al. Dapagliflozin a glucose regulating drug with diuretic properties in subjects with type 2 diabetes. Diabetes Obes Metab. 2013;15:853-62.
13. Mudaliar S, Alloju S, Henry RR. Can a shift in fuel energetics explain the beneficial cardiorenal outcomes in the EMPA-REG OUTCOM study? A unifying hypothesis. Diabetes Care. 2016;39:1115-22.
14. Ferrannini E, Muscelli E, Frascerra S, et al. Metabolic response to sodium-glucose cotransporter 2 inhibition in type 2 diabetic patients. J Clin Invest. 2014;124:499-508.
15. Daniele G, Xiong J, Solis-Herrera C, et al. Dapagliflozin enhances fatoxidation and ketone production in patients with type 2 diabetes. Diabetes Care. 2016;39:2036-41.
16. Jorgensen NB, Pedersen J, Vaag AA. EMPA-REG: glucose excretion and lipid mobilization—not storage—saves lives. J Diabetes Complications. 2016;30(4):753.
17. Newman JC, Verdin E. Ketone bodies as signaling metabolites. Trends Endocrinol Metab. 2014;25:42-52.
18. Maalouf M, Sullivan PG, Davis L, et al. Ketones inhibit mitochondrial production of reactive oxygen species production following glutamate excitotoxicity by increasing NADH oxidation. Neuroscience. 2007;145:256-64.
19. Wiviott SD, Raz I, Bonaca MP, et al. Dapagliflozin and Cardiovascular Outcomes in Type 2 Diabetes. N Engl J Med. 2019;380:347-57.
20. Kosiborod M, Cavender MA, Fu AZ, et al. Lower Risk of Heart Failure and Death in Patients Initiated on Sodium-Glucose Cotransporter-2 Inhibitors versus Other Glucose-Lowering Drugs The CVD-REAL Study. Circulation. 2017;136:249-59.
21. Birkeland KI, Jorgensen ME, Carstensen B, et al. Cardiovascular mortality and morbidity in patients with type 2 diabetes following initiation of sodium-glucose co-transporter-2 inhibitors versus other glucose-lowering drugs (CVD-REAL Nordic): a multinational observational analysis. Lancet Diabetes Endocrinol. 2017;5:709-17.

37

CHAPTER

Mineralocorticoid Antagonists in Heart Failure

Amrish Agrawal, Vishal Agrawal, Thair Al Jumaily

INTRODUCTION

Current guidelines have recommended the use of mineralocorticoid receptor antagonist (MRA) therapy in patients with heart failure (HF). However, many of HF patients have comorbidities such as diabetes mellitus (DM) and chronic kidney disease (CKD), which by themselves are well-known risk factors for the development of hyperkalemia and renal failure, an adverse effect linked to the use of MRA.[1] HF is characterized by high plasma levels of aldosterone, which has a well-documented role in the pathophysiology of cardiovascular (CV) diseases.[1,2] Apart from its direct renal effect on sodium retention and potassium excretion, MR overactivation within the heart causes coronary endothelial dysfunction, myocardial apoptosis, and reactive myocardial fibrosis and thereby contributing to cardiac remodeling and its adverse consequences.[3] Accordingly, blockade of mineralocorticoid receptor (MR) has proven efficacy in patients with HF with reduced ejection fraction (HFrEF), to some degree in HF with preserved ejection fraction (HFpEF), arterial hypertension and CKD.[2] Combining an angiotensin-converting enzyme (ACE) inhibitor with spironolactone may achieve more complete inhibition of the renin–angiotensin–aldosterone system (RAAS) and may produce further clinical benefits.[4-6]

PHARMACOLOGY OF MRA

Currently available MRA medications are summarized in Table 1. They can be divided into steroidal and nonsteroidal MRAs.

TABLE 1: Comparison of various mineralocorticoid receptor antagonist (MRA) available.

	Spironolactone	*Eplerenone*	*Finerenone*
MRA class	Steroidal	Steroidal	Nonsteroidal
Potency	High	Low	High
Selectivity	Low	Medium	High
Affinity to MR	High	Moderate	High
Affinity to other steroid hormone receptor	Moderate	Very low	Very low
Tissue distribution in heart vs kidney	Six-fold higher in kidney	Three-fold higher in kidney	Balanced between heart and kidney

Steroidal MRA

Spironolactone was the first anti-mineralocorticoid with high oral bioavailability introduced in 1960. It has characteristic adverse antiandrogenic and progestational symptoms such as gynecomastia, impotence, and menstrual irregularities. This fueled the development of a second generation of MRAs, a derivative of spironolactone called eplerenone in 1987. In vitro, eplerenone is ~40-fold less potent than spironolactone at MR inhibition but exhibits higher selectivity with respect to the other steroid hormone receptors. In clinical trials, eplerenone exhibited lower potency and efficacy versus spironolactone among hypertensive patients as well those with evidence of primary aldosteronism.[7]

Novel Nonsteroidal MRA

Further developments led to potential identification of several nonsteroidal MRAs belonging to the dihydropyridines (DHPs) class with an improved therapeutic index. Of these, BR-4628 was first of the potent and selective DHP-based MRAs. It was shown to block fibrotic remodeling in cardiac fibroblasts and demonstrated efficacy in preclinical models of cardiorenal diseases.[7] Developments in chemical optimization lead to the identification of a novel nonsteroidal MRA, finerenone. Finerenoneisa potent MRA with exceptional selectivity (~500-folds) and virtually no L-type Ca channel affinity. Finerenone has been investigated in different preclinical animal models and prevented rats from functional and structural heart and kidney damage at dosages which did not reduce systemic BP. Various mice animal models showed improved LV compliance and elastance when compared with infarcted control mice as well as reduced interstitial fibrosis.

PATHOPHYSIOLOGY OF MR OVERACTIVATION

Aldosterone, Mineralocorticoid Receptors, and Fibrosis

The heart contains mineralocorticoid receptors (MR) and levels of aldosterone are elevated in patients with HF even when on treatment with ACE inhibitors/ARB. Further, aldosterone is produced locally in the diseased heart in proportion to the severity of HF probably mediated by the induction of aldosterone synthase (CYP11B2) by angiotensin II in the failing ventricle. Chronically elevated aldosterone release leads to vascular, myocardial, and renal fibrosis and eventually end-organ damage and failure.

Aldosterone stimulates cardiac fibrosis and is one of the postulated mechanisms for heart failure progression, in both HFrEF and HFpEF.[8] Multiple animal models studies have shown increases in myocardial collagen and fibrosis in the presence of aldosterone,[8,9] which can be blocked in rats by treatment with spironolactone.[8,9] In a substudy of the RALES trial, in a group of 151 patients, blood samples were collected at baseline and at 6 months for analysis of markers of extracellular matrix (ECM) turnover.[10] Compared with baseline, these markers were significantly lower at 6 months in patients randomized to spironolactone but not seen in placebo. A hypothesis-generating subgroup analysis based on a small number of patients and events suggested that the effect of spironolactone on all-cause mortality was most apparent among patients with reduced ECM turnover markers above the median value.[10] Similarly, in a substudy of EPHESUS involving 476 patients, the procollagen peptides were significantly lower among patients randomized to eplerenone with values approaching those at baseline.[11]

Arrhythmia

Most common mode of death among patients with heart failure remains sudden cardiac death. Cardiac MR overexpression leads to ion channel remodeling, resulting in prolonged ventricular repolarization and in severe ventricular arrhythmias.[12] Transgenic mouse models have shown both spironolactone and eplerenone reduce inducible arrhythmias by reducing interstitial fibrosis and atrial fibrosis.

In the RALES trial,[4] spironolactone reduced sudden death [10 vs 13.1%, RR 0.71, $P = 0.02$] as well as heart failure death [15.5 vs 22.5%, RR 0.64, $P < 0.001$]. In EPHESUS,[5] eplerenone significantly reduced sudden death. There was significant reductions in sudden death and total mortality in the early post-MI period (first 30 days), when patients are at the greatest risk of sudden death. In EMPHASIS-HF, the incidence of new-onset atrial fibrillation (AF) or flutter was a pre-specified secondary endpoint. A subanalysis on patients without a history of atrial fibrillation or flutter at baseline[13] showed that incidence of new-onset AF was reduced by 42%, $p = 0.034$. Importantly, patients were already treated with a RAAS inhibitor (94%). The exact mechanism responsible for reduction in arrhythmogenic potential is not fully known.

Raising Serum Potassium

Mineralocorticoid receptor antagonist may preserve serum potassium concentration and thus counter the risk of hypokalemia and associated arrhythmic risk caused by nonpotassium-sparing diuretics. Support for this mechanism comes from SOLVD trial where increased arrhythmic mortality (relative risk 1.33) was observed with such nonpotassium-sparing diuretics after controlling for disease severity, comorbid illnesses, and concomitant medications, including ACE inhibitors. MRA therapy reduced the risk of hypokalemia in patients with systolic HF in clinical trials (e.g. in the EPHESUS trial,[5] serum potassium < 3.5 mEq/L occurred in 8.4% with eplerenone versus 13.1% with placebo).

REVIEW OF THE EVIDENCE IN HEART FAILURE

Spironolactone in Severe Heart failure of HFrEF: RALES

RALES[4] was the first large, prospective, randomized mortality trial of an MRA in patients with heart failure.

A total of 1,663 patients of HF with EF ≤ 35% and NYHA class III or IV symptoms were randomized to either spironolactone 25 mg OD (could be increased to 50 mg at 8 weeks based on potassium levels) or placebo. It is important to note that strict eligibility criteria and laboratory monitoring were used in RALES and all of the subsequent MRA heart failure trials (Table 2). The study was terminated early after a mean follow-up of 24 months as the primary endpoint—death from any cause—was significantly reduced in the spironolactone group (HR 0.70; CI 95% 0.60–0.82; $p < 0.001$). This extraordinary reduction of overall mortality was attributed to both a reduction in mortality from progressive HF and a reduction in SCD. Hospitalization for HF (HHF) was also significantly reduced with spironolactone (HR 0.65; CI 95% 0.54–0.77; $p < 0.001$). Beta-blocker use was low (11%). The incidence of serious hyperkalemia was not significantly different between two groups (2% vs 1%) as defined of serum potassium > 6 mmol/L ($p = 0.42$).

Eplerenone in Heart Failure with Mild Symptoms of HFrEF: EMPHASIS-HF

The Eplerenone in Mild Patients Hospitalization and Survival Study in Heart Failure (EMPHASIS-HF)[6] completed the investigation of eplerenone in mild symptomatic HF patients. In this trial, 2,737 patients with NYHA class II, an ejection fraction < 35% and a CV hospitalization within the last 6 months were randomized to eplerenone or placebo. Based on baseline eGFR, patients were starting with eplerenone 25 mg daily or 25 mg every other day (EOD) with a potential uptitration to the next higher dose level at 4 weeks. Patients had IHD as the leading cause for HF. The majority of the patients received SoC including ACEIs/ARBs as well as beta-blockers. This trial had a significant reduction in the primary composite endpoint—death from any cause or HFH (HR 0.63; 95% CI 0.34–0.74; $p < 0.001$) for patients being treated with eplerenone. The incidence of severe hyperkalemia serum potassium > 6 mmol/L was 2.5% versus 1.9% ($p = 0.29$) for eplerenone versus placebo, respectively.

Eplerenone in LV Systolic Dysfunction and Heart Failure after Acute Myocardial Infarction: EPHESUS Study

Eplerenone was investigated in patients with acute MI complicated by HF due to impaired LVSD-EPHESUS study.[5] The study was designed based on hypothesis of aldosterone as a mediator of ventricular remodeling and fibrosis. EPHESUS included 6,642 patients from 37 countries, who were randomized to eplerenone 25 mg per day or placebo for 4 weeks, after which the dose of eplerenone was increased to a maximum of 50 mg per day. After a mean follow-up of 16 months, the primary endpoint, death from any cause or hospitalization for CV events, was significantly reduced by eplerenone (HR 0.87; 95% CI 0.79–0.95; $p < 0.002$). This reduction was solely attributed to the prevention of sudden cardiac death. The majority of patients (86%) received concomitant background ACE-inhibitor or ARB therapy. Serious hyperkalemia (≥6 mmol/L) was reported more often in the eplerenone group (5.5 vs 3.9%,

TABLE 2: Exclusion and monitoring in clinical trials with mineralocorticoid receptor antagonist (MRA).

	Major exclusions				
Trial	*Renal exclusions*	*Potassium exclusions*	*Other relevant exclusions*	*Monitoring schedule*	*Dose adjustment*
RALES[4]	S-Cr > 2.5 mg/dL (221 µmol/L)	>5 mmol/L	Potassium-sparing diuretics, oral potassium supplements (unless hypokalemia, K < 3.5 mmol/L)	At weeks 1 and 5, and every 4 weeks for first 12 weeks, then every 3 months for 1 year, then every 6 months thereafter	Decrease dose to 25 mg every other
EPHESUS[5]	S-Cr > 2.5 mg/dL (221 µmol/L)	>5 mmol/L	Potassium-sparing diuretics	At 48 hours after initiation; at 1, 4, and 5 weeks; then every 3 months thereafter; and within 1 week after any dose change	Dose reduced or temporarily discontinued for serum potassium ≥ 5.5 mmol/L, until it fell below this value
EMPHASIS-HF[6]	eGFR < 30 mL/min/1.73 m^2	>5 mmol/L	Potassium-sparing diuretics	At 4 weeks, then every 4 months thereafter; within 72 hours of a dose adjustment due to hyperkalemia	Decrease dose for potassium 5.5–5.9 mmol/L Withhold drug for serum potassium ≥ 6 mmol/L, and restart when potassium < 5 mmol/L

P = 0.002); conversely, patients randomized to eplerenone had a lower incidence of serious hypokalemia (<3.5 mmol/L).

Spironolactone in Heart Failure with Preserved Ejection Fraction: TOPCAT

On the background of the role of MR overactivation in HFpEF, spironolactone was investigated in symptomatic HF patients with an EF ≥ 45% in TOPCAT trial, which randomized 3,445 patients to spironolactone or placebo.[14] The majority of them received diuretics, ACEIs/ARBs, and beta-blockers. After mean follow-up of 3.3 years, spironolactone missed to show a reduction in the primary composite endpoint of death from CV causes, aborted cardiac arrest or HHF compared to placebo (HR 0.89; 95% CI 0.77–1.04; p = 0.14). Only HHF had a significantly lower incidence in the spironolactone group. Interestingly, post hoc analyses demonstrated a ~four-fold difference in the composite event rate between the patients randomized from Russia and Georgia compared with those enrolled from the Americas and possible clinical benefits and reliable results with spironolactone in HFpEF patients from the Americas.[15]

CURRENT INDICATIONS AND RECOMMENDATIONS

The current indication and recommendation from guidelines are summarized in Table 3. There is strong

TABLE 3: Current recommendation for mineralocorticoid receptor antagonist (MRA) drugs in heart failure guidelines.

	ESC Guidelines 2016	*ACC/AHA Guidelines 2017*	*Canadian Heart Failure Guidelines 2017*
Chronic HFrEF	An MRA is recommended for patients with HFrEF, who remain symptomatic (NYHA Class II-IV) despite treatment with an ACE-I and a beta-blocker, to reduce the risk of HF hospitalization and death Class I, level of evidence A	MRA are recommended in patients with NYHA class II–IV HF and who have LVEF of 35% or less, unless contraindicated, to reduce morbidity and mortality. Patients with NYHA class II HF should have a history of prior CV hospitalization or elevated plasma natriuretic peptide levels to be considered for MRA. Class I, level of evidence A	We recommend that most patients with HFrEF be treated with triple therapy including an ACEi (or an ARB in those that are ACEi intolerant), a beta-blocker and a MRA unless specific contraindications exist. (Strong Recommendation, Moderate Quality Evidence)
Postmyocardial infarction		MRA are recommended to reduce morbidity and mortality following an acute MI in patients who have LVEF of 40% or less who develop symptoms of HF or who have a history of diabetes mellitus, unless contraindicated. Class I, level of evidence B	We recommend an MRA for patients with acute MI with EF < 40% and HF or with acute MI and an EF < 30% alone in the presence of diabetes (Strong Recommendation, High Quality Evidence)
HFpEF		In appropriately selected patients with stage C HFpEF (with EF ≥45%, elevated BNP levels or HF admission within 1 year, estimated glomerular filtration rate >30 mL/min, creatinine <2.5 mg/dL, potassium <5.0 mEq/L), aldosterone receptor antagonists might be considered to decrease hospitalizations. Class IIb, level of evidence B-R	We suggest that in individuals with HFpEF, serum potassium < 5.0 mmol/L, and an estimated (eGFR) > 30 mL/min, a MRA like spironolactone should be considered, with close surveillance of serum potassium and creatinine. (Weak Recommendation, Moderate Quality Evidence)

Source:

1. Ponikowski P, Voors AA, Anker SD, et al. 2016 ESC Guidelines for the diagnosis and treatment of acute and chronic heart failure: The Task Force for the diagnosis and treatment of acute and chronic heart failure of the European Society of Cardiology (ESC) Developed with the special contribution of the Heart Failure Association (HFA) of the ESC. Eur Heart J. 2016;37:2129-2200.
2. Yancy CW, Jessup M, Bozkurt B, et al. 2017 ACC/AHA/HFSA Focused Update of the 2013 ACCF/AHA Guideline for the Management of Heart Failure: A Report of the American College of Cardiology/American Heart Association Task Force on Clinical Practice Guidelines and the Heart Failure Society of America. Circulation. 2017;136:e137–e161.
3. Ezekowitz JA, O'Meara E, McDonald MA, et al. 2017 Comprehensive Update of the Canadian Cardiovascular Society Guidelines for the Management of Heart Failure. Can J Cardiol. 2017;33:1342-433.

(ACEi: angiotensin-converting enzyme inhibitor; ARB: angiotensin receptor blocker; HFpEF: heart failure with preserved ejection fraction) recommendation for addition of MRA therapy to ACE inhibitor or ARB or angiotensin receptor-neprilysin inhibitor and beta-blocker therapy to treat HF in patients who meet one or more of the following criteria, provided that they can be carefully monitored for changes in serum potassium and renal function. The serum potassium should be < 5 mEq/L and eGFR should be > 30 mL/min/1.73 m^2:

- Patients with NYHA functional class II to IV HF and LVEF < 35%.
- Patients' post-ST elevation myocardial infarction with an LVEF ≤ 40%, and either symptomatic HF or DM.

MRA IN PATIENTS PRONE TO HYPERKALEMIA

Despite the class IA recommendation in international guidelines to use an MRA, they are still being underutilized, especially in a background of CKD or DM where there is risk of hyperkalemia and/or worsening renal function. It is possible that the third-generation, MRA, finerenone may be better in this regard. The ARTS-HF Study[16] was a randomized, double-blind, comparator-controlled, six parallel group, multicenter phase 2b dose-finding study in a high-risk population (increased risk of postdischarge mortality and morbidity vis-a-vis prone to develop hyperkalemia and/or worsening renal function). A total of 1,066 patients with HFrEF and concomitant T2DM and/or CKD were randomized to receive finerenone or eplerenone. Results showed that all doses of finerenone had a similar safety profile and incidence of adverse effect as of eplerenone, though serum potassium concentration was greater in the eplerenone group (+0.262 mmol/L) than in each of the finerenone dose groups. These results show a promising safety and efficacy profile of the drug, corroborating evidence from the previous ARTS trial.

CONCLUSION

Four decades after the ascendency of ACE inhibitors and beta-blockers, with the publication of RALES, MR antagonism with spironolactone has found its way in patients with heart failure. Today, the two MRAs, spironolactone and eplerenone, have a grade 1A recommendation for patients with HFrEF as outlined in Table 3 and they consistently reduced morbidity and mortality in the investigated HF population. Despite proven benefit, the steroidal MRAs present some obstacles such as risk of developing hyperkalemia which makes the clinicians cautious to use them in everyday clinical practice. This has fueled research to develop potent and selective, nonsteroidal MRAs with a potential for a reduced risk of developing hyperkalemia and finerenone was identified and tested in phase 2b ARTS-HF trial.[16] Further research and clinical trials may establish its role and a useful addition to armamentarium of physicians.

REFERENCES

1. Pitt B, Ferreira JP, Zannad F. Mineralocorticoid receptor antagonists in patients with heart failure: current experience and future perspectives. Eur Heart J Cardiovasc Pharmacother. 2017;3:48-57.
2. Bauersaches J, Jaisser F, Toto R. Mineralocorticoid receptor activation and mineralocorticoid receptor antagonist treatment in cardiac and renal diseases. Hypertension. 2015;65:257-63.
3. Jaisser F, Farman N. Emerging roles of mineralocorticoid receptor in pathology: toward new paradigms in clinical pharmacology. Pharmacol Rev. 2016;68:49-75.
4. Pitt B, Zannad F, Remme WJ, et al. The effect of spironolactone on morbidity and mortality in patients with severe heart failure. Randomized Aldactone Evaluation Study Investigators. N Engl J Med. 1999;341:709-17.
5. Pitt B, Remme W, Zannad F, et al. Eplerenone, a selective aldosterone blocker, in patients with left ventricular dysfunction after myocardial infarction. N Engl J Med. 2003;348:1309-21.
6. Zannad F, McMurray JJ, Krum H, et al. Eplerenone in patients with systolic heart failure and mild symptoms. N Engl J Med. 2011;364:11-21.
7. Domanski MJ, Mehra MR, Pfeffer MA. Oxford Textbook of Advanced Heart Failure and Cardiac Transplantation, 1st Edition. UK: Oxford University Press; 2016. p. 283.
8. Brilla CG, Zhou G, Matsubara L, et al. Collagen metabolism in cultured adult rat cardiac fibroblasts: response to angiotensin II and aldosterone. J Mol Cell Cardiol. 1994;26:809-20.
9. Brilla CG. Aldosterone and myocardial fibrosis in heart failure. Herz. 2000;25:299-306.
10. Zannad F, Alla F, Dousset B, et al. Limitation of excessive extracellular matrix turnover may contribute to survival benefit of spironolactone therapy in patients with congestive heart failure: insights from the randomized aldactone evaluation study (RALES). Rales Investigators. Circulation. 2000;102:2700-6.
11. Iraqi W, Rossignol P, Angioi M, et al. Extracellular cardiac matrix biomarkers in patients with acute myocardial infarction complicated by left ventricular dysfunction and heart failure: insights from the Eplerenone Post-Acute Myocardial Infarction Heart Failure Efficacy and Survival Study (EPHESUS) study. Circulation. 2009;119:2471-9.
12. Ouvrard-Pascaud A, Sainte-Marie Y, Benitah JP, et al. Conditional mineralocorticoid receptor expression in the heart leads to life-threatening arrhythmias. Circulation 2005;111:3025-33.

13. Swedberg K, Zannad F, McMurray JJ, et al. Eplerenone and atrial fibrillation in mild systolic heart failure: results from the EMPHASIS-HF (Eplerenone in Mild Patients Hospitalization and Survival Study in Heart Failure) study. J Am Coll Cardiol. 2012;59:1598-603.
14. Pitt B, Pfeffer MA, Assmann SF, et al. Spironolactone for heart failure with preserved ejection fraction. N Engl J Med. 2014;370:1383-92.
15. Pfeffer MA, Claggett B, Assmann SF, et al. Regional variation in patients and outcomes in the Treatment of Preserved Cardiac Function Heart Failure with an Aldosterone Antagonist (TOPCAT) trial. Circulation. 2015;131:34-42.
16. Filippatos G, Anker SD, Böhm M, et al. A randomized controlled study of finerenone vs. eplerenone in patients with worsening chronic heart failure and diabetes and/or chronic kidney disease. E Eur Heart J. 2016;37:2105-14.

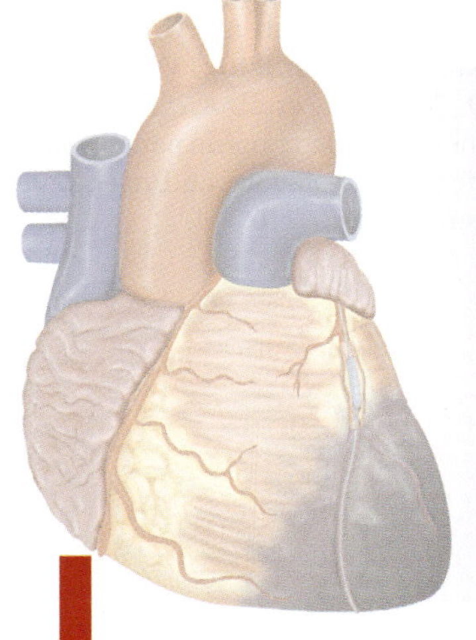

ACC/AHA/HFSA Guideline Update in Heart Failure Pharmacotherapy

Shraddha Ranjan, Manish Bansal, Ravi R Kasliwal, HK Chopra

INTRODUCTION

As defined by American College of Cardiology (ACC)/American Heart Association (AHA), the term guideline-directed management and therapy (GDMT) encompasses clinical evaluation, diagnostic testing, and pharmacological and procedural treatments. For last 30–40 years, ACC/AHA has translated clinical research into guidelines with recommendations to improve cardiovascular health. Around the same time when the first cardiovascular guidelines were published, CONSENSUS (Cooperative North Scandinavian Enalapril Survival) study[1] for the first time proved a definite role of pharmacotherapy in improving hitherto dismal outcomes in patients with heart failure (HF). Since then, number of drugs has been studied in the area of HF management. Few of them showed amazing results with mortality benefit and gained a position in GDMT, whereas many of them faded into oblivion due to lack of evidence. Angiotensin-converting enzyme inhibitors (ACEI), angiotensin receptor blockers (ARB), mineralocorticoid receptor antagonists (MRA) and beta-blockers have been the mainstay of HF medical management over the years. Recently, the PARADIGM-HF (Prospective comparison of ARNi with ACEi to Determine Impact on Global Mortality and Morbidity in Heart Failure) study[2] showed incremental mortality benefit with a new class of drug known as angiotensin receptor neprilysin inhibitor (ARNI). This has been a landmark development in the field of HF and it would not be wrong to say that, with the arrival of ARNI it is a very exciting and hopeful time in the challenging field of HF management.[3] The aim of this document is to review the recent (year 2017) evidence-based guidelines from the AHA/ACC/Heart Failure Society of America (HFSA) for management of HF (Fig. 1), focusing primarily on practical aspects of pharmacotherapy.[4] Table 1 summarizes guideline approved daily dosage of commonly used HF drugs.

WHAT IS NEW IN 2019?

- Angiotensin-converting enzyme inhibitors, ARB, and beta-blockers continue to be the mainstay of pharmacological therapy in HF management without any significant change in recommendations.
- Recent randomized clinical trials have shown benefit of two new pharmacological agents—ARNI and ivabradine, in treating HF with reduced ejection fraction (HFrEF), and hence they are included in the guidelines.
- Management of important comorbidities like anemia and hypertension has been given importance.

Pharmacological Treatment of Heart Failure

Renin-angiotensin-aldosterone System Inhibition with ACEI/ARB/ARNI

Angiotensin-converting enzyme inhibitors/ARB's interfere with renin-angiotensin-aldosterone system (RAAS) and as a result decrease peripheral resistance by preventing vasoconstriction, improve symptoms by decreasing sodium water retention and halt/prevent left ventricular (LV) remodeling though various hemodynamic and direct cellular effects. Collectively, all these beneficial effects

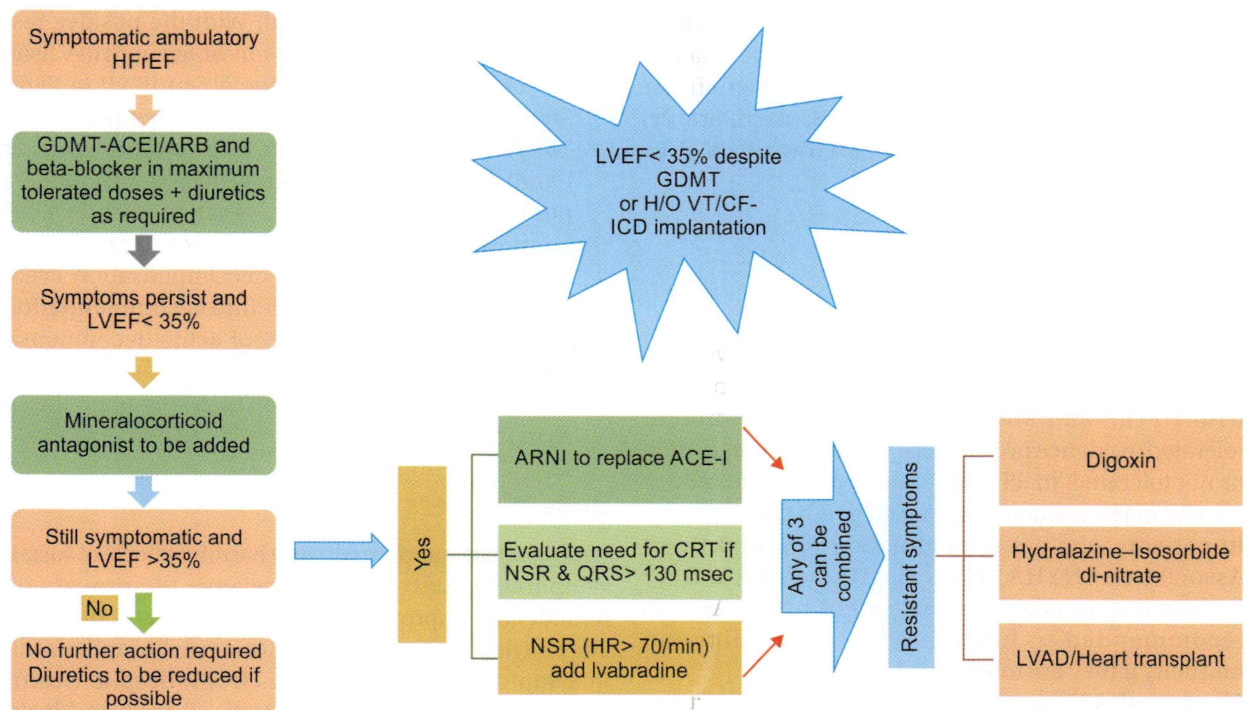

Fig. 1: Algorithm for management of heart failure with reduced ejection fraction as recommended by the American College of Cardiology/American Heart Association/Heart Failure Society of America.
(ACEI: angiotensin converting enzyme inhibitor; ARB: angiotensin receptor blocker; ARNI: angiotensin II receptor neprilysin inhibitor; CRT: cardiac resynchronization therapy; GDMT: guideline-directed management and therapy; HFrEF: heart failure with reduced ejection fraction; HR: heart rate; ICD: implantable cardioverter defibrillator; LVAD: left ventricular assist device; LVEF: left ventricular ejection fraction; NSR: normal sinus rhythm; VF: ventricular fibrillation; VT: ventricular tachycardia)

TABLE 1: Guideline approved daily dosage of commonly used heart failure drugs.

Drug	*Initial dose*	*Maximum dose*
Captopril	6.25 mg TDS	50 mg TDS
Enalapril	2.5 mg BD	10–20 mg BD
Ramipril	2.5 mg OD	10 mg OD
Perindopril	2 mg OD	8–16 mg OD
Lisinopril	2.5–5 mg BD	20–40 mg BD
Candesartan	4–8 mg BD	32 mg BD
Losartan	25–50 mg BD	50–150 mg BD
Valsartan	20–40 mg BD	160 mg BD
Sacubitril/Valsartan	24/26–49/51 mg BD	97/103 mg BD
Ivabradine	5 mg BD	7.5 mg BD
Spironolactone	12.5–25 mg OD	25 mg BD
Eplerenone	25 mg OD	50 mg OD
Bisoprolol	1.25 mg OD	10 mg OD
Carvedilol	3.125 mg BD	50 mg BD
Carvedilol CR	10 mg BD	80 mg BD
Metoprolol succinate CR/XL	12.5–25 mg OD	200 mg OD

lead to reduced hospitalization and improved survival. The efficacy of ACEI has been proven over several decades with overwhelming evidence. Enalapril is the only ACEI that has been used in placebo-controlled mortality trials of HF like CONSENSUS and SOLVD (Studies of left ventricular dysfunction).[1,5] However, many other ACEI have been shown to be beneficial if given in acute settings after an ischemic episode, as in myocardial infarction (MI) trials. These benefits have been shown to remain clinically significant throughout long courses of therapy.[1,5]

Angiotensin receptor blockers are as effective as ACEI, especially in those patients who are intolerant to ACEI due to its inhibitory action on kininase II which leads to upregulation of bradykinin causing more side effects. Candesartan and valsartan have been shown to have mortality benefit in CHARM (Candesartan in Heart Failure Assessment of Reduction in Mortality and morbidity[6,7] and VAL-HeFT (Valsartan Heart Failure Trial)[8] respectively. The VALIANT (VALsartan In Acute myocardial iNfarcTion) trial showed that valsartan was noninferior to captopril and their combination had more side effects with no additional benefits.[9]

Angiotensin receptor neprilysin inhibitor is a new class of agents that inhibits RAAS as well as neutral endopeptidase system. It is a combination of two drugs–valsartan, which is an ARB and sacubitril, which is a neprilysin inhibitor that slows down degradation of natriuretic peptides; thus, enhancing diuresis, natriuresis, and myocardial relaxation. In PARADIGM-HF trial,[2] this drug showed significant reductions in all-cause mortality, cardiovascular mortality, and HF hospitalizations when compared with an ACEI alone.

Recommendations

Class I

- Angiotensin-converting enzyme inhibitor have been shown to reduce mortality and morbidity in patients with HFrEF and are recommended in maximum tolerated/evidence proven dose unless contraindicated or not tolerated, in all symptomatic patients to reduce the risk of HF, hospitalization, and death.
- In patients who are symptomatic [New York Heart Association (NYHA) class II, III and ambulatory IV] despite on GDMT, replacement by an ARNI is recommended to further reduce morbidity and mortality if they are tolerating ACEI/ARB.
- The use of ARB to reduce morbidity and mortality is recommended in patients with prior or current symptoms of chronic HFrEF who are intolerant to ACEI because of cough and angioedema.
- Angiotensin-converting enzyme inhibitor is recommended in patients with asymptomatic LV systolic dysfunction with or without a history of MI in order to prevent or delay the onset of HF and prolong life.

Class IIa

Angiotensin-converting enzyme inhibitor should be considered in patients with stable coronary artery disease (CAD) even if they do not have LV systolic dysfunction, in order to prevent or delay the onset of HF.

Class III

- Angiotensin receptor neprilysin inhibitor should not be administered concomitantly with ACEI or within 36 hours of the last dose of an ACEI.
- Angiotensin receptor neprilysin inhibitor should not be given in patients with a history of angioedema.
- The addition of an ARB (or renin inhibitor) to the combination of an ACEI and an MRA is contraindicated in patients with HF, because of the increased risk of renal dysfunction and hyperkalemia.
- Angiotensin receptor neprilysin inhibitor has been included in GDMT for those who are already on an ACEI/ARB. It is advised to substitute ARNI for ACE/ARB in class II and III NYHA patients for symptomatic as well as mortality benefit. With the positive results of PIONEER-HF (Comparison of Sacubitril–Valsartan versus Enalapril on Effect on NT-proBNP in Patients Stabilized from an Acute Heart Failure Episode)[10] and TRANSITION (A Multicenter, Randomized, Open Label, Parallel Group Study Comparing Pre-discharge and posT-discharge tReatment Initiation With LCZ696 in heArt Failure patieNtS With Reduced ejectIon-fracTion hospItalized for an Acute decOmpensation eveNt)[11] trials, ARNI is expected to find recommendation in treatment of naive patients of acute decompensated heart failure (ADHF) also.
- The recommendations for ACEI/ARB remain the same as in previous guidelines.

Beta-blockers

Beta-blockers interfere with the harmful effects of sustained sympathetic activation and reverse the process of LV remodeling, improve patient symptoms and prolong life. They have been proven to reduce mortality and morbidity in symptomatic patients with HFrEF, despite treatment with an ACEI and, usually a diuretic. Three beta-blockers–bisoprolol, sustained release metoprolol succinate, and carvedilol, have shown mortality benefit in CIBIS II (Cardiac Insufficiency Bisoprolol Study II),[12] MERIT-HF (Effect of metoprolol CR/XL in chronic heart failure: Metoprolol CR/XL Randomised Intervention Trial in Congestive Heart Failure)[13] and COPERNICUS (Carvedilol Prospective Randomized Cumulative Survival)[14] trials respectively when used in patients with chronic HF. There is consensus that beta-blockers and ACEI are complementary and can be disease-modifying. These drugs should be started as soon a diagnosis of HFrEF is made, provided that the patient is hemodynamically stable.

Recommendations

Class I

- A beta-blocker is recommended in addition to an ACEI for patients with stable, symptomatic HFrEF to reduce the risk of HF hospitalization and death.
- Beta-blockers should be initiated in clinically stable patients at a low dose and gradually up-titrated to the maximum tolerated dose.
- Beta-blocker is recommended in patients with asymptomatic LV dysfunction and a history of MI, in order to prevent or delay the onset of HF and/or prolong life.

Beta-blockers remain an integral part of HF management with no new changes in guideline recommendations.

Mineralocorticoid Receptor Antagonists

Mineralocorticoid receptor antagonists (spironolactone and eplerenone), though classified as potassium sparing diuretics, have dominant effects through RAAS modification, mediated by aldosterone receptor blockade. This makes them beneficial over and above their sodium-related diuretic effects. ACEI though have some effect on reducing aldosterone, this action is not persistent and there is a rapid return of aldosterone levels, which is why MRA showed clinical benefits in trials like RALES (Randomized ALdactone Evaluation Study)[15] and EMPHASIS-HF (Eplerenone in Mild Patients Hospitalization and Survival Study in Heart Failure).[16]

Recommendations

Class I

- Spironolactone or eplerenone are recommended in all symptomatic patients (despite treatment with an ACEI and a beta-blocker) with HFrEF and LV ejection fraction (LVEF) ≤35%, to reduce mortality and HF hospitalization.
- Mineralocorticoid receptor antagonists should be used cautiously in patients with impaired renal function and in those with high-normal serum potassium levels. Regular monitoring is advisable.

WHAT IS NEW IN 2019?

Mineralocorticoid receptor antagonists hold their position in GDMT in addition to ACEI/ARB/ARNI and beta-blockers and no new change in recommendation has been made.

Ivabradine

Ivabradine slows the heart rate through inhibition of I_f channel in the sinus node. In patients with HFrEF, this heart rate slowing effect has been shown to result in improved clinical outcomes through prevention of heart rate mediated deleterious effects on cardiac myocytes. SHIFT (Systolic Heart failure treatment with the I_f inhibitor ivabradine Trial) was the main trial demonstrating clinical utility of ivabradine.[17] It enrolled patients with LVEF <35% who were symptomatic and had heart rate ≥70 beats/minute, despite being on GDMT including beta-blockers. Addition of ivabradine resulted in significant reduction in HF-hospitalization and HF-related deaths, though overall cardiovascular mortality was not reduced. This led to guideline recommendation as well as wide clinical acceptability of this drug in significant number of patients who are intolerant to high doses of beta-blockers due to various reasons, most common being low blood pressure. It should be noted that ivabradine is effective only in patients who are in sinus rhythm as the sinus node is the primary site of action for this drug.

Recommendations

Class IIa

- Ivabradine should be considered to reduce the risk of HF hospitalization or cardiovascular death in symptomatic patients with stable chronic HF (LVEF ≤35%), in sinus rhythm and a resting heart rate ≥70 beats/minutes despite treatment with a maximum tolerated dose of beta-blocker, ACEI (or ARB), and an MRA (or ARB).
- It is also suggested for patients of above category who are intolerant or have contraindications to beta-blockers and are already receiving ACEI/ARB and MRA.

SHIFT trial results were published in 2010 but the drug was approved by the United States Food and Drug Administration only in 2015 and therefore, has now been included in the ACC/AHA guidelines. However, the European guidelines had started recommending it several years back itself.[18]

Hydralazine and Isosorbide Dinitrate

The hemodynamic rationale behind this combination is to decrease both cardiac preload and afterload by causing arterial dilation (hydralazine) and venodilatation (nitrates). This reduces intracardiac filling pressures and prevents cardiac remodeling. This drug has not been tested formally in any large trial, nonetheless it remains a useful drug in patients of HF with renal insufficiency.[19]

Recommendations

- Hydralazine and isosorbide dinitrate may be considered in symptomatic patients with HFrEF who can tolerate neither an ACEI nor an ARB (or they are contraindicated) to reduce the risk of death (class IIb).
- In black patients, this carries a class IIa recommendation in the same scenario.

Diuretics

Diuretics (primarily loop-diuretics) mitigate most of the clinical manifestations of HF which usually result from sodium water retention causing volume overload in the body. Diuretics induce negative sodium-water balance which decreases LV dilation, functional mitral insufficiency, and subendocardial ischemia. In short-term clinical trials, diuretics have shown to reduce jugular venous pressure, pulmonary congestion, peripheral edema, body weight and subsequently symptoms and exercise tolerance.[19]

However, the long-term usage of loop-diuretics seems to be associated with increase cardiac mortality.[20] Therefore, they are recommended for short-term use to relieve HF symptoms.

Recommendations

- Diuretics are recommended in order to improve symptoms and exercise capacity in patients with signs and/or symptoms of congestion (class I).
- Diuretics should be considered to reduce the risk of HF hospitalization in patients with signs and/or symptoms of congestion (class IIa).

Miscellaneous Drugs

Drugs with Probable Benefit

- Digoxin may be considered in symptomatic patients in sinus rhythm despite treatment with an ACEI (or ARB), a beta-blocker and an MRA, to reduce the risk of hospitalization (both all-cause and HF-hospitalizations) (class IIb).
- N-3 polyunsaturated fatty acids preparation may be considered in symptomatic HF patients to reduce the risk of cardiovascular hospitalization and cardiovascular death (class IIb).

Drugs with Unproven Benefit/Harm

- Nonsteroidal anti-inflammatory drugs or cyclooxygenase-2 inhibitors are not recommended in patients with HF, as they increase the risk of worsening of HF and hospitalizations (class III).
- Diltiazem or verapamil are not recommended in patients with HFrEF as they have been shown to increase sympathetic tone and may be unsafe (class III).

Recommendations for Management of Important Comorbidities

Anemia

Anemia is independently associated with HF disease severity, and iron deficiency appears to be uniquely associated with reduced exercise capacity. FAIR-HF (Ferinject Assessment in Patients with Iron Deficiency and Chronic Heart Failure)[21] and CONFIRM-HF (Ferric CarboxymaltOse evaluatioN on perFormance in patients with IRon deficiency in coMbination with chronic Heart Failure)[22] trials demonstrated improvements in NYHA class and functional capacity with intravenous iron therapy over a short-term exposure, thus making a place in HF management. However, role of oral iron and strong recommendation for intravenous iron are still awaited and will depend on further trials.

- In patients with NYHA class II and III HF and iron deficiency (ferritin <100 ng/mL or 100–300 ng/mL if transferrin saturation is <20%), intravenous iron replacement might be reasonable to improve functional status and quality of life (class IIb).
- The strong evidence from STAMINA-HeFT (Study of Anemia in Heart Failure Trial)[23] and large randomized controlled trials such as RED-HF (Reduction of Events by Darbepoetin Alfa in Heart Failure)[24] suggests lack of benefit and increased adverse events with erythropoietin-stimulating agent therapy in HF. Therefore, erythropoietin-stimulating agent therapy cannot be recommended in patients with HF and anemia (class III).

Hypertension

A new section on hypertension has been included in the recent guidelines which highlights the importance of hypertension management in both prevention and treatment of HF.

- In patients at increased risk of HF (stage A) or hypertensives with symptomatic HFrEF, the optimal blood pressure should be less than 130/80 (class I).
- Angiotensin-converting enzyme inhibitor/ARB, beta-blocker or MRA (single drug or a combination) is recommended to reduce blood pressure in HF because of their associated benefits in HFrEF reducing death and HF hospitalization (class I).
- A diuretic/amlodipine/hydralazine is recommended to reduce blood pressure when hypertension persists despite treatment with a combination of above drugs (class I).
- Moxonidine, alpha-adrenergic antagonists, diltiazem and verapamil are not recommended to reduce blood pressure because of harmful effects like increased mortality, worsening of HF, neurohormonal activation, and negative inotropic action respectively (class III).

Sleep Disordered Breathing

- In patients with NYHA class II–IV HF and suspicion of sleep-disordered breathing or excessive daytime sleepiness, a formal sleep assessment is reasonable (class IIa).
- In patients with cardiovascular disease and obstructive sleep apnea, continuous positive airway pressure therapy may be reasonable to improve sleep quality and daytime sleepiness (class IIb).
- In patients with NYHA class II–IV HFrEF and central sleep apnea, adaptive servo-ventilation causes harm (class III).

Diabetes

- Metformin should be considered as first-line treatment for glycemic control in patients with diabetes and HF, unless contraindicated.
- Thiazolidinediones are not recommended in patients with HF, as they increase the risk of worsening of HF and hospitalizations (class III).

CONCLUSION

It is well documented that the diuretic especially Chlorthalidone, beta-blocker especially beta 1 selective beta-blocker bisoprolol, MRA, ARBs, and ACEi have shown morbidity and mortality benefits in heart failure. Recently, ARNI is a new class of agents that inhibits RAAS as well as neutral endopeptidase system. It is a combination of two drugs–valsartan, which is an ARB and sacubitril, which is a neprilysin inhibitor that slows down degradation of natriuretic peptides; thus enhancing diuresis, natriuresis, and myocardial relaxation. In PARADIGM-HF trial,[2] this drug showed significant reductions in all-cause mortality, cardiovascular mortality and HF hospitalizations when compared with an ACEI alone. Recent trials on sodium glucose co-transporter 2 (SGLT2) inhibitors like EMPAREG OUTCOME (Empagliflozin Cardiovascular Outcome Event Trial in Type 2 Diabetes Mellitus Patients), CANVAS (Canagliflozin Cardiovascular Assessment Study) and real-life data from CVD-REAL (Cardiovascular Events Associated with SGLT-2 Inhibitors versus Other Glucose-Lowering Drugs) have demonstrated benefit in diabetic patients with HF. However, translation of these findings in to guideline recommendations is awaited.[25]

REFERENCES

1. CONSENSUS Trial Study Group. Effects of enalapril on mortality in severe congestive heart failure. Results of the Cooperative North Scandinavian Enalapril Survival Study (CONSENSUS). N Engl J Med. 1987;316(23):1429-35.
2. McMurray JJ, Packer M, Desai AS, et al. Dual angiotensin receptor and neprilysin inhibition as an alternative to angiotensin-converting enzyme inhibition in patients with chronic systolic heart failure: rationale for and design of the Prospective comparison of ARNI with ACEI to Determine Impact on Global Mortality and morbidity in Heart Failure trial (PARADIGM-HF). Eur J Heart Fail. 2013;15(9):1062-73.
3. Ponikowski P, Voors AA, Anker SD, et al. 2016 ESC Guidelines for the diagnosis and treatment of acute and chronic heart failure: The Task Force for the diagnosis and treatment of acute and chronic heart failure of the European Society of Cardiology (ESC). Developed with the special contribution of the Heart Failure Association (HFA) of the ESC. Eur Heart J. 2016;37(27):2129-200.
4. Yancy CW, Jessup M, Bozkurt B, et al. 2017 ACC/AHA/HFSA Focused Update of the 2013 ACCF/AHA Guideline for the Management of Heart Failure: A Report of the American College of Cardiology/American Heart Association Task Force on Clinical Practice Guidelines and the Heart Failure Society of America. Circulation. 2017;136(6):e137-e161.
5. Investigators S, Yusuf S, Pitt B, et al. Effect of enalapril on survival in patients with reduced left ventricular ejection fractions and congestive heart failure. N Engl J Med. 1991;325(5):293-302.
6. Young JB, Dunlap ME, Pfeffer MA, et al. Mortality and morbidity reduction with Candesartan in patients with chronic heart failure and left ventricular systolic dysfunction: results of the CHARM low-left ventricular ejection fraction trials. Circulation. 2004;110(17):2618-26.
7. Wong CM, Hawkins NM, Jhund PS, et al. Clinical characteristics and outcomes of young and very young adults with heart failure: The CHARM programme (Candesartan in Heart Failure Assessment of Reduction in Mortality and Morbidity). J Am Coll Cardiol. 2013;62(20):1845-54.
8. Cohn JN, Tognoni G, Valsartan Heart Failure Trial I. A randomized trial of the angiotensin-receptor blocker valsartan in chronic heart failure. N Engl J Med. 2001;345(23):1667-75.
9. Pfeffer MA, McMurray JJ, Velazquez EJ, et al. Valsartan, captopril, or both in myocardial infarction complicated by heart failure, left ventricular dysfunction, or both. N Engl J Med. 2003;349(20):1893-906.
10. Velazquez EJ, Morrow DA, DeVore AD, et al. Angiotensin-neprilysin inhibition in acute decompensated heart failure. N Engl J Med. 2019;380(6):539-48.
11. Wachter R, Senni M, Belohlavek J, et al. Initiation of sacubitril/valsartan in hospitalized patients with heart failure with reduced ejection fraction after hemodynamic stabilization: primary results of the TRANSITION study. Abstract P6531. Presented at: European Society of Cardiology Congress; Aug. 25-29, 2018; Munich. 2018.
12. The Cardiac Insufficiency Bisoprolol Study II (CIBIS-II): a randomised trial. Lancet. 1999;353(9146):9-13.
13. Effect of metoprolol CR/XL in chronic heart failure: Metoprolol CR/XL Randomised Intervention Trial in Congestive Heart Failure (MERIT-HF). Lancet 1999;353(9169):2001-7.
14. Packer M, Fowler MB, Roecker EB, et al. Carvedilol Prospective Randomized Cumulative Survival (COPERNICUS) Study Group. Effect of carvedilol on the morbidity of patients with severe chronic heart failure: results of the carvedilol prospective randomized cumulative survival (COPERNICUS) study. Circulation. 2002;106(17):2194-9.
15. Pitt B, Zannad F, Remme WJ, et al. The effect of spironolactone on morbidity and mortality in patients with severe heart failure. Randomized Aldactone Evaluation Study Investigators. N Engl J Med. 1999;341(10):709-17.
16. Zannad F, McMurray JJ, Krum H, et al. EMPHASIS-HF Study Group. Eplerenone in patients with systolic heart failure and mild symptoms. N Engl J Med. 2011;364(1):11-21.
17. Swedberg K, Komajda M, Bohm M, et al. Ivabradine and outcomes in chronic heart failure (SHIFT): a randomised placebo-controlled study. Lancet. 2010;376(9744):875-85.

18. McMurray JJ, Adamopoulos S, Anker SD, et al. ESC Guidelines for the diagnosis and treatment of acute and chronic heart failure 2012: The task force for the diagnosis and treatment of acute and chronic heart failure 2012 of the European Society of Cardiology. Developed in collaboration with the Heart Failure Association (HFA) of the ESC. Eur Heart J. 2012;33(14):1787-847.
19. Mann D, Zipes D, Libby P, et al. Braunwald's Heart Disease: A Textbook of Cardiovascular Medicine, 10th edition. Amsterdam: Elsevier; 2015.
20. Kapelios CJ, Malliaras K, Kaldara E, et al. Loop diuretics for chronic heart failure: a foe in disguise of a friend? Eur Heart J Cardiovasc Pharmacother. 2018;4(1):54-63.
21. Anker SD, Comin Colet J, Filippatos G, et al. Ferric carboxymaltose in patients with heart failure and iron deficiency. N Engl J Med. 2009;361(25):2436-48.
22. Ponikowski P, van Veldhuisen DJ, Comin-Colet J, et al. Beneficial effects of long-term intravenous iron therapy with ferric carboxymaltose in patients with symptomatic heart failure and iron deficiency. Eur Heart J. 2015;36(11):657-68.
23. Ghali JK, Anand IS, Abraham WT, et al. Randomized double-blind trial of darbepoetin alfa in patients with symptomatic heart failure and anemia. Circulation. 2008;117(4):526-35.
24. Swedberg K, McMurray JJ, Young JB. Darbepoetin alfa in systolic heart failure. N Engl J Med. 2013;369:488-9.
25. Kosiborod M, Cavender MA, Fu AZ, et al. Lower risk of heart failure and death in patients initiated on sodium-glucose cotransporter-2 inhibitors versus other glucose-lowering drugs: The CVD-REAL Study (Comparative effectiveness of cardiovascular outcomes in new users of sodium-glucose cotransporter-2 inhibitors). Circulation. 2017;136(3):249-59.

CHAPTER 39

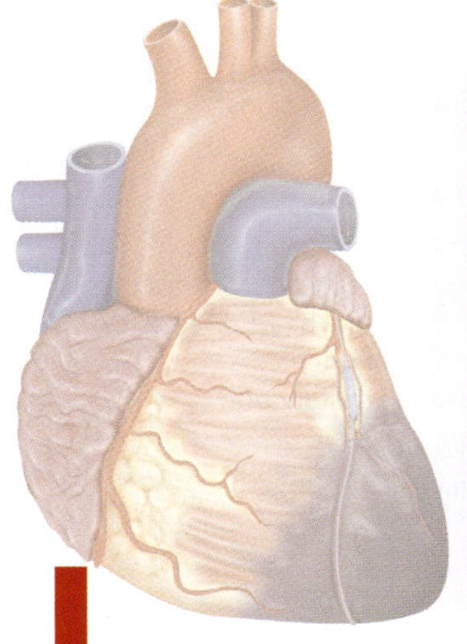

Clinical Guidelines for Heart Failure with Preserved Ejection Fraction

Dinkar Bhasin, Saurabh Mehrotra, Sundeep Mishra

INTRODUCTION

Heart failure with preserved ejection fraction (HFpEF) contributes to nearly 50% of patients presenting with heart failure (HF). However, guidelines specific to HFpEF are lacking because of the paucity of high-quality in this area. Recommendations regarding HFpEF have been made in the societal guidelines for HF. In this chapter, we summarize the recommendations pertaining to the diagnosis and management of HFpEF based on the ESC 2016, American College of Cardiology Foundation (ACCF)/American Heart Association (AHA) 2013 and ACCF/AHA/Heart Failure Society of America (HFSA) focused guidelines published in 2017.[1-3]

GUIDELINES FOR DIAGNOSIS OF HEART FAILURE WITH PRESERVED EJECTION FRACTION

Heart failure is a clinical diagnosis that is made based on the patient's symptoms and examination findings (Table 1). There are broadly two varieties: Heart failure with reduced ejection fraction (HFrEF) and HFpEF distinguishable on echocardiographic finding of reduced ejection fraction (EF) or not. However, it is difficult to distinguish between HFrEF and HFpEF purely on clinical grounds. Certain subtle clinical findings such as the absence of cardiomegaly or presence of S4 (and no S3) do suggest HFpEF but these are "soft" findings, the sensitivity and specificity being generally low. The ESC 2016 guidelines suggest an algorithmic approach to diagnose heart failure (Flowchart 1). This includes the use of natriuretic peptides (NP) levels and echocardiography. As a matter of fact, the plasma concentration of NP is a good rule-out test for HF. Plasma concentration of brain natriuretic peptide (BNP) <35 pg/mL and NT-pro-BNP <125 pg/mL can help in excluding HF.

TABLE 1: Signs and symptoms of heart failure syndrome.

Symptoms	*Examination findings*
Typical	*More specific*
• Ankle edema • Easy fatigability • Dyspnea • Orthopnea • Paroxysmal nocturnal dyspnea	• Ankle edema • Cardiomegaly • Elevated JVP • Hepatojugular reflux • Rales • S3
Less typical	*Less specific*
• Anorexia • Bendopnea* • Depression • Nocturnal cough or wheezing • Nocturia • Oliguria • Palpitations, dizziness, syncope • Weight loss	• Ascites • Cardiac cachexia • Cheyne–Stokes respiration • Cold extremities • Hepatomegaly • Narrow pulse pressure • Pleural effusion • Weight gain (>2 kg/week) • Weight loss on diuretic therapy • Sacral/scrotal edema

Source: Adapted from 2016 ESC Guidelines for the diagnosis and treatment of acute and chronic heart failure[1]

*Bendopnea is a newly described symptom of heart failure, **meaning** shortness of breath when leaning forward.

TABLE 2: Classification of heart failure (HF): preserved ejection fraction (HFpEF), mid-range ejection fraction (HFmrEF), and reduced ejection fraction (HfrEF).

Classification		*HFrEF*	*HFmrEF*	*HFpEF*
Diagnostic criteria	*Clinical features*	Signs and/or symptoms	Symptoms and/or signs*	Symptoms and/or signs*
	EF	LVEF < 40%	LVEF = 40–49%	LVEF ≥ 50%
	Additional features	Nil	• Increased NP levels** • Additional criteria (at least one) – Structural heart disease (LVH and/or LAE) • Diastolic dysfunction	• Increased NP levels** • Additional criteria (at least one) – Structural heart disease (LVH and/or LAE) • Diastolic dysfunction

(NP: natriuretic peptide; LAE: left atrial enlargement; LVEF: left ventricular ejection fraction; LVH: left ventricular hypertrophy)

* Patients in early stages may not manifest,may not be present in the early stages of HF and in patients treated with diuretics

** BNP > 35 pg/mL and/or NT-proBNP > 125 pg/mL

Source: Adapted from 2016 ESC Guidelines for the diagnosis and treatment of acute and chronic heart failure.[1]

Flowchart 1: Algorithmic approach to diagnosis of heart failure.

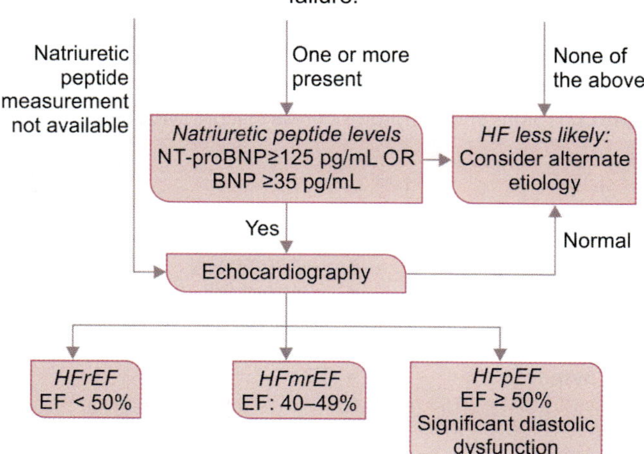

(BNP: brain natriuretic peptide; ECG: electrocardiogram; HF: heart failure; HFmrEF: heart failure with mid-range ejection fraction; HFpEF: heart failure with preserved ejection fraction; HFrEF: heart failure with reduced ejection fraction; JVP: jugular venous pressure; NP: natriuretic peptide)

Source: Adapted from 2016 ESC Guidelines for the diagnosis and treatment of acute and chronic heart failure.[1]

TABLE 3: AHA/ACC definitions of HF*r*EF and HF*p*EF.

Type of HF	*EF*	
HFrEF	≤40	Often described as systolic heart failure. Most RCTs have included such patients and there is good quality evidence with GDMT
HFpEF	≥50	Occasionally described as diastolic heart failure. Studies have used different criteria for diagnosis of HFpEF. Limited high-quality evidence with GDMT
HFpEF, borderline	41–49	These patients fall into a borderline or intermediate group. Although EF is mildly reduced, management is similar to HFpEF
HFpEF, improved	>40	Patients with HFrEF in whom EF has recovered on treatment. More research is required to guide treatment in this group of patients

(GDMT: guideline-mediated drug therapy; HFpEF: heart failure with preserved ejection fraction; HFrEF: heart failure with reduced ejection fraction; EF: ejection fraction; HF: heart failure; HFpEF: heart failure with preserved ejection fraction; HFrEF: heart failure with reduced ejection fraction)

Source: Adapted from 2013 ACCF/AHA Guideline for the Management of Heart Failure.[2]

Echocardiography is the single most important test which can rule in/rule out the diagnosis, suggest possible etiology and also classify HF. Conceptually, diagnosis of HFpEF requires demonstration of normal EF with significant diastolic dysfunction. Different trials related to HFpEF have used variable cut-offs for EF. To avoid any ambiguity in definition of HFpEF, the ESC 2016 guidelines have used the term heart failure with mid-range ejection fraction (HFmrEF) for patients with EF between 40% and 49%. Patients with EF ≥ 50% are classified as HFpEF. However, for practical purposes, it is reasonable to manage patients with HFmrEF as HFpEF. The recommended classifications of HF as per the ESC guidelines are summarized in Table 2. The AHA/ACC 2011 guidelines use the term heart failure with borderline ejection fraction for patients with EF between 40% and 49% (Table 3).

Assessment of diastolic dysfunction is perhaps the most important aspect in the diagnosis of HFpEF. The latest guidelines on the echocardiographic assessment of diastolic dysfunction were published by the American Society of Echocardiography and the European Association of Cardiovascular Imaging in 2016.[4] The definitive diagnosis of diastolic dysfunction requires presence of at least three of four qualifying criteria which include:

1. Mean E/e' > 14 (septal E/e' > 13 or lateral E/e' > 15)
2. Lateral e' velocity < 10 cm/sec or medial e' velocity < 7 cm/s
3. Tricuspid regurgitation velocity > 2.8 m/s
4. LA volume index > 34 mL/m^2 (Flowchart 2)

After the diagnosis has been established the diastolic dysfunction should be graded for I-III (Flowchart 3 and Table 4). Echocardiographic parameters can suggest elevated left atrial pressure or left ventricular (LV) filling pressure and help in guiding therapy especially regarding the use of diuretics.

BASIC DIAGNOSTIC TESTS

All patients with clinical diagnosis of HF syndrome should undergo certain basic tests to identify possible etiologies, detect comorbidities, and guide treatment. These include baseline renal function tests, serum electrolytes,

Flowchart 2: Approach to diagnosis of diastolic dysfunction.

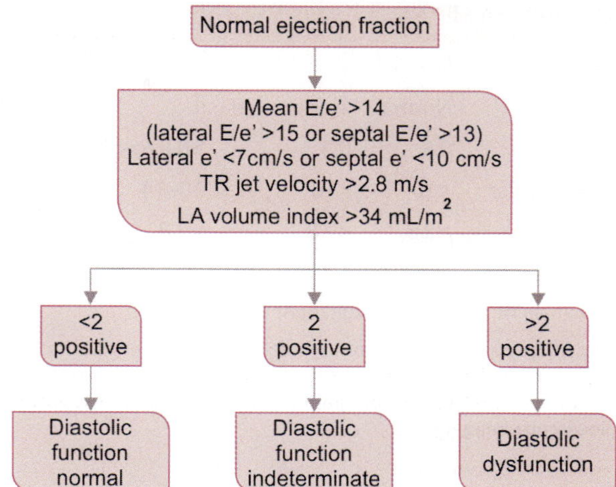

(LA: left atrial; TR: tricuspid regurgitation)
Source: Adapted from the recommendations for the evaluation of left ventricular diastolic function by echocardiography: An update from the American Society of Echocardiography and the European Association of Cardiovascular Imaging.[4]

Flowchart 3: Approach for estimating LA pressure and grading diastolic dysfunction.

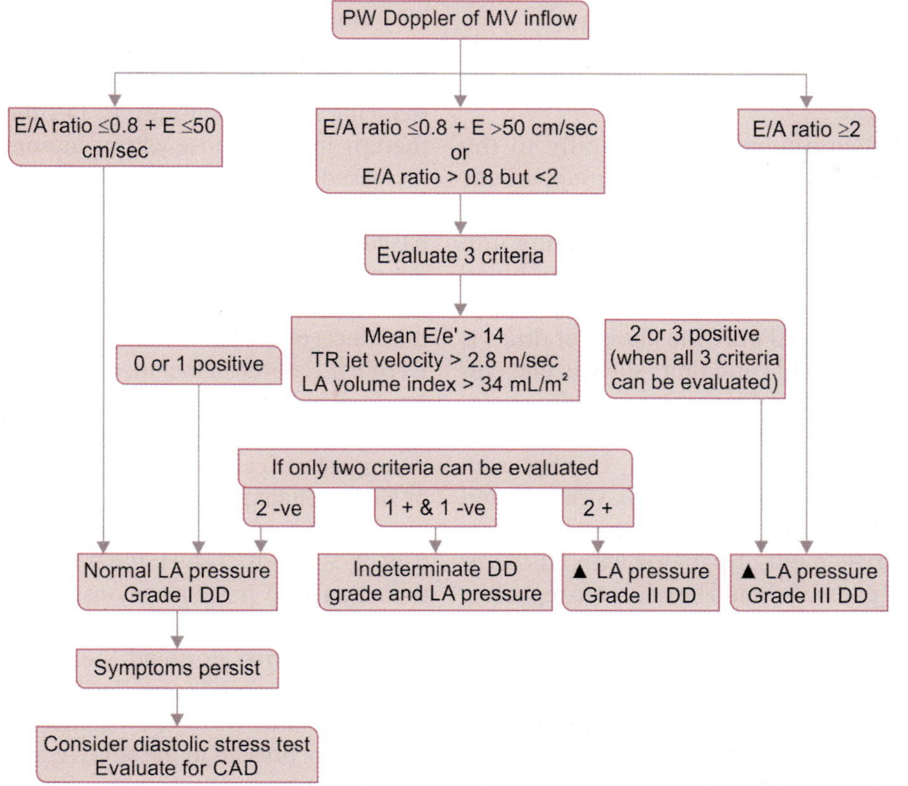

(DD: diastolic dysfunction; LA: left atrium; PW: pulsed wave; MV: mitral valve; TR: tricuspid regurgitation)
Source: Adapted from the recommendations for the evaluation of left ventricular diastolic function by echocardiography: An update from the American Society of Echocardiography and the European Association of Cardiovascular Imaging.[4]

TABLE 4: Grades of diastolic dysfunction.

	Normal	*Grade I*	*Grade II*	*Grade III*
Relaxation	Normal	↓	↓	↓
LA pressure	Normal	↓ or normal	↑	↑
E/A ratio	0.8	0.8	>0.8 to <2	>2
Mean E/e' ratio	<10	<10	10–14	>14
TR jet (m/sec)	<2.8	<2.8	>2.8	>2.8
LA volume index	Normal	Normal or ↑	↑	↑

(LA: left atrial; TR: tricuspid regurgitation)

Source: Adapted from the recommendations for the evaluation of left ventricular diastolic function by echocardiography: An update from the American Society of Echocardiography and the European Association of Cardiovascular Imaging.[4]

BOX 1: Common comorbidities in patients with heart failure with preserved ejection fraction (HFpEF).

- Atrial fibrillation
- Diabetes mellitus
- Obesity
- Pulmonary disorders such as COPD
- Pulmonary hypertension
- Renal dysfunction
- Sleep apnea
- Systemic hypertension

(COPD: chronic obstructive pulmonary disease)

Source: Adapted from 2016 ESC Guidelines for the diagnosis and treatment of acute and chronic heart failure.[1]

hemoglobin, fasting blood sugar, HbA1c, lipid profile, thyroid function tests, and serum ferritin. A 12-lead electrocardiogram and a chest radiograph should be done in all patients. Exercise testing may be done for diagnosis and risk stratification of coronary artery disease (CAD). Cardiac catheterization is not routinely indicated but may be done when there is doubt about the diagnosis and surgical revascularization is a possibility. Invasive hemodynamics with exercise testing or saline loading results in significant elevation of left-ventricular end-diastolic pressure.

TREATMENT

Guideline-based recommendations specific to the treatment of HFpEF are limited. Most hospitalizations in patients with HFpEF occur because of comorbidities. Guidelines stress the importance of identifying and managing such comorbidities (Box 1). Adequate blood pressure control remains a cornerstone for treatment in hypertensive patients with HFpEF. The choice of drugs is influenced by the co-existing conditions such as diabetes mellitus and CAD. All the first-line agents including beta-blockers, angiotensin-converting enzyme (ACE) inhibitors and angiotensin receptor blockers (ARB) can be used. Patients with co-existent CAD should be risk-stratified and revascularization should be advised as per guidelines.

The general management of patients with HFrEF or HFpEF is similar. All patients should be educated regarding self-care. This includes imparting knowledge about drug adherence, weight monitoring, regular follow-up, and lifestyle interventions. Restriction of dietary sodium can be considered in severely symptomatic patients while general advice to restrict sodium <3 g/day appears appropriate in most patients. Patients should be screened for sleep-related breathing disorders and the same managed with positive pressure ventilation. Exercise training should be prescribed for all symptomatic patients who can participate as it improves functional status. Specifically, cardiac rehabilitation improves outcomes and should be considered wherever feasible. Patients should be encouraged to maintain optimal weight. Pneumococcal vaccine and annual influenza vaccine should be prescribed to all patients with HF.

Options for pharmacological therapy of HFpEF are limited. Guideline-mediated drug therapy (GDMT) recommends the use of diuretics for symptomatic patients to decrease pulmonary venous congestion and loop diuretics are the drugs of the first choice. Use of mineralocorticoid receptors antagonists (MRAs) may be considered reasonable in patients with HFpEF for reducing HF hospitalizations. Eligible candidates for this therapy include those with symptoms and an EF ≥45%, increased levels of NP, serum creatinine <2.5 mg/dL, and normal serum potassium levels. This recommendation is based on the TOPCAT (Treatment of Preserved Cardiac Function Heart Failure with an Aldosterone Antagonist) trial which was a multicenter study designed to investigate the effects of spironolactone on outcomes in patients with HFpEF (EF ≥45%). It included over 3,000 patients who were randomized to receive either spironolactone or placebo and followed-up over 3.3 years. The primary outcome was a composite of cardiovascular death, aborted cardiac arrest, or HF hospitalizations. There was no difference in primary outcome between the two groups (18.6% vs. 20.4%; HR = 0.89, 95% CI = 0.77–1.94; P = 0.14). However, a significant reduction in HF hospitalizations (12.0% vs. 14.2%; HR = 0.83; 95% CI = 0.69–0.99; P = 0.04) was observed. The incidence of hyperkalemia doubled (18.7% vs. 9.1%) and serum creatinine increased more frequently in patients receiving spironolactone. However, significant recruitment related issues were present in the study. An important interaction was noted between the country of enrollment and outcomes in this study. In patients from Russia and Georgia, the event rates were observed to be similar to controls.[5] A post-hoc analysis showed that after excluding patients from these countries a significant reduction in the primary outcome was noted (HR = 0.82; 95% CI 0.69–0.98).[6]

Use of angiotensin receptor blockers (ARB) is a class IIB recommendation for patients with HFpEF. This evidence is derived from the CHARM-Preserved Randomized Trial which studied the utility of the ARB candesartan in over 3,000 patients with HFpEF (LVEF >40%). The primary outcome was cardiovascular death or hospitalization for CHF. After a median follow-up of 36.6 months, there was no difference in the primary outcome or cardiovascular deaths, but there was a significant reduction in hospitalization for CHF.[7]

Atrial fibrillation (AF) is a common complication in patients with HFpEF. Patients often deteriorate at the onset of AF. Management should be based on standard guidelines, but in patients with refractory HF, rhythm control should be preferred. Catheter ablation has emerged as an effective and safe alternative to pharmacological rhythm control, especially in patients with paroxysmal AF or early AF. Most of the patients are candidates for anticoagulation (elderly, heart failure, and often hypertension) and direct-acting oral anticoagulants remain the drugs of first choice.

REFERENCES

1. Ponikowski P, Voors AA, Anker SD, et al. 2016 ESC Guidelines for the diagnosis and treatment of acute and chronic heart failure: The Task Force for the diagnosis and treatment of acute and chronic heart failure of the European Society of Cardiology (ESC) developed with the special contribution of the Heart Failure Association (HFA) of the ESC. Eur Heart J. 2016;37(27):2129-200.
2. Yancy CW, Jessup M, Bozkurt B, et al. 2013 ACCF/AHA Guideline for the Management of Heart Failure. J Am Coll Cardiol. 2013;62(16):e147–239.
3. Yancy CW, Jessup M, Bozkurt B, et al. 2017 ACC/AHA/HFSA Focused Update of the 2013 ACCF/AHA Guideline for the Management of Heart Failure. J Am Coll Cardiol. 2017;70(6):e137-e161.
4. Nagueh SF, Smiseth OA, Appleton CP, et al. Recommendations for the evaluation of left ventricular diastolic function by echocardiography: An update from the American Society of Echocardiography and the European Association of Cardiovascular Imaging. J Am Soc Echocardiogr. 2016;29(4):277-314.
5. Pitt B, Pfeffer MA, Assmann SF, et al. Spironolactone for heart failure with preserved ejection fraction. N Engl J Med. 2014;370(15):1383-92.
6. Pfeffer MA, Claggett B, Assmann SF, et al. Regional variation in patients and outcomes in the Treatment of Preserved Cardiac Function Heart Failure With an Aldosterone Antagonist (TOPCAT) Trial. Circulation. 2015;131(1):34-42.
7. Yusuf S, Pfeffer MA, Swedberg K, et al. Effects of candesartan in patients with chronic heart failure and preserved left-ventricular ejection fraction: the CHARM-Preserved Trial. Lancet. 2003;362(9386):777-81.

CHAPTER

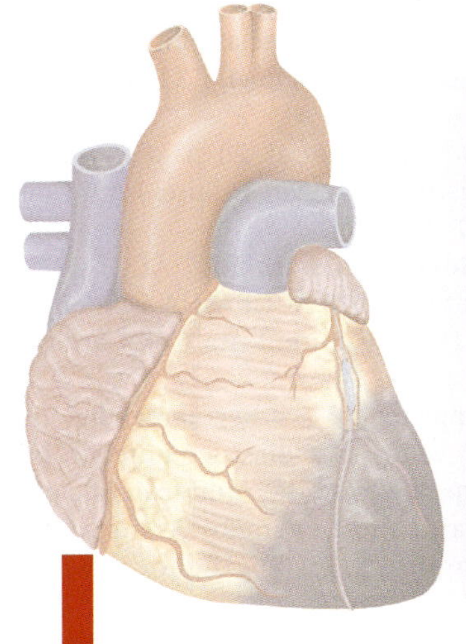

Clinical Guidelines for HFrEF: AHA, ACC and ESC

Tapan Sinha, Jayanta Sharma, Mrinal Kanti Das

INTRODUCTION

Despite remarkable advancements in our understanding of physiological basis of heart failure, our erudition on pathophysiological mechanism remained somewhat less comprehensive. Failure to achieve significant progress in improving outcome through treatment of heart failure is embedded in crevices of such knowledge. Since 1970s, huge and diverse range data regarding evidence-based treatment outcome on studies with heart failure are available. These researches exposed necessity of some form of standardization of available information through guidelines to put them in clinical practice. To this end, the American College of Cardiology (ACC) and the American Heart Association (AHA) in 1980 established a Task Force on Assessment of Diagnostic and Therapeutic Cardiovascular Procedures (now the ACC/AHA Task Force on Practice Guidelines) with the following charges:

- Develop guidelines for role of new therapeutic approaches and for noninvasive and invasive procedures in the diagnosis and management of cardiovascular disease.
- Estimation of contribution, uniqueness, sensitivity, specificity, indications, contraindications, and cost-effectiveness of such diagnostic procedures and therapeutic modalities.
- Emphasize the role and values of the developed guidelines as an educational resource.[1] Since those early days of guidelines, there has been significant progress in management of heart failure. However, the de-novo development of an evidence-based guideline requires considerable time, expertise, and resources, which are limited, even in developed countries.[2,3] It was therefore suggested that guideline development should be based on the adaptation and consolidation of existing information.[4]

"Under normal conditions, the research scientist is not an innovator but a solver of puzzles, and the puzzles upon which he concentrates are just those which he believes can be both stated and solved within the existing scientific tradition."

—Thomas S Kuhn, The Structure of Scientific Revolutions

In 1937, Fishberg defined modern concept of heart failure as "those forms of cardiac insufficiency which are due to inadequate diastolic filling of the heart (hypo-diastolic failure) [i.e. heart failure with preserved ejection fraction, (HFpEF)] and the far more common ones in which heart fills adequately but does not empty to the normal extent (hyposystolic failure) [i.e. heart failure with reduced ejection fraction (HFrEF)].[5,6] From definitions, it is apparent that for establishing the diagnosis of diastolic heart failure (DHF) or systolic heart failure (SHF), it is necessary to measure left ventricular ejection fraction (LVEF) after confirming the presence of clinical HF. It should be appreciated that signs and symptoms, radiologic and electrocardiographic findings, and neurohormonal profile may supplant but cannot distinguish between HFrEF and HFpEF.[7] Over last few decades, prodigious data has accumulated proving that these two entities are not only echocardiographically distinct but also have different pathophysiological basis and therapeutic outcome (Table 1).

Before 1990s, despite substantial advancement in treatment and investigations, about 60–70% of patients

TABLE 1: HFrEF versus HFpEF—salient differences.

HFrEF	*HFpEF*
• Basic pathophysiology—reduction of LV systolic function • Men > women • Younger (compared to HFpEF) • History of MI and DCM is more common • LV is dilated with eccentric remodeling • Vasodilators improves LV systolic performance • Myocardial stress/injury is more pronounced	• Alteration of LV filling • Women > men • More often older • History of hypertension, AF, and VHD is more common. Impact of comorbidities may be more profound • Concentric remodeling (with or without LVH) is present in many. LV end-diastolic volume is not increased relative to the stroke volume • Vasodilators have little impact on LV systolic performance • Myocardial inflammation and fibrosis are more prominent

(AF: atrial fibrillation; DCM: dilated cardiomyopathy; HFpEF: heart failure with preserved ejection fraction; HFrEF: heart failure with reduced ejection fraction; LV: left ventricular; LVH: left ventricular hypertrophy; MI: myocardial infarction; VHD: valvular heart disease)

Source: Adapted from Mishra S, Mohan JC, Nair T, et al. Consensus Document Management protocols for chronic heart failure in India. Indian Heart J. 2018;70:105-27.

with HFrEF, died within 5 years of diagnosis. Since then, adherence to clinical practice guideline (CPG)-based management improved outcome with relative reduction in hospitalization by about 30–50% and smaller but significant decrease in mortality.[8] Both international and Indian data show enormous burden of HF in the community with huge socioeconomic implications.[9,10] The 2012 European Society of Cardiology (ESC) Guideline on diagnosis and treatment of acute and chronic heart failure[10] introduced differential approach on diagnosis of HFrEF and HFpEF based on echocardiographic findings, leaving a gray area in between. Introduction of this approach in guideline is game changer not only because of its prognostic importance (the lower the EF the poorer the survival) but also because it was observed that most clinical trials selected patients based upon lower EF. The major trials in patients with HFrEF mostly enrolled patients with an EF ≤ 35%. Only in these patients, therapeutic benefit have been demonstrated to date.[11,12] There is a group of patients who had LVEF > 50% and yet suffered from clinical HF. Because of this, the term HF with "preserved" EF (HFpEF) was created to describe these patients. Thus, broadly, patients with an EF in the range 35–50% represent a "gray area" and most probably have primarily mild systolic dysfunction. The diagnosis of HFpEF is more difficult than the diagnosis of HFrEF because it is largely one of exclusion, i.e. potential noncardiac causes of the patient's symptoms (such as anemia or chronic lung disease) must first be discounted. This approach has been endorsed by both AHA, ACC and ESC in their latest guidelines.[13,14]

In September 2014, one single study (PARADIGM-HF) seems to have turned entire spectrum of treatment and approach toward HFrEF by its tail. It included HFrEF with LVEF 40–45% of ischemic etiology only. PARADIGM-HF not only changed the approach to treatment of HFrEF but also the way treatment guidelines may be written in future; by all means a *paradigm shift*.[15] Such has been the impact of this paradigm shift that even after more than 4 years, entire discipline of cardiology practice, though accepting it in clinical practice, yet struggling to come in terms with its philosophical content. Under this backdrop, we shall try to deconstruct recent HFrEF treatment guidelines of AHA, ACC, and ESC.[13,14] Emphasis of this review will be on treatment and its implications, though issues relating to investigation will be touched upon.

"...though the world does not change with a change of paradigm, the scientist afterward works in a different world. Nevertheless,"

—Thomas S Kuhn, The Structure of Scientific Revolutions

METHODOLOGY OF GUIDELINES REVIEW

In a seminal article published in 2009, Christiane Muth et al. conceived a method of systematic guidelines review of CPG involving method, rationale, and tests on chronic heart failure (Box 1).[16]

With some refinements, the basic structure remains valid till this date. Elaborating further on 2013 AHA/ACC guidelines frame, in 2014, ACC/AHA Task Force Statement "The Evolution and Future of ACC/AHA Clinical Practice Guidelines: A 30-Year Journey" was published.[17] The Task Force evaluated data from ADHERE (Acute Decompensated Heart Failure National Registry) and demonstrate that patients in HFrEF treated on line with Class I recommendations, according to heart failure performance indicators have a significant reduction in in-hospital mortality and length of stay.[18] The Class of Recommendation (COR—Class I, IIa, IIb) is a statement of the strength of the recommendation and continues to serve as the primary guide for clinicians. The choice of the COR involve consideration of an estimate of the

BOX 1: Structure of creation of guidelines.

- Assessment of quality of guidelines
- Data extraction
- Consistency analysis
- Information synthesis
- Validation
- Draft guideline
- Formal consensus
- Guideline review
- Authorization of new guideline

size and strength of the effect of the intervention (diagnostic test or therapeutic strategy, medication, device, procedure, or other intervention) and the magnitude of benefit in relation to risk. The level of evidence (LOE—Level A, B-R, B-NR, C) describes the certainty or precision of the information supporting the recommendation based on the type and quality of the evidence. COR-I and LOE-A recommendations are considered strong recommendations. COR-III is generally considered harmful and is not considered in this review.

For LOE, ESC guideline is limited to A, B and C whereas AHA/ACC guidelines have subclasses B-R, B-NR, L-LD, and C-EO. Authors of this review consider that such intricate subdivisions are of limited clinical use.

In 2012, a survey comprising 206 cardiologists who sat in different guidelines committees of ACC/AHA revealed some interesting results for evaluation of CPG in treatment of HFrEF (Table 2).

TABLE 2: 2012 Guidelines survey—summary of results and implications.

- COR and LOE (Class IIa and IIb and LOE C): More than two-thirds of cardiologists indicated that the weaker class/levels were helpful or very helpful when making informed diagnostic and therapeutic decisions. It indicates that clinicians seek guidance on important topics even in situations where the evidence base is weak. It also suggests that focusing CPGs only on strong evidence is not adequate for clinicians to deliver comprehensive best practices. These observations highlight the tension between the value of a comprehensive CPG and a more restricted CPG limited to a few recommendations informed by a strong scientific evidence base.
- More than 90% of cardiologists found the ACC/AHA CPGs routinely useful in clinical practice. In fact, > 80% of cardiologists apply CPGs in managing patients in most circumstances. The CPG features found most useful are clinical applicability and authority, brevity and clarity, comprehensiveness, ease of access and use, and currency.

(ACC/AHA: American College of Cardiology/American Heart Association; COR: class of recommendation; CPG: clinical practice guideline; LOE: level of evidence)

REVIEW OF AHA, ACC, AND ESC GUIDELINES ON HFrEF

ESC Guideline 2016[14]

Principal Changes from the 2012

- *Emphasis on new terminology of HF*: LVEF from 40% to 49%—"HF with midrange EF (HFmrEF)".
  Objective: Stimulate research into the underlying characteristics, pathophysiology, and treatment of this population.
- Clear recommendations on the diagnostic criteria for HFrEF, HFmrEF, and HFpEF.
  Objective: Standardization of diagnosis and treatment.
- A new algorithm for the diagnosis of chronic HF based on the evaluation of HF probability.
  Objective: Standardization of diagnosis criteria on basis of latest development.
- Recommendations aimed at prevention.
  Objective: Delay of the development of overt HF and prevention of death before the onset of symptoms.
- Indications for the use of the new compound sacubitril/valsartan, the first in the class of angiotensin receptor neprilysin inhibitors (ARNIs).
  Objective: Therapeutic translation of PARADIGM-HF study.
- Modified indications for cardiac resynchronization therapy (CRT).
  Objective: Interventions in selected cases of refractory HFrEF.
- Incorporation of concept of an early initiation "time to therapy" approach.
  Objective: Early treatment of chronic HF for reduction of mortality and morbidity, an approach as already well-established in acute coronary syndrome (ACS).
- Inclusion of hypertension.
  Objective: Further improvement of treatment outcome.
- A new algorithm for a combined diagnosis and treatment approach of acute HF.
  Objective: Further improvement on treatment outcome by evidence-based medical practice.

AHA/ACC Focused Updated Guidelines 2017[10]

Principal Changes from 2013

- Recommendations reflect the new 2015 COR/ LOE system, in which LOE B and C are subcategorized for the purpose of increased clarity.
  - *Objective*: To streamline available investigation and treatment choices based on evidence-based medicine.
- Update in areas in which new evidence has emerged since 2013:
  - Revision to the sections on biomarkers.
  - New therapies indicated for stage C HF with reduced ejection fraction (HFrEF).
  - Updates on HF with preserved ejection fraction (HFpEF).
  - New data on important comorbidities, including sleep apnea, anemia, and hypertension, and new insights into the prevention of HF.

- Guidance on new therapies:
  - Angiotensin receptor neprilysin inhibitor (valsartan/sacubitril)
  - Sinoatrial node modulator (ivabradine).
- Adoption of a "knowledge byte" format. This approach is to accommodate time constraints of clinicians and supports the evolution of guidelines as "living documents" that can be dynamically updated as needed.

In general, it is a policy of AHA/ACC to either issue a new Guideline or a Focused Update on the existing one on every 6 years based on recent developments.

ACC/AHA Heart Failure Classification

- *Stage A*: Patients at risk for heart failure who have not yet developed structural heart changes (i.e. those with diabetes, those with coronary disease without prior infarct)
- *Stage B*: Patients with structural heart disease (i.e. reduced ejection fraction, left ventricular hypertrophy, chamber enlargement) who have not yet developed symptoms of heart failure
- *Stage C*: Patients who have developed clinical heart failure
- *Stage D*: Patients with refractory heart failure requiring advanced intervention (i.e. biventricular pacemakers, left ventricular assist device, transplantation).

ESC Heart Failure Classification

HFrEF: Stage 1: Signs ± symptoms
Stage 2: LVEF < 40%.

HFmrEF: Stage 1: Signs ± symptoms
Stage 2: LVEF 40–49%.
Stage 3: a. Elevation of natriuretic peptides (NPs)
b. At least one additional criteria
i. Relevant structural heart disease
ii. Diastolic dysfunction

HFpEF: Stage 1: Signs ± symptoms
Stage 2: LVEF ≥ 50%
Stage 3: a. Elevation of natriuretic peptides
b. At least one additional criteria
i. Relevant structural heart disease
ii. Diastolic dysfunction

- ACC/AHA Guideline Writing Committee accepts importance of emphasis on HFrEF, HFmrEF and HFpEF and includes them in their 2017 focused update HF Guidelines.
- Unlike AHA/ACC classification, ESC does not include any *subclinical* stage of HF.
- The ESC HF classification does not have a class corresponding to Stage A of AHA/ACC classification.
- Stage B of AHA/ACC classification does not correspond to any ESC HF class.
- Stage C of AHA/ACC HF somehow fit in all stages of ESC HF classification.
- Patients refractory to medical treatment in HFrEF group of ESC may correspond to Stage D of AHA/ACC classification.
- Both ESC and AHA/ACC/HFSA (Heart Failure Society of America) follow identical COR and LOE criteria. However, two stage Focused Updates (2016 and 2017) on HF Guidelines of AHA/ACC/HFSA appears more comprehensive, though a little complex.

DIAGNOSIS OF HEART FAILURE WITH REDUCED EJECTION FRACTION

Table 3 describes biomarkers used in diagnosis of HFrEF.

- The use of NPs is recommended for ruling-out HF, but not to establish the diagnosis.
- Emphasis on Natriuretic Biomarkers in ESC 2016 is lower than in AHA/ACC guidelines 2017 (IIaC as opposed to IA) as specificity for HFrEF is low.
- European Society of Cardiology guidelines on HF recommend NP testing ahead of echocardiography in their diagnosis algorithm. This can be hardly justified in Indian condition.[9]
- Recommendations for utility of biomarkers in ambulatory and stable HFrEF are not very strong (ESC 2016 and AHA/ACC 2013) (Table 4).
- Transthoracic echocardiogram (TTE) is recommended to establish a diagnosis of HFrEF, HFmrEF, or HFpEF and to identify patients with HF who would be suitable for pharmacological and device [implantable cardioverter-defibrillator (ICD), cardiac resynchronization therapy

TABLE 3: Biomarkers in HFrEF in AHA/ACC and ESC guidelines.

Investigation	*COR*	*LOE*	*Guidelines*	*Remarks*
Natriuretic biomarkers (NP)	I	A	AHA/ACC 2017	In patients presenting with HFrEF, measurement of natriuretic peptide biomarkers is useful to support a diagnosis or exclusion of HF. They also have implications in predicting prognosis and prevention.
	IIa	C	ESC 2016	Diagnostic values apply similarly to HFrEF and HFpEF; on average, values are lower for HFpEF than for HFrEF.

(ACC/AHA: American College of Cardiology/American Heart Association; COR: class of recommendation; CPG: clinical practice guideline; ESC: European Society of Cardiology; HFpEF: heart failure with preserved ejection fraction; HFrEF: heart failure with reduced ejection fraction; LOE: level of evidence)

TABLE 4: Recommendations for cardiac imaging in patients with HFrEF.

Investigation	COR	LOE	Guidelines	Remarks
TTE	I	A	ESC 2016 AHA/ACC 2017	Same recommendations
CMR	I-II1	C	ESC 2016 AHA/ ACC 2017	Same recommendations
Non-invasive stress Imaging	IIb	B	ESC 2016 AHA/ACC 2017	Same recommendations
Invasive CAG	IIc	C	ESC 2016 AHA/ACC 2017	Same recommendations
Cardiac CT	IIb	C	ESC 2016 AHA/ACC 2017	Same recommendations

(ACC/AHA: American College of Cardiology/American Heart Association; CAG: coronary angiogram; CMR: cardiovascular magnetic resonance imaging; COR: class of recommendation; CT: computed tomography; ESC: European Society of Cardiology; LOE: level of evidence; TTE: transthoracic echocardiogram)

(CRT)] for treatment of HFrEF. TTE is recommended for the assessment of myocardial structure and function in subjects to be exposed to treatment which potentially can damage myocardium (e.g. chemotherapy). Doppler velocities and deformation indices, i.e. strain and strain rate should be considered in a TTE protocol.

- Cardiac magnetic resonance (CMR) imaging is recommended for the assessment of myocardial structure and function (including right heart) especially in subjects with poor acoustic window for TTE. CMR should be considered in patients with dilated cardiomyopathy in order to distinguish between ischemic and nonischemic myocardial damage by characterization of myocardial tissue.
- The CMR, cardiac CT, single photon emission computed tomography (SPECT), positron emission tomography (PET) may be considered for the assessment of myocardial ischemia and myocardial viability in patients with HFrEF and *coronary artery disease* (CAD) for coronary revascularization.
- Invasive coronary angiography should be considered in patients with HFrEF and intermediate to high pretest probability of CAD and the presence of ischemia but viable myocardium in noninvasive stress tests.

PREVENTION OF HEART FAILURE WITH REDUCED EJECTION FRACTION

Recommendation for prevention of HFrEF are given in Table 5.

- SPRINT (Systolic Blood Pressure Intervention Trial) study demonstrated that treating hypertension to a lower goal [systolic blood pressure (SBP) < 120 mm Hg versus > 140 mm Hg] in older hypertensive subjects (≥ 75 years of age) or high-risk hypertensive patients reduces the risk of cardiovascular disease, death, and hospitalization for HF.
- The AHA/ACC maintains that clinical trials evaluating goal blood pressure reduction and optimal blood pressure-lowering agents in the setting of HFrEF and concomitant hypertension have not been done. However, those patients at higher risk, blood pressure lowering is associated with fewer adverse cardiovascular events. Guideline-directed medical therapy (GDMT)

TABLE 5: Recommendations for prevention or delaying HFrEF.

Recommendations	COR	LOE	Guidelines	Remarks
Hypertension	I I	A C	ESC 2016 AHA/ACC 2017	New inclusion over 2013 guidelines New inclusion over 2013 guidelines
Statins	I I	A A	ESC 2016 AHA/ACC 2017	New inclusion over 2013 guidelines Same as in 2013
SGLT2 inhibitor	IIa	B	ESC 2016 AHA/ACC 2017	New inclusion over 2013 guidelines No recommendation
ACEI	I	A	ESC 2016 AHA/ACC 2017	Same as in 2013 Same as in 2013
Beta-blockers	I I	B B	ESC 2016 AHA/ACC 2017	Same as in 2013 Same as in 2013
Anemia	IIb	B-R	ESC 2016 AHA/ACC 2017	New inclusion over 2013 guidelines New inclusion over 2013 guidelines

(ACC/AHA: American College of Cardiology/American Heart Association; ACEI: angiotensin-converting-enzyme inhibitor; COR: class of recommendation; ESC: *European Society of Cardiology;* HFrEF: heart failure with reduced ejection fraction; LOE: level of evidence; SGLT2: sodium-glucose cotransporter-2) with agents known to lower blood pressure not yet proven by randomized controlled trials (RCTs) in a population with HFrEF.

- Angiotensin II receptor blockers (ARBs) have not been consistently proven to reduce mortality in patients with HFrEF and their use should be restricted to patients intolerant of an angiotensin-converting-enzyme inhibitor (ACEI) or those who take an ACEI but are unable to tolerate.
- Although smoking cessation has not been shown to reduce the risk of developing HF, the epidemiological associations with the development of cardiovascular disease suggest that such advice, if followed, would be beneficial.
- The association between alcohol intake and the risk of developing de novo HF is U-shaped, with the lowest risk with modest alcohol consumption (up to 7 drinks/week).
- An inverse relationship between physical activity and the risk of HF has been reported. A recent meta-analysis found that doses of physical activity in excess of the guideline recommended minimal levels may be required for more substantial reductions in HF risk.
- Neither aspirin nor other antiplatelet agents, nor revascularization, have been shown to reduce the risk of developing HF or mortality in patients with stable CAD. Obesity is also a risk factor for HF, but the impact of treatments of obesity on the development of HF is unknown.
- Studies examining correction of iron deficiency in HFrEF have demonstrated improvement in surrogate endpoints, such as quality of life, NT-proBNP, and LVEF; however, controlled trials have been underpowered to detect reductions in hard clinical endpoints. The FAIR-HF (Ferric Carboxymaltose Assessment in Patients With Iron Deficiency and Chronic Heart Failure) trial demonstrated improvements in NYHA class and functional capacity over a short term exposure. The CONFIRM-HF (Ferric Carboxymaltose Evaluation on Performance in Patients With Iron Deficiency in Combination with Chronic Heart Failure) trial demonstrated improvements in 6-minute walk test. However, a strong recommendation for oral iron repletion or intravenous iron repletion must await the results of an appropriately powered trial on morbidity and mortality.

SLEEP DISORDER AND BREATHING RECOMMENDATIONS FOR HEART FAILURE WITH REDUCED EJECTION FRACTION (TABLE 6)

- ESC as opposed to AHA/ACC does not recommend continuous positive airway pressure (CPAP) in HFrEF, though it has been shown to reduce the frequency of episodes of apnea and hypopnea, and improve LVEF and 6-minute walk test distance. However, improvement in prognosis or the rate of HF related hospitalizations appears limited.
- In a guarded statement, ESC guideline conclude that nocturnal oxygen supplementation, CPAP, bi-level positive airway pressure (BiPAP), and adaptive servo-ventilation (ASV) may be considered to treat nocturnal hypoxemia in obstructive sleep apnea as recommended in other guidelines.

TREATMENT RECOMMENDATIONS

Refer to Table 7 for treatment recommendations.

- No change (IA) in recommendations on ACEI and ARB on either guideline in AHA/ACC guidelines of 2013 and 2017, respectively.
- ESC 2016 Guideline place ARBs in IB and IIbC as they have not been consistently proven to reduce mortality in

TABLE 6: Sleep disorder and breathing recommendations for HFrEF.

Recommendations	*COR*	*LOE*	*Guidelines*	*Remarks*
In patients with NYHA class II–IV HF and suspicion of sleep-disordered breathing or excessive daytime sleepiness, a formal sleep assessment is reasonable.	IIa	C-LD	AHA/ACC 2017	New inclusion: Recommended
In patients with cardiovascular disease and obstructive sleep apnea, CPAP may be reasonable to improve sleep quality and daytime sleepiness	IIb	B-R	AHA/ACC 2017	New inclusion: Recommended
Adaptive servo-ventilation is not recommended in patients with HFrEF and a predominant central sleep apnea because of an increased all-cause and cardiovascular mortality	III	B	ESC 2016	New inclusion: Not recommended

(ACC/AHA: American College of Cardiology/American Heart Association; CPAP: continuous positive airway pressure; ESC: European Society of Cardiology; HF: heart failure; HFrEF: heart failure with reduced ejection fraction; LOE: level of evidence; NYHA: New York Heart Association)

TABLE 7: Treatment recommendations for HFrEF with ACEI, ARB and ARNI.

COR	LOE	Guidelines	Treatment	Remarks
I	A	AHA/ACC 2017	ACEI	The use of ACE inhibitors is beneficial for patients with prior or current symptoms of chronic HFr EF to reduce morbidity and mortality.
		ESC 2016	ACEI	Same as in AHA/ACC 2016 with addition comment on usefulness of a beta-blocker, for symptomatic patients with HFrEF to reduce the risk of HF hospitalization and death.
I	A	AHA/ACC 2016	ARB	The use of ARBs to reduce morbidity and mortality in patients with prior or current symptoms of chronic HFrEF who are intolerant to ACE inhibitors because of cough or angioedema.
I	B	ESC 2016	ARB	An ARB reduce the risk of HF hospitalization and cardiovascular death in symptomatic HFrEF patients unable to tolerate an ACEI (patients should also receive a beta-blocker and an MRA)
IIb	C	ESC 2016	ARB	An ARB may be considered to reduce the risk of HF hospitalization and death in patients who are symptomatic despite treatment with a beta-blocker who are unable to tolerate an MRA.
I	BR	AHA/ACC 2017	ARNI	In patients with chronic symptomatic HFrEF NYHA class II or III who tolerate an ACE inhibitor or ARB, replacement by an ARNI is recommended to further reduce morbidity and mortality.
I	B	ESC 2016	ARNI	Sacubitril/valsartan is recommended as a replacement for an ACEI to further reduce the risk of HF hospitalization and death in ambulatory patients with HFrEF who remain symptomatic despite optimal treatment with an ACEI, a beta-blocker and an MRA.

patients with HFrEF and their use should be restricted to patients intolerant of an ACEI or those who take an ACEI but fail to improve despite beta-blocker are unable to tolerate a mineralocorticoid receptor antagonist (MRA).

- Recommendations on ARB in HFrEF in ESC 2016 guidelines are not as convincing as that in AHA/ACC 2017 guidelines.
- Though ARNI is placed in same category of recommendations on both guidelines (on a marginally different nomenclature—I-BR of AHA/ACC and I-B of ESC), ESC guidelines place important caveat of failed treatment with ACEI + beta-blocker + MRA; whereas AHA/ACC recommend a more sweeping statement of replacement of ACEI/ARB by ARNI even in treatment responders for "further reduction of morbidity and mortality".
- It is interesting to note that though COR and LOE of ARNI is of I-B and I-BR, it is recommended to replace ACEI and ARB with IA and IB recommendations even in treatment responders. *This is a paradigm shift in treatment of HFrEF.* The paradigm shift is not only in therapeutic option but also in our approach to COR and LOE.

In the absence of a paradigm ... all of the facts ... seem equally relevant. .. Paradigms gain their status because they are more successful than their competitors in solving ... problems. .. A paradigm [provides] a criterion for choosing problems that ... can be assumed to have solutions. .. Rules ... derive from paradigms, .. but paradigms can guide research even in the absence of rules. .. There is no such thing as research in the absence of any paradigm.

—Thomas S Kuhn, The Structure of Scientific Revolutions

PARADIGM SHIFT WITH ANGIOTENSIN RECEPTOR NEPRILYSIN INHIBITOR IN TREATMENT OF HFrEF

Since 2012, medical treatment of HFrEF has been centered around ARBI. Issue was clinched following a number of clinical trials.[19-24] Paradigm shift with ARNI, especially in AHA/ACC 2017 guidelines was obtained for astonishing statistical significance of PARADIGM-HF (Prospective Comparison of ARNI with ACEI to Determine Impact on Global Mortality and Morbidity in Heart Failure) Trial. As Dr John McMurray, one of the principal investigators, states in a commentary on ARNI "The P-value for the primary endpoint (4×10^{-7}) in PARADIGM-HF is equivalent to having four to five trials each with $p < 0.05$ (for all-cause mortality, the equivalent number is two to three trials)". It can be emphasized with reasonable confidence that no medical research, across disciplines, has been able to produce such robust statistical power as witnessed in PARADIGM-HF trial. However, critics, with substantial veracity, have indicated at a significant number of issues in the trial, discussions of which are beyond the scope of this review article. Interestingly, though patients included

TABLE 8: Recommendations for ICD and CRT—ESC 2016 and AHA/ACC 2013.

Treatment	*Guideline*	*COR*	*LOE*	*Remarks*
ICD	AHA/ACC 2013	I	A	ICD therapy is recommended for primary prevention of SCD in selected patients with HFrEF at least 40 days post-MI with LVEF ≤ 35% and NYHA class II or III symptoms on chronic GDMT, who are expected to live > 1 year.
	ESC 2016	I	A	Same as above.
CRT	AHA/ACC 2013	I	A	CRT is indicated for patients who have LVEF ≤ 35%, sinus rhythm, LBBB with a QRS ≥ 150 ms, and NYHA class II, III, or ambulatory IV symptoms on GDMT
		IIa	B	CRT can be useful for patients who have LVEF ≤ 35%, sinus rhythm, LBBB with a QRS 120–149 ms, and NYHA class II, III, or ambulatory IV symptoms on GDMT
	ESC 2016	I	A	CRT is recommended for symptomatic patients with HF in sinus rhythm with a QRS duration ≥150 ms and LBBB QRS morphology and with LVEF ≤ 35% despite OMT in order to improve symptoms and reduce morbidity and mortality
		I	B	CRT is recommended for symptomatic patients with HF in sinus rhythm with a QRS duration of 130–149 ms and LBBB QRS morphology and with LVEF ≤ 35% despite OMT in order to improve symptoms and reduce morbidity and mortality

(ACC/AHA: American College of Cardiology/American Heart Association; CRT: cardiac resynchronization therapy; ESC: European Society of Cardiology; GDMT: guideline-directed medical therapy; HFrEF: heart failure with reduced ejection fraction; ICD: implantable cardioverter-defibrillator; LBBB: left bundle branch block; LVEF: left ventricular ejection fraction; MI: myocardial infarction; NYHA: New York Heart Association; OMT: optimal medical therapy; SCD: sudden cardiac death)

in the trial had CAD, in the concluding statement of PARADIGM-HF study and HFrEF guidelines a sweeping recommended use of ARNI in all cases of HFrEF regardless of etiology (Table 8).

- Beta-blockers reduce mortality and morbidity in symptomatic patients with HFrEF, despite treatment with an ACEI, but have not been tested in congested or decompensated patients. Beta-blockers and ACEIs are complementary and can be started together as soon as the diagnosis of HFrEF is made. There is no evidence for initiation of treatment with a beta-blocker before an ACEI has been started. Beta-blockers should be initiated in clinically stable patients at a low dose and gradually up-titrated to the maximum tolerated dose. In patients admitted due to acute HF, beta-blockers should be cautiously initiated in hospital, once the patient is stabilized. Meta-analysis of all the major beta blocker trials in HFrEF has shown no benefit on hospital admissions and mortality in the subgroup of patients with HFrEF who are in atrial fibrillation.
- Diuretics are recommended to reduce the signs and symptoms of congestion in patients with HFrEF, but their effects on reduction of mortality and morbidity has not been proven on RCT. The aim of diuretic therapy is to achieve and maintain euvolemia with the lowest achievable dose.
- Mineralocorticoid receptor antagonists (spironolactone and eplerenone) are recommended in all symptomatic patients (despite treatment with an ACEI and a beta-blocker) with HFrEF and LVEF ≤ 35%, to reduce mortality and HF hospitalization. Caution should be exercised when MRAs are used in patients with impaired renal function and in those with serum potassium levels 5.0 mmol/L.
- Ivabradine is a new therapeutic agent included in guidelines. One RCT demonstrated the efficacy of ivabradine in reducing the composite endpoint of cardiovascular death or HF hospitalization. The benefit of Ivabradine was driven by a reduction in HF hospitalization in HFrEF (LVEF) ≤ 35%, in sinus rhythm with a resting heart rate of ≥ 70 bpm. The target of Ivabradine is heart rate slowing (the presumed benefit of action).
- There is no clear evidence to suggest the use of this fixed-dose combination therapy or isolated use of hydralazine and nitrates in all patients with HFrEF. However, they may be used where AECI/ARB/ARNI are not well tolerated. Though included in 2013, focused update of AHA/ACC 2017 does not elaborate on use.
- Digoxin may be considered in patients in sinus rhythm with symptomatic HFrEF to reduce the risk of hospitalization (both all-cause and HF hospitalizations), although its effect on top of beta-blockers has never been tested. Recent studies have suggested potentially higher risk of events (mortality and HF hospitalization) in patients with AF receiving digoxin. However, this remains controversial, as another recent meta-analysis concluded on the basis of non-RCTs that digoxin has no deleterious effect on mortality in patients with AF and concomitant HF, most of whom had HFrEF. Though included in 2013, focused update of AHA/ACC 2017 does not elaborate on use.
- N-3 polyunsaturated fatty acid (N-3 PUFA) preparations containing 850–882 mg of eicosapentaenoic acid (EPA) and docosahexaenoic acid (DHA) as ethyl esters in the

average ratio of 1:1.2 may be considered as an adjunctive therapy in patients with symptomatic HFrEF who are already receiving optimized recommended therapy with an ACEI/ARB/ARNI, a beta-blocker, and an MRA. Though included in 2013, focused update of AHA/ACC 2017 does not elaborate on use (Table 8).

- The use of ICDs for primary prevention in patients with HFrEF should be considered only in the setting of optimal GDMT and with a minimum of 3–6 months of appropriate medical therapy.
- Since publication of the 2009 HF guideline, new evidence supports extension of CRT to patients with milder symptoms. Benefit appears confined largely to patients with a QRS duration of at least 150 ms and LBBB pattern.

Recommendations for other issues in HFrEF, e.g. comorbidities and multidisciplinary approaches, are same in both guidelines.

CONCLUSION

Clinicians always struggle to get the core substance out of the voluminous guideline materials. Even the executive summaries comprise of many pages. It is practically impossible for a busy clinician to remember intricate recommendations based on very subtle differences. To overcome this difficulty, Focus update of AHA/ACC 2017 Guidelines has developed App based program for convenient reference in clinical practice.

REFERENCES

1. Guidelines for the evaluation and management of heart failure. Report of the American College of Cardiology/American Heart Association Task Force on Practice Guidelines (Committee on Evaluation and Management of Heart Failure). Circulation. 1995;92:2764-84.
2. Feder G, Eccles M, Grol R, et al. Using clinical guidelines. BMJ. 1999;318:728-30.
3. Shekelle P, Eccles MP, Grimshaw JM, et al. When should clinical guidelines be updated? BMJ. 2001;323:155-7.
4. Council of Europe. [Developing a methodology for drawing up guidelines on best medical practices. (Recommendation (2001)13 and explanatory memorandum)]. Z Arztl Fortbild Qualitatssich. 2002;96 Suppl 3:5-59.
5. Fishberg AM. Heart failure. Philadelphia, PA: Lea and Febiger; 1937.
6. Brutsaert DL, Sys SU, Gillebert TC. Diastolic failure: pathophysiology and therapeutic implications. J Am Coll Cardiol. 1993;22(4):1272.
7. Chatterjee K, Massie B. Systolic and diastolic heart failure: differences and similarities. J Cardiac Fail. 2007;13:569-76.
8. Ponikowski P, Anker SD, AlHabib P, et al. Heart failure: preventing disease and death worldwide. ESC Heart Fail. 2014;1:4-25.
9. Mishra S, Mohan JC, Nair T, et al. Consensus document management protocols for chronic heart failure in India. Indian Heart J 2018;70:105-27.
10. McMurray JJ, Adamopoulos S, Anker SD, et al. ESC Committee for Practice Guidelines. ESC guidelines for the diagnosis and treatment of acute and chronic heart failure 2012: the Task Force for the Diagnosis and Treatment of Acute and Chronic Heart Failure 2012 of the European Society of Cardiology. Eur Heart J. 2012;33:1787-847.
11. Borlaug BA, Paulus WJ. Heart failure with preserved ejection fraction: pathophysiology, diagnosis, and treatment. Eur Heart J. 2011;32:670-79.
12. Paulus WJ, Tschope C, Sanderson JE, et al. How to diagnose diastolic heart failure: a consensus statement on the diagnosis of heart failure with normal left ventricular ejection fraction by the Heart Failure and Echocardiography Associations of the European Society of Cardiology. Eur Heart J. 2007;28:2539-50.
13. Yancy CY, Jessup M, Bozkurt B, et al. 2017 ACC/AHA/HFSA Focused Update of the 2013 ACCF/AHA Guideline for the Management of Heart Failure A Report of the American College of Cardiology/American Heart Association Task Force on Clinical Practice Guidelines and the Heart Failure Society of America. . Circulation. 2017;136:e137-61.
14. Ponikowski P, Voors AA, Anker SD, et al. 2016 ESC guidelines for the diagnosis and treatment of acute and chronic heart failure. The Task Force for the diagnosis and treatment of acute and chronic heart failure of the European Society of Cardiology (ESC). Eur Heart J. 2016;37:2129-200.
15. McMurray JV, Packer M, Desai AS, et al. Angiotensin–neprilysin inhibition versus enalapril in heart failure. N Engl J Med. 2014;371:11.
16. Muth C, Gensichen J, Beyer M, et al. The Systematic Guideline Review: Method, Rationale, and Test on Chronic Heart Failure. BMC Health Services Research 2009;9:74.
17. Jacobs AK, Anderson JL, Halperin JL. The Evolution and Future of ACC/AHA Clinical Practice Guidelines: A 30-Year Journey. J Am Coll Cardiol. 2014;64:13.
18. Fonarow GC. The Acute Decompensated Heart Failure National Registry (ADHERE): opportunities to improve care of patients hospitalized with acute decompensated heart failure. Rev Cardiovasc Med. 2003;4 (Suppl 7): S21-30.
19. The CONSENSUS Trial Study Group. Effects of enalapril on mortality in severe congestive heart failure. Results of the Cooperative North Scandinavian Enalapril Survival Study (CONSENSUS). N Engl J Med. 1987;316:1429-35.
20. The SOLVD Investigators. Effect of enalapril on survival in patients with reduced left ventricular ejection fractions and congestive heart failure. N Engl J Med. 1991;325:293-302.

21. Packer M, Poole-Wilson PA, Armstrong PW, et al. Comparative effects of low and high doses of the angiotensin-converting enzyme inhibitor, lisinopril, on morbidity and mortality in chronic heart failure. ATLAS Study Group. Circulation. 1999;100:2312-8.
22. Pfeffer MA, Moyé LA, Davis BR, et al. Effect of captopril on mortality and morbidity in patients with left ventricular dysfunction after myocardial infarction: results of the Survival and Ventricular Enlargement Trial. The SAVE Investigators. N Engl J Med. 1992;327:669-77.
23. The Acute Infarction Ramipril Efficacy (AIRE) Study Investigators. Effect of ramipril on mortality and morbidity of survivors of acute myocardial infarction with clinical evidence of heart failure. Lancet. 1993;342:821-8.
24. Kober L, Torp-Pedersen C, Carlsen JE, et al. A clinical trial of the angiotensin-converting-enzyme inhibitor trandolapril in patients with left ventricular dysfunction after myocardial infarction. Trandolapril Cardiac Evaluation (TRACE) Study Group. N Engl J Med. 1995;333:1670-6.

CHAPTER

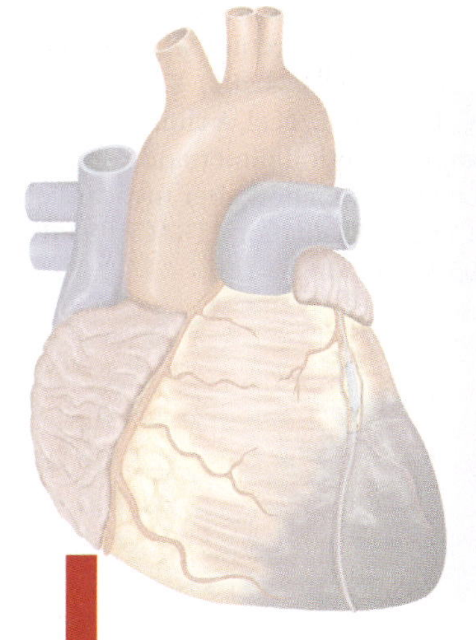

New Innovations in Systolic Assessment of Heart Failure

Samuel Kim, Bicky Vettichira, Smadar Kort

INTRODUCTION

Left ventricular ejection fraction (LVEF) has strong clinical implications that includes, but not limited to, diagnosis, conferring prognosis, and determining treatment regimen. While there is no gold standard for assessing left ventricular systolic function, cardiac magnetic resonance imaging (CMRI) is considered the reference standard while echocardiography is more frequently used due its portability, cost-effectiveness, and lack of ionizing radiation exposure. Current guidelines by the American Society of Echocardiography and the European Association of Cardiovascular Imaging recommend the use of three-dimensional echocardiography (3DE) if image quality is adequate, otherwise apply modified Simpson model for two-dimensional echocardiography (2DE) for the assessment of LVEF.[1]

CONTENTS AND DESCRIPTION

Two-dimensional Echocardiography

The modified Simpson method is based upon the idea that the mitral valve and papillary muscles trisect the left ventricle (LV). Its volume is calculated by the summation of discs derived from the visualization and tracing of the LV endocardial border during both end-diastole and end-systole. This method require some geometric assumptions regarding the LV chamber geometry in order to allow for the differences in biplane measurements derived at each point (end-diastole and end-systole) to in turn represent change in volume.[2] This therefore results in significant limitations in patients with abnormally shaped ventricle, such as the presence of an aneurysm, and is inaccurate in assessing LVEF or absolute LV volumes in patients with localized LV wall motion abnormalities.[3]

As manual tracing of the endocardial border is inconsistent and requires additional time, the practice of subjective visual assessment of ejection fraction (EF) has continued.[4] The challenges of EF evaluation and its clinical importance have led to renewed interest in image processing algorithms. While previously technical limitations have prevented its use in clinical practice, advancements in the field has shown promising results.[5,6] Recent improvements in automated boundary detections with newer algorithms and the addition of artificial intelligence in tracking techniques have demonstrated that fully automated assessment is able to accurately measure LV volume and EF within seconds.[4]

The introduction of contrast echocardiography further improved the evaluation of LV function and regional wall motion abnormalities, as well as in the assessment of myocardial perfusion.[7-9] Present day contrast contains microbubbles filled with high-molecular-weight gas that oscillates to the changes in acoustic pressure created by the transducer.[8,9] When coupled with harmonic imaging, it enhances the visualization of the LV cavity and endocardial border that is comparable to CMRI.[10] Current guidelines recommend contrast 2D echocardiography when two or more contiguous segments are poorly visualized and should be considered, irrespective of image quality, when clinical management is dependent on accurate LVEF measurement.[9] Such examples include in the evaluation for intracardiac defibrillator (ICD) or cardiac resynchronization therapy (CRT), and in the serial measurements for cardiotoxic effects of chemotherapy. Contrast echocardiography also can be used for the evaluation of intracardiac masses, identification of apical abnormalities, and currently is the only bedside method to evaluate for myocardial rupture. While contrast has been demonstrated in 2D echocardiography, there are limited studies regarding its use in 3D echocardiography and thus no official recommendations have been made thus far.[8,9]

Three-dimensional Echocardiography

The 3DE was introduced with the development of matrix transducers and allowed for the entire LV cavity to be visualized. It minimized the necessity for geometric assumptions[6] and have consistently demonstrated its superiority in measuring volume and EF and with higher test-retest variability as compared to 2DE.[3,11,12] With continued advancement in technology, such as the introduction of real-time 3D echocardiography (RT3DE), 3DE is becoming feasible for everyday clinical practice.[13]

While full-volume multi-beat 3DE provides the highest quality images for optimal assessment, certain patient factors (i.e. irregular cardiac rhythm, inability to adequately hold breath) do create challenges. As datasets are obtained over several beats, artifacts caused by breathing changes alter the endocardial border and are observed as various LV segments contracting at different times.[2] This has led to further investigation to minimize duration of imaging with results of two-beat modality demonstrating comparable accuracy in LV volume and EF measurements.[14] In addition, several studies have reported 3DE's underestimation of LV volume[11] and believed secondary to its inability to precisely differentiate between myocardial and trabecular tissue and based on imaging modality.[15] One potential solution to address this is the use of automated correction or the use of contrast agents to improve the endocardial border recognition.[6] Recently, a novel automated algorithm for the calculation of left ventricular volume, left atrial volumes, and the LVEF in 3DE was assessed with reports of good correlation when compared to manual measurements and CMRI.[16] The newest automated software provides greater simplicity with excellent reproducibility by automatically undergoing analysis once the 3DE dataset is loaded with similar results to CMRI with exception of slight underestimation of LV end-diastolic volume.[16]

In addition, evaluation of LV mass with 3DE was superior to that of 2DE as was demonstration by 3DE reconstruction that was validated in humans undergoing heart transplantation. 3DE was shown to have threefold lower test-retest variability as compared to 2DE and thus more significant for serial monitoring.[6] In addition to the LV chamber, 3DE also allows for improved visualization of various cardiac structures and its dynamic motions.[3] Several studies found 3DE provides accurate and reproducible evaluation of the right ventricle (RV) volume and EF that was difficult for 2DE to capture in one image due to the complex crescent shape of the RV as well as its location causing suboptimal image quality.[6,12]

SPECKLE TRACKING FOR STRAIN MEASUREMENT

The myocardial fibers in the heart are organized into a helical structure with the cardiac apex being relatively fixed. As the heart contracts during systole, the fibers shorten longitudinally and thicken transversely due to the heart's incompressible nature. This results in the approach of the basal LV to the apex, with the overall shape changing due to the movement of different segments at various velocities.[17] However, as contraction of the apical portion naturally pulls the ventricular base downward, motion can be detected due to displacement of segments even of those that are completely passive segments.[18] Deformation analysis allows for the differentiation between active and passive myocardial tissue movement and thus the ability to detect wall motion abnormalities.[19]

Strain refers to the myocardial fiber's ability to shorten or thicken relative to its baseline length, and the proportional change occurring within a specified time frame is referred as strain rate. These two terminologies characterize deformation and are used to describe the relative velocity differences of various segments over a period of time resulting in the overall shape to change.[17] Myocardial deformation imaging was first made possible with tissue Doppler, but recent advancements have allowed it to become possible with speckle-tracking using echocardiography. Speckles are natural acoustic markers that are statically distributed throughout the myocardium. It is then tracked to reflect the myocardial tissue's motion pattern and used to calculate the myocardial wall strain and strain rate.[19] The advantage of this imaging modality is that it is angle independent as it tracks along the direction of wall, and not along the ultrasound beam, with good reproducibility. It does, however, require high resolution image quality at high frame rate. It is important to note that while different tracking algorithms result in different measurements, 2D-strain echo correlated well when compared with tagged magnetic resonance imaging, the current gold standard for deformation analysis.[20]

Echocardiographic strain and strain-rate imaging allows for more accurate evaluation of myocardial function. Its clinical application is extensive due to its ability to differentiate between active and passive movements of myocardial segments. Strain and strain rate measurements are sensitive indicators in the detection and assessment of early myocardial involvement in asymptomatic patients with systemic disease (e.g. sarcoidosis, systemic sclerosis, amyloidosis, and Duchenne muscular dystrophy). Global longitudinal strain has also been demonstrated to be a stronger predictor factor compared to EF in patients with heart failure.[21] Speckle-tracking has been used to differentiate physiological hypertrophy (such as that seen in athletes) from asymptomatic nonobstructive hypertrophic cardiomyopathy as well as hypertensive cardiac hypertrophy.[19] It is a useful management tool in heart transplant recipients allowing for noninvasive monitoring for acute allograft rejection, transplant coronary artery disease in asymptomatic patients, and treatment efficacy.[19] 2D-strain was demonstrated to be highly sensitive in the early detection of doxorubicin-induced cardiac injury through the observation of reduced radial strain in combination with detection of associated histologic markers of doxorubicin-induced cardiomyopathy.[22] One of the most important aspects of 2D-strain is the high sensitivity and specificity for diagnosing myocardial infarction, assessing myocardial viability, and efficiency of myocardial revascularization.[19,23] It has also been useful in identifying patients that are more likely to benefit from CRT, as the main predictive factor of responsiveness to therapy is mechanical dyssynchrony (Figs. 1 to 7).[24,25]

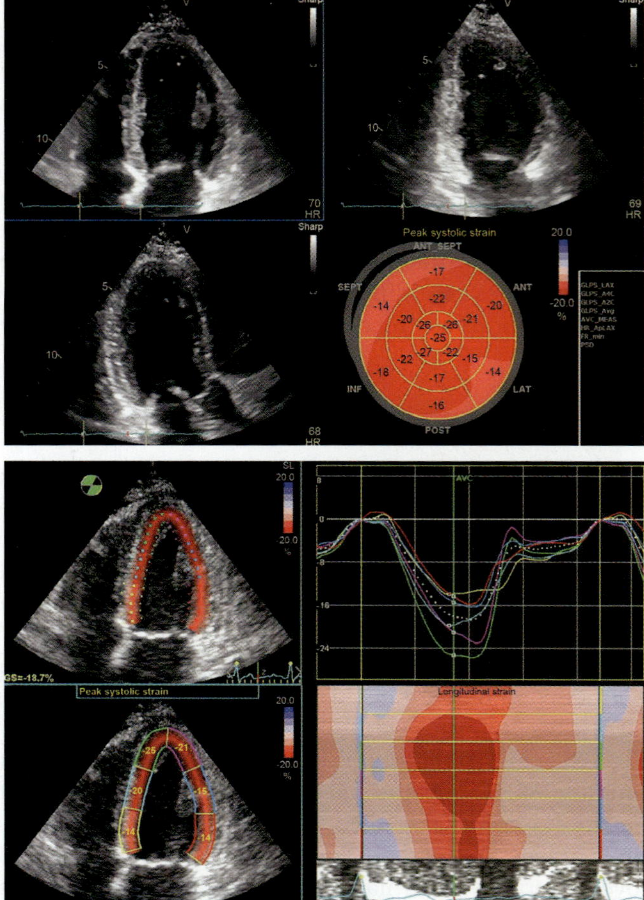

Fig. 1: Normal 2D speckle with normal LVEF.
(2D: two-dimensional; LVEF: left ventricular ejection fraction)

CONCLUSION

The 2D speckle-tracking echocardiography requires the assumption that speckles remain within the scan frame in consecutive frames. But in reality, speckles have complex 3D motions and are subjected to through-plane motion due to the simultaneous apex-to-base and twisting movements throughout the LV cardiac cycle.[19,26] But with the development of 3D echocardiography, 3D and 4D strain measurements have allowed acoustic markers be tracked without any out-of-plane motion and reduced the processing time because the entire LV data set can be collected from only one apical window.[26] The 4D echo has several advantages over 2D echo, as it is less influenced by apical foreshortening and minimizes errors in visual wall motion interpretation as the imaging plan can be corrected at any time after image acquisition. The 4D strain has been shown to be more accurate and reproducible for the assessment of LV volumes, EF, and mass compared to 2D strain, and also has led to newer methods for analyzing regional and systolic function. One such method is global area strain (GAS) which have shown GAS to be strongly correlated with LVEF and with a direct relationship with heart function.[6] The 3D and 4D area strain has been shown to correlate with severity and extent of transmural necrosis in coronary artery disease patients as well.[27] Other applications include amyloidosis, HOCM, diabetic patients, and untreated hypertensive patients where 4D area strain could detect early impairment in systolic function.[28] Current limitations of 4D strain include the technical limitations, lower feasibility due to reliance on good acoustic windows, regular rhythm and patient cooperation, relatively low temporal resolution, and lack of evidence on prognostic value in comparison with 2D strain.[29]

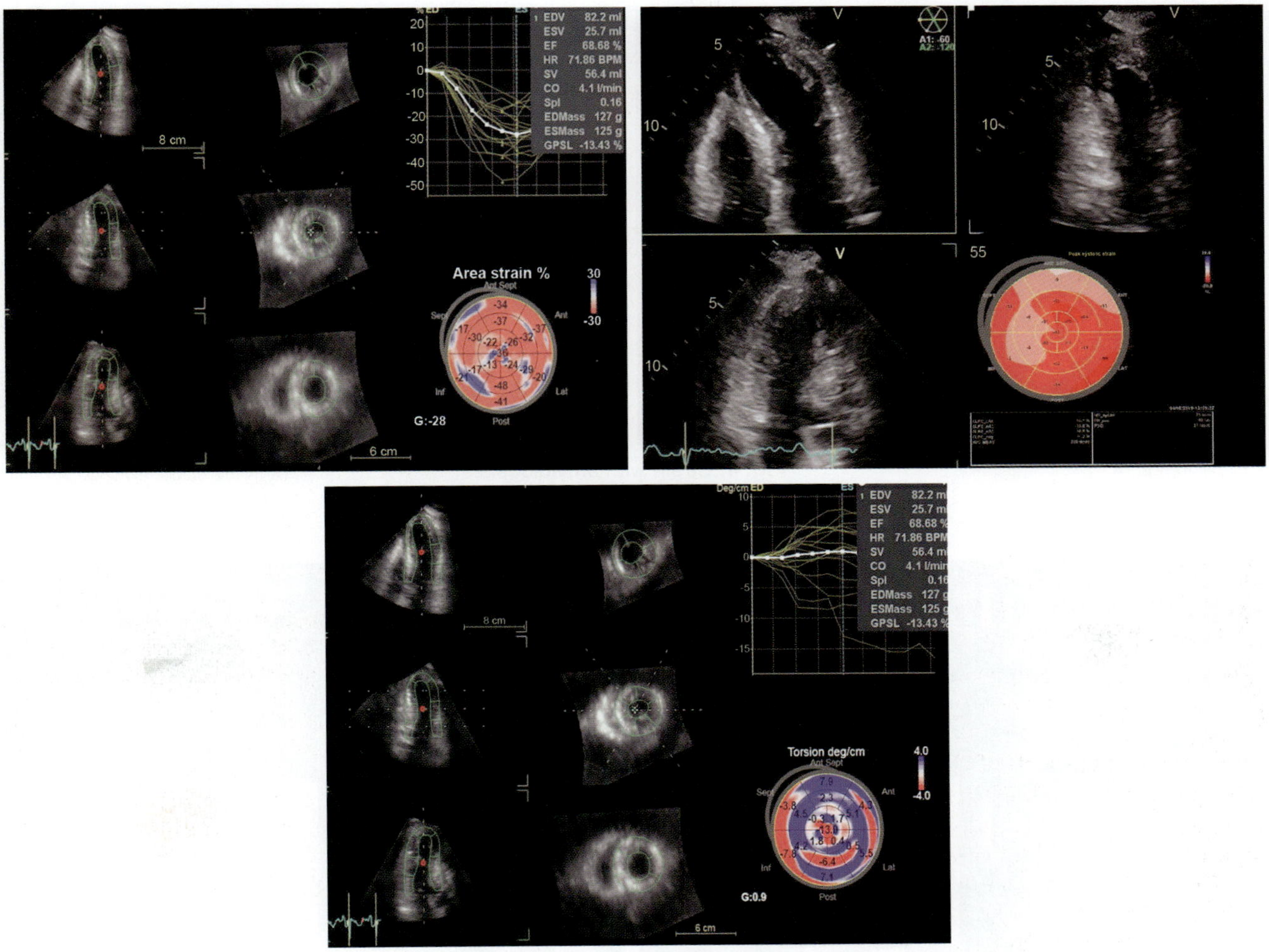

Fig. 2: 3D area strain, triplane strain and 3D torsion.
(3D: three-dimensional)

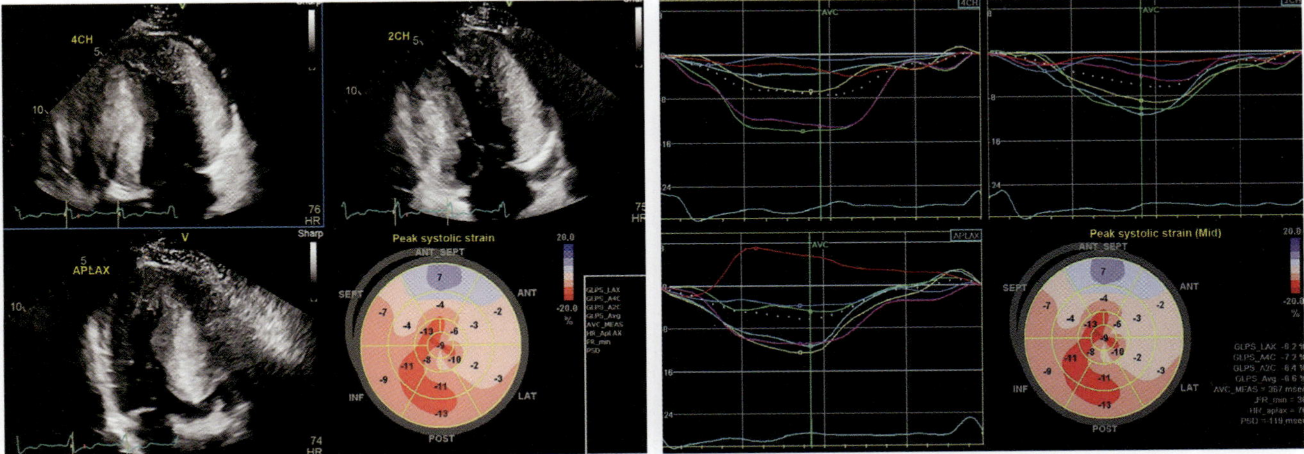

Fig. 3: Strain with HOCM.
(HOCM: hypertrophic obstructive cardiomyopathy)

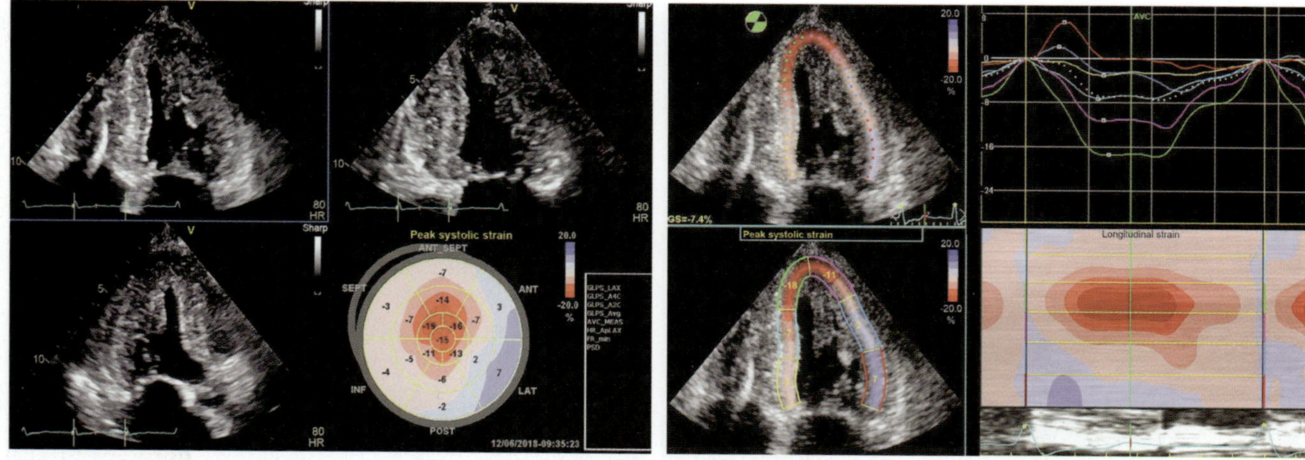

Fig. 4: Strain with amyloidosis.

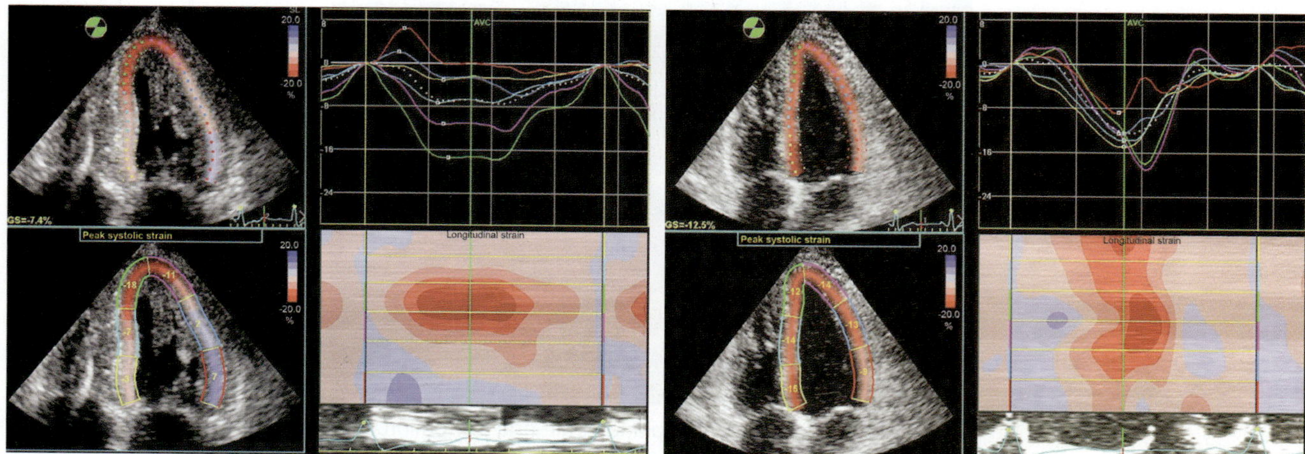

Fig. 5: Abnormal 2D strain with abnormal LVEF.
(2D: two-dimensional; LVEF: left ventricular ejection fraction)

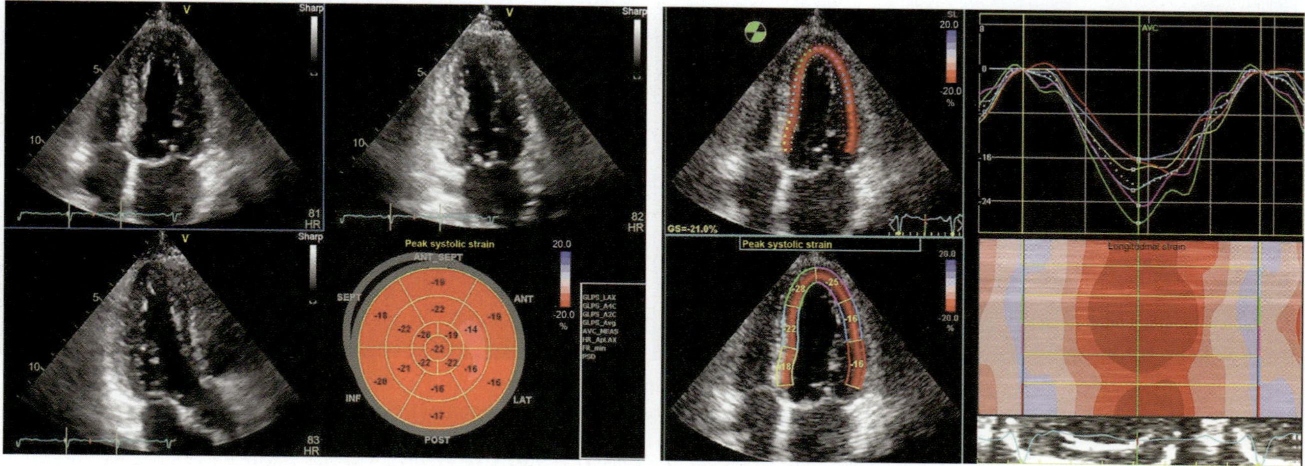

Fig. 6: Strain suggestive of focal sarcoid involvement.

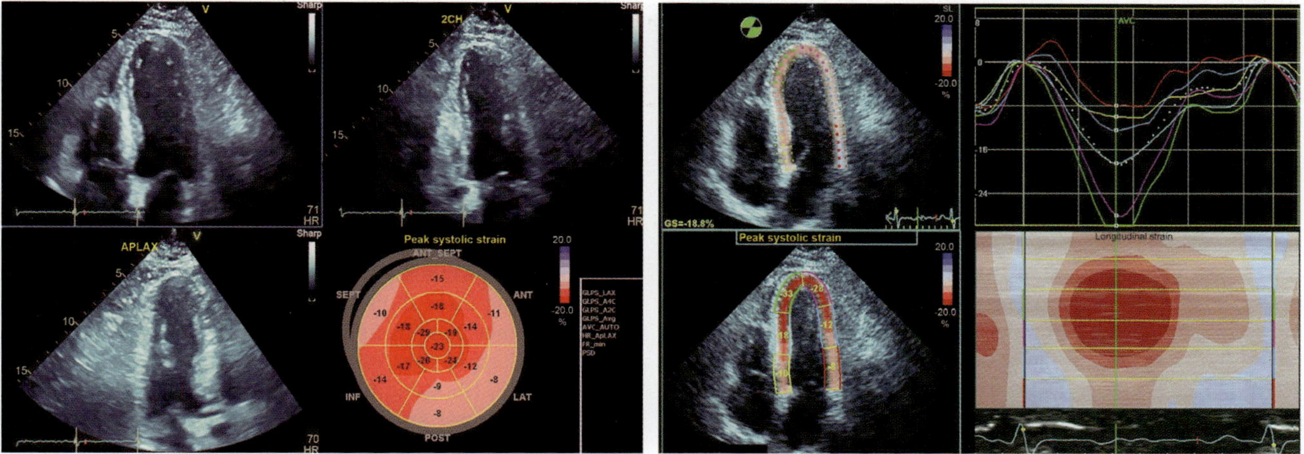

Fig. 7: Aortic stenosis with abnormal strain and preserved LVEF.
(LVEF: left ventricular ejection fraction)

REFERENCES

1. Lang RM, Badano LP, Mor-Avi V, et al. Recommendations for cardiac chamber quantification by echocardiography in adults: An Update from the American Society of Echocardiography and the European Association of Cardiovascular Imaging. J Am Soc Echocardiogr. 2015;28: 1-39.e14.
2. Foley TA, Mankad SV, Anavekar N, et al. Measuring left ventricular ejection fraction—techniques and potential pitfalls. Eur Cardiol. 2012;8(2):108-14.
3. Shiota T. 3D echocardiography: The present and the future. J Cardiol. 2008;52:169-85.
4. Knackstedt C, Bekkers SC, Schummers G, et al. Fully automated versus standard tracking of left ventricular ejection fraction and longitudinal strain: The FAST-EFs Multicenter Study. J Am Coll Cardiol. 2015;66:1456-66.
5. Asch FM, Abraham T, Jankowski M, et al. Accuracy and reproducibility of a novel artificial intelligence deep learning-based algorithm for automated calculation of ejection fraction in echocardiography. J Am Coll Cardiol. 2019;73:1447.
6. Kwon SH, Gopal AS. 3D and 4D Ultrasound: current progress and future perspectives. Current Cardiovascular Imaging Reports. 2017;10:43.
7. Yu EHC, Sloggett CE, Iwanochko RM, et al. Feasibility and accuracy of left ventricular volumes and ejection fraction determination by fundamental, tissue harmonic, and intravenous contrast imaging in difficult-to-image patients. J Am Soc Echocardiogr. 2000;13:216-24.
8. Mulvagh SL, Rakowski H, Vannan MA, et al. American Society of Echocardiography Consensus Statement on the Clinical Applications of Ultrasonic Contrast Agents in Echocardiography. J Am Soc Echocardiogr. 2008;21: 1179-201.
9. Senior R, Becher H, Monaghan M, et al. Clinical practice of contrast echocardiography: recommendation by the European Association of Cardiovascular Imaging (EACVI) 2017. Eur Heart J Cardiovasc Imag. 2017;18:1205-05af.
10. Hoffmann R, von Bardeleben S, Kasprzak JD, et al. Analysis of regional left ventricular function by cineventriculography, cardiac magnetic resonance imaging, and unenhanced and contrast-enhanced echocardiography: a multicenter comparison of methods. J Am Coll Cardiol. 2006;47:121-8.
11. Rigolli M, Anandabaskaran S, Christiansen JP, et al. Bias associated with left ventricular quantification by multimodality imaging: a systematic review and meta-analysis. Open Heart. 2016;3:e000388.
12. Jan MF, Tajik AJ. Modern imaging techniques in cardiomyopathies. Circul Res. 2017;121:874-91.
13. Hare JL, Jenkins C, Nakatani S, et al. Feasibility and clinical decision-making with 3D echocardiography in routine practice. Heart. 2008;94:440-5.
14. Macron L, Lim P, Bensaid A, et al. Single-beat versus multibeat real-time 3D echocardiography for assessing left ventricular volumes and ejection fraction: a comparison study with cardiac magnetic resonance. Circul Cardiovasc Imag. 2010;3:450-5.
15. Mor-Avi V, Jenkins C, Kühl HP, et al. Real-time 3-dimensional echocardiographic quantification of left ventricular volumes: multicenter study for validation with magnetic resonance imaging and investigation of sources of error. JACC: Cardiovasc Imag. 2008;1:413-23.
16. Tsang W, Salgo IS, Medvedofsky D, et al. Transthoracic 3D echocardiographic left heart chamber quantification using an automated adaptive analytics algorithm. JACC: Cardiovasc Imag. 2016;9:769-82.
17. Kurt M, Tanboga IH, Aksakal E. Two-dimensional strain imaging: basic principles and technical consideration. Eurasian J Med. 2014;46:126-30.
18. Stoylen A, Heimdal A, Bjornstad K, Torp HG, Skjaerpe T. Strain rate imaging by ultrasound in the diagnosis of regional dysfunction of the left ventricle. Echocardiography. 1999;16:321-9.

19. Dandel M, Lehmkuhl H, Knosalla C, et al. Strain and strain rate imaging by echocardiography—basic concepts and clinical applicability. Curr Cardiol Rev. 2009;5:133-48.
20. Amundsen BH, Helle-Valle T, Edvardsen T, et al. Noninvasive myocardial strain measurement by speckle tracking echocardiography: validation against sonomicrometry and tagged magnetic resonance imaging. J Am Coll Cardiol. 2006;47:789-93.
21. Marwick TH, Shah SJ, Thomas JD. Myocardial strain in the assessment of patients with heart failure: a review myocardial strain in the assessment of patients with heart failure myocardial strain in the assessment of patients with heart failure. JAMA Cardiology. 2019;4:287-294.
22. Migrino RQ, Aggarwal D, Konorev E, et al. Early detection of doxorubicin cardiomyopathy using two-dimensional strain echocardiography. Ultrasound Med Biol. 2008;34:208-214.
23. Perk G, Tunick PA, Kronzon I. Non-doppler two-dimensional strain imaging by echocardiography—2013; from technical considerations to clinical applications. J Am Soc Echocardiogr. 2007;20:234-43.
24. Gelzer ARM, Koller ML, Otani NF, et al. Dynamic mechanism for initiation of ventricular fibrillation in vivo. Circulation. 2008;118:1123-9.
25. Ammar KA, Paterick TE, Khandheria BK, et al. Myocardial mechanics: understanding and applying three-dimensional speckle tracking echocardiography in clinical practice. Echocardiography. 2012;29:861-72.
26. Muraru D, Niero A, Rodriguez-Zanella H, et al. Three-dimensional speckle-tracking echocardiography: benefits and limitations of integrating myocardial mechanics with three-dimensional imaging. Cardiovasc Diag Ther. 2017;8:101-17.
27. Hayat D, Kloeckner M, Nahum J, et al. Comparison of real-time three-dimensional speckle tracking to magnetic resonance imaging in patients with coronary heart disease. Am J Cardiol. 2012;109:180-6.
28. Abate E, Hoogslag GE, Antoni ML, et al. Value of three-dimensional speckle tracking longitudinal strain for predicting improvement of left ventricular function after acute myocardial infarction. Am J Cardiol. 2012;110(7):961-7.
29. Galderisi M, Esposito R, Schiano-Lomoriello V, et al. Correlates of global area strain in native hypertensive patients: a three-dimensional speckle-tracking echocardiography study. Eur Heart J Cardiovasc Imag. 2012;13(9):730-8.

CHAPTER

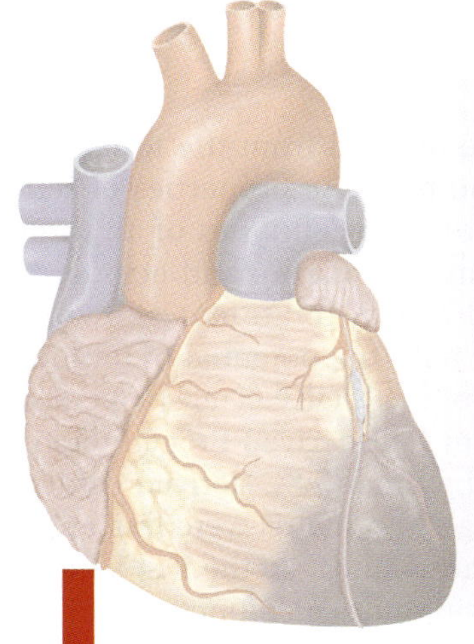

Stem Cells and Gene Therapy in Heart Failure

Sandeep Seth, Karishma Landge, Harshita Singh

INTRODUCTION

There are a number of therapies available for heart failure ranging from drugs like angiotensin-converting enzyme (ACE) inhibitors, beta-blockers, angiotensin receptor neprisyln inhibitors, ivabradine, and left ventricular assist devices (LVADs) and when all else fails there is the option of a heart transplant. Advanced options like heart transplant are limited due to lack of donor hearts and LV assist devices are expensive and out of reach of many.[1] There is, therefore, need for alternative forms of therapy and stem cell and gene therapy have been tried to repair the heart.[2-6] In this article, we will review in brief the various types of stem cell therapy and gene therapy tried in cardiac disorders, the results, the proposed mechanisms, and the future.

Stem cells are cells that have the ability to develop into different cell types. In some cases, they also have the ability to repair damaged tissues. The two broad types of stem cells are embryonic stem cells and adult stem cells. In a developing embryo, stem cells can differentiate into all of the specialized embryonic tissues. In adult organisms, stem cells act as a repair system for the body. Stem cell therapy was first established in the treatment of blood malignancies in the form of a bone marrow transplant. Two decades ago, this was extended to nonblood disorders in an attempt to repair nonblood disorders by using the pluripotent nature of stem cells to repair other organs.

STEM CELL THERAPY AND ITS TYPES

First Generation Cell Therapy

Skeletal Myoblasts

Skeletal myoblasts were the first cells tested in preclinical and clinical trials.[7,8] The advantages include that they have minimum ethical concerns, their expansion in-vitro is quick, resistant to ischemic conditions, and there will be minimal risk of tumorigenicity. Contrarily, disadvantages include that there will be no transdifferentiation into functional cardiomyocytes. Due to lack of electrochemical coupling, risks of ventricular arrhythmias are high.

After the initial promising preclinical and clinical trials, the large MAGIC trial was conducted and it showed no benefit and a high incidence of arrhythmias. Trials with myoblasts have since diminished.[7]

Bone Marrow-derived Cells

The bone marrow contains a mix of mature and immature cells. Experiments have shown that an injury causes the recruitment of bone marrow-derived cells to the injured/ inflamed area and they can aid in repair.[9-13] After the initial clinical experiments with bone marrow-derived cells, the interest shifted to bone marrow-derived mononuclear cells (MNCs). Trials with MNCs have shown mixed results showing a benefit of improvement in the ventricular function of about 2–5% in some trials[2,14-17] while not showing a benefit in some.[18]

Mesenchymal Stem Cells

Mesenchymal cells are nonhematopoietic stem cells, which are multipotent, and immune privileged. A number of clinical trials have shown a benefit of mesenchymal cells on ventricular function. In the PROCHYMAL [ejection fraction (EF) improved 7.3%] and the POSEIDON (EF improved 5–8%), the improvement was significant.[19-21]

Second Generation Cell Therapy

Cardiac Stem/Progenitor Cells/Propagated Cells

Several cardiac stem cells (CSCs) and cardiac progenitor cells (CPCs), such as cardiosphere-derived cells (CDCs), stem cell antigen (Sca)-1+ cells, and many other types of CSCs have been found. The clinical trials SCIPIO (*Cardiac Stem Cell Infusion in Patients With Ischemic* CardiOmyopathy), CADUCEUS (**CA**rdiosphere-**D**erived a**U**tologous Stem **CE**lls to reverse ventric**U**lar dy**S**function), ALLSTAR (**ALL**ogeneic Heart **ST**em Cells to **A**chieve Myocardial **R**egeneration), and DYNAMIC (**D**ilated cardiom**Y**opathy i**N**tervention with **A**llogeneic **M**yocard**I**ally-regenerative **C**ells) used an intracoronary infusion of propagated cells or autologous c-Kit + CSCs and CDCs grown from endomyocardial biopsy, respectively and showed improvements in regional ventricular function.[22,23]

Embryonic Stem Cells

Embryonic stem cells are derived from the inner cell mass of the blastocyst and have the properties of self-renewal and differentiation into cell types of all three germ layers, i.e. endoderm, mesoderm, and ectoderm. There is a demonstrated risk of teratomas shown in animal experiments. They have the potential of forming cardiomyocytes. In phase one ESCORT (Transplantation of Human Embryonic Stem Cell-derived Progenitors in Severe Heart Failure) trial, human ESC derived cardiac progenitors embedded in a fibrin matrix were implanted in patients with severe heart failure.[24] In the first patient, there was an improvement in ventricular function with no tumor formation or arrhythmia.

Mechanism of Action

A number of mechanisms (Fig. 1) have been proposed and these include direct cardiac differentiation of injected cells into cardiac muscle and the integration into the myocardium. However, this has been seen more in animal experiments and is probably a highly inefficient mechanism. However, data obtained from numerous *in vitro* and *in vivo* studies have shown paracrine signaling is the fundamental

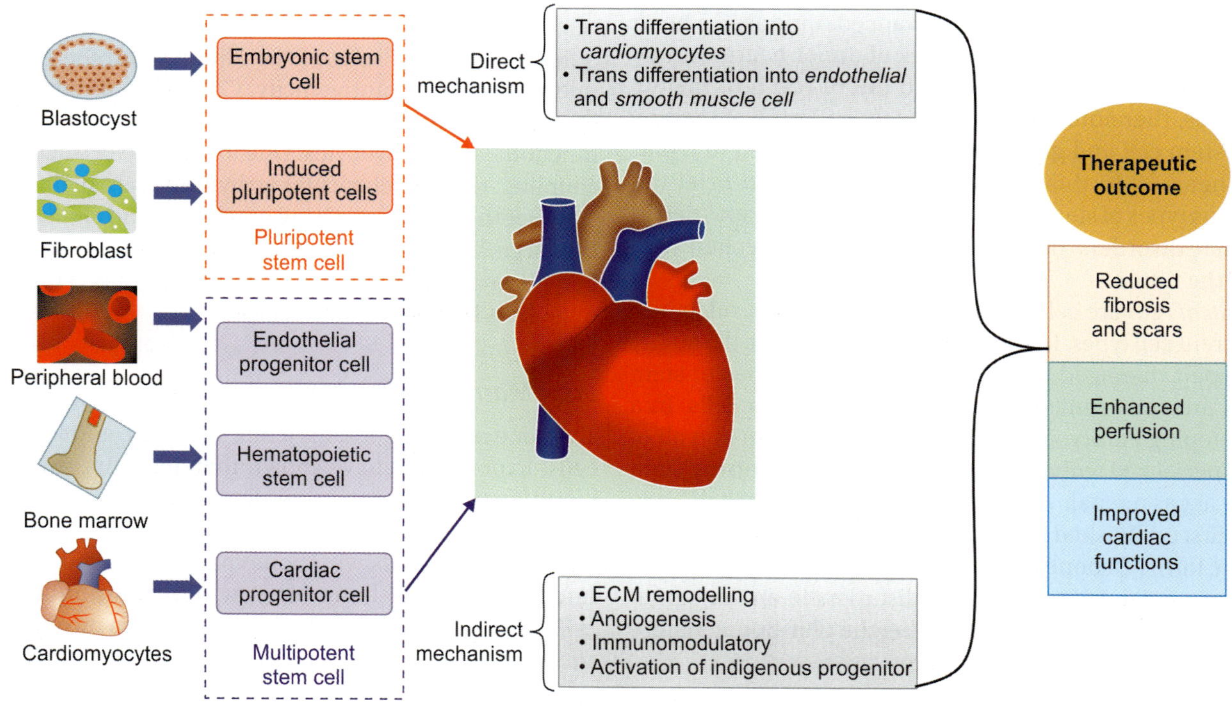

Fig. 1: Mechanism of action.
(ECM: extracellular matrix)

mechanism that mediates the beneficial effects of stem cell therapy.[25] They can have immunomodulatory and effects. They can also recruit resident CSCs.

IMPROVING STEM CELL THERAPY

Attempts are being made to improve the homing ability of the stem cells and the proangiogenic properties by incubating the stem cells with growth factors and cytokines.[26] Stem cells can also be modified to overexpress cytokines by transducing with a lentivirus construct.[27] Using machine learning, responders to stem cell therapy can be picked up based on clinical and biochemical markers leading toward personalized stem cell therapy.[28] Primarily to repair cardiocytes efficiently with the help of SCs, two considerable to formulate "next generation" is (1) genetic engineering modifications and (2) nongenetic modification.[29]

The interest in Stem Cell in India started to work that started in AIIMS (*All India Institute of Medical Sciences*), Delhi by Prof P Venugopal. This was a series of studies which was started in patients undergoing coronary artery bypass surgery who had a scar and had a nonviable myocardium which received a stem cell injection during the bypass surgery. This area showed improvement on subsequent evaluation on Echocardiograms and PET scan.[30] This study was followed by a study in patients with dilated cardiomyopathy [The ABCD (Appropriate Blood Pressure Control in Diabetes) trial] in which patients with dilated cardiomyopathy were injected with bone marrow-derived stem cells injected into the coronary arteries. They showed an improvement in ventricular function and quality of life at 3 and 6 months, which was sustained at 3 years.[31,32] The biopsies done in these patients showed that there was a trend toward increased vascularity but no new muscle seen. Subsequent studies done with labeling at AIIMS have shown interesting results with technetium-labeled stem cells showing inconsistent homing to the infarct area, which could be one reason why bone marrow-derived stem cells do not always result in an improvement in cardiac function after an intracoronary injection.[33] An *Indian Council of Medical Research* (ICMR) sponsored study was then done in patients with recent myocardial infarction where the infarct-related artery had not been opened up within 24 hours. The artery was opened between 24 hours and 30 days and then stem cells were injected. There was a significant improvement in ventricular function (article in press).

The ICMR also sponsored a multicentric study in India where stem cells were injected in patients who were successfully treated for myocardial infarction and were then injected with intracoronary stem cells. The study did not result in positive results.[34]

CURRENT STATUS OF STEM CELL THERAPY

The current status of research in stem cell therapy suggests that the therapy could reduce the risk of mortality in chronic ischemic heart disease with heart failure, and that there are no major adverse events associated with it. This benefit has not been shown in acute myocardial infarction These studies still need to be confirmed in larger clinical trials before cell-based treatment for these patients can be developed as standard treatment. The next studies have to focus on better understanding, and improvement of the cell therapies used (e.g. MNCs, circulating progenitor cells, mesenchymal stem cells, embryonal or hematopoietic progenitor cells). Predictors of responders, outcomes need to be carefully assessed and perhaps therapy needs to be tailored to each patient.

TARGETED GENE THERAPIES FOR HEART FAILURE PATIENTS

"Gene therapy" basically is a technology which includes manipulation of genes, small-sized DNA or RNA which are delivered in target cells, tissues, and organs.[35-37] The main goal of gene therapy is to either elevate or lower the level of distinct proteins at the cellular level, which indirectly cure or modify diseases which are incurable through pharmacological means.[38] Improvements in myocardial angiogenesis have been seen in the preclinical studies in which either vascular endothelial growth factors (VEGF) or fibroblast growth factors (FGF) level alterations were seen to improve myocardial contractility and bring down vulnerability to arrhythmia.[39-47]

Gene Delivery through Vectors

Vectors are specific molecular vehicles, which carry the gene. They are highly specific and are capable of releasing one or more genes efficiently into a stem cell, which are usually not identified by the immune system. Most importantly, a vector should be competent enough in the continuous expression of the gene throughout the life.[48,49] In the past few decades, a new flood of clinical trials has shown us how to select vectors and targeting relevant cells.[50] In late 1960, National Institute of Health (NIH) came to a conclusion that the discouraging results were due to deficient knowledge of vectors, cells, and tissues of interest, as well as pathology of diseases.[51] Vectors are gene delivery vehicles, which come under two categories: Viral and nonviral gene delivery vectors. Many viral vectors are derived from retroviruses, sendai virus, and adenoassociated virus (AAV) which have reached now at clinical trials. The most common reason for using viruses as a vector is that they are excellent nanostructured particles which invade and integrate into the genome of cells. The main target cell type in gene therapy is divided into two groups—gene therapies which include manipulating germline cells and gene therapy which manipulates somatic cell.[52,53]

Types of Vectors

An Introduction to Nonviral Vectors

Gene delivery methods of nonviral vectors include the transfer of gene using solely naked DNA or conjugated with liposomes.[54,55] Expression of recombinant genes in the myocardium in vivo after direct injection of DNA. A nonviral naked DNA vector is uncomplicated, enclosing circular DNA that at least contains a promoter which operates gene of interest and a region of polyadenylation.[56] The biggest disadvantage of using naked DNA is that they are inefficacious, as after transfection only few target cells express new incorporated gene.[57]

An Introduction to Viral Vectors

In cardiovascular diseases, viral vectors (Table 1) are most commonly used as the gene delivery agent, as they are specific and efficient as compared to nonviral vectors. In addition to this, their transmission efficiency into the cardiomyocytes is much higher than that of other "nonviral vectors". Frequently used viral vectors encompass retroviruses, adenoviruses (ADs), lentiviruses, and AAVs. Retroviruses have been a poor choice in the treatment of cardiac applications because they need an active dividing cell for their proper functioning and integration into the genome of the cell. The most commonly used viral vectors for cardiac applications are Lentiviruses as they do not require active cell division. But the major drawback with lentiviral includes they are unable to produce an adequate concentration of viruses for transmission by coronary perfusion. ADs and AAVs are capable of infecting nondividing cells. Both have reasonable transmission efficiency. But AAVs have much longer transmission efficiency as they do not trigger an immune response as compared to AD, which has much more ability in triggering immune responses.[58] A considerable limitation of AAVs is that they insert small size of the gene from 4.5 kb up to 5 kb and also they need helper virus or other miscellaneous methods for its amplification.[59] A major drawback of gene therapy is an immune response. Especially with ADs, toxicity is due to severe inflammation and sometimes organ failures are also reported.[60]

The major characteristics of HF involve numerous defects in Ca^{2+} related proteins, which basically help in excitation-contraction. Some of the therapies that targets Ca^{2+} which have a promising results are shown further in text.

TREATMENT OF HEART FAILURE: A NOVEL APPROACH

Some important genes like sarcoendoplasmic reticulum-ATPase 2a (SERCA2a), SDF-1 (stromal cell-derived factor-1), and adenylate cyclase (AC6) are the one in which clinical trials are completed (Table 2) or still going on.

TABLE 1: Characteristics of potential viral vectors.[61]

Features	*Retroviral*	*Lentiviral*	*Adenoviral*	*AAV*
Cell division required for the target cell	Yes	G1 phase	No	No
Viral genome	RNA	RNA	DNA	DNA
Packaging limitation	8 kb	8 kb	8–30 kb	5 kb
Immune response to vector	Few	Few	Extensive	Few
Duration of transgene expression	Long	Long	Transient	Long in postmitotic cells
Integration in the genome	Yes	Yes	Poor	Poor
Long-term expression	Yes	Yes	No	Yes
Adverse effects	Insertional mutagenesis	Insertional mutagenesis	Inflammatory response	Mild inflammatory response
Main advantages	Constant gene transfer in a dividing cell	Continuous gene transfer in transduced tissue	Favorably effective in transducing tissues	Elicits few inflammatory responses

(AAV: adenoassociated virus)

TABLE 2: Targets of gene therapy in heart failure.[62-73]

Molecular target	*Stage in development*	*Findings*	*Model organism*
SERCA2a	Clinical trial phase 2	Decreased HF symptom, increased functional status, and reversal of negative LV modeling	Human
SDF1	Clinical trial phase ½	Safe and improved 6-minute walk test, quality of life, and NHYA class	Human
ADCY6	Preclinical	Increased LV function, increased cAMP levels, reversal of dysfunctional, and increased survival Improved LV contractility	Mice Pig
BARKct-carboxy terminal peptide from GRK1	Preclinical	Increased reuptake SR Ca^{2+}, lowered Ca^{2+} leak, enhanced cardiac function, and reversed LV remodeling	Rat cardiomyocytes
PVALB	Preclinical	Increased rate of Ca^{2+} removal and improved relaxation rate	Rat

(ADCY6: adenylate cyclase type-6; BARKct: β-adrenergic receptor kinase C-terminal peptide; cAMP: cyclic adenosine monophosphate; HF: heart failure; LV: left ventricle; NYHA: New York Heart Association; SDF1: stromal-derived growth factor-1; SERCA2a: sarcoendoplasmic reticulum calcium ATPase 2a; SR: sarcoplasmic reticulum; PVALB: parvalbumin)

Clinical Programs of SERCA2a Gene

There were three clinical trials which began with AAV1 targeting SERCA2a , by percutaneous administration of gene therapy: CUPID (Calcium Upregulation by Percutaneous Administration of Gene Therapy in Cardiac Disease), AGENT-HF (AAV1-CMV-Serca2a GENe Therapy Trial in Heart Failure), and SERCA-LVAD (SERCA2a Gene Transfer in Patients With Chronic Heart Failure). In the CUPID trial first, a human study was done to study the clinical impression in the re-establishing expression of SERCA2a. The vector SERCA2a was AAV1, which was directly administered in a single intracoronary infusion.

Sarcoplasmic/endoplasmic reticulum calcium ATPase 2a (SERCA2a) was the target in the CUPID trial. Promising results were observed in the CUPID 1 trial, but the results of the CUPID 2 trial were negative.[74] The initial CUPID trial met a 6-month composite endpoint. In the CUPID-2 study, 243 subjects received either placebo or AAV1.SERCA2a. AAV1. SERCA2a administration, was safe, but failed to meet the primary or secondary endpoints.

During myocardial infarction, the expression of SDF-1 has been thought to act as a cellular signal to attract potentially beneficial stem cells to repair, and possibly regenerate, damaged myocardium via. In a phase I study, patients with ischemic cardiomyopathy received SDF-1 endomyocardial injection. The patients were followed for 12 months and patients receiving the highest doses were found to have an improvement in their clinical status including quality of life, 6-minute walk test, and New York Heart Association (NYHA) class.[75] The STOP-HF (Stromal Cell-Derived Factor-1 Plasmid Treatment for Patients with Heart Failure) used plasmid endocardial injection of stromal cell-derived factor-1 to promote stem-cell recruitment. In a trial of patients with ischemic etiology heart failure, the primary endpoints failed, but subgroup analyzes showed improvements in subjects with the lowest EFs.

The AC6 is part of β-adrenergic signaling, playing a role in converting adenosine triphosphate (ATP) to cyclic adenosine monophosphate (cAMP). In HF, activity of AC6 is decreased. Hammond et al. reported the results of a phase 2 clinical trial using adenovirus 5 encoding human AC6 (Ad5.hAC6).23AC6 gene transfer in patients with HF and demonstrated it to be safe and associated with increases in EF, however, the improvement in cardiac function was transient, as increase in EF was shown to fall off at 12 weeks.[76]

CONCLUSION

Both stem cell and gene therapy may be effective in only some subgroups of patients. It is necessary to develop methods to select the most suitable patients for each clinical intervention. Various products (types of stem cells and gene therapy) and endpoints (e.g. survival, exercise tolerance, biomarkers, recurrent HF hospitalizations) have been used in previous clinical trials. There is a clear need to develop validated therapeutic products and endpoints in future clinical trials.

REFERENCES

1. Mozaffarian D, Benjamin EJ, Go AS, et al. Heart disease and stroke statistics—2015 update: a report from the American Heart Association. Circulation. 2015;131(4):e29-322.
2. Jeevanantham V, Butler M, Saad A, et al. Adult bone marrow cell therapy improves survival and induces long-term

improvement in cardiac parameters: a systematic review and meta-analysis. Circulation. 2012;126:551-68.
3. Fisher Sa, Doree C,Mathur A, et al. Meta-analysis of cell therapy trials for patients with heart failure. Circ Res. 2015;116:1361-77.
4. Gyöngyösi M, Wojakowski W, Lemarchand P, et al. Meta-Analysis of Cell-based Cardiac studies (ACCRUE) in patients with acute myocardial infarction based on individual patient data. Circ Res. 2015;116:1346-60.
5. Delewi R, Hirsch A, Tijssen JG, et al. Impact of intracoronary bone marrow cell therapy on left ventricular function in the setting of ST-segment elevation myocardial infarction: a collaborative meta-analysis. Eur Heart J. 2014;35:989-98.
6. Wollert KC, Drexler H. Cell therapy for the treatment of coronary heart disease: a critical appraisal. Nature Reviews Cardiology. 2010;7:204-15.
7. Menasche P, Alfieri O, Janssens S, et al. The Myoblast Autologous Grafting in Ischemic Cardiomyopathy (MAGIC) trial: first randomized placebo-controlled study of myoblast transplantation. Circulation. 2008;117:1189-200.
8. Choudhury T, Mozid A, Hamshere S, et al. An exploratory randomized control study of combination cytokine and adult autologous bone marrow progenitor cell administration in patients with ischaemic cardiomyopathy: the REGENERATE-IHD clinical trial. Eur J Heart Fail. 2017;19:138-47.
9. Schachinger V, Erbs S, Elsasser A, et.al. Intracoronary bone marrow-derived progenitor cells in acute myocardial infarction. N Engl J Med. 2006;355:1210-21.
10. Wollert KC, Meyer GP, Lotz J, et.al. Intracoronary autologous bone-marrow cell transfer after myocardial infarction: The BOOST randomised controlled clinical trial. Lancet. 2004;364:141-8.
11. Huikuri HV, Kervinen K, Niemela M, et al. Effects of intracoronary injection of mononuclear bone marrow cells on left ventricular function, arrhythmia risk profile, and restenosis after thrombolytic therapy of acute myocardial infarction. Eur Heart J. 2008;29:2723-32.
12. Assmus B, Walter DH, Seeger FH, et.al. Effect of shock wave-facilitated intracoronary cell therapy on LVEF in patients with chronic heart failure: the CELLWAVE randomized clinical trial. JAMA. 2013;309:1622-31.
13. Malliaras K, Marban E. Cardiac cell therapy: where we've been, where we are, and where we should be headed. Br Med Bull. 2011;98:161-85.
14. Sadat K, Ather S, Aljaroudi W, et al. The effect of bone marrow mononuclear stem cell therapy on left ventricular function and myocardial perfusion. J Nucl Cardiol. 2014;21:351-67.
15. Wen Y, Chen B, Wang C, et al. Bone marrow-derived mononuclear cell therapy for patients with ischemic heart disease and ischemic heart failure. Expert Opin Biol Ther. 2012;12:1563-73.
16. Ye Z, Zhang BL, Zhao XX, et al. Intracoronary infusion of bone marrow-derived mononuclear cells contributes to longstanding improvements of left ventricular performance and remodelling after acute myocardial infarction: a meta-analysis. Heart Lung Circ. 2012;21:725-33.
17. Jong R de, Houtgraaf JH, Samiei S, et al. Intracoronary stem cell infusion after acute myocardial infarction: a meta-analysis and update on clinical trials. Circ Cardiovasc Interv. 2014;7:156-67.
18. Traverse JH, Henry TD, Moye' LA. Is the measurement of left ventricular ejection fraction the proper end point for cell therapy trials? An analysis of the effect of bone marrow mononuclear stem cell administration on left ventricular ejection fraction after ST-segment elevation myocardial infarction when evaluated by cardiac magnetic resonance imaging. Am Heart J. 2011;162:671-7.
19. Chen SL, Fang WW, Ye F, et al. Effect on left ventricular function of intracoronary transplantation of autologous bone marrow mesenchymal stem cell in patients with acute myocardial infarction. Am J Cardiol. 2004;94:92-5.
20. Lee JW, Lee SH, Youn YJ, et al. A randomized, open-label, multicenter trial for the safety and efficacy of adult mesenchymal stem cells after acute myocardial infarction. J Korean Med Sci. 2014;29:23-31.
21. Mathiasen AB, Qayyum AA, Jorgensen E, et al. Bone marrow-derived mesenchymal stromal cell treatment in patients with severe ischaemic heart failure: A randomized placebo-controlled trial (MSC-HF trial). Eur Heart J. 2015;36:1744-53.
22. Chugh AR, Beache GM, Loughran JH, et al. Administration of cardiac stem cells in patients with ischemic cardiomyopathy: The SCIPIO trial: surgical aspects and interim analysis of myocardial function and viability by magnetic resonance. Circulation. 2012;126:S54-64.
23. Makkar RR, Smith RR, Cheng K, et al. Intracoronary cardiosphere derived cells for heart regeneration after myocardial infarction (CADUCEUS): A prospective, randomised phase 1 trial. Lancet. 2012;379:895-904.
24. Menasché P, Vanneaux V, Fabreguettes JR, et al. Towards a clinical use of human embryonic stem cell-derived cardiac progenitors: a translational experience. Eur Heart J. 2015;36:743-50.
25. Gallina C, Turinetto V, Giachino C. A new paradigm in cardiac regeneration: the mesenchymal stem cell secretome. Stem Cells Int. 2015;2015:765846.
26. Pasha Z, Wang Y, Sheikh R, et al. Preconditioning enhances cell survival and differentiation of stem cells during transplantation in infarcted myocardium. Cardiovasc Res. 2008;77:134-42.
27. Tilokee EL, Latham N, Jackson R, et al. Paracrine engineering of human explant-derived cardiac stem cells to over-express stromal cell derived factor 1α enhances myocardial repair. Stem Cells. 2016;34:1826-35.
28. Steinhoff G, Nesteruk J, Wolfien M, et al. Cardiac function improvement and bone marrow response -: outcome analysis of the randomized PERFECT phase iii clinical trial of intramyocardial CD133(+) application after myocardial infarction. EBioMedicine. 2017;22:208-24.
29. Balram A, Talwar S, Choudhary SK, et al. Application of stem cell technology for coronary artery disease at the All India Institute of Medical Sciences. Heart Surg Forum. 2007;10(2):1-4.

30. Seth S, Narang R, Bhargava B, et al. Percutaneous intracoronary cellular cardiomyoplasty for nonischemic cardiomyopathy: clinical and histopathological results: the first-in-man ABCD (Autologous Bone Marrow Cells in Dilated Cardiomyopathy) trial. J Am Coll Cardiol. 2006;48:2350-1.
31. Seth S, Bhargava B, Narang R, et al. AIIMS Stem Cell Study Group. The ABCD (Autologous Bone Marrow Cells in Dilated Cardiomyopathy) trial a long-term follow-up study. J Am Coll Cardiol. 2010;55(15):1643-4.
32. Patel CD, Agarwal S, Seth S, et al. Detection of homing in of stem cells labeled with technetium-99m hexamethylpropyleneamine oxime in infarcted myocardium after intracoronary injection. Indian J Nucl Med. 2014;29(4):276-7.
33. Nair V, Madan H, Sofat S, et al. Efficacy of stem cell in improvement of left ventricular function in acute myocardial infarction - MI3 Trial. Indian J Med Res. 2015;142:165-74.
34. Friedmann T, Roblin R. Gene therapy for human genetic disease? Science. 1972;175:949-55.
35. Kullo IJ, Ding K. Mechanisms of disease: the genetic basis of coronary heart disease. Nat Clin Pract Cardiovasc Med. 2007;4:558-69.
36. Anguela XM, High KA. Entering the modern era of gene therapy. Ann Rev Med. 2019;70:273-88.
37. Donahue JK, Heldman AW, Fraser H, et al. Focal modification of electrical conduction in the heart by viral gene transfer. Nat Med. 2000;6:1395-8.
38. Hajjar RJ, Schmidt U, Matsui T, et al. Modulation of ventricular function through gene transfer in vivo. Proc Natl Acad Sci USA. 1998;95:5251-6.
39. Takeshita S, Zheng LP, Brogi E, et al. Therapeutic angiogenesis. A single intraarterial bolus of vascular endothelial growth factor augments revascularization in a rabbit ischemic hind limb model. J Clin Invest. 1994;93:662-70.
40. Harada K, Grossman W, Friedman M, et al. Basic fibroblast growth factor improves myocardial function in chronically ischemic porcine hearts. J Clin Invest. 1994;94:623-30.
41. Greener ID, Sasano T, Wan X, et al. Connexin43 gene transfer reduces ventricular tachycardia susceptibility after myocardial infarction. J Am Coll Cardiol. 2012;60:1103-10
42. Sundararaman S, Miller TJ, Pastore JM, et al. Plasmid-based transient human stromal cell-derived factor-1 gene transfer improves cardiac function in chronic heart failure. Gene Ther. 2011;18:867-73.
43. Igarashi T, Finet JE, Takeuchi A, et al. Connexin gene transfer preserves conduction velocity and prevents atrial fibrillation. Circulation. 2012;125:216-25.
44. Sasano T, McDonald AD, Kikuchi K, et al. Molecular ablation of ventricular tachycardia after myocardial infarction. Nat Med. 2006;12:1256-8.
45. Lau DH, Clausen C, Sosunov EA, et al. Epicardial border zone overexpression of skeletal muscle sodium channel SkM1 normalizes activation, preserves conduction, and suppresses ventricular arrhythmia: an in silico, in vivo, in vitro study. Circulation. 2009;119:19-27.
46. Misra S. Human gene therapy: a brief overview of the genetic revolution. J Assoc Physicians India. 2013;61(2):127-33.
47. Gardlík R, Pálffy R, Hodosy J, et al. Vectors and delivery systems in gene therapy. Med Sci Monit. 2005;11(4): RA110-21.
48. Lyon AR, Sato M, Hajjar RJ, et. al Gene therapy: targeting the myocardium. Heart. 2008:94:89-99.
49. Orkin SH, Motulsky AG. Report and recommendations of the panel to assess the NIH investment in research on gene therapy. Report to the NIH Director. 1995. Available from https://osp.od.nih.gov › uploads › 2014/11 › Orkin_Motulsky_Report [Last accessed November, 2019].
50. Mathews QL, Curiel DT. Gene therapy: human germline genetics modifications assessing the scientific, socioethical, and religious issues. South Med J. 2007;100(1):98-100.
51. Bank A. Human somatic cell gene therapy. Bioessays. 1996;18(12):999-1007.
52. Lin H, Parmacek MS, Morle G, et al. Circulation. 1990;82(6):2217-21.
53. Nabel EG, Plautz G, Nabel GJ. Site-specific gene expression in vivo by direct gene transfer into the arterial wall. Science. 1990;249(4974):1285-8.
54. Prazeres DM, Ferreira GN, Monteiro GA, et al. Large-scale production of pharmaceutical-grade plasmid DNA for gene therapy: problems and bottlenecks. Trends Biotechnol. 1999;17(4):169-74.
55. Nabel EG, Plautz G, Nabel GJ. Site-specific gene expression in vivo by direct gene transfer into the arterial wall. Science. 1990;249(4974):1285-8.
56. Flotte TR, Afione SA, Conrad C, et al. Stable in vivo expression of the cystic fibrosis transmembrane conductance regulator with an adeno-associated virus vector. Proc Natl Acad Sci USA. 1993;90(22):10613-7.
57. Dong JY, Fan PD, Frizzell RA. Quantitative analysis of the packaging capacity of recombinant adeno-associated virus. Hum Gene Ther. 1996;7(17):2101-12.
58. Muruve DA. The innate immune response to adenovirus vectors. Hum Gene Ther. 2004;15(12):1157-66.
59. Simmen RC, Pabona JM, Velarde MC, et al. The emerging role of Kruppel-like factors in endocrine-responsive cancers of female reproductive tissues. J Endocrinol. 2010;204:223-31.
60. Jessup M, Greenberg B, Mancini D, et al. Calcium Upregulation by Percutaneous Administration of Gene Therapy in Cardiac Disease (CUPID): a phase 2 trial of intracoronary gene therapy of sarcoplasmic reticulum ca2+-ATPase in patients with advanced heart failure. Circulation. 2011;124:304-13.
61. Penn MS, Mendelsohn FO, Schaer GL, et al. An open-label dose escalation study to evaluate the safety of administration of nonviral stromal cell-derived factor-1 plasmid to treat symptomatic ischemic heart failure. Circ Res. 2013;112: 816-25.
62. Rebolledo B, Lai NC, Gao MH, Takahashi T, et al. Adenylylcyclase gene transfer increases function of the failing heart. Hum Gene Ther. 2006;17:1043-8.
63. Roth DM, Gao MH, Lai NC, Drumm J, et al. Cardiac-directed adenylyl cyclase expression improves heart function in murine cardiomyopathy. Circulation. 1999;99:3099-102.

64. Roth DM, Bayat H, Drumm JD, et al. Adenylyl cyclase increases survival in cardiomyopathy. Circulation. 2002;105:1989-94.
65. Takahashi T, Tang T, Lai NC, et al. Increased cardiac adenylyl cyclase expression is associated with increased survival after myocardial infarction. Circulation. 2006;114:388-96.
66. Lai NC, Roth DM, Gao MH, et al. Intracoronary delivery of adenovirus encoding adenylyl cyclase VI increases left ventricular function and Camp-generating capacity. Circulation. 2000;102:2396-401.
67. Shah AS, White DC, Emani S, et al. In vivo ventricular gene delivery of a beta-adrenergic receptor kinase inhibitor to the failing heart reverses cardiac dysfunction. Circulation. 2001;103:1311-6.
68. Williams ML, Hata JA, Schroder J, et. al. Targeted beta-adrenergic receptor kinase (betaARK1) inhibition by gene transfer in failing human hearts. Circulation. 2004;109:1590-3.
69. Most P, Remppis A, Pleger ST, et al. S100a1: a novel inotropic regulator of cardiac performance. Transition from molecular physiology to pathophysiological relevance. Am J Physiol Regul Integr Comp Physiol. 2007;293:R568-R577.
70. Pleger ST, Most P, Boucher M, et al. Stable myocardial-specific AAV6-S100A1 gene therapy results in chronic functional heart failure rescue. Circulation. 2007;115:2506-15.
71. Szatkowski ML, Westfall MV, Gomez CA et. al. In vivo acceleration of heart relaxation performance by parvalbumin gene delivery. J Clin Invest. 2001;107:191-8
72. Jessup M, Greenberg B, Mancini D, et al. Calcium Upregulation by Percutaneous Administration of Gene Therapy in Cardiac Disease (CUPID): a phase 2 trial of intracoronary gene therapy of sarcoplasmic reticulum ca2+-ATPase in patients with advanced heart failure. Circulation. 2011;124:304-13.
73. Jessup M, Greenberg B, Mancini D, et al. Calcium Upregulation by Percutaneous Administration of Gene Therapy in Cardiac Disease (CUPID): a phase 2 trial of intracoronary gene therapy of sarcoplasmic reticulum ca2+-ATPase in patients with advanced heart failure. Circulation. 2011;124:304-13.
74. Hajjar RJ, Hulot JS. Myocardial delivery of SDF1 in patients with ischemic heart disease: safe & promising. Circ Res. 2013;112(5):746-7.
75. Pleger ST, Shan C, Ksienzyk J, et al Cardiac AAV9-S100A1 gene therapy rescues post ischemic heart failure in a preclinical large animal model. Most P Sci Transl Med. 2011;3(92):92ra64.
76. Hammond HK, Penny WF, Traverse JH, et al. Intracoronary gene transfer of adenylyl cyclase 6 in patients with heart failure. J JAMA Cardiol. 2016;1:163-71.

CHAPTER 43

Advances in Drug Therapy in Heart Failure

Rakesh Varma, Gunjan Garg

INTRODUCTION

The very essence of cardiovascular practice is the early detection of heart failure.

—Sir Thomas Lewis, 1933

An estimated 5.1 million Americans have heart failure and this is expected to increase 25% by 2030.[1] Heart failure results in nearly 1 million hospital admissions annually.[2] Heart failure is a clinical syndrome that results from either functional or structural changes in the ventricles, which leads to filling or ejection abnormalities. Heart failure can be classified on the basis of ejection fraction (EF). But, systolic and diastolic dysfunction can coexist in both these groups.

- Heart failure with reduced ejection fraction (HFrEF) describes patients with a dilated left ventricle (LV) and EF < 40%.
- Heart failure with preserved ejection fraction (HFpEF) indicates patients have EF > 50% and a normal LV size.
- Heart failure with midrange ejection fraction (HFmrEF) indicates patient having EF 40–49%.

HEART FAILURE IN ANCIENT LITERATURE

The oldest identified cases of heart failure come from the Egyptian mummies, dating back over 3,500 years. Egyptians also knew of other components of heart failure like cardiac hypertrophy, etc. As early as 2600 BC, the "*Yellow Emperor's Classic of Internal Medicine*" from China describes about dropsical swellings. Hippocrates described rales, as "When the ear is held to the chest, and one listens for some time, it may be heard to see the inside like the boiling of vinegar". He further described the technique of draining the fluid through hole drilled in the rib cage. Medieval Arab scholar Ibn Sina, had written "*The Books on Drugs for Cardiac Diseases*" in which he describes treatment for various cardiac symptoms. William Harvey's 1628 "*Description of Circulatory System*" set a foundation for our current understanding of heart failure.[3]

PATHOPHYSIOLOGY

Several mechanisms chip in to the advancement of heart failure. Neurohormonal activation, endothelial dysfunction, venous congestion, and myocardial remodeling are just a few that can be named. In the initial stages of heart failure, neurohormonal activation, such as the renin angiotensin-aldosterone system (RAAS) improves cardiac contractility, sodium and fluid retains, and peripheral vasoconstriction occurs to provide perfusion to organs.[4,5] Despite early benefits, these mechanisms lead to cardiac dysfunction and remodeling by fibroblast proliferation, oxidative stress, and extracellular matrix deposition ensuing in apoptosis and fibrosis (Figs. 1 and 2).[6]

NEWER RECOMMENDATION BY ACC/AHA FOR DIAGNOSIS OF HEART FAILURE

In patients presenting with dyspnea, measurement of natriuretic peptide biomarkers is useful to support a diagnosis or exclude HF (Class I). Measurement of brain natriuretic peptide (BNP) or NT-proBNP is useful for

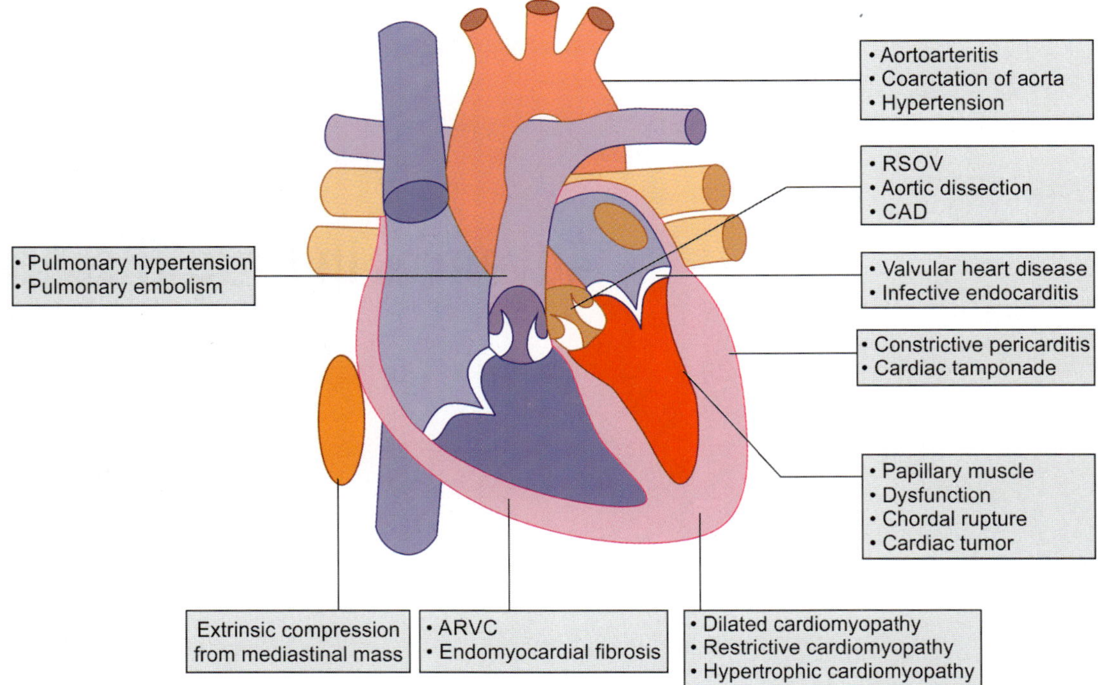

Fig. 1: Diagram showing various etiologies of heart failure.
(ARVC: arrhythmogenic right ventricular cardiomyopathy; CAD: coronary artery disease; RSOV: rupture of sinus of Valsalva)

establishing prognosis or disease severity in chronic HF (Class I). Measurement of baseline levels of natriuretic peptide biomarkers and/or cardiac troponin on admission to the hospital is useful to establish a prognosis in acutely decompensated HF (Class I). Higher levels of natriuretic peptide biomarkers on admission are usually associated with greater risk for clinical outcomes, including all-cause and cardiovascular mortality, morbidity, and composite outcomes, across different time intervals in patients with decompensated HF.[7] Similarly, abnormal levels of circulating cardiac troponin are commonly found in patients with acute decompensated HF, often without obvious myocardial ischemia or underlying coronary artery disease (CAD), and this is associated with worse clinical outcomes and higher risk of death.[8] Studies have demonstrated incremental prognostic value of these biomarkers to standard approaches of cardiovascular disease risk assessment.[9,10] During a HF hospitalization, a predischarge natriuretic peptide level can be useful to establish a postdischarge prognosis (Table 1).

PHARMACOLOGICAL ADVANCEMENT IN HEART FAILURE WITH REDUCED EJECTION FRACTION

Of the several new medicines, a combination was found to have remarkable effects in heart failure which effect were much bigger then effect of either sacubitril/valsartan.

Sacubitril/Valsartan

Sacubitril/Valsartan was developed to minimize the activation of renin-angiotensin-aldosterone system (RAAS) and enhance the natriuretic peptide system. It has two separate components. The first drug is valsartan, which blocks angiotensin type I. The second component is a neprilysin inhibitor (NEPI) prodrug, sacubitril. This is converted to an enzyme that inhibits NEP, the enzyme which breaks down atrial natriuretic peptide (ANP), BNP, and C-type natriuretic peptide.[11] In addition, it has the ability to decrease vasoconstriction, sodium retention, and maladaptive remodeling.

PARADIGM HF was a prospective trial comparing angiotensin receptor neprilysin inhibitor (ARNI) with angiotensin-converting-enzyme inhibitor (ACEI) to determine impact on mortality and morbidity in heart failure. The study was terminated early because of significant reductions in both primary end-point and cardiovascular death. Sacubitril/valsartan reduced cardiovascular death or heart failure-related hospitalization by 20% and all-cause mortality by 16%.[12] There was a higher risk of symptomatic hypotension in the valsartan/sacubitril group. It is the latest drug to get the United States Food and Drug Administration (USFDA) approval. It has class IA recommendation in latest American College of Cardiology/American Heart Association (ACC/AHA) guidelines, in patients who are symptomatic despite on tolerable doses of optimal medical therapy.

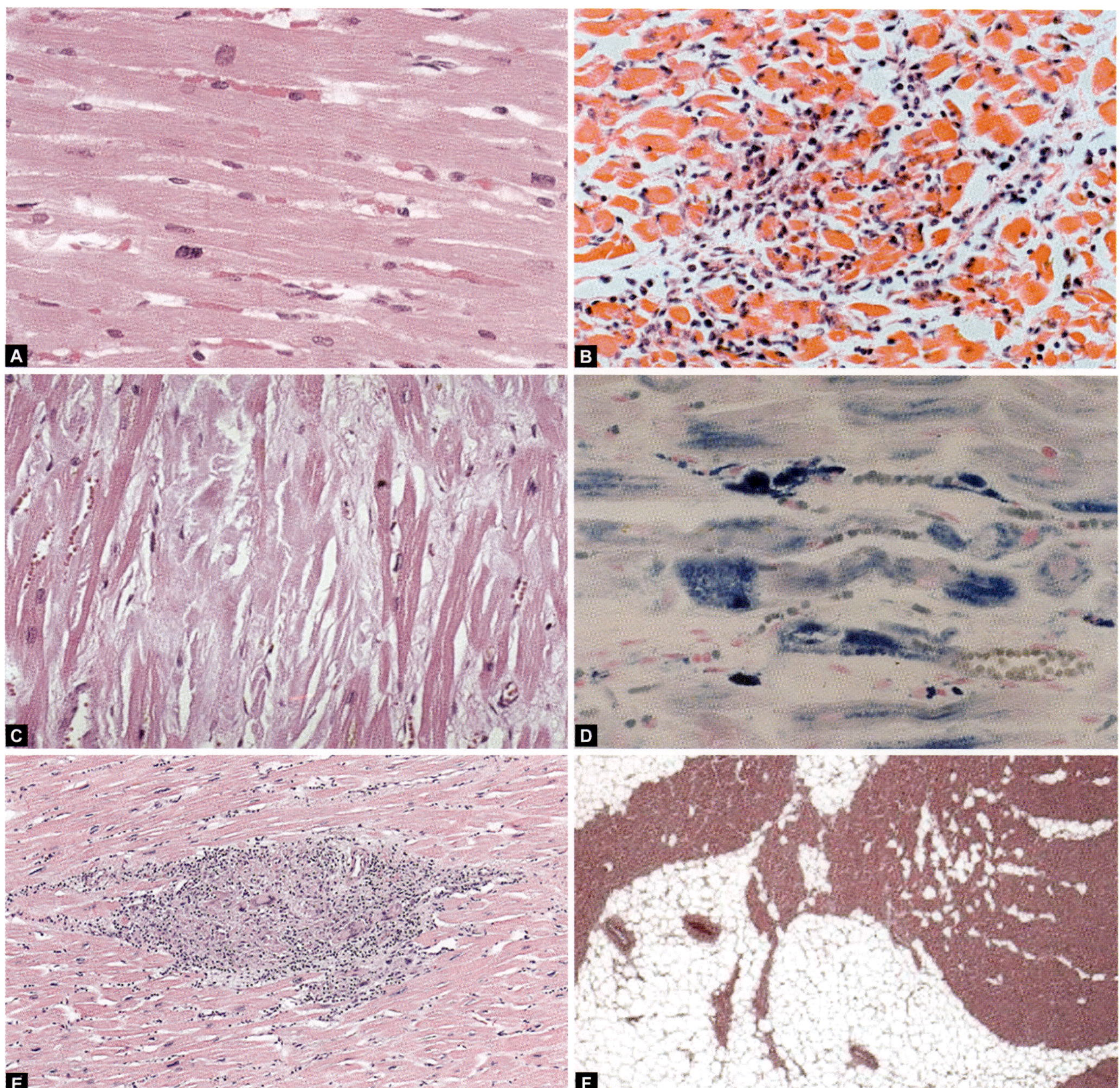

Figs. 2A to F: Histopathology of various myocardial disease: (A) Normal myocardium; (B) Lymphocytic infiltration in viral myocarditis; (C) Amyloid deposition in myocardium; (D) Iron deposition in hemochromatosis; (E) Granuloma in cardiac sarcoidosis; (F) Fatty infiltration in arrhythmogenic right ventricular cardiomyopathy (ARVC).

Ivabradine

Elevated heart rate contributes to increased morbidity and mortality in patients with heart failure.[13] A heart rate of 70 bpm or higher was associated with 34% increase in cardiovascular death and 53% increase in admission to the hospital for heart failure in patients with CAD and LV dysfunction. Ivabradine selectively inhibits I_f current in the sinoatrial node (SA), which is partially responsible for initiation of pacemaker activity. By reducing SA nodal discharge, this new drug is able to reduce the heart rate without affecting myocardial contractility or intracardiac conduction.

TABLE 1: Timeline of invention of heart failure management strategies.

Ancient times	Bloodletting and leech therapy— for heart failure
1628	William Harvey—described circulation
1755	William Withering—described the use of digitalis
1920	Organomercurial diuretics used
1954	Inge Edler and Hellmoth Hertz invented ultrasonogram to image cardiac structures
1958	Thiazide diuretics—discovered
1959	Furosemide—discovered
1963	First report of implant of artificial ventricle by Liotta
1966	DeBackey inserted first pneumatic LVAD
1967	Christian Bernard did first cardiac transplantation
1969	Denton Cooley implanted first total artificial heart (TAH) as bridge therapy
1982	JARVIC 7 first TAH as permanent therapy
1986	V-HEFT trial: ISDN/hydralazine in heart failure
1987	ACEI in heart failure CONSENSUS I trial
1994	First heart transplant in India: Dr P Venugopal
1999	Beta-blockers: MERIT HF, CIBIS trials
2001	Heart mate XVE: REMATCH trial
2003	CRT-P in heart failure: COMPANION/CARE HF trials
2004	Spironolactone: RALES trial
2007	Heart mate II first continuous flow LVAD
2009	MADIT CRT: CRT-D in heart failure
2010	SHIFT trial: Ivabradine in heart failure
2014	PARADIGM HF: ARNI
2017	MOMENTUM trial: Heart mate III
2018	Tafamidis in ATTR amyloidosis
2020 and beyond	Stem cell therapy, gene therapy , cell-based therapy

(ACEI: angiotensin-converting enzyme inhibitor; ARNI: angiotensin receptor neprilysin inhibitor; ATTR: transthyretin amyloid; COMPANION/CARE HF: Comparison of Medical Therapy, Pacing and Defibrillation in Heart Failure/ Cardiac Resynchronization in Heart Failure; CIBIS: Cardiac Insufficiency Bisoprolol Study; CONSENSUS: COoperative North Scandinavian ENalapril SUrvival Study; LVAD: left ventricular assist device; MADIT-CRT: multicenter automatic defibrillator implantation with cardiac resynchronization therapy; MERRIT HF: Metoprolol CR/XL Randomized Intervention Trial in-Congestive Heart Failure; PARADIGM HF: Prospective Comparison of ARNI with ACEI to determine impact on global mortality and morbidity in heart failure; REMATCH: Randomized Evaluation of Mechanical Assist Treatment for congestive heart failure; V-HeFT: vasodilator heart failure trial)

In the SHIFT (Systolic Heart failure treatment with the If inhibitor Ivabradine Trial) trial, ivabradine showed significant reduction in heart failure hospitalizations compared with placebo.[14] However, there were several problems with this trial including that not all patients were on β-blockers (89%) and only 56% of patients were receiving 50% or more of the targeted β-blocker dose. In April 2015, ivabradine was FDA approved for patients with chronic stable heart failure, with EF < 35% who are unable to tolerate β-blockers or are on maximally tolerated β-blockers with a resting heart rate > 70 bpm. It has class IIA recommendation in latest ACC/AHA guidelines.

- Sudden other medicines are in pipeline and are being evaluated.

ROLE OF DEVICES

- MIRACLE (Multicenter InSync Randomized Clinical Evaluation) trial showed that cardiac resynchronization therapy (CRT) in patients with New York Heart Association (NYHA) class III/IV heart failure provides beneficial effects in improving quality of life, 6-minute walk distance, NYHA functional class, peak VO_2, and treadmill exercise time, reduced QRS duration, improved cardiac structure and function, fewer hospitalizations over 6 months, and an improved clinical composite response. COMPANION (Comparison of Medical Therapy, Pacing and Defibrillation in Heart Failure) and CARE HF (Cardiac Resynchronization in Heart Failure) trials demonstrated mortality benefit from CRT. It has class IA recommendation in latest ACC/AHA guidelines.[15]
- The Multicenter Automatic Defibrillator Implantation Trial (MADIT) II enrolled the patients with ischemic cardiomyopathy and an EF < 35%. It showed significant reduction in all-cause mortality.[16] However, more research is needed on the use of ICDs in nonischemic cardiomyopathy (NICMP) as DANISH trial did not clearly showed beneficial effects in such patients. It has class IA recommendation in latest ACC/AHA guidelines.
- The Randomized Evaluation of Mechanical Assist Treatment for Congestive Heart failure (REMATCH) trial randomized patients who were not eligible for transplantation to left ventricular assist device (LVAD) implantation or medical therapy for end-stage heart failure. Trial showed a highly significant reduction in all-cause mortality in the LVAD population at 1 year compared with those who received medical therapy. Based on this data, USFDA designated this device as a destination therapy. Drawback of this device is its cost. Two major trials for LVADs were recently published. In the Endurance trial, the centrifugal-flow LVAD was tested against axial-flow LVAD (Heart-Mate II). The results were noninferior in terms of survival free from disabling stroke or need for device replacement in

patients with destination therapy. Six-month results from the MOMENTUM trial showed that the HMIII (HeartMate III) has better results compared with HMII, primarily because of lower rates of reoperation because of pump malfunction. The FDA has recently approved HMIII for patients as a bridge to transplant or recovery.[17] It has class IIA recommendation in latest ACC/AHA guidelines for refractory heart failure.

- The Coapsys device applies tension through a cable which passes through the middle of the LV chamber; from the lateral wall to septum. The results of trial involving coapsys device showed reduction in mitral regurgitation and wall stress with improved survival and reduced cardiovascular events. Another device, the Ancora submitral annular myocardial implant, clinches the LV free wall reducing the size of the mitral annulus and reducing the radius of curvature of the LV. These devices reduce the degree of mitral regurgitation, decrease myocardial wall stress, and induce reverse ventricular remodeling. In Device-based Therapy for Mitral Regurgitation and Ventricular Reshaping trial, involving ancora device showed reductions in MR followed by progressive improvements in ventricular size and function that plateaued at approximately 90 days and remained stable during the 1-year follow-up. Prior attempts to induce reverse remodeling by surgically removing a portion of the LV wall to decrease the radius of curvature and reduce wall stress (e.g. the Batista operation) have been unsuccessful. While early preclinical data are promising, the transition to the clinical environment proved challenging, with changes required in the delivery system, the implant, and procedural end-points.[18]

TREATMENT FOR SLEEP APNEA

Continuous positive airway pressure ventilation (CPAP) was associated with improvement of EF in patients with heart failure and obstructive sleep apnea (OSA) but mortality benefit is lacking; whereas, other modes of ventilation such as adaptive seroventilation (ASV) therapy were associated with increased mortality. In the SERVE-HF trial (Treatment of Predominant CSA by ASV in Patients with Heart Failure), the use of ASV in patients with HFrEF (EF < 45%), NHYA class II–IV, and predominantly CSA was not only proven to have no benefit but it was also associated with increased all-cause and cardiovascular mortality. Similarly, whenever both obstructive and central moderate-to severe sleep apnea patients hospitalized for heart failure in the CAT-HF trial (Cardiovascular Outcomes with Minute Ventilation-Targeted Adaptive Servo-Ventilation Therapy in Heart Failure), there was no benefit when ASV was added to optimal medical therapy. SERVE-HF trial showed reduction of sleep apnea with the use of ASV but without benefits on the study end-points.[19] Given the current evidence and in agreement with the current guidelines, it is reasonable to use CPAP to treated patients with OSA and heart failure to improve EF and the distance on 6MW (Class IIb).

GENE THERAPY

Identification of genetic derangements has spurred lot of interest in novel targets for genetic therapy. Three genes namely *SERCA2a* (sarcoplasmic/endoplasmic reticulum Ca2þ-ATPase), *SDF-1* (stromal cell-derived factor-1), and *AC6* (adenylyl cyclase-6) have now been studied in randomized clinical trials. CUPID 2 (Calcium upregulation by percutaneous administration of gene therapy in patients with cardiac disease) is a randomized, double blinded, placebo-controlled study to evaluate the safety and benefit of gene therapy with *SERCA2a*, which proved futile. STOP-HF (Screening to Prevent Heart Failure) is a randomized, placebo controlled trial of a plasmid encoding human SDF-1. SDF-1 activates tissue repair and angiogenesis. The primary composite end-point of 6-minute walk distance and Minnesota Living with Heart Failure Quality-of-Life Questionnaire (MLHFQ) score did not improve compared with the placebo arm. AC6 catalyzes the conversion of adenosine triphosphate (ATP) to cyclic adenosine monophosphate (cAMP). Increased AC6 content in animal studies after gene transfer increased the left ventricular function and reversed adverse remodeling.[20]

CELL-BASED THERAPY

Several recent advances in cell-based therapies have been made in treatment of heart failure. Human mesenchymal stem cells (MSC) have antifibrotic and pluripotential properties. A recent randomized trial compared autologous MSCs with allogeneic MSCs in patients with NICMP. Allogeneic cell therapy was found to be well-tolerated and more efficacious compared with autologous cell therapy. In another randomized, double blinded, placebo-controlled trial, transendocardial delivery of ixmyelocel-T resulted in reduction of cardiovascular mortality and hospitalizations within the 1st year. But, still this mode of treatment is novice.[21] Various stem cell techniques have tried like embryonal stem cells, induced pluripotent stem cells, skeletal muscle stem cells, MSCs, and bone marrow stem cells. Even though an innovative strategy, stem cell therapy did not translate into clinical outcomes. We are still in primitive stages in stem cell techniques and lots of studies are ongoing to improvise the techniques. In future, it is an viable strategy for managing patients with heart failure.

SURGICAL TREATMENT FOR HEART FAILURE

Various surgical techniques have tried for heart failure management, but without much success. Carpentier and Chachques came up with dynamic cardiomyoplasty, in which the latissimus dorsi muscle was wrapped around the heart and muscle was stimulated to assist contraction. However, symptomatic improvement was seen in only a few patients. Passive cardiomyoplasty is a procedure where an elastic net is slipped over the myocardium to reduce ventricular enlargement, which will further help in reducing ventricular strain. Partial left ventriculectomy introduced by Batista, was aimed at reverse remodeling of LV by removing lateral part of LV. Both these procedures did not show significant improvement in symptoms and was associated with high surgical mortality. Coronary artery bypass grafting in ischemic cardiomyopathy, left ventricular aneurysectomy in postmyocardial infarction LV aneurysm and mitral valve repair/replacement are the various techniques that are currently being practiced.[22]

Orthotropic heart transplant was first performed by Christian Bernard in 1967. Since then this has become a ray of hope for patients with end-stage heart failure. In India, the first successful heart transplant was done by Dr. P Venugopal at AIIMS, New Delhi. Since then more than 50 successful heart transplants have been done at AIIMS. Since the inception, the surgical techniques and quality of immunosuppression have improved by leaps and bounds. Currently, the 1-year and 5-year survival rates after transplant stand at 88% and 75%, respectively.[23]

TELEMONITORING

Pulmonary artery pressure monitoring continues to show a continued benefit with extended follow-up of patients with chronic heart failure with NHYA class III symptoms from the CHAMPION trial (the CardioMEMS Heart Sensor Allows Monitoring of Pressure to Improve Outcomes in NYHA Class III Heart Failure Patients).[24]

CONCLUSION

Despite plentiful of advances in heart failure therapy, it continues to be a deadly disease. β-blockers, ACEIs, aldosterone antagonists, and hydralazine isosorbide dinitrate combinations have been mainstay therapy. Newer therapies such as sacubitril/valsartan, ivabradine, CRT, and ICD have shown to improve morbidity and hospital readmission rates. Future directions likely include more pharmacological therapies, cardiac reshaping devices as well as gene therapy to reduce fatalities and improve quality of life of these patients. I strongly feel that next decade for newer invention and newer modalities for treatment of heart failure. I express my thanks to Dr Ahmad Basis for his valuable inputs.

REFERENCES

1. Go AS, Mozaffarian D, Roger VL. Heart disease and stroke statistics—2013 update: a report from the American Heart Association. Circulation. 2013;127:e6-245.
2. Roger VL. Epidemiology of heart failure. Circ Res. 2013;113:646-59.
3. Ferrari R, Balla C, Fucili A, et al. Heart failure a historical perspective. Eur Heart J Suppl. 2016;18(28):G3-10.
4. Yancy CW, Jessup M, Bozkurt B, et al. Writing Committee Members, American College of Cardiology Foundation/American Heart Association Task Force on Practice Guidelines. 2013 ACCF/AHA guideline for the management of heart failure: a report of the American College of Cardiology Foundation/American Heart Association Task Force on practice guidelines. Circulation. 2013;128:e240-327.
5. Mentz RJ, O'Connor CM. Pathophysiology and clinical evaluation of acute heart failure. Nat Rev Cardiol. 2016;13: 28-35.
6. Udelson JE, Stevenson LW. The future of heart failure diagnosis, therapy, and management. Circulation 2016;133: 2671-86.
7. Van Kimmenade RR, Pinto YM, Bayes-Genis A. Usefulness of intermediate amino-terminal pro-brain natriuretic peptide concentrations for diagnosis and prognosis of acute heart failure. Am J Cardiol. 2006;98:386-908.
8. Bettencourt P, Azevedo A, Pimenta J. N terminal-pro-brain natriuretic peptide predicts outcome after hospital discharge in heart failure patients. Circulation. 2004;110: 2168-74.
9. Santaguida PL, Don-Wauchope AC, Ali U. Incremental value of natriuretic peptide measurement in acute decompensated heart failure (ADHF): a systematic review. Heart Fail Rev. 2014;19:507-19.
10. Cohn JN, Archibald DG, Ziesche S, et al. Effect of vasodilator therapy on mortality in chronic congestive heart failure: result of a Veterans Administration Cooperative study. N Engl J Med. 1986;314:1547-52.
11. Vardeny O, Miller R, Solomon SD. Combined neprilysin and renin-angiotensin system inhibition for the treatment of heart failure. JACC Heart Fail. 2014;2:663-70.
12. McMurray JJ, Packer M, Desai AS. Angiotensin-neprilysin inhibition versus enalapril in heart failure. N Engl J Med. 2014;371:993-1004.
13. McAlister FA, Wiebe N, Ezekowitz JA, et al. Meta-analysis: beta-blocker dose, heart rate reduction, and death in patients with heart failure. Ann Intern Med. 2009;150:784-94.
14. Swedberg K, Komajda M, Böhm M, et al. Ivabradine and outcomes in chronic heart failure (SHIFT): a randomised placebo-controlled study. Lancet. 2010;376:875-85.

15. Abraham WT, Fisher WG, Smith AL, et al. Cardiac resynchronization in chronic heart failure. N Engl J Med. 2002;346:1845-53.
16. Moss AJ, Zareba W, Hall WJ, et al. Prophylactic implantation of a defibrillator in patients with myocardial infarction and reduced ejection fraction. N Engl J Med. 2002;346:877-83.
17. Raj L, Adhyaru B. An evidence-based review of recent advances in therapy for heart failure with reduced ejection fraction (HFrEF). Postgrad Med J. 2016;92:726-34.
18. Tenorio C, González N, Jaramillo JS, et al. Device-based therapy for mitral regurgitation and ventricular reshaping, structural heart. 2017;1:195-8.
19. Cowie MR, Woehrle H, Wegscheider K, et al. Adaptive servo-ventilation for central sleep apnea in systolic heart failure. N Engl J Med. 2015;373:1095-105.
20. Hammond HK, Penny WF, Traverse JH, et al. Intracoronary gene transfer of adenylyl cyclase 6 in patients with heart failure: a randomized clinical trial. JAMA Cardiol. 2016;1:163-71.
21. Patel AN, Henry TD, Quyyumi AA, et al. Ixmyelocel-T for patients with ischaemic heart failure: a prospective randomised double-blind trial. Lancet. 2016;387:2412-21.
22. Walter EMD, Hetzer R. Surgical treatment concepts for heart failure. HSR Proc Intensive Care Cardiovasc Anesth. 2013;5(2):69-75.
23. Airan B, Singh SP, Seth S, et al. Heart transplant in India: Lessons learnt. J Pract Cardiovasc Sci. 2017;3:94-9.
24. Abraham WT, Stevenson LW, Bourge RC, et al. Sustained efficacy of pulmonary artery pressure to guide adjustment of chronic heart failure therapy: complete follow-up results from the CHAMPION randomised trial. Lancet. 2016;387:453-61.

Cardiac Devices for Patients with Heart Failure

Rajendra Kumar Agarwal, Viveka Kumar

INTRODUCTION

Despite advances in medical therapy, heart failure (HF) is associated with high mortality. Unfortunately, we do not have a reliable data for prevalence of HF in India. The United Kingdom National Heart Failure Audit reported that during hospital admission for HF the in-patient mortality was 9.5%, with a 1-year mortality of 27% in 2013–14.[1] There is also huge morbidity associated with the condition, representing 5% of emergency admissions and almost 20% of readmissions to hospital. HF prevalence is more common in the elderly, with 10% of people over 75 being affected. HF due to reduced left ventricular ejection fraction (HFrEF) is treated mainly by medication, including angiotensin converting enzyme (ACE) inhibitors, beta-receptor blockers, and mineralocorticoid receptor antagonists. These treatments have a very good evidence base for improving symptoms and life expectancy. Despite this, many patients remain symptomatic. Advanced HF represents a stage of the disease where patients' symptoms are resistant to therapy and they remain very limited and at risk of lethal ventricular arrhythmia. In patients who meet the appropriate criteria, device therapy—either an implantable cardioverter-defibrillator (ICD), a cardiac resynchronization therapy pacemaker (CRT-P), or a cardiac resynchronization therapy defibrillator (CRT-D)—may offer substantial benefit. In patients with HFREF [particularly with a left ventricular ejection fraction (LVEF) under 35%], there is a risk of lethal arrhythmia (mainly ventricular arrhythmia) despite medical therapy. An ICD can detect these arrhythmias and treat them with antitachycardia pacing (ATP) and, if this is unsuccessful, defibrillation. In patients with HFREF who also have a QRS duration on their electrocardiogram (ECG) of greater than 120 milliseconds, a CRT-P can improve symptoms and prognosis. A CRT-D offers both CRT-P and ICD capability.

IMPLANTABLE CARDIOVERTER-DEFIBRILLATORS

Implantable cardioverter-defibrillators have been in use for the last 30 years. Initially, they were much larger than they are now and were implanted under general anesthesia with the generator in the abdomen with epicardial patches; however, over time, the generator has become smaller and can be placed subcutaneously in the pectoral region where pacemakers are implanted, and the leads are placed endocranially in the venous system. The devices can act as pacemakers, and can deliver ATP and shocks via the coils on the lead and the generator. The decision to implant ICDs should be discussed in detail with patients and their family. As well as being made aware of the risks associated with the actual procedure itself, the lifetime risks of the device itself, including the need for future generator replacements, lead failure, potential advisories, the potential risk of infection with these procedures, and the small but definite risk of inappropriate therapy. They should be aware that, when a patient is at the "end of life", the therapies for ventricular arrhythmia may be discontinued to prevent the distress of recurrent shocks.

INDICATIONS FOR IMPLANTABLE CARDIOVERTER-DEFIBRILLATOR IN PATIENTS WITH HEART FAILURE

Indications for ICD in patients with heart failure are as follows:

Secondary Prevention

Patients who have hemodynamically unstable ventricular tachycardia or ventricular fibrillation have a class I indication for a defibrillator in both the European Society of Cardiology (ESC) and American Heart Association (AHA) guidelines.[2,3] There are three randomized controlled trials (RCTs) where the efficacy of ICDs was examined in secondary prevention. When the results were combined in a meta-analysis, there was a statistically significant reduction in absolute mortality with ICDs.[4] The largest benefit was seen in patients who had a low ejection fraction.

Primary Prevention

The two large principal RCTs of patients with HF which suggest a benefit of ICDs in this category are MADIT-II (Multicenter Automatic Defibrillator Implantation Trial-II) and SCD-HeFT (Sudden Cardiac Death in Heart Failure Trial). Both demonstrated a statistically significant relative risk reduction in overall mortality (in the order of 20–30%) in patients with an ICD compared to those receiving medical treatment alone.[5,6] The ESC recommend that ICD implantation is a class I indication in patients with an ejection fraction under 35% who are in New York Heart Association (NYHA) Class II-III despite being on optimal medical therapy for 3 months and who are expected to live for more than 12 months.[2] The AHA guidelines are very similar to this.[3] The risk of sudden death is greater in ischemic cardiomyopathy (ICM) (10% over 20 months in the MADIT-II cohort) than in dilated cardiomyopathy (DCM); therefore, the risk reduction afforded by an ICD is greater in ICM. A meta-analysis of studies examining the efficacy of ICDs in patients with DCM demonstrated a mortality reduction with ICD; however, a recently published RCT demonstrated no benefit in such a group of patients with ICDs.[7,8] One possible explanation for this is that the medical therapy in the recent study was much better than that taken by patients in older studies which significantly decreased the risk of ventricular arrhythmia, mitigating the benefit of the ICD.

PROGRAMMING STRATEGIES

The most common indication for ICD implantation in patients with HF is the primary prevention of sudden death. Previously, the focus of ICD programming has been to have a short detection time for ventricular arrhythmias before therapy (through either ATP or shocks) is delivered. It has become apparent, however, that a large proportion of ventricular tachycardias within these detection zones self-terminate and therefore therapy is unnecessary. Furthermore, short detection times have been associated with a higher rate of inappropriate shocks. Several trials (and meta-analyses) have since suggested that having longer detection times or detection zones at higher rates (greater than 200 bpm) reduces both inappropriate and appropriate therapy, improving outcomes without increasing syncope, or mortality.[9] As a result, ICDs now being implanted for primary prevention are commonly programmed as a "shock box" with a single therapy zone above 200 bpm.

Right ventricular pacing in patients with impaired ventricular function is associated with worsening HF.[10] Therefore, these devices are only programmed to pace when the heart rate is low, for example 40 bpm.

CARDIAC RESYNCHRONIZATION THERAPY

The use of cardiac resynchronization therapy (CRT) was first described more than 30 years ago and multiple RCTs have since demonstrated an improvement in symptoms, exercise capacity, left ventricular function, and outcomes (including all-cause mortality) with this therapy. It is primarily aimed at patients with advanced HF (NYHA functional Class III and ambulatory Class IV) who have a LVEF under 35%, who are in sinus rhythm, and have a QRS duration above 120 ms. The procedure is more complicated than for an ICD because, as well as a right atrial and right ventricular lead, a pacing lead is placed in a branch of the coronary sinus, normally on the posterolateral surface of the heart. CRT targets patients who have abnormal electrical activation and therefore abnormal mechanical activation which in turn leads to further cardiac inefficiency and performance. The abnormal electrical activation is represented as a prolonged QRS duration on ECG and commonly left bundle branch block (LBBB). The abnormal activation pattern is termed dyssynchrony and can be intraventricular (delayed activation within the left ventricle—normally lateral wall contraction is significantly delayed), interventricular (delayed activation of one ventricle with respect to the other), and atrioventricular where atrial transport to the ventricle is impaired. The atrial synchronized pacing from the right ventricle and left ventricle provided by CRT allows the correction of this cardiac dyssynchrony and improvement of cardiac function.

Evidence for Cardiac Resynchronization Therapy

The patients who benefit most from CRT are those with very wide QRS durations (above 150 ms) and those with LBBB morphology.[11,12] In the ESC guidelines, symptomatic patients with LBBB with a QRS duration greater than 120 ms have a class I indication for CRT, whereas those who have non-LBBB morphology (with a QRS duration greater than 120 ms) have a class II indication.[13] COMPANION (Comparison of medical therapy, pacing and defibrillation in heart failure) and CARE-HF (Cardiac Resynchronization-Heart Failure) are the two large RCTs which demonstrated a beneficial effect of CRT (both CRT-P and CRT-D) on outcomes (HF hospitalization or all-cause mortality) in patients with advanced HF.[14,15] The majority of patients were in NYHA Class III. Further trials have evaluated the effect of CRT in patients with less symptomatic HF (mainly NYHA Class II). There was an improvement in hospitalization for HF in all studies. In a meta-analysis of these trials, there was also a statistically significant reduction in all-cause mortality.[16] The ESC guidelines therefore do not distinguish between patients with advanced or mild HF and state that patients in NYHA Class II, III, and ambulatory Class IV patients who fulfill the previously described criteria have an indication for CRT.[13] AHA guidelines strongly mirror the ESC guidelines.[17]

Cardiac Resynchronization Therapy in Patients with Atrial Fibrillation

Atrial fibrillation (AF) occurs in one of four patients undergoing CRT. Only a few patients with permanent AF have been included in RCTs evaluating CRT; however, in real-world practice, AF and HF frequently overlap and, correspondingly, CRT is implanted in a large number of patients. Without special therapy, the prognosis of AF patients with CRT has been generally worse than those in sinus rhythm. The importance of a high percentage of biventricular pacing (BIV%) was confirmed in a large study,[18] where the mortality was inversely associated with BIV% both in the presence of normal sinus and atrial paced rhythm and with AF. The greatest reduction in mortality was observed with BIV% > 98%.

Patients with BIV% > 99.6% experienced a 24% reduction in mortality ($p < 0.001$) while those with BIV% < 98.4% had a 19% increase in mortality. The optimal BIV% cutpoint was 98.7%. This cutoff would appear mandatory but it would be best to approach 100%. Careful evaluation of device interrogation data upon which the BIV% is based is essential because the memorized data can vastly overestimate the percentage of truly resynchronized beats since it does not account for fusion and pseudofusion between intrinsic (not paced) and paced beats. The randomized CERTIFY (Cardiac Resynchronization Therapy in Atrial Fibrillation Patients Multinational Registry) trial[19] for the value of AV junctional (AVJ) ablation in CRT patients with AF confirmed the favorable results of AVJ ablation by many other studies and two important meta-analyses and therefore established the firm recommendation that the procedure should be performed in most, if not all, patients with permanent AF as well as those with frequent and prolonged episodes of paroxysmal AF. Patients after AVJ have improved mortality with a mortality similar to those in sinus rhythm. The AVJ ablation procedure carries the theoretical risk of device failure and death in pacemaker dependent patients. An inappropriate first ICD shock for AF seems to increase mortality. Increased long-term mortality after an inappropriate shock may be due to the underlying atrial arrhythmia substrate as opposed to the effect of the shock itself.

The ESC guidelines recommend CRT (with a class IIA indication) in patients with AF who are in NYHA Class III or ambulatory Class IV and have a QRS duration greater than 120 ms with an LVEF under 35% despite optimal medical therapy, provided close to 100% BIV% is achieved. CRT is also recommended in patients who have AF with uncontrolled heart rates (despite medication), with reduced LVEF who will require AV junction ablation.[13]

Cardiac Resynchronization Therapy in Patients with Bradycardia

There is a clear detrimental effect of a high degree of right ventricular pacing in patients who already have LV dysfunction and HF.[10] In these patients who already have a conventional pacemaker or ICD, there is therefore an option to upgrade these devices to a CRT device where there is a large burden of right ventricular pacing. This practice is already widespread and represents a substantial proportion of CRT implants. Several RCTs have reported improvements in symptoms, cardiac function, and HF admissions in patients who have had CRT upgrades.[20] The ESC guidelines have therefore recommended CRT upgrade as a class I indication in patients with a high degree of RV pacing who have an LVEF under 35%, who are in NYHA Class III, and ambulatory Class IV.[13]

Given the harmful effects of RV pacing in patients with LV dysfunction, there is emerging evidence that, in patients who have an indication for pacing because of a slow heart rate (where there is anticipation of a high burden of RV pacing), CRT should be offered. The largest RCT to date in such a cohort of patients reported a reduction in HF admissions with patients assigned to CRT compared with those having conventional RV pacing.[21] ESC guidelines have therefore recommended this as a class II indication for CRT implantation in such patients.[13]

Complications

Despite the substantial benefits afforded by CRT, this comes at a price, namely an increased complication rate. There are two main reasons for this. The first is related to patient factors. Given that CRT is implanted in patients with HF, these patients tend to be more unwell and have more comorbidities (e.g., diabetes, renal impairment, increased age, and frailty), which increases the risk of complications, especially infection. A large proportion of these patients will also be on anticoagulation and/or antiplatelet medication, which will further increase the risk of hematoma and bleeding. The second reason is related to the procedure itself. CRT is a longer and technically more challenging procedure than conventional ICD and pacemaker implantation, and therefore the complication risk of the procedure is higher. A large meta-analysis of CRT trials looking at 9,000 patients has shown this, with a more than 5% rate of failure to implant the LV lead, a 3.2% risk of mechanical complication, a 1.4% risk of infection, and a 6% risk of lead problems.[16] The complication risk with CRT upgrade or revision procedures is even higher.

Therefore, given the risk of complications, it is important that the procedural risks and benefits are tailored to the individual patient and carefully discussed with the patient and their family before undertaking such a procedure, especially in cases where the outcome is less certain.

Cardiac Resynchronization Therapy Nonresponse

It has been consistently shown in CRT trials that 60–70% of patients respond positively but the other 30–40% of patients are unchanged or get worse. There has been a lot of research into identifying the reasons for "nonresponse". There are several causes for this, including those related to patients and those related to the cardiac phenotype and the device itself. In this review, some of these factors have already been discussed: low QRS duration, the presence of non-LBBB QRS morphology, and the presence of AF all increase the chance of nonresponse. Patients with DCM tend to have a better response than patients with ICM; this is probably related to a larger scar burden in ischemic heart disease, especially if the LV lead is overlying an area of scar. Response is higher in women than in men. Patients with more comorbidities, such as renal impairment and anemia, tend not to respond as well. LV lead position also probably influences response and the presence of the lead in an apical position is associated with worse outcomes.

Cardiac Resynchronization Therapy Defibrillator versus Cardiac Resynchronization Therapy Pacemaker

The decision whether to implant a CRT defibrillator or CRT pacemaker in patients with HF is not completely clear. There is the obvious benefit of CRT-D over CRT-P regarding the treatment of ventricular arrhythmia; however, there is no RCT comparing the two treatments. It is likely that CRT-D would offer a greater reduction in outcome if there was an RCT, but it would require the study to recruit a very large number of patients and may only demonstrate a small benefit. Furthermore, the complication rate and cost with CRT-D is higher than with CRT-P. Factors which may guide CRT-P implantation would be the presence of advanced HF and the presence of major comorbidities. CRT-D, on the other hand, may be of greater benefit in patients with less symptomatic HF and a lack of comorbidities. It is important that patients and their carers are given the appropriate information about both therapies so that an informed decision can be made.

VENTRICULAR ASSIST DEVICES

A ventricular assist device (VAD) is a percutaneous device/pump attached to the heart to help the weakened ventricle pump blood throughout the body. A VAD may be used in patients with advanced HFrEF as a final treatment option or as a "bridge to heart transplant", which means the device is in place until you can have a heart transplant. There are different types of VADs. The devices have transitioned from pulsatile to continuous flow design and are now smaller, with enhanced durability more suited for long-term support. The mean survival following left ventricular assist device implantation is nearly 5 years. However, some complications, including bleeding, infection, pump thrombosis, and stroke, limit the potential of the therapy. There are many innovations now under investigation that promise to further improve outcomes and enhance patient satisfaction.

CONCLUSION

Device therapy is now well established in pathways for treating patients with HF. It is important that all patients who are eligible can have these procedures made available to them.

REFERENCES

1. National Heart Failure Audit 2013-2014. [online] Available from https://www.nicor.org.uk/wp-content/uploads/2019/02/annual-report-2015-6-v8.pdf. [Last accessed November, 2019].
2. Priori SG, Blomström-Lundqvist C, Mazzanti A. 2015 ESC Guidelines for the management of patients with ventricular arrhythmias and the prevention of sudden cardiac death: The Task Force for the Management of Patients with Ventricular Arrhythmias and the Prevention of Sudden Cardiac Death of the European Society of Cardiology (ESC). Endorsed by: Association for European Paediatric and Congenital Cardiology (AEPC). Eur Heart J. 2015;36(41):2793-867.
3. Epstein AE, DiMarco JP, Ellenbogen KA, et al. ACC/AHA/HRS 2008 Guidelines for Device-Based Therapy of Cardiac Rhythm Abnormalities: a report of the American College of Cardiology/American Heart Association Task Force on Practice Guidelines (Writing Committee to Revise the

ACC/AHA/NASPE 2002 Guideline Update for Implantation of Cardiac Pacemakers and Antiarrhythmia Devices): developed in collaboration with the American Association for Thoracic Surgery and Society of Thoracic Surgeons. Circulation. 2008;117(21):e350-408.

4. Connolly SJ, Hallstrom AP, Cappato R. Meta-analysis of the implantable cardioverter defibrillator secondary prevention trials. AVID, CASH and CIDS studies. Antiarrhythmics vs Implantable Defibrillator study. Cardiac Arrest Study Hamburg. Canadian Implantable Defibrillator Study. Eur Heart J. 2000;21:(24):2071-8.
5. Moss AJ, Zareba W, Hall WJ; Multicenter Automatic Defibrillator Implantation Trial III Investigators. Prophylactic implantation of a defibrillator in patients with myocardial infarction and reduced ejection fraction. N Engl J Med. 2002;346(12):877-83.
6. Bardy GH, Lee KL, Mark DB. Sudden Cardiac Death in Heart Failure Trial (SCD-HeFT) Investigators. Amiodarone or an implantable cardioverter-defibrillator for congestive heart failure. N Engl J Med. 2005;352(3):225-37.
7. Desai AS, Fang JC, Maisel WH. Implantable defibrillators for the prevention of mortality in patients with nonischemic cardiomyopathy: a meta-analysis of randomized controlled trials. JAMA. 2004;292(23):2874-9.
8. Køber L, Thune JJ, Nielsen JC. Defibrillator Implantation in Patients with Nonischemic Systolic Heart Failure. N Engl J Med. 2016;375(13):1221-30.
9. Tan VH, Wilton SB, KuriachanV. Impact of programming strategies aimed at reducing nonessential implantable cardioverter defibrillator therapies on mortality: a systematic review and meta-analysis. Circ Arrhythm Electrophysiol. 2014;7(1):164-70.
10. Wilkoff BL, Cook JR, Epstein AE, Dual-chamber pacing or ventricular backup pacing in patients with an implantable defibrillator: the Dual Chamber and VVI Implantable Defibrillator (DAVID) Trial. JAMA. 2002;288(24):3115-23.
11. Stavrakis S, Lazzara R, Thadani U. The benefit of cardiac resynchronization therapy and QRS duration: a meta-analysis. J Cardiovasc Electrophysiol. 2012;23(2):163-8.
12. Sipahi I, Chou JC, Hyden M. Effect of QRS morphology on clinical event reduction with cardiac resynchronization therapy: meta-analysis of randomized controlled trials. Am Heart J. 2012;163(2):260-7.
13. Ponikowski P, Voors AA, Anker SD. 2016 ESC Guidelines for the diagnosis and treatment of acute and chronic heart failure. The Task Force for the diagnosis and treatment of acute and chronic heart failure of the European Society of Cardiology (ESC) Developed with the special contribution of the Heart Failure Association (HFA) of the ESC. Eur Heart J. 2016;37(27):2129-200.
14. Bristow MR, Saxon LA, Boehmer J; Comparison of Medical Therapy, Pacing, and Defibrillation in Heart Failure (COMPANION) Investigators. Cardiac-resynchronization therapy with or without an implantable defibrillator in advanced chronic heart failure. N Engl J Med. 2004;350(21): 2140-50.
15. Cleland JG, Daubert JC, Erdmann E; Cardiac Resynchronization-Heart Failure (CARE-HF) Study Investigators. The effect of cardiac resynchronization on morbidity and mortality in heart failure. N Engl J Med. 2005;352(15):1539-49.
16. Al-Majed NS, McAlister FA, Bakal JA. Meta-analysis: cardiac resynchronization therapy for patients with less symptomatic heart failure. Ann Intern Med. 2011;154(6):401-12.
17. Epstein AE, DiMarco JP, Ellenbogen KA. 2012 ACCF/AHA/HRS focused update incorporated into the ACCF/AHA/HRS 2008 guidelines for device-based therapy of cardiac rhythm abnormalities: a report of the American College of Cardiology Foundation/American Heart Association Task Force on Practice Guidelines and the Heart Rhythm Society. J Am Coll Cardiol. 2013;61(3):e6-75.
18. David LH, John PB, John DD, et al. Cardiac resynchronization therapy and the relationship of percent biventricular pacing to symptoms and survival. Heart Rhythm. 2011;8 (9):1469-75.
19. Maurizio G, Christophe L, Maurizio L. Cardiac resynchronization therapy in patients with atrial fibrillation: the CERTIFY study (Cardiac Resynchronization Therapy in Atrial Fibrillation Patients Multinational Registry). JACC Heart Fail. 2013;1 (6):500-7.
20. Leclercq C, Cazeau S, Lellouche D. Upgrading from single chamber right ventricular to biventricular pacing in permanently paced patients with worsening heart failure: The RD-CHF Study. Pacing Clin Electrophysiol. 2007;(Suppl 1): S23-30.
21. Curtis AB, Worley S, Adamson PB, et al. Biventricular versus Right Ventricular Pacing in Heart Failure Patients with Atrioventricular Block (BLOCK HF) Trial Investigators. Biventricular pacing for atrioventricular block and systolic dysfunction. N Engl J Med. 2013;368(17):1585-93.

Cardiogenic Shock: Diagnosis and Management

Charan Reddy KV, Vijay Bang

INTRODUCTION

Cardiogenic shock (CS) is characterized by a low cardiac output state leading to circulatory failure resulting in life-threatening end-organ hypoperfusion and tissue hypoxia.[1-3] It is often multifactorial, hemodynamically complex condition associated with high mortality. Despite advances in reperfusion and mechanical circulatory support (MCS), management remains highly variable with poor clinical outcomes.[4,5] However, with the advent of newer standardized team-based approach and risk assessment, the outcomes have improved with 30-day survival of 47% in 2016 to 57.9% and 76.6% in 2017 and 2018 respectively ($p < 0.01$).[3]

There were several reasons to account for poor outcomes in CS. The short-term stabilizing effects of vasopressors and inotropes are compensated by their adverse effects on afterload and oxygen demand leading to lactic acid accumulation, resulting in end-organ hypoperfusion and refractory heart failure (HF). In addition, the intra-aortic balloon pump (IABP) offers minimal hemodynamic benefit with no improvement in clinical outcomes.[6] Therefore, the limitations of these therapies have prompted the development of other MCS devices for use not only in CS but also in high-risk percutaneous coronary intervention (PCI).[7]

The most common cause of CS is acute myocardial infarction (AMI).[4,8,9] Despite advances in reperfusion therapy and MCS, morbidity and mortality among patients with CS remain high.[3,10] The subset of nonischemic HF often accounts for up to 30% of CS.[4] Among people with CS, the proportion of people with hypertension, renal dysfunction, and previous primary PCI has increased over the time, whereas the proportion of people with previous HF has declined. PCI is established as a standard therapy for revascularization in people with AMI complicated by CS. This has led to an increase of PCI from 19% to 60% over the years.

Therapeutic strategies in people with CS due to AMI depend predominantly on early and effective revascularization of the infarct related artery and to protect the myocardium.[11] Traditionally, drugs like dopamine, dobutamine, norepinephrine, or epinephrine have been used to increase perfusion pressure and cardiac output.[12,13] Recently, in a Cochrane Database of Systematic Review, Schumann et al.[14] have methodically updated clinical trial data on CS with regard to levosimendan, inotropic or vasodilative drugs [e.g. epinephrine, amrinone, dopexamine, enoximone, and nitric oxide (NO)]. New management strategies like treatment with phosphodiesterase (PDE) inhibitors or calcium sensitizers have been suggested, in addition to mechanical circulatory support (MCS) devices.[15]

DEFINITION OF CS

Various definitions, according to the clinical practice guidelines and operationalization have been described by various researchers. SHOCK (Should We Emergently Revascularize Occluded Coronaries for Cardiogenic Shock), IABP-SHOCK II (Intra-aortic Balloon Pump in Cardiogenic Shock II), and ESC-HF (European Society of Cardiology Heart Failure) trial have been the most commonly used definitions to describe CS (Table 1).[1,5,6]

These investigators have defined CS as a primary cardiac disorder that results in both clinical and biochemical evidence of tissue hypoperfusion. Clinical criteria include a systolic blood pressure (SBP) of <90 mm Hg for ≥ to

TABLE 1: Clinical criteria for the definition of cardiogenic shock (CS).

Clinical definition	*SHOCK trial*	*IABP SHOCK-II*	*ESC-HF*
Cardiac disorder that result in both clinical and biochemical evidence of tissue hypoperfusion	**Clinical criteria** SBP <90 mm Hg for ≥30 min or support to maintain SBP ≥90 mm Hg and end-organ hypoperfusion (urine output 30 mL/h or cold, clammy skin and extremities) hemodynamic criteria (CI: ≤2.2 L/mm/m² and PCWP: ≥15 mm Hg)	**Clinical criteria** SBP <90 mm Hg for ≥30 min or to catacholamines to maintain SBP >90 mm Hg and clinical pulmonary congestion and impaired end-organ perfusion (altered mental status, urine output <30 mL/h or lactate >2.0 mmol/L)	SBP <90 mm Hg for ≥30 min with adequate volume and clinical or laboratory signs of hypoperfusion clinical hypoperfusion, cold extremities, mental confusion, laboratory hypoperfusion metabolic acidosis, elevated serum lactate and creatinine

(CI: cardiac index; ESC: European Society of Cardiology; HF: heart failure; IABP: intra-aortic balloon pump; LV: left ventricular; PCWP: pulmonary capillary wedge pressure; SBP: systolic blood pressure; SHOCK: Should We Emergently Revascularize Occluded Coronaries for Cardiogenic Shock)

30 minutes or support to maintain SBP >90 mm Hg and urine output ≤30 mL/h or cool extremities. Hemodynamic criteria include a depressed cardiac index (≤2.2 L/min/m² of body surface area) and pulmonary capillary wedge pressure (PCWP) is >15 mm Hg.[3,16]

ETIOPATHOGENESIS OF CS

The pathophysiology of CS is complex with only a meager information currently available.[3]

Myocardial ischemia can cause systolic and diastolic ventricular dysfunction leading to depressed myocardial contractility. The most common causes of CS are: (1) AMI; (2) mechanical defects [rupture of both papillary muscle (acute mitral regurgitation) and ventricular wall (septal or free wall)], cardiac tamponade, left ventricular outflow obstruction (hypertrophic obstructive cardiomyopathy: HOCM), left ventricular inflow obstruction [mitral stenosis (MS), atrial myxoma and aortic stenosis (AS)]; (3) contractility defect (ischemic and nonischemic cardiomyopathy; (4) arrhythmias; (5) septic shock with myocardial depression; (6) myocarditis; (7) pulmonary embolism (right ventricular with or without left ventricular failure); (8) aortic dissection and (9) other causes include cardiotoxic drugs (doxorubicin), medication overdose (beta/calcium channel blockers), metabolic disorder (elevated lactate levels) and electrolyte abnormalities (calcium or phosphate).[17,18]

Systemic inflammation due to acute cardiac injury leads to pathological vasodilatation that can initiate and potentiate CS. Endothelial and inducible NO synthase may play a major role in the production of high NO levels, along with peroxynitrite, which not only has a negative inotropic effect but is also cardiotoxic.[19,20] Other inflammatory mediators such as interleukins and tumor necrosis factor can also contribute to systemic vasodilation and have been associated with mortality in CS (Flowchart 1). Chronic HF can present in an acute decompensated state

Flowchart 1: Pathophysiology of cardiogenic shock.

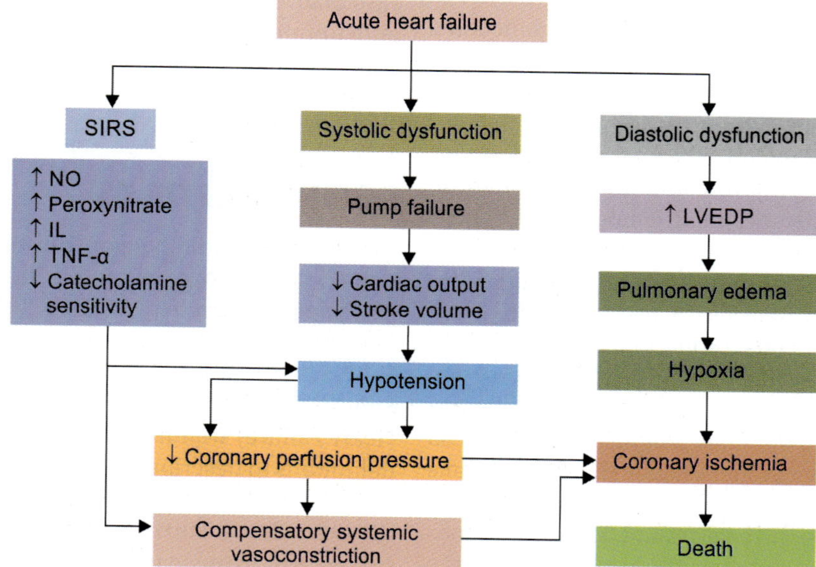

(IL: interleukin; LVEDP: left ventricular end-diastolic pressure; NO: nitric oxide; SIRS: systemic inflammatory response syndrome; TNF-α: tumor necrosis factor-alpha)

and may account for up to 30% of CS cases.[20] Among patients who had cardiac surgery, 2–6% of patients develop postcardiotomy shock.[21]

DIAGNOSIS OF CS

Cardiogenic shock is a condition that is often difficult to fully reverse even with an early diagnosis. Early initiation of inotropes, immediate PCI, MCS or a heart transplantation may improve clinical outcomes.[2] Though the diagnosis of CS is mainly based on clinical examination,[16] the advent of invasive hemodynamic measurements, patients are now characterized by cardiac index, systemic vascular resistance index (SVRI), and PCWP. The classic "cold and wet" (Table 2) profile is the most frequent CS phenotype, accounting for nearly two-third of patients with MI-associated CS.[3]

The diagnosis of CS is based on the presence of: (1) persistent hypotension defined as SBP <90 mm Hg or mean arterial pressure (MAP) 30 mm Hg below baseline or requirement of vasopressors to achieve a SBP ≥90 mm Hg and (2) signs of impaired organ perfusion (e.g. central nervous system abnormalities including confusion or lack of alertness or loss of consciousness, oliguria, cold, clammy skin and extremities, tachypnea, increased arterial lactate >2 mmol/L) despite normovolemia or hypervolemia (Table 1). Some clinical trials include hemodynamic parameters as diagnostic criteria, including low cardiac index (<1.8 L/min/m² without support or <2.2 L/min/m² with support) and adequate or elevated filling pressures (left ventricular end-diastolic pressure >15 mm Hg).

MANAGEMENT OF CS

The goal of medical management of CS is to restore cardiac output and prevent irreversible end-organ damage. Key to formulating reliable CS algorithm is to understand the importance of hemodynamic data to guide clinical decision making (Flowchart 2). Esposito et al.[22,23] have suggested three primary treatment objectives for managing AMI-CS: (1) coronary perfusion via revascularization; (2) circulatory support to achieve a viable MAP and (3) ventricular unloading to mitigate the deleterious effects of afterload and oxygen demand on failing heart.

Treatment of CS depends on the cause with the initial goal of improving tissue perfusion (Flowchart 2). This can be done in a number of ways: fluid resuscitation, vasopressors, ionotropes, and blood transfusions. Norepinephrine may be better in very low blood pressures, whereas dopamine or dobutamine may be more useful in slightly low blood pressure.[24]

If CS is due to AMI or acute coronary syndrome (ACS), attempts should be made to open the occluded coronary arteries immediately. Inotropes may also be helpful. However, it is unclear which is better.[14] Inotropic agents (such as dobutamine or milrinone), act on β1 receptors in the heart and improve myocardial contractility and correct the low blood pressure by improving cardiac output.[25] Milrinone, also a widely used inotrope, has been shown to reduce left ventricular filling pressures. Norepinephrine is preferred over dopamine in patients with severe hypotension (SBP <70 mm Hg) or hypotension unresponsive to other medication as dopamine has been associated with higher rates of arrhythmias and a higher risk of mortality. However, norepinephrine should be prescribed with a caution as it can cause tachycardia and elevate myocardial oxygen demand in patients with recent myocardial infarction.

TABLE 2: Hemodynamic presentations of cardiogenic shock (CS).

		Volume status	
		Wet	*Dry*
Peripheral ciculation	*Cold*	Classic cardiogenic shock (↓CI; ↑SVRI; ↑PCWP)	Euvolemic cardiogenic shock (↓CI; ↑SVRI; ↔PCWP)
	Warm	Vasodilatory cardiogenic shock or Mixed shock (↓CI; ↓/↔SVRI; ↑PCWP)	Vasodilatory shock (not cardiogenic shock) (↑CI; ↓SVRI; ↓PCWP)

(↑: increase; ↓: decrease; ↔: equivalence; CI: cardiac index; PCWP: pulmonary capillary wedge pressure; SVRI: systemic vascular resistance index)

Flowchart 2: Pathways in cardiogenic shock management.

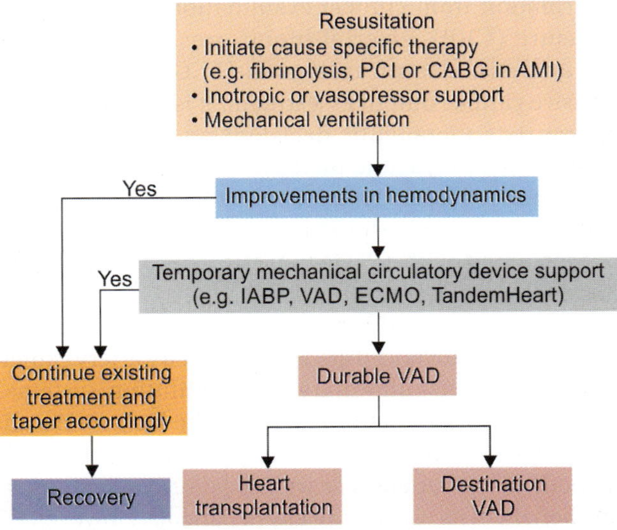

(AMI: acute myocardial infarction; CABG: coronary artey bypass grafting; ECMO: extracorporeal membrane oxygenation; IABP: intra-aortic balloon pumps; PCI: percutaneous coronary intervention; VAD: ventricular assist device)

Fibrinolytic therapy can be the choice for patients who are unsuitable for either PCI or coronary artery bypass grafting (CABG), if there are no contraindications. IABP (which reduces cardiac workload, and improves perfusion to the coronary arteries) or a left ventricular assist device (VAD) (which augments the pump-function and assists in unloading) can be considered in the event of inadequate response.[14] Unfortunately, even with revascularization, multiorgan failure is common, and the long-term survival is poor. Because CS affects almost every organ in the body, the condition is best managed by a multidisciplinary team that encompasses cardiologists, interventionalists, cardiothoracic surgeons, critical care physicians, emergency medical personnel, dedicated nursing staff, perfusionists, and cath laboratory staff. Although drugs and medical devices have been developed to treat CS, survival rates for patients with the condition have been uniformly poor for nearly two decades, at about 50%.

Revascularization remains the most important intervention for CS in settings of AMI and in patients with multivessel disease. Recent trial data recommend revascularization on a "culprit-lesion-only" rather than multivessel PCI. Although diverse types of MCS devices improve hemodynamics and organ perfusion in patients with CS, results from almost all randomized trials incorporating clinical end-points were inconclusive. However, development of new algorithms for utilization of MCS devices and progresses in technology has shown some benefit in selected patients.

The second step of the hemodynamic management of CS is to optimize the hemodynamic goals and stabilize the patient to prevent complications. After collecting information from clinical examination, central venous pressure (CVP), arterial blood pressure, heart rate, gas analysis, electrocardiogram (ECG) and minimally invasive cardiac output assessment, it is possible to make appropriate therapeutic decisions and select the most required hemodynamic therapy. It is also recommended that advanced hemodynamic monitoring should be used earlier when acute respiratory distress syndrome (ARDS) is associated with CS because in this situation fluid management is even more challenging.

The two hemodynamic monitoring parameters considered as advanced are the pulmonary artery catheter (PAC) and transpulmonary thermodilution systems.[26] PAC use has fallen out of favor over the last two decades because of the difficulty measuring and interpreting the hemodynamic variables as well as failure to demonstrate any benefit of its use in critically ill patients. However, PAC may still have a key role in the hemodynamic monitoring of critically ill patients.[27] Currently, the PAC is recommended in patients with refractory shock. Its advantage is that it can be used to measure the pulmonary artery pressure, and to provide an estimation of pulmonary vascular resistance and other potentially useful hemodynamic variables, such as right atrial pressure, pulmonary artery occlusion pressure (PAOP), mixed venous oxygen saturation (SvO_2), oxygen delivery, oxygen consumption and extraction.[26] The use of transpulmonary thermodilution is recommended in patients with severe shock, especially in the case of ARDS.[26] This technique measures cardiac output through pressure waveform analysis. In the third and final step, patients should be carefully evaluate the response to therapy. Clinical examination, hemodynamic variables, perfusion tissue markers and if possible, microcirculation should be assessed in an integrative approach to discern the circulatory status of patient. In the case of hemodynamic stability, vasoactive drug weaning may be started and deescalating therapies should be the goal. However, 10–15% of patients develop refractory shock needing increased doses of vasopressors and inotropes, with signs of tissue hypoxia, and in many cases already developing organ failure. In this setting, MCS should be considered.

Lactate levels have been identified as an important surrogate marker of poor clinical outcomes. A lactate level ≥3 mg/dL at 24 hours had a sensitivity of 45.9%, false-positive rate of 1.5%, and positive predictive value of 94.4% for mortality, similar to what has been reported in the National CS Initiative.[28] Cardiac power output (CPO) and pulmonary artery pulsatility index (PAPi) have been identified as two significant hemodynamic variables to assess response to therapy. Both can be included in risk scoring, highlighting the complementary role of hemodynamics and laboratory markers in tailoring therapies in CS.

Fluid and red blood cells transfusion maybe beneficial in patients who develop hypovolemia in CS. In these cases, dynamic assessment of fluid status should be performed, through echocardiographic parameters and cardiac output monitors.[29] Red blood cell transfusion is recommended on individual basis, according to hemodynamic parameters after the administration of inotropes, vasopressors, and fluid status assessment. Usually, hemoglobin levels >8 g/dL are needed to optimize oxygen delivery in patients with CS. However, the value is dependent on hemodynamic circumstances, patient age, comorbidities, and compensatory response to anemia and shock.[30]

Many uncertainties about CS management remain in clinical practice, and these relate to the intensity of invasive monitoring, the type and timing of vasoactive therapies, the risk-benefit ratio of MCS therapy and optimal ventilation mode. The focus of the treatment of CS is to prevent organ failure through hemodynamic resuscitation and optimization, and simultaneously to assess and treat a potential reversible cause. Depending on the type of CS, treatment involves infusion of fluids or in shock refractory to fluids, inotropic supports. In case of an abnormal heart rhythm several antiarrhythmic agents may be administered.

Approach in Acute Coronary Syndrome with CS

In the case of CS due to ACS, myocardial revascularization is the only evidence-based therapy with proven survival benefit. Fibrinolysis should be reserved for patients with ST-elevation myocardial infarction (STEMI) when timely PCI is not feasible.[31] The SHOCK trial is one of the milestone randomized trials in CS.[4] Although it failed to show a reduction in 30-day mortality by early revascularization-based management either with PCI or CABG.[4] More than 80% of patients with CS have multivessel or left main coronary artery disease.[25]

In recent years, immediate multivessel PCI of all significant lesions has been recommended in addition to the culprit lesion.[31] However, the randomized, multicenter culprit lesion only PCI vs multivessel PCI in CS (CULPRIT-SHOCK) trial showed a significant clinical benefit of a culprit-lesion-only strategy with a reduction in the primary endpoint of 30-day mortality or severe renal failure requiring renal replacement therapy [RRT; 45.9% culprit-lesion-only PCI vs 55.4% immediate multivessel PCI group, which was mainly due to an absolute 8.2% reduction in 30-day mortality (43.3% vs. 51.5%)].[7] Evidence comparing PCI vs. CABG showed that the type of revascularization did not influence the outcome of patients with CS.[25] These authors further reported that current clinical practice, immediate CABG is performed in less than 4% of patients. ECG and echocardiography should be performed in the initial assessment of patients with CS to promptly diagnose and treat mechanical complications of AMI, cardiac tamponade, acute valve insufficiency or pulmonary embolism. Independent of the phase of therapy, organ support and maintenance must be given according to shock severity.

Role of Levosimendan in CS

As a calcium sensitizer and inodilator that augments cardiac contractility without increasing myocardial oxygen demand or worsening ischemia, levosimendan can be used to deliver inotropic support in cases of acute heart failure (AHF). Effects of levosimendan on systemic hemodynamics include its significant, dose-dependent increases in cardiac output, stroke volume, and heart rate, and decrease in both right and left ventricular filling and total peripheral resistance. There is also a rapid and sustained reduction in levels of natriuretic peptides with favorable effect on other neurohormonal indicators of cardiac stress. Hence, levosimendan should be considered more often as a preferable alternative to conventional adrenergic inotropes. In Levosimendan Infusion versus Dobutamine (LIDO) study, levosimendan was compared with dobutamine in 203 patients with low-output heart failure. Patients in the levosimendan group of the LIDO study spent significantly more days alive and out of hospital than dobutamine-treated patients in a retrospective 180-day follow-up analysis.[32]

The RUSSLAN (Randomized Study on Safety and Effectiveness of Levosimendan in Patients with Left Ventricular Failure due to an AMI Study) was a safety evaluation of levosimendan in patients with left ventricular failure complicating an AMI. The combined risk of death and worsening HF was significantly lower as compared to the control group and at 24 hours. The SURVIVE (Survival of Patients with Acute Heart Failure in Need of Intravenous Inotropic Support) study compared the effects of levosimendan or dobutamine on mortality in patients with severe systolic HF.[33]

The REVIVE (Randomized Multicenter Evaluation of Intravenous Levosimendan Efficacy) studies evaluated the efficacy of levosimendan on symptoms of AHF based on a novel composite endpoint of clinically relevant measures expressed as "improved", "unchanged", or "worse" during 5 days of observation. Levosimendan was administered as a 24-hour intravenous infusion at a rate of 0.1–0.2 mg/kg/min. A greater percentage of patients treated with levosimendan were released within 5 days (46% vs. 37%) and the mean duration of the initial hospitalization was almost 2 days shorter in the levosimendan group than the placebo group (7 vs. 8.9 days).[34]

Role of IABP in CS

The IABP counterpulsation pump is currently the most commonly used assist device worldwide. The balloon is placed percutaneously in the descending aorta and requires a native beat and a stable rhythm. For more than four decades, IABP has been used to improve hemodynamic parameters in patients with CS. The IABP-SHOCK II trial randomized 600 patients with CS after AMI and early revascularization to IABP or conventional treatment and found no difference in 30-day mortality between the treatment groups. These results led to a downgrading of the IABP recommendation in the ESC guidelines with a current class IIIB recommendation for routine use of IABP in CS. The 2017 ESC STEMI guidelines now recommend IABP use only in patients with mechanical complications (class IIa, level C).[31] Another field of interest is the use of IABP in patients receiving extracorporeal membrane oxygenation (ECMO). There are data showing benefits of IABP in patients with ECMO, with a decrease in PAOP, less pulmonary edema, and increased survival rates.[35]

Role of Impella in CS

Since Food and Drug Administration (FDA) premarket approval (PMA), Abiomed (Danvers, MA, USA) has collected data on nearly 100% of US Impella patients in the observational IQ database. This clinical data, combined with the FDA postapproval studies embedded in Abiomed's prospective catheter-based VAD study, helped identify and validate best practices for Impella use and is associated with improved survival and native heart recovery. The Impella is a continuous, nonpulsatile, axial flow Archimedes-screw pump that provides active support by expelling aspirated blood from the left ventricle into the ascending aorta. Unlike an IABP, the Impella does not require ECG or arterial waveform triggering, facilitating stability even in the setting of tachyarrhythmias or electromechanical dissociation. Reported complications include limb ischemia due to sheath occlusion, device migration, device malfunction due to thrombosis, hemolysis, bleeding requiring transfusion, arrhythmias, tamponade, aortic or mitral valve injury, and stroke.[36]

Placement of Impella pre-PCI is associated with more complete revascularization and improved survival to discharge in the setting of AMI-CS (65% with Impella placed prePCI vs. 41% postPCI).[37] Initiation of Impella before PCI and prior to initiation of inotropes or vasopressors is independently associated with improved survival. Survival to discharge was 68%, 46%, 35%, 35%, and 26% for patients requiring 0, 1, 2, 3, and ≥4 inotropes before MCS, respectively, in an analysis of 281 AMI-CS patients.[37] It was also reported that a 48% survival at 30 days when Impella is implanted prePCI, compared to a 13% survival when Impella is implanted postPCI for left main in CS.[37] Further analysis of 15,259 US patients in the IQ database demonstrated an improvement in survival to explant from 52% to 59% when Impella was placed prePCI.[37] This study reinforces best practices of reduced use of inotropes and placement of Impella prePCI leads to improved survival rates. Survival benefit of Impella prePCI revealed trend vs. "matched" IABP-Shock: 57.3% vs. 46.7%. This study also revealed that significant survival to discharge benefit with Impella in patients who did not receive inotropes (56.6% vs. 29.4%). van Diepen et al.[38] study revealed that best practices are associated with improved survival in AMI-CS. Ouweneel et al.[39] reported the results from the IMPRESS (Initial Management of Patients Receiving a Single Shock) trial, which randomized 48 patients with CS postAMI to hemodynamic support with the Impella CP or an IABP. Device placement occur either prior to PCI, during PCI, or immediately after PCI. Notably, 92% of the study population had a history of recent cardiac arrest requiring resuscitation. At 30 days, mortality was similar (50% vs. 46% for patients receiving support with the Impella CP or IABP, respectively). More bleeding events occurred in patients receiving support with the Impella CP. In a recent meta-analysis including 148 patients, TandemHeart or Impella use was not associated with increased survival in patients with CS.[7] The most recent results that further validate that with early use of percutaneous MCS support, AMI-CS survival at 30 days rose from 44% to 82%.

Role of TandemHeart in CS

The TandemHeart is a small pump that delivers blood to the organs while allowing the heart's left ventricle to rest. The TandemHeart (TandemLife, Pittsburgh, PA, US) is a percutaneous centrifugal pump that provides MCS of up to 4 L/min via a continuous flow centrifugal pump. Oxygenated blood is withdrawn from the left atrium via a 21 Fr inflow cannula placed via transseptal puncture and then reinjected into the lower abdominal aorta or iliac arteries via a 15–17 Fr outflow cannula.[36] The TandemHeart is inserted through the femoral vein and is advanced across the interatrial septum into the left atrium. The need for transseptal puncture is a potential limitation to its widespread use. In 2005, Thiele et al. reported their experience with TandemHeart therapy in patients with CS postAMI.[40] In 2011, Kar et al.[41] reported outcomes following TandemHeart insertion in 80 patients with CS postAMI. Almost half of these patients had undergone cardiopulmonary resuscitation (CPR) immediately before or at the time of implantation. TandemHeart insertion was associated with significant improvements in hemodynamic indices. The 30-day and 6-month mortality rates were 40.2% and 45.3%, respectively. One patient died following wire-mediated perforation of the left atrium. Other complications included the need for blood transfusion (71%), sepsis/systemic inflammatory response syndrome (SIRS; 29.9%), bleeding around the cannula (29.1%), gastrointestinal bleeding (19.7%), coagulopathy (11%), stroke (6.8%), and device-related limb ischemia (3.4%).

Role of ECMO in CS

Extracorporeal membrane oxygenation (ECMO) temporarily replaces the function of the heart and lungs. ECMO uses a device to pump blood into an artificial lung and back into the bloodstream. Venoarterial (VA)-ECMO is a form of heart–lung bypass machine that offers extended support to patients whose heart and/or lungs are unable to sustain life in the acute setting. VA-ECMO provides cardiopulmonary support for patients in refractory CS as a bridge to myocardial recovery, bridge to decision, bridge to durable MCS, bridge to heart transplant or bridge to decision for palliative therapy.[42] In a VA-ECMO circuit, deoxygenated blood is pulled from the venous circulation by a pump via a large cannula. Patients may be cannulated centrally (open chest) or peripherally. Blood passes through the pump into an oxygenator where gas exchange occurs (carbon dioxide removal and oxygenation). Oxygenated blood returns via another cannula to the arterial circulation using a centrifugal pump. Modern centrifugal pumps cause less blood damage, reduced heat generation, cause less thrombogenicity, and are smaller than old roller pumps. Survival among patients on VA-ECMO support remains modest, with hospital mortality rates of 50–60% and 6-month survival as low as 30%.[36] This may be a consequence of inadequate selection of potential candidates and insufficient training of the involved medical support staff.

Russo et al.[43] (2018) reported that left ventricular unloading was associated with improved clinical outcomes when used in patients treated with VA-ECMO for CS. In the absence of a randomized controlled trial, the research suggests left ventricular unloading should be considered in appropriately selected patients undergoing VA-ECMO for CS. VA-ECMO is not an end goal, but rather a potential life-saving bridge to recovery or a more durable support strategy. VA-ECMO's efficacy, safety, and optimal implementation however have not been well-studied.

The next big leap in the battle against AMI-CS likely to be a comprehensive regional networks of smaller hospitals linked to large centers of excellence that are equipped to treat all levels of CS with team-based, multidisciplinary care, and rapidly deployable percutaneous MCS.

CONCLUSION

Cardiogenic shock caused by ACS is associated with significantly higher mortality risk compared with other causes of CS. Before routine use of early revascularization, MI associated CS had in-hospital mortality >80%. After advent of revascularization, mortality has reduced to 27-51%. Common physiology among all subtypes of CS is low cardiac index, but ventricular preload (PCWP or CVP), volume, and systemic vascular resistance may vary. All patients with CS should be evaluated with ECG, chest X-ray (CXR), and echocardiogram. CS is a complex syndrome that requires timely diagnosis and careful decision-making. Many advances have contributed to improve diagnosis and treatment of CS. Even though CS cannot be entirely prevented, patients must be educated on reducing risk factors for heart disease. In future, to obtain better results, one should learn how to deliver existing effective therapies within a timely and multifaceted strategy. Additional research is needed to establish triage algorithms and to clarify intensity and timing of pharmacological and mechanical therapies.

REFERENCES

1. Thiele H, Ohman EM, Desch S, et al. Management of cardiogenic shock. Eur Heart J. 2015;36:1223-30.
2. Van Diepen VS, Katz JN, Albert NM, et al. Contemporary management of cardiogenic shock. A scientific statement from the American Heart Association. Circulation. 2017;136:1-52.
3. Kosaraju A, Hai O. (2019). Cardiogenic Shock. [online] Available from https://www.ncbi.nlm.nih.gov/books/NBK482255 [Last accessed November, 2019].
4. Hochman JS, Sleeper LA, Webb JG, et al. Early revascularization in acute myocardial infarction complicated by cardiogenic shock: SHOCK Investigators: Should We Emergently Revascularize Occluded Coronaries for Cardiogenic Shock. N Engl J Med. 1999;341:625-34.
5. Wayangankar SA, Bangalore S, McCoy LA, et al. Temporal trends and outcomes of patients undergoing percutaneous coronary interventions for cardiogenic shock in the setting of acute myocardial infarction: a report from the Cath-PCI Registry. J Am Coll Cardiol Intv. 2016;9:341-51.
6. Thiele H, Zeymer U, Thelemann N, et al. Intraaortic balloon pump in cardiogenic shock complicating acute myocardial infarction: long-term 6-year outcome of the randomized IABP-SHOCK II trial. Circulation. 2018;139:395-403.
7. Thiele H, Jobs A, Ouweneel D, et al. Percutaneous short-term active mechanical support devices in cardiogenic shock: a systematic review and collaborative meta-analysis of randomized trials. Eur Heart J. 2017;38:3523-31.
8. Atti V, Patel NJ, Kumar V, et al. Frequency of 30-day readmission and its causes after percutaneous coronary intervention in acute myocardial infarction complicated by cardiogenic shock. Catheter Cardiovasc Interv. 2019;94:E67-77.
9. Goldberg RJ, Samad NA, Yarzebski J, et al. Temporal trends in cardiogenic shock complicating myocardial infarction. New Engl J Med. 1999;340:1162-8.
10. Maeda K, Takanashi S, Saiki Y. Perioperative use of the intra-aortic balloon pump: where do we stand in 2018? Curr Opin Cardiol. 2018;33:613-21.
11. Hochman JS, Sleeper LA, Webb JG, et al. Early revascularization and long-term survival in cardiogenic shock complicating acute myocardial infarction. JAMA. 2006;295:2511-15.
12. Dickstein K, Cohen-Solal A, Filippatos G, et al. ESC Guidelines for the diagnosis and treatment of acute and chronic heart failure 2008: the Task Force for the Diagnosis and Treatment of Acute and Chronic Heart Failure 2008 of the European Society of Cardiology. Developed in collaboration with the Heart Failure Association of the ESC (HFA) and endorsed by the European Society of Intensive Care Medicine (ESICM). Eur Heart J. 2008;29:2388-442.
13. Werdan K, Rus M, Buerke M, et al. Cardiogenic shock due to myocardial infarction: diagnosis, monitoring and treatment: a German Austrian S3 Guideline. Dtsch Arztebl Int. 2012;109:343-51.

14. Schumann J, Henrich EC, Strobl H, et al. Inotropic agents and vasodilator strategies for the treatment of cardiogenic shock or low cardiac output syndrome. Cochrane Database Syst Rev. 2018;1:CD009669.
15. Reyentovich A, Barghash MH, Hochman JS. Management of refractory cardiogenic shock. Nat Rev Cardiol. 2016;13:481-92.
16. Vahdatpour C, Collins D, Goldberg S. Cardiogenic shock. J Am Heart Assoc. 2019;8:43.
17. Ginwalla M, Tofovic DS. Current status of inotropes in heart failure. Heart Fail Clin. 2018;14:601-16.
18. Saleh M, Ambrose JA. Understanding myocardial infarction. F1000Res. 2018;7.
19. Prondzinsky R, Unverzagt S, Lemm H, et al. Interleukin-6, 7, 8 and 10 predict outcome in acute myocardial infarction complicated by cardiogenic shock. Clin Res Cardiol. 2012;101:375-84.
20. Nagpure BV, Bian JS. Interaction of hydrogen sulfide with nitric oxide in the cardiovascular system. Oxid Med Cell Longev. 2016;2016:6904327.
21. Hausmann H, Potapov EV, Koster A, et al. Prognosis after the implantation of an intra-aortic balloon pump in cardiac surgery calculated with a new score. Circulation. 2002;106:I203-6.
22. Nitasha S, Steven HM. "Cardiogenic Shock". Hospital Practice. 2015;38:74-83.
23. Esposito M, Bader Y, Pedicini R, et al. The role of acute circulatory support in ST-segment elevation myocardial infarction complicated by cardiogenic shock. Indian Heart J. 2017;69:668-74.
24. Joe K, Peter D. "Pressors and Inotropes". Emerg Med Clin North Am. 2014;32:823-34.
25. Mebazaa A, Combes A, Van Diepen S, et al. Management of cardiogenic shock complicating myocardial infarction. Intensive Care Med. 2018;44:760-73.
26. Jozwiak M, Monnet X, Teboul JL. Less or more hemodynamic monitoring in critically ill patients. Curr Opin Crit Care. 2018;24:309-15.
27. De Backer D, Bakker J, Cecconi M, et al. Alternatives to the Swan-Ganz catheter. Intensive Care Med. 2018;44:730-41.
28. Basir M, Isseh I, Schreiber T, et al. TCT-83 lactate and cardiac power output measurements at 12-24 hours predict outcomes in cardiogenic shock: insights from the National Cardiogenic Shock Initiative. J Am Coll Cardiol. 2018;72:B37.
29. Toscani L, Aya HD, Antonakaki D, et al. What is the impact of the fluid challenge technique on diagnosis of fluid responsiveness? A systematic review and meta-analysis. Crit Care. 2017;21:207.
30. Nakamura RE, Vincent JL, Fukushima JT, et al. A liberal strategy of red blood cell transfusion reduces cardiogenic shock in elderly patients undergoing cardiac surgery. J Thorac Cardiovasc Surg. 2015;150:1314-20.
31. Ibanez B, James S, Agewall S, et al. 2017-ESC guidelines for the management of acute myocardial infarction in patients presenting with ST-segment elevation: the Task Force for the management of acute myocardial infarction in patients presenting with ST-segment elevation of the European Society of Cardiology (ESC). Eur Heart J. 2018;39:119-77.
32. Mebazaa A, Nieminen MS, Packer M, et al. Levosimendan vs dobutamine for patients with acute decompensated heart failure: the SURVIVE Randomized Trial. JAMA. 2007;297:1883-91.
33. Gustafsson F, Guarracino F, Schwinger RHG. The inodilator levosimendan as a treatment for acute heart failure in various settings. Eur Heart J (Suppl). 2017;19:C2-7.
34. Harjola VP, Giannakoulas G, Lewinski DV, et al. Use of levosimendan in acute heart failure. Eur Heart J (Suppl). 2018;20:I2-110.
35. Aso S, Matsui H, Fushimi K, et al. The effect of intraaortic balloon pumping under venoarterial extracorporeal membrane oxygenation on mortality of cardiogenic patients: an analysis using a nationwide inpatient database. Crit Care Med. 2016;44:1974-9.
36. Mandawat A, Rao SV. Percutaneous mechanical circulatory support devices in cardiogenic shock. Circ Cardiovasc Interv. 2017;10:e004337.
37. Abiomed Inc. Cardiogenic shock survival rates improve significantly in three years since Impella FDA approval. [online] Available from https://www.businesswire.com/news/home/ 20190404005387/en/viewed [Last accessed November, 2019].
38. van Diepen S, Alemayehu WG, Zheng Y, et al. Temporal changes in biomarkers and their relationships to reperfusion and to clinical outcomes among patients with ST segment elevation myocardial infarction. J Thromb Thrombolysis. 2016;42:376-85.
39. Ouweneel DM, Eriksen E, Sjauw KD, et al. Percutaneous mechanical circulatory support versus intra-aortic balloon pump in cardiogenic shock after acute myocardial infarction. J Am Coll Cardiol. 2017;69:278-87.
40. Thiele H, Sick P, Boudriot E, et al. Randomized comparison of intra-aortic balloon support with a percutaneous left ventricular assist device in patients with revascularized acute myocardial infarction complicated by cardiogenic shock. Eur Heart J. 2005;26:1276-83.
41. Kar B, Gregoric ID, Basra SS, et al. The percutaneous ventricular assist device in severe refractory cardiogenic shock. J Am Coll Cardiol. 2011;57:688-96.
42. Kleeber ME, Haddad EV, Choi CW, et al. Venoarterial extracorporeal membrane oxygenation in cardiogenic shock. JACC Heart Fail. 2018;6:503-16.
43. Russo JJ, Aleksova N, Pitcher I, et al. Left Ventricular Unloading During Extracorporeal Membrane Oxygenation in Patients With Cardiogenic Shock. J Am Coll Cardiol. 2019;73:654-62.

CHAPTER

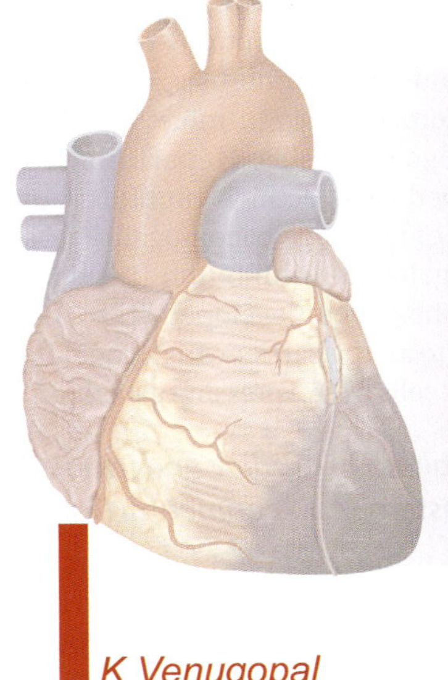

The Impact of Galectin-3 Inhibition on Aldosterone-induced Cardiac and Renal Injuries in Heart Failure

K Venugopal

INTRODUCTION

A major mechanism of heart failure and renal failure has been development of fibrosis and replacement of viable myocardial and renal tissues with fibrous tissue. Aldosterone role has been well-elucidated in development of fibrosis but the mediating agents and exact mechanisms responsible have not been clearly understood. Galectin-3, a carbohydrate-binding nonglycosylated protein, has been postulated to be responsible for mineralocorticoid receptor (MR)-mediated fibrosis. It has been thought that galectin-3 could act as a biomarker in heart failure and inhibition of galectin-3 could lead to prevention of fibrosis in cardiac and renal tissues and act as a new therapeutic modality in heart failure.

ALDOSTERONE IN CARDIOVASCULAR AND RENAL INFLAMMATION AND FIBROSIS

Aldosterone activation leads to vasoconstriction and volume expansion. Sodium chloride cotransporter (NCC) in the distal convoluted tubule and the epithelial sodium channel (ENaC) in the late distal convoluted tubules and collecting tubule and duct are involved in the aldosterone-mediated sodium reabsorption. Aldosterone also acts at the MR and increases the levels of serum-glucocorticoid-regulated kinase (SGK 1).[1] SGK1 prevents the degradation of ENaC. There are other mechanisms involving the NCC also, ultimately resulting in sodium retention and potassium excretion. Aldosterone also has direct effect on the vasculature, the heart, and the kidney. MRs are present in cardiomyocytes, endothelial cells and vascular smooth muscles, kidneys, adipocytes, and monocytes.[2] Aldosterone causes inflammatory changes initially leading to monocyte and macrophage infiltration, increased levels of cyclooxygenase-2, monocyte chemotactic protein and intercellular adhesion molecule 1 (ICAM1) in the heart, kidney, and the major blood vessels. This is followed by the proliferation of fibroblasts and myofibroblasts leading to excess collagen production and perivascular and interstitial fibrosis.[3] The RALES (Randomized Aldactone Evaluation Study) trial[4] and the EPHESUS (Epleronone Postacute Myocardial Infarction Heart Failure Efficacy and Survival Study) trial[5] showed that there was reduction in mortality in patients with heart failure in both patients receiving standard care and in those with postmyocardial left ventricular (LV) dysfunction when MR antagonist was added to treatment. There have been studies which showed reduction of proteinuria in patients already on angiotensin converting enzyme inhibitor/angiotensin receptor blockers (ACEI/ARBs) when MR antagonists have been administered.[6] Aldosterone and MR activation stimulates production of reactive oxygen species (ROS) which activates activator protein 1 (AP1) and nuclear factor kappa B and in the heart calmodulin-dependent protein kinase which is implicated in postmyocardial infarction (MI) LV remodeling.[7] Aldosterone-mediated myocardial inflammation and fibrosis can be influenced by a variety of agents. Aldosterone induces expression of molecules like the transforming growth factor beta 1 (TGF-β1), plasminogen activator inhibitor 1 (PAI-1), endothelin (ET), placental growth factor (PGF), connective tissue growth factor (CTGF), osteopontin, and galectin-3 which are profibrotic molecules.[8]

GALECTINS

Galectins are water-soluble nonglycosylated globular proteins that bind with carbohydrates.[9] They have an affinity for beta-galactoside derivatives. They are present in intracellular and extracellular compartments and intracellularly in the nucleus and cytoplasm and also in circulation and in the extracellular matrix. They are classified into three types: proto, chimera, and tandem repeat types. Galectin-3 is the only chimeric galectin member. It is involved in the pathogenesis of fibrosis, cardiovascular problems, and malignancies. It has a similarity to B cell lymphoma protein.[10] The levels of galectin-3 rise in various disease states and there is an interest in their role as a biomarker in various disease states. Galectin-3 has been known by different names, Mac 2 antigen, immunoglobulin E (IgE)-binding protein, carbohydrate-binding protein, and lectin (L-29). Different tissues have varying galectin-3 expressions with highest in lung, spleen, stomach, colon, uterus and ovary, moderate expression in liver, kidney, and adrenal glands, and low levels in heart, pancreas, and ileum. The expressions can vary during periods of injury and in cardiac tissue it can rapidly increase during myocardial injury. Sustained overexpression of galectin-3 can produce myocardial fibrosis.[11]

Functions of Galectin-3

Intracellular functions of galectin-3 are not clearly elucidated. It has a postulated role in growth and development of the embryo and in renal morphogenesis.[12] It may also play a part in inflammatory response through various mechanisms. There is some relation between type 1 diabetes mellitus (DM) by causing B cellular apoptosis. Extracellularly it binds with glycoproteins and glycolipids. Extracellular galectin-3 has role in embryogenesis, growth and development, and homeostasis.[13] Galectin-3 levels have been correlated with increased extracellular matrix turnover. This factor may be used in developing galectin-3 as a biomarker especially in heart failure with preserved ejection fraction.[14]

Inhibitors of Galectin-3

A variety of substances can act as inhibitors of galectin-3.[15] Simple sugars like lactose or N-acetyllactosamin (LacNAc) have been tried as inhibitors but cannot act as drugs as they are rapidly metabolized. Another group of drugs tried are galactomannans (GM) and citrus modified pectin (CMP). CMPs have been shown to inhibit galectin-3-mediated hemagglutination, reduction of organ fibrosis, reduction of inflammation, and atherosclerosis in mice. Another potential inhibitor is thiogalactosides. Heparin-based inhibitors are also developed as galectin-3 inhibitors but tested so far in vivo studies only. Neoglycoconjugates have also been shown to have galectin-3 inhibition. Peptide-based galectin-3 inhibitor has been developed (G3-C12) which could be conjugated to a drug carrier which could be used intracellularly to affect cells overexpressing galectin-3.

Impact of Galectin-3 Inhibition in Cardiac and Renal Injuries Mediated by Aldosterone: Experimental Data

There are no clinical trials using galectin-3 inhibitors to prove that galectin-3 inhibition could prevent or retard the progression of myocardial and renal injury and fibrosis. There are experimental animal studies. In the study by Calvier et al., CMP was used as the inhibitor in adult male Wistar rats. Monocyte chemoattractant protein (MCP) prevented aldosterone-induced myocyte hypertrophy. In this study, the role of galectin-3 in producing cardiac and renal fibrosis was demonstrated and the effect of inhibitor like CMP in preventing or reducing cardiac and renal injuries was also demonstrated.[16] The implications of this study could mean that a galectin-3 inhibitor like CMP can be used to clinically benefit patients who have aldosterone-mediated cardiac and renal fibrosis and could lead to a new avenue of treatment in the fight against cardiac failure and renal failure. Large scale clinical trials may be undertaken to establish this new strategy and to demonstrate patient benefits which after all is the major aim of these experimental studies. It would be interesting to see this approach in patients with heart failure and preserved ejection fraction where currently there are no specific drugs to reduce mortality and improve the quality of life.

CONCLUSION

Myocardial and renal injuries causing fibrosis leading to cardiac and renal failure have been well-documented as a result of aldosterone-mediated mechanisms. Various clinical trials including RALES and EPHESUS trials have demonstrated benefit of MRAs in retarding the progress of cardiac failure presumably by preventing cardiac fibrosis. Among the various agents which promote fibrosis, galectin-3 has been held responsible and attempts to produce fibrosis by galectin-3 and to reduce fibrosis by galectin-3 inhibition by CMP has been shown in experimental studies. It is a new avenue of therapy for cardiac failure and renal failure management and needs to be replicated in larger clinical trials for widespread application especially in the setting of heart failure with preserved ejection fraction. Another role of galectins could be as biomarker in heart failure with preserved ejection fraction.

REFERENCES

1. Naray-Fejes-Toth A, Canessa C, Cleaveland ES, et al. sgk is an aldosterone induced kinase in the renal collecting duct. Effects on epithelial Na+ channels. J Biol Chem. 1999;274:16973-8.
2. Sato A, Funder JW. High glucose stimulates aldosterone-induced hypertrophy via type 1 mineralocorticoid receptors in neonatal rat cardiomyocytes. Endocrinology. 1996;137:4145-53.
3. Gerling IC, Sun Y, Ahokas RA, et al. Aldosteronism: an immunostimulatory state precedes proinflammatory/fibrogenic cardiac phenotype. Am J Physiol Heart Circ Physiol. 2003;285:H813-21.
4. Pitt B, Zannad F, Remme WJ, et al. The effect of spironolactone on morbidity and mortality in patients with severe heart failure. N Engl J Med. 1993;341:709-17.
5. Pitt B, Remme W, Zannad F, et al. Eplerenone, a selective aldosterone blocker, in patients with left ventricular dysfunction after myocardial infarction. N Engl J Med. 2003;348:1309-21.
6. Volk MJ, Bomback AS, Klemmer PJ. Mineralocorticoid receptor blockade in chronic kidney disease. Curr Hypertens Rep. 2011;13:282-8.
7. Fiebeler A, Schmidt F, Muller DN, et al. Mineralocorticoid receptor affects AP-1 and nuclear factor-kappab activation in angiotensin II-induced cardiac injury. Hypertension. 2001;37:787-93.
8. Brown NJ. Contribution of aldosterone to cardiovascular and renal inflammation and fibrosis. Nat Rev Nephrol. 2013;9:459-69.
9. Drickamer K, Taylor ME. Biology of animal lectins. Annu Rev Cell Biol. 1993;9:237-64.
10. Leffler H, Masiarz FR, Barondes SH. Soluble lactose binding vertebrate lectins: a growing family. Biochemistry. 1989;28:9222-9.
11. Yu L, Ruifrok WP, Meissner M, et al. Genetic and pharmacological inhibition of galectin-3 prevents cardiac remodeling by interfering with myocardial fibrogenesis. Circ Heart Fail. 2013;6:107-17.
12. Koch A, Poirier F, Jacob R, et al. Galectin-3, a novel centrosome associated protein required for epithelial morphogenesis. Mol Biol Cell. 2010;21:219-31.
13. Van den Brule FA, Fernandez PL, Buicu C, et al. Differential expression of galectin 1 and galectin 3 during first trimester human embryogenesis. Dev Dyn. 1997;209:399-405.
14. de Boer RA, van der Velde AR, Mueller C, et al. Galectin-3: a modifiable risk factor in heart failure. Cardiovasc Drugs Ther. 2014;28:237-46.
15. Suthahar N, Meijers WC, Sillje HH, et al. Galectin-3 activation and inhibition in heart failure and cardiovascular disease: An update. Theranostics. 2018;8:593-609.
16. Calvier L, Martinez EM, Miana M, et al. The impact of galectin-3 inhibition on aldosterone-induced cardiac and renal injuries. JACC Heart Fail. 2015;1:59-67.

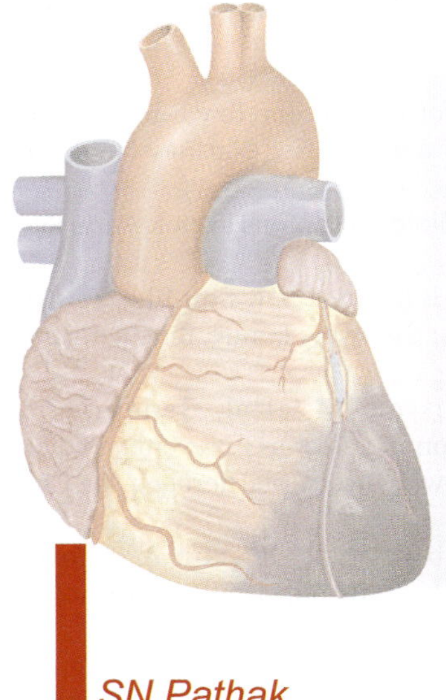

Sleep Apnea and Heart Failure

SN Pathak

INTRODUCTION

In spite of recent triumphs in pharmacological and device therapy, chronic heart failure (CHF) remains a major public health problem. CHF is associated with high morbidity, frequent hospitalizations and readmissions, huge economical cost, and excess mortality. Therefore, identification of comorbidities which contribute to progression of CHF, particularly if treatable, is our current challenge and needs to be pursued systematically and aggressively. Among multiple comorbidities, sleep-related disordered breathing (SRBD) is the most common and least recognized by cardiologists.

There are two major types of sleep apnea: Central and obstructive (Flowchart 1).

CENTRAL SLEEP APNEA

Central sleep apnea (CSA) is due to temporary failure in the pontomedullary pacemaker generating breathing rhythm. This is analogous to sinus node arrest for at least 10 seconds.

Flowchart 1: Types of sleep apnea.

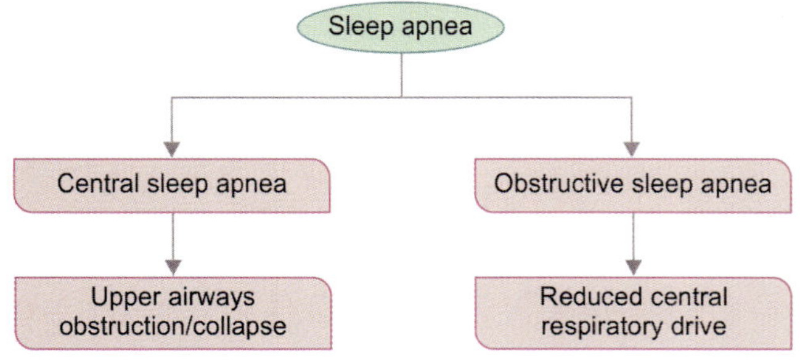

During central apnea, there is no brainstem inspiratory neural output through the nerves innervating the diaphragm and intercostal pump muscles. Therefore, polygraphically, central apnea is characterized by the absence of naso-oral airflow and thoracoabdominal excursions. Mechanistically, central apneas occur when the prevailing partial pressure of carbon dioxide (pCO_2) decreases below a certain level referred to as apneic threshold pCO_2. Due to cessation of breathing, pCO_2 rises and when it exceeds the apneic threshold pCO_2, breathing resumes.

OBSTRUCTIVE SLEEP APNEA

Obstructive sleep apnea (OSA) is due to upper airway occlusion secondary to neuromuscular failure, primarily involving hypoglossal nerve and genioglossus muscle. Normally, during sleep, genioglossus muscle activity decreases and during inspiration due to the negative airway pressure, the tongue falls backward. In susceptible individuals, this results in upper airway closure (obstructive apnea) or narrowing (obstructive hypopnea). Obesity is the major risk factor for OSA, in part due to excess fat deposition in the pharynx. OSA is 2–3 times more common in men than in women and in elderly than in young both in the general population and in patients with heart failure.[1] Obesity is regarded as one of the major risk factors for OSA. Nevertheless, OSA can occur in individuals of normal weight in whom other factors can contribute to pharyngeal collapsibility, such as macroglossia, and adenotonsillar hypertrophy. Anomalies of craniofacial structure, such as retrognathia, which can displace the tongue backward and narrow the pharynx, can be important in nonobese Asians.

PREVALENCE OF SLEEP APNEA IN PATIENT WITH HEART FAILURE

Sleep apnea and heart failure are common diseases affecting approximately 10%[2] and 2%[3] of the population, respectively. Literature to date suggests that sleep apnea is more common in patients with heart failure than in subjects with normal cardiac function.[2,4-7]

PATHOPHYSIOLOGY (FLOWCHARTS 2 AND 3)

Increased inspiratory efforts against the occluded pharynx during obstructive apneas and hypopneas generate exaggerated negative intrathoracic pressure[8] that increases left ventricular (LV) transmural pressure and hence afterload. Negative pressure also increases venous return causing distension of the right ventricle and leftward displacement of the interventricular septum during diastole. This impairs LV filling and reduces stroke volume.[9] Intermittent hypoxia during OSA may impair cardiac contractility directly or reduce cardiac output indirectly by increasing pulmonary artery pressure. In patients with ischemic heart disease, it may also precipitate myocardial ischemia. Intermittent apnea, hypoxia, carbon dioxide (CO_2) retention, and

Flowchart 3: Schema of intermittent hypoxia-induced vascular damage in obstructive sleep apnea.

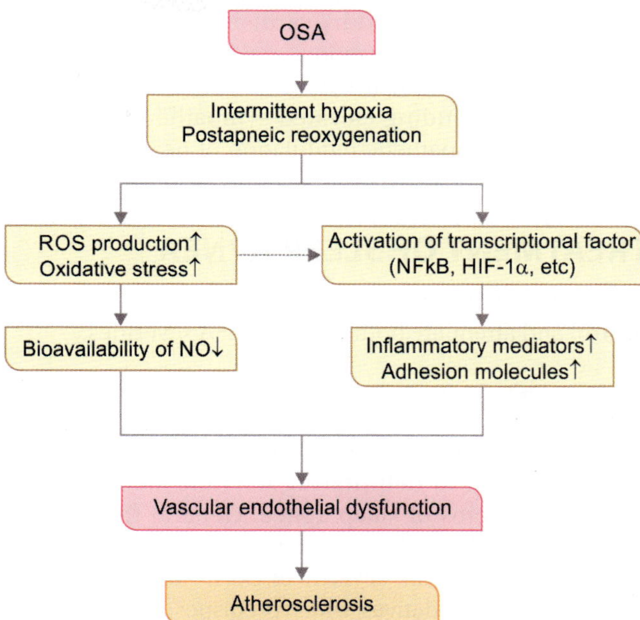

(HIF-1α: hypoxia induced factor-1-alpha; NFκB: nuclear factor kappa-light-chain-enhancer of activated B cells; NO: nitric oxide; OSA: obstructive sleep apnea; ROS: reactive oxygen species)
Source: Kasai T. Sleep apnea and heart failure. J Cardiol. 2012;60:78-85.

Flowchart 2: Pathogenesis of central sleep apnea in heart failure.

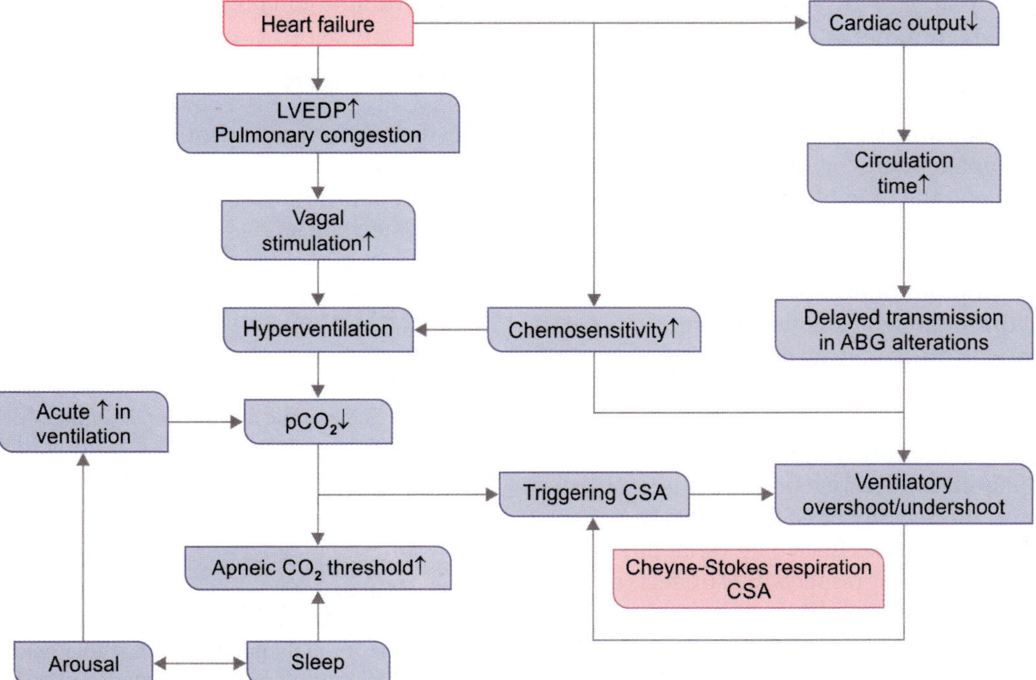

(ABG: arterial blood gas; CSA: central sleep apnea; LVEDP: left ventricular end-diastolic pressure; pCO_2: partial pressure of carbon dioxide)
Source: Yumino D, Bradley TD. Central sleep apnea and Cheyne-Stokes respiration. Proc Am Thorac Soc. 2008;5:226-36.

arousal from sleep trigger increases in sympathetic neural outflow that are accompanied by surges in systemic blood pressure acutely,[10,11] and by cardiac myocyte necrosis, β-adrenoceptor desensitization, and cardiac arrhythmias chronically.[12] These nocturnal cardiovascular stresses have after-effects, including elevated sympathetic activity,[11] reduced parasympathetic modulation of heart rate,[13] and hypertension, which are sustained into the daytime.[14]

TREATMENT OF SLEEP APNEA

Optimizing heart failure therapy can stabilize ventilatory control and attenuate both OSA and CSA severities.

Obstructive Sleep Apnea

Most compelling indication for treatment of OSA would be a complaint of debilitating daytime sleepiness or related symptoms of sleep apnea. General therapeutic considerations for such patients include weight reduction, which may reduce the severity of OSA,[15] and abstinence from alcohol and sedatives, which predispose to pharyngeal collapse during sleep.[16]

The standard treatment for OSA in patients with heart failure is continuous positive airway pressure (CPAP). CPAP splints the pharynx and maintains its patency, thereby preventing apneas and hypopneas and may have beneficial positive airway pressure effects on heart failure independent from treating OSA. In general population, oral appliances or surgery are less effective than CPAP. Randomized trials in patients with OSA and excessive daytime sleepiness but with normal cardiac function have demonstrated that CPAP applied via a nasal mask alleviates OSA, improves sleep quality, reduces daytime sleepiness, augments neurocognitive function, and may lower nocturnal and daytime blood pressure.[17,18] On the other hand, a randomized trial of patients with relatively severe OSA (apnea hypopnea index 30 per hour of sleep) but without a symptom of excessive daytime sleepiness demonstrated that although patients randomized to CPAP were compliant with it, they did not derive any symptomatic or neurocognitive benefit.[19] These findings support the use of CPAP for patients with symptomatic OSA, but do not support its use for those with asymptomatic OSA. There is no evidence that pharmacological agents used to treat HF have any influence on the severity of OSA.[20] In awake patients with HF, CPAP also increases heart rate variability and its vagal modulation.[21] In many respects, these effects of CPAP are analogous to the chronic effects of beta-blockade in heart failure,[22] but they are achieved nonpharmacologically by reducing oxygen demand and increasing oxygen supply and by attenuating central sympathetic outflow.

Mandibular advancement devices have been shown in randomized trials to improve OSA and its symptoms, but they are generally not as effective as CPAP.[23,24]

Central Sleep Apnea

In particular, first-line therapy for CSA patients should be optimization of heart failure treatment which can cause a reduction of systemic and pulmonary congestion since CSA is largely a consequence of heart failure and pulmonary congestion.

Specific Treatment of CSA

Respiratory stimulants:

Theophylline: Theophylline stimulates central respiratory drive, and augments cardiac contractility by antagonism of adenosine. However, theophylline, once widely used for therapy for acute heart failure, is no longer used for this purpose because it increased the incidence of cardiac arrhythmias[25] and sudden death.[26]

Carbonic anhydrase inhibitor: Carbonic anhydrase inhibitor acetazolamide stimulates respiration by causing metabolic acidosis. However, it cannot be recommended for therapy for CSA in heart failure at present.

CPAP: CPAP reduces LV transmural pressure and afterload in patients with heart failure by increasing intrathoracic pressure.[27] It also reduces LV preload by reducing end-diastolic volume and pressure.[28]

CONCLUSION

In a substantial proportion of patients with HF, sleep apnea may play a role in the pathogenesis and progression of cardiac failure through mechanical, adrenergic, and vascular mechanisms.

REFERENCES

1. Yumino D, Wang H, Floras JS, et al. Prevalence and physiological predictors of sleep apnea in patients with heart failure and systolic dysfunction. J Card Fail. 2009;15:279-85.
2. Young T, Palta M, Dempsey J, et al. The occurrence of sleep-disordered breathing among middle-aged adults. N Engl J Med. 1993;328:1230-5.
3. American Heart Association. Heart disease and stroke statistics: 2005 update. Dallas, Texas: American Heart Association; 2005.
4. Javaheri S, Parker TJ, Liming JD, et al. Sleep apnea in 81 ambulatory male patients with stable heart failure: types and their prevalences, consequences, and presentations. Circulation. 1998;97:2154-9.

5. Sin DD, Fitzgerald F, Parker JD, et al. Risk factors for central and obstructive sleep apnea in 450 men and women with congestive heart failure. Am J Respir Crit Care Med. 1999;160:1101-6.
6. Solin P, Bergin P, Richardson M, et al. Influence of pulmonary capillary wedge pressure on central apnea in heart failure. Circulation. 1999;99:1574-9.
7. Shahar E, Whitney CW, Redline S, et al. Sleep-disordered breathing and cardiovascular disease: cross-sectional results of the Sleep Heart Health Study. Am J Respir Crit Care Med. 2001;163:19-25.
8. Malone S, Liu PP, Holloway R, et al. Obstructive sleep apnoea in patients with dilated cardiomyopathy: effects of continuous positive airway pressure. Lancet. 1991;338:1480-4.
9. Tolle FA, Judy WV, Yu PL, et al. Reduced stroke volume related to pleural pressure in obstructive sleep apnea. J Appl Physiol. 1983;55:1718-24.
10. Tkacova R, Rankin F, Fitzgerald FS, et al. Effects of continuous positive airway pressure on obstructive sleep apnea and left ventricular afterload in patients with heart failure. Circulation. 1998;98:2269-75.
11. Somers VK, Dyken ME, Clary MP, et al. Sympathetic neural mechanisms in obstructive sleep apnea. J Clin Invest. 1995;96:1897-904.
12. Floras JS. Clinical aspects of sympathetic activation and parasympathetic withdrawal in heart failure. J Am Coll Cardiol. 1993;22:72A-84A.
13. Narkiewicz K, Montano N, Cogliati C, et al. Altered cardiovascular variability in obstructive sleep apnea. Circulation. 1998;98:1071-7.
14. Peppard PE, Young T, Palta M, et al. Prospective study of the association between sleep-disordered breathing and hypertension. N Engl J Med. 2000;342:1378-84.
15. Smith PL, Gold AR, Meyers DA, et al. Weight loss in mildly to moderately obese patients with obstructive sleep apnea. Ann Int Med. 1985;103:850-5.
16. Issa FG, Sullivan CE. Alcohol, snoring and sleep apnea. J Neurol Neurosurg Psychiatry. 1985;45:353-9.
17. Engleman HM, Martin SE, Deary IJ, et al. Effect of continuous positive airway pressure treatment on daytime function in sleep apnoea/hypopnoea syndrome. Lancet. 1994;343:572-5.
18. Pepperell JC, Ramdassingh-Dow S, Crosthwaite N, et al. Ambulatory blood pressure after therapeutic and subtherapeutic nasal continuous positive airway pressure for obstructive sleep apnoea: a randomized parallel trial. Lancet. 2002;359:204-10.
19. Barbe F, Mayoralas LR, Duran J, et al. Treatment with continuous positive airway pressure is not effective in patients with sleep apnea but no daytime sleepiness: a randomized controlled trial. Ann Int Med. 2001;134:1015-23.
20. Kraiczi H, Hedner J, Peker Y, et al. Comparison of atenolol, amlodipine, enalapril, hydrochlorothiazide, and losartan for antihypertensive treatment in patients with obstructive sleep apnea. Am J Respir Crit Care Med. 2000;161:1423-8.
21. Butler G, Naughton MT, Rahman A, et al. Acute effects of continuous positive airway pressure on heart rate variability in congestive heart failure. J Am Coll Cardiol. 1995;25:672-9.
22. Packer M, Coats AJ, Fowler MB, et al. Carvedilol Prospective Randomized Cumulative Survival Study Group. Effect of carvedilol on survival in severe chronic heart failure. N Engl J Med. 2001;344:1651-8.
23. Gotsopoulos H, Chen C, Qian J, et al. Oral appliance therapy improves symptoms in obstructive sleep apnea. Am J Respir Crit Care Med. 2002;166:743-8.
24. Engleman HM, McDonald JP, Graham D, et al. Continuous positive airway pressure and mandibular repositioning splint. Am J Respir Crit Care Med. 2002;166:855-9.
25. Bittar G, Friedman HS. The arrhythmogenicity of theophylline: a multivariate analysis of clinical determinants. Chest. 1991;99:1415-20.
26. Suissa S, Hemmelgarn B, Blais L, et al. Bronchodilators and acute cardiac death. Am J Respir Crit Care Med. 1996;154:1598-602.
27. Naughton MT, Rahman MA, Hara K, et al. Effect of continuous positive airway pressure on intrathoracic and left ventricular transmural pressures in patients with congestive heart failure. Circulation. 1995;91:1725-31.
28. Mehta S, Liu PP, Fitzgerald FS, et al. Effects of continuous positive airway pressure on cardiac volumes in patients with ischemic and dilated cardiomyopathy. Am J Respir Crit Care Med. 2000;161:128-34.

Emergency and Urgent Care in Heart Failure

Saumitra Ray, Biswarup Sarkar

INTRODUCTION

Acute heart failure (AHF) is among the most common causes for hospitalization in patients older than 65 years of age in the developed world.[1] The number of hospitalizations for heart failure has tripled during the past three decades and is projected to continue to increase because of a convergence of several epidemiologic trends. Previously considered part of the clinical history of chronic heart failure, AHF is increasingly recognized as a distinct disorder with unique epidemiology, pathophysiology, treatments, and outcomes. According to a study published in the National Medical Journal of India in 2010, the estimated prevalence of heart failure due to coronary artery disease (CAD), hypertension, obesity, diabetes, and rheumatic heart disease alone ranged from 1.3 million to 4.6 million.[2,3] The Trivandrum Heart Failure Registry (THFR) enrolled 1,205 admissions for heart failure (834 men, 69%). The mean age was 61.2 years. The most common etiology of heart failure was ischemic heart disease (72%). Heart failure with preserved ejection fraction (HFpEF) constituted 26%.[4] Other studies supported this.[5-7] Acute decompensated heart failure (ADHF) is defined as progression of heart failure necessitating urgent medical care. In-hospital mortality rates of ADHF in the US and Europe range from 4% to 7%. Data from the control arm of published Indian studies in heart failure intervention trials suggest a mortality rate of around 10% over 6 months.[8]

TYPICAL PRESENTATION OF ADHF[9]

Median age: 75 years; hypertension: 72%; diabetes mellitus (DM): 44%; chronic obstructive pulmonary disease (COPD): 31%; chronic kidney disease (CKD): 30%; atrial fibrillation (AF): 31%; reduced EF: ~50%; New York Heart Association (NYHA) class at admission: I: 2%; II: 11%; III: 40%; IV: 47%; systolic blood pressure (SBP) at admission: <90 mm Hg: 2%; 90-140 mm Hg: 48%; >140 mm Hg: 50%.

SENSITIVITY AND SPECIFICITY OF SYMPTOMS AND SIGNS IN AHF[10]

Table 1 summarizes the sensitivity and specificity of the signs and symptoms in acute heart failure.

TABLE 1: Sensitivity and specificity of signs and symptoms of acute heart failure.

	Sensitivity	*Specificity*	*PPV*	*NPV*
Rales (≥1/3 lung fields)	*15*	*89*	*69*	*38*
Ventricular filling murmur (S_3)	62	32	61	33
Ascites (moderate/ massive)	21	92	81	40
Edema (≥2)	41	66	67	40
Orthopnea (≥2 pillows)	*86*	*25*	*66*	*51*
Hepatomegaly (>4 finger breadths)	15	93	78	39
Hepatojugular reflux	*83*	*27*	*65*	*49*
JVP ≥12 mm Hg	*65*	*64*	*75*	*52*
JVP <8 mm Hg	4.3	81	28	33

(JVP: jugular venous pressure; NPV: negative predictive value; PPV: positive predictive value)

MORTALITY AFTER FIRST HOSPITALIZATION FOR HEART FAILURE[11]

In-hospital: 3%, 30 day: 10.4%, 1 year: 22%, 5 years: 40-60%.

Five-year mortality by stage: Stage A: 3%, Stage B: 4%, Stage C: 25%, and Stage D: 80%.

CLASSIFICATION AND COMMON CLINICAL CHARACTERISTICS OF AHF (TABLE 2)

Decompensated Heart Failure

This group is composed of patients with worsening signs and symptoms of congestion on a background of chronic heart failure. The time course of this progression may be acute, subacute, or indolent with gradually worsening symptoms over days to weeks. They may have either preserved or reduced ejection fraction, but cardiac output generally is preserved and blood pressure is within the normal range. Overall, this group represents the largest proportion of patients hospitalized for AHF.

Acute Hypertensive Heart Failure

Hypertension is increasingly recognized as a common feature of the AHF presentation, with 50% of patients presenting with SBP higher than 140 mm Hg and 25% with SBP higher than 160 mm Hg.[2] In this group, hypertension may be triggered by a high sympathetic tone related to dyspnea and accompanying anxiety (reactive hypertension) or acute hypertension with accompanying changes in afterload may be a trigger for decompensation. Both of these mechanisms may be operative in a given patient, and cause-and-effect relationships may be difficult to discern with precision. Epidemiologically, patients in whom acute hypertensive heart failure are more likely to have HFpEF, and women. Frank pulmonary edema is common. Although often strikingly ill at the time of initial presentation, these patients tend to respond well to therapy and have low in-hospital mortality.[3]

Cardiogenic Shock

This group presents with signs and symptoms of organ hypoperfusion despite adequate preload. SBP often (although not always) is decreased, and evidence of frank or impending end-organ dysfunction (renal, hepatic, central nervous system) is common. This type of AHF is relatively uncommon [4% of AHF presentations in EuroHeart Failure Survey II (EHFS II)] in broad community registries but is more common in tertiary care settings.

INITIAL EVALUATION (FIG. 1)[12]

Determine the ejection fraction (preserved or reduced); electrocardiography (ECG)—important to look for underlying ischemia, arrhythmia. Natriuretic peptides (NPs): They have high sensitivity, and normal levels in patients with suspected AHF makes the diagnosis unlikely

TABLE 2: Clinical classification and characterization of acute heart failure.

Clinical classification	*Symptom onset*	*Triggers*	*Signs and symptoms*	*Clinical assessment*	*Course*
Decompensated heart failure	Usually gradual	Noncompliance, ischemia, infections	Peripheral edema, orthopnea, dyspnea on exertion	SBP: Variable CXR: Often clear despite elevated filling pressures	Variable; high rehospitalization rate
Acute hypertensive heart failure	Usually sudden	Hypertension, atrial arrhythmias, ACS	Dyspnea (often severe), tachypnea, tachycardia, rales common	SBP: High (>180/100 mm Hg) CXR: Evidence of pulmonary edema Hypoxemia common	High acuity but often responds quickly to therapy with vasodilators, noninvasive ventilation; low postdischarge mortality
Cardiogenic shock	Variable	Progression of advanced HF or major myocaridal insult (e.g., large-infarct AMI, acute myocarditis)	End-organ hypoperfusion; oliguria, confusion, cool extremities	SBP: Low or low-normal LV function usually severely depressed RV dysfunction common Laboratory evidence of end-organ dysfunction (renal, hepatic)	High inpatient mortality; poor prognosis except with readily reversible cause or mechanical support/ transplantation

(ACS: acute coronary syndrome; AMI: acute myocardial infarction; CXR: chest X-ray; SBP: systolic blood pressure)

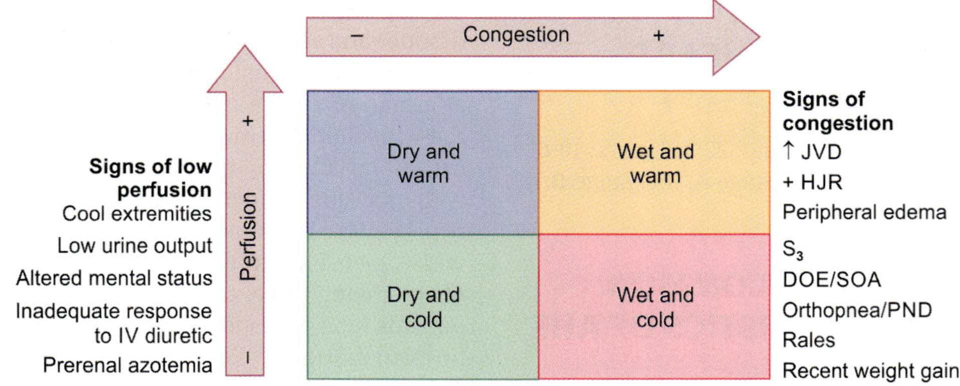

Fig. 1: Initial evaluation of AHF.[10,11]

(↑: increased; +: positive; –: negative; DOE: dyspnea on exertion; HJR: hepatojugular reflux; JVD: jugular venous distension; IV: intravenous; PND: paroxysmal nocturnal dyspnea; S_3: ventricular filling murmur; SOA: shortness of air)

[thresholds: brain natriuretic peptide (BNP) <100 pg/mL, N-terminal-proBNP (NT-proBNP) <300 pg/mL, midregional pro-atrial NP (MR-proANP) <120 pg/mL)]. However, elevated levels of NPs do not automatically confirm the diagnosis of AHF, as they may also be associated with a wide variety of cardiac and noncardiac causes.[13,14]

Troponins and procalcitonin: Measurement of cardiac troponins is useful for detection of acute coronary syndrome (ACS) as the underlying cause of AHF. In acute pulmonary embolism as the underlying cause of acute decompensation, elevated troponins are useful for risk stratification and decision-making. Assessment of procalcitonin levels may be considered in patients with AHF with suspected coexisting infection, particularly for the differential diagnosis of pneumonia and to guide antibiotic therapy.[15]

MANAGEMENT[16]

The overall aims of pharmacological interventions in managing AHF are as follows:

- Immediate aims:
  - To relieve symptoms and optimize the fluid volume status.
  - To restore the respiratory function, gas exchange, and systemic oxygenation.
  - To improve the hemodynamics and end-organ function.
  - To address any underlying cause or precipitant (e.g. myocardial ischemia, arrhythmia, infection, anemia, iatrogenic, etc.).
- Further aims:
  - To identify patients who may benefit from further nonpharmacological therapy in the short-term [e.g. invasive ventilation, ultrafiltration, percutaneous coronary intervention (PCI), and mechanical circulatory support] and medium-term [e.g. cardiac resynchronization therapy (CRT), transplantation).
  - To optimize oral therapy for chronic heart failure [i.e. angiotensin converting enzymes inhibitors (ACEIs) or angiotensin receptor/neprilysin inhibitors (ARNIs), β-blockers, and mineralocorticoid receptor antagonists], once stable and prior to discharge.

INITIAL TREATMENT[9]

Oxygen

Supplemental O_2 may be needed to treat hypoxemia due to pulmonary congestion and/or edema. There is no evidence base to support this approach. O_2 should not be used routinely in patients who are not hypoxic, as this causes vasoconstriction and a reduction in cardiac output, effects which are likely to be detrimental in AHF.

Opiates

Intravenous (IV) morphine (2.5–10 mg IV bolus) can provide a prompt symptomatic improvement, due to several pharmacological properties. First, opiates have a mild anxiolytic effect and reduce distress associated with symptoms. They also have a mild venodilator effect which can help reduce congestion and preload. However, opiates frequently induce nausea and require the coprescription of antiemetic drugs, some of which have undesirable actions, e.g. vasoconstriction. A further unwanted side effect of opiate therapy is a potential depression of the respiratory drive which may precipitate the requirement for invasive ventilation. There is no evidence base to support the use of opiates, and indeed there are some registry data suggesting that opiate use is associated with adverse outcomes.

BASIC TREATMENT STRATEGIES[9]

- *Warm and dry*: Continue PO outpatient treatment [Guideline Determined Medical Therapy (GDMT)]
- *Warm and wet*: Diuretics vasodilators
- *Cold and dry*: Inotropes +/- IV fluids
- *Cold and wet*: Diuretics, inotropes.

Diuresis

- Intravenous loop diuretics:
  - Institute early in the emergency room (ER)
  - Dose should equal or exceed PO dose
  - *Furosemide*: Renally excreted, ~50% orally absorbed; Variable absorption: 10-100% in various patients
  - *Torsemide and bumetanide*: More reliably absorbed in oral doses, most notably in patients with edema of gastrointestinal (GI) tract [right-sided (R) heart failure]. Torsemide/bumetanide is hepatically metabolized and 80-100% orally absorbed.
- Patients on torsemide have less hospitalization and a better quality of life (QOL) than patients treated with furosemide.
- Diuretic tolerance (causes):
  - *Braking*: Decreased response after first dose.
  - *Long-term*: Increased distal reabsorption of sodium; counteracted by concomitant use of thiazide diuretics.
- If a sulfa allergy exists, ethacrynic acid may be used—no sulfa moiety
- If all diuretic strategies are unsuccessful:
  - Ultrafiltration is reasonable (class 2b)
  - Low-dose dopamine (class 2b).

Inotropes

In patients with clinical evidence of hypotension associated with hypoperfusion and obvious evidence of elevated cardiac filling pressures (e.g. elevated jugular venous pressure; elevated pulmonary artery wedge pressure), IV inotropic or vasopressor drugs should be administered to maintain systemic perfusion and preserve end-organ performance while more definitive therapy is considered.

Two types of inotropes (Table 3):

1. *Traditional inotropes*: Dobutamine, milrinone or dopamine. Disadvantages of traditional inotropes—proarrhythmic, probably increase mortality in ischemic patients, ischemic or injured myocardium may "hibernate" as a protective mechanism, inotropes recruit hibernating myocytes and may hasten cell injury or apoptosis, short-term gains appear to be offset by higher mid- and long-term mortality.[17]

TABLE 3: Types of inotropes.

	CO	*PCWP*	*SVR*	*MAP*	*HR*
Dobutamine	↑↑↑	↓/↔	↓	↓/↔	↑/↔
Dopamine–moderate	↑↑	↑/↔	↑/↔	↑↑	↑
Dopamine–high	↑	↑	↑↑↑	↑↑	↑↑
Milrinone	↑↑	↓	↓↓	↓/↔	↑/↔
Levosimendan	↑↑↑	↓↓	↓↓	↓	↑

(CO: cardiac output; HR; heart rate; MAP: mean arterial pressure; PCWP: pulmonary capillary wedge pressure; SVR: systemic vascular resistance)

2. *New inotropes [not approved by Food and Drug Administration (FDA)]*: Levosimendan (calcium sensitizer), omecamtiv mecarbil (cardiac myosin activator), and istaroxime [sodium-potassium adenosine triphosphate (Na/K-ATPase) inhibitor].

Vasodilators

Class IIB recommendation for treatment of ADHF in hypertensive patients and in pulmonary congestion not responsive to initial diuretics and standard heart failure therapy.

Beneficial effects: Decrease BP and improve the efficiency of cardiac work, speed symptom relief, possibly decrease risk for coronary care unit (CCU), mechanical ventilation, and no proven change in mortality.

Nitroglycerin[18]

It is a primary venodilator. It decreased preload and decreased pulmonary congestion. May get rebound tachycardia and 20% patients develop resistance, preferred in ischemia; Less potent arteriolar dilator than nitroprusside.

Advantages: Effective, high comfort level, established safety profile, and cost.

Disadvantages: Rapid tachyphylaxis, frequently underdosed, requires titration in CCU or intermediate care unit (IMCU), dose-limiting toxicities (sx; 20%).

Nitroprusside[18]

It is the primary arteriolar dilator; most useful in patients with marked hypertension or hypertensive emergency; improves symptoms of pulmonary congestion, and signs of peripheral perfusion. Titration of infusion rate is initially based on invasive hemodynamic monitoring. *Nitroprusside toxicities*: Cyanide intoxication—metabolic acidosis; Thiocyanate toxicity—hyperreflexia, seizures, and altered mental status. Serum concentration assay available. *Advantages*: Potent, fine titration.

Disadvantages: Intensive care unit (ICU) and arterial line, thiocyanate toxicity (especially in renal or hepatic insufficiency), and no randomized trials.

Nesiritide

It is recombinant BNP. It has significant vasodilator effect (venous and arterial), natriuretic effect. It causes suppression of renin–angiotensin system (RAS) and catechols and causes indirect increase of cardiac output. It reduces LV filling pressure, variable effect on cardiac output, urine output, and sodium excretion. It is better than diuretics for dyspnea. It has longer half-life (t½) than nitroglycerin or nitroprusside.[19]

Advantages: Faster than nitroglycerin, easy dosing, few side effects, tested in a randomized controlled trial.

Summary

Table 4 summarizes the different treatment strategies for acute heart failure.

EMERGING PHARMACOLOGICAL THERAPIES FOR AHF

Serelaxin

Relaxin is a 53-amino acid endogenous peptide hormone which is a member of the insulin-like growth factor receptor family. In humans, relaxin produces dose-dependent vasodilatation in ex-vivo peripheral resistance arteries, but not pulmonary arteries. In vivo, it increases the renal blood flow and has a modest natriuretic effect in healthy humans. A large randomized placebo-controlled trial of serelaxin (recombinant relaxin-2), in addition to standard therapy, in patients with AHF revealed a significant improvement in one of the coprimary measures of dyspnea and the safety endpoint of 180-day mortality in patients receiving serelaxin. However, despite initial optimism surrounding this trial, this finding was not replicated in the adequately powered RELAX-AHF-2 trial which was presented at the European Society of Cardiology (ESC) Heart Failure Association in May 2017 but has not yet been published.[20]

TABLE 4: Summary of AHF treatment.

	ESC	ACC/AHA	HFSA
Supplemental oxygen	1 C	-	1 C
Opiates	2b B	-	-
IV diuretics	1 C	1 B	1 B
Vasopressin receptor antagonists	-	2b B	-
Nitroglycerin	2a B	2b A	2b B
Sodium nitroprusside	2b B	2b A	2b B
Nesiritide	-	2b A	2b B
Inotropes in cardiogenic shock	2b C	1 C	2b C
Thromboprophylaxis	1 B	1 B	1 B

(ACC: American College of Cardiology; AHA: American Heart Association; ESC: European Society of Cardiology; HFSA: Heart Failure Society of America; IV: intravenous)

Omecamtiv Mecarbil

Omecamtiv mecarbil is a myosin-activating agent which potentiates the excitation-contraction coupling and increases the systolic ejection time, contractility, and stroke volume. In theory, it has no arrhythmogenic potential, given its lack of effect on the phosphodiesterases, intracellular calcium (Ca^2+) concentrations, or myocardial O_2 consumption. Phase II studies in stable heart failure patients have confirmed its ability to increase the stroke volume. The randomized placebo-controlled ATOMIC-AHF (Acute Treatment with Omecamtiv Mecarbil to Increase Contractility in Acute Heart Failure) study examined three doses of omecamtiv mecarbil in patients with AHF given as a 48-hour infusion. The primary endpoint of reduction in dyspnea at 6, 24, and 48 hours was met only in the highest dose group. Tolerability and adverse events were no different to placebo but active treatment was associated with an increase in troponin concentrations.[21]

Ularitide

Ularitide is a synthetic analog of urodilatin, which is an endogenous NP expressed in the kidney. Phase I/II studies showed the parenteral administration of exogenous ularitide in AHF results in reductions in the right atrial pressure, pulmonary capillary wedge pressure (PCWP), and NT-proBNP, with no adverse effect on the renal function. The Trial of Ularitide's Efficacy and Safety in Patients with Acute Heart Failure (TRUE-AHF) was a large (>800 patients) international phase III event-driven trial of ularitide vs. placebo in patients with AHF and preserved blood pressure. Whist the ularitide group displayed a greater reduction in NT-proBNP concentrations, no difference was noted in the clinical course during index admission or in subsequent mortality over a follow-up period of 15 months.[22,23]

Istaroxime

Istaroxime is a novel inotropic agent with concomitant lusitropic properties. It has a dual action of increasing the cytosolic Ca^{2+} concentration through inhibition of the Na/K-ATPase. These effects are not oxygen-dependent, meaning that the myocardial O_2 demand is not increased. Infusion increases the cardiac index. In AHF patients, istaroxime significantly increases the SBP and decreases the heart rate (HR), whilst reducing the PCWP and the LV end diastolic dimension (LVEDD).[24]

GOALS AND STRATEGIES FOR DISCHARGE

During clinical evaluation, patients must maintain SBP ≥90 mm Hg, HR <80 bpm or <100 bpm in cases with AF, and oxygen saturation of ≥95% (≥90% in COPD), without the adverse events of the treatments used (e.g. dizziness or orthostatic hypotension).[25] Discontinuation of inotropes and vasodilators must take place at least 24 hours before disposition and at the same time the patient must maintain stable renal function and sufficient diuresis with oral diuretic regiments. Although NP levels are strongly associated with cardiac dysfunction, studies with NP-guided management have yield mixed results.[26] In all patients hospitalized with heart failure, both with preserved and low ejection fraction, transition from IV to oral diuretics prior to discharge (class I). Minimum 24 hours on PO regimen prior to discharge. Uptitration to recommended dose of guideline-based therapies [ACEI/angiotensin receptor blockers (ARBs), beta-blockers (BBs), aldosterone inhibitor, hydralazine or nitroglycerin as indicated], activity level, follow-up appointments, weight monitoring, what to do if heart failure symptoms worsen.[27,28]

A detailed postdischarge schedule of subsequent visits and further investigations, regarding evaluation for advanced therapies [implantable cardioverter-defibrillator (ICD), CRT, left ventricular assist device (LVAD), cardiac transplant].[29]

REFERENCES

1. Go AS, Mozaffarian D, Roger VL, et al. Heart disease and stroke statistics—2013 update: A report from the American Heart Association. Circulation. 2013;127:e6-e245.
2. Xavier D, Pais P, Devereaux PJ, et al. Treatment and outcomes of acute coronary syndromes in India (CREATE): a prospective analysis of registry data. Lancet. 2008;371:1435-42.
3. Joshi P, Islam S, Pais P, et al. Risk factors for early myocardial infarction in South Asians compared with individuals in other countries. JAMA. 2007;297:286-94.
4. Srinath RK, Shah B, Varghese C, et al. Responding to the threat of chronic diseases in India. Lancet. 2005;366:1744-9.
5. Gupta R, Guptha S, Sharma KK, et al. Regional variations in cardiovascular risk factors in India: India heart watch. World J Cardiol. 2012;4:112-20.
6. Patel V, Chatterji S, Chisholm D, et al. Chronic diseases and injuries in India. Lancet. 2011;377:413-28.
7. Office of the Registrar General of India, New Delhi. (2009). Report on causes of death in India 2001-03. [online] Available from http://censusindia.gov.in/Vital_Statistics/Summary_Report_Death_01_03.pdf. [LAst accessed November, 2019].
8. GBD 2013 Mortality and Causes of Death Collaborators. Global, regional, and national age-sex specific all-cause and cause-specific mortality for 240 causes of death, 1990-2013: a systematic analysis for the Global Burden of Disease Study 2013. Lancet. 2015;385:117-71.
9. Nieminen MS, Brutsaert D, Dickstein K, et al. EuroHeart Failure Survey II (EHFS II): a survey on hospitalized acute heart failure patients: description of population. Eur Heart J. 2006;27:2725-36.
10. Felker GM, Leimberger JD, Califf RM, et al. Risk stratification after hospitalization for decompensated heart failure. J Card Fail. 2004;10:460-6.
11. Nohria A, Tsang SW, Fang JC, et al. Clinical assessment identifies hemodynamic profiles that predict outcomes in patients admitted with heart failure. J Am Coll Cardiol. 2003;41:1797-804.
12. Adams KF Jr, Fonarow GC, Emerman CL, et al. Characteristics and outcomes of patients hospitalized for heart failure in the United States: rationale, design, and preliminary observations from the first 100,000 cases in the Acute Decompensated Heart Failure National Registry (ADHERE). Am Heart J. 2005;149:209-16.
13. Fonarow GC, Abraham WT, Albert NM, et al. Factors identified as precipitating hospital admissions for heart failure and clinical outcomes: findings from OPTIMIZE-HF. Arch Intern Med. 2008;168:847-54.
14. Ponikowski P, Jankowska EA. Pathogenesis and clinical presentation of acute heart failure. Rev Esp Cardiol. 2015;68:331-7.
15. Opasich C, Rapezzi C, Lucci D, et al. Precipitating factors and decision-making processes of short-term worsening heart failure despite "optimal" treatment (from the IN-CHF Registry). Am J Cardiol. 2001;88:382-7.
16. Nieminen MS, Bohm M, Cowie MR, et al. Executive summary of the guidelines on the diagnosis and treatment of acute heart failure: the Task Force on Acute Heart Failure of the European Society of Cardiology. Eur Heart J. 2005;26: 384-416.
17. Cuffe MS, Califf RM, Adams KF, et al. Short-term intravenous milrinone for acute exacerbation of chronic heart failure: a randomized controlled trial. JAMA. 2002;287:1541-7.
18. Cotter G, Metzkor E, Kaluski E. "Randomised trial of high-dose isosorbide dinitrate plus low-dose furosemide versus high-dose furosemide plus low-dose isosorbide dinitrate in severe pulmonary oedema". Lancet. 1998;351:389-93.
19. Kelly JP, Mentz RJ, Hasselblad V, et al. Worsening heart failure during hospitalization for acute heart failure: insights from the Acute Study of Clinical Effectiveness of Nesiritide in Decompensated Heart Failure (ASCEND-HF). Am Heart J. 2015;170:298-305.
20. Diez J. Serelaxin: a novel therapy for acute heart failure with a range of hemodynamic and non-hemodynamic actions. Am J Cardiovasc Drugs. 2014;14:275-85.
21. Teerlink JR, Felker GM, Mcmurray JJ, et al. Acute treatment with omecamtiv mecarbil to increase contractility in acute

heart failure: The ATOMIC-AHF Study. J Am Coll Cardiol. 2016;67:1444-55.
22. Mitrovic V, Lüss H, Nitsche K, et al. Effects of the renal natriuretic peptide urodilatin (ularitide) in patients with decompensated chronic heart failure: a double-blind, placebo-controlled, ascending-dose trial. Am Heart J. 2005;150:1239.
23. Mitrovic V, Seferovic PM, Simeunovic D, et al. Haemodynamic and clinical effects of ularitide in decompensated heart failure. Eur Heart J. 2006;27:2823-32.
24. Micheletti R, Palazzo F, Barassi P, et al. Istaroxime, a stimulator of sarcoplasmic reticulum calcium adenosine triphosphatase isoform 2a activity, as a novel therapeutic approach to heart failure. Am J Cardiol. 2007;99:24A-32.
25. Colucci WS. Pathophysiology of heart failure: Neurohumoral adaptations. UpToDate. 2008;15:3.
26. Colucci WS, Braunwald E. Pathophysiology of heart failure. In: Zipes DP (Ed). Braunwald's Heart Disease: A Textbook of Cardiovascular Medicine, 7th edition. Philadelphia: Elsevier Saunders; 2005. pp. 509-38.
27. Singer, AJ, RH Birkhahn, D Guss, et al. Rapid Emergency Department Heart Failure Outpatients Trial (REDHOT II): a randomized controlled trial of the effect of serial B-type natriuretic peptide testing on patient management. Circ Heart Fail. 2009;2:287-93.
28. Maisel, A, Hollander JE, Guss D, et al. Primary results of the Rapid Emergency Department Heart Failure Outpatient Trial (REDHOT). A multicenter study of B-type natriuretic peptide levels, emergency department decision making, and outcomes in patients presenting with shortness of breath. J Am Coll Cardiol. 2004;44:1328-33.
29. Keren, H, D Burkhoff, P Squara. Evaluation of a noninvasive continuous cardiac output monitoring system based on thoracic bioreactance. Am J Physiol Heart Circ Physiol. 2007;293:H583-9.

CHAPTER 49

Heart Failure Care in ICU

Sadanand Shetty, Milind Phadke, Md Talha Khan Abid

INTRODUCTION

Acute heart failure (AHF) is a complex heterogeneous condition, characterized by rapid onset or acute worsening of symptoms and/or signs of heart failure (HF), associated with elevated plasma levels of natriuretic peptides (NPs).[1] It can be a first occurrence of AHF (de novo) or more frequently, acute decompensation of chronic heart failure (ADHF). De novo AHF is mainly caused by primary cardiac dysfunction [mainly acute coronary syndrome (ACS)], while ADHF may be precipitated by infection, uncontrolled hypertension, rhythm disturbances or noncompliance with the prescribed drugs or diet.[1,2] AHF may present with impaired or preserved left ventricular ejection fraction, or disturbance of right ventricle function. Being a life-threatening medical condition, urgent diagnostic and treatment methods and intensive care (ICU) are of key importance. The critical aspects of management of AHF include rapid evaluation and establishment of diagnosis of AHF, prompt treatment for potentially life-threatening conditions (e.g. shock, respiratory failure), identification and treatment of relevant clinical triggers or conditions [e.g. ACS, acute pulmonary embolism (PE)], risk stratification and clinical profile assessment [based on blood pressure (BP), volume status, and renal function] to implement the most appropriate therapy on urgent basis (Flowchart 1).

MANAGEMENT OF THE PATIENT WITH AHF

Phases of Management

The management of AHF patients may be considered in the context of four phases of treatment with distinct goals.

Phase I: Urgent/Emergent Care

The initial goals in the management of a patient presenting with AHF are to expeditiously establish the diagnosis, treat life-threatening abnormalities, initiate therapies to rapidly provide symptom relief, and identify the etiology and precipitating triggers for the episode of AHF.

Phase II: Hospital Care

The goals for the management during this phase are to complete the diagnostic and acute therapeutic processes initiated at the initial presentation; optimize the patient's hemodynamic profile, volume status, and clinical symptoms; and to initiate or optimize chronic HF therapy.

Phase III: Predischarge Planning

This phase focuses on the goals of evaluating readiness for discharge, optimizing chronic oral therapy, minimizing

Flowchart 1: Algorithm for initial stabilization and management of patients with acute heart failure (AHF).[1]

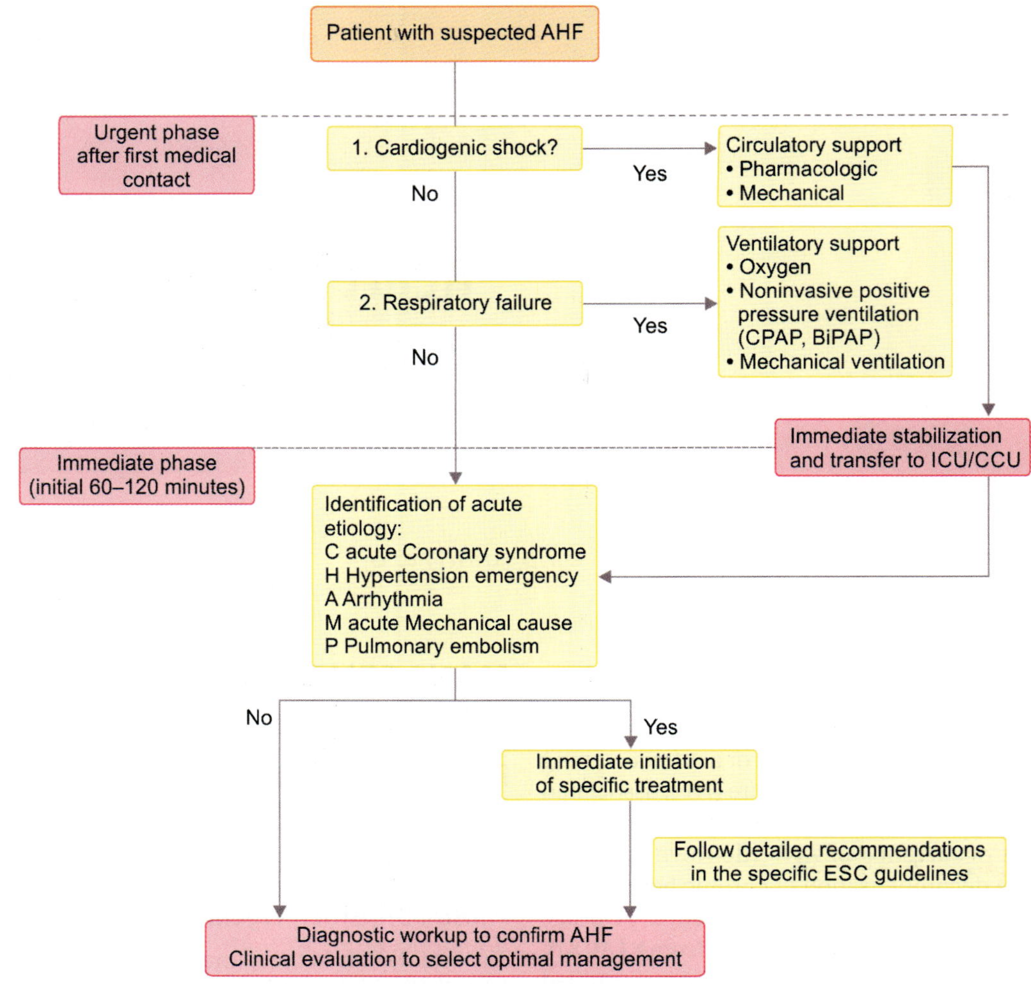

(BiPAP: bilevel positive airway pressure; CCU: coronary care unit; CPAP: continuous positive airway pressure; ESC: European Society of Cardiology; ICU: intensive care unit)

the side effects of treatments, and improving symptoms and survival.

Phase IV: Postdischarge Management

This phase focuses on preventing recurrence of signs and symptoms of HF likely to contribute to the high rates of readmission that are observed in AHF.

In this chapter, we shall be describing the phase I, and partly phase II of management that requires intensive care (ICU).

Managing Heart Failure in ICU

Immediate and concomitant investigation, diagnostic tests, pharmacologic, and nonpharmacologic treatment should be initiated on the arrival (Flowchart 1).

Initial Clinical Evaluation

In the earliest stages of diagnostic workup, emphasis should be given to determination of cardiopulmonary stability based on dyspnea severity, hemodynamic status, and heart rhythm.[1,3] This may be achieved by following assessments:

- Respiratory rate, orthopnea, accessory muscles use in respiration, visible cyanosis, pulse oximetry as objective measurements of respiratory distress.
- Audible rales as sign of pulmonary congestion.
- Systolic blood pressure (SBP) and diastolic BP.
- Heart rate and rhythm.
- Objective determination of body temperature and signs or symptoms of hypoperfusion.

Patients with respiratory failure or hemodynamic compromise or cardiogenic shock (CS) should be urgently transferred to ICU. Next, patient should be examined for

TABLE 1: Common presenting symptoms and signs of decompensated heart failure.

Symptoms	*Signs*
Predominantly related to volume overload	
Dyspnea (exertional, paroxysmal nocturnal dyspnea, orthopnea, or at rest), cough, wheezing	Rales, pleural effusion
Foot and leg discomfort	Peripheral edema (legs, sacral)
Abdominal discomfort/ bloating; early satiety or anorexia	Ascites/increased abdominal girth; right upper quadrant pain or discomfort; hepatomegaly/ splenomegaly; scleral icterus Increased weight Elevated jugular venous pressure, abdominojugular reflux Increasing S_3, accentuated P_2
Predominantly related to hypoperfusion	
Fatigue	Cool extremities
Altered mental status, daytime drowsiness, confusion, or difficulty concentrating	Pallor, dusky skin discoloration, hypotension
Dizziness, presyncope, or syncope	Pulse pressure (narrow) Proportional pulse pressure (low)
Other signs/symptoms of acute heart failure	
Depression	Orthostatic hypotension (hypovolemia)
Sleep disturbances	S_4
Palpitations	Systolic/diastolic cardiac murmurs

(P_2: pulmonic valve closure, S_3 and S_4: two abnormal heart sound)

signs of systemic congestion, such as peripheral edema, jugular venous dilatation, and others (Table 1). Bedside examination of symptoms or signs of congestion ("dry" vs "wet") and/or peripheral hypoperfusion ("warm" vs "cold"),[4] divides the patients into four groups, which helps guide the treatment in the initial phase and also has prognostic value (Flowchart 2).[4-6]

Additional tests used in patients with suspected AHF include:

- *Electrocardiogram (ECG)*: Will exclude ST-segment elevation myocardial infarction (STEMI), arrhythmias, and other high-risk changes.[1]
- *Imaging modalities*:
  - *Chest X-ray*: Identifies pulmonary venous congestion, pleural effusion, interstitial or alveolar edema and cardiomegaly[1] and other alternative etiology of dyspnea, such as pneumonia or other pulmonary infections.
  - *Echocardiography*: Should be done urgently in all patients with CS and when acute life-threatening structural or functional cardiac abnormalities (mechanical complications, aortic dissection, etc.) are suspected.[1] In other cases, it may be performed later during hospitalization.
  - *Chest computed tomography (CT)*: Required if PE is suspected as a precipitating factor of AHF.[7]
- *Laboratory tests*:
  - *Natriuretic peptides*: Plasma NP levels [B-type NP, N-terminal pro-brain NP (BNP), or midregional proatrial NP] have high sensitivity in ruling out AHF as an etiology of dyspnea.
  - *Cardiac troponins*: Useful for detection of ACS as the precipitator of AHF.[1]

The following laboratory assessments should be performed at admission in all patients with AHF—blood urea nitrogen (BUN)/urea, creatinine, electrolytes (sodium, potassium), liver function tests, glucose, complete blood count, thyroid-stimulating hormone (TSH) and arterial blood gas (in severe cases of hemodynamic instability and respiratory distress), and procalcitonin (PCT) for bacterial infections.

Initial Therapy

Oxygen therapy and/or ventilatory support: Oxygen therapy is indicated when peripheral capillary oxygen saturation (SpO_2) is below 90%. However, hyperoxia [fraction of inspired oxygen (FiO2) >0.4] causes vasoconstriction and may decrease coronary and cerebral blood flow and should be avoided.[8]

Noninvasive ventilation [continuous positive airway pressure (CPAP) and bilevel positive pressure ventilation (PPV)] is indicated in patients with respiratory distress and should be initiated urgently, since it reduces respiratory distress and rate of mechanical endotracheal intubation.

Specific Therapies

Diuretics: Loop diuretics (furosemide, torsemide, bumetanide, and ethacrynic acid; Table 2) can lead to excretion of up to 25% of the filtered sodium, and intravenous (IV) administration allows rapid onset of action, typically within 30-60 minutes, resulting in rapid symptom relief in most patients.[9] Based on Diuretic Optimization Strategies Evaluation (DOSE) study, initial doses of approximately 2.5 times the outpatient dose should be considered for patients receiving chronic oral diuretic therapy, with underlying renal dysfunction, or with severe volume overload followed by rapid uptitration,

Flowchart 2: Algorithm for management of patients admitted with acute heart failure (AHF) based on degree of congestion and perfusion.[1]

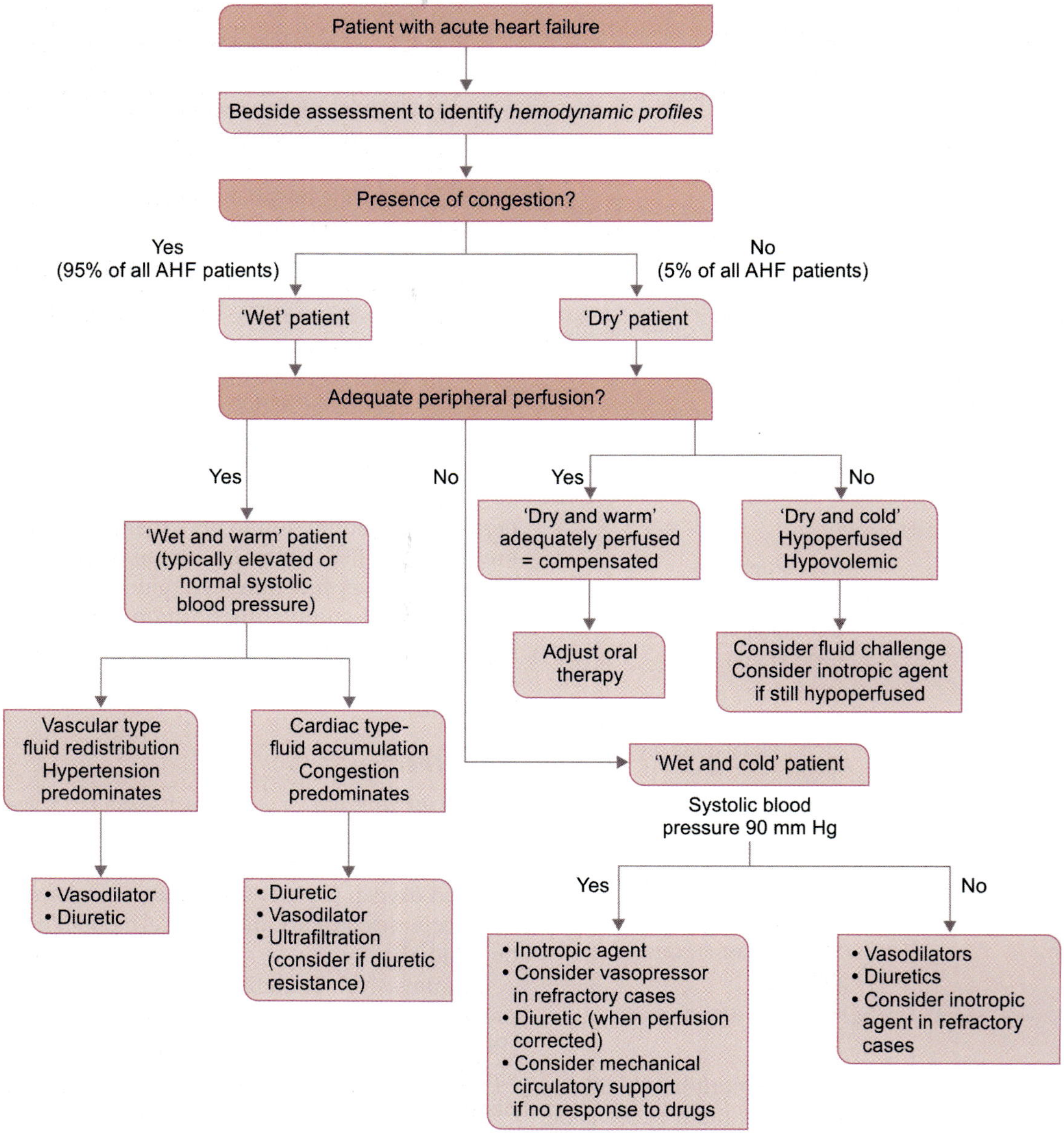

Patient with acute heart failure

Bedside assessment to identify *hemodynamic profiles*

Presence of congestion?

Yes (95% of all AHF patients) → 'Wet' patient

No (5% of all AHF patients) → 'Dry' patient

Adequate peripheral perfusion?

'Wet' patient – Yes → 'Wet and warm' patient (typically elevated or normal systolic blood pressure)

- Vascular type fluid redistribution Hypertension predominates
  - Vasodilator
  - Diuretic
- Cardiac type-fluid accumulation Congestion predominates
  - Diuretic
  - Vasodilator
  - Ultrafiltration (consider if diuretic resistance)

'Wet' patient – No → 'Wet and cold' patient

Systolic blood pressure 90 mm Hg

- Yes
  - Inotropic agent
  - Consider vasopressor in refractory cases
  - Diuretic (when perfusion corrected)
  - Consider mechanical circulatory support if no response to drugs
- No
  - Vasodilators
  - Diuretics
  - Consider inotropic agent in refractory cases

'Dry' patient – Yes → 'Dry and warm' adequately perfused = compensated → Adjust oral therapy

'Dry' patient – No → 'Dry and cold' Hypoperfused Hypovolemic → Consider fluid challenge Consider inotropic agent if still hypoperfused

with doubling of the dose until an effective response is noted. In the setting of diuretic resistance, administration of a thiazide-like diuretic [IV chlorothiazide (500-1,000 mg) or oral metolazone (2.5-10 mg)] that blocks the distal tubule can provide significant augmentation of the diuretic effect.[10] If hypokalemia is a persistent problem, potassium-sparing diuretic, such as spironolactone or eplerenone should be considered and it may also provide synergistic diuretic effects,[11] as well as long-term beneficial effects on outcomes.

Vasodilators: In the absence of hypotension, vasodilators can be used as first-line therapy in combination with diuretics in the management of AHF patients to improve congestive symptoms.[12] Currently available vasodilators include the organic nitrates [nitroglycerin (NTG) and isosorbide dinitrate], sodium nitroprusside, and nesiritide (Table 3). Vasodilators are contraindicated in shock and should be used cautiously when significant mitral or aortic valvular stenosis is suspected or in predominant right ventricular (RV) failure.[3]

TABLE 2: Therapeutic approaches for volume management in acute heart failure (AHF).

Severity of volume overload	*Diuretic*	*Dose (mg)*	*Comments*
Moderate	Furosemide, or	20–40, or up to 2.5 times oral dose	IV administration preferable in symptomatic patients
	Bumetanide, or	0.5–1.0	Titrate dose according to clinical response.
	Torsemide	10–20	Monitor Na^+, K^+ creatinine, BP
Severe	Furosemide, or	40–160, or 2.5 times oral dose 5–40 mg/h infusion	Intravenously
	Bumetanide, or	1–4/0.5–2 mg/h infusion (max, 2–4 mg/h, limit 2–4 h)	Bumetanide and torsemide have higher oral bioavailability than furosemide, but IV administration preferable in AHF.
	Torsemide	20–100/5–20 mg/h	
	Ultrafiltration	200–500 mL/h	Adjust ultrafiltration rate to clinical response; monitor for hypotension; consider hematocrit sensor.
Refractory to loop diuretics	Add HCTZ, or	25–50 twice daily	Combination with loop diuretic may be better than very high dose of loop diuretics alone.
	Metolazone, or	2.5–10 once daily	Metolazone more potent if creatinine clearance <30 mL/min
	Chlorothiazide, or	250–500 mg IV 500–1000 mg PO	
	Spironolactone	25–50 once daily	Spironolactone best choice if patient not in renal failure and normal or low serum K^+, although may not be very potent
In case of alkalosis	Acetazolamide	0.5	Intravenously
Refractory to loop diuretics and thiazides	Add dopamine (renal vasodilation), or dobutamine or milrinone (inotropic agent) Ultrafiltration, or hemodialysis if coexisting renal failure		

(AHF: acute heart failure; BP: blood pressure; HCTZ: hydrochlorothiazide; IV: intravenous; K^+: potassium ion; Na^+: sodium ion)

Nitrates: At low doses are potent venodilators, while at slightly higher doses, nitrates are also arteriolar vasodilators. The starting dose of nitroglycerin is usually 20 µg/min with rapid uptitration occurring every 5-15 minutes in either 20 µg/min increments or doubling of the dose, titrated to the goal of immediate symptom relief, while avoiding hypotension. Oral and sublingual forms can be used for emergent treatment before establishing IV access. The recent use of phosphodiesterase-5 (PDE5) inhibitors (sildenafil, tadalafil, vardenafil) should be ruled out before administration of nitrates, to avoid severe catastrophic hypotension.

Sodium nitroprusside: Sodium nitroprusside induces a balanced reduction in afterload and preload that is exquisitely titratable, because of a very short half-life (seconds to a few minutes), and is particularly effective in the setting of markedly elevated afterload (e.g. hypertensive AHF) and moderate-severe mitral regurgitation.

Nesiritide: Nesiritide (recombinant human BNP) causes potent venous and arterial vasodilation, resulting insignificant reductions in venous and ventricular filling pressures and mild increases in cardiac output.

Inotropes and inodilators: The inotropic drugs and inodilators (inotropic drugs with vasodilatory properties; Table 3) increase cardiac output through cyclic adenosine 3',5'-monophosphate (cAMP)-mediated inotropy and reduce pulmonary capillary wedge pressure (PCWP) through vasodilation. Even the short-term use (hours to few days) of IV inotropes (except for digoxin) is associated

TABLE 3: Intravenous vasoactive agents for treatment of acute heart failure.

Intravenous medication	*Initial dose*	*Effective dose range*	*Comments*
Vasodilators			
Nitroglycerin; glyceryl trinitrate	20 µg/min	40–400 µg/min	Hypotension, headache Tolerance with continuous use after 24 hours
Isosorbide dinitrate	1 mg/h	2–10 mg/h	Hypotension, headache Tolerance with continuous use within 24 hours
Nitroprusside	0.3 µg/kg/min	0.3–5 µg/kg/min (usually <4 µg/kg/min)	Caution in patients with active myocardial ischemia Hypotension; cyanide side effects (nausea, dysphoria); thiocyanate toxicity; light sensitive
Nesiritide	2 µg/kg bolus with 0.010–0.030 µg/kg/min infusion	0.010–0.030 µg/kg/min	Uptitration: 1 µg/kg bolus, then increase infusion rate by 0.005 µg/kg/min no more frequently than every 3 hours, up to maximum of 0.03 µg/kg/min Hypotension, headache (less than with organic nitrates)
Inotropes			
Dobutamine	1–2 µg/kg/min	2–20 µg/kg/min	For inotropy and vasodilation; hypotension, tachycardia, arrhythmias; ?mortality
Dopamine	1–2 µg/kg/min	2–4 µg/kg/min	For inotropy and vasodilation; hypotension, tachycardia, arrhythmias; ?mortality
	4–5 µg/kg/min	5–20 µg/kg/min	For inotropy and vasoconstriction; tachycardia, arrhythmias; ?mortality
Milrinone	25–75 µg/kg bolus over 10–20 min followed by infusion	0.10–0.75 µg/kg/min	For vasodilation and inotropy; hypotension, tachycardia, arrhythmias; renal excretion; ?mortality
Enoximone	0.25–0.75 mg/kg	1.25–7.5 µg/kg/min	For vasodilation and inotropy; hypotension, tachycardia, arrhythmias; ?mortality
Levosimendan	12–24 µg/kg bolus over 10 min followed by infusion	0.5–2.0 µg/kg/min	For vasodilation and inotropy; active metabolite present for ~84 hours; hypotension, tachycardia, arrhythmias; ?mortality
Epinephrine		0.05–0.5 µg/kg/min	For vasoconstriction and inotropy; tachycardia, arrhythmias, end-organ hypoperfusion; ?mortality
Norepinephrine		0.2–1.0 µg/kg/min	For vasoconstriction and inotropy; tachycardia, arrhythmias, end-organ hypoperiusion; ?mortality

with significant side effects, such as hypotension, atrial or ventricular arrhythmias, and an increase in in-hospital[13] and possibly long-term mortality.

Dobutamine: Dobutamine (agonist of both beta-1 and beta-2-adrenergic receptors with variable effects on the alpha receptors) is the most commonly used positive inotrope, despite evidence that it increases mortality.[14]

Dopamine: Dopamine is used as often as dobutamine, presumably as a vasoconstrictor and for its putative effects on renal vasodilation. Initiation of dopamine therapy causes a rapid release of norepinephrine (NE) that can precipitate tachycardia, as well as atrial and ventricular arrhythmias. In addition, intermediate to high doses can cause significant vasoconstriction, precipitating HF, and poor perfusion. Patients should be gradually weaned from higher doses down to 3-5 µg/kg/min and then discontinued, to avoid potential hypotensive effects of low-dose dopamine.

Epinephrine: Epinephrine (full beta receptor agonist with potent inotropic and balanced vasodilator and vasoconstrictor effects) directly increases inotropy independent of myocardial catecholamine stores making it useful in treatment of transplant patients with denervated hearts.

Phosphodiesterase inhibitors: Specific inhibitors of PDE III, such as milrinone and enoximone, have been developed to provide organ-specific improvements in hemodynamics through increasing myocardial and vascular smooth muscle cell cAMP concentrations.

Levosimendan: Levosimendan increases myocardial contractility and produces peripheral vasodilation, through cardiac myofilament calcium sensitization by calcium-dependent (systolic) troponin C binding and activation of vascular smooth muscle potassium channels, respectively.

Vasopressors: These agents should be reserved for patients with marked hypotension in whom central organ hypoperfusion is evident (Table 3). Vasopressors redistribute cardiac output centrally, decrease peripheral perfusion, and may induce end-organ hypoperfusion and tissue necrosis.

Norepinephrine: Norepinephrine (potent agonist of beta-1 and alpha-1 receptors and weaker agonist of beta-2 receptors) is preferred vasopressor for CS.[1] In the Sepsis Occurrence in Acutely Ill Patients II (SOAP II) trial, 1,679 patients with shock were randomized to either dopamine or NE showed a nonstatistical difference increase in mortality, with dopamine associated with a significant increase in arrhythmic events.[15]

Phenylephrine: Phenylephrine (selective alpha-1 receptor agonist with potent direct arterial vasoconstrictor effects) may be used in patients with severe hypotension, particularly due to systemic vasodilation, rather than to a decrease in cardiac output.

Other Pharmacologic Therapies

Digoxin: Digoxin rapidly improves hemodynamics without increasing heart rate or decreasing BP and may be considered in patients with a low BP caused by low cardiac output.[16] Digoxin may be used intravenously with an initial bolus of 0.5 mg, followed by an oral or IV dose of 0.25 mg at least 12 hours after the initial dose. In symptomatic HF patients, digoxin therapy should be continued in addition to other therapies. Ischemia, hypokalemia, or hypomagnesemia may increase the likelihood of developing digitalis intoxication even at the therapeutic doses. Digoxin should not be used in patients with moderate to severe renal impairment, ongoing ischemia, or advanced atrioventricular (AV) block.

Arginine vasopressin (AVP) antagonists: In patients with AHF, volume overload, and persistent hyponatremia at risk for or having active cognitive symptoms, therapy with an AVP antagonist (tolvaptan for oral and conivaptan for IV use) for short-term improvement in serum sodium concentration may be considered. They have not been shown to improve long-term outcomes in HF and are not currently approved for this indication.[17,18].

Calcium channel blockers: CCBs without significant myocardial depressant effects, such as nicardipine and clevidipine, may be used in patients with AHF presenting with severe hypertension refractory to other therapies.

SPECIFIC CLINICAL PRESENTATIONS

Atrial Fibrillation with Fast Ventricular Response

Atrial fibrillation (AF) is the most common tachyarrhythmia requiring treatment in patients with AHF. Ventricular response usually decreases in parallel with the relief of dyspnea, and decreased sympathetic drive, however additional therapy may be required. Immediate cardioversion is generally not indicated, except in the unstable patient, because of the high rate of recurrent AF in significantly decompensated patients. In patients with systolic dysfunction, IV digoxin (in the absence of an accessory pathway), cautious use of beta-adrenergic blocker therapy or amiodarone may be used.

Right Ventricular Heart Failure

The most common cause of right ventricular heart failure (RVHF) in AHF is left-sided failure. Isolated RVHF is relatively rare and is usually caused by acute RV infarction, acute PE, or severe pulmonary hypertension. Acute RV infarction is best treated with early reperfusion, whereas hemodynamically significant PE may be treated with thrombolytics. Hemodynamic stabilization by optimizing central venous pressure (CVP) with monitored fluid loading (target CVP, approximately 10-12 mm Hg), and increasing RV systolic function with IV inotropic support may be necessary.[19] Selective pulmonary artery vasodilation by inhaled [nitric oxide (NO), prostacyclin analogs] or IV (prostacyclin analogs, sildenafil) agents may improve RV function through decreased afterload. If the patient is mechanically ventilated, normoxia and hypocarbia should be the goals using moderate tidal volumes (approximately 8 mL/kg) and as low a positive end-expiratory pressure (PEEP) as possible (<12 cm H_2O) to maintain moderate plateau pressures.

Acute Coronary Syndromes

Acute coronary syndromes may be the underlying trigger in patients presenting with AHF, but the diagnosis is confounded by the high prevalence of elevated troponins in AHF itself. These patients may present with chest discomfort, electrocardiographic changes consistent with ischemia, and elevated serum troponin. Aggressive therapy for ACS should be rapidly instituted. In the absence of CS, inodilators should be avoided in patients with ACS and with significant asymptomatic coronary artery disease (CAD), as experimental data suggests that inodilators can cause necrosis of ischemic and hibernating myocardium.

Cardiogenic Shock

Cardiogenic shock is characterized by hypotension (SBP <80 mm Hg) lasting more than 30 minutes, associated with severe reduction of cardiac index (usually <1.8 L/min/m^2) despite adequate LV filling pressure (PCWP >18 mm Hg), resulting in organ hypoperfusion. CS occurs in less than 4% of the AHF patients in EuroHeart Failure Survey II (EHFSII),[20] most of whom had myocardial infarction (MI). Mechanical complications of acute myocardial infarction (AMI) such as mitral regurgitation, cardiac rupture with ventricular septal defect or tamponade, and isolated RV infarct may also be caused in this setting. IV inotropes, even vasoconstrictors may be required with mechanical circulatory support, such as intraaortic balloon pump (IABP) or left ventricular assist device (LVAD), for critical refractory cases, as a bridge to heart transplant or other mechanical intervention.

Cardiorenal Syndrome

Defined as an increase in serum creatinine of more than 0.3 mg/dL [or 25% decrease in glomerular filtration rate (GFR)] despite evidence of persistent clinical or hemodynamic congestion, the syndrome occurs in approximately 25-35% of patients admitted with AHF, and is associated with longer hospital stay and higher postdischarge mortality.[21] Though hypotension is an important factor, arterial underfilling from overdiuresis or low cardiac output does not appear to be the most frequent primary cause of worsening renal function. Estimated GFR should be calculated in AHF patients as absolute serum creatinine concentrations can be misleading. Vasodilators, either IV (nitroglycerin or nitroprusside) or oral (isosorbide dinitrate and hydralazine) should be used, and renin-angiotensin-aldosterone system (RAAS) inhibitors should be discontinued, if there is progressive deterioration of renal function [blood urea nitrogen (BUN) >80 mg/dL and creatinine >3 mg/dL] or hyperkalemia. Profound diuretic resistance is seen and increasing doses of diuretics are typically required. Ultrafiltration is often considered in this scenario, however clinical trial data have not supported the efficacy or safety of this approach. Overall, cardiorenal syndrome is one of the greatest therapeutic challenges in patients of AHF.

Peripartum Cardiomyopathy

Peripartum cardiomyopathy (PPCM) should be suspected in any female presenting in late pregnancy or, the early postpartum period with features of AHF. Patients usually have LV systolic dysfunction [left ventricular ejection fraction (LVEF) <45% or fractional shortening <30%, or both], though RV dysfunction can also be seen. Standard treatments for HF with reduced ejection fraction are indicated in PPCM, with special attention to avoiding adverse fetal effects in women who are still pregnant. If hemodynamics permit, β-blockers should be used, especially β1 selective ones (e.g. metoprolol tartrate) to avoid stimulating uterine contraction through β2 innervation. Currently, the addition of bromocriptine to standard treatments for HF may be best justified in women with PPCM who have severe cardiomyopathy (LVEF <25%) or CS (or both).[22] Thromboembolism is a relatively common complication and anticoagulation should be considered especially in patients who are on bromocriptine.

CONCLUSION

Acute heart failure is one of the most challenging and life-threatening cardiovascular problems, with unacceptably high postdischarge rehospitalization and mortality rates. Despite extensive research and advances, valid therapeutic options are still missing due to a lack of evidence, and most patients are still treated primarily with IV loop diuretics. Currently, management primarily consists of treating the manifestations of the syndrome rather than central pathophysiologic causes. AHF being a heterogeneous condition, it is unlikely that a "one therapy fits all", and treatment should be individualized. Continued efforts to improve and standardize process of care, optimize therapy, and postdischarge follow up, will potentially allow us to better utilize currently available therapies to improve outcomes from this highly morbid condition.

REFERENCES

1. Ponikowski P, Voors AA, Anker SD, et al. 2016 ESC Guidelines for the diagnosis and treatment of acute and chronic heart failure: The Task Force for the diagnosis and treatment of acute and chronic heart failure of the European Society of Cardiology (ESC) developed with the special contribution of the Heart Failure Association (HFA) of the ESC. Eur Heart J. 2016;37:2129-200.
2. Yancy CW, Jessup M, Bozkurt B, et al. 2013 ACCF/AHA guideline for the management of heart failure: a report of the American College of Cardiology Foundation/American Heart Association Task Force on practice guidelines. Circulation. 2013;128:e240-327.
3. Mebazaa A, Tolppanen H, Mueller C, et al. Acute heart failure and cardiogenic shock: a multidisciplinary practical guidance. Intensive Care Med. 2016;42:147-63.
4. Nohria A, Lewis E, Stevenson LW. Medical management of advanced heart failure. JAMA. 2002;287:628-40.
5. Stevenson LW. Design of therapy for advanced heart failure. Eur J Heart Fail. 2005;7:323-31.

6. Nohria A, Tsang SW, Fang JC, et al. Clinical assessment identifies hemodynamic profiles that predict outcomes in patients admitted with heart failure. J Am Coll Cardiol. 2003;41:1797-804.
7. Konstantinides SV, Torbicki A, Agnelli G, et al. 2014 ESC guidelines on the diagnosis and management of acute pulmonary embolism. Eur Heart J. 2014;35:3033-73.
8. Branson RD, Johannigman JA. Pre-hospital oxygen therapy. Respir Care. 2013;58:86-97.
9. Felker GM, Mentz RJ. Diuretics and ultrafiltration in acute decompensated heart failure. J Am Coll Cardiol. 2012;59:2145-53.
10. Jentzer JC, DeWald TA, Hernandez AF. Combination of loop diuretics with thiazide-type diuretics in heart failure. J Am Coll Cardiol. 2010;56:1527-34.
11. Bansal S, Lindenfeld J, Schrier RW. Sodium retention in heart failure and cirrhosis. Circ Heart Fail. 2009;2:370-6.
12. Singh A, Laribi S, Teerlink JR, et al. Agents with vasodilator properties in acute heart failure. Eur Heart J. 2017;38: 317-25.
13. Mebazaa A, Parissis J, Porcher R, et al. Short-term survival by treatment among patients hospitalized with acute heart failure: the global ALARM-HF registry using propensity scoring methods. Intensive Care Med. 2011;37:290-301.
14. Coletta AP, Cleland JG, Freemantle N, et al. Clinical trials update from the European Society of Cardiology Heart Failure meeting: SHAPE, BRING-UP 2 VAS, COLA II, FOSIDIAL, BETACAR, CASINO and meta-analysis of cardiac resynchronisation therapy. Eur J Heart Fail. 2004;6:673-6.
15. De Backer D, Biston P, Devriendt J, et al. Comparison of dopamine and norepinephrine in the treatment of shock. N Engl J Med. 2010;362:779-89.
16. Gheorghiade M, Braunwald E. Reconsidering the role for digoxin in the management of acute heart failure syndromes. JAMA. 2009;302:2146-7.
17. Gheorghiade M, Konstam MA, Burnett JC Jr, et al. Short-term clinical effects of tolvaptan, an oral vasopressin antagonist, in patients hospitalized for heart failure: the EVEREST clinical status trials. JAMA. 2007;297:1332-43.
18. Konstam MA, Gheorghiade M, Burnett JC Jr, et al. Effects of oral tolvaptan in patients hospitalized for worsening heart failure: the EVEREST outcome trial. JAMA. 2007;297:1319-31.
19. Green EM, Givertz MM. Management of acute right ventricular failure in the intensive care unit. Curr Heart Fail Rep. 2012;9:228-35.
20. Nieminen MS, Brutsaert D, Dickstein K, et al. EuroHeart Failure Survey II (EHFS II): a survey on hospitalized acute heart failure patients: description of population. Eur Heart J. 2006;27:2725-36.
21. Damman K, Testani JM. The kidney in heart failure: an update. Eur Heart J. 2015;36:1437-44.
22. Regitz-Zagrosek V, Roos-Hesselink JW, Bauersachs J, et al. ESC Scientific Document Group 2018 ESC Guidelines for the management of cardiovascular diseases during pregnancy. Eur Heart J. 2018;39:3165-241.

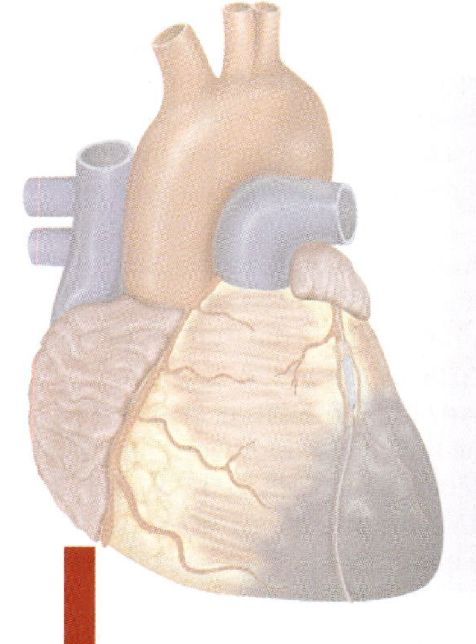

Heart Failure and Critical Care

Yatin Mehta, Ajmer Singh

INTRODUCTION

Heart failure (HF) is a complex clinical syndrome that results from any structural or functional impairment of ventricular filling or ejection of blood. HF is the most common cause of hospital admission after 65 years of age. 2013 American College of Cardiology Foundation (ACCF)/American Heart Association (AHA) guidelines for the management of HF have classified HF into two major categories: (1) HF with reduced (≤40%) ejection fraction (EF) or HFrEF; and (2) HF with preserved (≥50%) EF (HFpEF).[1] Patients with acute decompensated HF (ADHF) require an unplanned emergency room visit and/or hospitalization in an intensive care unit (ICU). The cardinal feature of ADHF, irrespective of underlying etiology, is pulmonary or systemic congestion due to increased filling pressure. A preliminary observation from the first 100,000 cases in ADHF National Registry (ADHERE) indicates that in-patient and post-discharge mortality rates after HF are 5% and 10% respectively.[2] In contrast to chronic HF, patients with *de-novo* HF are more likely to present with pulmonary edema or cardiogenic shock and need admission in an ICU.

CRITERIA FOR ADMISSION TO HOSPITAL AND ICU

The precipitating factors, etiology, pathophysiology, and clinical presentation of HF have been described in the previous chapters. Admission to the hospital should be considered in the event of—(1) worsened pulmonary or systemic congestion even without weight gain or dyspnea; (2) major electrolyte imbalance; (3) associated comorbid conditions like pneumonia, pulmonary embolism, diabetic ketoacidosis, transient ischemic attack or stroke; and (4) repeated implantable cardioverter-defibrillator (ICD) firings. Admission to ICU is recommended for patients with ADHF who have—(1) evidence of severely decompensated HF including hypotension [systolic blood pressure (BP) <90 mm Hg], hypertension (systolic BP >210 mm Hg), heart rate <40 or >130 beats/min, worsening renal function, or altered sensorium; (2) impending respiratory failure with oxygen saturation <90%; (3) hemodynamically significant arrhythmia including new-onset atrial fibrillation (AF); (4) acute coronary syndrome; and (5) need for continuous vasodilator/inotropic support/mechanical circulatory support (MCS).[3] Decompensation in HF due to a respiratory etiology, ischemia, or renal dysfunction is associated with a longer ICU stay and higher in-hospital mortality, compared to decompensation resulting from uncontrolled hypertension or medication nonadherence.

INITIAL AND FURTHER EVALUATION

Initial evaluation of a patient with HF includes a detailed clinical history (hypertension, use of diuretics, ischemic heart disease, and familial cardiomyopathy), physical examination, electrocardiogram (ECG), and chest X-ray. Cardiovascular examination may reveal narrow pulse pressure, displaced apical impulse, S_3 gallop, and jugular venous distension. A positive hepatojugular reflux suggests fluid overload and a pulmonary capillary wedge pressure (PCWP) of >15 mm Hg in the absence of right HF. BP should be measured in both supine and upright positions, because orthostatic hypotension suggests volume depletion or excess vasodilation from medications. Laboratory tests include measurement of plasma natriuretic peptide (NP) level, cardiac troponin, complete blood count, blood urea nitrogen, creatinine, electrolytes, glucose, liver function tests, and thyroid profile. In acute HF, patients <50 years of age typically have N-terminal pro-B-type natriuretic peptide (NT-proBNP) of >450 pg/mL, 50-75 years have NT-proBNP of >900 pg/mL, and patients >75 years old typically have NT-proBNP of >1,800 pg/mL.[4] Use of NPs is recommended to rule out HF, but not to establish the diagnosis of HF. Plasma NP levels may be disproportionately high in patients with AF, old age, and renal failure, while they may be low in obese patients. An abnormal ECG may provide clue to the etiology [e.g. myocardial infarction (MI)], and findings on the ECG might provide indications for therapy [e.g. anticoagulation for AF, pacing for bradycardia, cardiac resynchronized therapy (CRT) if broadened QRS complex]. Chest X-ray may show florid alveolar edema, interstitial edema, pulmonic vessel cephalization, Kerley B lines, basal pleural effusions, or cardiomegaly in a patient with HF, particularly in the acute setting. Two-dimensional echocardiography with Doppler is the most widely used test in patients with suspected HF to establish the diagnosis. It provides information on chamber volumes, ventricular function (systolic and diastolic), regional and global wall motion abnormalities, EF, wall thickness, valve function, and pulmonary hypertension.[5] For the assessment of LV systolic function, LVEF is measured using modified biplane Simpson's rule. Assessment of LV diastolic function is important in patients with HFpEF, and echocardiography is the best modality to assess diastolic dysfunction. Cardiac catheterization criteria for the diagnosis of diastolic HF include: an increase in LV end-diastolic pressure (LVEDP) >16 mm Hg with preserved LV systolic function and normal ventricular volumes. The key alterations that occur in diastolic HF include left atrial (LA) enlargement (LA volume index > 34 mL/m^2), LV hypertrophy, E/e' >14, septal e' velocity <7 cm/s, lateral e' velocity <10 cm/s, and tricuspid regurgitation systolic jet velocity >2.8 m/s.[6] Assessment of right ventricular (RV) function includes measurement of right atrium (RA)/RV dimensions, pulmonary artery pressure (PAP), and an estimation of RV systolic function. Echocardiography is helpful in patients with hemodynamic instability to rule out aortic dissection, pulmonary embolism, and mechanical complications of MI such as mitral regurgitation or ventricular septal rupture.

Coronary angiography is recommended in patients with HF who suffer from unstable angina despite medical therapy, and who have had an aborted cardiac arrest. Right heart catheterization with pulmonary artery catheter (PAC) is recommended in patients of severe HF being considered for cardiac surgery, heart transplantation or MCS. The ESCAPE (Evaluation Study of Congestive Heart Failure and Pulmonary Artery Catheterization) trial, which included 433 patients, showed that the addition of PAC to a careful clinical assessment increased adverse events, but did not affect hospitalization or overall mortality.[7] Invasive hemodynamic monitoring should be considered in selected patients admitted to ICU with persistent symptoms refractory to standard therapies or those who require parenteral vasoactive medications.

TREATMENT

Acute decompensated HF is life-threatening condition that requires urgent admission to the hospital, thorough evaluation, and initiation of appropriate therapy (Fig. 1). The goals of management include relief of symptoms, restoration of hemodynamic stability, ensuring oxygenation, and treatment of precipitating cause. Physical examination will reveal whether the patient has symptoms or signs of congestion (dry or wet if absent or present) or hypoperfusion (warm or cold if absent or present) to guide therapy. Oxygen therapy is recommended in patients with arterial oxygen saturation (SpO_2) of <90% or PaO_2 of <60 mm Hg.

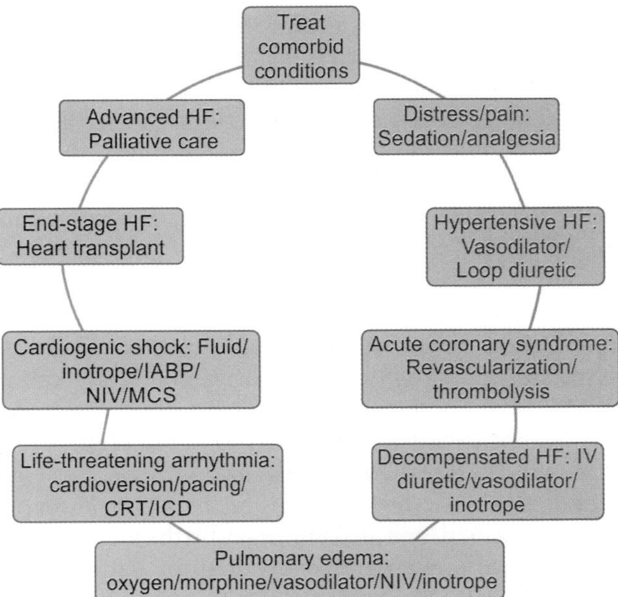

Fig. 1: Treatment options for hospitalized heart failure patients. (CRT: cardiac resynchronization therapy; HF: heart failure; IABP: intraaortic balloon pump; ICD: implantable cardioverter-defibrillator; IV: intravenous; MCS: mechanical circulatory support; NIV: noninvasive ventilation)

Noninvasive ventilation (NIV) in the form of continuous positive airway pressure (CPAP) or bilevel positive pressure ventilation (BiPAP) should be considered in patients with respiratory distress, pulmonary edema, and acidemia to improve minute ventilation. Endotracheal intubation and mechanical ventilation are recommended in patients with respiratory failure (PaO_2 <60 mm Hg, $PaCO_2$ >50 mm Hg, pH <7.35), reduced consciousness, and physical exhaustion who cannot be managed noninvasively. Use of opiates, such as morphine may be considered in patients of ADHF with dyspnea and pulmonary edema. However, in ADHERE trial, use of morphine was associated with greater frequency of mechanical ventilation, prolonged hospitalization, and higher mortality.[2] Intravenous loop diuretics (20-40 mg of furosemide or 10-20 mg of torasemide) are recommended for all patients of acute HF admitted with features of fluid overload. Diuretics increase renal sodium and water excretion and provide symptomatic relief in patients with fluid overload and congestion. In the Diuretic Optimization Strategies Evaluation (DOSE) trial, there were no statistically significant differences in symptom relief and creatinine levels in bolus vs continuous diuretic infusion and in high-dose vs low-dose groups.[8] Analysis of ADHERE trial showed that patients receiving the lower doses of loop diuretics had a lower risk of adverse renal effects, prolonged hospitalization, ICU stay, and in-hospital mortality. If diuretic agents do not provide the desired effect, ultrafiltration may be considered. Vasodilators are useful in hypertensive HF, but should be used with caution in patients with stenotic valvular lesions. The recommended drugs and dosages for vasodilators in HF include: nitroglycerine at the rate of 10-100 μg/min, isosorbide dinitrate at the rate of 1-10 mg/h, sodium nitroprusside at the rate of 0.3-5 μg/kg/min, nesiritide at the rate of 2 μg/kg bolus followed by 0.01 μg/kg/min. Vasopressin antagonist such as tolvaptan may be used to treat patients with fluid overload and hyponatremia. Among the newer drugs for treatment of HF, angiotensin receptor neprilysin inhibitor (ARNI) has shown beneficial effects in terms of BP lowering efficacy, improved cardiac biomarkers, cardiac remodeling, and improved prognosis.[9] Valsartan is the prototype ARNI drug, and is still known as LCZ696. A combination sacubitril with valsartan has been extensively used in both HFrEF and HFpEF. One such trial (PARADIGM), consisting of 8,442 patients, compared LCZ696 with enalapril and found 21% lower rate of hospitalization, and lesser mortality in the former group.

Inotropes are generally reserved for patients with hypotensive HF, associated with severe reduction in cardiac output and organ perfusion (cardiogenic shock). All patients with cardiogenic shock should be transferred to a tertiary care center which has a facility of cardiac catheterization, cardiac ICU and MCS. The routine use of inotropic agents in patients with acute HF is not recommended, as these agents may increase myocardial oxygen consumption, induce arrhythmia, and affect regional blood flow. Short-term use of inotropic agents, in the lowest possible doses, however may be considered for patients with hypotension and hypoperfusion until definitive therapy is available or the precipitating cause is removed. The commonly used inotropes include: dobutamine (2-20 μg/kg/min), dopamine (3-5 μg/kg/min), epinephrine (0.05-0.5 μg/kg/min), milrinone (0.375-0.75 μg/kg/min after a bolus of 50 μg/kg), and levosimendan (0.05-0.2 μg/kg/min). Dobutamine is the most commonly used agent, while phosphodiesterase (PDE) III-inhibitors may be another option in nonischemic patients. A comparison of dobutamine vs milrinone in hospitalized patients awaiting heart transplantation did not show any difference within two groups in terms of ventricular arrhythmia, need for additional vasodilator/inotrope/MCS therapy or death.[10] Levosimendan, a calcium-channel sensitizer, in combination with vasopressors may be used to improve cardiovascular hemodynamics without risk of producing hypotension. Vasopressors, such as norepinephrine (at the rate of 0.2-1 μg/kg/min) may be considered in patients with cardiogenic shock to increase BP and vital organ perfusion. Thromboprophylaxis with unfractioned heparin or low-molecular-weight heparin (LMWH) is recommended unless contraindicated, to reduce the risk of deep vein thrombosis and pulmonary embolism in patients who are not anticoagulated. Patients with HF and AF generally need anticoagulation; the risk–benefit ratio should be evaluated by CHA_2DS_2-VASc and HAS-BLED scores.[11]

Nonpharmacological treatment of HFrEF includes use of ICD, CRT, intraaortic balloon pump (IABP), and MCS. An ICD reduces the risk of sudden cardiac death in patients with HFrEF.[11] Secondary prevention of sudden cardiac death by use of ICD is recommended in patients who have recovered from ventricular arrhythmia causing hemodynamic instability, and who are expected to survive for >1 year. Primary prevention is recommended to reduce the risk of sudden death and all-cause mortality in patients with symptomatic HF despite optimum medical therapy, LVEF ≤35%, or those with dilated cardiomyopathy. CRT improves symptoms and cardiac performance in appropriately selected patients. CRT should be considered in symptomatic patients of HF in sinus rhythm with QRS duration of 130-149 ms; and is recommended in patients with QRS duration of ≥150 ms, left bundle branch block or high-degree atrioventricular block with LVEF ≤35%.[12]

An IABP is used to support the circulation in patients with myocardial ischemia or infarction before, during, or after percutaneous or surgical revascularization, to treat cardiogenic shock resulting from acute MI. Percutaneous or surgical revascularization is recommended in patients with HF, who present with angina and suitable coronary anatomy. Transcatheter aortic valve implantation (TAVI) should be considered if HF is caused by severe aortic stenosis in patients unsuitable for surgical aortic valve replacement.

Use of MCS is recommended for patients with HF who cannot be stabilized on medical therapy. The short-term MCS devices include IABP and extracorporeal membrane oxygenation (ECMO), while long-term devices include LA to femoral arterial bypass (TandemHeart), transvalvular aortic percutaneous assist device (Impella Systems), and ventricular assist device (VAD). MCS devices help unload the failing ventricles and maintain sufficient end-organ perfusion. The terms describing various indications for MCS include: (1) *bridge to decision*: use of short-term MCS in patients with cardiogenic shock until hemodynamics and end-organ perfusion are stabilized; (2) *bridge to candidacy*: use of long-term devices to make an ineligible patient eligible for heart transplantation; (iii) *bridge to transplantation*: use of MCS till donor organ becomes available; (iv) *bridge to recovery*: use of MCS until cardiac function improves sufficiently to remove MCS; (v) *destination therapy*: use of VAD as an alternative to transplantation in patients ineligible for transplantation.[13] Continuous-flow MCS devices are smaller, more durable, safer, and more effective for treating patients with severe HF than their pulsatile-flow predecessors.

Cardiac transplantation should be considered in patients with end-stage HF with severe symptoms, when no alternative therapeutic option is available. The patient should be motivated, well-informed, emotionally stable, and capable of complying with the intensive treatment and regular follow-up. Contraindication for cardiac transplantation include malignancy, active infection, severe peripheral arterial or cerebrovascular disease, pulmonary hypertension, irreversible renal dysfunction, and alcohol or drug abuse.[14]

For patients with HFpEF, no specific therapy has been convincingly shown to reduce morbidity and mortality. Most of these patients are elderly, highly symptomatic, and have poor quality of life, therefore the goals of treatment are to alleviate symptoms and to improve quality of life. General guidelines for patients with HFpEF include regular moderate activity, aerobic exercises, smoking cessation, weight reduction, fluid restriction (up to 1.5-2 L/day), sodium restriction, and management of comorbidities. The specific therapies include diuretics for systemic or pulmonary congestion, vasodilators for hypertensive HF, anticoagulation for chronic AF, and angiotensin converting enzyme inhibitors or angiotensin receptor blockers for control of BP.

CONCLUSION

Criteria for discharge from the ICU include euvolemia, transition from intravenous to oral diuretics, stable hemodynamics, absence of postural hypotension, normal electrolytes, and stable renal parameters for at least 24 hours. Patient and family must be educated about diet, medications, activity level, weight monitoring, self-care, and what to do if HF symptoms worsen. When life expectancy is limited, goals of care are palliative and focused on management of symptoms. End-of-life issues should be discussed with the patient, key members of the family, and primary care physician.[15] It is assumed that management of HF with nonpharmacological, modern pharmacological, and surgical therapies can substantially reduce the morbidity and mortality. Future research should be aimed to identify the monitoring and management strategies that improve quality of life and prolong survival in patients with HF.

REFERENCES

1. Yancy CW, Jessup M, Bozkurt B, et al. 2013 ACCF/AHA guideline for the management of heart failure: a report of the American College of Cardiology Foundation/American Heart Association Task Force on Practice Guidelines. Circulation. 2013;128:1810-52.
2. Adams KF Jr, Fonarow GC, Emerman CL, et al. Characteristics and outcomes of patients hospitalized for heart failure in the United States: rationale, design, and preliminary observations from the first 100,000 cases in the Acute Decompensated Heart Failure National Registry (ADHERE). ADHERE Scientific Advisory Committee and Investigators. Am Heart J. 2005;149:209-16.
3. Ponikowski P, Voors AA, Anker SD, et al. 2016 ESC guidelines for the diagnosis and treatment of acute and chronic heart failure: The task force for the diagnosis and treatment of acute and chronic heart failure of the European Society of Cardiology (ESC). Eur Heart J. 2016;37:2129-200.
4. Maisel A, Mueller C, Adams K, et al. State of the art: using natriuretic peptide levels in clinical practice. Eur J Heart Fail. 2008;10:824-39.
5. Paulus WJ, Tschope C, Sanderson JE, et al. How to diagnose diastolic heart failure: a consensus statement on the diagnosis of heart failure with normal left ventricular ejection fraction by the Heart Failure and Echocardiography Associations of the European Society of Cardiology. Eur Heart J. 2007;28:2539-50.
6. Nagueh SF, Smiseth OA, Appleton CP, et al. Recommendations for the evaluation of left ventricular diastolic function by echocardiography: An update from the American Society of Echocardiography and the European Association of Cardiovascular Imaging. J Am Soc Echocardiogr. 2016;29:277-314.
7. Binanay C, Califf RM, Hasselblad V, et al. Evaluation study of congestive heart failure and pulmonary artery catheterization effectiveness: the ESCAPE trial. JAMA. 2005;294:1625-33.

8. Felker GM, Lee KL, Bull DA, et al. Diuretic strategies in patients with acute decompensated heart failure. N Engl J Med. 2011;364:797-805.
9. Volpe M, Tocci G, Battistoni A, et al. Angiotensin II receptor blocker neprilysin inhibitor (ARNI): New avenues in cardiovascular therapy. High Blood Press Cardiovasc Prev. 2015;22:241-6.
10. Aranda JM Jr, Schofield RS, Pauly DF, et al. Comparison of dobutamine versus milrinone therapy in hospitalized patients awaiting cardiac transplantation: a prospective, randomized trial. Am Heart J. 2003;145:324-9.
11. Kirchof P, Benussi S, Kotecha D, et al. 2016 ESC Guidelines for the management of atrial fibrillation developed in collaboration with EACTS. Eur Heart J. 2016;37:2893-962.
12. Theuns DA, Smith T, Hunink MG, et al. Effectiveness of prophylactic implantation of cardioverter-defibrillators without cardiac resynchronization therapy in patients with ischaemic or non-ischaemic heart disease: a systematic review and meta-analysis. Europace. 2010;12: 1564-70.
13. Stewart GC, Givertz MM. Mechanical circulatory support for advanced heart failure: patients and technology in evolution. Circulation. 2012;125:1304-15.
14. Mehra MR, Canter CE, Hannan MM, et al. The 2016 International Society for Heart Lung Transplantation listing criteria for heart transplantation: a 10-year update. J Heart Lung Transplant. 2016;35:1-23.
15. Wiegand DL. Withdrawal of life-sustaining therapy after sudden, unexpected life-threatening illness or injury: interactions between patients' families, healthcare providers, and the healthcare system. Am J Crit Care. 2006;15:178-87.

SECTION 2

Echo, Imaging and Heart Failure

CHAPTER

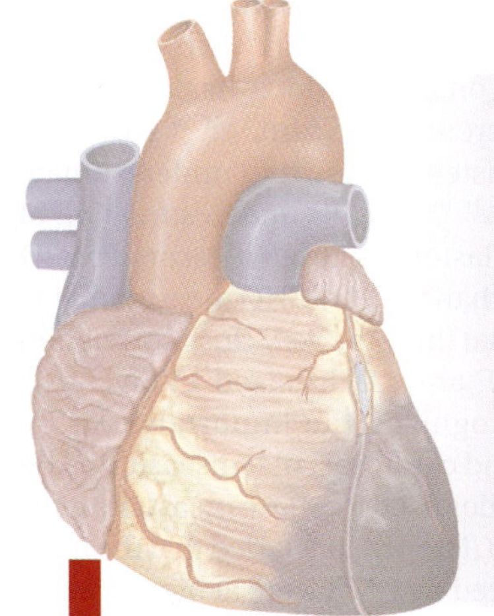

Usefulness of Three-dimensional Echocardiography in Heart Failure

Amit Nanda, Rami N Khouzam, Navin C Nanda, Mohamed K Ahmed, Ahmed Y Salama, Raziye E Akdogan, HK Chopra

INTRODUCTION

Heart failure (HF) has become a primary cause of morbidity and mortality across the world with 1–2% of adults having HF. The prevalence in people greater than 70 years of age has risen to 10% or higher.[1] In the United States, approximately 6.2 million adults had HF in 2013–2016, which is a 5.2% increase since the preceding 3 years. Newly diagnosed HF patients were almost evenly divided between those that had reduced ejection fraction and those with preserved ejection fraction. HF prevalence continues to rise due to the aging population and increasing pool of surviving coronary artery disease patients.[2] HF results in over 1 million hospital admissions annually, and carries a 5-year mortality of almost 50%.[3,4] HF has traditionally been a clinical diagnosis with laboratory data playing a very little role. The overall accuracy of the clinical presentation is limited to less than 25% due to its nonspecific nature.[5] Therefore, delineation of structural or functional abnormalities of the heart can corroborate clinical suspicion. Echocardiography (ECHO) has been the most frequently used noninvasive test due its easy use and safety. It provides significant information about the structure and function of the heart, and it plays a major role in guiding therapy and monitoring response to treatment of HF. Over the last 25 years, several advancements have been made in ECHO that have revolutionized our comprehension of the morphologic and functional basis of HF and hence tailor therapeutic efforts to the specific pathophysiology of HF. Three-dimensional (3D) ECHO is one such development that has enhanced our understanding of the basis of HF and holds promise to alter the way HF patients are evaluated and managed.

CLASSIFICATION OF HF OR HF PATHOGENESIS AND PHENOTYPING

Several classifications of HF have come to exist over the years, predominantly on the basis of clinical presentation and left ventricular (LV) function. HF has been categorized in various clinical settings as low-output failure or high-output HF, systolic HF or diastolic HF, HF with reduced ejection fraction (HFrEF) or HF with preserved ejection fraction (HFpEF). These entities have a significant overlap and this often makes the picture confusing. Recently, however, HF has also been classified based on the changes in the mechanical LV function that leads to HF.[6]

Since the ability to record and understand the relationship of volume, pressure, and flow changes during the cardiac cycle, our understanding of HF is evolved into three models of cardiac functions. Correlating the mechanical aspects of cardiac pump function has become the basis of (3D) ECHO. The contraction and relaxation phases result from the shortening and distortion of cardiac myocytes, which represent the mechanical/functional unit of the heart. A 3D structure is produced from the intricately connected myocytes, creating two oppositely oriented helices—endocardial helix and epicardial helix. Myocytes contracting in this helical conformation cause a synchronized deformation in various directions. This leads to the thickening in the radial directions and shortening in the longitudinal and circumferential directions.[7] When these forces are released during relaxation, it causes successive pump-suction action of the cardiac chambers, which is physiologically necessary for systolic and diastolic function. These mechanical changes in the myocardium could only be observed, and not quantified and recorded until recently, due to the nonavailability of technology to do so. The techniques used in the evaluation of myocardial function in these patients have significantly evolved during the past few decades, from invasive hemodynamic measurements to noninvasive assessment of the structure and function of the myocardium. Using ECHO to assess cardiac function has progressed rapidly from volumetric assessments and calculation of EF using geometric and structural parameters, to now looking at strain and torsion, which are parameters of myocardial deformation. These new imaging modalities, especially deformation imaging, allow for the understanding of the pathophysiology of myocardial dysfunction and resultant clinical HF.

While two-dimensional (2D) ECHO is the most frequently used modality for left ventricular ejection fraction (LVEF) assessment, it is susceptible to off-axis imaging and involves several geometric assumptions. These limitations render this test to significant test–retest variability as well as susceptible to frequent underestimation of the true volumes. Opacification of the LV cavity and enhanced recognition of the endocardium with ultrasound contrast minimizes these errors.[8] The automation of methods for image analysis also hold the potential of minimizing the variability in LVEF measurements.[9] Currently, 3D ECHO is the most accurate echocardiographic method for the measurement of LV volumes and EF.[8,10,11] Also, 3D ECHO is very precise and it also correlates well with cardiac magnetic resonance imaging (CMR). The ability to acquire volumetric data in real-time on 3D ECHO removes any geometric assumptions.[11] Real-time 3D ECHO also allows for the visualization of heart structures that contribute to the pathophysiology of HF with depth. It allows for the study of the interplay of these structures in HF and holds promise in defining appropriate management strategies in HF patients.

Left Ventricular Volume and Function

Assessing changes in LV volumes accurately throughout the cardiac cycle is the mainstay in assessing LV function. While 2D ECHO is the modality most often used to assess LV function and size, its accuracy in the presence of abnormal LV cavity geometries has been seriously questioned, due to the potential nonapplicability of the conventional geometric assumptions used for the 2D ECHO measurements. 3D ECHO allows for the calculation of absolute stroke volumes, EF, and LV volumes independent of such mathematical or geometric assumptions.[12-18] The LV volumes and EF by 3D ECHO correlate more precisely with the same measurements acquired on CMR, which has developed into an independent reference standard.[14,16-20] However, 3D ECHO has been consistently shown to underestimate CMR derived LV volumes.[14,16,19,21] This underestimation of LV end-systolic and end-diastolic volumes measured on 3D ECHO is significantly less than the 2D ECHO measurements and studies have shown that there is a very close correlation with the 3D ECHO LVEF and CMR based LVEF.[22] In a recent study, O'Dell recognized the importance of LV volume and LVEF in HF and cardiovascular disease, and he compared several modalities used for these measurements specifically CMR and 3D ECHO. He concluded that the most accurate results as validated by CMR were achieved when all available anatomical data from multiple views were incorporated on to a 3D conformal surface model resulting in <1% mean error in LV volume over the physiologic range, and also a LVEF error of less than 2.1%.[23] The recent addition of semiautomated and completely automated algorithms based on artificial intelligence has further enhanced the accuracy of 3D ECHO in assessing LVEF and volumes with low intra- and interobserver variability (Fig. 1).

3D speckle tracking methods have been recently reported to be used successfully to measure LVEF and volume.[24,25] 3D ECHO allows for better assessment of focal wall motion, regional function, and EF due to its improved image quality and better time resolution, and therefore holds promise to be used for assessing the effectiveness of resynchronization treatment in HF patients.[26-29] 3D ECHO analysis in ischemic cardiomyopathy with the current systems does not correlate with tissue Doppler imaging to assess LV dyssynchrony and further studies are ongoing.[30] Availability of new probes and software has significantly enhanced the accuracy and reproducibility of 3D ECHO, facilitating measurements, and calculations for assessing intraventricular mechanical dyssynchrony.[31] Efficacy of cardiac resynchronization therapy (CRT) can be studied by evaluating the segmental time–volume curves of the 16-17 LV segments individually, calculating and plotting then against time, hence calculating a systolic dyssynchrony index (SDI).[32]

Left Ventricular Mass Assessment

Left ventricular size and EF have been the conventional measures of LV function. LV mass has however, found a role as a prognosticator in various cardiac disease processes. The LV is assumed to be spherical on M-mode and bullet shape in 2D ECHO for calculating LV mass. This limits the reproducibility and accuracy of the measurement.

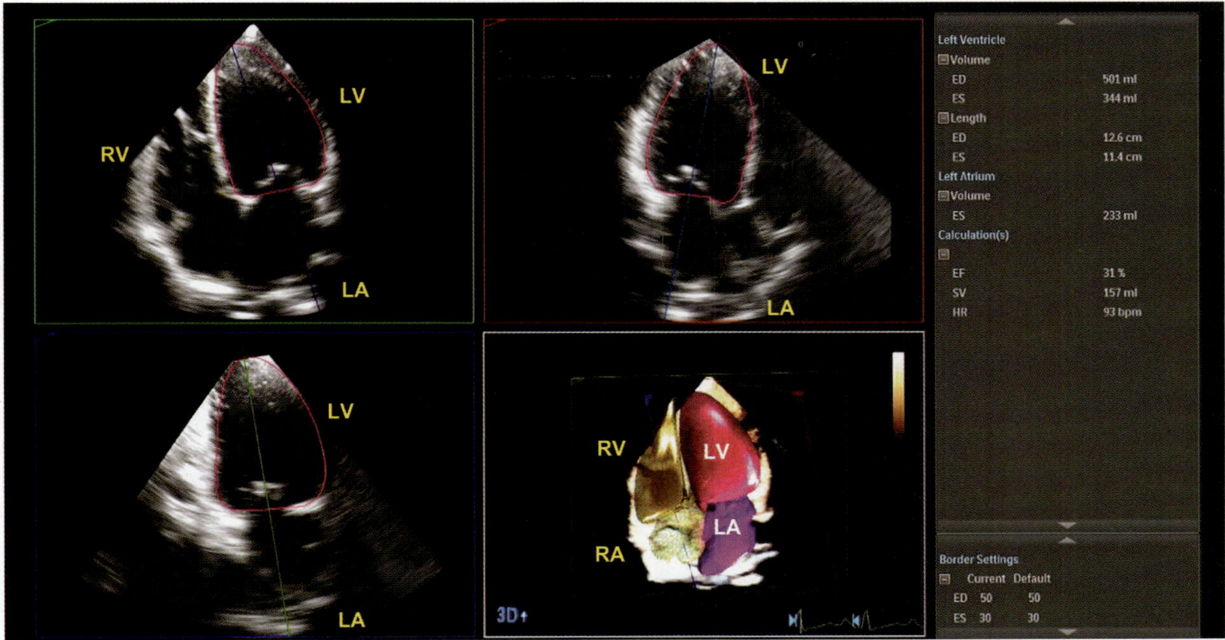

Fig. 1: Left ventricular (LV) and left atrial (LA) volumes and LV ejection fraction assessed by artificial intelligence aided three-dimensional transthoracic echocardiography in an adult patient with dilated cardiomyopathy. Both the end-diastolic (ED) and end-systolic (ES) LV volumes are very large measuring 501 mL and 344 mL, respectively. The LA ES volume is also high (233 mL). Both the LV stroke volume (SV) and ejection fraction (EF) are markedly reduced at 157 mL and 31%, respectively.
(RA: right atrium; RV: right ventricle)

3D ECHO is however, clearly able to define the epicardial and endocardial boundaries of the LV and measure the LV myocardial volume,[33,34] has allowed the development and validation of a polyhedral surface reconstruction algorithm to calculate LV volume and mass. Gopal et al. found that 3D ECHO provided the best correlation with CMR-derived LV mass.[35] Mor-Avi et al. used real-time 3D ECHO data sets to select nonforeshortened apical four and two-chamber views. M-mode LV mass measurements poorly correlated with both 3D ECHO and CMR measured LV mass.[36] In addition to LV mass, 3DE gives, accurate, and reproducible LV volume and EF assessment as mentioned earlier.[37]

Left Ventricular Volume and Systolic Function Assessment

The assessment of LVEF and volumes by using 2DE-based truncated ellipsoid method and area-length method is limited by errors due to image position, geometric assumption, and boundary tracing inaccuracies.[8,18,38] Ischemic cardiomyopathy with regional wall motion abnormalities, challenges the accuracy of this calculated measurement.[39,40] 3D ECHO is free of any LV-shape assumptions, hence, LVEF and LV volumes are expected to be more accurate and correlate better with that obtained by CMR than 2D ECHO-based measurements.[41] In LV aneurysm, the irregular geometry precludes accurate LV volume and EF assessment by 2D ECHO.[42,43]

3D ECHO Assessment of LV Regional Function

Live/real-time 3D ECHO has the advantage of capturing the entire LV in any arbitrary plane and assesses regional wall motion in all segments. Corsi et al. have shown a close correlation between 3D ECHO and CMR-based partial and global LV volumes and regional wall motion. However, they noted significant differences at various levels of the LV. In this study, they concluded that this correlation was stronger in the mid and basal ventricular levels compared to the apical level.[44]

Right Ventricular Volume and Function

Several 2D ECHO parameters, including tricuspid annular plane systolic excursion, Tei index, fractional area change, and strain as well as the speckle tracking-based strain rate have been used to look at right ventricular (RV) function and size. 3D ECHO imaging is more important in RV assessment than LV volume, because of the complex RV geometry. Shimada et al. in a meta-analysis on 23 studies with 807 subjects, showed 3D ECHO RV volume underestimation

($P < 0.00001$) as well as that of RVEF ($P = 0.03$) when compared with CMR values.[45]

The RV chamber's complex geometry makes it impossible to quantify volumes with 2D ECHO. Therefore, 3D ECHO imaging for measuring RV volumes including stroke volumes has been revolutionary. 3D ECHO has applied sophisticated software for RV volumes and function assessment the accuracy of which correlates well with CMR. These measurements use rapid acquisition, independent of geometric assumptions, utilizing semiautomated border detection and dynamic RV cast visualization.[46-51] Normal RV volumes and ejection fraction ranges have been proposed,[47,52,53] however, the prognostic values of these measurements for different clinical scenarios need to be defined.[54] Some limitations for RV quantification are encountered due to the close proximity of RV outflow wall to the sternum or chest wall, leading to occasional dropout of the wall that precludes accurate volumetric measurements. Also, severe RV dilatation may prevent imaging of the chamber even with 3D ECHO technology. Applying a newly developed offline tracing of RV borders in systole and diastole and a phase of semiautomatic contour detection using 3D ECHO data in the apical views, the RV is divided into the inflow, outflow and apical portions, which can be independently assessed, even in the presence of RV dilatation. This holds the promise of overcoming the traditional limitations of 2D ECHO and Doppler measurements used to assess RV function. This 3D ECHO algorithm facilitates noninvasive RV function and volume evaluation, which has a great potential in clinical practice while assessing acute and chronic right HF syndromes.[55]

3D Speckle-tracking Echo (STE) for Assessment of Myocardial Deformation: Advantages Over 2D STE

Speckle-tracking echocardiography is a gray scale-based technique to study myocardial deformation and depends on the fact that the myocardium has anisotropic acoustic properties. Mechanics of cardiac chambers is readily assessed by 2D STE but foreshortened views limit the accuracy of quantification of myocardial deformation. LV contraction is a complex 3D movement involving simultaneous twisting motion and movement of the LV base toward the apex. In 2D STE, speckles are lost during frame-by-frame speckle-tracking analysis due to planes cutting through one another. In 3D STE, speckles of the entire myocardium are tracked in all directions in 3D space, potentially eliminating out-of-plane motion speckle-tracking.[56] At the same time, it provides the three orthogonal strain values, radial strain, longitudinal strain (LS), circumferential strain (CS), as well as 3D area strain and area change ratio (ACR) that have developed as measures for area tracking-based deformation.[57] The 3D area strain and ACR to track myocardial motion are being increasingly used along with its components of CS and LS. ACR has been validated as a sensitive parameter defining early stage HF and detecting subtle LV systolic dysfunction in patients with aortic valve disease, hypertension, and those who have had chemotherapy. Nagata et al. have shown that the 3D global LS is the most reliable predictor of future adverse cardiovascular events in patients with asymptomatic aortic stenosis.[58]

Left Ventricular Twist and Torsion

Left ventricular myocardial fibers have helical orientation with the endocardium being right-handed obliquely oriented, the mid-myocardium is circumferentially orientated, and the epicardium is left-handed obliquely oriented. A spiral squeeze caused by concurrent apical counterclockwise rotation and basal clockwise rotation, represents LV contraction when visualized from the apex up.[7] The sum total of the apical rotated degree and the basal rotated degree measures the LV twist, while the LV torsion is a measure of the twist in degrees that is normalized by the long-axis distance between the apex and the base.[59] While 2D STE has studied the LV twist and torsion well for the wringing motion of the heart, the results are affected by limitations of tracking speckles in 2D imaging due to image foreshortening and loss of speckles due to intersecting planes. By the simultaneous measurement of rotations in the basal and apical and short-axis planes and the distance between these planes, 3D STE more accurately calculated LV torsion.[60] This allows for a better understanding of age-related changes in LV systolic twist, diastolic untwisting, and changes of LV mechanics.

Left Ventricular Wall Motion Abnormalities

Assessing wall motion abnormalities in coronary artery disease (CAD) with 2D ECHO is a subjective visual assessment with poor reproducibility. STE myocardial deformation index using strain and strain rate is believed to be superior for wall motion analysis.[61] The 2D STE assessment however, is limited by the aforementioned factors especially foreshortening. LV wall motion abnormality with 3D ECHO is more accurate as it analyzes all LV walls in several planes and incorporates this information in the calculation datasets. With simultaneous display of several short-axis tomographic slices, 3D ECHO allows subtle wall motion abnormality to be detected. These 3D STE data allow for reproducible quantification of wall motion and through the use of new myocardial deformation markers and 3D area strain its calculations are believed to closely correlate with LVEF.[62] Another advantage that 3D ECHO and 3D STE data present is that these LV deformation parameters can be studied using a single, full-volume beat and hence is reproducible irrespective of the rhythm. Volumetric 3D STE is a simple modality that assesses both regional and global longitudinal, circumferential, radial, and area strains that parallels regional and global LV function in CAD.

Left Ventricular Mechanical Dyssynchrony

Conduction abnormality, especially complete left bundle branch block, is encountered in one-fourth of patients with HF.[63] This interventricular and intraventricular conduction prolongation leads to regional mechanical delay and dyssynchronized LV contraction, worsening LV function with reduced LVEF. This also results in ventricular remodeling and increased mortality. LV septal-to-posterior wall motion dyssynchrony by 2D ECHO is an important criterion that defines the use CRT but has been associated with a 20–30% nonresponder rate, and its reliability has been questioned and more accurate measures of LV mechanical dyssynchrony (LVMD) are needed.[64] 3D ECHO has allowed the development of a SDI that uses the time taken to reach minimum regional volume for each segment as a percentage of the cardiac cycle and SDI is measured as the standard deviation of these timings calculated as a percentage of the duration of cardiac cycle.[65] The 3D ECHO measured LVMD has been shown to be reproducible between centers. In severe LV dysfunction, SDI is an excellent predictor of response to CRT in HF patients independent of QRS morphology and duration,[66] even though it has lower temporal and spatial resolution compared to 2D ECHO.[67]

3D ECHO Assessment of Functional Mitral Regurgitation Severity in Heart Failure: Advantages Over 2D ECHO

Mitral valve (MV) structure is complex and saddle-shaped that is better visualized by 3D ECHO than 2D ECHO imaging.[68] Mitral regurgitation (MR) is both a cause and effect of HF. Annular dilation and distortion of the MV annulus in HF patients leads to functional MR. In MV stenosis, planimetry measured MV area is more accurate on 3D ECHO compared to 2DE and correlates with MV orifice area calculated by the Gorlin formula on cardiac catheterization.[69] MR severity, assessed by vena contracta width (VCW) in different 2D views, has been found to be discordant. 3D ECHO quantifies the severity of MR using the size of vena contracta (VC), which is often irregular rather than circular and easily viewed enface by 3D ECHO and is more accurate to calculate effective regurgitant orifice area (EROA) to assess the severity of MR. Studies have shown that 3D ECHO is superior to conventional 2D ECHO when evaluating the MV anatomy in patients with both structural and functional MR.[70-74]

3D ECHO Assessment of Functional Tricuspid Regurgitation Severity in Heart Failure: Advantages Over 2D ECHO

3D ECHO for Assessment of Pacemaker-related Tricuspid Regurgitation

Functional tricuspid regurgitation (TR) results from abnormalities of structures that support the tricuspid valve (TV), including dilatation of tricuspid annulus, often due to RV dilation and dysfunction or pulmonary artery hypertension and often associated with right HF.[75-78] 3D ECHO has several advantages over 2D ECHO for assessment of the TV and TR. Primary TR can be due to various anatomical abnormalities which are better delineated when using 3D instead of 2D ECHO, including the apically "displaced" TV septal/posterior leaflet in Ebstein's anomaly, or the thickening and restricted movement of TV leaflets in carcinoid syndrome.[79,80] Fukuda et al. used 3D ECHO to document that dilation and flattening of the tricuspid annulus was the primary cause of secondary or functional TR.[81] In a 3D ECHO study of 54 patients, Park et al. showed that the degree of functional TR was primarily determined by the severity of pulmonary hypertension, septal-lateral annular dilatation, and extent of the septal leaflet tethering.[82]

3D ECHO is also superior in delineating pacemaker or defibrillator lead-associated TR. Studies have shown that 3D ECHO precisely located lead interference with TV leaflet motion as well as lead impaction leading to significant TR.[83,84] Lead impaction generally involves the septal tricuspid leaflet. Therefore, when assessing patients who are suspected to have significant TR due to lead interference, 3D ECHO should be used.[84]

Role of 3D ECHO in LV Assist Devices

In patients with HF and severe LV dysfunction and hypotension, a LV-assist device (AD) such as an Impella or Heart Mate may be needed. Extracorporeal membrane oxygenation (ECMO) has also been used in in HF patients presenting with acute myocardial infarction and cardiogenic shock.[85-87] While 2D ECHO is the standard for delineating the inflow cannula placement, 3D ECHO may add further to the optimization and hemodynamic advantage that the LVAD affords.[84,85]

3D images can confirm the appropriate positioning of the inflow cannula at the LV apex in context to the MV, as 3D ECHO has the ability to allow multiple views including enface views such that any adjacent tissue such as a papillary muscle which could obstruct the cannula inlet can be avoided.[86] It allows the assessment of the RV contour to rule out the impact of the LVAD on the interventricular septum as the LVAD can create an excessive amount of suction that can cause interventricular septal deviation, RV dilation and dysfunction and possibly lead to ventricular arrhythmia.[86] Thrombi in the LV which could be sucked into the cannula leading to stroke or other embolic events are also more accurately assessed by 3D ECHO than 2D ECHO.

Limitations of 3D ECHO

3D ECHO image acquisition is limited by the availability of acoustic windows to a somewhat greater extent compared to 2D ECHO. In its current state 3D ECHO spatial and temporal resolution are not superior to 2D ECHO. 3D ECHO is also prone to stitch artifacts in the setting of rhythm abnormality and respiratory motion. Real-time 3D ECHO imaging overcomes this drawback by capturing the entire movement of the heart during a single beat and allows overcoming the limitations encountered in multi-beat mode but at the expense of spatiotemporal resolution. New development in hardware technology is ongoing in order to overcome these limitations.

CONCLUSION

In conclusion, 3D ECHO confers significant incremental value over 2D ECHO in the assessment of patients with HF. It helps in delineating the etiology of HF, provides reliable and accurate assessment of both LV and RV function as well as severity of functional mitral and tricuspid regurgitation and assists in management strategies.

REFERENCES

1. Mosterd A, Hoes AW. Clinical epidemiology of heart failure. Heart. 2007;93:1137-46.
2. Benjamin EJ, Muntner P, Alonso A. et al. Heart disease and stroke statistics. Circulation. 2019;139(10).
3. Go AS, Mozaffarian D, Roger VL, et al. Heart disease and stroke statistics–2013 update: A report from the American Heart Association. Circulation. 2013;127:e6-e245.
4. Levy D, Kenchaiah S, Larson MG, et al. Long-term trends in the incidence of and survival with heart failure. N Engl J Med. 2002;347:1397-402.
5. McMurray JJ, Adamopoulos S, Anker SD, et al. ESC Guidelines for the diagnosis and treatment of acute and chronic heart failure 2012: The Task Force for the Diagnosis and Treatment of Acute and Chronic Heart Failure 2012 of the European Society of Cardiology. Developed in collaboration with the Heart Failure Association (HFA) of the ESC. Eur Heart J. 2012;33:1787-847.
6. Sengupta PP, Narula J. Reclassifying heart failure: Predominantly subendocardial, subepicardial, and transmural. Heart Fail Clin. 2008;4:379-82.
7. Lo CI, Lai YH, Wu JJ, et al. Cardiac systolic mechanics in heart failure with preserved ejection fraction: New insights and controversies. Acta Cardiol Sin. 2013;29:515-23.
8. Jenkins C, Moir S, Chan J, et al. Left ventricular volume measurement with echocardiography: A comparison of left ventricular opacification, three-dimensional echocardiography, or both with magnetic resonance imaging. Eur Heart J. 2009;30:98-106.
9. Knackstedt C, Bekkers SC, Schummers G, et al. Fully automated versus standard tracking of left ventricular ejection fraction and longitudinal strain: The FAST-EFs Multicenter Study. J Am Coll Cardiol. 2015;66:1456-66.
10. Lang RM, Bierig M, Devereux RB, et al. Chamber Quantification Writing Group; American Society of Echocardiography's Guidelines and Standards Committee; European Association of Echocardiography. Recommendations for chamber quantification: A report from the American Society of Echocardiography's Guidelines and Standards Committee and the Chamber Quantification Writing Group, developed in conjunction with the European Association of Echocardiography, a branch of the European Society of Cardiology. J Am Soc Echocardiogr. 2005;18: 1440-63.
11. Dorosz JL, Lezotte DC, Weitzenkamp DA, et al. Performance of 3-dimensional echocardiography in measuring left ventricular volumes and ejection fraction: A systematic review and meta-analysis. J Am Coll Cardiol. 2012;59:1799-1808.
12. Gopal AS, King DL, Katz J, et al. Three-dimensional echocardiographic volume computation by polyhedral surface reconstruction: In vitro validation and comparison to magnetic resonance imaging. J Am Soc Echocardiogr. 1992;5:115-24.
13. King DL, Harrison MR, King DL Jr, et al. Improved reproducibility of left atrial and left ventricular measurements by guided three-dimensional echocardiography. J Am Coll Cardiol. 1992;20:1238-45.
14. Kuhl HP, Schreckenberg M, Rulands D, et al. High-resolution transthoracic real-time three-dimensional echocardiography: Quantitation of cardiac volumes and function using semi-automatic border detection and comparison with cardiac magnetic resonance imaging. J Am Coll Cardiol. 2004;43:2083-90.
15. Gutierrez-Chico JL, Zamorano JL, Perez de Isla L, et al. Comparison of left ventricular volumes and ejection fractions measured by three-dimensional echocardiography versus by two-dimensional echocardiography and cardiac magnetic resonance in patients with various cardiomyopathies. Am J Cardiol. 2005;95:809-13.
16. Sugeng L, Mor-Avi V, Weinert L, et al. Quantitative assessment of left ventricular size and function: Side-by-side comparison of real-time three dimensional echocardiography and computed tomography with magnetic resonance reference. Circulation. 2006;114:654-61.

17. Pouleur AC, le Polain de Waroux JB, Pasquet A, et al. Assessment of left ventricular mass and volumes by three-dimensional echocardiography in patients with or without wall motion abnormalities: Comparison against cine magnetic resonance imaging. Heart. 2008;94:1050-7.
18. Qi X, Cogar B, Hsiung MC, et al. Live/real time three-dimensional transthoracic echocardiographic assessment of left ventricular volumes, ejection fraction, and mass compared with magnetic resonance imaging. Echocardiography. 2007;24:166-73.
19. Shiota T, McCarthy PM, White RD, et al. Initial clinical experience of real-time three-dimensional echocardiography in patients with ischemic and idiopathic dilated cardiomyopathy. Am J Cardiol. 1999;84:1068-73.
20. Corsi C, Lang RM, Veronesi F, et al. Volumetric quantification of global and regional left ventricular function from real-time three-dimensional echocardiographic images. Circulation. 2005;112:1161-70.
21. Jenkins C, Leano R, Chan J, et al. Reconstructed versus real-time 3-dimensional echocardiography: Comparison with magnetic resonance imaging. J Am Soc Echocardiogr. 2007;20:862-8.
22. Shimada YJ, Shiota T. A meta-analysis and investigation for the source of bias of left ventricular volumes and function by three-dimensional echocardiography in comparison with magnetic resonance imaging. Am J Cardiol. 2011;107:126-38.
23. O'Dell WG. J Am Heart Association: Cardiovascular and Cerebrovascular Disease. 2019;8(6):e009124.
24. Kawamura R, Seo Y, Ishizu T, et al. Feasibility of left ventricular volume measurements by three-dimensional speckle tracking echocardiography depends on image quality and degree of left ventricular enlargement: Validation study with cardiac magnetic resonance imaging. J Cardiol. 2014;63:230-8.
25. Kleijn SA, Aly MF, Terwee CB, et al. Reliability of left ventricular volumes and function measurements using three-dimensional speckle tracking echocardiography. Eur Heart J Cardiovasc Imaging. 2012;13:159-68.
26. Takeuchi M, Jacobs A, Sugeng L, et al. Assessment of left ventricular dyssynchrony with real-time 3-dimensional echocardiography: Comparison with Doppler tissue imaging. J Am Soc Echocardiogr. 2007;20:1321-9.
27. van Dijk J, Dijkmans PA, Gotte MJ, et al. Evaluation of global left ventricular function and mechanical dyssynchrony in patients with an asymptomatic left bundle branch block: A real-time 3D echocardiography study. Eur J Echocardiogr. 2008;9:40-6.
28. van Dijk J, Knaapen P, Russel IK, et al. Mechanical dyssynchrony by 3D echo correlates with acute haemodynamic response to biventricular pacing in heart failure patients. Europace. 2008;10:63-8.
29. Baker GH, Hlavacek AM, Chessa KS, et al. Left ventricular dysfunction is associated with intraventricular dyssynchrony by 3-dimensional echocardiography in children. J Am Soc Echocardiogr. 2008;21:230-33.
30. Burgess MI, Jenkins C, Chan J, et al. Measurement of left ventricular dyssynchrony in patients with ischaemic cardiomyopathy: A comparison of real-time three-dimensional and tissue Doppler echocardiography. Heart. 2007;93:1191-6.
31. Kapetanakis S, Kearney MT, Siva A, et al. Real-time three-dimensional echocardiography: A novel technique to quantify global left ventricular mechanical dyssynchrony. Circulation. 2005;112(7):992-1000.
32. Lang. European Cardiology. 2008;4(2):27-30.
33. Mor-Avi V, Sugeng L, Lang RM. Real-time 3-dimensional echocardiography: An integral component of the routine echocardiographic examination in adult patients? Circulation. 2009;119:314-29.
34. Yap SC, van Geuns RJ, Nemes A, et al. Rapid and accurate measurement of LV mass by biplane real-time 3D echocardiography in patients with concentric LV hypertrophy: Comparison to CMR. Eur J Echocardiogr. 2008;9:255-60.
35. Gopal AS, Keller AM, Shen Z, et al. Three-dimensional echocardiography: In vitro and in vivo validation of left ventricular mass and comparison with conventional echocardiographic methods. J Am Coll Cardiol. 1994;24:504-13.
36. Mor-Avi V, Sugeng L, Weinert L, et al. Fast measurement of left ventricular mass with real-time three-dimensional echocardiography: Comparison with magnetic resonance imaging. Circulation. 2004;110:1814-8.
37. van den Bosch AE, Robbers-Visser D, Krenning BJ, et al. Comparison of real-time three-dimensional echocardiography to magnetic resonance imaging for assessment of left ventricular mass. Am J Cardiol. 2006;97:113-7.
38. Chukwu EO, Barasch E, Mihalatos DG, et al. Relative importance of errors in left ventricular quantitation by two-dimensional echocardiography: Insights from three-dimensional echocardiography and cardiac magnetic resonance imaging. J Am Soc Echocardiogr. 2008;21:990-97.
39. Sapin PM, Gopal AS, Clarke GB, et al. Three-dimensional echocardiography compared to two-dimensional echocardiography for measurement of left ventricular mass anatomic validation in an open chest canine model. Am J Hypertens. 1996;9:467-74.
40. Abramov D, Helmke S, Rumbarger Lel K, et al. Overestimation of left ventricular mass and misclassification of ventricular geometry in heart failure patients by two-dimensional echocardiography in comparison with three-dimensional echocardiography. Echocardiography. 2010;27:223-9.
41. Gopal AS, Keller AM, Rigling R, et al. Left ventricular volume and endocardial surface area by three-dimensional echocardiography: Comparison with two-dimensional echocardiography and nuclear magnetic resonance imaging in normal subjects. J Am Coll Cardiol. 1993;22:258-70.
42. Qin JX, Jones M, Shiota T, et al. Validation of real-time three-dimensional echocardiography for quantifying left ventricular volumes in the presence of a left ventricular aneurysm: In vitro and in vivo studies. J Am Coll Cardiol. 2000;36:900-07.
43. Jahnke C, Foell D, Heinrichs G, et al. Three-dimensional echocardiography for quantitative analysis of left ventricular aneurysm. Echocardiography. 2010;27:64-8.

44. Corsi C, Lang RM, Veronesi F, et al. Volumetric quantification of global and regional left ventricular function from real-time three-dimensional echocardiographic images. Circulation. 2005;112:1161-70.
45. Shimada YJ, Shiota M, Siegel RJ, et al. Accuracy of right ventricular volumes and function determined by three-dimensional echocardiography in comparison with magnetic resonance imaging: A meta-analysis study. J Am Soc Echocardiogr. 2010;23:943-53.
46. Jenkins C, Chan J, Bricknell K, et al. Reproducibility of right ventricular volumes and ejection fraction using real-time three-dimensional echocardiography: Comparison with cardiac MRI. Chest. 2007;131:1844-51.
47. Graspa J, O'Regan DP, Pavlopoulos H, et al. Right ventricular remodeling in pulmonary arterial hypertension with three-dimensional echocardiography: Comparison with cardiac magnetic resonance imaging. Eur J Echocardiogr. 2010;11:64-73.
48. Sugeng L, Mor-Avi V, Weinert L, et al. Multimodality comparison of quantitative volumetric analysis of the right ventricle. JACC Cardiovasc Imaging. 2010;3:10-18.
49. Van der Zwaan HB, Helbing WA, McGhie JS, et al. Clinical value of real-time three-dimensional echocardiography for right ventricular quantification in congenital heart disease: Validation with cardiac magnetic resonance imaging. J Am Soc Echocardiogr. 2010;23:134-40.
50. Leibundgut G, Rohner A, Grize L, et al. Dynamic assessment of right ventricular volumes and function by real-time three-dimensional echocardiography: A comparison study with magnetic resonance imaging in 100 adult patients. J Am Soc Echocardiogr. 2010;23:116-26.
51. Medvedofsky D, Addetia K, Patel AR, et al. Novel approach to three-dimensional echocardiographic quantification of right ventricular volumes and function from focused views. J Am Soc Echocardiogr. 2015;28:1222-31.
52. Tamborini G, Marsan NA, Gripari P, et al. Reference values for right ventricular volumes and ejection fraction with real-time three-dimensional echocardiography: Evaluation in a large series of normal subjects. J Am Soc Echocardiogr. 2010;23:109-15.
53. Maffessanti F, Muraru D, Esposito R, et al. Age-, body size, and sex-specific reference values for right ventricular volumes and ejection fraction by three-dimensional echocardiography: a multicenter echocardiographic study in 507 healthy volunteers. Circ Cardiovasc Imaging. 2013;6:700-10.
54. Thavendiranathan P, Phelan D, Thomas JD, et al. Quantitative assessment of mitral regurgitation: Validation of new methods. J Am Coll Cardiol. 2012;60:1470-83.
55. Tamborini G, Brusoni D, Torres Molina J, et al. Feasibility of a new generation three-dimensional echocardiography for right ventricular volumetric and functional measurements. Am J Cardiol. 2008;102:499-505.
56. Wu VC, Takeuchi M, Otani K, et al. Effect of through-plane and twisting motion on left ventricular strain calculation: Direct comparison between two-dimensional and three-dimensional speckle-tracking echocardiography. J Am Soc Echocardiogr. 2013;26:1274-81.
57. Seo Y, Ishizu T, Atsumi A, et al. Three-dimensional speckle tracking echocardiography. Circ J. 2014;78:1290-1301.
58. Nagata Y, Takeuchi M, Wu VC, et al. Prognostic value of LV deformation parameters using 2D and 3D speckle-tracking echocardiography in asymptomatic patients with severe aortic stenosis and preserved LV ejection fraction. JACC Cardiovasc Imaging. 2015;8:235-45.
59. Takeuchi M, Nakai H, Kokumai M, et al. Age-related changes in left ventricular twist assessed by two-dimensional speckle-tracking imaging. J Am Soc Echocardiogr. 2006;19:1077-84.
60. Kaku K, Takeuchi M, Tsang W, et al. Age-related normal range of left ventricular strain and torsion using three-dimensional speckle-tracking echocardiography. J Am Soc Echocardiogr. 2014;27:55-64.
61. Stanton T, Leano R, Marwick TH. Prediction of all-cause mortality from global longitudinal speckle strain: comparison with ejection fraction and wall motion scoring. Cir Cardiovasc Imaging. 2009;2:356-64.
62. Hayat D, Kloeckner M, Nahum J, et al. Comparison of real-time three-dimensional speckle tracking to magnetic resonance imaging in patients with coronary heart disease. Am J Cardiol. 2012;109:180-86.
63. Eriksson P, Hansson PO, Eriksson H, et al. Bundle-branch block in a general male population: The study of men born 1913. Circulation. 1998;98:2494-2500.
64. Marcus GM, Rose E, Viloria EM, et al. VENTAK CHF/CONTAK-CD Biventricular Pacing Study Investigators. Septal to posterior wall motion delay fails to predict reverse remodeling or clinical improvement in patients undergoing cardiac resynchronization therapy. J Am Coll Cardiol. 2005;46:2208-14.
65. Kapetanakis S, Kearney MT, Siva A, et al. Real-time three-dimensional echocardiography: A novel technique to quantify global left ventricular mechanical dyssynchrony. Circulation. 2005;112:992-1000.
66. Kapetanakis S, Bhan A, Murgatroyd F, et al. Real-time 3D echo in patient selection for cardiac resynchronization therapy. JACC Cardiovasc Imaging. 2011;4:16-26.
67. Chan YH, Wang CL, Kuo CT, et al. Clinical assessment and implication of left ventricular mechanical dyssynchrony in patients with heart failure. Acta Cardiol Sin. 2013;29:505-14.
68. Cavalcante JL, Rodriguez LL, Kapadia S, et al. Role of echocardiography in percutaneous mitral valve intervention. JACC Cardiovasc Imaging. 2012;5:733-46.
69. Zamorano J, Cordeiro P, Sugeng L, et al. Real-time three-dimensional echocardiography for rheumatic mitral valve stenosis evaluation: an accurate and novel approach. J Am Coll Cardiol. 2004;43:2091-96.
70. Agricola E, Oppizzi M, Pisani M, et al. Accuracy of real-time 3D echocardiography in the evaluation of functional anatomy of mitral regurgitation. Int J Cardiol. 2008;127:342-49.
71. Zakkar M, Patni R, Punjabi PP. Mitral valve regurgitation and 3D echocardiography. Future Cardiol. 2010;6:231-42.
72. Shiota T, Sinclair B, Ishii M, et al. Three-dimensional reconstruction of color Doppler flow convergence regions and regurgitant jets: An in vitro quantitative study. J Am Coll Cardiol. 1996;27:1511-18.

73. De Simone R, Glombitza G, Vahl CF, et al. Three-dimensional color Doppler: A clinical study in patients with mitral regurgitation. J Am Coll Cardiol. 1999;33:1646-54.
74. Sugeng L, Spencer KT, Mor-Avi V, et al. Dynamic three-dimensional color flow Doppler: An improved technique for the assessment of mitral regurgitation. Echocardiography. 2003;20:265-73.
75. Lopez-Mattei JC, Ibrahim H, Shaikh KA, et al. Comparative assessment of mitral regurgitation severity by transthoracic echocardiography and cardiac magnetic resonance using an integrative and quantitative approach. Am J Cardiol. 2016;117:264-70.
76. Matsumura Y, Saracino G, Sugioka K, et al. Determination of regurgitant orifice area with the use of a new three-dimensional flow convergence geometric assumption in functional mitral regurgitation. J Am Soc Echocardiogr. 2008;21:1251-6.
77. Altiok E, Hamada S, van Hall S, et al. Comparison of direct planimetry of mitral valve regurgitation orifice area by three-dimensional transesophageal echocardiography to effective regurgitant orifice area obtained by proximal flow convergence method and vena contracta area determined by color. Am J Cardiol. 2011;107:452-8.
78. Chandra S, Salgo IS, Sugeng L, et al. A three-dimensional insight into the complexity of flow convergence in mitral regurgitation: Adjunctive benefit of anatomic regurgitant orifice area. Am J Physiol Heart Circ Physiol. 2011;301: H1015-24.
79. Patel V, Nanda NC, Rajdev S, et al. Live/real time three-dimensional transthoracic echocardiographic assessment of Ebstein's anomaly. Echocardiography. 2005;22:847-54.
80. Bhattacharyya S, Toumpanakis C, Burke M, et al. Features of carcinoid heart disease identified by 2-and 3-dimensional echocardiography and cardiac MRI. Circ Cardiovasc Imaging. 2010;3:103-11.
81. Fukuda S, Saracino G, Matsumura Y, et al. Three-dimensional geometry of the tricuspid annulus in healthy subjects and in patients with functional tricuspid regurgitation: A real-time, 3-dimensional echocardiographic study. Circulation. 2006;114:I492-98.
82. Park YH, Song JM, Lee EY, et al. Geometric and hemodynamic determinants of functional tricuspid regurgitation: A real-time three-dimensional echocardiography study. Int J Cardiol. 2008;124:160-65.
83. Seo Y, Ishizu T, Nakajima H, et al. Clinical utility of 3-dimensional echocardiography in the evaluation of tricuspid regurgitation caused by pacemaker leads. Circ J. 2008;72:1465-70.
84. Addetia K, Maffessanti F, Mediratta A, et al. Impact of implantable transvenous device lead location on severity of tricuspid regurgitation. J Am Soc Echocardiogr. 2014;27:1164-75.
85. Stainback RF, Estep JD, Agler DA, et al. Echocardiography in the Management of Patients with Left Ventricular Assist Devices: Recommendations from the American Society of Echocardiography. J Am Soc Echocardiogr. 28(8):853-909.
86. Chumnanvej S, Wood MJ, MacGillivray TE, et al. Perioperative echocardiographic examination for ventricular assist device implantation. Anesth Analg. 2007;105:583-601.
87. Haglund, NA, Maltais, S, Bick, JS, et al. Hemodynamic transesophageal echocardiography after left ventricular assist device implantation. J Cardiothorac Vasc Anesth. 2014;28:1184-90.

CHAPTER

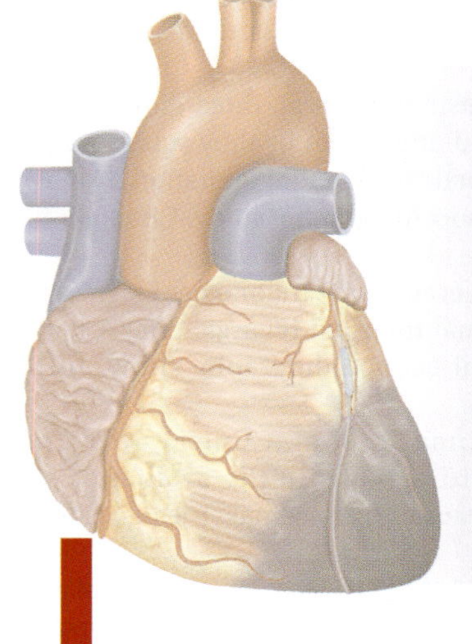

3D Echocardiography and BNP Screening in Heart Failure

V Amuthan, RVA Ananth

INTRODUCTION

Echocardiography since its inception from the days of Elder, has revolutionized the diagnosis and treatment in the management of cardiac patients. From the days of single crystal probe to M-mode, 2 dimensional (2D), color flow mapping, the advancement has reached the stage of 3D echocardiogram with added fourth dimension of time (4D echocardiography: The real-time 3D echocardiography) due to the advancement in the transducer technology to that of matrix array technology. The 3D matrix array transducer acquires a pyramidal cone of data set.

DIAGNOSIS OF HEART FAILURE

Heart failure can be defined as an abnormality of cardiac structure or function leading to failure of the heart to deliver oxygen at a rate commensurate with the requirements of the metabolizing tissues, despite normal filling pressures (or only at the expense of increased filling pressures). Based on ejection fraction, heart failure can be classified as:[1,2]

- HFrEF (reduced ejection fraction: EF <40%)
- HFmEF (mildly impaired EF: EF 40–49%)
- HFpEF (preserved ejection fraction: EF ≥50%).

Heart failure with preserved ejection fraction (HFpEF) is a clinical syndrome in patients with current or prior symptoms of HF with a left ventricular ejection fraction (LVEF) ≥50% and evidence of cardiac dysfunction as a cause of symptoms (e.g. abnormal LV filling and elevated filling pressures).[3] The echocardiography remains the single noninvasive modality of investigation which is beneficial in day-to-day management of heart failure which is a silently progressive disease (Fig. 1).[4-8] The echocardiographic measurement, indication, and modality used in the management of heart failure are summarized in Table 1. Evidence-based management of heart failure with 2D and 3D echocardiographic evidence of reducing filling pressure and pulmonary congestion along with evaluation of B-type natriuretic peptide (BNP) monitoring has proved to be a better way of controlling heart failure.[9] When compared to symptom-guided treatment, structured follow-up using echocardiography and BNP monitoring prolonged life by 2.5–4 years (Fig. 2).

CLINICAL APPLICATION OF 3D ECHOCARDIOGRAPHY IN HEART FAILURE

Examination of Left Ventricle and LV Function Assessment

Left ventricular ejection fraction: The cornerstone of the prognostication and treatment schedule for echocardiographic evaluation starts with evaluation of LVEF. Despite its limitations, ejection fraction has become part of the lingua franca of cardiology.[10] The evidence base for modern cardiology is so heavily based on this simple measurement that it is unlikely to disappear. The problems in calculating EF as the ratio between stroke volume and end-diastolic volume and their solutions are enumerated in Table 1. 3D imaging is available with

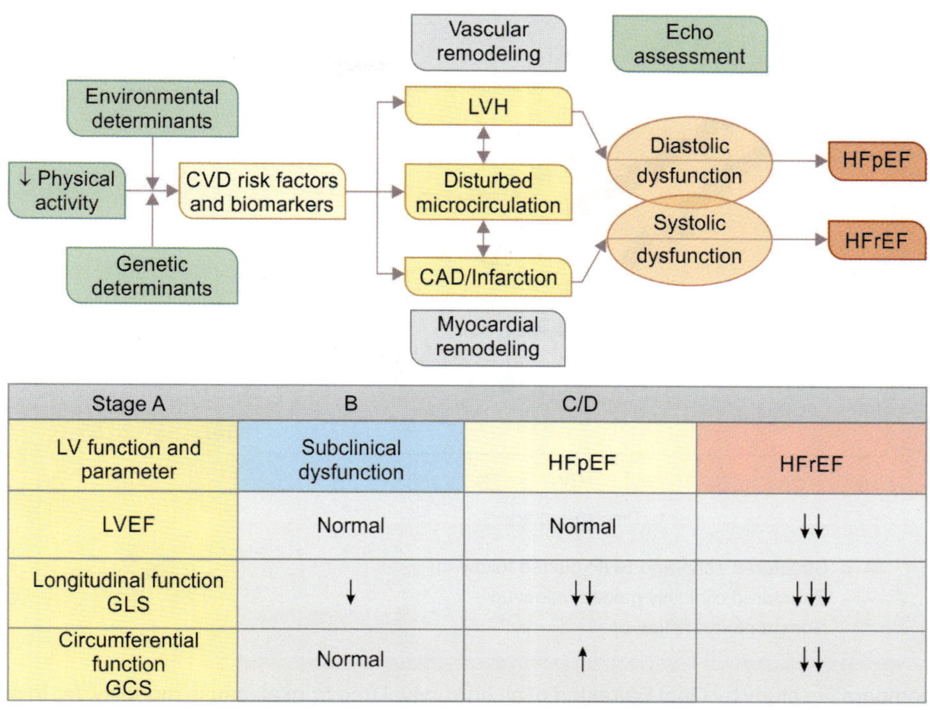

Stage A	B	C/D	
LV function and parameter	Subclinical dysfunction	HFpEF	HFrEF
LVEF	Normal	Normal	↓↓
Longitudinal function GLS	↓	↓↓	↓↓↓
Circumferential function GCS	Normal	↑	↓↓

Fig. 1: Schematic diagram showing the progress of heart failure time line and echocardiographic assessment in heart failure with preserved and reduced ejection fraction.

TABLE 1: Echocardiographic measurement, indication, and modality in evaluation of heart failure.

	Measurement	*Indication*	*Modality*
Systolic function	EF	Classification, risk assessment; selection for implantable cardioverter defibrillator and cardiac resynchronization therapy	2D or 3D echocardiography, contrast
	Non-EF indices of LV function	Risk assessment	GLS (Global longitudinal strain 2D and 3D) LV torsion and twist Doppler dP/dt
	RV assessment	Prognosis, evaluation for assist device	3D RV EF RV strain, tissue Doppler, tricuspid annular plane systolic excursion, fractional area change, etc.
	Mitral regurgitant orifice area	Quantification of mitral regurgitation	Color and CW Doppler
	LV regional function	Assessment of CAD	Wall motion analysis, strain
Diastolic function	Trans mitral and annular velocities	Assessment of diastolic function and filling pressure	Pulsed-wave tissue and blood-flow Doppler
	Left atrial volume	Prognosis, diastolic evaluation	2D or 3D echocardiography
	Tricuspid regurgitation	Diastolic function	TR peak velocity
	Regional timing	Site of greatest maximal delay	Cardiac resynchronization therapy selection

(CAD: coronary artery disease; CW: continuous wave; EF: ejection fraction; LV: left ventricular; RV: right ventricular; TR: tricuspid regurgitation)

echocardiography, magnetic resonance imaging (MRI), and computed tomography (CT). The main attraction and advantage of 3D imaging is to avoid geometric assumptions when calculations of LV volumes are being obtained, and to avoid errors created by cutting a 3D structure in two dimensions.[11-14] The current software for 3D evaluation of

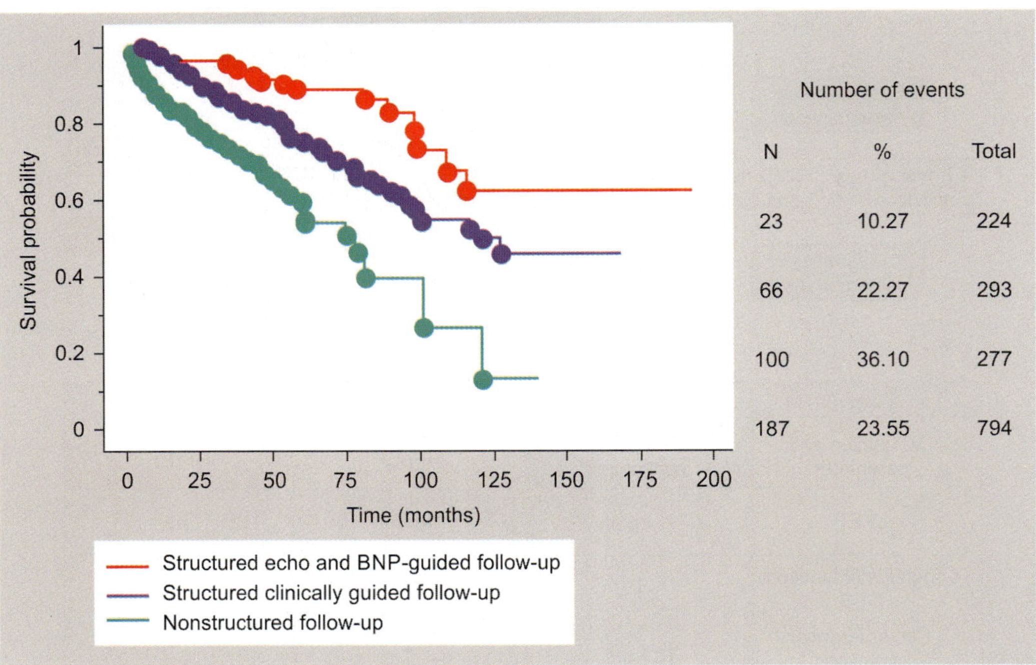

Fig. 2: Figure from comparative study by Gani Bajraktari et al. on survival free from all-cause mortality. (a) In patients of the echo- and BNP-guided follow-up, (b) In patients of the clinical follow-up, and in those who received no specific follow-up care (×2 53.5; $p < 0.0001$) showing life to be prolonged by an average of 2.5 years and 4 years, respectively, by the echo- and BNP-guided strategy.

LVEF is much easier and can be performed within minutes in the setting of emergency room (Figs. 3 and 4).

4D Left Ventricular Strain and Estimation of LV Torsional Deformation

Global Longitudinal, Circumferential and Radial Strain

Two-dimensional global longitudinal strain (GLS) has evolved as one of the most robust parameters, and this has been shown to identify subclinical LV dysfunction and improvement with cardiac resynchronization therapy (Figs. 5A and B). GLS is calculated using a variety of proprietary software (EchoPac, GE Medical Systems, Milwaukee, Wisconsin, USA; Syngo velocity vector imaging, Siemens, Mountain View, California, USA; LV analysis, Tomtec GmbH, Unterschleissheim, Germany). Three-dimensional echocardiography allows the calculation of global longitudinal, circumferential and radial strain in one-go, with their normal values recorded in healthy individuals as GLS –18% to –20%, systolic circumferential strain –20% to –22%, and systolic radial strain >+40%.[15-18] (Figs. 6A to D). Unlike 2D strain where speckles moving in three-dimensional space is recorded and are subjected to through plane artifacts, 3D strain analysis uses blocks. Because blocks are used, they can be followed in any direction. In one of the recent meta-analyses, Kalam et al have shown the independent prognostic significance of GLS in patients with mild LV global impairment. The prognostic value of this information seems likely to be superior to that provided by LVEF.[19] LV GLS before discharge after ST-segment-elevation myocardial infarction is independently associated with LV dilatation at follow-up.[20] In another study of 576 patients who underwent echocardiography ≤24 hours after primary percutaneous coronary intervention for STEMI, GLS, and Wall motion score index (WMSI) were comparable and both superior for early risk assessment compared with volume-based LV function indicators such as LVEF and end-systolic volume index (ESVI). Compared with WMSI, the advantage of GLS is the provision of a semiautomated quantitative measure.[21]

Shortening and lengthening which are the basic functions of the myocardial fibers result in a systolic twist followed by a diastolic untwisting of the left ventricle due to helical orientation of the fibers. In systole, the LV apex undergoes a counterclockwise rotation about its longitudinal axis as viewed from the apex, preceded by a brief clockwise rotation due to the earlier shortening of the subendocardial fibers during isovolumic contraction. Rotation of the LV base in systole is opposite in direction compared to apical rotation, with a brief counterclockwise rotation during isovolumic contraction followed by a clockwise rotation during LV ejection. This motion has

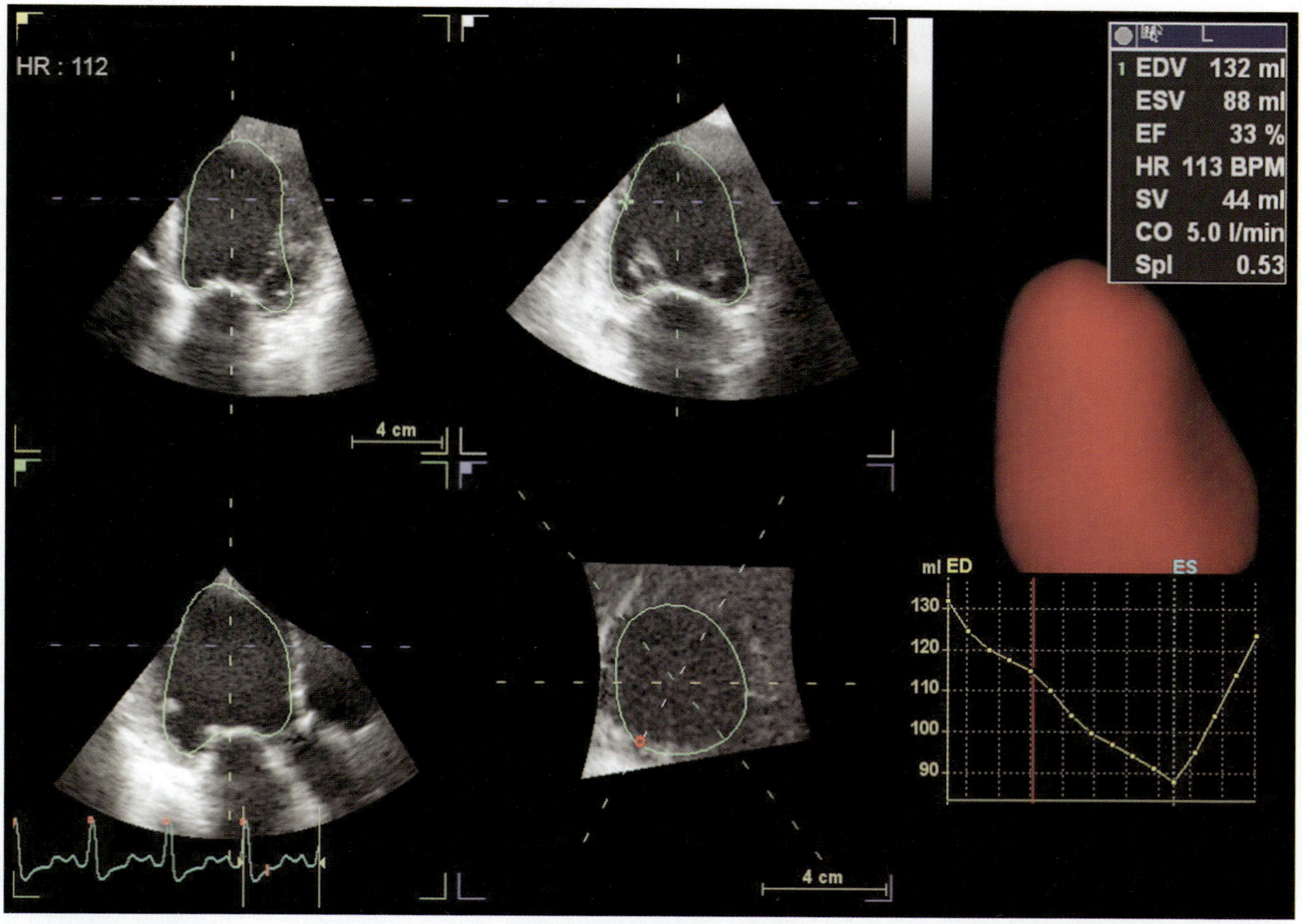

Fig. 3: 3D echocardiography calculation of left ventricular ejection fraction in a patient with dilated cardiomyopathy, increased end-diastolic and end-systolic volume and reduced ejection fraction with increased sphericity index more than >0.5 using GE Echo system (EchoPac software).

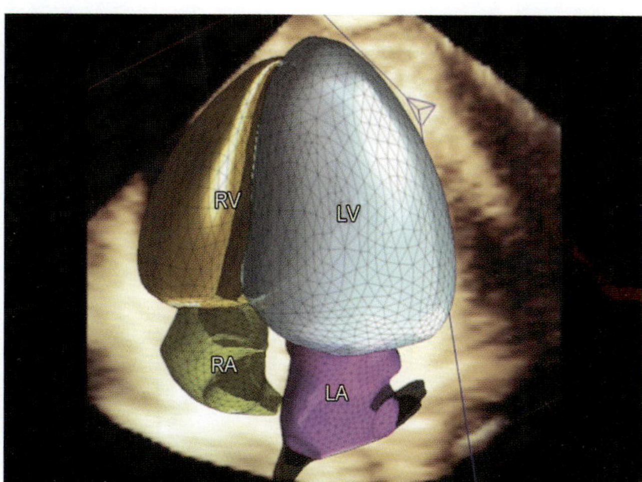

Fig. 4: 3D echocardiography and heart model in calculation of ejection fraction using Philips system.

been compared with that used to squeeze water out of a wet towel.[22] The main determinant of the LV twist is the apical rotation (Figs. 7A to C).

- Left ventricular rotation is defined as the myocardial rotation around the long axis of the left ventricle. It is rotational displacement and is expressed in degrees.
- Left ventricular twist is the absolute apex-to-base difference in LV rotation referred to as the net angle (LV twist = LV apical twist–LV basal twist) also expressed in degrees.
- Left ventricular torsion is defined as the base-to-apex gradient in the rotation angle along the long axis (LV torsion = LV twist/LV length), expressed in degrees per centimeter.
- Left ventricular twist rate is the systolic time derivative of LV twist. LV untwisting is usually defined as the peak diastolic time derivative of twist.

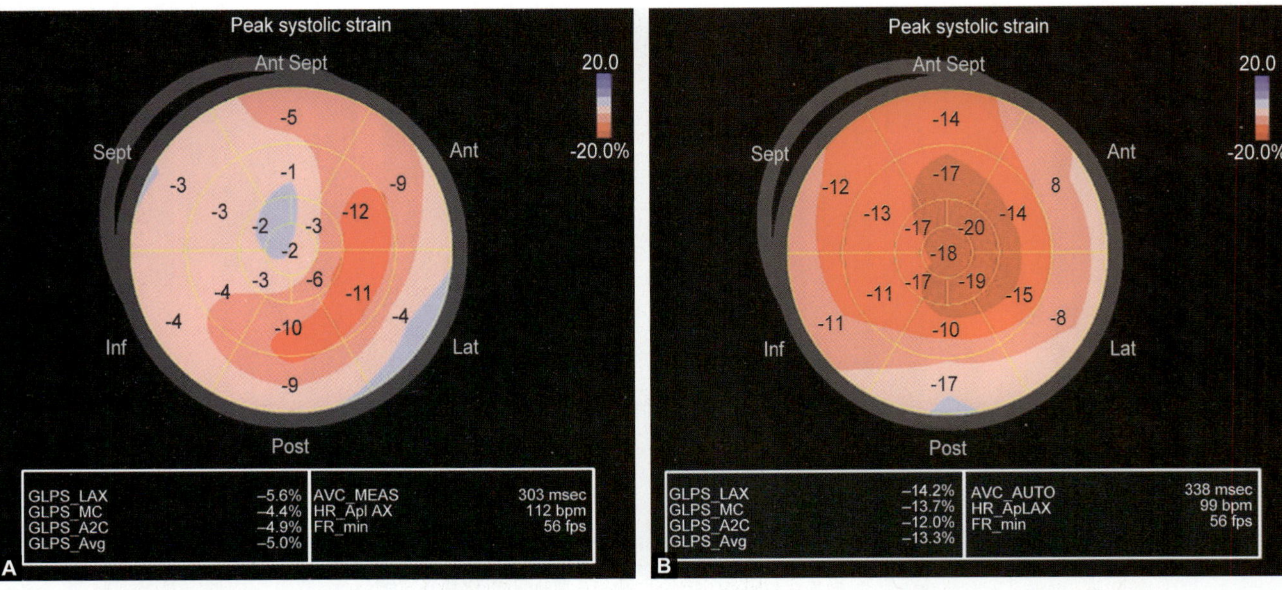

Figs. 5A and B: (A) Two-dimensional speckle tracking derived global longitudinal strain (GLS) of −5% in a patient with dilated cardiomyopathy; (B) GLS of −13% after cardiac resynchronization therapy.

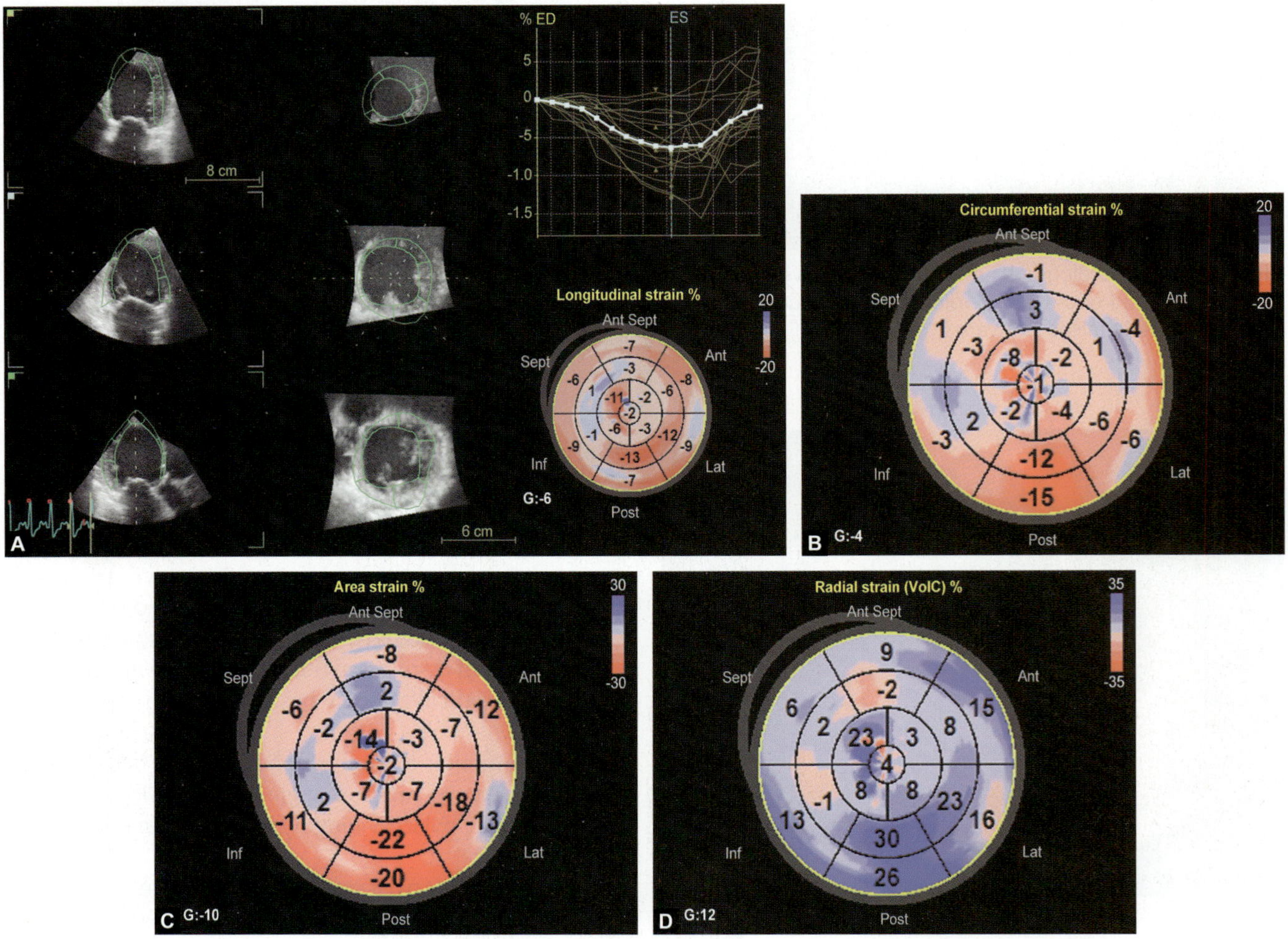

Figs. 6A to D: Three-dimensional speckle tracking derived. (A) Global longitudinal strain; (B) Global circumferential strain; (C) Global area strain; (D) Global radial strain.

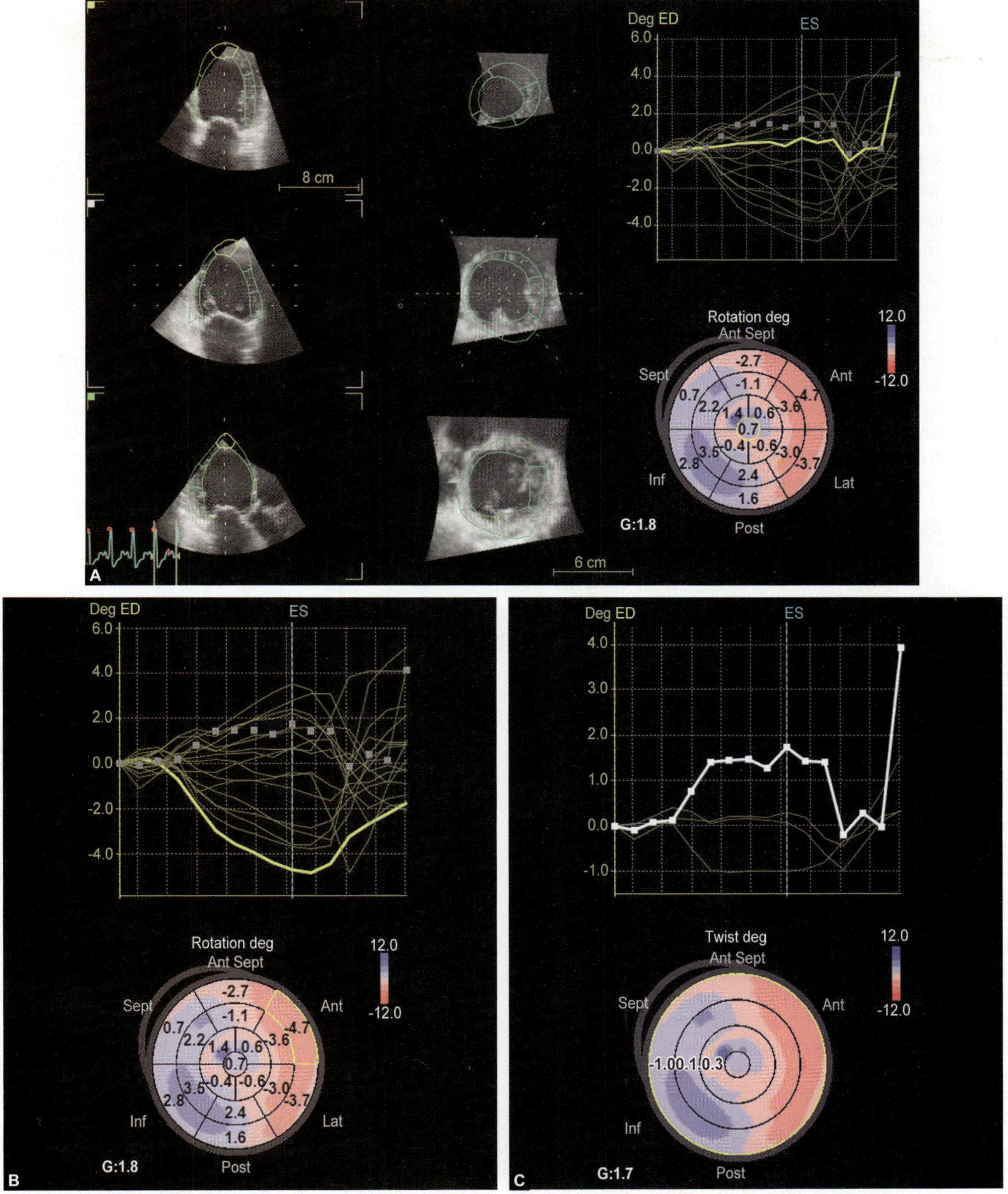

Figs. 7A to C: (A) Depicts the marked reduction in apical counter clockwise rotation to 0.7°; (B) Reduction in basal clockwise rotation to −4.7°; (C) Reduction in left ventricular twist to less than 2u in a patient with dilated cardiomyopathy.

TABLE 2: Comparison of 3D and 2 strain.

Characteristics	*3D strain*	*2D strain*
Acquisition	One apical 6 beat full volume	3 apical 2D views
Temporal resolution	34–50 volumes/sec	40–80 frames/sec
Area strain	Yes	No
Bull's eye map	Dynamic	Static
Global strain calculation	Simultaneous in all segments	Non-simultaneous
Radial strain	Calculated from area strain	Measured
Out of plane motion speckles	No	Yes
Definition of end systole	Time of left ventricular minimal volume	Time of aortic valve closure

Source: Adapted from Reference 18.

A recent study by Muhammad Ashraf et al to compute LV twist from 3D echocardiography concluded LV twist and torsion can be computed accurately. 3D speckle tracking has improved the accuracy of LV deformation imaging and torsion dynamics. To date, no prognostic information exists on the role of rotational parameters of LV function. The areas most likely to benefit are HFpEF and cardiac dyssynchrony resynchronization therapy (Table 2).[23-25.]

3D Evaluation of Left Ventricular Regional Function

The American Society of Echocardiography has recently recommended a 17-segment model for this.[26,27] In a 17-segment model, beginning at the anterior junction of the interventricular septum and the right ventricular (RV) free wall and continuing counter clockwise, basal and mid-ventricular segments should be labeled as anteroseptal, inferoseptal, inferior, inferolateral, anterolateral, and anterior. The apex is divided into five segments, including septal, inferior, lateral, and anterior segments, as well as the "apical cap," which is defined as the myocardium beyond the end of the LV cavity. A bull's eye plot can be constructed where the outer ring represents the basal segments, the middle ring represents the segments at mid-papillary muscle level, and the inner ring represents the distal level. The fact is that some manufacturers and many echocardiography laboratories never adopted these guidelines.[28] The severity of contractile dysfunction is scored visually in each segment as 1 for normal contraction or hyperkinesia, 2 for hypokinesia, 3 for akinesia, and 4 for dyskinesia. The global wall motion score is there after calculated by averaging the readings in all the segments. A score of 5 for aneurysmal segments has been deleted from the recent guidelines statement from American Society of Echocardiography.[28] A normal LV has a WMSI of 1, and the index increases as wall motion abnormalities increase in severity. A WMSI of 1.1–1.9 can predict a small infarct size, and an index equal to or greater than 2.0 can predict a larger infarct size. However, this approach is subjective and operator dependent, demands complete visualization of the endocardium, and is subject to the vicissitudes of cardiac loading and heart rate. The ability of 3D echocardiography in providing tomographic slicing of LV nine short axis tomographic slices with simultaneous display of LV in apical two-chamber, three-chamber, and four-chamber views greatly enhances the diagnostic accuracy. 4D strain analysis would help in this in depicting the bull's eye plot or the automated functional imaging of the longitudinal, circumferential, area and radial strain on a scale of –20 to +20 instead of the four-grade regional wall motion score analysis. Further myocardial deformation analysis by speckle-tracking echocardiography has been shown to accurately predict viability in patients with chronic ischemic LV dysfunction.[29]

3D Evaluation of RV Function

Echocardiographic assessment of the right ventricle is difficult because of its complex shape. RV performance is known to be a major determinant of clinical status and long-term outcomes in patients with pulmonary hypertension, cardiomyopathies, and congenital heart disease. Apical acquisition of volumes is recommended in the adult population. The modified RV apical four-chamber view is used. One way (the medial approach) is to move the transducer medially to get the RV-modified apical four-chamber view and then tilt the transducer cranially and anteriorly—and even rotate—to include the pulmonary valve in the guidance images. Because of the complicated structure and geometry of the right ventricle, conventional two-dimensional echocardiography is unable to correctly estimate RV volume using reasonable geometric assumptions. From the echocardiographer's perspective, the right ventricle is divided into four segments: The infundibulum (or outflow tract), anterior free wall,

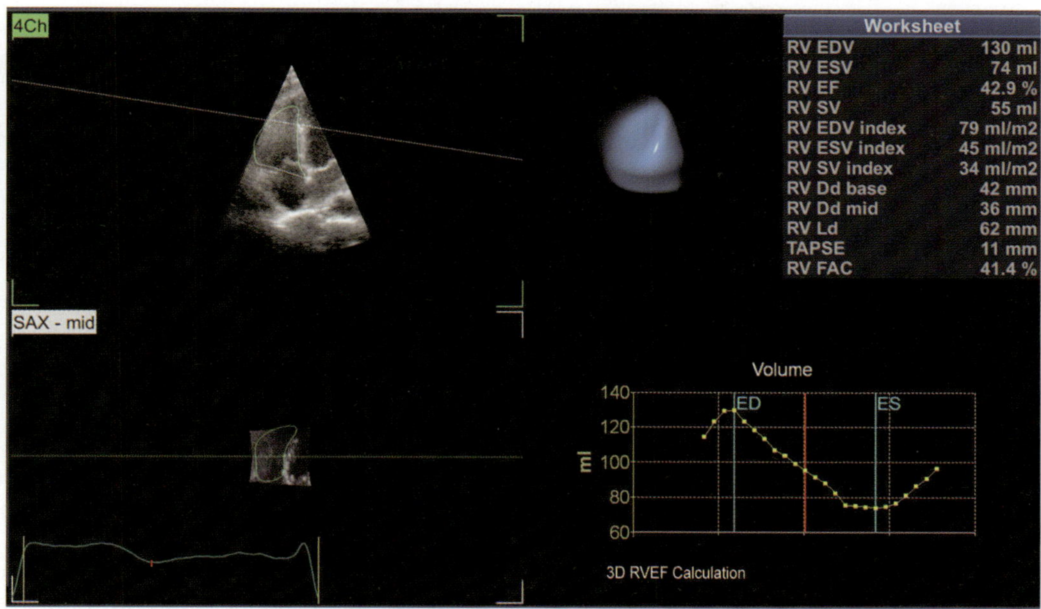

Fig. 8: 3D right ventricular (RV) volume calculation in a patient with acute mountain sickness showing reduced 3D RV ejection fraction (RVEF) and increased RV volumes.

lateral wall, and inferior wall.[30-32] The dual blood supply [right coronary artery (RCA) and left anterior descending (LAD)] of the infundibulum and the anterior wall makes these segments the most resistant to ischemia, while the inferior wall is the most susceptible and the lateral wall has an intermediate level of susceptibility to ischemia. Steps involved in 3D Evaluation of RV are shown in Figure 8.

3D Evaluation of Left Atrium

Although 2D assessment remains the current standard for left atrial volume assessment in clinical practice, the visualization of the left atrium in 3D shape, independent of geometric assumptions, favors its use, and it may be the preferred method for LA volume assessment.[33-35] The 3D LV quantification software can be used for calculation of left atrial end-diastolic volume and end-systolic volume manually from maximal minimal left atrial size. This is because, the left atrial systole occurs during ventricular diastole in steps elaborated earlier.

3D Evaluation for Structural Heart Disease Intervention in Heart Failure

Structural heart disease intervention in heart failure involves mainly mitral valve interventions for secondary mitral regurgitation. This requires knowledge of the 3D echocardiographic anatomy of interatrial septum to determine the exact position of Brockenbrough puncture of the interatrial septum and that of mitral valve. Interatrial septum is a three-dimensional structure, which is very important in structural and interventional cardiology. The landmarks on the left and right side of the interatrial septum are very well studied using three-dimensional transthoracic and transesophageal echocardiography.[36-38] Three-dimensional imaging of the left atrial side is characterized by a homogeneous, flat surface showing only small pits and dents.[39] From the right atrial perspective interatrial septum (IAS) is formed by the fossa ovalis and its surrounding rim. Figure 9 shows the superior vena cava (SVC) entering the cut open right atrium. Foramen ovale is in the center and anteriorly placed below which we can see the coronary sinus. The inferior vena cava (IVC) opening is situated posteriorly and inferiorly. The rim of the Foramen ovale often appears as a ridge of thicker muscle surrounding the oval-shaped depression (the fossa). The fossa ovalis is completely overlapped by its valve, a flap of thin tissue, which lies on the left side of the IAS and is continuous with left atrial wall. Now more recent advancements have led to fusion echocardiography and techniques of integration of 3D transesophageal images over the fluoroscopic screen.[40] The placement of septal puncture in the specific areas of interatrial septum is made possible with this technique. For example, puncture in foramen ovale area for balloon mitral valvuloplasty, superioposterior aspect of foramen ovale for MitraClip application and prosthetic mitral paravalvular leak interventions and inferoposterior aspect for left atrial appendage interventions are possible with this technique (Fig. 9).[41-45]

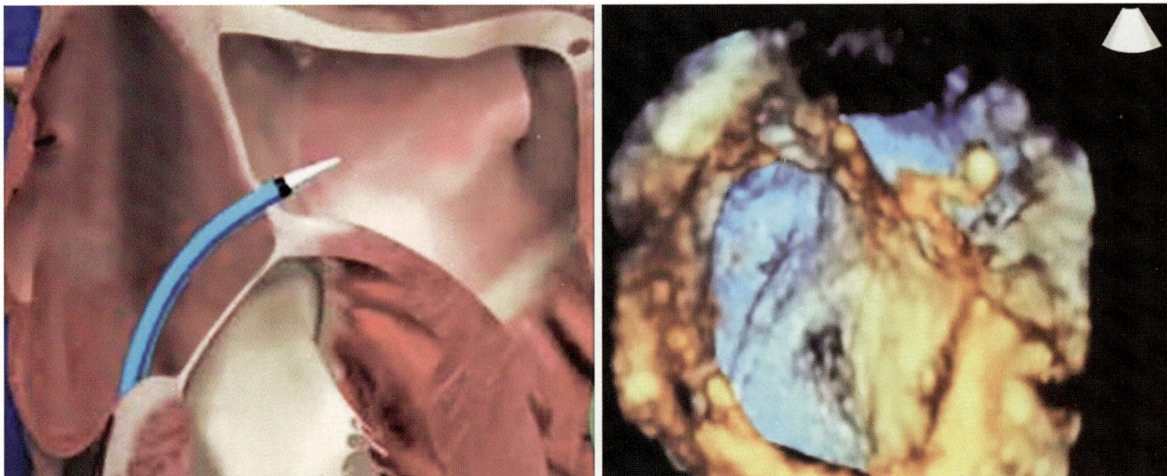

Fig. 9: Brockenbrough puncture: Diagrammatic representation and 3D echocardiography showing right atrial side of interatrial septum, aiding in selection of location of puncture.

The mitral valve is a complex structure ideally suited for examination by 3D echocardiography as mental makeup of the valve by two-dimensional echocardiography is difficult. Three dimensionally it consists of atrioventricular junction or the mitral annulus, anterior and posterior mitral leaflets with commissures in medial and lateral aspects, chordae tendineae, anterolateral and posteromedial papillary muscles and the ventricular myocardial attachments. The anterior leaflet comprises roughly two-thirds of the valve area, is about two-fold longer than the posterior leaflet, and is somewhat triangular. The posterior leaflet is more elongated and rectangular. The anterior leaflet is attached to the septum and fibrous annulus of the heart, and it is relatively nondistensible. Although the anterior leaflet accounts for two-thirds of the mitral valve area, its attachment to the mitral annulus accounts for only approximately one-third of the mitral annular circumference. The anterior mitral leaflet spans the distance between the two fibrous trigones and is in direct continuity with the noncoronary cusp of aortic valve. The posterior mitral valve leaflet is attached to the posterior two-thirds of the mitral annulus, which runs along the free wall of the left ventricle and is primarily muscular with little fibrous tissue (explaining its tendency to distend and elongate). The secondary mitral regurgitation is due dilatation of left atrium and left ventricle which in turn result in annular dilatation and increased tethering force. In echocardiographic four-chamber view, this increase in tethering force is seen as "Tenting sign" which is better seen in 3D echocardiography (Fig. 10). Percutaneous edge-to-edge repair of mitral valve regurgitation using MitraClip system mimics the surgical mitral repair introduced by Otavio Alfieri in the year 1991. The EVEREST I (Endovascular Valve Edge-to-Edge Repair Study) showed the safety and efficacy of the MitraClip system (Evalve Inc., Menlo Park, California). The procedure is shown in sequence in the following figures.

- In Figure 11A, transesophageal echocardiography shows bi-plane 2-dimensional and color flow image with MitraClip in situ, having been optimally "clipped" to the mitral leaflets.
- In Figure 11B, transesophageal echocardiography showing 3-dimensional image of the mitral valve from the left atrial side with Mitra Clip in place.

In EVEREST trial, the mortality was low and the severity of the mitral regurgitation was reduced remarkably.[45-49] The recent COAPT trial concluded that among patients with moderate-to-severe heart failure and secondary mitral regurgitation, transcatheter mitral valve repair resulted in lesser incidence of rehospitalization and mortality over a period of 24-month follow-up.[50-54]

CONCLUSION

The ever-increasing use and the literature on 3D echocardiography is a proof of the acceptance of this technique in the real world. However, with more and more development of techniques and transducer technology, special and temporal resolution of the 3D data sets are increased and there is single beat acquisition possible to avoid the stitch artifact. At present, the following are the areas where 3D echocardiography has demonstrated the usefulness. Major advantages of 3D echocardiography compared to traditional two-dimensional echocardiography in the evaluation of heart failure are the following:

- *Left ventricular function assessment*: Improved accuracy of evaluation of LV chamber volumes (by eliminating

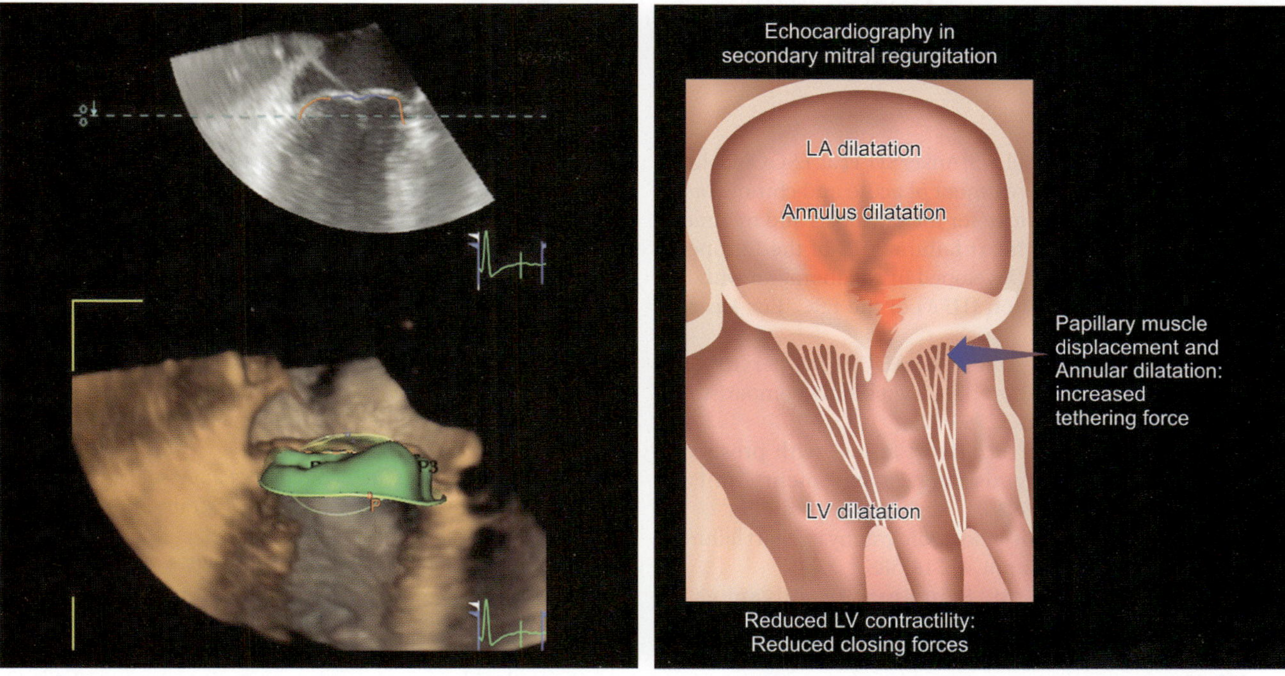

Fig. 10: The increase in tethering force on mitral valve is seen as "Tenting sign" well brought out by 3D echocardiography.

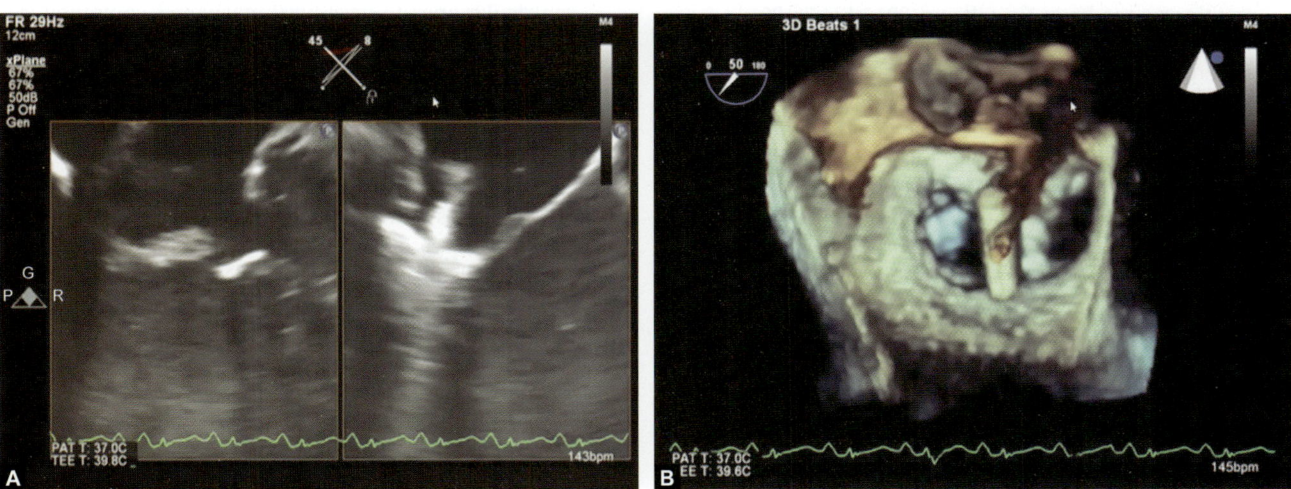

Figs. 11A and B: (A) Biplane view; (B) 3D enface view during ventricular systole and during diastole.

the need for geometric modeling as well as a reduction in errors caused by foreshortened views).

- Realistic visualization of cardiac valves especially mitral valve and mitral regurgitation. Volume rendered 3D displays of transthoracic or transesophageal images enable improved evaluation of the anatomy of the heart valves and their supporting structures. Accordingly, 3D imaging is particularly helpful to the cardiac surgeon or interventional cardiologist to provide the most detailed anatomic and functional information.
- RV volume assessment 3D echocardiography permits evaluation of regional LV function and objective detection of wall motion abnormalities.
- Data from 3D echocardiography can provide objective evidence of LV systolic dyssynchrony which may serve as an additional criterion for referral for cardiac resynchronization therapy.
- The improved echo fluoroscopic fusion images are very useful for the interventional cardiologist during structural heart interventions involving transseptal

puncture, mitral, aortic interventions, and left atrial appendage occlusion.

REFERENCES

1. McMurray JJ, Adamopoulos S, Anker SD, et al. ESC Guidelines for the diagnosis and treatment of acute and chronic heart failure 2012: The task force for the diagnosis and treatment of acute and chronic heart failure 2012 of the European Society of Cardiology. Developed in collaboration with the Heart Failure Association (HFA) of the ESC. Eur Heart J. 2012;33(14):1787-847.
2. Meer P, Gaggin HK, Dec GW. ACC/AHA versus ESC guidelines on heart failure: JACC guideline comparison. J Am Coll Cardiol. 2019;73:2756-68.
3. Gazewood JD, Turner PL. Heart failure with preserved ejection fraction: Diagnosis and management. Am Fam Physician. 2017;96(9):582-8.
4. Marwick TH. The role of echocardiography in heart failure. J Nucl Med. 2015;56(6 Suppl. 4):31S-38S.
5. Omar AMS, Bansal M, Sengupta PP. Advances in echocardiographic imaging in heart failure with reduced and preserved ejection fraction. Circ Res. 2016;119: 357-74.
6. Shah SJ, Kitzman DW, Borlaug BA, et al. Phenotype-specific treatment of heart failure with preserved ejection fraction: A multiorgan roadmap. Circulation. 2016;134:73-90.
7. Adigopula S, Grapsa J. Advances in imaging and heart failure: Where are we heading? Cardiac Fail Rev. 2018;4(2):73-7.
8. Girerd N, Seronde MF, Coiro S, et al. Integrative assessment of congestion in heart failure throughout the patient journey. J Am Coll Cardiol HF. 2018;6:273-85.
9. Bajraktari G, Pugliese NR, D'Agostino A, et al. Echo- and B-type natriuretic peptide-guided follow-up versus symptom-guided follow-up: Comparison of the outcome in ambulatory heart failure patients. Cardiol Res Pract. 2018:1-8.
10. Marwick TH. Methods used for the assessment of LV systolic function: Common currency or tower of Babel. Heart. 2013;99:1078-86.
11. Jenkins C, Bricknell K, Hanekom L, et al. Reproducibility and accuracy of echocardiographic measurements of left ventricular parameters using real-time three-dimensional echocardiography. J Am Coll Cardiol. 2004;44:878-86.
12. Albakri A. Heart failure with reduced ejection fraction: A review of clinical status and meta-analyses of diagnosis by 3D echocardiography and natriuretic peptides-guided heart failure therapy. Trends Res. 2018;1(4):1-2.
13. Jacobs LD, Salgo IS, Goonewardena S, et al. Rapid online quantification of left ventricular volume from real-time three-dimensional echocardiographic data. Eur Heart J. 2005;27:460-8.
14. Jenkins C, Chan J, Hanekom L, et al. Accuracy and feasibility of online 3-dimensional echocardiography for measurement of left ventricular parameters. J Am Soc Echocardiogr. 2006;19:1119-28.
15. Clinical applications—speckle tracking: EACVI 3D Echocardiography Box. European Society of Cardiology; 2019.
16. Ammar KA, Paterick TE, Khandheria BK, et al. Myocardial mechanics: Understanding and applying three-dimensional speckle tracking echocardiography in clinical practice. Echocardiography. 2012;29(7):861-72.
17. Ewer MS, Banchs JA. Strain echocardiography: Routine strain analysis is ready for clinical purpose. Expert analysis. Am Coll Cardiol. 2017.
18. Muraru D, Niero A, Rodriguez-Zanella H, et al. Three-dimensional speckle-tracking echocardiography: Benefits and limitations of integrating myocardial mechanics with three-dimensional imaging. Cardiovasc Diagn Ther. 2018;8(1):101-17.
19. Kalam K, Otahal P, Marwick TH. Prognostic implications of global LV dysfunction: A systematic review and meta-analysis of global longitudinal strain and ejection fraction. Heart. 2014;100:1673-80.
20. Joyce E, Hoogslag GE, Leong DP, et al. Association between left ventricular global longitudinal strain and adverse left ventricular dilatation after ST-segment–elevation myocardial infarction. Circ Cardiovasc Imaging. 2014;7:74-81.
21. Munk Kim, Andersen NH, Terkelsen CJ, et al. Global left ventricular longitudinal systolic strain for early risk assessment in patients with acute myocardial infarction treated with primary percutaneous intervention. J Am Soc Echocardiogr. 2012;25(6):644-51.
22. Ashraf M, Myronenko A, Nguyen T, et al. Defining left ventricular apex-to-base twist mechanics computed from high-resolution 3D echocardiography validation against sonomicrometry. J Am Coll Cardiol Imaging. 2010;3:227-34.
23. Beladan CC, Călin A, Roşca M, et al. Left ventricular twist dynamics: Principles and applications. Heart. 2014;100: 731-40.
24. Helle-Valle T, Crosby J, Edvardsen T, et al. New noninvasive method for assessment of left ventricular rotation: Speckle tracking echocardiography. Circulation. 2005;112:3149-56.
25. Kauer F, Geleijnse ML, van Dalen BM. Role of left ventricular twist mechanics in cardiomyopathies, dance of the helices. World J Cardiol. 2015;7(8):476-82.
26. Schiller NB, Shah PM, Crawford M, et al. Recommendations for quantitation of the left ventricle by two-dimensional echocardiography. American Society of Echocardiography Committee on Standards, Subcommittee on Quantitation of Two-Dimensional Echocardiograms. J Am Soc Echocardiogr. 1989;2:358-67.
27. Lang RM, Badano LP, Mor-Avi V, et al. Recommendations for cardiac chamber quantification by echocardiography in adults: An update from the American Society of Echocardiography and the European Association of Cardiovascular Imaging. J Am Soc Echocardiogr. 2015;28:1-39.
28. Feigenbaum H. Echocardiographic chamber quantification in the era of multimodality imaging: Beware of unintended consequences. Correspondence. J Am Soc Echocardiogr. 2015;28:847-50.
29. Altiok E, Tiemann S,Becker M, et al. Myocardial deformation imaging by two-dimensional speckle-tracking echocardiography for prediction of global and segmental functional changes after acute myocardial infarction: A

comparison with late gadolinium enhancement cardiac magnetic resonance. J Am Soc Echocardiogr. 2014;27(3) 249-57.

30. Rudski LG, Lai WW, Afilalo J, et al. Guidelines for the echocardiographic assessment of the right heart in adults: A report from the American Society of Echocardiography endorsed by the European Association of Echocardiography, a registered branch of the European Society of Cardiology, and the Canadian Society of Echocardiography. J Am Soc Echocardiogr. 2010;23:685-713.
31. Rallidis LS, Makavos G, Nihoyannopoulos P. Right ventricular involvement in coronary artery disease: Role of echocardiography for diagnosis and prognosis. J Am Soc Echocardiogr. 2014;27:223-9.
32. Ostenfeld E, Flachskampf FA. Assessment of right ventricular volumes and ejection fraction by echocardiography: From geometric approximations to realistic shapes. Echo Res Pract. 2015;2(1):R1-R11.
33. Miyasaka Y, Tsujimoto S, Maeba H, et al. Left atrial volume by real-time three-dimensional echocardiography: Validation by 64-slice multidetector computed tomography. J Am Soc Echocardiogr. 2011;24:680-6.
34. Marsan NA, Tops LF, Holman ER, et al. Comparison of left atrial volumes and function by real-time three-dimensional echocardiography in patients having catheter ablation for atrial fibrillation with persistence of sinus rhythm versus recurrent atrial fibrillation three months later. Am J Cardiol. 2008;102:847-53.
35. Delgado V, Vidal B, Sitges M, et al. Fate of left atrial function as determined by real-time three-dimensional echocardiography study after radiofrequency catheter ablation for the treatment of atrial fibrillation. Am J Cardiol. 2008;101:1285-90.
36. Faletra FF, Nucifora G, Ho SY. Imaging the atrial septum using real-time three-dimensional transesophageal echocardiography: Technical tips normal anatomy its role in transseptal puncture. J Am Soc Echocardiogr. 2011;24: 593-99.
37. Roberson DA, Cui W, Patel D, et al. Three-dimensional transesophageal echocardiography of atrial septal defect: A qualitative and quantitative anatomic study. J Am Soc Echocardiogr. 2011;24(6):600-10.
38. Saric M, Perk G, Purgess JR, et al. Imaging atrial septal defects by real-time three-dimensional transesophageal echocardiography: Step-by-step approach. J Am Soc Echocardiogr. 2010;23:1128-35.
39. Mahmoud HM, Al-Ghamdi MA, Ghabashi AE, et al. A proposed maneuver to guide transseptal puncture using real-time three-dimensional transesophageal echocardiography: Pilot study. Cardiol Res Pract. 2015;4.
40. Afzal S, Veulemans V, Balzer J, et al. Safety and efficacy of transseptal puncture guided by real-time fusion of echocardiography and fluoroscopy. Neth Heart J. 2017;25:131-6.
41. Altiok E, Hamada S, van Halla S, et al. Comparison of direct planimetry of mitral valve regurgitation orifice area by three-dimensional transesophageal echocardiography to effective regurgitant orifice area obtained by proximal flow convergence method and vena contracta area determined by color Doppler echocardiography. Am J Cardiol. 2011;107(3):452-8.
42. Siegel RJ, Luo H, Makar M, et al. Optimal use of echocardiography in valvular heart disease evaluation. Heart. 2015;101:977-86.
43. Eng MH, Salcedo EE, Quaife R, et al. Implementation of real time three-dimensional transesophageal echocardiography in percutaneous mitral balloon valvuloplasty and structural heart disease interventions. Echocardiography. 2009;26: 958-66.
44. Navarro MA, Kim M, Salcedo EE. Real-time 3D echocardiography in percutaneous balloon mitral valvuloplasty. 2013.
45. Cavalcante JL, Rodriguez L, Kapadia S, et al Role of echocardiography in percutaneous mitral valve interventions. JACC Cardiovasc Imaging. 2012;5:733-46.
46. Feldman T, Kar S, Rinaldi M, et al.; EVEREST investigators. Percutaneous mitral repair with the MitraClip system: Safety and midterm durability in the initial EVEREST (Endovascular Valve Edge-to-Edge REpair Study) cohort. J Am Coll Cardiol.2009;54:686-94.
47. Gopalamurugan AB, Pantazis A, Schievano S, et al. Percutaneous transvenous mitral valve implantation. J Am Coll Cardiol. 2013;61(7):e143.
48. Regueiro A, Granada JF, Dagenais F, et al. Transcatheter mitral valve replacement: Insights from early clinical experience and future challenges. J Am Coll Cardiol. 2017;69:2175-92.
49. Mor Avi V, Lang RM. Three-dimensional echocardiography. UpToDate. 2015;1-18
50. Stone GW, Lindenfeld J, Abraham WT, et al.; COAPT Investigators. Transcatheter mitral-valve repair in patients with heart failure. N Engl J Med. 2018;379(24):2307-18.
51. Lavall D, Hagendorff A, Schirmer SH, et al. Mitral valve interventions in heart failure. ESC Heart Fail. 2018;5:552-61.
52. Pinamonti B, Lenarda AD, Sinagra G, et al. Restrictive left ventricular filling pattern in dilated cardiomyopathy assessed by Doppler echocardiography: Clinical, echocardiographic and hemodynamic correlations and prognostic implications. J Am Coll Cardiol. 1993;22(3):808-15.
53. Park JH, Marwick TH. Use and limitations of E/e' to assess left ventricular filling pressure by echocardiography. J Cardiovasc Ultrasound. 2011;19(4):169-73.
54. Oh JK, Park SJ, Nagueh SF. Established and novel clinical applications of diastolic function assessment by echocardiography. Circ Cardiovasc Imaging. 2011;4:444-55.

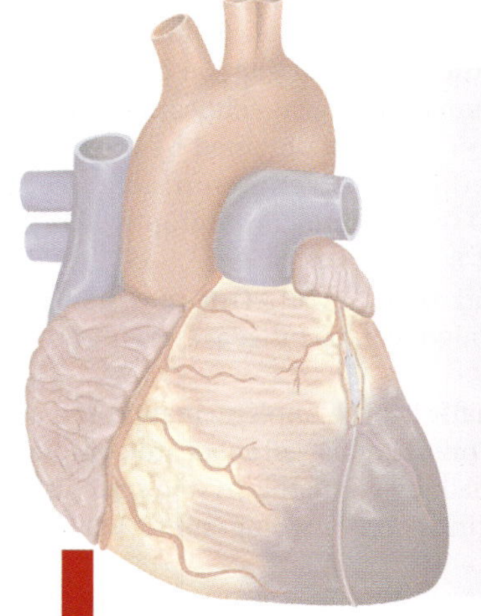

Echocardiographic Assessment of Left Ventricular Hypertrophy and Left Atrial Volume in Heart Failure

Manish Bansal, Ravi R Kasliwal, HK Chopra, Karishma Walia

INTRODUCTION

Development of left ventricular hypertrophy (LVH) and left atrial (LA) enlargement are common cardiac structural changes that occur in patients with heart failure. These changes either occur as the primary cardiac abnormality responsible for heart failure or result from the altered loading conditions that the left ventricle and left atrium are chronically exposed to. Their presence thus provides important pathophysiological insights into heart failure and has both diagnostic and prognostic implications. For this reason, assessment of LVH and LA size forms an important part of evaluation of patients with heart failure. Echocardiography is the most commonly used modality for this purpose, owing to its easy availability, simplicity, safety, and the ability to permit comprehensive cardiac assessment in virtually no time.

LEFT VENTRICULAR HYPERTROPHY

Left ventricular hypertrophy usually occurs as a response to chronic pressure or volume overload of the left ventricle. In some patients, such as those with cardiomyopathies or infiltrative myocardial disorders, LVH is the direct manifestation of the underlying etiological process. Although LVH can be detected on ECG also, echocardiography is more sensitive and specific than ECG alone for detection of LVH.[1] Additionally, echocardiography also permits quantification of LV mass, characterization of LVH pattern, and recognition of any hemodynamic or functional effects of LVH.

Echocardiographic Assessment of LVH

The diagnosis of LVH on echocardiography can be made based on increased left ventricular (LV) wall thickness, or more formally, by estimation of LV mass. Compared with LV wall thickness, LV mass assessment is more accurate and has superior prognostic value.[2] For this reason, LV mass estimation is the preferred method for diagnosis of LVH by echocardiography. There are several echocardiographic methods available for estimation of LV mass,[3] all of which rely on calculating LV myocardial volume by subtracting LV cavity volume from the total LV volume. Multiplying LV myocardial volume with density factor yields LV mass, which is then index to body surface area.

Linear Method

This is the simplest and the most commonly employed method for estimation of LV mass. The following equation is used for calculating LV mass:[4]

$$\text{LV mass (g)} = 1.04 \times [(\text{LVIDd} + \text{IVSd} + \text{PWd})^3 - \text{LVIDd}^3] \times 0.8 + 0.6$$

where 1.04 is the myocardial density, and 0.8 is the correction factor. LVIDd, IVSd, and PWd represent the end-diastolic LV internal diameter, interventricular septal thickness, and posterior wall thickness, respectively (Fig. 1). These chamber dimensions are obtained from the parasternal long-axis view. Traditionally, M-mode imaging has been used for obtaining these measurements. However, two-dimensional echocardiography (2DE) or 2DE-guided

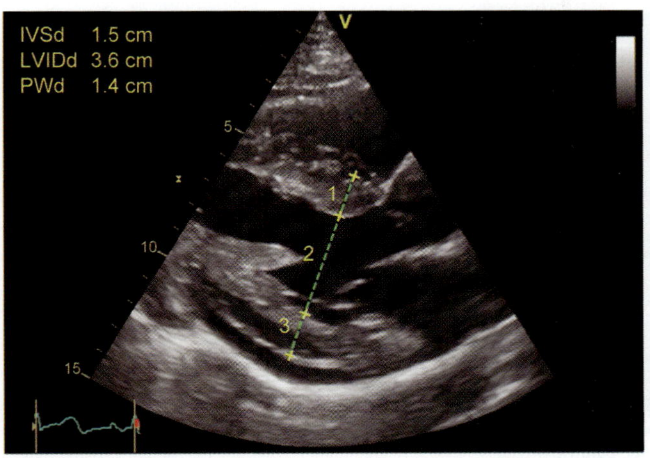

LV mass (gm) = 1.04 × [(LVIDd + IVSd + PWd)³ – LVIDd³] × 0.8 + 0.6
= 1.04 × [(3.6 + 1.5 + 1.4)³ – 3.6³] × 0.8 + 0.6
= 1.04 × [274.6 – 46.7] × 0.8 + 0.6
= 190.2 gm

Fig. 1: Estimation of left ventricular mass using the linear method. See text for more details.
(LV: left ventricular; IVSd: interventricular septal thickness; LVIDd: LV internal diameter; PWd: posterior wall thickness)

M-mode is currently preferred because they allow accurate alignment of measurement plane perpendicular to the long-axis of the left ventricle.

Despite its popularity, the linear method has several limitations because of which it is less preferred now a days (Table 1). The most important limitation is that it is based only on a single dimension and involves mathematical assumptions about LV geometry, which do not hold true if the LV shape is distorted. Furthermore, the method is error prone as any error in the measurement of LV dimension gets greatly amplified once the dimension is raised to power 3 for converting to volumes. Nonetheless, in uniformly enlarged left ventricles, it remains a reasonably accurate method for assessment of LVH.

2D Methods

Two different 2DE methods are currently available for estimation of LV mass—the area-length method and the truncated ellipsoid method.

For the area-length method, parasternal short-axis view is obtained at the papillary muscle level and the LV epicardial and endocardial cross-sectional areas (A_1 and

TABLE 1: Relative advantages and limitations of different echocardiographic methods for estimation of LV mass.

Method	Advantages	Limitations
Linear method (M-mode or 2D)	• Simple and quick method • Suitable for screening large populations • Fairly accurate in normally shaped ventricles • Most commonly used method in various studies; hence, it has demonstrated prognostic value with a wealth of published data	• Involves mathematical assumptions about LV shape which may not necessarily be correct • LV dimensions are measured only along one axis; therefore, not accurate in presence of asymmetric hypertrophy, distorted ventricles • Alignment of measurement plane perpendicular to the long-axis of the left ventricle is essential for accurate measurement • Even small measurement errors in dimensions or thickness result in significant error in LV mass as the measurements are cubed • Overestimates LV mass
2D methods (area-length method, truncated ellipsoid method)	• Provides partial correction for LV shape distortions • Less dependent on geometrical assumptions than the linear measurements	• Requires good image quality with good endocardial and epicardial definitions • Proper orientation of parasternal short-axis views (no oblique planes) is crucial • Cumbersome methodology • Higher measurement variability • Few published normative data • Limited prognostic data
3D echocardiography	• Direct measurement without geometrical assumptions about cavity shape and hypertrophy distribution • More accurate than the linear or the 2D measurements • Higher inter-measurement and test/retest reproducibility • Better discriminates small changes within a patient	• Highly dependent on image quality • Patient's cooperation required for acquisition of analysis quality images • Normal values less well established

(2D: two dimensional; 3D: three dimensional; LV left ventricular)
Source: Modified from Lang et al.[3]

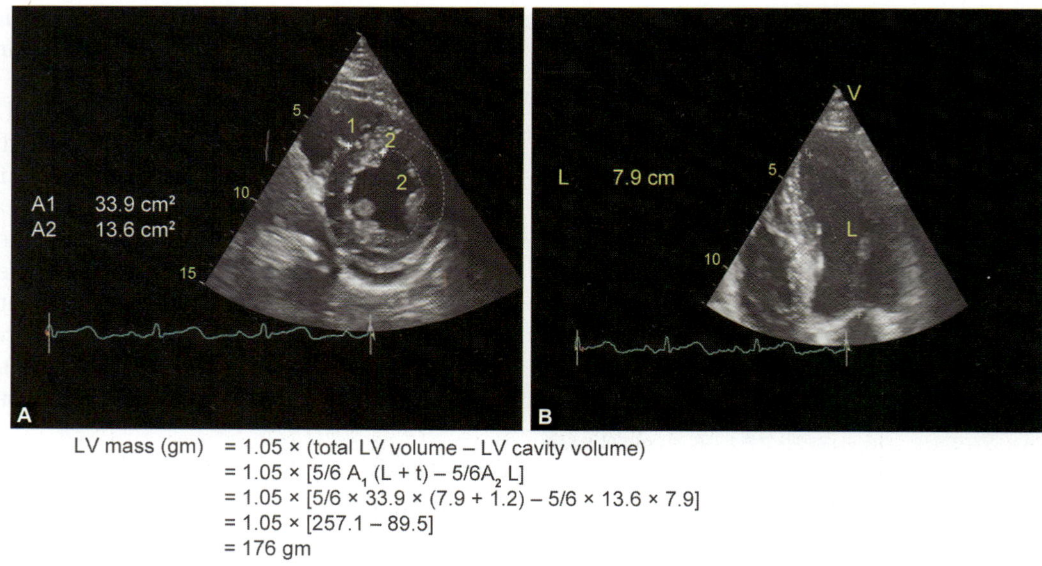

Figs. 2A and B: Estimation of the left ventricular (LV) mass using the area-length method. (A) measurement of LV cross-sectional areas from the parasternal short axis view; (B) LV length measurement from the apical four-chamber view. See text for more details.
(A1: total LV cross-sectional area; A2: LV cavity area; L: length of the left ventricle; t: mean wall thickness)

A_2) are measured by tracing the epicardium and the endocardium, respectively (Figs. 2A and B). Care should be taken to include the papillary muscles in the cavity and not in the myocardium. Next, the LV length (L) is measured from the apical four-chamber view and the LV mass is calculated using the following equation:

$$\text{LV mass} = 1.05 \times (\text{total LV volume} - \text{LV cavity volume})$$
$$= 1.05 \times [5/6\, A_1\, (L+t) - 5/6 A_2\, L]$$

where t is the mean wall thickness derived by subtracting the LV cavity radius from the LV radius as described below:

$$t = \sqrt{(A_1/\pi)} - \sqrt{(A_2/\pi)}$$

The echocardiographer does not have to perform these calculations manually as the analysis package on most of the currently available echocardiography machines includes this calculation. Thus, once the LV short-axis areas and LV length are measured, the inbuilt software automatically calculates LV mass.

The truncated ellipsoid method is somewhat more complex and hence, not discussed here in detail.

Three-Dimensional Echocardiography

Three-dimensional (3D) echocardiography (3DE) is currently the most accurate echocardiographic method for estimation of LV. The greater accuracy of 3DE relates to the fact that, unlike the 2D methods, the 3D method includes whole left ventricle in the image and analyzes it in toto, without resorting to any mathematical assumption. For 3DE estimation of LV mass, first a full-volume 3D dataset is acquired from apical position and then LV endocardial and epicardial borders are semiautomatically traced at end-diastole and end-systole in different LV projections. The border tracking is reviewed throughout the cardiac cycle and along different imaging planes and can be manually adjusted as required. Once satisfactory border tracking is achieved, the in-built software automatically calculates LV mass (Fig. 3). Compared with 2DE, 3DE-derived LV mass is more accurate and more reproducible with less interobserver variability.[5-7] Several studies have shown that LV mass measured by 3DE has excellent correlation with the measurements obtained using cardiac myocardial resonance imaging.[5-18] Furthermore, the accuracy is maintained even in the presence of regional wall motion abnormalities or abnormal LV geometry due to other causes.[13,14,19]. Keeping with these evidences, the American Society of Echocardiography (ASE) recommends 3DE as the preferred method for LV mass assessment, whenever feasible, and particularly in abnormally shaped ventricles or in patients with asymmetric or localized hypertrophy.[3] However, the practicality, feasibility, or prognostic value of 3DE-derived LV mass estimation in large-scale clinical environments has not been adequately assessed.[20]

Normal Values of LV Mass

The normal ranges and the partition values for LV mass using the linear and the 2DE methods are summarized in Table 2. However, only limited data are currently available for 3DE-derived LV mass,[21] which is insufficient for recommending normal reference values for healthy subjects at present.

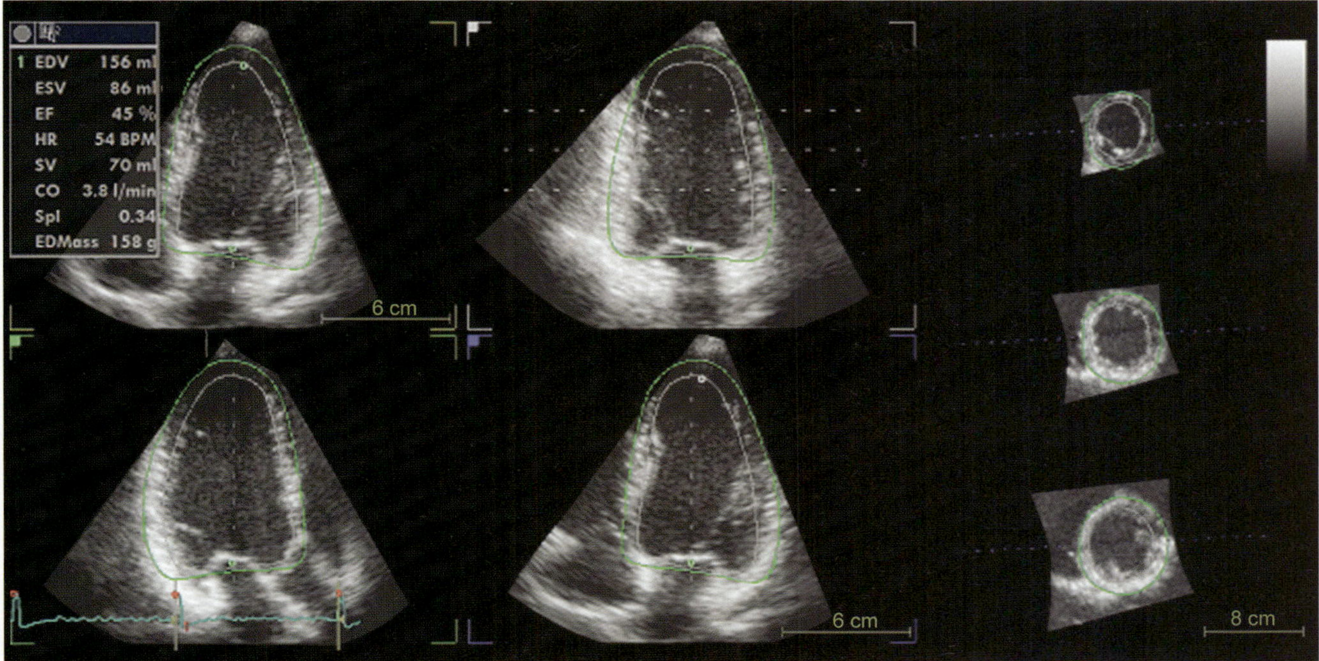

Fig. 3: Estimation of left ventricular mass by three-dimensional echocardiography. See text for more details. (CO: cardiac output; ED Mass: end-diastolic mass; EDV: end-diastolic volume; EF: ejection fraction; ESV: end-systolic volume; HR: heart rate; SpI: sphericity index; SV: stroke volume)

Pattern of LVH

Depending on whether the increase in LV wall thickness is proportionate to the LV cavity size or not, the LVH can be categorized as concentric or eccentric. When the wall thickness is increased out of proportion to LV cavity size, it is called concentric LVH, which typically occurs in response to pressure overload of the left ventricle as seen in longstanding hypertension, aortic stenosis, etc. Conversely, when the LV cavity size is enlarged in proportion to the increase in LV mass, it is known as eccentric LVH. Eccentric LVH usually occurs as a result of LV volume overload as in aortic regurgitation, mitral regurgitation, etc. The distinction between concentric and eccentric LVH is based on relative wall thickness (RWT).[3] RWT is a measure of myocardial thickness relative to the LV cavity size and is calculated using the following equation:

$$RWT = (2 \times PWd)/LVIDd$$

A value of >0.42 indicates increased RWT, supporting a diagnosis of concentric LVH, whereas a value of <0.42

TABLE 2: Reference ranges and partition values for left ventricular mass estimated by echocardiography.

	Men				*Women*			
	Reference range	*Mildly abnormal*	*Moderately abnormal*	*Severely abnormal*	*Reference range*	*Mildly abnormal*	*Moderately abnormal*	*Severely abnormal*
Linear method								
LV mass (g)	88–224	225–258	259–292	≥293	67–162	163–186	187–210	≥211
LV mass index* (g/m²)	49–115	116–131	132–148	≥149	43–95	96–108	109–121	≥122
Two-dimensional method								
LV mass (g)	96–200	201–227	228–254	≥255	66–150	151–171	172–192	≥193
LV mass index* (g/m²)	50–102	103–116	117–130	≥131	44–88	89–100	101–112	≥112

*Indexed to body surface area.
(LV: left ventricular)
Source: Lang et al.[3]

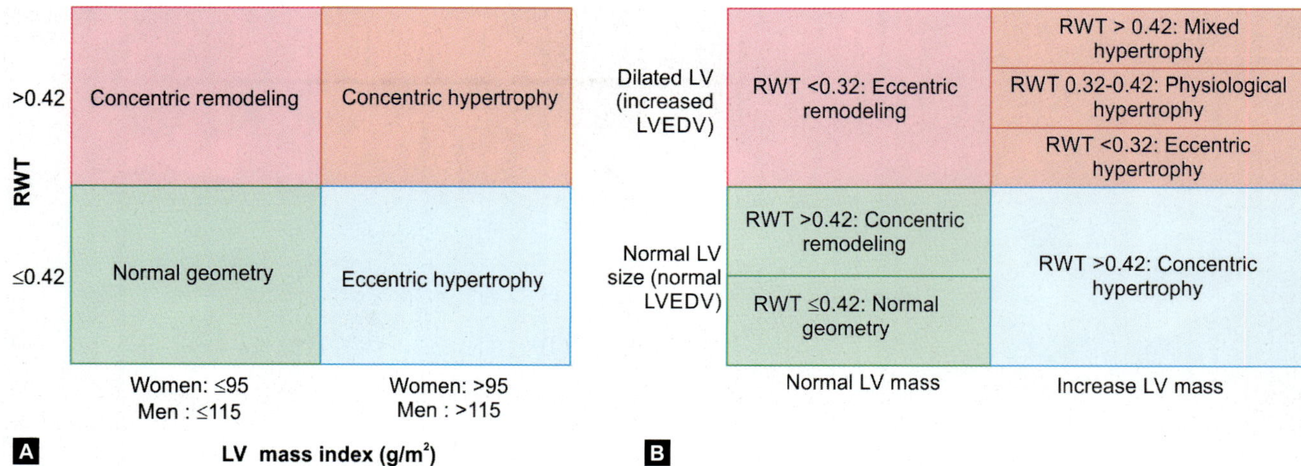

Figs. 4A and B: Classification of patterns of left ventricular geometry. (A) The classification recommended by the American Society of Echocardiography; (B) The alternate classification proposed by Gaasch and Zile.[24] See text for details.
(LV: left ventricular; LVEDV: left ventricular end-diastolic volume; RWT: relative wall thickness)

favors a diagnosis of eccentric LVH (Figs. 4A and B). In some individuals, RWT is increased, but the LV mass is either normal or the increase in LV mass is not sufficient to qualify for LVH. This is known as concentric remodeling, which usually occurs in response to pressure overload. Although concentric LVH is associated with a greater risk of cardiovascular mortality, concentric remodeling too has been shown to be an adverse prognostic marker.[22,23] Gaasch and Zile have proposed an alternative scheme for classification of LVH that takes into account LV cavity size as well.[24] Prognostic value of this classification was assessed in the Cardiovascular Health Study cohort in which it was found to have incremental predictive value for cardiovascular outcomes.[25]

Clinical Significance of LVH in Patients with Heart Failure

Concentric LVH or concentric remodeling are common in patients with heart failure with preserved ejection fraction (HFpEF), occurring in 30–35% patients each.[26-30]. Eccentric LVH occurs rarely, in 7–9% patients, whereas the remaining 30% patients have normal LV geometry. The high prevalence of concentric LVH/remodeling in HFpEF is due to increased radial thickness of LV myocardial fibers with increased deposition of extracellular collagen, which occur almost ubiquitously in HFpEF.[31-33] The development of concentric LVH leads to LV diastolic dysfunction which is the key pathophysiological abnormality in HFpEF. Hence, the finding of concentric LVH in a patient with HF symptoms with preserved LVEF serves as an important corroborative to support the diagnosis of HFpEF. In contrast, the patients with heart failure with reduced ejection fraction (HFrEF) have an elongation of cardiac myocytes with no increase in the width. There is also myocyte necrosis and degradation of extracellular collagen due to the increased activity of matrix metalloproteinase and other similar enzymes.[31-33] As a result, there is eccentric LV remodeling with an increase in LV cavity size but without any increase in LV wall thickness, or there may even be LV wall thinning. The overall LV mass may remain normal or may be increased. Apart from its diagnostic value in HFpEF, LVH has considerable prognostic significance as well. Being a marker of underlying structural adaptations and a precursor to LV diastolic dysfunction, LVH is associated with increased risk for incident heart failure, arrhythmias, stroke, and sudden death. The adjusted relative risk for cardiovascular mortality is estimated to be 1.5–3.5 in various studies.[34-36] For example, in the MAVI (The MAssaVentricolare sinistra nell'Ipertensione) study, each 39 g/m^2 increase in LV mass was associated with a 40% rise in the risk of major cardiovascular events and this association was independent of clinical parameters including age, cigarette smoking, and diabetes.[37]

LEFT ATRIAL VOLUME

Left atrial enlargement can occur in a variety of cardiac conditions including LV diastolic dysfunction of any cause, mitral valve diseases, atrial fibrillation, and atrial cardiomyopathy.

Echocardiographic Estimation of LA Volume

During echocardiography, LA size can be assessed by measuring LA linear diameter, LA area, or LA volume. Since

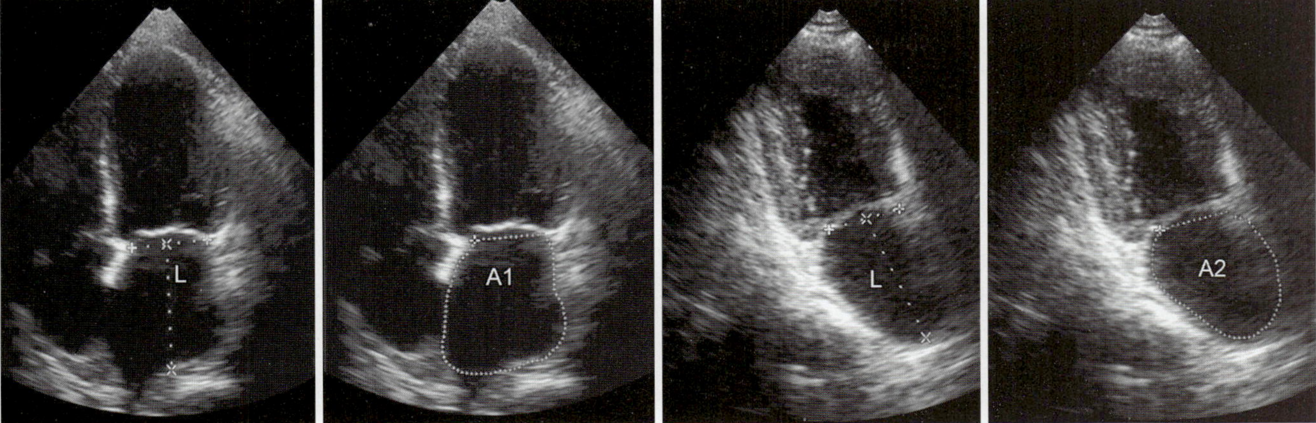

Fig. 5: Estimation of the left atrial volume by the biplane area-length method during transthoracic echocardiography. See text for details.
(A1 and A2: left atrial areas obtained by planimetry from the apical four-chamber and two-chamber views; L: left atrial length measured from the apical four-chamber and two-chamber views)

LA diameter or area reflect LA enlargement in only one or two dimensions respectively, they are inherently inaccurate and are currently not preferred.[38-41]

There are two commonly employed methods for estimation of LA volume by echocardiography--the biplane area-length method based on the ellipsoid model or the Simpson's method. Although most of the data has been derived using the biplane area-length method, the current guidelines recommend Simpson's method owing to its simplicity.[3] For area-length method, the left atrium needs to be planimetered in apical four-chamber and two-chamber views to obtain LA areas (A1 and A2 respectively, Fig. 5). The LA length (L) also needs to be measured in both these views, as the perpendicular distance from the mid-point of the mitral annular plane to the superior aspect of the left atrium. Shorter of the two measurements is used for subsequent calculations.

The following equation is used for calculating LA volume:

$$\text{LA volume} = 8/3p\ (A_1 \times A_2/L)$$

Certain precautions need to be taken when planimetering LA area. The confluences of pulmonary veins and LA appendage should be excluded from the area measurement. Additionally, foreshortening of the left atrium should be avoided by ensuring that the base of the left atrium is at its largest size in the views used for the measurements. The biplane Simpson's method for LA volume estimation is identical to the method used for LV volume estimation. The LA endocardial border is traced in apical four-chamber and two-chamber views and the inbuilt software automatically calculates LA volume.

Similar to the left ventricle, 3D echocardiography has been used for estimation of LA volume also, although it remains technically challenging. Recent studies have shown superiority of 3DE over 2DE for estimation of LA volumes (Fig. 6).[42,43] Compared with 2DE-derived LA volumes, the 3DE-derived LA volumes have been shown to be more reproducible and have better correlations with computed tomography and cardiac magnetic resonance imaging.[44-46]

Normal Values

The recommended upper limit of LA volume by 2DE methods is 34 mL/m^2. Compared with 2DE, 3DE generally provides larger values of LA volumes.[46] However, due to paucity of data,[47] reference ranges for 3DE-derived LA volume have not been recommended in the recent guidelines.[3]

Clinical Utility in Heart Failure Patients

Left atrial enlargement is quite common in heart failure, occurring in most patients with HFrEF and nearly 50–66% patients with HFpEF.[26,28] Persistent elevation of LV filling pressure is the main driving force for LA enlargement, though atrial fibrillation and mitral regurgitation also contribute to this.

Being a marker of chronic LV diastolic dysfunction, LA enlargement is an important supportive evidence for diagnosis of HFpEF. In absence of an alternate cause (such as atrial fibrillation or mitral regurgitation), LA enlargement is virtually diagnostic of LV diastolic dysfunction. Moreover, the size of the left atrium correlates with the severity and the chronicity of LV diastolic dysfunction.[48-50] For this reason, LA size is also considered to be the glycosylated hemoglobin of LV diastolic function.

Left atrial size is a strong predictor of adverse cardiovascular outcomes. It is associated with increased

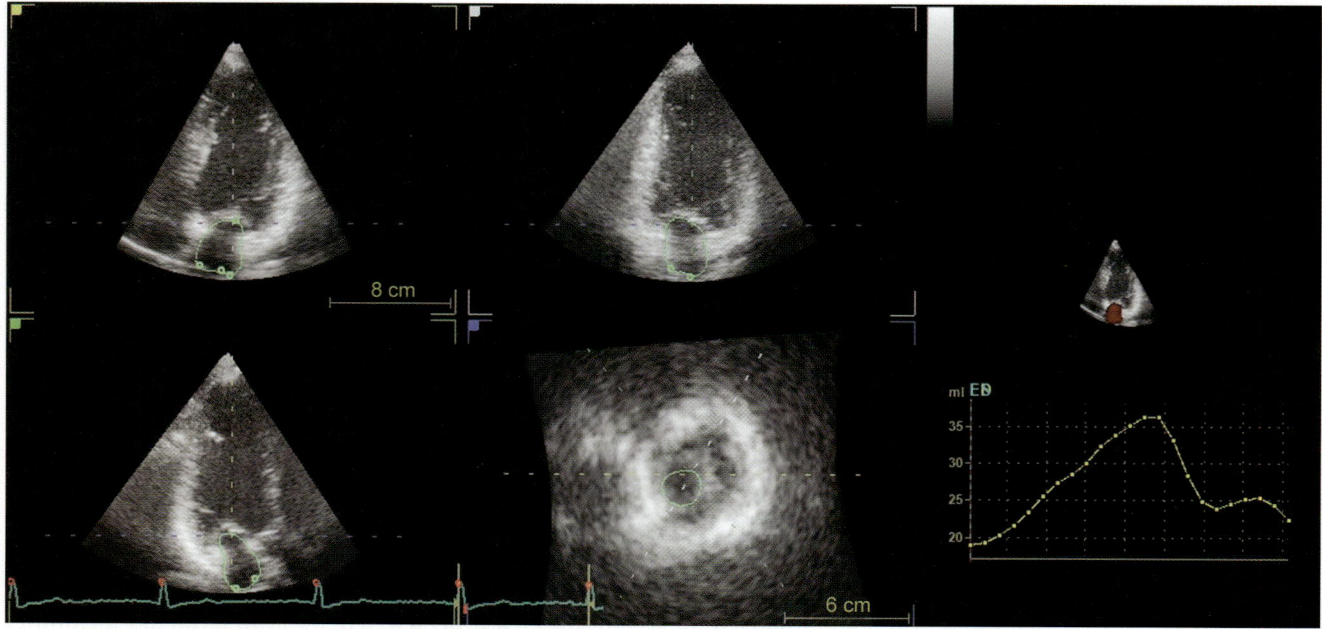

Fig. 6: Three-dimensional echocardiography for estimation of left atrial volume.

risk of atrial fibrillation, heart failure hospitalizations, stroke, and overall cardiovascular mortality.[26,28,40,48,51-62] In the Framingham Heart Study, prognostic value of LA size was assessed in a subset of 1,924 elderly subjects followed up for 7.2 years.[60] The LA size was found to be a strong independent predictor of the risk of nonrheumatic atrial fibrillation. Similarly, in yet another study involving elderly subjects with no prior atrial fibrillation, LA volume was independently predictive of first ischemic stroke and even death.[58] Several other studies have also reported similar findings.

CONCLUSION

Left ventricular hypertrophy and LA enlargement are common cardiac structural changes occurring in patients with heart failure. Their presence in HFpEF patients provides a confirmation of the underlying LV diastolic dysfunction and is thus helpful in establishing the diagnosis. Their diagnostic utility in HFrEF is relatively limited. Nonetheless, in both HFpEF and HFrEF, LVH and LA enlargement have significant prognostic value. Increase in the LV mass or LA size is strong predictors of adverse cardiovascular outcomes including heart failure hospitalizations, atrial fibrillation, stroke, and overall cardiovascular mortality. Echocardiography is the simplest and widely available diagnostic modality that can easily permit accurate assessment of LV mass and LA size. This further enhances the utility of echocardiography in heart failure.

REFERENCES

1. Victor RG, Kaplan NM. Systemic hypertension: Mechanisms and diagnosis. In: Libby P, Bonow RO, Mann DL, Zipes DP, editors. Braunwald's Heart Disease: A Text-book of Cardiovascular Medicine, 8th edition. Philadelphia: Saunders; 2008. pp. 1027-48.
2. Cuspidi C, Facchetti R, Bombelli M, et al. Differential value of left ventricular mass index and wall thickness in predicting cardiovascular prognosis: Data from the PAMELA population. Am J Hypertens. 2014;27(8):1079-86.
3. Lang RM, Badano LP, Mor-Avi V, et al. Recommendations for cardiac chamber quantification by echocardiography in adults: An update from the American Society of Echocardiography and the European Association of Cardiovascular Imaging. J Am Soc Echocardiogr. 2015;28:1-39e14.
4. Devereux RB, Alonso DR, Lutas EM, et al. Echocardiographic assessment of left ventricular hypertrophy: Comparison to necropsy findings. Am J Cardiol. 1986;57:450-8.
5. Mor-Avi V, Sugeng L, Weinert L, et al. Fast measurement of left ventricular mass with real-time three-dimensional echocardiography: Comparison with magnetic resonance imaging. Circulation. 2004;110:1814-8.
6. Yap SC, van Geuns RJ, Nemes A, et al. Rapid and accurate measurement of LV mass by biplane real-time 3D echocardiography in patients with concentric LV hypertrophy: comparison to CMR. Eur J Echocardiogr. 2008;9:255-60.
7. Pacileo G, Castaldi B, Di Salvo G, et al. Assessment of left-ventricular mass and remodeling in obese adolescents: M-mode, 2D or 3D echocardiography? J Cardiovasc Med. (Hagerstown, Md) 2013;14:144-9.

8. Jenkins C, Bricknell K, Hanekom L, et al. Reproducibility and accuracy of echocardiographic measurements of left ventricular parameters using real-time three-dimensional echocardiography. J Am Coll Cardiol. 2004;44:878-86.
9. Oe H, Hozumi T, Arai K, et al. Comparison of accurate measurement of left ventricular mass in patients with hypertrophied hearts by real-time three-dimensional echocardiography versus magnetic resonance imaging. Am J Cardiol. 2005;95:1263-7.
10. Mor-Avi V, Sugeng L, Weinert L, et al. Fast measurement of left ventricular mass with real-time three-dimensional echocardiography: Comparison with magnetic resonance imaging. Circulation. 2004;110:1814-8.
11. Bicudo LS, Tsutsui JM, Shiozaki A, et al. Value of real time three-dimensional echocardiography in patients with hypertrophic cardiomyopathy: Comparison with two-dimensional echocardiography and magnetic resonance imaging. Echocardiography. 2008;25:717-26.
12. Caiani EG, Corsi C, Sugeng L, et al. Improved quantification of left ventricular mass based on endocardial and epicardial surface detection with real time three dimensional echocardiography. Heart (British Cardiac Society). 2006;92:213-9.
13. Chang SA, Kim HK, Lee SC, et al. Assessment of left ventricular mass in hypertrophic cardiomyopathy by real-time three-dimensional echocardiography using single-beat capture image. J Am Soc Echocardiogr. 2013;26:436-42.
14. van den Bosch AE, Robbers-Visser D, Krenning BJ, et al. Comparison of real-time three-dimensional echocardiography to magnetic resonance imaging for assessment of left ventricular mass. Am J Cardiol. 2006;97:113-7.
15. Shimada YJ, Shiota T. A meta-analysis and investigation for the source of bias of left ventricular volumes and function by three-dimensional echocardiography in comparison with magnetic resonance imaging. Am J Cardiol. 2011;107:126-38.
16. Qin JX, Jones M, Travaglini A, et al. The accuracy of left ventricular mass determined by real-time three-dimensional echocardiography in chronic animal and clinical studies: A comparison with postmortem examination and magnetic resonance imaging. J Am Soc Echocardiogr. 2005;18:1037-43.
17. Lenstrup M, Kjaergaard J, Petersen CL, et al. Evaluation of left ventricular mass measured by 3D echocardiography using magnetic resonance imaging as gold standard. Scand J Clin Lab Invest. 2006;66:647-57.
18. Oe H, Hozumi T, Arai K, et al. Comparison of accurate measurement of left ventricular mass in patients with hypertrophied hearts by real-time three-dimensional echocardiography versus magnetic resonance imaging. Am J Cardiol. 2005;95:1263-7.
19. Pouleur AC, le Polain de Waroux JB, Pasquet A, et al. Assessment of left ventricular mass and volumes by three-dimensional echocardiography in patients with or without wall motion abnormalities: Comparison against cine magnetic resonance imaging. Heart. 2008;94:1050-7.
20. Marsan NA, Bleeker GB, Ypenburg C, et al. Real-time three-dimensional echocardiography as a novel approach to assess left ventricular and left atrium reverse remodeling and to predict response to cardiac resynchronization therapy. Heart Rhythm. 2008;5:1257-64.
21. Mizukoshi K, Takeuchi M, Nagata Y, et al. Normal values of left ventricular mass index assessed by transthoracic three-dimensional echocardiography. J Am Soc Echocardiogr. 2016;29:51-61.
22. Berger J, Ren X, Na B, et al. Relation of concentric remodeling to adverse outcomes in patients with stable coronary artery disease (from the Heart and Soul Study). Am J Cardiol. 2011;107:1579-84.
23. Verdecchia P, Schillaci G, Borgioni C, et al. Adverse prognostic significance of concentric remodeling of the left ventricle in hypertensive patients with normal left ventricular mass. J Am Coll Cardiol. 1995;25:871-8.
24. Gaasch WH, Zile MR. Left ventricular structural remodeling in health and disease: With special emphasis on volume, mass, and geometry. J Am Coll Cardiol. 2011;58:1733-40.
25. Zile MR, Gaasch WH, Patel K, et al. Adverse left ventricular remodeling in community-dwelling older adults predicts incident heart failure and mortality. JACC Heart Fail. 2014;2:512-22.
26. Shah AM, Shah SJ, Anand IS, et al. Cardiac structure and function in heart failure with preserved ejection fraction: Baseline findings from the echocardiographic study of the Treatment of Preserved Cardiac Function Heart Failure with an Aldosterone Antagonist trial. Circ Heart Fail. 2014;7:104-15.
27. Katz DH, Beussink L, Sauer AJ, et al. Prevalence, clinical characteristics, and outcomes associated with eccentric versus concentric left ventricular hypertrophy in heart failure with preserved ejection fraction. Am J Cardiol. 2013;112:1158-64.
28. Zile MR, Gottdiener JS, Hetzel SJ, et al. Prevalence and significance of alterations in cardiac structure and function in patients with heart failure and a preserved ejection fraction. Circulation. 2011;124:2491-501.
29. Gupta DK, Solomon SD. Imaging in heart failure with preserved ejection fraction. Heart Fail Clin. 2014;10:419-34.
30. Kraigher-Krainer E, Shah AM, Gupta DK, et al. Impaired systolic function by strain imaging in heart failure with preserved ejection fraction. J Am Coll Cardiol. 2014;63:447-56.
31. Aurigemma GP, Zile MR, Gaasch WH. Contractile behavior of the left ventricle in diastolic heart failure: With emphasis on regional systolic function. Circulation. 2006;113:296-304.
32. Komajda M, Lam CS. Heart failure with preserved ejection fraction: A clinical dilemma. Eur Heart J. 2014;35:1022-32.
33. van Heerebeek L, Borbely A, Niessen HW, et al. Myocardial structure and function differ in systolic and diastolic heart failure. Circulation. 2006;113:1966-73.
34. Levy D, Garrison RJ, Savage DD, et al. Prognostic implications of echocardiographically determined left ventricular mass in the Framingham Heart Study. N Engl J Med. 1990;322:1561-6.
35. Koren MJ, Devereux RB, Casale PN, et al. Relation of left ventricular mass and geometry to morbidity and mortality in uncomplicated essential hypertension. Ann Intern Med. 1991;114:345-52.
36. Muiesan ML, Salvetti M, Rizzoni D, et al. Association of change in left ventricular mass with prognosis during long-

term antihypertensive treatment. J Hypertens. 1995;13: 1091-5.
37. Verdecchia P, Carini G, Circo A, et al. Left ventricular mass and cardiovascular morbidity in essential hypertension: The MAVI study. J Am Coll Cardiol. 2001;38:1829-35.
38. Pritchett AM, Jacobsen SJ, Mahoney DW, et al. Left atrial volume as an index of left atrial size: A population-based study. J Am Coll Cardiol. 2003;41:1036-43.
39. Tani T, Tanabe K, Ono M, et al. Left atrial volume and the risk of paroxysmal atrial fibrillation in patients with hypertrophic cardiomyopathy. J Am Soc Echocardiogr. 2004;17:644-8.
40. Tsang TS, Abhayaratna WP, Barnes ME, et al. Prediction of cardiovascular outcomes with left atrial size: is volume superior to area or diameter? J Am Coll Cardiol. 2006;47: 1018-23.
41. Lester SJ, Ryan EW, Schiller NB, et al. Best method in clinical practice and in research studies to determine left atrial size. Am J Cardiol. 1999;84:829-32.
42. Muller H, Burri H, Shah D, et al. Evaluation of left atrial size in patients with atrial arrhythmias: comparison of standard 2D versus real time 3D echocardiography. Echocardiog. (Mount Kisco, NY) 2007;24:960-6.
43. Anwar AM, Soliman OI, Geleijnse ML, et al. Assessment of left atrial volume and function by real-time three-dimensional echocardiography. Int J Cardiol. 2008;123:155-61.
44. Miyasaka Y, Tsujimoto S, Maeba H, et al. Left atrial volume by real-time three-dimensional echocardiography: validation by 64-slice multidetector computed tomography. J Am Soc Echocardiogr. 2011;24:680-6.
45. Rohner A, Brinkert M, Kawel N, et al. Functional assessment of the left atrium by real-time three-dimensional echocardiography using a novel dedicated analysis tool: Initial validation studies in comparison with computed tomography. Eur J Echocardiogr. 2011;12:497-505.
46. Mor-Avi V, Yodwut C, Jenkins C, et al. Real-time 3D echocardiographic quantification of left atrial volume: Multicenter study for validation with CMR. JACC Cardiovasc Imaging. 2012;5:769-77.
47. Aune E, Baekkevar M, Roislien J, et al. Normal reference ranges for left and right atrial volume indexes and ejection fractions obtained with real-time three-dimensional echocardiography. Eur J Echocardiogr. 2009;10:738-44.
48. Tsang TSM, Barnes ME, Gersh BJ, et al. Left atrial volume as a morphophysiologic expression of left ventricular diastolic dysfunction and relation to cardiovascular risk burden. Am J Cardiol. 2002;90:1284-89.
49. Simek CL, Feldman MD, Haber HL, et al. Relationship between left ventricular wall thickness and left atrial size: Comparison with other measures of diastolic function. J Am Soc Echocardiogr. 1995;8:37-47.
50. Appleton CP, Galloway JM, Gonzalez MS, et al. Estimation of left ventricular filling pressures using two-dimensional and Doppler echocardiography in adult patients with cardiac disease. Additional value of analyzing left atrial size, left atrial ejection fraction and the difference in duration of pulmonary venous and mitral flow velocity at atrial contraction. J Am Coll Cardiol. 1993;22:1972-82.
51. Benjamin EJ, D'Agostino RB, Belanger AJ, et al. Left atrial size and the risk of stroke and death. The Framingham Heart Study. Circulation. 1995;92:835-41.
52. Moller JE, Hillis GS, Oh JK, et al. Left atrial volume: A powerful predictor of survival after acute myocardial infarction. Circulation. 2003;107:2207-12.
53. Meris A, Amigoni M, Uno H, et al. Left atrial remodelling in patients with myocardial infarction complicated by heart failure, left ventricular dysfunction, or both: The VALIANT Echo study. Eur Heart J. 2009;30:56-65.
54. Tsang TSM, Barnes ME, Gersh BJ, et al. Prediction of risk for first age-related cardiovascular events in an elderly population: The incremental value of echocardiography. J Am Coll Cardiol. 2003;42:1199-205.
55. Bolca O, Akdemir O, Eren M, et al. Left atrial maximum volume is a recurrence predictor in lone atrial fibrillation: An acoustic quantification study. Jpn Heart J. 2002;43:241-8.
56. Di Tullio MR, Sacco RL, Sciacca RR, et al. Left atrial size and the risk of ischemic stroke in an ethnically mixed population. Stroke. 1999;30:2019-24.
57. Tsang TS, Barnes ME, Bailey KR, et al. Left atrial volume: important risk marker of incident atrial fibrillation in 1655 older men and women. Mayo Clin Proc. 2001;76:467-75.
58. Barnes ME, Miyasaka Y, Seward JB, et al. Left atrial volume in the prediction of first ischemic stroke in an elderly cohort without atrial fibrillation. Mayo Clin Proc. 2004;79:1008-14.
59. Tsang TS, Barnes ME, Gersh BJ, et al. Risks for atrial fibrillation and congestive heart failure in patients ≥65 years of age with abnormal left ventricular diastolic relaxation. Am J Cardiol. 2004;93:54-8.
60. Vaziri SM, Larson MG, Benjamin EJ, et al. Echocardiographic predictors of nonrheumatic atrial fibrillation. The Framingham Heart Study. Circulation. 1994;89:724-30.
61. Flaker GC, Fletcher KA, Rothbart RM, et al. Clinical and echocardiographic features of intermittent atrial fibrillation that predict recurrent atrial fibrillation. Stroke Prevention in Atrial Fibrillation (SPAF) Investigators. Am J Cardiol. 1995;76:355-8.
62. Gardin JM, McClelland R, Kitzman D, et al. M-mode echocardiographic predictors of six- to seven-year incidence of coronary heart disease, stroke, congestive heart failure, and mortality in an elderly cohort (the Cardiovascular Health Study). Am J Cardiol. 2001;87:1051-7.

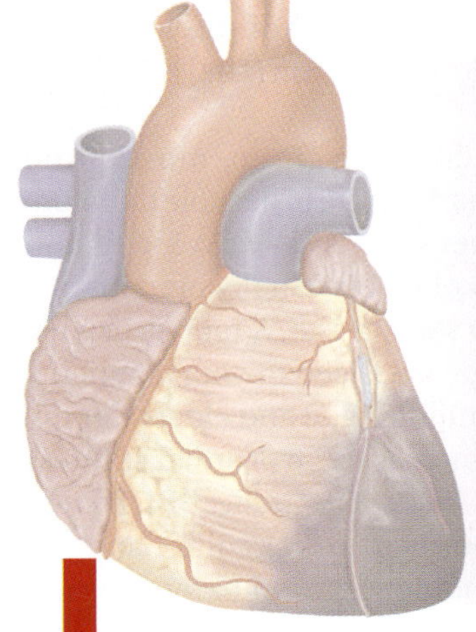

Diagnostic Prognostic and Therapeutic Implications of E/e' in Heart Failure

Naveen Garg, KK Kapur, HK Chopra

INTRODUCTION

Heart failure (HF) can be defined as inability of the left ventricle (LV) to maintain cardiac output (CO) commensurate with body needs for the physiological state with filling pressure less than 12 mm Hg. In the early stages of HF, stroke volume (SV) and CO can be maintained by increase in filling pressures. The filling pressure of LV is dependent on several active and passive processes that determine relaxation of the LV. When decreased contractility of LV is the prime component of the reduced SV, this is termed as systolic HF or more appropriately heart failure with reduced ejection fraction (HFrEF), however, when increased myocardial stiffness is the major mechanism for reduced CO and the myocardial contractility is well maintained; this condition is termed as heart failure with preserved ejection fraction (HFpEF) which was previously termed as diastolic HF. In HFrEF, increased LV filling pressure promotes stretching of the LV myocardium and this strives to maintain the LV-SV via Frank–Starling mechanism. In HFpEF, the increased LV filling pressures strive to overcome myocardial stiffness and thus maintain LV filling and thus the SV and CO. Therefore, increased filling pressure is an important feature of HF with both reduced and preserved myocardial contractility. Thus, the assessment of filling pressures is an important step in the noninvasive evaluation of HF.[1-4]

Heart failure with preserved ejection fraction is observed in almost half the cases of congestive cardiac failure. The usual causes of HF with relatively preserved ejection fraction are depicted in Table 1 and includes diabetes, hypertension, aging, obesity, anemia, atrial fibrillation (AF), chronic lung disease, chronic renal failure, etc. (Fig. 1).

The common garden etiological factors for HFrEF include valvular heart diseases, primary heart muscle disease, myocarditis, and coronary artery disease (Table 2).

In all these conditions noninvasive assessment of LV-filling pressures could facilitate early recognition and prompt treatment of HF.

ASSESSMENT OF LEFT VENTRICLE FILLING PRESSURES

The various methods to assess LV filing pressures include the following:

- Mitral inflow Doppler
- Mitral propagation velocity

TABLE 1: Determinants of HFpEF.

Aging	*Hypertension*	*Diabetes*
Anemia	Metabolic syndrome	Obesity
Aortic stenosis	Restrictive cardiomyopathy	Constrictive cardiomyopathy
Vascular stiffness	Pulmonary hypertension	Chronotropic incompetence
Sepsis	Organ failure	Dyssynchrony
COAD	Obstructive sleep apnea	Chronic kidney disease
AF	Coronary artery disease	

(AF: atrial fibrillation; COAD: chronic obstructive airway disease; HFpEF: heart failure with preserved ejection fraction)

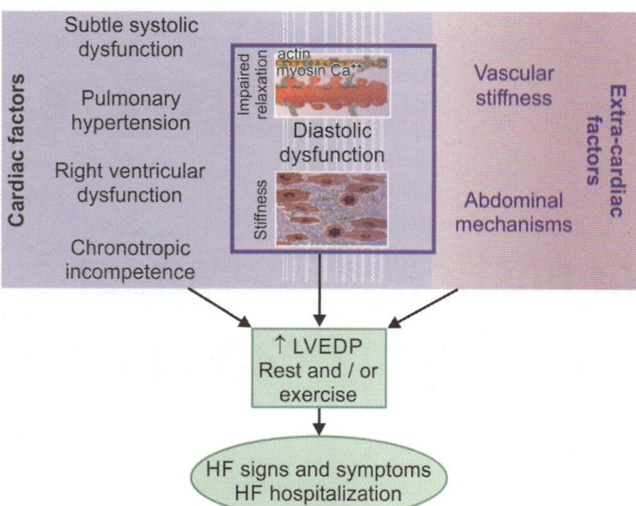

Fig. 1: Depicting the mechanism in development of diastolic dysfunction in HFpEF.
(HFpEF: heart failure with preserved ejection fraction; LVEDP: left ventricular end-diastolic pressure).

TABLE 2: Heart failure with reduced ejection fraction.

Myocardial infarction	*Myocarditis*	*Valvular heart diseases*
Cardiomyopathy	Arrhythmias	

- Tissue Doppler
- Pulmonary vein Doppler
- Peak velocities of mitral and aortic regurgitation jets
- Left atrial (LA) volume (in the absence of valvular pathologies)
- Estimation of pulmonary artery (PA) pressures.

Mitral Inflow Doppler

In the standard 4C apical view, the pulse Doppler sample volume (size 2–4 mm) is placed at the mitral tips. The mitral Doppler waveform comprises early diastolic filling wave (E-wave) as well as a late diastolic atrial contraction wave (A-wave). The time period between the E wave and A wave represents diastasis phase (slow filling) of diastole. Several factors affect the velocity of E-wave viz.:

- Mitral orifice area
- Left ventricular stiffness
- Cardiac output
- Heart rate and cardiac rhythm.

The atrial contraction A wave is primarily related to the booster-up pump function of LA. An increased A wave velocity implies a poorly compliant LV as seen in elderly population and indicates good boost-up pump function of LA. Increased A wave velocity is also seen in hypovolemia and other low CO states. A reduced A wave velocity is seen in restrictive physiology and poor LA booster pump function.

Occasionally, a positive wave is observed in diastasis period called L-wave, which could indicate impaired diastolic function. The quantitative significance of the L wave as regards the degree of diastolic dysfunction (DD) is however unclear.[5-9]

In the young to the middle age group, most of the diastolic filling occurs in the early phase of diastole therefore the E wave velocity is higher than A wave velocity and usually >50 m/sec. The ratio of E/A is usually more than 1 but less than 2.5. In high CO state, this E/A ratio is usually increased (akin to physiological S3 seen in young patients with high CO). However, in middle aged and elderly group, a high E/A ratio implies an increased myocardial stiffness and restrictive pathology (E/A >2–2.5, Grade-III DD). On the other hand, in impaired myocardial compliance as seen in normal ageing phenomenon or in early phase of myocardial ischemia or myocardial hypertrophy, the E/A ratio is generally less than 0.8 (grade-I DD). This pattern is also observed in hypovolemia and tachycardia (before E wave and A wave fusion occurs). When transition occurs from impaired relaxation to restrictive LV DD, a phase of normal E/A ratio (E/A >1 but <2) could occur. This pattern is also called pseudonormal pattern and implies elevated LV filling pressures (Grade-II) (Fig. 2).

Thus, the E/A ratio is dependent on age, loading conditions, heart rate as well as cardiac rhythm. When E and A wave fuse in tachycardia, the fusion wave has a high velocity. In AF, only E wave is observed.

Thus, the mitral diastolic filling pattern is affected by both diastolic and systolic functions and is highly dependent on loading conditions. Moreover, this method lacks adequate sensitivity and specificity for the diagnosis

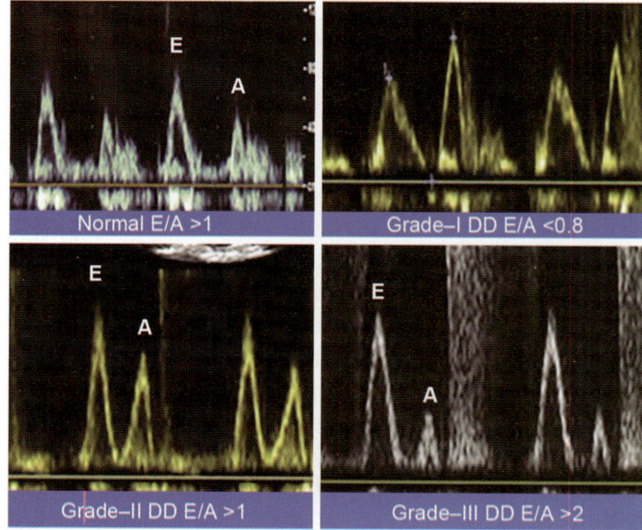

Fig. 2: Mitral inflow patterns depicted in different stages of diastolic dysfunction in HFpEF.
(HFpEF: heart failure with preserved ejection fraction)

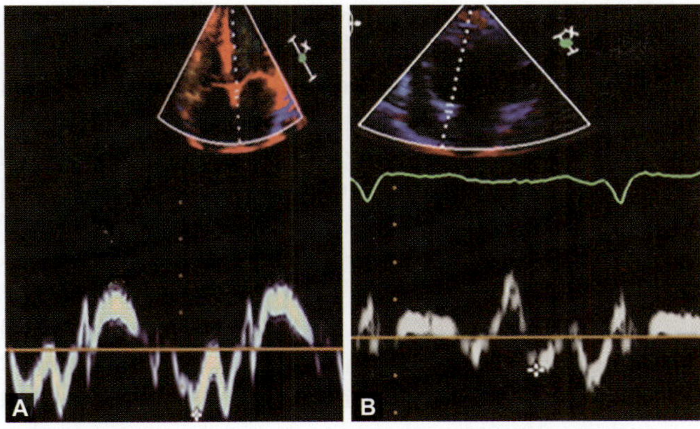

Figs. 3A and B: (A) Depicting septal tissue Doppler e' velocities in normal diastolic function (e' >7 cm/s). (B) In diastolic dysfunction (reduced velocity of septal e' <7 cm/s).

of restrictive physiology in patients with normal systolic function and elevated LV filling pressures.[8,9]

TISSUE DOPPLER IMAGING

With the advent of tissue Doppler imaging technology in the mid and late 1990s, it was possible to record myocardial velocities. These velocities are best recorded at the mitral annulus (medial and lateral). The myocardial systolic velocity is called *s'* and diastolic velocities are designated as *e'* and *a'* corresponding to the blood flow velocities during diastole (E and A). Although the systolic velocity *s'* has been shown to correlate with LV systolic function and could indicate very early systolic dysfunction [even in the presence of normal left ventricular ejection fraction (LVEF)], the diastolic velocities *e'* and *a'* (especially the former) have been found to be more useful in the diagnostic evaluation, treatment, and prognostication of myocardial dysfunction (Figs. 3A and B).[10,11]

The tissue velocity e' represents myocardial relaxation in early diastole while a' indicates late diastolic myocardial function. A reduced e'/a' ratio suggests Grade-I diastolic function or impaired myocardial compliance, while significantly reduced e' velocity is consistent with restrictive DD (Grade-III DD). Tissue Doppler velocities are relatively independent of loading conditions and therefore E/e' ratio for both medial and lateral annulus shows a better correlation with LV filling pressures as compared to e' velocity alone. Owing to greater number of longitudinal fibers at the lateral wall of the LV; the tissue Doppler systolic velocity s' and diastolic velocities e' and a' are higher at the lateral annulus. In middle-aged population, e' for medial annulus is >7 cm/sec while at the lateral annulus the cut-off value is 10 cm/sec. An E/e' ratio of <10 for the medial annulus and <8 for lateral annulus correlates with normal LV filling pressures, while averaged E/e' ratio for medial and lateral annulus of <14 implies normal LV filling pressures (Table 3).[12,13]

TABLE 3

Tissue Doppler	*Abnormal values*
e' septal	<7
e' lateral	<10 cm/sec
E/e'	>14
E/e' (septal) in AF	>11

(AF: atrial fibrillation)

Several regression equations derived from correlative studies using invasively measured LV filling pressures and simultaneously measured E/e' ratios have emerged for septal or lateral annulus alone or averaged both septal and lateral annulus.[14-17]

1. PCWP = 1.24 (E/e') + 1.9
2. Short-cut formula: PAWP = 4 + E/e'
3. PCWP= 1.47 (E/e') + 1.55
4. PCWP = 0.97(E/e') + 4.34

However, caution should be exercised while attempting to predict filling pressures from E/e' ratios using the above regression formulas owing to widely different correlation coefficient shown by different authors.

While interpreting high E/e' ratios, additional parameters of chronic DD such as LA volume index (>34 cm^3/m^2) and tricuspid regurgitation (TR) jet velocity (2.8 cm/sec) are also considered.[18-22] Therefore, according to recommendation of the American Society of Echocardiography/European Society of Cardiology (ASE/ESE)-2016, the criteria for restrictive LV DD implying significantly increased LV filling pressures are given below (Figs. 4A and B).[9,12,13]

LIMITATIONS OF E/e' IN THE ASSESSMENT OF FILLING PRESSURES

Although E/e' ratio as an index for LV filling pressures is considered a noninvasive gold standard or also called *"noninvasive Swan"*; there are several limitations which have tempered the initial enthusiasm and expectations.[23-25]

These limitations are as follows:

- Nonparallel alignment: Being a Doppler technique, the velocity estimation at both medial and lateral annulus is highly angle dependent. Ideally the Doppler interrogation angle should be less than 20°.
- Tachycardia causing fusion of e' and a' waveforms.
- Significant mitral annular calcification.
- Post-ring annuloplasty as well as post-mitral valve replacement (mitral prosthesis)
- Mitral valve diseases including both mitral stenosis (MS) as well as mitral regurgitation (MR). In nonvalvular MR as in dilated cardiomyopathy E/e' ratio could provide useful information of LV-filling pressures.
- Marked left ventricular hypertrophy (LVH), especially in cases of hypertrophic cardiomyopathy (HCM).

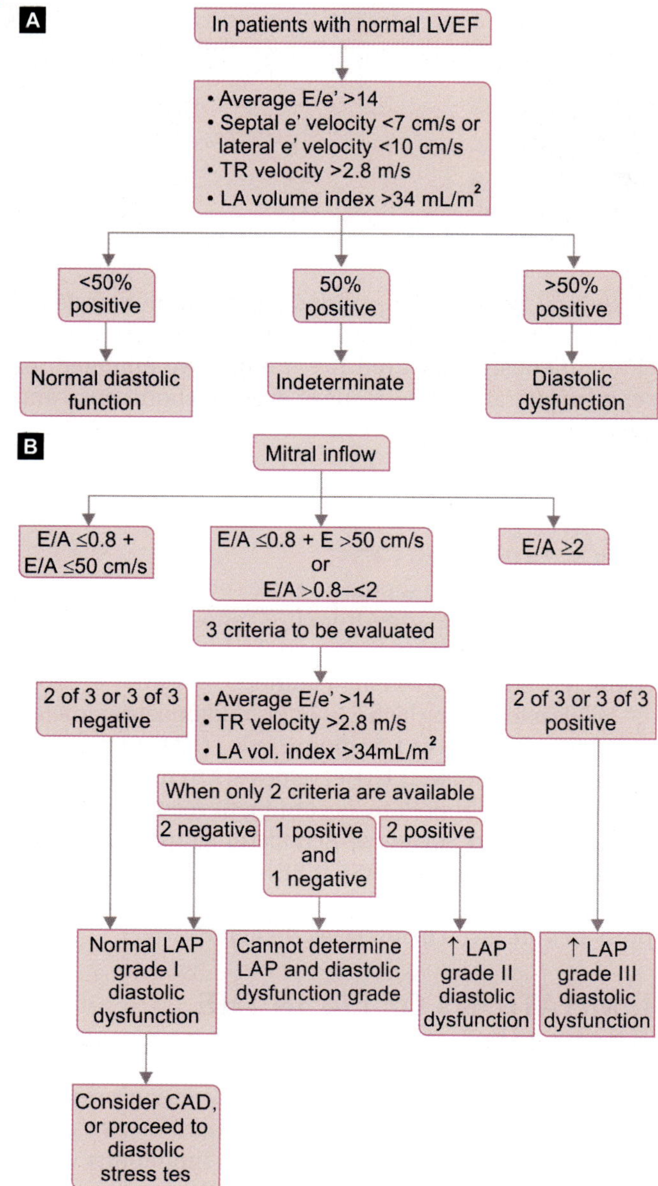

Figs. 4A and B: (A) Depicting 2016 criteria which include other parameters for diagnosing diastolic dysfunction; (B) Depicting algorithm for grading diastolic dysfunction.
(LVEF: left ventricular ejection fraction)

- Significant scarring of either the ventricular septum or the LV lateral wall or both.
- Unstable cardiac rhythm, including ventricular and supraventricular ectopic as well as AF with marked variability in cardiac cycle length. However, in well-controlled AF with fairly stable RR intervals, E/e' ratio could still provide useful information as regards LV filling pressures.[26-30]
- In patients with left bundle branch block (LBBB) as well as in patients with pacemaker rhythm, E/e' (septal) ratios could be falsely elevated; therefore, lateral annular velocities would be more reliable.[13,31]
- In constrictive pericarditis (CP): E/e' ratio does not reflect LV filling pressures owing to compensatory increased motion of longitudinal fibers at the medial and lateral annulus with restricted mediolateral expansion imposed by thickened pericardium.[32,33] This phenomenon is called annulus paradoxus (Fig. 5).
- Although ASE/ESE guidelines have advocated use of averaged E/e' ratio for medial and lateral annulus, there is conflicting opinion amongst several authors. However, there is a general agreement that in severe pulmonary arterial hypertension (PAH), right ventricular (RV) dysfunction, marked septal hypertrophy, and septal infarction, the septal annulus e/e' estimation should be avoided. Similarly, in lateral wall myocardial infarction (MI), the lateral annulus should not be used.[9,12,13]

Therefore, even though E/e' provides useful information about LV filling pressures and has fairly good correlation with the invasively determined left ventricular end-diastolic pressure (LVEDP), an expectation of one to one such correlations is unrealistic.[34-36]

PROGNOSTIC VALUE AND OTHER APPLICATIONS OF E/e'

Utility of E/e' in HFrEF

Although E/e' ratio is primarily an index of DD, it also has important prognostic implications in the management of HFrEF. It has been shown in several studies that a low E/e' ratio in patients with HFrEF implies a good prognosis while a high E/e' ratio indicates a worse prognosis.[10,11,35-41]

Utility of E/e' in Myocardial Infarction

In acute MI and LV dysfunction, E/e' ratio is a useful prognostic indicator. A high E/e' ratio is indicative of relatively poorer outcomes in such patients. A ratio of >15 is found to be a powerful predictor of mortality after MI (Fig. 6).[42-47]

UTILITY OF E/e' IN EVALUATING DRUG THERAPY IN PATIENTS WITH HEART FAILURE

In the serial follow-up of patients treated for HF, a lower E/e' ratio is one of the important indicators of a good response to drug therapy. This includes the use of diuretics, angiotensin-converting enzyme (ACE) inhibitors and beta-blockers.

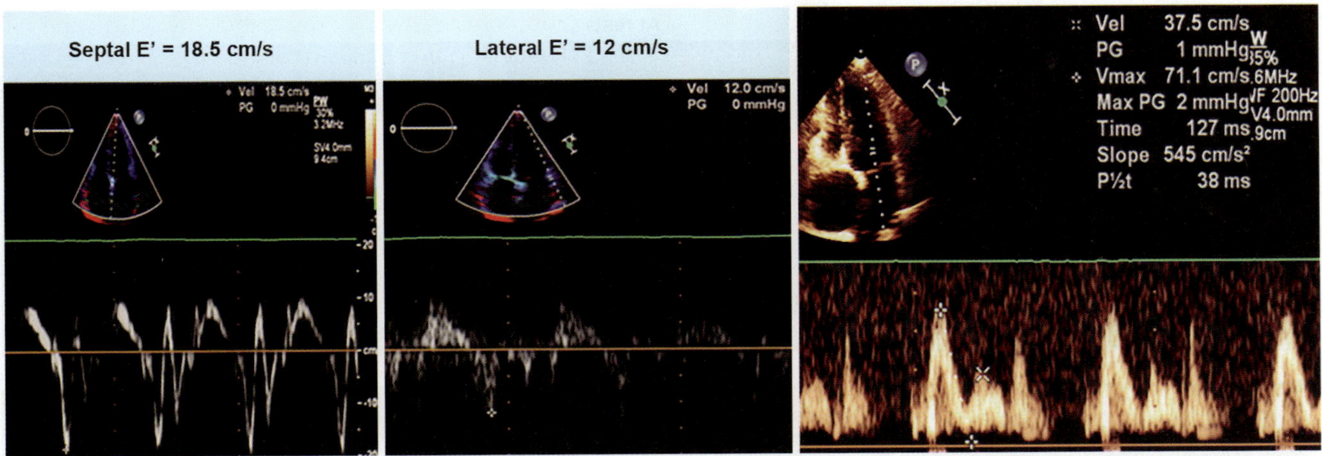

Fig. 5: Depicting annular paradox in constrictive pericarditis. E/e'**(average)** = 37.5/15.25 = 2.45 falsely indicate a normal LVEDP in CP.

(CP: constrictive pericarditis; LVEDP: left ventricular end-diastolic pressures)

However, in patients with on neprilysin inhibitors, an improvement in clinical parameters may not be accompanied by a concomitant decrease in E/e' ratio.[36,48,49]

Utility of E/e' in Diastolic Stress Test

In patients with dyspnea on exertion and having a normal resting E/A ratio or an impaired relaxation pattern, as well as a normal E/e', it is important to assess whether the etiology of the patient's dyspnea is based on DD (Table 4). In such situations, diastolic stress test (DST) could prove extremely useful. An elevated E/e' ratio in the immediate postexercise study helps in establishing the mechanism of dyspnea being due to elevated LV filling pressures (Fig. 7).[50-53]

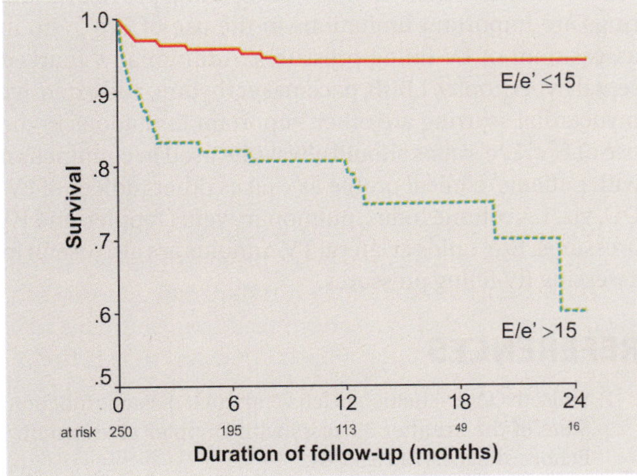

Fig. 6: E/e' >15 indicates high mortality after myocardial infarction during follow-up.

Source: Hillis GS, Møller JE, Pellikka PA, et al. Noninvasive estimation of left ventricular filling pressure by E/e is a powerful predictor of survival after acute myocardial infarction. J Am Coll Cardiol. 2004;43:360-7.

Utility of E/e' in Right Ventricular Diastolic Dysfunction

Similar to its role in LV DD, E/e' ratio has also been shown to be useful in the assessment of RV filling pressures. A pulse Doppler sample volume (5 mm) is placed on the lateral annulus of tricuspid valve (TV) and the tissue Doppler signals of RV longitudinal fibers are analyzed and e' and a' are estimated. The pulse Doppler sample volume is then positioned at the tip of TV to assess RV inflow E wave. The E/e' ratio thus obtained is then utilized to provide an estimation of right ventricular end-diastolic pressure (RVEDP). An E/e' ratio <4.7 has been shown to be consistent with normal RVEDP (<8 mm Hg) while E/e ratio >6 is associated with elevated RV filling pressures, usually more than 10 mm Hg.[54-60] The regression equations derived from invasive assessment of RVEDP or CVP and simultaneously estimated E/e' at lateral TV annulus are following:

- Right ventricular end-diastolic pressure = 1.62 × E/e' + 2.13
- E/e' >6 = RVEDP >10 (sensitivity 79% and specificity 73% for RVEDP >10 mm Hg).

TABLE 4: A patient with dyspnea on exertion with either normal E/A or G-1 DD.

	E	*e'*	*E/e'*	*Interpretation*
Pre-exercise	N	N	N	?
At peak exercise	↑	↑	N	Normal (noncardiac dyspnea)
	↑↑	↑/-	↑↑	Elevated LVEDP as cause of dyspnea (positive DST)

(DD: diastolic dysfunction; DST: diastolic stress test; LVEDP: left ventricular end-diastolic pressures)

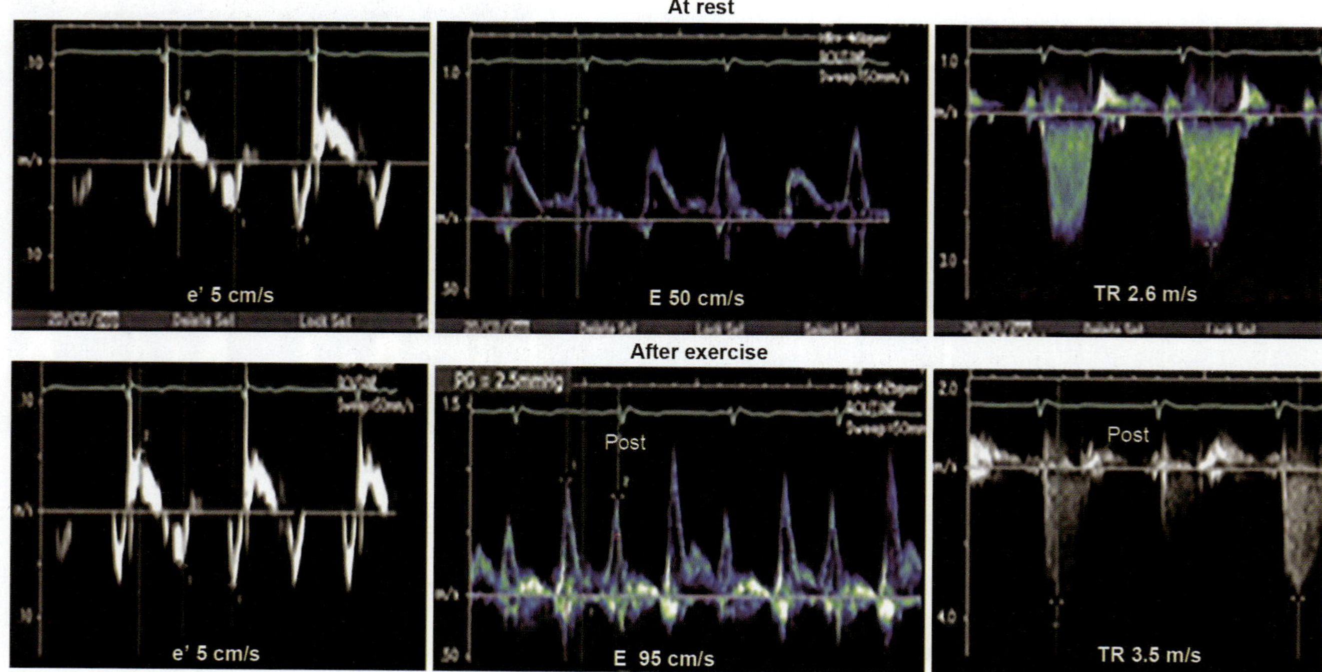

Fig. 7: Increase in E/e' on exercise from 10 to 19 and TR-velocity from 2.6 cm/sec to 3.5 cm/sec indicates impaired myocardial relaxation.

FUTURE TRENDS AND DIRECTIONS IN EVALUATING LEFT VENTRICLE FILLING PRESSURES IN HEART FAILURE

Speckle tracking echocardiography (STE) provides a noninvasive, operator independent and objective accurate assessment of LV systolic function and is a sensitive marker for myocardial dysfunction even in patients with normal ejection fraction (HFpEF). A significantly reduced LV global longitudinal strain (GLS) in patients with HFpEF implies elevated LVEDP. Additionally, use of STE in evaluating peak longitudinal LA strains (PALS) has been shown to have better correlations with LV-filling pressures when compared with E/e' ratio. However, LA strain values are also influenced by LA function which may not always correlate with LV filling pressures. Moreover STE-derived strain values are highly dependent on imaging quality as well as are subject to vendor variability. Therefore, at present LA strain (PALS) and GLS are not routinely used for evaluating LV filling pressures as per the current recommendations.[61-64]

CONCLUSION

Tissue Doppler echocardiography has been a significant advance in evaluation of myocardial dysfunction. Although e' and a' velocities have been found to be useful in evaluation of myocardial dysfunctions. E/e' ratios have shown a superior correlation with LV filling pressures in both HFpEF and HFrEF. Although some studies have shown good correlations of E/e' ratio with invasively derived filling pressures, several other such studies have shown inconsistent results. E/e' ratio has important prognostic implications in patients with acute MI, HFrEF, and HFpEF. In the serial follow-up of patients with HFpEF and HFrEF, E/e' ratio has been shown to have important therapeutic implications in guiding therapy and monitoring patients progress. Mitral annular calcifications, other mitral valve diseases including mitral prosthesis and rings are important limitations in the use of E/e' ratio in assessment of LV filling pressures. Additionally, marked septal hypertrophy, LBBB, pacemaker rhythm, and extensive myocardial scarring are other important limitations in the use of E/e'. E/e' ratios should always be used in conjunction with patients' clinical profile as well as other indices of LV-DD, viz. LA volume index, pulmonary vein Doppler, and PA pressures. E/e' ratios at lateral TV-annulus are also useful in assessing RV filling pressures.

REFERENCES

1. Smiseth OA. Evaluation of left ventricular diastolic function: State of the art after 35 years with Doppler assessment. J Echocardiogr. 2018;16:55-64.
2. Pfeffer MA, Shah AM, Borlaug BA. Heart failure with preserved ejection fraction in perspective. Circ Res. 2019; 124:1598-617.
3. Gazewood JD, Turner PL, et al. Heart failure with preserved ejection fraction: Diagnosis and management. Am Fam Phys. 2017;96(9):582-8.

4. Gori M, Iacovoni A, Senni M. Haemodynamics of heart failure with preserved ejection fraction: A clinical perspective. Card Fail Rev. 2016;2(2):102-5.
5. Andersen OS, Smiseth OA, Dokainish H, et al. Estimating left ventricular filling pressure by echocardiography. J Am Coll Cardiol. 2017;69(15):1937-48.
6. Nagueh SF, Middleton KJ, Kopelen HA, et al. Doppler tissue imaging: A noninvasive technique for evaluation of left ventricular relaxation and estimation of filling pressures. J Am Coll Cardiol. 1997;30:1527-33.
7. Rivas-Gotz C, Khoury DS, Manolios M, et al. Time interval between onset of mitral inflow and onset of early diastolic velocity by tissue Doppler: A novel index of left ventricular relaxation experimental studies and clinical application. J Am Coll Cardiol. 2003;42:1463-70.
8. Ie EH, Vletter WB, ten Cate FJ, et al. Preload dependence of new Doppler techniques limits their utility for left ventricular diastolic function assessment in hemodialysis patients. J Am Soc Nephrol. 2003;14:1858-62.
9. Nagueh SF, Smiseth OA, Appleton CP, et al. Recommendations for the evaluation of left ventricular diastolic function by echocardiography: An update from the American Society of Echocardiography and the European Association of Cardiovascular Imaging. J Am Soc Echocardiogr. 2016;29:277-314.
10. Mornos C, Crişan S, Petrescu L, et al. The prognostic value of a new tissue Doppler parameter in patients with heart failure with reduced ejection fraction. Romanian J Cardiol. 2017;27(1).
11. Arques S, Roux E, Luccioni R, et al. Current clinical applications of spectral tissue Doppler echocardiography (E/e' ratio) as a noninvasive surrogate for left ventricular diastolic pressures in the diagnosis of heart failure with preserved left ventricular systolic function. Cardiovasc Ultrasound. 2007;5:16.
12. Nagueh SF, Smiseth OA, Appleton CP, et al. Recommendations for the evaluation of left ventricular diastolic function by echocardiography: An update from the American Society of Echocardiography and the European Association of Cardiovascular Imaging. Eur Heart J Cardiovasc Imaging. 2016;7:1321-60.
13. Lancellotti P, Galderisi M, Edvardsen T, et al. Echo-Doppler estimation of left ventricular filling pressure: results of the multicentre EACVI Euro-Filling study. Eur Heart J Cardiovasc Imaging. 2017;18:961-8.
14. Nagueh SF, Mikati I, Kopelen HA, et al. Doppler estimation of left ventricular filling pressure in sinus tachycardia: A new application of tissue doppler imaging. Circulation. 1998;98:1644-50.
15. Bouhemad B, Nicolas-Robin A, Benois A, et al. Echocardiographic Doppler assessment of pulmonary capillary wedge pressure in surgical patients with postoperative circulatory shock and acute lung injury. Anesthesiology. 2003;98:1091-100.
16. López B, Sanchez V, Delgado JF, et al. Accuracy of noninvasive estimation of pulmonary wedge pressure by echocardiographic indices in heart transplant recipients. Transplant Proc. 2012;44(9):2639-41.
17. Nagueh SF, Kopelen HA, Zoghbi WA. Feasibility and accuracy of Doppler echocardiographic estimation of pulmonary artery occlusive pressure in the intensive care unit. AJC. 1995;75(17):1256-62.
18. Jeong EM, Dudley SC. New diagnostic and therapeutic possibilities for diastolic heart failure. RI Med J (2013). 2014;97(2):35-7.
19. Paulus WJ, Tschöpe C, Sanderson JE, et al. How to diagnose diastolic heart failure: A consensus statement on the diagnosis of heart failure with normal left ventricular ejection fraction by the Heart Failure and Echocardiography Associations of the European Society of Cardiology. Eur Heart J. 2007;28:2539-50.
20. Santos M, Rivero J, McCullough SD, et al. E/é ratio in patients with unexplained dyspnea lack of accuracy in estimating left ventricular filling pressure. Circ Heart Fail. 2015;8:749-56.
21. Dokainish H. Left ventricular diastolic function and dysfunction: Central role of echocardiography. Glob Cardiol Sci Pract. 2015;2015:3.
22. Tobushi T, Nakano M, Hosokawa K, et al. Improved diastolic function is associated with higher cardiac output in patients with heart failure irrespective of left ventricular ejection fraction. J Am Heart Assoc. 2017;6(3):pii: e003389.
23. Park JH, Marwick TH. Use and limitations of E/e' to assess left ventricular filling pressure by echocardiography. J Cardiovasc Ultrasound. 2011;19(4):169-73.
24. Previtali M, Chieffo E, Ferrario M, et al. Is mitral E/e' ratio a reliable predictor of left ventricular diastolic pressures in patients without heart failure? Eur Heart J Cardiovasc Imaging. 2012;13:588-95.
25. Kadappu KK, Thomas L. Tissue Doppler imaging in echocardiography: Value and limitations. Heart Lung Circ. 2015;24:224-33.
26. Okura H, Takada Y, Kubo T, et al. Tissue Doppler-derived index of left ventricular filling pressure, E/e', predicts survival of patients with nonvalvular atrial fibrillation. Heart. 2006;92:1248-52.
27. Nagueh SF, Kopelen HA, Quiñones MA. Assessment of left ventricular filling pressures by Doppler in the presence of atrial fibrillation. Circulation. 1996;94:2138-45.
28. Park SJ, Lee SC, Jang SY, et al. E/e' ratio is a strong prognostic predictor of mortality in patients with non-valvular atrial fibrillation with preserved left ventricular systolic function. Circ J. 2011;75:2350-56.
29. Kusunose K, Yamada H, Nishio S, et al. Clinical utility of single-beat E/e' obtained by simultaneous recording of flow and tissue Doppler velocities in atrial fibrillation with preserved systolic function. J Am Coll Cardiol Imaging. 2009;2:1147-56.
30. Popovic´ ZB, Klein AL. Cracking the mysteries of diastolic function in atrial fibrillation: New technology for an old problem. JACC Cardivasc Imaging. 2009;2(10);1157-8.
31. Nagueh SF. Non-invasive assessment of left ventricular filling pressure. Eur J Heart Fail. 2018;20:38-48.
32. Garcia MJ, Rodriguez L, Ares M, et al. Differentiation of constrictive pericarditis from restrictive cardiomyopathy: Assessment of left ventricular diastolic velocities in longitudinal axis by Doppler tissue imaging. J Am Coil Cardiol. 1996;27:108-14.
33. Ha JW, Oh JK, Ling LH, et al. Annulus paradoxus transmitral flow velocity to mitral annular velocity ratio is inversely

proportional to pulmonary capillary wedge pressure. Circulation. 2001;104:976-8.
34. Wang M, Yip GW, Wang AY, et al. Peak early diastolic mitral annulus velocity by tissue Doppler imaging adds independent and incremental prognostic value. J Am Coll Cardiol. 2003;41:820-6.
35. Yu CM, Sanderson JE, Marwick TH, et al. Tissue Doppler: Imaging a new prognosticator for cardiovascular diseases. J Am Coll Cardiol. 2007;49:1903-14.
36. Mitter SS, Shah SJ, Thomas JD. A test in context E/A and E/e' to assess diastolic dysfunction and LV filling pressure. J Am Coll Cardiol. 2017;69:1451-64.
37. Mullens W, Borowski AG, Curtin RJ, et al. Tissue Doppler imaging in the estimation of intracardiac filling pressure in decompensated patients with advanced systolic heart failure. Circulation. 2009;119(1):62-70.
38. Kim MK, Kim B, Lee JY, et al. Tissue Doppler-derived E/é ratio as a parameter for assessing diastolic heart failure and as a predictor of mortality in patients with chronic kidney disease. Korean J Intern Med. 2013;28:35-44.
39. Correale M, Totaro A, Ieva R, et al. Tissue Doppler imaging in coronary artery diseases and heart failure. Curr Cardiol Rev. 2012;8:43-53.
40. Lee EH, Yun SC, Chin JH, et al. Prognostic implications of preoperative E/e ratio in patients with off-pump coronary artery surgery. Anesthesiology. 2012;116(2):362-71.
41. Okura H, Kubo T, Asawa K, et al. Elevated E/e' predicts prognosis in congestive heart failure patients with preserved systolic function. Circulation. 2008;73(1):86-91.
42. Hillis GS, Møller JE, Pellikka PA, et al. Noninvasive estimation of left ventricular filling pressure by E/e is a powerful predictor of survival after acute myocardial infarction. J Am Coll Cardiol. 2004;43:360-7.
43. Hameed AK, Gosal T, Fang T, et al. Clinical utility of tissue Doppler imaging in patients with acute myocardial infarction complicated by cardiogenic shock. Cardiovasc Ultrasound. 2008;6:11.
44. Ramesh R, Rveeramani S, Shivakuma GS. Mitral valve Doppler E/e' as a prognostic marker in acute myocardial infarction. Int J Sci Study. 2017;5(1).
45. Kenawy MM, Saber HM, Al Akawaby HAH, et al. Role of tissue Doppler imaging in predicting left ventricular dysfunction after myocardial infarction. Egyptian J Crit Care Med. 2013;1:87-94.
46. Mogelvang R, Biering-Sørensen T, Jensen JS. Tissue Doppler echocardiography predicts acute myocardial infarction, heart failure, and cardiovascular death in the general population. Eur Heart J Cardiovasc Imaging. 2015;16:1331-7.
47. Møller JE, Pellikka PA, Hillis GS, et al. Prognostic importance of diastolic function and filling pressure in patients with acute myocardial infarction. Circulation. 2006;114:438-44.
48. Sharp AS, Tapp RJ, Thom SA, et al. Tissue Doppler E/e' ratio is a powerful predictor of primary cardiac events in a hypertensive population: An ASCOT substudy. Eur Heart J. 2010;31:747-52.
49. Barron AJ, Hughes AD, Sharp A, et al. Long-term antihypertensive treatment fails to improve E/é despite regression of left ventricular mass an Anglo-Scandinavian cardiac outcomes trial substudy. Hypertension. 2014;63:252-8.
50. Kovacs G, Herve P, Barbera JA, et al. An official European Respiratory Society statement: Pulmonary haemodynamics during exercise. Eur Respir J. 2017;50:1700578.
51. Holland DJ, Prasad SB, Marwick TH. Prognostic implications of left ventricular filling pressure with exercise. Circ Cardiovasc Imaging. 2010;3:149-56.
52. Dorfs S, Zeh W, Hochholzer W, et al. Pulmonary capillary wedge pressure during exercise and long-term mortality in patients with suspected heart failure with preserved ejection fraction. Eur Heart J. 2014;35:3103-12.
53. Dalsgaard M, Kjaergaard J, Pecini R, et al. Left ventricular filling pressure estimation at rest and during exercise in patients with severe aortic valve stenosis: Comparison of echocardiographic and invasive measurements. J Am Soc Echocardiogr. 2009;22:343-9.
54. Riley DC, Gerson S, Arbo J, et al. Emergency department right atrial pressure and intravascular volume estimation using right ventricular tissue Doppler bedside ultrasonography. Crit Ultrasound J. 2010;2:31-3.
55. Arbo JE, Maslove DM, Beraud AS, et al. Bedside assessment of right atrial pressure in critically ill septic patients using tissue Doppler ultrasonography. J Crit Care. 282013;1112.e1-5.
56. Sade LE, Gulmez O, Eroglu S, et al. Noninvasive estimation of right ventricular filling pressure by ratio of early tricuspid inflow to annular diastolic velocity in patients with and without recent cardiac surgery. J Am Soc Echocardiogr. 2007;20:982-8.
57. Beigel R, Cercek B, Luo H, et al. Noninvasive evaluation of right atrial pressure. J Am Soc Echocardiogr. 2013;26:1033-42.
58. DiLorenzo MP, Bhatt SM, Mercer-Rosa L. How best to assess right ventricular function by echocardiography? Cardiol Young. 2015;25(8):1473-81.
59. Pagourelias ED, Efthimiadis GK, Parcharidou DG, et al. Prognostic value of right ventricular diastolic function indices in hypertrophic cardiomyopathy. Eur J Echocardiogr. 2011;12:809-17.
60. Nagueh SF, Smiseth OA, Dokainisah H, et al. Mean right atrial pressure for estimation of left ventricular filling pressure in patients with normal left ventricular ejection fraction: Invasive and noninvasive validation. J Am Soc Echocardiogr. 2018;31:799-806.
61. Cameli M, Lisi M, Mondillo S, et al. Left atrial longitudinal strain by speckle tracking echocardiography correlates well with left ventricular filling pressures in patients with heart failure. Cardiovasc Ultrasound. 2010;8:14.
62. Collier P, Phelan D, Klein A. A test in context: Myocardial strain measured by speckle-tracking echocardiography. J Am Coll Cardiol. 2017;69(8):1043-56.
63. Leischik R, Littwitz H, Dworrak B, et al. Echocardiographic evaluation of left atrial mechanics: Function, history, novel techniques, advantages, and pitfalls. BioMed Res Int. 2015;2015:765921.
64. Rimbaş RC, Dulgheru RE, Vinereanu D, et al. Methodological gaps in left atrial function assessment by 2D speckle tracking echocardiography. Arq Bras Cardiol. 2015;105(6):625-36.

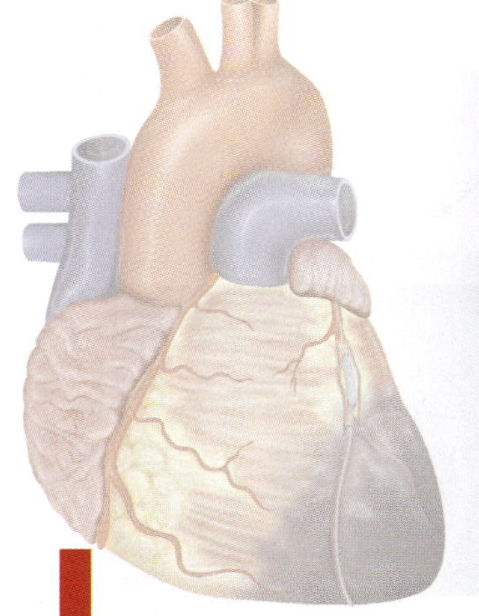

CHAPTER 55

Role of Echocardiography for Prognosis in Patients with Heart Failure

Keval D Patel, John Gorcsan

INTRODUCTION

Echocardiography is an important diagnostic tool for the diagnosis and management of patients with heart failure (HF). This review will focus on clinical applications of noninvasive echocardiographic measures for prognosis in HF. Items to be discussed include quantifying left ventricular (LV) volumes and ejection fraction (EF), routine Doppler and tissue Doppler measures of diastolic function, and the newer method of speckle tracking strain imaging. These measures may influence choices of therapy and anticipating which HF patients are at higher risk for clinical events. This information can be valuable to determine how often to follow patients clinically, and counsel patients and their families for prognosis.

IMPORTANCE OF LEFT VENTRICULAR EJECTION FRACTION

The left ventricular ejection fraction (LVEF) remains one of the most important metrics of cardiac function in the modern practice of cardiology. The contemporary approach to patients presenting with the clinical syndrome of pulmonary edema from HF is simply divided into two groups: HF with reduced EF (HFrEF) and HF with preserved EF (HFpEF). Because these syndromes may appear to be very similar at the patient's bedside, imaging most often with echocardiography is used for determination of LVEF to begin the appropriate diagnostic and therapeutic pathway. The evidence for pharmacological and device therapy in HF patients has come from randomized clinical trials that have enrolled patients based on LVEF (Fig. 1).[1] Mortality benefits for patients with HFrEF have been shown with angiotensin converting enzyme inhibitors, angiotensin II receptor blockers, beta-blockers, and spironolactone. More recently, ivabradine and sacubitril/valsartan have been shown to also benefit HFrEF patients in randomized clinical trials.[1] Furthermore, contemporary device therapy is assigned by LVEF. Patients with cardiomyopathies of ischemic or nonischemic origin may benefit from an implanted cardioverter-defibrillator with reduced EF below 30% or 35%.[2] In HFrEF patients with electrical delay shown by QRS widening by electrocardiography, cardiac resynchronization therapy (CRT) has been lifesaving, and randomized clinical trials selected patients with EF ≤35%.[2] On the other hand, there are currently no definitive studies of pharmacological agents that demonstrated benefit to patients with HFpEF, although spironolactone is suggested to be beneficial in subgroup analysis.[3] Other agents, such as sacubitril/valsartan are being studied for HFpEF.[4] In summary, a clinical approach to patients with HF must logically begin with determining LVEF and echocardiography plays an important diagnostic and prognostic role. Physiologically, one can understand the importance of LVEF as a measure of both pump function and LV remodeling. The LVEF is the ratio of the stoke volume over the end-diastolic volume. The numerator (stroke volume) is a fundamental measure of pump function of the left ventricle. The denominator (end-diastolic volume) is a measure of remodeling or chamber enlargement, which reflects disease progression (Fig. 2).

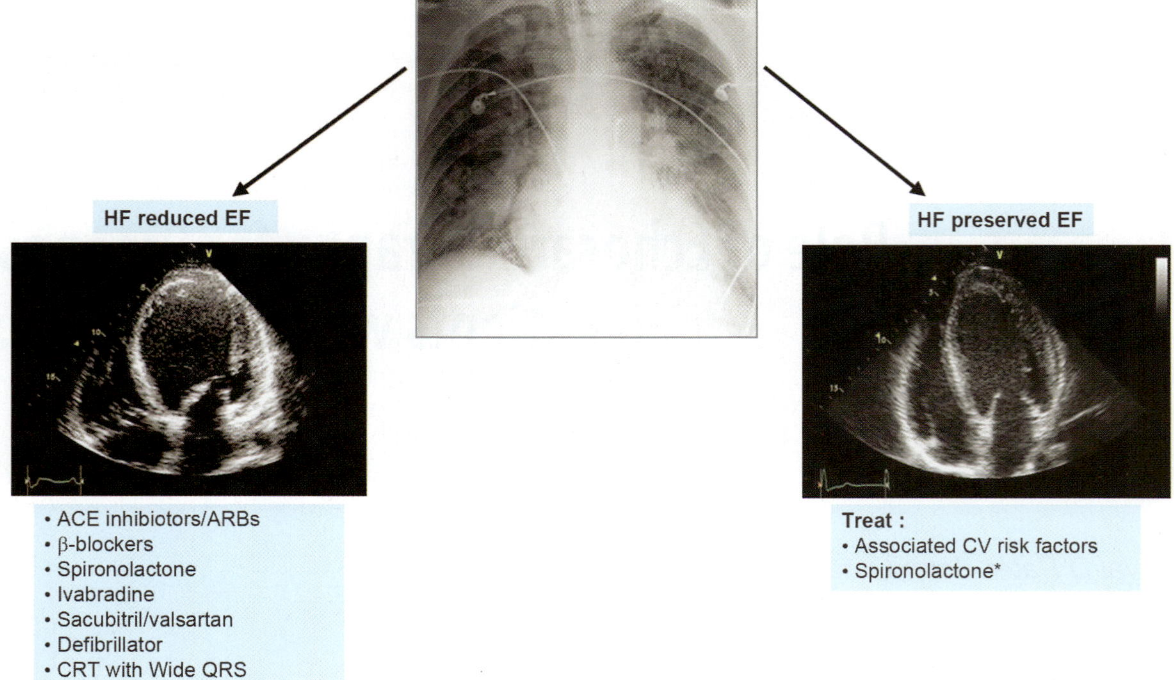

Fig. 1: An approach to a patient with clinical heart failure (HF) based on ejection fraction (EF). Clinical trials have supported pharmacological and device therapies listed for HF patients with reduced EF. Treatment of HF patients with preserved EF focuses on treating associated cardiovascular (CV) risk factors.
*Spironolactone is supported from clinical trial subgroup analysis.
(ACE: angiotensin converting enzyme; ARB: angiotensin receptor blocker; CRT: cardiac resynchronization therapy)

The LVEF combines these two parameters which have additive prognostic value in a clinically useful single number. LVEF first became established as having prognostic value from the multiple-gated acquisition (MUGA) scan using the radioactive isotope, technetium-99m-pertechnetate.[5]

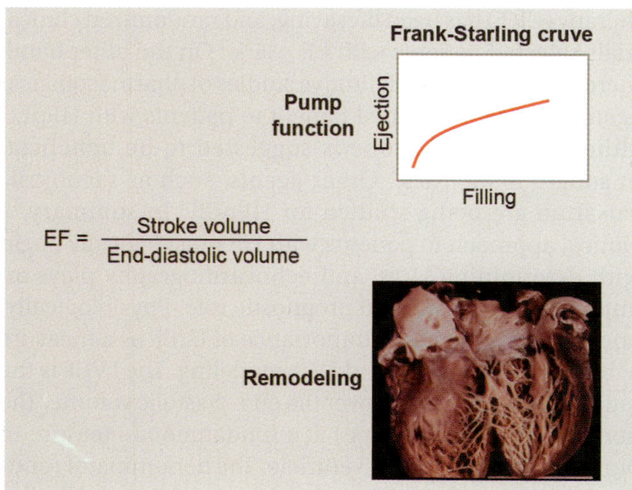

Fig. 2: A composite figure of left ventricular ejection fraction (EF) representing pump's function and remodeling.

A strong relationship between EF and 1-year mortality was demonstrated in patients after myocardial infarction.[6] An increase in mortality was observed if LVEF was <40%, and mortality sharply increased after LVEF dropped below 35%. The use of echocardiography to measure LVEF has supplanted radionuclide angiography due to its greater availability and lower cost.[7] Two-dimensional biplane measurements using the four-chamber and two-chamber views are the standard clinical approach for LVEF (Fig. 3).[8] The use of microbubble contrast agents can improve the accuracy and feasibility of LVEF in patients with technically difficult ultrasound windows and has made a significant clinical contribution.[8] While three-dimensional (3D) echo has an advantage of improved reproducibility, this technique is less commonly used by many centers currently. 3D LVEF has an advantage for serial assessment of LV volumes and EF and in patients with geometrical distortion, such as LV aneurysms.[8]

PROGNOSTIC VALUE OF DOPPLER MEASURES OF DIASTOLIC FUNCTION

Routine pulsed Doppler and tissue Doppler measures to assess LV diastolic function have prognostic significance in

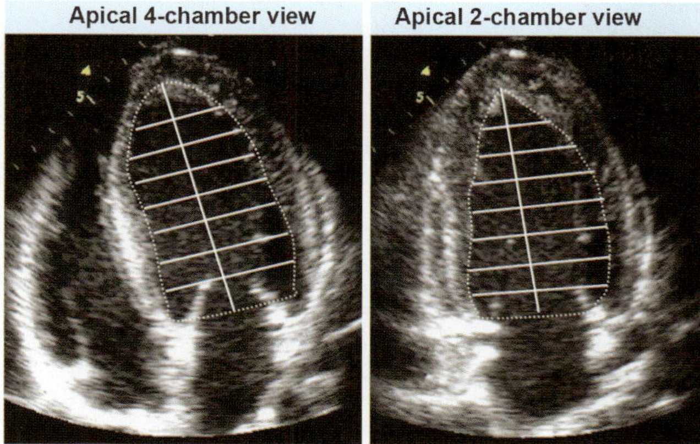

$$\text{Volume} = \Sigma\,(\tfrac{1}{4}\,\pi\,D^2)\,h$$

$$\text{Ejection fraction} = \frac{\text{End-diastolic volume} - \text{End-systolic volume}}{\text{End-diastolic volume}}$$

Fig. 3: Echocardiographic determination of left ventricular ejection fraction tracing end-diastolic and end-systolic frames from apical four-chamber and two-chamber views and using the modified Simpson's rule formula.

HF patients. The early diastolic E wave velocity is affected by several variables, but principally early diastolic active relaxation and left atrial (LA) pressure (Fig. 4). Mitral E deceleration time is measured from the peak of the E wave to the zero baseline. A shortened E deceleration occurs from a combination of impaired early diastolic relaxation and elevated LA pressure. A short E deceleration time is known as a restrictive pattern. A mitral E deceleration time ≤150 ms has been associated with increased mortality in HFrEF patients with cumulative mortality 55% over 2.5 years vs. 5% if mitral E was nonrestrictive.[9]

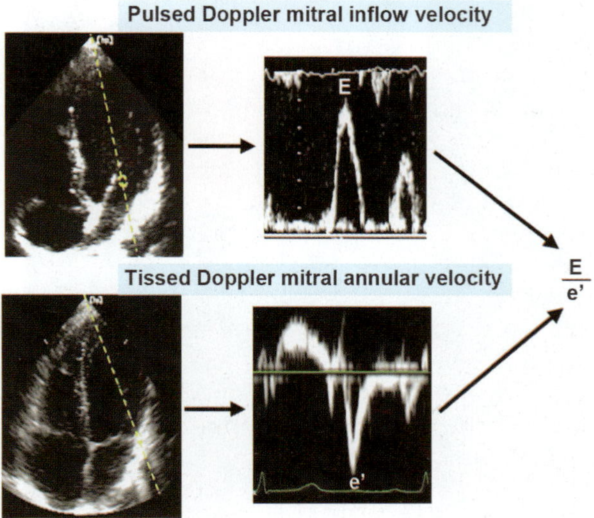

Fig. 4: Examples of mitral inflow velocity from puled Doppler (top) and later mitral annular velocity using tissue Doppler (bottom). To the right is the mitral inflow (E) to annular (e') ratio used to assess cardiac diastolic function.

Pulsed Doppler measures of LV early diastolic expansion velocity (e') reflect LV diastolic function. A normal LV diastolic e' velocity is approximately 10 cm/s, and is reduced in all forms of myocardial disease, including ischemic, idiopathic nonischemic, hypertrophic, and infiltrative cardiomyopathies. On the other hand, e' is elevated to supernormal levels >10 cm/s in individuals with athletic hearts and is a useful marker of LV early diastolic suction. Wang et al. studied 182 patients with LVEF <50% and demonstrated that e' <3 cm/s had striking prognostic value being associated with a decreased survival over approximately 5.5 years.[10] The mitral inflow to annular ratio (E/e') has been used as an estimate of LV filling pressures and is also a marker of clinical outcomes in patients with HF. Hillis et al. showed that patients with E/e' >15 had a 4.8-fold increased risk of mortality after myocardial infarction, (p <0.0002).[11] Dokainish et al. also showed in 116 HF patients that E/e' ≥15 was predictive of mortality (p <0.001).[12] Wang et al. showed that mitral E deceleration time ≤140 ms had additive prognostic value to clinical factors, which improved with the addition of E/e' >15 and further improved if mitral annular e' was <3 cm/s.[10] Accordingly, mitral inflow deceleration time, e' and mitral inflow to annular ratio provide additive prognostic information in HFrEF patients.

STRAIN IMAGING AND PROGNOSIS IN HEART FAILURE

Speckle tracking strain imaging is a more recent advance that has made an impact on assessing LV function in HF patients. Although radial, circumferential, rotational, and longitudinal vectors of myocardial contraction may be measured by strain imaging, the average longitudinal shortening, known as global longitudinal strain (GLS) is most often utilized clinically. Longitudinal strain is the change in length divided by the original length and expressed as % (Fig. 5). GLS is typically measured from apical four-chamber, two-chamber, and apical long-axis views with regions of interest placed on the LV walls. The average peak % shortening is calculated as GLS (Fig. 6). Although GLS has a negative sign, it may be easier to understand for clinicians in terms of its absolute value so that a larger GLS represents better cardiac function and a smaller GLS represents poorer cardiac function. Normal GLS is typically >17%, and GLS <15% is abnormal and GLS between 15% and 17% may be considered as borderline abnormal. It is believed that GLS is additive to LVEF because it also reflects wall properties, such as fibrosis, hypertrophy, and infiltration. Strain provides additional information to blood displacement within the chamber measured by LVEF.

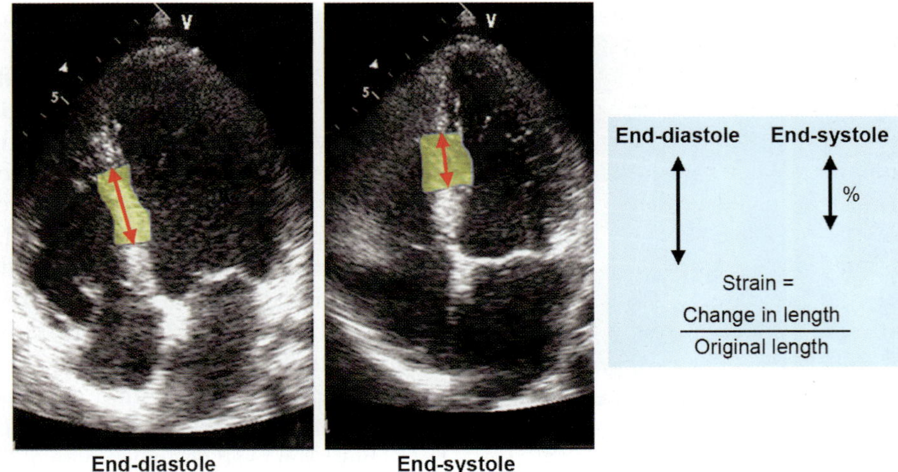

Fig. 5: A diagrammatic representation of longitudinal strain with % strain expressed as change in length from end-diastole to end-systole divided by its original length.

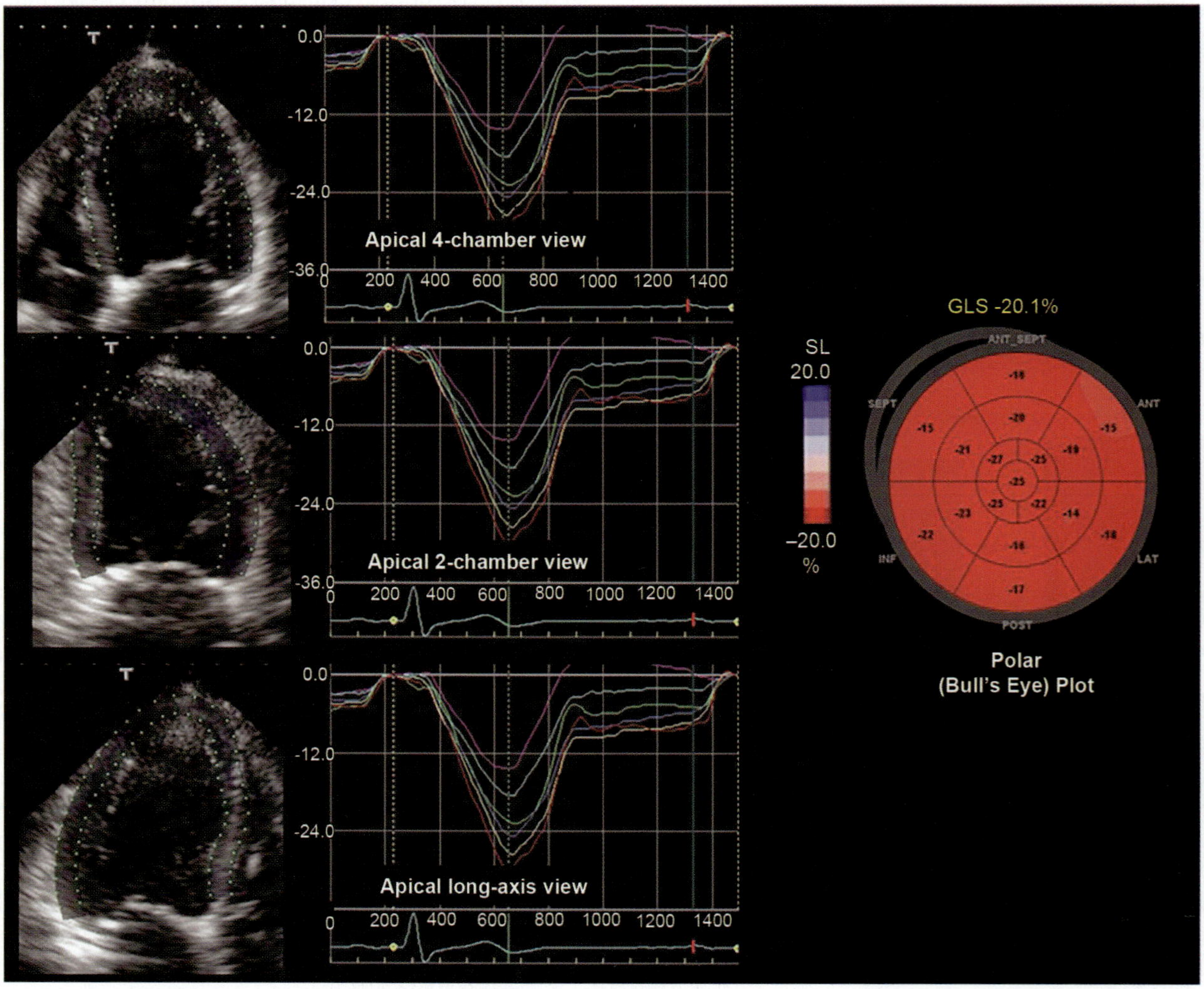

Fig. 6: An example of the calculation of global longitudinal strain (GLS) from apical four-chamber, apical two-chamber, and apical long-axis views. The peak segmental strain values from all three views are averaged (usually from 16 segments) for the GLS value.

Motoki et al. studied GLS in a series of 194 HFrEF patients showed that GLS <6.95% (absolute values) was significantly associated with the combined endpoint of death, heart transplant, or need for LV assist device (LVAD) placement and had additive prognostic value to LVEF.[13] Sengeløv et al. showed GLS was a superior predictor of survival in 1,065 HFrEF patients who were followed in the HF clinics.[14] They showed that GLS had additive prognostic value to all routine echocardiographic measures of systolic and diastolic function tested in the same patients. Delgado-Montero et al. showed in a group of HF patients with LVEF ≤35% who underwent CRT, that baseline GLS <9% before CRT was significantly associated with the risk of death, heart transplant or LVAD.[15] Park et al. in a landmark study of 4,172 patients with acute HF demonstrated the powerful prognostic value of GLS.[16] In patients with reduced (LVEF <40%), midrange (LVEF 40–49%), or preserved EF (LVEF ≥50%), they found risk of mortality to significantly increased with GLS <12%. HF patients with GLS <8% had the highest risk. Each 1% decrease in GLS was associated with a 5% increased risk for mortality (p <0.001). Sugahara et al. in a recent study of 89 patients with peripartum cardiomyopathy reported that GLS at presentation with a cutoff of 10.6% was associated with subsequent death, transplantation, LVAD or evidence of persistent LV dysfunction (LVEF <50%) at 1 year (sensitivity of 75% and specificity of 95%).[17] GLS has also been useful in patients with HFpEF. Kraigher-Krainer et al. in a substudy from a multicenter trial of HFpEF patients showed that GLS was decreased in patients with hypertensive heart disease compared to normal volunteers, and further decreased in patients with HFpEF compared to other groups.[18] Furthermore, GLS was correlated with increasing levels of the HF biomarker N-terminal probrain natriuretic peptide (NT-proBNP).

LIMITATIONS

There are limitations with each of the echocardiographic techniques described. LVEF remains of great importance, but there is approximately 5% variability by EF units among experts with biplane EF by echocardiography. Variability is increased further with visual estimation of LVEF. Doppler assessment of diastolic function is affected by many confounding variables. Arrhythmias, such as atrial fibrillation interfere with interpretation of these data. Finally, a limitation of speckle tracking strain imaging is that it cannot be applied to technically inadequate images, and approximately 10% of consecutive patients cannot be studied by strain imaging. There is variability among vendor software programs, although improvements are underway. Overall, the GLS measure appears to be stable and more reproducible than other strain measures.

CONCLUSION

Echocardiography is the most commonly employed imaging technique in patients with HF. It provides critically important information about cardiac function by LVEF. Routine Doppler and tissue Doppler measures of diastolic function provide additional prognostic information. Finally, GLS by speckle tracking strain imaging has emerged as a powerful new prognostic measure in HF patients with both reduced and preserved LVEF and is becoming a routine addition.

REFERENCES

1. Yancy CW, Jessup M, Bozkurt B, et al. 2017 ACC/AHA/HFSA Focused Update of the 2013 ACCF/AHA Guideline for the Management of Heart Failure: A Report of the American College of Cardiology/American Heart Association Task Force on Clinical Practice Guidelines and the Heart Failure Society of America. J Am Coll Cardiol. 2017;70:776-803.
2. Tracy CM, Epstein AE, Darbar D, et al. 2012 ACCF/AHA/HRS focused update of the 2008 guidelines for device-based therapy of cardiac rhythm abnormalities: a report of the American College of Cardiology Foundation/American Heart Association Task Force on Practice Guidelines. J Am Coll Cardiol. 2012;60:1297-313.
3. de Denus S, O'Meara E, Desai AS, et al. Spironolactone Metabolites in TOPCAT—New Insights into Regional Variation. N Engl J Med. 2017;376:1690-2.
4. Chandra A, Vaduganathan M, Lewis EF, et al. Health-Related Quality of Life in Heart Failure With Preserved Ejection Fraction: The PARAGON-HF Trial. JACC Heart Fail. 2019;7:862-74.
5. Zaret BL, Strauss HW. The past, present and future of nuclear cardiology. Rev Port Cardiol. 2000;19:I9-11.
6. Moss AJ. Prognosis after myocardial infarction. Am J Cardiol. 1983;52:667-9.
7. Rashid H, Exner DV, Mirsky I, et al. Comparison of echocardiography and radionuclide angiography as predictors of mortality in patients with left ventricular dysfunction (studies of left ventricular dysfunction). Am J Cardiol. 1999;84:299-303.
8. Lang RM, Badano LP, Mor-Avi V, et al. Recommendations for cardiac chamber quantification by echocardiography in adults: an update from the American Society of Echocardiography and the European Association of Cardiovascular Imaging. J Am Soc Echocardiogr. 2015;28:1-39.
9. Xie GY, Berk MR, Smith MD, et al. Prognostic value of Doppler transmitral flow patterns in patients with congestive heart failure. J Am Coll Cardiol. 1994;24:132-9.
10. Wang M, Yip G, Yu CM, et al. Independent and incremental prognostic value of early mitral annulus velocity in patients with impaired left ventricular systolic function. J Am Coll Cardiol. 2005;45:272-7.
11. Hillis GS, Moller JE, Pellikka PA, et al. Noninvasive estimation of left ventricular filling pressure by E/e' is a powerful

predictor of survival after acute myocardial infarction. J Am Coll Cardiol. 2004;43:360-7.

12. Dokainish H, Zoghbi WA, Lakkis NM, et al. Incremental predictive power of B-type natriuretic peptide and tissue Doppler echocardiography in the prognosis of patients with congestive heart failure. J Am Coll Cardiol. 2005;45:1223-6.
13. Motoki H, Borowski AG, Shrestha K, et al. Incremental prognostic value of assessing left ventricular myocardial mechanics in patients with chronic systolic heart failure. J Am Coll Cardiol. 2012;60:2074-81.
14. Sengeløv M, Jorgensen PG, Jensen JS, et al. Global longitudinal strain is a superior predictor of all-cause mortality in heart failure with reduced ejection fraction. JACC Cardiovasc Imaging. 2015;8:1351-9.
15. Delgado-Montero A, Tayal B, Goda A, et al. Additive prognostic value of echocardiographic global longitudinal and global circumferential strain to electrocardiographic criteria in patients with heart failure undergoing cardiac resynchronization therapy. Circ Cardiovasc Imaging. 2016;9.
16. Park JJ, Park JB, Park JH, et al. Global longitudinal strain to predict mortality in patients with acute heart failure. J Am Coll Cardiol. 2018;71:1947-57.
17. Sugahara M. Global left ventricular strain at presentation is associated with subsequent recovery in patients with peripartum cardiomyopathy. J Am Soc Echocardiogr. 2019.
18. Kraigher-Krainer E, Shah AM, Gupta DK, et al. Impaired systolic function by strain imaging in heart failure with preserved ejection fraction. J Am Coll Cardiol. 2014;63:447-56.

CHAPTER

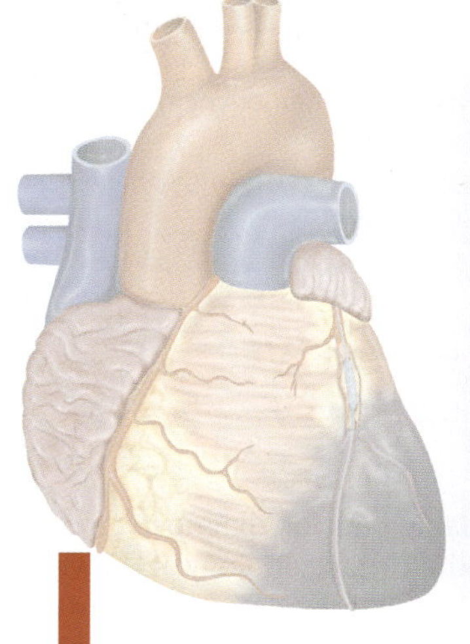

Echocardiographic Evaluation of Heart Failure in Emergency

Rekha Mishra, Uday S Yadav, Amitabh Poonia

INTRODUCTION

Heart failure (HF) is a complex clinical syndrome characterized by symptoms that may be accompanied by signs caused by structural and/or functional cardiac abnormality, resulting in reduced cardiac output and elevated intracardiac pressures at rest or during exertion. Echocardiography is the single most useful noninvasive bedside diagnostic test in the evaluation of patients with heart failure to accurately and noninvasively calculate left and right ventricular function, diagnosing structural heart disease, assessment of the hemodynamic and to guide therapy in HF. Echocardiography is noninvasive, cost-effective, portable, yields immediate result and can be done repeatedly for ongoing monitoring of the patient. Up to one-third of patients admitted to the hospital are of severe HF symptoms and early recognition of the condition is vital if subsequent injuries are to be avoided. It is recommended as the modality of first choice in consensus guidelines.[1] Acute heart failure (AHF) is among the most common causes for hospitalization in patients older than 65 years in the developed world. In the United States alone, 4 million patients are hospitalized each year with a primary or secondary diagnosis of heart failure (HF), and AHF contributes to more than 7 million hospital days annually.[2] Acute decompensation of heart failure can occur due to a wide range of precipitants (Table 1). Most of the cases of HF have both systolic and diastolic dysfunction. Depending on the severity of LV dysfunction, HF is classified in three categories by the European Society of Cardiology (ESC)-HF 2016 guideline:[3,4]

- HFpEF: HF with preserved ejection fraction (LVEF ≥50%)
- HFmrEF: HF with midrange ejection fraction (LVEF 40–49%)
- HFrEF: HF with reduced ejection fraction (LVEF <40%).

Coronary artery disease (CAD) is labeled as the most common underlying cause of LV dysfunction leading

TABLE 1: Common causes of heart failure and precipitants.

Common causes of heart failure	*Precipitants of heart failure*
Ischemic cardiomyopathy	Myocardial ischemia
Dilated cardiomyopathy	Acute valvular catastrophe
Valvular obstruction or insufficiency	Hypertension (malignant, crisis)
Hypertrophic cardiomyopathy	Acute myocarditis
Restrictive cardiomyopathy	Arrhythmias (rapid ventricular response)
Arrhythmogenic right ventricular cardiomyopathy	Acute pulmonary embolism (right heart failure)
Acute myocarditis, stress cardiomyopathy	Cardiac tamponade
Peripartum cardiomyopathy	Infections
Prosthetic valvular dysfunction	Medication noncompliance

to systolic HF but multiple other causes of pulmonary edema/HF symptoms like valvular regurgitations (AR, MR, TR) and severe stenotic lesions (aortic stenosis, mitral stenosis, pulmonic stenosis), dissection of aorta with acute AR, acute myocarditis, decompensated nonischemic dilated cardiomyopathy (DCMP), obstructive hypertrophic cardiomyopathy, restrictive cardiomyopathy, pericardial pathology like constrictive pericarditis, atrial and ventricular tachyarrhythmias, sepsis results in HF symptoms and echocardiography is the only bedside tool that can diagnose the underlying etiology of HF with great sensitivity and specificity.[5] Rapid cardiac assessment by echo (RACE) using just two-dimensional (2D) and M-mode echocardiography demonstrates major underlying abnormality in the acute HF symptoms with detailed echocardiographic assessment using Doppler after stabilization.[6] Left ventricular (LV) size and systolic function including left ventricular ejection fraction (LVEF), fractional shortening, regional wall motion abnormalities, myocardial thickness, interventricular septal thickness and motion, right ventricular size and function, valvular diseases, intravascular volume status, pericardial or pleural effusion, presence of intramural mass and aortic pathology can be easily identified by echo.[7] Introduction of 3D echo has enhanced the accuracy and reliability with which chamber volume and function are measured and also the evaluation of regurgitations.

Echocardiography along with spectral Doppler allows the measurement of several hemodynamics parameters such as stroke volume (SV), cardiac output (CO), central venous pressure (CVP), intracavitary pressures, systemic vascular resistance (SVR), pulmonary vascular resistance (PVR), myocardial contractility and biventricular interactions. This basic hemodynamic assessment enables proper and immediate hemodynamic support. Estimation of four parameters (CVP, pulmonary capillary wedge pressure, SV and CO) helps to ensure optimum balance of fluids, inotropes, and vasoconstrictors in the acute decompensated state.

ECHOCARDIOGRAPHIC EVALUATION OF HEART FAILURE IN EMERGENCY

Clinical studies have shown that standard physical examination have low sensitivity and specificity in detecting either systolic or diastolic LV dysfunction, especially in the preclinical phase. Moreover, physical examination has limitation to accurately characterize the volume status and cardiac output in patients with LV dysfunction.[8] Echocardiography is one of the most powerful diagnostic and monitoring tools available and its availability is fundamental to the management of patients with acute cardiovascular disease (Box 1).

BOX 1: Emergency echocardiographic assessment of patients with HF.

- Etiological causes of HF
- Systolic or diastolic dysfunction with hemodynamic grading of severity
- To assess for need of emergency medical or surgical therapy
- Response and monitoring of HF therapy
- Predicting prognosis in HF

Heart Failure with Reduced LVEF: Etiological Diagnosis of HF by Echocardiography

Echocardiography is a valuable bedside diagnostic tool in emergency to differentiate the various etiology of HF when clinical signs and symptoms are mixed with noncardiac etiology. "Eyeballing methods" is often used to calculate the LVEF in emergency room and detecting the hypokinetic, akinetic or dyskinetic LV segments where endocardial delineation is difficult to trace which is reasonably accurate by an experienced echocardiographer. Structural heart disease when detected in HF must be assessed in terms of severity of the disease and benefit and risk of urgent surgery or intervention therapy.

Coronary Artery Disease Presented with Heart Failure Symptoms

Two-dimensional echo along with Doppler is the diagnostic modality of choice that can provide detailed information about the patient's cardiovascular system. Immediately after the onset of ischemia, myocardial thickening ceases and depending on the severity of ischemia the wall becomes hypokinetic, akinetic or dyskinetic. This rapid diagnosis by echocardiography leads to early targeted therapy. Echo helps in estimation of infarct size, assessment of ventricular systolic as well as diastolic function, assessment of reperfusion, identification of location/severity of disease in patients with ongoing ischemia and evaluation of complications. Post-myocardial infarction (post-MI) complications like ventricular septal rupture, papillary muscle/chordal rupture leading to acute MR, thrombus formation, pericardial effusion and right ventricular infarct can be detected easily by echocardiography while in ICU stay (Figs. 1A to C).

HF Associated with Nonischemic Cardiomyopathy

All cardiomyopathies can lead to acute episodes of HF, either in the presence of reduced ejection fraction or when the ejection fraction is still normal since the main determinant of cardiac symptoms and prognosis is represented by the increase in LV filling pressure.[9] Heart

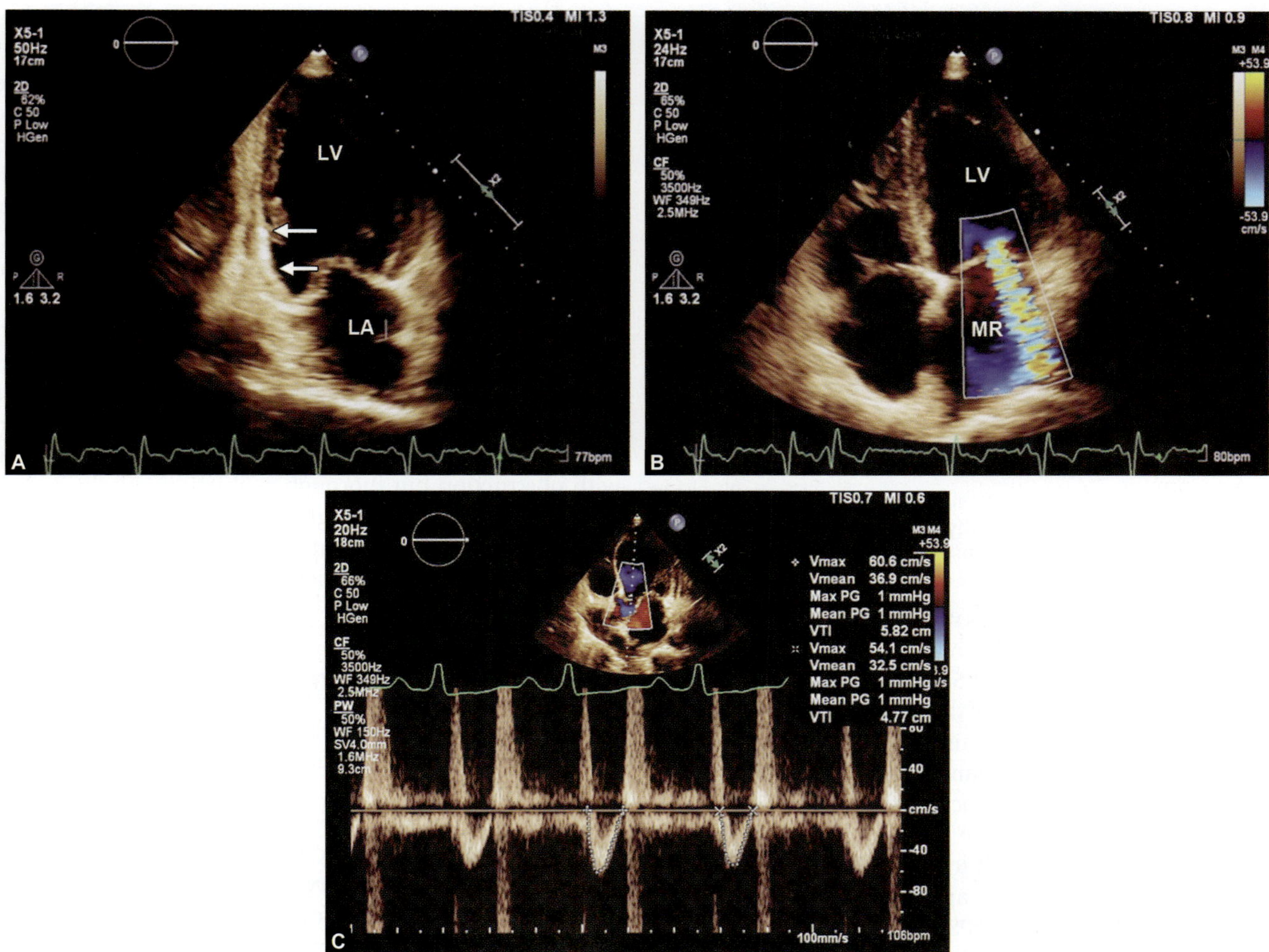

Figs. 1A to C: (A) Apical 2-C view shows akinetic and scarred LV inferior wall, tenting of mitral leaflets seen; (B) Apical 4-C view, color Doppler reveals severe MR; (C) PW Doppler across the LVOT reveals marked reduction in LVOT velocity time integral (VTI) consistent with severely reduced stroke volume.
(LVOT: left ventricular outflow tract; LV left ventricle; LA: left atrium; MR: mitral regurgitation)

failure due to systolic dysfunction is relatively easy to diagnose by echocardiography which demonstrates a dilated LV with reduced ejection fraction but echo has many other roles beyond the recognition of systolic dysfunction since dilatation of the LV results in alteration of intracardiac geometry and hemodynamics leading to increased morbidity and mortality.[10] It has been seen that LV volume is one of the most important prognostic indicators for the patients with ischemic or dilated cardiomyopathy.[11,12] In the BEST trial, Grayburn and his colleagues demonstrated that echo parameters like LV end-diastolic volume, deceleration time of early diastolic mitral inflow velocity which is a surrogate for pulmonary capillary wedge pressure, and severity of mitral valve regurgitation were the strongest predictors of survival in patients with ejection fraction of 35% or less cardiomyopathies caused by processes such as postviral myocarditis, postpartum cardiomyopathy, idiopathic/genetic, postchemotherapy (Adriamycin therapy), tachycardia induced, and toxins like alcoholic cardiomyopathy typically display diffuse LV hypokinesis. HF associated with septic myocarditis/chemotherapy typically display normal size or minimal dilatation of LV with global hypokinesis and mitral inflow velocities suggesting near normal LV filling pressures. There is often pronounced yet reversible RV dysfunction and RV dilatation.[13] Echo can rapidly rule out mimics of CAD/ACS. Takotsubo cardiomyopathy (stress cardiomyopathy) typically has apical ballooning with apical akinesia and basal hyperkinesia in the majority (>80%) of patients.[14] Complete resolution can take place days to weeks which can be detected with serial echoes. Rarer "reverse" stress cardiomyopathy in which basal or midventricular wall motion abnormalities occur with preservation of apical function presents with HF.[15] The degree of impairment in LV contractility is quantifiable by

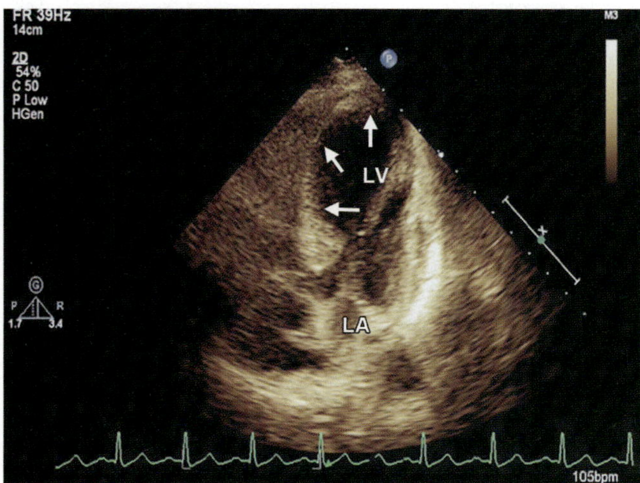

Fig. 2: Apical 4-C view, apical ballooning in a patient with Takotsubo cardiomyopathy (arrows).
(LV: left ventricle; LA: left atrium)

2D echo (modified Simpson's method) or M-mode findings such as increased separation of the mitral E point from the interventricular septum (EPSS), decreased mitral leaflet opening, and early closure of the aortic valve. The SV of the ventricle reflected by velocity time integral of left ventricular outflow tract (LVOT) less than 16 cm/sec and diminished tissue Doppler (systolic) velocity suggestive of low SV. RV size and contractility may be assessed by parallel means although it is more difficult to assess RV volume without the use of 3D echocardiography. One easily obtainable measure of RV function is TAPSE, which reflects shortening in the long-axis dimension of RV myocardial fibers; a TAPSE of less than 17 mm is considered abnormal, and 14 mm or less suggestive of worse prognosis in patients with dilated cardiomyopathy (Fig. 2).

Heart Failure Symptoms Associated with Stenotic and Regurgitant Valvular Pathology

Echocardiography helps in delineating the etiology, valvular pathology as well as grading of severity of valvular lesions causing HF symptoms. Acute volume overload due to renocardiac syndrome, severe degenerative aortic stenosis, acute aortic regurgitation due to aortic dissection at ascending aorta and acute mitral regurgitation due to post-MI rupture of a papillary muscle, perforation or rupture of valvular leaflets due to infective endocarditis, spontaneous chordal rupture in degenerative or rheumatic mitral valve can be diagnosed rapidly and accurately by echocardiography (Figs. 3A to F).[16]

HF Secondary to Prosthetic Valvular Dysfunction

Prosthetic valves are more difficult to evaluate than native valves, and therefore, in a case of suspected prosthetic related emergency, it should be evaluated by an expert in both transthoracic echocardiography (TTE) and transesophageal echocardiography (TEE).[17] HF in the presence of prosthetic valve replacement can occur in the presence of massive prosthetic obstruction or regurgitation in addition to prosthetic endocarditis in patients with sepsis. Prosthetic regurgitation is frequently paraprosthetic; however, in bioprosthetic valves sudden structural deterioration may cause severe transvalvular regurgitation. Abnormal mobility of the prosthesis sewing ring always implies severe paraprosthetic regurgitation. Obstruction is generally due to either thrombosis or pannus. Direct observation of the valve mechanism is usually feasible for mitral and tricuspid prostheses, but can be challenging in case of aortic position. Transprosthetic gradients increase with obstruction but thorough evaluation is indicated as concomitant prosthetic regurgitation, patient prosthesis mismatch, high cardiac output states or sepsis will also lead to abnormally high velocities without true mechanical obstruction (Figs. 4A to D).

Heart Failure with Preserved LVEF

It is a clinical syndrome characterized by symptoms and signs of heart failure, a preserved ejection fraction, and abnormal diastolic function. The term "preserved" EF refers to EFs that are normal or near normal. Approximately half of all patients with chronic heart failure have a normal or near normal (i.e. "preserved") left ventricular ejection fraction.[18,19] Because the dominant abnormality present in patients with HFpEF is abnormal diastolic function, this clinical syndrome is called "diastolic heart failure" (DHF). Patients with DHF are older, are more often female, have mostly hypertensive heart disease, and less often have ischemic heart disease than patients with systolic heart failure.[20,21]

The term *diastolic dysfunction* refers to abnormalities in LV filling secondary to altered compliance, relaxation, and/or recoil. Abnormalities in diastolic function can occur in the presence or absence of a clinical syndrome of heart failure and with normal or abnormal systolic function. Whereas *diastolic dysfunction* describes abnormal LV performance, *HFpEF* describes a clinical syndrome of heart failure.

Echocardiography with Doppler readily helps in assessing not only LV diastolic function but also in assessment of severity/grading, identification of etiology, important differential diagnosis and management of acute heart failure.[3] The assessment of diastolic dysfunction is complex, in exact science multiple factors must be assessed, and no one parameter can be used in isolation. According to the latest guidelines from American society of Echocardiography and European Association of

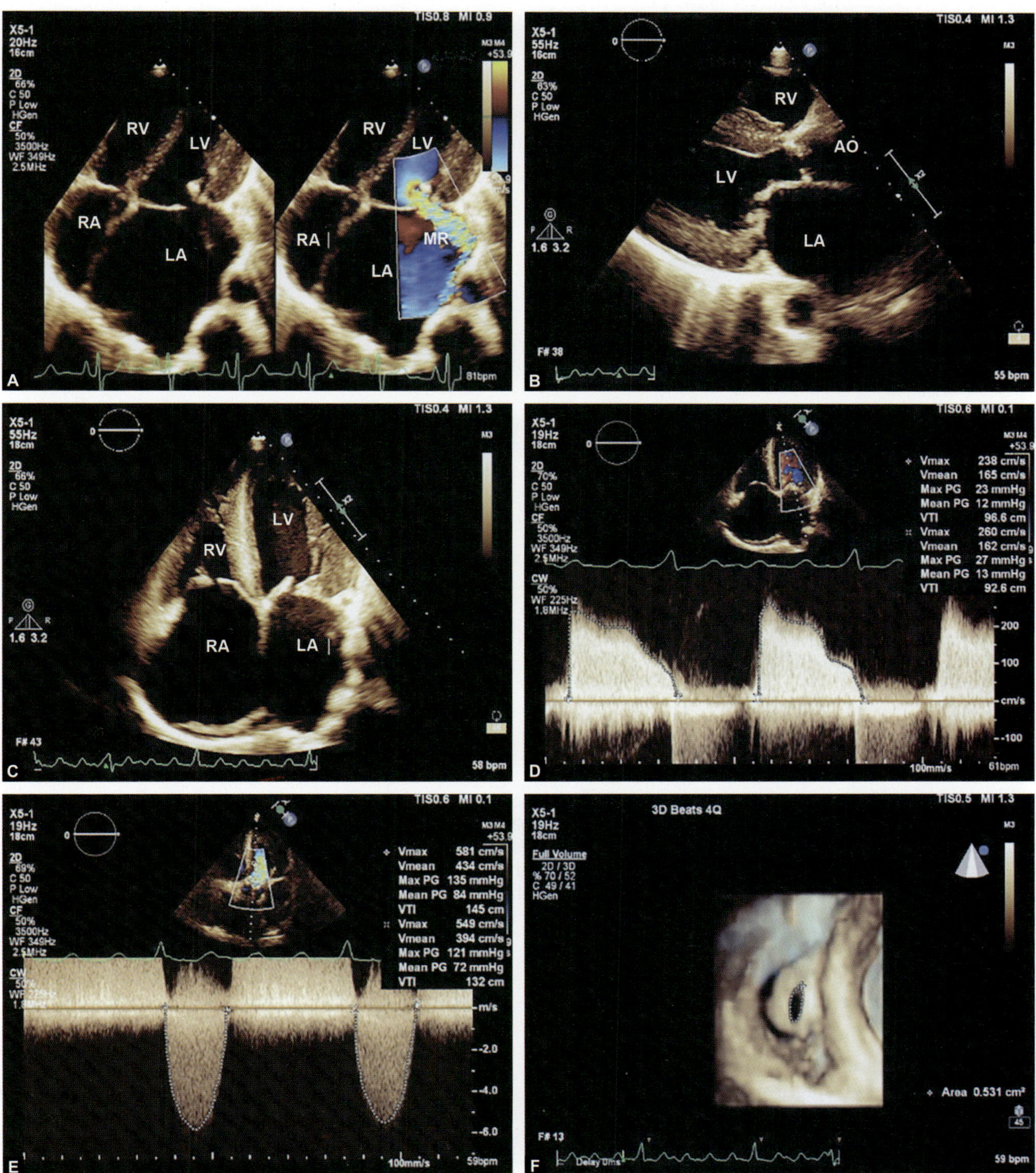

Figs. 3A to F: (A) Apical 4-C view shows marked dilatation of LA, posterior mitral leaflet is thickened and restricted with systolic non-coaptation of mitral leaflets leading to severe MR. The jet of MR is highly eccentric and directed posterolaterally; (B) PLAX view shows concentric LVH, dilatation of LA, thickening of MV as well as AoV with diastolic doming of AML consistent with rheumatic involvement of the valves; (C) Apical 4-C view shows dilatation of LA and RA, diastolic doming of mitral and tricuspid valve consistent with rheumatic mitral and tricuspid stenosis; (D and E) The peak instantaneous pressure gradient and mean pressure gradient across the MV and AoV was 27/13 mm Hg and 135/84 mm Hg respectively consistent with severe MS and AS; (F) 3-D en-face view of TV from RV aspect, TVA by 3D—0.53 cm^2.

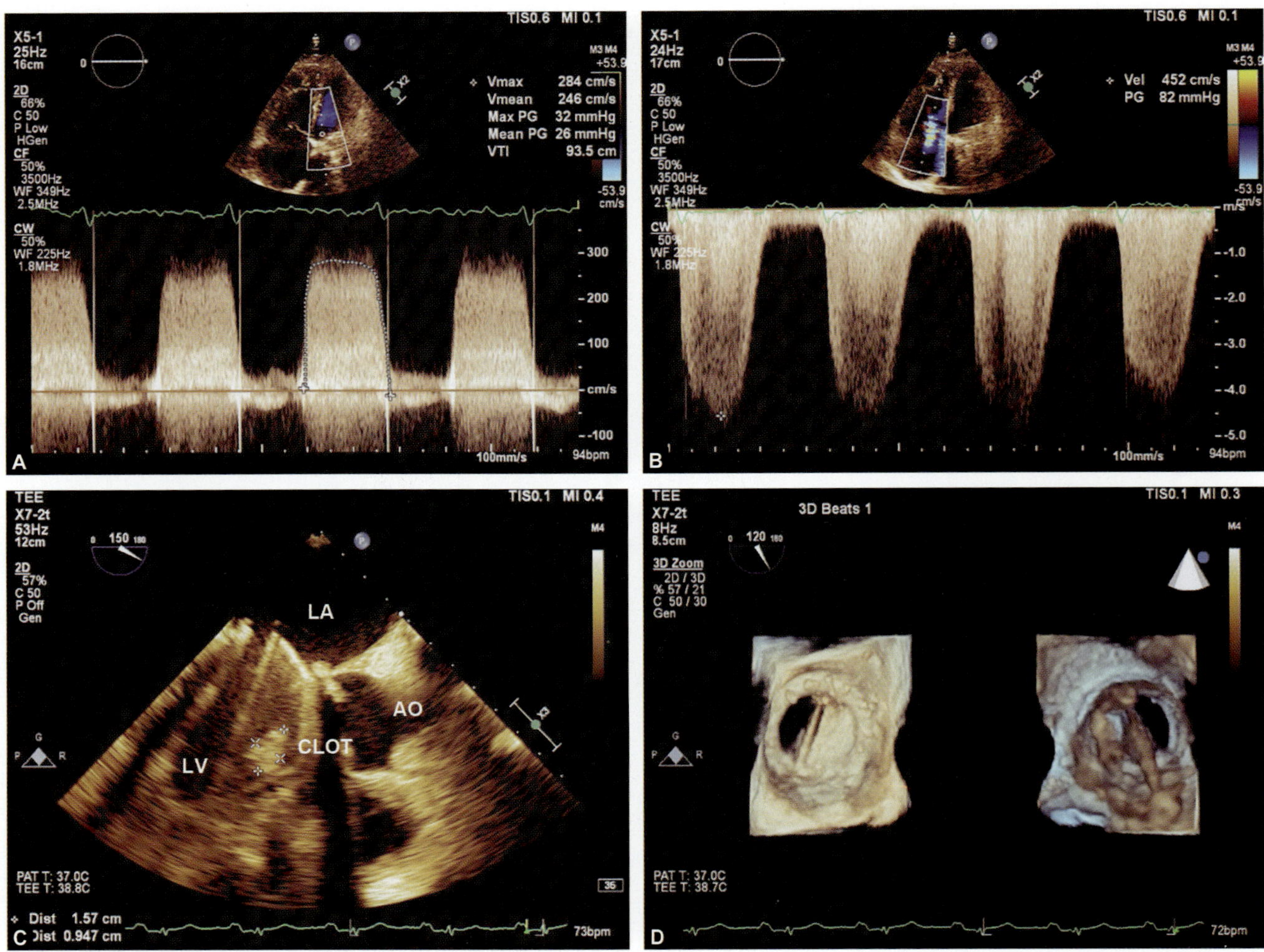

Figs. 4A to D: (A) Continuous-wave Doppler across the mitral mechanical prosthesis with markedly elevated peak instantaneous PG and mean gradient being 32/26 mm Hg, respectively; (B) Pulmonary artery systolic pressure using TR jet in the same patient −82 mm Hg + RAP; (C) TEE reveals mitral mechanical prosthesis in situ with restricted motion of one of the disks along with a well-defined clot toward LV aspect; (D) 3-D TEE en-face view of the same prosthesis clearly delineates one disk in closed position (LA aspect) and multiple layered clots in the vicinity of the prosthesis (LV aspect).
(LV: left ventricle; LA: left atrium; AO: aorta)

Cardiovascular imaging mainly four variables need to be evaluated in determining the diastolic function if LV systolic is preserved.[22]

These four variables and their abnormal variables are:

1. Annular e' velocity (septal e' velocity <7.0 cm/sec, lateral e' <10 cm/sec)
2. An average E/e' ratio of >14
3. LA maximum volume index of 34 mL/m^2
4. Peak TR velocity of >2.8 m/sec.

At times only the medial or lateral e' velocity is available and, in these circumstances, medial E/e' ratio >15 cm/sec or a lateral E/e' >13 cm/sec is considered abnormal.

According to the latest guidelines of European Society of Heart Failure, the diagnosis of HFpEF is made on the basis of clinical, echocardiographic, laboratory and invasive assessment (Fig. 5).

Identification of Etiology

Echocardiography is very helpful in ruling out the less common causes of HFpEF including hypertensive heart diseases, hypertrophic cardiomyopathy, constrictive pericarditis and restrictive cardiomyopathies which includes infiltrative cardiomyopathies such as amyloidosis, storage disorders, radiation-induced heart disease and endomyocardial fibrosis. Although, these diseases account for a small minority of cases of HFpEF, the clinical presentation in older persons with HFpEF may be identical. The main use of echocardiography in acute cardiac care of

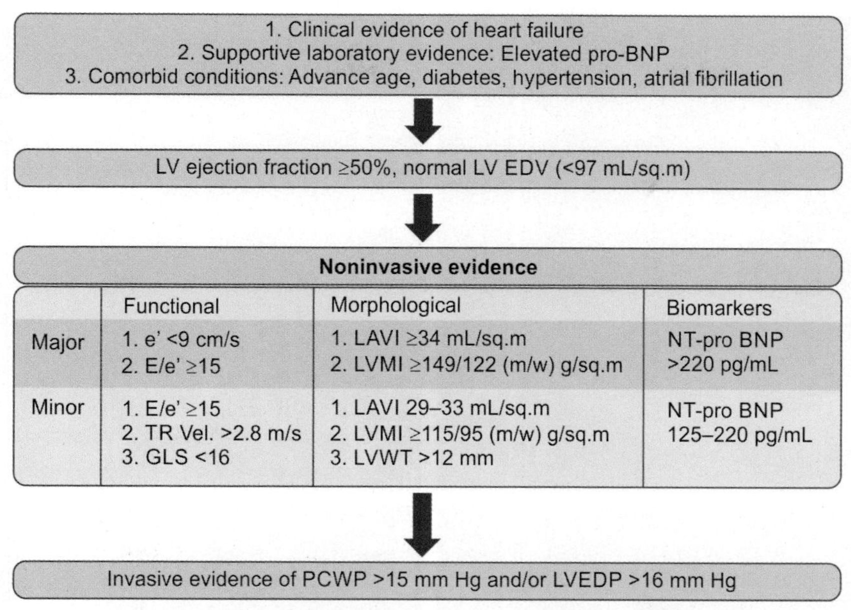

Fig. 5: Flow diagram for the diagnostic criteria of HFpEF.

(E: mitral inflow during early phase; e': mitral annular velocity; GLS: global longitudinal strain; LAVI: left atrial volume index; LVEDV: left ventricle end-diastolic volume; LVMI: left ventricle mass index; LVWT: left ventricle wall thickness; TR: tricuspid regurgitation; m: men; w: women)

Source: Modified from Ponikowski P, Voors AA, Anker SD, et al. 2016 ESC—Guidelines for the diagnosis and treatment of acute and chronic heart failure. Eur Heart J. 2016;37(27):2129-200.

patients affected by these cardiomyopathies relates to the diagnosis and management of acute HF.

Important Differential Diagnosis

Diastolic dysfunction is an important cause of heart failure symptoms in patients with normal ejection fraction. However, several other conditions may also lead to similar symptoms and must therefore be considered in the differential diagnosis. Pericardial disease, particularly constrictive pericarditis (CP) should be considered when heart failure and normal EF coexist. Pericardial thickening is a hallmark of constriction but is a relatively insensitive finding. The distinction between CP and other causes of diastolic heart failure is essential since the treatment is totally different. Findings that suggest CP include a normal or high e' velocity (medial anulus velocity > lateral anulus velocity), which is unusual in other causes of restrictive fillings.

HF Associated with Hypertension

Hypertension is frequently concomitant with diastolic heart failure and may precipitate acute decompensation. LVH is a marker for hypertensive heart disease which can be detected easily by echocardiography.[23] Hypertensive patients with HFpEF evolve to HF with a reduced EF remains a frequently debatable question (Figs. 6A to E).

HF Secondary to Pericardial Disease

Cardiac tamponade results from large and/or rapid accumulation of fluid in the pericardial space leading to increase in intrapericardial pressure, above intracavitary pressure, resulting in fall in transmural pressure. Therefore, ventricular filling is decreased and cardiac output is compromised. The most specific sign by 2D echo is diastolic RV collapse and is best appreciated by M-mode (Figs. 7A and B) or 2D echo from the parasternal or subcostal long axis views and short axis view at the base of the heart (Fig. 7C). Other important signs include dilated inferior vena cava with no respiratory variation, marked respiratory variation of transvalvular velocities and cyclic compression, inversion or collapse of the right atrium. Pericardial constriction occurs when there is thickening, with or without calcification of the pericardium, results in impaired cardiac diastolic filling. The clinical features mimic those of biventricular heart failure. The clinical differential diagnosis is "restrictive cardiomyopathy" versus pericardial constriction, since ejection fraction is generally preserved in both. The M-mode and 2D echocardiographic features of CP include a thickened pericardium, abnormal ventricular septal motion, flattening of the LV posterior wall during diastole, respiratory variation in ventricular size, and a dilated inferior vena cava (Figs. 8A and C). But to establish the diagnosis, Doppler echocardiography is extremely important. A

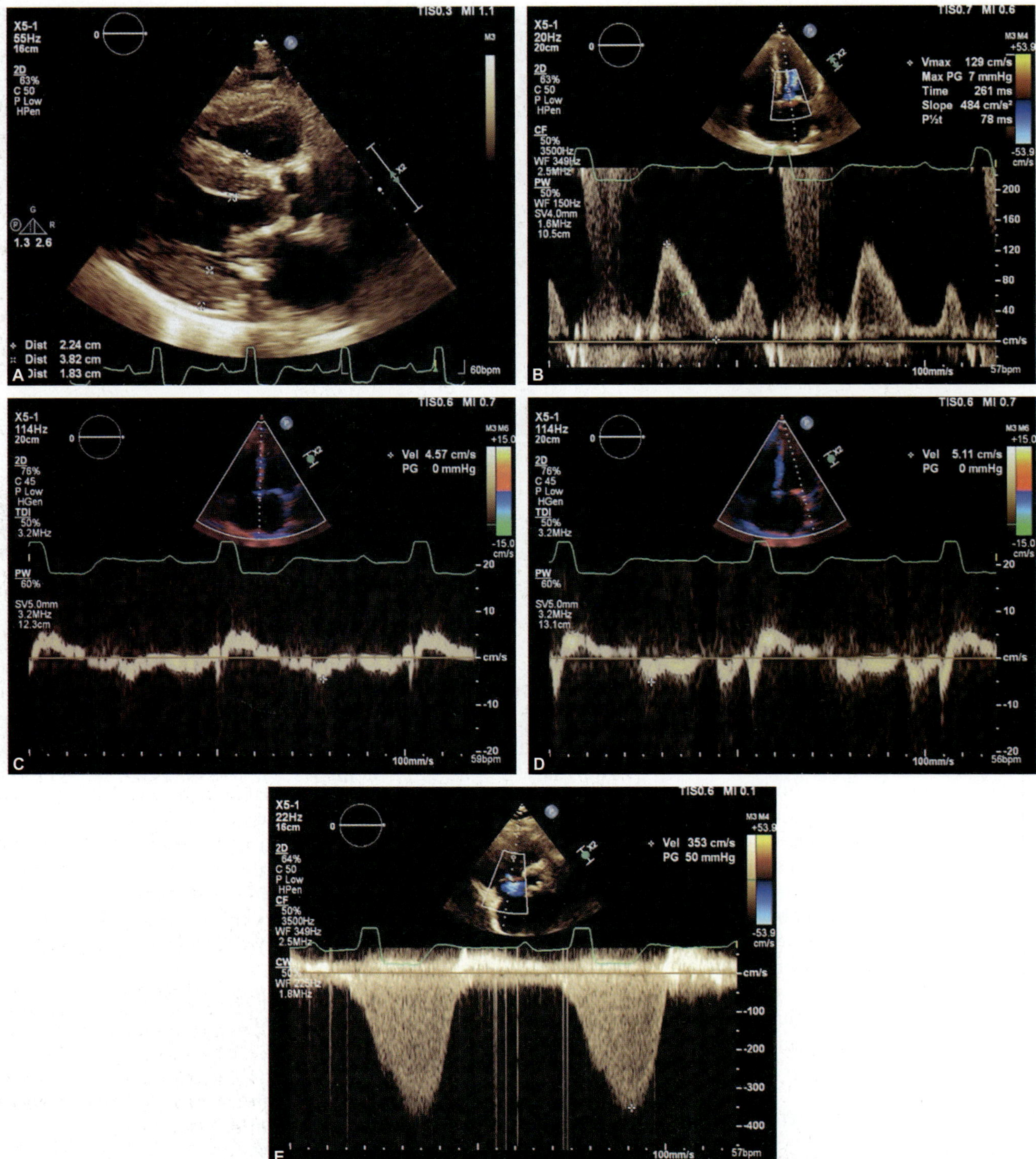

Figs. 6A to E: (A) PLAX view showing marked concentric LVH with dilatation of left atrium, mitral annular calcification in a patient of chronic renal disease; (B) Doppler of mitral inflow show E and A waves with E>A, but both medial and lateral mitral annular velocities; (C and D) are markedly reduced E/e'(Av) = 26.6 suggestive of severely elevated LV end-diastolic filling pressure; (E) Pulmonary artery systolic pressure using TR jet −50 mm Hg + RA pressure.

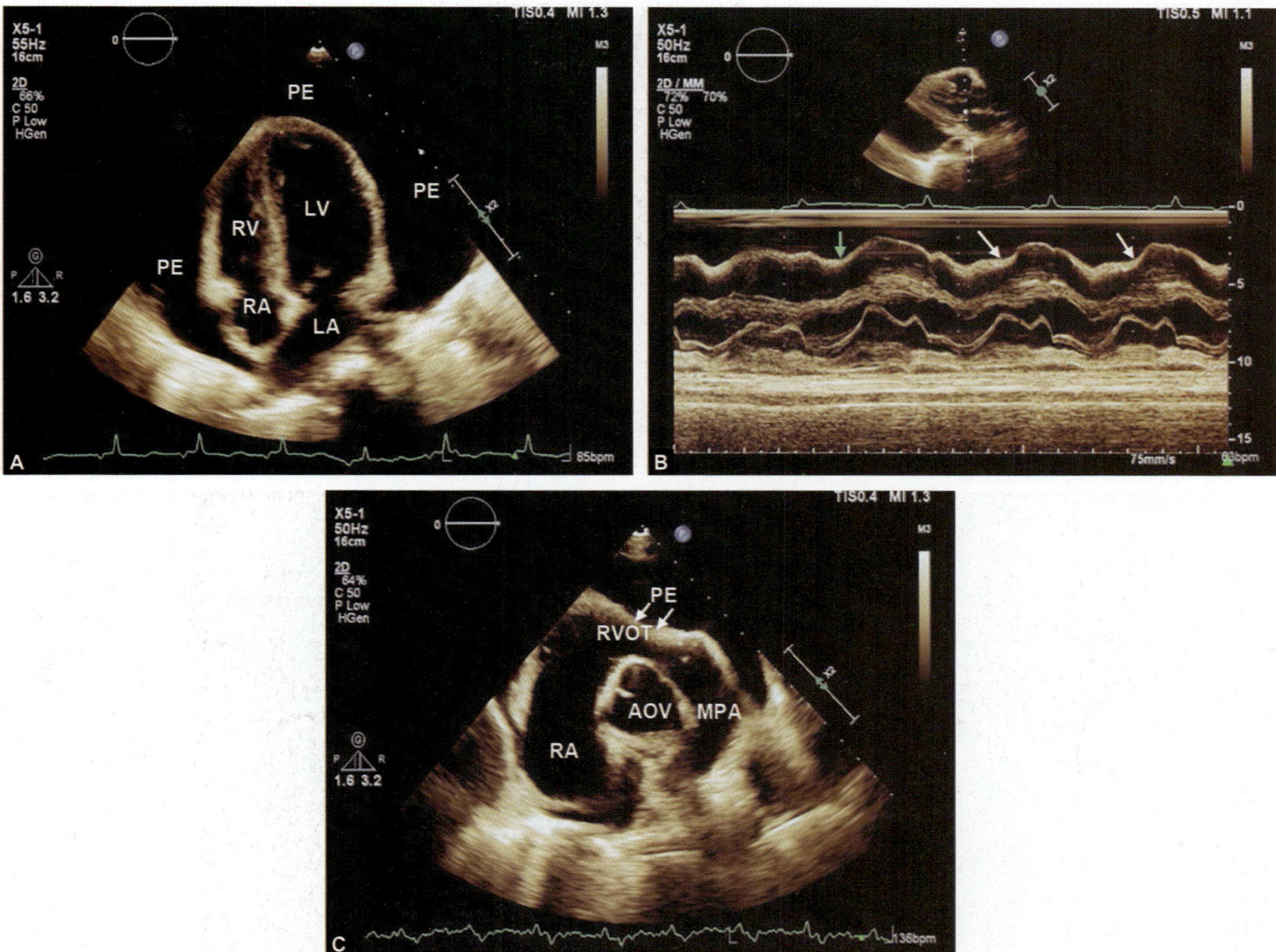

Figs. 7A to C: (A) Apical 4-C view showing large circumferential pericardial effusion; (B) 2D guided M-mode clearly delineating early diastolic collapse of RV consistent with cardiac tamponade; (C) SAX view showing diastolic collapse of RV free wall (arrow). (AOV: aortic valve; MPA: main pulmonary artery; PE: pericardial effusion; RA: right atrium; RVOT: right ventricular outflow tract)

respiratory variation of >25% in mitral E velocity, >40% in tricuspid E velocity and expiratory increased diastolic flow reversal in the hepatic vein need to be demonstrated (Figs. 8D and E).

HF with Restrictive Cardiomyopathy

The distinct morphological and hemodynamic characteristics of restrictive cardiomyopathy by echocardiography are: Nondilated ventricle (<40 mL/m^2) with normal wall thickness (<1–1.2 cm). Rigid ventricular walls with normal systolic function in majority of patients and severe LV diastolic dysfunction with restrictive filling leading to elevated filling pressures. Biatrial enlargement and normal pericardium. Echocardiography also helps to distinguish etiology of various restrictive cardiomyopathies, e.g. infiltrative disorders like amyloidosis, sarcoidosis, storage diseases like hemochromatosis, Fabry disease, and endomyocardial disease like endomyocardial fibrosis (EMF).[24]

HF with Hypertrophic Cardiomyopathy

Hypertrophic cardiomyopathy (HCMP) is the most common genetic cardiac disease with a prevalence of 1:5,000 in the general population.[25] HF is a common complication of HCMP and is most commonly due to dynamic mechanical impedance to left ventricular outflow produced by mitral valve systolic anterior motion, leading to high intracavitary pressures.[26] Profiles of advanced HF in HCMP are due to diverse pathophysiological mechanisms, as described by Paola Melacini which includes LV outflow obstruction, diastolic or global systolic ventricular dysfunction and echocardiography helps in evaluating all the parameters in detail (Table 2).[27]

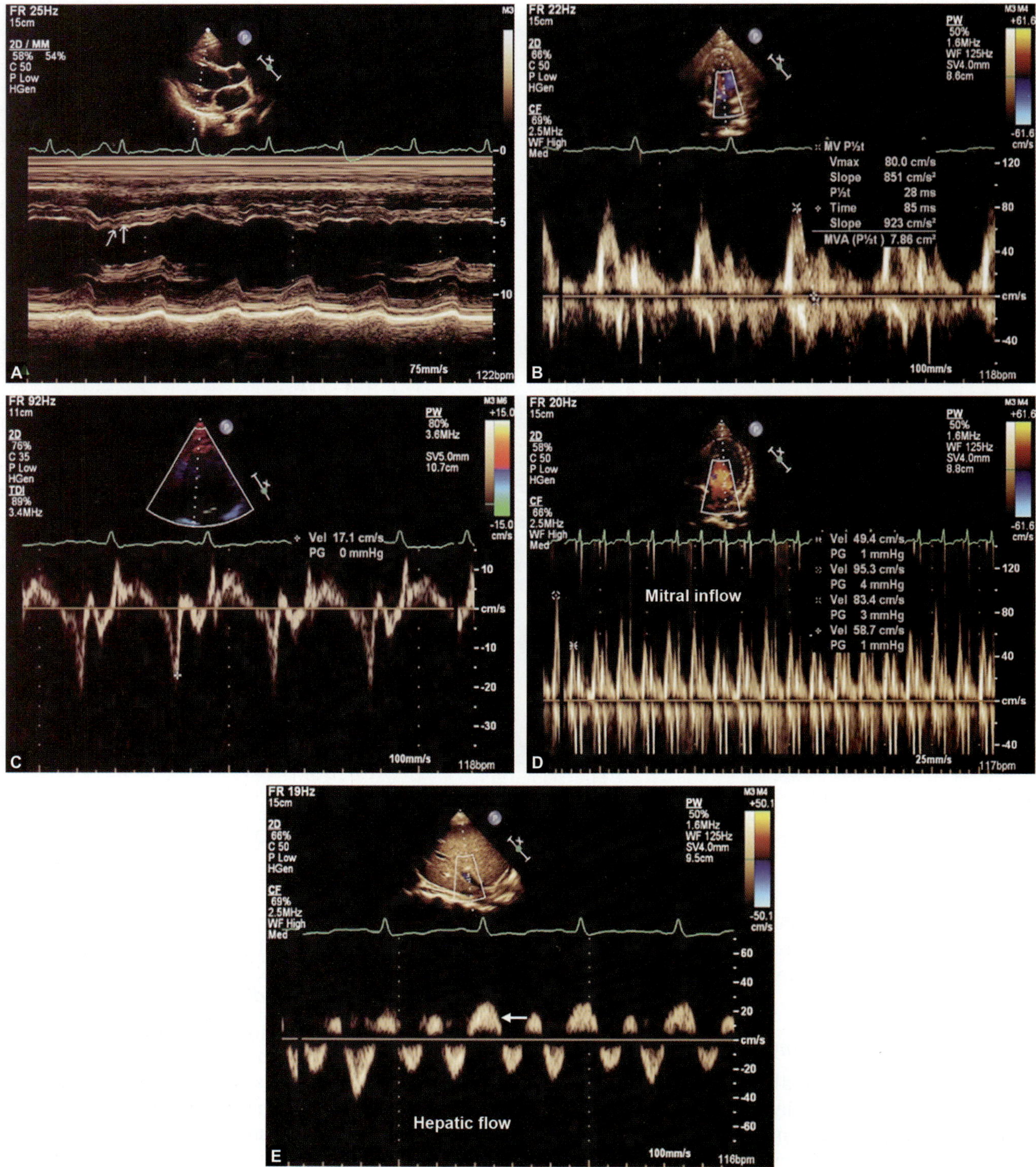

Figs. 8A to E: (A) M-mode shows diastolic flattening of the posterior wall endocardium, abrupt posterior motion of the IVS in early diastole with inspiration (septal shudder and bounce); (B and C) Transvalvular Doppler of mitral inflow and tissue Doppler medial mitral annulus, E/e' = 80/17.1 = 4.6 suggests annulus paradoxus; (D) Significant respiratory variation of mitral inflow with >40% inspiratory decrease in mitral inflow velocity; (E) Doppler of hepatic venous flow with expiratory increase in diastolic reflux (arrow) due to ventricular interaction and the dissociation of intracardiac and intrathoracic pressures.

TABLE 2: Echo distinction of cardiomyopathies.

	DCMP	HCMP	RCMP
LV volume	↑↑↑	↓↓	N
Wall thickness	N or ↓	IVS ↑↑	↑ or N
LV contractility	↓↓↓	↑↑↑	N or ↓
LVEDP	↑	↑	↑↑↑

(N: normal; ↑: increased; ↓: decreased; LV: left ventricle; IVS: intraventricular septum; LVEDP: left ventricular end-diastolic pressure; DCMP: dilated cardiomyopathy; HCMP: hypertrophic cardiomyopathy; RCMP: restrictive cardiomyopathy)

Heart Failure Secondary to RV Dysfunction

HF Secondary to Acute Pulmonary Embolism

Acute pulmonary embolism presents with classical right heart changes which can be demonstrated by echo in massive pulmonary embolism which includes acute RV dysfunction associated with RV dilatation, paradoxical motion of IVS, D-shaped LV in parasternal SAX view, elevated pulmonary artery pressure with high resistant flow (notched forward Doppler signal) in pulmonary artery, decreased cardiac output and rarely intracavitary emboli. The IVC may be dilated with minimal or no respiratory variation. McConnell's sign which is defined as mid RV free wall akinesia with sparing of the apex.[28] It is thought to be specific but not very sensitive sign for acute pulmonary embolism (sensitivity 77%; specificity 96%). This sign is believed to be caused by tethering of the RV to the hyperdynamic LV apex.[29] The acceleration time of the pulmonary ejection signal (PAcT) is often used in case of absence of a reliable TR jet.[30] PAcT of 70–90 msec indicates pulmonary artery systolic pressure of >70 mm Hg. The presence of mid-systolic notch in pulmonary ejection signal also indicates severe pulmonary hypertension

HF Secondary to Chronic Obstructive Pulmonary Disease

Chronic obstructive pulmonary disease is a leading cause of death and disability worldwide. It has considerable effects on cardiac functions, including those of the RV, LV and the pulmonary blood vessels. Approximately 25% of patients with COPD develop cor pulmonale.[31] Echocardiography provides a rapid and accurate method to assess the secondary changes leading to development of pulmonary hypertension, RV dilatation, RV hypertrophy and dysfunction and the left ventricular dysfunction too. PA systolic pressure can be estimated using TR jet, PA mean pressure and end-diastolic pressure can be estimated through pulmonary regurgitation jet (Table 3).

TABLE 3: Echocardiographic signs suggestive of the cause of clinical admission in acute cardiovascular conditions.

HFrEF	HFpEF	Pulmonary embolism	Tamponade
LVEF <45–50%	LVEF ≥50%	Thrombus into right chambers	Usually large pericardial effusion
LVEDD >55 mm or >32 mm/m²	LVEDV <97 mL/m²	Abnormal septal motion	Swinging heart
LVESD >45 mm or >25 mm/m²	LVESV <43 mL/m²	Dilated RA and RV (RVEDD/LVEDD >0.6 or area >1.0)	Diastolic collapse of the RV free wall (rarely LV)
LVEDV >97 mL/m²	E/e' >14 (Av)	Global RV hypokinesia	RA collapse (rarely LA)
LVESV >43 mL/m²	Ar: A ≥30 ms	McConnell sign hyperkinesia	IVC dilatation (no collapse with inspiration)
Abnormal wall motion	LA volume ≥34 mL/m²	Mid to severe TR	TV flow increases and MV flow decreases during inspiration (reverse in expiration)
Functional MR and TR	Peak tricuspid velocity >3 m/s	Pulmonary hypertension around 40–50 mm Hg (>60 mm Hg in the case of pre-existing pulmonary hypertension)	Systolic and diastolic flows are reduced in systemic veins in expiration and reverse flow with atrial contraction is increased
Peak tricuspid velocity >3 m/s			
Aortic time velocity integral <15 cm			
Diastolic dysfunction (E/A ≥2 + DT <150 ms)			

(A: duration of the A wave; DT: deceleration time; E: early mitral inflow velocity; e': early diastolic mitral annular velocity; Ar: duration of the pulmonary flow reversal; IVC: inferior vena cava; LVEDD: left ventricular end-diastolic diameter; LVEDV: left ventricular end-diastolic volume; LVEF: left ventricular ejection fraction; LVESV: left ventricular end-systolic volume; LVESD: left ventricular end-systolic diameter)

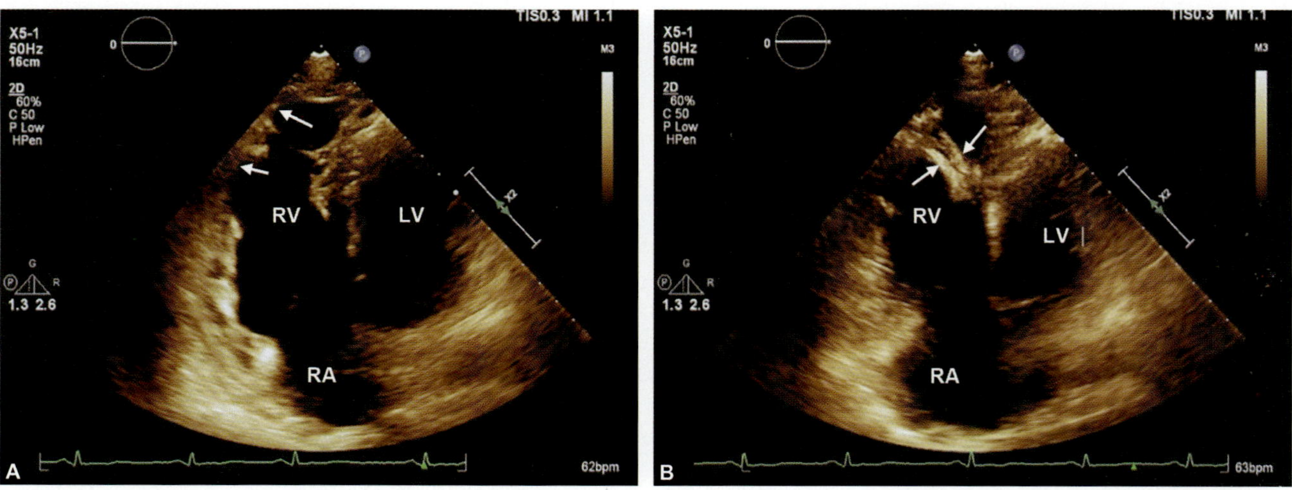

Figs. 9A and B: (A) Modified apical 4-C view showing multiple RV lateral wall aneurysms (arrows); (B) Prominent moderator band in RV apex (arrows).
(LV: left ventricle; RA: right atrium; RV: right ventricle)

HF Associated with Arrhythmogenic Right Ventricular Dysplasia

It is characterized by fibrofatty infiltration of RV myocardium, which often leads to ventricular arrhythmias, RV dilatation and dysfunction ultimately leading to RV failure.[32,33] Echocardiographic findings include parasternal long-axis right ventricular outflow tract (RVOT) (end-diastole) >32 mm or parasternal short-axis RVOT >36 mm or fractional area change <33%, thinning of RV wall, regional RV akinesia/dyskinesia/aneurysm (Fig. 9A) and hyper-reflective moderator band (Fig. 9B).[34]

CONCLUSION

Echocardiography is an invaluable modality to diagnose the various etiology and pathophysiology of heart failure and to rule out noncardiac diagnosis with high accuracy as well as to guide specific management. New HF guidelines recommend repeat echocardiography for HF patients with changes in symptoms, a clinical event, or a treatment likely to affect cardiac function. In properly trained hands, it provides valuable information for follow up and a very good noninvasive tool to assess the various cardiac diseases with rapid results.

REFERENCES

1. Cecconi M, De Backer A, Antonelli M, et al. Consensus on circulatory shock and hemodynamic monitoring. Task force of the European Society of Intensive Care Medicine. Intensive Care Med. 2014;40:1795-815.
2. Mozaffarian D, Benjamin EJ, Go AS, et al. Heart disease and stroke statistics—2016 update: A report from the American Heart Association. Circulation. 2016;133:e38–e60.
3. Ponikowski P, Voors AA, Anker SD, et al. 2016 ESC - Guidelines for the diagnosis and treatment of acute and chronic heart failure. Eur Heart J. 2016;37(27):2129-200.
4. McMurray JJ V, Adamopoulos S, Anker SD, et al. ESC Guidelines for the diagnosis and treatment of acute and chronic heart failure 2012: The Task Force for the Diagnosis and Treatment of Acute and Chronic Heart Failure 2012 of the European Society of Cardiology. EJHF. 2012;14: 803-69.
5. Lloyd-Jones DM, Larson MG, Leip EP, et al. Framingham Heart Study: Lifetime risk for developing congestive heart failure: The Framingham Heart Study. Circulation. 2002;106:3068-72.
6. McLean AS, Huang SH. Critical Care Ultrasound Manual, 1st edition. Churchill Livingstone, Australia: Elsevier; 2012.
7. Mok KL. Make it simple: Enhanced shock management by focussed cardiac ultrasound. J Intensive Care. 2016;4:51.
8. Badgett RG, Lucey CR, Mulrow CD. Can the clinical examination diagnose left-sided heart failure in adults? JAMA. 1997;277:1712-19.
9. Stevenson L, Tillisch J, Hailton M, et al. Importance of hemodynamic response to therapy in predicting survival with ejection fraction less than or equal to 20% secondary to ischemic or nonischemic dilated cardiomyopathy. Am J Cardiol. 1990;66:1348-54.
10. Oh JK. Echocardiography in heart failure: Beyond diagnosis. Eur J Echocardiogr. 2007;8(1):4-14.
11. Wong S, French J, Lyndon A, et al. Relation of left ventricular sphericity to 10-year survival after acute myocardial infarction, Am J Cardiol. 2004;94:1270-75.
12. Grayburn P, Appleton C, DeMaria A, et al. Echocardiographic predictors of morbidity and mortality in patients with advanced heart failure. The beta blocker evaluation of survival trial (BEST). J Am Coll Cardiol. 2005;45:1064-71.
13. Vieillard-Barron A. Septic cardiomyopathy. Ann Intensive Care. 2011;1(1):6.

14. Templin C, Ghadri JR, Diekmann J, et al. Clinical features and outcomes of takotsubo (stress) cardiomyopathy. N Engl J Med. 2015;373:929.
15. Omar AM, Bansal M, Sengupta PP. Advances in echocardiographic imaging in heart failure with reduced and preserved ejection fraction. Circ Res. 2016;119:357.
16. Foster E, Tseng ZH. Echocardiography in the coronary care unit: Management of acute myocardial infarction and, detection of complications and prognostic implications. In: Otto CM (Ed). The Practice of Clinical Echocardiography, 2nd edition. Philadelphia: WB Saunders; 2002. pp. 251-75.
17. Flachskampf FA, Wouters PF, Edvardsen T, et al. Transesophageal echocardiography: EACVI update 2014. Eur Heart J Cardiovasc Imaging. 2014;15:353-65.
18. Ramachandran SV, Larson MG, Benjamin EJ, et al. Congestive heart failure in subjects with normal versus reduced left ventricular ejection fraction. J Am Coll Cardiol. 1999;33:1948-55.
19. Lenzen MJ, Scholte op Reimer WJM, Boersma E, et al. Differences between patients with a preserved and a depressed left ventricular function: A report from the EuroHeart failure survey. Eur Heart J. 2004;25:1214-20.
20. Hogg K, Swedberg K, McMurray J. Heart failure with preserved left ventricular systolic function. Epidemiology, clinical characteristics, and prognosis. J Am Coll Cardiol. 2004;43:317-27.
21. Bhatia RS, Tu JV, Lee DS, et al. Outcome of heart failure with preserve ejection fraction in a popular-based study. N Engl J Med. 2006;355:260-69.
22. Nagueh SF, Smiseth OA, Appleton CP, et al. Recommendations for the evaluation of left ventricular diastolic function by echocardiography: An update from American Society of Echocardiography and the European Association of Cardiovascular Imaging. J Am Soc Echocardiogr. 2016:19:277-314.
23. Flather MD, Shibata MC, Coats AJ, et al. Randomized trial to determine the effect of nebivolol on mortality and cardiovascular hospital admission in elderly patients with heart failure (SENIORS). Eur Heart J. 2005;26:215.
24. Kushwaha SS, Fallon JT, Fuster V. Restrictive cardiomyopathy. N Engl J Med. 1997;336(4):267-76.
25. Maron BJ, Rowing EJ, Udelson JE, et al. Clinical spectrum and management of heart failure in hypertrophic cardiomyopathy. JACC Heart Fail. 2018; 6(5):353-63.
26. Maron BJ. Hypertrophic cardiomyopathy: A systemic review. JAMA. 2002;287:1308-20.
27. Melacini P, Basso C, Maron BJ. Clinicopathological profiles of progressive heart failure in hypertrophic cardiomyopathy. Eur Heart J. 2010;31(17):2111-23.
28. McConnell MV, Solomon SD, Rayan ME et al. Regional right ventricular dysfunction detected by echocardiography in acute pulmonary embolism. Am J Cardiol. 1996;78:469-73.
29. Lopez-Candales A, Edelman K, Candales MD. Right ventricular apical contractility in acute pulmonary embolism: The McConnell sign revisited. Echocardiography. 2010;27:614-20.
30. Tossavainen E, Soderberg S, Gronlund C, et al. Pulmonary artery acceleration time in identifying pulmonary hypertension patients with raised pulmonary vascular resistance. EHJ (Cardiovasc Imag). 2013;14:890-7.
31. Springhouse. Respiratory disorders. In: Springhouse (Ed). Professional Guide to Diseases, 9th edition. Philadelphia: Lippincott William and Wilkins; 2008. p. 120.
32. Basso C, Thiene G, Corrado D, et al. Arrhythmogenic right ventricular cardiomyopathy: Dysplasia, dystrophy, or myocarditis? Circulation. 1996;94(5):983-91.
33. Marcus FI, Fontaine GH, Guiraudon G, et al. Right ventricular dysplasia: A report of 24 adult cases. Circulation. 1982;65(2):384-98.
34. Lancellotti P, Price S, Edvardsen T, et al. The use of echocardiography in acute cardiovascular care: Recommendations of the European Association of Cardiovascular Imaging and the Acute Cardiovascular Care Association. Eur Heart J Cardiovasc Imaging. 2015;4(1):3-5.

CHAPTER 57

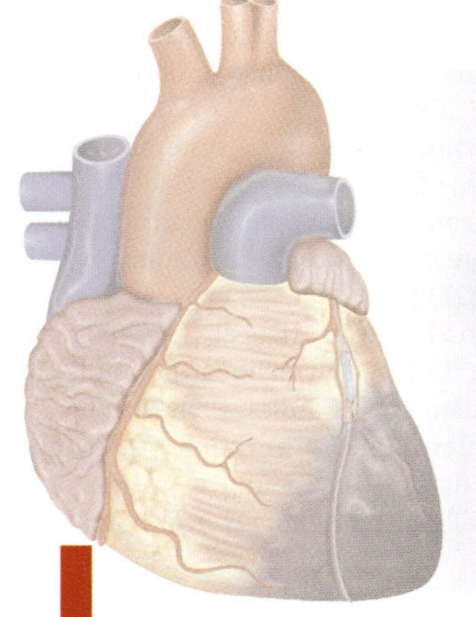

Echocardiographic Evaluation of LV, LA, RV, and RA Strain in Heart Failure

Nitin Burkule, Gautam Rege

INTRODUCTION

Heart failure (HF) is an illness that consumes significant health care resources, causes significant morbidity and mortality, and greatly impacts quality of life with a rapidly escalating prevalence.[1] HF is considered to be primarily a clinical diagnosis based on the patient's symptoms and clinical examination findings.[2] However, due to paucity of specific clinical manifestations of HF, its early diagnosis and management is challenging. Data from echocardiography provide a cornerstone in the evaluation and subsequent treatment of HF.[3] HF is currently classified according to left ventricular (LV) ejection fraction (LVEF).[4] Markers of LV function influence the recognition of HF phenotypes in HF guidelines[5] and the provision of treatment.[6] Among the markers of LV function, reduced LVEF is known to be associated with unfavorable outcomes in populations with established cardiovascular disease (CVD) but also in people without known CVD. However, it has various limitations like load dependency, low reproducibility and geometric assumptions.[7] The speckle-tracking echocardiography (STE) detects the LV myocardial deformation in longitudinal, radial and circumferential direction in systole and diastole. STE-based LV strain imaging has been shown to have an independent and additional prognostic value over conventional echocardiographic measures in a number of studies of populations with CVD.[7] Similarly, the STE can detect longitudinal myocardial deformation in the thin walled chambers like left atrium (LA), right atrium (RA) and the right ventricle (RV). This review focuses on chamber-wise evaluation of strain in managing patients with HF.

LEFT VENTRICULR STRAIN IN HEART FAILURE

The measurement of LV deformation in the longitudinal, circumferential, and radial planes with standard B-mode echocardiography has now been possible as a standard clinical test for more than a decade.[8,9] Strain is a dimensionless index of a change in length between 2 points and can be calculated using the formula $\varepsilon = (L-Lo)/Lo$, where ε indicates strain, L indicates length after deformation, and Lo indicates baseline length. Because of 3D cardiac geometry and complex myofiber arrangement, there may be multiple components of directions of strain (circumferential, longitudinal, and radial) that may be normal (i.e. orthogonal or perpendicular) or shear. The direction of greatest deformation is called as the principle strain. By convention strain can be either positive which indicates lengthening or negative which indicates shortening. Strain can be measured as global strain or regional strain. Global longitudinal strain (GLS), a metric that reflects the longitudinal strains of all myocardial segments in the apical views, has already been validated in multiple studies as a sensitive marker of systolic function (Fig. 1).[10-13] The average GLS in studies of normal ranges is –19.7%,[14] with a lower limit of normal being –18%.[15] LV GLS can be used for the following clinical situations in HF.

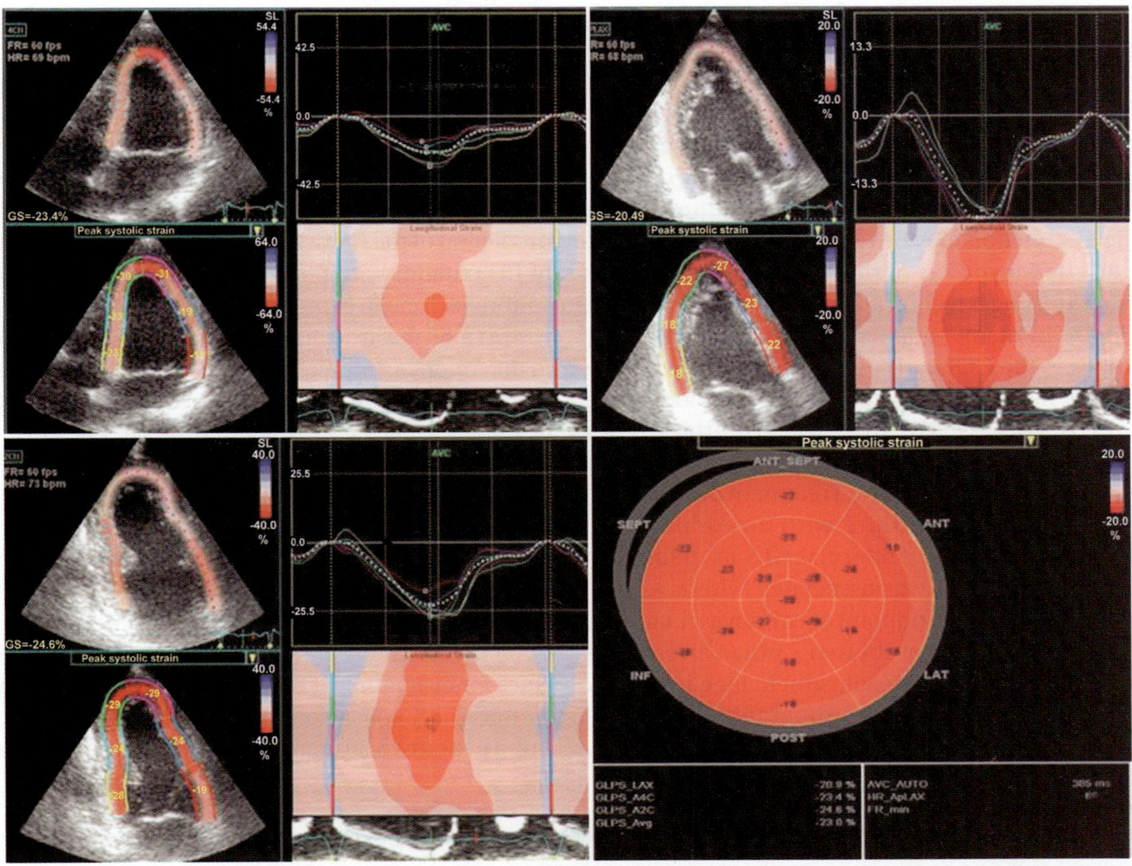

Fig. 1: Three apical projections; apical 4-chamber, 2-chamber and apical long-axis views shown with endocardial tracking with Bull's-eye plot of global longitudinal strain.

Role of GLS in Heart Failure with Reduced EF

The 2016 ESC guidelines define heart failure with reduced EF (HFrEF) as patients having clinical features of HF with LVEF <40%.[16] LVEF is a well-established and a widely used marker for identifying, managing, and predicting mortality of patients with HFrEF.[17] However, LVEF has limitations in the form of requirement of good quality images for endocardial visualization, geometric assumptions and reflects volumetric changes. GLS by STE partially overcomes these limitations as itis angle independent and reflects myocardial deformation. In patient with HFrEF without acute decompensation, GLS may be an independent predictor of mortality. In a study[18] of 1,065 HFrEF patients without acute decompensation found that GLS remained the only independent predictor of mortality among echocardiographic variables in a multivariable model after adjusting for age, sex, body mass index, total cholesterol, mean arterial pressure, heart rate, ischemic cardiomyopathy, percutaneous transluminal coronary angioplasty, coronary artery bypass graft surgery, noninsulin dependent diabetes mellitus, and conventional echocardiographic parameters [hazard ratio (HR): 1.15; 95% confidence interval (CI): 1.04 to 1.27; p = 0.008, per 1% decrease]. The relationship of GLS with mortality was however modified by atrial fibrillation and gender. In acute HF, GLS may have a higher prognostic value than LVEF.[4] GLS may also help in prognostication by identifying patients who may or may not improve with ARNI therapy.[19] Furthermore, in patients who have recovered their LVEF [LVEF increased by at least 10% and normalized (>50%) on guideline-directed optimal medical therapies], a normal GLS (>16%) on follow-up can identify patients who are more likely to have sustained recovery of LV function.[20]

Role of GLS in Heart Failure with Preserved EF

The 2016 ESC guidelines define heart failure with preserved EF (HFpEF) as patients having clinical features of HF with and LVEF >50%.[16] HFpEF currently accounts for approximately 50% of new cases of HF and its prevalence relative to HFrEF is increasing.[21,22] Currently, the guidelines propose that natriuretic peptides and markers of diastolic dysfunction should be abnormal for diagnosis of HFpEF.[16] However natriuretic peptides may not be elevated in minimally symptomatic patients and patients who are not dyspneic at rest as the stimulus for release in these patients is only intermittent. Hence, these patients may not be diagnosed in the early stages. Similarly, the markers of diastolic dysfunction may be normal or mildly impaired at rest, and diagnostic on performing stress. However diastolic stress testing is technically challenging and subject to signal noise in many patients of HFpEF with multiple comorbidities.[15] The GLS in resting echocardiography can be used to predict the exercise capacity or intolerance in this group of patients. A study[23] investigated the role GLS for prognosis in 447 patients with left ventricular EF ≥45% in the echocardiography substudy of the Treatment of Preserved Cardiac Function Heart Failure with an Aldosterone Antagonist (TOPCAT) trial. Abnormal GLS as defined by an absolute value <15.8% was associated with a >2-fold increase in the composite endpoint of cardiovascular (CV) death, HF hospitalization or aborted cardiac arrest. This association persisted following adjustment for clinical risk factors and conventional echocardiographic measures including EF, left ventricular size and diastolic dysfunction. When the cohort was restricted to those with EF ≥55% or in a subgroup with adjustment for natriuretic peptide level similar findings were observed. When the incremental value of impaired GLS for risk prediction was assessed through multivariate analysis, GLS provided marginal additive utility beyond conventional measures for predicting the composite outcome but yielded modest incremental values for the prediction of the CV death component. In a small subgroup of 131 patients with serial GLS assessment, treatment with spironolactone in comparison with placebo was associated with a trend toward improvement in GLS over 12–18 months in the America. Impaired LV GLS is common among HFpEF patients indicating the presence of early systolic dysfunction despite normal LV EF. Impaired LV GLS has been shown to be associated with elevated biomarkers of wall stress, collagen synthesis and diastolic dysfunction.[24]

Heart failure with preserved EF patients are older, hypertensive with female preponderance and have more often increase in LV mass and concentric remodeling.[25] In addition to the magnitude of depressed GLS, the pattern of LS involvement on GLS polar maps may provide vital clues for evaluating of the underlying etiology of increased LV mass, e.g. apical sparing in amyloidosis (Fig. 2), apical impairment in apical hypertrophic cardiomyopathy

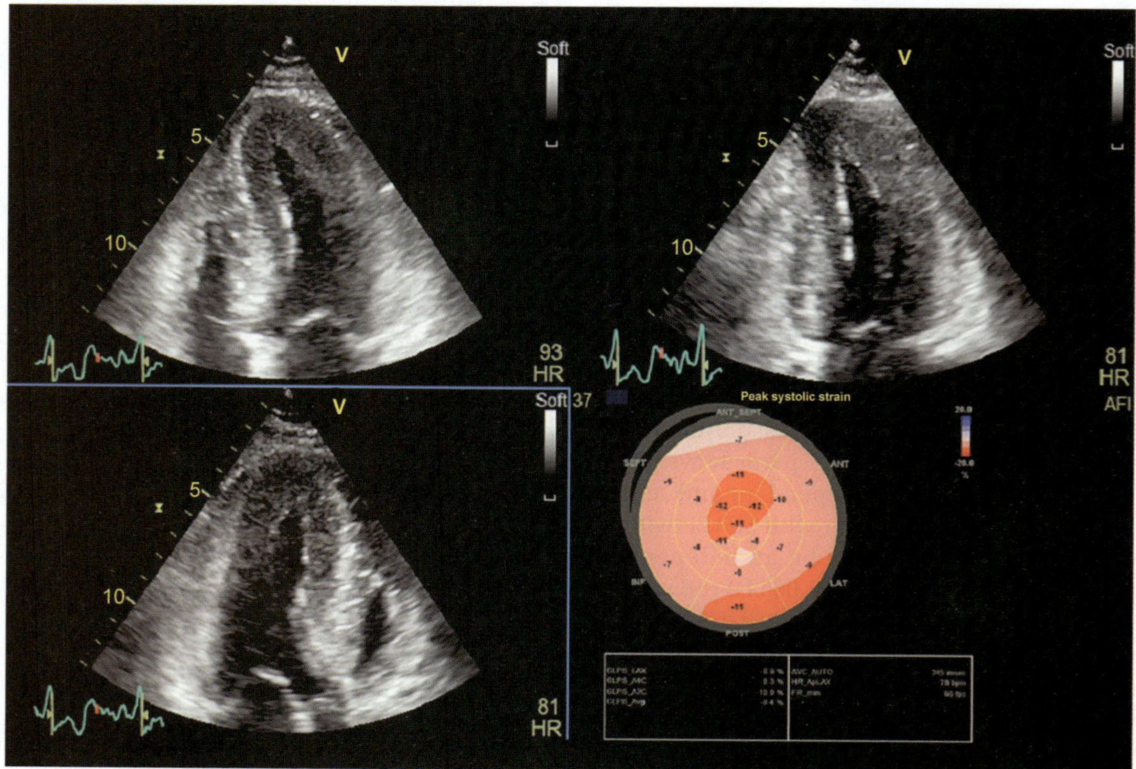

Fig. 2: Three apical projections; apical 4-chamber, 2-chamber and apical long-axis views with a Bull's eye plot of global longitudinal strain in a case of cardiac amyloidosis with typical apical sparing pattern.

(HCM), septal impairment in classical HCM, lateral wall involvement in Fabry disease.[26] In addition to identification of the underlying etiology, GLS can also help in prognostication of these patients. GLS is a strong predictor of survival in patients with AL amyloidosis undergoing autologous hematopoietic cell transplantation (HCT) and can provide incremental value over serum cardiac biomarkers for risk stratification.[27] In patients with hypertrophic cardiomyopathy, GLS along with left atrial volume index (LAVi) can identify the subset of patients who progress to develop overt HF.[28]

LEFT ATRIAL STRAIN IN HEART FAILURE

Heart failure with preserved EF has traditionally been thought of as a disorder of the left ventricle. However, now there is new interest in the evaluation of the left atrium as recent studies have shown that abnormalities in the LA play an important role in the pathophysiology and disease progression of HFpEF.[29] The LA function is traditionally assessed by LA volumetric assessment at end-systole, just before mitral valve opening when the LA volume is maximum and at end-diastole, when the mitral valve closes when the LA volume is at its minimum, and immediately before atrial systole (before the electrocardiographic P-wave). From these volumes, total (reservoir), passive (conduit), and active emptying (contractile) fractions can be calculated. However, calculating fractions in day to day clinical practice is technically challenging. The LA strain and strain rate can be used as surrogate markers for the LA volumetric analysis. Speckle tracking strain can be helpful for assessing the left atrial (LA) function by allowing measurement of LA performance at various phases of the cardiac cycle in a single beat.[30] LA strain is calculated as the global strain averaged in six segments, over three cardiac cycles, in the four-chamber and two-chamber views to calculate reservoir, conduit and booster strain (Fig. 3).[31] Atrial strain is measured using the QRS as the fiducial point given the inclusion of patients with permanent atrial fibrillation (AF) without P waves. Six different parameters may be used to evaluate the contractile (Sa, SRa), conduit (Scon, SRcon) and reservoir (SR, SRR) components of LA function.[32] The S and SR are measured either by Doppler tissue imaging (DTI) or more preferably by gray scale 2D strain imaging using 2D or 3D speckle tracking echocardiography (STE) or vector velocity imaging (VVI). Studies have shown a very good correlation of S and SR values with the LA phasic volume changes (fractional emptying), tissue Doppler and mitral and pulmonary venous Doppler flow velocities.[33] The LA

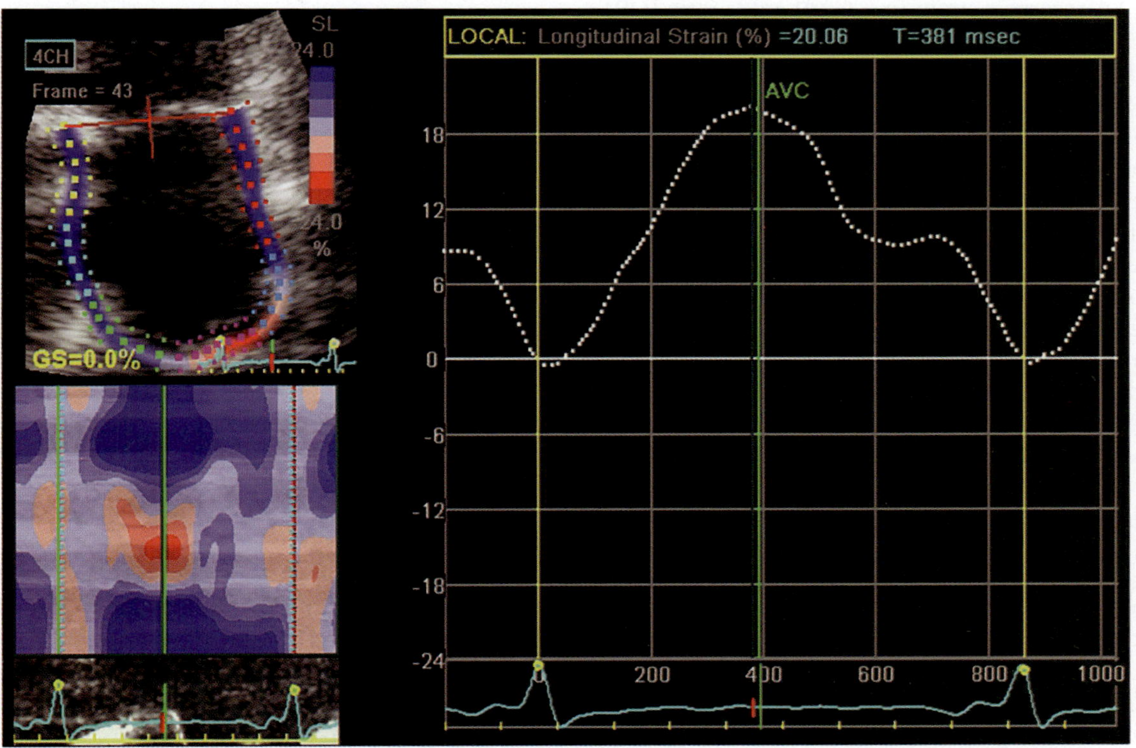

Fig. 3: Measurement of global longitudinal left atrial strain rate from an apical 4-chamber view demonstrating reservoir, conduit and booster functions.

S and SR measurements for LA function were comparable when measured with either VVI or 2D STE technique in a study of 127 patients.[34] The LA 3D STE-measured area strain values in 184 patients (at end systole and before atrial systole) were highly reproducible and compared favorably with LA emptying and active ejection fractions measured from phasic LAVs.[35]

The normal values of LA strain are as follows: Sa 15.3 + 2.9, SR 35.7 + 5.8, Scon 20.4 + 5.0. The normal values of LA Strain rate are as follows: SRa –1.95 + 0.33, SRR 1.43 + 0.24, SRcon –1.65 + 0.37. The reservoir, conduit, and contractile LA S decreases, while SR during the contractile phase increases with aging.[32]

For Identification of HFpEF

LA reservoir strain quantifies the deformation of the LA during atrial filling, whereby less deformation or a lower strain has been associated with adverse LA remodeling and increased fibrosis.[30] Impaired LA reservoir strain reflects the cumulative impact of adverse LV and LA remodeling over time from high filling pressures, which in turn occurs due to atrioventricular uncoupling and systemic inflammation.[36] LA reservoir strain may be particularly useful in patients where annular motion is altered, such as with pacing, bundle branch block and mitral annular calcification.[29] A study with 83 patients with suspected HFpEF found reduced LA reservoir strain [$p = 0.049$, odds ratio (OR) = 0.71, 95 % CI = 0.451–0.99], B-type natriuretic peptide ($p = 0.025$, OR = 1.08, 95 % CI = 1.01–1.14), and LAVi ($p = 0.042$, OR = 1.59, 95 % CI = 1.02–2.48), as independent prognostic indicators for identification of HFpEF. Moreover, the lack of augmentation of LA strain with increased preload (by performing passive leg raise) may be able to assist in the diagnosis of HFpEF.[37] A study done with 72 patients with suspected HFpEF found that the LA reservoir and pump strain correlated with exercise pulmonary capillary wedge pressure ($r = -0.64$ and $r = 0.72$, $p < 0.001$), and remained independent predictors after adjusting for left ventricular mass index, LA volume index, mean E/e' and systolic blood pressure ($B = -0.66$ and $B = 1.41$, respectively, $p < 0.001$). Reservoir strain at cut-off of ≤ 33% predicted invasively verified HFpEF diagnosis with 88% sensitivity and 77% specificity, which helped to provide a net reclassification improvement of 12% in comparison to the 2016 European Society of Cardiology criteria for noninvasive diagnosis of HFpEF.[38]

Prediction of Atrial Fibrillation

Frequently occurring together, HF can beget AF, and AF can beget HF.[39,40] AF and HF can act synergistically to confer a poor prognosis compared to those without these conditions or with either condition alone.[41] AF was common among both HFpEF and HFrEF, and its prevalence increases as age advances. Compared to those without AF, those with AF experienced higher in-hospital mortality regardless of HF subtype.[42] Hence, it is essential to identify patients who are high risk for atrial fibrillation. The LV systolic dysfunction as indicated by reduced GLS is a strong predictor of cardiovascular (CV) events and may even predict new-onset AF in a population setting. In Northern Manhattan Study[43] of 675 subjects in sinus rhythm with mean age 71 ± 9 years were followed for 63.6 ± 18.7 months. During the follow-up, 32 subjects (4.7%) developed new AF. Lower GLS and increased LAVi were significantly associated with incident AF but not the LV ejection fraction. Abnormal GLS (>–14.7%) was associated with 3.2-fold high risk of new-onset AF. Subjects with presence of both 'abnormal GLS and abnormal LAVi' had 28.6% incidence of AF compared to 2% in absence of both. AF incidence was intermediate in those with either abnormal GLS or abnormal LAVi. Three-dimensional (3D) speckle tracking echocardiography (3D STE) can measure LA longitudinal, circumferential (CS) and the area strain (AS). In a study[44] of 47 patients with AF (31 with paroxysmal AF and 16 with permanent AF) the LA strains were reduced in patients with PAF compared with controls and further reductions of these parameters were observed in patients with permanent AF. The standard deviations (SD) of strain, marker of LA dyssynchrony, were larger in patients with PAF and in those with permanent AF compared with controls. 2D STE, 3D STE strains were independent predictors of PAF irrespective of LA size. 3D STE may make it possible to identify patients with normal LA sizes but increased risk for PAF. 3D STE may be the most sensitive modality for the stratification of PAF risk.

Strain and SR Imaging for Predicting Heart Failure and Cardiovascular Mortality in AF

The thromboembolic risk and HF signs and symptoms in AF depend upon the advanced LA structural remodeling and fibrosis. The LA reservoir strain (S_R) with LA volume improve the accuracy of the $CHADS_2$ score to predict mortality and future hospitalization for cardiac causes in patients with AF.[45]

Studies have shown that the addition of LA S_R and LAVi to statistical models, incorporating clinical risk score, was incremental to the $CHADS_2$ score in predicting hospitalization and/or death in patients with AF.[46] In a study[47] of 190 persistent with AF patients, increased mitral inflow velocity (E)/LA reservoir strain (S_R) was associated with CV events. The addition of E/LA S_R to a model, containing CHA2DS2-VASc score, LA volume index, and LV systolic and diastolic function, had an incremental value in predicting CV events.

Similar to many CV disease conditions, the LV global longitudinal strain (GLS) is a powerful predictor of clinical adverse events in AF. Measuring LV-GLS in AF requires averaging of >13 beats and is too cumbersome to utilize in clinical practice. An index beat is defined as the cardiac cycle which has nearly equal preceding two cardiac cycles (RR1 and RR2). The RR1 and RR2 intervals of the index beat must be >500 msec and the difference between them must be <60 msec. Measuring LV-GLS in the index beat gives near identical values as measured by more laborious conventional method.[48] Compared with those with lower risk scores of stroke ($CHADS_2$ scores < 2 or CHA_2DS_2-VASc scores <2), patients with higher risk scores of stroke ($CHADS_2$ scores >2 or CHA_2DS_2-VASc scores >2) had lower LV-GLS measured by index beat.

The ratio of early mitral inflow velocity (E) to global LV early diastolic strain rate (E_{SR}) has been correlated with left ventricular filling pressure. In a study[49] of 190 patients with persistent AF, LV E_{SR} was calculated by using the index beat method. During a follow-up period of 20 months, 22 deaths and 28 hospitalizations for HF were registered. The old age, chronic HF, and increased E/E_{SR} ratio were associated with increased cardiac events. $E/E_{SR} > 64$ had the best performance in predicting adverse cardiac events. The addition of E/E_{SR} ratio had further incremental value to a clinical model including age, chronic HF, diabetes, hypertension, left atrial volume index, left ventricular ejection fraction, and E/e' to predict adverse cardiac events.

RIGHT VENTRICULAR STRAIN IN HEART FAILURE

Right ventricular remodeling has been long neglected as the RV was considered a dispensable cardiac chamber whose function had no influence on overall outcome in cardiac patients.[50] However, it is now been established that the RV plays a critical role in both the clinical expression and the prediction of adverse cardiovascular outcomes in cardiomyopathies, and congenital, ischemic, valvular, and pulmonary heart diseases.[51] Despite significant developments in cardiac imaging, assessing RV structure and function remains challenging, which can be attributed to the complicated geometry which require imaging in multiple views and striking load dependence of the RV. However, evaluation of the RV by echocardiography is most often used because of its easy availability, cost, repeatability, and its ability to image in real time. Echocardiographic indices of RV function include fractional area change, tricuspid annular plane systolic excursion, tricuspid annular systolic tissue velocity, tricuspid annular isovolumic acceleration, and RV myocardial performance index. These methods are limited by the asymmetrical shape and retrosternal location of the RV. Prominent trabeculations of the RV leading to poor endocardial definition and modest correlations with cardiac magnetic resonance-measured RV ejection fraction are additional challenges.[52] Many of these limitations are overcome by the application of deformational analysis (strain and strain rate imaging) of the RV.[53] Strain being a measure of deformation provides a method of contractile function assessment that corrects for translational error and is less dependent on imaging plane angle. Hence, 2D RV systolic longitudinal strain calculated using STE has emerged as a feasible and reproducible measure of RV systolic function.[54] RV longitudinal strain can be measured as average value of the longitudinal peak systolic strain only from the free wall (RV-fwLS) (Fig. 4) and from all segments of the free wall and septal wall of the RV (RV-GLS; (Fig. 5) in the apical 4-chamber view (AP4CH) focused in the RV.

A study[55] of 332 outpatients with chronic HF, found that Both RV-GLS and RV-fwLS were associated with all-cause mortality in univariate (HR: 1.16; 95% CI: 1.10–1.23; $p < 0.001$; C-index: 0.72; and HR: 1.10; 95% CI: 1.06–1.15; $p < 0.001$; C-index: 0.68, respectively) as well as multivariate analysis (HR: 1.13; 95% CI: 1.05–1.21; p: 0.001; C-index: 0.85; and HR: 1.07; 95% CI: 1.02–1.12; p: 0.004; C-index: 0.84, respectively). Another study[56] with 618 patients (age, 72 ± 13 years; 38% women; ejection fraction, 46 ± 16%) hospitalized for acute decompensated HF among echocardiographic parameters, only impaired RV-fwLS (≥13.1%; HR, 1.51; 95% CI, 1.12–2.04; $p = 0.01$) was independently associated with cardiac events in multivariate Cox models. Adding RV-fwLS to clinical risk evaluation (age, New York Heart Association class III/IV, blood urea nitrogen, and brain natriuretic peptide) also markedly improved prognostic utility and consequently increased net reclassification improvement by 0.30 ($p = 0.01$). While comparing STE -LS with CMR a study found that the additional predictive value of STE-RVGLS (chi-square to enter = 10.8; $p < 0.001$) was significantly ($p < 0.05$) higher than CMR-RVEF, Fwl - RV GLS, FAC, and TAPSE. Additionally, hazard ratio to predict overall mortality was 2.5 (95% CI: 1.6–3.9) for STE-RVGLS <–19%.[57]

RIGHT ATRIAL STRAIN IN HEART FAILURE

The RA plays important role in the electromechanical and endocrine function of the heart. RA dysfunction and remodeling can contribute to right ventricular filling and cardiac output, particularly when ventricular dysfunction is present.[58] With 2D echocardiography, the assessment of RA is limited due to viewing dependency and geometric

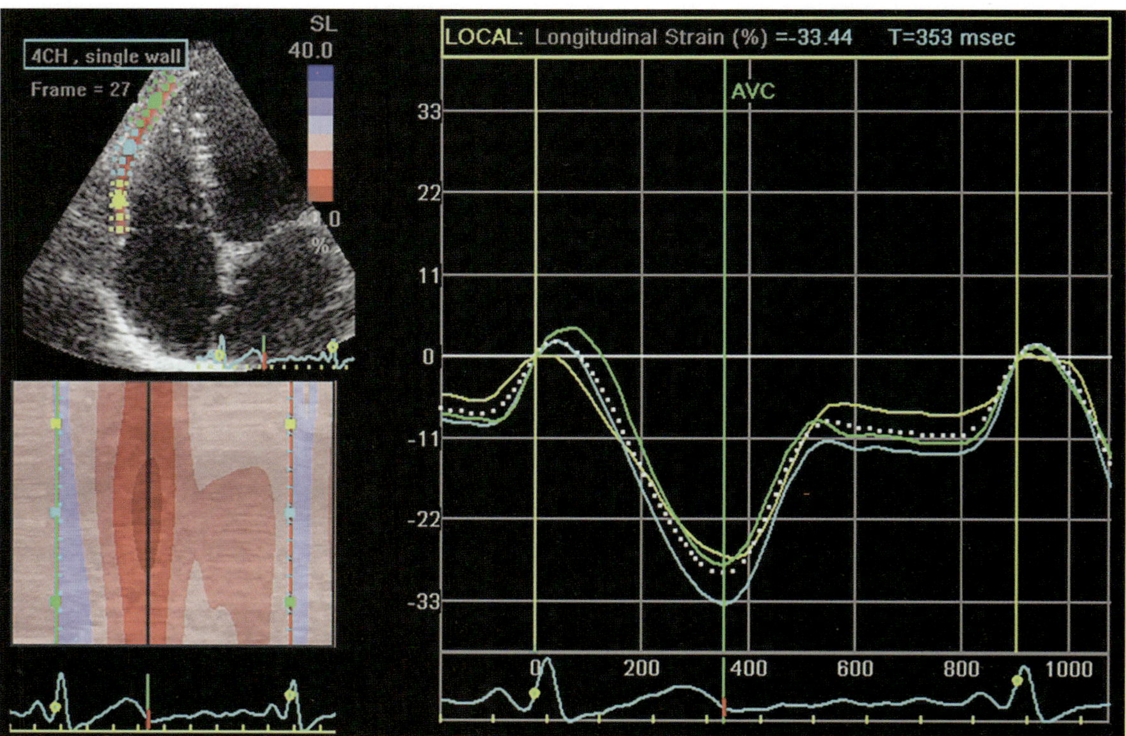

Fig. 4: Normal right ventricular free-wall strain measured from 2D speckle imaging in a normal patient.

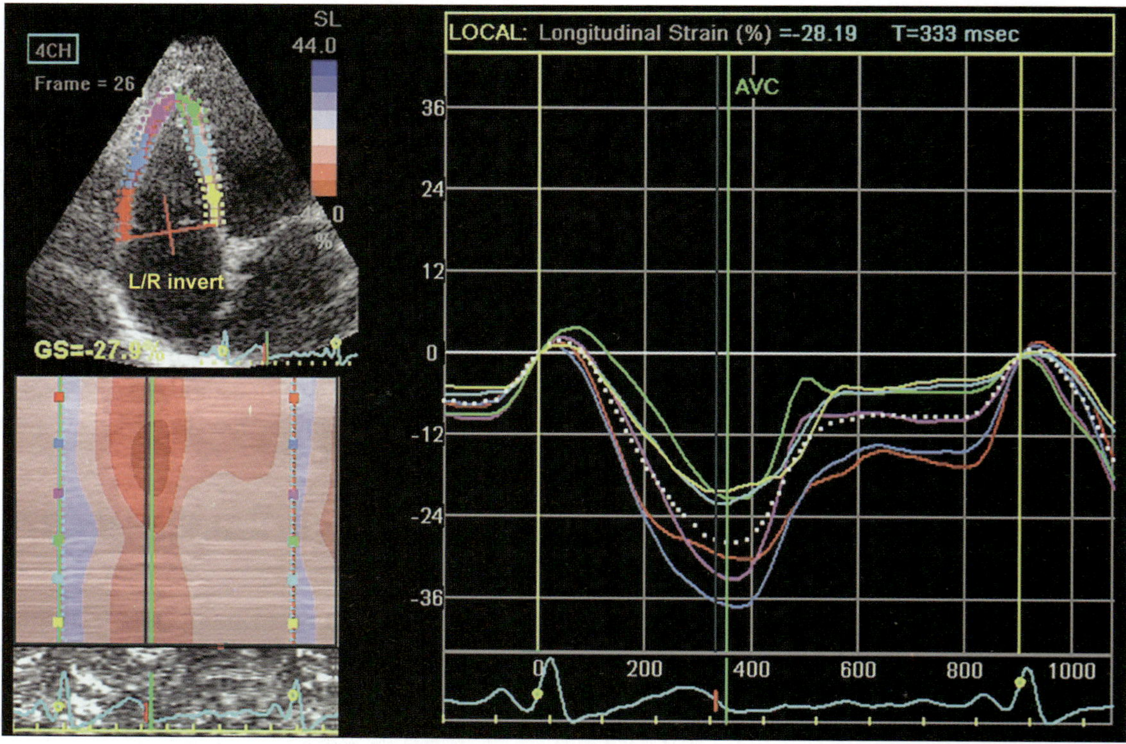

Fig. 5: Normal right ventricular global longitudinal strain measured from apical 4-chamber view with 2D speckle imaging in a normal patient.

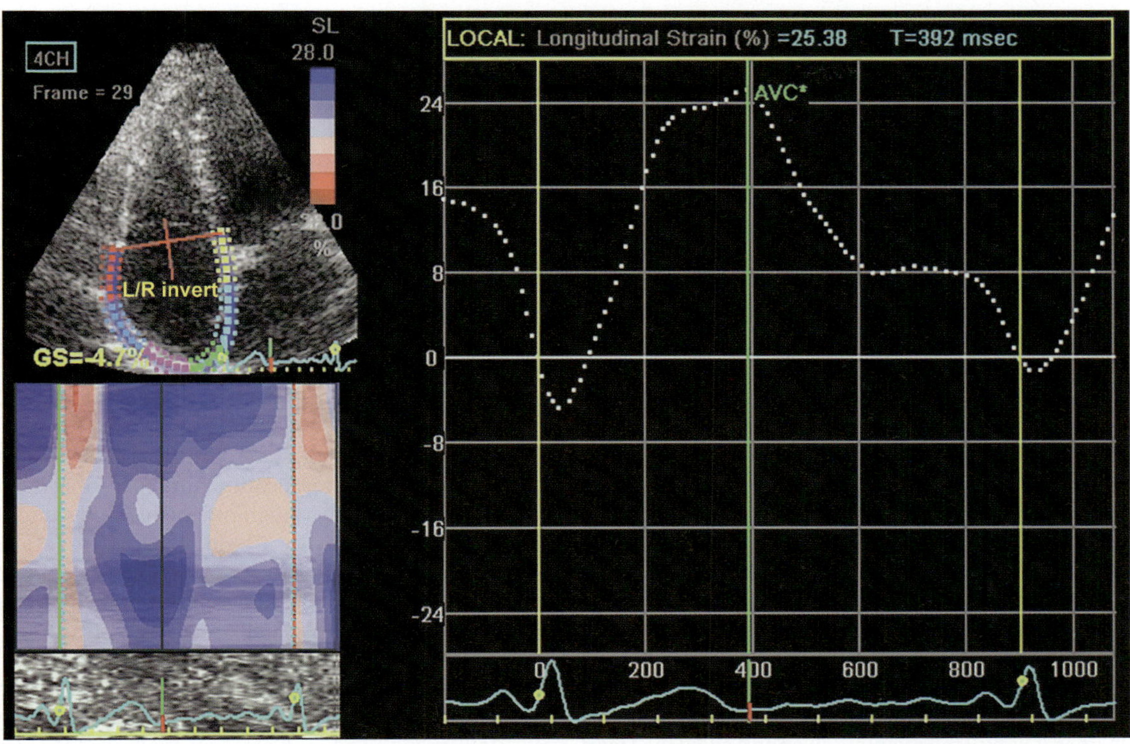

Fig. 6: Right atrial strain assessment with 2D speckle-tracking in the apical 4-chamber view. The atrium is divided into 6 segments and demonstrates reservoir, conduit and booster functions similar to the left atrium.

difficulties. RA diameter and area are measured in AP4CH view.[59,60]

Conventional parameters for assessment of RA function are load dependent. Similar to left atrial function, right atrial function has three components: reservoir (filling during ventricular systole and atrial diastole), conduit (allowing blood to flow passively into the ventricle), and pump (pushing blood into the right ventricle) function (Fig. 6). RA strain, as measured by transthoracic echocardiogram with speckle tracking, provides an accurate measure of all three components of RA function.[61] Most studies were focused on the pulmonary hypertension (PH) (35%) and HF (30%) with the remainder (35%) being studies of other cardiac diseases.[62] While measuring RA strain, the AP4CH view in which the RA free wall is best visualized is selected. Frame rates are generally in the 40–80 Hz range. Peak RA strain is measured using speckle-tracking software. The zero-strain reference point is set at the QRS (end-diastole), and peak RA strain was measured at end-systole. Using this method, the peak RA strain represents the reservoir function of the RA.[61] A study[63] compared RA strain in 32 patients diagnosed with HF (LVEF ≤35%) scheduled for right heart catheterization with a control group of 32 healthy adults matched for age and sex. The right atrial deformation indices were significantly compromised in the HF patients compared to the normal subjects (RAS: 68.5 ± 53.9 vs. 189.3 ± 61.2, p = 0.000; RASSR: 2.9 ± 1.9 vs. 5.3 ± 1.5, p = 0.000). There was a significant correlation between the RA strain and RA strain rate and cardiac output and cardiac index. Right atrial strain parameters could be deranged earlier in coronary artery disease (CAD) even before any changes in atrial volumes or dimensions.[64]

CONCLUSION

The STE has diagnostic, prognostic, and therapeutic implications in HFpEF and HFrEF in reference to evaluation of LV, LA and RV, RA strain parameters with or without CAD. It has tremendous prognostic implications which may help in guiding therapeutic to help in reducing the cardiac morbidity and mortality.

REFERENCES

1. Yancy CW, Januzzi JL, Allen LA, et al. 2017 ACC Expert Consensus Decision Pathway for Optimization of Heart Failure Treatment: Answers to 10 Pivotal Issues About Heart Failure with Reduced Ejection Fraction: A Report of the American College of Cardiology Task Force on Expert Consensus Decision Pathways. J Am Coll Cardiol. 2018;71(2):201-30.

2. McMurray JJ, Adamopoulos S, Anker SD, et al. ESC Committee for Practice Guidelines. ESC Guidelines for the diagnosis and treatment of acute and chronic heart failure 2012: The Task Force for the Diagnosis and Treatment of Acute and Chronic Heart Failure 2012 of the European Society of Cardiology. Developed in collaboration with the Heart Failure Association (HFA) of the ESC. Eur Heart J. 2012;33:1787-847.
3. Marwick TH. The role of echocardiography in heart failure. J Nucl Med. 2015;56:31S-38S.
4. Park JJ, Park JB, Park JH, et al. Global longitudinal strain to predict mortality in patients with acute heart failure. J Am Coll Cardiol. 2018;71(18):1947-57.
5. Hunt SA, Abraham WT, Chin MH, et al. American College of Cardiology; American Heart Association Task Force on Practice Guidelines; American College of Chest Physicians; International Society for Heart and Lung Transplantation; Heart Rhythm Society. ACC/AHA 2005 guideline update for the diagnosis and management of chronic heart failure in the adult: a report of the American College of Cardiology/American Heart Association Task Force on Practice Guidelines (Writing Committee to Update the 2001 Guidelines for the Evaluation and Management of Heart Failure): developed in collaboration with the American College of Chest Physicians and the International Society for Heart and Lung Transplantation: endorsed by the Heart Rhythm Society. Circulation. 2005;112(12):e154-e235.
6. Tracy CM, Epstein AE, Darbar D, et al. 2012 ACCF/AHA/HRS focused update of the 2008 guidelines for device-based therapy of cardiac rhythm abnormalities: A report of the American College of Cardiology Foundation/American Heart Association Task Force on Practice Guidelines. J Am Coll Cardiol. 2012;60(14):1297-313.
7. Al Saikhan L, Park C, Hardy R, et al. Prognostic implications of left ventricular strain by speckle-tracking echocardiography in population-based studies: a systematic review protocol of the published literature. BMJ Open. 2018;8:e023346.
8. Collier P, Phelan D, Klein A. A test in context: Myocardial strain measured by speckle-tracking echocardiography. J Am Coll Cardiol. 2017;69(8):1043-56.
9. Negishi K, Negishi T, Kurosawa K, et al. Practical guidance in echocardiographic assessment of global longitudinal strain. JACC Cardiovasc Imaging. 2015;8(4):489-92.
10. Buchalter MB, Weiss JL, Rogers WJ, et al. Noninvasive quantification of left ventricular rotational deformation in normal humans using magnetic resonance imaging myocardial tagging. Circulation. 1990;81(4):1236-44.
11. Maier SE, Fischer SE, McKinnon GC, et al. Evaluation of left ventricular segmental wall motion in hypertrophic cardiomyopathy with myocardial tagging. Circulation. 1992;86(6):1919-28.
12. Yeon SB, Reichek N, Tallant BA, et al. Validation of in vivo myocardial strain measurement by magnetic resonance tagging with sonomicrometry. J Am Coll Cardiol. 2001;38(2):555-61.
13. MacGowan GA, Shapiro EP, Azhari H, et al. Noninvasive measurement of shortening in the fiber and cross-fiber directions in the normal human left ventricle and in idiopathic dilated cardiomyopathy. Circulation. 1997;96(2):535-41.
14. Yingchoncharoen T, Agarwal S, Popović ZB, et al. Normal ranges of left ventricular strain: A meta-analysis. J Am Soc Echocardiogr. 2013;26(2):185-91.
15. Marwick TH, Shah SJ, Thomas JD. Myocardial strain in the assessment of patients with heart failure: A review. JAMA Cardiol. 2019;4(3):287-94.
16. Ponikowski P, Voors AA, Anker SD, et al. 2016 ESC Guidelines for the diagnosis and treatment of acute and chronic heart failure. The Task Force for the diagnosis and treatment of acute and chronic heart failure of the European Society of Cardiology (ESC). Developed with the special contribution of the Heart Failure Association (HFA) of the ESC. Eur Heart J. 2016;37(27):2129-2200.
17. Lang RM, Bierig M, Devereux RB, et al. Recommendations for chamber quantification: a report from the American Society of Echocardiography's Guidelines and Standards Committee and the Chamber Quantification Writing Group, developed in conjunction with the European Association of Echocardiography, a branch of the European Society of Cardiology. J Am Soc Echocardiogr. 2005;18: 1440-63.
18. Sengelov M, Jorgensen PG, Jensen JS, et al. Global longitudinal strain is a superior predictor of all-cause mortality in heart failure with reduced ejection fraction. JACC Cardiovasc Imaging. 2015;8(12):135159.
19. Pandey AC, Pelter M, Montgomery P, et al. J Am Coll Cardiol. 2019;73(9 Supplement 1):832.
20. Adamo L, Perry A, Novak E, et al. Abnormal global longitudinal strain predicts future deterioration of left ventricular function in heart failure patients with a recovered left ventricular ejection fraction. Circ Heart Fail. 2017;10(6):e003788.
21. Lam CSP, Donal E, Kraigher-Krainer E, et al. Epidemiology and clinical course of heart failure with preserved ejection fraction. Eur J Heart Fail. 2011;13:18-28.
22. Owan TE, Hodge DO, Herges RM, et al. Trends in prevalence and outcome of heart failure with preserved ejection fraction. N Engl J Med. 2006;355:251-9.
23. Shah AM, Clagget B, Sweitzer NK, et al. The prognostic importance of impaired systolic function in heart failure with preserved ejection fraction and the impact of spironolactone. Circulation. 2015;132:402-14.
24. DeVore AD, McNulty S, Alenezi F, et al. Impaired left ventricular global longitudinal strain in patients with heart failure with preserved ejection fraction: Insights from the RELAX trial. Eur J Heart Fail. 2017;19(7):893-900.
25. Lam CSP, Roger VL, Rodeheffer RJ, et al. Cardiac structure and ventricular-vascular function in persons with heart failure and preserved ejection fraction from Olmsted County, Minnesota. Circulation. 2007;115:1982-90.
26. Phelan D, Collier P, Thavendiranathan P, et al. Relative apical sparing of longitudinal strain using two-dimensional speckle-tracking echocardiography is both sensitive and specific for the diagnosis of cardiac amyloidosis. Heart. 2012;98(19):1442-48.

27. Pun SC, Landau HJ, Riedel ER, et al. Prognostic and added value of two-dimensional global longitudinal strain for prediction of survival in patients with light chain amyloidosis undergoing autologous hematopoietic cell transplantation. J Am Soc Echocardiogr. 2018;31(1):64-70.
28. Hiemstra YL, Debonnaire P, van Zwet EW, et al. Development of and progression of overt heart failure in nonobstructive hypertrophic cardiomyopathy. Am J Cardiol. 2018;122(4):656-62.
29. Reddy YN, Obokata M, Egbe A, et al. Left atrial strain and compliance in the diagnostic evaluation of heart failure with preserved ejection fraction. Eur J Heart Fail. 2019;21(7): 891-900.
30. Hoit BD. Left atrial size and function: Role in prognosis. J Am Coll Cardiol. 2014;63:493-505.
31. Freed BH, Daruwalla V, Cheng JY, et al. Prognostic utility and clinical significance of cardiac mechanics in heart failure with preserved ejection fraction: Importance of left atrial strain. Circ Cardiovasc Imaging. 2016;9:e003754.
32. Vieira MJ, Teixeira R, Goncalves L, et al. Left atrial mechanics: Echocardiographic assessment and clinical implications. J Am Soc Echocardiogr. 2014;27:46378.
33. Saraiva RM, Demirkol S, Buakhamsri A, et al. Left atrial strain measured by two-dimensional speckle tracking represents a new tool to evaluate left atrial function. J Am Soc Echocardiogr. 2010;23:172-80.
34. Motoki H, Dahiya A, Bhargava M. Assessment of left atrial mechanics in patients with atrial fibrillation: Comparison between two-dimensional speckle-based strain and velocity vector imaging. J Am Soc Echocardiogr. 2012;25:428-35.
35. Ebato M, Maezawa H, Tanabe A, et al. Left atrial area strain measured by three-dimensional speckle tracking echocardiography represents global and regional left atrial function at once. J Am Coll Cardiol. 2012;59:E1269.
36. Zakeri R, Moulay G, Chai Q, et al. Left atrial remodeling and atrioventricular coupling in a canine model of early heart failure with preserved ejection fraction. Circ Heart Fail. 2016;9:e003238.
37. Aung SM, Güler A, Güler Y, et al. Left atrial strain in heart failure with preserved ejection fraction. Herz. 2017;42(2): 194-9.
38. Telles F, Nanayakkara S, Evans S, et al. Impaired left atrial strain predicts abnormal haemodynamics in heart failure with preserved ejection fraction. Heart Lung Circ. 2018;27(suppl 2):S55.
39. Santhanakrishnan R, Wang N, Larson MG, et al. Atrial fibrillation begets heart failure and vice versa: temporal associations and differences in preserved versus reduced ejection fraction. Circulation. 2016;133(5):484-92.
40. Kotecha D, Lam CS, Van Veldhuisen DJ, et al. Heart failure with preserved ejection fraction and atrial fibrillation: vicious twins. J Am Coll Cardiol. 2016;68(20):2217-28.
41. Wang TJ, Larson MG, Levy D, et al. Temporal relations of atrial fibrillation and congestive heart failure and their joint influence on mortality: The Framingham Heart Study. Circulation. 2003;107(23):2920-25.
42. Goyal P, Almarzooq ZI, Cheung J, et al. Atrial fibrillation and heart failure with preserved ejection fraction: Insights on a unique clinical phenotype from a nationally-representative United States cohort. Int J Cardiol. 2018;266:112-8.
43. Russo C, Jin Z, Sera F, et al. Left ventricular systolic dysfunction by longitudinal strain is an independent predictor of incident atrial fibrillation: A community-based cohort study. Circ Cardiovasc Imaging. 2015;8:e003520.
44. Mochizuki A, Yuda S, Oi Y, et al. Assessment of left atrial deformation and synchrony by three-dimensional speckle-tracking echocardiography: Comparative studies in healthy subjects and patients with atrial fibrillation. J Am Soc Echocardiogr. 2013;26:165-74.
45. Shih JY, Tsai WC, Huang YY, et al. Association of decreased left atrial strain and strain rate with stroke in chronic atrial fibrillation. J Am Soc Echocardiogr. 2011;24:513-9.
46. Saha SK, Anderson PL, Caracciolo G, et al. Global left atrial strain correlates with CHADS2 risk score in patients with atrial fibrillation. J Am Soc Echocardiogr. 2011;24:506-12.
47. Su HM, Lin FH, Hsu PC. The ratio of transmitral E-wave velocity to left atrial strain and left atrial strain itself can respectively predict cardiovascular and subsequent stroke outcomes in patients with atrial fibrillation. JACC. 2015;65(10S).
48. Lee CS, Lin TH, Hsu PC. Measuring left ventricular peak longitudinal systolic strain from a single beat in atrial fibrillation: Validation of the index beat method. J Am Soc Echocardiogr. 2012;25:945-52.
49. Hsu PC, Lee WH, Chu CY. The ratio of early mitral inflow velocity to global diastolic strain rate as a useful predictor of cardiac outcomes in patients with atrial fibrillation. J Am Soc Echocardiogr. 2014;27:717-25.
50. Tadic M, Pieske-Kraigher E, Cuspidi C, et al. Right ventricular strain in heart failure: Clinical perspective. Arch Cardiovasc Dis. 2017;110(10):562-71.
51. Haddad F, Doyle R, Murphy DJ, et al. Right ventricular function in cardiovascular disease, part II: Pathophysiology, clinical importance, and management of right ventricular failure. Circulation. 2008;117:1717-31.
52. Cameli M, Righini FM, Lisi M, et al. Right ventricular strain as a novel approach to analyze right ventricular performance in patients with heart failure. Heart Fail Rev. 2014;19:603-10.
53. Hoit BD. Right ventricular strain comes of age. Circ Cardiovasc Imaging. 2018;11(10):e008382.
54. Ayach B, Fine NM, Rudski LG. Right ventricular strain: Measurement and clinical application. Curr Opin Cardiol. 2018;33(5):486-92.
55. Iacoviello M, Citarelli G, Antoncecchi V, et al. Right ventricular longitudinal strain measures independently predict chronic heart failure mortality. Echocardiography. 2016;33:992-1000.
56. Hamada-Harimura Y, Seo Y, Ishizu T, et al. Incremental prognostic value of right ventricular strain in patients with acute decompensated heart failure. Circ Cardiovasc Imaging. 2018;11:e007249.
57. Houard L, Benaets MB, de Meester de Ravenstein C, et al. Additional prognostic value of 2D right ventricular speckle-tracking strain for prediction of survival in heart failure and reduced ejection fraction. JACC Cardiovasc Imaging. 2019; pii: S1936-878X(19)30052-X.

58. Chirinos JA, Satija V, Gaddam S, et al. J Am Coll Cardiol. 2018:71(Suppl 11):A1604.
59. Lang RM, Bierig M, Devereux RB, et al. American Society of Echocardiography's nomenclature and Standards Committee; Task Force on Chamber Quantification; American College of Cardiology Echocardiography Committee; American Heart Association; European Association of Echocardiography, European Society of Cardiology. Recommendations for chamber quantification. Eur J Echocardiogr. 2006;7(2):79-108.
60. Rudski LG, Lai WW, Afilalo J, et al. Guidelines for the echocardiographic assessment of the right heart in adults: A report from the American Society of Echocardiography endorsed by the European Association of Echocardiography, a registered branch of the European Society of Cardiology, and the Canadian Society of Echocardiography. J Am Soc Echocardiogr. 2010;23(7):685-713.
61. Bhave NM, Visovatti SH, Kulick B, et al. Right atrial strain is predictive of clinical outcomes and invasive hemodynamic data in group 1 pulmonary arterial hypertension. Int J Cardiovasc Imaging. 2017;33(6):847-55.
62. Khan S, Alenezi F, Bloomfield G. Right atrial speckle tracking strain echocardiography in heart failure. J Card Fail. 2018;24 (Suppl 8):S38.
63. Haghighi ZO, Naderi N, Amin A, et al. Quantitative assessment of right atrial function by strain and strain rate imaging in patients with heart failure. Acta Cardiol. 2011;66(6):737-42.
64. Khedr L, Elasfar A, Hekal S, et al. Assessment of left and right atrial geometrical changes in patients with stable coronary artery disease: Left and right atrial strain and strain rate imaging study. Egypt Hear J. 2018;70(2):101-6.

CHAPTER

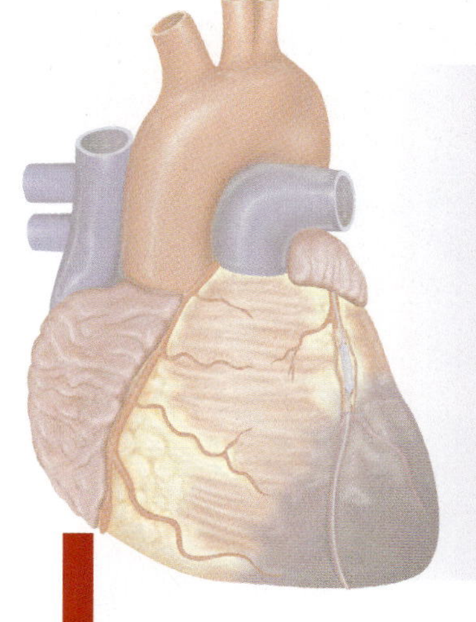

Echocardiographic Evaluation of LA Stiffness Index, RV and RA Strain in Heart Failure

Rahul Mehrotra, Raj Kumar

INTRODUCTION

Evaluation of systolic function of the left ventricle (LV) has largely depended on calculated left ventricular ejection fraction, a load dependent parameter with inherent limitations. Certain deformation parameters like strain and strain rate (SR) imaging have emerged as more sensitive parameters for this purpose in different clinical settings, in past few years. Strain is defined as percentage change in myocardial deformation, while its derivative, strain rate represents the rate of deformation of myocardium over time. Strain rate has been closely correlated with myocardial contractility in both, in vitro as well as in vivo experimental settings.[1] These simple parameters are largely load independent and quite simple. There has been increasing amount of literature being published with these parameters in different clinical settings with LV in focus. But deformation is also being studied for other chambers like the left atrium (LA), the right ventricle (RV) and the right atrium (RA). In this chapter, we briefly review the current status of strain and SR in LA, RA and RV and their current utility in heart failure.

LEFT ATRIAL DEFORMATION

Apart from LA dimension, assessment of LA function has become an actively investigated tool now since it is closely associated with LV function. One such parameter is the LA *stiffness*. It is now understood that a normally filling, flexible atrium which contracts normally, substantially improves the cardiac output as compared to a stiff LA. Left atrial stiffness is thus an important determinant of cardiac function. An increase in LA stiffness results in reduced stroke volume and forward flow, and reflects the structural remodeling and deterioration of the LA function. Also, there is potential association between LA stiffening and development of atrial fibrillation (AF), recurrences after AF ablation or after cardioversion. Doppler and volumetric approaches were the first methods used to assess LA function. Recently, strain imaging based speckle tracking echocardiography (STE), has been applied to assess LA deformation. STE measures LA strain and LA stiffness index for assessment of LA function. STE derived analysis of LA performance provides information about all phases of LA function (reservoir, conduit, and booster pump) and has shown prognostic significance in different pathological conditions.[2]

LEFT ATRIAL STRAIN

Strain (*S*) and SR can be used as surrogate markers for LA function.[2] The LAS (both S and SR) can be calculated either by Doppler tissue imaging or by gray-scale 2D imaging using STE or by velocity vector imaging (VVI) but generally, STE has been used. 3D STE derived strain has also been studied in LA. For analysis of left atrial strain (LAS), the region of interest LA is divided into 6 segments of in both the 4 and 2 chamber views and tracked frame by frame to maintain the position within the LA wall (Fig. 1). The LAS of the 6 segments is then averaged for analysis. Six parameters of strain (*S*) can be derived to evaluate the contractile (*S*a,

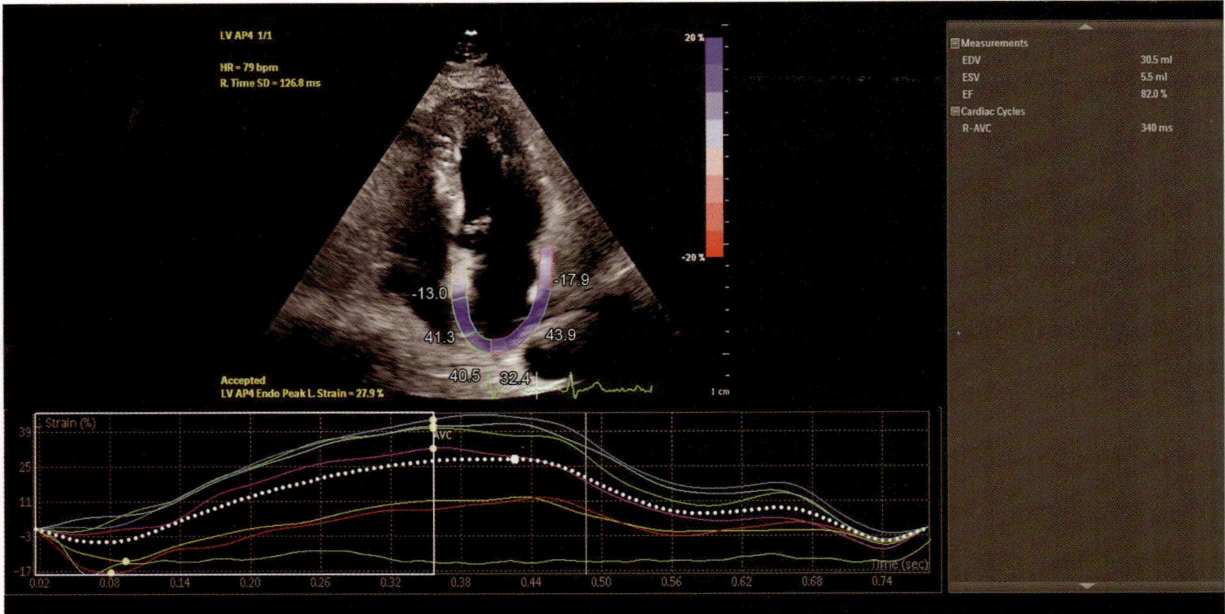

Fig. 1: Transthoracic echocardiographic image in apical 4 chamber view showing measurement of LA strain by 2D speckle tracking method. The left atrium is divided in six segments and peak longitudinal strain for each color coded segment are shown graphically. The dotted white line represents average of the six segments.

SRa), conduit (*S*con, SRcon), and reservoir (*S*R, SRR) function of the LA.[2] In a meta-analysis, Forty studies were included and normal reference ranges for three components of LA function were demonstrated. Analysis revealed a normal reference range for contractile strain of 17% (95% CI, 16–19% from 18 articles), for conduit strain of 23% (95% CI, 21–25%, from 14 articles) and for reservoir strain of 39% (95% CI, 38–41%, from 40 articles).[3] There are however no recommended cut-offs for all the different values of LAS owing to paucity of data from large scale studies, differences in the vendor specific software and differences observed in values due to age, gender, loading conditions, etc. Besides, the anatomy of LA with presence of pulmonary veins and LA appendage makes the assessment of LAS technically demanding and time-consuming.

Left atrial strain has also been studied in heart failure. In a study on 83 patients with suspected heart failure with preserved ejection fraction (HFpEF), parameters of diastolic dysfunction, such as left ventricular mass index (LVMI), LA volume index (LAVI), E/A ratio, deceleration time (DT), E/E', and global longitudinal LA strain during ventricular systole (GLAs-res) and strain during late diastole (GLAs-pump) were evaluated. It was concluded that LA function as assessed by 2D-STE is impaired in patients with HFpEF. A GLAs-res value of <17.5% was suggestive of impaired diastolic function of the LV and thus useful for the diagnosis of HFpEF.[4] In HF with reduced EF (HFrEF), assessment of LA reservoir function by peak atrial longitudinal strain (PALS) in systole, allows powerful prognostication, independently of LA volume and left ventricular longitudinal contraction. Impaired PALS was associated with greater left ventricular and LA volumes, worse left ventricular EF, left ventricular global longitudinal strain, right ventricular systolic function, and more severe diastolic dysfunction.[5] Besides, LA strain is also a predictor of AF occurrence and recurrence, and has an association with thromboembolic risk.[6]

LEFT ATRIAL STIFFNESS INDEX

Left atrial stiffness index (LASt) is defined as the amount of pressure (in mm Hg) required to induce a unit change in LA volume (in mL) during the passive filling phase ($\Delta P/\Delta V$).[7] It can be assessed by both invasive and noninvasive methods. Noninvasively, pressure and volume has been calculated by cardiac magnetic resonance (CMR) imaging volumetric data method. In a recent study, the validity and accuracy of LASt was examined using both invasive LA pressure, and noninvasive surrogates of left atrial pressure by echocardiography (E/A, E/E', and E/Vp). The calculation of LASt using E/E' had close correlation to LASt derived by invasively measured LA pressures [the formula used ratio of E/E' to LA strain, LAS measured by STE i.e. (E/E'/LAS]. LASt also increases with age and has been shown to be independently associated with recurrence of AF after LA ablation[7] and is higher in patients with persistent AF as compared to those with paroxysmal.[8] In a small study, in patients with AF, it was also shown that LASt is related to left ventricular diastolic dysfunction, LA dilatation, and collagen synthesis and may predict AF recurrences after pulmonary vein isolation and after cardioversion.[9,10] Small scale studies have been done in patients with HFpEF evaluating LA strain as well as stiffness index. In a study on 64 patients, LAS was significantly reduced, while LA strain index was increased and the authors concluded that LA strain index was most accurate in identifying patients with diastolic heart failure.[11] In another study also, it was observed that LA strain and strain index serve as useful markers of LV end diastolic pressure as well as help in prognostic stratification of patients who are likely to develop HFpEF.[12]

Right ventricle Strain imaging: Like on the left side, regional RV strain also represents a potential means to assess myocardial contractility that is less load dependent, and may be applicable across a wide range of pathologies. However, the complex anatomy of RV offers unique challenges in this regard. Also, there are very few studies and limited data available with the right side if heart. Usually, one-dimensional strain is acquired using Doppler tissue imaging in the apical 4-chamber view, interrogating the basal, mid, and apical segments of the RV free wall and it is limited mostly to the use of longitudinal strain.[13] A narrow imaging sector focusing on the RV free wall using high frame rates (ideally >/150 frames/s) are required. Care should be taken to align the segment in the center of the sector to avoid errors due to angle dependence of Doppler. A maximum tolerance of 10–15% off the axis of contraction is recommended.[14] Values for strain and SR are then derived by placing sample volume (s) or regions of interest of varying sizes in the mid portion of the segment (s).

Strain and SR values have been studied in a number of conditions affecting the right heart including arrhythmogenic RV dysplasia[15], pulmonary embolism[16], pulmonary hypertension[17], systemic RV[18], and amyloidosis.[19] There is a lack of normative data for strain and SR measures of the RV and most values in normal subjects have been obtained from small scale studies.

2D strain based on speckle tracking has also been studied on the RV. In addition to generating strain curves in individual segments, algorithms exist to average strain over the entire chamber. Advantage of 2D tracking methods is that it is relatively angle independent within the acquired imaging plane and possesses an improved signal-to-noise ratio, but proper alignment of image planes is still required (Fig. 2). There is a lack of normative data with this technique, and the "global" value is derived only from a single view (apical 4 chamber view), thus it is not a true global assessment of RV function. Finally, different algorithms in different vendors have resulted in different normal ranges. Because of these reasons, this technique is not recommended for routine clinical use and no reference limits can be recommended. In a small study, by Badano et al, the normal reference limit for speckle tracking strain of RV free wall was -23%.[20]

There have been few studies on RV in patients with PH and heart failure.

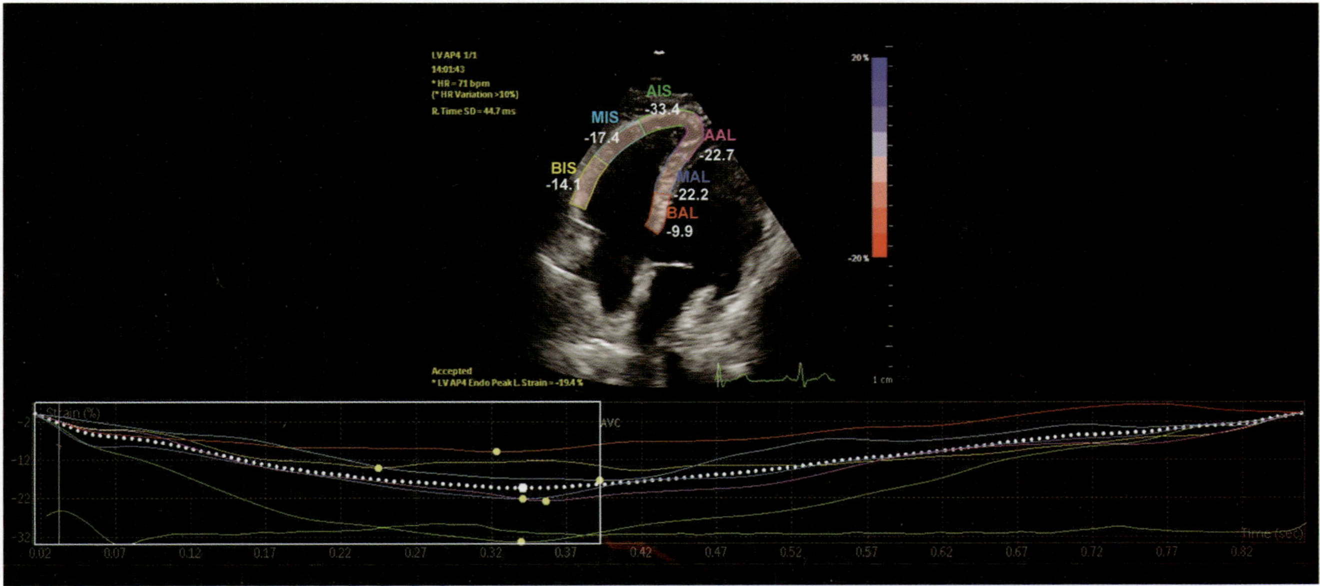

Fig. 2: Right ventricle focused apical 4 chamber view showing measurement of RV strain by 2D speckle tracking method. RV free wall strain is calculated by taking the average value of the three free wall segments.

In 575 patients with PH, free wall longitudinal strain by 2D-STE was predictive of functional capacity and 18-month mortality.[21]

In 200 patients with heart failure and normal RV systolic function tricuspid annular plane systolic excursion (TAPSE > 16 mm), a proportion of patients were found to have abnormal RV free wall strain indicative of subclinical RV dysfunction, which was also predictive of death and hospitalization in these patients.[22]

In patients presenting with acute myocardial infarction, RV free wall strain was superior to conventional echocardiographic parameters for picking up RV myocardial infarction.[23]

In another study, by Houard et al., it was demonstrated that RV global longitudinal strain by echo provided strong additional prognostic value, superior to CMR-derived RV measures [RVEF, FT-RVGLS, TAPSE, and fractional area change (FAC)] in predicting both overall and cardiovascular mortality.[24] In a relatively recent study on in patients with acute decompensated heart failure, RV free wall strain was an independent predictor of cardiac events and was of greater prognostic power than standard echocardiographic parameters.[25]

Right atrium strain imaging: Although, STE is able to assess the reservoir phase, passive conduit phase and active conduit phase of RA like in the LA, the role of speckle tracking imaging in assessment of RA deformation has not been defined and it remains a research tool. In a small study in healthy individuals, STE was found to be feasible for assessment of RA deformation and normal reference range of RA longitudinal strain indices were proposed. In this study PALS, peak atrial contraction strain (PACS) and time to peak longitudinal strain (TPLS) were measured by STE, using six-segment model of RA in apical 4 chamber view. The reference value proposed for global PALS was 49 + 13% and global TPLS was 363 + 59 msec.[26] These reference limits however, are not recommended because of very wide confidence intervals. In patients of heart failure, RA deformation indices have not been much studied.

In a recent study with MRI, RA strain was quantified in 407 subjects without HF, 106 with HFrEF and in 96 subjects with HFpEF. RA reservoir, conduit and booster pump functions were assessed. It was concluded that HFrEF was associated with significant RA dysfunction (lower reservoir and conduit strain and SR, reduced active emptying fraction), while HFpEF was associated with mildly reduced RA conduit strain with normal reservoir or booster pump function.[27]

In a study on pediatric population with PH, RA deformation properties were significantly altered. Progressive worsening of RA reservoir and conduit functions was related to changes in right ventricular diastolic dysfunction. RA reservoir function, pump function, the rate of atrial filling, and atrial minimum volume emerged as good predictors of outcome in pediatric PH.[28]

LIMITATIONS

Deformation imaging is a relatively new modality in echocardiography which is rapidly emerging as a useful; relatively load independent measure to assess myocardial contractile function. Large amount of data is available on strain and SR in LV in different clinical settings and pathologies. However, very limited data is available on the deformation indices of the LA, and on the right sided chambers. Few small scale studies are available in adults as well as pediatric population utilizing strain in normal subjects and normal cut-off values have been proposed. Thus, in pathological states like heart failure, there is very limited information available. Abnormal LA strain has been shown to be a good predictor of AF occurrence and prognosis in HFpEF as well as HFrEF. However, deformation imaging of atria and the RV is largely a research tool as of now and much more data is required before it is routinely recommended for interpretation in patients with heart failure. Besides, the thin walls of these chambers, the differences with age, gender, rapidly evolving softwares and variabilities in studies using different vendors make difficult to have simple, single cut-off values.

CONCLUSION

Two-dimensional echocardiography is a simple noninvasive tool of immense utility in heart failure. Deformation imaging in the form of strain and SR has emerged as sensitive measure of LV contractile function. Studies have established its role if several clinical settings including heart failure. However, there is very limited data with strain imaging of the atria and the RV and several limitations, as discussed above. More studies are needed in large number of patients to establish normal cut-off values and in different clinical scenarios like heart failure.

REFERENCES

1. Jamal F, Bergerot C, Argaud L, et al. Longitudinal strain quantitates regional right ventricular contractile function. Am J Physiol Heart Circ Physiol. 2003;285(6):H2842-7.
2. Burkule NJ. Advances in echocardiographic evaluation of left atrial strain in atrial fibrillation. Advances in Clinical Cardiovascular Imaging Echocardiography & Interventions (ACCI-EI). 2019;74:601-6.
3. Pathan F, Delia N, Nolan MT, et al. Normal ranges of left atrial strain by speckle-tracking echocardiography: A systematic review and meta-analysis. J Am Soc Echocardiogr. 2017;30(1):59-70.

4. Aung SM, Güler A, Güler Y, et al. Left atrial strain in heart failure with preserved ejection fraction. Herz. 2017;42(2):194-9.
5. Carluccio E, Biagioli P, Mengoni A, et al. Left atrial reservoir function and outcome in heart failure with reduced ejection fraction,the importance of atrial strain by speckle tracking echocardiography. Circ Cardiovasc Imaging. 2018;11(11):e007696.
6. Kosmala W, Saito M, Kaye G, Protect-Pace I, et al. Incremental value of left atrial structural and functional characteristics for prediction of atrial fibrillation in patients receiving cardiac pacing. Circ Cardiovasc Imaging. 2015;8(4):e002942.
7. Khurram IM, MaqboolF, Berger RD, et al. Association between left atrial stiffness index and atrial fibrillation recurrence in patients undergoing left atrial ablation. Circ Arrhythm Electrophysiol. 2016;9(3):e003163.
8. Rahman HA, Hassan AKM, Abosetta AHS, et al. Increased left atrial stiffness in patients with atrial fibrillation detected by left atrial speckle tracking echocardiography. Egyptian Heart J. 2015;67:217-23.
9. Machino-Ohtsuka T, Seo Y, Tada H, et al. Left atrial stiffness relates to left ventricular diastolic dysfunction and recurrence after pulmonary vein isolation for atrial fibrillation. J Cardiovasc Electrophysiol. 2011;22(9):999-1006.
10. Shaikh AY, Maan A, Khan UA, et al. Speckle echocardiographic left atrial strain and stiffness index as predictors of maintenance of sinus rhythm after cardioversion for atrial fibrillation: a prospective study. Cardiovasc Ultrasound. 2012;10:48.
11. Kurt M, Wang J, Torre-Amione G, et al. Left atrial function in diastolic heart failure. Circ Cardiovasc Imaging. 2009;2(1): 10-5.
12. Todaro MC. Left atrial morphology and function: a strong cardiovascular predictor of outcome. J Cardiovasc Echogr. 2017;27(3):118-9.
13. Rudski LG, Lai WW, Afilalo J, et al. Guidelines for the echocardiographic assessment of the right heart in adults: a report from the American Society of Echocardiography endorsed by the European Association of Echocardiography, a registered branch of the European Society of Cardiology, and the Canadian Society of Echocardiography. J Am Soc Echocardiogr. 2010;23(7):685-713.
14. Berg S. Myocardial strain rate by Doppler ultrasound methods. Angle dependency and error estimation. Master's thesis, Department of Engineering Cybernetics, NTNU, Trondheim, Norway. 2004.
15. Sutherland GR, Di Salvo G, Claus P, et al. Strain and strain rate imaging: a new clinical approach to quantifying regional myocardial function. J Am Soc Echocardiogr. 2004;17(7): 788-802.
16. Kjaergaard J, Sogaard P, Hassager C. Right ventricular strain in pulmo- nary embolism by Doppler tissue echocardiography. J Am Soc Echocardiogr. 2004;17(11):1210-2.
17. Kittipovanonth M, Bellavia D, Chandrasekaran K, et al. Doppler myocardial imaging for early detection of right ventricular dysfunction in patients with pulmonary hypertension. J Am Soc Echocardiogr. 2008;21(9):1035-41.
18. Chow PC, Liang XC, Cheung EW, et al. New two-dimensional global longitudinal strain and strain rate imaging for assessment of systemic right ventricular function. Heart. 2008;94(7):855-9.
19. Sun JP, Stewart WJ, Yang XS, et al. Differentiation of hypertrophic cardiomyopathy and cardiac amyloidosis from other causes of ventricular wall thickening by two-dimensional strain imaging echocardiography. Am J Cardiol. 2009;103(3):411-5.
20. Badano LP, Muraru D. Subclinical right ventricular dysfunction by strain analysis: Refining the targets of echocardiographic imaging in systemic sclerosis. Circ Cardiovasc Imaging. 2016;9(6):e005009.
21. Fine NM, Chen L, Bastiansen PM, et al. Outcome prediction by quantitative right ventricular function assessment in 575 subjects evaluated for pulmonary hypertension. Circ Cardiovasc Imaging. 2013;6(5):711-21.
22. Carluccio E, Biagioli P, Alunni G, et al. Prognostic value of right ventricular dysfunction in heart failure with reduced ejection fraction: Superiority of longitudinal strain over tricuspid annular plane systolic excursion. Circ Cardiovasc Imaging. 2018;11(1):e006894.
23. Lemarié J, Huttin O, Girerd N, et al. Usefulness of speckle-tracking imaging for right ventricular assessment after acute myocardial infarction: A magnetic resonance imaging/ echocardiographic comparison within the relation between aldosterone and cardiac remodeling after myocardial infarction study. J Am Soc Echocardiogr. 2015;28(7):818-27.
24. Houard L, Benaets MB, de Meester de Ravenstein C, et al. Additional prognostic value of 2D right ventricular speckle-tracking strain for prediction of survival in heart failure and reduced ejection fraction: a comparative study with cardiac magnetic resonance RV strain for prediction of survival in HFrEF. JACC Cardiovasc Imaging. 2019;pii: S1936-878X(19)30052-X.
25. Harimura-Hamada Y, Seo Y, Ishizu T, et al. Incremental prognostic value of right ventricular strain in patients with acute decompensated heart failure. Circ Cardiovasc Imaging. 2018;11(10):e007249.
26. Padeletti M, Camelli M, Lisi M, et al. Reference values of right atrial longitudinal strain imaging by two dimensional speckle tracking. Echocardiography. 2012;29(2):147-52.
27. Chirinos JA, Satija V, Gaddam S, et al. RA function in heart failure with reduced and preserved ejection fraction. JACC. 2018;71:11.
28. Jone PN, Schafer M, Li L, et al. Right atrium deformation in predicting outcomes in pediatric pulmonary hypertension. Circ Cardiovasc Imaging. 2017;10(12):e006250.

CHAPTER

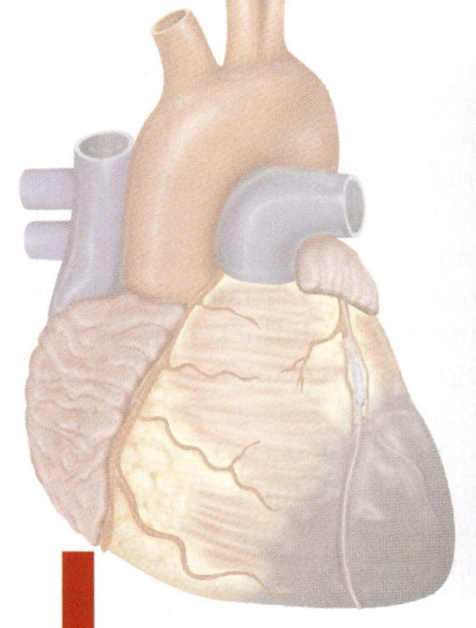

Left Ventricular Dyssynchrony: Echocardiographic Evaluation and Treatment in Heart Failure

Qiangjun Cai, Masood Ahmad

INTRODUCTION

Left ventricular (LV) contraction is induced by myocardial excitation through a highly coordinated electrical-mechanical coupling. LV systolic performance is affected not only by the contractile status of the myocardium, but also by the synchronicity of the myocardial segments. The asynchronous electrical activation of the LV due to intraventricular conduction disturbance is reflected in QRS widening on the electrocardiogram termed as electrical dyssynchrony. LV mechanical dyssynchrony, on the other hand, refers to the mechanical effects of asynchronous ventricular contraction and relaxation, which may or may not be associated with electrical conduction disturbance. Mechanical dyssynchrony presents as simultaneous contraction and stretch in different segments of the LV, and delays in the time to peak contraction from one segment to another. In healthy hearts without conduction abnormalities, the electrical activation occurs within 70 msec and all LV segments contract almost simultaneously. However, in left bundle branch block (LBBB), the posterolateral basal LV is the last segment to depolarize and contract. The hemodynamic consequences of dyssynchronous LV contraction include energy waste, decreased stroke volume, and systolic mitral regurgitation. We will discuss the echocardiographic evaluation of LV dyssynchrony and the available treatment options in the setting of heart failure.

CARDIAC RESYNCHRONIZATION THERAPY

Despite advances in evidence-based pharmacological therapy for patients with heart failure (HF) with reduced ejection fraction (HFrEF), a significant percentage of patients remain symptomatic with persistently reduced EF, resulting in increased morbidity and mortality. Substantial prolongation of the QRS duration is found in approximately one-third of such patients associated with worse clinical outcome. Cardiac resynchronization therapy (CRT) has been an important therapeutic breakthrough for patients with HFrEF and wide QRS complex (ideally LBBB morphology) who remain symptomatic despite optimal medical treatment. The rationale is that such patients are expected to have some degree of LV mechanical dyssynchrony due to their prolonged depolarization and if optimally targeted by multisite pacing (biventricular pacing), a more synchronous LV contraction may result leading to higher stroke volume and cardiac output. The most common treatment is to use biventricular pacing to create two activation wave fronts, originating from opposite walls. Large multicenter randomized trials have demonstrated that CRT can improve HF symptoms, improve exercise capacity and quality of life, induce LV reverse remodeling and improve LVEF with consequent reduction in all-cause mortality.[1] The current American College of Cardiology (ACC) guideline recommendations on patient selection for CRT are based on QRS duration, morphology, and HF functional classification (Table 1)[2].

Electrocardiographic Criteria for Cardiac Resynchronization Therapy

Current ACC guidelines have established electrocardiographic QRS duration and morphology, as a surrogate of electrical dyssynchrony, as an essential criterion for selecting HF patients eligible for CRT. However, 30–40% of patients fulfilling these traditional inclusion criteria do not demonstrate significant improvement in symptoms, EF, or survival following this costly therapy, the so-called nonresponders. This observation suggests that additional measures beyond QRS duration and morphology are needed to identify patients who will benefit from CRT. One of the postulated etiologies for nonresponder is that electrical dyssynchrony may not reflect LV mechanical dyssynchrony in patients with HF. Several studies have demonstrated a high prevalence of LV mechanical dyssynchrony in HF patients independent of the QRS duration and morphology. In 1,680 HF patients with QRS duration <130 msec enrolled in the Echocardiography Guided Cardiac Resynchronization Therapy (EchoCRT) trial, 74% showed echocardiographic LV mechanical dyssynchrony.[3] Patients with similar QRS duration may show different magnitudes of LV mechanical dyssynchrony. In addition, about 30% of patients with LBBB do not have mechanical dyssynchrony by echocardiography particularly those with QRS <150 msec. Therefore, the association between QRS duration, as a measure of LV electrical dyssynchrony, and echocardiographic LV mechanical dyssynchrony is not straightforward. Assessing LV mechanical dyssynchrony may provide additional prognostic information to characterize CRT candidates and predict CRT response. This assessment may be particularly helpful for those patients with QRS between 120 msec and 149 msec and/or nonLBBB morphology.

TABLE 1: Recommendations for CRT in patients with systolic heart failure.

COR	*Indications*	*LOE*
I	LVEF ≤35%, sinus rhythm, LBBB, QRS ≥150 ms, NYHA III or ambulatory IV	A
	LVEF ≤35%, sinus rhythm, LBBB, QRS ≥150 ms, NYHA II	B
IIa	LVEF ≤35%, sinus rhythm, LBBB, QRS 120 to 149 ms, NYHA II, III, or ambulatory IV	B
	LVEF ≤35%, sinus rhythm, non-LBBB, QRS ≥150 ms, NYHA III or ambulatory IV	A
	LVEF ≤35%, atrial fibrillation requires ventricular pacing or otherwise meets CRT criteria, and allows near 100% ventricular pacing with CRT	B
	LVEF ≤35%, new or replacement device placement with anticipated >40% ventricular pacing	C
IIb	LVEF ≤30%, ischemic etiology, sinus rhythm, LBBB, QRS ≥150 ms, NYHA I	C
	LVEF ≤35%, sinus rhythm, nonLBBB, QRS 120 to 149 ms, NYHA III or ambulatory class IV	B
	LVEF ≤35%, sinus rhythm, nonLBBB, QRS ≥150 ms, NYHA II	B
III	NYHA I or II, nonLBBB, QRS <150 ms	B
	Comorbidities and/or frailty limit survival with good functional capacity to less than 1 year	C

(COR: class of recommendation; LOE: level of evidence; LBBB: left bundle branch block; LVEF: left ventricular ejection fraction; NYHA: New York Heart Association; CRT: cardiac resynchronization therapy)

Echocardiographic Assessment of Dyssynchrony

Echocardiography has provided several parameters to quantify LV mechanical dyssynchrony.

- *M-mode imaging*: Early research in identifying segmental LV dyssynchrony focused on the time difference between peak shortening of septal and posterior walls. Septal to posterior wall motion delay (SPWMD) is a standard dyssynchrony parameter measurement from M-mode imaging. SPWMD is the difference in timing of septal and posterior wall contraction. SPWMD ≥130 msec has been proposed as a cut-off value in predicting LV reverse remodeling and long-term clinical improvement after CRT with about 85% accuracy. M-mode imaging allows quick analysis with high temporal resolution. However, M-mode imaging has a number of limitations. It is difficult to obtain optimal alignment of the M-mode cursor perpendicular to the posterior wall and the septum. This method is also adversely affected by myocardial scar and passive motion.
- *Tissue Doppler*: Using pulsed wave tissue Doppler, the time interval from the beginning of the QRS complex to the Sm peak (mitral annular peak systolic velocity), and the time interval from the beginning of the QRS to the onset of Sm can be derived. Mechanical dyssynchrony has been defined as differences of >65 msec of time to Sm peak between segments. A dyssynchrony index can be calculated as the standard deviation (SD) of the average values of time to peak systolic velocities. Tissue Doppler parameters predict LV reverse remodeling after CRT with high specificity, sensitivity and accuracy. Tissue Doppler offers high frame rates with excellent temporal resolution. It can also color-code the timing of cardiac events allowing for a snapshot of synchrony or dyssynchrony.

- Multiple single-center studies have demonstrated that LV mechanical dyssynchrony indices assessed by echocardiography can predict response to CRT and long-term outcome. Unfortunately, the large multicenter Predictors of Response to CRT (PROSPECT) trial[4], which compared 12 indices obtained with conventional echocardiography and tissue Doppler imaging, found that none of these indices could predict CRT response better than the electrocardiogram. Poor reproducibility of various two-dimensional (2D) parameters and controversial cutoff values of tissue Doppler measurements might have contributed to their low predictive values. Research has therefore, shifted toward finding novel, more automated, and more reproducible echocardiographic indices and modalities.

Emerging Echocardiographic Modalities

- *Two-dimensional strain speckle tracking*: 2D strain has inherent advantages over tissue Doppler including angle independence and the ability to differentiate between active deformation and passive motion. This speckle tracking technique is applicable to over 90% patients. Radial and longitudinal strain analyses have been used to characterize LV mechanical dyssynchrony. High inter- and intraobserver agreements with superior reproducibility have been reported. Mechanical dyssynchrony is assessed using the standard deviation of multiple time-to-peak longitudinal myocardial strain with a cutoff value of 60 msec separating CRT responders from nonresponders. This index of dyssynchrony was named "mechanical dispersion index". From the midventricular short-axis view, LV mechanical dyssynchrony is measured as the time difference between peak radial strain of the anteroseptal and posterolateral segments. A cutoff value of >130 msec has been shown to be highly predictive of echocardiographic response to CRT with a sensitivity and specificity of 83 and 80%. Studies have shown that the LV lead position is generally not located at the most delayed segment with a concordance of only 30–40% in real world practice. Using speckle tracking to target LV lead placement yielded significantly improved clinical response and lower rates of combined death and heart failure-related hospitalization. One of the limitations of speckle tracking analysis is the low frame rate.
- *Septal flash and apical rocking*: In normal subjects, all LV walls move in a homogeneous fashion towards or away from the apex. In contrast, in patients with dyssynchrony (such as LBBB), early activation of the septum without the corresponding contraction of the posterolateral wall, results in the early contracting septum moving away from the apex, while the posterolateral wall is pulled towards the apex. Septal flash is an early inward motion of the interventricular septum during the isovolumic contraction period. Later on during the systole, the posterolateral wall contracts and pulls the apex laterally and induces a typical apex motion pattern described as apical rocking. Septal flash and apical rocking are qualitative variables that can be easily identified without specific software. Both are highly reproducible and applicable even without any expertise. The presence of apical rocking and/or septal flash was strongly associated with better echocardiographic volumetric response and predicted long-term outcome better than guideline Classes I, IIa, IIb, and Doppler velocity-based assessments. About 40% of the patients who were not recommended for CRT according to current guidelines, showed a volume response based on septal flash and apical rocking. Septal flash and apical rocking are considered two specific myocardial signatures of mechanical dyssynchrony and could be a valuable supplement to the current guidelines.[5]
- *Three-dimensional echocardiography*: LV dyssynchrony is a complex 3D electrical and mechanical phenomenon and therefore it may be better assessed using a 3D approach. Using a matrix array transducer, 3D echocardiography allows fast acquisition of a dynamic 3D data set that encompasses the entire heart from a single acoustic window.[6] This technique offers an accurate and a quantitative means of assessing global LV function and is uniquely capable of providing precise information about segmental LV function. 3D echocardiography avoids geometric assumptions and uses automated quantification tools which are more accurate and reproducible than 2D echocardiography.

Semi-automated analysis of LV volume using 3D echocardiography allows simultaneous assessment of the time-to-minimum volume of all LV segments. The systolic dyssynchrony index (SDI) has been developed to quantify the severity of cardiac dyssynchrony. SDI is measured as a standard deviation of the time taken to reach minimum regional volume for each segment. The value is expressed as a percentage of the cardiac cycle (Fig. 1). SDI is highly reproducible with good inter- and intraobserver correlation. After the patients received CRT, the SDI exhibited an immediate significant decrease at 24–48 hours, and a progressive decrease during 6 months of follow-up. There was a significant positive correlation between baseline SDI and the decrease in LV volume 6 months after CRT. A more pronounced reduction in SDI immediately after CRT was independently associated with superior long-term survival. A newly developed 3D speckle tracking system can quantify LV strain and dyssynchrony by measuring the endocardial area change ratio (area strain). Area strain dyssynchrony index (ASDI) was calculated as the average difference between peak and end-systolic area strain derived from 16 segments.

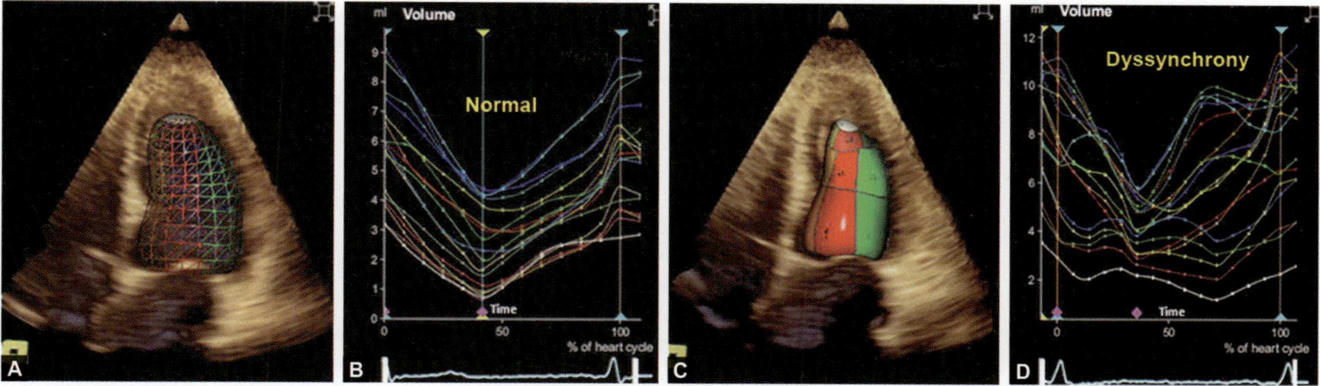

Figs. 1A to D: Example from our laboratory showing 3-dimensional echocardiography assessment of left ventricular (LV) mechanical dyssynchrony. (A) Full-volume acquisition. (B). Regional volume curves in a normal control with all segments reaching a minimum volume at the same time. (C) LV cast produced by quantitative analysis. (D) Regional volume curves in a patient with severe intraventricular dyssynchrony. There is a disarray of the time-volume curves signifying LV dyssynchrony.

ASDI ≥3.8% was the best predictor of response to CRT with a specificity of 100% and a response rate of 100%.

3D echocardiography is feasible in >90% of studied subjects. It is superior to tissue Doppler imaging in assessing LV reverse remodeling, identifying the optimal pacing site for the LV lead, and predicting response to CRT. Potential limitations of 3D echocardiography for the assessment of dyssynchrony include substandard image quality and relatively low temporal and spatial resolution, which may compromise the sensitivity.

MECHANICAL DYSSYNCHRONY WITH NARROW QRS

3D echocardiography demonstrated significant mechanical dyssynchrony in >50% HFrEF patients with narrow QRS. Among those patients, about one-third have their earliest contracting segment located in areas conventionally for delayed segment targeted for LV pacing, i.e. lateral, posterior, or inferior segments. This finding may explain why patients with narrow QRS do not respond to CRT despite the presence of mechanical dyssynchrony.

CONCLUSION

Based on the review of the current literature and our own experience, we have the following conclusions. First, there is an unmet need for patient selection for CRT. Emerging echocardiographic modalities have provided indices which are more robust, reproducible, and predictive. Among those, 3D echocardiography particularly 3D strain speckle tracking seems more accurate and efficient due to its ability to interrogate all LV segments simultaneously. Large multicenter prospective studies with long-term follow-up and hard endpoints will be needed to support routine application of these echocardiographic modalities in clinical practice. Second, the detection of LV mechanical dyssynchrony should be translated into more accurate LV lead placement. Newer echocardiographic modalities especially speckle tracking and 3D echocardiography may provide better guidance in LV lead placement. Finally, LV mechanical dyssynchrony is affected by multiple factors, such as the loading conditions, heart rate, and degree of LV remodeling, dynamic changes during exercise, and the size and location of myocardial scar. Not all of these factors are amenable to CRT. An integrated approach combining clinical, electrocardiographic and echocardiographic variables may offer additional value to the selection of CRT candidates.

REFERENCES

1. Abraham WT, Fisher WG, Smith AL, et al. Cardiac resynchronization in chronic heart failure. N Engl J Med. 2002;346(24):1845-53.
2. Tracy CM, Epstein AE, Darbar D, et al. 2012 ACCF/AHA/HRS focused update of the 2008 guidelines for device-based therapy of cardiac rhythm abnormalities: a report of the American College of Cardiology Foundation/American Heart Association Task Force on Practice Guidelines. J Am Coll Cardiol. 2012;60(14):1297-313.
3. Ruschitzka F, Abraham WT, Singh JP, et al. Cardiac-resynchronization therapy in heart failure with a narrow QRS complex. N Engl J Med. 2013;369(15):1395-405.
4. Chung ES, Leon AR, Tavazzi L, et al. Results of the Predictors of Response to CRT (PROSPECT) trial. Circulation. 2008;117(20):2608-16.
5. Stankovic I, Prinz C, Ciarka A, et al. Relationship of visually assessed apical rocking and septal flash to response and long-term survival following cardiac resynchronization therapy (PREDICT-CRT). Eur Heart J Cardiovasc Imaging. 2016;17(3):262-9.
6. Hung J, Lang R, Flachskampf F, et al. 3D echocardiography: a review of the current status and future directions. J Am Soc Echocardiogr. 2007;20(3):213-33.

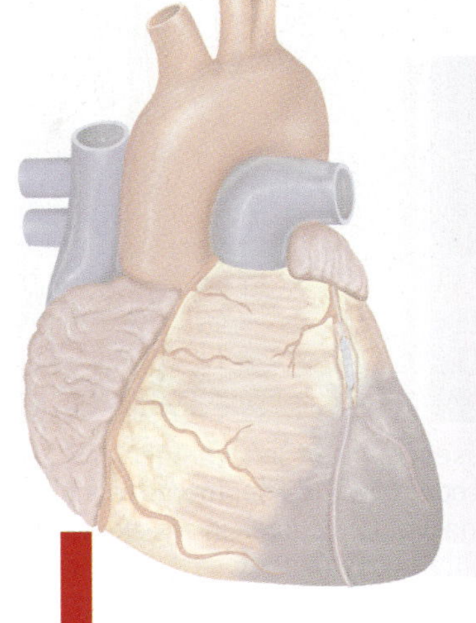

Echocardiography in Dilated Cardiomyopathy

S Shanmugasundaram

INTRODUCTION

Heart failure is a common disorder affecting 1–2% of the general population. With increasing life expectancy, the disease is on the rise, affecting as much as 5–10% of elderly beyond 65 years. It carries an ominous prognosis, with an overall annual mortality of nearly 10%. Those in class IV have actually a 50% risk of dying within the next year. Apart from the high mortality risk, the need for repeated hospitalizations for worsening of heart failure, arrhythmias and systemic embolism impair the quality of life of patients. In a developing country like ours, rheumatic valvular heart disease (RHD) is still an important cause of heart failure. But with the decline in rheumatic fever, roughly 10–20% of hospital admissions for heart failure may be caused by RHD. Among the rest, roughly half may have heart failure with preserved ejection fraction (HFpEF) and the other half have heart failure with reduced ejection fraction (HFrEF). Virtually in all those with HFrEF, dilated cardiomyopathy (DCM) is the cause—two-thirds of them have coronary artery disease and the rest may have idiopathic DCM.

Dilated cardiomyopathy is the most common type of cardiomyopathies encountered in practice, almost to a proportion of 90%. An astute physician could diagnose DCM, based on the typical symptoms like dyspnea on effort, paroxysmal nocturnal dyspnea, orthopnea, edema feet and typical signs like elevated jugular venous pressure, displaced apex beat and third heart sound with or without murmurs of mitral and tricuspid regurgitation. ECG may be nonspecific, showing left atrial (LA) enlargement and left ventricular (LV) hypertrophy with ST-T changes. Bundle branch blocks are not uncommon. Q waves, if present may suggest the diagnosis of ischemic DCM. Chest X-ray may show enlargement of left ventricle and left atrium with evidence of increased pulmonary venous pressure. But none of these basic investigations could be diagnostic of DCM. One would definitely need an appropriate imaging technique to diagnose DCM and echocardiography has proved to be the ideal method because of its extremely high sensitivity to detect the hallmarks of the disease namely dilated ventricles and impaired contractility. Widespread availability of echocardiograms and trained personnel, portability for bedside testing and low cost also make it an attractive choice.

Cardiomyopathies are diseases which primarily affect the myocardium leading to altered ventricular performance (heart failure) and or electrical disturbances (arrhythmias or conduction abnormalities). Phenotypically, cardiomyopathies are classified into dilated, hypertrophic, restrictive, arrhythmogenic and noncompaction types. Such a comprehensive classification is essentially based on the echocardiographic appearances. DCM is the most common type characterized by varying degrees of dilatation and systolic dysfunction of left ± right ventricle with or without mitral and or tricuspid regurgitation, in the absence of chronic volume or pressure overload. This characteristic expression of the disease may result from various disease processes, like infections (as a sequel to myocarditis), toxins (alcohol, cocaine), drugs (anthracyclines, trastuzumab), auto immune disorders systemic lupus erythematosus

[(SLE), giant cell and Takayasu arteritis], endocrine and metabolic disorders (thyroid dysfunction, diabetes mellitus, Cushing's, pheochromocytoma, hypophosphatemia, hypocalcemia, deficiency of thiamine, carnitine, selenium etc.), infiltrative diseases like sarcoidosis and amyloidosis, iron overload states, tachyarrhythmias [incessant atrial tachycardia, ventricular premature depolarizations (VPDs) of huge burden], as a peripartum disease or due to stress (Takotsubo cardiomyopathy). Roughly 25% of cases are idiopathic and another 25–35% of DCM could be due to single gene defects (autosomal dominant or recessive or X linked; more than 30 genes have been implicated). Some may have syndromic presentation (mostly muscular dystrophies, rarely mitochondrial type).[1] Except in few conditions, etiology cannot be identified by echocardiography.

DIAGNOSIS BY 2D, M-MODE AND DOPPLER ECHOCARDIOGRAPHY

A comprehensive study should be performed using 2-D, M-mode and Doppler echo techniques. An eyeballing of LV size and performance should be done quickly in parasternal long axis view, parasternal short axis views at basal, mid LV and apical levels, A4C and A2C views. It should be followed by quantification of LV dilatation and dysfunction, detection of LV hypertrophy (LVH) and LV remodeling, assessment of diastolic function, RV function, mitral and tricuspid regurgitation, measurement of pulmonary artery (PA) pressure, identification of LV and LA thrombi and finally measurement of different dyssynchrony indices.[2]

Documenting LV dilatation: As the name implies, DCM is characterized by increased LV dimensions, though the degree of dilatation is variable depending on the etiology and the time course of the disease. In a patient with uniform dilatation of LV with near uniform impairment of contractility, an M-mode study done at the level of tip of mitral valve may yield LV dimensions that can be measured at end-diastole [at peak of R wave in electrocardiogram (ECG)] and end-systole (the most minimum dimension). In such circumstances, these simple measurements may provide excellent indices for follow-up assessment which are likely to be better than serial ejection fraction (EF) measurement. Generally, LV end-diastolic (LVED) dimension exceeding 112% of the age and body surface area (BSA) derived upper limit of normal value, is supposed to indicate LV dilatation. In middle aged, Indian adults the upper limit of LV (ULN) at end-diastole is 25 mm/m^2 for men and 27 mm/m^2 for women and at end-systole is 16 mm/m^2 for both men and women.[3] Adding 2 SD to the ULN, LV diastolic dimension exceeding 28 mm/m^2 and end-systolic dimension exceeding 18 mm/m^2 can be taken as LV dilatation in our population. M-mode has the advantage of providing better temporal resolution (Fig. 1). However, with nonuniform enlargement of LV cavity and nonuniform pattern of contractile disturbances, it is better to measure LV volumes in end-diastole and at end-systole by modified Simpson method using biplane (A4C and A2C) imaging (Fig. 2). The upper limit of LV end-diastolic volume (LVEDV) in normal middle aged adult Indians is 46 mL/m^2 in men and 44 mL/m^2 in women. LVEDV of >52 mL/m^2 may indicate LV enlargement in our population. LV end-systolic volume (LVESV) appears to be a better predictor of outcomes in various studies and in a population of heart failure patients, LVESV of >25 mL/m^2 proved to a better prognosticator than LVEDV or LV dimensions or even LV EF.[4] LVESV of >25 mL/m^2 predicted an increase

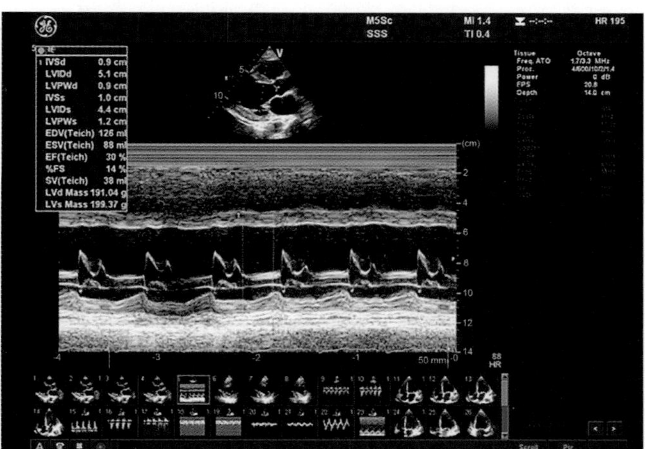

Fig. 1: M-mode study of a patient with dilated cardiomyopathy (DCM), documenting dilated LV with reduced motion and systolic thickening of septum and posterior wall.

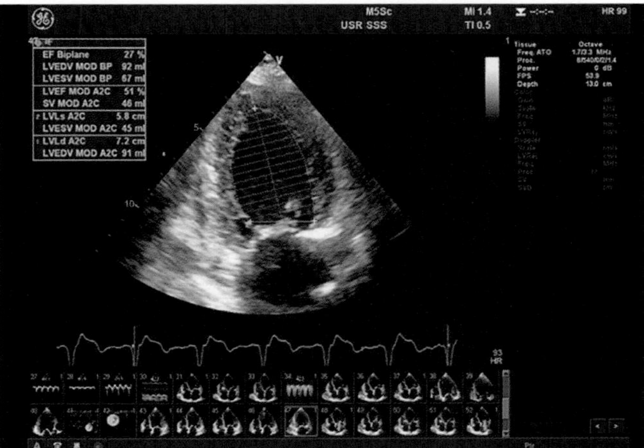

Fig. 2: Estimation of left ventricular (LV) volumes and ejection fraction (EF) by biplane Simpson's method.

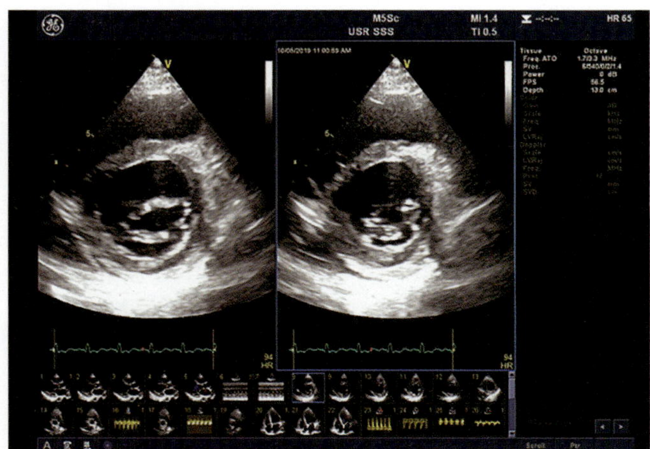

Fig. 3: Minimally dilated cardiomyopathy: Parasternal short axis images in diastole and systole. Mild dilatation of LV but with little change in cavity size in systole indicating impaired contractility.

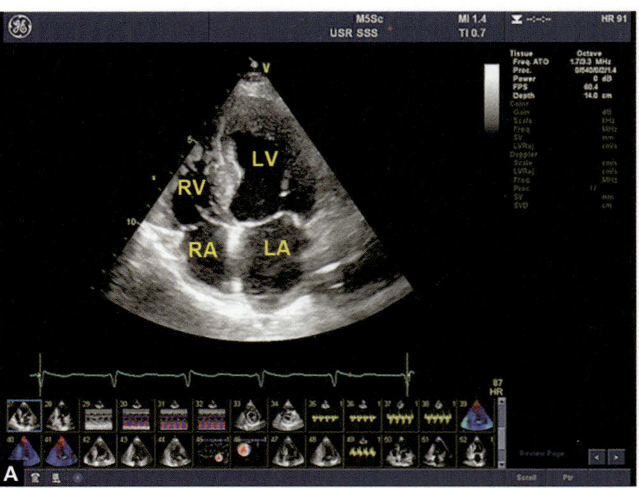

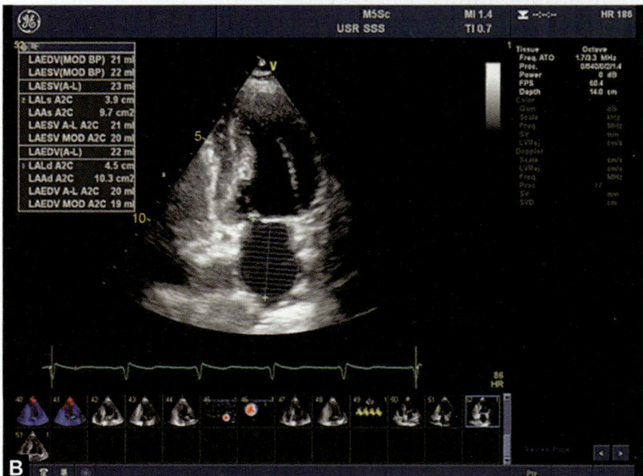

Figs. 4 A and B: Calculation of left atrial (LA) volume by biplane area length method.

in heart failure hospitalizations by nearly 5-fold. Since, LV diastolic dimension, LV diastolic volume and EF may be altered by the coexisting MR, LVESV is obviously a better index. Another practical advantage of measuring LVESV is that endocardial definition is better in systole rather than in diastole. In dilated heart, LV endocardium may be poorly defined and even be outside the sector of imaging.

Roughly 5% of those with DCM may not exhibit dilatation significant enough to fulfill the diagnostic criteria. LVED diameter may be within 15% of the ULN. For want of better terminology, this is often referred to as minimally DCM (Fig. 3). Myocarditis, genetically, mediated DCM and diabetic cardiomyopathy are known to have such presentations. Prognosis may still be poor in at least some of them despite lack of dilatation.

Left atrial dilatation: Considerable degree of LA dilatation is a common feature and is due to elevated LV filling pressures, mitral regurgitation (MR), atrial fibrillation and possibly atrial muscle disease. Since, left atrium may dilate either in anteroposterior or superoinferior or mediolateral directions, estimate of LA volume is a better method of quantification of LA enlargement, rather than relying on single dimension. LA volume is measured by biplane area length method from A4C and A2C images obtained in end-systole (Fig. 4). LA volume = 0.85 x (A1 x A2)/L (L=shortest vertical length). Normal range is 16–28 mL/m^2 in the Western population and 18.7 ± 2 mL/m^2 for Indians. LA volume is a predictor of adverse prognosis.

Documenting impaired LV contractility: Conventionally, EF is being viewed as the gold standard of systolic performance measurement. EF is stroke volume indexed to end-diastolic volume measured as the ratio of (LVEDV-LVESV)/LVEDV and the normal value is 62 ± 5%. A value of < 50% is generally, considered to indicate LV systolic dysfunction. EF of < 45% has been conventionally used to diagnose DCM in early days. The recent European guidelines classify systolic function based on EF as follows:

Normal when EF is > 50%, reduced when it is < 40% and midrange when the value is 40–50%. Arbitrarily, LV dysfunction is considered to be severe if it is below 30–35%. LV EF is an ejection phase index that is affected by preload, afterload, contractility and heart rate. Coexistent MR may falsely give higher values for the degree of contractile dysfunction because of reduced afterload and increased preload in this condition. On the contrary, increased afterload as in hypertension may falsely give lower EF values despite mild reduction in contractility. End-systolic volume (ESV) is affected by afterload and contractility and end-diastolic volume (EDV) by preload and contractility.

Left ventricular ejection fraction has been proven to be a good determinant of prognosis but a poor indicator of symptomatic status. The reasons for lack of correlation between EF and symptoms is that, there are many other determinants of symptoms (dyspnea and fatigue), namely heart rate, presence of arrhythmias which may cause AV dissociation or loss of atrial booster function, diastolic dysfunction, presence of anemia, skeletal muscle perfusion, status of neurohormonal activation and autonomic nerve function. In addition, EF by virtue of the principle of measurement, mainly takes into account the radial function of LV and does not consider many other altered parameters of systolic performance like, long axis function, intraventricular dyssynchrony, rapidity of contraction, twisting and untwisting function, etc. However, measuring LVEF has gained popularity because of the simplicity of measurement. It is used to discriminate patients with heart failure as those with preserved EF and those with reduced EF. Such a simple approach has been well validated in terms of response to drug therapy. Beta-blockers, angiotensin-converting-enzyme inhibitors (ACEI) and mineralocorticoid receptor antagonists have been found to decrease mortality only in those with reduced EF. Moreover, the decision regarding the need for devices like implantable cardioverter-defibrillator (ICD) and cardiac resynchronization therapy (CRT) is based solely on the presence of an EF < 30–35%.

In diseased and deformed ventricles, EF calculation has to be done either by 2D biplane imaging (Fig. 2) or more ideally by 3D echo. Automated LV function assessment is possible with recently available systems and beat by beat values are obtained in real time. The major limitations of 2D estimate of LV EF are that, it is operator dependent and reliable only when endocardial border definition is precise. In 15% of individuals, endocardial border is poorly defined due to body habitus and associated lung disease. For better endocardial delineation, second harmonic imaging should invariably be used. Left heart contrast may also be considered, if the endocardial delineation is poor. Despite all such efforts, LVEF values obtained by the same observer or different observers may show significant variations, as much as a standard deviation of 8.5% around the mean value. Calculation of EF by M-mode is most unreliable, even in normal persons and hence discouraged. Documentation of EF has to be done along with observation on volume status, heart rate and afterload (blood pressure as a simple surrogate) in order to use it for serial studies. Eye balling for estimation of LV EF is unreliable in the presence of very fast or very slow heart rate, irregular heart rhythm and when LV is too small or too large. Every effort has to be made to measure EF by standard techniques.

Fractional shortening (FS) of LV is at times used as a surrogate for LVEF, but the limitations of using single dimension of LV for estimating the global function have to be understood. It is calculated by the formula: FS = left ventricular internal dimension (LVIDd – LVIDs)/LVIDd. A value of < 25% is used to indicate systolic dysfunction.

Yet another method of quantifying LV dysfunction is calculation of Wall Motion Score. Depending on the severity of disease process, LV segments may show hypokinesia or akinesia. Dyskinesia is generally a feature of ischemic cause. Wall motion is assessed not by the amplitude of endocardial excursion but the degree of systolic thickening. Because of excellent temporal resolution, M-mode or anatomical M-mode may define the magnitude of wall motion changes more precisely. Though DCM is characterized by global reduction of wall motion, there may be subtle differences in the extent of involvement of different segments in idiopathic DCM. In most of them, basal inferior or inferolateral segment may continue to show normal contractility until the disease is well advanced. Apart from coronary artery disease, myocarditis and muscular dystrophies are the causes of pronounced differential involvement of various segments of LV. Wall motion index is calculated by assigning values for altered wall motion (normal 1, hypokinesia 2, Akinesia 3 and dyskinesia 4) for each of the 17 segments of LV and get an average.

Calculating isovolumic acceleration in tissue Doppler may be better than EF for assessing intrinsic contractile function of LV, as it is relatively load independent. It is measured by dividing peak velocity in isovolumic contraction phase in TDI obtained from septum or lateral wall by the time taken to reach the maximal velocity. It is generally around 1.2 ± 0.5 m/s^2 in normal.

Measures of LV remodeling: When myocardium is insulted by disease or drug or toxin, the depressed contractility leads to lowering of stroke volume and LV dilatation occurs as an adaptive process to exploit Frank Starling principle in order to achieve near normal stroke volume. However, this process becomes maladaptive with the progression of the disease and activation of neurohormonal systems. Progressive enlargement of LV changes the shape of LV from an ellipsoid to a sphere. Spherical LV is hemodynamically disadvantageous as it results in increased wall stress. This adverse remodeling is calculated by echo in the form of sphericity index (SI). The ratio between the maximal transverse dimension of LV and the base to apex dimension (midpoint of mitral annulus to apex) is measured both in end-diastole and in end-systole. The normal value is 0.52 ± 0.06 in diastole and 0.45 ± 0.06 in systole (Fig. 5). The sphericity index increases with progressive remodeling and approaches 1 as the severity increases.[5] Ideally, the sphericity index is calculated by the ratio of LVEDV to the theoretical sphere volume calculated as $1/6\ \Pi \times L^3$, where L is the long axis dimension of LV. Normal value for SI with this method is 0.36 ± 0.08 in diastole and 0.28 ± 0.07 in systole. SI is not only a predictor of prognosis but a sensitive index of exercise performance in patients with LV dysfunction.[6]

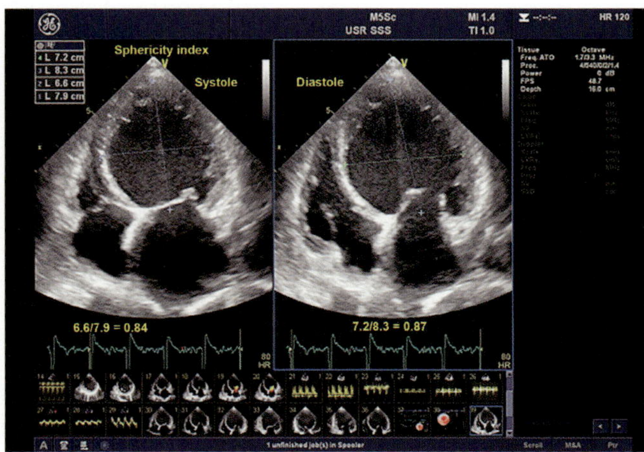

Fig. 5: Sphericity index–ellipsoid LV remodeling into a spherical chamber.

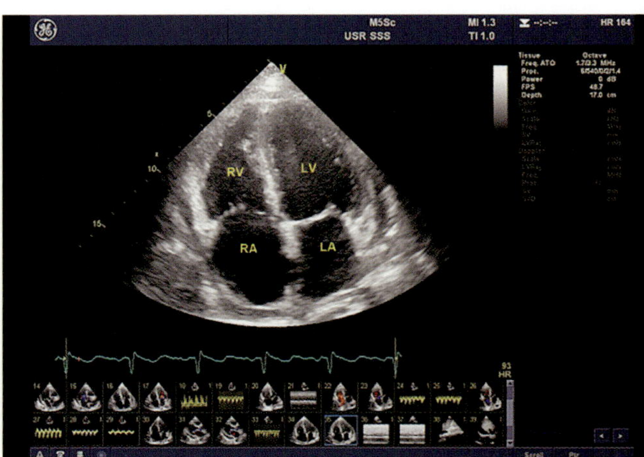

Fig. 6: Dilated right atrium and right ventricle–biventricular involvement in DCM.

Right ventricular involvement: RV involvement may occur as a part of biventricular disease, occurring in roughly 30% of DCM patients (Fig. 6) or may be secondary to pulmonary hypertension caused by elevated left heart filling pressures. Pulmonary hypertension, when present is usually modest and may resolve with optimal medical therapy of heart failure. In some, elevation of PA pressure as detected from tricuspid regurgitation velocity, may be severe as a result of combined postcapillary and precapillary pulmonary hypertension. RV dysfunction may be identified by RV fractional shortening (<35%), RV EF by 3D echo (<45%), reduced tricuspid annular plane systolic excursion (TAPSE) (<16 mm), prolonged Tei Index [> 0.40 by pulsed wave Doppler (PWD) method > 0.55 by tissue Doppler imaging (TDI) method], lower TDI s' (< 10 cm/s), lower IVA (< 2.2 m/s^2) and lower 2D strain (< -20%) (Fig. 7).

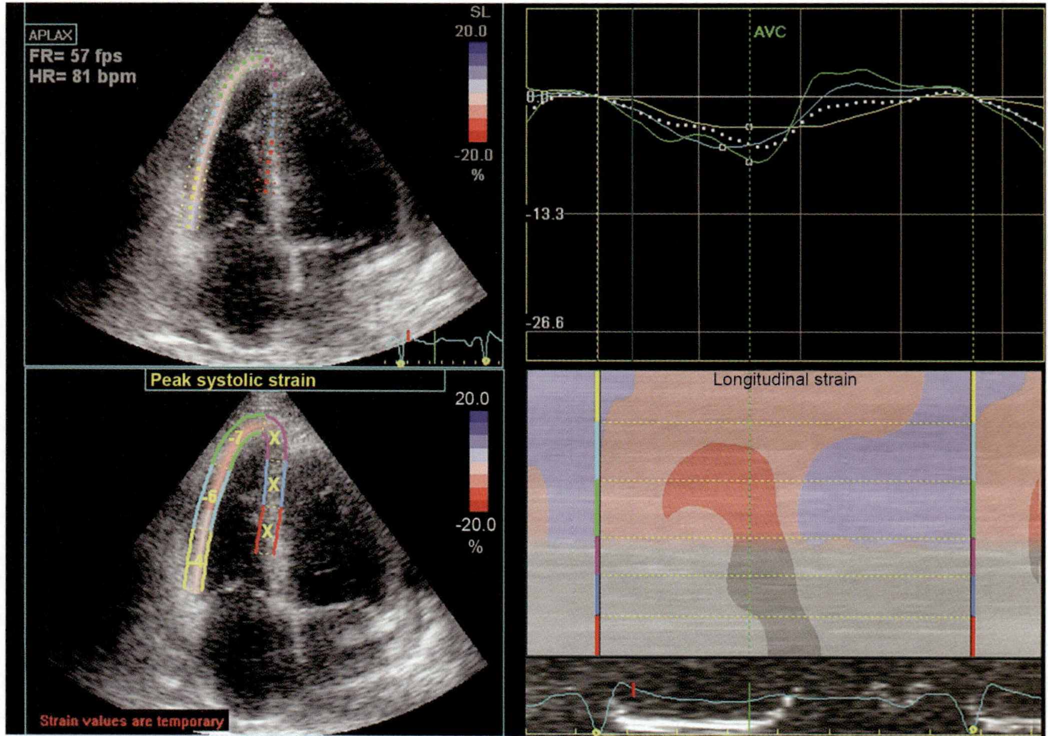

Fig. 7: Very low RV strain by speckle tracking, implying poor RV function.

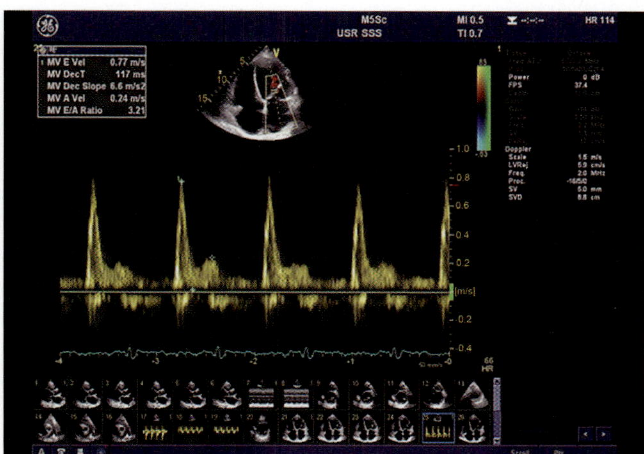

Fig. 8: Transmitral Doppler showing features of type III diastolic dysfunction: E/A = 3.2; DT 117 mms.

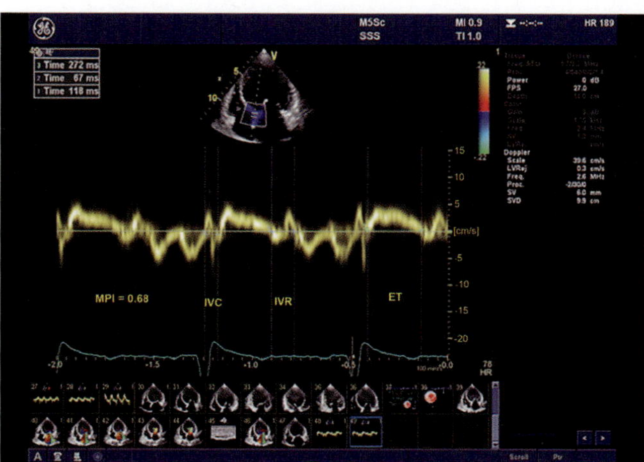

Fig. 9: Calculation of Tei Index from Tissue Doppler isovolumetric contraction time + isovolumic relaxation time/ejection time (IVCT+IVRT)/ET.

Assessment of diastolic function: Almost all with DCM will have some degree of diastolic dysfunction. Transmitral E/A ratio obtained by PWD with the sample volume kept at the tip of mitral leaflets in open position is the simplest one to assess diastolic function. If >2, it directly identifies grade III diastolic dysfunction. Deceleration time is often short < 140 ms. LA pressures are markedly elevated in them. Grade III diastolic dysfunction implies poor prognosis, particularly when it is not reversible with drug therapy (Fig. 8).

On the other hand, if E/A ratio is < 0.8 with E wave measuring < 50 cm/s, diastolic dysfunction grade I may be diagnosed. LA pressure is often normal in them. If E/A is 0.8 - 2.0 or if E/A is < 0.8 but with E amplitude > 50 cm/s, the following 3 criteria may be assessed: Average E/e' > 14, tricuspid regurgitation (TR) velocity >2.8 m/s, LA volume index > 34 mL/m^2. If 2 out of 3 or all 3 are positive, grade II diastolic dysfunction exists. LA pressure is modestly elevated in this stage. If 2 out of 3 or all the 3 are negative, the diastolic dysfunction is graded I. In case only 2 criteria could be calculated and if both are positive it is grade III, if both are negative, it is grade I and 1 positive 1 negative it is indeterminate.[7]

Myocardial performance index: Tei Index aims at calculating the sum of isovolumic contraction and isovolumic relaxation times. It may be obtained by PWD study with the cursor kept midway between left ventricle outflow tract (LVOT) and mitral flow (mitral closing to opening time–LV ejection time/LV ejection time) or directly from tissue Doppler (Fig. 9). With the former technique, the normal values are 0.39 ± 0.05 and in DCM it is often around 0.59 ± 0.10. This parameter is somewhat load independent, reproducible, easily obtainable and independent of LV geometry.

Measurement of LV mass: Though not required for diagnosis, measurement of LV mass helps in prognostication. DCM is typically characterized by eccentric hypertrophy–dilatation with normal wall thickness. In many of the patients with DCM, particularly in advanced disease state, LV wall may show thinning. Prognosis is poor when dilatation is severe and LV wall thickness is reduced. On the contrary, presence of increased LV mass is predictive of better outcome.[8] In a study, that used the septal or posterior wall thickness of ≥ 13 mm as a measure of LVH, contractile reserve was better in those with LVH and exercise induced elevation of catecholamines was lower.[9] LV mass may be calculated easily from M-Mode (Fig. 1) using the formula: LV mass = $0.8 \times 1.04\,[(IVSd + LVIDd + PWTd)^3 - LVID^3] + 0.6$. The normal value indexed to BSA is 49–115 g/m^2 (men) and 43–95 g/m^2 (women). However, M-mode estimate is unreliable in the presence of dilated left ventricle. Ideally, in DCM, LV mass may be calculated by area length method: LV mass = $1.05 \times \{[5/6 \times A_1 \times (l+t)] - (5/6 \times A_2 \times l)\}$. A1 refers to the total area of LV in short axis at papillary muscle level by tracing the epicardium; A2 is the area of LV in short axis view by tracing the endocardium excluding the papillary muscle; l is the length of LV in apical view from apex to annulus and t is the mean thickness of LV wall. Measurements are done in end-diastolic frame. Normal values are 44–88 g/m^2 (women) and 50–100 g/m^2 (men).

Left ventricular thrombus: Diligent search should be made to identify thrombus, as early recognition and institution of anticoagulant therapy may prevent systemic embolism. Presence of autocontrast in LV should make us spend extra -time to locate a thrombus. The thrombus shows a predilection to the apical part of LV, although, any segment that is akinetic or dyskinetic may be involved. The size, echo density, extent of mobility, etc. should be documented. Newly formed thrombi, as identified by the free mobility,

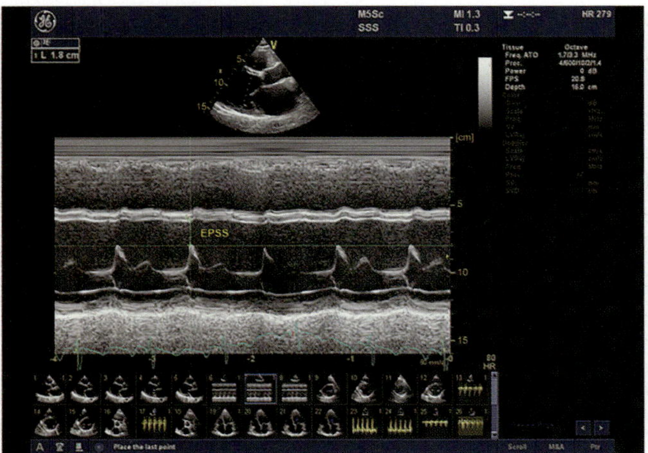

Fig. 10: E Point septal separation indicating LV dilatation and dysfunction.

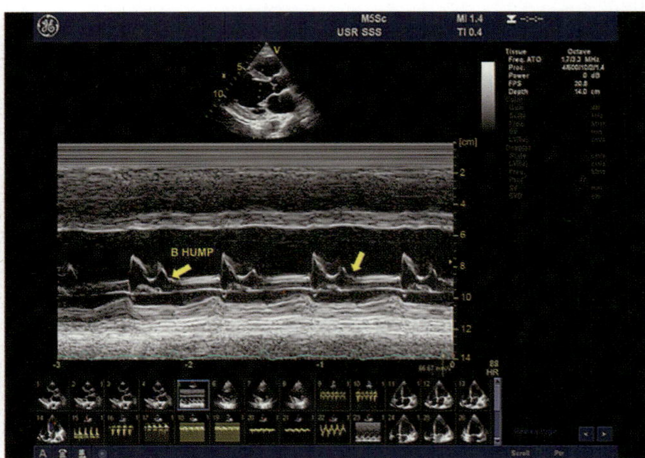

Fig. 11: B Hump in mitral valve M-mode, caused by elevated left ventricular end-diastolic pressure (LVEDP).

protrusion into LV cavity and variegated or generalized echo lucency, are more likely to respond to anticoagulant therapy. Older thrombi are firmly adherent over the endocardium with a flat surface, have no free mobility and exhibit greater and more uniform echo density. Interestingly, a study had looked at the strain rate of the thrombus by deformational imaging and concluded that a strain rate value of >1 S^{-1} might indicate that the thrombus is likely to be newly formed one, as the higher strain rate indicates more elasticity or compressibility of a fresh thrombus.[10]

M-mode Echocardiography: M-mode echo still has a place in evaluating patients with DCM. A simple parameter namely (E Point Septal Separation) (EPSS) measured as the distance between the E point of anterior leaflet and the corresponding point of left side of septum in M-mode echo may give useful information. Normally, it ranges from 0 mm–3 mm. It generally exceeds 7 in LV dysfunction but absence of this finding does not rule out the diagnosis (Fig. 10). B hump (a hump seen on the a-c slope) of the mitral leaflet M-mode echo indicates, that there is elevated filling pressure (Fig. 11). Smaller amplitude of opening of mitral leaflets may give a diamond like configuration. Gradual closure of aortic valve towards end of systole in M-mode may imply low cardiac output. Mitral annulus plane systolic excursion (MAPSE), obtained by placing the cursor on the mitral annulus might identify impaired long axis function. The magnitude of apical displacement of annulus measures the global change in the size of the cavity in the long axis direction. It may be obtained as an average of values obtained from four regions of the annulus namely, septal, lateral (A4C) anterior and posterior (A2C). In normal, it ranges from 12 mm to 15 mm. A value of <8 mm is associated with a depressed EF of <50%. It is valid in normal or dilated ventricles but may not show correlation to EF in hypertrophied ventricles.[11]

Tissue Doppler imaging: Subendocardium mostly contains longitudinally oriented myocardial fibers. Since, various disease processes involve sub-endocardium at an early stage and to a greater extent, myocardial performance in long axis is affected early and to a greater extent. Regional and global long axis function is derived from Tissue Doppler obtained from various segments of LV in A4C and A2C view. The velocities indicate the speed with which various segments of LV contract resulting in annulus descent towards apex in systole. Septal and lateral velocities both in systole(s') and early diastole (e') show a decrease quite early in disease. Since, elevated LA pressure increases transmitral E velocities, E/e' ratio is significantly, increased in the presence of LV dysfunction and elevated filling pressures (Figs. 12 A and B). There is a linear correlation of the ratio E/e' with LA pressure. If the ratio exceeds 14 (when septal and lateral e' are averaged) or > 15 (septal e' alone used) or 13 (when lateral e' alone is used), it indicates elevated LA pressures. In a study of 33 patients with DCM, systolic velocity of lateral annulus of < 5 cm/s and the ratio of E/e' of > 15, identified those with higher BNP values, lower VO_2 max and 6-fold increase in cardiac events.[12] In another study, E/e' was found to correlate with VO_2 max and VE/VCO_2 slope, the determinants of exercise performance.[13] The distinct advantage of using tissue Doppler velocities to assess LV systolic function is that, it can be accurately calculated even in those with poor endocardial definition. Normal values depend on the method of measuring the tissue velocities; if done by PWD technique, the values are slightly higher than those obtained by color coded velocities, as the former measures peak velocities while the later measures mean velocities. When done by color

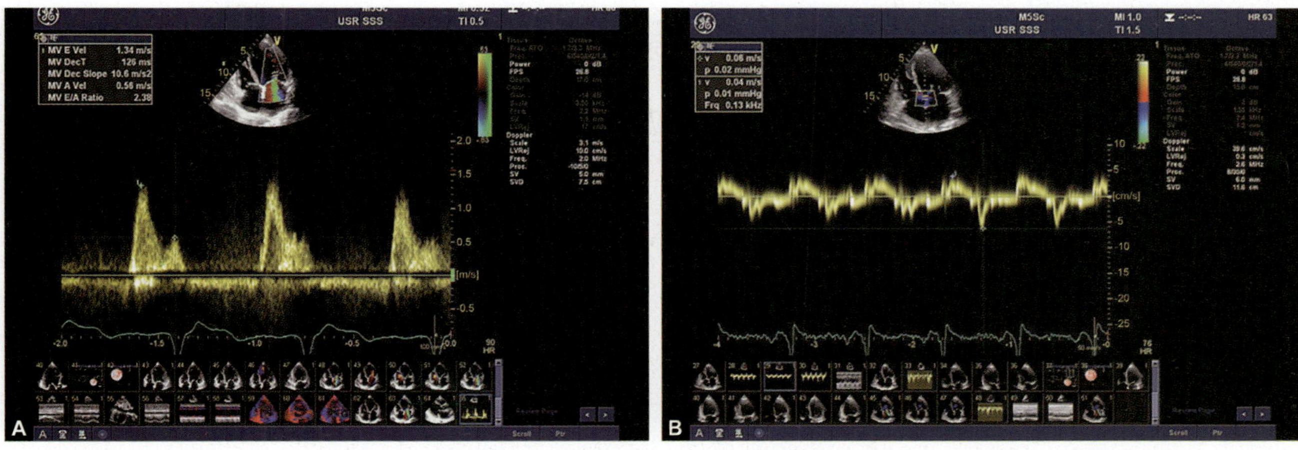

Figs. 12A and B: (A) Transmitral Doppler by PWD for measuring E/e'; (B) Septal tissue Doppler for measuring e'. E/e' = 22.

coded tissue Doppler method, six site (basal inferoseptal, lateral wall, anterior, inferior, anteroseptal and inferolateral) average s' of > 5.4 cm/s correlated well with an EF of > 50%, with a sensitivity of 88% and specificity of 97%).[14] An average of septal and lateral velocities also fared well, when compared to 6 site average in predicting EF. LVEF can be calculated by a regression equation EF = (8 x 6 site average s') + 3%. In another study, medial annulus systolic velocities were measured using PWD technique. With this method, medial annulus s' of < 6.8 cm/s identified subjects with 3D echo calculated EF of < 50% with a sensitivity of 94.1% and a specificity of 87%.[15]

Mitral regurgitation: In a dilated hypofunctioning left ventricle, some degree of MR is common and is caused by tethering of mitral leaflets, dilated hypo-functioning annulus and papillary muscle displacement. 35–50% of patients with DCM manifest MR and is severe in one-third of them. Assessment of mechanism and severity of MR is important in the present era, as salvaging procedures like MitraClip are available. In DCM in which LV is uniformly dilated assuming a globular shape, mitral valve leaflets may show symmetrical tethering of leaflets and coaptation occurs close to the free margin rather than at the usual coaptation line. Tenting distance and area are larger than normal. Inter papillary distance is increased. Mitral annulus is flat, dilated and shows decreased systolic narrowing. Dyssynchrony may also contribute to defective closure of mitral leaflets. All these mechanisms are responsible for MR, to a variable extent in different individuals. The MR jet is often centrally directed (Figs. 13 A and B). There are some in whom LV dysfunction is severe but MR is only mild to moderate and on the other end of the spectrum some may have mild to moderate LV dysfunction but with severe MR. Preliminary data suggest that it is the second category of patients that will benefit from mitraClip procedure.

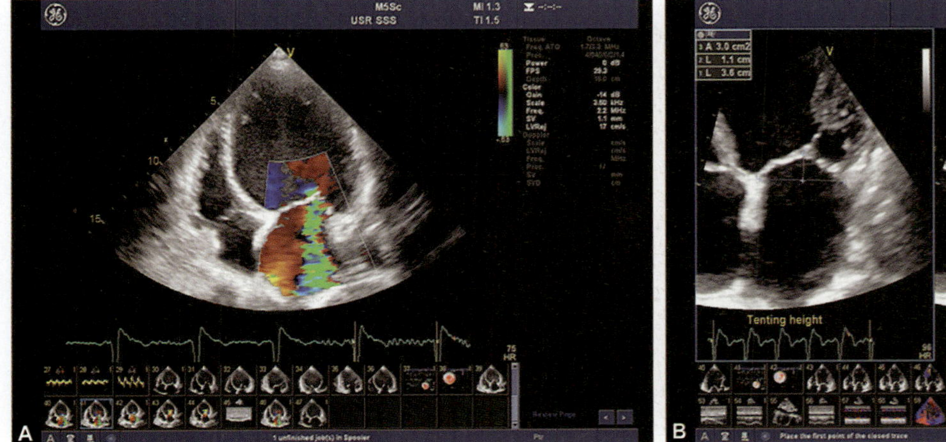

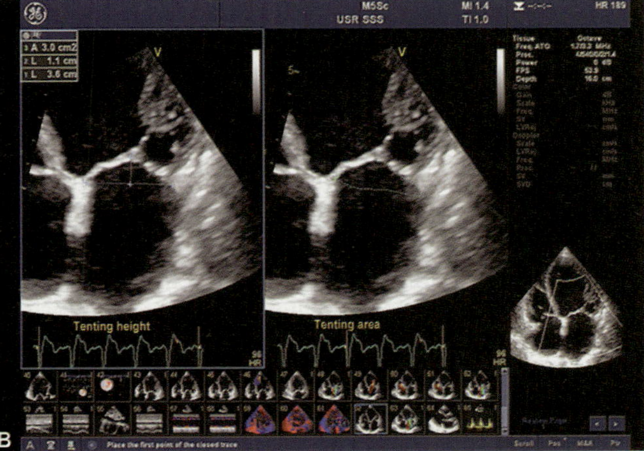

Figs. 13 A and B: (A) Remodeled spherical LV with dilated annulus and symmetrical tethering of mitral leaflets causing a central jet of mitral regurgitation; (B) Measurement of tethering height and tethering area in functional MR.

In view of poor prognosis of functional MR, echo Doppler values for defining severe MR are kept at a lower threshold level. For example, ERO of > 20 mm^2 and regurgitant volume of > 30 mL/beat are considered to indicate severe functional MR, requiring some form of valve intervention at this threshold level.

Interrogation of MR jet by continuous wave Doppler (CWD) may help us to noninvasively calculate LV dP/dt. The time taken for the MR velocity to change from 1–3 m/s is used to derive this value. This is equivalent to increase of LV-LA pressure gradient of 32 mm Hg, used as a surrogate of LV pressure rise considering that LA pressure is uniform in this period. 32 divided by the time measured in seconds gives dP/dt, derived noninvasively. Normal value is 1,000–1,200 mm Hg/s and a value of <600 mm Hg/s is a poor prognostic marker.

Rarely, in those with significantly elevated filling pressures, diastolic MR has been found to occur.

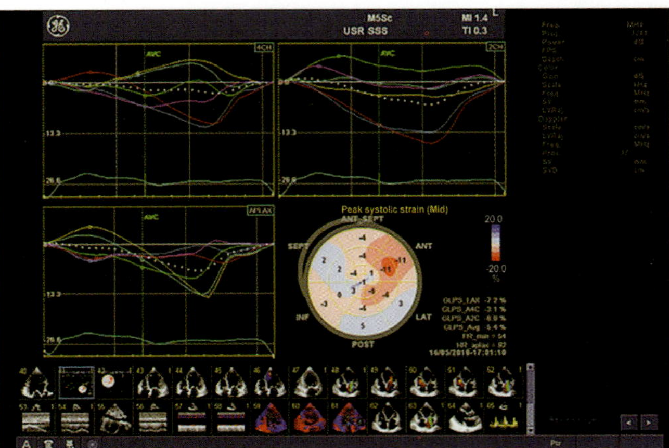

Fig. 14: Grossly lowered global longitudinal systolic strain in DCM.

Deformational imaging: Speckle tracking (2D strain) echocardiography measures regional and global myocardial strain (extent of deformation i.e., shortening or lengthening) and strain rate (rate at which deformation occurs) by tracking the myocardial speckles throughout the cardiac cycle. This method has the advantage of being angle independent and noise free. In contrast to 2D, M-mode and tissue Doppler assessment of contraction and relaxation, strain and strain rate are least affected by translational movements and tethering effects of adjacent myocardial segments. Though, strain analysis can be done along longitudinal, circumferential and radial directions, it is the LS that has gained popularity, because of the simplicity of its measurement and the fact that long axis function gets affected early in disease processes. Global LS (GLS), is obtained by averaging the peak systolic strain values obtained from basal, mid and apical segments of LV along the longitudinal axis in A4C, A2C and Apical long axis vies. GLS varies with age, gender and loading conditions and is > (more negative than) -18% in normals. A value of < (less negative than) 16% is abnormal and is considered borderline when it is between -16 and -18%. In DCM the GLS is markedly reduced (Fig. 14) and actually it declines even before EF decreases, thereby making it as an ideal tool for detection of preclinical disease. GLS has a linear correlation to LVEF and actually LVEF may be derived using GLS using a formula: EF = 3 x (GLS) + 8. Even in patients with advanced heart failure with reduced EF, GLS appears to be an independent predictor of mortality with a hazard ratio of 1.22 per 1% reduction of GLS.[16] In a study of 94 patients with nonischemic DCM, much lower values of GLS (≤ -7.1%) and greater degree of myocardial dispersion, i.e. standard deviation of time to peak negative strain from the 16 LV segments (> 72 ms) predicted ventricular arrhythmias and may serve as an additional marker for selecting patients for ICD for primary prevention.[17] Left atrial strain (LAS) is emerging as a new tool in evaluation of heart failure patients. LAS during "reservoir" phase may give an idea about the wall stiffness and hence, indirectly the LA pressure. LAS during "pump function" phase is predictive of exercise capacity and more often depressed in idiopathic DCM rather than in ischemic DCM.

Dyssynchrony: Atrioventricular, Interventricular and Intraventricular mechanical dyssynchrony is a common feature of DCM. It occurs more often with prolonged QRS (electrical dyssynchrony), particularly in those with left bundle branch block (LBBB), that too when the QRS duration is more than 150 ms. Roughly one-third of patients with narrow QRS may manifest mechanical dyssynchrony and roughly one-third of patients with broad QRS may not exhibit mechanical dyssynchrony. Mechanical dyssynchrony tends to perpetuate adverse remodeling and worsen EF, because of the stretch stimulus of contracting segment exerted on the noncontracting segment and due to wasted work of LV–a part of LV ejecting blood into another part of LV without achieving forward ejection into aorta. Mechanical dyssynchrony predicts poor prognosis and also identifies patients who are more prone to develop complex ventricular arrhythmias. Recently, dyssynchrony induced cardiomyopathy is recognized as an important entity in those who have LBBB. A number of studies have pointed out that documentation of mechanical dyssynchrony is not useful to identify CRT responders. However, echo may play an important role in programming CRT parameters after implantation in such a way to permit optimal filling of LV and improved stroke volume. Though not for selection of

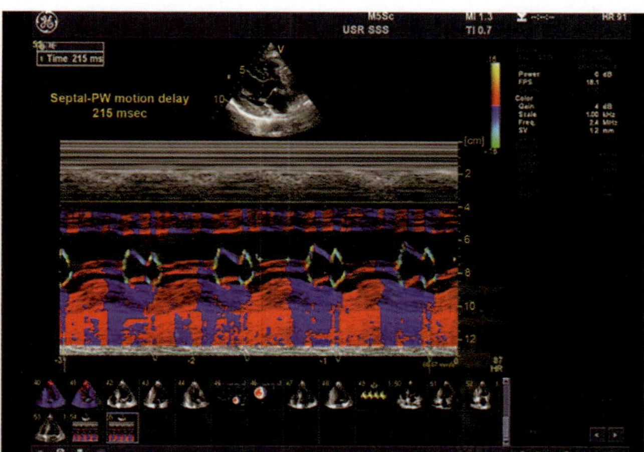

Fig. 15: Color TD M-mode for measuring septal posterior wall motion delay.

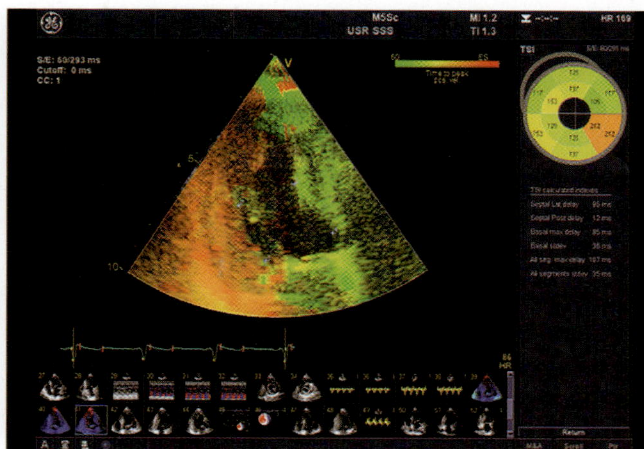

Fig. 16: Color coded tissue Doppler for dyssynchrony indices (Tissue Synchronization Index).

ideal candidates for CRT, every effort should be undertaken to document dyssynchrony for overall risk assessment.

Basically, in all with DCM, the following parameters should be calculated to document dyssynchrony.[18] Interventricular dyssynchrony: Time delay between onset of pulmonary flow to aortic flow, measured from Q to onset of flow by PWD. If it is > 40 ms it is abnormal. Interventricular Dyssynchrony: 1. Septal posterior wall motion delay either from M-Mode or Color coded M-mode (Fig. 15) at mid cavity level: a value of > 130 ms (time interval from peak of septal movement to the peak of posterior wall movement) indicates dyssynchrony. 2. Septolateral delay measured by TDI PWD (Time delay between beginning of septal s' to that of lateral wall s') of > 60 ms is abnormal. Color coded TDI (time to peak systolic velocity) may also be used to calculate this parameter (> 65 ms is abnormal). 3. Color coded TDI velocities (Fig. 17) from 12 segments of LV (mid and basal in 3 views) may be used to calculate maximal wall delay i.e., time interval between the earliest peak to the latest peak (> 100 ms), Yu Index, i.e. SD of time to peak of 12 segments (> 33 ms) (Fig. 16).

Radial dyssynchrony calculated from short axis is abnormal when it is > 130 ms. Systolic dyssynchrony index calculated from the dispersion of time to minimum regional volume for all 16 LV segments by 3D echo (3.5 ± 1.8% in normal). An arbitrary cut-off for significant dyssynchrony is defined as > 3 SD above the mean of normal subjects, i.e. >8.3%.[19] Septal flash and apical rocking motion readily indicate the presence of dyssynchrony. Atrioventricular dyssynchrony is diagnosed when the diastolic filling time measured by transmitral Doppler is < 40% of cardiac cycle and in the presence of diastolic MR. Truncated A of mitral Doppler and Fused E and E of mitral Doppler in the absence of tachycardia are the other markers of AV dyssynchrony.

Value of 3D echocardiography: 3D echo is superior to 2D echo in precisely measuring LV volumes and EF and the values obtained by 3D echo match with that obtained by cardiac MR imaging. 3D echo derived LV volumes are more precise because there is geometric assumption in calculation and there is no problem of apical foreshortening. Moreover, 3D strain calculation can be done very quickly which is useful for prognostication.

Noncompaction: There are some who present clinically, as DCM may have noncompaction of LV myocardium often affecting the apical segments. Echocardiography is often helpful in identifying this condition and a ratio of noncompacted to compacted myocardium of > 2 is used for diagnosis. LV noncompaction is characterized by LV trabeculations, deep intertrabecular recesses, and a thin layer of normal myocardium. This cardiomyopathy accounts for 5–9% of childhood cardiomyopathies. Adults do manifest this process of noncompaction as an acquired phenomenon in an otherwise typical DCM phenotype (Fig. 17).

Left ventricular reverse remodeling: There are certain situations where LV dilatation and systolic dysfunction are entirely reversed with medical treatment. This phenomenon is more likely to happen when there is an identifiable cause that can be corrected, e.g. alcoholic or peripartum cardiomyopathy, tachycardiomyopathy, thyroid dysfunction, deficiency of selenium or carnitine, metabolic causes like hypophosphatemia or hypocalcemia. Apart from total reversibility of the disease, there are many with DCM who may show improvement of EF and reduction of LV volumes–the so called reverse remodeling. It has been reported in as many as 35–45% of individuals.[20] Optimal medical therapy, Cardiac resynchronization therapy or revascularization when DCM is due to ischemia could

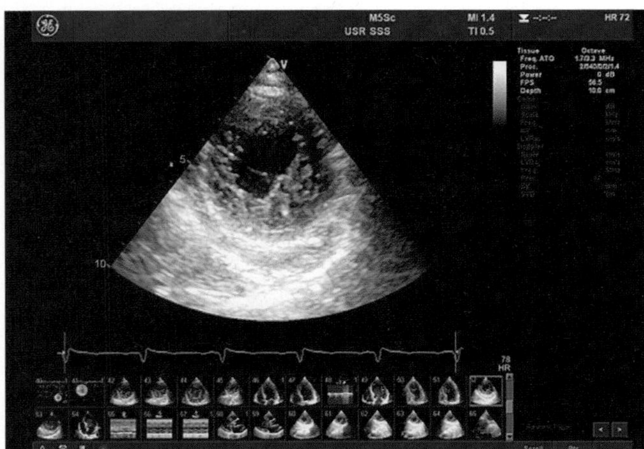

Fig. 17: Parasternal short axis view at apex depicting noncompacted myocardium.

result in such beneficial reverse remodeling, which is often associated with good prognosis. Moreover, this phenomenon may happen comprehensively in the form of reduction of MR, regression of pulmonary hypertension and improvement of RV function. Favorable response to CRT may be identified by echo in the form of reduction of LVEDV > 15% of baseline, improvement of LVEF > 5% of baseline, any decrease in MR, any decrease in LV mass and any decrease of LV myocardial performance index. LBBB, atrial fibrillation, grossly dilated spherical ventricles and thinned out myocardium may identify those who may not show this phenomenon.

Stress echocardiography: Stress echo is rarely needed for diagnosis but it can help us to refine prognostication. Assessment of contractile reserve is generally done by using low dose dobutamine echocardiography (DSE). In those with DCM, myocardial beta-receptors are downregulated and desensitized, more so with advanced LV dysfunction. Hence, if there is improvement of contractile performance after dobutamine challenge, it may indicate adequacy of beta-receptor density and sensitivity and serve as a good prognostic marker. On similar grounds, it is suggested that DSE may identify those who may favorably response to beta-blocker therapy. Moreover, those with contractile reserve are more likely to improve and may even normalize their LV function with optimal medical therapy.[21] Among the patients with recent onset DCM, those who had their EF improved to > 40% in follow-up showed an increase of EF of >14% with DSE and those who did not reach their follow-up of 40% had manifested <6% improvement of EF with DSE.

Ideally, a low dose dobutamine infusion is administered-starting with 5 μg/kg/min and then increasing the dose to 10, 15 and 20 μg/kg/min with each stage for 3 minutes. It has to be terminated if the patient complaints of angina or develops hypotension or ventricular tachyarrhythmias. Ideally, beta-blocker therapy may be withheld for three days prior to testing. Presence of contractile reserve is diagnosed when the LVEF calculated by biplane Simpson method, increases by an absolute value of 5% at least or by > 20% of the baseline value. An improvement of wall motion index of > 0.44 may also indicate, the presence of contractile reserve. A more sophisticated but time consuming method is to calculate the LV cardiac power output, the advantage being that, it is not sensitive to afterload and if preload is optimized, it may truly reflect the intrinsic contractile properties of the myocardium. It is calculated by the formula–Cardiac Power Output (Watts) = (Cardiac output × mean arterial pressure) × 2.2 × 10^{-3}. Cardiac output is measured from LVOT VTI (HR × stroke volume; stroke volume = LVOT VTI × LVOT area). If the value increases by > 1 Watt, good prognosis is implied.[22]

Another small study used a simple exercise, squatting and standing up in succession for 30 times, and defined contractile reserve, if there is an increase of EF > 4%. Failure of EF to increase by at least 4% predicted death and cardiac events.[23]

Excluding secondary causes of LV dysfunction: Chronic pressure overload states like aortic stenosis and hypertension may result in LV dysfunction. In these conditions, significant LV hypertrophy is invariably present. Thickened, often calcified, aortic valve with restricted mobility of the leaflets could be readily identified by echo. However, the underestimated pressure gradient due to reduced flow across the valve may pose diagnostic difficulties. In difficult situations, low dose DSE may be performed. If the mean gradient increases by at least 10 mm Hg without increase in Doppler derived aortic valve or increase of valve area by not more than 0.3 cm^2, true aortic stenosis with secondary LV dysfunction can be diagnosed. The other features that may suggest aortic stenosis with LV dysfunction are, an increase of peak velocity > 0.6 m/s with DSE, mean gradient of 40 mm Hg with the valve area of ≤ 1 cm^2 at any flow rate and velocity index (LVOT VTI/aortic valve VTI) of < 0.25.

Chronic volume overload states like Aortic or MR may progress to LV dysfunction. At times, it may be difficult to say whether, it is the sick ventricle that has made the valve dysfunctional (secondary MR) or it is the abnormal valve that has made the ventricle sick (primary MR with secondary LV dysfunction). Significant leaflet thickening, redundancy of the leaflets, prolapsing or flailing cusps, fused commissures or sub valvular disease may suggest primary valve disease. On the contrary, focal remodeling of LV (usually inferolateral wall) with tethering of posterior leaflet resulting in eccentric MR implies ischemic MR (Figs. 18A and B). Similarly, gross dilatation of LV, dilated flat annulus, symmetrical tethering of

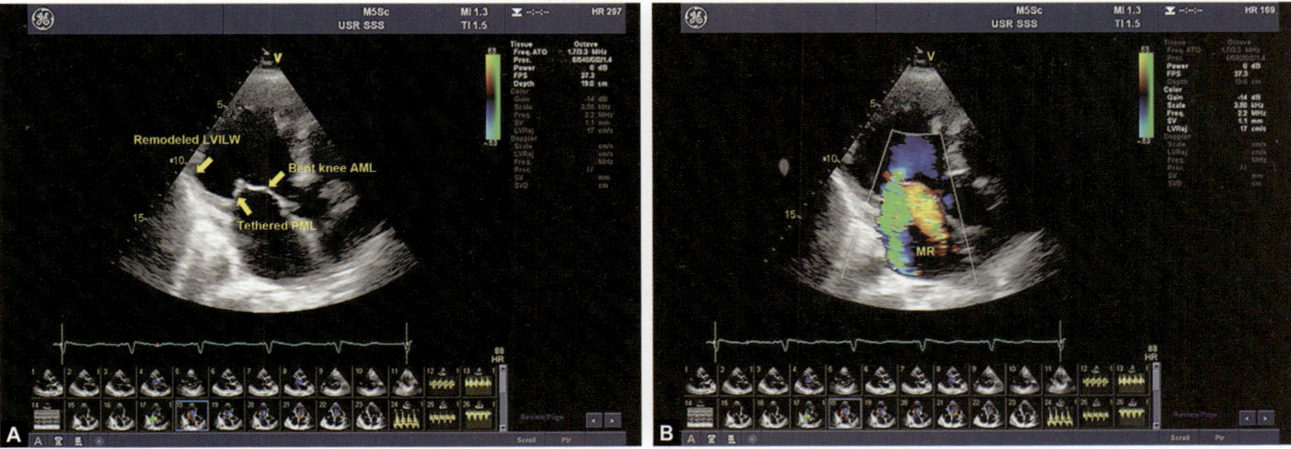

Figs. 18A and B: (A) 2D appearance of asymmetrical tethering of anterior mitral leaflet (AML) induced by dyskinetic LV posterior wall; (B) Color Doppler showing typical eccentric MR due to posterior mitral leaflet (PML) tethering.

both leaflets causing central MR is likely to indicate that MR is functional (after a large anterior wall infarction or in DCM).

Nearly, 10% of patients with hypertrophic cardiomyopathy (HCM) may exhibit progressive wall thinning, dilatation of LV with impairment of systolic performance-the so called burnt out phase of HCM. Diagnosis of this condition will be straight forward, if previously done echocardiograms are available for comparison.

Ischemic cardiomyopathy (ICM), if strictly defined, refers to only those who manifest global hypokinesia of LV after a focal infarction, without documented ischemia in other territories. For example, after a small inferior wall MI as an initial insult, rest of the left ventricle may develop remodeling in the absence of coronary artery disease of these remote segments of LV, possibly in response to mechanical stretch and or activated neurohormonal system. However, the term is now loosely applied to any DCM phenotype occurring in patients with coronary artery disease-after multiple infarctions involving different coronary artery territories or as a result of hibernation induced by chronic diffuse ischemia (without infarction) in a patient with multivessel disease. Differentiation from idiopathic DCM is not always possible. But the presence of regional thinning or scarring (Figs. 19A and B) or differential wall motion in relation to the respective coronary artery territories (for e.g. one segment hypokinetic, other segment akinetic) may suggest ICM. DSE may help to identify ICM, if at least 2 segments of LV demonstrate biphasic response i.e., initial improvement followed by worsening of wall motion. Atherosclerotic narrowing of proximal coronaries if demonstrable by echo may at times be helpful. Presence of dyskinetic segments or LV aneurysm makes the diagnosis of ICM more likely. If there is regional remodeling of LV associated with typical features of asymmetrical tethering

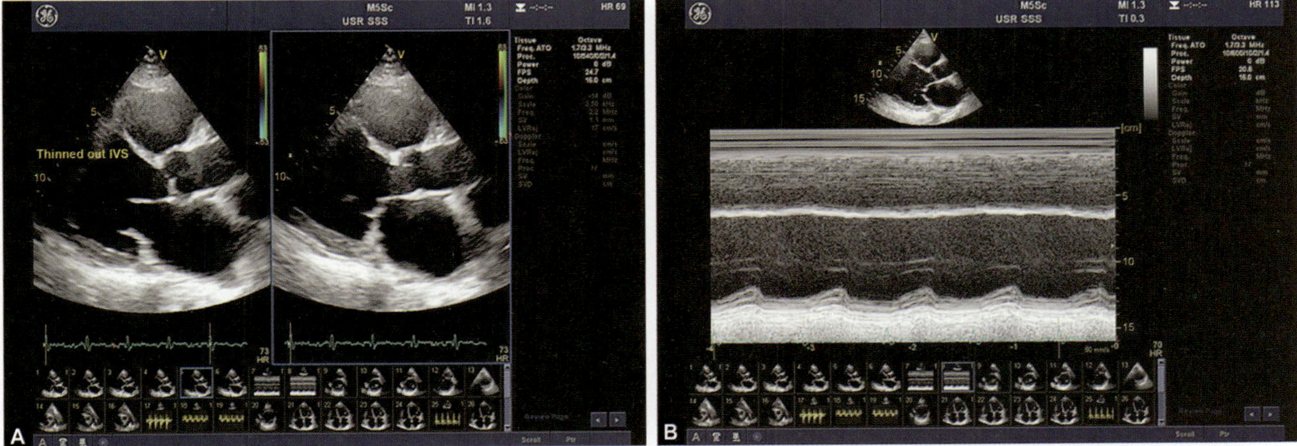

Figs. 19A and B: Thinned scarred interventricular septum (IVS) in ischemic DCM; (B) M-mode depiction of thinned scarred IVS in a patient with ischemic cardiomyopathy.

of mitral leaflets with an eccentric MR jet, ICM may be considered. Because of the potential for near total reversal of disease by revascularization, ICM should be ruled out at any cost in all those who manifest as DCM. To this effect, coronary angiography should be considered as a part of evaluation to identify ICM even if there are no clues in echo, particularly in the presence of multiple atherosclerotic risk factors. It should be noted that reverse remodeling with routine disease modifying agents of heart failure, does not rule out ICM.

The following echo findings should alert the physician regarding the possibility of conditions that could mimic idiopathic DCM. Significant LVH may be due to hypertensive heart disease, transition phase of HCM to DCM phenotype or infiltrative diseases like amyloid. Segmental wall motion abnormalities corresponding to coronary artery distribution, regional thinning and fibrosis, Dyskinesia or aneurysm, and biphasic response in at least 2 segments in DSE or extensive ischemic response in high dose DSE, may suggest ischemic DCM. Regional wall motion abnormalities not corresponding to coronary artery distribution or aneurysms in unusual locations may suggest myocarditis, sarcoidosis, left dominant arrhythmogenic cardiomyopathy. When there is poor LV function with near normal sized ventricles, one should consider restrictive cardiomyopathy in differential diagnosis. Combined phenotype of restrictive cum minimally DCM may raise the possibility of hemochromatosis.

Screening family members: All the first degree relatives of probands with idiopathic DCM should have echo screening once in 3–5 years or earlier if symptoms appear. Those who manifest mild LV dilatation but preserved EF need close follow-up as this could represent an early phase of the disease. In such circumstances abnormal tissue Doppler and 2D strain imaging parameters identify preclinical disease.

Detection of latent (preclinical) disease: This is required to identify those who are likely to develop LV dysfunction during cancer chemotherapy as well as while screening family members. A reduction of global longitudinal systolic strain of > 10% identify those who are likely to develop decline in LV function during cancer chemotherapy. Similarly, the gene carriers in families with DCM may exhibit reduction of strain. Moreover, 15–25% of family members of DCM proband may exhibit LV dilatation without alteration of LV function and 10–20% of such individuals develop DCM in the next 5 years.

Poor prognostic markers: Marked LV dilatation with LVESV > 25 mL/m^2, Involvement of basal inferior and inferolateral wall which is usually spared in the early phase of disease, very low EF < 25%, thinning of myocardial segments, abnormal sphericity index, irreversible grade III diastolic dysfunction of LV, abnormally, low TDI s' < 4 cm/s, increased LA volume, Presence of severe MR, pulmonary hypertension, RV dysfunction and inter and intraventricular dyssynchrony are some of the poor prognostic markers identified by echo.

CONCLUSION

Echocardiography plays a comprehensive role in prompt diagnosis of the disease, identification of complications like MR and LV thrombus and prognostication. Newer, echo parameters like 2D strain may help in identifying the disease in preclinical phase which has practical implications in family screening and identifying myocardial vulnerability to cancer chemotherapeutic agents. Serial studies help us to refine prognosis, and to identify reverse remodeling. Though not having an essential role in identifying responders to CRT, echo may be of help in appropriate programming of CRT to achieve optimal hemodynamic status.

REFERENCES

1. Japp AG, Gulati A, Cook SA. The diagnosis and evaluation of dilated cardiomyopathy. J Am Coll Cardiol. 2016;67(25): 2996-3010.
2. Mathew T, Williams L, Navaratnam G. Diagnosis and assessment of dilated cardiomyopathy: a guideline protocol from the British Society of Echocardiography. Echo Res Pract. 2017;4(2):G1-13.
3. Bansal M, Mohan JC, Sengupta SP. Normal echocardiographic measurements in Indian adults: How different are we from the western populations? A pilot study. Indian Heart J. 2016;68(6):772-5.
4. McManus DD, Shah SJ, Fabi MR. Prognostic value of left ventricular end-systolic volume index as a predictor of heart failure hospitalization in stable coronary artery disease: data from the heart and soul study. J Am Soc Echocardiogr. 2009;22(2):190-7.
5. Di Donato M, Dabic P, Castelvecchio S. Left ventricular geometry in normal and post-anterior myocardial infarction patients: sphericity index and 'new' conicity index comparisons. Euro J Cardio-Thorac Surg. 2006;29(Suppl 1): S225-30.
6. Tischler MD, Niggel J, Borowski DT, et al. Relation between left ventricular shape and exercise capacity in patients with left ventricular dysfunction. J Am Coll Cardiol. 1993;22:751-7.
7. Nagueh SF, Otto AS, Appleton CP. Recommendations for the evaluation of left ventricular diastolic function by echocardiography: an update from the American Society of Echocardiography and the European Association of Cardiovascular Imaging. J Am Soc Echocardiogr. 2016;29(4):277-314.
8. Naqvi TS, Goel RK, Forrester JS, et al. Myocardial contractile reserve on dobutamine echocardiography predicts late

spontaneous improvement in cardiac function in patients with recent onset idiopathic dilated cardiomyopathy. J Am Coll Cardiol. 1999;34(5):1537-44.
9. Ida K, Sersu MF, Fujieda K. Pathologic significance of left ventricular hypertrophy in dilated cardiomyopathy. Clin Cardiol. 1996;19(9):704-8.
10. Niemann M, Gaudron PD, Bijnens B. Differentiation between fresh and old left ventricular thrombi by deformation imaging. Cir Cardiovasc Imag. 2012;5(5):667-5.
11. Dan Liu KH, Herrmann S, Niemann M. Clinical implication of mitral annular plane systolic excursion for patients with cardiovascular disease. Eur Heart J Cardiovasc Imag. 2013;14(3):205-12.
12. Galrinho A, Branco L, Soares R. Prognostic implications of tissue Doppler in patients with dilated cardiomyopathy. Rev Port Cardiol. 2006;25(9):781-93.
13. Zambon E, Lorio A, Berton E. Tissue Doppler imaging and cardiopulmonary testing: insight into idiopathic dilated cardiomyopathy. Eur Heart J. 2013;34:1190.
14. Gulati VK, Katz WE, Follansbee WP, et al. Mitral annular descent velocity by tissue Doppler echocardiography as an index of global left ventricular function. Am J Cardiol. 1996;77(11):979-84.
15. Park YS, Park JH, Ahn KT. Usefulness of mitral annular systolic velocity in the detection of left ventricular systolic dysfunction: comparison with three dimensional echocardiographic data. J Cardiovasc Ultrasound. 2010;18(1):1-5.
16. Sengeløv M, Jørgensen PD, Jensen JS, et al. Global longitudinal strain is a superior predictor of all-cause mortality in heart failure with reduced ejection fraction. JACC Cardiovasc Imaging. 2015;8(12):1351-9.
17. Haugaa KH, Goebel B, Dahlslett T. Risk assessment of ventricular arrhythmias in patients with nonischemic dilated cardiomyopathy by strain echocardiography. J Am Soc Echocardiogr. 2012;25(6):667-73.
18. Gorcsan J 3rd, Abraham T, Agler DA, et al. Echocardiography for cardiac resynchronization therapy: Recommendations for performance and reporting–a report from the American Society of Echocardiography Dyssynchrony Writing Group Endorsed by the Heart Rhythm Society. J Am Soc Echocardiogr. 2008;21(3):191-213.
19. Kapetanakis S, Kearney MT, Siva A, et al. Real-time three-dimensional echocardiography: A novel technique to quantify global left ventricular mechanical dyssynchrony. Circulation. 2005;112(7):992-1000.
20. Merlo M, Caiffa T, Gobbo M. Reverse remodeling in dilated cardiomyopathy: Insights and future perspectives. Int J Cardiol Heart Vasc. 2018;18:52-7.
21. Naqvi TS, Goel RK, Forrester JS, et al. Myocardial contractile reserve on dobutamine echocardiography predicts late spontaneous improvement in cardiac function in patients with recent onset idiopathic dilated cardiomyopathy. J Am Coll Cardiol. 1999;34(5):1537-44.
22. Neskovic AN, Otasevic P. Stress-echocardiography in idiopathic dilated cardiomyopathy: instructions for use. Cardiovasc Ultrasound. 2005;3:3.
23. Sveric KM, Ulbrich S, Rady M. Repetitive squatting exercise as a diagnostic predictor in patients with dilated cardiomyopathy. BMJ Open Heart. 2018;10:1136.

CHAPTER

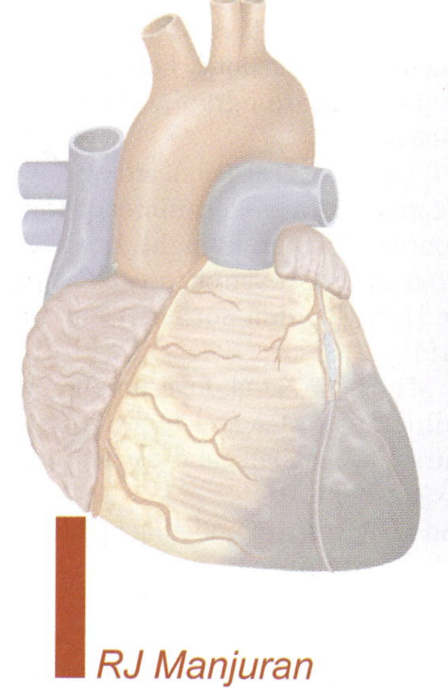

Hypertrophic Obstructive Cardiomyopathy with Heart Failure: Echocardiographic Evaluation

RJ Manjuran

INTRODUCTION

Hypertrophic cardiomyopathy (HCM) is the most common inherited structural heart disease. It is the most important underlying heart disease in young adults who die suddenly. Next to sudden cardiac death, the most important complication of HCM is heart failure (HF).[1] Echocardiography is the simplest, at the same time most useful, investigation to evaluate HF in patients of HCM.

HEART FAILURE IN HYPERTROPHIC CARDIOMYOPATHY

Heart failure in HCM may be due to one of the following mechanisms:[2]

- Progressive systolic left ventricular (LV) dysfunction leading to reduced ejection fraction (EF) and systolic heart failure
- Left ventricular outflow obstruction leading to HF
- Nonobstructive HCM presenting as diastolic HF or heart failure with preserved EF.

Echocardiographic Features of Hypertrophic Cardiomyopathy with Heart Failure

The main echocardiographic features of HCM are thickened interventricular septum with speckled appearance, dynamic LV outflow obstruction, reduced LV end systolic volume, LV diastolic dysfunction, dilated left atrium, and systolic anterior motion of mitral valve with mitral regurgitation (Figs. 1 to 4).

A small percentage of patients of HCM with severe myocardial fibrosis and microvasculopathy can progress to LV wall thinning, LV dilatation, reduced EF, and systolic heart failure.[3] Some patients can have preserved EF till quite late in the progression of the disease process. In few of these patients, the LV outflow gradient can reduce or even disappear. These patients are burned out cases of HCM and have poor prognosis and are candidates for cardiac transplantation. Systolic dysfunction and heart failure in HCM can be with/without LV chamber remodeling.[4]

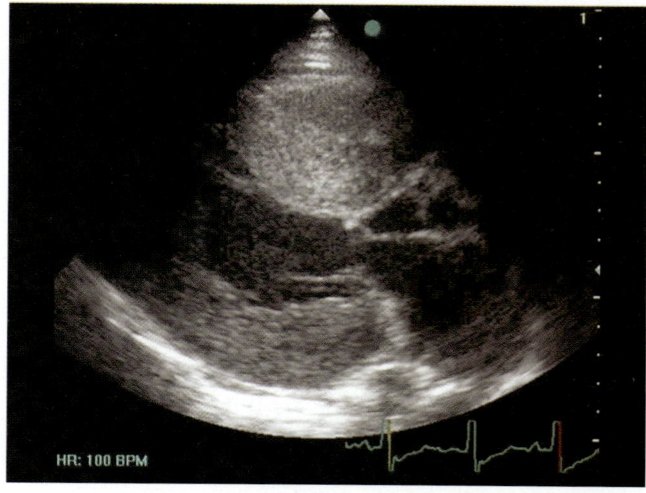

Fig. 1: Hypertrophic cardiomyopathy showing hypertrophied myocardium and systolic anterior motion of mitral valve.

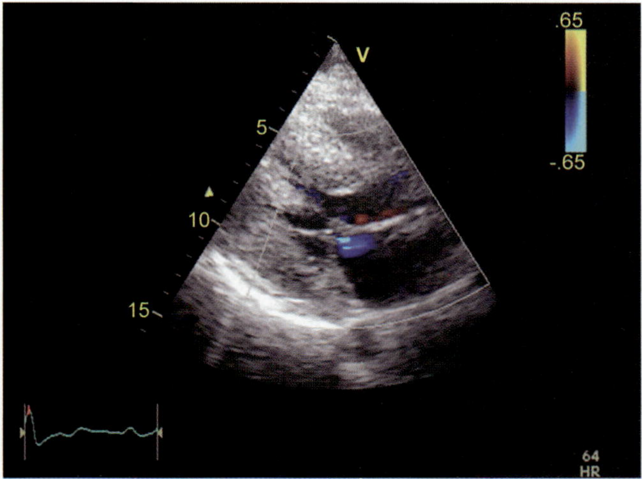

Fig. 2: Mitral regurgitation in hypertrophic cardiomyopathy.

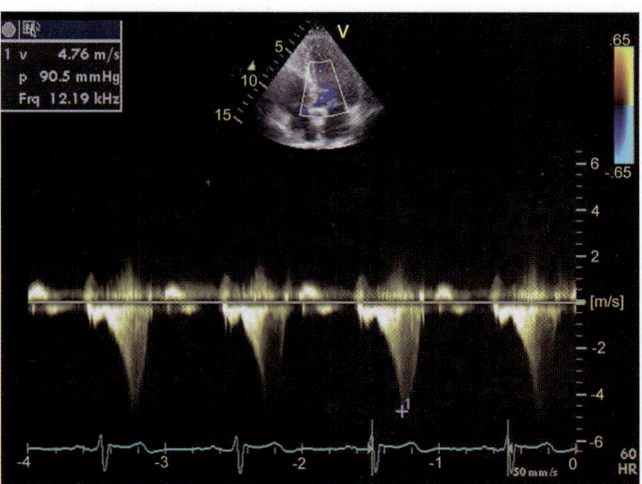

Fig. 3: Hypertrophic cardiomyopathy showing LV outflow gradient.

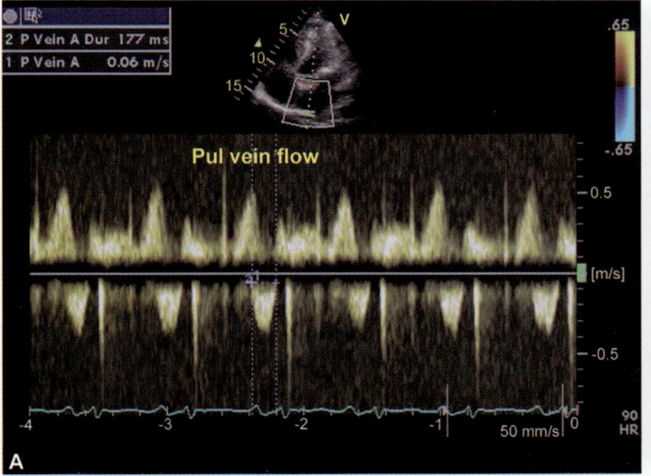

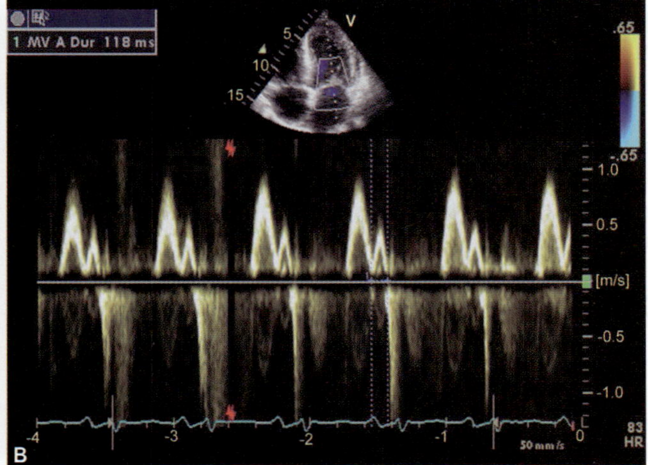

Figs. 4A and B: Mitral (M) flow and pulmonary venous (PV) flow. "a" reversal in PV flow is longer than "A" wave in M flow indicating LV diastolic dysfunction.

In 90% of patients of HCM, the main echocardiographic observation predisposing for HF is LV outflow obstruction at rest and/or with exercise. These patients will have elevated LV systolic pressure. This can result in increase in already existing mitral regurgitation and further worsening of HF.[5,6] However, there is no direct correlation between LV outflow gradient and development of HF in HCM as patients with significant resting gradients (>50 mm of Hg) can remain asymptomatic for long periods.[7,8] However, most of the patients of HCM who develop HF have resting and/or exercise LV outflow tract gradient of >50 mm of Hg. In view of associated LV diastolic dysfunction resulting in elevated LV end diastolic pressure and left atrial (LA) pressure, these patients can develop pulmonary arterial hypertension.

Third group of patients with HCM developing HF are those with preserved LV function without obstruction.[9] These patients have echocardiographic evidence of diastolic dysfunction. E/e' ratio can be elevated >15 indicating elevated LV filling pressures. Echocardiographic assessment of LV filling pressures can be done during exercise in those with normal diastolic function in the resting state. Approximately 50% patients of HCM with end stage heart failure have diastolic dysfunction with preserved systolic function.[8] Patients of this group have greater LA size compared to patients with LV outflow obstruction.[2]

Echocardiography can detect LA clots attached to LA appendage in patients of HCM in HF.[2]

Left Atrial Volume Index

Various factors like LV diastolic dysfunction, LV systolic dysfunction, LV outflow obstruction, LV chamber hypertrophy, atrial fibrillation and/or mitral regurgitation contribute to increased LA volume index in patients of HCM. LA volume index if >27 mL/m^2 BSA is correlated with adverse outcome in HCM including development of HF.[10,11] LA anteroposterior dementia >48 mm is associated with HF.[11]

Global Longitudinal Strain by Speckle Tracking

Global longitudinal strain (GLS) in HCM is correlated with the degree of fibrosis and LV wall thickness. Patients of HCM with greater degree of fibrosis have reduced GLS.[12] LV fibrosis in HCM predispose for LV dysfunction and development of HF.[13] GLS can be abnormal even in patients with normal EF.

Role of Transesophageal Echocardiography

In patient of HCM, transthoracic echocardiography can provide most of the information related to structural abnormality. However, transesophageal echocardiography (TEE) is useful to assess the mitral valve apparatus-systolic anterior motion, mitral regurgitation, and chordal and leaflet abnormalities.[14] In these patients of HCM suspected to have structural abnormality of mitral valve, TEE may be performed.

CONCLUSION

Next to sudden cardiac death, HF is the most important complication of HCM. Three pathological mechanisms predispose for HF in HCM. Echocardiography can detect the structural abnormalities associated with HF. GLS can be abnormal in patients of HCM with normal EF. These patients have increased myocardial fibrosis and future HF. TEE can be of use in patients of HCM with structural abnormality of mitral valve. Echocardiography with Doppler and GLS evaluation is the simplest and most useful investigation for the assessment of patients of HCM in HF.

REFERENCES

1. Maron BJ. Hypertrophic cardiomyopathy: a systematic review. JAMA. 2002;287:1308-20.
2. Melacini P, Basso C, Angelini A, et al. Clinicopathological profiles of progressive heart failure in hypertrophic cardiomyopathy. Eur Heart J. 2010;31(17):2111-23.
3. Ciro E, Maron BJ, Bonow RO, et al. Relation between marked changes in left ventricular outflow gradient and disease progression in hypertrophic cardiomyopathy. Am J Cardiol. 1984;53(8):1103-9.
4. Harris KM, Spirito P, Maron MS, et al. Prevalence, clinical profile, and significance of left ventricular remodeling in the end-stage phase of hypertrophic cardiomyopathy. Circulation. 2006;114:216-25.
5. Maron BJ, Rowin EJ, Casey SA, et al. How hypertrophic cardiomyopathy became a contemporary treatable genetic disease with low mortality: shaped by 50 years of clinical research and practice. JAMA Cardiol. 2016;1(1):98-105.
6. Authors/Task Force members, Elliott PM, Anastasakis A, et al. 2014 ESC Guidelines on diagnosis and management of hypertrophic cardiomyopathy: the Task Force for the Diagnosis and Management of Hypertrophic Cardiomyopathy of the European Society of Cardiology (ESC). Eur Heart J. 2014;35(39):2733-79.
7. Gersh BJ, Maron BJ, Bonow RO, et al. 2011 ACCF/AHA guideline for the diagnosis and treatment of hypertrophic cardiomyopathy: executive summary: a report of the American College of Cardiology Foundation/American Heart Association Task Force on Practice Guidelines. Circulation. 2011;124(24):2761-96.
8. Maron MS, Olivotto I, Betocchi S, et al. Effect of left ventricular outflow tract obstruction on clinical outcome in hypertrophic cardiomyopathy. N Engl J Med. 2003;348(4):295-303.
9. Maron MS, Rowin EJ, Olivotto I, et al. Contemporary natural history and management of nonobstructive hypertrophic cardiomyopathy. J Am Coll Cardiol. 2016;67(12):1399-409.
10. Yang WI, Shim CY, Kim YJ, et al. Left atrial volume index: A predictor of adverse outcome in patients with hypertrophic cardiomyopathy. J Am Soc Echocardiogr. 2009;22(12):1338-43.
11. Chun S, Woo A. Echocardiography in hypertrophic cardiomyopathy: In with strain, out with straining? J Am Soc Echocardiogr. 2015;28(2):204-9.
12. Popovic ZB, Kwon DH, Mishra M, et al. Association between regional ventricular function and myocardial fibrosis in hypertrophic cardiomyopathy assessed by speckle tracking echocardiography and delayed hyperenhancement magnetic resonance imaging. J Am Soc Echocardiogr. 2008;21(12):1299-305.
13. Moon JC, McKenna WJ, McCrohon JA, et al. Toward clinical risk assessment in hypertrophic cardiomyopathy with gadolinium cardiovascular magnetic resonance. J AM Coll Cardiol. 2003;41(9):1561-7.
14. Widimsky P, Ten Cate FJ, Vletter W, et al. Potential applications for transesophageal echocardiography in hypertrophic cardiomyopathies. J Am Soc Echocardiogr. 1992;5(2):163-7.

CHAPTER

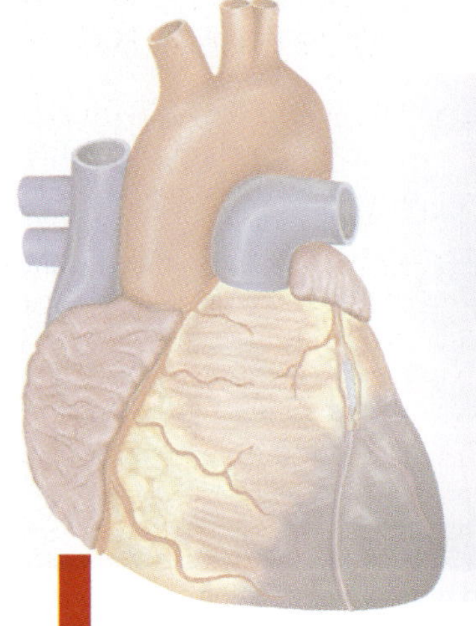

Echocardiographic Pericardial Effusion Evaluation in Heart Failure

Bantwal Vivek Baliga, Satish C Govind

INTRODUCTION

Pericardial effusion (PE) is an infrequent finding in patients with heart failure, while pleural effusions are more common (87%). Small PE's can be seen in about 12–20% of patients with heart failure during echocardiography while moderate PE is uncommon.[1] Clinical presentation can range from patients being asymptomatic (even with moderate effusion) to presenting as cardiac tamponade. In chronic heart failure the size of the PE correlates poorly with the hemodynamic effect it has on the heart.[2] Even small PE is associated with adverse events like all-cause mortality, cardiac mortality and indication for heart transplantation. In patients who present with acute heart failure, presence of significant PE (moderate) with no hemodynamic impact has increased mortality at 1 year.[3] To further complicate matters, there are numerous other conditions that lead to PE which can coexist in heart failure patients. In this chapter, we discuss PE in heart failure by looking at it from different perspectives and focusing on some of its unresolved issues. The pericardium of the heart consists of two layers—the inner visceral pericardium, attached to the epicardial surface of the heart and—the outer parietal pericardium. In between these two layers is present less than 50 mL of plasma ultrafiltrate in normal individuals. Any amount above this value is considered abnormal and characterized as mild, moderate or severe PE (Figs. 1 and 2) depending on the amount that accumulates (Table 1). As an initial investigative test, echocardiography is the preferred imaging modality to screen and detect individuals for PE. In fact, the need for diagnosis of PE to be differentiated from a dilated heart was the main object of interest when echocardiography was first introduced.[4,5] Estimation of an approximate quantity of PE through echocardiography has become standard practice. When seen, grading of severity of PE can be of help in assessing prognosis of patients. PE can present as circumferential, localized (Fig. 3) or loculated, while it can also be characterized as transudate (hydropericardium or noninflammatory fluid) or exudate. Less often the nature of the effusion as seen on echocardiography may provide a clue towards its etiology.

PATHOPHYSIOLOGY

Pericardial effusion in heart failure can present as an isolated entity or it can be associated with systemic disorders like hypothyroid, cancer, etc. and myocardial abnormalities like infarction, myocarditis, etc. One should

TABLE 1: Assessment of pericardial effusion by echocardiography.

Severity	*Pericardial fluid thickness (mm)*	*Estimated pericardial fluid (mL)*
Trivial	Seen in systole alone	<50
Measured in diastole		
Mild (small)	<10	50–100
Moderate	10–20	100–500
Severe (large)	>20	>500
Very large	>25	>700

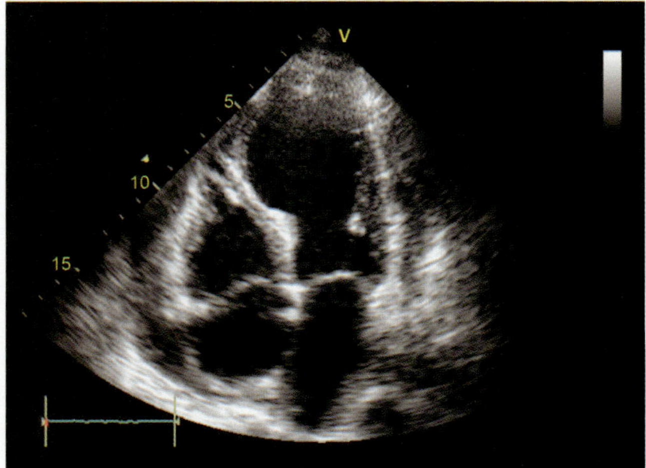

Fig. 1: Mild pericardial effusion.

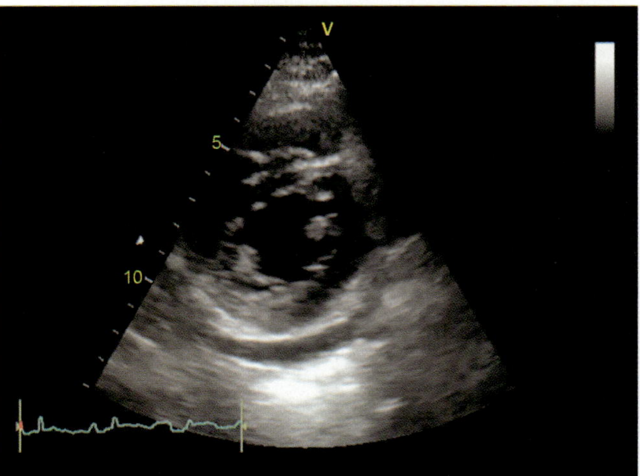

Fig. 3: Localized pericardial effusion.

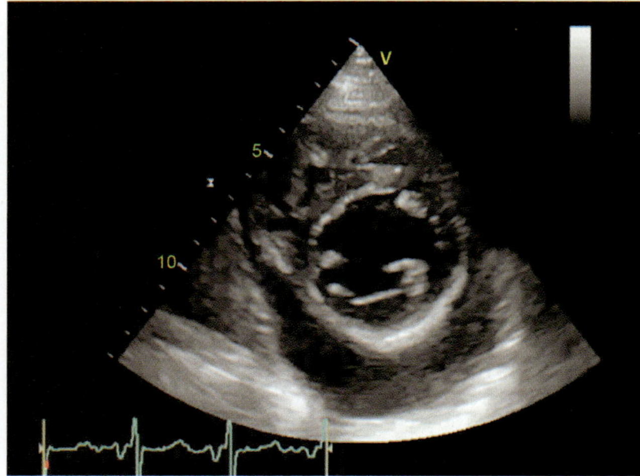

Fig. 2: Large pericardial effusion.

note that PE associated with congestive heart failure (CHF) is rarely severe. When inflammation of the pericardium occurs as in tuberculosis, it usually leads to exudative PE, while in severe hypoalbuminemia and CHF transudate is seen. Normally, fluid movement in and out of the pericardial space happens among numerous microvascular exchange barriers involving circulatory and lymphatic systems.[6] The formation of pericardial fluid happens with ultrafiltration of plasma across the capillaries of the epicardium and pericardium along with the fluid of the interstitium of the myocardium which courses through the epicardium. On the other hand, the pericardial fluid is drained out by the lymphatic system mainly along the parietal layer and to a lesser extent from the epicardial surface. The pathophysiology behind the production and drainage of pericardial fluid is that abnormal PE's are a consequence of imbalance between the rates of fluid accumulation in the pericardial cavity to the rate of fluid resorption. In CHF, abnormal pericardial fluid accumulation is explained as secondary to altered production and drainage of fluid via the venous and lymphatic channels when exposed to higher hemodynamic pressures.

MECHANISMS

- Congestive heart failure is often attributed to left ventricular (LV) dysfunction, where advanced cases eventually result in chronic pulmonary venous hypertension. Over time, this leads to pulmonary arterial hypertension (PAH) and right ventricular (RV) dysfunction, both of which are predictors of worsening prognosis.
- Available literature suggests that in CHF, PE is associated with more of increased RV filling pressures (higher pressures are present more on the right side) rather than the increased LV filling pressure.
- Pericardial effusion in CHF is a common accompaniment in patients with coexistent PAH. While the exact mechanisms remain unclear, right heart catheterization evaluations have demonstrated a direct correlation between mean right atrial pressures (RAP) and PE.
- Elevated RAP of >13 mm Hg causes increased pressure in the coronary sinus. This leads to increase in the filtration with consequent increase in the volume of pericardial fluid.
- Similarly, elevated systolic blood pressure increases filtration of plasma across the parietal pericardium capillaries, while raised diastolic blood pressure increases filtration of plasma across the coronary capillaries.
- Increased systemic venous pressure can cause higher pressure in the lymphatic ducts and thoracic ducts, thus

BOX 1: Proposed mechanisms causing pericardial effusion in heart failure.

Mechanisms causing pericardial effusion
- Increased right atrial pressure
- Increased systemic venous pressure
- Increased right ventricular filling pressure
- Increased systemic systolic and diastolic blood pressure
- Pulmonary hypertension
- Right ventricular dilatation and dysfunction
- Significant tricuspid regurgitation

reducing the amount of lymphatic drainage from the pericardial cavity.

- Thus, two or more factors (Box 1) can alter the dynamics and influence fluid movement in the pericardial space (also the pleural space as both share a common pathway). Interestingly, one study looking at patients with LV systolic dysfunction with or without PE found a good correlation between increased RV diastolic internal dimension with increased RV filling pressure and the presence of pericardial effusion. The dilated RV likely alters the pressure and volume dynamics affecting the venous and lymphatic drainage.[7]
- Pericardial effusion when present in CHF has also been looked as representative of RV dysfunction and this is generally associated with severe or advanced phase of heart failure.
- Frohlich and his group[2] in their study of 897 patients having chronic heart failure due to LV failure showed that even PE's with no hemodynamic effects had an increased risk of death and need for transplantation.

OTHER PARAMETERS

Looking at other parameters, heart failure patients with PE are seen having higher levels of N-terminal-probrain natriuretic peptide (NT-proBNP) which increases their risk levels which in turn exposes them to more unfavorable events. Increased levels of BNP in pericardial fluid has also been studied where worse grades of LV diastolic dysfunction and also mild LV dilatation in heart failure were associated with higher levels of BNP.[8] Associated systemic diseases with their inflammatory responses (reflected by increased leukocyte count and C-reactive proteins) increase capillary permeability adding one more causative layer to the complex mechanism causing PE.

ASSOCIATED PLEURAL EFFUSION

Significant PE when associated with significant pleural effusion has been shown to have no quantitative association between the two.[1] There is scant data on this, with one experimental study showing that increased pericardial effusion is more likely to be seen with systemic venous hypertension, increased RAP, increased RV filling pressure and right heart failure than pulmonary venous hypertension caused by increased LV filling pressure. An acute increase in RV filling pressure (>15 mm Hg) or LV filling pressure (>18 mm Hg) is explained as the likely cause for pleural effusion. An exact mechanism of how fluid accumulates in both pericardial and pleural cavities is still not known. It has been suggested that CHF with PE is more likely to be associated with right pleural effusion or bilateral effusion, while presence of left pleural effusion especially in the absence of heart disease favors PE due to a pericardial cause. Increased RV filling pressure is less commonly observed, than elevated LV filling pressure which explains the reason why PE occurs less often than pleural effusion.

IMAGING MODALITIES

Multiple imaging modalities are available to evaluate PE. Echocardiography remains to date the preferred approach and a convenient way to detect PE. It is widely available, an easy method and a reliable way to make an initial assessment of the location and severity of the effusion. It also provides for physiological and hemodynamic effects it might exert on the cardiac function. Other imaging modalities include cardiac computed tomography and cardiac magnetic resonance imaging, and a detailed discussion regarding these is beyond the scope of this chapter.

Assessment by Echocardiography

The primary advantage of echocardiography in evaluating a PE lies in the simplicity and speed it brings with it. Bedside evaluations can be performed even in emergency situations, and accurate assessments can dictate life-saving therapies. PE can be defined as an echo free space between the epicardium and pericardium. In patients with heart failure, an anterior echo free space with no posterior PE is unlikely to be effusion and more likely to be epicardial fat.[9] PE can be hemodynamically significant when it is characterized by paradoxical movement of the interventricular septum, chamber compression and increased respiratory variation of Doppler velocities of inflow into the ventricles.

When performing echocardiographic evaluation of PE, certain points need to be borne in mind:

- Quantifying PE is helpful in not just making a diagnosis but also in determining prognosis. Trivial PE's when seen during ventricular systole have no clinical significance. However, small and persistent PE's in heart failure are independently associated with an increased risk of adverse events. It is, therefore, important that this finding is identified, monitored during follow-up and mentioned in the echocardiography report. Typically, PE's in heart failure are mild.

- The parasternal long axis view (PLAX) is a good view to estimate quantity posteriorly and anteriorly, though subcostal views are also helpful. However, care must be taken when using the latter view as the size of the effusion may be overestimated. Additionally, parasternal short axis and apical views are also of value when making a comprehensive evaluation.
- Bear in mind that pleural effusions often mimic PE's, and care must be taken to notice this especially in an emergency. Echocardiography in PLAX view can clearly delineate the space between the epicardium and the parietal pericardium where the presence of fluid between the descending thoracic aorta and the heart indicates a PE. In contrast, a pleural effusion can be seen to be outside the descending thoracic aorta.
- In an emergency, using a subcostal view is often enough to achieve a goal of establishing presence or absence of PE and detecting any possible chamber compression.
- M-mode echocardiography may also be used when assessing the thickness of the echo free space.
- Doppler velocities of mitral and tricuspid inflow should be observed for significant variation which may suggest tamponade. Coexisting inferior vena cava dilatation and its noncollapsing nature further reinforces the diagnosis of tamponade.
- When evaluating any PE, signs of cardiac tamponade (Figs. 4 and 5) must be always be carefully observed. While uncommon in CHF, the presence of both right atrial and RV collapse is an important sign of tamponade.

While linear measures of PE volume estimation remain standard practice, the biplane disc method has been utilized as another technique of quantification. In one study of 126 patients scheduled to undergo pericardiocentesis, the pericardial and epicardial borders were traced in the 4-chamber view, and the difference in the two values was estimated as the quantity of effusion. These values were compared with the quantity of fluid drained. Compared to linear measurement, the biplane disc method demonstrated better correlation to the quantity of fluid.[10] Besides quantification, location of PE as either global or localized effusions and the nature of the fluid around the heart (transudative, exudative with intrapericardial fibrin and clotted blood) can be made based on the echo density of the fluid.

Presence of PE even if it has no hemodynamic effect is associated with 2-fold increase in death.[2] PE which continues to be present for long periods is associated with bad outcome (increased cardiac events) when compared with patients where PE has resolved. Heart failure patients with PE have a more reduced biventricular ejection fraction, increased atrial size with worse functional class. They especially have larger RV and right atrial dimensions, significant tricuspid regurgitation and more likely to have pulmonary hypertension.

CONCLUSION

The mechanism of PE is still debated, while its impact on prognosis is an area that is not well explained. The pathogenesis of PE is unclear, with most studies showing that it may be due to increased right heart pressures rather than the impact of elevated left sided pressures. To further

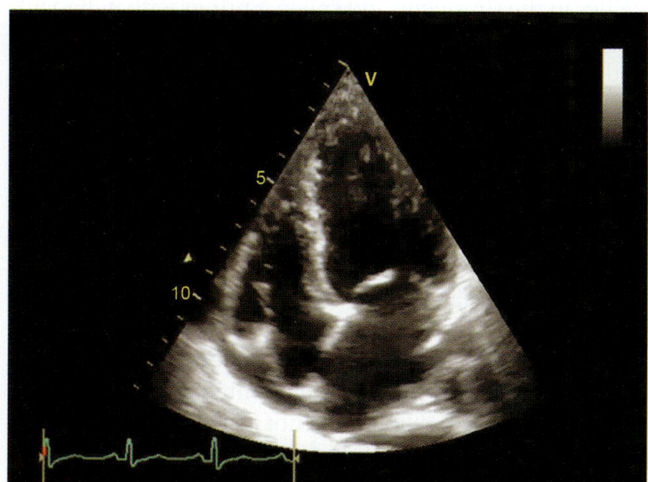

Fig. 4: Pericardial effusion with right atrial compression.

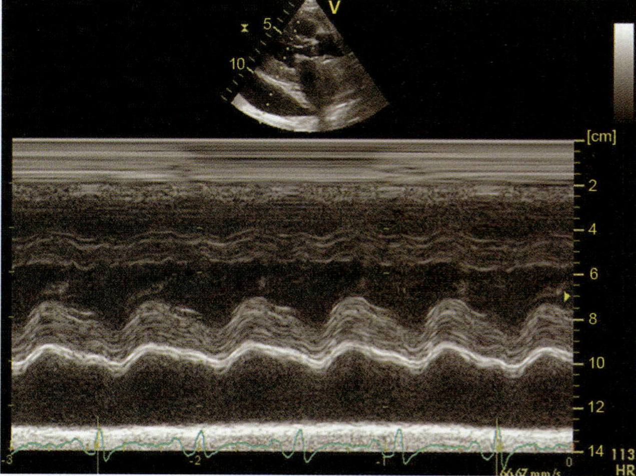

Fig. 5: M-mode showing large pericardial effusion with right ventricular diastolic collapse and paradoxical septal motion suggesting tamponade.

add complexity, PE in heart failure can be sometimes due to other systemic causes which coexist along with the disease specific associated inflammatory responses. Presence of PE is a marker of the underlying disease of CHF.[11]

The actual percentage of PE on echocardiography in heart failure patients is less with mild PE being seen more often. Adverse prognosis is more often associated with moderate PE, rather than small PE though there are reports that show even small effusions are associated with adverse prognosis. Even hemodynamically insignificant PE in heart failure patients has a worse prognosis when compared with those who do not have PE especially when they are persistent over a long period of time. What is not sure is whether larger effusions which tend to persist more are just associated mechanical sequelae caused by RV dysfunction and overloading or whether it has a deeper implication on the worsening prognosis of these high-risk patients. When seen PE has to be documented, co-related clinically and closely monitored for better management of CHF patients.

REFERENCES

1. Kataoka H. Pericardial and pleural effusions in decompensated chronic heart failure. Am Heart J. 2000;139(5):918-23.
2. Fröhlich GM, Keller P, Schmid F, et al. Haemodynamically irrelevant pericardial effusion is associated with increased mortality in patients with chronic heart failure. Eur. Heart J. 2013;34(19):1414-23.
3. Santas E, Sandino J, Chorro FJ, et al. Prognostic implications of pericardial effusion in acute heart failure: does size matter? Int J Cardiol. 2015;184:259-61.
4. Feigenbaum H, Waldhausen JA, Hyde LP. Ultrasound diagnosis of pericardial effusion. JAMA. 1965;191:711-14.
5. Winters WL Jr, Carter BL, Stauffer HM, et al. Pericardial effusion in congestive heart failure. Dis Chest. 1961;40:82-6.
6. Natanzon A, Kronzon I. Pericardial and pleural effusions in congestive heart failure-anatomical, pathophysiologic, and clinical considerations. Am J Med Sci. 2009;338(3):211-6.
7. Kessler KM, Rodriguez D, Rahim A, et al. Echocardiographic observations regarding pericardial effusions associated with cardiac disease. Chest. 1980;78(5):736-40.
8. Watanabe M, Kawaguchi S, Nakahara H, et al. The roles of natriuretic peptides in pericardial fluid in patients with heart failure. Clin Cardiol. 2009;32(3):159-63.
9. Yu SB, Zhao QY, Huang H, et al. Prognosis investigation in patients with chronic heart failure and pericardial effusion. Chin Med J (Engl). 2012;125(5):882-7.
10. DeMaria D, Waring A, Gregg D, et al. Echocardiographic assessment of pericardial effusion size: time for a quantitative approach. J Am Coll Cardiol. 2018;71(11):A1622.
11. De Filippo O, Gatti P, Rettegno S, et al. Is pericardial effusion a negative prognostic marker? Meta-analysis of outcomes of pericardial effusion. J Cardiovasc Med (Hagerstown). 2019;20(1):39-45.

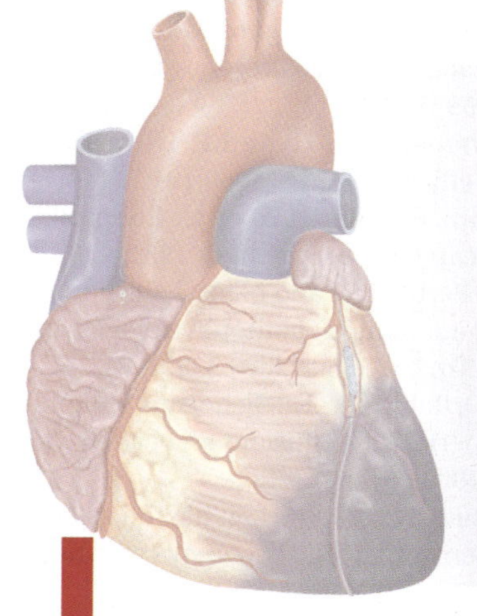

Echocardiographic Endomyocardial Fibrosis: Evaluation with Heart Failure

G Vijayaraghavan, S Sivasankaran

INTRODUCTION

Endomyocardial fibrosis (EMF) or Davies disease is a neglected tropical disease affecting subjects in low income countries with geographical predisposition, predominantly presenting as heart failure.[1] Endomyocardial deposition of fibrous tissue, leads to restrictive filling of the heart resulting in atrial dilatation and heart failure.[2] Though an acute, subacute and chronic phases are described in the natural history, most of the subjects come to clinical recognition in the late burnt-out phase or, are incidentally detected.[3] Recent community surveys with echocardiographic scanning has identified this disorder as the most common cardiac disorder in certain endemic areas. Improvement in socio-economic status has resulted in its virtual disappearance from the southern state of Kerala, India.[1,3] Prognosis is poor for subjects presenting with heart failure but the disease has generated lot of research in understanding the reaction pattern of the endocardium to circulating insults, and newer modalities of surgical treatment like endocardiectomy.[4] Public health efforts in improving the living standards can prevent the occurrence of this distressing malady but late presentation warrants, cardiac transplantation for improving survival.[5,6]

CONTENTS AND DESCRIPTION

Tropical EMF is a form of restrictive cardiomyopathy commonly found in some parts of the tropics and sporadically in other parts of the world.[3] It is an obliterative cardiomyopathy characterized by fibrotic thickening and obliteration of either right ventricle (RVEMF), left ventricle (LVEMF) or both ventricles (BVEMF) with a predilection to selectively involve the ventricular apices and inflow region and sparing the outflow tract.[7] The fibrotic process does not involve the valve leaflets per se, the atria, or the great vessels. Involvement of the atrioventricular sub-valvar apparatus in the fibrotic process plasters and hinders the leaflet mobility leading to progressive regurgitation. Figure 1 reflects the classical four chamber view of a subject with biventricular

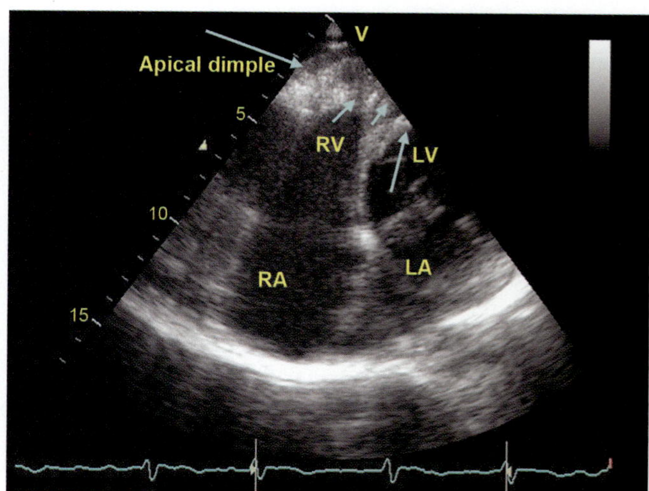

Fig. 1: Apical 4 chamber view from a patient with biventricular EMF. Note the fibrotic obliteration of both ventricular apices (short arrows). Endocardial calcification of the left ventricular apex is diagnostic of EMF (long arrow inside LV). Both atria are dilated.
(RA: right atrium; LA: left atrium: RV: right ventricle; LV: left ventricle)

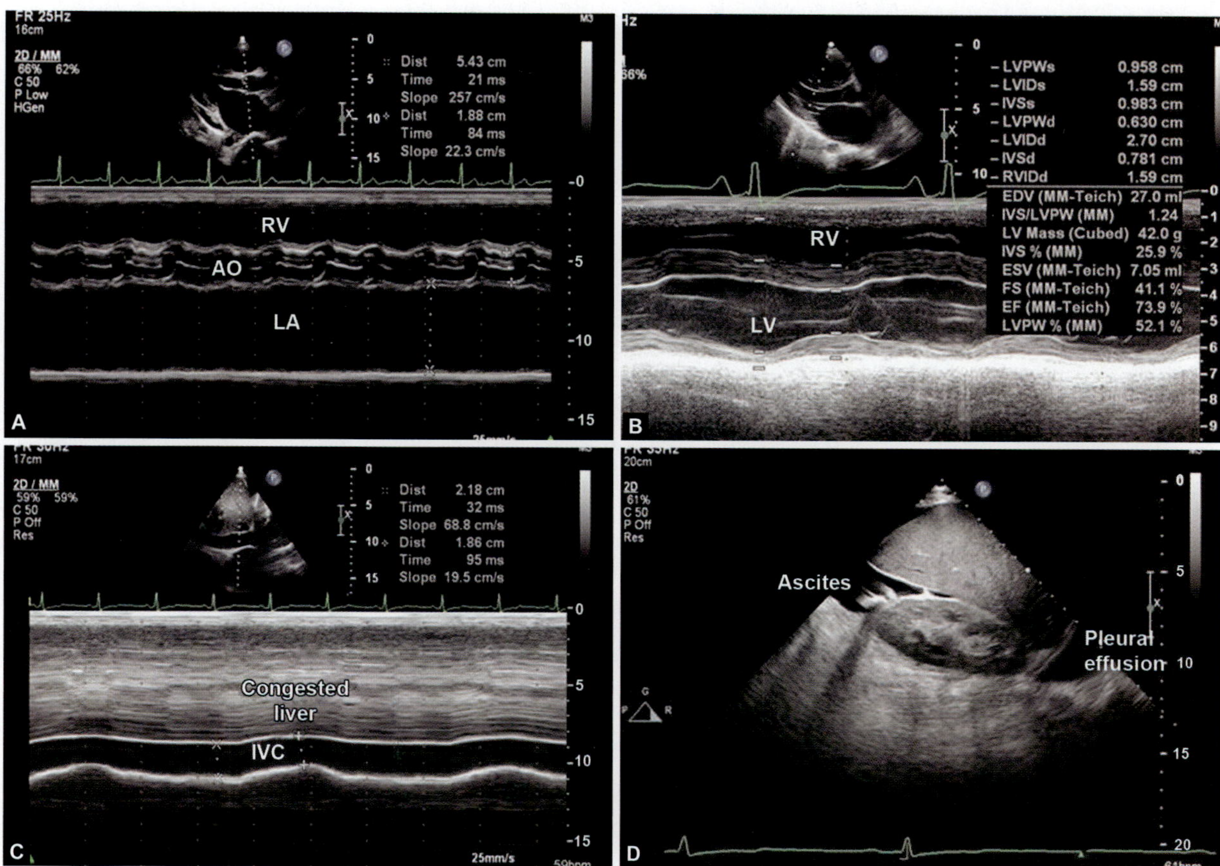

Figs. 2A to D: Typical echocardiographic features of left ventricular endomyocardial fibrosis. (A) The M-mode across the aorta (AO) and left atrium (LA) showing normal aortic valve and dilated left atrium; (B) The M-mode of the nondilated nonhypertrophied left ventricle (LV) with normal mitral valve movement and good systolic function; (C) The congested liver with dilated inferior vena cava (IVC) secondary to pulmonary arterial hypertension and right heart failure; (D) The other consequences like ascites and pleural effusion on tilting the transducer to abdomen.

endomyocardial fibrosis. The atria are disproportionately dilated giving an inverted owl-eye appearance and because of the dilated atria. The ventricular endocardium is thick and echogenic but the overall systolic function is good. Figure 2 shows the good left ventricular (LV) function on M-mode echocardiogram. Figure 3 shows 3D echocardiogram, unusually dilated atrial chambers with normal ventricular function. Finer aspects of M-mode echocardiography and Doppler interrogation are described in Figures 2 and 4.

Right Ventricular Endomyocardial Fibrosis

Right ventricular EMF, the most common form of the disease in many published report is readily diagnosed at the bedside in countries where, it is commonly seen.[8] The autopsy-proven cases had similar incidence of right ventricular (RV), LV and biventricular involvement.[3] When either of the ventricles are involved long-term follow up have not shown further extension of the disease to the other ventricle, possibly because of the abbreviated natural history. Atrial fibrillation, thromboembolic complications. Infective endocarditis and incidentally detected calcification on the skiagram are rare presentation which bring the patient to the clinician's attention (Figs. 5A to C). Isolated cases of RV inflow or outflow tract obstruction by fibrosis can occur, but are seen in occasional case reports.[3] Dominant or isolated RVEMF presents in an emaciated adolescent with cachexia, massive pericardial effusion and gross ascites (Fig. 5C). These types of early onset disease with aggressive clinical course is currently not seen in India but are reported elsewhere, in the world.[9] An occasional patient can have cyanosis with digital clubbing because of stretched open foramen ovale. This type of presentation needs to be differentiated from Ebstein's anomaly and the former from constrictive pericarditis.[10,11] The clinical presentation of the disorder can vary from asymptomatic incidental detection

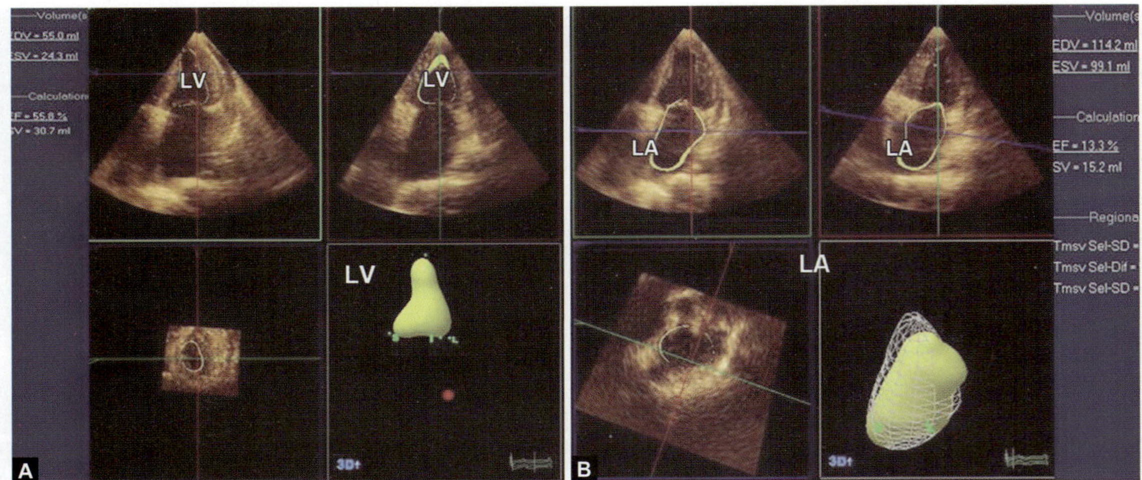

Figs. 3A and B: Three-dimensional volume rendered images in left ventricular (LV) endomyocardial fibrosis. Left ventricular volume measurements in panel A shows good left ventricular function and the left atrial (LA) volume measures on the right panel B shows the disproportionate atrial dilatation with left atrial systolic volume index more than 30 mL/m^2.

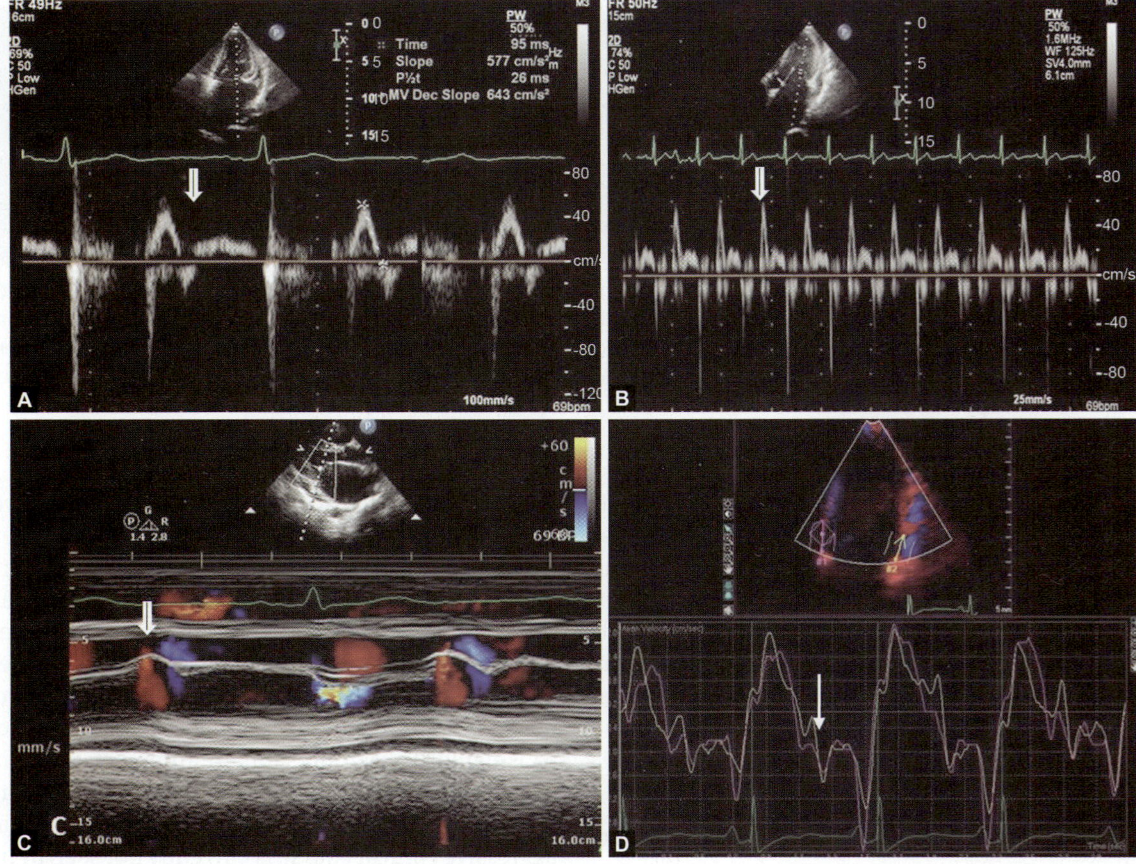

Figs. 4A to D: Mitral valve Doppler features of restrictive ventricular filling. Panel A shows prominent filling E waves (broad arrow) and declaration time is less than 130 milliseconds. Panel B shows a slow speed recording to document minimal variation in mitral inflow during respiration. Panel C: Colour M-mode across the mitral valve, shows monophasic mitral flow only in early diastole though the valve is open during most of the diastole reflecting pressure equalization between the atria and the ventricle. Panel D shows the tissue Doppler characteristics of the septal (violet) and lateral (yellow) mitral annulus. Contrary to blood flow, the tissue movement during early diastole (e') (slender arrow) is minimal with high E/e' ratio is > 15 reflecting high filling pressures which rapidly drives the initial blood flow into the ventricle.

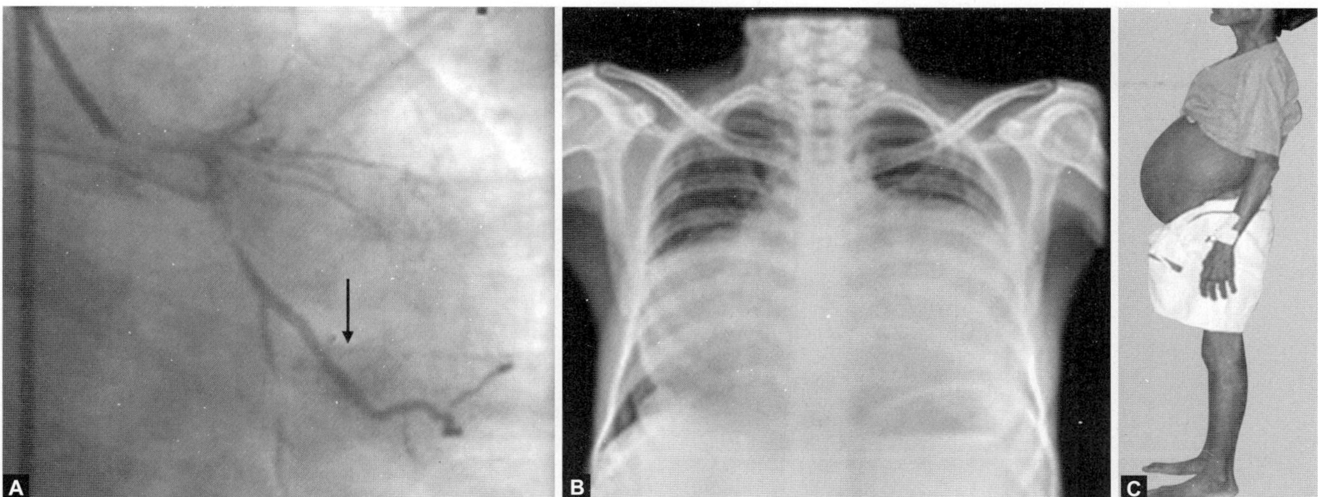

Figs. 5A to C: (A) Incidentally detected endocardial calcification in a 50-year-old male evaluated for coronary artery disease. EMF was confirmed at catheterization and angiography; (B) Massive cardiomegaly and pericardial effusion noted in the lady shown in the adjacent clinical picture; (C) Cardiac cachexia in a 30-year-old lady suffering from right ventricular EMF. Note the massive ascites and minimal pedal edema and dilated neck veins.

to massive ascites and cardiac cachexia. Development of ascites is out of proportion to the degree of pedal edema, as seen in Figure 5C, which could be inflammatory, could be a marker of a systemic disorder.[3]

In the initial report of EMF from Kerala, RV involvement was seen in 60% of patients, LV and biventricular involvement in 20% each.[12] There was slight female preponderance, and 50% of patients were in the second decade of life. Stunting of growth was prominent when the age group was below 20 years. Onset was insidious with facial puffiness and abdominal distention and half had leg edema. The classical clinical triad of RVEMF, viz. distended jugular veins, hepatomegaly and ascites was present in all the symptomatic subjects. Dependant edema when present did not bear any relation to the degree of ascites. The hepatomegaly was smooth, firm and nonpulsatile. Upper level of the distended neck veins could not be made out in many and prominent 'a' waves were present when in sinus rhythm. Cardiomegaly was massive extending from one midclavicular line to the other in 15% of the subjects. RV third sound and systolic murmur of tricuspid regurgitation were the auscultatory features.

Two-dimensional echocardiographic findings (Figs. 6A to D), are dominated by the aneurysmal right atrium. RV apex will be filled by dense fibrous mass which encroaches on to the inflow tract involving the chordopapillary structures of the tricuspid valve. RV cavity is shrunken with an apical notch to the right of interventricular groove due to the apical fibrosis pulling the RV apex inwards. Apex to tricuspid valve distance is reduced because of the apical obliteration and fibrosis. RV endocardial calcification is diagnostic. Fibrosis does not involve the outflow tract which becomes dilated and hyperdynamic. Late stages of the disease will show a common right atrial and ventricular cavity with low pressure tricuspid regurgitation as in Ebstein's anomaly. Slowing of the circulation with dynamic intracavitary echoes and right atrial thrombi are not uncommon. Inferior vena cava is markedly dilated and nonpulsatile. M-Mode of pulmonary valve may show atrial systolic opening of the pulmonary valve. Doppler reveals low pressure tricuspid regurgitation, which is often difficult to quantify.

Advanced RVEMF presents as severe systemic venous hypertension and right heart failure with ascites and pericardial effusion. Thin walled right ventricle allows the fibrotic retraction of the free wall which can now be identified as the RV dimple by imaging, and by morphology (Fig. 7).

Pulmonary arterial blood flow patterns can also be utilized to understand the RV function in isolated RVEMF as shown in Figure 8. Elevation of RV end diastolic pressures above the pulmonary arterial diastolic pressures will push open the pulmonary valve in atrial systole causing presystolic opening and forward flow into pulmonary artery which can be demonstrated by M-mode, pulse Doppler and color M-mode Doppler (Figs. 8A to C). In end stage RVEMF because of severe systemic venous congestion, RV diastolic pressures are more than pulmonary arterial diastolic pressures and early diastolic or pan diastolic forward flow into pulmonary artery can be demonstrated which is consistent with the paradox of Fontan circulation.[13]

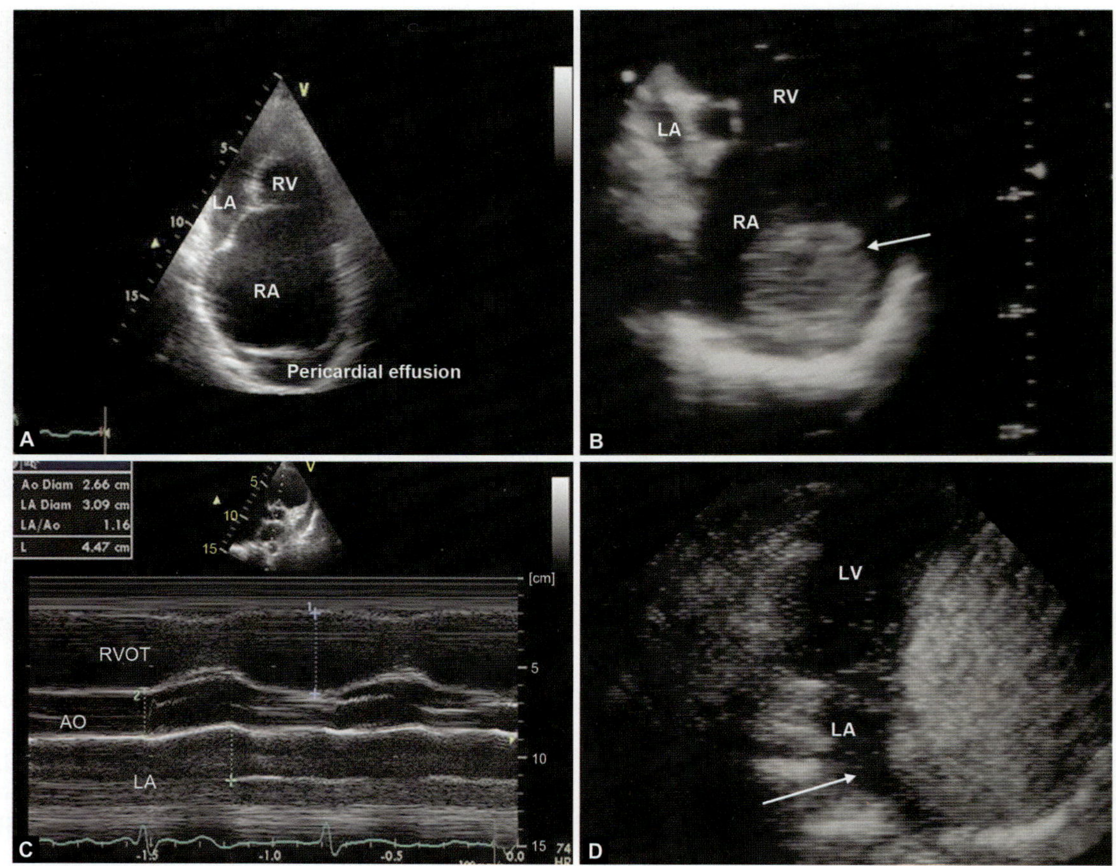

Figs. 6A to D: Echocardiographic features of right ventricular endomyocardial fibrosis. (A) Note the aneurysmal right atrium (RA); distorted right ventricle (RV), and the small pericardial effusion; (B) Thin white arrow shows a large right atrial thrombus; (C) Dilated hyperdynamic right ventricular outflow tract (RVOT); (D) Contrast filled large right atrium with stretched open foramen ovale with small right to left shunt.

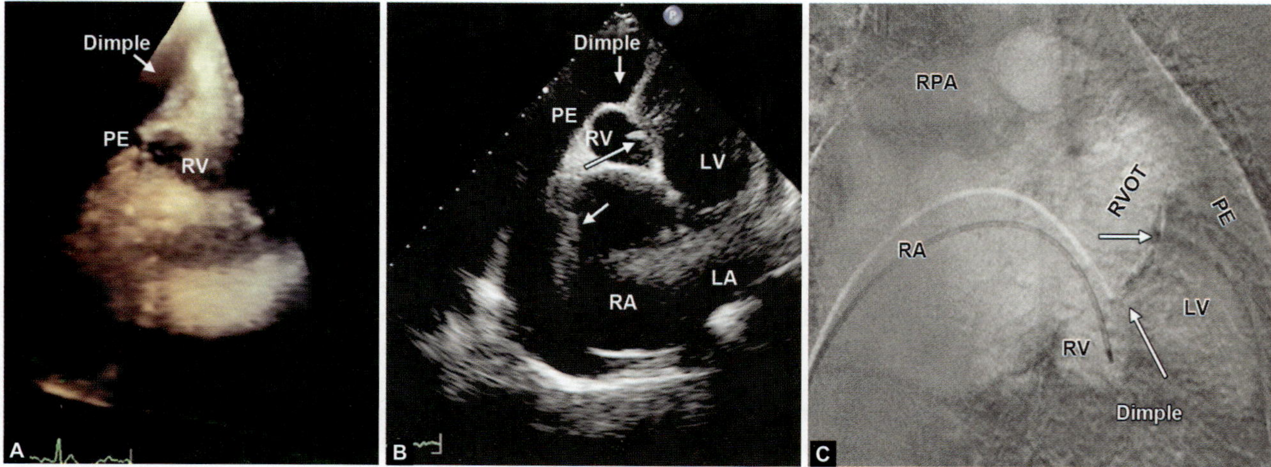

Figs. 7A to C: Ventricular dimple in right ventricular endomyocardial fibrosis. (A and B) The reduction of long axis of the right ventricle because of fibrotic obliteration from apex leads to dimple like retraction of the free wall which can be delineated by 3 (A) and 2-dimensional (B) echocardiography in presence of moderate pericardial effusion; (C) The digital subtraction of the right ventricular angiogram in levo phase to delineate the relation of the dimple to the cardiac apex. Horizontal dense arrows in Figures B and C show the right ventricular calcium and the small arrow in the right atrium in Figure B shows the layered thrombus in the free fall.

(RA: right atrium; RV: right ventricle; LA: left atrium; LV: left ventricle; RPA: right pulmonary artery; RVOT: right ventricular outflow tract; PE: pericardial effusion)

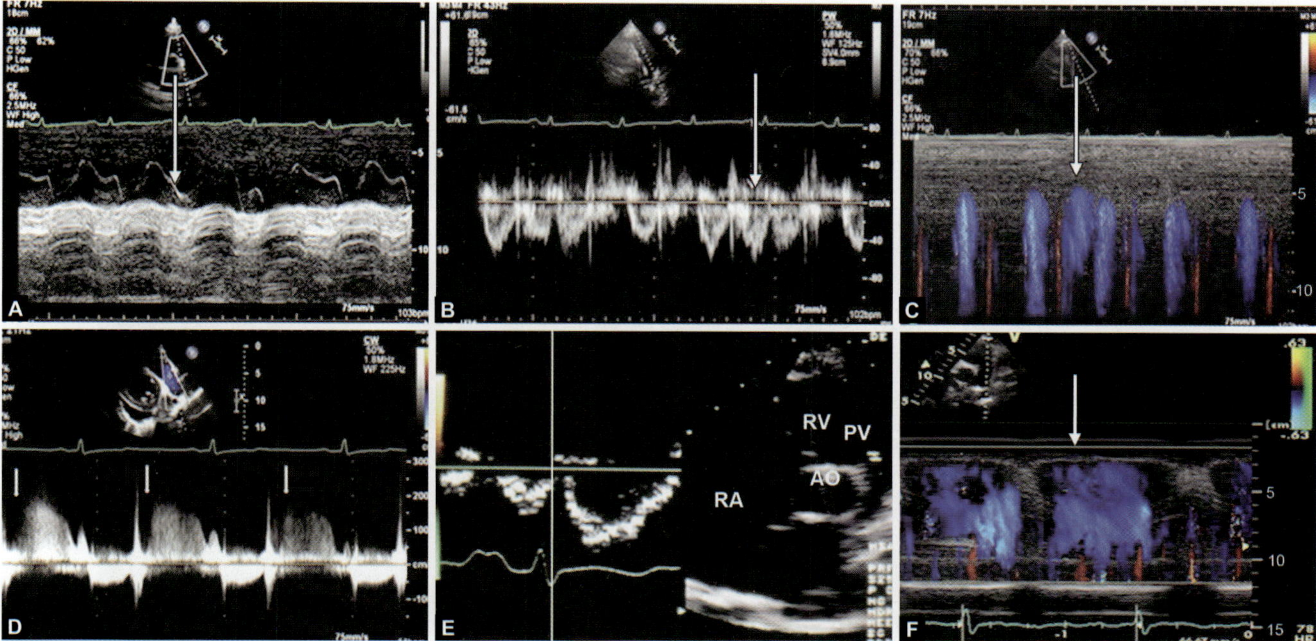

Figs. 8A to F: M-mode and Doppler flow across the pulmonary valve in right ventricular endomyocardial fibrosis. (A) The presystolic opening of the pulmonary valve indicated by the long white arrows demonstrated by M-mode; (B and C) Pulse Doppler in panel B and color Doppler M-mode across the pulmonary valve in Figure C shows the presystolic forward flow; (D) Continuous wave Doppler signal of pulmonary regurgitation showing early diastolic loss of gradient, reflecting the sudden increase in the right ventricular diastolic pressures (short arrows); (E) Expanded single beat Doppler forward flow into pulmonary artery to illustrate the atrial systolic forward flow into pulmonary artery preceding the QRS complex (vertical line); (F) The pan diastolic forward flow into pulmonary artery, illustrating elevation of systemic venous pressures above the pulmonary artery diastolic pressures, the Fontan paradox which is peculiar for isolated right ventricular cardiomyopathy.

Left Ventricular Endomyocardial Fibrosis

Isolated LVEMF often presents as mitral regurgitation or severe pulmonary hypertension.[2] Moderate cardiomegaly, well felt apex beat, left parasternal heave, loud pulmonary component of the second heart sound, loud LV third heart sound and varying degrees of mitral regurgitation are the salient clinical features. Onset of atrial fibrillation herald profound clinical deterioration. Left atrial P waves and LV hypertrophy with strain are often seen in the electrocardiogram. Plain X-ray film closely resembles that of patients with rheumatic mitral valve disease. LV calcification when present is diagnostic. Biventricular EMF can be recognized in an equal subset of patients with EMF, but their signs and symptoms overlap and at times is dominated by the dominant chamber involvement.

Many patients presenting with atypical chest pain and palpitations, with electrocardiographic abnormalities are often referred for coronary angiogram, when in fact they have LVEMF detected by 2D echo study.[14] Endocardial fibrosis involves the entire inflow tract or be patchy involving the papillary muscles and chordae. The apical fibrotic thickening of endocardium may be mistaken apical hypertrophic cardiomyopathy. Endocardial calcification is specific for EMF and is easily recognized by 2D Echo.[15] Fibrotic process spares the outflow tract and a distinct ridge is seen at the junction of the inflow and outflow tracts.[16] Posterior mitral leaflet is often plastered on the posterior LV wall as the papillary muscle is entangled in the fibrotic process. Anterior mitral leaflet appears normal. Mitral valve pathology and incompetence can be accurately quantified to plan surgical intervention. Significant left atrial dilatation is common. Color-coding of regional echo amplitude can reveal high intensity echoes at areas of early fibrosis (Figs. 9A to D). Doppler studies reveal mitral regurgitation and restrictive LV filling pattern (Fig. 9D). Tissue Doppler imaging can be used to assess diastolic LV function.

M-Mode echocardiography may show abrupt posterior motion of the LV posterior wall with a notch in the opposite direction in the interventricular septum consistent with the rapid early filling. The posterior wall motion is subsequently flat reflecting the dip and plateau phase of the pressure tracings. The mitral valve movements will look normal with a fast-initial EF slope (Fig. 10).

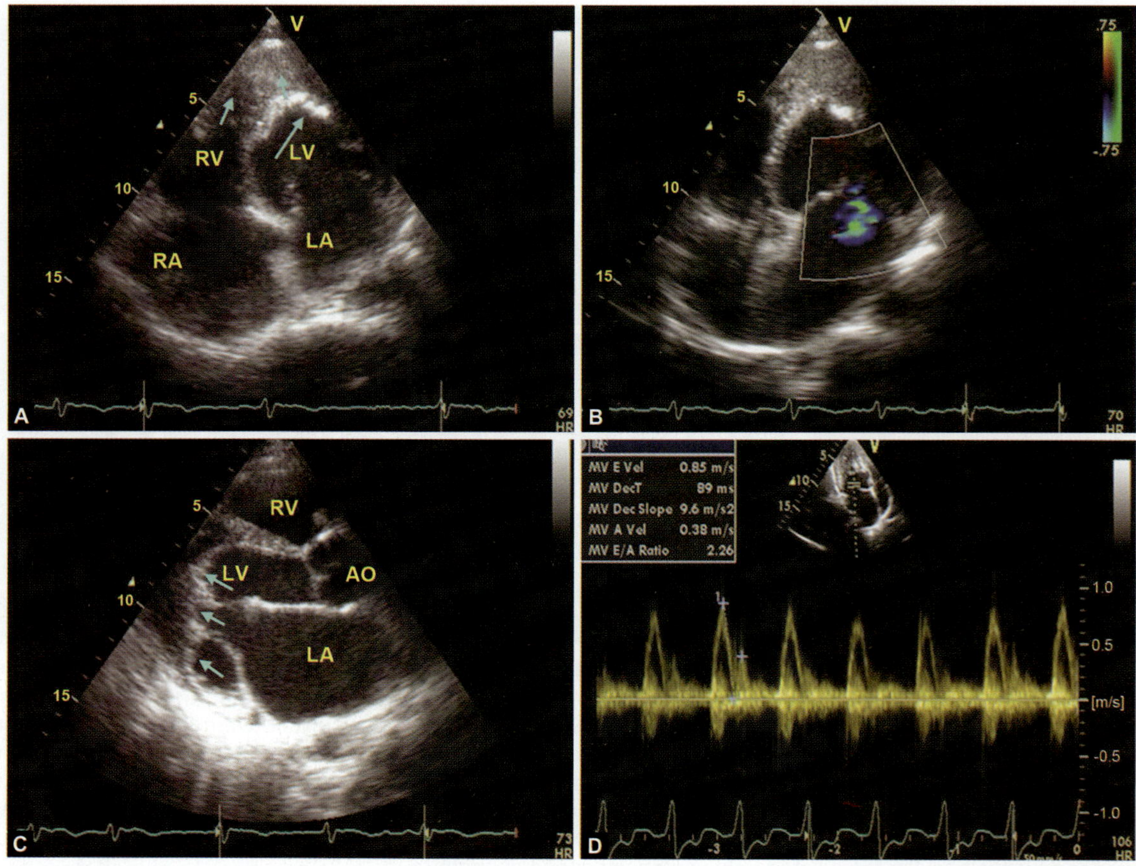

Figs. 9A to D: Echo Doppler features of left ventricular endomyocardial fibrosis. (A) Apical 4 chamber view showing apical fibrosis (short arrows) and endocardial calcification (long arrows). (B and C) Mitral valve leaflets are only minimally involved with mild regurgitation. (D) Restrictive filling pattern with e/a ratio > 2 and mitral deceleration time of 89 msec.
(RA: right atrium; LA: left atrium; RV: right ventricle; LV: left ventricle)

Speckle tracking echocardiography is the new addition in understanding ventricular function in EMF (Fig. 11). Mapping the Bull's eye plot results in a regional pattern with good systolic strain of the basal segments similar to Takotsubo syndrome.[17] But simultaneous 2D imaging will decipher the absence of apical ballooning and apical obliteration, typical of EMF.

LIMITATIONS

Restrictive cardiomyopathies and EMF are rare and need meticulous and systematic echocardiography for diagnosis and therapeutic evaluation.[7,11,18] Unlike other modalities, echocardiography is cost-effective and is available at the bed side for multiple interrogations but the detailed evaluation of diastolic function is time consuming and hampered by tachycardia, atrial fibrillation, atrioventricular valve regurgitation and pericardial effusions. If the echo window is good, the high temporal resolution provides finer details for evaluation and understanding of this enigmatic disease but needs a trained echocardiographer to decipher the finer details.

CONCLUSION

Endomyocardial fibrosis as a cause of restrictive cardiomyopathy is the most common cause of cardiac failure in certain geographical hot spots, but is uncommon in the rest of the world.[19] Echocardiography forms the mainstay for the diagnosis and clinical staging of the disease and in understanding the hemodynamic consequences of the disease. Echocardiographic recognition can help in utilizing specific surgical procedures like endocardiectomy, valve replacement and creation of Fontan circulation to postpone or avoid a more challenging surgical intervention like cardiac transplant.[20] Current efforts at early recognition by community screening will define the natural history and progression of the disease better.[1]

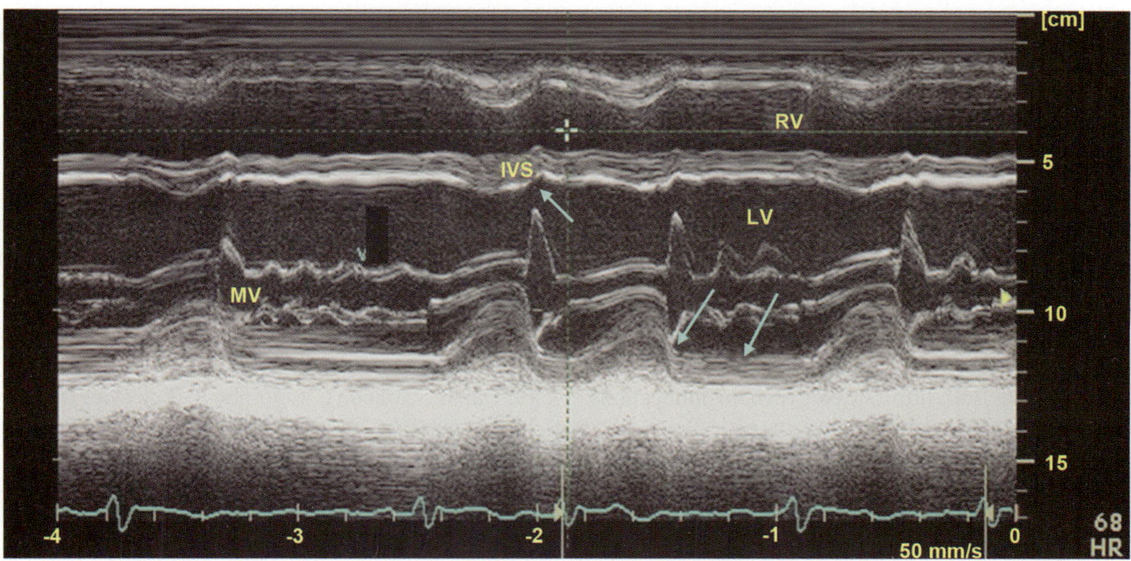

Fig. 10: M-mode echocardiographic pattern in left ventricular endomyocardial fibrosis. The upward directed arrow shows the early abrupt septal movement. The downward directed arrows show the early abrupt motion followed by the plateauing of the LV posterior wall.
(RV: right ventricle; LV: left ventricle; IVS: interventricular septum; MV: mitral valve)

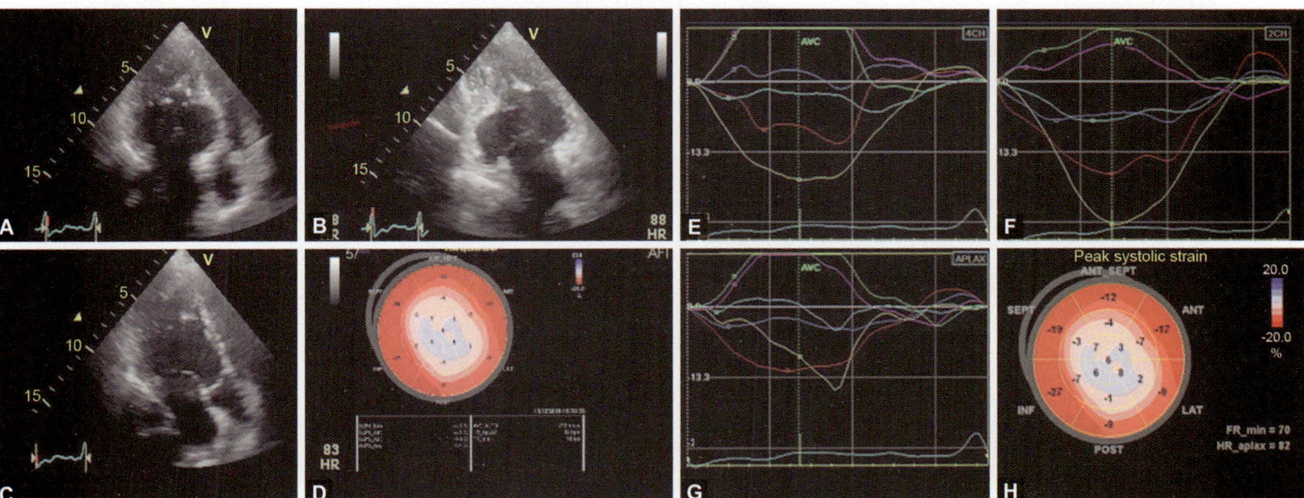

Figs. 11A to H: Quad screen formats of the left ventricular strain imaging in a subject with left ventricular endomyocardial fibrosis. The 3 views utilized for generating the strain image (moving images can be depicted in the video mode) with the Bull's eye map of the peak systolic strain. Note that the reduced strain values of the fibrosed and calcified apical segments and the blue color indicating the systolic lengthening of apical segments.

REFERENCES

1. Antonio G, Olga MA, Juergen F, et al. Tropical Endomyocardial Fibrosis. Circulation. 2016;133(24):2503-15.
2. Sivasankaran S. Restrictive cardiomyopathy in India: the story of a vanishing mystery. Heart. 2009;95(1):9-14.
3. Vijayaraghavan G, Sivasankaran S. Tropical endomyocardial fibrosis in India: a vanishing disease! Indian J Med Res. 2012;136(5):729-38.
4. Kartha CC. Endomyocardial fibrosis, a case for the tropical doctor. Cardiovasc Res. 1995;30(5):636-43.
5. Akinwusi PO, Odeyemi AO. The changing pattern of endomyocardial fibrosis in South-west Nigeria. Clin Med Insights Cardiol. 2012;6:163-8.
6. de Freitas HFG, de Castro PPN, Chizzola PR, et al. Heart transplantation in a patient with endomyocardial fibrosis. Arq Bras Cardiol. 2005;84(1):49-50.
7. Bukhman G, Ziegler J, Parry E. Endomyocardial fibrosis: still a mystery after 60 years. PLoS Negl Trop Dis. 2008;2(2):e97.
8. Mocumbi AO. Right ventricular endomyocardial fibrosis (2013 Grover Conference series). Pulm Circ. 2014;4(3): 363-9.

9. Marijon E, Hausse AO, Ferreira B. Typical clinical aspect of endomyocardial fibrosis. Int J Cardiol. 2006;112(2): 259-60.
10. Balakrishnan KG, Sapru RP, Sasidharan K, et al. A comparison of the clinical, haemodynamic and angiographic features in right ventricular endomyocardial fibrosis and Ebstein's anomaly of the tricuspid valve. Cardiology. 1982;69(5):265-75.
11. Hassan WM, Fawzy ME, Al Helaly S, et al. Pitfalls in Diagnosis and Clinical, Echocardiographic, and Hemodynamic Findings in Endomyocardial Fibrosis: a 25-year experience. Chest. 2005;128(6):3985-92.
12. Vijayaraghavan G. Clinical, Electrocardiographic and Radiological features. in "Endomyocardial fibrosis in India". [online] Available from http://www.gvr.co.in/publications.php. [Last Accessed November, 2019].
13. Narayan GS, Sivasubramonian S. Spontaneous Fontan Physiology in Burnt-Out Endomyocardial Fibrosis. Circulation. 2012;125(4):e296–7.
14. Indian Academy of Science. Current perspective on endomyocardial fibrosis. [online] Available from www.ias.ac.in/currsci/aug102009/405.pdf. [Last Accessed November, 2019].
15. Vijayaraghavan G, Balakrishnan M, Sadanandan S, et al. Pattern of cardiac calcification in tropical endomyocardial fibrosis. Heart Vessels Suppl. 1990;5:4-7.
16. Davies JN. The ridge in endomyocardial fibrosis. Lancet. 1968;1(7543):631-2.
17. Dias A, Franco E, Rubio M, et al. Usefulness of left ventricular strain analysis in patients with takotsubo syndrome during acute phase. Echocardiography. 2017;35(2):179-83.
18. Pereira NL, Grogan M, Dec GW. Spectrum of Restrictive and Infiltrative Cardiomyopathies: Part 2 of a 2-Part Series. J Am Coll Cardiol. 2018;71(10):1149-66.
19. Dabas N, Macon C, Colombo R, et al. Does Endomyocardial Fibrosis Exist in the United States? A Challenging Case. J Am Coll Cardiol. 2019;71(11 Supplement):A2430.
20. Kumar N, Prabhakar G, Fawzy ME, et al. Total cavopulmonary connection for right ventricular endomyocardial fibrosis. Eur J Cardiothorac Surg. 1992;6(7):391-2.

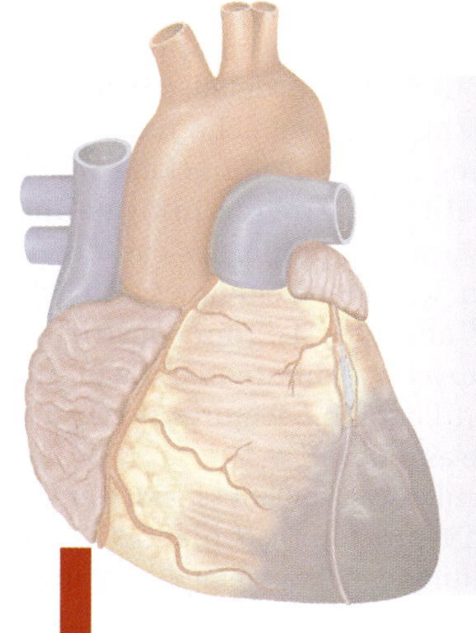

Noninvasive Evaluation of Cardiac Amyloidosis and Sarcoidosis

Chandramukhi Sunehra, P Krishnam Raju

INTRODUCTION

Amyloidosis and sarcoidosis are systemic disorders which frequently involve the heart. Cardiac involvement in these disorders dictates the treatment and the prognosis. Amyloidosis occurs as a result of extracellular deposition of fibrillar protein while sarcoidosis occurs as a result of inflammatory response with formation of granulomas. The clinical manifestations of both these disorders range from asymptomatic state to overt heart failure. A very high index of clinical suspicion is required for the diagnosis. Early diagnosis facilitates early institution of specific therapy and improves symptoms and prolongs the survival. The initial diagnosis is usually picked up by echocardiography and can be complemented by cardiac magnetic resonance imaging (MRI) and radionuclide imaging.

AMYLOIDOSIS

Amyloidosis is a multisystem disorder involving skin, nerves, liver, kidney, heart and tongue with interstitial aggregation of fibrillar protein. It is the most frequent cause of restrictive cardiomyopathy. Cardiac involvement determines the course of the disease and usually associated with poor prognosis and short survival. Cardiac involvement is primarily encountered in immunoglobulin amyloid light-chain (AL) and transthyretin-associated (hereditary/familial and senile) amyloidoses. The commonly occurring clinical types of cardiac amyloidosis are light chain amyloidosis, wildtype transthyretin amyloidosis (ATTRwt), and mutant transthyretin amyloidosis (ATTRm). Early detection of cardiac amyloidosis is frequently missed or delayed due to nonspecific systemic symptoms in the early course of the disease. The initial evaluation in suspected case should include routine investigations like complete blood picture with erythrocyte sedimentation rate (ESR) liver function tests and kidney function tests, serum electrolytes, thyroid profile, urine analysis and blood sugars. In addition, serum and urine analysis for the presence of a monoclonal immunoglobulin should be done. The standard serum protein electrophoresis may fail to detect a monoclonal band in a significant number of cases, hence immunofixation which is more sensitive and should be performed whenever amyloidosis is suspected.[1]

The basic evaluation should be followed by electrocardiography (ECG) and echocardiography for identification of cardiac involvement. The type of amyloid, extent of organ involvement and the individual mutation determine treatment options. The management of amyloidosis should include a team approach and multidisciplinary management involving cardiologist, neurologist, nephrologist, rheumatologist and hematologist.

DIAGNOSIS

The diagnosis of cardiac amyloidosis requires a very high degree of clinical suspicion and should be suspected in a patient with unexplained heart failure, in the presence or absence of systemic manifestations of amyloidosis. In suspected cases cardiac evaluation should include ECG, multimodality echocardiographic assessment, cardiac MRI and radionuclide imaging in selected cases, if required. The presence of low-voltage complexes on ECG, despite ventricular wall thickening on echocardiography is highly suggestive of cardiac amyloidosis, and should raise the alarm to search for features of amyloidosis during echocardiographic evaluation. The diagnosis of amyloidosis is confirmed by biopsy specimen which stains with Congo red dye to produce an apple-green birefringence when viewed under polarized light. Endomyocardial biopsy is the gold standard for diagnosis of cardiac amyloidosis. A screening biopsy should be taken from an easily accessible, safe and likely site of involvement, e.g. abdominal fat pad biopsy or rectal biopsy.

Electrocardiography

The characteristic ECG patterns diagnostic of cardiac amyloidosis are:

- *Low voltage complexes*: The low voltage complexes in precordial and limb leads is primarily due to the destruction and replacement of myocytes by the electrically inert amyloid. This ECG pattern is exhibited by approximately 70% of AL-associated cardiac amyloidosis and only one-third of patients with hereditary amyloidosis and senile systemic amyloidosis show low voltage.
- *Pseudoinfarction pattern*: It is evidenced by QS waves in two consecutive leads and commonly seen in AL amyloid. It usually involves the precordial ECG leads (V1-V3), but can also occur in the inferior leads (II, III, and aVF).[2]
- Large P waves due to biatrial enlargement
- *Conduction abnormalities*: Intraventricular conduction delays or blocks like incomplete right bundle branch block or left anterior fascicular block may be present
- *Arrhythmia and long QTc*: Usually, the rhythm is sinus rhythm but atrial fibrillation usually occurs in the advanced stages and may be responsible for rapid clinical deterioration.
- Fragmented QRS complexes
- Reduced heart rate variability on a 24-hour Holter predicts high short-term mortality
- Late after potentials on signal averaged ECG
- Fragmented QRS complexes on ECG.

Echocardiography

Cardiac involvement in amyloidosis with amyloid deposition in interstitial space results in disruption of the structure and function. Cardiac amyloidosis is characterized by diastolic dysfunction in the early course of disease. Despite preserved left ventricular (LV) ejection fraction in early stages, systolic dysfunction is common and unmasked by advanced imaging techniques like tissue velocity imaging and strain rate imaging. A thorough echocardiographic evaluation including two-dimensional (2D) imaging, motion (M) mode, Doppler evaluation and color Doppler imaging gives a comprehensive description of cardiac involvement with detailed structural and hemodynamic assessment. Novel echo techniques like tissue velocity imaging and speckle tracking which analyses strain and strain rate provide information regarding ventricular myocardial properties can detect the disease in its early course. These techniques also help in differentiating cardiac amyloidosis from constrictive pericarditis which is a very close differential diagnosis. The characteristic echocardiographic features suggestive of cardiac amyloidosis are as follows:

- Increase in the ventricular wall thickness with normal size ventricles or small ventricles. Discordant ECG and echocardiographic features with low voltage complexes on ECG despite increased thickness of interventricular septum and LV posterior wall on the echocardiogram are highly specific for cardiac amyloidosis. Low voltage on ECG and interventricular septal thickness of >19.8 mm on echocardiography together have a sensitivity of 72% and specificity of 91% for cardiac amyloidosis.[3] Associated right ventricular (RV) wall thickening >7 mm will also be noticed.
- "Granular" or "sparkling" (ground glass) appearance of the myocardium: Hyperechogenicity of the myocardium, with granular or "sparkling" echotexture, has been reported to be highly specific for cardiac amyloidosis in many studies (Fig. 1A). However, one has to keep in mind that granular echotexture applies only to standard echocardiographic imaging, without tissue harmonics being applied. Tissue harmonic imaging enhances the appearance of myocardium generally and may render this finding less noticeable. Though highly specific for amyloidosis, the sparkling echotexture can occur in other conditions like hypertensive heart disease with renal failure, infiltrative diseases, e.g. Anderson Fabry's disease, mucopolysaccharidosis, etc. Myocardial sparkling, a qualitative sign of amyloid infiltration is subjective and highly dependent on the imaging technique (harmonic imaging).[3]
- Thickening of the atrioventricular valves–mitral and tricuspid valves, papillary muscles and interatrial septum. Mild valvular regurgitation is a common finding, though severe regurgitation rarely occurs (Fig. 1C). Interatrial septal thickening is a characteristic feature of cardiac amyloidosis, though it can be better appreciated by Cardiac MRI.
- Ventricular function: LV systolic function is usually preserved in early stages of the disease. It may be normal in early stages but it is reduced in advanced stages. Segmental tissue imaging and strain rate imaging show impairment in long-axis contraction even when the

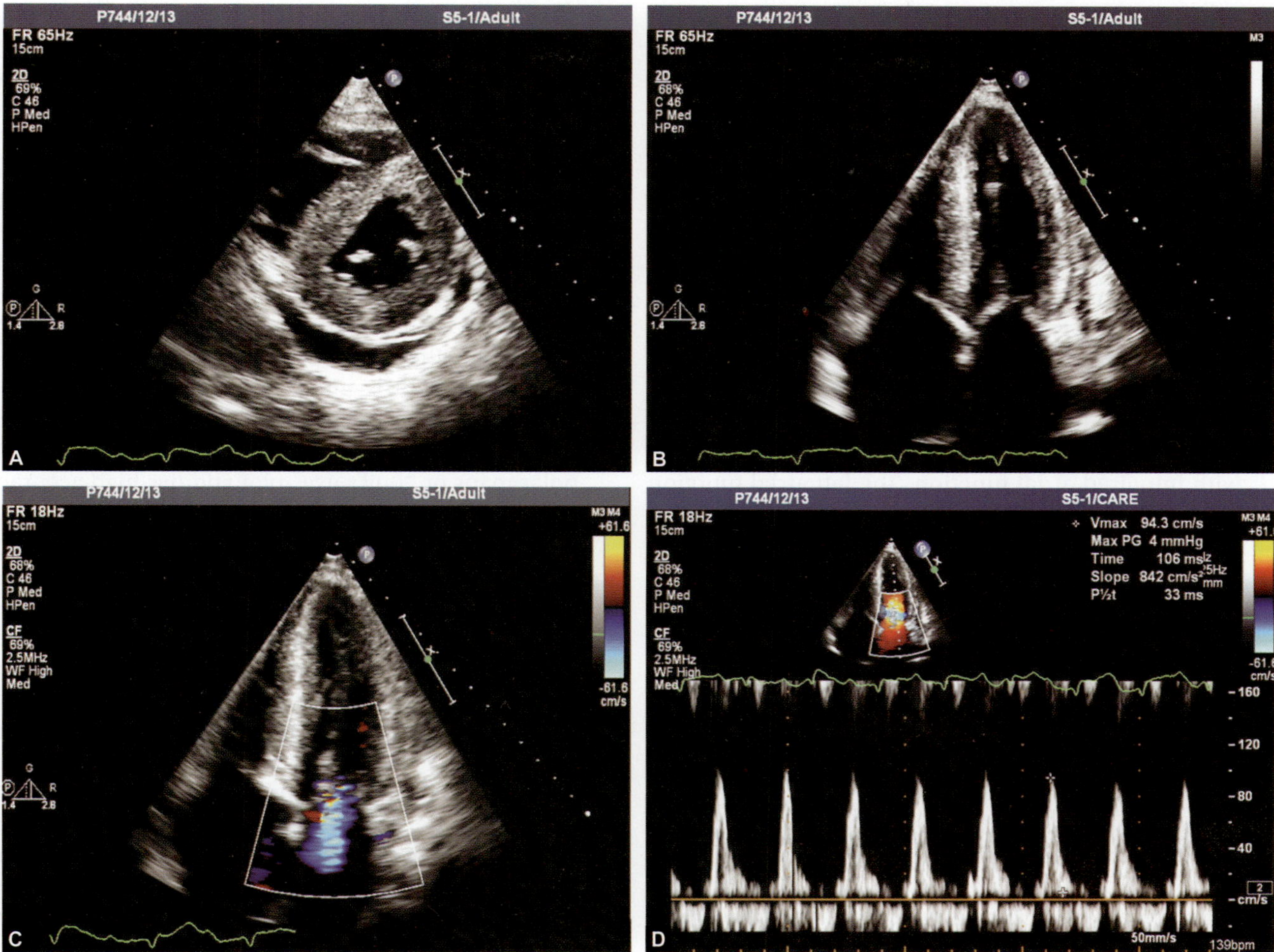

Figs. 1A to D: Echocardiographic features of cardiac amyloidosis. (A) Parasternal short axis view shows thickened left ventricle with sparkling appearance of myocardium and small posterior pericardial effusion; (B) Apical 4 chamber view shows normal size LV and RV, dilated atria, thickened and sparkling interventricular septum. Mitral valve leaflets are thickened; (C) Color Doppler interrogation across the mitral valve in apical 4 chamber view shows mild mitral regurgitation; (D) Restrictive filling pattern is evident on the transmitral pulsed wave Doppler interrogation with high early diastolic (E-wave) and low late diastolic (A-wave) filling wave, i.e. high E/A ratio and short deceleration time suggestive of elevated left atrial filling pressures.

LV ejection fraction is normal and thus facilitate the identification of LV systolic dysfunction at an earlier stage. Similarly, tricuspid annular peak systolic velocity on tissue velocity imaging and RV strain rate imaging may demonstrate RV dysfunction at an early stage of the disease.

- Diastolic dysfunction is the hallmark of cardiac amyloidosis and cardiac amyloidosis should be suspected in patients with heart failure with preserved LV ejection function but diastolic dysfunction. The echocardiographic features of LV diastolic dysfunction depend on the stage of the disease. In the early stage of cardiac amyloidosis, the diastolic dysfunction is evident as impaired relaxation of LV which progresses to restrictive filling pattern in advanced stage. Restrictive filling pattern (Fig. 1D) is evident on the transmitral pulsed wave Doppler interrogation with high early diastolic (E-wave) and low late diastolic (A-wave) filling wave, i.e. high E/A ratio and short deceleration time suggestive of elevated left atrial filling pressures. Pulmonary venous flow velocity interrogation with the pulsed wave Doppler sample placed at the opening of the pulmonary vein into left atrium shows a lower systolic and higher diastolic velocities (severely blunted systolic flow) and increased atrial reversals (unless atrial systolic failure). Diastolic dysfunction can be assessed with the help of tissue velocity imaging which provides relatively load independent variables like e'. Reduced e' velocity for age is suggestive of impaired relaxation-septal e' velocity <7 cm/sec and lateral e' velocity <10 cm/sec is suggestive of diastolic dysfunction. E/e' ratio gives an estimation of LV filling pressures. E/e' ratio >14 mm Hg is suggestive of elevated LV end diastolic pressure.[4]

In clinical practice, it is important to remember that in some patients with restrictive cardiomyopathy (RCM), treatment with diuretics may normalize the filling pattern. In this situation, restrictive filling pattern can be unmasked after a fluid challenge.

Similar changes in RV diastolic function can be evident and assessed by the transtricuspid pulsed wave Doppler interrogation, superior vena cava, and hepatic vein flow velocities.

- Biatrial enlargement: Left atrium (LA) and right atrium (RA) are dilated and relatively immobile (Fig. 1B). There is increase in the left and right atrial volumes with impaired atrial function. The left atrial function can be assessed by left atrial ejection fraction, and also novel echocardiographic modalities, e.g. segmental tissue velocity imaging and left atrial strain rate imaging.
- Small pericardial effusion is often present followed by the right atrial appendages are the common sites for thrombus formation.[5] LV diastolic dysfunction, lower left atrial appendage emptying velocity and atrial fibrillation were independently associated with increased risk for intracardiac thrombosis.
- Intracardiac thrombi: There is a high prevalence of intracardiac thrombus in cardiac amyloidosis as identified by echocardiography, especially transesophageal echocardiography. More frequently, the atrial thrombi are noted at the autopsy.
- Hepatic vein Doppler interrogation reveals diastolic flow reversal which is exaggerated during inspiration.
- *Tissue velocity imaging* facilitates the identification of systolic and diastolic dysfunction at an early stage. Color tissue Doppler imaging enables the assessment of myocardial tissue velocities of various segments of LV and RV in apical views. It reveals significantly reduced segmental myocardial tissue velocities of LV and RV and it provides information on subclinical ventricular dysfunction before any changes in ejection fraction occur. It also helps in distinguishing amyloid and other restrictive cardiomyopathies from constrictive pericarditis, with a mitral annular diastolic velocity E ≤ 8 cm/s, a good discriminator for restrictive physiology.[6] While annulus reversus and normal myocardial tissue velocities favor the diagnosis of constrictive pericarditis.
- *Characteristic strain rate imaging pattern diagnostic of cardiac amyloidosis*: Strain rate imaging reveals markedly reduced global strain–both longitudinal and circumferential strain of LV. However, there is overlap of disease states with reduced global strain which poses difficulty in differentiating cardiac amyloidosis from other infiltrative disorders like Fabry's disease or hypertrophic cardiomyopathy. Phelan et al.[7] studied the pattern of regional longitudinal strain (LS) using 2-D speckle-tracking echocardiography in patients with cardiac amyloidosis in comparison to patients with hypertrophic cardiomyopathy and aortic stenosis who also had hypertrophied left ventricle. The authors documented characteristic regional patterns in LS in cardiac amyloidosis with severe impairment of LS in the basal and mid segments of LV with relative sparring of LS in the apical segments of LV. This relative *"apical sparing"* pattern of LS can be easily appreciated on strain polar maps or "Bull's eye" plot and has high accuracy and reproducibility.
  This characteristic pattern was also described as "cherry on the top" on "Bull's eye" plot (Fig. 2). This pattern was integrated into a relative apical LS formula as:
  Relative apical LS = average apical LS/(average of basal + mid LS)

A score of >1 was associated with high sensitivity (93%) and specificity (82%) for the diagnosis of cardiac amyloidosis. However, patients with known coronary artery disease were excluded from this study.

None of the echocardiographic characteristics are specific for cardiac amyloidosis. The diagnosis of cardiac amyloidosis is challenging in early stages. However, there are many echocardiographic features which are commonly seen in cardiac amyloidosis, combining these features with the clinical signs and usually a low voltage ECG will assist in the early diagnosis of cardiac amyloidosis.

Key point 1: Echocardiography is the preferred non-invasive diagnostic modality for the evaluation of cardiac amyloidosis. The characteristic features include ventricular wall thickning, "granular sparkling" appearance of the myocardium, atrioventricular valve thickening with regurgitation, interatrial septal thickening, nondilated ventricles, biatrial enlargement, and pericardial effusion. Restrictive LV filling pattern occurs in the advanced disease state and hence, its absence should not exclude the diagnosis of cardiac amyloid. Tissue velocity imaging, myocardial strain and strain rate imaging are more sensitive and facilitate early diagnosis. A relative **"apical sparing"** pattern of LS is an easily recognizable, accurate and reproducible sign of cardiac amyloidosis.

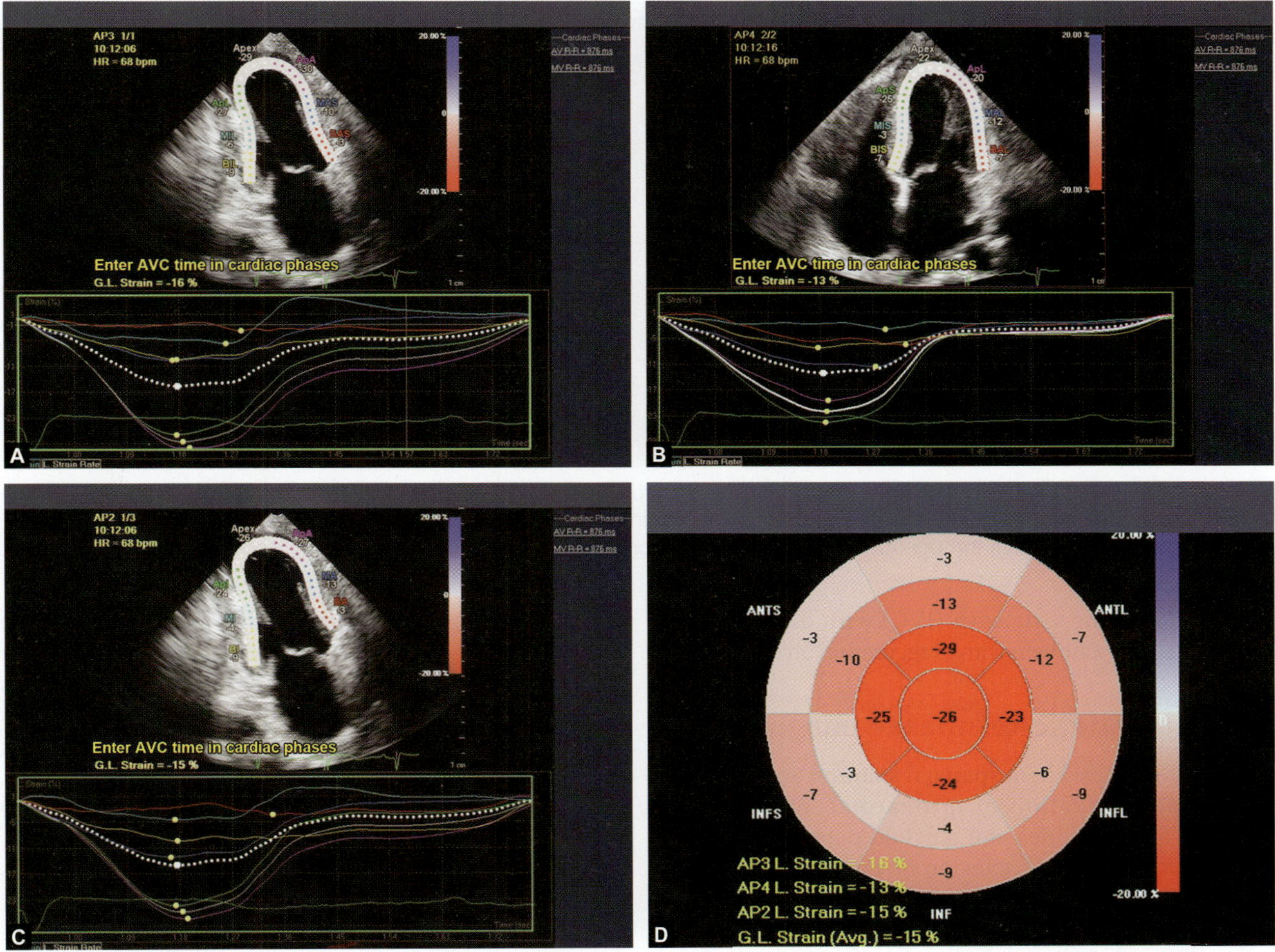

Figs. 2A to D: Strain rate imaging depicting the longitudinal strain and Bull's eye map in a patient with cardiac amyloidosis. Strain rate imaging shows reduced longitudinal peak systolic strain in the (A) apical long axis view, (B) apical 4 chamber view and (C and D) apical 2 chamber view and also shows reduced longitudinal peak systolic strain of basal and mid-segments and preserved longitudinal peak systolic strain in the apical segments. The average global longitudinal strain of left ventricle is reduced at 15% with characteristic sparing in the apical segments. This is the characteristic relative *"apical sparing"* pattern of longitudinal strain also called as "Cherry on the top" pattern which is diagnostic of cardiac amyloidosis.

LV wall thickness ≥ 15 mm, restrictive filling on Doppler echocardiography with an early mitral inflow (E) deceleration time <150 ms and reduced LV ejection fraction have been associated with poor prognosis.[8,9] Reduced global LS has been shown to be a strong predictor of reduced survival.

Checklist for Echocardiographic Evaluation in a Patient with Suspected Cardiac Amyloidosis

- Increased LV wall thickness even in the absence of hypertension or LV hypertrophy on ECG
- Sparkling appearance of myocardium, though not specific for cardiac amyloidosis
- Diastolic dysfunction which varies according to the stage of the disease and restrictive filling pattern of LV is seen in advanced stage
- Biatrial enlargement with reduced atrial function
- Thickening of the atrioventricular valves with regurgitation. Thickening of the interatrial septum
- Pericardial effusion
- Reduced segmental myocardial tissue velocities of left ventricle
- Impaired average LS of LV with relative apical sparing
- Impaired RV function which can be assessed by tricuspid annular peak systolic velocity on tissue Doppler imaging or tricuspid annular peak systolic excursion on M-mode

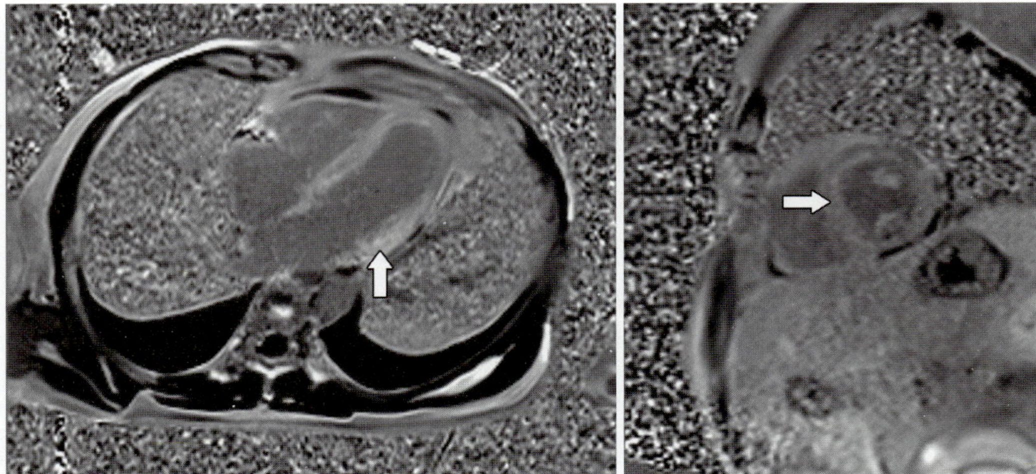

Fig. 3: Cardiac magnetic resonance imaging features of cardiac amyloidosis. Four-chamber and short-axis views of late gadolinium enhancement cardiac magnetic resonance imaging in a patient with cardiac amyloidosis. There is diffuse transmural late gadolinium enhancement throughout the left ventricle with pronounced at the base of the left ventricle as indicted by arrow.

- Dilated inferior vena cava (IVC) with diastolic flow reversal in hepatic vein with exaggeration on inspiration.

Cardiac Magnetic Resonance Imaging

Cardiac MRI has excellent spatial resolution and provides better characterization of myocardial involvement, functional abnormalities and amyloid deposition. It aids in the identification or exclusion of various etiologies of RCM. It is highly sensitive for diagnosing the infiltrative cardiomyopathy, even in the very early stage without any ventricular wall thickness. In cardiac amyloidosis there is increase in the interstitial cardiac volume as a result of interstitial deposition of amyloid fibrils. Thus, gadolinium stays longer in the tissue, which explains the late gadolinium enhancement. Delayed postgadolinium enhancement images reveal the characteristic diffuse subendocardial enhancement with diffuse LV subendocardial or transmural late gadolinium enhancement (LGE) (Fig. 3), which may also involve the RV and atrial walls and aid in the diagnostic confirmation of cardiac amyloidosis. This characteristic pattern of global transmural or diffuse subendocardial LGE can detect the disease early when significant increase in LV wall thickness is not present and it correlates with disease severity.[10]

Late gadolinium enhancement enables identification of myocardial fibrosis, scar, necrosis or infiltration. In cardiac amyloidosis, the interstitial amyloid deposit avidly picks up and retains gadolinium resulting in signal enhancement of the tissue and there is relatively faster washout of gadolinium from myocardium and blood pool. The degree of enhancement depends on the ventricular mass and global ventricular systolic function. Thus, these patients exhibit abnormal myocardial and blood-pool gadolinium kinetics. Together, these findings have 97% accuracy for diagnosing cardiac amyloidosis.[11] RV enhancement is seen in transthyretin related (ATTR) amyloidosis and less commonly in AL amyloidosis. Austin et al.[12] showed that LGE Cardiac MRI had a sensitivity of 88%, specificity 95%, positive predictive value of 93%, and negative predictive value of 90% in patients with biopsy proven amyloidosis. Left atrial LGE is a useful evidence of cardiac amyloidosis and predicts atrial fibrillation.

In cardiac amyloidosis, gadolinium kinetics are abnormal with a faster washout of gadolinium from blood pool as compared to the amyloid myocardium. An especially unique feature of LGE appearances in this population is the blood pool appearing atypically dark. This reflects the similar myocardial and blood T1 values due to high myocardial uptake and fast blood pool washout of the contrast agent. This occurs as a result of myocardial amyloid deposition with increase in extracellular space resulting in gadolinium accumulation.

Novel parametric mapping technique with noncontrast, native T1 mapping captures a combined signal from the intracellular and extracellular compartments and allows the estimation of extracellular volume. Amyloid deposition results in the increase in the cardiac longitudinal relaxation time (T1) magnetic property. This results in longer myocardial noncontrast T1 values in cardiac amyloidosis in comparison with normal controls. This finding has higher sensitivity for detecting early subclinical cardiac involvement than LGE. Novel technique of pre- and postcontrast T1 mapping is emerging as a promising tool for quantification of cardiac amyloid burden over time. The estimated extracellular volume fraction which quantifies the amyloid burden has a strong correlation with N-terminal pro-B-type natriuretic peptide (pro-BNP) levels and troponin T levels, which are strong prognostic indicators of cardiac amyloidosis. Extracellular volume fraction is found to be increased in cases with systemic amyloidosis even in the absence of ventricular thickening on echocardiography or LGE on CMR. This implies that extracellular volume fraction might be a very sensitive test, which may allow for earlier detection of cardiac amyloidosis than other methods of diagnosis.[13] Thus, extracellular volume measurement facilitates early diagnosis, disease monitoring, and, potentially, as a much needed cardiac surrogate endpoint for the various promising new therapies of amyloidosis.

Interstitial amyloid deposition appears to be more extensive in transthyretin amyloidosis (TTR) than in immunoglobulin AL. The addition of parametric mapping to standard CMR images is a powerful quantitative diagnostic tool that differentiates cardiac amyloidosis from other causes of RCM.[14]

However, there are few limitations to LGE-CMR:

- Patchy myocardial involvement is also seen in some cases and can be easily missed.
- Underestimation of the degree of disease burden as compared to 99mTc-diphosphonate nuclear imaging due to diffuse nature of LGE conventional CMR. This can happen because normal reference myocardium—used to provide context for setting pulse sequence parameters and for visual interpretation—may be absent.[15]
- Does not differentiate AL amyloidosis from ATTR amyloidosis. However, one characteristic feature is that ATTR subtype almost always has LGE of the right ventricle, while almost one-third of patients with AL do not.[13]

Key point 2: CMR aids in the confirmation of diagnosis once echocardiogram shows features of the cardiac amyloidosis. Delayed postgadolinium enhancement images reveal the characteristic diffuse subendocardial enhancement and atrial and valvular uptake as well. This characteristic pattern of global transmural or diffuse subendocardial LGE can detect the disease early.

Checklist for Cardiac Magnetic Resonance Evaluation in a Patient with Suspected Cardiac Amyloidosis

- Characteristic global transmural or diffuse subendocardial LGE involving LV, RV and the atrial walls. It correlates with disease severity. RV enhancement is seen in ATTR amyloidosis and less commonly in AL amyloidosis
- Abnormal myocardial and blood-pool gadolinium kinetics with faster washout of gadolinium from myocardium and blood pool as compared to the normal healthy myocardium
- Longer myocardial noncontrast T1 values
- The addition of parametric mapping to standard CMR images is a powerful quantitative diagnostic tool that differentiates cardiac amyloidosis from other causes of RCM.

Radionuclide Imaging

Radionuclide imaging for myocardial perfusion scintigraphy utilizes molecular-targeted radiolabelled compounds for detection of interstitial amyloid deposit in the heart (Fig. 4). It is helpful in patients with an inconclusive CMR study for the diagnosis of cardiac amyloidosis.

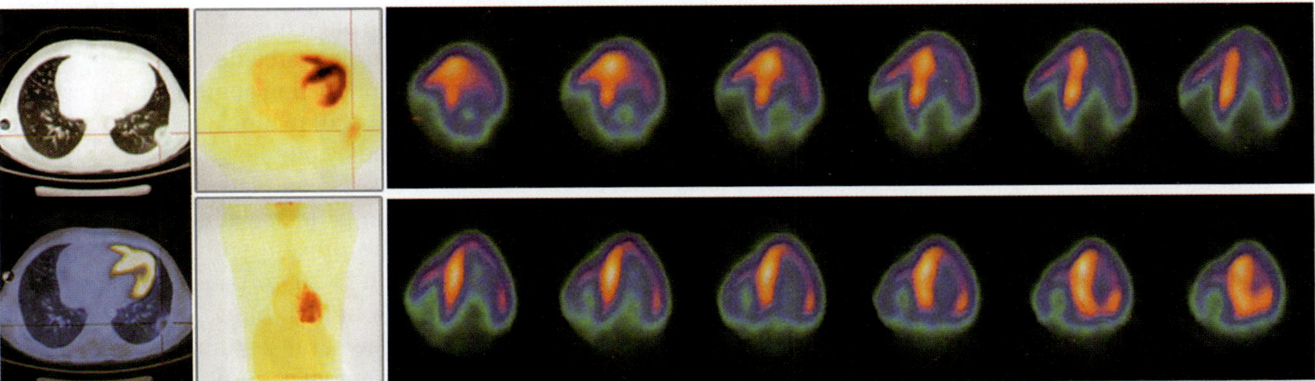

Fig. 4: Positron emission tomography-computed tomography (PET-CT) images in a patient with cardiac amyloidosis. Radionuclide imaging with ^{18}F-Fluorodeoxyglucose (FDG): PET-CT scan images in a patient with cardiac amyloidosis. It revealed tracer uptake in thickened LV and RV myocardium. Patchy low grade uptake is seen in thickened wall of dilated RA.

The prognosis and therapeutic options vary drastically in the two cardiac phenotypes—AATR and AL-of cardiac amyloidosis. Hence, early differentiation between the two subtypes of cardiac amyloidosis is as important as the early recognition of the disease itself.

^{99m}Tc-Phosphate derivatives-technetium-3, 3-diphosphono-1, 2-propanodicarboxylic acid (^{99m}Tc-DPD) and technetium pyrophosphate (^{99m}Tc-PYP)-selectively bind ATTR,[16] but not AL subtype. Myocardial perfusion scintigraphy has a very high sensitivity for detection of ATTR amyloidosis. Positive scans on myocardial perfusion scintigraphy of cardiac amyloid can, therefore, be used to identify wild-type and mutant ATTR amyloidosis. By contrast, cardiac localization of amyloid deposits occurs in only a small proportion of patients with AL amyloidosis, and usually to a lesser degree than in patients with ATTR amyloidosis. Consequently, negative scans are predictive of AL amyloidosis[17] and negative phenotype, warrants further evaluation. In the presence of positive myocardial uptake, endomyocardial biopsy may not be needed; genetic testing, however, is helpful to differentiate ATTR mutant from wild type, and if a mutation is identified, family screening should be performed.

Another potential role for nuclear imaging is monitoring disease progression, and more importantly, response to therapy.

Cardiac Catheterization and Endomyocardial Biopsy

Although endomyocardial biopsy (EMB) with immunohistochemistry is the gold standard for diagnosis, it is recommended in selected patients with inconclusive noninvasive imaging. Definitive diagnosis of cardiac amyloidosis is established by the mere demonstration of apple-green birefringence with Congo red under polarized light microscopy. Cardiac catheterization reveals the characteristic pattern with elevated LV enddiastolic pressure and "dip and plateau" or "square root" pattern diastolic pressure tracings, similar to those in constrictive pericarditis, are seen on hemodynamic pressure recordings. Endomyocardial biopsy can help to identifying or excluding cardiac amyloidosis from sarcoidosis and hemochromatosis. However, there are certain limitations of endomyocardial biopsy like low yield due to uneven distribution of amyloid deposition and deadly complications like cardiac rupture and cardiac tamponade.

In patients with suspected ATTR (based on clinical presentation, ECG, and echocardiographic findings), radionuclide imaging with either 99mTc-DPD or 99mTc-PYP can be used as a noninvasive screening method to differentiate between ATTR versus AL. In the presence of positive myocardial uptake, endomyocardial biopsy may not be needed; genetic testing, however, is helpful to differentiate ATTR mutant from wild type, and if a mutation is identified, family screening should be performed (Flowchart 1).[15] Such a workflow scheme, however, needs to be tested prospectively for efficiency, diagnostic accuracy, and more importantly cost effectiveness.

CARDIAC SARCOIDOSIS

Sarcoidosis is a multisystem granulomatous disorder of unknown etiology. Cardiac involvement is associated with poor prognosis if left untreated. Early and definitive diagnosis of cardiac involvement in sarcoidosis is challenging. Cardiac sarcoidosis is readily treatable with corticosteroids and other modalities of treatment, hence prompt diagnosis and treatment can prevent adverse outcome.

Granulomatous inflammation, which is the hallmark of sarcoidosis, may involve myocardium, endocardium or pericardium. Cardiac involvement is often patchy with the most common locations of granulomas found in the LV free wall and basal ventricular septum, often involving the conducting system. Clinical presentation may range from asymptomatic conduction abnormalities to fatal ventricular arrhythmias, depending upon the location and extent of granulomatous inflammation. The diagnostic evaluation of cardiac sarcoidosis has evolved over the past few decades and includes ECG, echocardiography, LGE CMR and positron emission tomography computed tomography (PET-CT)

Electrocardiogram

Patients with cardiac sarcoidosis often have ECG abnormalities, the prevalence of which depends on the severity of disease. ECG should be done in every patient with suspected cardiac sarcoidosis to detect subtle or overt conduction or repolarization abnormalities. Even though ECG abnormalities are frequently seen in cardiac sarcoidosis, these may be often nonspecific, and a normal ECG does not exclude cardiac sarcoidosis.

The most common conduction abnormality in cardiac sarcoidosis is atrioventricular block, which occurs in 26–62% of cases, followed by bundle branch block, which occurs in 12–61% of cases. Complete heart block is the most common finding in patients with clinically evident cardiac sarcoidosis who present with heart failure or syncope and is reported in 23–30% of patients.[18] First degree heart block and bundle branch block also often occur, due to involvement of the basal septum by scar tissue or granulomas or the involvement of the nodal artery causing ischemia in the conduction system. Sarcoid granulomas in the ventricular myocardium can become foci for abnormal automaticity, increasing the likelihood of re-entrant tachyarrhythmias. Ventricular tachycardia (VT) is the most

Flowchart 1: Schematic diagram of the steps in evaluation of cardiac amyloidosis.[15]

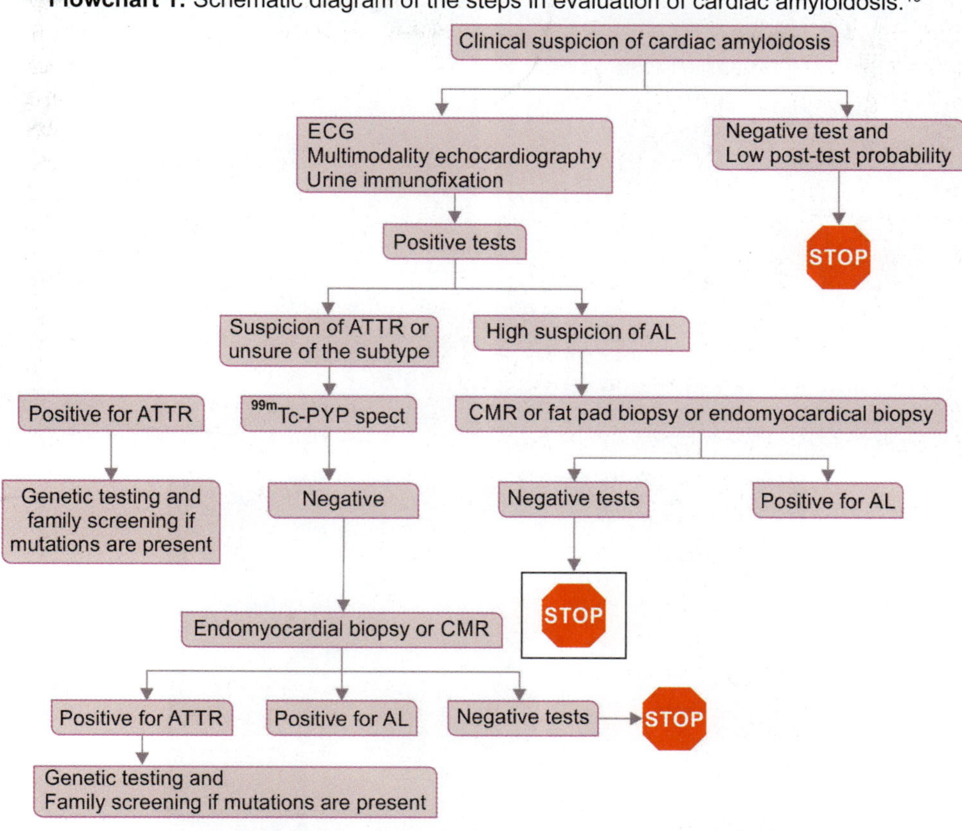

(CMR: cardiac magnetic resonance imaging; PYP: pyrophosphate; SPECT: single-photon emission computerized tomography; ECG: electrocardiogram)

frequent arrhythmia noted in cardiac sarcoidosis with a reported incidence of 23%.[19]

Splintered QRS complexes are another common ECG abnormality in cardiac sarcoidosis.

The subtle ECG abnormalities may be missed on routine baseline resting ECG. Signal averaged ECG and 24-hour ECG monitoring increase the sensitivity for detection of subclinical rhythm disturbances[20] and also, aid in risk estimation of sudden death.

Echocardiography

Echocardiography has been recommended as the diagnostic and screening tool in the evaluation of cardiac sarcoidosis. Early in the course of disease echocardiographic abnormalities may be subtle and nonspecific. But later in advanced stages typical findings are present such as focal thinning and akinesia of LV segments not consistent with coronary vascular distribution. Novel techniques, including tissue velocity imaging, and strain and strain rate imaging, help in early detection of subclinical disease by demonstration of reduced average global LS or reduced regional strain of particular LV segments. Cardiac sarcoidosis may present as dilated cardiomyopathy with dilated cardiac chambers, global hypokinesia but with patchy thinning and scarring of LV-mainly in the basal septum. Valvular dysfunction occurs due to papillary muscle involvement and results in significant regurgitation. Diastolic dysfunction and pulmonary arterial hypertension are other manifestations of cardiac sarcoidosis. Cardiac sarcoidosis can involve any cardiac structure, the myocardium being most frequently affected. The pericardial and endocardial involvements usually reflect direct extensions of myocardial disease.[20] The granulomatous inflammation in the myocardium occurs in unusual locations and results in fibrosis. Myocardial scars in unusual locations, not typical for ischemic injury, in the absence of coronary artery disease, should raise the suspicion of cardiac sarcoidosis. Cardiac sarcoidosis responds favorably to corticosteroid therapy alone or in combination with immunosuppressive therapy.

Characteristic Echocardiographic Findings in Cardiac Sarcoidosis

- Ventricular wall thinning with focal hyperechogenicity or scarring of myocardium, usually affecting the basal

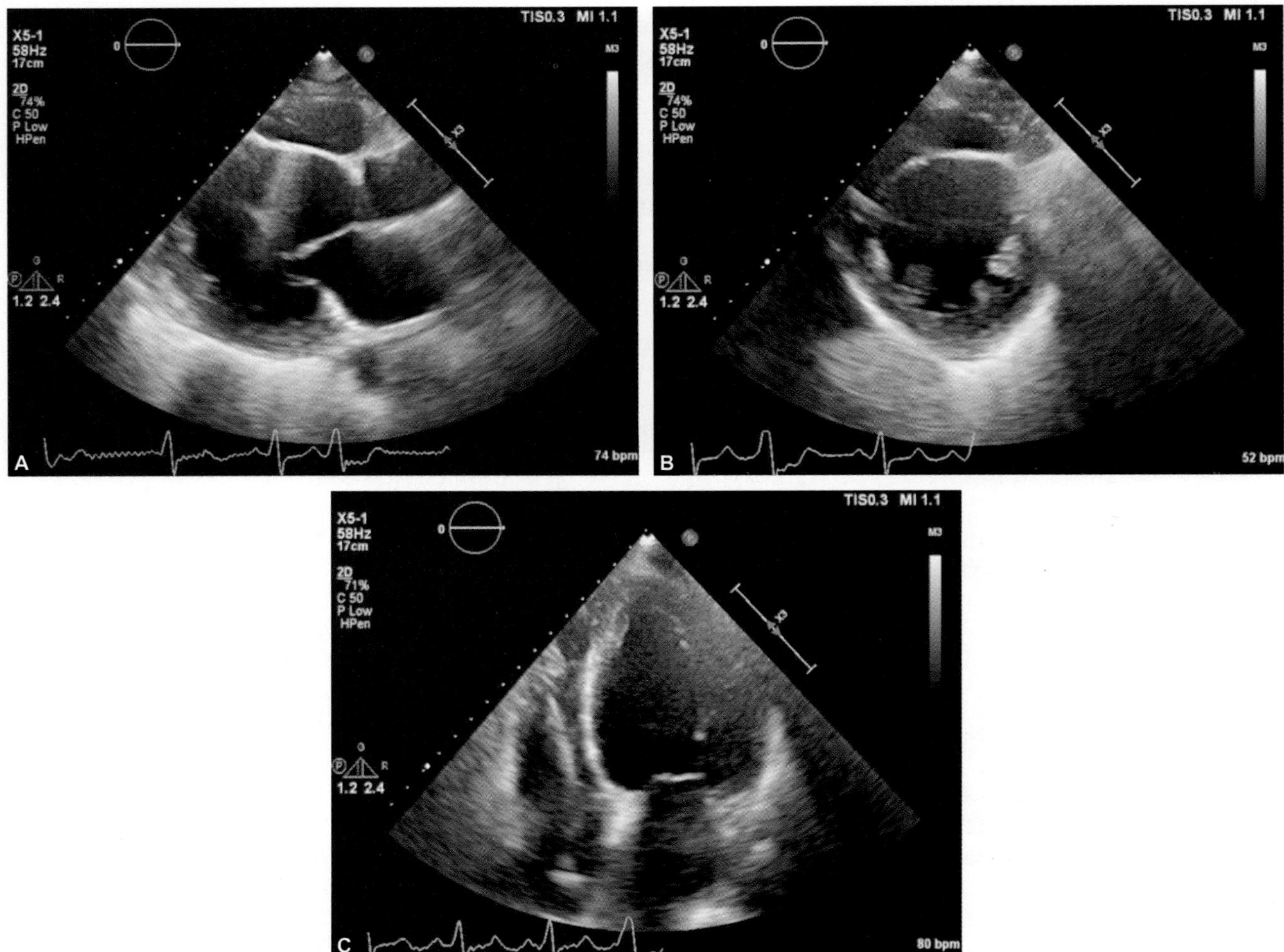

Figs. 5A to C: Echocardiographic features diagnostic of cardiac sarcoidosis. (A) Parasternal long axis view shows dilated LA and LV with hyperechoic and thinned out basal and mid anterior septum; (B) Parasternal short axis view of LV at the level of papillary muscles shows dilated LV with thinning of inferior and anterior septum; (C) Apical 4 chamber view shows dilated all 4 cardiac chambers with focal thinning and hyperechogenicity of basal and mid inferior septum. This focal thinning and hyperechogenicity is not consistent with any vascular territory and is diagnostic of cardiac sarcoidosis.

anterior and inferior septum while sparing the apex (Fig. 5). This patchy thinning and scarring may involve the LV free wall, papillary muscles, right ventricle or the atria. Ventricular aneurysms may be formed.

- Initially during the phase of early inflammation there is myocardial edema which may be appreciated as subtle wall thickening relating to tissue swelling. However, these changes may be difficult to appreciate on echocardiographic imaging and are better visualized on cardiac MRI
- Global hypokinesia of LV or regional wall motion abnormalities not consistent with vascular territory
- Systolic function may be normal initially but it is usually severely impaired late in the course of the disease when it usually comes to clinical attention due to symptoms of heart failure. Novel echocardiographic techniques of tissue velocity imaging, and strain and strain rate imaging, facilitate early detection of subclinical LV and RV dysfunction[21] by demonstration of reduced average global LS or reduced regional strain of particular LV or RV segments. LV systolic function is an important prognostic indicator. Reduced LV and RV function carries a grave prognosis with increased morbidity and mortality and also associated with poor response to immunosuppressant therapy.
- Diastolic dysfunction of LV: Initially during the phase of early inflammation, diastolic dysfunction typically predominates even in the presence of normal contractility.[22] But as the disease progresses with granuloma formation and myocardial fibrosis, the diastolic dysfunction progresses to grade III.
- Dilated cardiac chambers

- Pulmonary involvement is frequently noted in patients with cardiac sarcoidosis and there will be resultant pulmonary hypertension or right heart failure
- Mitral regurgitation due to papillary muscle involvement
- Pericardial effusion may be seen in few cases. Usually, it will be small but occasionally large with hemodynamic instability, typically with granulomatous involvement of pericardium.[22]

Echocardiography also plays an important role in assessing the response to therapy through assessment of the following parameters:

- Reduction in LV end-diastolic dimension–LVEDD, LV volumes
- Improvement in LV systolic function as assessed by LV ejection fraction, myocardial tissue velocities and average global LS
- Improvement in segmental myocardial tissue velocities and regional LS
- Diastolic dysfunction also reverses.

Checklist for Echocardiographic Evaluation in a Patient with Suspected Cardiac Sarcoidosis

- Ventricular wall thinning with focal hyperechogenicity or scarring of myocardium
- Subtle wall thickening relating to tissue swelling in the early stages of the disease
- Regional wall motion abnormalities not consistent with vascular territory
- Reduced LV and RV function as indicated by reduced LVEF and reduced fractional area change for RV.
- Novel techniques like tissue velocity imaging and average global LS or regional strain detect ventricular dysfunction in early stage of the disease.
- Diastolic dysfunction is predominant in early sage and progresses to grade III in the advanced stage.
- Pulmonary hypertension or right heart failure
- Mitral regurgitation due to papillary muscle involvement
- Pericardial effusion.

Cardiac Magnetic Resonance Imaging

Cardiac MRI has high spatial and soft tissue resolution, and currently, it is the preferred imaging modality for the diagnosis and evaluation of cardiac sarcoidosis. CMR is useful in evaluation of patients with a cardiomyopathy of unexplained origin and also in identification of cardiac involvement in patients with pulmonary disease. The CMR features of cardiac sarcoidosis vary according to the disease stage. The early stage of acute inflammation is potentially reversible and associated with myocardial edema, which can be identified as focal areas of thickening and high intensity signals on T2- weighted images[23] (Fig. 6A). T1-weighted (cine) imaging illustrates wall motion abnormalities, hypertrophy due to possible infiltrative disease, wall thinning or heart failure.

The advanced stage of cardiac sarcoidosis is characterized by focal myocardial thinning and scarring[24] and LV dysfunction. LGE CMR demonstrates typical patterns of patchy areas of enhancement in a nonvascular territory (Fig. 6B). The LGE pattern can be mid-myocardial, and subepicardial with linear or nodular areas of enhancement. The delayed enhancement may be noticed in any of the cardiac

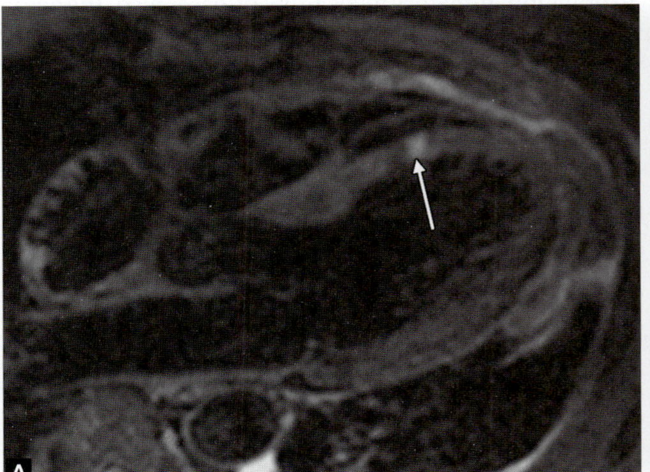

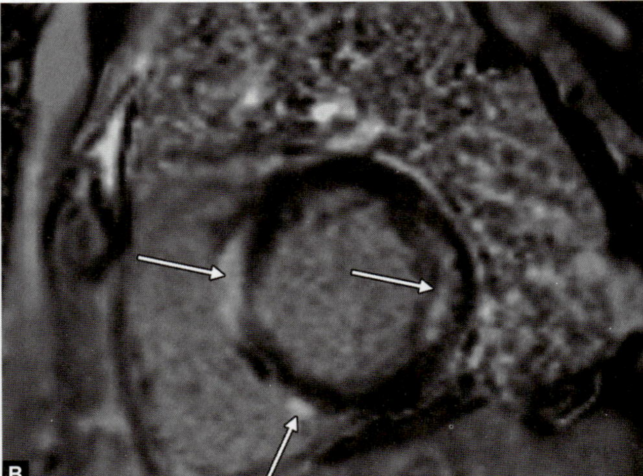

Figs. 6A and B: Cardiac magnetic resonance imaging features of cardiac sarcoidosis. (A) T2 weighted cardiac magnetic resonance image demonstrates focus of inflammation (indicated by arrow) in the interventricular septum; (B) Late gadolinium enhancement cardiac magnetic resonance image demonstrates multiple focal areas of myocardial fibrosis and scarring (indicated by arrows) in the left ventricle not consistent with the vascular distribution.

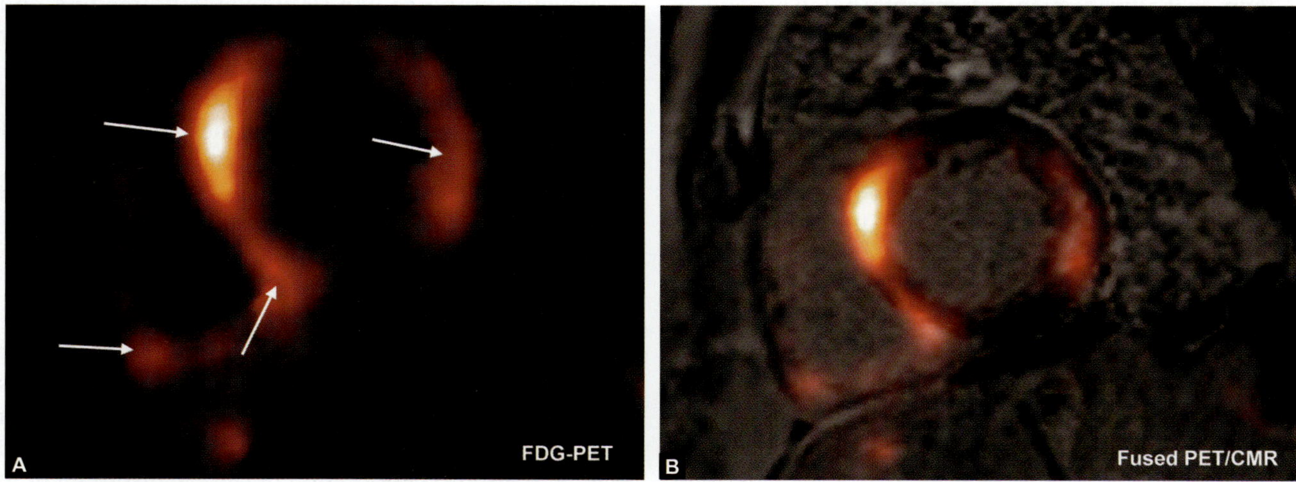

Figs. 7A and B: Positron emission tomography (PET)/computed tomography (CT) and fused PET/cardiac magnetic resonance (CMR) images in a patient with cardiac sarcoidosis.[30] (A) PET/CT scan demonstrates abnormal areas of fluorodeoxyglucose (FDG) uptake in several of the nodules with patchy uptake in the heart as indicated by arrows; (B) Fused PET/CMR demonstrates matched the areas of patchy uptake.

chambers—LV, RV, LA or the RA. CMR may demonstrate fibrosis or edema of basal anteroseptal and inferoseptal region of LV, apical inferoseptal area of both ventricles, moderator band or the papillary muscles. LGE has a very high sensitivity of 100% and moderate specificity of 78% for diagnosing cardiac sarcoidosis.[25]

Myocardial scar detected by LGE is an independent predictor of sudden cardiac death in patients with suspected cardiac sarcoidosis.[25] The new Japanese guidelines consider LGE as a major criterion in the diagnosis of cardiac sarcoidosis. CMR imaging enables fast, accurate, high-resolution, and noninvasive diagnosis of subclinical or clinical cardiac sarcoidosis, and is currently the technique of choice in the evaluation of sarcoidosis.

Checklist for Cardiac Magnetic Resonance Evaluation in a Patient with Suspected Cardiac Sarcoidosis

- Early stage of acute inflammation shows focal areas of thickening and high intensity signals on T2- weighted images
- Wall motion abnormalities or hypertrophy on T1-weighted images
- Patchy areas of enhancement in a nonvascular territory on LGE CMR in any of the cardiac chambers—LV, RV, LA or the RA.

Positron Emission Tomography

^{18}F-Fluorodeoxyglucose (FDG) positron emission tomography (PET)/computed tomography (CT) has become a key technique in the diagnosis of active cardiac sarcoidosis. It has been used to diagnose and "stage" cardiac sarcoidosis.[20] PET scans demonstrating patchy and focal uptake patterns (Fig. 7A) within the heart are most specific for cardiac sarcoidosis. Increased 18FDG uptake is observed most frequently in the basal and mid-anteroseptal lateral wall of the LV; while involvement of the apex is rare. Less commonly RV involvement may be seen.

Fluorodeoxyglucose PET is more sensitive than gallium-67 scintigraphy, thallium-201, or technicium-99m single-photon emission computed tomography (SPECT).[26] It can also be combined with myocardial perfusion imaging to detect fibrogranulomatous replacement. However, PET is non-specific for sarcoidosis and uptake of 18F-FDG is seen in other inflammatory myocardial diseases also. The actual specificity of FDG PET perfusion imaging is uncertain. Reported specificity has ranged from 38% to 90%, in which the lower range may be due to detection of early subclinical disease. Serial PET-CT scans are useful in evaluating response to immunosuppressive therapy in cardiac sarcoidosis.[27] Improvement in PET scans (i.e. reduction in 18FDG uptake) has been noted following therapy.

Cardiac Magnetic Resonance Imaging versus Positron Emission Tomography/ Computed Tomography

Cardiac MR and PET-CT are the key imaging modalities in the evaluation of cardiac sarcoidosis. A normal CMR study has a high negative predictive value to exclude significant cardiac involvement and patient may be monitored clinically. However, select patients with high clinical suspicion of cardiac sarcoidosis and normal CMR might be considered for 18F-FDG PET. CMR may be preferable to 18F-FDG PET as a first line test to minimize ionizing radiation.[28]

PET-CT has the advantage over CMR of evaluating the extent of systemic disease. PET-CT is also useful in patients with glomerular filtration rate below 30 mL/min, ferromagnetic devices such as defibrillators or pacemakers (with the exception of a few approved devices), or other contraindication to CMR. PET-CT has the disadvantage of exposing patients to ionizing radiation and it requires, careful patient preparation.[28]

Patients with inflammation by 18F-FDG PET should be considered for anti-inflammatory therapy and repeat 18F-FDG PET imaging in 3–6 months to evaluate response to therapy.

With the emergence of hybrid PET-CMR system, the unique strengths of PET and CMR may be combined. The simultaneous use of PET and CMR has the ability to demonstrate regions of active inflammation by increased FDG uptake bordering regions of fibrosis identified by CMR LGE (Fig. 7B).[29,30] Combined PET-CMR offers the advantage of an accurate assessment of function by CMR, identification of fibrosis/scar by CMR using LGE, and assessment of inflammation via 18F-FDG PET. Hybrid PET-CMR will soon become preferred imaging modality for the early diagnosis of cardiac sarcoidosis.

Endomyocardial Biopsy

The gold standard foe diagnosis of cardiac sarcoidosis is noncaseating granuloma with limited lymphocyte infiltration and patchy fibrosis on endomyocardial biopsy. However, EMB is invasive and has low sensitivity due to patchy distribution of disease with predilection to basal and lateral LV wall regions difficult to biopsy. Hence, EMB is indicated only in the absence of histological confirmation of noncaseating granulomas from any other source like paratracheal or other lymph nodes.

> **Key point 3:** Cardiac sarcoidosis is usually detected late in the stages of heart failure in daily clinical practice. The echocardiographic features typical of cardiac sarcoidosis are focal thinning and scarring of myocardium which is not consistent with vascular territory and the diagnosis can be confirmed by CMR or nuclear imaging--PET scan. PET appears to be more sensitive but less specific than CMR.

CONCLUSION

In conclusion, diagnosis of cardiac sarcoidosis requires high index of suspicion and multidisciplinary teamwork. Identification of early cardiac dysfunction with noninvasive modalities among subjects with systemic sarcoidosis is pivotal in risk stratification and early intervention. Integrated echocardiography with tissue velocity imaging and strain rate imaging, CMR and PET-CT are the key imaging modalities for the early diagnosis of cardiac sarcoidosis and for monitoring the response to immunosuppressive therapy.

REFERENCES

1. Gertz MA, Comenzo R, Falk RH, et al. Definition of organ involvement and treatment response in immunoglobulin light chain amyloidosis (AL): a consensus opinion from the 10th International symposium on Amyloid and Amyloidosis. Am J Hematol. 2005;79(4):319-28.
2. Dubrey SW, Hawkins PN, Falk RH. Amyloid diseases of the heart: assessment, diagnosis, and referral. Heart. 2011;97(1):75-84.
3. Rahman JE, Helou EF, Gelzer-Bell R, et al. Noninvasive diagnosis of biopsy-proven cardiac amyloidosis. J Am Coll Cardiol. 2004;43(3):410-5.
4. Nagueh SF, Smiseth OA, Appleton CP, et al. Recommendations for the Evaluation of Left Ventricular Diastolic Function by Echocardiography: An Update from the American Society of Echocardiography and the European Association of Cardio-vascular Imaging. J Am Soc Echocardiogr. 2016;29(4):277-314.
5. Feng D, Syed IS, Martinez M, et al. Intracardiac thrombosis and anticoagulation therapy in cardiac amyloidosis. Circulation. 2009;119(18):2490-7.
6. Ha JW, Ommen SR, Tajik AJ, et al. Differentiation of constrictive pericarditis from restrictive cardiomyopathy using mitral annular velocity by tissue Doppler echocardiography. Am J Cardiol. 2004;94(3):316-9.
7. Phelan D, Collier P, Thavendiranathan P, et al. Relative "apical sparing" of longitudinal strain using 2-dimensional speckle-tracking echocardiography is both sensitive and specific for the diagnosis of cardiac amyloidosis. Heart. 2012;98(19):1442-8.
8. Cueto-Garcia L, Reeder GS, Kyle RA, et al. Echocardiographic findings in systemic amyloidosis: spectrum of cardiac involvement and relation to survival. J Am Coll Cardiol. 1985;6(4):737-43.
9. Klein AL, Hatle LK, Taliercio CP, et al. Prognostic significance of Doppler measures of diastolic function in cardiac amyloidosis. A Doppler echocardiography study. Circulation. 1991;83(3):808-16.
10. Syed IS, Glockner JF, Feng D, et al. Role of cardiac magnetic resonance imaging in the detection of cardiac amyloidosis. JACC Cardiovasc Imaging. 2010;3(2):155-64.
11. Maceira AM, Joshi J, Prasad SK, et al. Cardiovascular magnetic resonance in cardiac amyloidosis. Circulation. 2005;111(2):186-93.
12. Austin BA, Tang WH, Rodriguez ER, et al. Delayed hyper-enhancement magnetic resonance imaging provides incremental diagnostic and prognostic utility in suspected cardiac amyloidosis. JACC Cardiovasc Imaging. 2009;2(12):1369-77.

13. Banypersad SM, Sado DM, Flett AS, et al. Quantification of myocardial extracellular volume fraction in systemic AL amyloidosis: An equilibrium contrast cardiovascular magnetic resonance study. Circ Cardiovasc Imaging. 2013;6(1):34-9.
14. Habib G, Bucciaarelli-Ducci C, Caforio ALP, et al. Multimodality Imaging in Restrictive Cardiomyopathies: An EACVI expert consensus document in collaboration with the "Working Group on myocardial and pericardial diseases" of the European Society of Cardiology Endorsed by The Indian Academy of Echocardiography. Eur Heart J Cardiovas Imaging. 2017;18(10):1090-121.
15. Aljaroudi WA, Desai MY, Tang WH, et al. Role of imaging in the diagnosis and management of patients with cardiac amyloidosis: State of the art review and focus on emerging nuclear techniques. J Nucl Cardiol. 2014;21(2):271-83.
16. Sachchithanantham S, Wechalekar AD. Imaging in systemic amyloidosis. Br Med Bull. 2013;107:41-56.
17. Bokhari S, Castano A, Pozniakoff T, et al. 99mTc-pyrophosphate scintigraphy for differentiating light-chain cardiac amyloidosis from the transthyretin-related familial and senile cardiac amyloidoses. Circ Cardiovasc Imaging. 2013;6(2):195-201.
18. Roberts WC, McAllister HA Jr, Ferrans VJ. Sarcoidosis of the heart. A clinicopathologic study of 35 necropsy patients (group 1) and review of 78 previously described necropsy patients (group 11). Am J Med. 1977;63(1):86-108.
19. Sekiguchi M, Numao Y, Imai M, et al. Clinical and histopathological profile of sarcoidosis of the heart and acute idiopathic myocarditis. Concepts through a study employing endomyocardial biopsy. I. Sarcoidosis. Jpn Circ J. 1980;44(4):249-63.
20. Lynch JP III, Hwang J, Bradfield J, et al. Cardiac involvement in sarcoidosis: evolving concepts in diagnosis and treatment. Semin Respir Crit Care Med. 2014;35(3):372-90.
21. Aggeli C, Felekos I, Tousoulis D, et al. Myocardial mechanics for the early detection of cardiac sarcoidosis. Int J Cardiol. 2013;168(5):4820-1.
22. Evanchan JP, Crouser ED, Kalbfleisch SJ. Cardiac Sarcoidosis: Recent Advances in Diagnosis and Treatment and an Argument for the Need for a Systematic Multidisciplinary Approach to Management. J Innovat Cardiac Rhyth Manag. 2013;4:1160-74.
23. Dubrey SW, Falk RH. Diagnosis and Management of Cardiac Sarcoidosis. Prog Cardiovasc Dis. 2010;52(4):336-46.
24. Said SAM, Post S, Nooijer R de, et al. Multimodality Diagnostic Approach in Cardiac Sarcoidosis: from ECG to Magnetic Resonance Imaging. Curr Cardiol Rev. 2016;3:54-62.
25. Greulich S, Deluigi CC, Gloekler S, et al. CMR imaging predicts death and other adverse events in suspected cardiac sarcoidosis. JACC Cardiovasc Imaging. 2013;6(4):501-11.
26. Ishimaru S, Tsujino I, Sakaue S, et al. Combination of 18F-fluoro-2-deoxyglucose positron emission tomography and magnetic resonance imaging in assessing cardiac sarcoidosis. Sarcoidosis Vasc Diffuse Lung Dis. 2005;22(3):234-5.
27. Braun JJ, Kessler R, Constantinesco A, et al. 18F-FDG PET/CT in sarcoidosis management: review and report of 20 cases. Eur J Nucl Med Mol Imaging. 2008;35(8):1537-43.
28. Hulten E, Aslam S, Osborne M. Cardiac sarcoidosis—state of the art review. Cardiovasc Diagn Ther. 2016;6(1):50-63.
29. White JA, Rajchl M, Butler J, et al. Active cardiac sarcoidosis: first clinical experience of simultaneous positron emission tomography–magnetic resonance imaging for the diagnosis of cardiac disease. Circulation. 2013;127(22):e639-41.
30. Srichai MB, Addrizzo-Harris DJ, Friedman K. Cardiac Sarcoidosis. J Am Coll Cardiol. 2011;58(4):438.

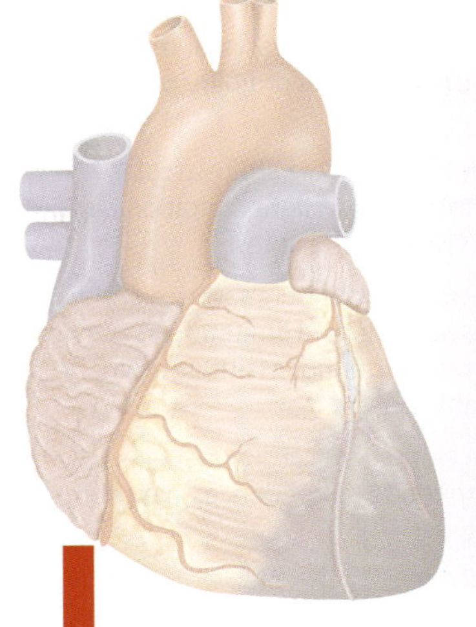

Telemedicine and Internet of Things Technology for Management of Heart Failure

P Krishnam Raju, SG Prasad

INTRODUCTION

The increasing cost of healthcare services has made it imperative for adopting innovative ways for healthcare delivery by application of technology. This has particular relevance for chronic diseases wherein hospital visits can be minimized by the utilization of appropriate technologies. One of the most common and growing health problem today is heart failure which is generally associated with high healthcare costs, mainly due to frequent hospitalizations. The advances in the field of information and communication technology (ICT) over the last decade have helped in balancing the supply and demand in the healthcare services in quite an effective way. The emerging paradigm of Internet of Things (IoT) has further ensured that a continuum in care can be maintained, with patients having the opportunity to have wearable devices at their homes and using the telemedicine platform for transmission of medical data from these devices for consultations. The IoT techniques gives viable solutions that help in solving the problem of heart disease patients care as they can change the service model into a pervasive way, and trigger the healthcare service based on patient's physical status rather than their feelings. Telemedicine as a technology, thus, finds its application in assisting patients with providing consultations and also to have clinical data from these integrated IoT devices for ensuring quality services without requiring hospital visits and continuity in care that is much needed for chronic diseases like heart failure. The impact of social networking platforms and mobile technologies in the healthcare domain needs further work especially in their utility to serving the underserved and remote populations.[1]

As per the World Bank, the life expectancy in India has grown from 41 years in 1960 to 68 years in 2015.[2] As the life expectancy is steadily increasing, the requirement for self-health monitoring and preventive medicine is also increasing due to the projected dramatic increase in the number of elderly people (by 2020). Among the main challenges faced by patients in India are accessibility, affordability and quality healthcare services. The need of the hour is to explore how we can address these issues most efficiently using innovative and disruptive digital health solutions. With innovative digital healthcare solutions, patients can have a better outcome to treatment focusing on prevention and providing independence and freedom to communicate with doctors and caregivers. As the number of smartphone users in India increases, patients are taking ownership of their personal health and wellness. There is an increasing demand from people for technologies to go beyond trend and actually work toward assisting them in reaching their health and fitness goals, and specific health-monitoring requirement, especially in older age groups.

The evolving list of IoT-based medical devices has increased the opportunities for monitoring patients with chronic diseases like hypertension, diabetes, heart failure, etc. Heart failure is a chronic disorder that leaves patients prone to exacerbations and hospital readmissions.

There is always a demand on clinicians to find alternatives to hospitalizations for worsening heart failure. Remote patient management for patients with heart failure can facilitate early detection of signs and symptoms of cardiac decompensation, allowing care providers to quickly respond to their patient's needs and subsequently reduce the likelihood of hospitalization. Heart failure is a complex syndrome and the final common pathway of many different pathological processes, often resulting in unplanned emergency hospitalization (Fonarow, 2008; Cleland et al., 2011). Upon discharge, the health trajectory of such patients is variable, with many having a persistently impaired quality of life and high rates of readmission (McMurray et al., 2012).

HEART FAILURE—ASSESSMENT AND MONITORING

One of the most common chronic ailments globally is heart failure that has a major impact on healthcare costs, due to frequent hospitalizations that are required. Patients' heart failure classifications are determined by a doctor based on their heart failure symptoms and functional limitations. The severity of heart failure depends on how well the heart is able to pump blood to various organs and tissues of the body. The most common measure of heart failure severity is based on the NYHA (New York Heart Association) Class guidelines (Table 1).

TABLE 1: NYHA functional classication.

NYHA Class	*Patients with cardiac disease (Description of heart failure related symptoms)*
Class I	Patients with cardiac disease but without resulting in limitation of physical activity. Ordinary physical activity does not cause undue fatigue, palpitation (rapid or pounding heartbeat), dyspnea (shortness of breath), or anginal pain (chest pain)
Class II	Patients with cardiac disease resulting in slight limitation of physical activity. They are comfortable at rest. Ordinary physical activity results in fatigue, palpitation, dyspnea, or anginal pain
Class III	Patients with cardiac disease resulting in marked limitation of physical activity. They are comfortable at rest. Less than ordinary activity causes fatigue, palpitation, dyspnea, or anginal pain
Class IV	Patients with cardiac disease resulting in the inability to carry on any physical activity without discomfort. Symptoms of heart failure or the anginal syndrome may be present even at rest. If any physical activity is undertaken, discomfort is increased

(NYHA: New York Heart Association)

TABLE 2: Objective assessment classification of heart failure.

Rating	*Description*
Stage A	No objective evidence of cardiovascular disease. No symptoms and no limitation in ordinary physical activity
Stage B	Objective evidence of minimal cardiovascular disease. Mild symptoms and slight limitation during ordinary activity. Comfortable at rest
Stage C	Objective evidence of moderately severe cardiovascular disease. Marked limitation in activity due to symptoms, even during less-than-ordinary activity. Comfortable only at rest
Stage D	Objective evidence of severe cardiovascular disease. Severe limitations. Experiences symptoms even while at rest

In 2001, the American Heart Association and American College of Cardiology developed a rating system to evaluate the progression of heart failure symptoms. The points (Table 2) provide a description of the patient as heart failure progresses.

The most recent heart failure guidelines have emphasized the role of daily monitoring of body weight and vital signs.[3] Online consultations through the telemedicine platform, integrated with educational interventions, can provide optimized home-based clinical management of heart failure patients by reducing hospitalizations and emergency department access, while improving outcomes and quality of life.[3] Currently available devices show adequate levels of efficiency and safety and allow for easy implementation of home-based telemedicine programs and high-quality patient care.

Congestive heart failure (CHF) occurs when the heart cannot provide the necessary cardiac output for the metabolic needs of the human body. It is a frequent cause of disability, emergency hospital admission and premature death.[4,5] The prevalence and incidence rates of heart failure increase with age.[6] Due to demographic changes and the increasing probability to survive an acute myocardial infarction and diseases of the heart valves and the myocardium, the number of CHF patients will continue to increase in the next years.[7] One more reason for the increase in the incidence of CHF is because of improved cardiovascular interventions for disease processes that reduce early mortality but may result in cardiac changes that lead to heart failure (Fig. 1).

The most prominent symptoms are increased venous pressure, abnormal heart and breathing rate, tiredness and leg swelling. Most important pathogenesis influences are age, gender, high blood pressure, alcohol and smoking, sedentary lifestyle and diet, genetic predisposition and family history, diabetes, and atherosclerosis. Common

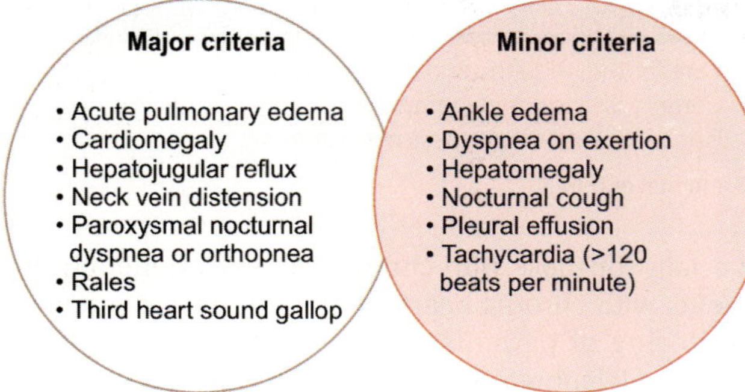

Fig. 1: Framingham diagnostic criteria (major and minor) for heart failure.

causes are considered to be valvular heart disease, coronary heart disease and hypertension. CHF diagnosis can be achieved through physical examination, ECG, chest X-ray, biomarkers and echocardiography.

The initial evaluation includes a history and physical examination, chest radiography, electrocardiography, and laboratory assessment to identify causes or precipitating factors. A displaced cardiac apex, a third heart sound, and chest radiography findings of venous congestion or interstitial edema are useful in identifying heart failure. Figure 1 shows the Framingham diagnostic criteria (major and minor) for heart failure.

It is important to understand that there is no single diagnostic test for heart failure. Therefore, it remains a clinical diagnosis requiring a history, physical examination, and laboratory testing. Symptoms of heart failure can be caused by systolic or diastolic dysfunction. Heart failure is associated with a wide spectrum of left ventricular functional abnormalities. These range from preserved left ventricular ejection fraction (EF) and normal left ventricular size to severely reduced EF and marked dilation of the left ventricle. Echocardiography with Doppler studies is arguably the most important single diagnostic test in evaluating a patient with heart failure. Table 3 shows the classification of heart failure based on left ventricular EF.

Inferior vena cava (IVC) ultrasonography (ECHO) is a simple and useful tool in patients with heart failure. An increase in IVC diameter or a reduction of IVC inspiratory collapse allows detection of volume overload. Therefore, these parameters have been proposed in the management of heart failure, based on their capacity to detect hemodynamic congestion. The evaluation of the right internal jugular vein (RIJV) allows assessment of central venous pressure and is a direct measure of right atrial pressure (RAP). The majority of patients with acute decompensated heart failure (ADHF) have elevated RAP, which reflects elevated left ventricular filling pressures. Therefore, measurement of RAP is a fundamental part of the bedside heart failure evaluation. In certain clinical scenarios, a patient with

TABLE 3: Classification of heart failure based on left ventricular ejection fraction (EF).

Type	*Ejection Fraction (%)*
HFpEF (Heart failure with preserved EF) – Asymptomatic	>50
HFpEF (Heart failure with preserved EF) – Symptomatic	
HFmrEF (Heart failure with mid-range EF) – Asymptomatic	40–49
HFmrEF (Heart failure with mid-range EF) – Symptomatic	
HFrEF (Heart failure with reduced EF) – Asymptomatic	<40
HFrEF (Heart failure with reduced EF) – Symptomatic	
HFrEF Severe	<35
HFcontEF	HF on treatment and controlled with reduced EF

(EF ejection fraction; HF: heart failure)

chronic heart failure and established echocardiographic findings of poor left ventricular function and currently presenting with acute pulmonary edema, or in a patient presenting with undifferentiated dyspnea, an immediate full echocardiographic exam may not be indicated. In such instances, lung ultrasound can provide timely data sufficient to support or refute the diagnosis of ADHF. Lung ultrasonographic multiple B-lines are a good indicator of the alveolar interstitial syndrome but are not specific for ADHF. The absence of multiple B-lines can be used to rule out ADHF as a causative etiology and in clinical scenarios where the assessment of acute dyspnea boils down to single or dichotomous pathologies, lung ultrasound can help rule in ADHF. Appropriate diagnosis and therapy for heart failure are important given the poor prognosis. Telemedicine integrated with IoT devices can play a vital role for patients with CHF by detecting early signs and symptoms of cardiac decompensation, thus enabling a prompt initiation of the appropriate treatment and care before a full manifestation of a heart failure decompensation.

HEART FAILURE: EPIDEMIOLOGY

Heart failure is a common clinical syndrome associated with high morbidity and mortality. It is a major public health problem, with a prevalence of over 5.8 million people affected in the US, and over 26 million people worldwide.[8] In the US and in Europe, heart failure prevalence ranges from 1.1% to 2.2% in the general population. Most of the heart failure burden is situated in people aged over 65 years, who account for more than 80% of deaths and prevalent cases in

BOX 1: Facts

- Chronic HF is a cardiovascular disorder affecting approximately 1-2% of adult population worldwide.
- Lack of good surveillance system in India to predict the incidence and prevalence of HF.
- Lifetime risk of HF increases with age, so the burden likely to increase with aging population.

(HF: heart failure)

the US and Europe.[9,10] The lifetime probability of developing heart failure is believed to be one in five.

The lack of a good surveillance system has made it difficult to estimate the incidence and prevalence estimates of heart failure in India. However, this issue is not unique to India as in 2001, Mendez and Cowie found no population-based heart failure studies in all developing countries, (Box 1)[11] making global prevalence estimates also very difficult. The lack of standard definition has further hampered estimating the burden of heart failure. In fact, the WHO Global Burden of Disease study places heart failure in several categories within the cardiovascular disease, including ischemic, hypertensive, inflammatory and rheumatic heart disease (RHD).[12]

Based on disease-specific estimates of prevalence and incidence rates of heart failure, we conservatively estimate the prevalence of heart failure in India due to coronary heart disease, hypertension, obesity, diabetes and rheumatic heart disease to range from 1.3 to 4.6 million, with an annual incidence of 4.916–1.8 million.[13] The double burden of rising cardiovascular risk factors and persistent "pretransition" diseases such as rheumatic heart disease, limited healthcare infrastructure and social disparities contribute to these estimates.

India's economic development, industrialization and urbanization have been accompanied by transitions that contribute to the increase in the overall risk of heart failure. First, the population of India is aging due to recent successes against communicable diseases such that the number of people >60 years old increased from 62 million in 1996 to 113 million in 2016.[14] Heart failure is predominantly a disease of the elderly, as the lifetime risk for heart failure increases with age, so the burden of heart failure is likely to increase with the aging population.[15] Managing heart failure symptoms is complex and often requires changes in patients' diets, daily activities, and medications to optimize symptom control and prevent acute decompensation.[16]

ROLE OF TECHNOLOGY IN MANAGEMENT OF HEART FAILURE

The emergence of the ICT platform and IoT medical devices have opened up many opportunities for the healthcare platform to assist in providing healthcare at the doorstep,

BOX 2: Applications—IoT based medical devices

- Care for the pediatric and the aged.
- Chronic disease management.
- Personal health and fitness management.

(IOT: Internet of Things)

especially for those with chronic ailments. Generally, for patients with chronic heart failure, non-invasive remote monitoring of patients involves regularly scheduled structured telephone contact between patients and health care providers and/or the electronic transfer of physiologic data using IoT-based medical devices (Box 2). This approach allows for the assessment of symptoms, vital signs, and daily weights, and other select non-invasive parameters of interest. The efficacy of such non-invasive monitoring methods remains uncertain, although a growing body of evidence suggesting that the advent of IoT medical devices which help in providing the vitals have made monitoring of these patients easier and far more effective in their management.

NEED OF INTERNET OF THINGS IN HEALTHCARE

The emerging paradigm of IoT is especially focused on collecting and processing data everywhere and all the time.[17-20] This expansion of the IoT is allowing to use all type of objects beyond their basic functions, or at least, for those they were designed for a wide range of applications. IoT-based medical devices help in vital parameters being monitored irrespective of their location, thereby enabling patients to lead a normal life in familiar surroundings with the satisfaction of their vital parameters being monitored. Additionally, the data acquired can be sent to remote physicians with low cost, which ensures these experts be aware of patients' physical status continuously and in real-time. This IoT-based monitoring system is particularly suitable for patients with chronic heart failure. Telemedicine in heart failure can be of great support to guarantee the patient's continuity of care between hospitals and the clinician. It allows:

- Monitor weight and fluid balance and adjust diuretic therapy to avoid over-diuresis and hypotension
- Control HR (heart rate), BP (blood pressure), and arrhythmias
- Better titrate therapy after hospital discharge
- Enhance educational interventions to promote empowerment and self-management.

IoT-based devices in remote health monitoring systems are not only capable of the conventional sensing tasks but can also exchange information with each other (Fig. 2),

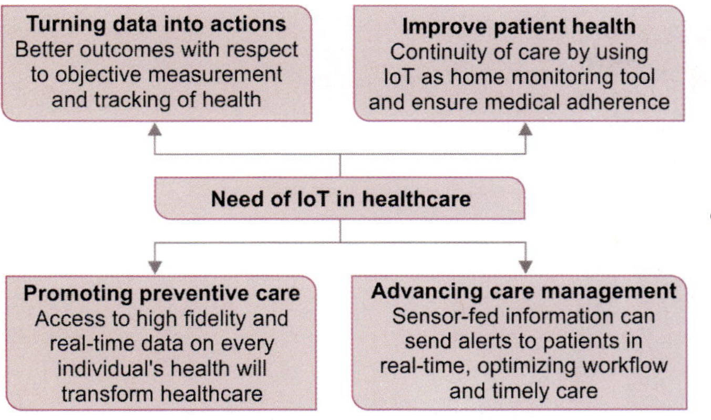

Fig. 2: Importance of IoT in healthcare and management.
(IoT: Internet of Things)

automatically connect to and exchange information with health institutes through the Internet, significantly simplifying set up and administration tasks. As exemplified in, such systems are able to provide services such as an automatic alarm to the nearest healthcare institute in the event of a critical event for a supervised patient. The system architecture for this remoted-based pervasive monitoring essentially consists of the following three components:

1. Acquisition
2. Transmission.
3. Visualization.

The system architecture for a remote health monitoring system are (Fig. 3):

- *Data acquisition* is performed by multiple wearable sensors that measure physiological biomarkers, such as ECG, skin temperature, respiratory rate, EMG muscle activity, and gait (posture). The sensors (as shown in the diagram below) connect to the network through an intermediate data aggregator or concentrator, which is typically a smartphone or a tablet located in the vicinity of the patient (Fig. 4).
- *The data transmission:* Components of the system are responsible for conveying recordings of the patient from the patient's house (or any remote location) to the data center of the Healthcare Organization (HCO) with the assured security and privacy, ideally in near real-time. Typically, the sensory acquisition platform is equipped with a short-range radio such as Zigbee or low-power Bluetooth, which it uses to transfer sensor data to the concentrator. Aggregated data is further relayed to an HCO for long-term storage using Internet connectivity on the concentrator, typically via a smartphone's Wi-Fi or cellular data connection. Sensors in the data acquisition part form an IoT-based architecture as each individual sensor's data can be accessed through the Internet. Often a storage/processing device in the vicinity of a mobile client, sometimes referred to as a cloudlet, is used to augment its storage/processing capability whenever the local mobile resources do not fulfil the application's requirements. The cloudlet can be a local processing unit (such as a desktop computer) which is directly accessible by the concentrator through Wi-Fi network. In addition to providing temporary storage prior to the communication of data to the cloud, the cloudlet can also be used for running time critical tasks on the patient's aggregated data. Moreover, the cloudlet can be used to transmit the aggregated data to the cloud in case of limitations on the mobile device such as a temporary lack of connectivity or energy.
- *Cloud processing* has three distinct components: storage, analytics, and visualization. The system is designed for long-term storage of patient's biomedical information as well as assisting health professionals with diagnostic information. Cloud-based medical data storage and the upfront challenges have been extensively addressed in the literature *Analytics* that use the sensor data along with e-Health records that are becoming prevalent can help with diagnoses and prognoses for a number of health conditions and diseases. Additionally, V*isualization* is a key requirement for any such system because it is impractical to ask physicians to pore over the voluminous data or analyses from wearable sensors. Visualization methods that make the data and analyses accessible to them in a readily digestible format are essential if the wearable sensors are to impact clinical practice.

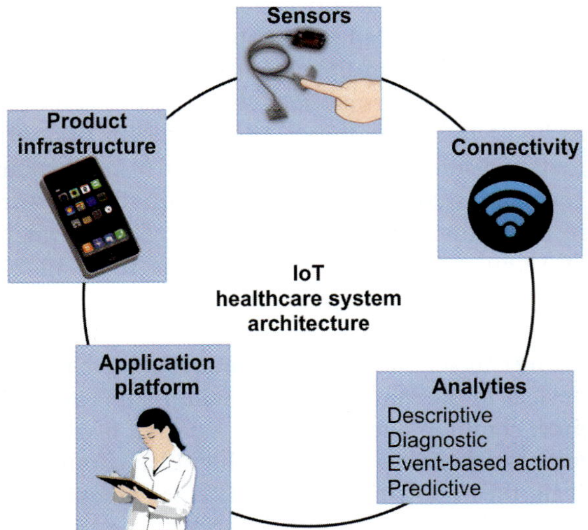

Fig. 3: System architecture for a remote health monitoring system.
(IoT: Internet of Things)

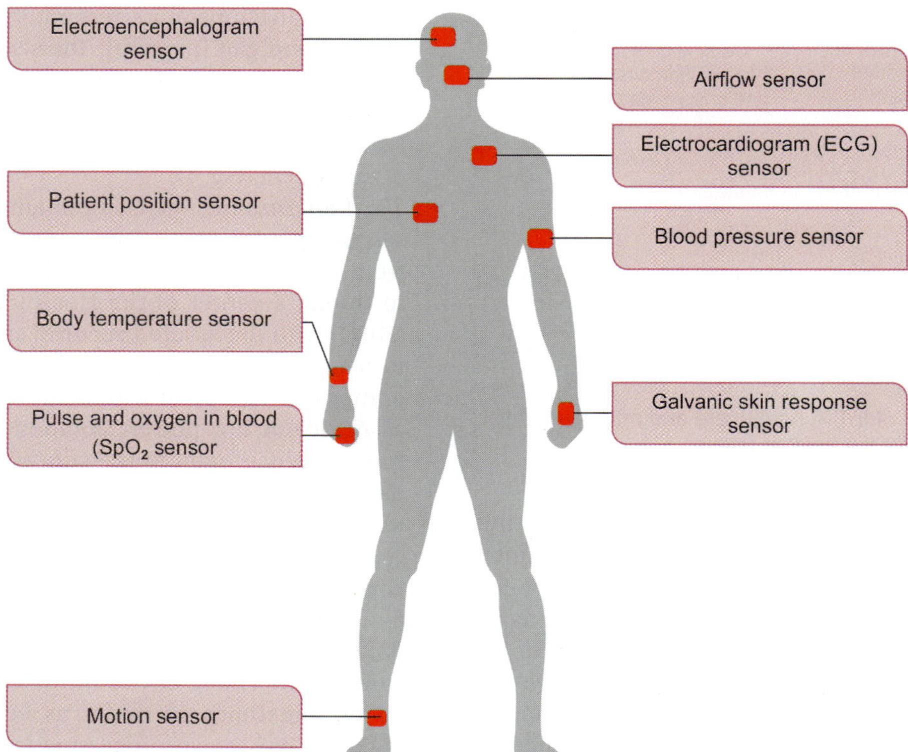

Fig. 4: Remote health monitoring system based on wearable sensors.

REMOTE MONITORING METHODOLOGIES

Remote monitoring has been designed to facilitate early detection of adverse events and to minimize regular follow-up visits for heart failure patients (Tables 4 and 5). The following are the methodologies of remote monitoring for the management of heart failure

- *Telephonic support:* One of the easiest approaches of monitoring involves periodic telephonic calls to patients by trained nurses to assess patient's symptoms and get body weight parameters followed by a conversation with a clinician as and when required. However, it should be noted that measurement of weight also needs to be done in a systematic manner involving the usage of the same weighing machine and also noting the weight first thing in the morning after passing urine. The telephonic follow up's may be designed on a monthly basis in order to ensure continuity of progress in these patients.
- *IoT-based smart monitoring:* With a surge of IoT-based medical devices in the market, it has become lot easier to get some clinical data from these devices and corroborate the same with symptoms to make an assessment for change in treatment plan or for a planned hospital visit, rather than making it on an emergency basis. With real-time monitoring of the condition in place by means of a smart medical device connected to a smartphone application, connected devices can collect medical and other required health data and use the data connection of the smartphone to transfer collected information to a physician. For chronic heart failure patients, it is important to monitor for other cardiac conditions that may eventually lead to heart failure patients. Identification of cardiac rhythm disorders like atrial fibrillation (AF), premature ventricular complexes (PVCs) is equally important in the patient's daily management. The prevalence of AF among heart failure patients is about 13–27%. Early diagnosis and management of AF may prevent AF-associated complications and worsen of the heart failure course.[21-25] There are a number of IoT-based ECG devices in the market that can address this issue. The most common devices used as a part of telemedicine for heart failure patients are the pulse oximeter, the scale, the BP/HR monitor, the ECG (one or more leads), the detector of motion and fall and the personal alarm services. Some of the available devices which help in acquisition and communication of the data through Wi-Fi or Bluetooth and that provide useful clinical

TABLE 4: Devices used in the remote monitoring for the management of heart failure.

Sl. No.	Device	Functionality
1.	AliveCor	Sensor-embedded watchband in an effort to have a real-time display of the cardiac rhythm which is created by conversion of an electrical signal into ultrasound and is captured by the smartphone microphone. Helps in the assessment of rhythm disorders
2.	TeleSense Remote Cardiac Monitor	Wi-Fi based remote and local communication Live patient visibility and wireless transmission of arrhythmia events
3.	External Memory Loop recorder	Automatic, manually and time triggered event recording and ECG transmission
4.	Electronic stethoscope	Most heart diseases are associated with and reflected by the sounds that the heart produces. The emergence of digital stethoscopes have made it possible to identify conditions like murmurs remotely and give the treating physician vital clinical information of the patient
5.	Blood pressure and oxygen saturation	A number of Internet of Things (IoT) devices have emerged which are Wi-Fi and bluetooth enabled for transmission of data for measurement of blood pressure and oxygen saturation
6.	Mobile-based handheld echocardiography	A new device called the Butterfly iQ replaces the conventional piezo crystals with a single silicon chip and helps in providing ultrasound images of the heart on a mobile platform. Butterfly's semiconductor technology can emulate all three-wave patterns in one probe, and the app includes presets that are tuned to the depth and size of specific body parts, like the heart or bladder

information of the patient's condition and help in the management of heart failure are listed in Table 4.

- *Implanted therapeutic devices:* The use of implantable cardioverter-defibrillators (ICDs) and cardiac resynchronization therapy (CRT) devices are expanding in the treatment of heart failure. Most of the current devices are equipped with remote monitoring functions, including bioimpedance for fluid status monitoring. However, there are still questions if the clinical outcomes are impacted positively from these bioimpedance measurements. Cardiac resynchronization therapy (CRT) devices and implantable cardioverter-defibrillators (ICDs) are guideline-recommended treatments for heart failure with reduced EF, left bundle branch block and very wide QRS complex (>150 ms). Several manufacturers have marketed thoracic impedance measurement algorithms integrated into their devices. Changes in bioimpedance measurements reflect changes in intrathoracic fluid status and are evaluated based on a vendor-specific computer algorithm. Early investigations reported an inverse correlation with pulmonary capillary wedge pressure and fluid balance[26] and higher sensitivity and lower unexplained detection rate compared to acute weight changes.[27] In addition, a decrease in bioimpedance happened even before clinical manifestation of heart failure worsening and before hospital admission for fluid overload.[26] These algorithms are therefore very promising for the early detection of impending decompensated heart failure and enable the possibility to adjust treatment strategies in order to prevent heart failure hospitalization.[28,29] The number of CIED implantations among heart failure patients has increased exponentially. For terminal heart failure, the treatment of choice used to be heart transplantation during the last three decades. But this is changing, largely due to a decreasing supply of donor organs. Left ventricular assist devices (LVAD) are emerging as alternative therapy for heart failure. The latest generation of LVADs has an ultrasonic flow probe incorporated in the actual pump that allows it not only to monitor and report speed and power consumption but also to report the actual flow of blood. Remote monitoring of the three key parameters namely speed, power consumption and blood flow has now become possible and alerts to the cardiac center of any abnormality abnormalities via the Internet has brought about a remarkable improvement in the overall function of the device and something that will inevitably allow for better care of these patients.
- *Hemodynamic deterioration in heart failure:* Implanted monitoring-only devices are hemodynamic monitors measuring intracardiac or intravascular pressures. These monitors presented by right ventricular, pulmonary artery and left atrial pressure monitors. The basic pathophysiology of heart failure (i.e. cardiac filling pressures determine the clinical symptoms and course of heart failure) lies behind the idea of using such monitors in clinical practice.[30] Medtronic Inc. has

developed the Chronicle, implantable hemodynamic monitor, which is a long-term implanted device consisting of a subcutaneously implanted generator and a unipolar transvenous pacemaker lead, carrying a pressure sensor, positioned in the RV outflow tract that records right ventricular systolic pressure (RVSP), RV developed pressure (RVDP) and estimation of PAP.

STUDIES RELATED TO THE APPLICATION OF TECHNOLOGY IN HEART FAILURE

A number of studies have been carried out to understand the effectiveness of remote monitoring for patients with heart failure.[31]

TABLE 5: Impact of telemonitoring on heart failure management.

Sl. No.	*Description*	*Remarks*
Telephonic Support		
1.	Tele-HF study: Telemonitoring care for 1653 patients with interactive voice response system	Readmission: Not significant Deaths: Not significant Hospitalization rates: Not significant
2.	TIM-HF study: Telemedical care (portable devices transferred encrypted data including electrocardiography, blood pressure and body weight vs. usual care for 710 patients	
Implanted therapeutic devices to detect rhythm disorders		
1.	ASSERT study: 2,580 patients with implanted CIEDs, 2.5 years of follow-up. Newly detected AF episodes (with more than 6 min of duration) were counted	Newly detected AF episode has been detected in 34.7% of the involved population
2.	TRENDS trial: 1,368 Patients with no history of AF were included. Newly detected AF episodes (with more than 5 min of duration) were counted	Newly detected AF episode has been detected in 30% of the involved population
3.	TRUST trial: 1339 patients Remote monitoring vs. standard follow-up	AF detection occurred at 5.5 days in the remote monitoring group compared with 40 days in the standard follow-up group
4.	CONNECT trial: 1997 patients Patients with implanted ICDs were involved	3 vs. 24 days interval between AF episodes detection and clinical response in the remote monitoring vs. standard follow-up groups
Detection and management of system-related complications in patients with implanted CIEDs		
1.	ECOST trial: 40 patients with high-voltage leads were involved, with 22 ± 4 months of follow-up after implantation	Lead failure was registered in 7.5% of patients
Detection of heart failure worsening in hemodynamics		
1.	SENSE-HF trial : 501 patients Intracardiac impedance-derived fluid index measurement	Low sensitivity and positive predictive value in the early period after implantation (6 months), though sensitivity improved within the first 6 months after implantation
2.	DOT-HF study: 335 patients with implanted CIEDs were involved and randomized to have information available to physicians and patients as an audible alert in case of preset threshold crossings (access arm) or not (control arm)	Routine monitoring of intrathoracic impedance was not associated with a better outcome and was associated with an increased likelihood of HF hospitalization
3.	PARTNERS-HF trial: 694 patients with implanted CRTDs were involved and followed-up for 11.7 ± 2 months	Reduced impedance (or increased fluid index) has been demonstrated to be the most sensitive parameter to predict HF hospitalizations
4.	IN-TIME trial: 664 with NYHA class II and III and implanted ICDs and CRTDs were enrolled and randomized to standard vs. remote monitoring (in response to telemonitoring observations the investigators did a standardized telephone interview to establish whether patient's overall condition or symptoms had worsened or not, whether there was a sudden increase in body weight (>2 kg within the preceding 3 days) or scheduled visit to family doctor) arms	• 63 patients (18.9%) with a worsened composite clinical score in the telemonitoring group vs. 90 patients (27.2%) in the control group ($P = 0.013$) • Mortality was lower in the telemonitoring group compared to the control group ($n = 10$ vs. 27) • No significant differences in hospitalization among these groups were demonstrated

Contd...

Contd...

Sl. No.	*Description*	*Remarks*
5.	REM-HF trial: 1,650 patients with implanted CIEDs (ICD, CRTP, and CRTD) with remote monitoring were enrolled in the study and randomized to usual care or remote monitoring, with 2.8 years of median follow-up. Management of patients with remote monitoring was based on the data healthcare professional has received on a weekly basis from the device. Patients in the usual care group had a usual care from heart failure service and remote monitoring of the device (once per 3–6 months)	No significant differences in the primary (death from any cause or unplanned hospitalization for cardiovascular reasons) and secondary (death from any cause, death from cardiovascular reasons, unplanned hospitalization) end points were demonstrated
6.	MORE-CARE trial: 865 patients with implanted CRTDs were enrolled and randomized into remote and standard follow-up arms	• No significant differences in the composite of death and hospitalization due to cardiovascular and device-related reasons between these two groups were demonstrated • A significant 38% reduction in healthcare resources utilization in the remote arm (2-year rates of cardiovascular hospitalizations, cardiovascular emergency department admissions, and cardiovascular in-office follow-ups) as compared with the standard arm was demonstrated
Remote monitoring with implanted monitoring-only devices		
1.	CHAMPION trial: 550 patients with NYHA Class II were included and randomized into the CardioMEMs and usual monitoring groups	• Statistically significant reduction in HF hospitalization (regardless of LV ejection fraction) by 28% and 37% in the CardioMEMS group over 6- and 15-months of follow up, respectively. • Rates of non-HF-related hospitalizations were similar in both groups • Patients included in the CardioMEMS group had a significant reduction in the mean pulmonary artery pressure and better quality of life during the 6-month of follow-up based on the Minnesota Living with Heart Failure Questionnaire

(AF: atrial fibrillation; CIEDs: cardiovascular implantable electronic devices; CRTDs: cardiac resynchronization therapy defibrillators; CRTP: cardiac resynchronization therapy pacemaker; ICD: implantable cardioverter defibrillator; NYHA: New York Heart Association)

OUR EXPERIENCE

Vital Sign Monitoring Solution

Vios Medical and CARE Foundation have codeveloped a wireless physiological vital signs monitoring platform (the Vios Monitoring System, or VMS,) to optimize patient management throughout the continuum of care, including in-hospital and home applications. While the initial application for the VMS is focused on step-down monitoring of cardiology patients especially for chronic ailments like CHF, the broader goal is to extend vigilance into environments beyond the hospital and leverage the value of the continuous, synchronized data to unlock clinical informatics and remote patient management services. VMS is comprised of wireless, reusable physiological vital sign sensors (Vios Chest Sensor and Pulse Oximeter) coupled with bedside monitor software (BSM) and central station monitor software (CSM).

The VMS allows for continuous monitoring of a patient's ECG (7 leads), heart rate, respiration rate, oxygen saturation, pulse rate, axillary temperature and spot checking of non-invasive blood pressure. The Vios Chest Sensor is a low power Bluetooth device that is placed on the patient's chest via standard electrodes, and the embedded pulse oximeter in the sensor enable measurement of oxygen saturation; these sensors continuously acquire vital signs and wirelessly transmit them to the BSM. The BSM software runs proprietary algorithms that process the received data for display of the patient's vitals, and generates an alarm if physiological signs fall outside of selected threshold parameters or if cardiac arrhythmias occur.

The wireless sensor transmits data through bluetooth to the tablet which houses the software application as an "APP" and further from the tablet transmits data to the server (housed within hospital or cloud based) through a Wi-Fi network. The application has the capability for real-time analysis and display on any tablet-based (7")

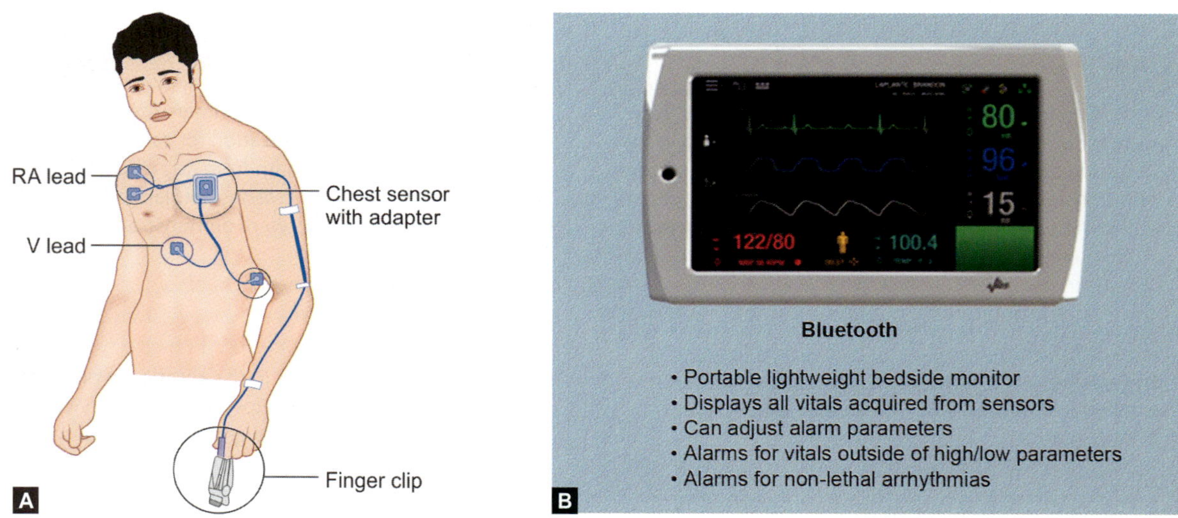

Figs. 5Aand B: (A) Monitoring of a patient for vital signs; (B) Cardiac monitor.

TABLE 6: IoT based VMS at CARE (Jan 2017–March 2019)

Description	Number
Total number of patients	401
Total number of monitoring days	1506
Number of males: Number of females	305:96
Mean age—Males (Max: Min)	63(92:22)
Mean age—Females (Max: Min)	54(89:25)

monitor and is synchronized for remote viewing from any global location. Continuous vital sign monitoring with standalone bedside monitors is a standard practice in ICUs and operating rooms, however, these systems are expensive and constrained to certain environments (Fig. 5). The main objective of this device is to facilitate and provide a cost-effective platform for continuous monitoring of patients in the step down ICUs, patient rooms. But, the portability and ease of use of this device have opened an opportunity to facilitate patients with chronic heart failure or arrhythmia problems as a home-based care solution.

Every time a patient with chronic heart failure is readmitted, the hospitalization costs per day which includes the ICCU/ward charges, consultancy charges, investigations (ECG, ECHO) and blood tests [Natriuretic peptides (BNP and pro-BNP), serum electrolytes, hemoglobin, lipid profile, serum creatinine] ranges between 12,000 and 15,000 per day (this cost however depends on the service provider, patient location in the hospital (ICCU/ward) and geographical location of the center. This however does not include medications being given. It is therefore imperative that IoT-based device technology is used effectively for such patients at home so that there is continuous monitoring about the wellbeing of the patient and thereby reducing rehospitalization as far as possible.

About 401 patients have availed services of this technology and it has immensely helped in the following ways (Tables 7 and 8):

- Reduced the average length of stay (ALOS) in ICCU with this device thereby giving a direct benefit to the patient in terms of expenditure involved.
- Ability to give timely treatment on the occurrence of adverse events like ventricular tachycardia (VT), VF,

TABLE 7: Use of telemonitoring in heart failure reduced length of hospital stay.

Sl. No.	Patient shifted from	Number
1.	ICCU → ward	221
2.	MICU → ward	32
3.	Post-catheterization → ward	20
4.	CTICU → ward	120
5.	ER → ward	8

(CTICU: cardiothoracic intensive care unit; ER: emergency room; ICCU: intensive cardiac care unit; MICU: medical intensive care unit)

TABLE 8: Effect on number of death due to continuous monitoring of patient with adverse effects.

Sl. No.	Patient shifted from	Number	Adverse event
1.	Ward → ICCU	03	Ventricular tachycardia
2.	Ward → ICCU	04	Ventricular fibrillation
3.	Ward → ICCU	05	Cardiac arrest
4.	Ward → MICU	20	SpO_2 drop
5.	Ward → CTICU	03	Post-CABG complications

(CTICU: cardiothoracic intensive care unit; CABG: coronary artery bypass graft; ICCU: intensive cardiac care unit; MICU: medical intensive care unit)

TABLE 9: Heart failure clinic at CARE (November 2014–March 2016)

Description	Number
Total number of patients	798
Number of males: Number of females	530:208
Mean age—Males (Max : Min)	59 (92:15)
Mean age—Females (Max : Min)	56 (83:10)
Atrial fibrillation (M : F)	20 (18:2)
Paroxysmal	8 (7:1)
Permanent	6 (5:1)
Persistent	6 (6:0)

(HF: heart failure)

cardiac arrest when in the ward. This was feasible only because there was continuous monitoring system available which was being viewed by duty doctors in the ICCU.

- The effectiveness achieved at CARE has prompted us to avail this technology for monitoring patients at home.

HEART FAILURE CLINIC AT CARE (TABLE 9)

CARE hospitals has set up a heart failure clinic in association with Medtronic since November 2014. The table below gives us an insight on the data collected. 20 patients were diagnosed with AF based on the findings of the 12 lead ECG showing the prevalence of AF in this population study was 2.5% of which paroxysmal AF was 1%, permanent AF was 0.75% and persistent AF was 0.75% (Unpublished data).

FUTURE SCENARIO

The advent of IoT-based medical devices will further enhance patients getting acclimatized to technology platform as the benefit it provides to them to avoid unnecessary hospital visits is immense. Wearable sensors are becoming promising due to the fact that these sensors are low cost, easily available, user friendly, accurate, and reliable. Many studies explored the clinical applications of wearable sensors in cardiovascular, neurological, asthma, and hypertension diseases.[32,33] For instance, a system has been developed to monitor congestive heart failure in patients, comprising a biosensor in the form of a ring that monitors heart data.[34] Smartphone-based ECG rhythm monitoring is definitely a valuable tool for diagnosing arrhythmias and early indicator of asymptomatic left ventricular dysfunction, a precursor to heart failure. Asymptomatic left ventricular dysfunction is characterized by the presence of a weak heart pump with a risk of overt heart failure. Mayo Clinic researchers hypothesized that asymptomatic left ventricular dysfunction could be reliably detected in the EKG by a properly trained neural network. These artificial intelligence (AI) based algorithms can be used as an effective tool with proper alert based mechanism to identify early onset of heart failure condition (Flowchart 1). The continuous data available because of the smart sensors have enabled creating a repository of data leading to the development of fairly ruggedized algorithms based on deep machine learning techniques for detection of specific conditions and triggering alerts. Machine learning essentially involves a set of techniques that enable AI. Physicians have long needed to identify, quantify, and interpret relationships among variables to improve patient care. AI and machine learning comprise a variety of methods that allow computers to do this, by algorithmically learning efficient representations of data. Machine learning uses essentially focuses on algorithmically representing data structure and making predictions or classifications by the application of advanced statistical methods. Machine learning programs incorporate data from a variety of sources (clinical measurements and observations, biological-omics, experimental results, environmental information, wearable devices) into sensible models for describing and predicting human disease. Flowchart 1 typically illustrates the machine learning workflow which begins from acquisition of data to feature extractions based on the inputs of the data leading to algorithm selection and model development, and finally results in model evaluation and application.

With increasing number of IoT-based sensors finding applications in healthcare, interoperability of the wide range of sensors and systems used will pose a challenge. However, the advent of blockchain technology has the potential to transform health care, placing the patient at the center of the health care ecosystem and increasing the security, privacy, and interoperability of health data. This technology could provide a new model for health information exchanges (HIEs) by making electronic medical records more efficient, disintermediated, and secure. The emergence of the fifth generation of mobile internet connectivity 5G will deliver significant improvement is healthcare quality and patient experience. 5G technology has the potential to help healthcare organizations meet the growing demands of IoT-focused transformation by providing a pathway for more significant amounts of data to be shared in a faster way and across networks. The lower latency associated with 5G will allow for new and more advanced IoT applications that require rapid responsiveness, such as remote equipment control or monitoring of patient data/images where the file sizes are very large in an efficient manner. With immediate access to substantial data files, the people and machines, critical decisions about patient's health can be done faster and in the much-required timely manner. AI systems need a massive amount of data to learn and improve in real-time,

Flowchart 1: Artificial intelligence in management of heart failure.

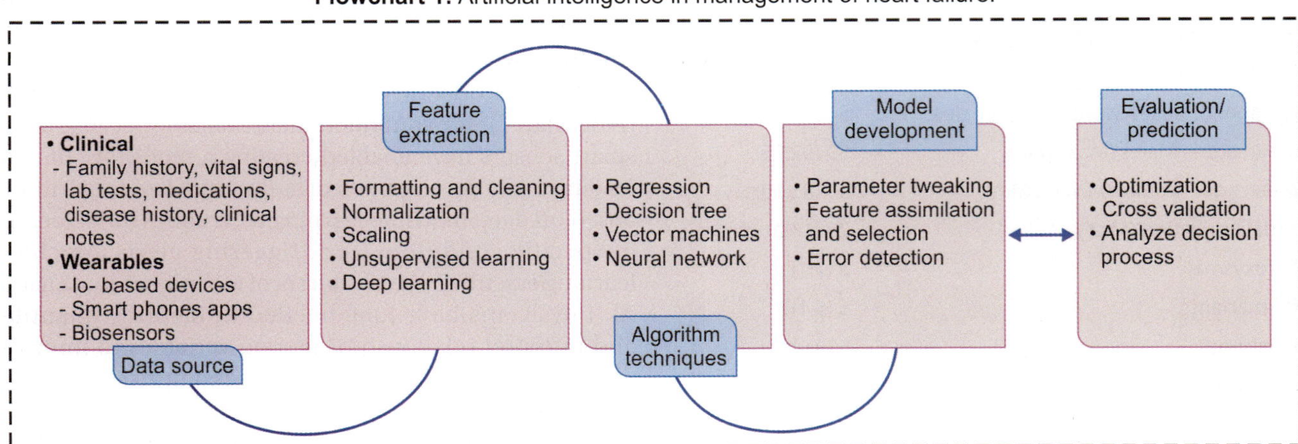

and that data typically comes from disparate sources and can deliver via mobile devices especially if 5G technology becomes completely operational. AI will likely become an integrative system to all smart sensors thereby prompting information to the clinicians and patients as and when required based on a set of conditions programmed per patient for alerts. While smartphone-based ECG rhythm monitoring applications provide physicians with the ability to diagnose patients with intermittent symptoms, there is one caveat: the magnitude of this potentially limitless source of data is enormous. The big question that emerges is whether the healthcare system in place is able to handle this huge amount of information. Unless strategies are adopted to appropriately manage this wealth of information, the ability to remotely diagnose heart conditions may not be as helpful as it originally sounds. There is always the potential of encountering false positives based on the sensitivities of these algorithms and hence more the data that can be obtained the better the effectiveness of the algorithms can be achieved. With these tools in our hands, the future of telemedicine in the smartphone era will definitely be bright, leading to improved patient care. The biggest challenge is to provide a platform which will allow the rapid and simple interpretation of the remote monitoring data that produces a targeted and effective response. The diagnostic, therapeutic and preventive potential of remote monitoring remains undefined in terms of cost/risk/benefit ratio. This is currently one of the limitations of such devices. Another major area of concern in the management of heart failure especially in India has been the compliance to the prescribed medication. It is therefore important to put the treatments together for each patient, and disease management programs, heart failure nurses, and heart failure clinics are useful in this direction.[35,36] A small number of heart failure clinics have been started all over India in a number of government and private hospitals and they need to be increased. Heart failure clinics can provide all the necessary IoT-based sensors for evaluating patient's condition wherein patients can walk in anytime to the clinic and get an assessment with the help of heart failure nurse. This information can be transmitted to the clinician and appropriate advice on treatment can be taken. This will be much more cost effective for the patient than visiting the hospital for the same set of investigations and it also helps in reducing the usually long waiting times at hospitals for investigations. Mobile-based ultrasound (echo) machines can also be positioned in these clinics and heart failure nurses can be trained to provide live echocardiographic views to clinicians through the ICT platform thereby maintaining a continuity in the care given to the patient without them having to visit hospitals.

CONCLUSION

One of the challenges for patients with CHF is to prevent acute decompensation and/or readmission to hospitals. Chronic heart failure can be viewed as "oncological" cardiac disease with grave prognosis, unless appropriate optimal medical and device-based therapies are instituted. The progression of heart failure is usually irreversible once the period of decompensation/instability begins. Consequently, efforts should be made to decrease heart failure incidence and prevalence and improve survival among heart failure patients by the early detection of disease deterioration and timely changes in the treatment of affected patients. The advent of IoT-based medical devices and the easy availability of internet across most geographical locations have enabled remote monitoring as a spectacular tool in the arsenal of cardiologists to facilitate an early detection of adverse events and to minimize regular follow-up visits of heart failure patients. Although there still seems to be an air of controversy with the data collected because of significant differences in IoT devices design, interoperability and acquisition capabilities, the emergence of blockchain technology and 5G technology will possibly ensure that remote monitoring can still be considered a reliable mechanism for early detection of heart failure.

Points to note

- One of the most common and growing health problem today is heart failure (HF) which is generally associated with high healthcare costs, mainly due to frequent hospitalizations.
- Chronic HF is a cardiovascular disorder affecting approximately 1–2% of adult population worldwide. However, there is lack of good surveillance system in India to predict the incidence and prevalence of HF.
- Lifetime risk of HF increases with age, so the burden likely to increase with aging population.
- Remote monitoring has gained fair success in managing patients with heart failure by avoiding unnecessary hospital visits/hospitalization.
- IoT-assisted wearable sensor-based medical devices have made it relatively easy to monitor patients and have the information sent to cloud server which is accessible to physicians along with necessary alert mechanism embedded into the application.
- Blockchain technology has the potential to transform health care, placing the patient at the center of the health care ecosystem and increasing the security, privacy, and interoperability of health data.
- Low latency associated with 5G technology will allow for new and more advanced IoT applications that require rapid responsiveness, such as remote equipment control or monitoring of patient data/images where the file sizes are very large in an efficient manner.
- Artificial intelligence (AI)-based algorithms can be used as an effective tool with proper alert-based mechanism to identify early onset of heart failure condition.

REFERENCES

1. Fjeldsoe BS, Marshall AL, Miller YD. Behavior change interventions delivered by mobile telephone short-message service. American journal of preventive medicine. 2009;36(2):165-73.
2. The World Bank. Life expectancy at birth, total (years). [online] Available from https://data.worldbank.org/indicator/sp.dyn.le00.in. [Last accessed November, 2019].
3. Ponikowski P, Voors AA, Anker SD, et al. ESC 2016 sobre el diagnóstico y tratamiento de la insuficiencia cardiaca aguda y crónica. Revista Espanola de Cardiologia. 2016;69(12):1167-e1.
4. Statistisches Bundesamt, editor. Diagnosedaten der Patienten und Patientinnen in Krankenhäusern. Fachserie 12 Reihe 6.2.1. Wiesbaden; 2012. p. 103.
5. Statistisches Bundesamt, editor. Todesursachen in Deutschland. Fachserie 12 Reihe 4. Wiesbaden; 2013. p. 53.
6. Mozaffarian D, Benjamin EJ, Go AS, et al. Heart disease and stroke statistics-2016 update a report from the American Heart Association. Circulation. 2016;133(4):e38-48.
7. Roger VL. Epidemiology of heart failure. Circ Res. 2013;113(6):646-59.
8. [online] Available from http://www.has-sante.fr/portail/upload/docs/application/pdf//2012-04/guideparcoursdesoinsicweb.pdf.
9. Croft JB, Giles WH, Pollard RA, et al. Heart failure survival among older adults in the United States: a poor prognosis for an emerging epidemic in the Medicare population. Archives of internal medicine. 1999;159(5):505-10.
10. Rich MW. Heart failure in the 21st century: a cardiogeriatric syndrome. J Gerontol A Biol Sci Med Sci. 2001;56(2):M88-96.
11. Mendez GF, Cowie MR. The epidemiological features of heart failure in developing countries: a review of the literature. Int J Cardiol. 2001;80(2-3):213-9.
12. World Health Organization. Global burden of disease—2004 update. Geneva: WHO; 2004.
13. Huffman MD, Prabhakaran D. Heart failure: epidemiology and prevention in India. Natl Med J India. 2010;23(5):283.
14. National Commission on Population, Government of India. (2010). [online] Available at http://populationcommission.nic.in/. [Last accessed November, 2019].
15. Lloyd-Jones DM, Larson MG, Leip EP, et al. Lifetime risk for developing congestive heart failure: the Framingham Heart Study. Circulation. 2002;106(24):3068-72.
16. Hall AK, Dodd V, Harris A, et al. Heart failure patients' perceptions and use of technology to manage disease symptoms. Telemedicine and e-Health. 2014;20(4):324-31.
17. Gil D, Ferrández A, Mora-Mora H, et al. Internet of things: A review of surveys based on context aware intelligent services. Sensors. 2016;16(7):1069.
18. Colom JF, Mora H, Gil D, et al. Collaborative building of behavioural models based on internet of things. Comput Electr Eng. 2017;58:385-96.
19. Lanza J, Sotres P, Sánchez L, et al. Managing Large Amounts of Data Generated by a Smart City Internet of Things Deployment. Int J Semant Web Inf Syst. 2016;12(4):22-42.
20. Llaves A, Corcho O, Taylor P, et al. Enabling RDF stream processing for sensor data management in the environmental domain. Int J Semant Web Inf Syst. 2016;12(4):1-21.
21. Middlekauff HR, Stevenson WG, Stevenson LW. Prognostic significance of atrial fibrillation in advanced heart failure. A study of 390 patients. Circulation. 1991;84(1):40-8.
22. Carson PE, Johnson GR, Dunkman WB, et al. The influence of atrial fibrillation on prognosis in mild to moderate heart failure. The V-HeFT Studies. The V-HeFT VA Cooperative Studies Group. Circulation. 1993;87(6 Suppl):VI102-10.
23. Mahoney P, Kimmel S, DeNofrio D, et al. Prognostic significance of atrial fibrillation in patients at a tertiary medical center referred for heart transplantation because of severe heart failure. Am J Cardiol. 1999;83:1544-7.
24. Senni M, Tribouilloy CM, Rodeheffer RJ, et al. Congestive heart failure in the community: a study of all incident

cases in Olmsted County, Minnesota, in 1991. Circulation. 1998;98:2282-9.
25. Deedwania PC, Singh BN, Ellenbogen K, et al. Spontaneous conversion and maintenance of sinus rhythm by amiodarone in patients with heart failure and atrial fibrillation: observations from the Veterans Affairs Congestive Heart Failure Survival Trial of Antiarrhythmic Therapy (CHF-STAT): the Department of Veterans Affairs CHF-STAT Investigators. Circulation. 1998;98:2574-9.
26. Yu C, Wang L, Chau E, et al. Intrathoracic impedance monitoring in patients with heart failure: correlation with fluid status and feasibility of early warning preceding hospitalization. Circulation. 2005;112(6):841-8.
27. Abraham WT, Compton S, Haas G, et al. Intrathoracic impedance vs daily weight monitoring for predicting worsening heart failure events: results of the Fluid Accumulation Status Trial (FAST). Congest Heart Fail. 2011;17(2):51-5.
28. Vollmann D, Nägele H, Schauerte P, et al. Clinical utility of intrathoracic impedance monitoring to alert patients with an implanted device of deteriorating chronic heart failure. Eur Heart J. 2007;28(15):1835-40.
29. Ypenburg C, Bax JJ, van der Wall EE, et al. Intrathoracic impedance monitoring to predict decompensated heart failure. Am J Cardiol. 2007;99(4):554-7.
30. Kuck KH, Bordachar P, Borggrefe M, et al. New devices in heart failure: an European Heart Rhythm Association report. Developed by the European Heart Rhythm Association; Endorsed by the Heart Failure Association. Europace. 2014;16:109-28.
31. Martirosyan M, Caliskan K, Theuns DAMJ, et al. Remote monitoring of heart failure: benefits for therapeutic decision making. Expert Rev Cardiovasc Ther. 2017;15:503-15.
32. Patel S, Park H, Bonato P, et al. A review of wearable sensors and systems with application in rehabilitation. J Neuroeng Rehabil. 2012;9(1):21.
33. Palumbo F, Ullberg J, Štimec A, et al. Sensor network infrastructure for a home care monitoring system. Sensors. 2014;14(3):3833-60.
34. Taplidou SA, Hadjileontiadis LJ. Wheeze detection based on time-frequency analysis of breath sounds. Comput Biol Med. 2007;37(8):1073-83.
35. Yancy CW, Jessup M, Bozkurt B, et al. 2017 ACC/AHA/HFSA focused update of the 2013 ACCF/AHA guideline for the Management of heart failure: A Report of the American college of cardiology/American heart association task force on clinical practice guidelines and the heart failure society of America. J Card Fail. 2017;23:628-51.
36. Gandhi S, Mosleh W, Sharma UC, et al. Multidisciplinary heart failure clinics are associated with lower heart failure hospitalization and mortality: systematic review and meta-analysis. Can J Cardiol. 2017;33(10):1237-44.

CHAPTER

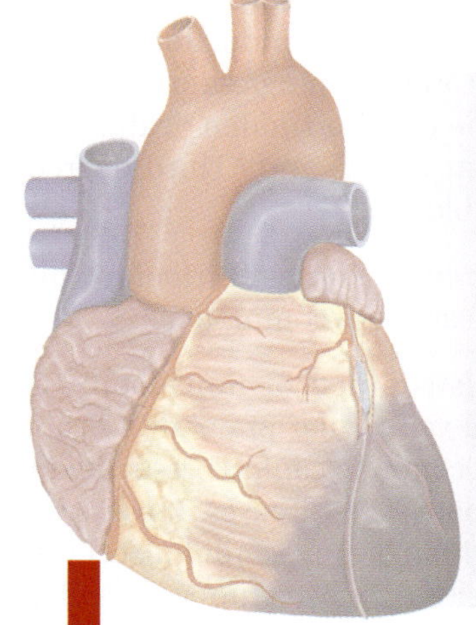

Cardiac Sarcoidosis: Diagnosis, Imaging, and Management

Surendra K Chutani, Arun Chutani, Arti Shah, Jui Shah, Bharat Kantharia

INTRODUCTION

Sarcoidosis is a granulomatous disease of unknown etiology. Noncaseating granulomas are diagnostic Hallmark on pathology examination. It is most often associated with pulmonary involvement and may involve heart, liver, peripheral lymph nodes, spleen, skin, eyes, pharyngeal bones, parotid gland and other organs. A recent studies indicates that disease may be an immunological response to an unidentified antigen or trigger.

HISTORY OF SARCOIDOSIS

An English skin specialist, Dr Johnathan Hutchinson, first recognized sarcoidosis in 1877. He reported a case of a woman who had unusual skin symptoms to the Dermatological Society of London in 1895. It was then named "Mortimer's Malady" after the patient's name. In the turn of the century, a Norwegian skin specialist named Boeck called the condition "Sarkoid" as it was thought to be a form of sarcoma, a form of tumor. It was then named "Boecks Sarcoid" in honor of his name, which was then used widely throughout the century. It is now known as "sarcoidosis".

CLINICAL MANIFESTATIONS AND DIAGNOSIS OF CARDIAC SARCOIDOSIS

The clinical presentation of cardiac sarcoidosis (CS) ranges from an incidentally discovered condition to heart failure (HF) and sudden death. The key clinical manifestations of CS are conduction system disease, tachyarrhythmia, cardiomyopathy, HF, and rarely coronary artery disease (CAD).

The diagnosis of CS is difficult to establish, and as a result, CS is often under-recognized in clinical practice. CS most often occurs as a manifestation of systemic sarcoidosis, although isolated CS can occur in patients who do not have evidence of sarcoidosis in other organs. Yet, commonly used clinical criteria require the diagnosis of extracardiac disease in order to establish the diagnosis of CS in the absence of having a positive endomyocardial biopsy. While endomyocardial biopsy provides a high specificity for diagnosing CS, this invasive test has a limited sensitivity. Furthermore, there is limited understanding of disease progression and a lack of consensus on the optimal methods for disease detection.

PREVALENCE

The true prevalence of CS remains unknown and is potentially underestimated since many individuals with CS may have nonspecific symptoms or subclinical disease. CS can affect patients of all racial backgrounds and ages, with an average age at presentation of approximately 50 years old. The prevalence of CS among patients with systemic sarcoidosis has been reported to be 20–27% in the United States and as high as 58% in Japan. Yet, autopsy studies indicate that subclinical cardiac involvement may be present in up to 70% of cases. In the United States, 13–25% of deaths from sarcoidosis have been attributed to CS, while in Japan, 47–85% of deaths from sarcoidosis have been attributed to cardiac involvement. Isolated CS may occur in up to 25% of CS cases, and thus the absence of extracardiac sarcoidosis does not rule out CS. Several reports have suggested that the incidence of CS may be increasing; however, it is unclear if such an increase is due to a true increase in the prevalence of a disease or to increased awareness and detection of this condition.

PATHOGENESIS

Sarcoidosis is a heterogeneous disorder of unknown etiology whose signature lesions are Noncaseating granulomata. Sarcoidosis may involve any part of the heart. While the ventricular myocardium is most commonly affected, involvement by the atria, papillary muscles, valves, coronary arteries, and pericardium has been described. Similar to other involved organs, cardiac disease generally progresses from areas of focal inflammation to scar. However, the natural history of CS is not well characterized and is highly variable. Some individuals may only have a small area of inflammation or scar and will not experience any significant clinical sequelae. On the other hand, some patients will progress to develop a pattern of extensive inflammation and scar. Given the limited data on how this disease progresses, it may be preferable to refer to different patterns of CS rather than stages, as use of stages implies a linear progression across different stages.

CLINICAL MANIFESTATIONS

The most frequent clinical manifestations of CS are atrioventricular (AV) block, arrhythmias, HF, and sudden cardiac death.

Symptoms and signs: This includes palpitations, presyncope, syncope, fatigue, dyspnea, orthopnea, and sudden cardiac death. Palpitations may be caused by either supraventricular or ventricular arrhythmias. Presyncope or syncope can be caused by AV block, ventricular tachycardia, or supraventricular tachycardia. Fatigue, dyspnea, and orthopnea can reflect HF caused by CS. However, fatigue and dyspnea are nonspecific symptoms that may also result from lung disease in patients with pulmonary sarcoidosis. Angina symptoms are generally considered more suggestive of atherosclerotic CAD, as CS only rarely causes angina.

Conduction system disease: AV block is the most common clinical presentation in patients with clinically evident CS. In a retrospective study of 110 patients with histologically confirmed CS, symptomatic heart block was present in 44% of patients. Complete AV block occurs at a younger age in patients with CS than in individuals with complete AV block due to other etiologies. Prolongation of the PR interval (first-degree AV block) due to disease of the AV node or bundle of His and intraventricular conduction defects is common and may progress. Thus, conduction system disease may initially be silent and then progress to complete AV block and cause syncope or even sudden death. [see "Etiology of atrioventricular block" and "Third degree (complete) atrioventricular block"].

Arrhythmias/tachyarrhythmias: Supraventricular and ventricular tachyarrhythmia are both common in CS.

Ventricular arrhythmias [sustained or nonsustained ventricular tachycardia and ventricular premature beats (VPBs)] are the second most common clinical presentation of CS, occurring in approximately 30% of cases. These arise when sarcoid granulomas within the myocardium become foci for abnormal automaticity, or may disrupt ventricular activation and recovery, causing re-entrant arrhythmias. Scar within the myocardium may also cause re-entrant arrhythmias.

Supraventricular arrhythmias seen with CS include paroxysmal atrial tachycardia, atrial flutter, atrial fibrillation, and sinus arrest secondary to granulomatous involvement of the sinus node. In a retrospective study that included 100 patients with definite or probable CS, the prevalence of supraventricular arrhythmias over a mean follow-up of 5.8 years was 32%, with atrial fibrillation being the most common arrhythmia. The presence of left atrial enlargement by echocardiography was most strongly associated with the development of supraventricular arrhythmias.

Sudden cardiac death: Due to ventricular tachyarrhythmia or conduction block accounts for 25–65% of deaths caused by CS. Some patients with known systemic sarcoidosis develop symptomatic or electrocardiographically evident arrhythmias or conduction abnormalities prior to sarcoid-related sudden death, assisting diagnosis and therapeutic management. However, sudden death can occur in the absence of symptoms or a previous cardiac event. Thus, a key diagnostic challenge is to identify individuals at risk for sudden death to enable preventive therapies.

Cardiomyopathy and heart failure: Presence of cardiomyopathy or HF in a patient with known extracardiac sarcoidosis should prompt an evaluation for CS. HF is less common than arrhythmia at initial presentation and is the first clinical manifestation of CS in fewer than 20% of cases. However, CS may even be diagnosed after transplant in the explanted hearts of patients thought to have an idiopathic cardiomyopathy. CS is a cause of cardiomyopathy, which may manifest with symptoms and signs of HF, e.g. orthopnea, edema. CS can cause either a dilated cardiomyopathy [with dilated left ventricular (LV) volumes and depressed LV ejection fraction (LVEF), which can lead to HF with reduced ejection fraction (HFrEF)] or a restrictive cardiomyopathy (with normal LV volumes and preserved LVEF), which can lead to HF with preserved ejection fraction.

Fewer data are available on the prevalence and clinical significance of right ventricular dysfunction attributable to CS. Some patients with CS present with signs of predominantly right-sided HF, which can be caused by sarcoid-related inflammation or scar affecting the right ventricle or less commonly secondary to CS involving the tricuspid valve. Right HF due to CS involving the right ventricle should be distinguished from other causes of right HF including pulmonary hypertension secondary to lung disease.

Coronary artery disease: Sarcoidosis can involve the coronary arteries with a vasculitis, which has been reported as a rare cause of unstable angina or myocardial infarction. However, patients with CS may also be more likely to have CAD.

CLINICAL DIAGNOSIS

The diagnosis of CS requires appropriate clinical suspicion and often requires integrating clinical and pathologic data together with the results of advanced cardiac imaging.

Electrocardiographic (ECG) findings in patients with CS include PR interval prolongation, second- or third-degree AV block, QRS prolongation (with or without right bundle branch block or left bundle branch block), frequent VPBs, atrial arrhythmias, pathologic Q waves, and nonspecific ST-segment and T-wave abnormalities. However, none of these features is specific for CS. The 12-lead ECG has low sensitivity (generally reported as <50%) for detection of CS. A chest radiograph is not required to diagnose CS, but it is a component of the diagnosis of pulmonary sarcoidosis. Findings suggestive of HF include cardiomegaly, cephalization of the pulmonary vessels, Kerley B-lines, and pleural effusions. However, these findings are not specific for CS, and absence of these findings does not exclude CS.

Although elevated levels of serum angiotensin converting enzyme, serum lysozyme, and urinary calcium have been reported in patients with CS, these biomarkers do not have a role in screening for CS or in assigning diagnostic probability.

DIAGNOSTIC CRITERIA FOR DIAGNOSIS OF CARDIAC SARCOIDOSIS

Only absolute test for organ involvement in sarcoidosis is histological examination of tissue for the presence of granulomatous inflammation, procurement of historical tissue may not always be easy and recognizable. They are to proposed diagnostic guidelines, viz.

1. *Japanese ministry of health and welfare criteria for diagnosis of cardiac sarcoidosis*

A. *Histological diagnosis group*: Cardiac sarcoidosis is confirmed when endomyocardial biopsy demonstrate noncaseating epithelioid granuloma with histological or clinical diagnosis of extracardiac sarcoidosis.

B. *Clinical diagnosis group*: Although endomyocardial biopsy specimens do not demonstrate noncaseating epithelioid granulomas, extracardiac sarcoidosis is diagnosed histologically or clinically and satisfies the following condition and more than one of the six basic diagnostic criteria:
   - Two or more of the four major criteria status
   - One in four of the major criteria and two or more of the five minor criteria are satisfied:

   Major criteria:
   1. Advanced AV block
   2. Basal thinning of the interventricular septum
   3. Positive gallium 67 uptakes in the heart
   4. Depressed left ventricular ejection fraction less than 50%.

   Minor criteria:
   1. *Abnormal EKG findings*: Ventricular arrhythmias like VT or multifocal or frequent PVCs, complete right bundle branch block, axis deviation or abnormal Q-waves.
   2. *Abnormal echo*: Wall motion abnormality or morphology curl abnormality (aneurysm or wall thickening or ventricular dilatation).
   3. *Perfusion defects on nuclear imaging*: Thallium 201, technetium 99 M SPECT.
   4. Delayed gadolinium enhancement on cardiac magnetic resonance (CMR).
   5. Interstitial fibrosis or monocyte infiltration on cardiac biopsy.

2. *Heart rhythm society consensus statement for diagnosis of cardiac sarcoidosis*

A. *Histological diagnosis of cardiac sarcoidosis*: Endomyocardial biopsy specimens with noncaseating epithelioid granulomas and no alternative cause identified.

B. *Clinical diagnosis of probable cardiac sarcoidosis*:
   a. Histological diagnosis of extra-cardiac sarcoidosis and one or more of the following is present while reasonable alternative cardiac causes other than CS have been excluded.
   b. Corticosteroid or immunosuppressive therapy responsive cardiomyopathy or heart block.
   c. Unexplained reduced LVEF less than 40%.

d. Mobitz type 2 second-degree heart block or third-degree heart block.
e. Depressed left ventricular ejection fraction less than 50%.
f. Patchy uptake on cardiac FDG-PET in a pattern consistent with cardiac sarcoidosis.
g. Late gadolinium enhancement (LGE) on cardiac MRI in a pattern consistent with cardiac sarcoidosis.
h. Positive gallium uptake in a pattern consistent with cardiac sarcoidosis.

IMAGING IN DIAGNOSIS OF SARCOIDOSIS

Echocardiographic Findings and Cardiac Sarcoidosis

Findings include regional wall motion abnormalities not consistent with CAD pattern, aneurysms, thinning of the basal septum, dilated left ventricle, and impaired right or left ventricular function both systolic and diastolic.

Echo is insensitive for detecting early stages of the disease and many patients with cardiac involvement can have normal findings. Further studies are required in order to determine whether more sensitive methods for identifying abnormal myocardial contractility for example strain imaging could improve clinical outcomes to earlier detection and treatment.

Cardiac Magnetic Resonance Imaging for Diagnosis and Prognosis

Cardiac magnetic resonance imaging really offers a multidimensional assessment of cardiac involvement of systemic sarcoidosis, thereby allowing noninvasive detection of scar, biventricular function, cellular edema and myocardial perfusion defects. The best advantage of CMR imaging is the lack of ionizing radiation, viz. nuclear imaging. In addition, gadolinium has a very low chance of serious adverse events like nephrogenic systemic fibrosis, which occurs in patients with acute or chronic very severe renal impairment with GFR less than 30 mL/minute.

The main diagnostic finding on CMR is a presence of late gadolinium enhancement, i.e. LGE which signifies presence of fibrosis. There are many different patterns of LGE the most typical being subepicardial and mid wall LV GE along the basal septum and or inferolateral wall. Sometimes septum is involved. Conte was involvement of right ventricular insertion point which is often present. Interestingly, the marked edema can also increase interstitial space, thereby increasing LGE. Therefore, the intensity and size of LGE may decrease following immunosuppressive therapy. Future research will include CMR T1 or T2 mapping techniques to further characterize myocardial disease in CS and potentially as therapeutic and point to evaluate response to anti-inflammatory therapy. Location of scar on and LGE imaging has been used as a guide to endomyocardial biopsy.

FDG-PET [Positron-emission Tomography (PET) with 18F-labeled Fluoro-2-deoxyglucose (18F-FDG)] for Diagnosis and Prognosis

If CMR cannot be performed, FDG-PET study is the alternative initial diagnostic test.

FDG-PET is recommended after CMR in the following clinical settings:

- If CMR is negative and high clinical suspicion for CS persists. As an example, FDG-PET is suggested for a patient with known extracardiac sarcoidosis and typical signs and/or symptoms of CS with negative CMR
- If CMR is inconclusive due to image quality or nonspecific findings, e.g. midwall LGE in a pattern consistent with myocarditis or sarcoidosis, or right ventricular involvement in a pattern that is consistent with arrhythmogenic right ventricular cardiomyopathy (ARVC) or sarcoidosis).

Additional tests: EP study or coronary angiography is indicated in the evaluation of only selected patients with suspected or known CS.*Coronary angiography*: Cardiac catheterization with coronary angiography (or in younger patients with a lower likelihood of CAD, coronary CT angiography) is useful in excluding the diagnosis of atherosclerotic CAD when other testing such as CMR or PET reveals regional myocardial abnormalities that could be caused by coronary disease or sarcoidosis.Primary sarcoidosis rarely involves the coronary arteries. Although granulomatous vasculitis may cause partial or complete narrowing of the epicardial coronary arteries, thrombosis and aneurysm formation are rare. Perfusion defects in patients with known systemic sarcoidosis strongly suggest cardiac involvement if coronary angiography has excluded significant atherosclerosis.

Electrophysiology study: While EP studies are not routinely performed for the diagnosis of CS, many patients with suspected CS undergo EP studies for risk stratification as discussed separately.

DIFFERENTIAL DIAGNOSIS

The differential diagnosis of CS includes other causes of AV block such as idiopathic progressive cardiac conduction disease and myocarditis, including Lyme disease, and genetically determined arrhythmias such as SCN5A and lamin A/C disease.

The differential diagnosis of CS also includes other etiologies of nonischemic cardiomyopathy, as well as myocarditis. Distinguishing between myocarditis and sarcoidosis is partially based upon clinical presentation, as myocarditis may have a viral prodrome associated with fever and myalgia. Myocarditis is also more likely to present with elevated cardiac biomarkers than CS.

Giant cell myocarditis, often presenting with AV block, unstable ventricular arrhythmias, and acute HF should be considered particularly when there is a more acute or fulminant clinical presentation. Patients with myocarditis may have evidence of scar on magnetic resonance imaging (MRI) indistinguishable from that seen with CS. Endomyocardial biopsy may be required to distinguish these conditions.

Arrhythmogenic right ventricular cardiomyopathy can also mimic CS. ARVC is often isolated to the right ventricle and spares the septum, while patients with CS and right heart myocardial involvement often also have significant septal and/or left heart infiltration. While some patients can have left-sided arrhythmogenic cardiomyopathy, the pattern of LGE on MRI between this condition and CS is different, e.g. left-sided arrhythmogenic cardiomyopathy often has a large amount of circumferential and often contiguous subepicardial LGE. While not a criterion on the 2010 Task Force Criteria for ARVC, the presence of significant fat in the myocardium would favor the diagnosis of ARVC. ARVC may also have a familial component as well as characteristic ECG findings, both features that are not present in CS. It is important to recognize that the 12-lead ECG in patients with CS may also meet many of the ECG criteria for ARVC. One of the most useful distinguishing ECG features is first-degree or higher AV block is extremely uncommon in ARVC but is a common feature of CS.

Fabry disease, a rare inherited disorder of fat metabolism, can present with concentric or asymmetric left ventricular hypertrophy, and on MRI often has midwall LGE of the basal inferolateral. While such LGE findings can also be seen in CS, CS is more likely to have multifocal LGE and focal areas of left ventricular hypertrophy. Left ventricular noncompaction may present with ventricular arrhythmia and increased wall thickness much like CS, but in noncompaction increased trabeculations of the ventricular myocardium are detected on echocardiography or cardiac magnetic resonance.

Hereditary hemochromatosis: Cardiac iron overload from hereditary hemochromatosis can present with conduction disease, arrhythmia, and HF much like CS, but hemochromatosis may be accompanied by diabetes and bronze skin and can be diagnosed by reduced T2* signal on CMR.

Cor pulmonale secondary to pulmonary sarcoidosis should be distinguished from CS involving the right ventricle. Pulmonary hypertension is a complication in some patients with pulmonary sarcoidosis and often occurs in the absence of CS. Some patients with pulmonary hypertension may develop right HF. Patients who have pulmonary sarcoidosis with cor pulmonale can have areas of focal LGE on MRI at the right ventricular insertion points. Such findings are well described in patients with pulmonary hypertension should be distinguished from CS where the LGE involvement is more extensive, and often extends beyond the insertion points to involve the right, and left ventricles.

Coronary artery disease: While most patients with CS have subepicardial or midwall LGE involvement on MRI, some can have subendocardial LGE, which is a pattern most commonly seen in patients who have had prior myocardial infarctions. Similarly, CS may be detected on 18F-fluorodeoxyglucose-positron emission tomography (FDG-PET) by a rest perfusion defect associated with increased FDG uptake. However, such a pattern can also be seen in patients with hibernating myocardium, and thus the presence of obstructive CAD should be ruled out in such scenarios.

Other diseases that can mimic CS include Chagas disease and tuberculosis. Both can cause cardiac aneurysms and ventricular arrhythmias.

Genetic cardiomyopathies, including those caused by mutations in desmosomes and lamin A/C protein genes, share some clinical characteristics with CS but have differing histologic characteristics.

CONCLUSION

Cardiac sarcoidosis is common, occurring in 20% or more of patients with systemic sarcoidosis, but the true prevalence remains unknown and is likely underestimated since many individuals with CS may have nonspecific symptoms or subclinical disease. Up to 25% of cases of CS are isolated without extracardiac involvement, and thus the absence of extracardiac sarcoidosis does not exclude CS. The clinical presentation of CS ranges from an incidentally discovered condition to syncope, HF, and sudden death. The diagnosis of CS requires appropriate clinical suspicion and often requires integrating clinical and pathologic data together with the results of advanced cardiac imaging. Diagnostic certainty of CS ranges from "definite" to "probable". In patients who have known extracardiac sarcoidosis, characteristic CMR imaging or FDG-PET findings can be used to confirm the diagnosis of CS. Endomyocardial biopsy is often not required. In the absence of biopsy-proven extracardiac sarcoidosis, or when data are inconclusive, integrating data from CMR imaging and FDG-PET may be useful for establishing the likelihood of CS.

BIBLIOGRAPHY

1. Adlan AM, Prasad SK, Varnava AM. Sarcoidosis presenting as dilated cardiomyopathy. Heart. 2011;97:1896.
2. Agarwal A, Sulemanjee NZ, Cheema O, et al. Cardiac sarcoid: a chameleon masquerading as hypertrophic cardiomyopathy and dilated cardiomyopathy in the same patient. Echocardiography. 2014; 31:E138-41.
3. Ammenwerth W, Wurps H, Klemens MA, et al. Reduced oxygen uptake efficiency slope in patients with cardiac sarcoidosis. PLoS One. 2014;9:e102333.
4. Baughman RP, Engel PJ, Taylor L, et al. Survival in sarcoidosis-associated pulmonary hypertension: the importance of hemodynamic evaluation. Chest. 2010;138:1078-85.
5. Birnie DH, Sauer WH, Bogun F, et al. HRS expert consensus statement on the diagnosis and management of arrhythmias associated with cardiac sarcoidosis. Heart Rhythm. 2014;11:1305-23.
6. Butany J, Bahl NE, Morales K, et al. The intricacies of cardiac sarcoidosis: a case report involving the coronary arteries and a review of the literature. Cardiovasc Pathol. 2006;15: 222-7.
7. Cain MA, Metzl MD, Patel AR, et al. Cardiac sarcoidosis detected by late gadolinium enhancement and prevalence of atrial arrhythmias. Am J Cardiol. 2014;113:1556-60.
8. Chapelon-Abric C, de Zuttere D, Duhaut P, et al. Cardiac sarcoidosis: a retrospective study of 41 cases. Medicine (Baltimore). 2004;83:315-34.
9. Chareonthaitawee P, Beanlands RS, Chen W, et al. Joint SNMMI-ASNC expert consensus document on the role of 18F-FDG PET/CT in cardiac sarcoid detection and therapy monitoring. J Nucl Med. 2017;58:1341-53.
10. Chareonthaitawee P, Beanlands RS, Chen W, et al. Joint SNMMI-ASNC Expert Consensus Document on the role of 18F-FDG PET/CT in cardiac sarcoid detection and therapy monitoring. J Nucl Med. 2017;58:1341-53.
11. Fleming H. Cardiac Sarcoidosis. In: James DG (Ed). Sarcoidosis and Other Granulomatous Disorders. New York: Dekker; 1994. p.323.
12. Freeman AM, Curran-Everett D, Weinberger HD, et al. Predictors of cardiac sarcoidosis using commonly available cardiac studies. Am J Cardiol. 2013;112:280-5.
13. Goyal SB, Aragam JR. Cardiac sarcoidosis with primary involvement of the tricuspid valve. Cardiology Rev. 2006;14:e12-3.
14. Greulich S, Deluigi CC, Gloekler S, et al. CMR imaging predicts death and other adverse events in suspected cardiac sarcoidosis. JACC Cardiovasc Imaging. 2013;6:501-11.
15. Hamzeh N, Steckman DA, Sauer WH, et al. Pathophysiology and clinical management of cardiac sarcoidosis. Nat Rev Cardiol. 2015;12:278-88.
16. Huitema MP, Grutters JC, Rensing BJ, et al. Pulmonary hypertension complicating pulmonary sarcoidosis. Neth Heart J. 2016;24:390-9.
17. Hulten E, Aslam S, Osborne M, et al. Cardiac sarcoidosis—state of the art review. Cardiovasc Diagn Ther. 2016;6:50-63.
18. Ishimaru S, Tsujino I, Sakaue S, et al. Combination of 18F-fluoro-2-deoxyglucose positron emission tomography and magnetic resonance imaging in assessing cardiac sarcoidosis. Sarcoidosis Vasc Diffuse Lung Dis. 2005;22:234-5.
19. Joyce E, Kamperidis V, Ninaber MK, et al. Prevalence and Correlates of Early Right Ventricular Dysfunction in Sarcoidosis and Its Association with Outcome. J Am Soc Echocardiogr. 2016;29:871-8.
20. Judson MA, Baughman RP, Teirstein AS, et al. Defining organ involvement in sarcoidosis: the ACCESS proposed instrument. ACCESS Research Group. A Case Control Etiologic Study of Sarcoidosis. Sarcoidosis Vasc Diffuse Lung Dis. 1999;16:75-86.
21. Judson MA, Costabel U, Drent M, et al. The WASOG Sarcoidosis Organ Assessment Instrument: An update of a previous clinical tool. Sarcoidosis Vasc Diffuse Lung Dis. 2014;31:19-27.
22. Kandolin R, Lehtonen J, Airaksinen J, et al. Cardiac sarcoidosis: epidemiology, characteristics, and outcome over 25 years in a nationwide study. Circulation. 2015;131:624-32.
23. Kandolin R, Lehtonen J, Graner M, et al. Diagnosing isolated cardiac sarcoidosis. J Intern Med. 2011;270:461-8.
24. Kim JS, Judson MA, Donnino R, et al. Cardiac sarcoidosis. Am Heart J. 2009;157:9-21.
25. Kouranos V, Tzelepis GE, Rapti A, et al. Complementary role of CMR to conventional screening in the diagnosis and prognosis of cardiac sarcoidosis. JACC Cardiovasc Imaging. 2017;10:1437-47.
26. Lam CS, Tolep KA, Metke MP, et al. Coronary sarcoidosis presenting as acute coronary syndrome. Clin Cardiol. 2009;32:E68-71.
27. Langah R, Spicer K, Gebregziabher M, et al. Effectiveness of prolonged fasting 18f-FDG PET-CT in the detection of cardiac sarcoidosis. J Nucl Cardiol. 2009;16:801-10.
28. Lønborg J, Ward M, Gill A, et al. Utility of cardiac magnetic resonance in assessing right-sided heart failure in sarcoidosis. BMC medical imaging. 2013;13:2.
29. Matsui Y, Iwai K, Tachibana T, et al. Clinicopathological study of fatal myocardial sarcoidosis. Ann N Y Acad Sci. 1976;278:455-69.
30. Mehta D, Lubitz SA, Frankel Z, et al. Cardiac involvement in patients with sarcoidosis: diagnostic and prognostic value of outpatient testing. Chest. 2008;133:1426-35.
31. Milman N, Andersen CB, Mortensen SA, et al. Cardiac sarcoidosis and heart transplantation: a report of four consecutive patients. Sarcoidosis Vasc Diffuse Lung Dis. 2008;25:51-9.
32. Murtagh G, Laffin LJ, Patel KV, et al. Improved detection of myocardial damage in sarcoidosis using longitudinal strain in patients with preserved left ventricular ejection fraction. Echocardiography. 2016;33:1344-52.

33. Nery PB, Beanlands RS, Nair GM, et al. Atrioventricular block as the initial manifestation of cardiac sarcoidosis in middle-aged adults. J Cardiovasc Electrophysiol. 2014;25:875-81.
34. Nihoyannopoulos P, Dawson D. Restrictive cardiomyopathies. Eur J Echocardiogr. 2009;10:iii23-33.
35. Okada DR, Bravo PE, Vita T, et al. Isolated cardiac sarcoidosis: A focused review of an under-recognized entity. J Nucl Cardiol. 2018;25:1136-46.
36. Okumura W, Iwasaki T, Toyama T, et al. Usefulness of fasting 18F-FDG PET in identification of cardiac sarcoidosis. J Nucl Med. 2004;45:1989-98.
37. Patel AR, Klein MR, Chandra S, et al. Myocardial damage in patients with sarcoidosis and preserved left ventricular systolic function: an observational study. Eur J Heart Fail. 2011;13:1231-7.
38. Patel MB, Mor-Avi V, Murtagh G, et al. Right Heart Involvement in Patients with Sarcoidosis. Echocardiography. 2016;33:734-41.
39. Patel MR, Cawley PJ, Heitner JF, et al. Detection of myocardial damage in patients with sarcoidosis. Circulation. 2009;120:1969-77.
40. Philips B, Madhavan S, James CA, et al. Arrhythmogenic right ventricular dysplasia/cardiomyopathy and cardiac sarcoidosis: distinguishing features when the diagnosis is unclear. Circ Arrhythm Electrophysiol. 2014;7:230-6.
41. Roberts WC, Chung MS, Ko JM, et al. Morphologic features of cardiac sarcoidosis in native hearts of patients having cardiac transplantation. Am J Cardiol. 2014;113:706-12.
42. Schaedel H, Kirsten D, Schmidt A, et al. Sarcoid heart disease--results of follow-up investigations. Eur Heart J. 1991;12 (Suppl D):26-7.
43. Schulte W, Kirsten D, Drent M, et al. Cardiac involvement in sarcoidosis. Eur Respir Mon. 2005;32:130.
44. Sekiguchi M, Yazaki Y, Isobe M, et al. Cardiac sarcoidosis: diagnostic, prognostic, and therapeutic considerations. Cardiovasc Drugs Ther. 1996;10:495-510.
45. Sharma OP, Maheshwari A, Thaker K. Myocardial sarcoidosis. Chest. 1993;103:253-9.
46. Sharma S. Cardiac imaging in myocardial sarcoidosis and other cardiomyopathies. Curr Opin Pulm Med. 2009;15:507-12.
47. Silverman KJ, Hutchins GM, Bulkley BH. Cardiac sarcoid: a clinicopathologic study of 84 unselected patients with systemic sarcoidosis. Circulation. 1978;58:1204-11.
48. Smedema JP, Snoep G, van Kroonenburgh MP, et al. Evaluation of the accuracy of gadolinium-enhanced cardiovascular magnetic resonance in the diagnosis of cardiac sarcoidosis. J Am Coll Cardiol. 2005;45:1683-90.
49. Soejima K, Yada H. The work-up and management of patients with apparent or subclinical cardiac sarcoidosis: with emphasis on the associated heart rhythm abnormalities. J Cardiovasc Electrophysiol. 2009;20:578-83.
50. Statement on sarcoidosis. Joint Statement of the American Thoracic Society (ATS), the European Respiratory Society (ERS) and the World Association of Sarcoidosis and Other Granulomatous Disorders (WASOG) adopted by the ATS Board of Directors and by the ERS Executive Committee, February 1999. Am J Respir Crit Care Med. 1999;160:736-55.
51. Uemura A, Morimoto S, Hiramitsu S, et al. Histologic diagnostic rate of cardiac sarcoidosis: evaluation of endomyocardial biopsies. Am Heart J. 1999;138:299-302.
52. Vignaux O, Dhote R, Duboc D, et al. Clinical significance of myocardial magnetic resonance abnormalities in patients with sarcoidosis: a 1-year follow-up study. Chest. 2002;122:1895-901.
53. Viles-Gonzalez JF, Pastori L, Fischer A, et al. Supraventricular arrhythmias in patients with cardiac sarcoidosis: prevalence, predictors, and clinical implications. Chest. 143:1085-90.
54. Vita T, Okada DR, Veillet-Chowdhury M, et al. Complementary value of cardiac magnetic resonance imaging and positron emission tomography/computed tomography in the assessment of cardiac sarcoidosis. Circ Cardiovasc Imaging. 2018;11:e007030.
55. Ward EV, Nazari J, Edelman RR. Coronary artery vasculitis as a presentation of cardiac sarcoidosis. Circulation. 2012;125:e344-6.
56. Yigla M, Badarna-Abu-Ria N, Tov N, et al. Sarcoidosis in northern Israel; clinical characteristics of 120 patients. Sarcoidosis Vasc Diffuse Lung Dis. 2002;19:220-6.
57. Yoshida Y, Morimoto S, Hiramitsu S, et al. Incidence of cardiac sarcoidosis in Japanese patients with high-degree atrioventricular block. Am Heart J. 1997;134:382-6.
58. Youssef G, Beanlands RS, Birnie DH, et al. Cardiac sarcoidosis: applications of imaging in diagnosis and directing treatment. Heart. 2011;97:2078-87.
59. Youssef G, Leung E, Mylonas I, et al. The use of 18F-FDG PET in the diagnosis of cardiac sarcoidosis: a systematic review and metaanalysis including the Ontario experience. J Nucl Med. 2012;53:241-8.
60. Zhou Y, Lower EE, Li HP, et al. Cardiac Sarcoidosis: The Impact of Age and Implanted Devices on Survival. Chest. 2017;151:139-48.

CHAPTER 67

Echocardiographic Pulmonary Embolism Evaluation with Heart Failure

Soumitra Kumar, Abhijit Biswas

INTRODUCTION

Pulmonary embolism (PE) is the third leading cause of cardiovascular deaths[1] and is a major health problem. The incidence of venous thromboembolism (VTE), which includes PE and deep vein thrombosis (DVT), has remained relatively constant, with age- and sex-adjusted rates of 117 per 100,000 person-years.[2] VTE incidence increases sharply after age 70 in both men and women, with PE accounting for the majority of the increase and having an incidence of up to 700 per 100,000 As a rule of thumb risk of VTE approximately double with each decade after age of 40 years.[3] All-cause mortality rate is 5.4% in PE at 30 days for patients diagnosed with PE in EMPEROR registry.[4] The dramatic mortality reduction with treatment makes the need for accurate diagnosis and expeditious treatment strongly compelling. Majority of preventable deaths due to PE can be ascribed to missed diagnosis rather than failure of therapy.[5] The value of echocardiography in the diagnosis of PE has been extensively investigated since 1970s. Early studies focused mainly on direct visualization of right cardiac thrombi,[6] but later studies focused on echocardiographic manifestations to the area of the affected pulmonary vasculature.[7] Recent studies are more elaborate on evaluation of RV dysfunction as a predictor of mortality.[8] Though no single noninvasive diagnostic test is specific or sensitive enough. Imaging is a key component in diagnostic evaluation of suspected PE, since clinical evidence is neither specific nor sensitive. Early diagnosis in acute PE is needed to prevent fatality and to institute definitive treatment.

Pulmonary embolism is classified as follows:

- Present diagnostic algorithm uses electrocardiographic (ECG), chest X-ray (CXR), V/Q scan, CT scan and echocardiography in initial evaluation for diagnosis of PE.
- Echocardiogram is helpful in diagnosis in those subsets of population who have high pretest probability of PE. Transthoracic echocardiography (TTE) is insensitive in diagnosing PE but provides essential information for risk stratification, hemodynamic status, right ventricular (RV) function and pulmonary hypertension.
- The American Society of Echocardiography guidelines for evaluation of cardiac source of embolic state are not a diagnostic modality of choice for the diagnosis of PE per se but are for risk stratification. 2014 ESC Guidelines do not recommend echocardiography as a part of diagnostic workup in non-high risk "hemodynamically stable, normotensive patients with suspected (not high risk) PE" (Tables 1 and 2).[9,10]

TABLE 1: American Heart Association classification of pulmonary embolism (PE).[9]

Risk	*Hemodynamic instability*	*RV function*	*Cardiac biomarkers*
Massive	Yes	NA	NA
Submassive	No	Abnormal	Abnormal
Low	No	Normal	Normal

TABLE 2: Classification of patients with acute pulmonary embolism (PE) based on early mortality risk.

Early mortality risk		*Risk parameters and scopes*			
		Shock or Hypotensin	*PESI Class III-V or sPESI ≥1[a]*	*Signs of RV dysfunction on an imaging test[b]*	*Cardiac laboratory biomarkers[c]*
High		+	(+)[d]	+	(+)[d]
Intermediate	Intermediate–high	–	+	Both positive	
	Intermediate–low	–	+	Either one (or none) positive	
Low		–	–	Assessment optional, if assessed both nagative[e]	

PE: pulmonary embolism; PESI: pulmonary embolism severity index; RV : right ventricular; sPESI: simlified pulmonay embolism severity index.

[a]PESI Class III to V indicates moderate to very high 30 day mortality risk; sPESI ≥ 1 point(s) indicate high 30 day mortality risk.

[b]Echocardiographic criteria of RV dyfunction include RV dysfunction include RV ditation and/or an increased end-diastolic RV-LV diameter ratio (in most studies, the reported threshold value was 0.9 or 1.0); hypokinesia of the free RV wall; Increased velocity of the tricuspid regurgitation jet or combinations of the above. On computed tomographic (CT) angiography (four-chamber views of the heart). RV dystuntion is defined as an increased end-diastolic RV/LV (left ventricular) diameter ratio (with a threshold of 0.9 or 1.0).

[c]Markers of mycocaridal injury (e.g. elevated caridac troponin I or –T concentrations in plasma), or of heart failure as a result of (right) ventricular dysfunction (elecated natriuretic peptide concentratons in plasma).

[d]Neither calculation of the PESI (or sPESI) nor laboratory resting are considered necessay in patients with hypotension or shock.

[e]Patients in the PESI class I–II, or with sPESI of O, and elevated cardiac biomarkers or signs of RV dysfunction on imaging tests, are also to be classified into the intermediate-low risk category. This might apply to situation in which imaging or biomarker results become available before calculation of the clinical severity index.

SUGGESTIVE MECHANISMS OF ECHOCARDIOGRAPHIC FINDINGS

Acute PE can interfere with both circulation and gas exchange. The abrupt increase in pulmonary vascular resistance results in RV dilatation altering contractile properties. Increased RV pressure and load leads to dilated RV and decreased contraction. This ultimately leads to reduced LV preload, cardiogenic shock and death.[11] So, evaluation of right ventricle (RV) is most important in PE. The echocardiographic evaluation is based on size and function of RV. RV size and RV function are most evaluated by transthoracic echocardiographic parameters in PE. The severity of hemodynamic compromise is directly related to:

- Thrombotic burden
- Extent of affected pulmonary vasculature
- Time of pulmonary embolization
- Location of PE
- Coexistent cardiovascular and respiratory abnormalities.

ROLE OF ECHOCARDIOGRAPHY IN PULMONARY EMBOLISM

- Diagnosis
- Indirect assessment of size or extent of PE
- Prognosis
- Monitoring therapy.

The extent of PE correlated with:

- RV systolic impairment
- RV end-diastolic dilatation
- *RA*: LA end-systolic area ratio
- *RV*: LV end-diastolic area ratio
- Tricuspid annulus motion and basal late diastolic velocity independently predicted the extent of PE on lung scintigraphy
- *RV apical*: Basal systolic velocity ratio correlated strongly with size of PE.[12,13]

Kjaergaard et al., however, proved that RV dysfunction is only found in patients with >25% perfusion defects.[13]

RV diameter, RV systolic pressure and RV systolic function correlated with size of PE in their study, but RV myocardial performance index (RV-MPI) or peak tricuspid annulus systolic velocity were unrelated to the size of PE.[12]

PA acceleration time was however shortened even in patients with small emboli.

ECHOCARDIOGRAPHIC FINDINGS IN ACUTE PULMONARY EMBOLISM

- Right ventricular dilatation and hypokinesis (apical, subcostal or transesophageal 4-chamber view) and subsequent TR.
  (Parameters of RV dilatation is RVEDD > 30 mm in parasternal view or RV/LV end-diastolic ratio > 1)
- *Septal flattening and paradoxical motion*: Right ventricular contraction continues even after left ventricle starts relaxing at end systole leading to septal bulging toward left ventricle (D-shaped septum on short axis).
- Pulmonary arterial hypertension detected by Doppler flow velocity in right ventricular outflow tract—

shortened acceleration time < 90 m/sec with peak velocity occurring close to onset of ejection. Biphasic ejection curve with mid-systolic reduction in velocity.

- *Diastolic left ventricular impairment*: Doppler mitral flow exhibits prominent A wave which is much higher than E wave.
- *Direct visualization pulmonary embolism*: Only if large and centrally located embolus. Much better visualized with transesophageal echocardiography (TEE) than transthoracic echo.
- *Right ventricular hypertrophy*: Mild increase in right ventricular thickness as much as up to 6 mm with prominent right ventricular trabeculations.
- *Patent foramen ovale*: When right atrial pressure exceeds left atrial pressure foramen ovale may open and worsen hypoxemia.
- TR velocity > 2.8 m/s or TR velocity > 2.5 m/s in absence of inspiratory collapse of IVC.
- Right pulmonary artery dilatation of >12 mm/ m^2.
- Decreased LV size and the ratio of right ventricular end-diastolic area to left ventricular end-diastolic area >0.6.
- *McConnell sign*: It was described by McConnell and colleagues.[14] It is a distinct pattern of regional RV dysfunction in patients with acute PE presenting as hypokinesia or akinesia of the mid-RV free wall with normal or hyperkinetic RV apex (Figs. 1A and B).

This finding has sensitivity, specificity, positive predictive and negative predictive value of 70%, 33%, 67%, and 36% respectively. So the sign is considered as nonspecific as two-thirds of patients with normally contracting RV apex may be seen in RV infarction.[15] No clear explanation available for this finding, but several mechanisms have been put forward:

- Tethering of RV apex to a contracting and often hyperdynamic LV preserving the contractility of LV

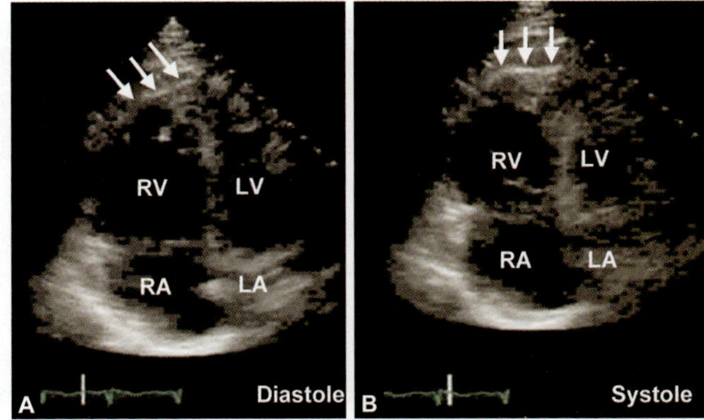

Figs. 1A and B: Dilated right ventricle (RV) and McConnell's sign.

- Mid RV free wall systolic bulging is caused by abrupt rise in afterload and increased regional stress
- Segmental ischemia of the RV free wall secondary to increased wall stress.

- The "60/60" sign (Figs. 2A and B) using Doppler echocardiography is defined as an acceleration time ≤ 60 milliseconds in the presence of a tricuspid regurgitation pressure gradient < 60 mm Hg. This sign has sensitivity, specificity, positive predictive and negative predictive values of 25%, 94%, 90%, and 38% respectively.[16]

When RVEF, RV systolic pressure and RV size were evaluated TTE had 56% sensitivity and 90% specificity for acute PE. TAPSE was evaluated in several studies and was found to be significantly different with controls its sensitivity was 72% and specificity was 66%.[17]

McConnell's sign and acute pulmonary embolism are not synonymous. The impression of normal RV apical motion in patients with McConnell's sign is likely due to RV tethering by the contracting left ventricular apex that occurs

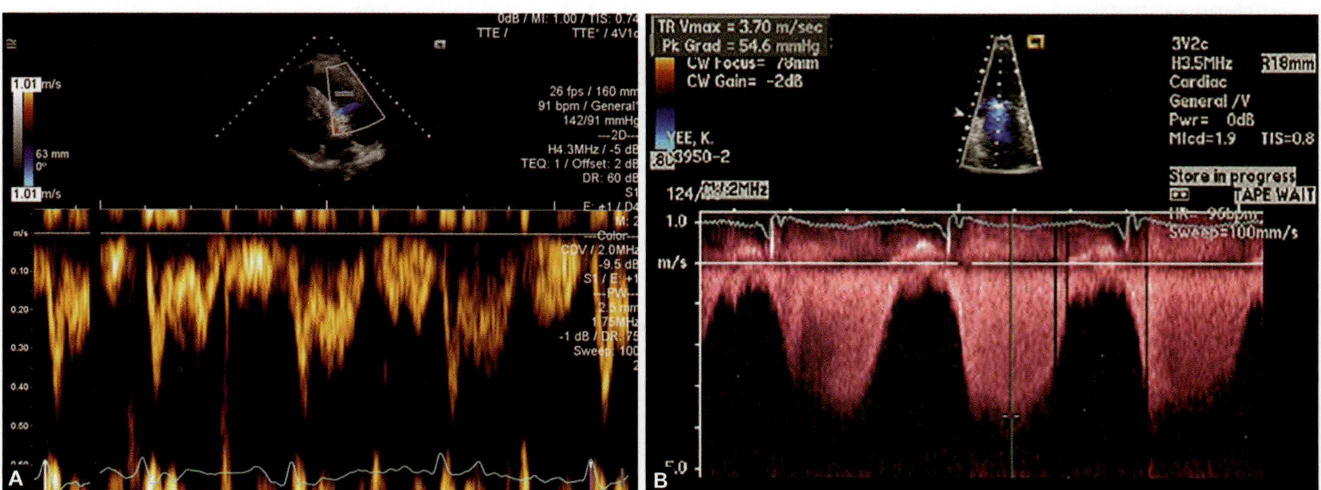

Figs. 2A and B: "60-60" sign.

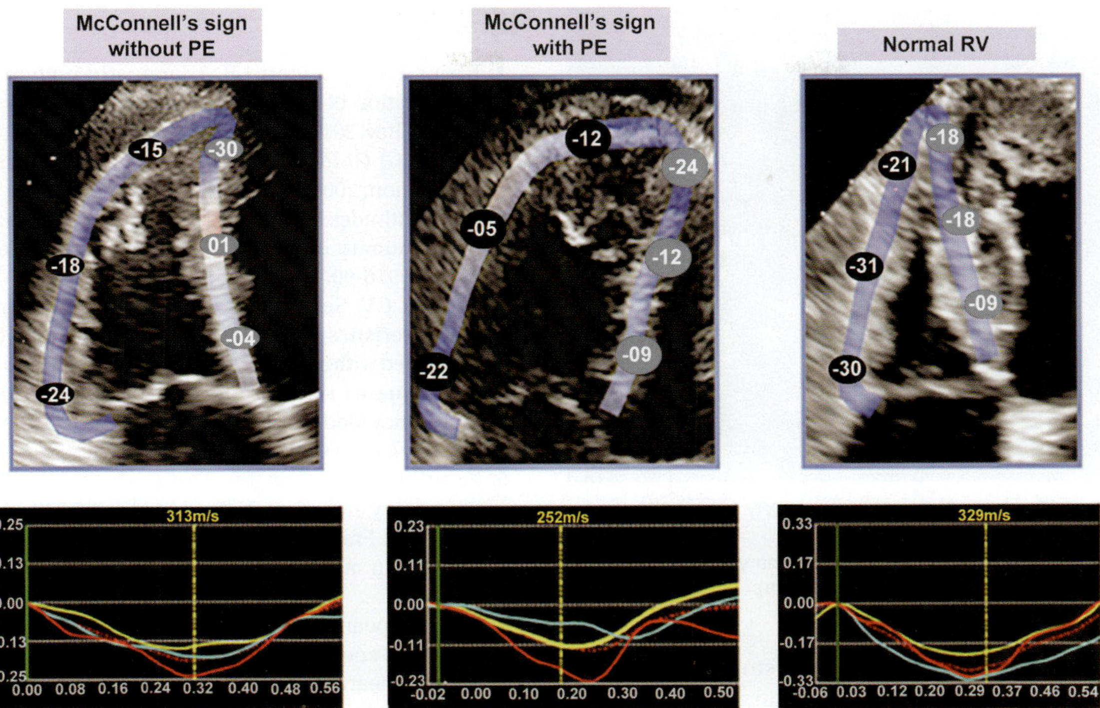

Fig. 3: Right ventricular free wall longitudinal strain measurements in two patients with McConnell's sign: one without pulmonary embolism (left) and the other with pulmonary embolism (middle), and in a normal subject (right), along with the corresponding free wall segmental strain curves (bottom). Note the difference in the magnitude of the segmental peak strain among the three patients (see text for details).
(PE: pulmonary embolism; RV: right ventricle)

in both acute pulmonary processes such as acute PE and more chronic conditions such as pulmonary hypertension. However, RV free wall strain measurements in patients with McConnell's sign can aid in differential diagnosis of patients with acute PE, because reduced magnitude of apical strain in absence of evidence of pulmonary hypertension indicated higher likelihood of acute PE[18] (Fig. 3). Another study showed mid-free wall RV strain is lower in patients with acute PE than in controls.[19]

However in a study presented by Benck et al. found that intermediate-to-high-risk PE and RV strain correlated with traditional abnormalities of RV dysfunction. But classical parameters improved with treatment, strain measurements did not show improvement in early posttreatment phase.[20]

Three-dimensional (3D) RV ejection fraction has been shown to be statistically significantly parameter in acute PE[19] as well; however, its clinical adoption in multicenter setting or certain cardiac diseases awaits further study.

ROLE OF TRANSESOPHAGEAL ECHOCARDIOGRAPHY

Transesophageal echocardiography is invaluable for direct visualization of proximal pulmonary artery and thrombus instead of relying on indirect signs such as right ventricular dilatation and hypokinesia. Although the main PA, PA bifurcation, and right PA can be easily visualized in mid-esophageal views of the ascending aorta, left PA is often obscured by the overlapped left main bronchus, whereas peripheral branches are not visible. The sensitivity and specificity of TEE for imaging intracavitary thrombi in patients with acute PE is 80% and 100% respectively[21] (Fig. 4).

PROGNOSIS

The mortality in patients with PE with coexistent echocardiographic RV dysfunction is estimated to be between 4% and 5%, whereas patients with normal echocardiographic findings on admission carry an in-hospital mortality of <1%. Patients with moderate to severe RV impairment possess sixfold increased death and 2.4-fold increased relative risk during first year.[22] Combination of RV dysfunction on echocardiography and a positive lower extremity complete compression ultrasound (CCUS) had higher prognostic value for PE related death.[23] Patients with baseline pulmonary systolic pressure > 50 mm Hg on admission have threefold increase risk of persistent hypertension and a lower 5-year survival

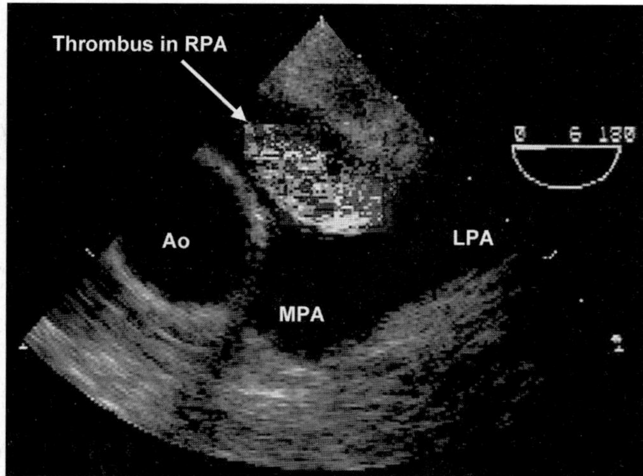

Fig.4: Transesophageal echocardiography (TEE) showing thrombus in RPA.
(MPA: main pulmonary artery; LPA: left pulmonary artery; RPA: right pulmonary artery; Ao; aorta)

rate.[24] PA acceleration time and LV systolic function are independent predictors of event-free survival.[25] Presence of patent foramen ovale (PFO) >4 mm size increased risk of embolic events.[26] In high risk PE, PFO is found in 35% of the patients and is associated with a 10-fold increase in-hospital mortality and increased incidence of embolic stroke and peripheral embolism. Detection of PFO by TTE or TEE in high-risk PE patients calls for aggressive thrombolysis.[27]

MONITORING THERAPY

Thrombolytic therapy appears to yield greatest benefit in massive PE manifested by hypotensive shock and RV dysfunction on echocardiography. Impact of thrombolysis can be assessed by echocardiography. Complete dissolution of right heart thrombus and significant reduction in RV end-diastolic diameter. RV/LV ratio, and tricuspid regurgitant flow velocity in first hour of treatment.[28,29]

CONCLUSION

Areas of confusion still exist. There are a few prospective studies related to diagnostic role of echocardiography in PE. Difference among studies exists in relation to patient selection, severity of PE, preexisting cardiorespiratory illness and parameters of diagnosis by echocardiogram. Sometimes the enrolled patients were not representative sample of the severity spectrum. In unselected patients, with suspected PE TTE failed to identify nearly 50% patients with angiographically proved PE.[30] So echocardiogram should not be used for PE screening due to low sensitivity in unselected subjects, but identifies patients with poor prognosis in acute PE.

REFERENCES

1. Burns KS, Haramati LB. Diagnostic imaging and risk stratification of patients with acute pulmonary embolism. Cardiol Rev. 2012;20:15-24.
2. Piazza G, Goldhaber SZ. Acute pulmonary embolism. Circulation. 2006;114:e28-e32.
3. Konstantinides SV, Barco S, Lankeit M, et al. Management of pulmonary embolism: An update. J Am Coll Cardiol. 2016;67:976-90.
4. Pollack CV, Screiber D, Goldhaber SZ, et al. Clinical characteristics, management and outcomes of patients diagnosed with acute pulmonary embolism in the emergency department: initial report of EMPEROR (Multicentre Emergency Medicine Pulmonary Embolism in the Real World Registry). J Am Coll Cardiol. 2011;57:700-6.
5. Fedullo PF, Tapson FF. The evaluation of suspected pulmonary embolism. N Eng J Med. 2003;349:1247-56.
6. Alpert JS, Francis GS, Vieweg WV, et al. Left ventricular function in massive pulmonary embolism. Chest. 1977;71: 108-11.
7. The European Working Group on Echocardiography. The European cooperative study on the clinical significance of the right heart thrombi. Eur Heart J. 1989;10:1046-59.
8. Ribeiro A, Juhlin-Dannfelt A, Brodin LA, et al. Pulmonary embolism: relation between degree of right ventricle overload and extent of perfusion defects. Am Heart J. 1998;135: 868-74.
9. Jaffe MR, McMurtry MS, Archer SL, et al. Management of massive and submassive pulmonary embolism, iliofemoral deep vein thrombosis, and chronic thromboembolic pulmonary hypertension: a scientific statement from the American Heart Association. Circulation. 2011;123:1788-830.
10. Konstantinides SV, Torbicki A, Agnelli G, et al. Task Force for the Diagnosis and Management of Acute Pulmonary Embolism of the European Society of Cardiology (ESC). 2014 ESC guidelines on the diagnosis and management of acute pulmonary embolism. Eur Heart J. 2014;35:3033-69.
11. Tapson VF. Acute pulmonary embolism. N Eng J Med. 2008;358:1037-105.
12. Pavlidis AN, Kallistratos MS, Karamasis GV, et al. Diagnosis and risk stratification in acute pulmonary embolism: the role of echocardiography. Rev Cardiovasc Med. 2013;14: 1-10.
13. Kjaergaard J, Schaad BK, Lund JO, et al. Quantification of right ventricular function in acute pulmonary embolism: relation to extent of pulmonary perfusion defects. Eur J Echocardiogr. 2008;9:641-5.
14. McConnell MV, Solomon SD, Rayan ME, et al. Regional right ventricular dysfunction detected by echocardiography in acute pulmonary embolism. Am J Cardiol. 1996;78:469-73.
15. Casazza F, Bongarzoni A, Capozi A. Right ventricular dysfunction in acute pulmonary embolism and right ventricular infarction. Eur J Echocardiogr. 2005;6:11-4.
16. Kurzyna M, Torbicki A, Pruszczyk P, et al. Disturbed right ventricular ejection pattern as a new Doppler echocardiographic sign of acute pulmonary embolism. Am J Cardiol. 2002;90: 507-11.

17. Dutta T, Frishman WH, Aronow WS. Echocardiography in the evaluation of pulmonary embolism. Cardiol Rev. 2017;25:309-14.
18. Mediralta A, Addetia K, Medvedofsky D, et al. Echocardiographic diagnosis of acute pulmonary embolism in patients with McConnell's sign. Echocardiography. 2016;33: 696-702.
19. Vitarelli A, Barilla F, Capotosto L, et al. Right ventricular function in acute pulmonary embolism: a combined assessment by three dimensional and speckle tracking echocardiography. J Am Soc Echocardiogr. 2015;28:355-62.
20. Benck L, Schimmel D, Puthumana J, et al. Right ventricular strain in intermediate to high-risk pulmonary embolism. Chest. 2016;150:1192A.
21. Pruszcuk P, Torbicki A, Kuch-Wocial A, et al. Transesophageal echocardiography for definitive diagnosis of hemodynamically significant pulmonary embolism. Eur Heart J. 1995;16:534-8.
22. Ribero A, Lindmaker P, Johnson H, et al. Pulmonary embolism: one-year follow-up with echocardiography Doppler and five year survival analysis. Circulation. 1999;99: 1325-30.
23. Aujesky D, Obrosky DS , Stone RA, et al. Derivation and validation of a prognostic model for pulmonary embolism. Am J Respir Crit Care Med. 2005;172:1041-6.
24. Ribero A, Lindmaker P, Johnson H, et al Pulmonary embolism: one-year follow-up with echocardiography Doppler and five year survival analysis. Circulation. 1999;99: 1325-30.
25. Jaergard J, Iverson KK, Vejlstrup NG, et al. Impacts of acute pulmonary regurgitation on right ventricular geometry and contractility assessed by tissue-Doppler echocardiography. Eur J Echocardiogr. 2010;11:1806-9.
26. Kronik G, Mosslacher H. Positive contrast echocardiography in patients with patent foramen ovale and abnormal right heart hemodynamics. Am J Cardiol. 1982;49:1806-9.
27. Konstantinides S, Geibel A, Kasper W, et al. Patent foramen ovale is an important predictor of adverse outcome of patients with major pulmonary embolism. Circulation.1998;97:1946-51.
28. Greco E, Bisignani G, Serafini O, et al. Successful treatment of right heart thromboemboli with IV recombinant tissue-type plasminogen activator during continuous echocardiographic monitoring: a case series report. Chest. 1999;83:78-82.
29. Nass N, McConnell MV, Goldhaber SZ, et al. Recovery of regional right ventricular function after thrombolysis for pulmonary embolism. Am J Cardiol. 1999;83(5):804-6.
30. Miniati M, Monti S, Pratali L, et al. Value of transthoracic echocardiography in the diagnosis of pulmonary embolism: results of a prospective study in unselected patients. Am J Med. 2001;110:528-35.

CHAPTER

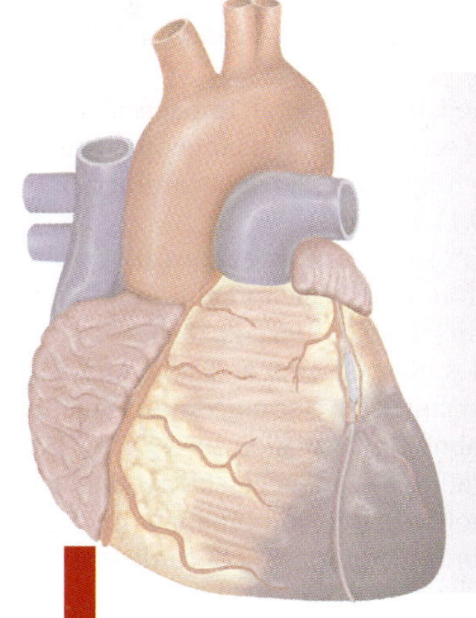

Computed Tomography Angiography in Heart Failure

Priya Jagia, Niraj Pandey

INTRODUCTION

Heart failure (HF) is a complex clinical syndrome that can be consequent to any structural or functional disorder which impairs ventricular filling or ejection of blood.[1] Over the last two decades, computed tomography (CT) technology has evolved from 4-slice acquisition systems to the modern 320-slice systems and dual-source scanners which allow for improved temporal and spatial resolution. The scan time has decreased allowing entire examinations to be completed in a single breath-hold while the contrast media requirement has also decreased considerably. Cardiac CT angiography (CTA) has evolved as an indispensable tool in the diagnosis as well as management of heart failure.

COMPUTED TOMOGRAPHY EVALUATION OF VARIOUS CARDIOVASCULAR STRUCTURES PATIENTS WITH HEART FAILURE

Coronary Arteries

Patients with newly diagnosed HF, patients who are known cases of HF with history of revascularization, patients with recurrent angina and patients with increasing symptoms may entail diagnostic evaluation of the coronary arteries. Calculation of coronary artery calcium alone can provide critical diagnostic and prognostic information with multiple studies emphasizing the importance of calcium scoring in excluding coronary artery disease (CAD) as the underlying cause of HF.[2-4] In diagnosed HF patients, a "zero calcium score" can exclude a "high-risk CAD" with 100% specificity highlighting the role of coronary artery calcium scoring as a first step in excluding an ischemic etiology for HF.[2-4] Over and above calcium scoring, CTA offers a comprehensive noninvasive evaluation of the lumen as well as wall of the coronary arteries. It has a high sensitivity and specificity and importantly, very high negative predictive value approaching 99%, for detection of obstructive CAD (Figs. 1A to D). CTA has been shown to be a highly accurate diagnostic modality for excluding an ischemic etiology in patients with cardiomyopathy of undetermined cause, with a sensitivity of 98% and a specificity of 97%.[5] Consequently, CTA has now been accepted as a substitute to invasive coronary angiography for coronary evaluation (as part of etiological assessment) in patients with new-onset HF.[5] With the advent of fractional flow reserve measurement on CT, evaluation of hemodynamic significance of the stenosis is possible as well utilizing the same datasets.

- *Cardiac veins*: Heart failure patients frequently require invasive interventions including biventricular pacing lead placement in the coronary sinus and various ablation procedures. Imaging of the cardiac veins can help establish the feasibility as well as determine the approach for these invasive procedures, curtailing the time and risk involved (Fig. 2).
- *Left ventricle*: An important step in determining the management and in prognosticating HF patients is

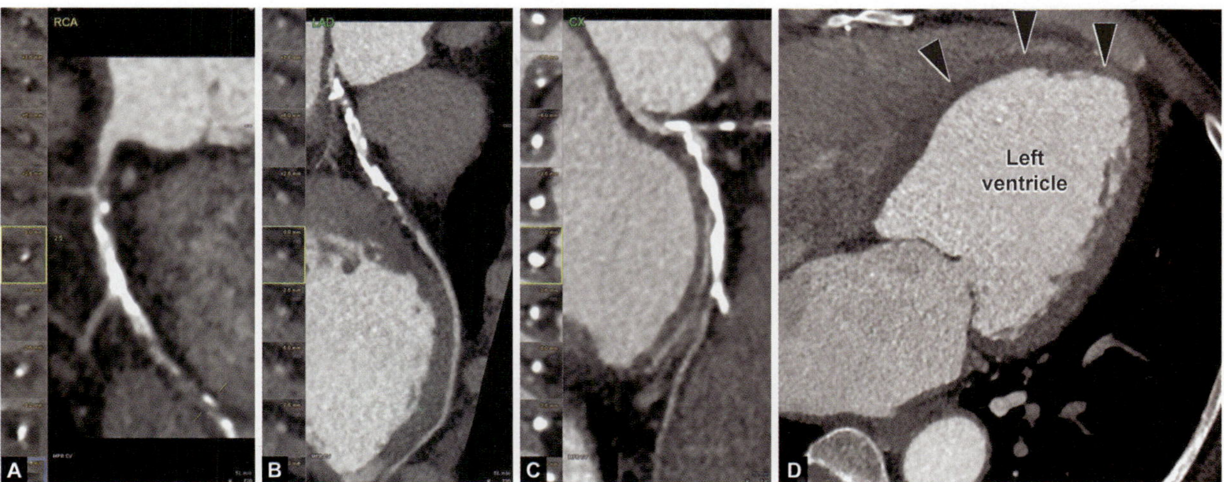

Figs. 1A to D: Curved multiplanar reconstruction of the (A) Right coronary artery (RCA); (B) Left anterior descending (LAD) artery; (C) Left circumflex (LCx) artery shows a heavily calcified plaques causing significant stenosis. Four-chamber view (D) shows dilated left ventricle with a broad-based aneurysm (arrowheads) involving the anteroseptal wall in the mid-ventricular region to apical segment and the left ventricular apex.

the structural and functional evaluation of the LV, especially the ejection fraction (EF) (Fig. 3A).[6] Volumes calculated on CT show good correlation to those calculated by magnetic resonance imaging (MRI) and echocardiography.[7] Since CT employs a true volumetric method for calculations, accuracy is not influenced by remodeling of the chambers. While CT is still not the first-line modality for assessment of the LV structure and function, it has potential for detailed LV assessment and can be considered as a substitute in specific scenarios. It is also prudent to note that a retrospectively gated CT performed for coronary evaluation can also provide this ancillary information from the same acquisition. With first-pass imaging of the myocardium after contrast administration, CTA also has the capability to ascertain myocardial perfusion defects, if any, in patients with ischemic cardiomyopathy (Figs. 3B to E). In a study comparing CTA with SPECT as the reference standard for evaluation of myocardial perfusion, CTA accurately identified perfusion defects in 93% of the involved segments while correctly ruled it out in 98% of the normal segments.[8]

Fig. 2: Volume rendered images of a delayed phase CT acquisition demonstrates the coronary sinus and the draining cardiac veins.

In HF patients of ischemic etiology, the size of infarct is a significant prognostic marker of clinical consequence and long-term LV function. The phenomenon of "delayed enhancement" is central in differentiating a scar from viable myocardium and is well established on MRI.[9] CTA can also differentiate between normal and infarcted myocardium with accurate depiction of the size of infarct on the basis of attenuation differences.[10-12] Recovery in chronic infarcted states is better evaluated on a dual-phase CTA; however, the increased radiation dose is a concern. While MRI remains the gold standard for evaluation of the LV myocardium, CTA evaluations as described above may be considered in patients with contraindications to MRI, such as patients with metallic devices.

- *Right ventricle*: Right ventricular (RV) function is a strong prognostic indicator in HF patients. Reconstruction of images at any point in the cardiac cycle in multiplanar orientations helps accomplish optimal evaluation of the complex shape of RV.[13]

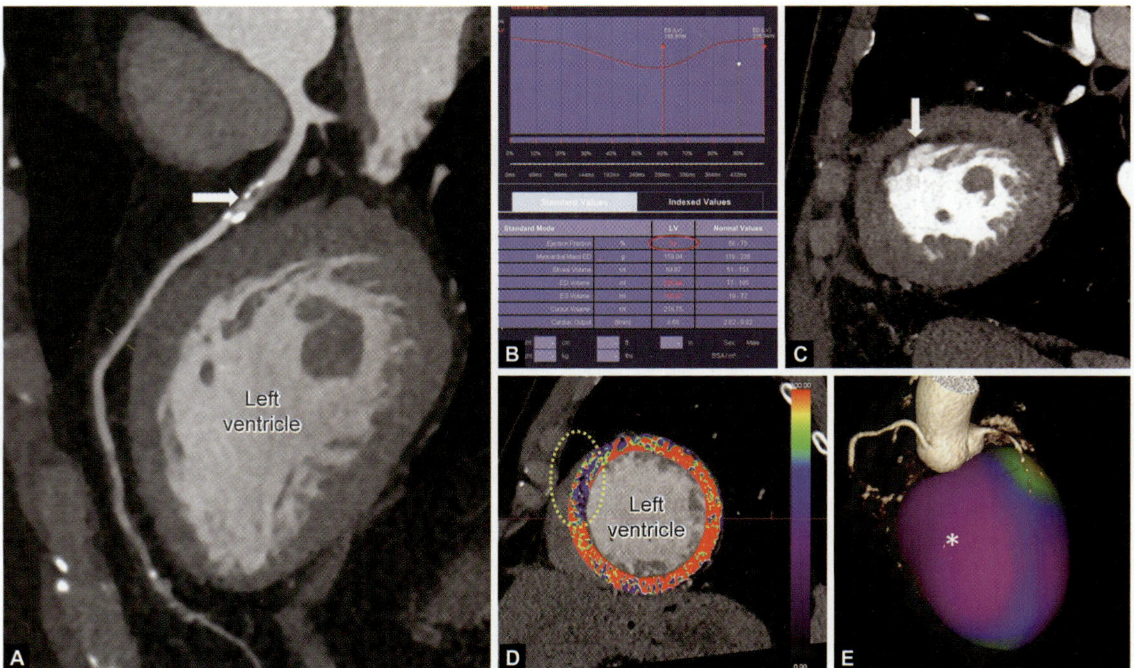

Figs. 3A to E: In the same patient as Figure 1, functional evaluation (A) of the left ventricle shows moderate dysfunction with an ejection fraction of 31%. Short axis image (B) of the left ventricular mid-segment shows subendocardial hypodensity (white arrow) in the anterior and anteroseptal region. Computed tomography perfusion imaging (C and D) shows territorial perfusion deficit in the same region (yellow circle in D; * in E).

- *Pulmonary veins*: Atrial fibrillation (AF) is common in HF patients and is a negative prognostic marker. CT helps in accurate delineation of arrhythmogenic foci which are usually at the pulmonary vein—left atrial junctions. Cardiac MRI has also been used for mapping; however, in HF patients with implanted devices, MRI might be contraindicated. High spatial resolution, multiplanar reconstructions, and volume rendering techniques providing endoscopic and surface shaded images make CT an ideal technique for preprocedural assessment as well as for evaluation of postprocedure complications (Figs. 4A and B).[14,15]

COMPUTED TOMOGRAPHY EVALUATION FOR DIAGNOSIS OF HEART FAILURE

- *HF with reduced EF*: Demonstrating reduced LV function is at the base of diagnosing HF with reduced EF. In addition to the commonly used diagnostic modalities such as echocardiography (most commonly used), cardiac MRI, LV injections during cardiac catheterization, single-photon emission computed tomography and multiple-gated acquisition (MUGA) scan, CTA can also effectively quantify reduced LV function. Using retrospective ECG-gated CTA, reconstruction of images at multiple phases across the cardiac cycle is possible using which the LV function may be calculated. Calculate of ventricular volumes and EF on CTA is not just limited to the LV as the same can be utilized for the functional evaluation of the RV also which is technically difficult to evaluate on echocardiography. With the calculations showing good correlations with values obtained on cardiac MRI, CTA is currently recommended for RV evaluation in patients with limited acoustic window or in patients contraindicated for cardiac MR imaging secondary to device placement.[16,17]
- *HF with preserved EF*: Heart failure embodies are more than just reduced LV function. About half the patients with clinical HF may show normal EF.[1] HF with preserved EF is frequently secondary to abnormal myocardial diastolic function. While echocardiographic indices, including tissue Doppler velocities and mitral valve flow velocities, are frequently used in diagnosing HF with preserved EF, it may be possible to evaluate the diastolic function using CTA as well (especially in the patients already undergoing CTA for coronary evaluation). However, it is not recommended to perform CTA for this sole purpose and MRI is preferred.

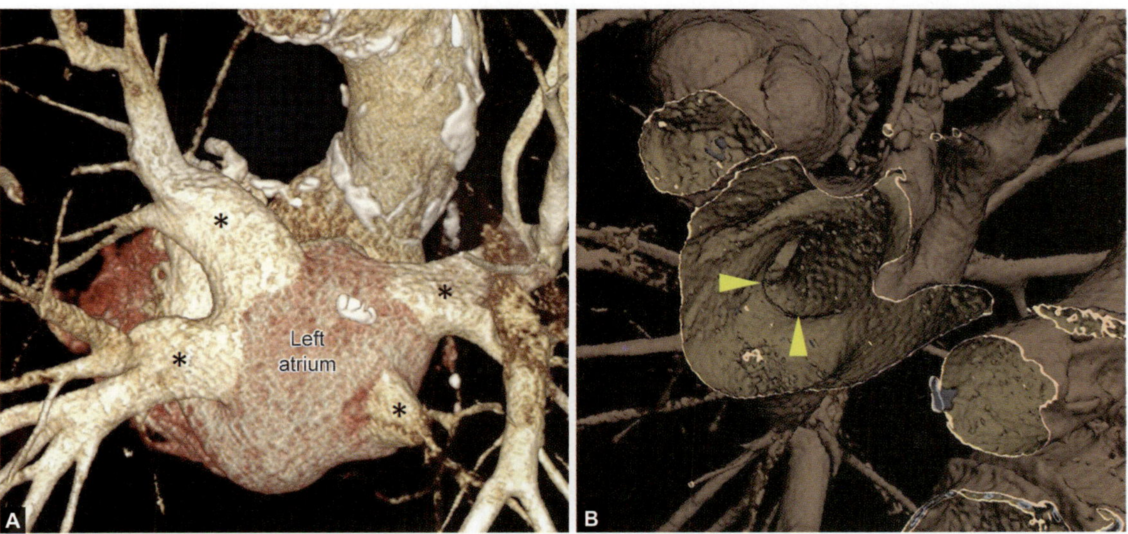

Figs. 4A and B: Surface shaded display image (A) demonstrates the left atrium with the four normally draining pulmonary veins (*). Virtual endoscopic view (B) delineates the ostium (arrowheads) of the right superior pulmonary vein.

- *Regional wall motion abnormalities*: Computed tomography angiography can also be useful for detecting regional wall motion abnormalities (RWMAs). Evaluation of retrospective ECG-gated images in a cine loop allows detection of RWMAs with high specificity approaching the accuracy of cardiac MRI.[18,19]

COMPUTED TOMOGRAPHY IN ESTABLISHING ETIOLOGY OF HEART FAILURE

Along with establishing the diagnosis of HF, it is also imperative to identify the underlying etiology as some of the conditions are potentially reversible or treatable.

- *Ischemic versus nonischemic cardiomyopathy*: Distinction between ischemic and nonischemic cardiomyopathy is an important initial diagnostic step in the workup of HF. As CAD may be the primary cause in about two-thirds patients with HF, revascularization can improve LV function in the subset of patients with impaired yet viable myocardium.[20,21] CT can provide an assessment of coronary calcium as well as allow a direct anatomical evaluation of the coronary arteries using contrast medium. CTA is accurate and safe for detecting CAD in patients with dilated cardiomyopathy and has been accepted as an alternative to invasive coronary angiography for evaluating coronaries in patients with new-onset HF to determine etiology.[22,23] Along with coronary arterial evaluation, CTA has the ability to determine resting myocardial perfusion defects with first-pass perfusion imaging. As described previously, although not conclusively established, CTA may be considered for scar evaluation as well. CTA can also help in diagnosis of other nonischemic cardiomyopathy subtypes, e.g. such as hypertrophic cardiomyopathy, LV noncompaction and arrhythmogenic RV dysplasia along with in the evaluation of adult patients with congenital heart defects (Figs. 5A and B).
- *Valvular heart disease*: Valvular heart disease is another common cause of HF. CTA plays an important role in the assessment of aortic valve lesions including aortic stenosis and aortic regurgitation as the area of the stenotic or regurgitant aortic valve orifice can be calculated using planimetry, which is comparable with transesophageal echocardiography.[5,24] CTA can also evaluate mitral valve lesions where it can show thickened leaflets in mitral stenosis, while it can demonstrate noncoaptation of the mitral valve cusps in mitral regurgitation along with detection of mitral valve prolapse and flail leaflets. It can also accurately pick up calcification in the valves (Figs. 6A and B).

ROLE OF COMPUTED TOMOGRAPHY IN THE FOLLOW-UP OF PATIENTS WITH HEART FAILURE

Computed tomography angiography is beneficial in the diagnostic evaluation of patients who have undergone various HF treatment modalities.

- *Post-heart transplant*: Coronary allograft vasculopathy is a feared complication in post-heart transplant patients. It affects up to half of the post-heart transplant patients within 10 years, and is associated with a poor prognosis.[25] Invasive catheter angiography may underestimate early

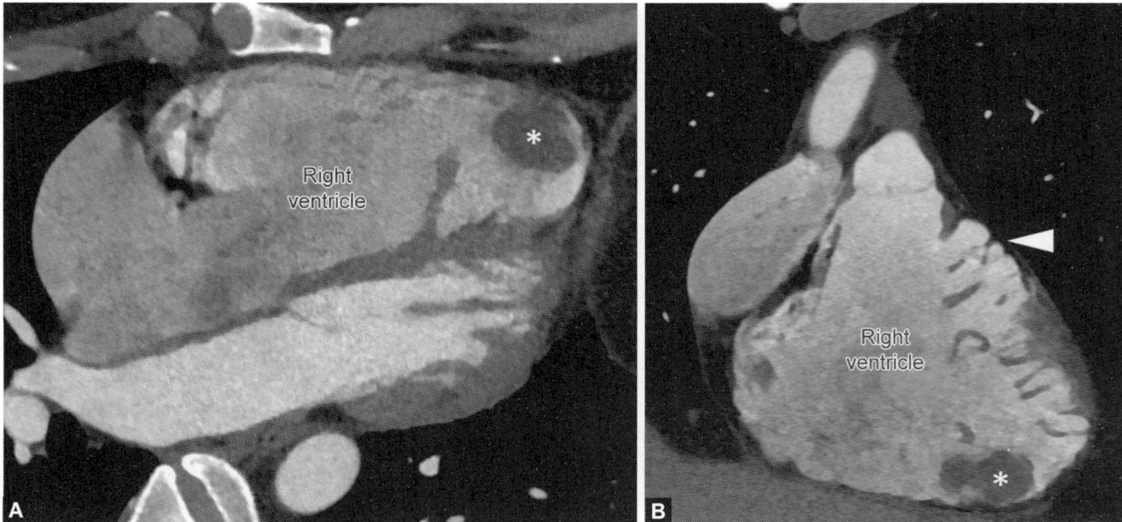

Figs. 5A and B: Four-chamber view (A) and oblique coronal view (B) shows dilated right ventricle with thinning of the walls. The free wall of the right ventricle and right ventricular outflow tract shows irregular margin with microaneurysms (arrowhead). There is a well-defined thrombus in the right ventricle apex (*).

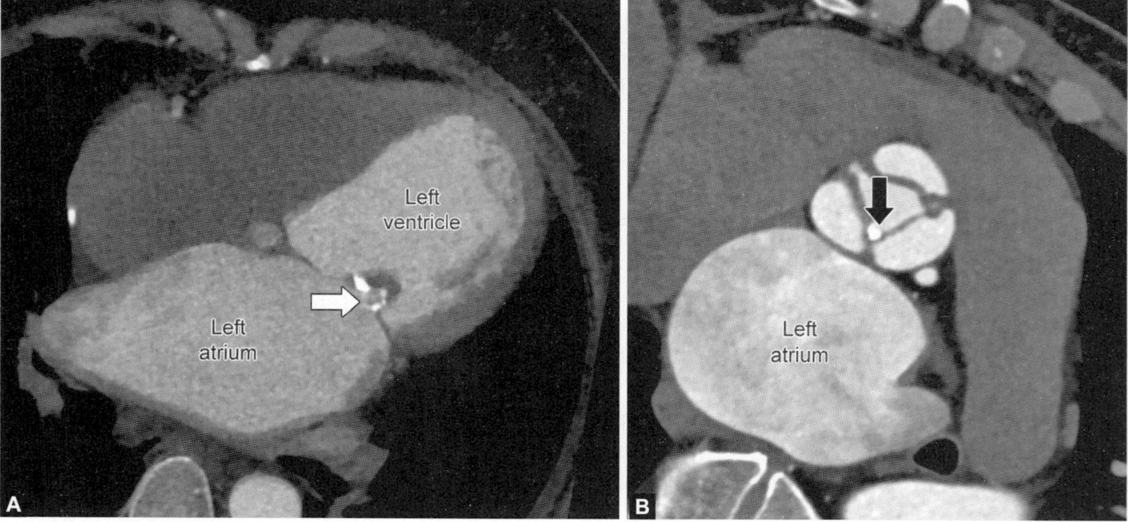

Figs. 6A and B: Four-chamber view (A) shows thickened and calcified mitral valve leaflets (white arrow). Planimetric view at the level of the aortic valve (B) in a different patient shows thickened aortic valve leaflets with a focus of calcification (black arrow).

lesions with <25% luminal stenosis as the evaluation is limited to the lumen outlined by contrast which may miss a concentric wall thickening.[26,27] This is less likely with CTA as it allows both luminal and mural evaluation of the coronaries and consequently compares favorably with intravascular ultrasound, in the detection of coronary allograft vasculopathy (Fig. 7).[28]

- *Cardiac resynchronization therapy*: Cardiac resynchronization therapy (CRT) entails the recoordination of regional wall contraction with LV dyssynchrony and cardiac venous anatomy is critical in determining its success. Presence of LV dyssynchrony at baseline is a crucial predictor of the response to CRT.[29] While conventionally echocardiography has been used to evaluate LV dyssynchrony, CTA is also capable of providing an assessment of mechanical dyssynchrony with an accuracy similar to echocardiography.[30] CTA is also helpful in guiding CRT therapy by delineating

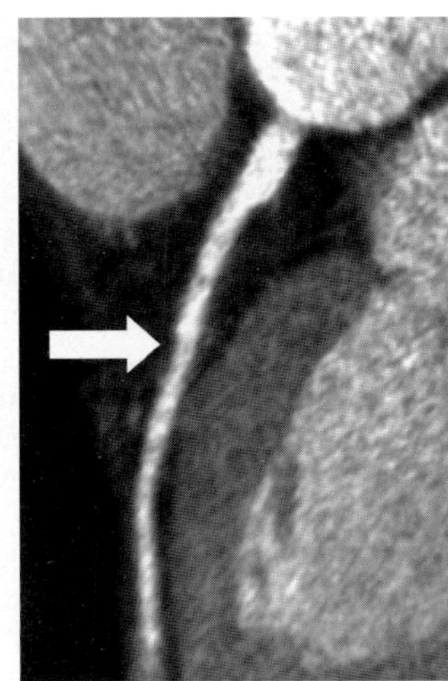

Fig. 7: In a post-heart transplant patient, curved multiplanar reconstruction of the left anterior descending artery shows concentric wall thickening (white arrow), most pronounced in the mid-segment causing mild luminal stenosis.

coronary venous anatomy. It is imperative for the success of LV lead implantation by ensuring whether the latest area of ventricular activation can be accessed with the pacing lead or not. CT can also help to improve efficacy of CRT by enabling avoidance of areas of myocardial scar.

- *Assessment of left ventricular assist devices*: Left ventricular assist devices (LVADs) are an increasingly used sustainable therapy for patients with advanced HF and provide significant mortality benefit over medical therapy. However, with more prevalent use of LVADs, various associated complications have come to the fore, and early detection and evaluation of the same have major therapeutic consequences. CTA allows high-resolution imaging of the entire LVAD with direct visualization of inflow and outflow cannulas with precise detection of any thrombus or deformation. CTA can also determine the cardiac output in presence of a continuous flow LVAD by using dynamic acquisition with mathematic analyses of flow.[31]

LIMITATIONS

Computed tomography is evolving with increasing applicability in HF patients; however, it is imperative to outline the risks associated with it and its limitations. CTA requires the injection of iodinated contrast medium which has risks of allergic reactions and nephrotoxicity. Low and regular heart rates are central to optimal image quality in cardiac CTA; however, HF patients frequently have arrhythmias like premature atrial/ventricular beats and AF. Use of CT also entails exposure to ionizing radiation. While evolution of dose reduction techniques has reduced the radiation exposure considerably, risks inherent to radiation exposure should be considered, especially in patients requiring repeated imaging.

CONCLUSION

Computed tomography has great utility in patients with clinical HF as it allows for a precise and comprehensive structural and functional evaluation of the heart, which may assist management. Evaluation with CT can help in the diagnosis of HF, its etiology, and in planning and monitoring of the treatment modalities including evaluation of implanted devices and post-heart transplant patients.

REFERENCES

1. Yancy CW, Jessup M, Bozkurt B, et al. 2013 ACCF/AHA guideline for the management of heart failure: a report of the American College of Cardiology Foundation/American Heart Association Task Force on practice guidelines. Circulation. 2013;128:e240-e327.
2. Abunassar JG, Yam Y, Chen L, et al. Usefulness of the Agatston score 5 0 to exclude ischemic cardiomyopathy in patients with heart failure. Am J Cardiol. 2011;107:428-32.
3. Budoff MJ, Shavelle DM, Lamont DH, et al. Usefulness of electron beam computed tomography scanning for distinguishing ischemic from non-ischemic cardiomyopathy. J Am Coll Cardiol. 1998;32:1173-8.
4. Sousa PA, Bettencourt N, Dias FN, et al. Role of cardiac multidetector computed tomography in the exclusion of ischemic etiology in heart failure patients. Rev Port Cardiol. 2014;33:629-36.
5. Bhatti S, Hakeem A, Yousuf MA, et al. Diagnostic performance of computed tomography angiography for differentiating ischemic vs non-ischemic cardiomyopathy. J Nucl Cardiol. 2011;18:407-20.
6. Hunt SA, Abraham WT, Chin MH, et al. ACC/AHA 2005 Guideline Update for the Diagnosis and Management of Chronic Heart Failure in the Adult: a report of the American College of Cardiology/American Heart Association Task Force on Practice Guidelines (Writing Committee to Update the 2001 Guidelines for the Evaluation and Management of Heart Failure): developed in collaboration with the American College of Chest Physicians and the International Society for Heart and Lung Transplantation: endorsed by the Heart Rhythm Society. Circulation 2005;112:e154-235.
7. Juergens KU, Fischbach R. Left ventricular function studied with MDCT. Eur Radiol. 2006;16:342-57.
8. Henneman MM, Schuijf JD, Jukema JW, et al. Comprehensive cardiac assessment with multislice computed tomography: evaluation of left ventricular function and perfusion in addition to coronary anatomy in patients with previous myocardial infarction. Heart. 2006;92:1779-83.

9. Kim RJ, Wu E, Rafael A, et al. The use of contrast-enhanced magnetic resonance imaging to identify reversible myocardial dysfunction. N Engl J Med. 2000;343:1445-53.
10. Baks T, Cademartiri F, Moelker AD, et al. Assessment of acute reperfused myocardial infarction with delayed enhancement 64-MDCT. Am J Roentgenol. 2007;188:W135-7.
11. Sato A, Hiroe M, Nozato T, et al. Early validation study of 64-slice multi-detector computed tomography for the assessment of myocardial viability and the prediction of left ventricular re-modelling after acute myocardial infarction. Eur Heart J. 2008;29:490-8.
12. Cury RC, Nieman K, Shapiro MD, et al. Comprehensive assessment of myocardial perfusion defects, regional wall motion, and left ventricular function by using 64-section multi-detector CT. Radiology. 2008;248:466-75.
13. Raman SV, Shah M, McCarthy B, et al. Multi-detector row cardiac computed tomography accurately quantifies right and left ventricular size and function compared with cardiac magnetic resonance. Am Heart J. 2006;151:736-44.
14. Niinuma H, George RT, Arbab-Zadeh A, et al. Imaging of pulmonary veins during catheter ablation for atrial fibrillation: the role of multi-slice computed tomography. Europace. 2008;10(suppl 3):iii14-21.
15. Lacomis JM, Wigginton W, Fuhrman C, et al. Multi-detector row CT of the left atrium and pulmonary veins before radiofrequency catheter ablation for atrial fibrillation. Radiographics. 2003;23:S35-48.
16. Plumhans C, Muhlenbruch G, Rapaee A, et al. Assessment of global right ventricular function on 64-MDCT compared with MRI. AJR. 2008;190:1358-61.
17. Taylor AJ, Cerqueira M, Hodgson JM, et al. ACCF/SCCT/ACR/AHA/ASE/ASNC/NASCI/SCAI/SCMR 2010 appropriate use criteria for cardiac computed tomography: a report of the American College of Cardiology Foundation Appropriate Use Criteria Task Force, the Society of Cardiovascular Computed Tomography, the American College of Radiology, the American Heart Association, the American Society of Echocardiography, the American Society of Nuclear Cardiology, the North American Society for Cardiovascular Imaging, the Society for Cardiovascular Angiography and Interventions, and the Society for Cardiovascular Magnetic Resonance. J Am Coll Cardiol. 2010;56:1864-94.
18. Lessick J, Mutlak D, Rispler S, et al. Comparison of multi-detector computed tomography versus echocardiography for assessing regional left ventricular function. Am J Cardiol. 2005;96:1011-5.
19. Yamamuro M, Tadamura E, Kubo S, et al. Cardiac functional analysis with multi-detector row CT and segmental reconstruction algorithm: comparison with echocardiography, SPECT, and MR imaging. Radiology. 2005;234:381-90.
20. Allman KC, Shaw LJ, Hachamovitch R, et al. Myocardial viability testing and impact of revascularization on prognosis in patients with coronary artery disease and left ventricular dysfunction: a meta-analysis. J Am Coll Cardiol. 2002;39:1151-5.
21. Wallis DE, O'Connell JB, Henkin RE, et al. Segmental wall motion abnormalities in dilated cardiomyopathy: a common finding and good prognostic sign. J Am Coll Cardiol. 1984;4:674-9.
22. Andreini D, Pontone G, Pepi M, et al. Diagnostic accuracy of multidetector computed tomography coronary angiography in patients with dilated cardiomyopathy. J Am Coll Cardiol. 2007;49:2044-50.
23. Zeb I, Hamirani YS, Mao S, et al. Detection of aortic regurgitation with 64-slice multidetector computed tomography (MDCT). Acad Radiol. 2010;17:1006-11.
24. Shah RG, Novaro GM, Blandon RJ, et al. Aortic valve area: meta-analysis of diagnostic performance of multi-detector computed tomography for aortic valve area measurements as compared to transthoracic echocardiography. Int J Cardiovasc Imaging. 2009;25:601-9.
25. Keogh AM, Valantine HA, Hunt SA, et al. Impact of proximal or midvessel discrete coronary artery stenoses on survival after heart transplantation. J Heart Lung Transplant. 1992;11:892-901.
26. Johnson DE, Alderman EL, Schroeder JS, et al. Transplant coronary artery disease: histopathologic correlations with angiographic morphology. J Am Coll Cardiol. 1991;17:449-57.
27. St Goar FG, Pinto FJ, Alderman EL, et al. Intracoronary ultrasound in cardiac transplant recipients. In vivo evidence of "angiographically silent" intimal thickening. Circulation. 1992;85:979-87.
28. Gregory SA, Ferencik M, Achenbach S, et al. Comparison of sixty-four-slice multidetector computed tomographic coronary angiography to coronary angiography with intravascular ultrasound for the detection of transplant vasculopathy. Am J Cardiol. 2006;98:877-84.
29. Yu CM, Bax JJ, Monaghan M, et al. Echocardiographic evaluation of cardiac dyssynchrony for predicting a favourable response to cardiac resynchronisation therapy. Heart. 2004;90 (suppl 6):vi17-22.
30. Buss SJ, Schulz F, Wolf D, et al. Quantitative analysis of left ventricular dyssynchrony using cardiac computed tomography versus three-dimensional echocardiography. Eur Radiol. 2012;22:1303-9.
31. Raman SV, Tran T, Simonetti OP, et al. Dynamic computed tomography to determine cardiac output in patients with left ventricular assist devices. J Thorac Cardiovasc Surg. 2009;137:1213-7.

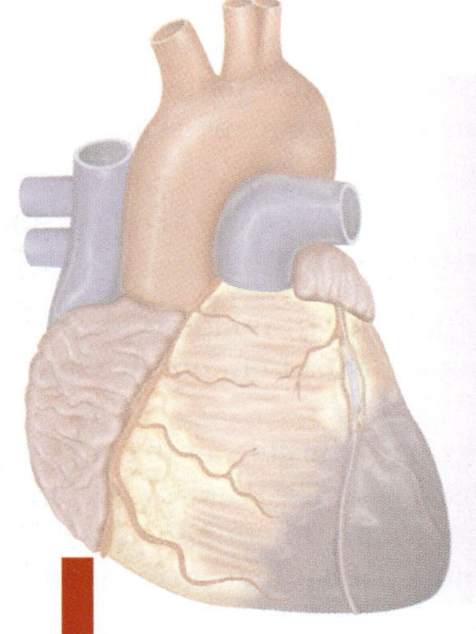

Role of Cardiac Magnetic Resonance Imaging in Heart Failure

Mona Bhatia, Amit Garg, Shashank Jain, Parveen Batra

INTRODUCTION

Heart failure (HF) is a growing global epidemic associated with a significant morbidity and mortality and financial consequences for healthcare. HF is a complex hemodynamic condition where as a result of abnormalities of cardiac structure and function, the heart is unable to meet the systemic oxygen demands. While classically HF entailed left ventricular (LV) systolic dysfunction, the gamut of HF now includes acute and chronic HF, right-sided HF, abnormalities of diastolic dysfunction, valvular, pericardial, endocardial, and heart rhythm conduction abnormalities. The spectrum includes HF with preserved, midrange or reduced ejection fraction (EF) [HF with preserved ejection fraction (HFpEF), HF with midrange ejection fraction (HFmrEF), and HF with reduced ejection fraction (HFrEF), respectively] with EF varying from ≥50%, 41–49%, and ≤40%, respectively.[1] Patients may transit from one to the other. Since various factors may be responsible for the onset of HF, it becomes imperative that all steps are taken to establish an early diagnosis and confirm the etiology as myocarditis, ischemic heart disease, hypertension, primary myocardial disorders, pericardial disorders, and valvular heart disease. Further aim is to assess the severity of HF based on ventricular morphology and function, assess severity of valvular lesions and cardiac shunts, and assist to guide management, prognosticate and follow-up, not only to relieve symptoms but also reduce risk of death. Primary evaluation of patients with suspected HF entails a good medical history, physical examination, ECG, chest X-ray, and transthoracic echocardiography[2-4] (TTE). Echocardiography (Echo) is the first-line imaging tool being widely available, portable, noninvasive, cost-effective, and capable of real-time dynamic imaging with comprehensive systolic and diastolic functional evaluation with no risks. Cardiovascular magnetic resonance (CMR) imaging plays an important complementary role in assessing the underlying etiologies, risk stratification, and prognostication and guides decision-making in patients particularly where Echo is inconclusive.[5]

CARDIOVASCULAR MAGNETIC RESONANCE IMAGE ACQUISITION PROTOCOL

Typical image acquisitions by CMR in patients with HF include T1W black blood spin-echo sequences for anatomy; cine imaging using segmented, breath-held steady-state free precession (SSFP) gradient echo sequences to acquire chamber volumes; morphologic imaging using turbo spin-echo (TSE) based sequences; perfusion imaging; inversion-recovery gradient echo sequences with appropriate nulling of normal myocardium to look for late gadolinium enhancement (LGE); phase-contrast flow imaging; and 3D SSFP coronary angiography.

Also, specific pulse sequences to evaluate diffuse fibrosis assessment [using T1 mapping and extracellular volume (ECV) measurement], iron overload (using $T2^*$ and "native" T1 measurements), tissue edema (using T2W images), fatty infiltration (using fat saturation sequences), and metabolism assessment (using MR Spectroscopy) are employed when required.[6-9] Most CMR images are generated with fast sequences gated to the R wave of the ECG to prevent artifacts from cardiac motion and acquired in end-expiratory breath hold to eliminate artifacts from respiratory motion.

CARDIOVASCULAR MAGNETIC RESONANCE VERSUS COMPETITION

Cardiovascular magnetic resonance has multiple advantages over other noninvasive imaging modalities. When compared to Echo, CMR is nonoperator dependent, with lack of restrictions due to poor acoustic windows and patient body habitus. CMR also allows myocardial assessment and tissue characterization with accurate scar detection and the images are reproducible.[10,11] CMR is the gold standard for assessment of LV volumes, ejection fraction[12,13] (EF), LV thrombi,[14-16] LA volumes,[17] and RV assessment.[18] On comparison with computed tomography (CT), single photon emission computed tomography (SPECT), and partial exchange transfusion (PET), CMR is nonionizing with superior myocardial assessment and capability to assess cardiac function and valves. Limitations of CMR, however, include availability, cost, exclusion of patients with non-MR compatible devices, renal dysfunction, and patients who are too breathless to lie flat or who have claustrophobia.

CARDIOVASCULAR MAGNETIC RESONANCE APPROACH IN CHRONIC HEART FAILURE

A systematic stepwise approach is recommended to ensure timely diagnosis, differentiation of etiology, choice of appropriate management strategy, risk stratification, and prognostication of HF.

Step 1: Diagnosis of Heart Failure

The diagnosis of HF is dependent on cardiac structure and function. CMR today is an excellent tool with a high spatial and temporal resolution to assess and evaluate both these components. As far as cardiac structure is concerned, CMR enables evaluation of LV/RV architecture (normal/ regional or diffuse wall thinning/concentric or asymmetric hypertrophy or noncompaction), evaluation of atria, cardiac valves, and pericardium. CMR is also the gold standard for functional assessment. Its high spatial and temporal resolution allows accurate, nonobserver dependent, objective and reproducible assessment of the end-diastolic volume (EDV), end-systolic volume (ESV), Cardiac output, EF, and myocardial mass. Thus, CMR today has achieved the status of gold standard for assessment of regional/global systolic function, quantitative assessment of chamber dimensions, valvular flow abnormalities, cardiac shunts, flow imaging of aortic outflow (Stroke volume and cardiac output), and transmitral inflow patterns, all of which are relevant in HF patient assessment, evaluation, management, and follow-up.

Step 2: Differentiating Etiology

Late gadolinium enhancement CMR imaging plays a critical role in differentiating ischemic from nonischemic cardiomyopathies.

Ischemic cardiomyopathy is responsible for the largest number of patients who present with HF. When evaluating HF, the three critical questions are function, perfusion, and viability, which determine patient management and prognostication.

The first step in CMR evaluation is T2W imaging which helps to determine reversible from nonreversible myocardial injury. This also gives a good estimation of area at risk.[19] The percentage of T2W edematous acute ischemic myocardial injury in excess of nonreversible injury is an indication of area at risk and reversibility/likely progression.[20]

The second step is evaluation of perfusion on dynamic imaging with assessment of stress induced ischemia. This can be performed with adenosine as the vasodilator followed by first pass CMR perfusion. The method has a high diagnostic accuracy for the detection of coronary artery disease[21-26] (CAD). Other methods of stress as exercise, dobutamine, etc. can also be used depending on the local capability. Following first pass perfusion, the next step is evaluation of scar tissue, i.e. irreversible myocardial injury. This is done by LGE, which typically is imaged 15–20 minutes post-dynamic first pass perfusion. LGE images are acquired following inversion recovery images performed to nullify the myocardial signal and enhance the scar signal. CMR is not only excellent and accurate in detection of scar tissue but also enables quantification of the same. Ischemic scars start as subendocardial scars which progress in a wave like pattern to attain transmurality[27,28] (Fig. 1). Percentage transmurality of scar is a prognostic feature to recovery. The high spatial resolution of CMR supersedes other modalities like SPECT.[29] Associated studies have shown an inverse relationship between the transmural extent of infarct and recovery of segmental contractile function post revascularization,[30] thus validating the ability of LGE CMR to prognosticate segmental functional recovery post revascularization. CMR is an extremely useful modality to evaluate various post myocardial infarction (MI) complications, as LV mural and intra-cavitatory thrombi, LV aneurysm, and papillary muscle involvement causing mitral regurgitation (MR) and rupture of the interventricular

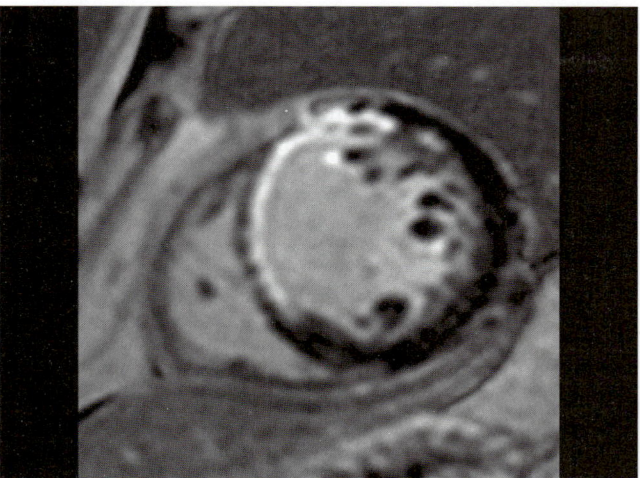

Fig. 1: Short-axis LGE CMR image at mid-ventricular level demonstrating mid-septal wall thinning and subendocardial enhancement along mid anterior and mid anterior-septal walls in a case of myocardial infarction.
(CMR: cardiovascular magnetic resonance; LGE: late gadolinium enhancement)

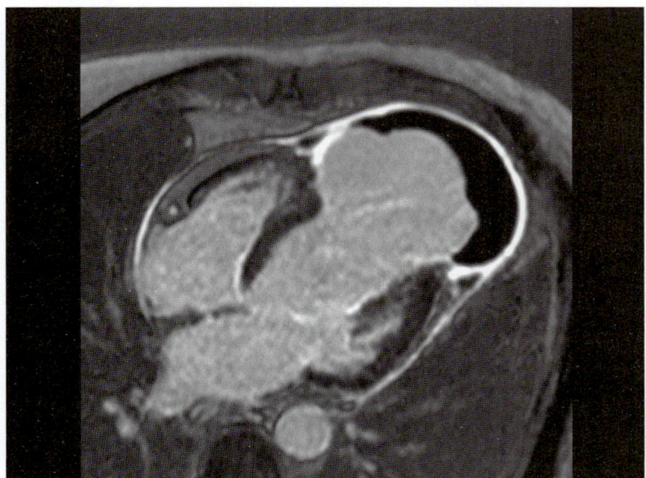

Fig. 2: Horizontal long-axis LGE CMR image in a post MI patient, showing LV apical aneurysm with transmural enhancement and large nonenhancing thrombus.
(CMR: cardiovascular magnetic resonance; LV: left ventricular; MI: myocardial infarction; LGE: late gadolinium enhancement)

septum (Fig. 2). The only area where CMR is limited is in evaluation of coronary stenosis. Currently, CMR coronary angiography is restricted and utilized for the assessment of coronary artery origins and course.[31]

Nonischemic Cardiomyopathy

The largest question while imaging cardiomyopathies (CMPs) in HF is to differentiate ischemic and nonischemic

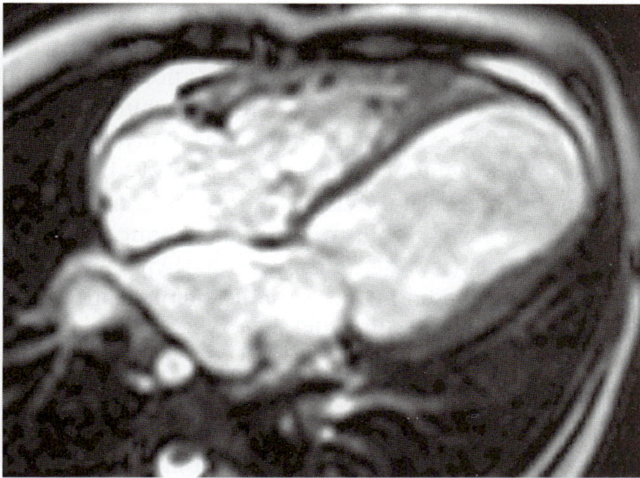

Fig. 3: Four chamber cine MR image demonstrating biventricular dilatation with global myocardial thinning and reduced ejection fraction in a case of dilated cardiomyopathy.

CMP. LGE and scar localization is extremely reliable to make this differentiation.

Dilated Cardiomyopathy

Dilated cardiomyopathy (DCM) comprises a group of conditions characterized by diastolic and systolic dysfunction of LV or both ventricles, unexplained by coronary artery disease or abnormal loading conditions.[32] While the LGE in ischemic CMP begins subendocardially to extend to transmurality with increasing severity, LGE in nonischemic, dilated CMP typically shows patchy or longitudinal striae of mid-wall enhancement.[33,34] Additional subendocardial or transmural LGE may symbolize concurrent/underlying infarction. Localization and quantification of this mid-wall LGE fibrosis and scars predispose patients to ventricular tachycardia and are arrhythmogenic substrates which guide therapeutic ablation[35,36] (Fig. 3).

Myocarditis

Myocarditis is inflammation of myocardial tissue secondary to infection, immune or toxic etiology and may manifest as new onset HF. Although the gold standard for diagnosing and characterizing myocarditis is endomyocardial biopsy (EMB), the success of the same is limited by sampling errors due to patchy involvement, besides the invasive need for diagnosis. CMR is the primary noninvasive imaging modality in clinically stable patients suspected of myocarditis.[37,38] T2W imaging followed by early and delayed LGE CMR has a high diagnostic accuracy in detecting acute myocarditis.[39] Subepicardial and mid-wall increased signal intensity on T2W images suggests myocardial edema. LGE shows a typical pattern of subepicardial extending to mid-wall involvement with relative subendocardial sparing, and lateral and infero-lateral wall predisposition.[40] The 2009 "Lake Louise Consensus CMR Criteria" requires two of the following three criteria for diagnosis of myocarditis—(1) increased regional/global signal on T2W images as compared with skeletal muscle (representing myocardial edema), (2) early global myocardial enhancement on Gd+T1W images (representing myocardial hyperemia), and (3) ≥1 focal lesion on LGE with nonischemic distribution (representing necrosis/fibrosis).[41]

Hypertrophic Cardiomyopathy

While echo has enjoyed the first-line imaging modality for hypertrophic CMP (HCMP), given the variable pattern, site of involvement and risk of missing the condition in echo-poor windows, CMR has evolved as a complementary and supplementary tool in evaluation of HCMP.

Hypertrophic cardiomyopathy (HCM) may be circumferential, regional or focal, most commonly presenting as asymmetric interventricular septum hypertrophy; however, other variants include symmetric, apical, and mass like LV hypertrophy (Fig. 4). CMR, due to its high spatial and temporal resolution, can not only detect but also determine the magnitude of LV hypertrophy superior to echocardiography.[42-45] This has important clinical significance, as wall thickness in excess of 30 mm is an independent and strong predictor of sudden cardiac death.[46] Papillary muscle abnormalities as anterolateral displacement and double bifid papillary muscles may be associated with LV outflow track obstruction in patients of HCM. Early detection by CMR is particularly essential in HCM patients to quantify myocardial disarray and scarring. LGE is usually patchy, typically mid-wall in localization, commonly involving the LV-RV junctions or cardiac apex in the apical variant,[47,48] Burnt-out HCM shows a thinned out LV wall with transmural enhancement, typically not conforming to a particular coronary arterial territory. CMR also detects LV apical aneurysms that are associated with increased risk of adverse events.[49]

Arrhythmogenic Right Ventricular Cardiomyopathy

While the title encompasses RV, biventricular affections are known. Arrhythmogenic right ventricular cardiomyopathy (ARVC) is a progressive cardiomyopathy with fibro-fatty replacement, enlargement, and arrhythmogenic dysfunction of the right ventricle.[50] CMR outscores echocardiography in better visualization of the right ventricle in orthogonal planes besides accurate functional and structural assessment. Functional irregularities in ARVC include focal aneurysms, global right ventricular dilatation, regional wall motion abnormalities, and dysfunction. Major criteria for diagnosis of ARVC include localized aneurysms, severe global/segmental RV dilatation, global systolic dysfunction; and minor criteria include mild global/segmental RV dilatation, regional contraction abnormalities, and global diastolic dysfunction.[51] Prior criteria of demonstration of fatty deposits in the right ventricular myocardium is no longer in the criteria, due to its poor sensitivity and specificity. On the contrary, detection of regional/global RV wall motion defects has a high specificity.[52] When associated with fibrosis, areas of increased enhancement on LGE CMR is evident involving the RV free wall and interventricular septum (Fig. 5).

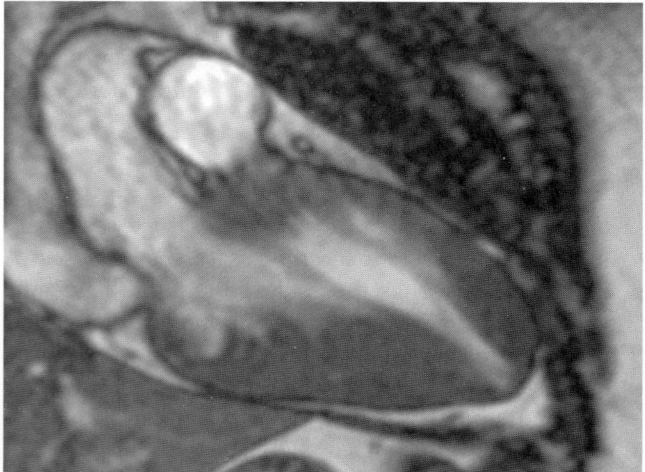

Fig. 4: Two chamber SSFP cine MR image showing apical hypertrophy and obliteration of LV apical cavity at end diastole, consistent with hypertrophic cardiomyopathy.
(LV: left ventricular; SSFP: Steady-state free precession)

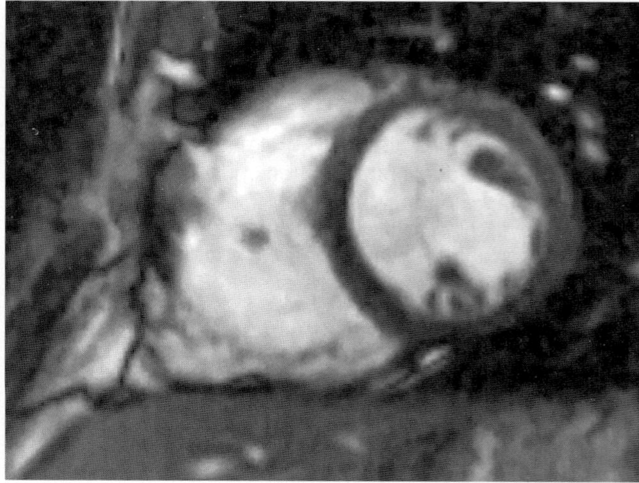

Fig. 5: Short-axis cine MR image showing global RV dilatation and pseudosacculations along free wall of RV in a case of arrhythmogenic right ventricular cardiomyopathy.
(RV: right ventricular)

Iron Overload Cardiomyopathy

Cardiac siderosis is seen in patients with beta-thalassemia major, primary hemochromatosis, and other transfusion dependent anemias. Iron overload cardiomyopathy is diagnosed by quantitative assessment of myocardial T2-star (T2*). Myocardial T2* <20 ms is a specific indicator of significant cardiac iron content.[53] Serial T2* measurements can be used to guide chelation therapies and monitor treatment response.[54,55]

Cardiac Amyloidosis

Amyloidosis is a systemic disease and the heart muscle is not exempt. When the heart is involved, most common presenting symptom is chronic heart failure (CHF) and if left untreated, fast progression may render the median survival to <6 months. Hence, early recognition and therapeutic intervention is important. CMR findings in amyloidosis include concentric hypertrophy with reduced contractility, bi-atrial dilatation, and thickened IAS[56] (interatrial septum). LGE CMR imaging is rather classic with circumferential subendocardial enhancement and an occasional patchy transmural pattern[56-58] (Fig. 6). A unique zebra-stripe appearance may be seen with LV/RV subendocardial enhancement and sparing of the mid-wall of the IVS. Recent studies have shown high diagnostic accuracy of noncontrast T1 mapping for detecting and differentiating the nature of amyloid deposition in patients of cardiac amyloidosis with higher sensitivity than LGE and significant correlation with markers of systolic/diastolic dysfunction.[59]

Sarcoidosis

Cardiac sarcoidosis can lead to progressive HF and may be fatal in one-fourth of patients with cardiac sarcoidosis.[60,61] T2W images with LGE CMR are extremely useful in detection of sarcoidosis besides LV/RV dilatation with systolic dysfunction, septal thinning, and pericardial effusion. LGE CMR imaging shows mid-wall or epicardial pattern of enhancement, nonischemic in distribution with anteroseptal and infero-lateral wall predisposition (Fig. 7).

Anderson-Fabry Disease

Anderson-Fabry disease (AFD) is an X-linked disorder with deficiency of alpha-galactosidase A resulting in accumulation of cellular glycosphingolipid in blood vessels and heart.[62] CMR demonstrates left ventricular hypertrophy (LVH) and can localize areas of fibrosis. LGE CMR in AFD demonstrates involvement of basal inferolateral LV with subendocardial sparing.

Constrictive Pericarditis

The differentiation of restrictive from constrictive cardiac involvement is often challenging on echo. CMR can demonstrate normal pericardium as an approx. 2 mm thin hypointense line. Constrictive pericarditis is characterized by an abnormally thickened pericardium (>4 mm) (Fig. 8). Calcifications, if present, appear dark on all pulse sequences. Segmented SSFP cine CMR frequently demonstrates the characteristic septal "bounce" appearing as early inspiratory

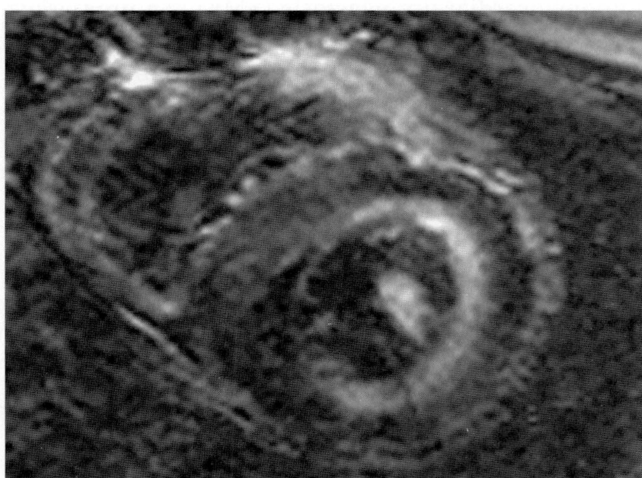

Fig. 6: Short-axis LGE CMR image at mid-ventricular level demonstrating global subendocardial LGE with dark blood pool, consistent with amyloidosis.
(CMR: cardiovascular magnetic resonance; LGE: late gadolinium enhancement)

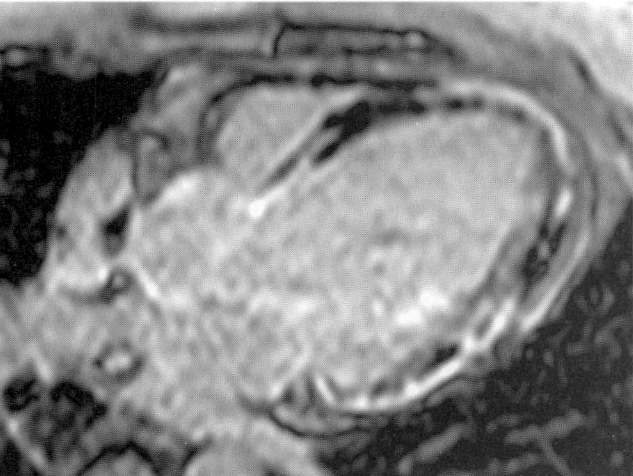

Fig. 7: Horizontal long-axis LGE CMR image demonstrating LV dilatation with septal thinning and mid-wall enhancement along apical septal, apical lateral, mid-lateral and basal lateral walls of LV in a case of sarcoidosis.
(CMR: cardiovascular magnetic resonance; LGE: late gadolinium enhancement; LV: left ventricular)

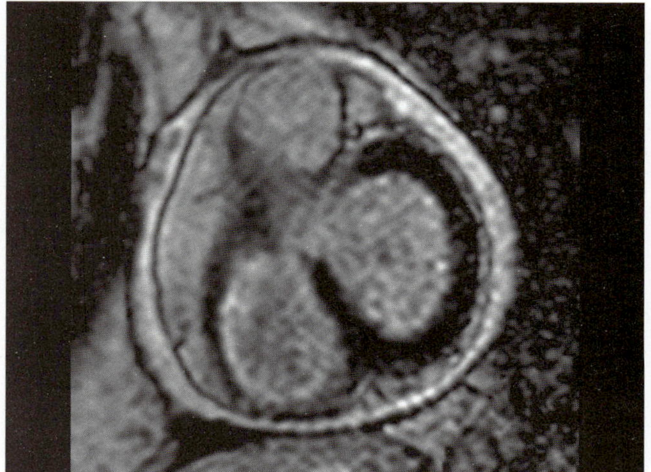

Fig. 8: Short-axis LGE CMR image at basal ventricular level demonstrating abnormally thickened enhancing pericardium, consistent with constrictive pericarditis.
(CMR: cardiovascular magnetic resonance; LGE: late gadolinium enhancement)

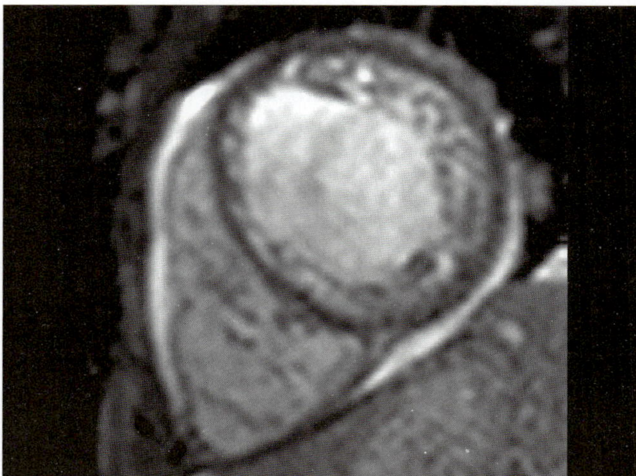

Fig. 9: Short-axis cine MR image at mid-ventricular level demonstrating increased trabeculations with deep intra-trabecular recesses in LV myocardium, consistent with noncompaction.
(LV: left ventricular)

flattening of IVS in diastole with ventricular coupling and dilatation of inferior vena cava (IVC).[63]

Noncompaction

Left ventricular noncompaction is a myocardial disorder due to failure of myocardial compaction during embryogenesis. While most frequently the LV is involved, biventricular involvement is known to occur with the congenital abnormality. The condition results in a two-layered myocardium with subendocardial noncompacted hypertrabeculated layer and a compacted epicardial component. The condition presents as a progressive systolic dysfunction, ventricular arrhythmias, and embolic events from LV thrombi trapped within the trabeculation of the noncompacted myocardium.[64,65] CMR shows varying degree of ventricular trabeculations and intertrabecular recesses, with the noncompacted to compacted myocardial ratio of >2.3:1, diagnostic of this condition[66] (Fig. 9).

Chagas Disease

Chagas disease is becoming a global health burden with cardiovascular deaths in endemic areas. The condition is characterized by progressive myocardial fibrosis, most commonly involving the LV apex and inferolateral walls demonstrating hyperenhancement on LGE CMR. In addition, sequelae to myocardial damage, such as regional hypokinesis/wall thinning, aneurysms, and global hypokinesia are well depicted by CMR.[67]

Tako-tsubo Cardiomyopathy

Tako-tsubo (stress) cardiomyopathy is a stress-induced transient weakness of the cardiac muscle with characteristic wall motion abnormalities resembling anteroapical infarction, manifesting as edema on T2W images without evidence of scarring on LGE CMR.[68-70]

Endomyocardial Fibroelastosis

Endomyocardial fibroelastosis (EMF) is a progressive disease of unknown origin causing restrictive CMP. It is characterized by diffuse thickening and fibrosis of the endocardium with adherent thrombus. CMR identifies extent of fibrosis and thrombus allowing identification and monitoring of patients with this condition associated with sudden cardiac death.

Step 3: Prognostication

Following diagnosis of HF, prognostication of the condition is essential to guide management. CMR plays a critical role in prognostication based on its pivotal position in being the gold standard for evaluation of function and assessment of scarring, both detection and quantification.

Ischemic Cardiomyopathy

Prognostication of ischemic CMP is based on function, wall thinning, wall motion abnormalities, scar evaluation, and complications. Infarct size, extent, and transmurality on LGE CMR is a better predictor of inducible ventricular tachycardia than LVEF.[71] RVEF late after MI is an important prognostic indicator and can be accurately determined by CMR.[72] CMR has the capability to predict ventricular remodeling and adverse cardiac events following acute MI,[73] evaluate, and quantify myocardial scarring on LGE CMR, which are arrhythmogenic substrates.[71,74] Stress CMR using adenosine, dobutamine or dipyridamole is useful to stratify patients suspected of CAD at high risk for CHF or sudden cardiac death (Flowchart 1).[75-77]

Dilated Cardiomyopathy

In patients with DCM, presence and extent of mid-wall fibrosis is associated with a higher rate of mortality and hospitalization.[78]

HYPERTROPHIC CARDIOMYOPATHY

Management of HCM alters significantly based on prognostication and risk of sudden cardiac death. The presence of LGE is an independent predictor of ventricular tachyarrhythmias in asymptomatic or mildly symptomatic patients.[79,80] A 7 times increased risk of nonsustained ventricular tachycardia was associated in patients with LGE. CMR can quantify scars and risk stratification of sudden cardiac death by CMR guides patients who are in need of an ICD device. LGE involving more than 15% of LV myocardium, is associated with increased incidence of sudden cardiac death, and ICD placement may be considered in these patients for primary prevention.[81]

Flowchart 1: Imaging algorithm in heart failure.

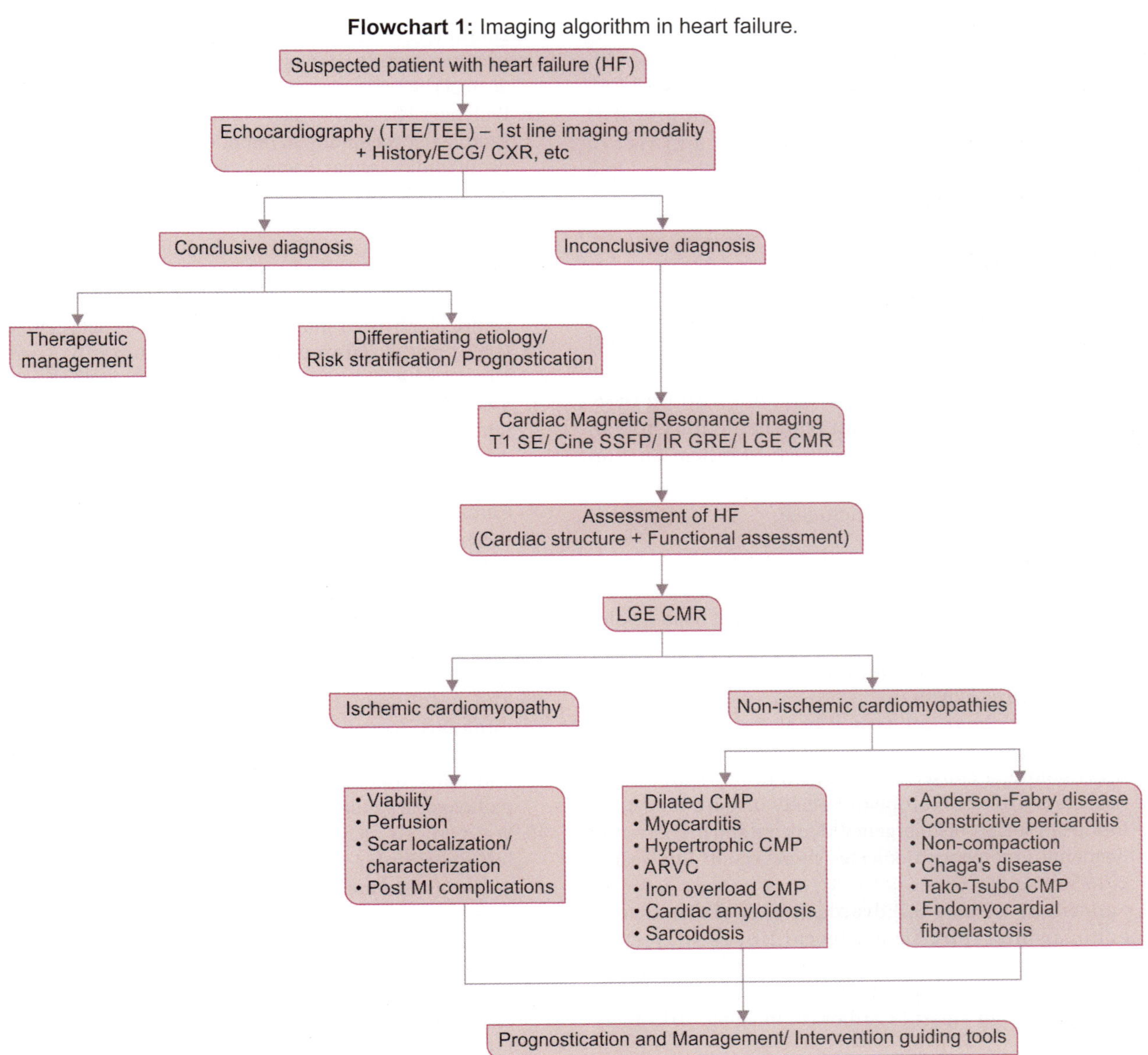

Further, myocardial wall thickness in excess of 3 cm is an independent predictor in HCM.

Amyloidosis

Presence of LGE in patients with proven cardiac amyloidosis is associated with notable survival differences.[82] Positive correlation has also been obtained between severity of HF and presence of LGE in patients with systemic amyloidosis.[83]

Thalassemia

Quantitative myocardial iron overload ($T2^* < 10$ ms) is associated with a higher risk of developing HF.[84]

Step 4: Role in Management/Interventions

Cardiovascular magnetic resonance is an important tool in guiding management and intervention. Following the diagnosis of HF and establishment of its etiology, LGE CMR plays a crucial role in scar localization, estimation, and quantification which guide management and ICD placement depending on prognostication and risk of sudden cardiac death, and are important findings guiding tools to ablative therapy.

CONCLUSION

Echocardiography (echo) is the first-line imaging tool being widely available, portable, noninvasive, cost-effective, and capable of real time dynamic imaging with comprehensive systolic and diastolic functional evaluation with no risks. CMR imaging plays an important complementary role in assessing the underlying etiologies, risk stratification, and prognostication, and guides decision-making in patients, particularly where echo is inconclusive.

REFERENCES

1. Teng TK, Tay WT, Dahlstrom U, et al. Different relationships between pulse pressure and mortality in heart failure with reduced, mid-range and preserved ejection fraction. Int J Cardiol. 2018;254:203-9.
2. Mebazaa A, Yilmaz MB, Levy P, et al. Recommendations on pre-hospital and early hospital management of acute heart failure: a consensus paper from the Heart Failure Association of the European Society of Cardiology, the European Society of Emergency Medicine and the Society of Academic Emergency Medicine--short version. Eur Heart J. 2015;36(30):1958-66.
3. Lancellotti P, Price S, Edvardsen T, et al. The use of echocardiography in acute cardiovascular care: Recommendations of the European Association of Cardiovascular Imaging and the Acute Cardiovascular Care Association. Eur Heart J Cardiovasc Imaging. 2015;16(2): 119-46.
4. Garbi M, McDonagh T, Cosyns B, et al. EACVI Imaging Task Force. Appropriateness criteria for cardiovascular imaging use in heart failure: report of literature review. Eur Heart J Cardiovasc Imaging. 2015;16(2):147-53.
5. Peterzan MA, Rider OJ, Anderson LJ. The role of cardiovascular magnetic resonance imaging in heart failure. Card Fail Rev. 2016;2(2):115-22.
6. Iles L, Pfluger H, Phrommintikul A, et al. Evaluation of diffuse myocardial fibrosis in heart failure with cardiac magnetic resonance contrast-enhanced T1 mapping. J Am Coll Cardiol. 2008;52(19):1574-80.
7. Sado DM, Flett AS, Banypersad SM, et al. Cardiovascular magnetic resonance measurement of myocardial extracellular volume in health and disease. Heart. 2012;98(19):1436-41.
8. Maestrini V, Treibel TA, White SK, et al. T1 mapping for characterization of intracellular and extracellular myocardial diseases in heart failure. Curr Cardiovasc Imaging Rep. 2014;7:9287.
9. Hudsmith LE, Neubauer S. Magnetic resonance spectroscopy in myocardial disease. JACC Cardiovasc Imaging. 2009;2(1):87-96.
10. Bellenger NG, Davies LC, Francis JM, et al. Reduction in sample size for studies of remodeling in heart failure by the use of cardiovascular magnetic resonance. J Cardiovasc Magn Reson. 2000;2(4):271-8.
11. Grothues F, Smith GC, Moon JC, et al. Comparison of interstudy reproducibility of cardiovascular magnetic resonance with two-dimensional echocardiography in normal subjects and in patients with heart failure or left ventricular hypertrophy. Am J Cardiol. 2002;90(1):29-34.
12. Greupner J, Zimmermann E, Grohmann A, et al. Head-to-head comparison of left ventricular function assessment with 64-row computed tomography, biplane left cineventriculography, and both 2- and 3-dimensional transthoracic echocardiography: comparison with magnetic resonance imaging as the reference standard. J Am Coll Cardiol. 2012;59(21):1897-907.
13. Bellenger NG, Burgess MI, Ray SG, et al. Comparison of left ventricular ejection fraction and volumes in heart failure by echocardiography, radionuclide ventriculography and cardiovascular magnetic resonance: Are they interchangeable? Eur Heart J. 2000;21(6):1387-96.
14. Srichai MB, Junor C, Rodriguez LL, et al. Clinical, imaging, and pathological characteristics of left ventricular thrombus: A comparison of contrast-enhanced magnetic resonance imaging, transthoracic echocardiography, and transesophageal echocardiography with surgical or pathological validation. Am Heart J. 2006;152(1):75-84.
15. Weinsaft JW, Kim HW, Shah DJ, et al. Detection of left ventricular thrombus by delayed-enhancement cardiovascular magnetic resonance prevalence and markers in patients with systolic dysfunction. J Am Coll Cardiol. 2008;52(2):148-57.
16. Weinsaft JW, Kim RJ, Ross M, et al. Contrast-enhanced anatomic imaging as compared to contrast-enhanced tissue characterization for detection of left ventricular thrombus. JACC Cardiovasc Imaging. 2009;2(8):969-79.

17. Habibi M, Chahal H, Opdahl A, et al. Association of CMR-measured LA function with heart failure development: results from the MESA study. JACC Cardiovasc Imaging. 2014;7(6):570-9.
18. Kawut SM, Barr RG, Lima JA, et al. Right ventricular structure is associated with the risk of heart failure and cardiovascular death: The Multi-Ethnic Study of Atherosclerosis (MESA)--right ventricle study. Circulation. 2012;126(14):1681-8.
19. Aletras AH, Tilak GS, Natanzon A, et al. Retrospective determination of the area at risk for reperfused acute myocardial infarction with T2-weighted cardiac magnetic resonance imaging: histopathological and displacement encoding with stimulated echoes (DENSE) functional validations. Circulation. 2006;113(15):1865-70.
20. Abdel-Aty H, Cocker M, Meek C, et al. Edema as a very early marker for acute myocardial ischemia: a cardiovascular magnetic resonance study. J Am Coll Cardiol. 2009;53(14):1194-201.
21. Nandalur KR, Dwamena BA, Choudhri AF, et al. Diagnostic performance of stress cardiac magnetic resonance imaging in the detection of coronary artery disease: a meta-analysis. J Am Coll Cardiol. 2007;50(14):1343-53.
22. Cheng AS, Pegg TJ, Karamitsos TD, et al. Cardiovascular magnetic resonance perfusion imaging at 3-Tesla for the detection of coronary artery disease: a comparison with 1.5-Tesla. J Am Coll Cardiol. 2007;49(25):2440-9.
23. Nagel E, Klein C, Paetsch I, et al. Magnetic resonance perfusion measurements for the noninvasive detection of coronary artery disease. Circulation. 2003;108(4):432-7.
24. Plein S, Radjenovic A, Ridgway JP, et al. Coronary artery disease: myocardial perfusion MR imaging with sensitivity encoding versus conventional angiography. Radiology. 2005;235(2):423-30.
25. Schwitter J, Wacker CM, van Rossum AC, et al. MR-IMPACT: comparison of perfusion-cardiac magnetic resonance with single-photon emission computed tomography for the detection of coronary artery disease in a multicenter, multivendor, randomized trial. Eur Heart J. 2008;29(4): 480-9.
26. Karamitsos TD, Arnold JR, Pegg TJ, et al. Tolerance and safety of adenosine stress perfusion cardiovascular magnetic resonance imaging in patients with severe coronary artery disease. Int J Cardiovasc Imaging. 2009;25(3):277-83.
27. Kim RJ, Fieno DS, Parrish TB, et al. Relationship of MRI delayed contrast enhancement to irreversible injury, infarct age, and contractile function. Circulation. 1999;100(19):1992-2002.
28. Wagner A, Mahrholdt H, Thomson L, et al. Effects of time, dose, and inversion time for acute myocardial infarct size measurements based on magnetic resonance imaging-delayed contrast enhancement. J Am Coll Cardiol. 2006;47(10):2027-33.
29. Wagner A, Mahrholdt H, Holly TA, et al. Contrast-enhanced MRI and routine single photon emission computed tomography (SPECT) perfusion imaging for detection of subendocardial myocardial infarcts: an imaging study. Lancet. 2003;361(9355):374-9.
30. Kim RJ, Wu E, Rafael A, et al. The use of contrast-enhanced magnetic resonance imaging to identify reversible myocardial dysfunction. N Engl J Med. 2000;343(20):1445-53.
31. Bluemke DA, Achenbach S, Budoff M, et al. Noninvasive coronary artery imaging: Magnetic resonance angiography and multidetector computed tomography angiography: a scientific statement from the American Heart Association Committee on Cardiovascular Imaging and Intervention of the Council on Cardiovascular Radiology and Intervention, and the Councils on Clinical Cardiology and Cardiovascular Disease in the Young. Circulation. 2008;118(5):586-606.
32. Elliott P, Andersson B, Arbustini E, et al. Classification of the cardiomyopathies: a position statement from the European Society of Cardiology Working Group on myocardial and pericardial diseases. Eur Heart J. 2008;29(2):270-6.
33. McCrohon JA, Moon JC, Prasad SK, et al. Differentiation of heart failure related to dilated cardiomyopathy and coronary artery disease using gadolinium-enhanced cardiovascular magnetic resonance. Circulation. 2003;108(1):54-9.
34. Mahrholdt H, Wagner A, Judd RM, et al. Delayed enhancement cardiovascular magnetic resonance assessment of non-ischemic cardiomyopathies. Eur Heart J. 2005;26(15):1461-74.
35. Nazarian S, Bluemke DA, Lardo AC, et al. Magnetic resonance assessment of the substrate for inducible ventricular tachycardia in nonischemic cardiomyopathy. Circulation. 2005;112(18):2821-5.
36. Bogun FM, Desjardins B, Good E, et al. Delayed-enhanced magnetic resonance imaging in nonischemic cardiomyopathy: utility for identifying the ventricular arrhythmia substrate. J Am Coll Cardiol. 2009;53(13):1138-45.
37. Friedrich MG, Marcotte F. Cardiac magnetic resonance assessment of myocarditis. Circ Cardiovasc Imaging. 2013;6(5):833-9.
38. Yilmaz A, Ferreira V, Klingel K, et al. Role of cardiovascular magnetic resonance imaging (CMR) in the diagnosis of acute and chronic myocarditis. Heart Fail Rev. 2013;18(6):747-60.
39. Abdel-Aty H, Boyé P, Zagrosek A, et al. Diagnostic performance of cardiovascular magnetic resonance in patients with suspected acute myocarditis: comparison of different approaches. J Am Coll Cardiol. 2005;45(11):1815-22.
40. Mahrholdt H, Wagner A, Deluigi CC, et al. Presentation, patterns of myocardial damage, and clinical course of viral myocarditis. Circulation. 2006;114(15):1581-90.
41. Friedrich M, Sechtem U, Schulz-Menger J, et al. International Consensus Group on Cardiovascular Magnetic Resonance in Myocarditis. Cardiovascular magnetic resonance in myocarditis: A JACC white paper. J Am Coll Cardiol. 2009;53(17):1475-87.
42. Pons-Lladó G1, Carreras F, Borrás X, et al. Comparison of morphologic assessment of hypertrophic cardiomyopathy by magnetic resonance versus echocardiographic imaging. Am J Cardiol. 1997;79(12):1651-6.
43. Rickers C, Wilke NM, Jerosch-Herold M, et al. Utility of cardiac magnetic resonance imaging in the diagnosis of hypertrophic cardiomyopathy. Circulation. 2005;112(16):855-61.
44. Olivotto I, Maron MS, Autore C, et al. Assessment and significance of left ventricular mass by cardiovascular

magnetic resonance in hypertrophic cardiomyopathy. J Am Coll Cardiol. 2008;52(7):559-66.
45. Moon JC, Fisher NG, McKenna WJ, et al. Detection of apical hypertrophic cardiomyopathy by cardiovascular magnetic resonance in patients with non-diagnostic echocardiography. Heart. 2004;90(6):645-9.
46. Spirito P, Bellone P, Harris KM, et al. Magnitude of left ventricular hypertrophy and risk of sudden death in hypertrophic cardiomyopathy. N Engl J Med. 2000;342(24):1778-85.
47. Rudolph A, Abdel-Aty H, Bohl S, et al. Noninvasive detection of fibrosis applying contrast-enhanced cardiac magnetic resonance in different forms of left ventricular hypertrophy relation to remodeling. J Am Coll Cardiol. 2009;53(3):284-91.
48. Yamada M, Teraoka K, Kawade M, et al. Frequency and distribution of late gadolinium enhancement in magnetic resonance imaging of patients with apical hypertrophic cardiomyopathy and patients with asymmetrical hypertrophic cardiomyopathy: a comparative study. Int J Cardiovasc Imaging. 2009;25(Suppl 1):131-8.
49. Maron MS, Finley JJ, Bos JM, et al. Prevalence, clinical significance, and natural history of left ventricular apical aneurysms in hypertrophic cardiomyopathy. Circulation. 2008;118:1541-9.
50. Ferrari VA, Scott CH, Basso C. Arrhythmogenic right ventricular dysplasia/cardiomyopathy. Curr Cardiol Rep. 2005;7:70-5.
51. McKenna WJ, Thiene G, Nava A, et al. Diagnosis of arrhythmogenic right ventricular dysplasia/cardiomyopathy. Task Force of the Working Group Myocardial and Pericardial Disease of the European Society of Cardiology and of the Scientific Council on Cardiomyopathies of the International Society and Federation of Cardiology. Br Heart J. 1994;71(3):215-8.
52. Tandri H, Castillo E, Ferrari VA, et al. Magnetic resonance imaging of arrhythmogenic right ventricular dysplasia: sensitivity, specificity, and observer variability of fat detection versus functional analysis of the right ventricle. J Am Coll Cardiol. 2006;48(11):2277-84.
53. Anderson LJ, Holden S, Davis B, et al. Cardiovascular T2-star (T2*) magnetic resonance for the early diagnosis of myocardial iron overload. Eur Heart J. 2001;22(23):2171-9.
54. Tanner MA, Galanello R, Dessi C, et al. A randomized, placebo-controlled, double-blind trial of the effect of combined therapy with deferoxamine and deferiprone on myocardial iron in thalassemia major using cardiovascular magnetic resonance. Circulation. 2007;115(14):1876-84.
55. Anderson LJ, Wonke B, Prescott E, et al. Comparison of effects of oral deferiprone and subcutaneous desferrioxamine on myocardial iron concentrations and ventricular function in beta-thalassaemia. Lancet. 2002;360(9332):516-20.
56. Selvanayagam JB, Hawkins PN, Paul B, et al. Evaluation and management of the cardiac amyloidosis. J Am Coll Cardiol. 2007;50(22):2101-10.
57. Maceira AM, Joshi J, Prasad SK, et al. Cardiovascular magnetic resonance in cardiac amyloidosis. Circulation. 2005;111(2):186-93.
58. Cheng AS, Banning AP, Mitchell AR, et al. Cardiac changes in systemic amyloidosis: visualization by magnetic resonance imaging. Int J Cardiol. 2006;113(1):E21-3.
59. Karamitsos TD, Piechnik SK, Banypersad SM, et al. Noncontrast T1 mapping for the diagnosis of cardiac amyloidosis. JACC Cardiovasc Imaging. 2013;6(4):488-97.
60. Doughan AR, Williams BR. Cardiac sarcoidosis. Heart. 2006;92(2):282-8.
61. Roberts WC, McAllister HA Jr, Ferrans VJ. Sarcoidosis of the heart. A clinicopathologic study of 35 necropsy patients (group 1) and review of 78 previously described necropsy patients (group 11). Am J Med. 1977;63(1):86-108.
62. Clarke JT. Narrative review: Fabry disease. Ann Intern Med. 2007;146(6):425-33.
63. Francone M, Dymarkowski S, Kalantzi M, et al. Assessment of ventricular coupling with real-time cine MRI and its value to differentiate constrictive pericarditis from restrictive cardiomyopathy. Eur Radiol. 2006;16(4):944-51.
64. Ritter M, Oechslin E, Sutsch G, et al. Isolated Noncompaction of the myocardium in adults. Mayo Clin Proc. 1997;72(1):26-31.
65. Oechslin EN, Attenhofer Jost CH, Rojas JR, et al. Long-term follow-up of 34 adults with isolated left ventricular noncompaction: a distinct cardiomyopathy with poor prognosis. J Am Coll Cardiol. 2000;36(2):493-500.
66. Petersen SE, Selvanayagam JB, Wiesmann F, et al. Left ventricular non-compaction: insights from cardiovascular magnetic resonance imaging. J Am Coll Cardiol. 2005;46(1):101-5.
67. Rochitte CE, Nacif MS, de Oliveira Júnior AC, et al. Cardiac magnetic resonance in Chagas' disease. Artif Organs. 2007;31(4):259-67.
68. Haghi D, Fluechter S, Suselbeck T, et al. Cardiovascular magnetic resonance findings in typical versus atypical forms of the acute apical ballooning syndrome (Takotsubo cardiomyopathy). Int J Cardiol. 2007;120(2):205-11.
69. Karamitsos TD, Bull S, Spyrou N, et al. Tako-tsubo cardiomyopathy presenting with features of left ventricular non-compaction. Int J Cardiol. 2008;128(1):e34-6.
70. Abdel-Aty H, Cocker M, Friedrich MG. Myocardial edema is a feature of Tako-Tsubo cardiomyopathy and is related to the severity of systolic dysfunction: insights from T2-weighted cardiovascular magnetic resonance. Int J Cardiol. 2009;132(2):291-3.
71. Bello D, Fieno DS, Kim RJ, et al. Infarct morphology identifies patients with substrate for sustained ventricular tachycardia. J Am Coll Cardiol. 2005;45(7):1104-8.
72. Larose E, Ganz P, Reynolds HG, et al. Right ventricular dysfunction assessed by cardiovascular magnetic resonance imaging predicts poor prognosis late after myocardial infarction. J Am Coll Cardiol. 2007;49(8):855-62.
73. Wu KC, Zerhouni EA, Judd RM, et al. Prognostic significance of microvascular obstruction by magnetic resonance imaging in patients with acute myocardial infarction. Circulation. 1998;97(8):765-72.
74. Yan AT, Shayne AJ, Brown KA, et al. Characterization of the peri-infarct zone by contrast-enhanced cardiac magnetic

resonance imaging is a powerful predictor of post-myocardial infarction mortality. Circulation. 2006;114(1):32-9.
75. Jahnke C, Nagel E, Gebker R, et al. Prognostic value of cardiac magnetic resonance stress tests: adenosine stress perfusion and dobutamine stress wall motion imaging. Circulation. 2007;115(13):1769-76.
76. Dall'Armellina E, Morgan TM, Mandapaka S, et al. Prediction of cardiac events in patients with reduced left ventricular ejection fraction with dobutamine cardiovasc. J Am Coll Cardiol. 2008;52(4):279-86.
77. Bodi V, Sanchis J, Lopez-Lereu MP, et al. Prognostic value of dipyridamole stress cardiovascular magnetic resonance imaging in patients with known or suspected coronary artery disease. J Am Coll Cardiol. 2007;50(12):1174-9.
78. Assomull RG, Prasad SK, Lyne J, et al. Cardiovascular magnetic resonance, fibrosis, and prognosis in dilated cardiomyopathy. J Am Coll Cardiol. 2006;48(10):1977-85.
79. Adabag AS, Maron BJ, Appelbaum E, et al. Occurrence and frequency of arrhythmias in hypertrophic cardiomyopathy in relation to delayed enhancement on cardiovascular magnetic resonance. J Am Coll Cardiol. 2008;51(14):1369-74.
80. Kwon DH, Setser RM, Popovic ZB, et al. Association of myocardial fibrosis, electrocardiography and ventricular tachyarrhythmia in hypertrophic cardiomyopathy: a delayed contrast enhanced MRI study. Int J Cardiovasc Imaging. 2008;24(6):17-25.
81. Chan RH, Maron BJ, Olivotto I, et al. Prognostic value of quantitative contrast-enhanced cardiovascular magnetic resonance for the evaluation of sudden death risk in patients with hypertrophic cardiomyopathy. Circulation. 2014;130(6):484-95.
82. Maceira AM, Prasad SK, Hawkins PN, et al. Cardiovascular magnetic resonance and prognosis in cardiac amyloidosis. J Cardiovasc Magn Reson. 2008;10:54.
83. Ruberg FL, Appelbaum E, Davidoff R, et al. Diagnostic and prognostic utility of cardiovascular magnetic resonance imaging in light-chain cardiac amyloidosis. Am J Cardiol. 2009;103(4):544-9.
84. Kirk P, Roughton M, Porter JB, et al. Cardiac T2* magnetic resonance for prediction of cardiac complications in thalassemia major. Circulation. 2009;120(20):1961-8.

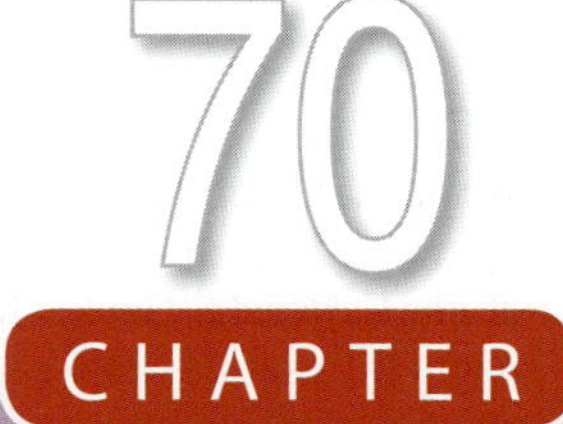

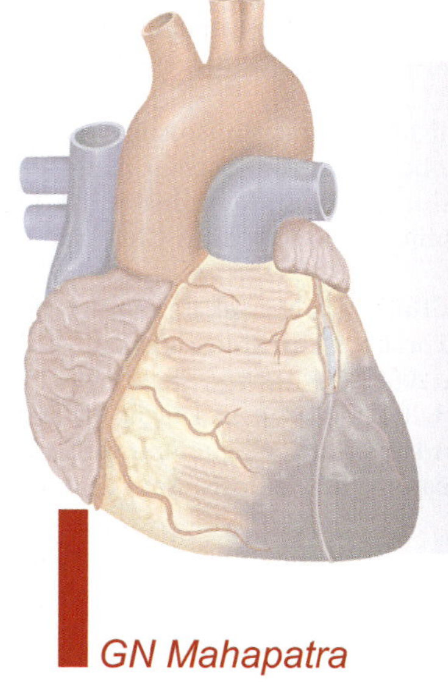

Nuclear Imaging and Heart Failure: New Frontiers

GN Mahapatra

INTRODUCTION

Heart failure is a major worldwide health problem and represents a common disease affecting approximately 5 million patients in the United States. The incidence of heart failure is increasing day by day and it remains the only area in a cardiovascular disease wherein hospitalization rates and associated mortalities have worsened in the past 25 years. Several conditions play an important role in the development and progression of heart failure including abnormalities in myocardial blood flow and sympathetic innervation. The focus is on three aspects—the value of nuclear imaging to distinguish ischemic from nonischemic etiologies, risk stratification of patients with heart failure with an evaluation of candidates for specific treatment strategies, and the role of cardiac neuronal imaging in patients with heart failure. Distinguishing ischemic from nonischemic cardiomyopathy is important because patients with ischemic cardiomyopathy can potentially have dramatic improvement with revascularization. Nuclear imaging represents the only imaging modality with sufficient sensitivity to assess myocardial blood flow and sympathetic innervation of the failing heart. Although nuclear imaging with single photon emission computed tomography (SPECT) is most commonly used for the evaluation of myocardial perfusion, positron emission tomography (PET) detects the gold standard technique in the assessment of myocardial viability as well as allows absolute quantification of myocardial blood flow beyond the assessment of relative myocardial perfusion. Both techniques can be used for evaluation of diagnosis, treatment options and prognosis in heart failure patients. Besides myocardial blood flow, cardiac sympathetic innervation represents another important parameter in patients with heart failure. Cardiac neuronal imaging of metaiodobenzylguanidine (MIBG) I-131 or I-123 is particularly helpful in risk stratification of patients with heart failure. This nuclear imaging modality can be used to monitor the response to therapy as dysfunctional MIBG uptake may show improvement with pharmacological treatment. A large number of studies have shown that an abnormal myocardial sympathetic innervation as assessed with I-123 MIBG imaging is associated with increased mortality and morbidity rates in patients with heart failure. Also, cardiac I-123 MIBG imaging can be used to risk-stratify patients for ventricular arrhythmias or sudden cardiac death. Furthermore, novel nuclear imaging techniques are developed that may provide more detailed information for the detection of heart failure in an early phase as well as for monitoring the effects of new therapeutic interventions in patients with heart failure.

POTENTIALITIES OF NUCLEAR IMAGING PROCEDURES IN HEART FAILURE

Myocardial perfusion imaging (MPI) represents the main stay of cardiovascular radionuclide applications for the diagnostic and prognostic workup of patients with coronary artery disease (CAD) and heart failure (Fig. 1). In addition, sympathetic innervation imaging is increasingly used in patients with heart failure predominantly for risk stratification.

Several technical advances have been introduced that contribute to the current trend toward molecular targeted imaging in clinical cardiology. The availability of high-end scanner systems with improved detection of sensitivity and image resolution allow the detection of weak signal coming from tissue specific molecular targeted tracers. The availability of PET system has substantially increased in the recent years due to its success in oncology. Moreover, an increasing number of molecular targeted radiotracers is now being introduced which may extend the current possibilities for molecular imaging of biologic processes. Finally, it is important to note that molecular targeted imaging is of growing interest as nuclear systems are increasingly integrated with computed tomography (CT) systems into SPECT-CT or PET-CT hybrid imaging devices which facilitate localization of a molecular signal by fusion with high-resolution morphologic image (Fig. 2).

Potentially, these dedicated nuclear imaging techniques having their superior detection sensitivity can play an important role in the evaluation of patients with heart failure by providing valuable information on several biological processes of the failing heart, including myocardial blood flow and sympathetic innervation of the myocardium.

Use of Radionuclide Imaging to Differentiate Ischemic from Nonischemic Heart Failure

Standard stress or pharmacological stress gated SPECT MPI or resting SPECT with F-18 fluorodeoxyglucose (FDG) PET study is based on its excellent diagnostic capabilities for detection of CAD and ischemia and is being used for initial evaluation to determine heart failure etiology. Present data suggests excellent negative predictive value (NPV) with normal imaging findings indicating the likely absence of CAD. There are some frequent false-positive MPI study results in NICMs including thinned walls that appear to have less tracer uptake owing to partial volume effect, soft tissue attenuation from blood pool in large hearts, scar or fibrosis that may occur in the settings of NICM particularly of hypertrophic cardiomyopathy (HCM) and extensive small vessel or microvascular CAD not appreciated in coronary angiogram. In general, defects in ischemic cardiomyopathies are more extensive and severe than in NICM.

A prevailing view among practicing cardiac physicians is that radionuclide MPI can usually exclude CAD in patients with heart failure, but that perfusion defects often do not indicate CAD and at the same time with a normal scan with frequent concerns for the potential occurrence of "balanced ischemia" in which ischemia of equivalent severity and all coronary territories leads to the absence of relative perfusion defect.

Ancillary markers such as transient ischemia dilatation of the LV cavity can potentially identify the situation of balanced ischemia in higher risk patients. Alternatively, quantitative blood flow techniques such as coronary flow reserve (CFR) using cardiac PET with rubidium-82 (Rb-82) or nitrogen-13 ammonia (NH-3). Abnormal CFR measurements can also potentially identify patients without known heart disease but who are at risk for developing clinical heart failure. Although CFR abnormalities may identify early nonclinical CAD that may progress to obstructive disease, many patients with nonischemic heart failure on cardiomyopathy have CFR abnormalities due to disease in the microvasculature. Such disease, although nonamenable to revascularization, predicts worsened outflow.

Use of Radionuclide Imaging to Evaluate Benefit from Revascularization

Once CAD is established as the probable cause of heart failure, radionuclide imaging is the choice of noninvasive techniques used to predict whether a patient is likely to benefit from revascularization procedure. A use of radionuclide imaging to access viability began with delayed thallium-201 or reinjection thallium-201 or augmented IV nitroglycerin-drip on patients with severe coronary stenosis showing redistribution defects even without stress imaging being performed.

Over the years, there have been numerous investigations of the best radionuclide techniques for assessing viability combined Tc-99m sestamibi/tetrofosmin and F-18 FDG study in a single day or two days protocol have been the mainstay of day to day nuclear cardiology practice.

RADIONUCLIDE IMAGING IN PATIENTS NOT AMENABLE TO REVASCULARIZATION

Many patients with heart failure cannot benefit from revascularization, particularly those with CAD having past history of old myocardial infarction (MI) with less than 15% of viable myocardium estimated by our various nuclear imaging procedures (Fig. 3). Patients having non-CAD particularly of NICM, radionuclide imaging though differentiates nonischemic from ischemic variety, still nonischemic patients cannot be benefitted following revascularization.

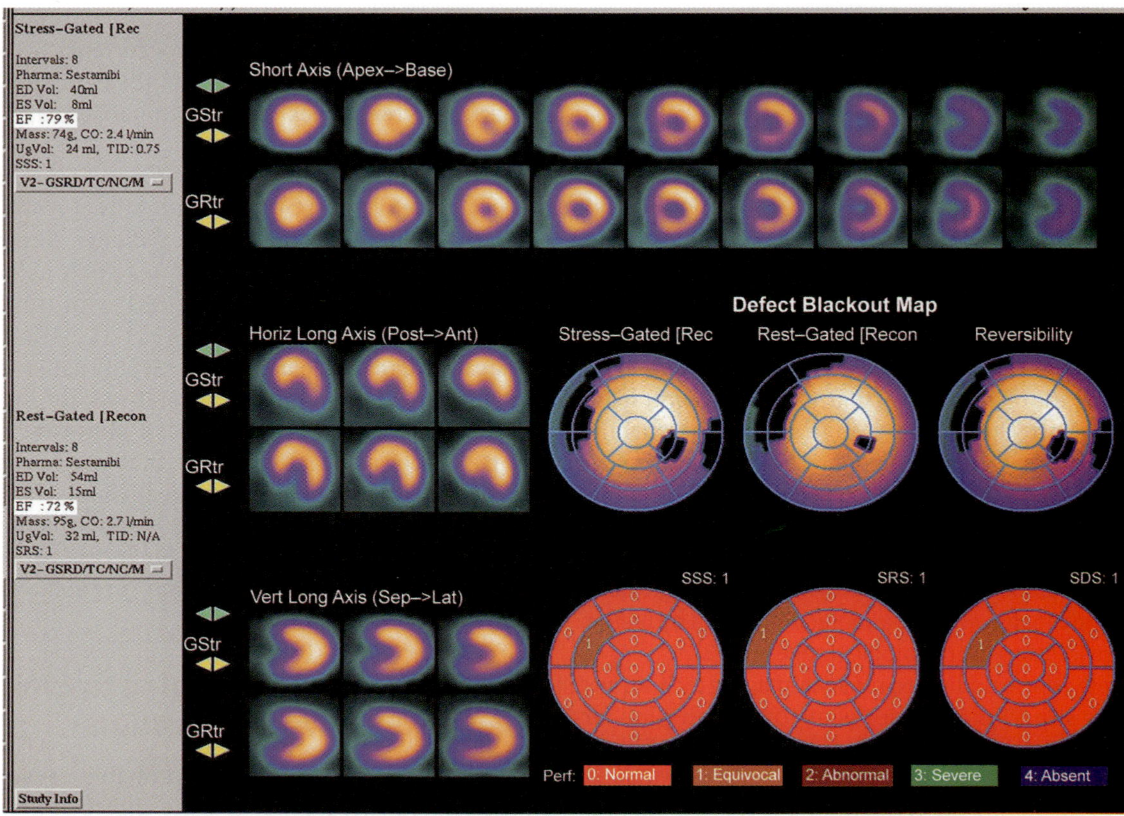

Fig. 1: Normal stress gated single photon emission computed tomography (SPECT) myocardial perfusion imaging scan showing uniform stress perfusion pattern involving all the defined myocardial segments.

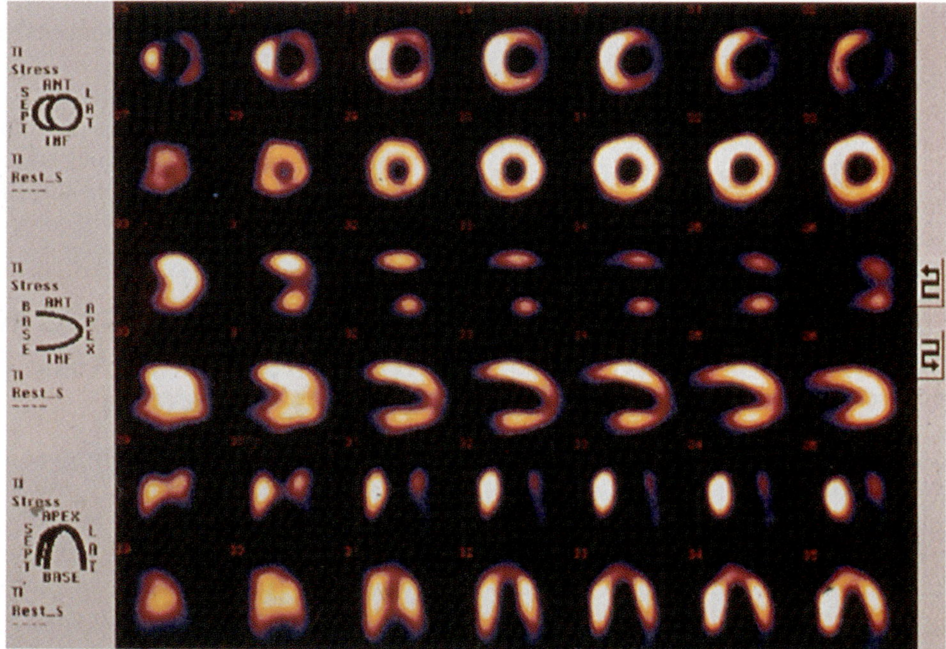

Fig. 2: Stress thallium myocardial perfusion scan showing a large area of stress perfusion defect involving anterolateral myocardial segments which shows a fair amount of reperfusion in resting image suggestive of anterolateral myocardial ischemia.

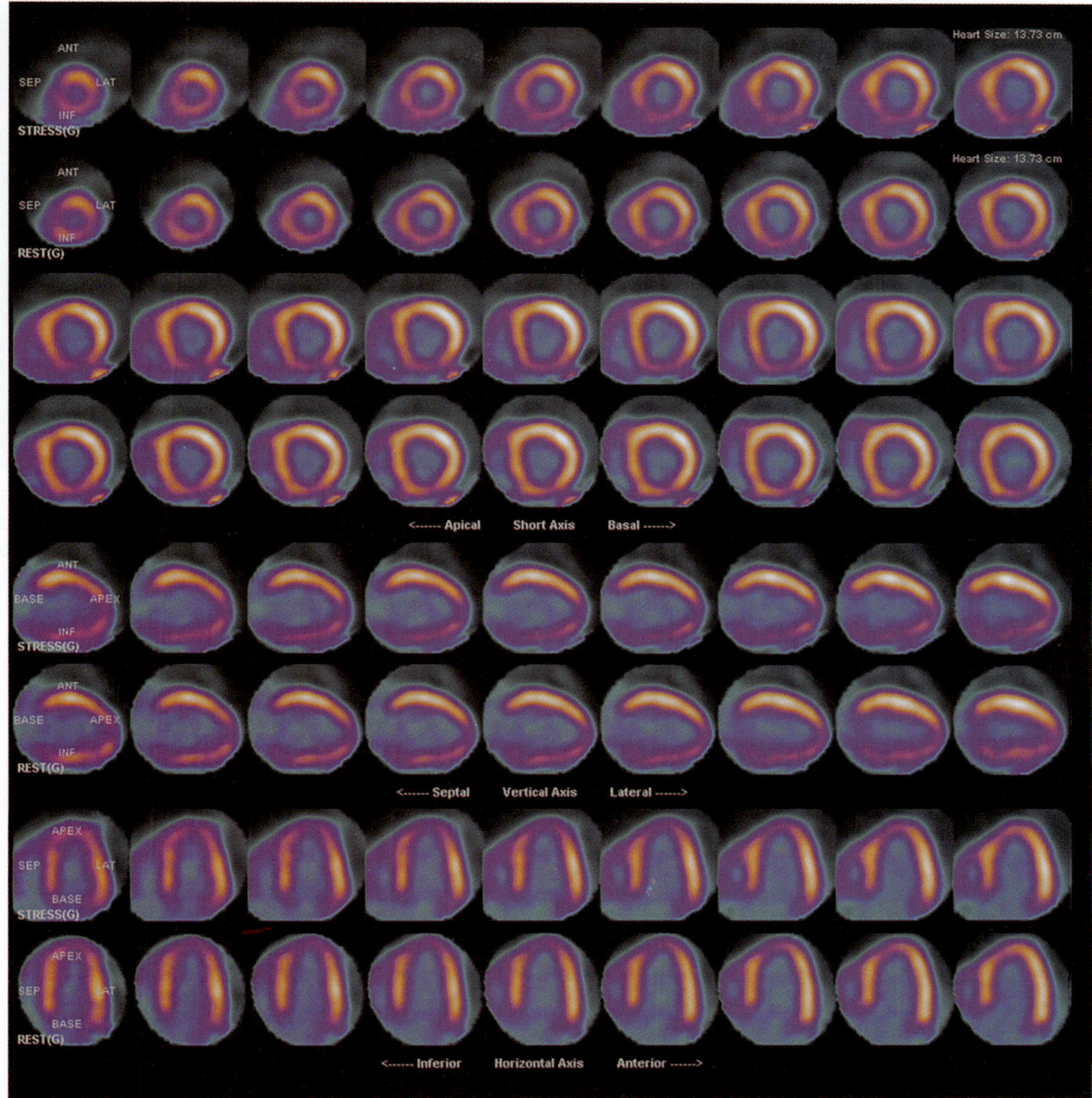

Fig. 3: Rest-dipyridamole stress Rb-82 myocardial perfusion scintigraphy showing dilated left ventricle with uniform stress perfusion pattern showing strong diagnostic information of nonischemic cardiomyopathy with heart failure.

RADIONUCLIDE IMAGING OF CARDIAC AUTONOMIC INNERVATION

The heart is an organ with a dense distribution of the sympathetic nerve. The sympathetic nervous system plays an important role in controlling the heart rate, blood pressure, capacity to cause myocardial contraction/dilatation and coronary tone. Hyperactivity of cardiac sympathetic nerves is known to cause exacerbation of myocardial ischemia, exacerbation of heart failure and induction of severe arrhythmia, and sympathetic functional disorder which has important clinical significance in heart diseases.

Iodine-123 MIBG myocardial scintigraphy is one of the few methods available for objective evaluation of a cardiac sympathetic function at the clinical level and provides an abundance of information useful for the evaluation of various heart diseases.

IMAGING METHODS OF METAIODOBENZYLGUANIDINE (FIGS. 4 TO 6)

Metaiodobenzylguanidine, an analog of norepinephrine, was developed as a sympathetic nerve imaging agent. Before

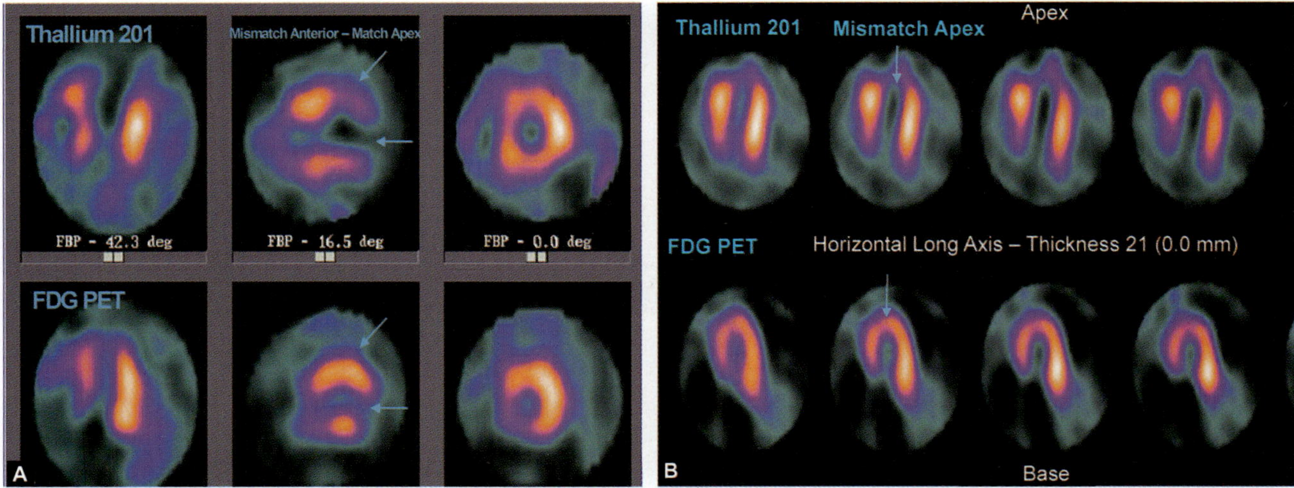

Figs. 4A and B: (A) Dual isotope myocardial imaging shows a resting perfusion defect involving part of anterior and apical myocardial segments which shows adequate metabolism involving anterior segments only. However, apical segment seems to have no metabolism suggesting scarred myocardium as evidenced from F-18 FDG metabolism study; (B) Resting myocardial perfusion imaging with thallium-201 perfusion showing an apical defect which shows adequate metabolism with F-18 FDG metabolism.

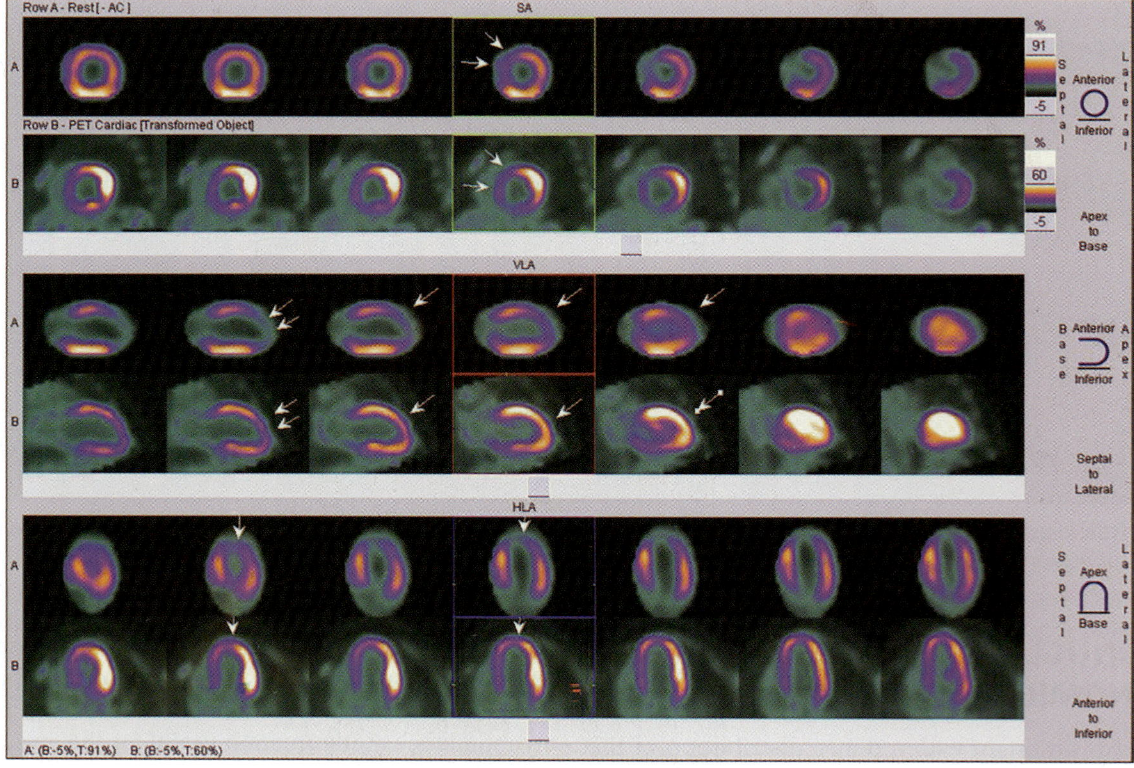

Fig. 5: Resting myocardial perfusion image shows multiple perfusion defects seen in anterior, septal and apical myocardial segments (1st row of images), which shows significant evidence of hibernating myocardium involving anterior and apical myocardial segments in the form of mismatch defects without any evidence of hibernating myocardium in septal segment in the form of match defect (scarred myocardium).

conducting the examination, it is necessary to know whether the patient has taken a drug that has an influence on the accumulation of MIBG. Regarding reserpine and tricyclic antidepressant agents, it is necessary to establish drug withdrawal for an appropriate period taking into account their blood half-life. As I-123 has a short half-life of 13 hours and is a nuclide, which emits only gamma rays, it does not necessarily require the blockage of thyroid accumulation.

Metaiodobenzylguanidine 111 MBq is intravenously administered at rest, and the early and delayed images

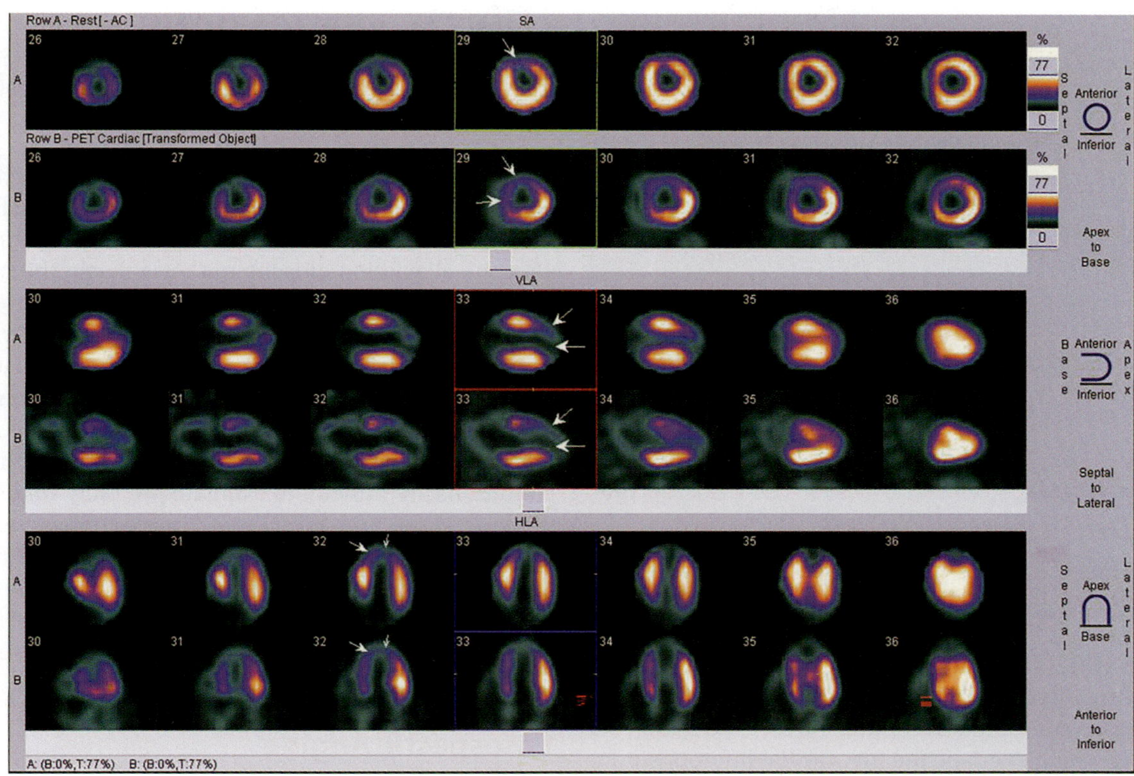

Fig. 6: Resting myocardial perfusion image shows multiple perfusion defects in anteroseptal and apical myocardial segments (1st row of images) without any evidence of hibernating myocardium in the form of match defects on fluorodeoxyglucose (FDG) images (2nd row).

are obtained 15–30 minutes later and from 3–4 hours later, respectively. It is desirable to prepare a gamma camera with sufficient visual field to cover most of the chest, and more than two detectors. In addition, it is necessary to use a collimator for low energy or I-123 only and to set the energy window to 159 keV±10%. Planar images have been used in many ways for the evaluation of cardiac sympathetic function, while SPECT images are advantageous for evaluating abnormalities in local distribution in myocardium. Practically, both of the above images are used in combination.

In the case of planar images, the anterior view is imaged for roughly 3 minutes, using a 128 × 128 or 256 × 256 matrix. If possible, further views in two directions are obtained at a left anterior oblique angle of 35–40° and at a 70° angle to the left lateral plane. The SPECT images are collected using a 64 × 64 matrix over a 360° range or over 180° from the right anterior oblique plane to left posterior oblique plane.

ANALYSIS AND INTERPRETATION OF METAIODOBENZYLGUANIDINE IMAGES

The most common indices are the heart to mediastinum ratio (H/M ratio) and the washout rate obtained from the anterior planar images. These indices represent simple semiquantitative measures, but have been widely used resulting in many reports which support its usefulness in severity and prognosis evaluation for heart failure. Regions of interest (ROIs) are set in the heart (H) and the mediastinum (M) to obtain the mean count in each ROI after which the H/M ratio is calculated. Based on the resulting ratio, the degree of accumulation in the heart is evaluated. It is desirable to set the mediastinal ROI as much as possible at an upper site that is unaffected by the thyroid gland and the cardiac ROI so as to surround the entire heart. The washout rate is an index that indicates the rate at which MIBG is washed out between the early image and the delayed image via comparison with the cardiac count in the early image. In this calculation, the mediastinal count is subtracted from the cardiac count as a background correction, in principle. A correction for decay due to the half-life of ^{123}I may be performed, as required. The accumulation on the early MIBG image reflects the distribution of cardiac sympathetic nerves and the uptake function at the nerve endings while the washout rate is an index of the degree of sympatheticotonia. The delayed image is a result of washout from the early image and thus is considered to contain combined information regarding both the accumulation on the early image and the washout rate (Fig. 7).

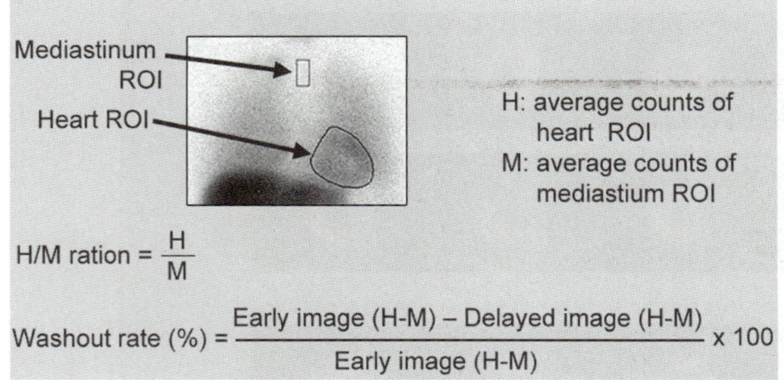

Fig. 7: Calculation of meta-iodobenizylguanidine.

$$\text{Washout rate (\%)} = \frac{\text{Early image (H-M) - delayed image (H-M)}}{\text{Early image (H-M)}} \times 100$$

Regarding the SPECT images, a method is available for visually scoring the degree of accumulation by division into segments which is similar to that used in MPI. The rate of uptake of MIBG in the myocardium is as low as 1–2% and the image quality is inferior compared with Tl-201 images. In some cases, substantial accumulation of MIBG may occur in the liver which overlaps the myocardial inferoposterior wall and scattering from the lung field to the lateral wall then exerts a considerable influence on the image, requiring careful interpretation.

CLINICAL UTILITY OF AUTONOMIC PERFUSION MISMATCH—A NEW FRONTIER IN THE ASSESSMENT OF PATIENTS OF HEART FAILURE

The clinical utility of interpretation of tomographic I-123 MIBG images remains unclear owing in part to frequent poor image quality. A potential strength of SPECT is that the identification of a regional autonomic tracer defects especially in the same myocardial defined region shows preserved tracer uptake on a standard rest perfusion image using Tc-labeled sestamibi/Myoview which is an autonomic-perfusion mismatch may represent a potential for electrical heterogeneity and myocardial denervation increasing the likelihood of a potentially lethal arrhythmias. It indicates that even in the presence of adequate myocardial viability using Tc-99m labeled sestamibi/tetrofosmin tracer and at the same time defects produced by I-123 MIBG tracer with low HMR, patients should be subjected to cardiac resynchronization therapy (CRT) using biventricular pacing which ultimately improves symptoms and mortality rather than only subjecting the patient for myocardial revascularization.

CLINICAL APPLICATIONS

Metaiodobenzylguanidine in Ischemic Heart Diseases

Sympathetic nerve ending is easily damaged by ischemia in comparison to myocardial cells and sympathetic function disorders are known to persist for a certain period even after the alleviation of ischemia. As a result, the potential exists for use of MIBG to detect ischemia with extreme sensitivity providing images that memorize transient ischemia. MPI as a nuclear cardiological examination has been used in many ways for ischemic heart diseases and sufficient evidence regarding the usefulness of this method had been established. However, in some cases, pathological conditions are difficult to evaluate precisely via perfusion imaging alone and MIBG may then be effective. In this group of patient, MIBG shows a decreased or reduced accumulation in the involved myocardium on the delayed image and increased washout is usually observed in the involved regions of the myocardium and the abnormal findings become more marked (Fig. 8).

Vasospastic Angina

In vasospastic angina, the practice of MPI during nonseizure results in normal accumulation and ordinary exercise loading rarely induces coronary spasms. Accordingly, the ability of MPI to diagnose these diseases is not clinically satisfactory.

According to a report by Taki et al., a small proportion of case of vasospastic angina shows abnormal early MIBG images while a high percentage shows increased washout in the region of the culprit coronary artery on delayed images indicating a clearly abnormal accumulation. In other words, delayed images are highly useful for diagnosis. Taki et al. found the positive and negative accuracy rate to be favorable at 83% and 81%, respectively. Sakata et al. reported MIBG to be more useful than stress myocardial perfusion SPECT in the prediction of cardiac events in patients with vasospastic angina having no dominant coronary stenosis.

Unstable Angina

A loading test is not indicated for unstable angina, although MPI at rest is unable to diagnose these diseases in many cases. MIBG makes it possible to identify culprit coronary artery with a high probability via findings at rest and it is of diagnostic value. In a study by Tsutsui et al., MIBG was demonstrated to have the ability to diagnose the culprit coronary artery in these diseases with a sensitivity of 71% and a specificity of 78%.

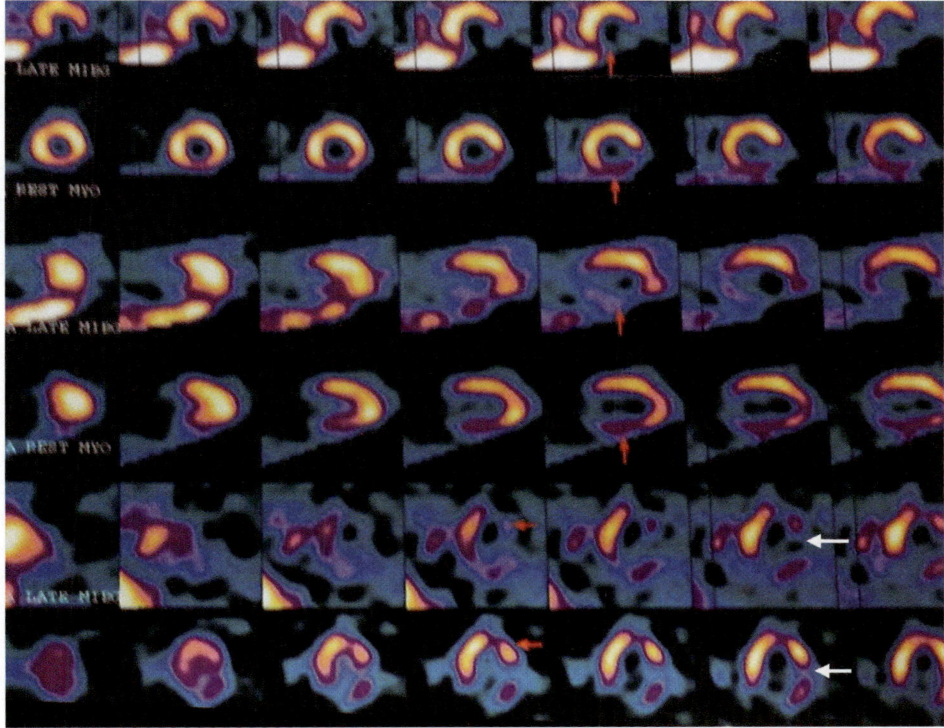

Fig. 8: Iodine-123 metaiodobenzylguanidine (MIBG) and Tc-99m tetrofosmin single photon emission computed tomography (SPECT) images in a patient with advanced heart failure showing large I-123 MIBG defects involving the inferior and lateral walls which shows almost normal resting perfusion which indicates an autonomic-perfusion mismatch.

EVALUATION OF RISK AREAS IN ACUTE CORONARY SYNDROME

Recently percutaneous coronary intervention (PCI) has been generally conducted for acute coronary syndrome in emergency situations. ^{99m}Tc agents are highly retained in the myocardium and exhibit almost no redistribution as is observed in the case of Tl-201. Thus, intravenous injection of such an agent prior to the practice of PCI enables evaluation of the state myocardium perfusion before reperfusion treatment, even if the imaging is conducted after the completion of PCI (this is referred to as freeze image). The defect range indicated on the image obtained via this method is called the risk area (i.e. the area at risk of infarction if not treated appropriately) and is clinically important. A second MPI procedure conducted in the subacute phase makes it possible to quantitatively measure the infarcted myocardium. The difference between the risk area and the infarcted area corresponds to the myocardium rescued by PCI.

While evaluation of risk area by means of ^{99m}Tc agents is an excellent method with high objectivity, it is not necessarily easy to conduct nuclear medical examinations in emergency during the acute phase. MIBG memorizes ischemia and thus reveals a wider range of defects compared with MPI, if used in the subacute phase. This results in a mismatch between two methods. It has been reported that the range of defects for MIBG corresponds more closely to the risk area obtained using ^{99m}Tc agents and that MIBG is useful in evaluating the risk area in acute coronary syndrome.

Non-Q Wave Myocardial Infarction

Between 30% and 50% of cases of myocardial infarction are considered to be non-Q wave infarction. In general, in such cases, myocardial disorders are slight and cardiac functions are maintained compared with cases of Q wave infarction. However, no difference in prognosis has been reported between these and non-Q wave infarction has been reported to have a rather high risk of leading to sudden cardiac death.

For non-Q wave infarction, the detection rate via MPI is regarded to be roughly 50%. While it is also reportedly possible to identify the culprit coronary lesions using MIBG in nearly all cases. According to a reported comparative investigation into "Q" wave infarction and non-"Q" wave infarction, ^{99m}Tc-sestamibi (MIBI) myocardial perfusion SPECT and MIBG SPECT, MIBI defects in non-Q wave infarction were significantly smaller than those in Q wave infarction, while MIBG defects showed no difference between these two types of infarction. In addition, the size of MIBG defects in Q wave infarction was proportional to that of MIBI defects while such a tendency was not observed in non-Q wave infarction. In other words, in non-Q wave infarction, a wide mismatch area is recognized between perfusion SPECT and MIBG SPECT. This mismatch area is said to be denervated but viable and is considered to be in an unstable state which easily results in lethal arrhythmia. This situation may be one of the reasons for many cases of cardiac sudden death in non-Q wave infarction.

Heart Failure

It has been reported that increased washout rate and the decreased H/M ratio on delayed MIBG image become marked with an increase in hypofunction in the left ventricle in cases of heart failure, regardless of the underlying diseases. Similar results have been reported from studies on dilated cardiomyopathy (DCM), HCM, valvular heart disease, pulmonary hypertension, amyloidosis and diabetes. As described above, the relationship between cardiac hypofunction and abnormal MIBG indices has been revealed in various diseases, and MIBG is, thus, useful for severity evaluation of heart failure.

Cardiac Neuronal Imaging using Positron Emission Tomography

Positron emission tomography is a highly specific tool for quantifying physiologic events. Compared with SPECT and conventional scintigraphy, it has a higher spatial and temporal resolution, and attenuation correction is readily available and established. In addition, many autonomic PET tracers more closely resemble the endogenous neurotransmitter than ^{123}I-MIBG used for SPECT imaging and the variety of available tracers may allow for more detailed analysis of neuronal signaling. For practical application, specific activity and radiochemical purity are critical factors. These may expose myocardium to unlabeled catecholamine, which competes with the labeled tracer and may not only limit image quality but also cause pharmacologic action via adrenoceptor activation.

^{11}C-Hydroxyephedrine

^{11}C-hydroxyephedrine (HED) is the most widely used PET tracer for cardiac neuronal imaging. In a healthy heart, there is an even distribution of HED over the left ventricle making it a valuable tracer for detecting specific regional defects of the presynaptic sympathetic system in disease. Denervation studies in an animal model and in human heart transplantation patients have shown that HED has a high affinity for the presynaptic neuronal catecholamine transporter (NET also known as uptake-1) and there exists negligible nonspecific binding. In addition, HED is not metabolized by monoamine oxidase (MAO) or catechol-O-methyl transferase (COMT). Recently it has been confirmed that HED retention is dependent on the NET density of the heart. When desipramine is used as a specific inhibitor of the uptake-1 system after HED administration, gradual HED washout may be seen; thus it has been suggested that HED retention is dependent on continuous release and reuptake.

^{11}C-Ephinephrine

Epinephrine also functions as a true neurotransmitter but only to a small extent. Epinephrine may be enzymatically labelled to ^{11}C, producing ^{11}C-epinephrine (EPI). Unlike HED is degraded by MAO; however, its storage in the vesicle is very efficient causing its slow clearance from the heart. Therefore, EPI reflects the whole cascade of uptake, metabolism and storage of neurotransmission while the primary target for HED is the uptake-1 system. It has been suggested that these properties make it superior as a ligand truly tracing neuronal dysfunction in the heart.

^{11}C-Phenylephrine

Phenylephrine is commonly used as a nasal decongestant. It may be labeled with ^{11}C, thus making it a PET tracer, ^{11}C-phenylephrine (PHEN). It is metabolized by MAO forming radiolabeled metabolite of PHEN, ^{11}C-methylamine. The metabolite rapidly diffuses out of the nerve terminals. PHEN is gradually washed from myocardium having a half-life of 60 minutes.

The importance of vesicular leakage as a contributor to PHEN washout in addition to MAO metabolism has been emphasized.

^{18}F-Flurodopamine

Dopamine may be labeled with ^{18}F-fluorine to obtain ^{18}F-flurodopamine which has been used in humans to assess cardiac and extracardiac sympathetic innervation using PET. In humans, ^{18}F-flurodopamine scanning visualized sympathetic innervation in the heart, renal cortex, thyroid gland. Its early clinical application was mainly for the identification of abnormalities in neuronal transmission in patients suffering from neurological diseases. The half-life of ^{18}F-flurodopamine is 110 minutes, which enables PET scanning for longer periods as compared with ^{11}C-labeled compounds. After tracer injection, sympathetic nerve terminals take up ^{18}F-flurodopamine via uptake-1, after which it is rapidly internalized into vesicles and beta-hydroxylated, forming radiolabeled norepinephrine. During sympathetic neurotransmission, labeled norepinephrine

is released similar to the endogenous norepinephrine. ^{18}F-flurodopamine uptake may be blocked with desipramine. Owing to the nature of the radiolabel and the similarity of the metabolic pathways compared with the endogenous norepinephrine, ^{18}F-flurodopamine may be used to assess the uptake and clearance of norepinephrine; however, the production of ^{18}F-flurodopamine is relatively difficult and, furthermore, owing to the complex fate of dopamine in plasma and the heart, it is not widely used as the tracer of choice in assessing cardiac neuronal function.

In Coronary Artery Disease

Myocardial ischemia and infarction result in nerve injury. This may be followed by sympathetic nerve sprouting and regional hyper-innervation, leading to environmental changes favorable to electrical imbalance. It has been observed that after myocardial infarction beta-adrenoceptor density is decreased as measured with ^{11}C-CGP12177. In humans, chronic CAD caused a reduction in HED uptake in patients with CAD but without myocardial infarction. Furthermore, the decrease in HED uptake is most prominent in regions of significant coronary stenosis. After myocardial infarction, there is an abnormal distribution of HED, showing impaired sympathetic activity in the heart when compared with HED distribution in healthy subjects. These defects remained the same after 8 months, showing no re-innervation process in these patients. Thus, though there is unarguable evidence of dysinnervation after ischemic insult, there is no clinical evidence as to whether this affects the prognosis of these patients, and further studies are warranted to determine the clear cut clinical value of the innervation in ischemic heart disease.

In Heart Failure

Heart failure as such is an end-stage form of several cardiac diseases. It is associated with neurohormonal activation causing impaired neurotransmission. Neuronal cardiac imaging with PET is an attractive method to study the failing heart since the sympathetic involvement in heart failure is extensive. A study employing ^{11}C-CGP12177 showed that in patients with idiopathic dilated cardiomyopathy, there is a significant reduction in the amount of left ventricular beta-adrenoceptor. These PET results were compared with results obtained from cardiac biopsies in the same study. Furthermore, Choudhary and associates presented a similar reduction of beta-adrenoceptor density in both primary and secondary left ventricular hypertrophy with sustained systolic function.[50] Various other studies have also presented results of reduced HED uptake in heart failure caused by end-stage coronary disease or dilated cardiomyopathy. Hartmann and coworkers found that there are a significant regional reductions in HED uptake in apical and inferoapical segments in these patients. In another study, patients with end-stage heart disease were scanned with HED before heart transplantation and after surgery the diseased heart was investigated for uptake-1 density and NE content. They found to have a significant correlation of uptake-1 and NE content with HED uptake, but not with uptake-1 affinity. According to these results, they concluded that in dilated cardiomyopathy there is loss of neurons or down regulation of uptake-1 in humans; furthermore, in the technical perspective, they showed that PET imaging with HED is valid in human heart failure imaging.

CONCLUSION

Heart failure is a major problem in day-to-day clinical cardiology practice having a high prevalence, morbidity, mortality and is expected to become more widespread in the near future. Radionuclide imaging plays an important role in evaluating these patients and giving substantial information towards the diagnosis and further treatment planning. MPI with SPECT as well as PET radiotracers is commonly used to differentiate ischemic from nonischemic etiology of heart failure and cardiomyopathy. Further developments in measuring quantitative blood flow promise to provide a more accurate determination of heart failure etiology. MPI or PET myocardial viability has been established as a gold standard for the assessment of myocardial viability and identification of patients likely to benefit from revascularization. In patients with heart failure who are not candidates for revascularization, myocardial remodeling often leads to poor patient's outcome. Newer Nuclear tests of the myocardial shape of dyssynchronous contraction or relaxation can risk stratify patients and may help CRT therapy. New molecular imaging techniques promise to better understand underlying pathophysiology such as in absence of significant area of resting perfusion defect in an MPI scan with an area of absence of either I-123 MIBG uptake or C-11-HED uptake which is otherwise known as autonomic perfusion mismatch indicates a significant amount of sympathetic denervation which warrants immediate CRT therapy.

BIBLIOGRAPHY

1. Almutairi A, Rossin R, Shokeen M, et al. Biodegradable dendritic positron-emitting nanoprobes for the noninvasive imaging of angiogenesis. Proc Natl Acad Sci USA. 2009;106(3):685-90.
2. Botvinick EH, Frais MA, Shosa DW, et al. An accurate means of detecting and characterizing abnormal patterns of ventricular activation by phase image analysis. Am J Cardiol. 1982;50:289-98.
3. Camici P, Chiriatti G, Lorenzoni R, et al. Coronary vasodilation is impaired in both hypertrophied and non-hypertrophied

myocardium of patients with hypertrophic cardiomyopathy: A study with nitrogen-13 ammonia and positron emission tomography. J Am Coll Cardiol. 1991;17(4):879-86.
4. Choudhury L, Elliott P, Rimoldi O, et al. Transmural myocardial blood flow distribution in hypertrophic cardiomyopathy and effect of treatment. Basic Res Cardiol. 1999;94(1):49-59.
5. Cohn JN. Behalf of an International Forum on Cardiac Remodeling. Cardiac remodeling: Concepts and clinical implications: A consensus paper from an international forum on cardiac remodeling: On Behalf of an International Forum on Cardiac Remodeling. J Am Coll Cardiol. 2000;35:569-82.
6. Danias PG, Ahlberg AW, Clark BA III, et al. Combined assessment of myocardial perfusion and left ventricular function with exercise technetium-99m sestamibi gated single-photon emission computed tomography can differentiate between ischemic and nonischemic dilated cardiomyopathy. Am J Cardiol. 1998;82:1253-8.
7. Drakos SG, Athanasoulis T, Malliaras KG, et al. Myocardial sympathetic innervation and long-term left ventricular mechanical unloding. J Am Coll Cardiol Imaging. 2010;3: 64-70.
8. Flotats A, Carrio I, Agostini D, et al. Proposal for standardization of ^{123}I–metaiodobenzylguanidine (MIBG) cardiac sympathetic imaging by the EANM Cardiovascular Committee and the European Council of Nuclear Cardiology. Eur J Nucl Med Mol Imaging. 2010;37:1802-12.
9. Gheorghiade M, Sopko G, De Luca L, et al. Navigating the crossroads of coronary artery disease and heart failure. Circulation. 2006;114(11):1202-13.
10. Herzog BA, Husmann L, Valenta I, et al. Long-term prognostic value of ^{13}N-ammonia myocardial perfusion positron emission tomography. J Am Coll Cardiol. 2009;54:150-6.
11. Iskandrian AS, Hakki A, Kane SA, et al. Rest and redistribution thallium-201 myocardial scintigraphy to predict improvement in left ventricular function after coronary arterial bypass grafting. Am J Cardiol. 1983; 51:1312-6.
12. Iskandrian AS, Hakki AH, Kane S. Resting thallium-201 myocardial perfusion patterns in patients with severe left ventricular dysfunction: differences between patients with primary cardiomyopathy, chronic coronary artery disease, or acute myocardial infarction. Am Heart J. 1986;111(4): 760-7.
13. Kasama S, Toyama T, Hatori T, et al. Evaluation of cardiac sympathetic nerve activity and left ventricular remondeling carvedilol. Eur Heart J. 2007;28:989-95.
14. Kauffman GJ, Boyne TS, Watson DD, et al. Comparison of rest thallium-201 imaging and rest technetium-99m sestamibi imaging for assessment of myocardial viability in patients with coronary artery disease and severe left ventricular dysfunction. J Am Coll Cardiol. 1996;27:1592-97.
15. Kiat H, Berman DS, Maddahi J, et al. Late reversibility of tomographic myocardial thallium-201, defects: An accurate marker of myocardial viability. J Am Coll Cardiol. 1988;12:1456-63.
16. Marcassa C, Galli M, Cuocolo A, et al. Rest-redistribution thallium-201 and rest technetium-99 m sestamibi SPECT in patients with stable coronary artery disease and ventricular dysfunction. J Nucl Med. 1997;38:419-24.
17. Mody FV, Brunken RC, Stevenson LW, et al. Differentiating cardiomyopathy of coronary artery disease from nonischemic dilated cardiomyopathy utilizing positron emission tomography. J Am Coll Cardiol. 1991;17(2):373-83.
18. Mori T, Yamabe H, Yokota Y, et al. Clinical significance of dipyridamole Tl-201 emission computed tomography perfusion abnormality for evaluating pathophysiological and pathological aspects in hypertrophic cardiomyopathy. Circ J. 1988;52(2):111-8.
19. Paulus WJ, Tscope C, Sanderson JE, et al. How to diagnose diastolic heart failure: A consensus statement on the diagnosis of heart failure with normal left ventricular ejection fraction by the Heart Failure and Echocardiography Associations of the European Society of Cardiology. Eur Heart J. 2007;28:2539-50.
20. Prakash R, deKemp RA, Ruddy TD, et al. Potential utility of rubidium 82 PET quantification in patients with 3-vessel coronary artery disease. J Nucl Cardiol. 2004;11:440-9.
21. Shah AM, Bourgoun M, Narula J, et al. Influence of ejection fraction on the prognostic value of sympathetic innervation imaging with iodine-123 MIBG in heart failure. JACC: Cardiovasc Imaging. 2012;5(11):1139-46.
22. Simoes MV, Barthel P, Matsunari I, et al. Presence of sympathetically denervated but viable myocardium and its electrophysiologic correlates after early revascularized, acute myocardial infarction or phenol application. Circulation. 1988;78:1008-19.
23. Somsen GA, Verberne HJ, Fleury E, et al. Normal values and within-subject variability of cardiac I-123 MIBG scintigraphy in healthy individuals: implications for clinical studies. J Nucl Cardiol. 2004;11(2):126-33.
24. Taylor AL, Ziesche S, Yancy C, et al. Combination of isosorbide dinitrate and hydralazine in blacks with heart failure. N Engl J Med 2004;351(20):2049-57.
25. Tillisch J, Brunken R, Marshall R, et al. Reversibility of cardiac wallmotion abnormalities predicted by positron tomography. N Engl J Med. 1986;314:884-8.
26. Udelson JE, Shafer CD, Carrio I. Radionuclide imaging in heart failure: Assessing etiology and outcomes and implications for management. J Nucl Cardiol. 2002;9:S40-52.
27. von Dohlen TW, Prisant LM, Frank MJ. Significance of positive or negative thallium-201 scintigraphy in hypertrophic cardiomyopathy. Am J Cardiol. 1989;64(8):498-503.
28. Weber KT. Extracellular Matrix remodeling in heart failure: A role for denovo angiotensin-II generation. Circulation. 1997;96:4065-82.
29. Ziadi MC, deKemp RA, Williams KA, et al. Impaired myocardial flow reserve on rubidium-82 positron emission tomography imaging predicts adverse outcomes in patients assessed for myocardial ischemia. J Am Coll Cardiol. 2011;58:740-8.

CHAPTER 71

Pulmonary Artery Catheter Guided Therapy in Heart Failure

Andrew Thai Nguyen, Anju Nohria

INTRODUCTION

Most symptoms of heart failure (HF) are related to congestion.[1] The presence of congestion, rather than impaired perfusion, is associated with adverse outcomes.[2] Lowering filling pressures not only improves symptoms and exercise tolerance in patients with HF, but also leads to decreased neurohormonal activation[3] that is known to be deleterious in HF. Thus, the ability to accurately assess filling pressures is important to optimally treat HF.

The bedside physical examination can be used to determine four hemodynamic profiles based on signs and symptoms of congestion and adequate perfusion (Fig. 1).[4] These hemodynamic profiles are routinely used to guide therapy in patients with HF.[5] The pulmonary artery catheter (PAC) provides quantitative measurements of filling pressures and cardiac output (CO) that are estimated by the bedside hemodynamic profiles. PAC use has traditionally been accepted as a diagnostic tool in patients with dyspnea of unclear etiology, to assess treatment response in patients with pulmonary hypertension, and to evaluate patients with advanced HF for cardiac transplantation. Historically, attempts to optimize hemodynamics in patients considered for transplantation led to the management strategy of "tailored therapy," where an indwelling PAC was used to guide diuretic and intravenous vasoactive therapies with a monitored transition to an oral regimen aimed at maintaining normal filling pressures and vascular resistance.[6] However, in randomized clinical trials, the routine use of PAC has not been shown to improve outcomes compared to a clinical assessment strategy in patients hospitalized with severe and recurrent HF.[7] In this chapter, we will review the current indications for the use of PAC in patients hospitalized with HF. We will also review data regarding the use of implantable hemodynamic monitors to manage HF in the ambulatory setting.

PULMONARY ARTERY CATHETER GUIDED "TAILORED" THERAPY

The pulmonary artery catheter or the Swan Ganz catheter allows simultaneous measurement of filling pressures, CO, and vascular resistance. This is most helpful in patients where congestion is accompanied by hypoperfusion (Fig. 1). In patients with elevated filling pressures and a high systemic vascular resistance (SVR), intravenous vasodilators (nitroprusside or nitroglycerin) can be used in combination with diuretics to achieve hemodynamic targets—right atrial pressure (RAP) ≤ 8 mm Hg, pulmonary capillary wedge pressure (PCWP) ≤ 16 mm Hg, and SVR 1000–1200 dynes. sec.cm^{-5} while maintaining a systolic blood pressure (SBP) ≥ 80 mm Hg.[4,6] Once target filling pressures are achieved, oral agents are added as intravenous vasodilators are weaned. Renin-angiotensin aldosterone (RAAS) inhibitors are preferred, but the combination of hydralazine and nitrates may be used in those who cannot tolerate RAAS blockade or in those with persistent vasoconstriction despite RAAS inhibition.[4,6] While intravenous inotropes (dobutamine, milrinone, low dose dopamine, or levosimendan) are discouraged due to the increased mortality associated with their use,[8] they may be needed temporarily in patients with

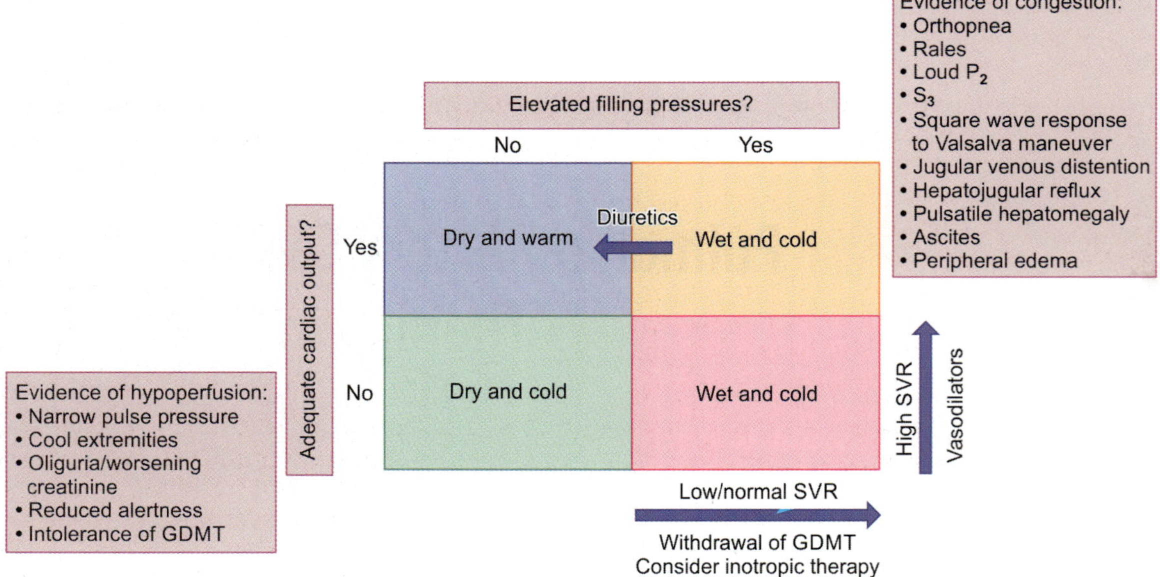

Fig. 1: Management based on hemodynamic profiles in heart failure.
(GDMT: Guideline-directed medical therapy; SVR: systemic vascular resistance)

cardiogenic collapse or in those with persistently elevated filling pressures and evidence of end-organ hypoperfusion, despite adequate vasodilation.[4,6] In general, attempts should be made to wean inotropes once clinical stability and hemodynamic targets have been achieved. Patients intolerant of inotrope withdrawal, should be evaluated for advanced therapies or palliation.

THE EVALUATION STUDY OF CONGESTIVE HF AND PAC EFFECTIVENESS TRIAL

Initial success with PAC-guided tailored therapy led to design of the evaluation study of congestive HF and PAC effectiveness (ESCAPE) trial. The ESCAPE trial compared the efficacy of a PAC-guided HF management strategy to management based on clinical assessment alone in 433 patients hospitalized with severe and recurrent symptomatic systolic HF.[7] The protocol did not specify drug choice or dose and investigators were encouraged to follow guidelines regarding intravenous diuretic and vasodilator use.[9] The goal of therapy in both groups was resolution of clinical congestion (jugular venous distention, edema, and orthopnea) with additional targets of RAP ≤8 mm Hg and PCWP ≤15 mm Hg in the PAC group.

Pulmonary artery catheter use did not affect the primary end point of days alive and out of the hospital during the first 6 months (HR 1.0, $p = 0.99$).[7] Additionally, PAC use was associated with increased inhospital adverse events (21.9% vs. 11.5%) including infection, bleeding, pulmonary infarct or hemorrhage, and ventricular tachycardia.[7] Analysis of secondary end points showed that exercise and quality of life improved in both groups, with a trend toward greater improvement in the PAC arm.[7] PAC use was also associated with a greater reduction in mitral regurgitation[10] and lesser increase in serum creatinine[11] during hospitalization, but these changes were not sustained after discharge. A subsequent meta-analysis of 13 randomized clinical trials enrolling 5,051 critically ill patients similarly showed no improvement in mortality or reduction in days hospitalized with PAC use.[12] Based on these results, the routine use of PAC is not recommended in patients hospitalized with acute systolic HF.[9]

Indications for Pulmonary Artery Catheter Use in Hospitalized Patients (Table 1)

Acute Hemodynamic Collapse

Concomitant with the ESCAPE trial, 439 patients were enrolled in the ESCAPE Registry if they were felt to be too sick to be randomized, if PAC use was considered necessary by the treating physician, or if they did not meet the inclusion/exclusion criteria of the trial.[13] In 40.5% of registry patients, PAC use was considered necessary for management by the treating physician and registry patients in general had a higher mortality than those enrolled in the clinical trial.[13] Some of the reasons cited included requirement for mechanical ventilatory support, high dose inotropic support, and intra-aortic balloon pump or other mechanical circulatory support. Patients

TABLE 1: Guideline-based indications for pulmonary artery catheter use in heart failure.

• Invasive hemodynamic monitoring with a PA catheter should be used to guide therapy in patients with respiratory distress or impaired systemic perfusion when clinical assessment is inadequate (COR I, LOE C)
• Invasive hemodynamic monitoring can be useful in acute HF with persistent symptoms despite seemingly appropriate adjustments of standard therapies if any of the following is true (COR IIa, LOE C): – Uncertain fluid status, perfusion, systemic vascular resistance, or pulmonary vascular resistance – Systolic pressure that remains low or is associated with symptoms despite initial therapy – Worsening renal function with therapy – Requiring IV inotropic agents – May need mechanical circulatory support or transplantation
• Routine invasive monitoring of hemodynamics is not recommended in normotensive patients with acute decompensated HF responding symptomatically to diuretics and vasodilators (COE III, LOE B)

(COR = Class of recommendation; HF = Heart failure; LOE = Level of evidence; PA = Pulmonary artery catheter)

presenting acutely with cardiac or respiratory arrest, shock or arrhythmias are often in this category and may need PAC guidance to identify the underlying etiology for their acute decompensation and to restore hemodynamic stability and end-organ perfusion.[1]

Uncertainty Regarding Hemodynamic Status

In the ESCAPE Registry, investigators were unable to assess jugular venous pressure (JVP) at the bedside in about 18% of patients compared to 2% in the trial.[13] Investigators also used PAC in 6.4% of registry patients to distinguish whether symptoms were related to HF or other comorbidities.[13] Thus, PAC can be helpful to define hemodynamics and guide therapy where there is clinical uncertainty.

Lack of Improvement with Empiric Treatment in Hospitalized Patients with Heart Failure

The recent American College of Cardiology (ACC) consensus statement on the management of patients hospitalized with HF describes three inpatient trajectories observed with empiric diuretic therapy—(1) improving toward target, (2) stalled after initial response, and (3) not improved/worsening.[1] In patients with the latter two trajectories, invasive hemodynamic monitoring can be helpful to establish goals of treatment.[1]

Discordance between right and left sided filling pressures should be considered in patients with an inadequate response to empiric therapy. In approximately 75% of patients who undergo PAC for transplant evaluation, the ratio of JVP to PCWP is approximately 1:2, where a JVP of 10 mm Hg corresponds to a PCWP of 22 mm Hg.[14] Thus, we commonly rely on JVP to estimate PCWP and define the limits of diuresis (JVP $\leq$ 10 cm H_2O). However, among patients with elevated filling pressures approximately 40% have right-left discordance making reliance on JVP misleading.[15] In cases where JVP << PCWP, diuresis based on JVP can lead to inadequate decongestion and persistent dyspnea. In these patients, the optimal JVP may be in the lower range of normal. Conversely, in patients with JVP >> PCWP, over-diuresis can lead to worsening renal function or hypotension. These patients may not be able to undergo diuresis to a normal JVP and may be more likely to need inotropic support. Thus, in these instances, invasive hemodynamic assessment with PAC can better define the right-left relationship and limits of diuresis.[1]

Approximately 15–20% of clinical trial patients have worsening HF during hospitalization that requires consideration of advanced therapies including inotropic support, mechanical circulatory support, or transplantation.[7] These patients often have a history of recurrent hospitalizations for refractory New York Heart Association (NYHA) Class III–IV symptoms, diuretic resistance with worsening renal function, borderline SBP with progressive intolerance to guideline-directed medical therapy (GDMT), and persistently elevated biomarkers despite escalating diuretics (brain natriuretic peptide and troponin).[1] In these patients, invasive hemodynamic monitoring should be considered to assess prognosis and the need for advanced therapies or palliative care.[1]

Implantable Hemodynamic Monitoring in Ambulatory Patients

While routine PAC guided therapy did not improve outcomes in hospitalized patients, invasive hemodynamic monitoring in the outpatient setting has shown promise. A retrospective analysis of 496 patients enrolled in the diuretic optimization strategy evaluation (DOSE-AHF) and cardiorenal rescue study in acute decompensated heart failure (CARRESS-HF) trials demonstrated that approximately one-half of patients admitted with acute systolic HF have residual symptoms of congestion at the time of discharge and the presence of residual congestion is associated with higher rates of death, readmission and need for urgent visits at 60 days.[16] Furthermore, of the 185 patients free from congestion at discharge, 65% developed recurrent congestion at 60 days follow-up.[16] Thus, the use of implantable hemodynamic monitors to remotely monitor filling pressures and optimize HF therapy in the ambulatory setting has been tested as a strategy to reduce HF readmissions (Table 2).

Of the existing outpatient implantable hemodynamic monitors, the CardioMEMS device has shown the greatest promise. The CardioMEMS™ device is an implantable wireless pulmonary artery (PA) pressure monitor. The

TABLE 2: Implantable hemodynamic monitors in ambulatory setting.

Device class	*Device name*	*Device system*	*Clinical application*	*Reference*
Impedance cardiography	Optivol™	Noninvasive assessment of thoracic electrical impedance to determine thoracic fluid content, changes in the duration of cardiac ejection, and the velocity of blood flow within the aorta	Pulmonary congestion due to elevated ventricular filling pressures results in decreased impedance across the lung, predicting cardiac output and cardiac filling pressures.	Packer M, Abraham WT, Mehra MR, et al. Prospective Evaluation and Identification of Cardiac Decompensation by ICG Test (PREDICT) Study Investigators and Coordinators. Utility of impedance cardiography for the identification of short-term risk of clinical decompensation in stable patients with chronic heart failure. J Am Coll Cardiol. 2006;47(11):2245-52.
Left atrial pressure monitor	HeartPOD™	Pressure sensor lead implanted transvenously into the left atrium through the inter-atrial septum	Physician-directed, patient self-management based on left atrial pressure recordings	Abraham WT, Adamson PB, Costanzo MR, et al.-emodynamic monitoring in advanced heart failure: results from the LAPTOP-HF trial. J Card Fail. 2016;22(11):940.
Left atrial pressure monitor	V-LAP™	Wireless and leadless device implanted directly in the atrial septum using a transseptal approach	Direct measurement of daily left atrial pressure providing daily hemodynamic feedback to guide therapy	NCT03775161
Pulmonary artery pressure monitor	Chronicle® implantable hemodynamic monitor (IHM)	Long-term programmable implanted device placed in pectoral area and transvenous electrode pressure sensor placed in right ventricular outflow tract.	Continuous measurements of right ventricular systolic and diastolic pressures, estimated pulmonary artery diastolic pressure, and maximum change in pressure over time (dP/dt) to guide therapy	Bourge RC, Abraham WT, Adamson PB, et al. COMPASS-HF Study Group. Randomized controlled trial of an implantable continuous hemodynamic monitor in patients with advanced heart failure: the COMPASS-HF study. J Am Coll Cardiol. 2008;51(11):1073-9.
Pulmonary artery pressure monitor	CardioMEMS™	Wireless pressures sensor implanted during right heart catheterization into a branch of the left pulmonary artery	Provides pulmonary artery pressure waveform tracings, heart rate, and systolic, diastolic, and mean PA pressures to guide therapy	Abraham WT, Adamson PB, Bourge RC, et al. CHAMPION Trial Study Group. Wireless pulmonary artery haemodynamic monitoring in chronic heart failure: a randomised controlled trial. Lancet. 2011;377(9766):658-66.

(PA = Pulmonary artery)

CardioMEMS™ heart sensor allows monitoring of pressure to improve outcomes in NYHA (CHAMPION) Class III heart failure patients trial was a prospective, randomized control trial that enrolled 550 patients with NYHA class III symptoms and a recent hospitalization for HF, irrespective of left ventricular ejection fraction.[17] All patients received the device and were randomized to either the treatment group where daily PA pressures from the device were used to guide medical therapy or the control group where daily uploaded pressures were not made available to investigators. Both groups also received standard care based on signs and symptoms of congestion. Unlike prior hemodynamic monitoring trials, CHAMPION provided specific recommendations for how to use PA pressures to guide HF management in the treatment arm. The protocol recommended lowering PA pressures to target ranges using a combination of diuretics and vasodilators. In patients with stable PA pressures, the protocol recommended up-titration of GDMT to target doses.

In the CHAMPION trial, the treatment group experienced a 28% reduction in HF hospitalizations over the 6-month study period compared to the control arm (HR 0.72, $p = 0.013$).[17] This reduction in HF hospitalizations was observed in both patients with HF with reduced ejection fraction (HFrEF) and in those with HF with preserved ejection fraction.[17] Furthermore, there was a trend toward reduced mortality in HFrEF patients randomized to the treatment arm over the extended follow-up period of 18 months (HR 0.68, $p = 0.06$).[18] The reduction in HF hospitalizations with ambulatory PA pressure monitor guided therapy has been further validated in a real-world sample of 1,114 patients who have undergone CardioMEMS™ guided HF management (HR 0.55, $p < 0.001$).[19] Thus, remote monitoring of intracardiac and PA pressures via implantable hemodynamic monitors provides serial hemodynamic data that can be acted upon by physicians to lower filling pressures and improve outcomes in ambulatory HF patients.

CONCLUSION

Symptoms of HF are most often related to congestion and inadequate relief of congestion is associated with adverse outcomes. Hemodynamic profiles based on a simple bedside evaluation can be used to guide therapy in most patients with HF. Therefore, routine use of PAC-guided tailored therapy is not recommended in patients hospitalized with HF. However, PAC use may be considered in patients with acute hemodynamic or respiratory compromise, those with diagnostic uncertainty, or in those who fail to improve or worsen with empiric HF therapy. Because many patients remain congested or develop recurrent volume overload shortly after hospital discharge, the use of implantable hemodynamic monitors that allow serial monitoring of filling pressures in the ambulatory setting has gained interest. Therapy based on the information derived from these devices could be a way to improve symptoms, reduce HF hospitalizations, and improve mortality in HF patients.

REFERENCES

1. Hollenberg SM, Warner Stevenson L, Ahmad T, et al. 2019 ACC Expert Consensus Decision Pathway on Risk Assessment, Management, and Clinical Trajectory of Patients Hospitalized With Heart Failure: A Report of the American College of Cardiology Solution Set Oversight Committee. J Am Coll Cardiol. 2019;74(15):1966-2011.
2. Cooper LB, Mentz RJ, Stevens SR, et al. Hemodynamic predictors of heart failure morbidity and mortality: Fluid or flow? J Card Fail. 2016;22(3):182-9.
3. Johnson W, Omland T, Hall C, et al. Neurohormonal activation rapidly decreases after intravenous therapy with diuretics and vasodilators for class IV heart failure. J Am Coll Cardiol. 2002;39(10):1623-9.
4. Nohria A, Lewis E, Stevenson LW. Medical management of advanced heart failure. JAMA. 2002;287(5):628-40.
5. Ponikowski P, Voors AA, Anker SD, et al.; Authors/Task Force Members; Document Reviewers. 2016 ESC Guidelines for the diagnosis and treatment of acute and chronic heart failure: The Task Force for the diagnosis and treatment of acute and chronic heart failure of the European Society of Cardiology (ESC). Developed with the special contribution of the Heart Failure Association (HFA) of the ESC. Eur J Heart Fail. 2016;18(8):891-975.
6. Stevenson LW. Tailored therapy to hemodynamic goals for advanced heart failure. Eur J Heart Fail. 1999;1(3):251-7.
7. Binanay C, Califf RM, Hasselblad V, et al.; ESCAPE Investigators and ESCAPE Study Coordinators. Evaluation study of congestive heart failure and pulmonary artery catheterization effectiveness: the ESCAPE trial. JAMA. 2005;294(13):1625-33.
8. Abraham WT, Adams KF, Fonarow GC, et al.; ADHERE Scientific Advisory Committee and Investigators; ADHERE Study Group. In-hospital mortality in patients with acute decompensated heart failure requiring intravenous vasoactive medications: an analysis from the Acute Decompensated Heart Failure National Registry (ADHERE). J Am Coll Cardiol. 2005;46(1):57-64.
9. Yancy CW, Jessup M, Bozkurt B, et al.; American College of Cardiology Foundation; American Heart Association Task Force on Practice Guidelines. 2013 ACCF/AHA guideline for the management of heart failure: a report of the American College of Cardiology Foundation/American Heart Association Task Force on Practice Guidelines. J Am Coll Cardiol. 2013;62(16):e147-239.
10. Palardy M, Stevenson LW, Tasissa G, et al.; ESCAPE Investigators. Reduction in mitral regurgitation during therapy guided by measured filling pressures in the ESCAPE trial. Circ Heart Fail. 2009;2(3):181-8.

11. Nohria A, Hasselblad V, Stebbins A, et al. Cardiorenal interactions: insights from the ESCAPE trial. J Am Coll Cardiol. 2008;51(13):1268-74.
12. Shah MR, Hasselblad V, Stevenson LW, et al. Impact of the pulmonary artery catheter in critically ill patients: meta-analysis of randomized clinical trials. JAMA. 2005;294(13):1664-70.
13. Allen LA, Rogers JG, Warnica JW, et al.; Escape Investigators and Coordinators. High mortality without ESCAPE: the registry of heart failure patients receiving pulmonary artery catheters without randomization. J Card Fail. 2008;14(8):661-9.
14. Drazner MH, Brown RN, Kaiser PA, et al. Relationship of right- and left-sided filling pressures in patients with advanced heart failure: a 14-year multi-institutional analysis. J Heart Lung Transplant. 2012;31(1):67-72.
15. Campbell P, Drazner MH, Kato M, et al. Mismatch of right- and left-sided filling pressures in chronic heart failure. J Card Fail. 2011;17(7):561-8.
16. Lala A, McNulty SE, Mentz RJ, et al. Relief and Recurrence of Congestion During and After Hospitalization for Acute Heart Failure: Insights From Diuretic Optimization Strategy Evaluation in Acute Decompensated Heart Failure (DOSE-AHF) and Cardiorenal Rescue Study in Acute Decompensated Heart Failure (CARESS-HF). Circ Heart Fail. 2015;8(4):741-8.
17. Abraham WT, Adamson PB, Bourge RC, et al.; CHAMPION Trial Study Group. Wireless pulmonary artery haemodynamic monitoring in chronic heart failure: a randomised controlled trial. Lancet. 2011;377(9766):658-66.
18. Givertz MM, Stevenson LW, Costanzo MR, et al.; CHAMPION Trial Investigators. Pulmonary artery pressure-guided management of patients with heart failure and reduced ejection fraction. J Am Coll Cardiol. 2017;70(15):1875-86.
19. Desai AS, Bhimaraj A, Bharmi R, et al. Ambulatory hemodynamic monitoring reduces heart failure hospitalizations in "real-world" clinical practice. J Am Coll Cardiol. 2017;69(19):2357-65.

CHAPTER

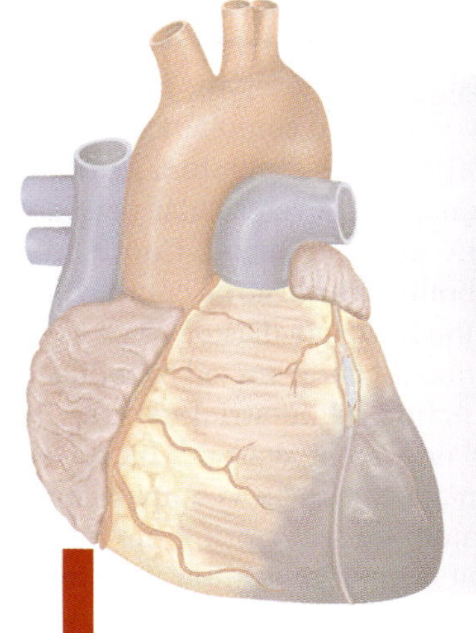

Myocardial Mechanics of Heart Failure with Preserved Ejection Fraction

Christopher M Bianco, Peter D Farjo, Partho P Sengupta

INTRODUCTION

Heart failure with preserved ejection fraction (HFpEF) is responsible for approximately half of all heart failure hospitalizations, with mean survival similar to those with heart failure with reduced ejection fraction.[1] Common conditions including hypertension, diabetes, chronic kidney disease, obesity, and increasing age predispose to preclinical structural heart disease, which is present in one fourth of the adult US population.[2] The evolution of subsequent symptomatic heart failure occurs with significant heterogeneity of cardiac structural and functional abnormalities.[3] With an increasing burden of comorbid states and the growing elderly population, the prevalence of HFpEF is projected to increase further. Diastolic dysfunction is found within most HFpEF patients, and although ejection fraction may be preserved, subtle systolic dysfunction is typically present as evidenced by deformation imaging.[4] Dysfunctional mechanics of the right and left ventricles, as well as both the right and left atria are common in HFpEF. Furthermore, myocardial dysfunction may initially only occur during exercise. Therefore, assessment during both rest and exercise plays an important role in diagnosis and prognostication. In addition to myocardial mechanical impairments, those with HFpEF may suffer from a multitude of associated conditions including endothelial dysfunction, ventricular-arterial uncoupling, chronotropic incompetence, tachyarrhythmias, renal dysfunction, pulmonary dysfunction, anemia, and maladaptive peripheral vascular and skeletal abnormalities.

LEFT VENTRICULAR MYOCARDIAL MECHANICS

Each myocardial layer contributes to longitudinal, circumferential, and radial motion. The subendocardial fibers largely contribute to longitudinal shortening, while subepicardial fiber contraction causes a dominant circumferential and twisting deformation of the left ventricle (LV).[5] Left ventricular untwisting during diastole releases stored mechanical energy from systolic deformation and create a centrifugal force for aspirating left atrial blood. Traditional imaging biomarkers may be normal in early subclinical disease, however, subendocardial dysfunction is commonly present and evident by reduced global longitudinal strain (GLS). The prevalence of reduced GLS in asymptomatic metabolic disease has been reported to range from 37% to 54%.[6] Reduced longitudinal strain may exist despite normal conventional diastolic functional indices.[7] Preclinical reduction in GLS is independently associated with a worse prognosis and should prompt more aggressive risk mitigation strategies.[8] Despite decreased longitudinal mechanics, the ejection fraction remains preserved due to retained circumferential and twist mechanics provided by the relatively unaffected subepicardial layer. If compensation is not possible due to concomitant dysfunction of the subepicardial region, the ejection fraction falls and ventricular dilatation ensues.[9] Patients with predominant subepicardial disease or constrictive pericarditis display impaired circumferential and twist mechanics, while longitudinal function remains relatively preserved. These patients retain a normal ejection fraction, but have significant mechanical impairment related to a dysfunctional and/or tethered subepicardial layer[10] (Table 1). A reduction in GLS may be present prior to the onset of LV remodeling and hypertrophy.[11] In those with subendocardial dysfunction that are able to compensate, myocardial hypertrophy of the subepicardial region may develop in an attempt to reduce subendocardial wall stress and preserve left ventricular ejection fraction (LVEF).[12]

With further clinical deterioration into symptomatic heart failure, global circumferential strain (GCS), LV twist, and twist/untwist rates may remain normal or even increase to supranormal values.[13] Although GCS, LV twist, and twist/untwist rates may remain normal or increase early in HFpEF, time to peak twist and peak untwist are often delayed, which impacts both systolic and diastolic performance.[14] Despite impaired resting longitudinal deformation, those with subclinical disease can augment longitudinal mechanics during exertion to a greater extent than those with symptomatic heart failure (Fig. 1). This may explain the initial onset of exertional symptoms during the transition from preclinical to clinical heart failure.[15] Therefore, deformation imaging and diastolic assessment during exercise has been utilized in the diagnosis of HFpEF. Progressive deterioration of circumferential, radial, and longitudinal strain, as well as LV twist and untwist, characterize the myocardial mechanics found in advanced HFpEF.[16,17] In the treatment of preserved cardiac function heart failure with an aldosterone antagonist (TOPCAT) trial, impaired longitudinal strain (GLS >–15.8%) was present in 52% of patients and predictive of both cardiac death and heart failure hospitalizations.[18]

LEFT ATRIAL MYOCARDIAL MECHANICS

The left atrium (LA) functions as a reservoir for pulmonary venous return during ventricular systole, as a conduit for pulmonary venous return during early ventricular diastole, and as a booster pump that augments late ventricular filling (Fig. 2).[19] LA deformation does not occur in isolation, and the interrelated nature of phasic atrial and ventricular deformation must be considered.[20] Reservoir function is dependent on both atrial volume and compliance, as well as LV systolic longitudinal annular excursion. Conduit function is dependent upon the atrioventricular pressure gradient created during LV diastolic recoil. Contractile function is dependent on both intrinsic atrial contractility and afterload imposed by the LV in late diastole.

Preclinical LA dysfunction is characterized by reduced reservoir and conduit function while atrial contractile function remains normal[21] or even increased.[22] Increased LA contractile deformation appears to be a compensatory mechanism to increase late filling, mirroring the mitral inflow pattern typical of abnormal relaxation. LA strain abnormalities occur prior to overt LA enlargement, and reduced reservoir function may occur in the absence of overt diastolic dysfunction or LV hypertrophy.[23] In an at-risk population, impaired LA reservoir function is associated with an increased risk of future heart failure hospitalization even adjusting for age and sex, and in patients with normal LAVI.[24] Overt clinical heart failure onset occurs when atrial contractile function fails to compensate for reservoir and/or conduit dysfunction[25] (Fig. 1). Therefore, abnormal LA deformation is useful in differentiating non-heart failure related dyspnea from HFpEF. A failure of compensatory conduit function in the setting of impaired reservoir function may also lead to early exercise-induced symptoms.[26] Those with atrial fibrillation may be at particular risk given failure of compensatory atrial contractile function, and the adequacy of compensatory conduit function is a large determinant of symptom onset.[27] Advanced symptomatic HFpEF is characterized by a decrement in all three atrial strain phases.[28] Impaired resting LA reservoir strain is associated with decreased peak oxygen consumption[29] and impaired LA reservoir augmentation with exercise leads to right ventricular (RV)-pulmonary circulation uncoupling and exercise ventilatory inefficiency.[30] LA reservoir strain

TABLE 1: Left ventricular cardiac mechanics of heart failure.

Functional state	*Longitudinal mechanics*	*Circumferential/ Torsional mechanics*	*Global LV ejection fraction*	*Clinical consequences*
Normal mechanics	Preserved	Preserved	Preserved	Normal patient
Predominant subendocardial dysfunction	Impaired	Preserved	Preserved	HFpEF, restrictive cardiomyopathy
Predominant subepicardial dysfunction	Preserved	Impaired	Preserved	Myopericardial disease, constrictive pericarditis
Transmural dysfunction	Impaired	Impaired	Reduced	HFrEF

(HFpEF: heart failure with preserved ejection fraction; HFrEF: heart failure with reduced ejection fraction)

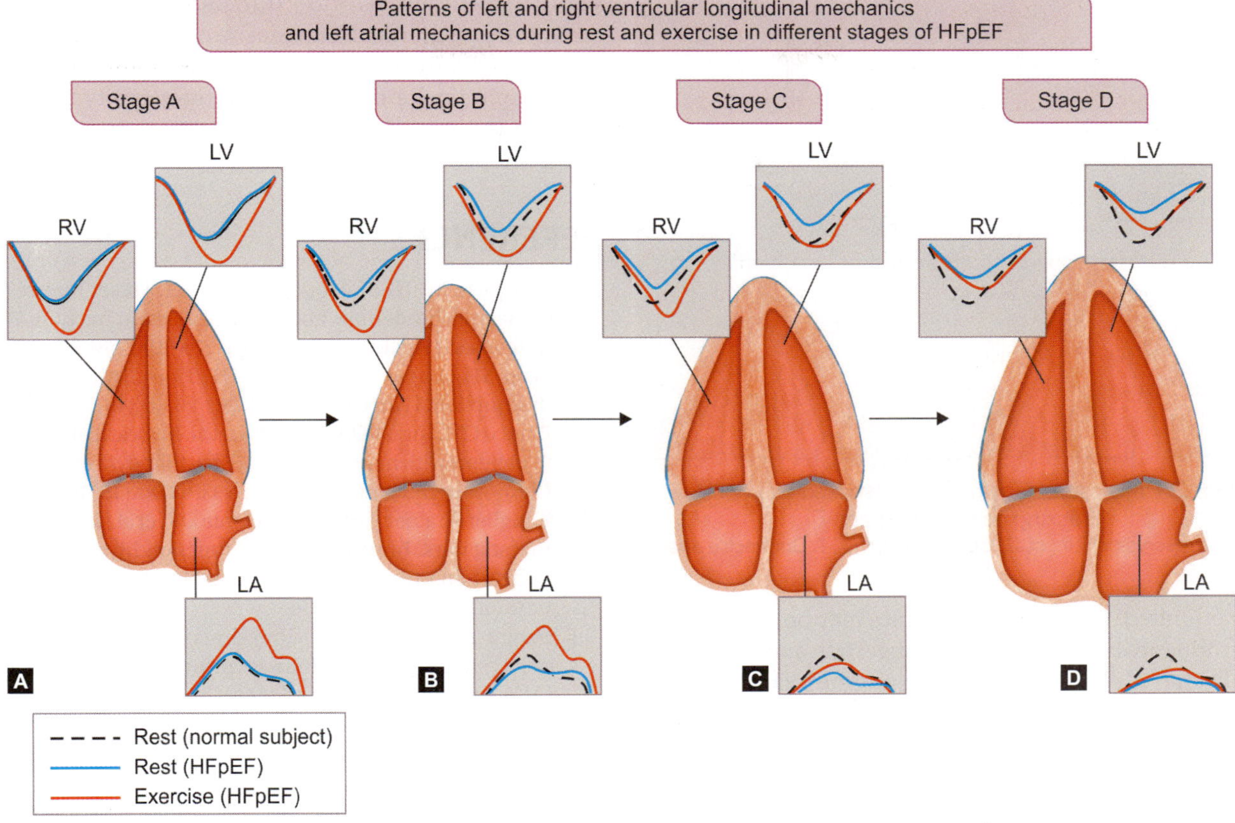

Figs. 1A to D: Pattern of myocardial mechanics during rest and exercise in different stages of HFpEF[3]. (A) Stage A is characterized by normal or nearly normal resting LV and RV GLS (blue), normal or nearly normal LA reservoir function, and normal LA conduit and booster functions (blue). All parameters augment adequately with exercise (red); (B) Stage B is characterized by mildly depressed resting LV and RV GLS, mildly depressed LA reservoir and conduit function, and increased LA booster function (blue). LV and RV GLS augment to nearly normal with exercise (red). LA conduit function increases significantly with exercise (red); (C) Stage C is characterized by moderately depressed resting LV and RV GLS (blue) with significantly impaired augmentation during exercise (red). Resting LA reservoir, conduit function, and booster function are impaired at rest (blue), and all parameters augment to suboptimal levels with exercise (red); (D) Stage D is characterized by markedly depressed resting LV and RV GLS (blue) with little augmentation during exercise (red). Similarly, all atrial functional phases are impaired at rest (blue) with little augmentation during exercise (red).

(GLS: global longitudinal strain; LA: left atrium; LV: left ventricle; RV: right ventricle).

may outperform LV GLS and RV free wall longitudinal strain in its prognostic and discriminative utility above and beyond traditional risk markers for prediction of heart failure hospitalization.[29]

RIGHT HEART MYOCARDIAL MECHANICS

The thin right ventricular free wall is composed predominantly of transversely oriented fibers. Circumferential compression of the RV free wall results in a bellows motion normally contributing approximately 20% of RV systolic function. Shearing forces of the oblique interventricular septal fibers result in systolic twisting of the base toward the apex.[31] Interventricular septal mechanics are responsible for RV longitudinal motion, contributing approximately 80% of RV systolic function. Infundibular fiber contraction results in a minor peristalsis like contribution to late RV ejection.[32] Asymptomatic patients with diabetes, hypertension, metabolic syndrome, and obesity commonly exhibit reduced RV longitudinal strain.[33,34] With disease progression into symptomatic heart failure, at least one-fifth of HFpEF patients have RV dysfunction by conventional parameters and almost half by deformation indices.[29,35,36] RV global longitudinal early-diastolic strain rate (RV-SRe) and RV GLS function are both more significantly impaired in patients with HFpEF than in those with asymptomatic diastolic dysfunction[37] (Fig. 1). Impairment of right atrial deformation has also been appreciated in HFpEF patients compared to asymptomatic controls,[38] however, the study of right atrial mechanics to

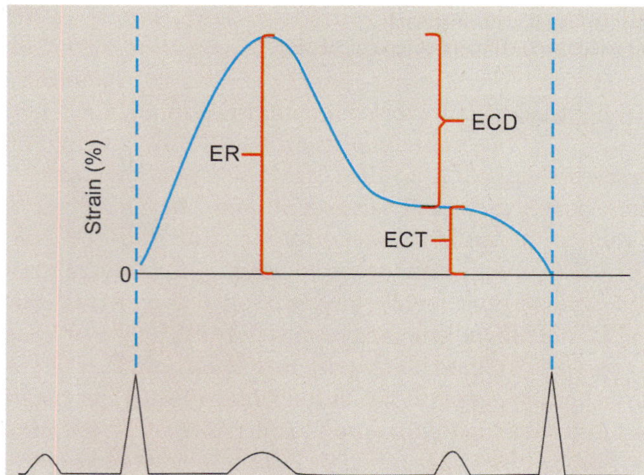

Fig. 2: Phasic left atrial function assessed by speckle-tracking echocardiography.
(εR: LA reservoir strain; εCD: Conduit strain, εCT: Contractile strain.

date is limited. Right atrial mechanics may be an important determinant of systemic venous congestion and cardiorenal syndrome. A distinct HFpEF phenogroup characterized by extensive remodeling with prominent pulmonary hypertension and right heart failure exists.[39] This phenogroup more often includes elderly patients with chronic kidney disease and appears to be at particularly high risk.

At least two-third of patients will exhibit evidence of resting pulmonary hypertension (PH), and pulmonary pressures may increase substantially during exercise leading to conditional right heart failure.[35,40] RV dilatation is present in almost a third of cases. RV dilatation leads to altered septal geometry, which impairs septal contractility and RV performance.[35] Although the right ventricle has been traditionally viewed as a nonessential conduit, RV performance becomes increasingly important when faced by the pulsatile resistive afterload characteristic of HFpEF related PH.[41] Exercise-induced LA dysfunction may play an important role in exercise-induced RV-pulmonary circulation uncoupling leading to exercise ventilatory inefficiency.[30] Furthermore, RV mechanics may suffer independent of pulmonary hypertension and in some may be more closely related to LV GLS than pulmonary pressures, supporting a common myocardial disease link coupling both ventricles.[37,42]

CONCLUSION

Abnormal myocardial mechanics evolve throughout each cardiac chamber as a patient progresses through the heart failure continuum. The development of HFpEF involves complex interactions between cardiac chambers during both systole and diastole. Certain deformation parameters conditionally deteriorate during exercise. Although common mechanical changes are present, significant heterogeneity in structure and function exist. In addition to multiple image biomarkers, heterogeneity of clinical features and associated medical conditions compound this syndromes complexity.

REFERENCES

1. Shah KS, Xu H, Matsouaka RA, et al. Heart failure with preserved, borderline, and reduced ejection fraction: 5-year outcomes. J Am Coll Cardiol. 2017;70(20):2476-86.
2. Wan SH, Vogel MW, Chen HH. Pre-clinical diastolic dysfunction. J Am Coll Cardiol. 2014;63(5):407-16.
3. Bianco CM, Farjo PD, Ghaffar YA, et al. Myocardial mechanics in patients with normal LVEF and diastolic dysfunction. JACC Cardiovasc Imaging. 2019. pii: S1936-878X(19)30363-8.
4. Kraigher-Krainer E, Shah AM, Gupta DK, et al.; PARAMOUNT Investigators. Impaired systolic function by strain imaging in heart failure with preserved ejection fraction. J Am Coll Cardiol. 2014;63(5):447-56.
5. Sengupta PP, Tajik AJ, Chandrasekaran K, et al. Twist mechanics of the left ventricle: principles and application. JACC Cardiovasc Imaging. 2008;1(3):366-76.
6. Wang Y, Marwick TH. Update on echocardiographic assessment in diabetes mellitus. Curr Cardiol Rep. 2016;18(9):85.
7. Ernande L, Bergerot C, Rietzschel ER, et al. Diastolic dysfunction in patients with type 2 diabetes mellitus: is it really the first marker of diabetic cardiomyopathy? J Am Soc Echocardiogr. 2011;24(11):1268-75.e1.
8. Wang Y, Yang H, Nolan M, et al. Variations in subclinical left ventricular dysfunction, functional capacity, and clinical outcomes in different heart failure aetiologies. ESC Heart Fail. 2018;5(3):343-54.
9. Sengupta PP, Narula J. Reclassifying heart failure: predominantly subendocardial, subepicardial, and transmural. Heart Fail Clin. 2008;4(3):379-82.
10. Sengupta PP, Krishnamoorthy VK, Abhayaratna WP, et al. Disparate patterns of left ventricular mechanics differentiate constrictive pericarditis from restrictive cardiomyopathy. JACC Cardiovasc Imaging. 2008;1(1):29-38.
11. Szelényi Z, Fazakas Á, Szénási G, et al. The mechanism of reduced longitudinal left ventricular systolic function in hypertensive patients with normal ejection fraction. J Hypertens. 2015;33(9):1962-9.
12. Zhang J. Myocardial energetics in cardiac hypertrophy. Clin Exp Pharmacol Physiol. 2002;29(4):351-9.
13. Wang J, Khoury DS, Yue Y, et al. Preserved left ventricular twist and circumferential deformation, but depressed longitudinal and radial deformation in patients with diastolic heart failure. Eur Heart J. 2008;29(10):1283-9.
14. Stohr EJ, Shave RE, Baggish AL, et al. Left ventricular twist mechanics in the context of normal physiology and cardiovascular disease: a review of studies using speckle tracking echocardiography. Am J Physiol Heart Circ Physiol. 2016;311(3):H633-44.

15. Kosmala W, Rojek A, Przewlocka-Kosmala M, et al. Contributions of nondiastolic factors to exercise intolerance in heart failure with preserved ejection fraction. J Am Coll Cardiol. 2016;67(6):659-70.
16. Yip GW, Zhang Q, Xie JM, et al. Resting global and regional left ventricular contractility in patients with heart failure and normal ejection fraction: insights from speckle-tracking echocardiography. Heart. 2011;97(4):287-94.
17. Nguyen JS, Lakkis NM, Bobek J, et al. Systolic and diastolic myocardial mechanics in patients with cardiac disease and preserved ejection fraction: impact of left ventricular filling pressure. J Am Soc Echocardiogr. 2010;23(12):1273-80.
18. Shah AM, Claggett B, Sweitzer NK, et al. Prognostic importance of impaired systolic function in heart failure with preserved ejection fraction and the impact of spironolactone. Circulation. 2015;132(5):402-14.
19. Pathan F, D'Elia N, Nolan MT, et al. Normal ranges of left atrial strain by speckle-tracking echocardiography: A systematic review and meta-analysis. J Am Soc Echocardiogr. 2017;30(1):59-70.e8.
20. Vieira MJ, Teixeira R, Goncalves L, et al. Left atrial mechanics: echocardiographic assessment and clinical implications. J Am Soc Echocardiogr. 2014;27(5):463-78.
21. Fang NN, Sui DX, Yu JG, et al. Strain/strain rate imaging of impaired left atrial function in patients with metabolic syndrome. Hypertens Res. 2015;38(11):758-64.
22. Brecht A, Oertelt-Prigione S, Seeland U, et al. Left atrial function in preclinical diastolic dysfunction: Two-dimensional speckle-tracking echocardiography-derived results from the BEFRI trial. J Am Soc Echocardiogr. 2016;29(8):750-8.
23. Cameli M, Lisi M, Righini FM, et al. Left atrial strain in patients with arterial hypertension. Int Cardiovasc Forum J. 2013;1(1):31-6.
24. Morris DA, Belyavskiy E, Aravind-Kumar R, et al. Potential usefulness and clinical relevance of adding left atrial strain to left atrial volume index in the detection of left ventricular diastolic dysfunction. JACC Cardiovasc Imaging. 2018;11(10):1405-15.
25. Sanchis L, Gabrielli L, Andrea R, et al. Left atrial dysfunction relates to symptom onset in patients with heart failure and preserved left ventricular ejection fraction. Eur Heart J Cardiovasc Imaging. 2015;16(1):62-7.
26. von Roeder M, Rommel KP, Kowallick JT, et al. Influence of left atrial function on exercise capacity and left ventricular function in patients with heart failure and preserved ejection fraction. Circ Cardiovasc Imaging. 2017;10(4). pii: e005467.
27. Goette A, Kalman JM, Aguinaga L, et al. EHRA/HRS/APHRS/SOLAECE expert consensus on atrial cardiomyopathies: Definition, characterization, and clinical implication. Heart Rhythm. 2017;14(1):e3-40.
28. Santos AB, Kraigher-Krainer E, Gupta DK, et al.; PARAMOUNT Investigators. Impaired left atrial function in heart failure with preserved ejection fraction. Eur J Heart Fail. 2014;16(10):1096-103.
29. Freed BH, Daruwalla V, Cheng JY, et al. Prognostic utility and clinical significance of cardiac mechanics in heart failure with preserved ejection fraction: Importance of left atrial strain. Circ Cardiovasc Imaging. 2016;9(3). pii: e003754.
30. Sugimoto T, Bandera F, Generati G, et al. Left atrial function dynamics during exercise in heart failure: Pathophysiological implications on the right heart and exercise ventilation inefficiency. JACC Cardiovasc Imaging. 2017;10(10 Pt B):1253-64.
31. Buckberg G, Hoffman JI, Nanda NC, et al. Ventricular torsion and untwisting: further insights into mechanics and timing interdependence: a viewpoint. Echocardiography. 2011;28(7):782-804.
32. Buckberg G, Hoffman JI. Right ventricular architecture responsible for mechanical performance: unifying role of ventricular septum. J Thorac Cardiovasc Surg. 2014;148(6):3166-71.e1-4.
33. Wong CY, O'Moore-Sullivan T, Leano R, et al. Association of subclinical right ventricular dysfunction with obesity. J Am Coll Cardiol. 2006;47(3):611-6.
34. Kosmala W, Przewlocka-Kosmala M, Mazurek W. Subclinical right ventricular dysfunction in diabetes mellitus--an ultrasonic strain/strain rate study. Diabet Med. 2007;24(6):656-63.
35. Gorter TM, Hoendermis ES, van Veldhuisen DJ, et al. Right ventricular dysfunction in heart failure with preserved ejection fraction: a systematic review and meta-analysis. Eur J Heart Fail. 2016;18(12):1472-87.
36. Gorter TM, van Veldhuisen DJ, Bauersachs J, et al. Right heart dysfunction and failure in heart failure with preserved ejection fraction: mechanisms and management. Position statement on behalf of the Heart Failure Association of the European Society of Cardiology. Eur J Heart Fail. 2018;20(1):16-37.
37. Morris DA, Gailani M, Vaz Pérez A, et al. Right ventricular myocardial systolic and diastolic dysfunction in heart failure with normal left ventricular ejection fraction. J Am Soc Echocardiogr. 2011;24(8):886-97.
38. Jain S, Kuriakose D, Edelstein I, et al. Right atrial phasic function in heart failure with preserved and reduced ejection fraction. JACC Cardiovasc Imaging. 2019;12(8 Pt 1):1460-70.
39. Shah SJ, Katz DH, Selvaraj S, et al. Phenomapping for novel classification of heart failure with preserved ejection fraction. Circulation. 2015;131(3):269-79.
40. Lam CS, Roger VL, Rodeheffer RJ, et al. Pulmonary hypertension in heart failure with preserved ejection fraction: a community-based study. J Am Coll Cardiol. 2009;53(13):1119-26.
41. Tedford RJ, Hassoun PM, Mathai SC, et al. Pulmonary capillary wedge pressure augments right ventricular pulsatile loading. Circulation. 2012;125(2):289-97.
42. Bosch L, Lam CS, Gong L, et al. Right ventricular dysfunction in left-sided heart failure with preserved versus reduced ejection fraction. Eur J Heart Fail. 2017;19(12):1664-71.

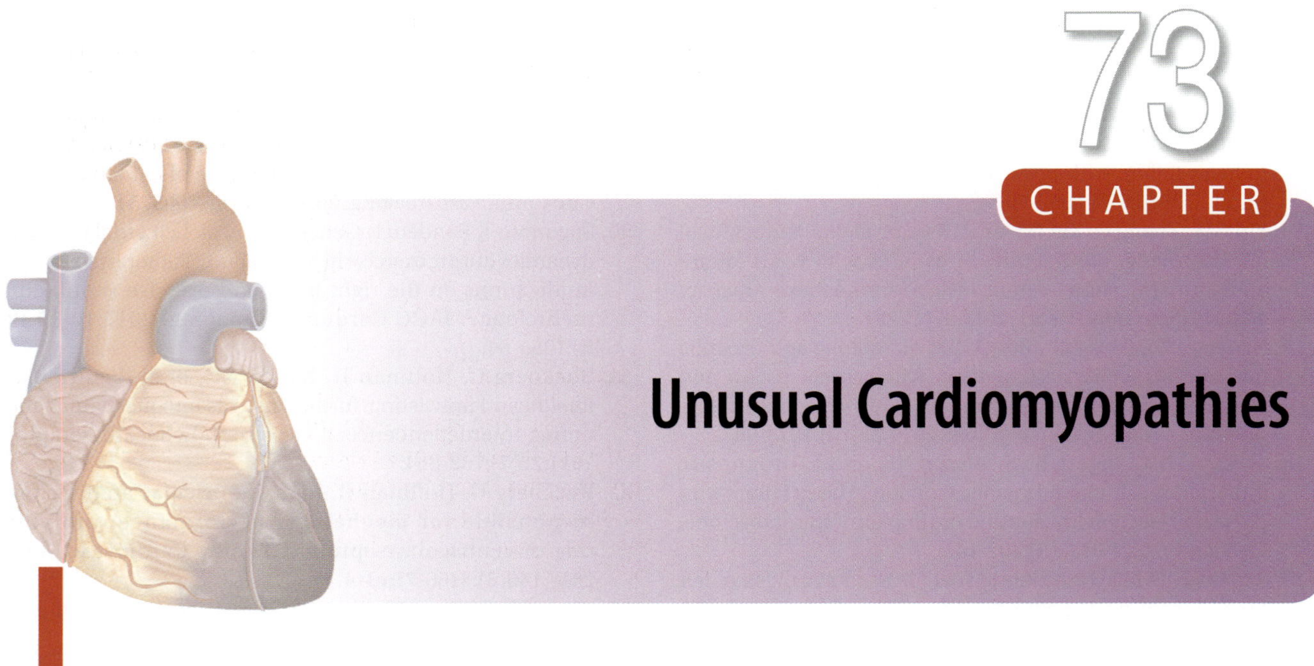

73

CHAPTER

Unusual Cardiomyopathies

Smadar Kort, Clive Goulbourne, Bicky Vettichira

NONCOMPACTION CARDIOMYOPATHY

INTRODUCTION

Noncompaction cardiomyopathy (NCM), also called left ventricular noncompaction cardiomyopathy (LVNC), is a rare congenital disorder hypothesized to result from the arrest of trabecular compaction of the left ventricular (LV) cavity during embryogenesis. It is characterized by a thin compacted epicardial layer and an extensive noncompacted endocardial layer, with prominent trabeculations and deep recesses which communicate with the LV cavity. This may lead to heart failure, atrial or ventricular arrhythmias, sudden cardiac death (SCD), or thromboembolic events.[1,2]

CONTENTS AND DESCRIPTION

The prevalence of LVNC is estimated to be 0.014–1.3% in the general population[3-5] and 3–4% among heart failure patients.[6] Mortality rates vary from 2% to 38%[2-4,7-9] with arrhythmias and systolic dysfunction carrying the greatest risks.[10] Patients with LVNC may present asymptomatically with incidental findings on cardiac imaging. The most common presenting symptoms are dyspnea, palpitations, chest pain, and syncope.[9] The electrocardiogram (EKG) may be normal or show nonspecific changes. LV systolic dysfunction is present in about two-thirds of patients at diagnosis, with a median ejection fraction (EF) of 30–35% (range 15–66%)[3,5] and continues to decline throughout the clinical course of the disease (Table 1 and Fig. 1).

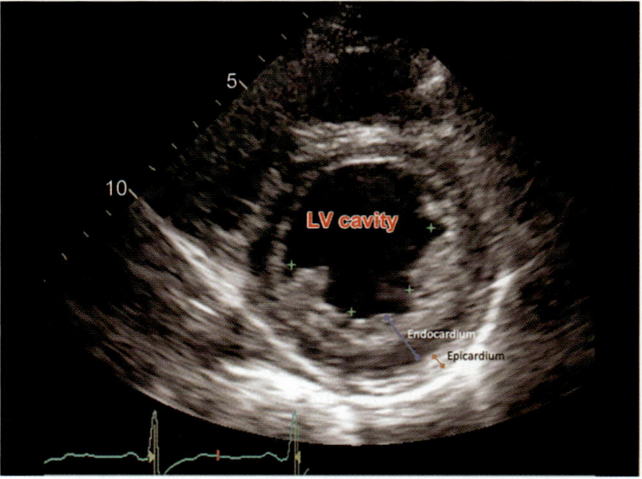

Fig. 1: Parasternal short axis view in end-systole comparing non-compacted thick endocardial layer of the LV to the thin epicardial layer, ratio >2:1 (Jenni criteria).
+Depicts areas of trabeculation.
(LV: left ventricle)

LIMITATIONS

Echocardiography is the first-line diagnostic tool for LVNC but has limited sensitivity (60–70%) and specificity (70–80%).[11-13] The addition of a contrast agent improves the diagnostic yield (sensitivity 80–90%) and reproductivity of the study.[14,15] Cardiac magnetic resonance imaging (CMRI) has sensitivity 86% and specificity 99%.[16] With the introduction of balanced steady state free precession (SSFP) cine imaging, it provides better visualization of

TABLE 1: Morphologic diagnostic criteria for noncompaction cardiomyopathy.

Echocardiographic criteria	
*Jenni criteria** • The presence of all four criteria are required for diagnosis • Image acquisition parasternal short axis view at end systole	• Ratio of non-compacted/ compacted myocardium >2.0 (>1.4 in children) • In trabecular recesses filled with blood from LV cavity on color flow Doppler • Predominant localization of non-compaction in the lateral apical or inferior walls of the LV • Absence of coexisting cardiac abnormalities
Chin criteria Image acquisition: apical 4 chamber or parasternal short axis views of the LV apex at end distole	Ration of X/Y <0.5**
Stöllberger criteria Image acquisition: oblique views	• >3 trabeculations protruding from the LV wall, apically to the papillary muscles, visible in a single image plane • Intertrabecular spaces perfused from the ventricular cavity on color doppler imaging
Cardiac MRI criteria	
Petersen criteria Image acquisition: end diastole	Ratio of non-compacted/ compacted myocardium >2.3
Jacquier criteria Image acquisition: end diastole	Trabecular lV mass >20% of global LV mass

(LV: Left ventricular)

*Compacted wall thickness ≤8.1 mm has been added to aid with diagnosis in patients with aortic valve stenosis

**X is the distance from the epicardial surface to the trough of the trabecular recess

**Y is the distance from the epicardial surface to peak of trabeculation

the LV apex and is more reliable at differentiating LVNC from apical hypertrophic cardiomyopathy, thrombus, eosinophilic endomyocardial disease, or fibroelastosis.[17] If CMR is not available or contraindicated, a cardiac computed tomography (CT) may be pursued, though this uses ionizing radiation and is less capable of characterizing myocardial tissue. The right ventricle is better visualized with CMR and cardiac CT allowing identification of concomitant or isolated right ventricular noncompaction, if present. Speckle-tracking echocardiography (STE) has identified abnormal ventricular mechanics in patients with LVNC by demonstrating that the basal and apical rotations occur in the same direction, resulting in the near absence of the normal LV twist termed "LV rigid body rotation". Real-time three-dimensional (3D) STE is an accurate method for the evaluation of LV rotation mechanics; these findings are promising for diagnosing LVNC.[18,19]

GUIDELINES

Several criteria have been put forth for the diagnosis of LVNC utilizing various imaging modalities (Table 1). The criteria validated by Jenni et al.[12] is perhaps the most widely accepted echocardiographic criteria while the two most common used for CMR are from Petersen et al.[16] and Jacquire et al.[20]

CONCLUSION

In general, medications for LVNC should include evidence-based, guideline-directed medical therapy for patients with cardiomyopathy. The objectives of management are the prevention and treatment of complications with thromboembolism, heart failure, and arrhythmias being the most common. The implantation of a cardiac defibrillators (ICD) should be based on the current guidelines for implantation for the primary or secondary prevention of lethal arrhythmias and not solely on the presence of LVNC. The available literature justifies prophylactic therapeutic anticoagulation in LVNC with low left ventricular ejection fraction (LVEF) <40% and/or atrial fibrillation (A. fib)[21] with warfarin preferred due to lack of data using the direct oral anticoagulants (DOAC) in these patients.

CHAGAS CARDIOMYOPATHY

INTRODUCTION

Chagas disease (CD) is caused by infection with the protozoan parasite *Trypanosoma cruzi* (*T. cruzi*). It is endemic to Latin America; however, there are numerous cases worldwide mainly due to international travel.[22] Chagas cardiomyopathy (CCM) ranges from benign changes on the EKG to acute myopericarditis, dilated cardiomyopathy with chronic heart failure, cardioembolic events, arrhythmias and sudden death.

CONTENTS AND DESCRIPTION

The triatomine bug, a subfamily of the reduviidae, is the main vector which transmits *T. cruzi*. In the absence of successful treatment, infection is lifelong and may cause cardiac complications in one-third of individuals.[23] It may also affect the digestive system. Nonvector-borne routes of infection include transmission between mother and child, blood transfusion or organ donation. Based on WHO estimates, over 8 million people have CD worldwide.

The incubation period for *T. cruzi* ranges from 1 week to 2 weeks after vector-borne transmission[24] and up to 3–4 months after transfusion or transplant transmission.[25] In the acute phase patients may be asymptomatic or have mild nonspecific symptoms but rarely present as florid myocarditis. Clinical manifestations of CCM result from electric conduction abnormalities, myocardial contractile dysfunction, arrhythmias, or thromboembolism.[26-28] Depending on the population, sudden death is the most common overall cause of death (55%–60%), sometimes, in the absence of previous significant symptoms or signs of advanced CCM,[29] followed by heart failure (25%–30%) and embolic events (10%–15%) (Figs. 2A and B).[29,30]

LIMITATIONS AND GUIDELINES

After a thorough history looking for evidence of exposure, the EKG is one of the most important initial tests if CCM is suspected. During mild acute disease, the EKG may show sinus tachycardia, first degree AV block, QT prolongation or low-voltage QRS complexes. The presence of a right bundle branch block (RBBB) with or without left anterior hemiblock usually indicates chronic disease and is associated with risk of progression to more severe cardiomyopathy.[31-34] There is no single gold standard laboratory test for diagnosing chronic CD. Polymerase chain reaction (PCR) testing is used to confirm infection with *T. cruzi* in the acute phase.[35,36] On echocardiography, the most common findings are pericardial effusion (42%–50%), regional wall motion abnormalities (0%–28%), and globally decreased LVEF (0%–35%).[37-39] LV aneurysms are common and 3D echocardiography with contrast injection can delineate and measure aneurysms that are small or atypically located. STE assessing LV strain, can be used to detect subtle changes in regional and global contractility and has the potential for detecting early myocardial impairment in asymptomatic patients with CD.[40] CMR can be used to evaluate the extension of fibrosis which can be seen in patients with normal global LV systolic function.[41] The typical predominant distribution of fibrosis to the posterior and apical regions of the LV and involvement of the sinus node and electric conduction system distinguishes CD from other cardiomyopathies.

CONCLUSION

The antiprotozoal drug benznidazole is first-line treatment of *T. cruzi* infection. Nifurtimox can be used as a second-line agent. These are the only drugs with proven efficacy against CD.[42] Treatment is indicated for all patients with acute infection with cure rates of 60–90%, but the efficacy in chronic infection is uncertain.[43] If there is symptomatic bradyarrhythmias a pacemaker can be placed, as the fibrosis in this condition has a predilection for the heart's conduction system. Heart failure is treated as per current management guidelines along with the need for ICD to treat lethal ventricular arrhythmias or SCD. Chagas cardiomyopathy carries a poor prognosis compared with other forms of cardiomyopathy. Poor outcomes have been attributed to the aggressive ventricular remodeling observed in these patients.[44]

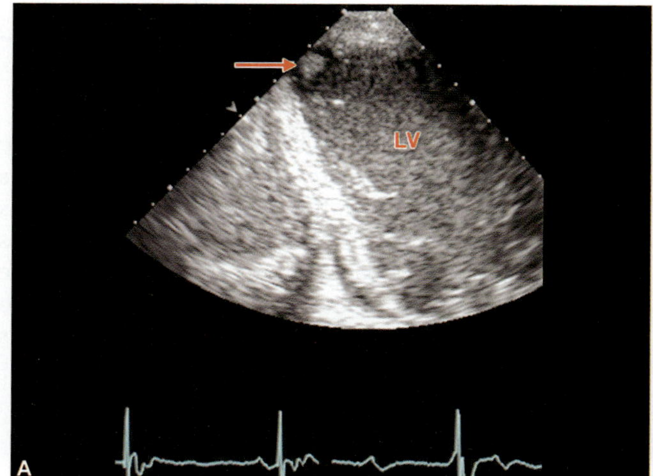

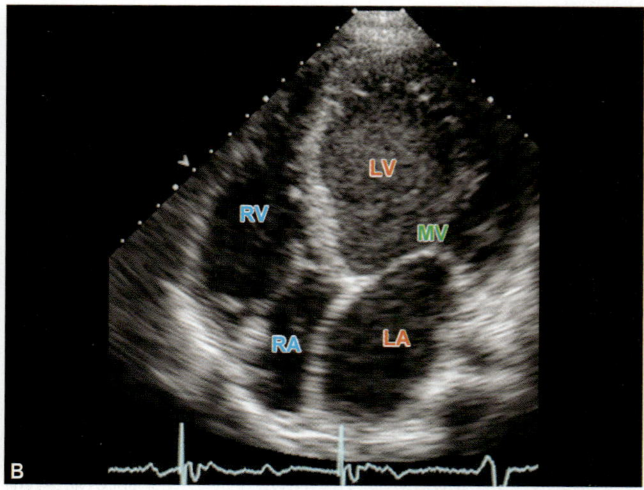

Figs. 2A and B: (A) LV cavity in apical 2 chamber view depicting apical thrombus with aneurysmal dilatation (red arrow); (B) 4 chamber apical view showing dilation of all 4 chambers and tethered mitral valve leaflets due annular dilatation.
(LV: left ventricle; LA: left atrium; RV: right ventricle; RA: right atrium; MV: mitral valve)

TAKOTSUBO CARDIOMYOPATHY

INTRODUCTION

Takotsubo cardiomyopathy (TCM) also known as stress-induced cardiomyopathy, is characterized by reversible segmental systolic dysfunction of the LV, mimicking myocardial infarction (MI), but in the absence of angiographic evidence of obstructive coronary artery disease (CAD) or acute plaque rupture.[45-48]

The Mayo Clinic diagnostic criteria for TCM includes: (all four are required for diagnosis)[45,49,50]

- Transient LV systolic dysfunction (hypokinesis, akinesis, or dyskinesis) with regional wall motion abnormalities (WMA) that extend beyond a single epicardial coronary distribution.
- Absence of obstructive CAD or angiographic evidence of acute plaque rupture. If coronary disease is found, the diagnosis of TCM can be made if the WMA are not in the distribution of the coronary disease. This exception is made as up to 15% of patients with TCM may have concurrent CAD.
- New EKG abnormalities ST elevation (STE) and/or T wave inversion or modest elevation in cardiac troponin.
- Absence of pheochromocytoma or myocarditis.

CONTENTS AND DESCRIPTION

Approximately 1–2% of patients who present with an acute coronary syndrome (ACS) [troponin positive or ST-elevation myocardial infarction (STEMI)] have been found to have TCM[51,52] with postmenopausal women more likely affected. The pathogenesis is not completely understood but postulated mechanisms include catecholamine excess, microvascular dysfunction, and coronary artery spasm.[53,54]

There can be apical or midventricular pattern of WMA and the typical apical WMA (apical ballooning) is only seen in 60% of cases.[51] LV dysfunction is transient and resolves in 80% of cases by 7 days.[55]

Takotsubo cardiomyopathy can be precipitated by intense emotional or physical stress or acute illness;[46,48] up to one-third of patients may have no recognizable trigger.[49] The most common symptoms are chest pain (68%) and dyspnea (18%); 4.2% of patients may present in cardiogenic shock or ventricular fibrillation (VF) in 1.5% of cases. The in-hospital mortality is low at about 1% and there is a 0–8% chance of recurrence.[45] Long-term follow-up of patients with TCM revealed a rate of death from any cause of 5.6% per patient-year and a rate of major adverse cardiac and cerebrovascular events of 9.9% per patient-year (Figs. 3A and B).[49]

LIMITATIONS AND GUIDELINES

The EKG shows STE in up to 90% of cases,[46] most commonly in the anterior precordial leads. ST depression may be seen in 8% of cases.[49,56] The cardiac biomarkers are elevated with median initial troponin of 7.7 times the upper limit of normal. Brain natriuretic peptide (BNP) is elevated in 83% of cases, median levels of 6 times upper limit of normal.[49]

Coronary artery obstruction should be ruled out in all suspected cases. Echocardiography shows LV dysfunction with typical apical WMA in 82% of cases. However, variations to this pattern exist (mid ventricular type 14%, basal/reverse or inverted takotsubo with sparing of the mid-ventricle and apex 2%, focal type; usually anterolateral wall 1.5%, global type; diffuse hypokinesis <1%). The mean LVEF ranges

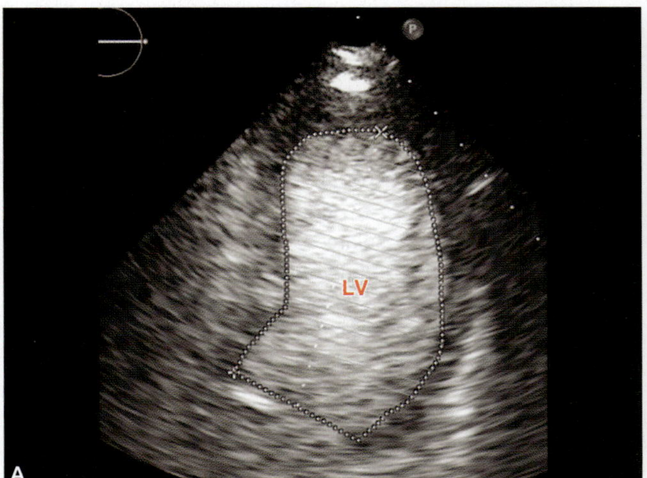

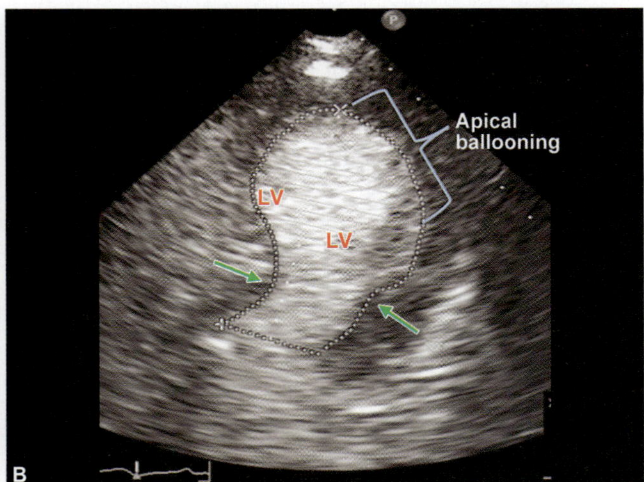

Figs. 3A and B: (A) Contrast echocardiography showing the LV in diastole, apical 2 chamber view; (B) LV now seen in systole showing basal hyperdynamic contraction (green arrows) with apical ballooning (bracket).
(LV: left ventricle)

from 20% to 49%.[52] In some patients, both the LV and right ventricle (RV) may be involved.[57] CMR may be helpful when the images from echocardiography are suboptimal; it may also assist in the differential diagnosis such as myocarditis, delineating the full extent of ventricular abnormalities, and identifying associated complications.

CONCLUSION

Probably the most important question to answer in the acute setting is whether or not the patient suspected of having TCM is in fact suffering from an ACS. Patients presenting with STE on EKG should undergo urgent cardiac catheterization to rule out obstructive CAD as the cause. If cardiac catheterization is not readily available, then these patients should be considered for fibrinolytic therapy and then undergo cardiac catheterization once available. Those who present with non-STEMI should undergo cardiac catheterization within 48 hours; until that is achieved standard therapy as per guidelines for the treatment of ACS is provided. Other conditions should also be excluded such as cocaine-induced coronary spasm; a toxicology screen is helpful in this setting. Myocarditis may present similarly with regional WMA and elevated cardiac biomarkers. The clinical course differs as the LV systolic dysfunction does not resolve rapidly as it does in TCM. Patients should have repeat echocardiography to confirm the resolution of systolic dysfunction.

REFERENCES

1. Yin L. Non-compact cardiomyopathy or ventricular non-compact syndrome? J Cardiovasc Ultrasound. 2014;22(4):165-72.
2. Oechslin EN, Attenhofer Jost CH, Rojas JR, et al. Long-term follow-up of 34 adults with isolated left ventricular noncompaction: a distinct cardiomyopathy with poor prognosis. J Am Coll Cardiol. 2000;36(2):493-500.
3. Pignatelli RH, McMahon CJ, Dreyer WJ, et al. Clinical characterization of left ventricular noncompaction in children: a relatively common form of cardiomyopathy. Circulation. 2003;108:2672-8.
4. Aras D, Tufekcioglu O, Ergun K, et al. Clinical features of isolated ventricular noncompaction in adults long-term clinical course, echocardiographic properties, and predictors of left ventricular failure. J Card Fail. 2006;12(9):726-33.
5. Stanton C, Bruce C, Connolly H, et al. Isolated left ventricular noncompaction syndrome. Am J Cardiol. 2009;104(8):1135-8.
6. Kovacevic-Preradovic T, Jenni R, Oechslin EN, et al. Isolated left ventricular noncompaction as a cause for heart failure and heart transplantation: a single center experience. Cardiology. 2009;112(2):158-64.
7. Wang C, Takasaki A, Watanabe Ozawa S, et al. Long-term prognosis of patients with left ventricular noncompaction-comparison between infantile and juvenile types. Circ J. 2017;81(5):694-700.
8. Goud A, Padmanabhan S. A rare form of cardiomyopathy: left ventricular non-compaction cardiomyopathy. J Community Hosp Intern Med Perspect. 2016;6(1):29888.
9. Bhatia NL, Tajik AJ, Wilansky S, et al. Isolated noncompaction of the left ventricular myocardium in adults: a systematic overview. J Card Fail. 2011;17(9):771-8.
10. Brescia ST, Rossano JW, Pignatelli R, et al. Mortality and sudden death in pediatric left ventricular noncompaction in a tertiary referral center. Circulation. 2013;27(22):2202-8.
11. Saleeb SF, Margossian R, Spencer CT, et al. Reproducibility of echocardiographic diagnosis of left ventricular noncompaction. J Am Soc Echocardiogr. 2012;25(2):194-202.
12. Jenni R, Oechslin E, Schneider J, et al. Echocardiographic and pathoanatomical characteristics of isolated left ventricular non-compaction: a step toward classification as a distinct cardiomyopathy. Heart. 2001;86(6):666-71.
13. Chin TK, Perloff JK, Williams RG, et al. Isolated noncompaction of left ventricular myocardium. A study of eight cases. Circulation. 1990;82(2):507-13.
14. Jorge C, Marques JS, Miltenberger-Miltényi G, et al. Hypertrophic cardiomyopathy or non-compaction? How the first impression can be wrong. Int J Cardiol. 2012;158(3):e53-4.
15. Zhang X, Yuan L, Qiu L, et al. Incremental value of contrast echocardiography in the diagnosis of left ventricular noncompaction. Front Med. 2016;10(4):499-506.
16. Petersen SE, Selvanayagam JB, Wiesmann F, et al. Left ventricular non-compaction: insights from cardiovascular magnetic resonance imaging. J Am Coll Cardiol. 2005;46(1):101-5.
17. Zuccarino F, Vollmer I, Sanchez G, et al. Left ventricular noncompaction: Imaging findings and diagnostic criteria. AJR Am J Roentgenol. 2015;204(5):W519-30.
18. van Dalen BM, Caliskan K, Soliman OI, et al. Diagnostic value of rigid body rotation in noncompaction cardiomyopathy. J Am Soc Echocardiogr. 2011;24(5):548-55.
19. Nemes A, Kalapos A, Domsik P, et al. Identification of left ventricular "rigid body rotation" by three-dimensional speckle-tracking echocardiography in a patient with noncompaction of the left ventricle: a case from the MAGYAR-Path Study. Echocardiography. 2012;(9):E237-40.
20. Jacquier A, Thuny F, Jop B, et al. Measurement of trabeculated left ventricular mass using cardiac magnetic resonance imaging in the diagnosis of left ventricular non-compaction. Eur Heart J. 2010;31(9):1098-104.
21. Kido K, Guglin M. Anticoagulation therapy in specific cardiomyopathies: Isolated left ventricular noncompaction and peripartum cardiomyopathy. J Cardiovasc Pharmacol Ther. 2019;24(1):31-6.
22. Nunes MC, Beaton A, Acquatella H, et al.; American Heart Association Rheumatic Fever, Endocarditis and Kawasaki Disease Committee of the Council on Cardiovascular Disease in the Young; Council on Cardiovascular and Stroke Nursing; and Stroke Council. Chagas cardiomyopathy: An Update of current clinical knowledge and management: A scientific statement from the American Heart Association. Circulation. 2018;138(12):e169-209.
23. Chagas disease in Latin America: an epidemiological update based on 2010 estimates. Wkly Epidemiol Rec. 2015;90(6):33-43.

24. Rassi A Jr, Rassi A, Marin-Neto JA. Chagas disease. Lancet. 2010;375(9723):1388-402.
25. Kun H, Moore A, Mascola L, et al.; Chagas Disease in Transplant Recipients Investigation Team. Transmission of Trypanosoma cruzi by heart transplantation. Clin Infect Dis. 2009;48(11):1534-40.
26. Rocha MO, Ribeiro AL, Teixeira MM. Clinical management of chronic Chagas cardiomyopathy. Front Biosci. 2003;8:e44-54.
27. Samuel J, Oliveira M, Correa De Araujo RR, et al. Cardiac thrombosis and thromboembolism in chronic Chagas' heart disease. Am J Cardiol. 1983;52(1):147-51.
28. Köberle F. The causation and importance of nervous lesions in American trypanosomiasis. Bull World Health Organ. 1970;42(5):739-43.
29. Yancy CW, Jessup M, Bozkurt B, et al.; American College of Cardiology Foundation; American Heart Association Task Force on Practice Guidelines. 2013 ACCF/AHA guideline for the management of heart failure: a report of the American College of Cardiology Foundation/American Heart Association Task Force on Practice Guidelines. J Am Coll Cardiol. 2013;62(16):e147-239.
30. Rassi A Jr, Rassi SG, Rassi A. Sudden death in Chagas' disease. Arq Bras Cardiol. 2001;76(1):75-96.
31. Maguire JH, Hoff R, Sherlock I, et al. Cardiac morbidity and mortality due to Chagas' disease: prospective electrocardiographic study of a Brazilian community. Circulation. 1987;75(6):1140-5.
32. Manzullo EC, Chuit R. Risk of death due to chronic chagasic cardiopathy. Mem Inst Oswaldo Cruz. 1999;94(Suppl 1):317-20.
33. Prata A. Clinical and epidemiological aspects of Chagas disease. Lancet Infect Dis. 2001;1(2):92-100.
34. Rosenbaum MB, Alvarez AJ. The electrocardiogram in chronic chagasic myocarditis. Am Heart J. 1955;50(4):492-527.
35. Schijman AG, Vigliano C, Burgos J, et al. Early diagnosis of recurrence of Trypanosoma cruzi infection by polymerase chain reaction after heart transplantation of a chronic Chagas' heart disease patient. J Heart Lung Transplant. 2000;19(11):1114-7.
36. Gomes ML, Galvao LM, Macedo AM, et al. Chagas' disease diagnosis: comparative analysis of parasitologic, molecular, and serologic methods. Am J Trop Med Hyg. 1999;60(2):205-10.
37. Parada H, Carrasco HA, Añez N, et al. Cardiac involvement is a constant finding in acute Chagas' disease: a clinical, parasitological and histopathological study. Int J Cardiol. 1997;60(1):49-54.
38. Carme B, Aune I, Nguyen G, et al. Four cases of acute chagasic myocarditis in French Guiana. Am J Trop Med Hyg. 2001;64(3-4):162-3.
39. Pinto AY, Valente SA, Valente Vda C. Emerging acute Chagas disease in Amazonian Brazil: case reports with serious cardiac involvement. Braz J Infect Dis. 2004;8(6):454-60.
40. Barbosa MM, Costa Rocha MO, Vidigal DF, et al. Early detection of left ventricular contractility abnormalities by two-dimensional speckle tracking strain in Chagas' disease. Echocardiography. 2014;31(5):623-30.
41. Mello RP, Szarf G, Schvartzman PR, et al. Delayed enhancement cardiac magnetic resonance imaging can identify the risk for ventricular tachycardia in chronic Chagas' heart disease. Arq Bras Cardiol. 2012;98(5):421-30.
42. Rodriques Coura J, de Castro SL. A critical review on Chagas disease chemotherapy. Mem Inst Oswaldo Cruz. 2002;97(1):3-24.
43. Wegner DH, Rohwedder RW. The effect of nifurtimox in acute Chagas' infection. Arzneimittelforschung. 1972;22(9):1624-35.
44. Shen L, Ramires F, Martinez F, et al.; PARADIGM-HF and ATMOSPHERE Investigators and Committees. Contemporary characteristics and outcomes in chagasic heart failure compared with other nonischemic and ischemic cardiomyopathy. Circ Heart Fail. 2017;10(11). pii: e004361.
45. Bybee KA, Kara T, Prasad A, et al. Systematic review: transient left ventricular apical ballooning: a syndrome that mimics ST-segment elevation myocardial infarction. Ann Intern Med. 2004;141(11):858-65.
46. Tsuchihashi K, Ueshima K, Uchida T, et al.; Angina Pectoris-Myocardial Infarction Investigations in Japan. Transient left ventricular apical ballooning without coronary artery stenosis: a novel heart syndrome mimicking acute myocardial infarction. Angina Pectoris-Myocardial Infarction Investigations in Japan. J Am Coll Cardiol. 2001;38(1):11-8.
47. Goulbourne C, et al. Can broken bones lead to a broken heart? J Am Coll Cardiol. 2019;73(9 Suppl 1):2540.
48. Abe Y, Kondo M, Matsuoka R, et al. Assessment of clinical features in transient left ventricular apical ballooning. J Am Coll Cardiol. 2003;41(5):737-42.
49. Templin C, Ghadri JR, Diekmann J, et al. Clinical features and outcomes of takotsubo (Stress) cardiomyopathy. N Engl J Med. 2015;373(10):929-38.
50. Prasad A, Lerman A, Rihal CS. Apical ballooning syndrome (Tako-Tsubo or stress cardiomyopathy): a mimic of acute myocardial infarction. Am Heart J. 2008;155(3):408-17.
51. Kurowski V, Kaiser A, von Hof K, et al. Apical and midventricular transient left ventricular dysfunction syndrome (tako-tsubo cardiomyopathy): frequency, mechanisms, and prognosis. Chest. 2007;132(3):809-16.
52. Gianni M, Dentali F, Grandi AM, et al. Apical ballooning syndrome or takotsubo cardiomyopathy: a systematic review. Eur Heart J. 2006;27(13):1523-9.
53. Wittstein IS, Thiemann DR, Lima JA, et al. Neurohumoral features of myocardial stunning due to sudden emotional stress. N Engl J Med. 2005;352(6):539-48.
54. Paur H, Wright PT, Sikkel MB, et al. High levels of circulating epinephrine trigger apical cardiodepression in a β2-adrenergic receptor/Gi-dependent manner: a new model of Takotsubo cardiomyopathy. Circulation. 2012;126(6):697-706.
55. Park JH, Kang SJ, Song JK, et al. Left ventricular apical ballooning due to severe physical stress in patients admitted to the medical ICU. Chest. 2005;128(1):296-302.
56. Parkkonen O, Allonen J, Vaara S, et al. Differences in ST-elevation and T-wave amplitudes do not reliably differentiate takotsubo cardiomyopathy from acute anterior myocardial infarction. J Electrocardiol. 2014;47(5):692-9.
57. Haghi D, Athanasiadis A, Papavassiliu T, et al. Right ventricular involvement in Takotsubo cardiomyopathy. Eur Heart J. 2006;27(20):2433-9.

74

CHAPTER

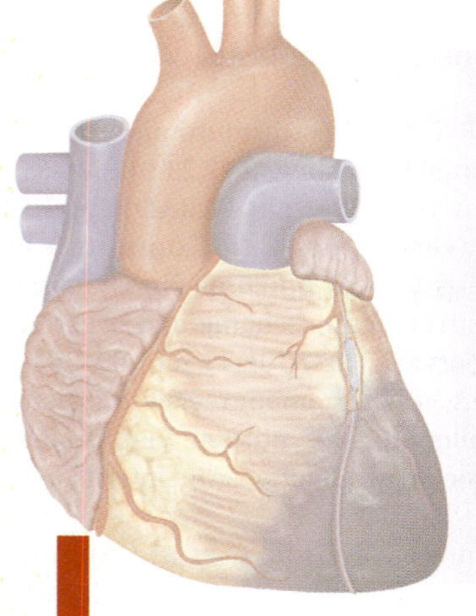

Artificial Intelligence: Its Impact in the Management of Heart Failure

Vidur Mahajan, Vasanthakumar Venugopal

INTRODUCTION

Artificial intelligence (AI) is a term first coined by John McCarthy in 1956. It has been used for any technology that can perform human-like tasks, or, the ability of machines to program themselves, without the need for explicit human instruction. Despite the existence of the concept for the better part of last century, practical applications of AI were enabled by a boom in the computing power at the turn of this decade. It is a well-known fact that a smartphone today has a million times more computing power than all of NASA combined in 1969, when Apollo 11 landed on the moon. Additionally, in the year 2015, Yann Lecun, Yoshua Bengio, and Geoffrey Hinton published a seminal paper on deep learning, a technique that allows computational models composed of multiple processing layers to learn representations of data with multiple levels of abstraction.[1] We will go a little deeper into what deep learning is, and why it is important, further ahead in this chapter. Since 2015, deep learning is being applied across industries that involve either speech recognition or computer vision, with attempts to find correlations between higher-dimensional datasets. In healthcare, it had been proven by many groups to be very effective in domains like radiology, pathology, pharmacology and genomics. More recently, researchers have started exploring the impact of deep learning and other machine learning techniques in the field of cardiology, and more specifically, heart failure. This chapter will give an overview of AI, as it stands today, some examples from literature, and some limitations of current AI techniques that any practicing cardiologist should be aware of. The attempt also is to give a framework for reading and judging any research article on AI, from a clinician's perspective.

HEART FAILURE: DISEASE BURDEN AND CLINICAL PRESENTATION

Heart failure is a global epidemic with increasing incidence in recent years. It affects 26 million patients worldwide with 3.5 million new patients added every year.[2] The diagnosis of heart failure is made by interpretation of multiple symptoms resulting from reduced ability of the heart to pump and/or fill with blood. The New York Heart Association (NYHA) classification of heart failure is widely used in practice to quantify clinical assessment of heart failure. Dyspnea is a cardinal sign of cardiac failure; it can present in progressively increasing levels of severity ranging from exertional dyspnea and orthopnea, to dyspnea at rest and/or in the most severe form as acute pulmonary edema (Table 1).

Heart failure has recently been classified into three subtypes, namely—heart failure with reduced ejection fraction (HFrEF), heart failure with preserved ejection fraction (HFpEF), and heart failure with midrange ejection fraction (HFmrEF), according to the ejection fraction, natriuretic peptide levels, and the presence of structural heart disease and diastolic dysfunction.

ARTIFICIAL INTELLIGENCE AND DEEP LEARNING

Deep learning is a machine learning technique where, simply put, machines can find patterns in data themselves,

TABLE 1: NYHA functional classification of heart failure.

Class	Functional capacity
I	Patients without limitation of physical activity
II	Slight limitation of physical activity. Comfortable at rest. Ordinary physical activity results in fatigue, palpitation, dyspnea (shortness of breath)
III	Marked limitation of physical activity. Comfortable at rest. Less than ordinary activity causes fatigue, palpitation, or dyspnea
IV	Unable to carry on any physical activity without discomfort. Symptoms of heart failure at rest. If any physical activity is undertaken, discomfort increases

(NYHA: New York Heart Association)

as opposed to the user or developer defining patterns. The unique feature of deep learning is that it uses multiple layers of abstraction (generally exceeding a hundred) to "learn" features in a dataset. From a clinician's point of view, it is important to know that there are two types of "learning"—supervised and unsupervised.

Supervised learning is best understood using an example of images accompanied by their labels. For instance, consider the chest X-ray 14 dataset released by the National Institutes of Health in 2017.[3] This is a massive dataset of about 1,00,000 chest X-rays which contains an image of the X-ray and a corresponding label of the radiologist report, for example, whether pleural effusion is present or absent. Earlier, using most traditional machine learning techniques, one would need to first "teach" the computer "what" pleural effusion looks like, i.e. first find the costophrenic angle, then see if it is sharp or not, and then decide whether pleural effusion exists there or not. Today, with deep learning, if one has enough examples of X-rays with and without pleural effusion, the computer can itself figure out what the location of pleural effusion is and what its features are—this power is what is being used today. This process of "teaching" a computer using examples where corresponding labels exist, is called supervised learning and most healthcare AI research today focuses on this aspect. It is becoming very easy to start applying these techniques to any dataset-we will discuss this democratization of AI further in the chapter.

The other form of "learning" is called unsupervised learning—this is best understood using an example of how a child learns. Children do not need to be explicitly taught how to do things; they learn simply by doing. We do not need to show a child 1,000 balls (with their labels!) for them to know what a ball is—humans are great at "transferring" what they have learnt from one part of their life to another. This mechanism is called unsupervised learning, where simply exposure to a huge amount of data enables one to learn patterns within the data. AlphaGo, which is a computer system by Deepmind Inc (a Google Company), uses reinforcement learning to learn how to play games without having to be taught how to play them—it simply learns by observation! In fact, Deepmind has gone on to claim that their computers can now beat the world's best players of ANY strategy game within a span of a day.[4]

APPLICATIONS OF AI—A FRAMEWORK

As we dive deeper into applications of AI in the medical world, we propose a framework using which one can categorize AI applications. There are two broad applications of AI, both of which are again best illustrated by examples:

1. *That what humans can do, but machines can do better:* Chilamkurthy et al.[5] showed how CT scans of the head can be automatically read by deep learning algorithms saving precious time in emergency situations. While reading CT scans is something that radiologists can do, reading scans immediately in the middle of the night with very high accuracy is difficult and costly. Another example is by Venugopal et al.[6] where they propose that all "normal" chest X-rays may be read by machines instead of radiologists, freeing up valuable time for radiologists to focus on more difficult and critical cases.
2. *That what humans cannot do:* Mahajan et al.[7] demonstrated that there is enough data in T2-weighted images of the brain to create diffusion-weighted images of the brain from them, using deep learning. Diffusion-weighted imaging is used to differentiate between acute and chronic infarcts, which are otherwise not discernible on T2-weighted images by radiologists demonstrating the ability of machines to "see" what humans cannot. Another similar example is by Venugopal et al.[8] where they created PET images from CT images—something which humans cannot do.

Generally, one will be able to fit most applications involving AI into one of these two buckets and going forward we will use this classification as we dive into examples of AI in heart failure.

APPLICATIONS OF ARTIFICIAL INTELLIGENCE IN HEART FAILURE

The applications of AI in management of heart failure can be broadly classified into two types:

1. *Diagnosis of heart failure:* These applications will enable early diagnosis and effective management of the symptoms, thereby reducing the mortality and morbidity.
2. *Prediction of heart failure beforehand:* These applications involve the "prediction" of heart failure,

enabling appropriate prognostication and therapeutic modification.

DIAGNOSTIC ARTIFICIAL INTELLIGENCE APPLICATIONS

There are several applications developed with the purpose of automatically diagnosing heart failure with a high degree of accuracy and using simple clinical, laboratory parameters or radiology tools like chest X-ray and echocardiography. We will discuss these studies in detail. The performance of these tools is practically easier to evaluate as compared to the prediction tools since establishing "ground truth" for these tools is easier as there is always a gold standard test available for diagnosis of heart failure. Moreover, for such diagnostic applications, it is relatively easier for developers to tune the algorithm to improve the accuracy.

DIAGNOSIS OF HEART FAILURE FROM CHEST X-RAYS

Conventional radiographic features of congestive heart failure (CHF) include cardiomegaly, pulmonary venous congestion, septal lines, airspace opacification, and bilateral pleural effusions. Scientists from Royal Melbourne Hospital have developed an AI algorithm that can diagnose cardiac failure from chest X-rays with a high accuracy.[9] Interestingly the ground truth used to train the algorithm was established not from radiological reports but using laboratory reports of serum B-type natriuretic peptide (BNP) levels. It is commonly used to diagnose and monitor CHF. At the threshold of 100 ng/L, serum BNP has a sensitivity of 0.95 and specificity of 0.63 for acute CHF. This cutoff was used to assign the labels for the chest X-rays. This approach has two advantages. First it enables training of deep learning models without human bias. Second, it allows the comparison of features the model had learned *de novo* with the traditional radiologically described features of heart failure on chest X-ray. This algorithm was trained using a labeled dataset comprising 7,390 radiographs from 5,232 unique patients with a paired BNP result within 36 hours of image acquisition. At a cutoff BNP of 100 ng/L as a marker for the presence of CHF, the correctly trained model obtained a good area under the curve (AUC) of 0.82. But the downside of this study, the reported results of the test cases were derived from the same dataset that was used for training. Note that it is always important to test any AI model on data that is not a subset of data that the algorithm was developed on. AI models, and more importantly deep learning models, are heavily prone to overfitting and hence this independent testing is critical.

DIAGNOSIS OF HEART FAILURE USING WHOLE SLIDE H&E IMAGES

Endomyocardial biopsy (EMB) is the gold standard for the evaluation of disease, when cause of heart failure cannot be identified. However, manual EMB interpretation has high inter-rater variability. Researchers from the University of Pennsylvania and Case Western University have developed an AI algorithm that can detect heart failure from H&E stained whole-slide images.[10] This algorithm was able to identify patients with heart failure or severe pathology with a 99% sensitivity and 94% specificity on the test set, outperforming conventional feature-engineering approaches. Importantly, it outperformed two expert pathologists by nearly 20%. AI algorithms like this can be used effectively to establish consensus in observations with high interobserver variability (Fig. 1).

SCREENING FOR ATRIAL FIBRILLATION FROM SINGLE LEAD SHORT ECHOCARDIOGRAPHY

Atrial fibrillation (AF) is the most common arrhythmia in elderly leading to morbidity and mortality usually from heart failure. Early detection of AF can help avert this possibility, but it is difficult due to its episodic occurrence. Xiaomao Fan et al. developed an algorithm that can identify AF from single lead ECG recordings of durations as short as 5 seconds.[11] They were able to identify the presence or absence of AF in these recordings with nearly 97% accuracy. Such algorithms can enable real-time monitoring of elderly patients for occurrence of AF through wearable devices, such as the newly launched Apple Watch.

PREDICTIVE ARTIFICIAL INTELLIGENCE APPLICATIONS

Applications under this category are developed with the aim of predicting the occurrence of heart failure well ahead in time, take corrective measures and hence prevent the occurrence of the event itself. For most skeptics, this might sound like science fiction. Robust pre-deployment validation of these applications has certain challenges that center around ethical dilemmas like whether to intervene or not intervene in positive predictions of control cases. Also, there are challenges of addressing false negative and false positive predictions. Nevertheless, such applications if deployed in the right manner will have the greatest impact on improving the chances of realization of the ideals of precision medicine and personalized healthcare.

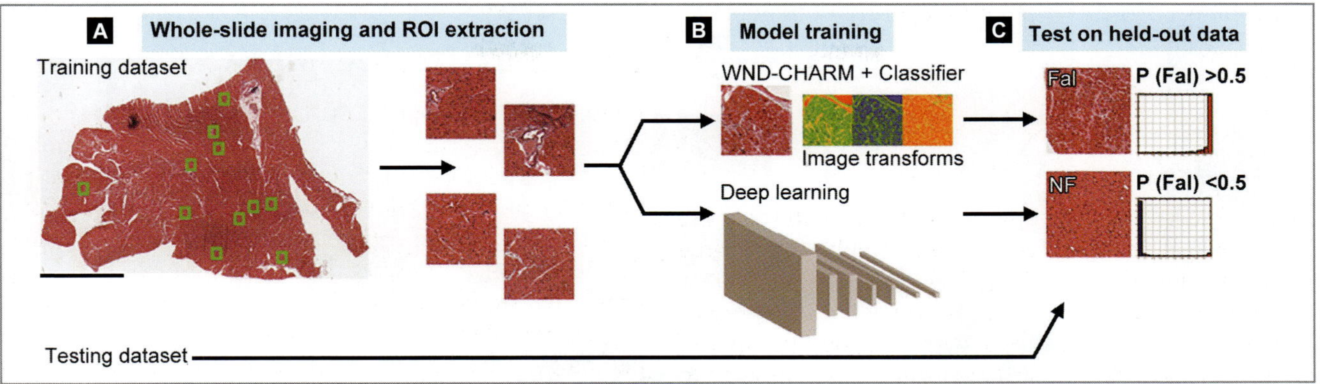

Figs. 1A to C: Schematic overview of digital pathology workflow to detect heart failure. (A) Patients were divided into a training and test dataset. Whole slide imaging (WSI) were scanned and regions of interest (ROI) were extracted for image analysis. All ROIs from the same patient were given the same label, which was determined by whether the patient had clinical or pathological evidence of heart disease; (B) Three-fold cross validation was used to train heart failure classifiers using a deep learning model or engineered features in WND-CHARM + a random decision forest classifier; (C) Trained models were evaluated at the image and patient-level on a held-out test dataset.

Source: Nirschl JJ, Janowczyk A, Peyster EG, et al. A deep-learning classifier identifies patients with clinical heart failure using whole-slide images of H&E tissue. PLoS One. 2018;13(4):e0192726.

PREDICTION OF LONG-TERM HEART FAILURE BY MACHINE LEARNING

X Zhuang et al. developed a machine learning technique using a "random forest" classifier to predict the occurrence of heart failure by using 625 variables from imaging and noninvasive tests, questionnaires, and biomarker panels. "Random forests", a statistical classification model, was used to identify the top predictors of heart failure.[12] Age, blood glucose levels, and body mass index were the most important predictors for heart failure. The Harrell concordance index or C-index (a surrogate measure for measuring of prediction accuracy concordance among various models) for the long-term heart failure prediction was 0.76 in this study.

PREDICTING ADHERENCE OF PATIENTS WITH HEART FAILURE THROUGH MACHINE LEARNING TECHNIQUES

There are many low risks but high-value applications of AI in management of heart failure. One of them that was addressed by G. Karanasiou et al. was estimating future adherence of patients to heart failure treatment.[13] These techniques were able to predict not only the probability of the patient being adherent to medication but also the probability of adherence to other medical advice like nutrition and physical activity. About 11 classification algorithms were employed and combined with feature selection and resampling techniques. They were able to predict with 82% and 91% accuracy the probability of the patient being globally adherent or adherent to medication only, respectively. Such lower-risk models offer a great starting point for applying AI in the management of heart failure.

PREDICTION OF MORTALITY FROM 12-LEAD ELECTROCARDIOGRAM

There are certain applications proposed by the data science community which can qualify for the previously described science fiction category. One such application was described by Raghunath S. et al., wherein they propose an algorithm which can predict future clinical event (one-year all-cause mortality) from ECG voltage-time traces.[14] The algorithm was developed and tested leveraging a large set of nearly 1.8 million ECGs collected from ~400 thousand patients over a period of 34 years and demonstrated good performance for predicting one-year mortality with an average AUC of 0.85. A blinded survey of three cardiologists suggested that the patterns captured by the model were generally not visually apparent to cardiologists even after being shown 240 paired examples of labelled true positives and true negatives. Such AI applications, although currently exploratory, demonstrate the ability of AI to add significant prognostic information to the interpretation of simple investigations like ECGs, X-rays or echocardiograms, even in cases that are interpreted as "normal" by physicians.

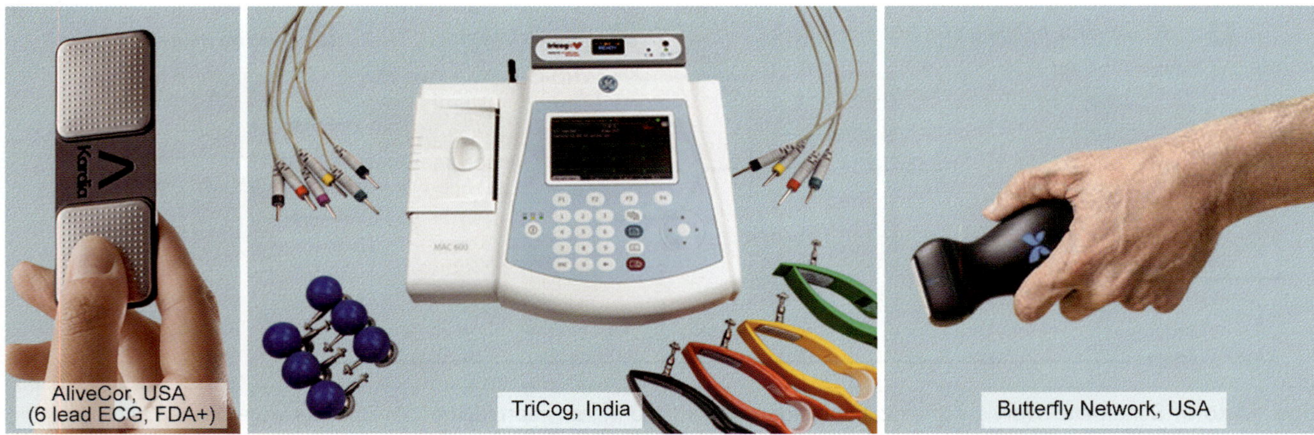

Fig. 2: New hardware technologies that complement the AI revolution.
(AI: artificial intelligence; ECG: echocardiography; FDA: Food and Drug Administration)

NEW HARDWARE TECHNOLOGIES THAT COMPLEMENT THE AI REVOLUTION

Apart from the rapid advancements happening in the field of AI and deep learning, there are similar technology developments and advancements happening on the hardware front also. There are mobile devices that complement the screening processes in remote, inaccessible locations. In the context of management of heart failure, there are three such commercially available devices which are worth mentioning (Fig. 2).

Tricog Insta Echocardiography

This is a mobile 12 lead ECG device, approved by the Food and Drug Administration (FDA) for clinical use. It is portable, works with a battery and has a mobile sim card built in that can upload the ECGs to cloud for expert opinion, which is typically available in less than a minute.

Alivecor KardiaMobile Six-lead Wireless Echocardiography Device

The Kardia mobile six-lead device has two electrodes on the top of the device and one additional electrode on the bottom. The user places his/her thumbs on each of the two top electrodes, and places the bottom electrode on the left knee or ankle. This formation, known in cardiology as the Einthoven triangle, allows cardiologists to view electrical activity in the heart from six perspectives or "leads." A six-lead ECG provides physicians with a far superior view of the heart than a single lead ECG, giving them ability to detect a far broader range of arrhythmias and other heart conditions, all without the hassle of gels or wires.

Butterfly IQ Ultrasound Probes

The Butterfly iQ is a convex, linear, and sector ultrasound transducer that connects to an iPhone or iPad with the Butterfly app to serve as a full ultrasound machine. The transducer is a multipurpose probe that uses a silicon chip instead of a piezoelectric crystal, which allows it to function as a multipurpose transducer. Such hand-held devices can bring cardiac imaging to remote locations and communities, improving the quality of care in these areas. Additionally, many tout these devices to be the "stethoscope of the future", given the pace at which cardiac imaging device prices are falling.

CONCLUSION

Artificial intelligence in the management of heart failure has promise and is showing great results in various academic settings. However, the adoption of AI in cardiology, and more specifically heart failure, is bound to be slow given the serious consequences associated with the role that AI will play. As AI starts percolating this field, it is important to practitioners to ask questions about the robustness of algorithms, think about appropriate clinical testing scenarios, and last and most importantly, be open and accepting to the changes that AI will bring about in the clinical realm.

REFERENCES

1. LeCun Y, Bengio Y, Hinton G. Deep learning. Nature. 2015;521(7553):436-44.
2. Savarese G, Lund LH. Global public health burden of heart failure. Card Fail Rev. 2017;3(1):7-11.
3. NIH Clinical Center Provides One of the Largest Publicly Available Chest X-ray Datasets to Scientific Community.

National Institutes of Health (NIH); (2017). [online] Available from: https://www.nih.gov/news-events/news-releases/nih-clinical-center-provides-one-largest-publicly-available-chest-x-ray-datasets-scientific-community. [Last accessed Nov., 2019].

4. Powles J, Hodson H. Google DeepMind and healthcare in an age of algorithms. Health Technol (Berl). 2017;7(4):351-67.
5. Chilamkurthy S, Ghosh R, Tanamala S, et al. Deep learning algorithms for detection of critical findings in head CT scans: a retrospective study. 2018;392(10162):2388-96.
6. Venugopal V. Automated classification of chest X-rays as normal/abnormal using a high sensitivity deep learning algorithm. European Congress of Radiology; 2019.
7. Mahajan V. Toward virtual MR imaging: predicting diffusion-weighted brain MR images from T2-weighted images using convolutional neural networks. European Congress of Radiology; 2019.
8. Venugopal V. Synthetic PET Generator: A Novel Method to Improve Lung Nodule Detection by Combining Outputs from a Pix2pix Conditional Adversarial Network and a Convolutional Neural Network Based Malignancy Probability Estimator. Annual Congress of Radiology Society of North America RSNA; 2019.
9. Seah JC, Tang JS, Kitchen A, et al. Chest radiographs in congestive heart failure: Visualizing neural network learning. Radiology. 2019;290(2):514-22.
10. Nirschl JJ, Janowczyk A, Peyster EG, et al. A deep-learning classifier identifies patients with clinical heart failure using whole-slide images of H&E tissue. PLoS One. 2018;13(4):e0192726.
11. Fan X, Yao Q, Cai Y, et al. Multiscaled fusion of deep convolutional neural networks for screening atrial fibrillation from single lead short ECG recordings. IEEE J Biomed Health Inform. 2018;22(6):1744-53.
12. Zhuang X, Sun X, Zhong X, et al. Deep phenotyping and prediction of long-term heart failure by machine learning. J Am Coll Cardiol. 2019;73(9 Suppl 1):690.
13. Karanasiou GS, Tripoliti EE, Papadopoulos TG, et al. Predicting adherence of patients with HF through machine learning techniques. Healthc Technol Lett. 2016;3(3):165-70.
14. Raghunath S, et al. Deep neural networks can predict mortality from 12-lead electrocardiogram voltage data. 2019.

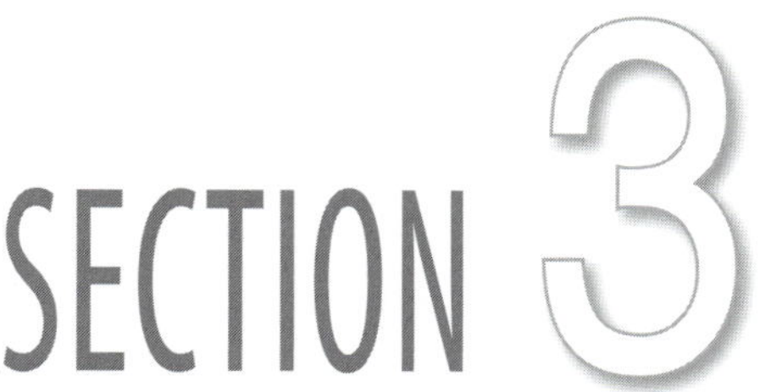

Coronary Artery Disease and Heart Failure

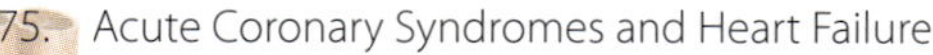

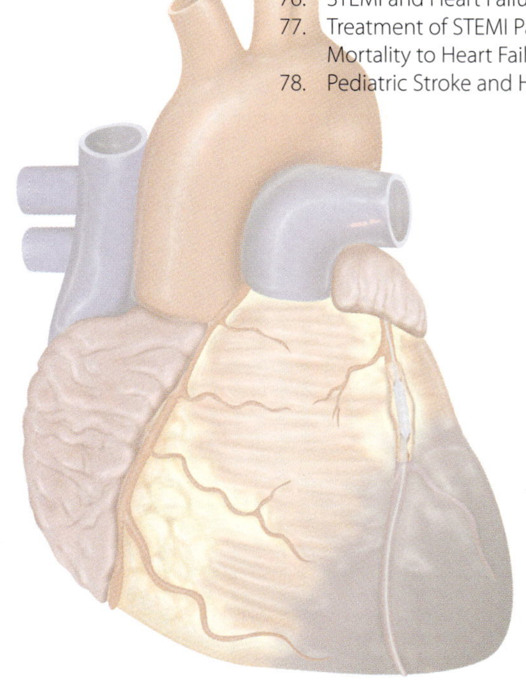

Acute Coronary Syndromes and Heart Failure

Brian Pinto, Bhavik Dhirawani, Neeraj A Desai

INTRODUCTION

Acute heart failure syndromes (AHFS) can be defined as a rapid or gradual change in signs and symptoms in patients with chronic heart failure (HF) or new-onset HF that necessitates urgent therapy.[1] Acute HF syndromes are a leading and increasingly common cause of hospitalization worldwide. Despite considerable expenditures and intensive investigational efforts, hospitalization for AHFS continues to be associated with a poor prognosis.[2-5] AHFS represent a heterogeneous group of patients in terms of their clinical presentation, pathophysiology, prognosis, and therapeutic options.[1] The majority of patients presenting with AHFS have coronary artery disease (CAD). These patients may present in one of two ways—acute coronary syndromes (ACS) complicated by HF or AHFS with underlying CAD. The cornerstone of the evaluation of CAD in ACS is coronary angiography. The evaluation of CAD in AHFS with coronary angiography, often in conjunction with noninvasive functional imaging to detect ischemic or dysfunctional but viable myocardium may represent an emerging approach to the assessment and management of AHFS patients.

EPIDEMIOLOGY

Acute heart failure syndromes account for more than one million hospitalizations per year in the US and a similar number in Europe.[6] AHFS is also the most common overall cause of hospitalization in adults 65 years and older, accounting for more than 5–10% of all admissions.[7] Approximately 80% of patients hospitalized with AHFS carry a previous diagnosis of HF. In 15% of patients, the diagnosis of HF is new, and the remaining 5% are admitted with advanced or refractory HF. The highest relative risk for mortality occurs within 30–60 days after discharge.

As the burden of AHFS increases with the aging population, the importance of evidence-based strategies to prevent HF exacerbations, decrease hospitalizations, contain costs, and improve outcomes has become an urgent public health issue.

PATHOPHYSIOLOGY: ACS COMPLICATED BY HF

Approximately 10–20% of patients with ACS have concomitant HF, and up to 10% of ACS patients develop HF during hospitalization.[8-13] In the EuroHeart Survey II on HF, 37% of patients had de novo HF, 42% of which was attributable to ACS.[14] Patients with ACS and ST-segment elevation typically have high levels of cardiac biomarker elevation, corresponding to high levels of myocardial injury. Of ACS patients with HF but without ST-segment elevation, more than two-third have significant cardiac enzyme elevation (troponin >3 times the upper limit of normal), a proportion similar to those presenting without HF. The majority of these patients do not have a history of HF and have preserved systolic function. The short-term risk of adverse clinical outcomes in patients with ACS complicated by HF is directly proportional to the level of troponin elevation.

Patients with ACS complicated by HF have markedly increased short- and long-term mortality rates compared with those without HF.[15-22]

Patients who develop HF after presentation have even higher mortality than those presenting with ACS and HF.[9,13] The prognosis of ACS complicated by HF is directly related to the degree of HF as measured by the Killip classification.[9,11,13] Compared with those with Killip class I HF, patients with an ACS in Killip class II or III HF are four times more likely to die during the index hospitalization, whereas those with cardiogenic shock (class IV) have a 10-fold higher mortality.[10,13] Furthermore, among ACS patients who recover from transient HF, the majority develop recurrent HF.[23]

ASSESSMENT OF CAD IN AHFS

Electrocardiography and echocardiography are the most common cardiac diagnostic tests obtained in patients with AHFS.[24] Patients with LV systolic dysfunction and electrocardiographic Q waves usually have significant CAD.[25] However, most patients with HF and CAD do not have Q waves, whereas those with nonischemic cardiomyopathies can have Q waves.[25] Similarly, segmental wall motions identified by echocardiography are predictive of CAD, but not its extent and severity.

Coronary Angiography

Coronary angiography is the gold standard for the diagnosis and reassessment of CAD against which all other modalities are compared.[26] In patients with HF, the long-term prognosis is directly related to the angiographic extent and severity of CAD.[26,27] This has been demonstrated in HF patients with LV systolic dysfunction and preserved systolic function.[28]

Patients with ACS complicated by HF are less likely to undergo coronary angiography and revascularization and to receive pharmacological therapy for CAD than ACS patients without HF.[22,29,30] In the Organized Program to Initiate Lifesaving Treatment in Hospitalized Patients with Heart Failure (OPTIMIZE-HF) registry,[31] it has been preliminarily reported that performance of coronary angiography during the index hospitalization for AHFS was associated with an increased utilization of aspirin, statins, and myocardial revascularization and a reduced risk of death in 60–90 days after discharge. This raises the hypothesis that the knowledge of the extent and severity of CAD in AHFS patients will have an important role in treatment decisions.

Multidetector coronary computed tomography angiography (CTA) has been shown to be highly accurate to determine the presence or absence of CAD in patients with HF.[32] However, when CAD is present, the ability of CTA to define its extent and severity is hampered by unseen segments and artifacts caused by motion and calcium.[33]

Management

Patients with acute decompensated heart failure (ADHF) often have CAD with or without an ACS.[34] The acute onset of severe myocardial ischemia can lead to a sudden impairment in systolic and/or diastolic function, resulting in a decreased cardiac output, elevated filling pressures, and the development of pulmonary edema. Flash pulmonary edema can result from myocardial ischemia with or without myocardial infarction (MI) and may occur in the absence of chest pain. Specific considerations apply to treatment of ADHF in patients presenting with ACS.

REVASCULARIZATION

Urgent revascularization is a major component of therapy for patients presenting with ST elevation myocardial infarction (STEMI), and is particularly important for those with HF. Early revascularization is indicated for patients presenting with unstable angina/non-ST elevation MI (UA/NSTEMI) and HF. As recommended in the 2016 ESC guidelines for heart failure, urgent cardiac catheterization and revascularization is reasonable when it is likely to prolong meaningful survival in patients with acute HF and known or suspected acute myocardial ischemia due to occlusive coronary disease, especially when there are signs and symptoms of systemic hypoperfusion.

- Primary percutaneous coronary intervention (PCI) is recommended in patients with STEMI when it can be performed within 90 minutes of first medical contact.[35,36] In addition, it is reasonable to promptly (within 30 minutes of arrival) transfer patients with STEMI with severe HF to facilities capable of rapid revascularization.
- Fibrinolytic therapy is recommended for patients with STEMI when timely primary PCI cannot be performed.[35,36] The routine performance of PCI within 3–24 hours after fibrinolytic therapy has been referred to as pharmacoinvasive strategy. For patients who have received fibrinolytic therapy, a strategy of coronary angiography with intent to perform PCI (or emergency coronary artery bypass graft surgery) is recommended for patients in the following clinical settings:
  - Cardiogenic shock who are <75 years of age who are candidates for revascularization
  - Severe HF and/or pulmonary edema
  - Hemodynamically compromising ventricular arrhythmias.

In addition, a pharmacoinvasive strategy is a reasonable option in the following settings:
 - Cardiogenic shock with ≥75 years of age and who are suitable candidates for revascularization
 - Hemodynamic instability and/or persistent ischemic symptoms.
- A strategy of early coronary angiography with intent to perform revascularization is indicated in certain UA/NSTEMI patients (without serious comorbidities or contraindications to such procedures) including those with the following (as well as others discussed separately):
 - Hemodynamic instability
 - Refractory or recurrent angina
 - Signs or symptoms of HF or new or worsening mitral regurgitation
 - Reduced left ventricular systolic function [left ventricular ejection fraction (LVEF) <40%].

MEDICAL THERAPY

Diuretic Use

A diuretic (low- to intermediate-dose furosemide, torsemide, or bumetanide) should be administered to treat pulmonary congestion if there is associated volume overload. However, caution is advised to avoid unnecessary or excessive diuresis since some patients are normovolemic, or even hypovolemic particularly those without prior left ventricular dysfunction and those who have not received fluid loading. In such patients, diuresis may lead to hypotension and potentially a worsening of ischemia.

- If respiratory distress, respiratory acidosis, and/or hypoxia persist, we suggest noninvasive ventilation (NIV) as the preferred initial modality of assisted ventilation as long as the patient does not have a contraindication.

Once initial therapy has begun, oxygen supplementation can be titrated in order to keep the patient comfortable and arterial oxygen saturation above 90%.

Morphine Sulfate

In the setting of STEMI, morphine sulfate is recommended as the analgesic of choice for ischemic pain relief provided that additional therapy is used to manage the underlying ischemia. In UA/NSTEMI, it is reasonable to administer morphine if there is uncontrolled ischemic pain provided that additional therapy is used to manage the underlying ischemia.

Vasodilator Therapy

Nitroglycerin is recommended for MI patients to treat ischemic pain, hypertension, or pulmonary congestion unless the systolic blood pressure is <100 mm Hg or ≥30 mm Hg below baseline.

Nitroprusside is often used when pronounced afterload reduction is required (as in the setting of ventricular septal rupture).

The adverse effect of nitroprusside in patients with acute MI may be attributable to reflex tachycardia and/or coronary steal.

Beta-blocker Therapy

Although initiation of beta-blocker therapy within the first 24 hours is generally recommended for patients presenting with MI, such therapy is contraindicated in patients with signs of HF, evidence of a low-output state, increased risk of cardiogenic shock, or other contraindications, such as heart block or reactive airways disease.

Beta-blocker therapy should be initiated before discharge for secondary prevention and continued indefinitely in all patients who have had an MI or ACS, unless contraindicated. For those who remain in HF throughout the hospitalization, low doses should be initiated with gradual titration on an outpatient basis.

Angiotensin Converting Enzyme Inhibitor and Angiotensin II Receptor Blocker Therapy

Initiation of an oral angiotensin converting enzyme (ACE) inhibitor is recommended in patients with an acute MI who have HF or systolic dysfunction (LVEF ≤ 40%) unless the systolic blood pressure is <100 mm Hg or >30 mm Hg below baseline or there are other contraindications. Therapy should be administered orally and titrated starting with a low initial dose. It should be noted that aggressive ACE inhibitor therapy prior to percutaneous intervention for acute MI or prior to hemodynamic stabilization has been associated with an increased risk of cardiogenic shock.

Angiotensin converting enzyme inhibitors should be initiated before discharge for secondary prevention and continued indefinitely in certain MI patients including those with HF, LVEF ≤40%, hypertension, diabetes, or chronic kidney disease.

An angiotensin II receptor blocker (ARB) should be administered to MI patients with HF, LVEF ≤40, or hypertension who are intolerant of ACE inhibitors.

Angiotensin converting enzyme inhibitor or ARB therapy should continue indefinitely. Careful blood pressure monitoring is required when using either agent.

Aldosterone Antagonists

Inpatient initiation of long-term aldosterone blockade (spironolactone or eplerenone) is recommended in post-MI patients with LVEF ≤40 and symptomatic HF and/or diabetes without significant renal dysfunction [serum creatinine ≤2.5 mg/dL (221 micromol/L) in men and ≤2.0 mg/dL (177 micromol/L) in women] or hyperkalemia who are already receiving therapeutic doses of ACE inhibitor.

MANAGEMENT OF LOW OUTPUT STATES

A low output state may manifest as hypotension or preserved blood pressure with evidence of hypoperfusion and is not always accompanied by pulmonary congestion. Recommended treatments include inotropic support, intra-aortic counterpulsation, revascularization, and surgical correction of mechanical complications (such as ventricular septal rupture or papillary muscle rupture).

Inotropic Agents

Patients with myocardial infarction (MI), pulmonary congestion, and marginal or low blood pressure often require circulatory support with inotropic and vasopressor agents and/or intra-aortic balloon counterpulsation to relieve pulmonary congestion and maintain adequate perfusion.

SUMMARY AND RECOMMENDATIONS

Patients with acute decompensated heart failure (ADHF) often have CAD with or without an ACS. Acute onset of myocardial ischemia with or without infarction can cause systolic and/or diastolic dysfunction, resulting in decreased cardiac output, elevated filling pressures, and/or the development of pulmonary edema.

- Urgent revascularization is a major component of therapy for patients presenting with STEMI and is particularly important for those with HF. Early revascularization is indicated for patients presenting with UA/NSTEMI and HF.
- Medical therapy of ADHF with ACS includes judicious use of diuretics, supplemental oxygen and ventilatory support as needed, and vasodilator therapy.
- Initiation of oral angiotensin converting enzyme inhibitor is recommended within the first 24 hours of an acute MI in patients with pulmonary congestion or an LVEF ≤40%. Beta-blocker therapy within the first 24 hours is generally recommended for patients presenting with MI but initiation should be deferred in patients with HF. Inpatient initiation of long-term aldosterone antagonist therapy is also recommended in selected patients.
- Patients with MI, pulmonary congestion, and marginal or low blood pressure often require circulatory support with inotropic and vasopressor agents and/or intra-aortic balloon counterpulsation to relieve pulmonary congestion and maintain adequate perfusion.
- In the setting of STEMI, dopamine is recommended in hypotensive patients with clinical evidence of shock and dobutamine is recommended in hypotensive patients without clinical evidence of shock.

CONCLUSION

Acute heart failure syndromes have emerged as a leading public health problem worldwide, accounting for a substantial number of hospitalizations and a high utilization of resources. A significant number of patients admitted with AHFS have CAD and can be divided into those who present with or without ACS. Both groups have high early after-discharge mortality and rehospitalization rates. Knowledge of the extent and severity of CAD and the presence of ischemic and/or stunned/hibernating myocardium may influence the initial and in-hospital management of these patients. Although specific guidelines exist for patients with ACS complicated by HF, prospective studies of the assessment and treatment of CAD in the setting of acute HF are urgently needed.

REFERENCES

1. Gheorghiade M, Zannad F, Sopko G, et al. International Working Group on Acute Heart Failure Syndromes. Acute heart failure syndromes: current state and framework for future research. Circulation. 2005;112(25):3958-68.
2. Solomon SD, Dobson J, Pocock S, et al. Candesartan in Heart failure: Assessment of Reduction in Mortality and morbidity (CHARM) Investigators. Influence of nonfatal hospitalization for heart failure on subsequent mortality in patients with chronic heart failure. Circulation. 2007;116(13):1482-7.
3. Ahmed A, Allman RM, Fonarow GC, et al. Incident heart failure hospitalization and subsequent mortality in chronic heart failure: a propensity-matched study. J Card Fail. 2008;14(3):211-8.
4. Jong P, Vowinckel E, Liu PP, et al. Prognosis and determinants of survival in patients newly hospitalized for heart failure: a population-based study. Arch Intern Med. 2002;162(15):1689-94.

5. Goldberg RJ, Ciampa J, Lessard D, et al. Long-term survival after heart failure: a contemporary population-based perspective. Arch Intern Med. 2007;167(5):490-6.
6. Rosamond W, Flegal K, Friday G. American Heart Association Statistics Committee and Stroke Statistics Subcommittee. et al. Heart disease and stroke statistics—2007 update: a report from the American Heart Association Statistics Committee and Stroke Statistics Subcommittee. Circulation. 2007;115(5):e69-171.
7. DeFrances CJ, Podgornik MN. 2004 National Hospital Discharge Survey. Adv Data. 2006;(371):1-19.
8. Roe MT, Chen AY, Riba AL, et al. CRUSADE Investigators. Impact of congestive heart failure in patients with non-ST-segment elevation acute coronary syndromes. Am J Cardiol. 2006;97(12):1707-12.
9. Khot UN, Jia G, Moliterno DJ, et al. Prognostic importance of physical examination for heart failure in non-ST-elevation acute coronary syndromes: the enduring value of Killip classification. JAMA. 2003;290(16):2174-81.
10. Steg PG, Dabbous OH, Feldman LJ, et al.; Global Registry of Acute Coronary Events Investigators. Determinants and prognostic impact of heart failure complicating acute coronary syndromes: observations from the Global Registry of Acute Coronary Events (GRACE). Circulation. 2004;109(4):494-9.
11. Di Chiara A, Fresco C, Savonitto S, et al. BLITZ-2 Investigators. Epidemiology of non-ST elevation acute coronary syndromes in the Italian cardiology network: the BLITZ-2 study. Eur Heart J. 2006;27(4):393-405.
12. Shibata MC, Collinson J, Taneja AK, et al. Long term prognosis of heart failure after acute coronary syndromes without ST elevation. Postgrad Med J. 2006;82(963):55-9.
13. Spencer FA, Meyer TE, Gore JM, et al. Heterogeneity in the management and outcomes of patients with acute myocardial infarction complicated by heart failure: the National Registry of Myocardial Infarction. Circulation. 2002;105(22):2605-10.
14. Nieminen MS, Brutsaert D, Dickstein K, et al. EuroHeart Survey Investigators, Heart Failure Association, European Society of Cardiology. EuroHeart Failure Survey II (EHFS II): a survey on hospitalized acute heart failure patients: description of population. Eur Heart J. 2006;27(22):2725-36.
15. Emanuelsson H, Karlson BW, Herlitz J. Characteristics and prognosis of patients with acute myocardial infarction in relation to occurrence of congestive heart failure. Eur Heart J. 1994;15(6):761-8.
16. O'Connor CM, Hathaway WR, Bates ER, et al. Clinical characteristics and long-term outcome of patients in whom congestive heart failure develops after thrombolytic therapy for acute myocardial infarction: development of a predictive model. Am Heart J. 1997;133(6):663-73.
17. Hasdai D, Topol EJ, Kilaru R, et al. Frequency, patient characteristics, and outcomes of mild-to-moderate heart failure complicating ST-segment elevation acute myocardial infarction: lessons from 4 international fibrinolytic therapy trials. Am Heart J. 2003;145(1):73-9.
18. Ali AS, Rybicki BA, Alam M, et al. Clinical predictors of heart failure in patients with first acute myocardial infarction. Am Heart J. 1999;138(6 Pt 1):1133-9.
19. Spencer FA, Meyer TE, Goldberg RJ, et al. Twenty year trends (1975-1995) in the incidence, in-hospital and long-term death rates associated with heart failure complicating acute myocardial infarction: a community-wide perspective. J Am Coll Cardiol. 1999;34(5):1378-87.
20. Wu AH, Parsons L, Every NR, et al. Second National Registry of Myocardial Infarction. Hospital outcomes in patients presenting with congestive heart failure complicating acute myocardial infarction: a report from the Second National Registry of Myocardial Infarction (NRMI-2). J Am Coll Cardiol. 2002;40(8):1389-94.
21. Segev A, Strauss BH, Tan M, et al. Canadian Acute Coronary Syndrome Registries Investigators. Prognostic significance of admission heart failure in patients with non-ST-elevation acute coronary syndromes (from the Canadian Acute Coronary Syndrome Registries). Am J Cardiol. 2006;98(4):470-3.
22. Haim M, Battler A, Behar S, et al. Acute coronary syndromes complicated by symptomatic and asymptomatic heart failure: does current treatment comply with guidelines? Am Heart J. 2004;147(5):859-64.
23. Torabi A, Cleland JG, Khan NK, et al. The timing of development and subsequent clinical course of heart failure after a myocardial infarction. Eur Heart J. 2008;29(7):859-70.
24. Cleland JG, Swedberg K, Follath F, et al. Study Group on Diagnosis of the Working Group on Heart Failure of the European Society of Cardiology. The EuroHeart Failure survey programme--a survey on the quality of care among patients with heart failure in Europe: Part 1: Patient characteristics and diagnosis. Eur Heart J. 2003;24(5):442-63.
25. Whellan DJ, Tuttle RH, Velazquez EJ, et al. Predicting significant coronary artery disease in patients with left ventricular dysfunction. Am Heart J. 2006;152(2):340-7.
26. Bart BA, Shaw LK, McCants CB Jr, et al. Clinical determinants of mortality in patients with angiographically diagnosed ischemic or nonischemic cardiomyopathy. J Am Coll Cardiol. 1997;30(4):1002-8.
27. Felker GM, Shaw LK, O'Connor CM. A standardized definition of ischemic cardiomyopathy for use in clinical research. J Am Coll Cardiol. 2002;39(2):210-8.
28. O'Connor CM, Gattis WA, Shaw L, et al. Clinical characteristics and long-term outcomes of patients with heart failure and preserved systolic function. Am J Cardiol. 2000;86(8):863-7.
29. Srichai MB, Jaber WA, Prior DL, et al. PURSUIT Investigators. Evaluating the benefits of glycoprotein IIb/IIIa inhibitors in heart failure at baseline in acute coronary syndromes. Am Heart J. 2004;147(1):84-90.
30. Lewis EF, Velazquez EJ, Solomon SD, et al. Predictors of the first heart failure hospitalization in patients who are stable survivors of myocardial infarction complicated by pulmonary congestion and/or left ventricular dysfunction: a VALIANT study. Eur Heart J. 2008;29(6):748-56.

31. Flaherty JD, Rossi JS, Davidson CJ, et al. OPTIMIZE-HF Investigators. Influence of coronary angiography on therapy utilization and survival in acute heart failure: A report from the OPTIMIZE-HF registry (abstr). Am J Cardiol. 2008;102(Suppl 1):25I.
32. Andreini D, Pontone G, Pepi M, et al. Diagnostic accuracy of multidetector computed tomography coronary angiography in patients with dilated cardiomyopathy. J Am Coll Cardiol. 2007;49(20):2044-50.
33. Shapiro MD, Butler J, Rieber J, et al. Analytic approaches to establish the diagnostic accuracy of coronary computed tomography angiography as a tool for clinical decision making. Am J Cardiol. 2007;99(8):1122-7.
34. Flaherty JD, Bax JJ, De Luca L, et al. Acute Heart Failure Syndromes International Working Group. Acute heart failure syndromes in patients with coronary artery disease early assessment and treatment. J Am Coll Cardiol. 2009;53(3):254-63.
35. Ibanez B, James S, Agewall S, et al. ESC Scientific Document Group. 2017 ESC Guidelines for the management of acute myocardial infarction in patients presenting with ST-segment elevation: The task force for the management of acute myocardial infarction in patients presenting with ST-segment elevation of the European Society of Cardiology (ESC). Eur Heart J. 2018;39(2):119-77.
36. Ponikowski P, Voors AA, Anker SD; Authors/Task Force Members, Document Reviewers, et al. 2016 ESC Guidelines for the diagnosis and treatment of acute and chronic heart failure: The task force for the diagnosis and treatment of acute and chronic heart failure of the European Society of Cardiology (ESC). Developed with the special contribution of the Heart Failure Association (HFA) of the ESC. Eur J of Heart Fail. 2016;18(8):891-975.

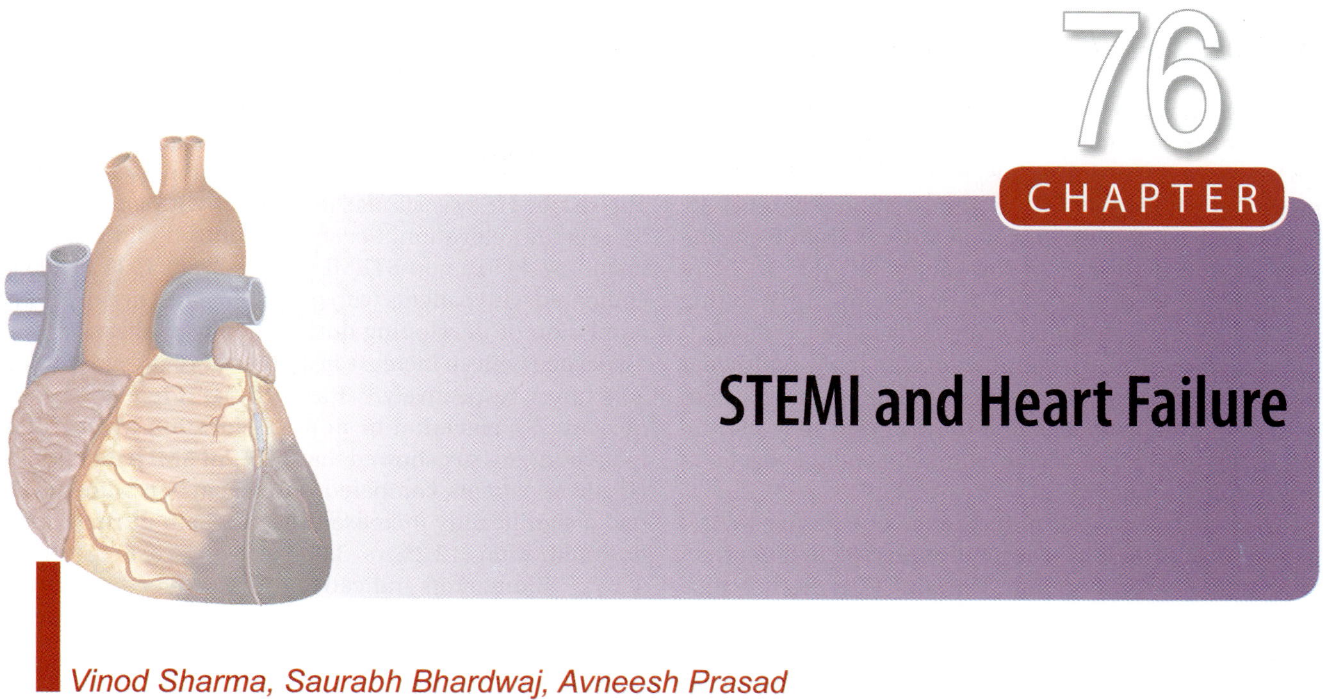

76

CHAPTER

STEMI and Heart Failure

Vinod Sharma, Saurabh Bhardwaj, Avneesh Prasad

The best physician for a patient with HF would be one with "*Excellent Training, Extensive Experience and Superb Judgment*" with regards to all aspect of disease. He or she "*would not necessarily follow guidelines slavishly*".

—*JN Cohn, Cir Heart Fail 2008*

HEART FAILURE—A MAJOR EPIDEMIC OF 21ST CENTURY

Heart failure (HF) complicating acute myocardial infarction (AMI) is common. Among patients with AMI, HF is the most powerful predictor of death[1] and it has important implications for treatment.

DEFINING HEART FAILURE AFTER MYOCARDIAL INFARCTION

Heart failure is defined as "a clinical syndrome resulting from any structural or functional cardiac disorder that impairs the ability of the ventricle to fill or eject blood".[2] The primary definition of HF as a clinical syndrome has led to differing clinical, imaging, and biomarker definitions coexisting in clinical practice and research. There is no "universal definition" and consequently, the diagnosis of HF is often heterogeneous between studies and over time.[3] Early studies of HF following myocardial infarction (MI) used clinical criteria such as the Killip and New York Heart Association (NYHA) classifications.[4,5] Though crude, Killip class has retained prognostic value in more recent cohorts such as the Global Registry of Acute Coronary Events (GRACE) registry: patients in Killip Class I had an in-hospital mortality of 3%, rising to 20% for those in class III.[6] The timing of HF following MI is important clinically, mechanistically and for research. Three key time periods need to be distinguished: HF at the index MI presentation, during the course of the first admission, and after discharge (Table 1).

TABLE 1: Three key time periods of HF following MI.

HF during index MI (A)	*HF during hospitalization (B)*	*Late HF*
• Myocyte necrosis • Myocardial stunning • Decompensation of preexisting HF • Acute mitral regurgitation due to PMD	A+ • Fluid or contrast overload • Renal dysfunction • VSD and cardiac tamponade	• Cardiomyocyte death • Scar formation • Ventricular remodeling

(HF: heart failure; MI: myocardial infarction; PMD: papillary muscle dysfunction; VSD: ventricular septal defect)

Incidence of Heart Failure Postmyocardial Infarction

Incidence of HF among patients hospitalized for an AMI varies among studies,[7] ranging from 14% to 36%. HF can be present on admission or develop during hospitalization. 4% presented with signs of HF on admission and another 39% developed HF during hospitalization.[8] In GRACE, 13% had HF on admission, and another 5.6% developed HF during the hospital stay.[6] Spencer et al.[9] found that 20.4% of patients presented with signs of HF, whereas another 8.6% developed HF during hospitalization. 12% of patients presented with signs of HF at admission and another 4% developed HF during hospitalization.[10] Data from the Cardiovascular Disease in Norway Project that 18.7% of the patients presented with HF or developed HF during hospitalization, and HF occurrence increased with age.[11] Comorbidities like atrial fibrillation with rapid ventricular rate and hypertensive emergency that often occurs in patients with normal ejection fraction (EF) may play an important role in both the development and management of HF complicating MI.

Data on the long-term incidence of HF after STEMI (ST-segment elevation myocardial infarction) in the current percutaneous coronary intervention (PCI) era is scarce and also historically varies among different studies. For example, in a recent nationwide Swedish Registry Study (SWEDEHEART), HF incidence during index hospitalization declined from 50% to 28% in the subgroup including STEMI patients between 1996 and 2008. Among others, this might indeed partly reflect the changes that occurred in the reperfusion treatment during the study period (from predominantly thrombolysis to predominantly primary PCI.[12] In comparison, in a Canadian cohort study, 13.6% of the STEMI patients were diagnosed with HF during index MI hospitalization with a 1-year cumulative HF incidence of 23.4% between 2002 and 2008.[13] In the same study, development of HF was associated with a 1-year mortality of 9.9% in the subset of STEMI patients.[13]

Prognosis

The prognostic significance of HF complicating MI has been assessed in many studies. In Canadian Acute Coronary Syndrome Registry enrolling 4,825 patients with non-STEMI, the presence of HF on admission increased the odds of in-hospital mortality by 1.87 times.[14] Observation from the GRACE revealed that HF on admission increased the odds of in-hospital mortality by 2.2 times among 13,707 patients enrolled in the GRACE registry.[6] In the GRACE risk score model, Killip class (Table 2) was found to be the most important predictor of mortality when compared with no HF; rales and/or S3 had two times, pulmonary edema three times, and cardiogenic shock four times the risk of death.[1] The risk of HF was similar in patients with and without ST-segment elevation. Seven randomized clinical trials including 46,519 non-STEMI patients from 1994 to 2008, compared with patients with no HF, the presence of HF on admission or developing during the hospitalization was associated with an increase in 30-day mortality of 1.74 and 2.34 times, respectively.[15] The FAST-MI (French Registry of Acute ST elevation or non-ST elevation Myocardial infarction) registry showed that 37.5% of AMI patients had HF; these patients, compared with MI patients without HF, had a significantly increased risk of death during index hospitalization (12.2% vs. 3.0%) and at 1 year (26.6% vs. 5.2%).[16] Biomarkers indicative of HF, B-type natriuretic peptide (BNP) and nonterminal pro-BNP, have also been shown to be strong independent predictors of risk.[17]

TABLE 2: Killip classification.

Class	Features	Hospital mortality rates (%)
1	No signs of HF	6
2	S3, rales, gallop, and radiographic HF	17
3	Pulmonary edema	38
4	Cardiogenic shock	81

(HF: heart failure)

Pathophysiology of Myocardial Infarction-induced Heart Failure

Heart failure manifests as an abnormality of the cardiac structure and/or function that impairs the heart to maintain adequate blood flux to peripheral tissues or to do it at the expense of increased filling pressures.[18] Several post-MI factors influence the appearance of left ventricular (LV) systolic dysfunction and reduced left ventricular ejection fraction (LVEF), thereby impairing cardiac function and structure. These factors include recurrent myocardial ischemia, infarct size, LV remodeling, myocardium mechanical complications, and hibernating myocardium (Flowchart 1).[19,20]

Several overlapping mechanisms contribute to HF after MI. HF during the index MI occurs due to a combination of myocardial stunning, myocyte necrosis, decompensation of preexisting HF or acute mitral regurgitation due to papillary muscle dysfunction. HF during the hospitalization may also be due to any of the above, compounded by fluid or contrast overload, renal dysfunction, or complications such as ventricular septal defect or cardiac tamponade. Late HF reflects the consequences of cardiomyocyte death and scar formation occurring alongside ventricular remodeling. Within 30 minutes of ischemia, cardiomyocyte structural changes and edema develop, leading to progressive cell death in 3 hours. Acute contractile dysfunction occurs due to oxidative stress and calcium overload, which is reversible if flow is restored.[21] Reperfusion itself causes a second wave of injury, by production of reactive oxygen species (ROS). Despite successful epicardial reperfusion, embolization of thrombotic debris, plugging by inflammatory cells, and release of vasoactive mediators from damaged endothelium

Flowchart 1: Factors contributing to heart failure in acute coronary syndromes. Loss of contractile tissue is the main determinant for heart failure after acute myocardial infarction. Other factors include diastolic dysfunction secondary to ischemia and edema, mechanical complications that impair the performance of the heart as a pump, stunning and hibernation, and activation of the neurohormonal system. Increase in left ventricular filling pressure and reduction in cardiac output are the main hemodynamic abnormalities responsible for symptoms of pulmonary congestion and hypoperfusion.

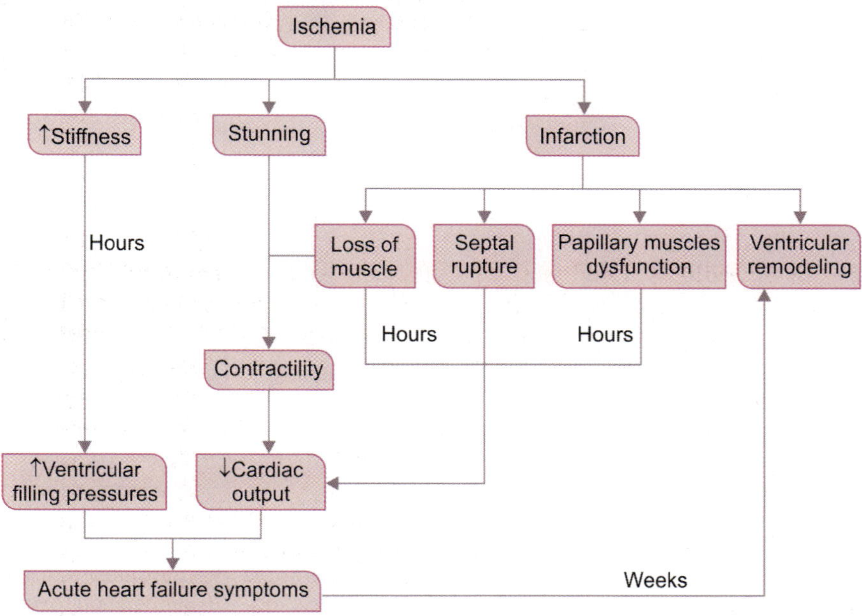

leads to ongoing microvascular dysfunction in up to 50% of patients.[22] Myocardial injury leads to activation of a stereotyped inflammatory cascade, comprised of early neutrophil ingress followed by monocyte-macrophage infiltration. Between 3 days and 5 days following MI, there is a transition from inflammation to repair, with activation of fibroblasts and progressive scar deposition (Fig. 1).[23]

Cardiovascular (CV) alterations due to MI before the establishment of HF can be divided into two periods: (1) an acute and beneficial compensatory phase that is followed by (2) a chronic maladaptive phase, in which compensatory mechanisms progressively contribute to the worsening of the disease.

Acute Compensatory Adaptations after Myocardial Infarction

Two main mechanisms are involved in the acute response of the body as it moves toward the establishment of hemodynamic homeostasis after MI: (1) the Frank–Starling mechanism and (2) the hyperactivation of neurohumoral systems. The Frank–Starling is an intrinsic mechanism of the heart that is activated in response to a decrease in cardiac output (CO). In the Frank–Starling mechanism, cardiac contractility changes according to tissue stretching and left ventricular end-diastolic volume (LVEDV).[24] Therefore, the heart responds with high contractile force rates when is stretched and with low contractile force rates when is either under- or overstretched. During an acute failure of cardiac pumping, the LVEF decreases abruptly drops the CO and increases the LVEDV. As a result, a higher LVEDV enhances the contractile force of the next systole and reestablishes the CO (Fig. 2).[24] Although the Frank–Starling mechanism acutely restores failed cardiac pumping, it is still insufficient to maintain CO over a long period. Therefore, other mechanisms must be activated to compensate CO for prolonged periods. Both the sympathetic nervous system (SNS) and the renin-angiotensin-aldosterone system (RAAS) are involved in this process.

The SNS is activated in response to the decreased systemic blood pressure (BP) and the subsequent stimulation of the baroreceptor complex.[25] SNS activation helps reestablish CO and BP by enhancing both cardiac contractility and peripheral resistance. The increase in contractile force is a consequence of cardiac cytosolic Ca^{2+} accumulation after continuous high-frequency depolarization (Treppe phenomenon).[26] By contrast, enhanced peripheral resistance is attained by the increase of both arterial and venous constriction. Vasoconstriction not only influences BP but also redistributes blood flow to vital organs and increases venous return and diastolic filling pressures.[27-29] Therefore, both the enhanced cardiac contractility status and peripheral resistance contribute to the acute stabilization of hemodynamic parameters after MI. Similar to the SNS, the RAAS also responds simultaneously to decreased CO and BP. However, the

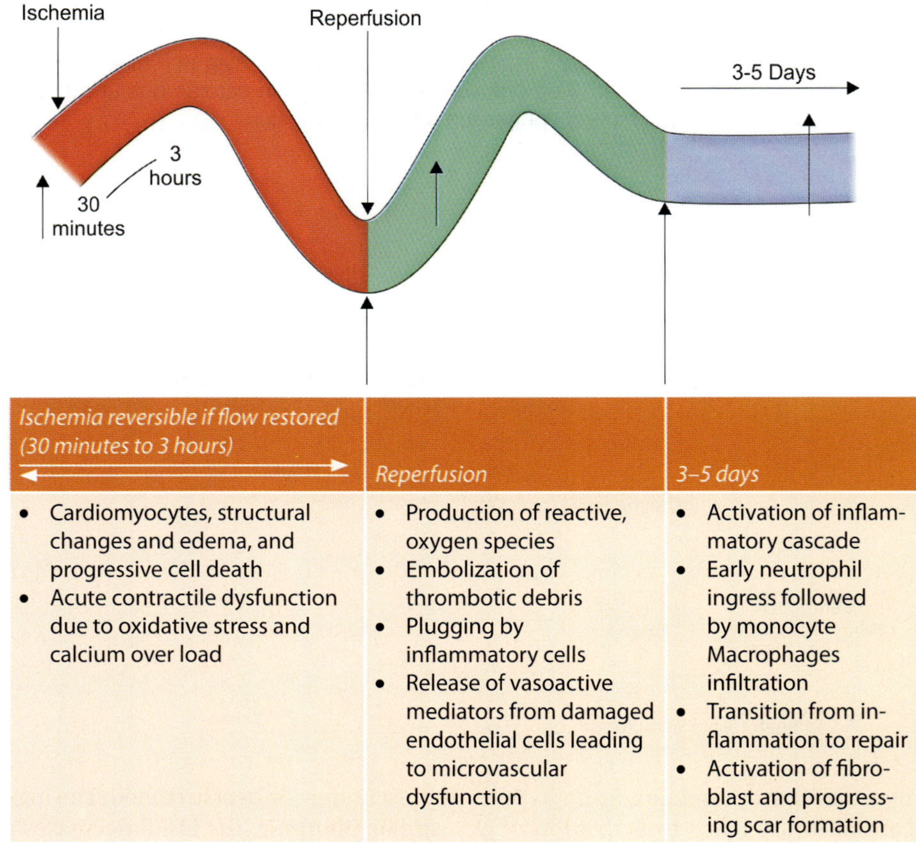

Fig. 1: Pathological basis of heart failure–Timeline.

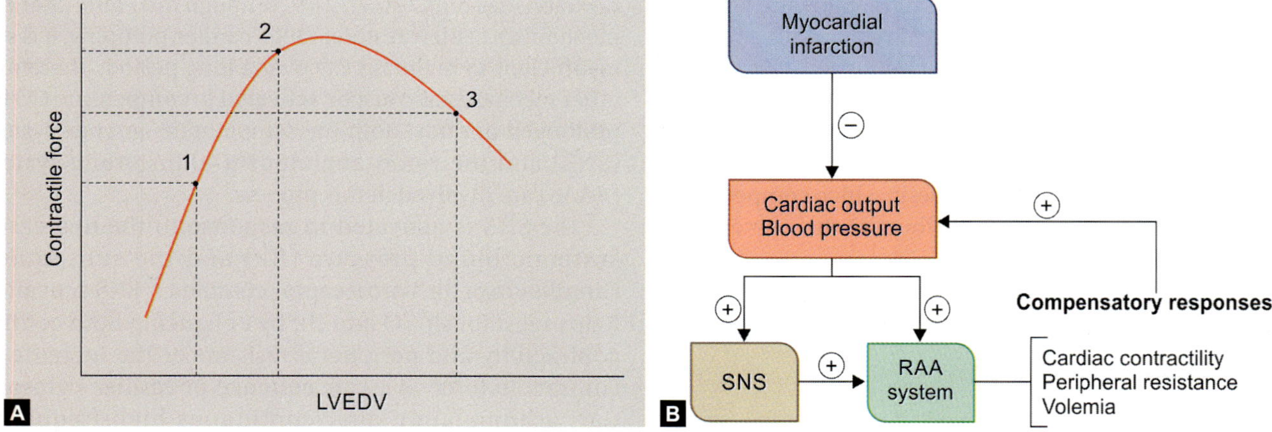

Figs. 2A and B: Representation of the acute responses of the cardiovascular system after myocardial infarction (MI). MI is characterized by the necrosis of the cardiac cells due to low oxygen supply as a consequence of the occlusion of coronary arteries, it reduces cardiac output (CO) and blood pressure (BP) and induces compensatory mechanisms that acutely rescue the hemodynamics from collapse. (A) It is a representation of the pressure × volume curve showing the Frank–Sterling mechanism. It states that cardiac contractility varies in the function of the left ventricular end-diastolic volume (LVEDV), so that when left ventricle (LV) stretches due to an increase of the LVEDV (point 1–2), the cardiac contractile force also increases. However, when the LV overstretches (point 2–3) cardiac contractility decreases. During an acute failure of cardiac pumping, left ventricular ejection fraction decreases abruptly, decreasing the CO and increasing the LVEDV. As a result, a higher LVEDV enhances the contractile force of the next systole and reestablishes the CO. (B) It represents the acute neurohumoral responses after MI. The sympathetic nervous system (SNS) and the renin-angiotensin-aldosterone system (RAAS) are activated in response to decrease in BP and CO. On the other hand, the SNS and RAAS increase cardiac contractility, peripheral resistance, and volemia, improving and reestablishing BP and CO.

response is slower than that observed after SNS activation because it involves the synthesis of effectors such as renin, angiotensin II (Ang II), and aldosterone and because its effects depend on the increase in mRNA and protein levels. The main response to the activation of the RAAS is an antidiuretic effect. The activation of the RAAS causes the retention of sodium (Na+) and water and increases volemia, assisting in the establishment of systemic BP levels.[30] In addition, Ang II induces vasoconstriction and blood redistribution and increases heart contractility.[31] On the other hand, the RAAS is directly modulated by the SNS, which further stimulates the release of renin from juxtaglomerular cells in the kidneys.[32,33] Both the SNS and RAAS act together to restore hemodynamic homeostasis and maintain the appropriate perfusion of vital organs for prolonged periods. Other paracrine factors and hormones also rescue acute CV function after MI, e.g. the antidiuretic hormone and endothelin; however, the SNS and the RAAS seem to have greater influence on this process.[34]

Chronic Compensatory Adaptation after Myocardial Infarction

The reduction in contractile cardiac mass after MI is irreversible, and mitosis-induced hyperplasia rarely occurs in differentiated cardiac cells.[28,35] To avoid failure of cardiac function and hemodynamic collapse, neurohumoral adaptive responses might be constantly activated to maintain adequate blood perfusion of the tissues. Chronic activation of these mechanisms is usually maladaptive and progressively converges to the global failure of the CV system and the development of HF.[23] Key mechanisms that trigger the progression of MI to HF are: (1) the hyperactivity of the SNS, with the subsequent and progressive desensitization of the β-adrenergic receptors, (2) the hyperactivity of the RAAS, (3) the development of an inflammatory process that culminates in the deposition of fibrotic tissue, (4) oxidative stress, (5) cardiac remodeling and dilated hypertrophy, (6) the modification of protein profiles and cardiac contractile dynamics, and (7) energetic substrate remodeling.[23,36-40]

Sympathetic Nervous System and Renin-angiotensin-aldosterone System Hyperactivity

Heart failure was known as a disease developed solely due to the impairment of the cardiac pump function, and its consequence was the congestion of the CV system.[28] More recently, CV research has challenged this knowledge and has demonstrated the involvement of neurohumoral activity in HF pathogenesis. Neurohumoral hyperactivation contributes to the development of HF in many ways.

One of the hallmarks of SNS hyperactivation is the loss of responsiveness to noradrenaline stimulus. Prolonged hyperactivity of the SNS leads to the desensitization of β1-adrenergic receptors and the reduction of β1-adrenergic receptor density in heart tissue, decreasing its activation and signaling.[41,42] The consequence is a decrease of the β1:β2 ratio and a reduction of cardiac force in response to sympathetic stimulation. This condition induces a harmful cycle, in which the sympathetic activity becomes more intense and further desensitizes more receptors.[43] Sustained stimulation of β-adrenergic receptors in the heart also activates signaling pathways related to protein expression patterns in the remaining cardiac cells.[44] These proteins are related to the modulation of the excitation–contraction coupling mechanism, Ca^{2+} handling and contractile processes, and the modifications of their expression progressively impairs the cardiac contractile status. Sustained SNS stimulus impairs cardiac contractility and further decreases CO. Finally, SNS hyperactivation also induces cardiac cell growth via the stimulation of mitogen-activated protein kinases (MAPKs) and calcineurin-nuclear factor of activated T-cells (calcineurin-NFAT) signaling pathways, leading to cardiac remodeling, and the development of dilated cardiac hypertrophy.

Chronic stimulation of molecular signaling via the RAAS, especially the stimulation of Ang II and aldosterone, produces similar effects to those of the β-adrenergic receptors.[45] After MI, cardiac angiotensin-converting enzyme (ACE) and mast cell produced chymase increase the local synthesis of Ang II, independent of renal renin.[45,46] Ang II has autocrine and paracrine effects on cardiac cells that after cardiac contractility and tissue remodeling, contributing to pathological heart hypertrophy.[47-52] Ang II activates the A1 receptor and the Gq-PKC-IP3/DAG (Gq-protein kinase C-inositol trisphosphate/diacylglycerol) signaling pathway. The activation of the Gq protein signaling pathway contributes to the development of pathological myocardial hypertrophy. Ang II also increases the synthesis of ROS, inflammatory cytokines, and collagen, further influencing the development of cardiac fibrosis and remodeling aldosterone has similar effects.[53-55]

The systemic consequences of chronic neurohumoral activation are increased end-diastolic LV pressure, LV wall stress, and the impairment of LV filling during diastole due to prolonged vasoconstriction.[56] Cardiac O_2 consumption also increases in response to elevated LV wall stress and overloads the CV system. These alterations impair cardiac pumping and LVEF. On the other hand, prolonged water retention induces edema and increases plasma Na+ levels in patients without dietary salt restriction. In more severe cases, the congestion can cause pulmonary edema.[57,58] Volume overload also contributes to the dilation of the LV chamber and dilated hypertrophy. Collectively, increased filling pressures, decreased CO, and dilated cardiac hypertrophy progressively result in the main symptoms of HF: weakness, dyspnea, fatigue, and exercise intolerance.[59,60]

INFLAMMATORY PROCESS, OXIDATIVE STRESS, AND CARDIAC REMODELING

After MI, the loss of cardiac cells must be compensated for by the deposition of scar tissue to maintain the integrity of the LV chamber. This is obtained by the activation of inflammatory and reparative responses that culminate in collagen deposition and the development of fibrosis. The first phase of cardiac tissue repair involves the activation of the innate immune response and the infiltration of leukocytes. On the other hand, the infiltration of immune cells clears matrix debris and dead cells from the infarct site. Second phase is marked by a reduction of the inflammatory activity and increase in the synthesis of growth factors and the activation/differentiation of mesenchymal cells into myofibroblasts. In turn, the secretion of extracellular matrix proteins by myofibroblasts repairs the infarct tissue, thereby preserving the structural integrity of the infracted heart. These fibrosis deposition is essential for the repair of cardiac tissue; however, it also compromises contractility, as it increases heart stiffness and impairs tissue elasticity. Both cardiac contraction and relaxation processes depend on the potential energy accumulated during systole and diastole, and fibrosis reduces this energy, contributing to the impairment of cardiac contractility.[28,61] Increased cardiac stiffness also enhances LV chamber wall stress. In contrast, the elevation of wall stress, filling pressures, and volume overload induce a pattern of dilated cardiac hypertrophy that is marked by LV wall thinning due to the deposition of sarcomeres arranged in series[61] and the enlargement of the LV. Dilated cardiac hypertrophy is thought to be regulated by cytoskeletal proteins, such as cadherins, integrins, and adhesion molecules (Fig. 3).[28,62-65]

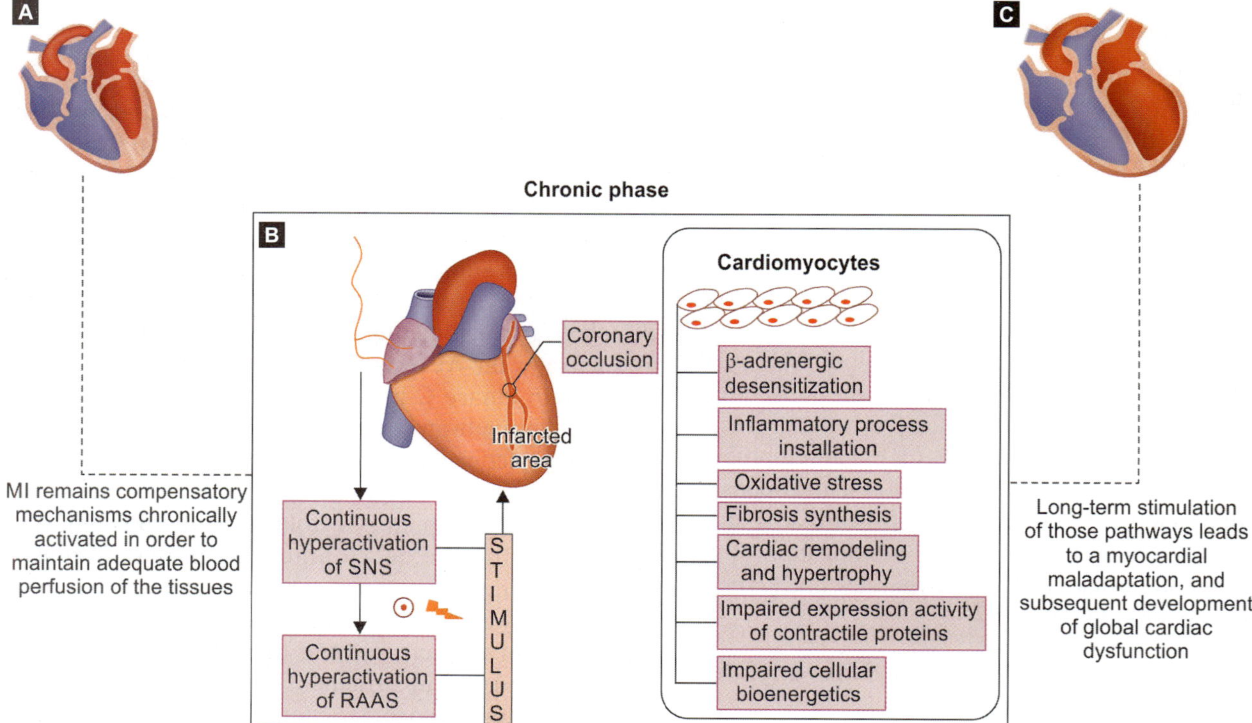

Figs. 3A to C: Chronic events after myocardial infarction (MI) and the subsequent progression to heart failure: (A) The normal heart is able to pump enough blood for the systemic circulation due to its regular ejection fraction; (B) MI chronically triggers the activation of both the sympathetic nervous system (SNS) and the renin-angiotensin-aldosterone system (RAAS) in order to maintain adequate blood tissue perfusion, and this leads to a harmful circle, wherein those factors are responsible for the development of global cardiac dysfunction through the desensitization of cardiomyocytes to adrenergic stimulus, myocardial inflammation, oxidative stress, the exacerbated synthesis of growth factors with subsequent remodeling and left ventricular hypertrophy, the impaired expression/activity of contractile proteins, and further debilitated cellular bioenergetics; (C) Chronically, the myocardium becomes weak and the heart cannot pump enough blood for the systemic circulation, an event called MI-induced heart failure.

Modification of Protein Profiles and Cardiac Contractile Dynamics

Myocardial infarction promotes qualitative and quantitative changes in the expression and activity of cardiac proteins involved in the systolic and diastolic processes. Mackiewicz et al.[66] observed the reduction in the expression/activity of SERCA2a (sarcoplasmic/endoplasmic reticulum Ca2+ ATPase 2a), with the concomitant increase in LV filling pressure 4 weeks after MI in rats. SERCA2a activity is responsible for sarcoplasmic reticulum (SR) Ca^{2+} uptake and the relaxation of heart tissue. Reduction of its expression/activity increases relaxation times and contributes to the enhancement of the end-diastolic pressure and to the reduction of LV filling (diastolic dysfunction). This process represents a progressive disorder of hemodynamics, which aggravates the symptoms of HF.[67] Expression of plasma membrane Ca^{2+} adenosine triphosphatase (ATPase) [plasma membrane Ca2+ ATPase (PMCA)] is also reduced after MI.[66] In the SR, Ca^{2+} uptake and extrusion are reduced by SERCA and PMCA, respectively. These alterations increase the cytosolic Ca^{2+} levels and intensify the operation of the Na^+/Ca^{2+} exchanger.[68] In addition, cardiac remodeling damages the excitation–contraction coupling process.

The fetal gene program is reactivated during HF development with the expression of genes that are normally only active during the fetal and postnatal periods.[69] One consequence of this reprogramming is the expression of the alpha-cardiac myosin heavy chain (α-MHC) isoform, which is associated with low ATPase activity, and the downregulation of the β-MHC isoform, which is associated with high ATPase activity.[70] This change in protein expression patterns seems to be highly relevant in humans, as the predominant isoform for this species is α-MHC.

The reactivation of the fetal gene program after MI leads to the synthesis of atrial and brain natriuretic peptides (ANP and BNP, respectively). This synthesis is speculated to occur as a compensatory mechanism to limit the infarct area, given that ANP and BNP induce vasodilation and decrease cardiac work.[71] Consistent with this hypothesis, the serum concentrations of ANP and BNP are significantly correlated with the extent of ischemic injury. ANP and BNP are considered markers of MI and progressive HF.[72,73] In addition to their effects on the vascular bed, both peptides have direct natriuretic effects. They reduce Na^+ and water reuptake in the distal nephrons. These peptides indirectly inhibit aldosterone synthesis in the adrenal zona glomerulosa cells by reducing sympathetic stimulation and releasing antidiuretic hormones from the pituitary gland. BNP mimetics, such as nesiritide, improve hemodynamic function in patients with decompensated HF.[74,75]

Energetic Substrate Remodeling

Energy substrates suffer alteration after MI and might be implicated in the pathogenesis of HF. The normal heart usually oxidizes fatty acids rather than glucose and other energy sources such as lactate to synthesize adenosine triphosphate (ATP). After MI, a change toward glucose and lactate utilization with a decrease in lipid oxidation has been observed. Glucose oxidation is more efficient than fatty acid utilization; therefore the changes are considered a compensatory mechanism to benefit cardiac performance.[76] However, as HF progresses, an uncoupling between glycolysis and oxidation occurs in cardiac cells.[38] This leads to a further decrease in ATP synthesis and the accumulation of protons as lactate is synthesized.[76] At the same time, there is a severe uncoupling of mitochondrial function, leading to ROS accumulation and a decrease in ATP synthesis. The shuttle systems also collapse, and energy transfer becomes impaired, with reductions in creatine phosphate and ATP levels in the latest phases of HF.[77] These alterations, in turn, may be linked to the reduction of contractile force and cardiac performance, contributing to the pathogenesis of HF.[38]

DIABETES AND HEART FAILURE IN THE POSTMYOCARDIAL INFARCTION PATIENTS: DANGEROUS INTERSECTION

Although a variety of clinical risk factors have been associated with the development of HF in the acute and more chronic phase following MI, multiple studies have consistently demonstrated that diabetes is a powerful risk factor for the development of HF in this setting. Importantly, the presence of diabetes in those who develop HF after MI is associated with increased risk of death. Given the increasing prevalence of diabetes, this dangerous intersection of diabetes and HF post-MI has significant health implications.

In those patients who develop HF early post-MI, the prevalence of diabetes is approximately 22–30% and is higher than in those individuals who do not develop HF.[6,78-80] Using multivariable analyses to adjust for comorbidities, the presence of diabetes is associated with an approximately 30% increased risk of developing HF early after MI compared with those without diabetes.[6,78,79]

In stable survivors of remote MI without previous HF symptoms, diabetes was associated with a 42% increased risk of developing HF compared with those without diabetes.[81] Similarly, in stable patients with reduced LVEF following acute MI, the risk of developing symptomatic HF, after adjusting for comorbidities, was 65% greater

Flowchart 2: Potential mechanisms leading to increased heart failure in patients with diabetes postmyocardial infarction.

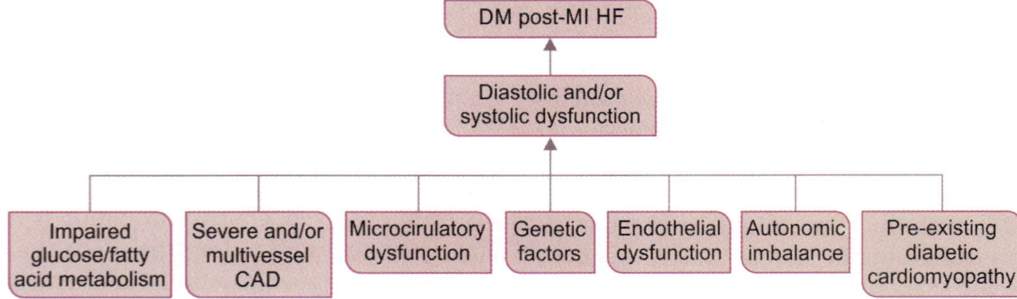

in those patients with diabetes compared with those without diabetes over a follow up period of 3–5 years.[82] Additionally, in the SOLVD (Studies of Left Ventricular Dysfunction) Prevention Study, the presence of diabetes in patients with ischemic cardiomyopathy was associated with an approximately 50% increased risk of transitioning from asymptomatic LV dysfunction to symptomatic HF compared with patients with ischemic cardiomyopathy without diabetes.[83]

Patients with diabetes and post-MI HF represent a high risk group. In a sub-study of the VALIANT (Valsartan in Acute Myocardial Infarction) trial, the presence of diabetes in patients presenting with an acute MI complicated by clinical signs and symptoms of HF and/or LV dysfunction was associated with a 40% to 50% increased risk of death in the first year following MI when compared with patients without diabetes, a finding that was present in those with both previously diagnosed and newly diagnosed diabetes.[84] Similarly, in the SAVE (Survival and Ventricular Enlargement) trial of stable survivors of acute MI with reduced LV systolic function, the presence of diabetes was associated with an approximately 40% higher total mortality and 50% more adverse CV events over a follow up period of 3.5 years, even after adjusting for differences in comorbidities.[82] The impact of HF in patients with diabetes presenting with MI was highlighted in DIGAMI (Diabetes Mellitus Insulin-Glucose Infusion in Acute Myocardial Infarction), a study of diabetic patients presenting with acute MI.[85] In DIGAMI, HF accounted for 66% of total mortality during the first year following acute MI. Because of these adverse outcomes, efforts to understand the pathophysiology and appropriate treatment are critical.

Potential Mechanisms Leading to Increased Heart Failure in Patients with Diabetes Following Myocardial Infarction

Potential explanations for the interaction between diabetes and the development of post-MI HF include increased comorbidities, more severe atherosclerosis, impaired endothelial and microvascular dysfunction, greater diastolic dysfunction, alterations in myocardial metabolism, dysregulation of the autonomic nervous system, and, potentially, genetic factors (Flowchart 2).

Previous studies have demonstrated more diffuse and severe coronary artery disease in diabetic patients than nondiabetic patients presenting with acute MI.[86-88] Despite these angiographic findings, clinical infarct size, as measured by creatinine kinase,[87,89] and LVEF[86,88,89] are similar in those patients with and without diabetes in the acute MI setting. In addition, infarct-related coronary artery patency rate following thrombolysis[86,88] and PCI[90] for treatment of acute MI is also similar in those with and without diabetes. These findings support the notion that the increased incidence of post-MI HF in diabetic patients is not due to larger infarct size, lower LVEF, or reduced infarct artery patency. Despite similar infarct-related coronary artery patency rates between those patients with and without diabetes, recent data have demonstrated that microvascular perfusion following reperfusion therapy is diminished in diabetic patients which may lead to worse outcomes.[90] Also despite similar LVEF in the acute MI period, reduced regional function in the noninfarct zone has been demonstrated, which may contribute to more HF.[86,88] This reduced noninfarct zone function is likely multifactorial, resulting from concomitant coronary artery disease, microvascular and endothelial dysfunction, and/or abnormalities of relaxation/compliance.

Perhaps more importantly than abnormalities of LV systolic function, diastolic dysfunction appears to be playing a significant role in the development of HF both in the acute and more chronic phase following MI. Multiple studies have suggested that diabetes is associated with a cardiomyopathy independent from associated hypertension and coronary artery disease.[91,92] Several causative mechanisms for this cardiomyopathy have been postulated including microangiopathy, metabolic disturbances, myocardial fibrosis, autonomic neuropathy, and insulin resistance. The phenotype of diabetic cardiomyopathy is often characterized by significant abnormalities of diastolic function.[91,92] Acute MI period, the similar LVEF, and infarct size suggest that abnormalities in compliance of the noninfarct myocardium is playing a significant role in the greater burden of HF in the acute setting. Similarly, more long-term studies demonstrate that despite a two- to threefold increase in the crude incidence of HF 4 months to 5 years following MI, LV systolic function is similar in those with and without diabetes.[89,93,94] In addition, the adverse remodeling that has been implicated in the development of post-MI HF[95] does not appear to be an independent predictor of the development of HF in the diabetic patient[94] as studies have shown that LV enlargement is not greater[93] and perhaps less[94] in diabetic patients than nondiabetic patients following MI. Echocardiographic analyses 6 months following acute MI have shown higher chamber stiffness (using mitral inflow velocities, tissue Doppler imaging, and color M-Mode propagation velocity.[93] In whole, these studies suggest that diastolic dysfunction plays a significant role in the development of HF in the post-MI diabetic patient.

Diabetes and post-MI HF may also result from the adverse effects of diabetes on cardiac energy metabolism. Although the normal heart can rapidly switch its energy substrate in the setting of different physiologic or patholophysiologic conditions, fatty acid oxidation accounts for approximately 70% of energy production under normal conditions. Under hypoxic periods, such as ischemia, the normal heart shifts energy metabolism to glucose, which requires less oxygen consumption. Diabetes is characterized by a profound reliance on fatty acids and suppression of cardiac glucose utilization.[96,97] Emerging data have suggested that this perturbed cardiac energy metabolism may play a role in the development of myocardial dysfunction both in the acute setting and more long-term setting following MI. Acutely, the diminished ability of the diabetic heart to switch from fatty acid oxidation to glucose oxidation leads to inefficient ATP production, generation of oxygen free radicals, and alterations in calcium metabolism which adversely affect the heart. Additionally, long-term reliance on fatty acid oxidation may potentially lead to adverse cardiac function via direct effects of lipids or fatty acid moieties on myocyte function (lipotoxicity) or activation of signaling pathways or gene transcription that leads to myocyte hypertrophy and/or dysfunction.[97,98] Peroxisome proliferator-activated receptor (PPAR) α, a nuclear receptor transcription factor involved in the control of genes involved in cardiac fatty acid uptake and oxidation, produces metabolic cardiac derangements similar to the diabetic heart and structural changes of cardiac hypertrophy and LV dysfunction.[99]

Other potential mechanisms for a greater degree of HF include increased markers of inflammation and alterations of the SNS. Recent data suggest that patients with type 2 diabetes have more elevated markers of inflammation, including tumor necrosis factor-α several months following MI.[100] Additionally, although circulation (systemic) renin-angiotensin system is suppressed in diabetic patients, tissue levels may be activated which may worsen outcomes.[101] Abnormalities of the SNS, including blunted sympathetic response in diabetic patients with decompensated HF, may also contribute to the higher incidence of HF in diabetic patients following MI.[102]

Genetic factors may also be playing a role in the development of post-MI HF in the diabetic patient. An example of one such genetic factor appears to be a functional allelic polymorphism in the haptoglobin (Hp) gene. A recent study has showed that diabetic patients who are homozygous for the Hp 1 allele (Hp 1-1) were at markedly reduced risk of death or development of HF at 30 days.[103] It has been proposed that the protection may be in part due to greater antioxidant properties conferred by the Hp 1-1 protein products.

CARDIAC BIOMARKERS AND HEART FAILURE

Despite significant overlaps, biomarkers can be loosely arranged into the following categories: (1) myocardial stress/injury, (2) neurohormonal activation, (3) remodeling, and (4) comorbidities (Table 3 and Fig. 4).

Myocardial Stress/Injury

B-type natriuretic peptide and N-terminal pro-brain natriuretic peptide (NT-proBNP) are considered the benchmarks against which other biomarkers are compared.

B-type Natriuretic Peptide and N-terminal Pro-brain Natriuretic Peptide

The most potent inducer of BNP gene transcription is LV wall stretch from increased pressure or volume. A prohormone (proBNP) is cleaved to BNP and NT-proBNP, resulting in a serologic evidence of BNP, NT-proBNP, and proBNP.

Stimulation of the natriuretic peptide (NP) receptor by BNP triggers natriuresis, diuresis, vasodilation, inhibition of renin and aldosterone, and inhibition of fibrosis. BNP is removed from circulation by a receptor-mediated mechanism as well as degradation by neutral endopeptidases such as neprilysin. Importantly, administration of LCZ696 significantly increases BNP (but not NT-proBNP) values as part of the effect of the drug. Therefore, interpretation of BNP in a patient taking LCZ696 will be challenging, if not impossible. Beyond these modes of clearance, both

TABLE 3: Biomarkers in heart failure.

Myocardial insult	*Neurohormonal activation*
• Myocyte stretch: – NT-proBNP, BNP, and MR-proANP • Myocardial injury: – Troponin T, troponin I, myosin light-chain I, heart-type fatty-acid protein, and CKMB • Oxidative stress: – Myeloperoxidase, uric acid, oxidized low-density lipoproteins, urinary biopyrrins, urinary and plasma isoprostanes, and plasma malondialdehyde	• Renin angiotensin system: – Renin, angiotensin II, and aldosterone • Sympathetic nervous system: – Norepinephrine, Chromogranin A, and MR-proADM • Arginine vasopressin system: – Arginine vasopressin and copeptin • Endothelins: – ET-1 and big proET-1
Remodeling	*Comorbidities*
• Inflammation: – C-reactive protein, TNF-α, soluble TNF receptors, Fas, interleukins (1, 6, and 18), osteoprotegerin, and adiponectin • Hypertrophy/ Fibrosis: – Matrix metalloproteinases, collagen propeptides, galectin-3, soluble ST2 • Apoptosis: – GDF-15 • Miscellaneous: – MicroRNA, quiescin Q6, and VEGFR-1	• Renal biomarkers: – Renal function: ◆ Creatinine, BUN, eGFR, cystatin C, and β-trace protein – Renal injury markers: ◆ NGAL, KIM-1, NAG, liver-type fatty acid binding protein, and IL-18 – Hematologic biomarkers: ◆ Hemoglobin, RDW, and iron deficiency (ferritin and transferring sat) – Liver function tests – Albumin

(NT-proBNP: N-terminal pro-brain natriuretic peptide; BNP: B-type natriuretic peptide; MR-proANP: mid-regional pro-atrial natriuretic peptide; CKMB: creatine kinase-MB; TNF: tumor necrosis factor; BUN: blood urea nitrogen; eGFR: estimated glomerular filtration rate; NGAL: neutrophil gelatinase-associated lipocalin; KIM-1: kidney injury molecule-1; NAG: N-acetyl-β-D-glucosaminidase; IL: interleukin; RDW: red cell distribution width; GDF: growth differentiation factor; VEGFR: vascular endothelial growth factor receptor)

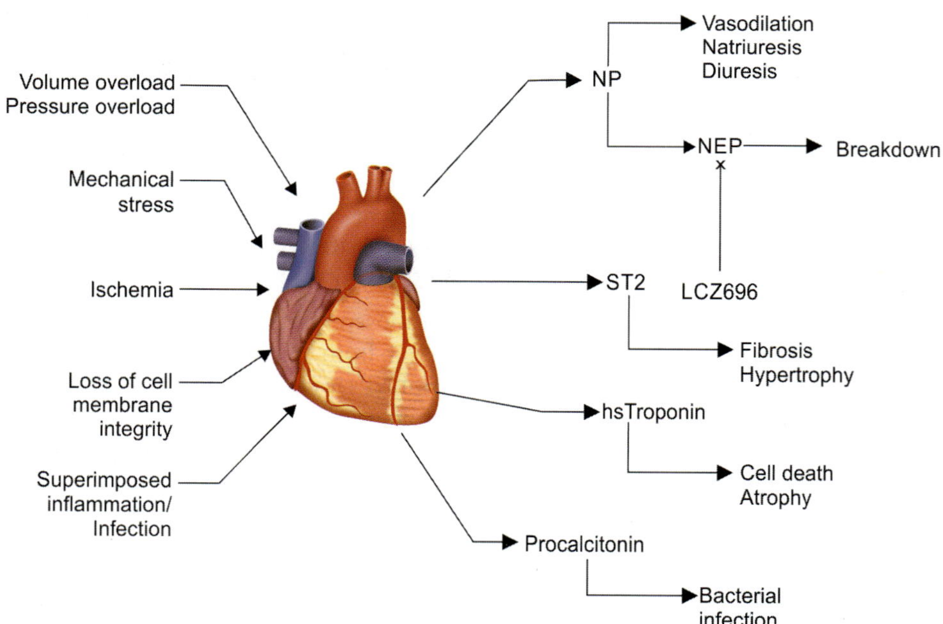

Fig. 4: Pathophysiologic factors leading to alterations in levels of biomarkers used in the assessment and management of heart failure. Note procalcitonin is not actually released from the heart, while natriuretic peptides, ST2, and high sensitivity troponin are released from the heart.
(NEP: neutral endopeptidase)

BNP and NT-proBNP are passively cleared by a number of organs including kidneys. The half-life of BNP is significantly shorter than that of NT-proBNP (approximately 20 vs. 60–120 minutes).

Diagnostic Evaluation of Acute Heart Failure (Table 4)

Normally, circulating BNP and NT-proBNP levels are quite low, but in the setting of HF, their concentrations rise dramatically. The Breathing Not Properly Multinational Study[104] demonstrated that BNP values >100 pg/mL diagnosed acute HF with high accuracy at 85% and strongly predicted of HF, outperforming clinical criteria. Similar findings were seen for NT-proBNP in the proBNP investigation of Dyspnea in the Emergency Department (PRIDE) Study[105] in which elevated NT-proBNP concentrations were the strongest predictor of HF compared with traditional assessment. A single NT-proBNP cutoff of 900 pg/mL provided similar diagnostic performance as BNP of 100 pg/mL, but age-stratified cutoff points for NT-proBNP (≥450 for ages <50 years, ≥900 for 50–75 years, and ≥1,800 pg/mL for >75 years) performed the best.[106] The best diagnostic approach for use of either BNP or NT-proBNP is to support clinical judgment. Both biomarkers are particularly useful when diagnostic indecision is present.

Caveats of Natriuretic Peptides

Beyond "HF", a number of cardiopulmonary disorders are associated with elevated BNP or NT-proBNP values: acute coronary syndrome (ACS), myocarditis, valvular heart disease, hypertrophic cardiomyopathy, cardiotoxic drugs, atrial fibrillation or flutter, and right ventricular dysfunction in the setting of significant pulmonary disease (pulmonary hypertension and pulmonary embolism), and many comorbidities such as advanced age, renal dysfunction, stroke, and critical illness also, and high output states. Lastly, use of neprilysin inhibitors (such as that within LCZ696) leads to pharmacologic "raising" of BNP values, notably these drugs do not affect NT-proBNP levels. When neprilysin inhibition becomes more widespread, the ability to interpret BNP will be substantially challenged in those patients so treated. Some conditions are associated with lower than expected NP levels: heart failure with preserved ejection fraction (HFpEF) compared with heart failure with reduced ejection fraction (HFrEF) and obesity. Obesity has been associated with lower than expected BNP or NT-proBNP values, likely due to the suppression of NP synthesis or release.

TABLE 4: Confounders of NP interpretation.

High NP levels than expected	*Lower NP levels than expected*
Increasing age* ACS* Renal insufficiency RV dysfunction* Atrial fibrillation Pulmonary hypertension* Pulmonary embolism* Anemia/high output states* Sepsis Mitral regurgitation*	Obesity Flash pulmonary edema Pericarditis/tamponade Genetic polymorphisms "Burned-out" cardiomyopathy

*Delineates likely elevation from ventricular stretch

(NP: natriuretic peptide)

Prognosis and Treatment of Heart Failure

B-type natriuretic peptide and NT-proBNP were strong predictors of clinical outcomes in all stages of HF in the Acute Decompensated Heart Failure National Registry (ADHERE).[107] Admission BNP values for acute HF decompensation in the highest quartile (BNP ≥1,730 pg/mL) was associated with 2.23-fold increase in in-hospital mortality compared with BNP in the lowest quartile (<430 pg/mL), even after adjustment for potential confounders and regardless of EF. NT-proBNP concentrations are strongly predictive of short- and long-term clinical outcomes; admission NT-proBNP >986 pg/mL was associated with almost threefold increase in 1 year mortality (adjusted hazard ratio 2.88).[106,108] Importantly, both absolute NP concentrations at discharge as well as percent change from admission to discharge provide substantially greater information regarding risk for subsequent mortality and/or rehospitalization than admission values. In the organized program to initiate lifesaving treatment in hospitalized patients with Heart Failure (OPTIMIZE-HF) trail,[109] the discharge (rather than admission) BNP was the most important predictor of 1-year mortality [hazard ratio (HR) of 1.34] and 1-year death or rehospitalization (HR 1.15). This suggests a strategy of admission/discharge level should be incorporated in routine care. Serial measurement in chronic HF patients also strongly predicts prognosis (Table 5).

Troponins

Beyond their ability to diagnose MI, troponin T (TnT) and I (TnI) are frequently detectable in HF.[110] In the ADHERE

TABLE 5: Measuring NP levels during hospitalization.

When to measure	*Reason to measure*
• After several days of treatment • In anticipation of discharge • At discharge	• Is the "wet NP" level dropping? (like following WBC for an infection) • Has the "euvolemic" NP been achieved? • Used as a basis to judge future decompensation or therapy titration

(NP: natriuretic peptide; WBC: white blood cell)

Registry,[111] 6.2% of patients with acute decompensated HF had an elevated troponin (as defined by conventional troponin assays as ≥1.0 μg/L for troponin I or ≥0.1 μg/L for troponin T), which was associated with worse in-hospital mortality. Using high sensitivity (hs) troponin assays, substantially more patients with acutely decompensated HF had abnormal concentrations.[112] Elevated hsTnT was independently predictive of all-cause mortality in a multivariable model including NT-proBNP as well as ST2 (HR = 1.16). As acute decompensation of HF may be a part of the presentation of acute MI, guidelines from major societies recommend troponin measurement in all patients presenting acutely, in order to exclude or diagnose ischemia as a cause.[113]

In patients with chronic HF, 92% of patients were found to have measurable or elevated hsTnT (detection limit ≤0.001 ng/mL)[114] and hsTnT >0.012 ng/mL was closely linked with poor clinical outcomes (adjusted HR = 2.08 for mortality and adjusted HR = 1.55 for first HF hospitalization). Serial measurement may add to a baseline value; in a large cohort of chronic HF patients,[114] increase in hsTnT over 3 or 4 months was strongly predictive of all-cause mortality (HR 1.88 after adjustment for traditional risk factors, baseline hsTnT, and baseline NT-proBNP).

Neurohormonal Activation

Cardiac injury leads to the activation of a number of biologically active proteins that attempts to compensate for reduced MI.

Mid-regional Proadrenomedullin

One of the first responses to cardiac dysfunction is the activation of the SNS. Mid-regional proadrenomedullin (MR-proADM) is a precursor to a potent vasodilator with inotropic properties, adrenomedullin, originally isolated from pheochromocytoma cells. MR-proADM is elevated in patients with acute and chronic HF and is a strong predictor of clinical outcomes such as mortality and HF hospitalization, even when added to BNP or NT-proBNP.[115-117]

Copeptin

Copeptin is a stable C-terminal propeptide fragment of arginine vasopressin (AVP); AVP is centrally involved in the regulation of free water clearance and plasma osmolality by regulating absorption of water from the kidneys. In the Biomarkers in acute Heart Failure (BACH) trial,[118] elevated copeptin level strongly predicted mortality, and in those with hyponatremia, elevated copeptin level was more predictive, even after adjusting for NT-proBNP and traditional variables.

Markers of Myocardial Remodeling

Myocardial remodeling is the pivotal process leading to progressive myocardial dysfunction and risk in HF. While BNP, NT-proBNP and hsTn are all also linked to remodeling risk, other biomarkers are worth mentioning.

ST2

ST2 gene is strongly induced in the setting of cardiomyocyte or cardiac fibroblasts stretch. ST2 is closely involved in LV hypertrophy, fibrosis, and remodeling via its interaction with interleukin (IL)-33, a protein with antifibrotic and antiremodeling properties.[119] Increasing ST2 concentrations are powerfully associated with adverse clinical outcomes in HF, compared with BNP or NT-proBNP, ST2 is not affected by age, renal function or BMI (Fig. 5).

In a multivariable model that included traditional markers of risk in acute HF patients, ST2 had independent and additive prognostic information beyond NT-proBNP (HR = 9.3) regardless of LVEF.[120] In addition, serial measurement of ST2 after acute HF therapy provided incremental information beyond a single value, and was superior to that provided by NT-proBNP.[121] In a multimarker panel, ST2 value was one of the strongest predictors of mortality at 30 days and 1-year in a reclassification analysis,[122] and was associated with more than threefold risk in adverse outcomes. Its ability to predict long-term outcomes appeared to be similar to that of NT-proBNP in chronic HF patients. In head-to-head studies, ST2 is often the most powerful biomarker predictor of risk. ST2 was recently shown to be superior to galectin-3 in patients with chronic HF.[123] ST2 can change significantly over time and serial measurement of ST2 adds independent and additive information to the baseline value and traditional risk factors in chronic HF if a rise and/or fall around the cut-off of 35 ng/mL is seen.[124] ST2 levels may interact with specific HF therapies. Beta-blockers, angiotensin II receptor antagonists, and mineralocorticoid receptor antagonists (MRAs) may influence ST2 values, opening the door for the possibility of guided HF therapy using serial measurement.[125-127] Large, prospective trials are needed to evaluate this further. In lower risk populations, those with acute MI[128] or in healthy community-based population,[129] elevated ST2 predicted future development of HF even after adjusting for traditional and novel markers of risk.

Soluble ST2 (sST2) is associated with adverse outcomes in HF, MI, pulmonary disease, infection, and rheumatologic disorders.[130] The recommended cut-off for sST2 in chronic HF is 35 ng/mL.[130] sST2 does not have the same caveats that NPs do when it comes to age, sex, body mass index, and renal function.[130] sST2 levels show less variability over the long-term compared with NPs.[130] sST2 performs well in both

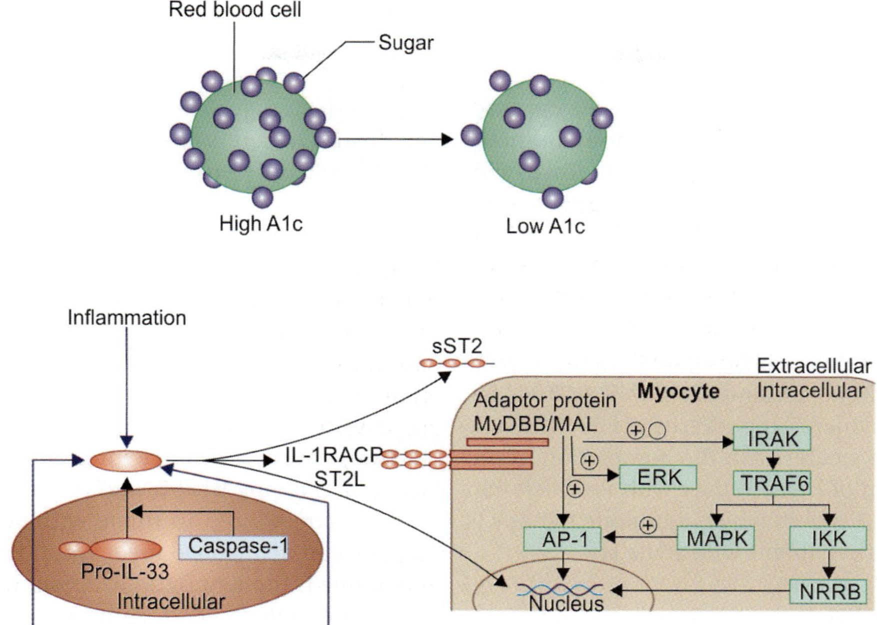

Fig. 5: Soluble ST2 (sST2) acts as a decoy receptor that, when elevated, binds interleukin (IL)-33. This effectively reduces the concentration of IL-33 that is available to bind the ST2 ligand (ST2L) and diminishes the cardioprotective effects of IL-33. Higher levels of sST2 reflect increased inflammation, fibrosis, and wall stress and thus serves like a hemoglobin A1c (HbA1c) for heart failure.

HFpEF and HFrEF.[131] From presentation in the emergency department, through hospitalization, and in the clinic, sST2 is strongest at predicting mortality risk in HF. It has beat out other biomarkers in both acute and chronic HF.[123,124] Furthermore, it works synergistically with NPs, enhancing mortality prediction in acute and chronic HF.[131-133]

In the PRIDE study, sST2 values were significantly higher in patients with HF.[120] HF patients with an sST2 ≥0.20 ng/mL had an increased risk of death at 1 year (this cut-off was from an older ST2 assay, newer assays have a cut-off >35 ng/mL).[120] Similar findings were seen in other cohorts of patients with dyspnea or acute HF.[132,134] Serial sampling of sST2 during a HF hospitalization can help predict mortality.[121] In outpatients with chronic HF, large cohort studies confirmed that an elevated sST2 value is associated with increased mortality.[135,136] Besides its prognostic ability for mortality, sST2 may help guide medical therapies in the future. Beta-blockade can mitigate some risk in patients with an elevated sST2, suggesting physicians should maximize β-blockers in patients with an elevated sST2.[125] Similarly, mineralocorticoid inhibitors may be especially effective in patients with an elevated sST2.[137] Another possible use is serial measurements in outpatients. One study found an increased risk of mortality and hospitalization in patients with increasing sST2 values on serial samples.[127] Further studies are needed to determine if serial sampling is helpful and if a similar biomarker-guided strategy can be applied to sST2 as it has been with NPs.

Galectin-3

Galectin-3 is involved in the inflammatory pathway following injury and ventricular remodeling via tissue repair, myofibroblast proliferation, and fibrogenesis. Galectin-3 is elevated in patients with acute or chronic HF.[138-140] Serial measurement of galectin-3 in chronic HF patients may add to a single measurement,[141] but to date, there are no known therapies that can alter galectin-3 values.

Procalcitonin

The chief complaint of shortness of breath requires a rapid and accurate assessment with regards to etiology with HF and pneumonia being top considerations that require timely treatment. However, misdiagnoses may result in delayed or erroneous treatment, potentially increasing adverse outcomes, mortality, and costs.[115,142] Accordingly, a biomarker to either help differentiate a bacterial pneumonia from acute HF in patients presenting with dyspnea, or to elucidate the presence of a concomitant bacterial infection in the setting of acute HF would be welcomed. This is where procalcitonin (PCT) serves as a valuable clinical aid.

Under normal physiologic conditions, PCT is produced in the C cells of the thyroid and cleaved into calcitonin with scant PCT detected in serum.[143] In pathologic states, PCT is produced in extrathyroidal tissues.[143] Serum levels increase, and with a half-life of approximately 24 hours, remain elevated for extended periods of time.[143] PCT increases with bacterial infections but not with viral.[143] This latter feature makes it a useful biomarker in acute HF. PCT has a high sensitivity and can help exclude pneumonia in patients with HF at a cut-off of 0.1 ng/mL.[144,145] Low levels of PCT strongly indicate that antibiotics should not be given. However, as the value of PCT increases, bacterial infection is far more likely and antibiotics should be administered.[144,146] PCT values can also increase with increasing severity of HF.[147] The use of PCT in HF will be clearer with the completion of the improve Management of Heart Failure with Procalcitonin (IMPACT-EU) Study, a trial in which antibiotic therapy is guided by PCT values in patients with acute HF.

MANAGEMENT OF HEART FAILURE POSTMYOCARDIAL INFARCTION

Initial Management

Despite efforts to find novel therapies, treatment of HF has progressed very little over the past 10 years; decongestion and fluid removal with diuretics, vasodilatation, and inotropes remains the cornerstone of management in acute pulmonary edema. Patients in acute HF are usually best managed in a high dependency setting where heart rate, oxygen saturations, and BP can be monitored continuously. Supplemental oxygen should be given to those who have peripheral oxygen saturation of less than 90%.[148]

Intravenous (IV) loop diuretics such as furosemide or bumetanide are the mainstay of treatment and offer quick symptomatic relief from pulmonary edema and congestion through removal of fluid. Diuretics should be given at a dose higher than the usual total daily dose-often double or triple the normal dose. The DOSE trial[149] suggested that diuretics given at 2.5 times the normal oral dose led to better diuresis and symptom relief although with transient deterioration of renal function. This trial also suggested that there was no difference between bolus diuretic regimes versus continuous infusion. A thiazide diuretic can be added which will act synergistically with the loop diuretic in order to promote fluid loss. Diuretics should be continued even if an acute kidney injury develops in a patient who remains fluid overloaded as long as the creatinine is <3 times baseline. If the creatinine rises >3 times baseline then dialysis should be considered. There is little evidence for ultrafiltration unless there is confirmed diuretic resistance with a 2B recommendation in the ESC guidelines.[148] Morphine can offer some symptomatic relief from dyspnea, although this is not routinely recommended due to the risk of respiratory depression and decreased conscious level.[150]

Vasodilators such as IV nitrate reduce both preload and afterload, but there is no evidence that they relieve dyspnea. They should not be used in people with a systolic BP of less than 110 mm Hg or those with severe aortic stenosis.

Dobutamine, a positive inotropic agent stimulating both β1 and β2 adrenoreceptors, should be reserved for those who are hypotensive with end organ hypoperfusion due to the risk of tachycardia and increased myocardial oxygen demand leading to myocardial ischemia. Other inotropes such as noradrenaline, a positive inotropic and vasoconstrictor agent stimulating β1 and α adrenoreceptors and adrenaline, a positive inotropic and vasoconstrictor agent stimulating β1, β2, and α adrenoreceptors should only be considered in those with severe hypotension as they can also cause myocardial ischemia. Low dose dopamine is thought by some to improve renal perfusion through stimulation of dopamine receptors but can cause hypoxemia and should not be used routinely as the ROSE trial[151] showed no superiority in decongestion compared to diuretics alone.

NOVAL INTRAVENOUS TREATMENT FOR ACUTE HEART FAILURE

There have been several trials exploring advanced IV therapy in addition to diuretics, nitrates, and vasopressors in order to improve symptoms and outcomes in HF, but widespread use has been limited due to safety concerns and lack of robust evidence.

- Milrinone has both positive inotropic and vasodilatory properties through inhibition of phosphodiesterase 3 which improves CO and reduces peripheral resistance. It can be used as an adjunct to standard therapy and does not increase myocardial oxygen consumption and ischemia in contrast to standard inotropes. OPTIME-CHF[152] sought to assess whether a short course of Milrinone in addition to standard therapy decreased length of hospital stay or reduced readmission within 60 days. Milrinone did not reduce length of hospital stay or reduce readmission within 60 days, it also did not improve dose titration of ACE inhibitors or improve symptoms of HF and as such is not routinely recommended. There was no mortality benefit with milrinone.
- Levosimendan is both a calcium sensitizer and a vasodilator which improves CO independent of beta adrenergic receptors. The SURVIVE[153] trial compared levosimendan to dobutamine with survival at 180 days as the primary endpoint. There was no difference

in mortality at 180 days between the two groups although BNP levels were significantly reduced in those who were treated with levosimendan and there was some symptomatic benefit. REVIVE I and II[154] was a randomized, double-blinded, prospective study which compared levosimendan plus standard therapy to standard therapy alone. Those treated with levosimendan had significant short-term clinical improvement in symptoms, but were more likely to have adverse CV outcomes such as atrial and ventricular arrhythmia including an increase in number of deaths.

- Nesiritide is a recombinant form of BNP which has vasodilatory effects and reduces pulmonary capillary wedge pressures. The ASCEND-HF[155] trial, a placebo randomized trial examined the effect of nesiritide on top of standard therapy on self-reported dyspnea at 6 hours and 24 hours, rehospitalization for HF, renal failure, and death from any cause at 30 days. A trend toward an improvement in patient reported dyspnea was observed, there was no significant difference in renal dysfunction, mortality or readmission for HF at 30 days.
- Serelaxin is a recombinant human relaxin 2 peptide; this has a role in regulating maternal adaptation to pregnancy by increase arterial compliance, CO, and renal blood flow. RELAX-AHF[156] was a prospective double-blinded randomized control trial which compared serelaxin to placebo for patients admitted to hospital with acute HF. Serelaxin or placebo were infused for up to 48 hours, other treatments were left to physician discretion. Primary endpoints were patient reported dyspnea from admission to day 5 and decrease in dyspnea at 6, 12, and 24 hours. Second endpoints were days alive and out of hospital at day 60 and CV death, renal failure or readmission to day 60. Serelaxin significantly improved symptoms of dyspnea, decreased length of stay and reduced CV deaths, and all-cause mortality. However, it did not reduce readmission to hospital for HF or renal failure. These findings have to be interpreted with caution as mortality was not the primary endpoint and there were few overall deaths. In addition, a lot of the patients had diastolic dysfunction so results may not necessarily be extrapolated to those with systolic dysfunction. Interestingly, serelaxin has not been approved by either National Institute for Health and Care Excellence or the Food and Drug Administration (FDA).

NONPHARMACOLOGICAL THERAPIES IN ACUTE HEART FAILURE

Continuous positive airway pressure (CPAP) can be used in patients who are hypoxemic and to relieve dyspnea. 3CPO[157] randomized patients to standard oxygen therapy, CPAP, or noninvasive positive-pressure ventilation (NIPPV) as well as diuretics, IV nitrates, and opiates according to physician discretion. There was improvement in respiratory distress and metabolic abnormalities, but no improvement in mortality to 7 days and 30 days. Therefore, CPAP should be offered to those who fail initial medical therapy in order to relive dyspnea but should not be offered to those who are hypotensive, have a depressed conscious level or are vomiting. These patients may require invasive ventilation in an intensive care setting. Critically-ill patients could also be considered for transfer to a regional transplant center.

Fluid and/or salt restriction is often used in patients presenting with acute HF, although there is no firm evidence for this.

Coronary Revascularization

Patients with acute HF who present with acute STEMI or new left bundle branch block (LBBB) should be offered immediate revascularization in line with established practice.[158] The role of intervention in those who present with predominantly HF symptoms without ischemia is less certain. The Surgical Treatment for Ischemic Heart Failure (STICH)[159] trial was a multicenter, international, randomized control trial comparing optimal medical therapy to optimal medical therapy plus coronary artery bypass grafting (CABG) in patients with an EF of <35% and coronary artery disease excluding those with left main stem disease. All-cause mortality was not significantly reduced by CABG, however, secondary outcomes of CV death and CV hospitalization were reduced. While a second on-treatment analysis indicated a benefit from surgical intervention, in terms of both mortality and secondary outcomes of hospitalization for CV disease,[160] this has obvious limitations. A substudy of myocardial viability also failed to demonstrate improved survival.[161] It is possible that the mortality benefit from CABG is offset by high procedural deaths. The recently published STITCHES study[162] reports the 10-year outcomes of the surgical revascularization versus optimal medical therapy arm of the STITCH[159] trial. All cause death, CV death, and death from any cause or hospitalization for CV causes were significantly lower among patients who underwent CABG in addition to receiving medical therapy than among those who received medical therapy alone. This is in contrast to the results of the 5-year follow up in the original STITCH trial and should lead to a change in practice so that an ischemic cause for LV systolic dysfunction is sought early. Percutaneous revascularization may carry less procedural risk than CABG, the REVIVED-BCIS2[163] trial is currently recruiting and will compare PCI to optimal medical therapy in ischemic cardiomyopathy therefore negating early postoperative mortality.

Cardiogenic shock is a leading cause of death in patient presenting to hospital with ACS. The SHOCK trial[164] sought to determine if emergency revascularization would improve outcomes in patients presenting with MI and cardiogenic shock. Patients were randomized to either early revascularization within 6 hours of randomization or intensive medical stabilization followed by revascularization if clinically appropriate. The primary endpoint was mortality at 30 days, secondary endpoints were mortality at 6 and 12 months. The study showed a nonsignificant trend toward improved mortality at 30 days, but by 6 months there was evidence of benefit in those who had emergent revascularization.

IABP-SHOCK II[165] trial examined whether placement of an intra-aortic balloon pump (IABP) would improve mortality outcomes in patients with cardiogenic shock complicating MI. This showed that there is no improvement in mortality to 30 days in patients who have an IABP placed. Therefore, there is no role for IABP in acute MI and HF and it therefore should be reserved for patients with a mechanical complication of acute MI or as a bridge to transplant.

PHARMACOLOGICAL THERAPY AFTER INITIAL STABILIZATION

Once patients have received initial therapy to remove congestion and improve dyspnea, then the focus of treatment should switch to disease modifying drugs which improve mortality and long-term outcomes such as hospitalization for HF, and recurrent MI. HF activates the renin-angiotensin system which increases aldosterone, and BP, promotes vasoconstriction, fibrosis, and LV hypertrophy. The majority of therapies such as ACE inhibitors, β-blockers, and MRAs work by blocking this pathway.

TREATMENT—POSTMYOCARDIAL INFARCTION HEART FAILURE

Patient with HF complicating AMI require different treatments than those without HF (Table 6, Figs. 6 and 7).

TABLE 6: Treatments for myocardial infarction complicated by heart failure.

Treatment	*Key points*	*Key trials*
Beta-blockers	Early use (within 24 hours) of high-dose β-blockers is harmful and should be avoided for MI patients in HF or high risk for cardiogenic shock defined as age >70 years, systolic blood pressure <120 mm Hg, sinus tachycardia >110 beats/min, heart rate <60 beats/min Patients with initial contraindications to β-blocker in first 24 hours should be reevaluated to assess eligibility	CAPRICON COMMIT-CCS2
ACEIs	ACEIs should be administered within first 24 hours for HF patients of EF <40%. HF patients or EF <40%. Significant survival benefit (40%) conferred on first day of treatment; early initiation is important. Contraindications systolic blood pressure <90–100 mm Hg, shock, acute kidney injury, renal failure, and drug allergy	SAVE AIRE TRACE
ARBs (as an alternative to ACEIs)	ARBs are indicated for patients intolerant to ACE inhibitors. Specifically, valsartan was noninferior to captopril in VALIANT	OPTIMAAL VALIANT
Aldosterone antagonist	Early initiation of eplerenone (<7 days) for patients with EF <40% and HF (or diabetes) had reduction in mortality and sudden cardiac death. Effect of eplerenone was time dependent and attenuated if the drug was added 7 days after index MI Contraindications: Creatinine >2.5 mg/dL in men and >2.0 mg/dL in women Potassium >5.0 mEq/L	EPHESUS ALBATROSS
Early revascularization	Early revascularization (as soon as possible) is the only therapy proven to reduce mortality in MI patients presenting with cardiogenic shock	SHOCK
Mechanical circulatory support	In the MI setting, routine use of IABP is not indicated to reduce infarct size or to manage cardiogenic shock	IABP SHOCK II IMPRESS

(ACEI: angiotensin-converting enzyme inhibitor; AIRE: Acute Infarction Ramipril Efficacy; ALBATROS: Aldosterone Lethal effects Blocked in Acute MI Treated with or without Reperfusion to improve Outcome and Survival at Six month follow up; ARB: angiotensin II receptor blocker; CAPRICORN: Carvedilol Post-Infarct Survival Control in Left Ventricular Dysfunction Study, COMMIT-CCS2: Clopidogrel and Metoprolol in Myocardial Infarction Trial/Second Chinese Cardiac Study; EF: ejection Fraction; EPHESUS: Eplerenone Postacute Myocardial Infarction Heart Failure Efficacy and Survival; HF: heart failure; IABP: Intra-aortic Balloon Pump; IABP SHOCK II: Intra-aortic Balloon Pump Should We Emergently Revascularize Occluded Coronaries for Cardiogenic Shock II; IMPRESS: Impella Versus IABP reduces Mortality in STEMI patients treated with primary PCI in severe cardiogenic shock; MI: myocardial infarction; OPTIMAAL: Optimal Trial in Myocardial Infarction with Angiotensin II Antagonist Losartan; SAVE: Survival and Ventricular Enlargement; SHOCK: Should We Emergently Revascularize Occluded for Cardiogenic Shock; TRACE: TRAndolapril Cardiac Evaluation; VALIANT: VALsartan in Acute Myocardial INfarction Trial)

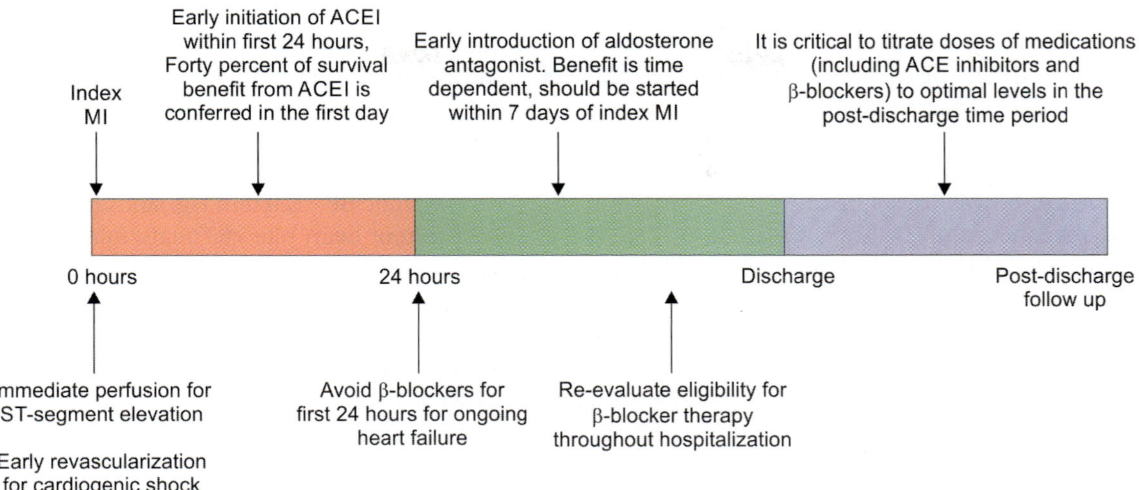

Fig. 6: Central illustration: Time-dependent therapies for post-myocardial infarction heart failure.
(ACE: angiotensin-converting enzyme; ACEI: angiotensin-converting enzyme inhibitor; MI: myocardial infarction)
Source: Bhait MC, et al. J Am Coll Cardiol HF. 2018;6(3):179-86.

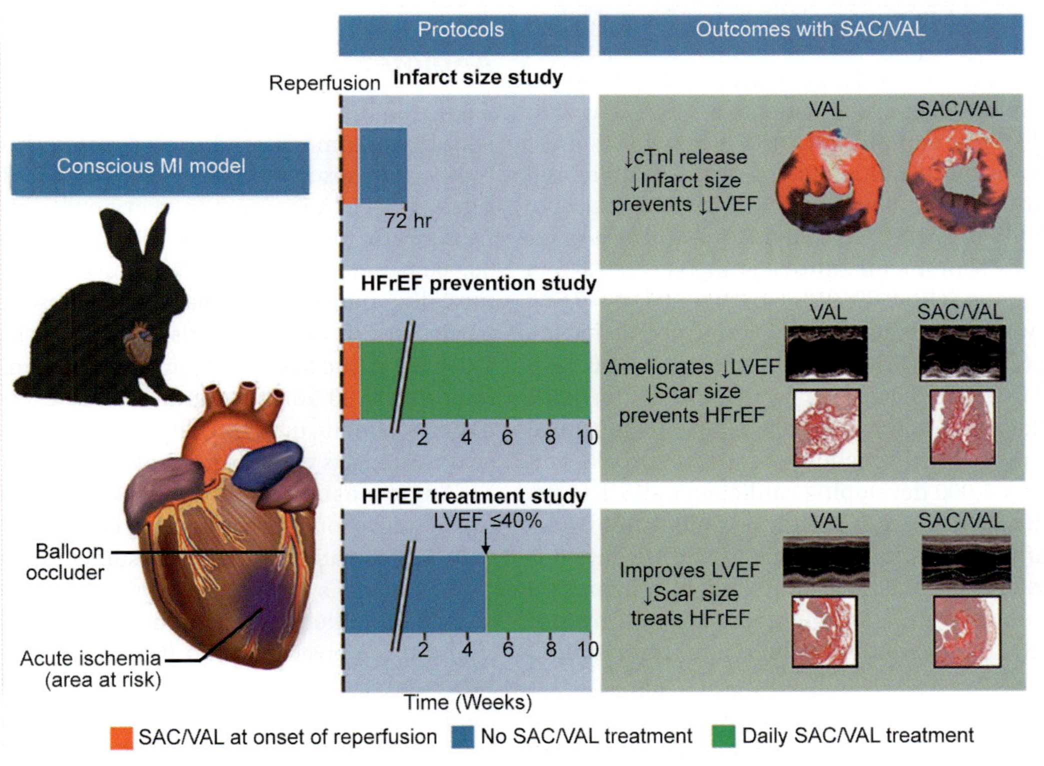

Fig. 7: Central illustration: Sacubitril/Valsartan protects against myocardial infarction-induced heart failure.

Beta-blockers

The benefits of long-term β-blockers in the years after MI have been well established.[166-169] In a meta-analysis of 31 randomized trials that included approximately 25,000 patients with a history of MI, the long-term use of β-blockers reduced the risk of reinfarction and death by approximately 20–25% after a mean of 2 years of treatment during an average of 2 years of follow-up.[170] The long-term efficacy of carvedilol on morbidity and mortality in patients with LV dysfunction after AMI was assessed in the CAPRICORN (Carvedilol Post Infarct Survival Control in Left Ventricular Dysfunction Study).[171] A total of 1,959 patients with AMI (3–21 days) and a LVEF of ≤40% were randomly assigned 6.25 mg carvedilol (maximum 25 mg/day) or placebo. The primary outcome (all-cause mortality and CV hospitalization) was not different between carvedilol (35%) and placebo (37%) cohorts. However, all-cause mortality was lower in the carvedilol group than in the placebo group [12% vs. 15%; HR: 0.77; 95% confidence interval (CI): 0.60–0.98; p = 0.03]. Similarly, in a meta-analysis of 29 randomized trials including more than 40,000 patients with suspected MI, during the first week in the hospital, IV followed by oral β-blocker seemed to reduce the relative risk of death by 13%, reinfarction by 22%, and ventricular fibrillation by 15%.[172] However, it is unknown if these findings were related to the use of IV β-blocker.

The COMMIT-CCS2 (Clopidogrel and Metoprolol in Myocardial Infarction Trial/Second Chinese Cardiac Study) included 45,852 patients admitted to 1,250 hospitals in China within 24 hours of suspected AMI who were randomly assigned to metoprolol (up to 15 mg IV then 200 mg oral daily) or placebo.[172] One-fifth of the patients presented with Killip class II and nearly 5% Killip Class III; approximately one-half of the patients were treated with fibrinolysis. Metoprolol did not show a beneficial effect in neither co-primary endpoints: for death, reinfarction, or cardiac arrest [9.4% metoprolol vs. with 9.9% placebo; odds ratio (OR): 0.96; 95% CI: 0.90–1.01; p = 0.10], and for death alone, 7.7% in the metoprolol group versus 7.8% in the placebo group (OR: 0.99; 95% CI: 0.92–1.05; p = 0.69). Metoprolol was associated with five fewer people having reinfarction (2.0% vs. 2.5% (OR: 0.82; 95% CI: 0.72–0.92; p = 0.001) and five fewer having ventricular fibrillation (2.5% vs. 3.0%; OR: 0.83; 95% CI: 0.75–0.93; p = 0.001) per 1,000 treated. Overall, these reductions were counterbalanced by 11 more per 1,000 developing cardiogenic shock (5.0% vs. 3.9%; OR: 1.30: 95% CI: 1.19–1.41; p <0.00001). This excess of cardiogenic shock was mainly during days 0–1 after admission, whereas the reductions in reinfarction and ventricular fibrillation emerged at day 2 onward. Consequently, the overall effect on death, reinfarction, arrest, or shock was significantly adverse during days 0–1 and significantly beneficial thereafter. When assigned to metoprolol as opposed to placebo, patients with pulmonary edema (Killip class III) were more likely to suffer cardiogenic shock (15.6% vs. 9.9%; absolute increase of 6%) and death (19.7% vs. 16.5%; absolute increase of 3.2%). This study shows that early use of high-dose β-blocker appears harmful for patients who present in HF. The American College of Cardiology (ACC)/American Heart Association (AHA) guidelines has incorporated these results to recommend, as a Class I recommendation which is as follows:[173,174]

- Oral β-blockers should be initiated in the first 24 hours in patients with STEMI who do not have any of the following: signs of HF, evidence of a low output state, increased risk for cardiogenic shock (age >70 years, systolic BP <120 mm Hg, sinus tachycardia >110 beats/min or heart rate <60 beats/min, and increased time since onset of symptoms of STEMI), or other contraindications to use of oral β-blockers (PR interval more than 0.24 seconds, second- or third-degree heart block, active asthma, or reactive airways disease) (Level of Evidence: B)
- Beta-blockers should be continued during and after hospitalization for all patients with STEMI and with no contraindications to their use (Level of Evidence: B)
- Patients with initial contraindications to the use of β-blockers in the first 24 hours after STEMI should be reevaluated to determine their subsequent eligibility (Level of Evidence: C).

Angiotensin-converting Enzyme Inhibitors

Angiotensin-converting enzyme inhibitors (ACEIs) should be administered to patients with impaired EFs (≤40%) or those who have experienced HF in the early phase of MI. A systematic overview[175] of four trials of ACEIs early (0–36 hours) in STEMI including more than 98,000 patients, showed a 7% relative reduction in 30-day mortality compared with placebo. The absolute benefit was particularly greater in high risk groups (such as Killip Class II/III, heart rate >100 beats/min at entry) and anterior MI. Importantly, 40% of the survival benefit occurred on the first day of treatment, underscoring the value of initiating ACEIs early, as long as patients have adequate BP.

Angiotensin-converting enzyme inhibitors were tested in five long-term randomized trials including more than 12,000 patients with LV dysfunction or HF after MI. A prospective systematic over[176] with pooled data from individual patients showed long-term benefit of ACEIs. In the three postinfarction trials; SAVE[177], AIRE (Acute Infarction Ramipril Efficacy)[178] and TRACE (TRAndolapril Cardiac Evaluation),[179] ACEIs were started between 3 days and 16 days post-MI. Overall, there was a 26% relative risk reduction (RRR) in mortality comparing ACEIs with placebo (OR: 0.74; 95% CI: 0.66–0.83). There was also a 27% RRR in readmission for HF (OR: 0.73; 95% CI: 0.63–0.85), 20% RRR in reinfarction (OR: 0.80; 95% CI: 0.69–0.94), and 25% RRR in the composite of these events. The SOLVD trials[180,181] evaluated the treatment effect of enalapril on mortality clinical HF in patients with an EF ≤35%. The outcomes were similar, with no apparent heterogeneity in results between symptomatic and asymptomatic patients when the data were examined at the same time.

The ACC/AHA guidelines recommend[173] based on this evidence, as a Class I, Level of Evidence: A, recommendation: "An angiotensin-converting enzyme (ACE) inhibitor should be administered within the first 24 hours to all patients with STEMI with anterior location, HF, or EF ≤0.40%, unless contraindicated".

Angiotensin Receptor Blockers

Angiotensin receptor blockers as alternatives to ACEIs in the context of STEMI have been evaluated in two clinical trials, OPTIMAAL (Optimal Trial in Myocardial Infarction with the Angiotensin II Antagonist Losartan)[182] included 5,477 patients with confirmed AMI and HF during the acute phase or a new Q-wave anterior infarction or reinfarction to receive either losartan 50 mg three times a day or captopril 50 mg three times a day. The losartan arm failed to show either superiority or noninferiority when compared with captopril for the primary endpoint (18% vs. 16% at 2.7 years follow-up). Conversely, in VALIANT,[183] 14,703 patients with AMI (0.5 and 10 days) and HF or evidence of LV systolic dysfunction ≤40% were randomly assigned to valsartan alone (160 mg twice daily), full-dose captopril (50 mg three times daily) or both (80 mg twice daily and 50 mg three times daily). The primary endpoint of all-cause mortality was similar in the three groups (valsartan 19.9%, captopril 19.5%, and both 19.3%). Therefore, valsartan, in the dosages used in the trial, represents an alternative to ACEIs (ACC/AHA Class I, Level of Evidence: B recommendation) in patients who have clinical signs of HF and/or an EF ≤40%, particularly in patients who do not tolerate ACEIs.

Aldosterone Antagonist

The EPHESUS (Eplerenone Postacute Myocardial Infarction Heart Failure Efficacy and Survival) study established the benefit of an aldosterone antagonist, eplerenone, added to optimal medical therapy in patients between 3 days and 14 days after STEMI with EF ≤0.40 and either symptomatic HF or diabetes mellitus versus placebo. Eplerenone was initiated at 25 mg/day, then titrated to a maximum dose of 50 mg/day. There was a 15% RRR of all-cause mortality with eplerenone compared with placebo. A similar treatment benefit was seen for the other co-primary endpoint of CV death or hospitalization for CV events, death from CV causes, and sudden death from cardiac causes. A post hoc analysis of the EPHESUS study[184] assessed the timing of eplerenone initiation and outcomes. Earlier eplerenone initiation (<7 days) reduced the risk of all-cause mortality by 31% ($p = 0.001$) when compared with the "earlier" placebo. Earlier eplerenone initiation also reduced the risks of CV hospitalization or CV mortality by 24% ($p = 0.0001$) and sudden cardiac death by 34% ($p = 0.0001$). Later eplerenone initiation (≥7 days) had no significant effect on outcomes. Interactions between time to randomization and treatment for mortality were significant ($p = 0.02$).

The ALBATROSS (Aldosterone Lethal effects Blocked in Acute MI Treated with or without Reperfusion to improve Outcome and Survival at Six months follow up) trial investigated the clinical effects of a rapid and prolonged MRA regimen initiated early after the onset of STEMI or high-risk non-STEMI plus standard therapy versus standard therapy alone in 1,603 subjects. Patients assigned to the MRA regimen received a 200 mg IV bolus of potassium canrenoate followed by 25 mg oral dose of spironolactone administered 12–24 hours after the IV injection. There was no difference in the combined primary endpoint of death, resuscitated cardiac arrest, significant ventricular arrhythmia, indication for implantable defibrillator, or new or worsening HF at 6-month follow-up. In a nonprespecified exploratory analysis, the use of MRA was associated with reduction in mortality compared with placebo (0.5% vs. 2.4%; HR: 0.20; 95% CI: 0.06–0.70) in the subgroup of STEMI, but not in non-STEMI.

Guidelines recommend that "an aldosterone antagonist should be given to patients with STEMI and no contraindications who are already receiving an ACE inhibitor and beta-blocker and who have an EF ≤0.40 and either symptomatic HF or diabetes mellitus (Level of Evidence: B).[173]

Sacubitril/Valsartan after Acute Myocardial Infarction

Post-myocardial infarction cardiac remodeling has a major role to play in the development of HF which then progresses with continued cardiac remodeling. In experimental animal models of HFrEF, LCZ696 ameliorated cardiac remodeling and improved LVEF compared with vehicle and valsartan.[185,186] These effects were hypothesized to be from angiotensin II receptor blocker neprilysin inhibitor (ARNI)-mediated inhibition of hypertrophy and fibrosis and suppression of local transforming growth factor-β by the sacubitril moiety of LCZ696.[185,186]

Sacubitril/Valsartan Averts Adverse Postinformation Ventricular Remodeling and Preserves Systolic Function in Rabbits

Sacubitril/Valsartan (SAC/VAL) is approved by the US FDA for HFrEF. New Zealand Whit rabbits were sedated and underwent conscious MI (45-minute ischemia) by balloon inflation (previously implanted surgically) followed by 72 hours (acute protocol) or 10 weeks (chronic protocols) of reperfusion. "Infarct-sparing" protocol: SAC/VAL, VAL, or placebo were randomly allocated and administered at reperfusion. "HFrEF-treatment" protocol: rabbits were randomized, and treatment commenced after echocardiography-confirmed LVEF ≤40%. "HFrEF-prevention" protocol: treatment started at reperfusion and continued daily throughout the study.

Compared with placebo, SAC/VAL and VAL significantly reduced infarct size [triphenyltetrazolium chloride (TTC) staining] and plasma troponin levels; however, only SAC/VAL preserved LVEF at 72 hours post-MI. In the HFrEF treatment protocol, LVEF improvement was observed with SAC/VAL compared with both placebo and VAL starting 2 weeks post-treatment, a benefit that persisted throughout study duration. In the HFrEF prevention protocol, SAC/VAL and VAL attenuated the decline in LVEF post-MI, although SAC/VAL offered better functional protection. The functional improvement observed in both treatment protocols was paralleled by significant reduction in LV scar size (Picrosirius red staining) in the SAC/VAL groups.

Reperfusion therapy with SAC/VAL or VAL offers robust acute infarct-sparing benefits; however, SAC/VAL treatment offered superior short-term and long-term benefits in preventing MI-induced LV dysfunction compared with VAL. SAC/VAL also significantly attenuated LV scar size following MI compared with placebo, whereas VAL did not reach statistical significance in scar reduction.

DEVICES

Both implantable cardiac defibrillators (ICDs) and cardiac resynchronization therapy (CRT) have survival benefit for those with LV systolic dysfunction. The SCD-HEFT[187] and MADIT-II[188] trials showed that implantation of an ICD for primary prevention reduces the risk of sudden cardiac death in both ischemic and nonischemic cardiomyopathy in those with EF <35% and with NYHA II–III symptoms. They should not be offered to those with class IV symptoms and patients need to be appropriately counseled regarding driving advice.

Cardiac resynchronization therapy should be offered to those with EF less than 35% with a broad QRS. The greatest benefit is seen with those who have a LBBB morphology with a QRS >150 msec, this benefit occurs with those who have NYHA II-IV HF. There is no benefit from CRT for those with a narrow QRS. Both the COMPANION[189] trial and CARE-HF[190] showed improvements in mortality and a decrease in hospital admissions for those with NYHA class III-IV symptoms. MADIT-CRT[191] showed a similar benefit for those with milder symptoms.

Device implantation should only be considered in those who have been on optimal medical therapy for 3 months as the LV function may improve. The DINAMIT[192] and IRIS[193] studies also showed that when ICDs were implanted within 40 days post-MI, then although sudden cardiac deaths from arrhythmia decreased they were offset by an increase in nonarrhythmic deaths. Therefore, device implantation should not be offered within 40 days post-MI.

Left Ventricular Restoration Devices Postmyocardial Infarction (Fig. 8)

Despite continuous improvements in acute and long-term treatment of MI over recent decades, the resulting myocardial injury remains an important cause of adverse LV remodeling, which over time progresses into the clinical syndrome of HF.[194] Typical for post-MI LV remodeling is dilatation, geometric change (from ellipsoid to spherical), and scar formation.[195] Both functional and structural measures of adverse LV remodeling, such as LVEF and LV dimensions, are associated with mortality and CV events after MI.[196-199] The beneficial effects of drugs or medical devices on LV remodeling measures have been associated with reduced long-term mortality.[200] Numerous devices have been developed that attempt to restore the LV shape and revert adverse post-MI changes, intended to provide long-term benefits in terms of survival and functional status (Table 7).

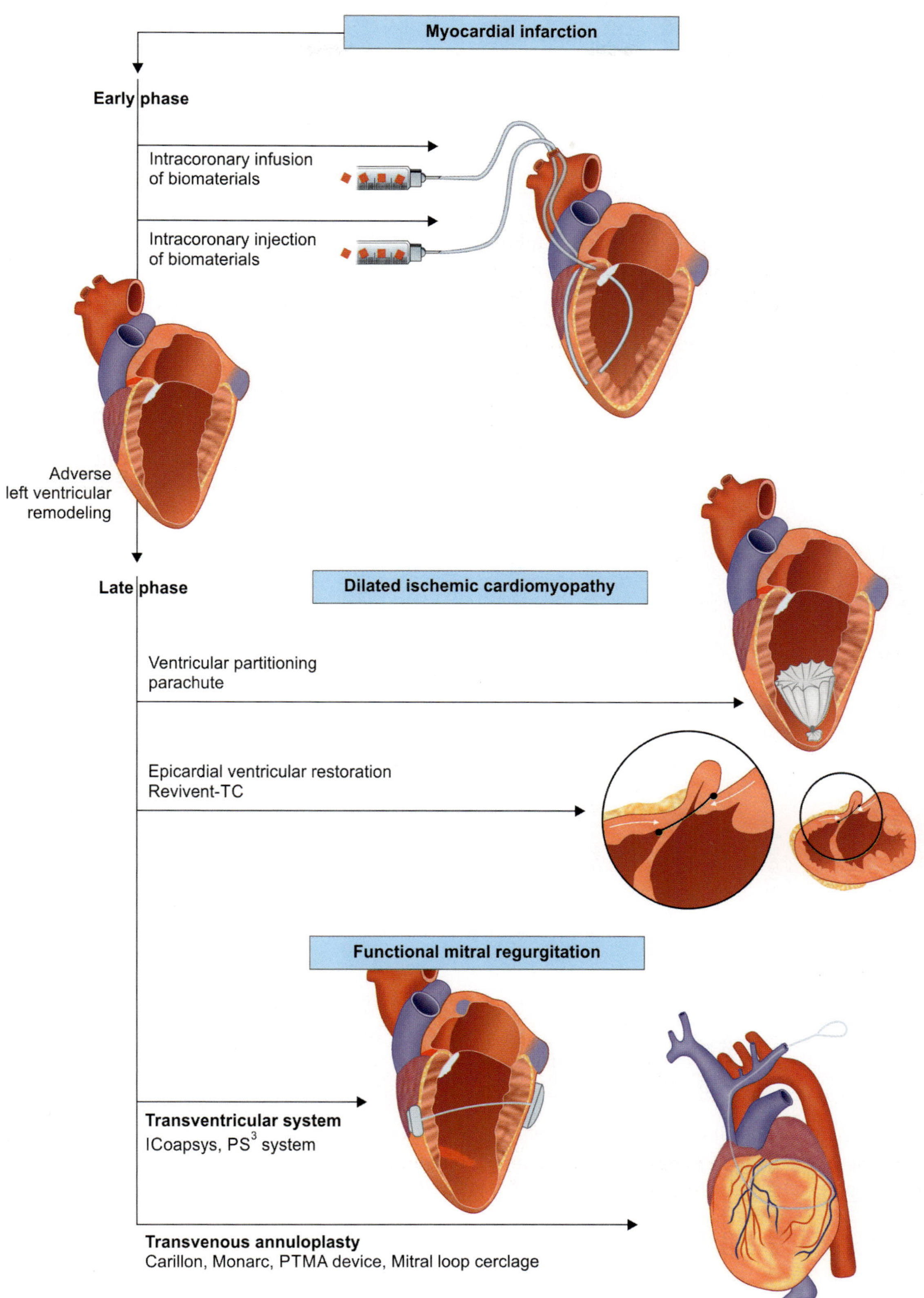

Fig. 8: An overview of the discussed transcatheter left ventricular restoration devices, grouped by indication for use based on the stage of adverse left ventricular remodeling postmyocardial infarction. The represented transvenous annuloplasty device is the mitral loop cerclage, the other devices are differently shaped.

TABLE 7: Left ventricular restoration devices used in various stages after MI.

	Type of device	*Device*	*Indication*	*Trials*	*Status*	*Primary endpoints*	*No of subject (nonischemic)*
Early phase	Intracoronary infusion of biomaterial	Sodium alginate + calcium + gluconate BCM	2–5 days after large STEMI and successful revascularization	first-in-human	Completed	180-day symptomatic heart failure (3.7%), renal failure 6 month ΔLVEDVi (BCM 14.1 ± 28.9 mL/m^2 vs saline 11.7 + 26.9 mL/m^2; p = 0.49)	27 (0)
				PRESERVATION 1	Completed		306 (0)
	Intramyocardial injection of biomaterial	Calcium hydroxyapatite microspheres (CHAM)	Directly post-MI	Animal studies	Completed	Infarct expansion, proteolytic pathways, LVEF, regional contractile strain, MR severity	-
		Injectable hyaluronic acid-based hydrogel	Directly post-MI	Animal studies	Completed	Global LV remodeling, infarct thinning and expansion, and infarct stiffness	-
		Myocardial matrix hydrogel (VentriGel)	60 days–3 years after STEMI, LVEF 25–45%	Fist in human	Recruiting	6 months SAE	18 (0)
Late phase	Ventricular partitioning	Parachute	LVEF <40%, abnormal LV wall motion, suitable LV anatomy	PARACHUTE first in human	Completed	Implantation success and 6 month	39 (0)
				PARACHUTE III	Completed	1 year procedural or device related MACCE (7%)	100 (0)
				PARACHUTE IV	Terminated	Death or rehospitalization for worsening heart failure	331 (0)
				PARACHUTE V	Terminated	Quality of life	85 (0)
	Epicardial ventricular restoration	Revivent–TC	LVEF <45%, dilated LV, acontractile scar, NYHA class II-IV	Revivent TCI	Recruiting	6 months SAE and ΔLVESVi	50 (0)
				Revivent-TC System Clinical Study	Recruiting	Effectiveness, compared to surgical treatment and medical therapy	126 (0)
	Transventricular system	iCoapsys	Severe FMR, NYHA class II – III	First in human	Terminated	Intra- and periprocedural safety and MR reduction	? (?)
		Percutaneous septal sinus shortening (PS^3) system	FMR	Animal studies	Completed	Septal–lateral dimension (–17%), mean force on bridge (1.16–1.87N)	-

Contd...

Contd...

Type of device	Device	Indication	Trials	Status	Primary endpoints	No of subject (nonischemic)
			First in human	Completed	Septal-lateral dimension (–29%), MR grade reduction (1 and 2)	2(1)
Transvenous annuloplasty	Monarc	Moderate to severe FMR, dilated LV, LVEF > 25%	EVOLUTION	Completed	30-day freedom from death, tamponade, and MI (91%, 82% at 1 year)	72 (23)
	Percutaneous transvenous mitral annuloplasty (PTMA)	Moderate to severe FMR, NYHA class II-IV, LVEF 20–50%	PTOLEMY-2	Terminated	30-day freedom from MACEs and 6 month MR reduction	43 (13–26)
	Carillon	Moderate to severe FMR, dilated LV, LVEF <50% 6MWT distance 150–450 m	AMADEUS	Completed	30-day MAE (13%)	48 (?)
			TITAN	Completed	30-day MAE (1.9%)	53 (19)
			TITAN II	Completed	30-day MAE (2.8%)	43 (15)
			REDUCE FMR	Active, not recruiting	1 year Δ regurgitant volume	180 (?)
			CARILLON	Recruiting	1 year freedom from MAE, Δ regurgitant volume, and clinical composite of death, time to first HF hospitalization and improvement in 6MWT distance	400 (?)
	Mitral loop cerclage		First in human	Completed		5 (2–4)
		Severe FMR, NYHA class III-IV			1-month freedom from MACE (80%) reduction of regurgitant volume (66%) and effective regurgitant orifice area (76%)	
Direct mitral valve annuloplasty (ventriculoplasty)	AccuCinch	Moderate to severe FMR, NYHA class II-IV, LVEF >20%	Safety and efficacy trials	Recruiting	30-day device related or procedure related MAE, MACE, acute and 30-day MR reduction	197 (?)

(BCM: bioabsorbable cardiac matrix; MI: myocardial infarction; STEMI: ST-segment elevation myocardial infarction; LVEF: left ventricular ejection fraction; MR: mitral regurgitation; LV: left ventricular; SAE: serious adverse events; MACCE: major adverse cardiac and cerebrovascular events; FMR: functional mitral regurgitation; NYHA: New York Heart Association; MACE: major adverse cardiac events; MAE: major adverse event; 6MWT: 6-minute walk test)

REFERENCES

1. Granger CB, Goldberg RJ, Dabbous OM, et al. Predictors of hospital mortality in the global registry of acute coronary events. Arch Intern Med. 2003;163:2345-53.
2. Yancy CW, Jessup M, Bozkurt B, et al. 2013 ACCF/AHA guideline for the management of heart failure: a report of the American College of Cardiology Foundation/American Heart Association Task Force on Practice Guidelines. J Am Coll Cardiol. 2013;62:e147-239.
3. Thygesen K, Alpert JS, Jaffe AS, et al. Third universal definition of myocardial infarction. Circulation. 2012;126:2020-35.
4. Killip T, Kimball JT. Treatment of myocardial infarction in a coronary care unit. A two year experience with 250 patients. Am J Cardiol. 1967;20:457-64.
5. Spencer FA, Meyer TE, Goldberg RJ, et al. Twenty year trends (1975-1995) in the incidence, in-hospital and long-term death rates associated with heart failure complicating acute myocardial infarction: a community-wide perspective. J Am Coll Cardiol. 1999;34:1378-87.
6. Steg PG, Dabbous OH, Feldman LJ, et al. Determinants and prognostic impact of heart failure complicating acute coronary syndromes: observations from the Global Registry of Acute Coronary Events (GRACE). Circulation. 2004;109:494-9.
7. Hellermann JP, Jacobsen SJ, Gersh BJ, et al. Heart failure after myocardial infarction: a review. Am J Med. 2002;113:324-30.
8. Ali AS, Rybicki BA, Alam M, et al. Clinical predictors of heart failure in patients with first acute myocardial infarction. Am Heart J. 1999;138:1133-9.
9. Spencer FA, Meyer TE, Gore JM, et al. Heterogeneity in the management and outcomes of patients with acute myocardial infarction complicated by heart failure the National Registry of Myocardial Infarction. Circulation. 2002;105:2605-10.
10. Shah RV, Holmes D, Anderson M, et al. Risk of heart failure complication during hospitalization for acute myocardial infarction in a contemporary population insights from the National Cardiovascular Data ACTION Registry. Circ Heart Fail. 2012;5:693-702.
11. Sulo G, Igland J, Vollset SE, et al. Heart Failure complicating acute myocardial infarction, burden and timing of occurrence a nation-wide analysis including 86771 patients from the Cardiovascular Disease in Norway (CVDNOR) Project. J Am Heart Assoc. 2016;5:e002667.
12. Desta L, Jernberg T, Lofman I, et al. Incidence, temporal trends, and prognostic impact of heart failure complicating acute myocardial infarction. The SWEDEHEART Registry (Swedish Web-System for Enhancement and Development of Evidence-based Care in Heart Disease Evaluated according to Recommended Therapies): a study of 199,851 patients admitted with index acute myocardial infarctions, 1996 to 2008. JACC Heart Fail. 2015;3:234-42.
13. Kaul P, Ezekowitz JA, Armstrong PW, et al. Incidence of heart failure and mortality after acute coronary syndromes. Am Heart J. 2013;165:379-85.
14. Segev A, Strauss BH, Tan M, et al. Prognostic significance of admission heart failure in patients with non-ST elevation acute coronary syndromes (from the Canadian Acute Coronary syndrome Registries). Am J Cardiol. 2006;98:470-3.
15. Bahit MC, Lopes RD, Clare RM, et al. Heart failure complicating non-ST-segment elevation acute coronary syndrome: timing, predictors, and clinical outcomes. JACC Heart Fail. 2013;1:223-9.
16. Juilliere Y, Cambou JP, Bataille V, et al. Heart failure in acute myocardial infarction: a comparison between patients with or without heart failure criteria from the FAST-MI registry. Rev Esp Cardiol. 2012;65:326-33.
17. James SK, Lindahl B, Siegbahn A, et al. N-terminal pro-brain natriuretic peptide and other risk markers for the separate prediction of mortality and subsequent myocardial infarction in patients with unstable coronary artery disease. A Global Utilization of Strategies To Open occluded arteries (GUSTO)-IV substudy. Circulation. 2003;108:275-81.
18. McMurray JJ, Adamopoulos S, Anker SD, et al. ESC Committee for Practice Guidelines. ESC guidelines for the diagnosis and treatment of acute and chronic heart failure 2012: the task force for the diagnosis and treatment of acute and chronic heart failure 2012 of the European Society of Cardiology. Developed in collaboration with the Heart Failure Association (HFA) of the ESC. Eur J Heart Fail. 2012;33(14):803-69.
19. Cleland JG, Torabi A, Khan NK. Epidemiology and management of heart failure and left ventricular systolic dysfunction in the aftermath of a myocardial infarction. Heart. 2005;91(Suppl 2):ii7-ii13.
20. Pfeffer MA, Braunwald E. Ventricular remodeling after myocardial infarction. Experimental observations and clinical implications. Circulation. 1990;81(4):1161-72.
21. Tennant R, Wiggers CJ. The effect of coronary occlusion on myocardial contraction. Am Heart J. 1935;112:351-61.
22. Niccoli G, Burzotta F, Galiuto L, et al. Myocardial no-reflow in humans. J Am Coll Cardiol. 2009;54:281-92.
23. Braunwald E. Heart failure. JACC Heart Fail. 2013;1:1-20.
24. Ertl G, Gaudron P, Eilles C, et al. Compensatory mechanisms for cardiac dysfunction in myocardial infarction. Basic Res Cardiol. 1991;86:159-65.
25. Sutton MG, Sharpe N. Left ventricular remodeling after myocardial infarction: pathophysiology and therapy. Circulation. 2000;101:2981-8.
26. Lilly LS. Braunwald's Heart Disease: a Textbook of Cardiovascular Medicine. Philadelphia: Saunders/Elsevier; 2012.
27. Francis J, Weiss RM, Wei SG, et al. Progression of heart failure after myocardial infarction in the rat. Am J Physiol Regul Integr Comp Physiol. 2001;281:R1734-45.
28. Katz AM. Physiology of the Heart. Philadelphia: Lippincott Williams & Wilkins; 2010.
29. Pina IL, Apstein CS, Balady GJ, et al. American Heart Association Committee on exercise, rehabilitation, and prevention. Exercise and heart failure: a statement from the American Heart Association Committee on exercise, rehabilitation, and prevention. Circulation. 2003;107:1210-25.
30. Chiong JR, Cheung RJ. Loop diuretic therapy in heart failure: the need for solid evidence on a fluid issue. Clin Cardiol. 2010;33:345-52.

31. Ma TK, Kam KK, Yan BP, et al. Renin-angiotensin-aldosterone system blockade for cardiovascular diseases: current status. Br J Pharmacol. 2010;160:1273-92.
32. Damkjaer M, Isaksson GL, Stubbe J, et al. Renal renin secretion as regulator of body fluid homeostasis. Pflugers Arch. 2013;465:153-65.
33. DiBona GF, Kopp UC. Neural control of renal function. Physiol Rev. 1997;77:75-197.
34. Riegger GA, Liebau G, Kochsiek K. Antidiuretic hormone in congestive heart failure. Am J Med. 1982;72:49-52.
35. Nadal-Ginard B, Kajstura J, Leri A, et al. Myocyte death, growth, and regeneration in cardiac hypertrophy and failure. Circ Res. 2003;92:139-50.
36. Bers DM. Altered Cardiac myocyte Ca regulation in heart failure. Physiology (Bethesda). 2006;21:380-7.
37. Dhalla NS, Rangi S, Babick AP, et al. Cardiac remodeling and subcellular defects in heart failure due to myocardial infarction and aging. Heart Fail Rev. 2012;17:671-81.
38. Fukushima A, Milner K, Gupta A, et al. Myocardial energy substrate metabolism in heart failure: from pathways to therapeutic targets. Curr Pharm Des. 2015;21:3654-64.
39. Munzel T, Gori T, Keaney JF Jr, et al. Pathophysiological role of oxidative stress in systolic and diastolic heart failure and its therapeutic implications. Eur Heart J. 2015;36:2555-64.
40. van Berlo JH, Maillet M, Molkentin JD. Signaling effectors underlying pathologic growth and remodeling of the heart. J Clin Invest. 2013;123:37-45.
41. Bristow MR, Ginsburg R, Umans V, et al. Beta 1- and beta 2-adrenergic-receptor subpopulations in nonfailing and failing human ventricular myocardium: coupling of both receptor subtypes to muscle contraction and selective beta 1-receptor down-regulation in heart failure. Circ Res. 1986;59:297-309.
42. Lymperopoulos A. The Cardiovascular Adrenergic System. New York: Springer International Publishing; 2015.
43. Brum PC, Rolim NP, Bacurau AV, et al. Neurohumoral activation in heart failure: the role of adrenergic receptors. An Acad Bras Cienc. 2006;78:485-503.
44. Swynghedauw B. Molecular mechanisms of myocardial remodeling. Physiol Rev. 1999;79:215-62.
45. E Gullo C, de Almeida Zia VA, Vilela-Martin JF. Blockade of renin angiotensin system in heart failure post-myocardial infarction: what is the best therapy? Recent Pat Cardiovasc Drug Discov. 2014;9:28-37.
46. Jin D, Takai S, Yamada M, et al. Possible roles of cardiac chymase after myocardial infarction in hamster hearts. Jpn J Pharmacol. 2001;86:203-14.
47. Bisping E, Wakula P, Poteser M, et al. Targeting cardiac hypertrophy: toward a causal heart failure therapy. J Cardiovasc Pharmacol. 2014;64:293-305.
48. Kim S, Ohta K, Hamaguchi A, et al. Angiotensin II induces cardiac phenotypic modulation and remodeling in vivo in rats. Hypertension. 1995;25:1252-9.
49. Pang XF, Zhang LH, Bai F, et al. Dual ACE-inhibition and angiotensin II AT1 receptor antagonism with curcumin attenuate maladaptive cardiac repair and improve ventricular systolic function after myocardial infarction in rat heart. Eur J Pharmacol. 2015;746:22-30.
50. Struthers AD. Mineralocorticoid receptor blockade in chronic heart failure. J Hum Hypertens. 1995;9:443-6.
51. Uehara Y, Miura S, Yahiro E, et al. Non-ACE pathway-induced angiotensin II production. Curr Pharm Des. 2013;19:3054-9.
52. Chrysant SG, Chrysant GS. Dual renin-angiotensin-aldosterone blockade: promises and pitfalls. Curr Hypertens Rep. 2015;17:511.
53. Ferrario CM, Schiffrin EL. Role of mineralocorticoid receptor antagonists in cardiovascular disease. Circ Res. 2015;116:206-13.
54. Abareshi A, Norouzi F, Asgharzadeh F, et al. Effect of angiotensin-converting enzyme inhibitor on cardiac fibrosis and oxidative stress Status in lipopolysaccharide-induced inflammation model in rats. Int J Prevent Med. 2017;8:69.
55. Zhang WW, Bai F, Wang J, et al. Edaravone inhibits pressure overload-induced cardiac fibrosis and dysfunction by reducing expression of angiotensin II AT1 receptor. Drug Des Dev Ther. 2017;11:3019-33.
56. Sciarretta S, Paneni F, Palano F, et al. Role of the renin-angiotensin-aldosterone system and inflammatory processes in the development and progression of diastolic dysfunction. Clin Sci (Lond). 2009;116:467-77.
57. Bekheirnia MR, Schrier RW. Pathophysiology of water and sodium retention: edematous states with normal kidney function. Curr Opin Pharmacol. 2006;6:202-7.
58. Kee K, Naughton MT. Heart failure and the lung. Circ J. 2010;74:2507-16.
59. Clark A, Coats A. Mechanisms of exercise intolerance in cardiac failure: abnormalities of skeletal muscle and pulmonary function. Curr Opin Cardiol. 1994;9:305-14.
60. Kelder JC, Cramer MJ, van Wijngaarden J, et al. The diagnostic value of physical examination and additional testing in primary care patients with suspected heart failure. Circulation. 2011;124:2865-73.
61. Weber KT, Sun Y, Bhattacharya SK, et al. Myofibroblast-mediated mechanisms of pathological remodelling of the heart. Nat Rev Cardiol. 2013;10:15-26.
62. Chopra A, Tabdanov E, Patel H, et al. Cardiac myocyte remodeling mediated by N-cadherin-dependent mechanosensing. Am J Physiol Heart Circ Physiol. 2011;300:H1252-66.
63. Cooper G. Cytoskeletal networks and the regulation of cardiac contractility: microtubules, hypertrophy, and cardiac dysfunction. Am J Physiol Heart Circ Physiol. 2006;291:H1003-14.
64. Lin L, Liu X, Xu J, et al. High-density lipoprotein inhibits mechanical stress-induced cardiomyocyte autophagy and cardiac hypertrophy through angiotensin II type 1 receptor-mediated PI3K/Akt pathway. J Cell Mol Med. 2015;19:1929-38.
65. Souders CA, Bowers SL, Baudino TA. Cardiac fibroblast: the renaissance cell. Circ Res. 2009;105:1164-76.
66. Mackiewicz U, Maczewski M, Konior A, et al. Sarcolemmal Ca2+-ATPase ability to transport Ca2+ gradually diminishes

after myocardial infarction in the rat. Cardiovasc Res. 2009;81(3):546-54.
67. Ferreira-Martins J, Leite-Moreira AF. Physiologic basis and pathophysiologic implications of the diastolic properties of the cardiac muscle. J Biomed Biotechnol. 2010;807084.
68. Lehnart SE, Maier LS, Hasenfuss G. Abnormalities of calcium metabolism and myocardial contractility depression in the failing heart. Heart Fail Rev. 2009;14:213-24.
69. Dirkx E, da Costa Martins PA, De Windt LJ. Regulation of fetal gene expression in heart failure. Biochim Biophys Acta. 2013;1832:2414-24.
70. Gupta MP. Factors controlling cardiac myosin-isoform shift during hypertrophy and heart failure. J Mol Cell Cardiol. 2007;43:388-403.
71. Kishimoto I, Tokudome T, Horio T, et al. Natriuretic peptide signaling via guanylyl cyclase (GC)-A: an endogenous protective mechanism of the heart. Curr Cardiol Rev. 2009;5:45-51.
72. Asakura M, Jiyoong K, Minamino T, et al. J-WIND Investigators. Rationale and design of a large-scale trial using atrial natriuretic peptide (ANP) as an adjunct to percutaneous coronary intervention for ST-segment elevation acute myocardial infarction: Japan-Working groups of acute myocardial infarction for the reduction of necrotic damage by ANP (J-WIND-ANP). Circ J. 2004;68:95-100.
73. Tsai SH, Lin YY, Chu SJ, et al. Interpretation and use of natriuretic peptides in non-congestive heart failure settings. Yonsei Med J. 2010;51:151-63.
74. Colucci WS, Elkayam U, Horton DP, et al. Intravenous nesiritide, a natriuretic peptide, in the treatment of decompensated congestive heart failure. Nesiritide study group. N Engl J Med. 2000;343:246-53.
75. Owan TE, Chen HH, Frantz RP, et al. The effects of nesiritide on renal function and diuretic responsiveness in acutely decompensated heart failure patients with renal dysfunction. J Card Fail. 2008;14:267-75.
76. Doenst T, Nguyen TD, Abel ED. Cardiac metabolism in heart failure: implications beyond ATP production. Circ Res. 2013;113:709-24.
77. Weiss RG, Gerstenblith G, Bottomley PA. ATP flux through creatine kinase in the normal, stressed, and failing human heart. Proc Natl Acad Sci U S A. 2005;102:808-13.
78. O'Connor CM, Hathaway WR, Bates ER, et al. Clinical characteristics and long-term outcome of patients in whom congestive heart failure develops after thrombolytic therapy for acute myocardial infarction: development of a predictive model. Am Heart J. 1997;133:663-73.
79. Velazquez EJ, Francis GS, Armstrong PW, et al. An international perspective on heart failure and left ventricular systolic dysfunction complicating myocardial infarction: the VALIANT registry. Eur Heart J. 2004;25:1911-9.
80. Wu AH, Parsons L, Every NR, et al. Hospital outcomes in patients presenting with congestive heart failure complicating acute myocardial infarction: a report from the Second National Registry of Myocardial Infarction (NRMI-2). J Am Coll Cardiol. 2002;40:1389-94.
81. Lewis EF, Moye LA, Rouleau JL, et al. Predictors of late development of heart failure in stable survivors of myocardial infarction: the CARE study. J Am Coll Cardiol. 2003;42:1446-53.
82. Murcia AM, Hennekens CH, Lamas GA, et al. Impact of diabetes on mortality in patients with myocardial infarction and left ventricular dysfunction. Arch Intern Med. 2004;164:2273-9.
83. Das SR, Drazner MH, Yancy CW, et al. Effects of diabetes mellitus and ischemic heart disease on the progression from asymptomatic left ventricular dysfunction to symptomatic heart failure: a retrospective analysis from the Studies of Left Ventricular Dysfunction (SOLVD) Prevention trial. Am Heart J. 2004;148:883-8.
84. Aguilar D, Solomon SD, Kober L, et al. Newly diagnosed and previously known diabetes mellitus and 1-year outcomes of acute myocardial infarction: the VALsartan In Acute myocardial iNfarcTion (VALIANT) trial. Circulation. 2004;110:1572-8.
85. Malmberg K, Ryden L, Hamsten A, et al. Effects of insulin treatment on cause-specific one-year mortality and morbidity in diabetic patients with acute myocardial infarction. DIGAMI Study Group. Diabetes Insulin-Glucose in Acute Myocardial Infarction. Eur Heart J. 1996;17:1337-44.
86. Granger CB, Califf RM, Young S, et al. Outcome of patients with diabetes mellitus and acute myocardial infarction treated with thrombolytic agents. The Thrombolysis and Angioplasty in Myocardial Infarction (TAMI) Study Group. J Am Coll Cardiol. 1993;21:920-5.
87. Mak KH, Moliterno DJ, Granger CB, et al. Influence of diabetes mellitus on clinical outcome in the thrombolytic era of acute myocardial infarction. GUSTO-I investigators. Global Utilization of Streptokinase and Tissue Plasminogen Activator for Occluded Coronary Arteries. J Am Coll Cardiol. 1997;30:171-9.
88. Woodfield SL, Lundergan CF, Reiner JS, et al. Angiographic findings and outcome in diabetic patients treated with thrombolytic therapy for acute myocardial infarction: the GUSTO-I experience. J Am Coll Cardiol. 1996;28:1661-9.
89. Stone PH, Muller JE, Hartwell T, et al. The effect of diabetes mellitus on prognosis and serial left ventricular function after acute myocardial infarction: contribution of both coronary disease and diastolic left ventricular dysfunction to the adverse prognosis. The MILIS Study Group. J Am Coll Cardiol. 1989;14:49-57.
90. Prasad A, Stone GW, Stuckey TD, et al. Impact of diabetes mellitus on myocardial perfusion after primary angioplasty in patients with acute myocardial infarction. J Am Coll Cardiol. 2005;45:508-14.
91. Fang ZY, Prins JB, Marwick TH. Diabetic cardiomyopathy: evidence, mechanisms, and therapeutic implications. Endocr Rev. 2004;25:543-67.
92. Asbun J, Villarreal FJ. The pathogenesis of myocardial fibrosis in the setting of diabetic cardiomyopathy. J Am Coll Cardiol. 2006;47:693-700.
93. Carrabba N, Valenti R, Parodi G, et al. Left ventricular remodeling and heart failure in diabetic patients treated

with primary angioplasty for acute myocardial infarction. Circulation. 2004;110:1974-9.
94. Solomon SD, St John Sutton M, Lamas GA, et al. Ventricular remodeling does not accompany the development of heart failure in diabetic patients after myocardial infarction. Circulation. 2002;106:1251-5.
95. St John Sutton M, Pfeffer MA, Plappert T, et al. Quantitative two-dimensional echocardiographic measurements are major predictors of adverse cardiovascular events after acute myocardial infarction. The protective effects of captopril. Circulation. 1994;89:68-75.
96. An D, Rodrigues B. The role of changes in cardiac metabolism in the development of diabetic cardiomyopathy. Am J Physiol Heart Circ Physiol. 2006, 291:H1489-H1506.
97. Finck BN. The role of the peroxisome proliferators-activated receptor alpha pathway in pathological remodeling of the diabetic heart. Curr Opin Clin Nutr Metab Care. 2004;7:391-6.
98. Young ME, McNulty P, Taegtmeyer H. Adaptation and maladaptation of the heart in diabetes: Part II: potential mechanisms. Circulation. 2002;105:1861-70.
99. Finck BN, Lehman JJ, Leone TC, et al. The cardiac phenotype induced by PPARalpha overexpression mimics that caused by diabetes mellitus. J Clin Invest. 2002;109:121-30.
100. Nystrom T, Nygren A, Sjoholm A. Increased levels of tumour necrosis factor-alpha (TNF-alpha) in patients with Type II diabetes mellitus after myocardial infarction are related to endothelial dysfunction. Clin Sci (Lond). 2006;110:673-81.
101. Giacchetti G, Sechi LA, Rilli S, et al. The rennin-angiotensin-aldosterone system, glucose metabolism and diabetes. Trends Endocrinol Metab. 2005;16:120-6.
102. Burger AJ, Aronson D. Blunted sympathetic response in diabetic patients with decompensated congestive heart failure. Int J Cardiol. 2001;81:243-9.
103. Suleiman M, Aronson D, Asleh R, et al. Haptoglobin polymorphism predicts 30-day mortality and heart failure in patients with diabetes and acute myocardial infarction. Diabetes. 2005;54:2802-6.
104. Maisel AS, Krishnaswamy P, Nowak RM, et al. Rapid measurement of B-type natriuretic peptide in the emergency diagnosis of heart failure. N Engl J Med. 2002;347:161-7.
105. Januzzi JL Jr, Camargo CA, Anwaruddin S, et al. The N-terminal Pro-BNP. Investigation of Dyspnea in the Emergency department (PRIDE) study. Am J Cardiol. 2005;95:948-54.
106. Januzzi JL, van Kimmenade R, Lainchbury J, et al. NT-proBNP testing for diagnosis and short-term prognosis in acute destabilized heart failure: an international pooled analysis of 1256 patients The International Collaborative of NT-proBNP Study. Eur Heart J. 2006;27:330-7.
107. Fonarow GC, Peacock WF, Phillips CO, et al. Admission B-type natriuretic peptide levels and in-hospital mortality in acute decompensated heart failure. J Am Coll Cardiol. 2007;49:1943-50.
108. Januzzi JL Jr, Sakhuja R, O'Donoghue M, et al. Utility of amino-terminal pro-brain natriuretic peptide testing for prediction of 1-year mortality in patients with dyspnea treated in the emergency department. Arch Intern Med. 2006;166:315-20.
109. Kociol RD, Horton JR, Fonarow GC, et al. Admission, discharge, or change in B-type natriuretic peptide and long-term outcomes: data from Organized Program to Initiate Lifesaving Treatment in Hospitalized Patients with Heart Failure (OPTIMIZE-HF) linked to Medicare claims. Circ Heart Fail. 2011;4:628-36.
110. Januzzi JL Jr, Filippatos G, Nieminen M, et al. Troponin elevation in patients with heart failure: on behalf of the third Universal Definition of Myocardial Infarction Global Task Force: Heart Failure Section. Eur Heart J. 2012;33:2265-71.
111. Peacock WFt, De Marco T, Fonarow GC, et al. Cardiac troponin and outcome in acute heart failure. N Engl J Med. 2008;358:2117-26.
112. Xue Y, Clopton P, Peacock WF, et al. Serial changes in high-sensitive troponin I predict outcome in patients with decompensated heart failure. Eur J Heart Fail. 2011;13:37-42.
113. Latini R, Masson S, Anand IS, et al. Prognostic value of very low plasma concentrations of troponin T in patients with stable chronic heart failure. Circulation. 2007;116:1242-9.
114. Masson S, Anand I, Favero C, et al. Serial measurement of cardiac troponin T using a highly sensitive assay in patients with chronic heart failure: data from 2 large randomized clinical trials. Circulation. 2012;125:280-8.
115. Maisel A, Mueller C, Nowak R, et al. Mid-region pro-hormone markers for diagnosis and prognosis in acute dyspnea: results from the BACH (Biomarkers in Acute Heart Failure) trial. J Am Coll Cardiol. 2010;55:2062-76.
116. Shah RV, Truong QA, Gaggin HK, et al. Mid-regional pro-atrial natriuretic peptide and pro-adrenomedullin testing for the diagnostic and prognostic evaluation of patients with acute dyspnoea. Eur Heart J. 2012;33:2197-205.
117. Richards AM, Doughty R, Nicholls MG, et al. Plasma N-terminal pro-brain natriuretic peptide and adrenomedullin: prognostic utility and prediction of benefit from carvedilol in chronic ischemic left ventricular dysfunction. Australia-New Zealand Heart Failure Group. J Am Coll Cardiol. 2001;37:1781-87.
118. Maisel A, Xue Y, Shah K, et al. Increased 90-day mortality in patients with acute heart failure with elevated copeptin: secondary results from the Biomarkers in Acute Heart Failure (BACH) study. Circ Heart Fail. 2011;4:613-20.
119. Sanada S, Hakuno D, Higgins LJ, et al. IL-33 and ST2 comprise a critical biomechanically induced and cardioprotective signaling system. J Clin Invest. 2007;117:1538-49.
120. Januzzi JL Jr, Peacock WF, Maisel AS, et al. Measurement of the interleukin family member ST2 in patients with acute dyspnea: results from the PRIDE (Pro-Brain Natriuretic Peptide Investigation of Dyspnea in the Emergency Department) study. J Am Coll Cardiol. 2007;50:607-13.
121. Boisot S, Beede J, Isakson S, et al. Serial sampling of ST2 predicts 90-day mortality following destabilized heart failure. J Card Fail. 2008;14:732-8.
122. Lassus J, Gayat E, Mueller C, et al. Incremental value of biomarkers to clinical variables for mortality prediction in acutely decompensated heart failure: the Multinational Observational Cohort on Acute Heart Failure (MOCA) study. Int J Cardiol. 2013;168:2186-94.

123. Bayes-Genis A, de Antonio M, Vila J, et al. Head-to-head comparison of 2 myocardial fibrosis biomarkers for long-term heart failure risk stratification: ST2 versus galectin-3. J Am Coll Cardiol. 2014;63:158-66.
124. Gaggin HK, Szymonifka J, Bhardwaj A, et al. Head-to-head comparison of serial soluble ST2, growth differentiation factor-15, and highly-sensitive troponin T measurements in patients with chronic heart failure. JACC Heart Fail. 2014;2:65-72.
125. Gaggin HK, Motiwala S, Bhardwaj A, et al. Soluble concentrations of the interleukin receptor family member ST2 and β-blocker therapy in chronic heart failure. Circ Heart Fail. 2013;6:1206-13.
126. Weir RA, Miller AM, Murphy GE, et al. Serum soluble ST2: a potential novel mediator in left ventricular and infarct remodeling after acute myocardial infarction. J Am Coll Cardiol. 2010;55:243-50.
127. Anand IS, Rector TS, Kuskowski M, et al. Prognostic value of soluble ST2 in the Valsartan Heart Failure Trial. Circ Heart Fail. 2014;7:418-26.
128. Kohli P, Bonaca MP, Kakkar R, et al. Role of ST2 in non-ST-elevation acute coronary syndrome in the MERLIN-TIMI 36 trial. Clin Chem. 2012;58:257-66.
129. Wang TJ, Wollert KC, Larson MG, et al. Prognostic utility of novel biomarkers of cardiovascular stress: the Framingham Heart Study. Circulation. 2012;126:1596-604.
130. Daniels LB, Bayes-Genis A. Using ST2 in cardiovascular patients: a review. Future Cardiol. 2014;10:525-39.
131. Manzano-Fernandez S, Mueller T, Pascual-Figal D, et al. Usefulness of soluble concentrations of interleukin family member ST2 as predictor of mortality in patients with acutely decompensated heart failure relative to left ventricular ejection fraction. Am J Cardiol. 2011;107:259-67.
132. Rehman SU, Mueller T, Januzzi JL Jr. Characteristics of the novel interleukin family biomarker ST2 in patients with acute heart failure. J Am Coll Cardiol. 2008;52:1458-65.
133. Bayes-Genis A, de Antonio M, Galan A, et al. Combined use of high-sensitivity ST2 and NT-proBNP to improve the prediction of death in heart failure. Eur J Heart Fail. 2012;14:32-8.
134. Mueller T, Dieplinger B, Gegenhuber A, et al. Increased plasma concentrations of soluble ST2 are predictive for 1-year mortality in patients with acute destabilized heart failure. Clin Chem. 2008;54:752-6.
135. Ky B, French B, McCloskey K, et al. High-sensitivity ST2 for prediction of adverse outcomes in chronic heart failure. Circ Heart Fail. 2011;4:180-7.
136. Felker GM, Fiuzat M, Thompson V, et al. Soluble ST2 in ambulatory patients with heart failure: Association with functional capacity and long-term outcomes. Circ Heart Fail. 2013;6:1172-9.
137. Maisel A, Xue Y, van Veldhuisen DJ, et al. Effect of spironolactone on 30-day death and heart failure rehospitalization (from the COACH Study). Am J Cardiol. 2014;114:737-42.
138. Gullestad L, Ueland T, Kjekshus J, et al. Galectin-3 predicts response to statin therapy in the Controlled Rosuvastatin Multinational Trial in Heart Failure (CORONA). Eur Heart J. 2012;33:2290-6.
139. Lok DJ, Van Der Meer P, de la Porte PW, et al. Prognostic value of galectin-3, a novel marker of fibrosis, in patients with chronic heart failure: data from the DEAL-HF study. Clin Res Cardiol. 2010;99:323-8.
140. van Kimmenade RR, Januzzi JL Jr, Ellinor PT, et al. Utility of amino-terminal pro-brain natriuretic peptide, galectin-3, and apelin for the evaluation of patients with acute heart failure. J Am Coll Cardiol. 2006;48:1217-24.
141. Motiwala SR, Szymonifka J, Belcher A, et al. Serial measurement of galectin-3 in patients with chronic heart failure: results from the ProBNP Outpatient Tailored Chronic Heart Failure Therapy (PROTECT) study. Eur J Heart Fail. 2013;15:1157-63.
142. Wuerz RC, Meador SA. Effects of prehospital medications on mortality and length of stay in congestive heart failure. Ann Emerg Med. 1992;21:669-74.
143. Picariello C, Lazzeri C, Valente S, et al. Procalcitonin in acute cardiac patients. Intern Emerg Med. 2011;6:245-52.
144. Christ-Crain M, Jaccard-Stolz D, Bingisser R, et al. Effect of procalcitonin-guided treatment on antibiotic use and outcome in lower respiratory tract infections: cluster-randomised, single-blinded intervention trial. Lancet. 2004;363:600-7.
145. Alba GA, Truong QA, Gaggin HK, et al. Diagnostic and prognostic utility of procalcitonin in patients presenting to the emergency department with dyspnea. Am J Med. 2016;129:96-104.e7.
146. Maisel A, Neath SX, Landsberg J, et al. Use of procalcitonin for the diagnosis of pneumonia in patients presenting with a chief complaint of dyspnoea: results from the BACH (Biomarkers in Acute Heart Failure) trial. Eur J Heart Fail. 2012;14:278-86.
147. Wang W, Zhang X, Ge N, et al. Procalcitonin testing for diagnosis and short-term prognosis in bacterial infection complicated by congestive heart failure: a multicenter analysis of 4,698 cases. Crit Care. 2014;18:R4.
148. McMurray JJ, Adamopouslos S, Anker DS, et al. ESC guidelines for the diagnosis and treatment of acute and chronic heart failure 2012. Eur Heart J. 2012;33:1787-847.
149. Felker GM, Lee KL, Bull DA, et al. Diuretic strategies in patients with acute decompensated heart failure. N Engl J Med. 2011;364:797-805.
150. National Institute for Health and Clinical Excellence. Acute Heart Failure: Diagnosis and management. Clinical guidelines. 2014;187.
151. Chen HH, Anstrom KJ, Givertz MM, et al. Low dose dopamine or low dose nesiritide in acute heart failure with renal dysfunction the ROSE acute heart failure randomized trial. J Am Med Assoc. 2013;310:2533-43.
152. Cuffe MS, Califf RM, Adams KF, et al. Short-term intravenous milrinone for acute exacerbation chronic heart failure: a randomized controlled trial. J Am Med Assoc. 2002;287: 1541-7.
153. Mebazaaa A, Niemien MS, Packer M, et al. Levosimendan vs dobutamine for patients with acute decompensated heart

failure: the SURVIVE randomized trial. J Am Med Assoc. 2007;197:1883-91.
154. Packer M, Colucci W, Fisher L, et al. Effector of levosimendan on short-term clinical course of patients with acutely decompensated heart failure. JACC Heart Fail. 2013;1:103-11.
155. Gottlieb SS, Stebbins A, Voors AA, et al. Effects of nesiritide and predictors of urine output in acute decompensated heart failure: results from ASCEND- HF (Acute Study of Clinical Effectiveness of Nesiritide and Decompensated Heart Failure). J Am Coll Cardiol. 2013;62:1177-83.
156. Teerlink, JR, Cotter G, Davison BA, et al. Serelaxin recombinant human relaxin-2 for treatment of acute heart failure (RELAX-AHF): a randomized, placebo-controlled trial. Lancet. 2013;381:29-39.
157. Gray AJ, Goodacre S, Newby DE, et al. A multicentre randomized controlled trial of the use of continuous positive airway pressure and non-invasive positive pressure ventilation in the early treatment of patients presenting to the emergency department with severe acute cardiogenic pulmonary oedema: the 3CPO trial. Health Technol Assess. 2009;13:1-106.
158. Steg G, James SK, Atar D, et al. ESC guidelines for the management of acute myocardial infarction in patients presenting with ST-segment elevation. Eur Heart J. 2012;33:2569-619.
159. Velazquez EJ, Lee KL, Deja MA, et al. Coronary-artery bypass surgery in patients with left ventricular dysfunction. N Engl J Med. 2011;364:160716.
160. Doenst T, Cleland JG, Rouleau JL, et al. Influence of crossover on mortality in a randomized study of revascularization in patients with systolic heart failure and coronary artery disease. Circ Heart Fail. 2013;6:443-50.
161. Bonnow RO, Maurer G, Lee KL, et al. Myocardial viability and survival in ischemic left ventricular dysfunction. N Engl J Med. 2011;364:1617-25.
162. Velazquez EJ, Lee KL, Jones RH, et al. Coronary artery bypass surgery in patients with ischemic cardiomyopathy. N Engl J Med. 2016;374:1511-20.
163. REVIVED-BCIS2 Clinical Trials Unit. 2013. Revascularization for ischemic ventricular dysfunction trial protocol version 7. [Online] Available from lshtm.ac.uk/revived/files/2015/05/Revived-BC152-protocol_v7_May-2015.pdf [Last Accessed, November, 2019]
164. Hochman JS, Sleeper LA, Webb JG, et al. Early revascularization in acute myocardial infarction complicated by cardiogenic shock. N Engl J Med. 1999;341:625-34.
165. Thiele H, Zeymer U, Neumann F-J, et al. Intraaortic balloon support for myocardial infarction with cardiogenic shock. N Engl J Med. 2012;367:1287-96.
166. Yusuf S, Peto R, Lewis J, et al. Beta-blockade during and after myocardial infarction: an overview of the randomized trials. Prog Cardiovasc Dis. 1985;27:335-71.
167. Smith SC Jr, Blair SN, Bonow RO, et al. AHA/ACC Guidelines for preventing heart attack and death in patients with atherosclerotic cardiovascular disease: 2001 update. A Statement for healthcare professionals from the American Heart Association and the American College of Cardiology. J Am Coll Cardiol. 2001;38:1581-3.
168. De backer G, Ambrosioni E, Borch-Johnsen K, et al. European guidelines on cardiovascular disease prevention in clinical practice. Third joint Task Force of European & other Societies on Cardiovascular Disease Prevention in Clinical Practice. Eur Heart J. 2003;24:1601-10.
169. Lopez-Sendo J, Swedberg K, McMurray J, et al. Expert consensus document on beta-adrenergic receptor blockers. Eur Heart J. 2004;25:1341-62.
170. Freemantle N, Cleland J, Young P, et al. beta blockade after myocardial infarction: systematic review and meta-regression analysis. BMJ. 1999;318:1730-7.
171. Dargie HJ. Effect of carvedilol on outcome after myocardial infarction in patients with left ventricular dysfunction: the CAPRICORN randomized trial. Lancet. 2001;357:1385-90.
172. Chen ZM. Early intravenous then oral metoprolol in 45,852 patients with acute myocardial infarction: randomized placebo-controlled trial. Lancet. 2005;366:1622-32.
173. O'Gara PT, Kushner FG, Ascheim DD, et al. 2013 ACCF/AHA guideline for the management of ST-elevation myocardial infarction: a report of the American College of Cardiology Foundation/American Heart Association Task Force on Practice Guidelines. J Am Coll Cardiol. 2013;61:e78-140.
174. Ponikowski P, Voors AA, Anker SD, et al. 2016 ESC Guidelines for the diagnosis and treatment of acute and chronic heart failure: the Task Force for the diagnosis and treatment of acute and chronic heart failure of the European Society of Cardiology (ESC) Developed with the special contribution of the Heart Failure Association (HFA) of the ESC. Eur Heart J. 2016;37:2129-200.
175. Indications for ACE inhibitors in the early treatment of acute myocardial infarction. Systematic overview of individual data from 100,000 patients in randomized trials. ACE inhibitor Myocardial infarction Collaborative Group. Circulation. 1998;97:2202-12.
176. Flather MD, Yusuf S, Køber L, et al. Long-term ACE-inhibitor therapy in patients with heart failure or left ventricular dysfunction; a systematic overview of data from individual patients. Lancet. 2000;355:1575-81.
177. Pfeffer MA, Braunwald E, Moye L, et al. Effect of captopril on mortality and morbidity in patients with left ventricular dysfunction after myocardial infarction: results of the survival and ventricular enlargement trial. N Engl J Med. 1992;327:669-77.
178. Effect of ramipril on mortality and morbidity of survivors of acute myocardial infarction with clinical evidence of heart failure. Acute infarction Ramipril Efficacy (AIRE) Study Investigators. Lancet. 1993;342:821-8.
179. Kober L, Torp-Pedersen C, Carisen JE, et al. A clinical trial of the angiotensin-converting-enzyme inhibitor trandolapril in patients with left ventricular dysfunction after myocardial infarction. N Engl J Med. 1995;333:1670-6.
180. The SOLVD Investigators. Effect of enalapril on survival in patients with reduced left ventricular ejection fractions and congestive heart failure. N Engl J Med. 1991;325;293-302.

181. The SOLVD Investigators. Effect of enalapril on mortality and the development of heart failure in asymptomatic patients with reduced left ventricular ejection fractions. N Engl J Med. 1992;327:685-91.
182. Dickstein K, Kjekshus J. OPTIMAAL Steering Committee of the OPTIMAAL Study Group. Effects of losartan captopril on mortality morbidity in high-risk patients after acute myocardial infarction: the OPTIMAAL randomized trial. Optimal Trial in Myocardial Infarction with Angiotensin II Antagonist Losartan. Lancet. 2002;360:752-60.
183. Pfeffer MA, McMurray JJ, Velazquez EJ, et al. Valsartan, captopril, or both in myocardial infarction complicated by heart failure, left ventricular dysfunction, or both. N Engl J Med. 2003;349:1893-906.
184. Adamopoulos C, Ahmed A, Fay R, et al. Timing of eplerenone initiation and outcomes in patients with heart failure after acute myocardial infarction complicated by left ventricular systolic dysfunction: insights from the EPHESUS trial. Eur J Heart Fail. 2009;11:1099-105.
185. Von Lueder TG, Wang BH, Kompa AR, et al. Angiotensin receptor neprilysin inhibitor LCZ696 attenuates cardiac remodelling and dysfunction after myocardial infarction by reducing cardiac fibrosis and hypertrophy. Circ Heart Fail. 2015;8:71-8.
186. Suematsu Y, Miura S, Goto M, et al. LCZ696, an angiotensin receptor-neprilysin inhibitor, improves cardiac function with the attenuation of fibrosis in heart failure with reduced ejection fraction in streptozotocin-induced diabetic mice. Eur J Heart Fail. 2016;18:386-93.
187. Bardy GH, Lee KL, Mark D, et al. Amiodarone or an implantable cardioverter-defibrillator for congestive heart failure. N Engl J Med. 2005;374:1521-32.
188. Moss AJ, Hall WJ, Cannom DS, et al. Improved survival with an implanted defibrillator in patients with coronary disease at high risk for ventricular arrhythmia: multicenter automatic Defibrillator implantation trial investigators. N Engl J Med. 1996;335:1933-44.
189. Bristow MR, Saxon LA, Boehmer J, et al. Cardiac resynchronization therapy with or without an implantable defibrillator in advanced chronic heart failure. N Engl J Med. 2004;350:2140-50.
190. Cleland J, Daubert JC, Erdmann E, et al. The Effect of cardiac resynchronization on morbidity and mortality in heart failure. N Engl J Med. 2005;352:1539-49.
191. Moss, AJ, Hall WJ, Cannom DS, et al. Cardiac resynchronization therapy for the prevention of heart failure events. N Engl J Med. 2009;361:1329-38.
192. Hohnloser SH, Kuck KH, Dorisan P, et al. Prophylactic use of an implantable cardioverter-defibrillator after acute myocardial infarction. N Engl J Med. 2004;351:2481-8.
193. Steinbeck G, Andresen D, Seidl K, et al. Defibrillator implantation early after myocardial infarction. N Engl J Med. 2009;361:1498-9.
194. Cohn JN, Ferrari R, Sharpe N. Cardiac remodelling–concepts and clinical implications: a consensus paper from an international forum on cardiac remodelling. Behalf of an International Forum on Cardiac Remodeling. J Am Coll Cardiol. 2000;35:569-85.
195. Bhatt AS, Ambrosy AP, Velazquez EJ. Adverse remodelling and reverse remodelling after myocardial infarction. Curr Cardiol Rep. 2017;19(8):71.
196. White HD, Norris RM, Brown MA, et al. Left ventricular end-systolic volume as the major determinant of survival after recovery from myocardial infarction. Circulation. 1987;76:44-51.
197. Solomon SD, Skali H, Anavekar NS, et al. Changes in ventricular size and function in patients treated with valsartan, captopril or both after myocardial infarction. Circulation. 2005;111:3411-9.
198. Bolognese L, Neskovic AN, Parodi G, et al. Left Ventricular remodelling after primary coronary angioplasty: patterns of left ventricular dilation and long-term prognostic implications. Circulation. 2002;106;2351-7.
199. Moller JE, Hillis GS, Oh JK, et al. Wall motion score index and ejection fraction for risk stratification after acute myocardial infarction. Am Heart J. 2006;151:419-25.
200. Kramer DG, Trikalinos TA, Kent DM, et al. Quantitative evaluation of drug or device effects on ventricular remodelling as predictors of therapeutic effects on mortality in patients with heart failure and reduced ejection fraction: a meta-analytic approach. J Am Coll Cardiol. 2010;56: 392-406.

Treatment of STEMI Paradigm Shift from Mortality to Heart Failure

VK Shah, SV Shah, KK Shalia

INTRODUCTION

Reperfusion by catheter-based methods or by fibrinolysis, made available within the first few hours (4 hours) to acute myocardial infarction (AMI) patients, is the standard treatment. However, those patients who are treated with same methods of reperfusion beyond this time span, do survive the index episode, but they now live with a significantly damaged heart or in more precise term, infarcted heart evident with reduced left ventricular ejection fraction (LVEF).[1,2] This is counteracted by dilatation of the LV leading to congestive heart failure (CHF) and repeated hospitalization.

Clinical research has led to interventions for heart failure with reduced ejection fraction (EF) that includes drugs, heart assist devices, and pacemaker. But, these interventions have shown not to prolong the survival and are not cost-effective. Cardiac transplant, due to lack of donor hearts, cannot meet even a partial demand of it. Moreover, these strategies are economically costly, precluding their universal implementation. Chronic treatment of heart failure represents a huge socioeconomic burden on individuals and healthcare systems.[3]

The strong relationship between infarct size and all-cause mortality, reinfarction, and hospitalization for heart failure suggested infarct size as an important prognostic measure when caring for patients with ST-segment elevation myocardial infarction (STEMI).[4] Therapies able to reduce infarct size are, therefore, urgently sought under the hypothesis that smaller infarctions will result in better long-term heart performance and that this will translate into fewer adverse clinical events. The stunning success of reperfusion therapies has resulted in a paradigm shift now, in clinical research in the treatment of STEMI. Attention is no longer solely aimed toward reducing mortality (already very low), but toward dealing with the parallel pathogenesis of improved survival which is postinfarction heart with reduced EF. The identification of therapies, supplemented to reperfusion or new therapies better able to reduce infarct size, is a major challenge of treatment of STEMI in the 21st century.

In the first stage of AMI, myocardial cells are injured as the result of anoxia and the absence of new essential metabolic substrates. In the absence of timely reperfusion and an inadequate collateral circulation, these injured cells die and scar tissue is formed. In the presence of reperfusion, either spontaneous or consequent to reperfusion therapy, ischemic injury is halted, but additional injury occurs as a result of reperfusion.[5] Clinical and experimental trials have shown that ischemic injury causes 50% of myocardial death and another 50% is caused by the reperfusion which is called reperfusion injury (RI).[6,7] This RI is characterized by myocardial, vascular, or electrophysiological dysfunction that is induced by the restoration of blood flow to previously ischemic tissue (Fig. 1).[8] *Thus, the main goals of salvaging the myocardium after AMI are:*

- *Decreasing ischemic injury*
- *Decreasing RI*
- *Regenerating myocardium.*

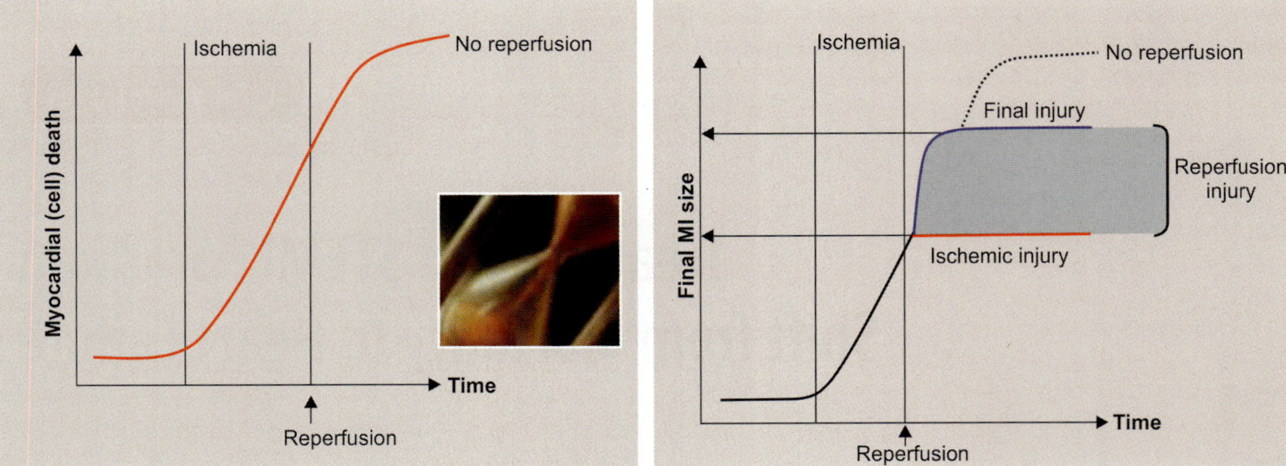

Fig. 1: Ischemia and reperfusion injury.[6]

DECREASING ISCHEMIC INJURY

It is important to note that 85% of muscle damage takes place within the first hour of AMI. This is often referred to as the "golden hour". It is within this time frame that the heart vessel needs to be opened. If time is lost and the vessel is opened after this time frame, the benefit is much less. Therefore, it is of the utmost importance that action be taken early. Thus, the central dogma of reperfusion therapy for STEMI is "Time is Muscle".[9] The total ischemic time is of paramount importance and often is overlooked in discussions about time to reperfusion. The importance of total ischemic time holds true regardless of whether reperfusion is attempted with a fibrinolytic or by PCI.[10] *It involves two steps: (1) reducing the symptoms to door time and (2) reducing the door-to-balloon time.*

Reducing the Symptoms to Door Time

Treatment regimens for AMI should aim to open the artery as soon as possible and as wide as possible. Early initiation of reperfusion therapy in STEMI improves outcome. It is also very much established that patients who received primary percutaneous coronary intervention (PPCI) as compared to thrombolysis have lower mortality and reinfarction rates. But there are regions where distance from to PPCI is more, which, in turn, consumes more time. In such instances, patients suitable for thrombolytic treatment and reperfusion should be initiated as soon as possible with some adjunctive antiplatelet agent such as aspirin and clopidogrel. *Prehospital thrombolysis (PHT)* is one strategy to deliver earlier reperfusion. PHT can begin with the nearest point of availability of trained paramedics with electrocardiogram (ECG) telemetry in consultation with hospital-based physicians, and need not wait till patient reaches hospital.[11] It is significantly superior to in-hospital thrombolysis (IHT). RIKS-HIA (The Swedish Register of Cardiac Intensive Care, also known as the Register of Information and Knowledge About Swedish Heart Intensive Care Admissions) and the NRMI (National Registry of Myocardial Infarction) trials have concluded that within 2 hours of symptom onset, patients should receive PHT only if PPCI is not available within 4 hours. Thus, when the total ischemic time is >120 minutes, PHT with immediate transport to a PCI-capable hospital is a more practical and effective approach (Fig. 2).[10]

The American Heart Association (AHA) and the American College of Cardiology (ACC) favor the use of PHT over PCI, placing the emphasis on the time factor rather than on the method of reperfusion. In CAPTIM (Comparison of primary angioplasty and prehospital fibrinolysis in acute myocardial infarction), which compared PPCI and PHT followed by PCI if thrombolysis failed and in GRACIA-1 (Grupo de Analisis de la Cardiopatia Isquemica Aguda) trial, which tested the role of systematic PCI within 24 hours of thrombolysis. The policy of systematic PCI following thrombolysis yielded better results than conservative management and proved to be a good backbone to subsequent in-hospital treatment. National Institute for Clinical Excellence supports reperfusion with fibrinolytics, recommending PHT using the newer agents, reteplase and tenecteplase, whose bolus application simplifies administration. PHT constitutes one of the means to administer reperfusion therapy without any delay.[11,12]

Prehospital thrombolysis is common in many parts of Europe. This includes a call center to dispatch a cardiac intensive care unit ambulance. The mobile ambulances include an onboard doctor/physician experienced in emergency assessment and treatment which comprises

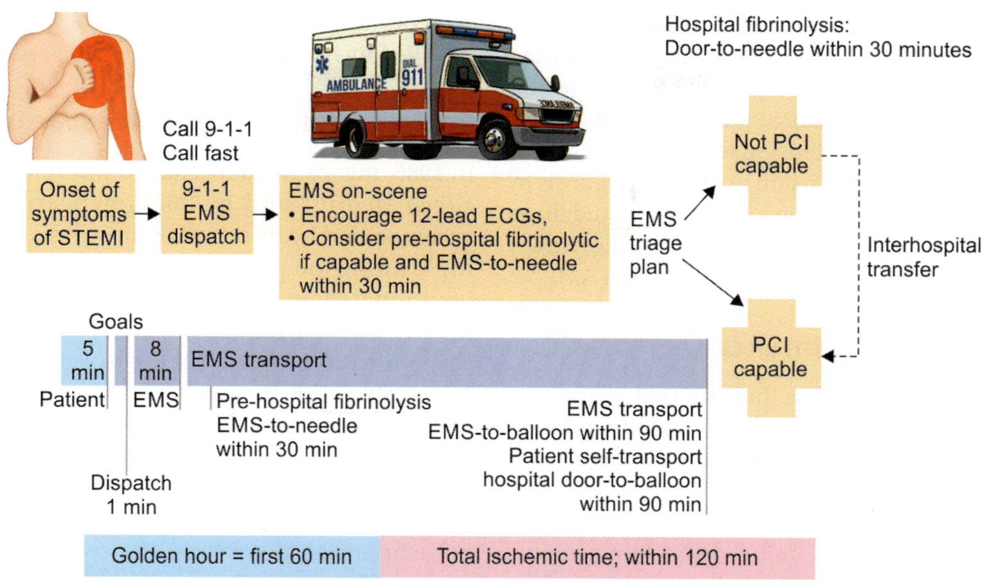

Fig. 2: Options for transportation of STEMI patients and initial reperfusion treatment goals.[9]
(EMS: emergency medical service; PCI: percutaneous coronary intervention; STEMI: ST-segment elevation myocardial infarction)

ECG diagnosis of STEMI, subsequent decision-making and administration of thrombolysis in the absence of contraindications. This eliminates the need for ECG telemetry and trained paramedic.[12] Based on studies conducted in higher income countries, McCaul et al. concluded that PHT reduced time to treatment and can be safely and correctly administered by trained staff. They have further suggested PHT could be of great help in low- and middle- income countries, especially in individuals who have limited access to PCI. There are no randomized controlled trials (RCTs) so far, which have evaluated the efficacy of PHT for STEMI in lower- and middle-income countries.[13]

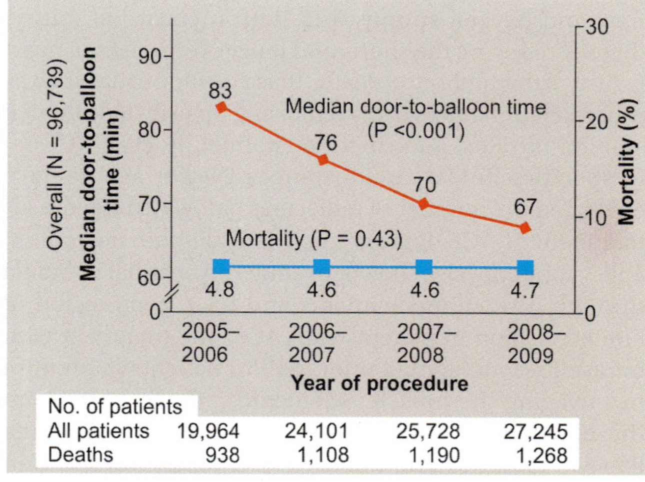

Fig. 3: Despite improvement in door-to-balloon time no change in mortality.[14]

Reducing the Door-to-Balloon Time

Door-to-balloon time has become a performance measure and is the focus of regional and national quality improvement initiatives. In a study carried out by Menees et al., 2013,[14] it was observed that Median door-to-balloon times declined significantly, from 83 minutes in the 12 months from July 2005 through June 2006 to 67 minutes in the 12 months from July 2008 through June 2009 (P < 0.001). Similarly, the percentage of patients for whom the door-to-balloon time was 90 minutes or less increased from 59.7% in the first year to 83.1% in the last year (P < 0.001). Despite improvements in door-to-balloon times, there was no significant overall change in unadjusted in-hospital mortality (4.8% in 2005–2006 and 4.7% in 2008–2009, P = 0.43 for trend) or in risk-adjusted in-hospital mortality (5.0% in 2005–2006 and 4.7% in 2008–2009, P = 0.34), nor was a significant difference observed in unadjusted 30-day mortality (P = 0.64) (Fig. 3).

The inference concluded from the study was that door-to-balloon time is one component of total ischemic time. As door-to-balloon time is reduced, it becomes a smaller fraction of total ischemic time, making the time before arrival at a hospital a more important factor. Therefore, efforts with potential to improve outcomes may include increasing patients' awareness of symptoms, patient's education with social responsible programs, and reaching at earliest to the chest pain centers, reducing the interval from the time of symptom onset to treatment, and shortening the transfer time between medical facilities. Thus, longer duration of coronary artery occlusion leads to larger infarct size, and therefore, early reperfusion improves prognosis by reducing infarct size and morality.[15-17] Current guidelines strongly recommends within 90 minutes coronary angioplasty as timely reperfusion for ST elevation AMI.[15]

Pharmacological Treatments

Current antiplatelet medications that are used in addition to aspirin include the thienopyridines, clopidogrel, and prasugrel, but there are several limitations to the use of these medications. Ticagrelor is a drug in a new chemical class that reversibly binds the P_2Y_{12} receptor and noncompetitively blocks adenosine diphosphate-induced platelet activation. It was specifically designed to address the limitations of the available antiplatelet agents while maintaining comparable or better antiplatelet effects.[18]

Other nonthrombotic treatments include decreasing myocardial oxygen demand, increasing coronary blood flow and oxygen supply, and limit myocardial injury, thereby reducing the short- and longer-term risks of heart failure, arrhythmia, and death. These include drugs such as β-blockers, inhibitors of the renin–angiotensin–aldosterone system, nitrates, and calcium channel blockers (CCBs) in specific clinical circumstances. Newer agents have expanded the number of molecular pathways targeted for treatment of ACS. Ranolazine, trimetazidine, nicorandil, and ivabradine have shown to reduce myocardial ischemia through diverse mechanisms and have been tested in limited fashion in patients with ACS. The treatment with intravenous metoprolol prior to PPCI has shown promise in salvaging the muscle (Metocard 2 trial). Apart from these primary measures, secondary measures include lifestyle modification, intensive risk-factor intervention and guideline-directed medical management with antithrombotic agents, and high-intensity statins to reduce the morbidity and mortality associated with ACS.[19]

DECREASING REPERFUSION INJURY

Myocardial injury in the setting of an AMI is the result of ischemic injury and RI. Reperfusion therapies, including PPCI and fibrinolytic therapy, promptly restore blood flow to ischemic myocardium and limit infarct size. Paradoxically, however, the return of blood flow can result in additional cardiac damage and complications; this is referred to as RI.[6,7] Even, timely reperfusion is not enough to solve the RI-related problems, as there is a dissociation seen between the coronary angiographic patency and the salvaged myocardium.

Reperfusion Injury to Myocardium

In 1985, myocardial reperfusion was referred as *a double-edged sword*[20] and by 2007 myocardial reperfusion accompanied by myocardial injury, was considered lethal RI.[21] During the past decade, three paradoxes have been incriminated as playing a role in lethal myocardial RI: (1) The *calcium paradox*, which raises intracytoplasmic calcium concentration, (2) the *oxygen paradox*, in which reperfusion raises myocardial pO_2, causing the formation of toxic reactive oxidants, and (3) *the pH paradox*, in which a physiologic pH is suddenly restored in the ischemic zone in which the pH had declined. It has been postulated that these paradoxes are involved in opening a channel in the inner mitochondrial membrane, the so-called *mitochondrial permeability transition pore (mPTP)*. This causes rapid influx of calcium and reactive oxygen species (ROS) through these pores and damages mitochondria. Now, mitochondria fail to synthesize high energy phosphate, thereby leading to myocyte death.[21] The pathogenesis of unique phenomenon, "No Reflow" is thought to be due to prolonged ischemia and extensive myocardial damage to microvascular (capillary) bed and distal embolization of the plaque/thrombus following reperfusion therapies.[5] The typical morphological features of reperfused myocardial infarction are contraction bands, karyolysis, mitochondrial swelling, disruption, membrane disruption in cardiomyocytes, and myocyte death accompanied by microvascular obstruction, interstitial hemorrhage, and inflammation.[22,23] Thus, RI accounts for up to 50% of the final myocardial damage in the setting of AMI.[23] Clinical manifestations of ischemic RI include arrhythmias, microvascular dysfunction, and myocardial stunning.[20]

Reperfusion injury can be prevented by an intervention applied at the time of reperfusion. However, effective therapies to reduce or prevent RI have proven elusive. Despite an improved understanding of the pathophysiology of this process and encouraging preclinical trials of multiple agents, most of the clinical trials to prevent RI have been disappointing due to many reasons. Multiple mechanisms contribute to the consequences of myocardial infarction (MI) and RI. Therefore, the impact of a therapy targeted to a single component of the pathophysiology may be diluted in clinical practice. Some mechanisms, such as neutrophil stimulation, may be mediators of injury, but also play important roles in the healing process. Targeting such mechanisms would have complex and unpredictable implications on outcomes. It may not be possible to administer a therapy at the optimal time in clinical practice. The presence of comorbidities, such as diabetes, hypercholesterolemia, and age, may impact the efficacy of a new treatment.[24] Identification of patients at highest risk of RI may be an important component of bringing therapies into clinical practice. As an example, myocardial blush grade has been used as a tool to evaluate myocardial level perfusion, wherein low blush grades correlate with myocardial dysfunction.[25] Such tools may also allow for better clinical assessment of therapeutic effectiveness of drugs tested in clinical trials. Despite these problems, adjunctive therapies to limit RI remain an active area of investigation.

Treatments that protect from RI should generally be applied before or as early as possible during reperfusion, because most cell death occurs during the first minutes of reflow. Over the past three decades, many cardioprotective strategies against myocardial ischemia-reperfusion injury (IRI) have been proposed.[26,27] Many interventions to prevent or diminish lethal myocardial RI have been studied. These can be broadly divided into several categories based on the protective modality.[28] These cardioprotective modalities that have been the most studied are based on either:

- The controlled application of episodes of brief ischemia and reperfusion (ischemic conditioning)
- Aspiration thrombectomy prior to coronary stenting
- The administration of pharmacological substances
- The application of physical measures, such as hypothermia, hyperoxemia/hyperoxia.

The Controlled Application of Episodes of Brief Ischemia and Reperfusion (Ischemic Conditioning)

Strategies based on ischemic conditioning include local ischemic preconditioning (IPC), remote ischemic conditioning (RIC), local ischemic post-conditioning (IPost), and perconditioning.

In *preconditioning*, brief cycles of alternating ischemia and reflow prior to a sustained occlusion have shown to reduce the size of the subsequent infarct.[29] Local IPC delays recovery of pH, prevents uncoupling of nitric oxide synthases (NOS) and subsequent generation of reactive oxygen and nitrogen species, and increases protein kinase G (PKG), RI salvage kinase (RISK), and survivor activating factor enhancement (SAFE), signaling in reperfused cardiomyocytes.[29] It has been observed that this cyclic ischemia can be induced in an organ or tissue other than the heart, yet remain cardioprotective, an intervention termed *remote ischemic preconditioning*.[30-32] RIC appears to share with IPC an effect on nitrotyrosylation and preservation of protein kinase G (PKG),[33] but also acts on mitochondrial function and activates the RISK and SAFE pathways.[34,35] However, the clinical value of ischemic preconditioning local or remote is useful only when the timing of the prolonged ischemia, such as that induced by cardiac surgery or a PCI, is known. It is not applicable to patients with the usual AMI, in whom the time when the coronary occlusion will occur, is of course not known. "Postconditioning" in which the cyclic periods of ischemia and reflow are begun immediately after the prolonged occlusion is relieved, has also been shown to reduce ischemic injury,[36,37] and it too can be effective when carried out remotely.[38] Conditioning can also be begun during the occlusion and it is then referred to as "*perconditioning*".[39]

Aspiration Thrombectomy Prior to Coronary Stenting

Another technique used to overcome RI was *aspiration thrombectomy prior to coronary stenting* to overcome RI. After the initial enthusiasm created by the single center TAPAS (Thrombus Aspiration During Percutaneous Coronary Intervention in Acute Myocardial Infarction), the other multicentric TASTE (Thrombus Aspiration in ST-Elevation Myocardial Infarction in Scandinavia), and TOTAL (Trial of Routine Aspiration Thrombectomy with PCI Versus PCI Alone in Patients with STEMI), each with more than 1,000 patients, undertook an individual patient-level meta-analysis to determine the effect of thrombus aspiration (TA) on 30-day cardiovascular mortality and stroke or transient ischemic attack (TIA).[40] The trial investigators concluded that there was no significant difference in recurrent myocardial infarction, stent thrombosis, heart failure, or target vessel revascularization between manual thrombus aspiration plus PCI and PCI alone in patients with STEMI. Similar results have been documented by Taglieri et al. (2019) wherein a meta-analysis of 25 randomized controlled trials was carried out.[41] Wu et al. (2018) performed meta-analysis of results from prospective or randomized control trials on intracoronary (IC) glycoprotein IIb/IIIa inhibitors (GPIs) after TA for patients STEMI, as compared with PCI alone and concluded that IC GPIs may have a synergistic effect with TA on short-term mortality, reinfarction, and cardiac functional recovery.[42] A single center experience on thrombo-aspiration during PCI by Manolis et al. (2019) have also concluded that selective thrombo-aspiration for angiographically visible thrombi in MI patients undergoing PCI, as an adjunct to mechanical reperfusion and to IIb/IIIa-inhibitors, may be an option, since this maneuver may improve procedural and clinical outcome. Although their literature survey revealed that several early observational and RCTs and meta-analyses favored manual, not mechanical, thrombectomy, they concluded that newer RCTs and meta-analyses significantly curtailed the initial enthusiasm for the clinical benefits of routine use of thromboaspiration.[43] The reason for no benefit can be traced back in 2005 in the study by Salloum, et al.,[44] who have demonstrated that during PCI of Saphenous Vein Grafts, in spite of using distal protection devices, i.e. filters to capture the insoluble particulate matter, there were soluble factors which may have injured the distal microvascular bed. This may explain the additional myocardial injury occurring post-PCI therapy. These soluble factors were evaluated during PCI and it was inferred that at 24 hours, there were increased soluble inflammatory and thrombotic components following reperfusion by intervention. Modulation of these components may protect the heart from RI over and above the conventional management of RI for insoluble particulate matter.[45]

The Administration of Pharmacological Substances

Cardioprotective strategies may be further categorized by their end targets. These molecular targets are ion exchangers and channels, proteases, ROS, contractile elements, or constituents of the mPTP involved mainly in necrotic cell death. These strategies have generally been based on the use of preexisting pharmacological tools. Other forms of cell death may occur during acute myocardial IRI, including apoptosis, autophagy, necroptosis, and pyroptosis, all of which may contribute in varying degrees to final MI size following acute IRI and provide new targets for cardioprotection.[24]

Other targets include activation of endogenous cardioprotective signaling pathways, including the NO/cGMP/PKG cascade, RISK and SAFE pathways, mitochondrial morphology, and cardiomyocyte metabolism.[46] Inflammation contributes to post-MI injury and forms an additional target for its reduction.[47] Translation of these individual targets to patients has met with variable success, but they could form part of a multitarget strategy.[48,49]

Finally, cardioprotective strategies may be aimed at either protecting cardiomyocytes or noncardiomyocyte cells, such as platelets or leukocytes.[47,48] Although cardiomyocytes are the working cells in the heart and the most susceptible to IRI, the myocardium also contains a large number of other cell types that are important players in myocardial IRI, including endothelial cells, fibroblasts, smooth muscle cells, and neuronal cells. Some factors released by the endothelium and fibroblasts (i.e. the "secretome") such as microRNA (miRNA) and exosomes, may contribute to cardioprotective signaling.[49,50] IRI may cause the death of noncardiomyocytes by various pathways including apoptosis.[51] Furthermore, IRI may disrupt the endothelial barrier favoring myocardial edema,[52,53] and may activate endothelial cells causing them to interact with circulating blood cells that may plug the microvessels, release molecules that affect cardiomyocyte function and tolerance to IRI, and infiltrate the myocardium. Platelets are some of the first hematopoietic cells to respond to IRI. Although activated platelets release factors that may exert cardioprotective effects during ischemia[54] strong evidence indicates that they may exacerbate RI by mechanisms not dependent on vessel obstruction.[55,56] They also form coaggregates with white blood cells (mainly neutrophils), and these plugs are distally embolized upon reperfusion contributing to microvascular obstruction (MVO).[44] MVO can also be caused by embolization from the recanalized coronary plaque and extrinsic compression secondary to edema formation upon reperfusion.[57,58] Furthermore, areas of no-reflow and intramyocardial hemorrhage may develop due to extreme myocardial devastation.[59] MVO and no-reflow have the potential to cause further cardiomyocyte necrosis[60] and are clearly associated with adverse prognosis in patients with AMI.[54] Table 1 lists some of the drugs against RI and their outcome.

Thus, erythropoietin, adenosine, etc. have not proved efficient for alleviation of lethal RI. A significant benefit has been reported for cyclosporine, nicorandil, ANP, insulin, and exenatide. However, each of these drugs needs more substantial evidence in larger clinical trials. For example, FX-06 significantly reduced the necrotic core zone compared with placebo in STEMI patients undergoing PCI. Whether FX-06 treatment can have a clinical benefit remains to be established. Nonetheless, the unique mechanism of action and short half-life that distinguish FX-06 from competitive pharmacological agents would allow its use in combination with other drugs, potentially contributing to a successful pharmacological therapy for the prevention of ischemia/RI after decades of disappointing results. Other new pharmacological agents also needed to be identified and tested in phase II trials.[85]

The sharp timing and the narrow time window for myocardial protection against reperfusion necrosis have two important consequences. First, it makes mandatory that the therapeutic intervention be performed before reopening of the culprit coronary artery. In terms of practical aspects, administration of the pharmacological treatment must, therefore, be started at any time before angioplasty (or thrombolysis), i.e. as early as first medical care but no later than before coronary reflow. It is likely that, in the future, many treatments aimed at not only opening the culprit artery but also preventing RI, will be started in the ambulance, before hospital admission. Second, it imposes that we consider the pharmacokinetics of the drug with specific attention to its availability at an optimal concentration within the reperfused myocardium at the onset of reperfusion. However, while we know that the drug must be active during the first minute of reperfusion, we do not yet know how long after reflow the exposure to this protective treatment should continue in order to optimize the prevention of myocardial injury.[86,87]

TABLE 1: Pharmacological treatments to combat IRI and ischemic events.

Drug	*Mechanism*	*Author/Trial*	*Remark*
Erythropoietin (EPO)	EPO displays anti-inflammatory properties, promotes neovascularization, and induces mobilization of endothelial progenitor cells from bone marrow, activates the RISK pathway and reduce infarct size in animal models of myocardial IRI.[61]	Lipsic et al. (2006),[62] Binbreck et al. (2009)[63] Ferrario et al. (2011)[64]	These trials showed discrepancy with preclinical studies and demonstrated no change in infarct size in the group of patients who received EPO.
Adenosine	Vasodilator, inhibitor of platelet aggregation and leukocyte adherence to the endothelium, direct cardioprotective effect on the cardiomyocytes. Protect from RI through RISK pathway and subsequent inhibition of the opening of mPTP.[65]	AMISTAD-I (Acute Myocardial Infarction STudy of ADenosine) AMISTAD II PREVENT (Prevention of Recurrent Venous Thromboembolism) and ICARUS (Intraperitoneal Chemotherapy After cytoReductive Surgery) trials.[65]	Demonstrated no reduction in a combined clinical end point of heart failure or overall mortality at 6 months.[65]
KAI-9803	Is a novel peptide that inhibits protein kinase C delta activity. Protein kinase C delta is an isoenzyme of the protein kinase C family that has been identified as a mediator of lethal RI through its binding to mitochondria. Therefore, inhibiting it will reduce the RI.[66]	DELTA-MI[66]	One before and one after primary PCI, of KAI-9803 has been recently established in the Protein Kinase C Enzyme to Limit Total Infarct Size in AMI trial conducted in patients with anterior STEMI.[66] However, cardioprotection seen in experimental models has not been translated into clinical trials.
Cyclosporin A (CsA)	Cyclosporin, a potent immunosuppressor through its binding to cyclophilin A and the subsequent inhibition of the calcineurin-nuclear transcription factor of activated T cells pathway and has also been recognized as an inhibitor of the opening of the mPTP, via its binding to the mitochondrial D isoform of cyclophilin.[67]	Griffiths et al.[67]	In a three-center clinical trial showed that cyclosporin A reduced infarct size.
		Piot et al.[68]	They demonstrated that cyclosporine-A inhibited mPTP at reperfusion.
		Cyclosporin and Prognosis in Acute Myocardial Infarction Patients (CIRCUS)[69] and Cyclosporine A in Reperfused Acute Myocardial Infarction (CYCLE)[70]	These trials failed to show any benefits
		Ikeda G, (2016)[71]	Demonstrated that poly-lactic/glycolic acid (PLGA) nanoparticle-mediated cyclosporine A (CsA), enhances CsA-induced cardioprotection.
Nicorandil	A Potassium-ATP (K-ATP) channel opener is involved in ischemic preconditioning and microvascular vasodilation.[72]	Krombach GA et al. (2005)[72]	Better perfusion and left ventricular wall motion, reduction in adverse events and improved microvascular obstruction by CMR imaging data.
Atrial natriuretic peptide	Reduced the RI through activation of known prosurvival signaling pathways.[73]	Kitakaze M (2007)[74]	In a large clinical trial administering carperitide (an ANP analog) at a time of PPCI demonstrated 14.7% reduction in enzymatic MI size.

Contd...

Contd...

Drug	*Mechanism*	*Author/Trial*	*Remark*
Insulin	Experimental animal studies have shown that promoting glucose metabolism using insulin during acute myocardial ischemia is beneficial for the heart. Insulin administration also acts through the cGMP/PKG pathway (via Akt and PI3P), as well as by increasing glucose use.[75,76]	CREATE-ECLA trial[77]	No benefit was observed.
		In IMMEDIATE trial[78]	In IMMEDIATE randomized, controlled double-blind study demonstrated, that glucose-insulin-potassium can reduce infarct size and serious electrical complications when administered in the ambulance to patients with STEMI who will receive primary angioplasty.
Glucagon-like peptide-1 (Exenatide)	Glucagon-like peptide-1 regulate glucose homeostasis, attenuate lethal RI in an animal model, possibly via the activation of several signaling pathways, e.g. cGMP/PKG.[79,80]	Lonborg J et al., 2012.[81,82]	These two clinical trials have evaluated the effect of a glucagon-like peptide-1 agonist, exenatide, in patients with STEMI who underwent primary angioplasty, and both studies have shown reduced infarct size[81,82]
Beta-blocker-metoprolol	Anti-ischemic effects of the beta-blockers are not only due to their negative inotropic/chronotropic effects but also due to a lipid peroxidation reducing mechanism.[83]	METOCARD-CNIC study[83] and Ndrepepa et al. (2013)[84]	These blinded studies aimed to determine the effect of intravenous metoprolol, administered immediately before primary angioplasty, demonstrated protection via salvage of myocardium without any major complications wherein infarct size was analyzed by magnetic resonance imaging (MRI).
FX-06	Competitively binds to vascular endothelial (VE)-cadherin, thereby inhibiting leukocyte transmigration and initiating VE-cadherin-mediated signaling, which tightens the endothelial barrier and reduces capillary leakage.[83]	Ahrens and Peter et al. (2009)[85]	In a phase II trial in patients with acute STEMI who were undergoing PCI, FX-06 significantly reduced the necrotic core zone compared with placebo.

(ANP: atrial natriuretic peptide; ATP: adenosine triphosphate; cGMP: cyclic guanosine monophosphate; IRI: ischemia-reperfusion injury; PCI: percutaneous coronary intervention; PKG: protein kinase G; RISK: reperfusion injury signaling kinase)

The Application of Physical Measures, Such as Hypothermia and Hyperoxemia/Hyperoxia

Hypothermia: *Major concept of cooling-induced cardioprotection is energy preservation*—(1) reduced metabolic demands of myocardium and preserved adenosine triphosphate and glycogens, (2) enhanced cellular membrane stability from reduced acidosis, (3) reduction of Na^+ and Ca^{2+} overload,[88-90] and (4) enhanced mitochondrial membrane stability by inhibition of calcium-induced mPTP opening, maintained ion homeostasis during ischemia and reperfusion, and preserved microvascular structures.[90] Therapeutic hypothermia during reperfusion prevents microvascular damage, obstruction and no-reflow phenomenon. The initial two trials, the Cooling as an Adjunctive Therapy to Percutaneous Intervention in patients with AMI (COOL-MI trial, n = 392) and The Intravascular Cooling Adjunctive to Percutaneous Coronary Intervention for AMI (ICE-IT trial, n = 228) showed no significant reduction of infarct size at 30 days. However subsequent pooled analysis of RCTs of Therapeutic Hypothermia (TH) in Patients with Acute Myocardial Infarction (Rapid MI-ICE, CHILL-MI, and VELOCITY) showed feasibility and safety of TH for cardioprotection in AMI, i.e. reduced infarct size and decreased incidence of postinfarction HF. In addition, TH was found to be more effective in large myocardium at risk and anterior wall infarction.[91-93]

Hence, rapid cooling, i.e. achieving target temperature of 32°, without delaying reperfusion therapy, was observed to be the most important for successful outcomes. The efforts now required are toward obtaining target temperature as low as 32°C to achieve maximum infarct size reduction in patients with AMI. The important topics to achieve target 32°C are: (1) Invention of clinically applicable devices and medications, (2) optimization of protocols and medical support during cooling and rewarming periods, and (3) diversification of cooling devices and dealing with safety issues, e.g. local cooling device.[94]

Hyperoxemia/Hyperoxia: In theory, increased availability of oxygen might increase ROS production and thus aggravate the RI. Furthermore, it has been shown that hyperoxia induces coronary vasoconstriction and decreases coronary flow in both healthy volunteers and patients with coronary artery disease (CAD).[95,96] Hypoxic or controlled reperfusion alleviates postischemic injury in skeletal muscle[96] and stomach.[97] In principle, oxygen supplementation during reperfusion by thrombolysis or PCI might be harmful. The optimal oxygenation strategy of patients with AMI undergoing reperfusion has not been studied in large randomized investigations. In a systematic review, *Wijesinghe and coworkers concluded that* the limited evidence that does exist suggests that the routine use of high-flow oxygen in uncomplicated AMI may result in a greater infarct size and possibly increase the risk of mortality.[98] *The Cochrane collaboration recently concluded:* "nonetheless, since the evidence suggests that oxygen may in fact be harmful, we think it is important to evaluate this widely used treatment in a large trial, as soon as possible, to make sure that current practice is not causing harm to people who have had a heart attack."[99] *A recent editorial in the British Medical Journal stated*: "The potential dangers of hyperoxia need to be recognized," and that "Oxygen therapy remains a cornerstone of modern medical practice. To further quantify the risks associated with hyperoxia more trials are needed."[100] In cardiac surgery using cardiopulmonary bypass and cardioplegia, there is a postcardioplegic reperfusion of the ischemic myocardium. Studies in different models have suggested that normoxia during reoxygenation of the hypoxic or cardioplegic heart reduces RI.[101-103] Lars Henrik Mariero, et al., 2012 demonstrated in a rat model that normobaric hyperoxia during early reperfusion did not increase ischemia/RI.[104]

It has been estimated that timely reperfusion can salvage approximately 50% of severely ischemic myocardium[105] and that prevention of lethal myocardial RI should prevent the necrosis of an additional 40%. If the latter is successful, it would further substantially reduce the mortality from AMI.[21] Many other trials have been carried out with each modality for reducing RI in patients presenting with STEMI. Despite 30–50% reduction of infarct size in animal models, no benefits were observed in clinical trials of these agents.[8,87]

NEW UPDATES

Emerging data suggest that optimal cardioprotection may require the combination of additive or synergistic multitarget therapies. These include interventions with single or multiple cardioprotective agents, targeting the cardiomyocyte and noncardiomyocytes at distinct time-points during ischemia and reperfusion.[27] Davidson et al. (2019*)* hypothesize that the ideal multitargeted therapy might be one that can target MVO (e.g. intravenous cangrelor or ANGPL4), target cardiomyocytes (e.g. remote ischemic per-conditioning), and target inflammation (e.g. metoprolol). The timing of administration of these modalities could potentially be separated over time.[27] Although more research is much needed in this area and the precise pathophysiology is still to be determined, the simple application of the current standard-of-care can help prevent the development of no-reflow.

Modern reperfusion strategies and advances in pharmacological management that resolve the ischemia, but not the infarct zone have resulted in an increasing proportion of AMI survivors at heightened risk of developing

LV remodeling and heart failure. None of our current therapies address the underlying cause of the remodeling process, that is, the damage of cardiomyocytes and the vasculature in the infarcted area.[87]

REGENERATING MYOCARDIUM

When there is no road ahead, one has to look left and right and if these turns also have dead end, then one has to take U-turn. After immense efforts toward protecting the myocytes from death, one group of irreverent thinkers at the end of the 20th century took this U-turn and started to question, the very fundamental concept of heart, i.e. "heart is a postmitotic organ incapable of regeneration". Their argument was that "if adult stem cells can restore blood and immune system then why not regenerate myocytes?" Supporting experimental evidences were endogenous cell recruitment form the systemic circulation within the myocardium, evidences that not only exogenously administered cell population home to the injured heart but also they can reconstitute infarcted myocardium, existence of cardiac stem cells, and regenerative potential of native human myocardium.[106]

The encouragement to this hypothesis was obtained by the revolutionary paper of Orlic et al. in 2001,[107] which suggested that directly injecting hematopoietic stem cells (HSCs) in an animal experiment, resulted in extensive myocardial regeneration. And subsequently, path breaking clinical study by Strauer et al. (2002)[108] who reported not only improved left ventricular function (LVF) in human trial but also safety and efficacy of infusing bone marrow mononuclear fraction (BMMNCs) through IC route, although in a very small study population. This began the journey of stem cells as therapy in regenerating the human myocardium. However, several trials although with positive outcome or no benefit, raised several questions on types of cells and number of cells to be injected, which cell application method to be used, when cells should be transferred, identification of specific cues and understanding the signaling pathways that direct stem cells to targeted destination and improve stem cell homing efficiency, what should be the clinical endpoints, etc.[109-113]

These questions brought diversion from the main bedside trials to the benchside experiments. These have included evaluating the possibilities of using induced pluripotent stem cells (IPSCs) as they can differentiate into multiple cell types of the adult body, in direct cardiac reprogramming, of endogenous cardiac fibroblasts into induced cardiomyocyte-like cells using transcription factors, Gata4, Mef2c, and Tbx5.[114-119] Other avenues explored are the Wnt/β-catenin signaling pathway to enhance cardiac tissue proliferation in mature cardiomyocytes,[120] three-dimensional (3D) printed scaffolds and 3D bioprinting technique have potential to develop fully functional heart construct that can integrate with native tissues rapidly,[121] the potential utility of extracellular matrix (ECM) in improving the therapeutic effect of transplanted cells,[122] combination of cell-cycle regulators that induce stable cytokinesis in adult postmitotic cells for reentering the cell cycle for regenerative repair,[123] allogeneic cell combination therapy (ACCT) [combination of mesenchymal stem cells (MSCs) and cardiac stem cells (CSCs)] demonstrates synergistic effects to enhance cardiac regeneration and LVF recovery.[124] Use of nanomaterials, to increase the retention and survival rate of engrafted cells is also explored.[125,126]

Stem cell potency is a double-aged sword, and therefore, although the initial experimental studies confirmed that the infusion of bone marrow stem cells (BMSCs) do not cause major side effects, several potential issues were raised such as electrical stability, increased restenosis, or progression of atherosclerotic disease. However, none of the clinical studies with BMSCs so far have reported an increased incidence of arrhythmias (as have been seen in some of the myoblast trials), bleeding complications, additional ischemic injury, or promoted inflammatory reaction as no further increase in C-reactive protein (CRP), and troponin was observed including in our study.[12] Cardiac regenerative medicine is promising, and a number of clinical trials in humans have already shown its indisputable safety. However, after initial rise in the hope with each trial, today stem cell therapy now is at plateau and requires to find answers on its mechanism and standardizing its parameters for its accommodation under conventional treatment.[111]

CONCLUSION

After a span of a centuries work on hypothesizing and demonstrating the pathogenesis of AMI and its treatment, new clinical era demands focus not only on epicardial coronary artery patency but also on MVO to salvage more myocardium. One will have to treat from all sides at all-time points to salvage the damaged infarcted myocardium. Initially prior to AMI, by pharmacologically inhibiting thrombotic ischemic injury at least in known and high-risk population. At the time of AMI, by using conventional modalities with additional physiological and pharmacological conditioning, during interventional stage (thrombolysis or PCI), by TA or by pharmacological and physical therapies, further, regenerating the myocardium by stem cells and last by post-hospitalization care. All these steps need to be standardized and included under conventional treatment. Current modalities have been able to open up macrovascular obstructions. Now the therapeutic arrow will have to be pointed at MVO to conquer the "no reflow", the main reason for the postinfarction reduced LVEF and save the myocardium.

REFERENCES

1. Antonelli L, Katz M, Bacal F, et al. Heart failure with preserved left ventricular ejection fraction in patients with acute myocardial infarction. Arq Bras Cardiol. 2015;105(2):145-50.
2. Braunwald E, Kloner RA. Myocardial reperfusion: a double-edged sword? J Clin Invest. 1985;76(5):1713-9.
3. Shah VK, Shalia KK. Reperfusion to regeneration and beyond. Ind J Cardio Biol Clin Sci. 2014;1(1):1-6.
4. Stone GW, Selker HP, Thiele H, et al. Relationship between infarct size and outcomes following primary PCI: Patient-level analysis from 10 randomized trials. J Am Coll Cardiol. 2016;67(14):1674-83.
5. Kloner RA, Ganote CE, Jennings RB, et al. The "no-reflow" phenomenon after temporary coronary occlusion in the dog. J Clin Invest. 19745;54(6):1496-508.
6. Reimer KA, Lowe JE, Rasmussen MM, et al. The wavefront phenomenon of myocardial ischemic cell death. 1: Myocardial infarct size vs duration of coronary occlusion in dogs. Circulation. 1977;56(5):786-94.
7. Reimer KA, Jennings RB. The "wavefront phenomenon" of myocardial ischemic cell death. II: Transmural progression of necrosis within the framework of ischemic bed size (myocardium at risk) and collateral flow. Lab Invest. 1979;40(6):633-44.
8. Kloner RA, Rude RE, Carlson N, et al. Ultrastuctural evidence of microvascular damage and myocardial cell injury after coronary artery occlusion: Which comes first? Circulation. 1980;62(5):945-52.
9. Antman EM. Time is muscle: Translation into practice. J Am Coll of Cardiol. 2008;52:(15):1216-21.
10. Ibáñez B, Heusch G, Ovize M, et al. Evolving therapies for myocardial ischemia/reperfusion injury. J Am Coll Cardiol. 2015;65(14):1454-71.
11. Vaishnav A, Vaishnav A, Khandekar S, et al. Pre-hospital thrombolysis. J Assoc Physicians India. 2011;59(Suppl):14-8.
12. Fletcher PJ, Stewart P, Savage L. Pros, cons, and organization of prehospital thrombolysis. Clin Ther. 2013;35(8):1058-63.
13. McCaul M, Lourens A, Kredo T. Pre-hospital versus in-hospital thrombolysis for ST-elevation myocardial infarction. Cochrane Database Syst Rev. 2014;(9):CD010191.
14. Menees DS, Peterson ED, Wang Y, et al. Door-to-balloon time and mortality among patients undergoing primary PCI. N Engl J Med. 2013;369(10):901-9.
15. Antman EM, Anbe DT, Armstrong PW, et al. American College of Cardiology; American Heart Association; Canadian Cardiovascular Society. ACC/AHA guidelines for the management of patients with ST-elevation myocardial infarction--executive summary. A report of the American College of Cardiology/American Heart Association Task Force on Practice Guidelines (Writing Committee to revise the 1999 guidelines for the management of patients with acute myocardial infarction). J Am Coll Cardiol. 2004;44(3):671-719.
16. Armstrong PW, Bogarty P, Buller CE, et al.; Canadian Cardiovascular Society Working Group. The 2004 ACC/AHA Guidelines: A perspective and adaptation for Canada by the Canadian Cardiovascular Society Working Group. Can J Cardiol. 2004;20(11):1075-9.
17. 1999 Update: ACC/AHA Guidelines for the Management of Patients With Acute Myocardial Infarction: Executive Summary and Recommendations : A report of the American College of Cardiology/American Heart Association Task Force on Practice Guidelines (Committee on Management of Acute Myocardial Infarction). Circulation. 1999;100(9): 1016-30.
18. Spinthakis N, Farag M, Rocca B, et al. More, more, more: Reducing thrombosis in acute coronary syndromes beyond dual antiplatelet therapy-current data and future directions. J Am Heart Assoc. 2018;7(3). Pii: e007754.
19. Soukoulis V, Boden WE, Smith SC Jr, et al. Nonantithrombotic medical options in acute coronary syndromes: Old agents and new lines on the horizon. Circ Res. 2014;114(12):1944-58.
20. Braunwald E, Kloner RA. Myocardial reperfusion: a double-edged sword? J Clin Invest. 1985;76(5):1713-9.
21. Yellon DM, Hausenloy DJ. Myocardial reperfusion injury. N Engl J Med. 2007;357(11):1121-35.
22. Reimer KA, Jennings RB, Tatum AH. Pathobiology of acute myocardial ischemia: Metabolic, functional and ultrastructural studies. Am J Cardiol. 1983;52(2):72A-81A.
23. Kloner RA, Rude RE, Carlson N, et al. Ultrastructural evidence of microvascular damage and myocardial cell injury after coronary artery occlusion: Which comes first? Circulation. 1980;62(5):945-52.
24. Pinto DS, Gibson M. Reperfusion Injury of the Heart. Topic 1511 Version 22.0 UpToDate. [online] Available from: https://www.uptodate.com/contents/search. [Last accessed Nov., 2019].
25. Hoffmann R, Haager P, Arning J, et al. Usefulness of myocardial blush grade early and late after primary coronary angioplasty for acute myocardial infarction in predicting left ventricular function. Am J Cardiol. 2003;92(9):1015-9.
26. Hausenloy DJ, Garcia-Dorado D, Bøtker HE, et al. Novel targets and future strategies for acute cardioprotection: Position paper of the European Society of Cardiology Working Group on Cellular Biology of the Heart. Cardiovasc Res. 2017;113:564-85.
27. Davidson SM, Ferdinandy P, Andreadou I, et al.; CARDIOPROTECTION COST Action (CA16225). Multitarget strategies to reduce myocardial ischemia/reperfusion injury: JACC review topic of the week. J Am Coll Cardiol. 2019;73(1):89-99.
28. Schwartz Longacre L, Kloner RA, Arai AE, et al.; National Heart, Lung, and Blood Institute, National Institutes of Health. New horizons in cardioprotection: Recommendations from the 2010 National Heart, Lung and Blood Institute Workshop. Circulation. 2011;124(10):1172-9.
29. Murry CE, Jennings RB, Reimer KA. Preconditioning with ischemia: A relay of lethal cell injury in ischemic myocardium. Circulation. 1986;74(5):1124-36.
30. Hausenloy DJ, Yellon DM. Remote ischemic preconditioning: Underlying mechanisms and clinical application. Cardiovasc Res. 2008;79(3):377-86.
31. Bøtker HE, Kharbanda R, Schmidt MR, et al. Remote ischemic conditioning before hospital admission, as a complement to angioplasty, and effect on myocardial salvage in patients with acute myocardial infarction: A randomized trial. Lancet. 2010;375(9716):727-34.

32. Giricz Z, Varga ZV, Baranyai T, et al. Cardioprotection by remote ischemic preconditioning of the rat heart is mediated by extracellular vesicles. J Mol Cell Cardiol. 2014;68:75-8.
33. Alburquerque-Bejar JJ, Barba I, Inserte J, et al. Combination therapy with remote ischemic conditioning and insulin or exenatide enhances infarct size limitation in pigs. Cardiovasc Res. 2015;107(2):246-54.
34. Kleinbongard P, Skyschally A, Heusch G. Cardioprotection by remote ischemic conditioning and its signal transduction. Pflugers Arch. 2017;469:159-81.
35. Heusch G. Molecular basis of cardioprotection: Signal transduction in ischemic pre-, post-, and remote conditioning. Circ Res. 2015;116:674-99.
36. Zhao ZQ, Corvera JS, Halkos ME, et al. Inhibition of myocardial injury by ischemic postconditioning during reperfusion: Comparison with ischemic preconditioning. Am J Physiol Heart Circ Physiol. 2003;285(2):H579-88.
37. Inserte J, Hernando V, Vilardosa Ú, et al. Activation of cGMP/protein kinase G pathway in postconditioned myocardium depends on reduced oxidative stress and preserved endothelial nitric oxide synthase coupling. J Am Heart Assoc. 2013;2(1):e005975.
38. Kerendi F, Kin H, Halkos ME, et al. Remote postconditioning: Brief renal ischemia and reperfusion applied before coronary artery reperfusion reduces myocardial infarct size via endogenous activation of adenosine receptors. Basic Res Cardiol. 2005;100(5):404-12.
39. Kleinbongard P, Amanakis G, Skyschally A, et al. Reflection of cardioprotection by remote ischemic perconditioning in attenuated ST-segment elevation during ongoing coronary occlusion in pigs: Evidence for cardioprotection from ischemic injury. Circ Res. 2018;122(8):1102-8.
40. Jolly SS, James S, Džavík V, et al. Thrombus aspiration in ST-segment-elevation myocardial infarction: An individual patient meta-analysis: Thrombectomy trialists collaboration. Circulation. 2017;135(2):143-52.
41. Taglieri N, Bacchi Reggiani ML, Ghetti G, et al. Efficacy and safety of thrombus aspiration in ST-segment elevation myocardial infarction: An updated systematic review and meta-analysis of randomized clinical trials. Eur Heart J Acute Cardiovasc Care. 2019;8(1):24-38.
42. Wu J, Hao P, Chen Y, et al. Intracoronary. Glycoprotein IIb/IIIa inhibitors improve short-term mortality and reinfarction in East Asian patients with ST-segment elevation myocardial infarction after thrombus aspiration: A meta-analysis. Evidence-Based Complementary and Alternative Medicine. 2018.
43. Manolis AS. Is Atherothromboaspiration a possible solution for the prevention of no-reflow phenomenon in acute coronary syndromes? Single centre experience and review of the literature. Curr Vasc Pharmacol. 2019;17(2):164-79.
44. Salloum J, Tharpe C, Vaughan D, et al. Release and elimination of soluble vasoactive factors during percutaneous coronary intervention of saphenous vein grafts: Analysis using the PercuSurge GuardWire distal protection device. J Invasive Cardiol. 2005;17(11):575-9.
45. Shah VK, Shalia KK, Nabar A, et al. Analysis of soluble factors during percutaneous coronary intervention in ST elevated MI. Enliven: Clin Cardiol Res. 2015;1(4):007.
46. Doukas J, Wrasidlo W, Noronha G, et al. Phosphoinositide 3-kinase gamma/delta inhibition limits infarct size after myocardial ischemia/reperfusion injury. Proc Natl Acad Sci U S A. 2006;103:19866-71.
47. Garcia-Prieto J, Villena-Gutierrez R, Gomez M, et al. Neutrophil stunning by metoprolol reduces infarct size. Nat Commun. 2017;8:14780.
48. Hausenloy DJ, Botker HE, Engstrom T, et al. Targeting reperfusion injury in patients with ST-segment elevation myocardial infarction: trials and tribulations. Eur Heart J. 2017;38:935-41.
49. Hausenloy DJ, Garcia-Dorado D, Bøtker HE, et al. Novel targets and future strategies for acute cardioprotection: position paper of the European Society of Cardiology Working Group on Cellular Biology of the Heart. Cardiovasc Res. 2017;113:564-85.
50. Abrial M, Da Silva CC, Pillot B, et al. Cardiac fibroblasts protect cardiomyocytes against lethal ischemia-reperfusion injury. J Mol Cell Cardiol. 2014;68:56-65.
51. Giricz Z, Varga ZV, Baranyai T, et al. Cardioprotection by remote ischemic preconditioning of the rat heart is mediated by extracellular vesicles. J Mol Cell Cardiol. 2014;68:75-8.
52. Jose Corbalan J, Vatner DE, Vatner SF. Myocardial apoptosis in heart disease: does the emperor have clothes? Basic Res Cardiol. 2016;111:31.
53. García-Prieto J, Villena-Gutiérrez R, Gómez M, et al. Myocardial edema: a translational view. J Mol Cell Cardiol. 2012;52:931-9.
54. Heusch G. The coronary circulation as a target of cardioprotection. Circ Res. 2016;118(10):1643-58
55. Russo I, Penna C, Musso T, et al. Platelets, diabetes and myocardial ischemia/reperfusion injury. Cardiovasc Diabetol. 2017;16(1):71.
56. Barrabés JA, Inserte J, Mirabet M, et al. Antagonism of P2Y12 or GPIIb/IIIa receptors reduces platelet-mediated myocardial injury after ischaemia and reperfusion in isolated rat hearts. Thromb Haemost. 2010;104(1):128-35.
57. Vilahur G, Gutiérrez M, Casani L, et al. Protective effects of ticagrelor on myocardial injury after infarction. Circulation. 2016;134(22):1708-19.
58. Fernández-Jiménez R, Barreiro-Pérez M, Martin-García A, et al. Dynamic edematous response of the human heart to myocardial infarction: Implications for assessing myocardial area at risk and salvage. Circulation. 2017;136(14):1288-300.
59. Garcia-Dorado D, Théroux P, Solares J, et al. Determinants of hemorrhagic infarcts. Histologic observations from experiments involving coronary occlusion, coronary reperfusion, and reocclusion. Am J Pathol. 1990;137(2):301-11.
60. Heusch G, Kleinbongard P, Böse D, et al. Coronary microembolization: From bedside to bench and back to bedside. Circulation. 2009;120(18):1822-36.
61. Lipsic E, Schoemaker RG, van der Meer P, Vet al. Protective effects of erythropoietin in cardiac ischemia: From bench to bedside. J Am Coll Cardiol. 2006;48(11):2161-7.
62. Lipsic E, van der Meer P, Voors AA, et al. A single bolus of a long-acting erythropoietin analogue darbepoetin alfa in patients with acute myocardial infarction: A randomized

feasibility and safety study. Cardiovasc Drugs Ther. 2006;20(2):135-41.

63. Binbrek AS, Rao NS, Al Khaja N, et al. Erythropoietin to augment myocardial salvage induced by coronary thrombolysis in patients with ST segment elevation acute myocardial infarction. Am J Cardiol. 2009;104(8):1035-40.
64. Ferrario M, Arbustini E, Massa M, et al. High-dose erythropoietin in patients with acute myocardial infarction: A pilot, randomised, placebo-controlled study. Int J Cardiol. 2011;147(1):124-31.
65. Headrick JP, Lasley RD. Adenosine receptors and reperfusion injury of the heart. Handb Exp Pharmacol. 2009;193:189-214.
66. Bates E, Bode C, Costa M, et al. Direct Inhibition of delta-Protein Kinase C Enzyme to Limit Total Infarct Size in Acute Myocardial Infarction (DELTA MI) Investigators. Intracoronary KAI-9803 as an adjunct to primary percutaneous coronary intervention for acute ST-segment elevation myocardial infarction. Circulation. 2008;117: 886-96.
67. Griffiths EJ, Halestrap AP. Protection by Cyclosporin A of ischemia/reperfusion-induced damage in isolated rat hearts. J Mol Cell Cardiol. 1993;25(12):1461-9.
68. Piot C, Croisille P, Staat P, et al. Effect of cyclosporine on reperfusion injury in acute myocardial infarction. N Engl J Med. 2008;359(5):473-81.
69. Cung TT, Morel O, Cayla G, et al. Cyclosporine before PCI in patients with acute myocardial infarction. N Engl J Med. 2015;373(11):1021-31.
70. Ottani F, Latini R, Staszewsky L, et al. CYCLE Investigators. Cyclosporine A in reperfused myocardial infarction: The multicenter, controlled, open-label CYCLE trial. J Am Coll Cardiol. 2016;67(4):365-74.
71. Ikeda G, Matoba T, Nakano Y, et al. Nanoparticle-mediated targeting of cyclosporine A enhances cardioprotection against ischemia-reperfusion injury through inhibition of mitochondrial permeability transition pore opening. Sci Rep. 2016;6:20467.
72. Krombach GA, Higgins CB, Chujo M, et al. Gadomer-enhanced MR imaging in the detection of microvascular obstruction: Alleviation with nicorandil therapy. Radiology. 2005;236(2):510-8.
73. Yang XM, Philipp S, Downey JM, et al.; J-WIND investigators. Atrial natriuretic peptide administered just prior to reperfusion limits infarction in rabbit hearts. Basic Res Cardiol. 2006;101(4):311-8.
74. Kitakaze M, Asakura M, Kim J, et al. J-WIND investigators. Human atrial natriuretic peptide and nicorandil as adjuncts to reperfusion treatment for acute myocardial infarction (J-WIND): Two randomised trials. Lancet. 2007;370(9597):1483-93.
75. Gao F, Gao E, Yue TL, et al. Nitric oxide mediates the antiapoptotic effect of insulin in myocardial ischemia-reperfusion: The roles of PI3-kinase. Akt, and endothelial nitric oxide synthase phosphorylation. Circulation. 2002;105(12):1497-502.
76. Opie LH, Bruyneel K, Owen P. Effects of glucose, insulin and potassium infusion on tissue metabolic changes within first hour of myocardial infarction in the baboon. Circulation. 1975;52(1):49-57.
77. Mehta SR, Yusuf S, Díaz R, et al.; The CREATE-ECLA Trial Group Investigators. Effect of glucose-insulin-potassium infusion on mortality in patients with acute ST-segment elevation myocardial infarction: the CREATE-ECLA randomized controlled trial. JAMA. 2005;293(4):437-46.
78. Selker HP, Beshansky JR, Sheehan PR, et al. Out-of-hospital administration of intravenous glucose-insulin-potassium in patients with suspected acute coronary syndromes: The IMMEDIATE randomized controlled trial. JAMA. 2012;307(18):1925-33.
79. Timmers L, Henriques JP, de Kleijn DP, et al. Exenatide reduces infarct size and improves cardiac function in a porcine model of ischemia and reperfusion injury. J Am Coll Cardiol. 2009;53(6):501-10.
80. Ban K, Noyan-Ashraf MH, Hoefer J, et al. Cardioprotective and vasodilatory actions of glucagon-like peptide 1 receptor are mediated through both glucagon-like peptide 1 receptor-dependent and -independent pathways. Circulation. 2008;117(18):2340-50.
81. Lønborg J, Kelbæk H, Vejlstrup N, et al. Exenatide reduces final infarct size in patients with ST-segment-elevation myocardial infarction and short-duration of ischemia. Circ Cardiovasc Interv. 2012;5(2):288-95.
82. Lønborg J, Vejlstrup N, Kelbæk H, et al. Exenatide reduces reperfusion injury in patients with ST-segment elevation myocardial infarction. Eur Heart J. 2012;33(12):1491-9.
83. Ibanez B, Macaya C, Sánchez-Brunete V, et al. Effect of early metoprolol on infarct size in ST-segment-elevation myocardial infarction patients undergoing primary percutaneous coronary intervention: The Effect of Metoprolol in Cardioprotection During an Acute Myocardial Infarction (METOCARD-CNIC) trial. Circulation.2013;128(14):1495-503.
84. Ndrepepa G, Kastrati A. Intravenous β-blockers in primary percutaneous coronary intervention: New hope for an old therapy. Circulation. 2013;128(14):1487-9.
85. Ahrens I, Peter K. FX-06, a fibrin-derived beta peptide for the potential treatment of reperfusion injury following myocardial infarction. Curr Opin Investig Drugs. 2009;10(9):997-1003.
86. Dirksen MT, Laarman GJ, Simoons ML, et al. Reperfusion injury in humans: A review of clinical trials on reperfusion injury inhibitory strategies. Cardiovasc Res. 2007;74(3):343-55.
87. Morel O, Perret T, Delarche N, et al. Pharmacological approaches to reperfusion therapy. Cardiovasc Res. 2012;94(2):246-52.
88. Duncker DJ, Klassen CL, Ishibashi Y, et al. Effect of temperature on myocardial infarction in swine. Am J Physiol. 1996;270(4 Pt 2):H1189-99.
89. Tissier R, Couvreur N, Ghaleh B, et al. Rapid cooling preserves the ischemic myocardium against mitochondrial damage and left ventricular dysfunction. Cardiovasc Res. 2009;83(2):345-53.
90. Simkhovich BZ, Hale SL, Kloner RA. Metabolic mechanism by which mild regional hypothermia preserves ischemic tissue. J Cardiovasc Pharmacol Ther. 2004;9(2):83-90.

91. O'Neill WW, Dixon SR. The year in interventional cardiology. J Am Coll Cardiol. 2004;43(5):875-890.
92. O'Neill WW, Dixon SR, Grines CL. The year in interventional cardiology. J Am Coll Cardiol. 2005;45(7):1117-34.
93. Erlinge D, Götberg M, Grines C, et al. A pooled analysis of the effect of endovascular cooling on infarct size in patients with ST-elevation myocardial infarction. EuroIntervention 2013;8(12):1435-40.
94. Kang IS, Fumiaki I, Pyun WB. Therapeutic hypothermia for cardioprotection in acute myocardial infarction. Yonsei Med J. 2016;57(2):291-7.
95. Ganz W, Donoso R, Marcus H, et al. Coronary hemodynamics and myocardial oxygen metabolism during oxygen breathing in patients with and without coronary artery disease. Circulation. 1972;45(4):763-8.
96. Korthuis RJ, Smith JK, Carden DL. Hypoxic reperfusion attenuates postischemic microvascular injury. Am J Physiol. 1989;256(1 Pt 2):H315-9.
97. Perry MA, Wadhwa SS. Gradual reintroduction of oxygen reduces reperfusion injury in cat stomach. Am J Physiol. 1988;254 (3 Pt 1):G366-72.
98. Wijesinghe M, Perrin K, Ranchord A, et al. Routine use of oxygen in the treatment of myocardial infarction: Systematic review. Heart. 2008;95(3):198-202.
99. Cabello JB, Burls A, Emparanza JI, et al. Oxygen therapy for acute myocardial infarction. Cochrane Database Syst Rev. 2016;12:CD007160.
100. Thomson AJ, Webb DJ, Maxwell SR, et al. Oxygen therapy in acute medical care. BMJ. 2002;324(7351):1406-7.
101. Ihnken K, Moita K, Buckberg GD, et al. Reduced oxygen tension during cardiopulmonary bypass limits myocardial damage in acute hypoxic immature piglet hearts. Eur J Cardiothorac Surg. 1996;10(12):1127-35.
102. Inoue T, Ku K, Kaneda T, et al. Cardioprotective effects of lowering oxygen tension after aortic unclamping on cardiopulmonary bypass during coronary artery bypass grafting. Circ J. 2002;66(8):718-22.
103. Morita K, Ihnken K, Buckberg GD. Studies of hypoxemic/reoxygenation injury: With aortic clamping: XII. Delay of cardiac reoxygenation damage in the presence of cyanosis: A new concept of controlled cardiac reoxygenation. J Thorac Cardiovasc Surg. 1995;110(4 Pt 2):1265-73.
104. Mariero LH, Rutkovskiy A, Stensløkken KO, et al. Hyperoxia during early reperfusion does not increase ischemia/reperfusion injury. Eur J Cardiothorac Surg. 2012;41(1):149-53.
105. Miura T, Miki T. Limitation of myocardial infarct size in the clinical setting: Current status and challenges in translating animal experiments into clinical therapy. Basic Res Cardiol. 2008;103(6):501-13.
106. Shah VK, Shalia KK. Regeneration of myocardium--dawn of a new era! J Assoc Physicians India. 2009;57:312-31.
107. Orlic D, Kajstura J, Chimenti S, et al. Bone marrow cells regenerate infarcted myocardium. Nature. 2001;410(6829):701-5.
108. Strauer BE, Brehm M, Zeus T, et al. Repair of infarcted myocardium by autologous intracoronary mononuclear bone marrow cell transplantation in humans. Circulation. 2002;106(15):1913-8.
109. Shah VK, Desai AJ, Vasvani JB, et al. Bone marrow cells for myocardial repair-a new therapeutic concept. Indian Heart J. 2007;59(6):482-90.
110. Shah VK, Shalia KK. Stem cell therapy for acute myocardial infarction-long term 24 months follow-up. J Clin Trial Cardiol. 2014;1(2):1-5.
111. Shah VK, Shalia KK. Stem cell therapy in acute myocardial infarction: A pot of gold or Pandora's Box. Stem Cells Int. 2011;2011:536758.
112. Shah VK, Shalia KK. Looking beyond reperfusion. J Cardiol Curr Res. 2016;7(3):253.
113. Miao C, Lei M, Hu W, et al. A brief review: The therapeutic potential of bone marrow mesenchymal stem cells in myocardial infarction. Stem Cell Res Ther. 2017;8(1):242.
114. Martin U. New muscle for old hearts: engineering tissue from pluripotent stem cells. Hum Gene Ther. 2015;26(5):305-11.
115. Iyer D, Gambardella L, Bernard WG, et al. Robust derivation of epicardium and its differentiated smooth muscle cell progeny from human pluripotent stem cells. Development. 2015;142(8):1528-1.
116. Thavandiran N, Dubois N, Mikryukov A, al. Design and formulation of functional pluripotent stem cell-derived cardiac microtissues. Proc Natl Acad Sci U S A. 2016;110(49):E4698-4707.
117. Masumoto H, Yamashita JK. Human iPS cell-engineered three-dimensional cardiac tissues perfused by capillary networks between host and graft. Inflamm Regen. 2018;38:26.
118. Ieda M, Fu JD, Delgado-Olguin P, et al. Direct reprogramming of fibroblasts into functional cardiomyocytes by defined factors. Cell. 2010;142(3):375-86.
119. Isomi M, Sadahiro T, Ieda M. Progress and challenge of cardiac regeneration to treat heart failure. J Cardiol. 2019;73(2):97-101.
120. Fan Y, Ho BX, Pang JK, et al. Wnt/β-catenin-mediated signaling re-activates proliferation of matured cardiomyocytes. Stem Cell Res Ther. 2018;9(1):338.
121. Qasim M, Haq F, Kang MH, et al. 3D printing approaches for cardiac tissue engineering and role of immune modulation in tissue regeneration. Int J Nanomedicine. 2019;14:1311-33.
122. Hematti P. Role of extracellular matrix in cardiac cellular therapies. Adv Exp Med Biol. 2018;1098:173-88.
123. Mohamed TM, Ang YS, Radzinsky E, et al. Regulation of cell cycle to stimulate adult cardiomyocyte proliferation and cardiac regeneration. Cell. 2018;173(1):104-16.e12.
124. Natsumeda M, Florea V, Rieger AC, et al. A combination of allogeneic stem cells promotes cardiac regeneration. J Am Coll Cardiol. 2017;70(20):2504-515.
125. Yao Y, Liao W, Yu R, et al. Potentials of combining nanomaterials and stem cell therapy in myocardial repair. Nanomedicine (Lond). 2018;13(13):1623-38.
126. Nazari-Shafti TZ, Kempfert J, Falk V, et al. Regenerative medicine/cardiac cell therapy: Adult/somatic progenitor cells. Thorac Cardiovasc Surg. 2018;66(1):42-52.

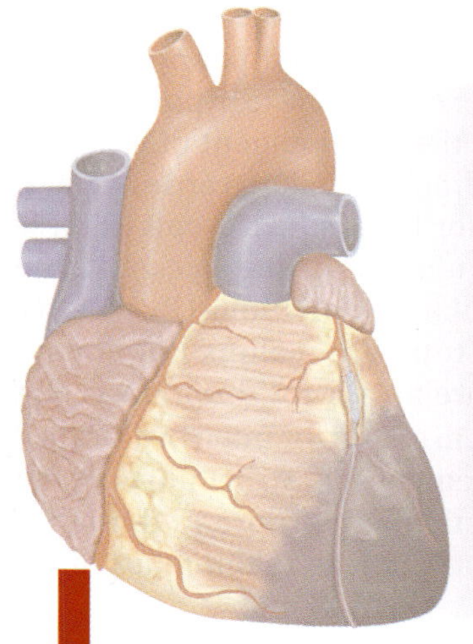

Pediatric Stroke and Heart Failure

Prabhakar Dorairaj, Raja Vijendra Reddy Janke, Anuradha Sridhar

INTRODUCTION

Heart failure (HF) is an important healthcare issue in both adults and children because of its high morbidity, mortality, and cost of care.The most common cause for heart failure in children is structural heart disease. The exact incidence of heart failure in children is unclear as there is a lot of under-reporting. Incidence of HF in children is 0.97–7.4 per 1,00,000.[1] Stroke, the leading cause of adult disability is relatively uncommon in children. Recent data has shown an increase in the incidence of stroke in the younger population where the conventional risk factors are absent. The prevalence of congenital heart disease (CHD) is 1% of live births. Among strokes in children, 20% have CHD.

EPIDEMIOLOGY OF HEART FAILURE AND STROKE

The most common cause for HF in children is a structural heart lesion. The exact incidence is unclear as there is significant under-reporting and patients reaching definitive treatment is doubtful in developing countries like India. Incidence of HF in children is 0.97–7.4 per 100,000. HF related hospitalizations occur in 11,000–14,000 children annually in the United States with an overall mortality of 7%.[1] Overall incidence of stroke in children is 1 in 1,600–4,000 neonates at birth and 2.3–13 per 1 lakh older children per year.[2] The risk of developing ischemic stroke was almost 11 times higher in young patients with CHD than in the general population.[3] The incidence of arterial ischemic stroke (AIS) in children is estimated at 2–8 per 100,000 children per year. Although many cases of AIS have a multifactorial etiology, cardiac disorders are associated with 10–30% of strokes in children.[4] Incidence of acute ischemic stroke will be around 132 per 1 lakh population in children with cardiac disease. These variable prevalence data clearly indicate the wide variability in the population studied. Analysing acute ischemic stroke in pediatric patients with cardiac disease, the prevalence of cardiac diseases was cyanotic CHD in 42 (55%), acyanotic heart disease in 24 (29%), cardiomyopathies/myocarditis in 6 (8%), infective endocarditis in 3 (4%), and primary arrhythmias in 3 (4%) (Fig. 1).[5]

Occurrence of stroke after cardiac procedures was noted in 52 patients (68%): 41 postcardiac surgery (4.6 strokes per 1,000 surgical procedures) and 11 postcardiac catheterization (1.7 strokes per 1,000 catheterizations).[6] International Paediatric Stroke Registry has noticed that most of the strokes are in the anterior circulation and in 30% multiple areas were involved.[4] Children with mechanical circulatory support devices including extracorporeal membrane oxygenation (ECMO) and ventricular assist devices (VADs) are at particularly high-risk of stroke. Neurological complications most commonly ischemic stroke about 29% was leading cause in children with ECMO.[7,8]

PATHOPHYSIOLOGY OF STROKE IN HEART FAILURE

There is still a controversy whether HF is a cause of stroke. Recently there are studies with evidence that HF itself is

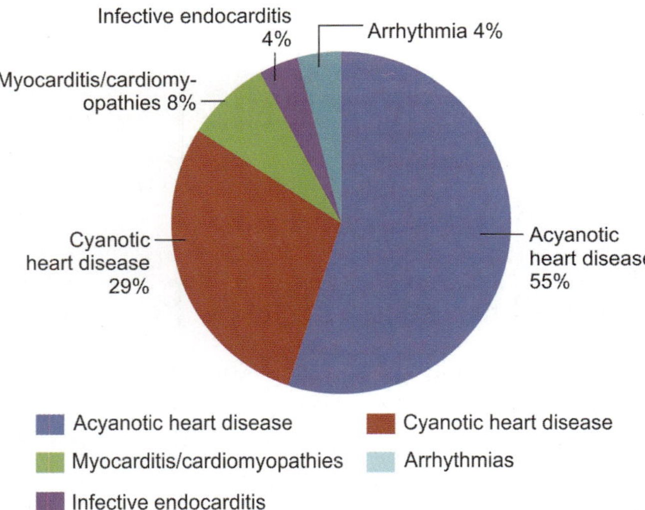

Fig. 1: Prevalence of cardiac disorders in acute ischemic stroke in pediatric patients.

a reason for stroke. The risk of ischemic stroke is higher in children with HF.[9,10] Multivariate analyses of factors associated with ischemic stroke in 25,985 patients with CHD showed the highest hazard ratio of HF (HR 6.94, 95% CI 4.70–10.34, p value <0.001). The other factors studied were atrial fibrillation, age, sex, systemic hypertension, and diabetes mellitus.[3] The exact pathophysiology is not known but there are few theories for the occurrence of stroke. There are multiple factors which lead to stroke in children with HF. About 1/3–2/3 of children with cardiac disease have stroke in the periprocedural period, cardiac surgery or intervention.[4,11] Cerebrovascular accidents in children occur at any stage of HF. Virchow's triad describes three variables that contribute to thrombosis—alterations in blood flow, injury to the vessel wall, and alterations in blood components. In children with cardiac disease, some or all of these factors may play a role in thrombosis.

Severe valvular regurgitation leads to volume overload and subsequent dysfunction of chamber based on pathology. This leads to stasis, thrombus formation, and thromboembolic stroke. Severe obstructive valvular lesion, such as mitral stenosis produces stasis in the proximal chamber. Vascular obstructive lesion, such as coarctation of aorta leads to ventricular dysfunction, stasis of blood, and thrombus formation.

Acyanotic heart disease, such as VSD which leads to shunting from left to right ventricle there is some risk of paradoxical embolism. Small defects, such as VSD carry a risk for infective endocarditis which further leads to embolic cerebrovascular event. Congenital coronary abnormalities, such as anomalous left coronary artery from the pulmonary artery (ALCAPA), in due course of time lead to ischemic heart diseases, HF and carry the risk of thrombosis. Same will be reason for primary myocardial diseases causing ventricular dysfunction.

Duct dependent lesion in neonatal period leads to ventricular dysfunction; ischemia is due to hypoxia as duct starts to close and favors the development of ischemic stroke. Eisenmengers syndrome in failure carries highest risk for thrombotic or hemorrhagic stroke events as these patients are on anticoagulants; further accentuation is due to severe ventricular dysfunction. Obstructive venous lesions, such as total anomalous pulmonary venous return (TAPVC) are at risk for thrombosis due to venous stasis. A shunt from patent foramen ovale (PFO) can produce paradoxical embolism. Arrhythmias which cause ventricular dysfunction, predispose to thrombus formation. Atrial fibrillation can lead to thrombus in left atrial appendage.

Acquired heart diseases, such as rheumatic heart disease and cardiomyopathies are also risk for thrombosis as there is ventricular dysfunction, valvular regurgitation. Other causes include atrial myxomas, mechanical valves, pacemakers devices will lead to thrombotic events. The implantable cardioverter defibrillator, left ventricle assist devices (LVAD) and ECMO are high-risk for thrombus formation and stroke. Some children have coexisting genetic and acquired prothrombotic disorders in children with cardiac disease. The exact incidence is not known. Lipoprotein (a) levels >30 mg/dL, protein C deficiency, anticardiolipin antibodies and combined prothrombotic disorders seem to be important risk factors for manifestation of ischemic strokes in children with underlying cardiac disorders.[12] Prothrombotic tests were performed infrequently in studies. But among those tested one-third had congenital prothrombotic tendencies. The prothrombotic tests must be routinely performed in pediatric stroke.

Data regarding the stroke recurrence is limited; predictors were mechanical valves, genetic or acquired prothrombotic states and acute infection. Cerebral vasculopathy was present in 25.8% of children with cardiac disorders.[13] Syndromes with both cardiac disorders and cerebral vasculopathy include Down syndrome, William syndrome, neurofibromatosis type I, Alagille syndrome.

DIFFICULTIES IN CLINICAL PRESENTATION AND INVESTIGATIONS

Symptoms of stroke are nonspecific in infancy. There are several factors that may delay the diagnosis. In the neonatal period hemiparesis is often difficult to diagnose initially, lack of picking up the subtle seizures are major hurdles which are present in childhood. Older children usually present with focal neurological deficits—hemiplegia, gross or focal motor deficit. Symptoms are based on the vascular territory involved. In sick children who are ventilator dependent there are hurdles for neuroimaging like MRI, herein neurosonogram in infants can give an idea to some extent. Studies show that about two-third of strokes are under reported by cranial ultrasound.[14,15] CT cranium is another option where MRI is not feasible, but about 50–80% of strokes are missed compared to MRI.[16,17] There is need for parents, patients, and healthcare practitioner to be aware of the risk of stroke in children with HF and to be vigilant toward early identification.

APPROACH

Good clinical history is very important in approach to diagnosis. Complete physical and neurological examinations are important in localizing lesion.

- *CT brain:* It can be done quickly in an emergency. It is useful to differentiate stroke or mass effect that causes the lesion. CT usually will be normal in first 12 hours. MRI is gold standard investigation due to its greater sensitivity and specificity. MR angiography detects vascular abnormalities.
- *Cardiac MRI:* It is the gold standard imaging to assess volumes, mass, EF both RV and LV. Assessment of myocardial fibrosis/ischemia, to rule out alternative diagnosis—amyloidosis, sarcoidosis, noncompaction, hemochromatosis, etc.
- *Brain MRI:* The extent and location of thrombus can be identified. MRI has greater benefit over CT in imaging the extent of the lesion. The major hurdles are the long duration of study and availability.

TREATMENT

Goals of therapy are to maintain stability, prevent progression and as soon as patients diagnosed to have stroke institute neuroprotective measures. Maintain normotension, euvolumia, euglycemia, and normothermia. Seizure control is important in management in stroke. Antiepileptic therapy should be started as soon as the patient is suspected to have seizure activity or when clinically indicated. Guidelines are sparse and inconclusive that are unique to the pediatric population with heart disease, hence large RCT are required. Current guidelines for prevention and treatment of stroke in pediatric age group with cardiac disease are based on low level of evidence.

Treatment of acute HF is to be done as per guidelines in concurrence with the start of treatment for stroke.

RECOMMENDATIONS OF TREATMENT

Early identification of stroke is important in management and prognosis of child. It is known that when stroke diagnosed within 4.5 hours thrombolytic therapy can be started.[13] Early administration of tissue plasminogen activator (tPA) facilitates early recanalization of an artery.[18,19] There is insufficient data in children to make definitive recommendation, such as tPA or endovascular therapy. There is a need for studies on the recommendation of tissue plasminogen activator therapy. As of now, few studies suggest to start tPA when onset less than 4.5 hours and age more than 2 years, but it is not recommended if age is less than 2 years. Recommended dosage is 0.9 mg/kg, first 10% is given as bolus over 5 minutes and later remaining is given as infusion over 1 hour. Monitor for response and further stroke episodes. Tissues plasminogen activators should be given in a tertiary care setup with ongoing care with cardiologist, neurologist, and intensivist.

RECOMMENDATIONS FOR PRIMARY PREVENTION OF THROMBOSIS

It is recommended to start anticoagulants in children with cardiac embolism and to continue for at least 1 year or until the cardiac lesion is corrected. Routine anticoagulant therapy is not recommended for patients with endocarditis who have native valve lesion. Child with reasonably sized atrial septal defect has to be recommended closure of the ASD by device or surgery. Recommendation for isolated PFO closure in children with risk factors requires further studies in pediatric age group. In patients with VAD there is need for anticoagulation.[19,20]

CONCLUSION

Presence of CHD is associated with higher incidence of pediatric stroke and vice versa. There is need to identify that the presence of HF is a very important risk factor for stroke. There is need for early identification and treatment of congenital cardiac diseases, appropriate management of HF. Further studies are lacking in preventive measures for stroke in HF. Role of anticoagulation in HF needs more data as a preventive measure. There is limited data on thrombolysis with tPA. Management of pediatric stroke requires a multispecialty team.

REFERENCES

1. Rossano JW, Kim JJ, Decker JA, et al. Prevalence, morbidity, and mortality of heart failure-related hospitalizations in children in the United States: A population based study. J Card Fail. 2012;18(6):459-70.
2. Bernson-Leung ME, Rivkin MJ. Stroke in neonates and children. Pediatr Rev. 2016;37(11):463-77.
3. Mandalenakis Z, Rosengren A, Lappas G, et al. Ischemic stroke in children and young adults with congenital heart disease. J Am Heart Assoc. 2016;5(2):e003071.

4. Dowling MM, Hynan LS, Lo W, et al.; International Paediatric Stroke Study Group. International paediatric stroke Study: Stroke associated with cardiac disorders. Int J Stroke. 2013;8(Suppl A100):39-44.
5. Lipshultz SE, Sleeper LA, Towbin JA, et al. The incidence of pediatric cardiomyopathy in two regions of the United States. N Engl J Med. 2003;348(17):1647-55.
6. Asakai H, Cardamone M, Hutchinson D, et al. Arterial ischemic stroke in children with cardiac disease. Neurology. 2015;85(23):2053-9.
7. Fraser CD Jr, Jaquiss RD, Rosenthal DN, et al.; Berlin Heart Study Investigators. Prospective trial of a pediatric ventricular assist device. N Engl J Med. 2012;367(6):532-41.
8. Almond CS, Morales DL, Blackstone EH, et al. Berlin Heart EXCOR pediatric ventricular assist device for bridge to heart transplantation in US children. Circulation. 2013;127(16):1702-11.
9. Pullicino PM, McClure LA, Wadley VG, et al. Blood pressure and stroke in heart failure in the REasons for Geographic and Racial Differences in Stroke (REGARDS) study. Stroke. 2009;40(12):3706-10.
10. Kannel WB, Wolf PA, Verter J. Manifestations of coronary disease predisposing to stroke. The Framingham Study. JAMA. 1983;250(21):2942-6.
11. Rodan L, McCrindle BW, Manlhiot C, et al. Stroke recurrence in children with congenital heart disease. Ann Neurol. 2012;72(1):103-11.
12. Sträter R, Vielhaber H, Kassenböhmer R, et al. Genetic risk factors of thrombophilia in ischaemic childhood stroke of cardiac origin. A prospective ESPED survey. Eur J Pediatr. 1999;158(Suppl 3):S122-5.
13. Aho K, Harmsen P, Hatano S, et al. Cerebrovascular disease in the community: Results of a WHO collaborative study. Bull World Health Organ. 1980;58(1):113-30.
14. Golomb MR, Dick PT, MacGregor DL, et al. Cranial ultrasonography has a low sensitivity for detecting arterial ischemic stroke in term neonates. J Child Neurol. 2003;18(2):98-103.
15. Cowan F, Mercuri E, Groenendaal F, et al. Does cranial ultrasound imaging identify arterial cerebral infarction in term neonates? Arch Dis Child Fetal Neonatal Ed. 2005;90(3):F252-6.
16. Srinivasan J, Miller SP, Phan TG, et al. Delayed recognition of initial stroke in children: Need for increased awareness. Pediatrics. 2009;124(2):e227-34.
17. McGlennan C, Ganesan V. Delays in investigation and management of acute arterial ischaemic stroke in children. Dev Med Child Neurol. 2008;50(7):537-40.
18. Demaerschalk BM, Silver B, Wong E, et al. ASPECT scoring to estimate >1/3 middle cerebral artery territory infarction. Can J Neurol Sci. 2006;33(2):200-4.
19. Intracerebral hemorrhage after intravenous t-PA therapy for ischemic stroke. The NINDS t-PA Stroke Study Group. Stroke. 1997;28(11):2109-18.
20. Giglia TM, Massicotte MP, Tweddell JS, et al.; American Heart Association Congenital Heart Defects Committee of the Council on Cardiovascular Disease in the Young, Council on Cardiovascular and Stroke Nursing, Council on Epidemiology and Prevention, and Stroke Council. Prevention and treatment of thrombosis in pediatric and congenital heart disease: A scientific statement from the American Heart Association. Circulation. 2013;128(24):2622-703.

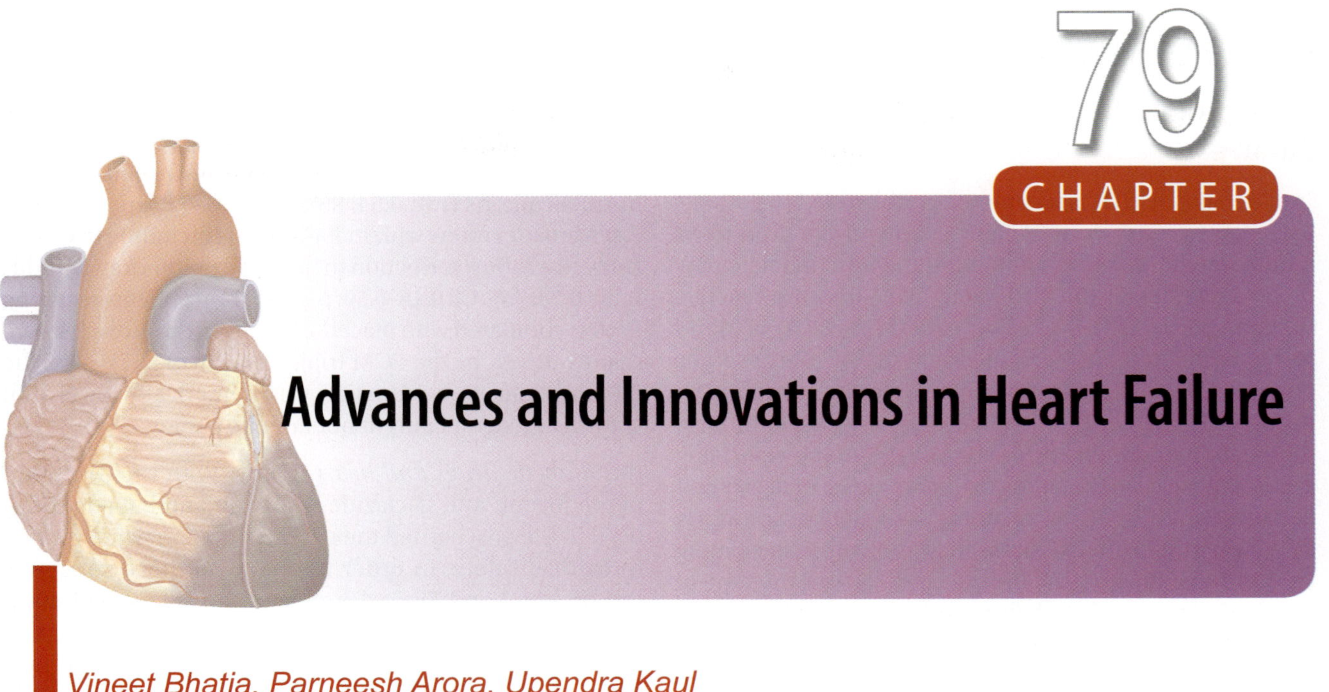

Advances and Innovations in Heart Failure

Vineet Bhatia, Parneesh Arora, Upendra Kaul

INTRODUCTION

Despite the fact that our knowledge about heart failure (HF) has grown by leaps and bounds, it continues to impact humans globally in epidemic proportions creating a significant impact on the lives and economy of the people affected. In the United States alone, there are more than 5.8 million patients affected by HF and the global estimates are to the tune of 23 million.[1] This highly morbid condition carries a grim prognosis with survival estimates at 50% at 5 years and 10% at 10 years.[1] Recent advances in pharmacotherapies, mechanical technologies in the form of device-based therapies, transplantation, and novel multidisciplinary approaches have substantially contributed to the care of this evergrowing patient population. This chapter intends to present a comprehensive review of various advances and innovations in the treatment of HF.

ADVANCES IN PHARMACOTHERAPY

Treatment with angiotensin-converting enzyme inhibitors (ACEI)/angiotensin receptor blockers (ARBs), beta-blockers, and mineralocorticoid receptor antagonists (MRAs) has substantially improved quality and quantity of life for patients with heart failure with reduced ejection fraction (HFrEF). The most recent addition to the drug armamentarium is the angiotensin receptor-neprilysin inhibitor (ARNI) which has shown great promise in such patients. The role of iron in HF has been revisited and intravenous (IV) iron replacement has emerged as an important means to improve the quality of life in certain subsets of HF patients. Similarly, there has been a great focus on the role of antidiabetic drugs in HF.

Angiotensin Receptor–neprilysin Inhibitor

The drug is a combination of valsartan (an ARB) and sacubitril (a neprilysin inhibitor) referred to as LCZ 696 and is indicated for use in symptomatic HFrEF [left ventricular ejection fraction (LVEF) <35%]. The Prospective Comparison of ARNI and ACEI to determine Impact on Global Mortality and Morbidity in Heart failure (PARADIGM-HF) trial was a landmark study comparing the novel agent ARNI with the standard of care ACEI, enalapril in symptomatic New York Heart Association (NYHA) class II-IV patients.[2] The primary objective of the trial was to determine whether LCZ 696 was superior to ACEI alone in reducing combined endpoint of cardiovascular (CV) death or hospitalization for HF. The trial was stopped prematurely at 27 months of planned 4-year duration in the light of significant benefits with ARNI. There was a 20% incremental reduction in CV death with ARNI beyond that achieved with enalapril and an absolute risk reduction of 4.7%. The PARADIGM-HF trial, thus demonstrated that ARNI is superior to enalapril in reducing the combined end point of CV death or hospitalization for HF, based on time to event analysis (P <0.001). Reduction in both CV death and HF hospitalization were reflected. However, it must be noted that only 1.5% of randomized patients were in NYHA class IV. Hypotension may be a limiting factor for use in ARNI in patients with advanced HF.

Emerging Role of Iron Deficiency in Heart Failure

Iron deficiency (ID) is a common problem in HF patients and may seriously impact their quality of life. Iron plays a fundamental role in maintaining the functional activity of key enzymes of the citric acid cycle and the reactive oxygen species (ROS) scavenging enzymes.[3] ID is found to be associated with reduced activity of all these key enzymes. Lower citric acid cycle activity impairs the normal bioenergetics in the cardiomyocytes, similar to the phenomenon observed in myocytes of the exercising skeletal muscle in HF leading to impaired maximal exercise capacity.[4] With regard to decreased ROS scavenging enzymes, local oxidative stress may intensify with ensuing myocardial damage.[5] The incidence of ID is to the tune of 30–50% in chronic heart failure and up to 70–80% in acute heart failure (AHF) situations. While iron replacement has no benefit in patients presenting with AHF, asymptomatic and advanced HF patients as well as heart failure with preserved ejection fraction (HFpEF) subsets, it is found to be beneficial in HFrEF patients who are in NYHA class II and III. The 2017 ACC/AHA/HFS (American College of Cardiology/American Heart Association/Heart Failure Society) guidelines[6] state that IV iron may be reasonable in selected NYHA functional class II to III patients with HF (recommendation level II-B), and the 2016 ESC guidelines[7] recommend (II-A) IV iron in symptomatic HFrEF to alleviate symptoms and improve functional status.

Oral iron supplementation: The available evidence [oral iron repletion effects on oxygen uptake in heart failure (IRONOUT HF)] does not support a role for oral iron in ID HFrEF patients, and one should refrain from futile polypharmacy causing unwanted adverse events (AEs).[8]

IV iron supplementation, on the other hand has shown remarkable results. The FAIR-HF (ferric carboxymaltose in patients with HF and iron deficiency) randomized controlled trial (RCT)[9] has shown symptomatic improvement in patients receiving ferric carboxymaltose (FCM) compared with placebo. The CONFIRM-HF (A Study to Compare the Use of Ferric Carboxymaltose with Placebo in Patients with Chronic Heart Failure and Iron Deficiency)[10] RCT strengthened these findings using higher single iron doses and extending the observed benefits to 1 year in patients with hemoglobin <15 g/dL. Both trials found benefits regardless of anemia. A meta-analysis including 839 patients with chronic HF enrolled in four double-blinded RCTs [FER-CARS-01, FAIR-HF[9] EFFICACY-HF (EFfect of Ferric Carboxymaltose on exercIse CApacity and Cardiac Function in Patients With Iron deficiencY and Chronic Heart Failure) (NCT00821717), and CONFIRM-HF][10] suggested that, compared with placebo, FCM reduced recurrent HF hospitalizations [relative risk (RR): 0.41; 95% confidence interval (CI): 0.23–0.73; p = 0.003] and recurrent CV hospitalizations (RR: 0.54; 95% CI: 0.36–0.83; p = 0.004).[11] A systematic review with meta-analysis including five RCTs showed a robust reduction in hospitalizations for HF (odds ratio: 0.28; 95% CI: 0.16–0.50; p <0.0001) in patients receiving IV iron compared with placebo. However, these results were mainly driven by the FCM trials (n = 760 of 851). Also, the HF hospitalization reduction was numerically lower (not statistically significant) in nonanemic patients.[12]

Antidiabetic drugs and heart failure: With the exception of metformin and gliclazide nearly all antidiabetic drugs used in the past earned the nasty reputation when it came to cardiac safety. In order to deal with these concerns, the US Food and Drug Administration (FDA) and other regulatory bodies mandated all new diabetes drugs to demonstrate CV safety. It is now required that all new drugs be approved for marketing only after adequately powered RCTs demonstrate that such treatment would not be associated with unacceptably high rates of CV events in the phase III clinical trials (upper bound of the 95% CI for major adverse CV event not to exceed 1.8). Postapproval, a phase IV CV safety outcome trial in high-risk patients [with preexisting cardiovascular disease (CVD)] would need to further demonstrate a CV event rate not exceeding the upper bound of the 95% CI of 1.3. A minimum of 2-year follow-up data would be required with independent adjudication of CV outcomes.[13,14] Four DPP4 inhibitors, namely saxagliptin, alogliptin, sitagliptin, and linagliptin have been tested in CVOTs [SAVOR-TIMI 53 (Does Saxagliptin Reduce the Risk of Cardiovascular Events When Used Alone or Added to Other Diabetes Medications)], EXAMINE (Cardiovascular Outcomes Study of Alogliptin in Patients With Type 2 Diabetes and Acute Coronary Syndrome), TECOS (Sitagliptin Cardiovascular Outcomes Study), CAROLINA: cardiovascular outcome study of linagliptin versus glimepiride in patients with type 2 diabetes respectively and Cardiovascular and Renal Microvascular outcome study with LINAgliptin in patients with type 2 diabetes mellitus (CARMELINA).[15-19] Recent data suggests higher rates of HF for saxagliptin and alogliptin. Sitagliptin and linagliptin were neutral with regards to HF.

The subtype 2 sodium-glucose transport proteins (SGLT-2) inhibitors are a new class of drugs which have shown impressive CV safety. The EMPA-REG OUTCOME [(Empagliflozin) Cardiovascular Outcome Event Trial in Type 2 Diabetes Mellitus Patients] trial evaluated the CV effects of empagliflozin added to standard therapy in diabetic patients with known CVD.[20] The primary composite outcome of CV death, myocardial infarction (MI), and stroke occurred less frequently with empagliflozin (10.5% compared to 12.1% in the placebo group; P = 0.04 for superiority). Most interestingly, empagliflozin reduced HF admissions by 35% (2.7% vs. 4.1%; P = 0.002). There was rapid separation of survival curves suggesting acute benefit of the drug. The robustness of HF outcomes in the EMPA-REG OUTCOME trial have been debated due to the lack of cardiac function and biomarker assessment (such as brain natriuretic peptide) which are otherwise a norm in most HF trials. Additionally, in subgroup analysis, HF hospitalizations were statistically significantly reduced in patients without HF at baseline but not in those with HF.[21] Trials specifically evaluating HF outcomes are now underway. Regardless, prior to these findings, no glucose-lowering drug had shown an improvement in HF outcomes in patients with diabetes.

Canagliflozin was the second SGLT-2 inhibitor to undergo a CV safety trial [CANVAS (CANagliflozin cardioVascular Assessment Study)],[22] and consistent with results of EMPA-REG OUTCOME, showed reduction in HF hospitalization (5.5% vs. 8.7%). Canagliflozin was shown to be superior to placebo in reducing the primary combined outcome of CV death, MI, and stroke (26.9% vs. 31.5%; P = 0.02) but did not improve any of these outcomes individually. However, the reduction in the HF-related outcome was identical to that observed with empagliflozin in the EMPA-REG OUTCOME trial.

Lixisenatide, liraglutide, semaglutide and most recently exenatide have been tested in CV outcome trials [ELIXA (Evaluation of Cardiovascular Outcomes in Patients With Type 2 Diabetes After Acute Coronary Syndrome During Treatment With AVE0010), LEADER (Liraglutide Effect and Action in Diabetes: Evaluation of Cardiovascular Outcome Results), SUSTAIN-6 (Trial to Evaluate Cardiovascular and Other Long-term Outcomes With Semaglutide in Subjects With Type 2 Diabetes), and EXSCEL (Exenatide Study of Cardiovascular Event Lowering Trial), respectively],[23-26] while dulaglutide is currently being tested [REWIND (Researching Cardiovascular Events With a Weekly Incretin in Diabetes)]. It is apparent from the results of the published trials that the benefits of glucagon-like peptide-1 (GLP-1) analogs may not be a class effect. While LEADER and SUSTAIN-6 were able to demonstrate CV event reduction, the results of ELIXA were not as encouraging and EXSCEL showed borderline beneficial effects. Neither liraglutide nor semaglutide had a significant effect on HF admissions, suggesting a different mechanism of action than SGLT2 inhibitors.

Trials like EMPagliflozin outcomE tRial in Patients With chrOnic heaRt Failure with Reduced Ejection Fraction (EMPEROR-Reduced) are underway and likely to be completed by 2020. The aim of the study is to investigate the safety and efficacy of empagliflozin versus placebo on top of guideline-directed medical therapy (GDMT) in patients with HFrEF in absence of associated diabetes.

Mechanical Circulatory Support (MCS) devices are mechanical pumps designed to assist or replace the function of either the left [left ventricular assist device (LVAD)] or the right [right ventricular assist device (RVAD)], both ventricles [biventricular support (BiVAD)], or replace both ventricles [total artificial heart (TAH)] of the heart. These devices may be placed outside the body (extracorporeal), adjacent to the body (paracorporeal), within the body (intracorporeal) or in normal position of the heart (orthotopic as TAH). The pumps may be planned for short-term use [days to weeks as bridge to recovery (BTR)] or long-term (months to years as [bridge-to-transplant (BTT) or destination therapy (DT)]. They may be further classified as those based on pulsatile flow or continuous flow. Typically short-term devices are extracorporeal while long-term devices are intracorporeal.

Three indications for MCS are approved by the US FDA and reimbursed by the Centers for Medicare and Medicaid Services (CMS): BTR, BTT and DT.

Bridge-to-recovery (BTR): It refers to the use of MCS in patients with cardiogenic shock or acute decompensated HF where it is reasonably believed that myocardial function will recover in a short period of time. Devices used include the intra-aortic balloon pump (IABP), extracorporeal life support (ELS), CentriMag ventricular assist device (VAD) (St. Judes, Minneapolis), Tandemheart pVAD (Cardiac Assist, Pittsburgh), and Impella 2.5, CP 5.0 or RP (Abiomed Corp., Denver, Mass). When cardiogenic shock complicates long-standing HF temporary MCS can provide the time needed by patients, family members, and physicians to make a critical decision for long-term MCS and heart transplantation (HT). Patients with HF severe enough to warrant long-term MCS but with reversible clinical characteristics (e.g. coagulopathy from hepatic congestion, acute renal failure from low cardiac output and high right atrial pressure, hypoalbuminemia resulting from cardiac cachexia or bowel edema) that put them at high risk for perioperative death with long-term device may benefit from temporary MCS, if their risk profile could be substantially improved with temporary MCS to the extent that they become good candidates for durable MCS device.

Bridge-to-transplant (BTT) and destination therapy (DT): MCS devices may be used in cases where myocardial recovery is unlikely. The devices which fall under this category, are the VADs and the TAH. Significant advances have been made in the VAD category in the last few years and deserve special mention.

Ventricular Assist Device

Supporting the circulation with a VAD has proved to be a safe and effective way in managing patients with end-stage HF who are refractory to optimal medical management (OMM).[27] The US FDA has approved these devices for two indications—as a BTT and DT.

These VADs were initially developed as a BTT; however, as the number of donor hearts is limited, there was an exponential increase in the number of people on these devices awaiting transplant. The proportion of HF patients who received a VAD as BTT increased from 19.1% in 2000 to 41.0% in 2012 in the United States.[28]

Ventricular assist devices have also emerged as DT in end-stage HF patients who are unable to undergo transplant due to chronological age and comorbid conditions. Typically, approximately 75% of such patients are on continuous inotropes, are NYHA functional class IV despite optimal medical therapy for >60–90 days, have LVEF <25% and have peak oxygen consumption <12 mL/kg/min. The REMATCH (Randomized Evaluation of Mechanical Assistance for the Treatment of Congestive Heart Failure) trial in 2001 by Rose et al. first demonstrated the potential of using VADs as a durable DT platform with superior survival outcomes compared with conventional medical therapy alone.[29] LVAD therapy halved [relative risk (RR), 0.52; 95% CI 0.34–0.78] the mortality seen in the control population (92% at 2 years) treated with OMM. Quality of life was also better in the device group.

In the US alone about 22,000 such devices have been implanted till date and about 2,500 new devices are implanted each year.[30]

There exists a third undifferentiated category of patients who fall under the "Bridge to decision" subgroup. Essentially, these patients are very sick with comorbidities which may preclude an immediate decision regarding transplant candidacy. With successful LVAD support, many patients improve and become eligible for cardiac transplant consideration.

Devices Available

The first generation VADs (HeartMate XVE and Novacor LVAS) were pneumatically driven and provided pulsatile flow. Many of the AEs noted with these devices were thought to be design related. The newer devices have the continuous-flow (CF) design which has helped to:

- Miniaturize these devices
- Enhance their durability
- Redefine their AE profile.

The two most commonly implanted CF design VADs are:

1. The axial-flow HeartMate II device (Abbott Laboratories, Abbott Park, IL) where axial flow is generated by a propeller in a pipe. The device has a cylindrical body and placed in the upper abdomen.
2. The centrifugal-flow HeartWare HVAD device (Medtronic, Minneapolis, MN) where the flow is generated by a bladed disk spinning in a cavity. The HVAD is a smaller device that is circular and entirely intrapericardial.

Both devices are designed to directly unload the left ventricle and augment the cardiac output into the ascending aorta and can provide full cardiac output, nearing 10 L/min.[27] Both devices are connected to an external power source via a driveline that is tunneled subcutaneously and exits at the level of the abdomen.

The most advanced centrifugal-flow device is the HeartMate 3 (Abbott Laboratories), which has several advanced features which are as follows:

- A fully magnetically levitated rotor (does not require hydrodynamic or mechanical bearings)
- Larger consistent blood-flow paths (helps reduce shear stress)
- Artificial pulsatility (reduces stasis and minimizes thrombosis).

The MOMENTUM 3 trial (The Multicenter Study of MagLev Technology in Patients Undergoing Mechanical Circulatory Support Therapy with HeartMate 3) data demonstrated superiority of this device over the HeartMate II.[31] More than 1,000 patients with NYHA Class IIIB or IV HF participated in the study. Patients were followed for a short-term end point of 6 months and a long-term end point of 2 years.

The principal findings of this trial are:

- *Superior rates of event-free survival*: The long-term cohort met its primary end point with 77.9% event-free survival (survival free from disabling stroke and device removal due to malfunction), showing superiority over the HeartMate II LVAD at 56.4%.
- *Improved survival*: Patients with the HeartMate 3 LVAD had a survival rate of 82.8% at two years compared to 76.2% for those with the HeartMate II LVAD.
- *Low pump thrombosis*: Rates remained very low at 1.2% suspected thrombosis for the HeartMate 3 LVAD, with no reoperations, pump replacements or urgent transplants occurring at 2 years.
- *Lower stroke rate:* Stroke rate was significantly lower (10%) for the HeartMate 3 LVAD compared to the HeartMate II LVAD (19%).

In addition, patients receiving HeartMate 3 LVAD had significant improvements compared to the HeartMate II LVAD in functional capacity and quality of life scores at 2 years compared to baseline.

Patient Selection and Risk Stratification

The ACC and the AHA guidelines advocate VAD implantation for patients who have Stage D HFrEF, which is estimated to include 100,000–250,000 patients. However, choosing the right candidates for this therapy which is highly invasive and expensive is vital.[27] Several patient characteristics are associated with adverse effects and poor outcomes. These broadly include factors which limit life expectancy at the onset, such as ongoing malignancy or irreversible end-organ failure [end-stage renal disease (ESRD) requiring renal replacement therapy, advanced emphysema, cirrhosis with elevated model for end-stage liver disease score, extensive cerebrovascular disease and those at an increased risk of stroke], those which may precipitate AEs postimplantation such as significant pulmonary hypertension or right ventricular (RV) dysfunction at baseline, inability to receive prolonged anticoagulation and antiplatelet therapy, and those which preclude adequate follow-up care such as psychosocial limitations. These boundaries are continually being redrawn as technological progress continues to improve patient outcomes and to diminish the burdens of AE. Several scoring systems are available which may help risk stratify patients such as INTERMACS scale (Interagency Registry for Mechanically Assisted Circulatory Support), HeartMate score, and the Penn Columbia risk score.

In order to assist with optimal patient selection for placement of an LVAD, the INTERMACS registry has developed seven clinical profiles to identify patients:

1. Level 1 includes patients who are in critical cardiogenic shock requiring mechanical support.
2. Level 2 includes patients who are declining despite inotropic support.
3. Level 3 includes patients who are stable on inotropic support.
4. Level 4 includes patients with resting symptoms.
5. Level 5 includes patients who are intolerant to exertion.
6. Level 6 includes patients who are able to engage in limited exertion.
7. Level 7 includes patients who have advanced NYHA III HF.

In the early years of LVAD implementation, the first two profiles (Level 1 and 2) comprised 60–80% of the LVAD candidates who were considered to be candidates for BTT. More recently, a shift has occurred in response to improved patient selection and risk stratification such that the majority of patients implanted are now INTERMACS 3 and 4 profiles. Currently, 80% of patients who are being implanted with LVAD fall within INTERMACS Levels 2–4.[32]

Survival Patterns

The CF design devices have been able to achieve 1- and 2-year survival rates of 81% and 70%, respectively. The results are more favorable in the BTT group rather than the DT groups, with 30% receiving HT at 1 year and 77% surviving to 2 years. The DT cohort includes a much sicker population, which precludes them to undergo transplantation and the long-term survival rates are at an encouraging 68% at 2 years. These figures are consistent across the HeartWare HVAD and HMII trials; 46–59% of them were able to reach the primary composite outcome of survival without disabling stroke or reoperation at 2 years. The HeartMate 3 cohort recently achieved a 79.5% rate of the same composite outcome, owing to significantly reduced stroke and pump thrombosis (PT) burden. These figures, compared with the trial in 2009 by Slaughter et al., where only 11% of the pulsatile-flow VAD patients were able to reach the composite outcome, convey a narrative of remarkable progress. Although long-term VAD outcomes with 30% survival at 5 years are still inferior to HT, VAD therapy is on the right path to becoming an equivalent alternative in the future.

Functional Status and Quality of Life

Patients with advanced HF have a very limited and poor quality of life. The VADs help improve their functional status such that 80% patients are in NYHA class 1 or 2 at the end of 24 months post-implant. Their 6-minute walk test distances are found to double in this time period. Quality of life estimated using available standard questionnaires also shows favorable results.

Complications Associated with Ventricular Assist Device

- Infections
- Pump thrombosis
- Right heart failure (RHF)
- Gastrointestinal bleed
- Aortic insufficiency
- Stroke.

TOTAL ARTIFICIAL HEART: SYNCARDIA TOTAL ARTIFICIAL HEART-TEMPORARY

Another option for MCS is the TAH. The 70 mL stroke volume version of the SynCardia Cardiowest Total Artificial Heart-temporary (TAH-t) was evaluated in a large, prospective, and nonrandomized clinical trial conducted in five centers for BTT indication in 81 patients at risk of imminent death from irreversible biventricular HF.[33] The study cohort was compared with a nonrandomized, observational control cohort of 35 patients. The primary study endpoints included the rates of survival to HT and survival after transplantation. The rate of survival to transplantation was 79%. Of the 35 patients in the control cohort who met the same entry criteria but did not receive the TAH-t, 16 (46%) survived to transplant ($p < 0.001$). Overall, 1-year survival rate among the patients who received the TAH-t was 70%, compared to 31% for controls ($p < 0.001$). After transplantation, 1-year and 5-year survival rates among patients who received the TAH were 86% and 64%, respectively. The SynCardia TAH was approved by the FDA for BTT in 2007 and is currently being evaluated for DT indication in the US. A smaller 50 cc version is also under evaluation.

The HeartMate II and III along with the HVAD are the commercially available devices in the United States. In addition to INTERMACS, international research efforts based on high-volume experiences, such as those captured in the EUROMACS (European Registry for Patients with Mechanical Circulatory Support), have led to significant contributions to the field. Rapid technological advances have helped introduce several newer devices with each exhibiting a technological edge over the other.[27] While refinements will continue the common aims are to provide devices which are smaller in size, easy to implant, durable and biocompatible. Some of the other VADs in use in other parts of the world are: INCOR (approved in EU; Berlin Heart, Berlin, Germany), Jarvik 2000 (approved in EU; ongoing DT trial in US; Jarvik Heart, Inc, New York, NY), EVAHEART LVAS (ongoing BTT trial in US; EVAHEART, Houston, TX), and more.

OVERCOMING PROBLEMS AND FUTURE DIRECTIONS

- The miniaturization of these devices deserves special mention as it eases the implantation process and makes it less invasive. An ongoing clinical trial is investigating the efficacy of the HeartWare miniature ventricular assist device (MVAD) system, which is an axial-flow device that can generate full cardiac output despite being a third of the size of the HVAD device. Perioperative morbidity has been shown to be lower when devices are implanted and exchanged by thoracotomy-based approaches. The LATERAL trial has finished enrollment and is awaiting publication on the safety and efficacy of HVAD implantation via thoracotomy instead of median sternotomy.[27] The Impella device can be installed percutaneously, though in its current state it comes at the cost of reduced durability, stability, and strength. In the near future miniature, minimally invasive VADs will become the standard of care, rendering it widely available to patients at considerably lower risks.
- *Lowering of PT rates*: PT is a major problem with these devices. If left untreated, it may lead to rapid clinical deterioration and prompt the device to be replaced. In the initial trials, the incidence of this complication was low. However, there was a spurt in such cases beyond 2011 (PT cases rose from 2.2% in 2011 to 8.4% in 2013). Most recent clinical trial data suggest that 10.7% to 12.2% of HeartMate II patients and 4.2–6.4% of HeartWare HVAD patients experience PT requiring device exchange in 2 years. Recent trial data from MOMENTUM 3 (studying the HeartMate III VAD) have shown very promising results with no case of PT being reported at 6 months while the incidence at 2 years was 1.1%. The fully magnetically levitated flow technology referred to as Full MagLev reduces trauma to blood passing through the pump, improves flow in a pulsatile fashion thereby reducing thrombosis rates.[31]
- *Lowering infection rates*: Infection of the driveline which is tunneled subcutaneously to an external power source is a cause of grave concern in patients receiving VADs. This may lead to sepsis and at times pocket infection necessitating prolonged antibiotics and at times even device change. Devices are being developed which shall be totally implantable batteries with transcutaneous recharging capabilities. This is bound to be a significant breakthrough in curbing the menace of infection. Several device companies are currently working to develop a wireless VAD power delivery system, using technologies such as magnetic resonance coupling.[34] Battery capabilities are also improving rapidly enabling greater efficiency even at more compact scales. Although it is not clear when VADs will become fully wireless, once available, their impact on patient care will be immediate.[27]
- To date a majority of devices are designed to provide complete cardiac output or full support. As MCS therapy moves into populations of patients with less advanced HF, the concept of small partial assist MCS devices has been developed to reverse HF symptoms with only limited assist of cardiac function. The C Pulse is a counterpulsation device similar to the concept of IABP but is implanted around the ascending aorta, rather than being placed in the circulation.[35] The major feature of the device is the reduction in the potential for stroke as the device is not incorporated into the circulation and can be turned on and off without risk of device thrombosis (nonobligatory). The intraventricular ventricular assist system (iVAS; NuPulse CV, Raleigh, NC) is a small IABP for partial circulatory support that is placed with a minimally invasive approach in the descending aorta via subclavian access. As with the C Pulse the iVAS is designed to be nonobligatory. A small, wearable pneumatic driver allows full ambulation.

- While the SynCardia TAH-t is the only approved total artificial heart approved at present. Similar devices such as the CARMAT Bioprosthetic artificial heart (CARMAT, Vélizy-Villacoublay), which is a hydraulic, pulsatile device comprising two ventricles and four bioprosthetic valves, and BiVACOR TAH (BiVACOR Inc, Houston, TX), which is a rotary pump with two centrifugal impellers, are currently in the pipeline undergoing clinical investigation and may immensely expand the potential of artificial heart technology. These technologies may reduce or prevent RHF altogether and potentially offer MCS therapy to patients with anatomic contraindications to VAD placement such as diastolic HF, noncompaction HF, or other congenital abnormalities. In a cohort of predominantly INTERMACS class I (91%) patients, TAH successfully bridged 68% to HT with reasonable long-term outcomes post-HT (41% at 10 years).[36]

DEVICES FOR LEFT ATRIAL DECOMPRESSION IN HEART FAILURE

These are a group of innovative devices which help reduce the elevated left atrial pressures in HF patients thereby relieving pulmonary vascular congestion. Therapies that aim to reduce total body volume and intravascular pressure have been associated with improved outcomes among patients who have HFrEF, but not HFpEF (EF >55%).[37] This may be partly because the latter group is not necessarily total body volume overloaded, but exhibits exertional increases in left atrial pressure.[38] Accordingly, more selective reductions in left atrial pressure, if achievable, may confer symptomatic benefits without the potentially negative sequelae of pharmacologic volume removal and additionally mitigate concerns regarding drug adherence and resistance.

Balloon septostomy has been reported in cases of recalcitrant HF and hypoxemia,[39] and the utilization of a fenestrated Amplatzer Septal Occluder (Abbott Vascular, formerly St. Jude Medical) to maintain a durable Fontan fenestration and interatrial communication was described more than 15 years ago.[40] Mechanical devices that aim to reduce left atrial pressure have been developed and evaluated in HFpEF and HFrEF patients. Recently three devices have been developed and studied that work on this principle.

- *Interatrial shunt device (IASD)*: Maximum clinical experience is with this device developed by Corvia medical. This device is made of nitinol and composed of right and left atrial disks (19 mm outer diameter) while the communication between the two is of 8 mm and delivered via a 16 F venous sheath. The device is delivered across the inter atrialseptum after transseptal puncture in the area of fossa ovalis and disks deployed serially much akin to the ASD device deployment using fluoroscopic, intracardiac, and transesophageal guidance. Based on the success of the First-in-Man experiences in 2014, the device has undergone evaluation in trials.
- The REDUCE LAP-HF trial, was a phase 1, open-label, single-arm trial[41] in which 66 patients underwent the procedure. Implantation success was high (97%), without major periprocedural AEs. At 6-month follow-up, most patients had reductions in pulmonary capillary wedge pressure (PCWP) at rest and with exertion (52% and 58%, respectively), along with significant improvements in NYHA class and 6-minute walk distance (from 313 m to 345 m; P = 0.023). These changes occurred in tandem with sustained left-to-right interatrial flow and pulmonary to systemic blood flow ratio (Qp:Qs ~1.3:1). At 1-year follow-up, there was a persistent and significant reduction in the pressure difference between the left and right atrium at rest and with exertion, again with improved NYHA class and 6-minute walk distance, as well as sustained shunt Qp/Qs ratio. In addition, fewer HF hospitalizations were observed in the year after implantation (mean, 1.5–0.8 per year; $P < 0.05$).[9,10] Based on this study, the IASD system received CE mark approval for the treatment of HFpEF and heart failure with midrange ejection fraction (HFmrEF) (EF, 40%–55%). Patients have been randomized in the United States, Australia, and Europe (N = 44) in the REDUCE LAP-HF I trial. 1-month outcomes were recently reported; there were no periprocedural AEs, and treated patients exhibited greater reductions in exercise-associated PCWP.
- *V device*: The V-wave device (V-Wave Ltd.) includes an hourglass-shaped nitinol frame that is partially covered with expanded polytetrafluoroethylene (ePTFE) that serves as an anchor for a porcine trileaflet pericardial valve. The valve is designed to prevent right-to-left atrial flow and delivered using a 14 F venous sheath.[42] First-in-human experience was reported in 10 patients with HFrEF (all NYHA III; mean EF, 25%). The device was successfully implanted in all enrolled patients. At 3 months, there were significant reductions in mean PCWP with improvements in the 6-minute walk test distance and most experiencing improved NYHA class.[28] At 1-year follow-up, resting shunt fraction had declined from a mean of 1.2:1–1.1:1, with 14% of patients having no interatrial flow. This occurred in conjunction with pannus thickening of the bioprosthetic leaflets and lumen loss, which prompted the creation of a second-generation device without the one-way valve component, extended the ePTFE coating, and included a hood to prevent potential thromboemboli

from apposing the right atrial side of the implant. This version of the device has been evaluated histologically, and late lumen loss has not been observed at 6 months.[43]

- *Atrial flow regulator (AFR)*: Occlutech International AB has developed an AFR that is a nitinol mesh device composed of two flat disks and a 1- to 2-mm connecting neck with a central fenestration that enables bidirectional flow.[44] It is manufactured in fenestration sizes of 6 mm, 8 mm, or 10 mm and is delivered via femoral venous approach with a 10- to 12-F sheath after an atrial septostomy. The first clinical utilization of the device followed a compassionate use approval from the US FDA and showed favorable results. A human international trial is forthcoming via the PRELIEVE trial. It is an open-label, nonrandomized trial including up to 30 patients with symptomatic HF (HFpEF or HFrEF) and a HF admission in the past 12 months (NCT03030274).

Concerns With Left Atrial Decompression Devices

Three major concerns have been raised with the use of these devices. The first is regarding right atrial and RV volume overload due to the left to right shunt with consequent RV dysfunction but present data has been favorable. The degree of shunting can be altered by altering the shunt diameter and companies are working on techniques whereby these shunts could be closed if right HF develops.[37] The second concern is regarding atrial arrhythmias and as these may worsen, the HF they need to be watched for. Lastly paradoxical embolism is a theoretical possibility but no such case has been reported to date with these devices.

MitraClip in Heart Failure

Heart failure patients develop functional mitral regurgitation (FMR) over time due to left ventricular (LV) remodeling. Functional mitral regurgitation has been associated with poor prognosis in patients with HF. Medical therapy has its own limitations in treating such patients. It helps provide symptomatic relief, however, is not very successful halting disease progression. While patients with degenerative mitral regurgitation (MR) have satisfying outcomes post valve replacement, patients those with FMR have far from optimal long-term outcomes most likely due to multiple comorbidities and high surgical risk. For these patients, transcatheter therapy could be a valuable therapeutic option. MitraClip (Abbott Laboratories, Abbott Park, Illinois) is a transcatheter-delivered device based on the original surgical technique known as edge-to-edge leaflet repair, described by Alfieri et al. in 1991. With the help of a cobalt/chromium-based implant, the anterior and posterior MV leaflets are opposed and relocated until the desirable hemodynamic effect is achieved. Echocardiography is performed to assess the severity of the MR, the mechanism involved (Carpentier classification), and the suitability for transcatheter treatment. In addition, it is used to guide the procedure and evaluate the postinterventional outcome. Although, currently, there is no sufficient evidence that FMR correction confers a survival benefit, several studies have demonstrated that mitral valve surgery, especially annuloplasty, reverses LV remodeling and improves HF-related symptoms. In this context, the percutaneous implantation of a MitraClip device appears to be a promising and reasonable therapeutic option that improves patients' quality of life.

Chatzistergiou et al. recently published an excellent systematic review of 28 studies and 2,383 patients with FMR treated with the MitraClip device.[45] They concluded that this device seems to be a safe therapeutic option for the treatment of secondary MR (30-day mortality rate: 2.3%, 1-year mortality rate: 18.9%) with excellent implantation rate success. The results are of major importance, considering that the patients who underwent the MitraClip procedure had severe MR (MR ≥ 3+: 98%) and were characterized by severe symptoms and high surgical risk (NYHA III-IV: 91%, mean Euroscore: 24.6%).

Two recent trials looked at the role of MitraClip in secondary MR with diametrically opposite results.

The MITRA-FR study (Percutaneous Repair with the MitraClip Device for Severe Functional/Secondary Mitral Regurgitation)[46] randomized 304 patients with symptomatic systolic HF and severe secondary MR defined as an effective regurgitant orifice area (EROA) >20 mm^2 and/or a regurgitant volume >30 mL, and LVEF between 15% and 40%, in a 1:1 ratio, to percutaneous mitral valve repair with MitraClip in addition to OMM (intervention group) or to OMM alone (control group). The primary efficacy endpoint was a composite of death from any cause or hospitalization for heart failure (HHF) at 1 year. There was no difference between the intervention vs. control groups for the rate of the primary composite end point (54.6% vs. 51.3%, respectively; P = 0.53), the rate of mortality (24.3% vs. 22.4%) or the rate of unplanned HF hospitalization (48.7% vs. 47.4%). The authors concluded that MitraClip is safe and effective in reducing secondary MR but does not improve prognosis (as compared with optimized medical therapy) in patients with secondary MR and systolic HF.

On the other hand, encouraging data in favor of MitraClip emerged from the COAPT Trial (Cardiovascular Outcomes Assessment of the MitraClip Percutaneous Therapy for Heart Failure Patients with Functional Mitral Regurgitation).[47] At 78 sites in the United States and Canada, 614 patients with ischemic or nonischemic cardiomyopathy (LVEF 20–50% and LV end systolic dimension ≤70 mm) and moderate-to-severe or severe secondary MR who remained symptomatic (NYHA class II–IVa) despite the use of maximal doses of GDMT were recruited. Patients were randomly assigned to transcatheter mitral-valve repair plus medical therapy (device group, N = 302) or medical therapy alone (control group, N = 302). The primary effectiveness endpoint was all HHF within 24 months of follow-up. The primary safety endpoint was freedom from device-related complications at 12 months; the rate for this endpoint was compared with a prespecified objective performance goal of 88.0%. The annualized rate of all hospitalizations for HF within 24 months was 35.8% per patient-year in the device group as compared with 67.9% per patient-year in the control group (hazard ratio, 0.53; 95% CI, 0.40–0.70; P <0.001). The rate of freedom from device-related complications at 12 months was 96.6% (lower 95% confidence limit, 94.8%; P <0.001 for comparison with the performance goal). Death from any cause within 24 months occurred in 29.1% of the patients in the device group as compared with 46.1% in the control group (hazard ratio, 0.62; 95% CI, 0.46–0.82; P <0.001).

The reasons for varying outcomes have been extensively debated. Pibarot et al. have brilliantly discussed the same.[48] They state that differences in the inclusion/exclusion criteria for MR severity, LV dimensions and dysfunction are the main reasons for the discrepancies in the outcomes observed between MITRA-FR and COAPT [patients with more severe MR (EROA >30 mm^2 in COAPT vs. >20 mm^2 in MITRA-FR) and less dilated ventricles (LVEDV 101 vs. 135, respectively)]. In MITRA-FR, the underlying cardiomyopathy was likely the predominant cause of the HF and thus the main determinant of the poor clinical outcome. And in this context, the MR was probably more a bystander than an actor of the HF. On the other hand, in COAPT HF was, in large part, related to the valvular disease (the MR was more severe), while LV disease (smaller size and higher LVEF) was less advanced. Hence, in COAPT, MR was an important contributor to the HF and the clinical outcomes, whereas in MITRA-FR the LV disease (dysfunction) was the main determinant of clinical outcomes. Possibly, because of these differences in baseline characteristics, the COAPT patients were more likely to benefit from the MitraClip procedure compared with the MITRA-FR patients.

In light of the results of the MITRA-FR and COAPT trials, it thus appears reasonable to conclude that the MitraClip procedure reduces HF hospitalization and mortality in patients meeting the following criteria:

- ≥ moderate-to-severe (3+) secondary MR defined as EROA ≥30 mm^2 and/or regurgitant volume >45 mL
- Left ventricular ejection fraction between 20% and 50% and LV end-systolic diameter <70 mm
- Persistent HF symptoms (NYHA ≥ II) despite optimal (maximally tolerated) GDMT with cardiac resynchronization and coronary revascularization if appropriate.
- Furthermore, the goal of the procedure should be to obtain an acute reduction of the MR severity to ≤mild (1+) and the implantation of additional clips should be considered to achieve this goal.

ROLE OF GENE THERAPY IN HEART FAILURE

Sarcoplasmic/endoplasmic reticulum (SERCA2a) activity is deficient in HF. It was postulated that if SERCA 2a levels could be increased in the failing heart, the cardiac contractility and relaxation would favorably improve. Encouraging data was noted in the CUPID 1 (Calcium upregulation by percutaneous administration of gene therapy in patients with cardiac disease) trial and paved the way for the CUPID 2 trial.[49] Patients with HF were randomized to gene transfer therapy (n = 123) versus placebo injection (n = 127). Gene therapy was performed by adeno-associated virus 1/SERCA2a. The primary outcome, recurrent events (defined as hospital readmission for HF or ambulatory treatment for worsening HF), occurred in 62.8% of the gene transfer group versus 73.9% of the placebo group (p = 0.81). The secondary outcome, death, was 21% versus 16% (p = not significant), respectively, for gene transfer versus placebo. The authors concluded that among HF patients, gene transfer therapy was not beneficial. Although there were no notable safety concerns, gene transfer therapy failed to improve clinical events. The trial results cast several uncertainties about future for this therapy. However, some recent research seems to point toward revival of this therapy using a new technique. Scientists have discovered a micropeptide called Dwarf Open Reading Frame (DWORF), which binds directly to SERCA and enhances its activity.[50] DWORF works by displacing a molecule that inhibits SERCA, called phospholamban (PLN). Experiments have shown that mice engineered to have higher levels of DWORF showed enhanced calcium cycling. Conversely, heart muscle cells from the mice with higher levels of PLN showed the opposite and had reduced contractility. In the mice engineered to have high levels of both DWORF and PLN, the adverse effects of excess PLN were completely prevented, suggesting that DWORF could protect against its pathological activity. Researchers have looked at the effects of increasing the levels of DWORF in mice with dilated cardiomyopathy. Higher levels of DWORF significantly improved LV function. Mice that had DWORF removed entirely had even more of a decline in heart function than the normal mice with cardiomyopathy. High levels of DWORF also prevented the physical hallmarks of cardiomyopathy in the mice-like chamber enlargement, thinning of the chamber wall, and increase in the cardiac volume. The build-up of scar tissue in the heart is also characteristic of myopathy, and this was also prevented in the mice with elevated levels of DWORF.

Taken together, the results show that DWORF can prevent both the functional and structural effects of cardiomyopathy in mice. So rather than directly enhancing SERCA 2a levels by gene transfer, enhancing them by inhibiting PLN may be the way forward.

CONCLUSION

Heart failure is a common problem with a high mortality and increasing incidence. In spite of several spectacular advances in the management of these patients, the problem continues to pose challenges. These advances include development of several drugs, devices, and innovative treatment algorithms including totally mechanical heart. This review gives a comprehensive detail of all these developments and also a peep into the future.

REFERENCES

1. Acker MA, Bolling S, Shemin R, et al.; Acorn Trial Principal Investigators and Study Coordinators. Mitral valve surgery in heart failure: Insights from the Acorn clinical trial. J Thorac Cardiovasc Surg. 2006;132(3):568-77.e1-4.
2. McMurray JJ, Packer MP, Desai AS, et al.; PARADIGM-HF Investigators and Committees. Angiotensin–neprilysin inhibition versus enalapril in heart failure. N Engl J Med. 2014;371(11):993-1004.
3. Jankowska EA, Kasztura M, Sokolski M, et al. Iron deficiency defined as depleted iron stores accompanied by unmet cellular iron requirements identifies patients at the highest risk of death after an episode of acute heart failure. Eur Heart J. 2014;35(36):2468-76.
4. Martens P, Verbrugge FH, Nijst P, et al. Limited contractile reserve contributes to poor peak exercise capacity in iron-deficient heart failure. Eur J Heart Fail. 2018;20(4):806-8.
5. Dai DF, Johnson SC, Villarin JJ, et al. Mitochondrial oxidative stress mediates angiotensin II-induced cardiac hypertrophy and Galphaq over expression-induced heart failure. Circ Res. 2011;108(7):837-46.
6. Yancy CW, Jessup M, Bozkurt B, et al. 2017 ACC/AHA/HFSA focused update of the 2013 ACCF/AHA Guideline for the Management of Heart Failure: A Report of the American College of Cardiology/American Heart Association Task Force on Clinical Practice Guidelines and the Heart Failure Society of America. J Am Coll Cardiol. 2017;70(6):776-803.
7. Ponikowski P, Voors AA, Anker SD, et al.; ESC Scientific Document Group. 2016 ESC guidelines for the diagnosis and treatment of acute and chronic heart failure: the Task Force for the Diagnosis and Treatment of Acute and Chronic Heart Failure of the European Society of Cardiology (ESC) Developed with the special contribution of the Heart Failure Association (HFA) of the ESC. Eur Heart J. 2016;37(27):2129-200.
8. Lewis GD, Malhotra R, Hernandez AF, et al.; NHLBI Heart Failure Clinical Research Network. Effect of oral iron repletion on exercise capacity in patients with heart failure with reduced ejection fraction and iron deficiency: the IRONOUT HF randomized clinical trial. JAMA. 2017;317(19):1958-66.
9. Anker SD, Comin CJ, Filippatos G, et al.; FAIR-HF Trial Investigators. Ferric Carboxymaltose in patients with heart failure and iron deficiency. N Engl J Med. 2009;361(25):2436-48.
10. Ponikowski P, van Veldhuisen DJ, Comin-Col J, et al.; CONFIRM-HF Investigators. Beneficial effects of long-term intravenous iron therapy with ferric carboxymaltose in patients with symptomatic heart failure and iron deficiency. Eur Heart J. 2015;36(11):657-68.
11. Anker SD, Kirwan BA, van Veldhuisen DJ, et al. Effects of ferric carboxymaltose on hospitalisations and mortality rates in iron-deficient heart failure patients: an individual patient data meta-analysis. Eur J Heart Fail. 2018;20(1):125-33.
12. Jankowska EA, Tkaczyszyn M, Suchocki T, et al. Effects of intravenous iron therapy in iron-deficient patients with systolic heart failure: a meta-analysis of randomized controlled trials. Eur J Heart Fail. 2016;18(7):786-95.
13. Department of Health and Human Services, Food and Drug Administration. Guidance for Industry: Diabetes Mellitus - Evaluating Cardiovascular Risk in New Anti-diabetic Therapies to Treat Type 2 Diabetes. [online] Available from: http://www.fda.gov/downloads/drugs/guidancecomplianceregulatory-formation/guidances/ucm071627.pdf. [Last accessed November, 2019].
14. European Medicines Agency Guideline on Clinical Investigation of Medicinal Products in the Treatment or Prevention of Diabetes Mellitus. London: Committee for Medicinal Products for Human Use; 2012.
15. Scirica BM, Bhatt DL, Braunwald E, et al.; SAVOR-TIMI 53 Steering Committee and Investigators. Saxagliptin and cardiovascular outcomes in patients with type 2 diabetes mellitus. N Engl J Med. 2013;369(14):1317-26.
16. White WB, Cannon CP, Heller SR, et al.; EXAMINE Investigators. Alogliptin after acute coronary syndrome in patients with type 2 diabetes. N Engl J Med. 2013;369(14):1327-35.
17. Green JB, Bethel MA, Armstrong PW, et al.; TECOS Study Group. Effect of sitagliptin on cardiovascular outcomes in type 2 diabetes. N Engl J Med. 2015;373(3):232-42.
18. Boehringer Ingelheim. CAROLINA: Cardiovascular Outcome Study of Linagliptin Versus Glimepiride in Patients with Type 2 Diabetes. In: ClinicalTrials.gov Bethesda, MD: National Library of Medicine. [online] Available from: https://clinicaltrials.gov/show/NCT01243424. NLM. [Last accessed November, 2019].
19. Boehringer Ingelheim. Cardiovascular and Renal Microvascular Outcome Study with Linagliptin in Patients with Type 2 Diabetes Mellitus (CARMELINA). In: ClinicalTrials.gov. Bethesda, MD: National Library of Medicine. [online] Available from: https://clinicaltrials.gov/show/NCT01897532. NLM Identifier: NCT01897532. [Last accessed November, 2019].
20. Zinman B, Wanner C, Lachin JM, et al.; EMPA-REG OUTCOME Investigators. Empagliflozin, cardiovascular

outcomes, and mortality in type 2 diabetes. N Engl J Med. 2015;373(22):2117-28.
21. Fitchett D, Zinman B, Wanner C, et al. EMPA-REG OUTCOME® trial investigators. Heart failure outcomes with empagliflozin in patients with type 2 diabetes at high cardiovascular risk: results of the EMPA-REG OUTCOME® trial. Eur Heart J. 2016;37(19):1526-34.
22. Neal B, Perkovic V, Mahaffey KW, et al.; CANVAS Program Collaborative Group. Canagliflozin and cardiovascular and renal events in type 2 diabetes. N Engl J Med. 2017;377(7): 644-57.
23. Pfeffer MA, Claggett B, Diaz R, et al.; ELIXA Investigators. Lixisenatide in patients with type 2 diabetes and acute coronary syndrome. N Engl J Med. 2015;373(23): 2247-57.
24. Marso SP, Daniels GH, Brown-Frandsen K, et al.; LEADER Steering Committee; LEADER Trial Investigators. Liraglutide and cardiovascular outcomes in type 2 diabetes. N Engl J Med. 2016;375(4):311-22.
25. Marso SP, Bain SC, Consoli A, et al.; SUSTAIN-6 investigators. Semaglutide and cardiovascular outcomes in patients with type 2 diabetes. N Engl J Med. 2016;375(19):1834-44.
26. Holman RR, Bethel MA, Mentz RJ,et al.; EXSCEL Study Group. Effects of once-weekly exenatide on cardiovascular outcomes in type 2 diabetes. N Engl J Med. 2017;377(13):1228-39.
27. Han JJ, Acker MA, Atluri P. Left ventricular assist devices. Circulation. 2018;138(24):2841-51.
28. Stehlik J, Edwards LB, Kucheryavaya AY, et al. International Society of Heart and Lung Transplantation. The Registry of the International Society for Heart and Lung Transplantation: 29th official adult heart transplant report—2012. J Heart Lung Transplant. 2012;31(10):1052-64.
29. Rose EA, Gelijns AC, Moskowitz AJ, et al. Randomized Evaluation of Mechanical Assistance for the Treatment of Congestive Heart Failure (REMATCH) Study Group. Long-term use of a left ventricular assist device for end-stage heart failure. N Engl J Med. 2001;345(20):1435-43.
30. Kirklin JK, Pagani FD, Kormos RL, et al. Eighth annual intermacs report: special focus on framing the impact of adverse events. J Heart Lung Transplant. 2017;36(10):1080-6.
31. Mehra MR, Goldstein DJ, Uriel N, et al.; MOMENTUM 3 Investigators. Two-year outcomes with magnetically levitated cardiac pump in heart failure. N Eng J Med. 2018;378(15):1386-95.
32. Kirklin JK, Naftel DC, Pagani FD, et al. Seventh INTERMACS annual report: 15,000 patients and counting. J Heart Lung Transplant. 2015;34(12):1495-504.
33. Copeland JG, Smith RG, Arabia FA, et al.; CardioWest Total Artificial Heart Investigators. Cardiac replacement with total artificial heart as a bridge to transplant. N Eng J Med. 2004;351(9):859-67.
34. Kassif Y, Zilbershlag M, Levi M, et al. A new universal wireless transcutaneous energy transfer (TET) system for implantable LVADs: Preliminary in vitro and in vivo results. J Heart Lung Transplant. 2013;32(4):S140-1.
35. Hayward CS, Peters WS, Merry AF, et al. Chronic extra-aortic balloon counterpulsation: First-in-human pilot study in end-stage heart failure. J Heart Lung Transplant. 2010;29(12):1427-32.
36. Copeland JG, Copeland H, Gustafson M, et al. Experience with more than 100 total artificial heart implants. J Thorac Cardiovasc Surg. 2012;143(3):727-34.
37. Lillie S, Burkoff D. Technologies for treating left atrial decompression in heart failure. Cardiac Interventions Today. 2018;12(1):59-61.
38. Borlaug BA, Nishimura RA, Sorajja P, et al. Exercise hemodynamics enhance diagnosis of early heart failure with preserved ejection fraction. Circ Heart Fail. 2010;3(5): 588-95.
39. Seib PM, Faulkner SC, Erikson CC, et al. Blade and balloon atrial septostomy for left heart decompression in patients with severe ventricular dysfunction on extracorporeal membrane oxygenation. Catheter Cardiovasc Interv. 1999;46(2)179-86.
40. Amin Z, Danford DA, Pedra CA. A new amplatzer device to main patency of Fontan fenestrations and atrial septal defects. Catheter Cardiovasc Interv. 2002;57(2):246-51.
41. Hasenfuss G, Hayward C, Burkhoff D, et al.; REDUCE LAP-HF study investigators. A transcatheter intracardiac shunt device for heart failure with preserved ejection fraction (REDUCE LAP-HF): a multicentre, open-label, single-arm, phase 1 trial. Lancet. 2016;387(10025):1298-304.
42. Amat-Santos IJ, Bergeron S, Bernier M, et al. Left atrial decompression through unidirectional left-to-right interatrial shunt for the treatment of left heart failure: First-in-man experience with the V-Wave device. EuroIntervention. 2015;10(9):1127-31.
43. Stone GW R-CJ, Amat-Santos IJ, Ben Gal T, et al. Interatrial Shunting for Heart Failure: The V-Wave Shunt. Presented at Transcatheter Therapeutics (TCT). Denver, Colorado: 2017.
44. Patel MB, Samuel BP, Girgis RE, et al. Implantable atrial flow regulator for severe, irreversible pulmonary arterial hypertension. EuroIntervention. 2015;11(6):706-9.
45. Chatzsitergiou KT, Papanastasiou CS, Kokkinidis DG, et al. MitraClip device for patients with functional Mitral regurgitation: A systematic review. Hellenic J Cardiol. 2019;60(2):101-7.
46. Obadia JF, Messika-Zeitoun D, Leurent G, et al.; MITRA-FR Investigators. Percutaneous repair or medical treatment for secondary mitral regurgitation. N Engl J Med. 2018;379(24):2297-306.
47. Stone GW, Lindenfeld JA, Abraham WT, et al. COAPT Investigators. Transcatheter mitral-valve repair in patients with heart failure. N Engl J Med. 2018;379(24):2307-18.
48. Pibarot P, Delgado V, Bax JJ. MITRA-FR vs. COAPT: Lessons from two trials with diametrically opposed results. Eur Heart J Cardiovasc Imaging. 2019;20(6):620-4.
49. Greenberg B, Butler J, Felker GM, et al. Calcium upregulation by percutaneous administration of gene therapy in patients with cardiac disease (CUPID 2): A randomized, multinational, double-blind, placebo-controlled, phase 2b trial. Lancet. 2016;387(10024):1178-86.
50. Makarewich CA, Munir AZ, Schiattarella GG, et al. The DWORF micropeptide enhances contractility and prevents heart failure in a mouse model of dilated cardiomyopathy. Elife. 2018;7. pii: e38319.

CHAPTER 80

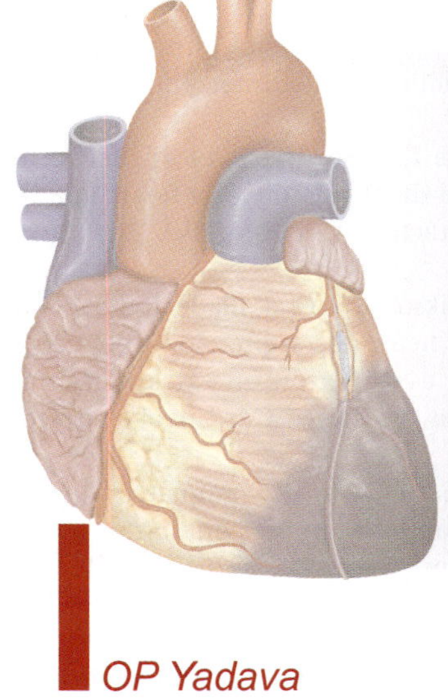

Coronary Artery Bypass Graft in Heart Failure

OP Yadava

INTRODUCTION

The epidemic of heart failure (HF) is blossoming into a public health issue in India. The available data are tenuous and scarce, but a conservative estimate of the prevalence of HF in India is in the range of 1.3–4.6 million with an annual incidence of 0.4–1.8 million.[1] Though rheumatic heart disease is a major contributor, ischemic heart disease (IHD) is the most common etiology.[2] These patients are an altogether different subset, presenting at a younger age with more left ventricular (LV) dysfunction and having higher atherosclerotic burden, mainly driven by the higher prevalence of diabetes mellitus (DM), thereby impacting their prognosis.[2] Velazquez and Bonow sum it succinctly, "This more aggressive course represents the convergence of ischemia, myocardial fibrosis, and endothelial dysfunction, which are super imposed on the inherent progressive nature of LV dysfunction, often with associated comorbidities, such as diabetes, which accelerate the adverse clinical trajectory".[3] HF may even develop after coronary artery bypass graft (CABG) surgery, either as a continuum of preoperative LV dysfunction or because of perioperative myocardial injury/stunning due to the reperfusion injury. Even early postoperative graft failure, which may occur in up to 10% of cases, may contribute to this and may call for aggressive treatment in form of angiography and reintervention, most often percutaneous. Cardiac arrhythmias, infections, postcardiotomy syndrome, and acute kidney injury (AKI) too may contribute to postoperative cardiac failure.

EVALUATION

Besides a good clinical history and physical examination, especially looking for signs of fluid overload, certain routine investigations would need an interpretation with a hawk's eye, as they may impact surgical outcomes. Electrocardiogram (ECG) should be specifically looked for P-R interval, QRS duration, and bundle branch blocks. Chest X-ray should be evaluated for signs of fluid overload and cardiomegaly. Echocardiography is usually the cornerstone of HF diagnosis. Its iterations in form of transesophageal echocardiography (TOE), especially to look for intracardiac thrombi and stress echocardiography to evaluate myocardial viability and hibernation, as also to look at exercise capacity, can be definitive. Though biomarkers, like B-type natriuretic peptide (BNP)/N-terminal (NT) Pro-BNP, have a role in a difficult case, echocardiography takes precedence in India.[2] On echocardiography, both systolic and diastolic function and the left and the right heart should be specifically examined and subjected to advanced technologies such as Tissue Doppler Imaging, Speckle Tracking, and Tricuspid Annular Plane Systolic Excursion (TAPSE) for adequate risk assessment. 3D echocardiography, contrast echocardiography and dobutamine stress echocardiography (DSE) are complementary. Cardiac magnetic resonance (CMR) imaging is the gold standard for left ventricular ejection fraction (LVEF). It can also be used to assess myocardial viability and transmurality of infarction, using delayed gadolinium enhancement, and for assessing the contractile reserves. This helps in predicting survival and all-cause mortality, independent of the LVEF.[4,5] Positron emission tomography (PET) and single photon emission computed tomography (SPECT) too may be helpful in assessing ischemia and myocardial viability. Obviously coronary angiography, computed tomography (CT) based or cine, are mandatory tests and would be required in all cases to assess coronary anatomy.

PREOPERATIVE PREPARATION

These patients are sick and at times cachexic, and their preoperative clinical state should be optimized. Anemia should be corrected and iron stores repleted. Left ventricular end diastolic pressure (LVEDP) should be normalized, as far as possible, with use of diuretics, and anticoagulants and antiplatelets stopped according to accepted guidelines.[6] However, aspirin should be continued as it reduces early mortality and morbidity in form of AKI and myocardial infarction (MI).[7,8] Beta-blockers and statins too should be continued, and in fact started in patients not already on them.[8] Oral antidiabetics must give way to sliding scale insulin and peripheral blood vessels should be screened for any probable use of mechanical support post-CABG. Atrial fibrillation, a common accompaniment of these sick elderly patients, should be adequately controlled.

VIABILITY TESTING

Viable hibernating myocardium must have preserved cell membrane integrity (as assessed by uptake of thallium 201 or 99-m technetium), preserved metabolism [uptake of 18 F-fluorodeoxyglucose (FDG)], contractile reserve during stimulation (DSE or stress CMR imaging) and absence of scar (late gadolinium enhancement on CMR). Out of these modalities, none is foolproof, but nuclear modalities have higher sensitivity and wall motion imaging have greater specificity. Therefore, all these techniques are complementary and more than one may be needed to demonstrate hibernating myocardium.[9] Though viability testing is routinely used to detect hibernating myocardium and finds support in observational studies, randomized data and high level of evidence (LOE) is lacking. In a meta-analysis of 24 observational studies, myocardial revascularization was associated with a reduction in annual mortality from 16% to 3.2% (p <0.0001) with medical treatment in patients with viability, as compared to no difference in those without viability (7.7% vs. 6.2%, p-NS).[10] A Cleveland Clinic study found a threshold of 10% of hibernating myocardium, beyond which, there was incremental benefit from revascularization.[11] However, PARR-2 (PET and recovery following revascularization) Trial, which is in fact the only randomized controlled trial (RCT) available on the subject, found no benefit of FDG-PET imaging, with the primary composite end point of cardiac mortality/MI/recurrent hospitalization at 1 year being exactly the same [FDG-PET Arm 30% vs. 36%, risk ratio (RR) 0.82, 95% confidence interval (CI) 0.59–1.14, p -0.16].[12] This study has been challenged by a subgroup analysis and the subsequent 5 years follow-up, where a significant reduction in the primary endpoint was demonstrated in the PET-guided therapy group [hazard Ratio (HR) 0.73, 95% CI 0.54–0.99, p -0.042].[13] The viability substudy of the STICH (Surgical Treatment for Ischemic Heart Failure) Trial, consisting of 601 patients, used SPECT or DSE and univariate analysis found viability to the associated with a reduced mortality (HR 0.64, p -0.003). However, on multivariate analysis, though there was a numerical trend toward lower mortality and cardiovascular hospitalization with viability, it did not assume statistical significance [55.2% CABG vs. 72.1% optimum medical therapy (OMT), p -0.3903].[14] The AIMI-HF (Alternative Imaging Modalities in Ischemic Heart Failure) is an ongoing study which may address this question more definitely.[15]

The American College of Cardiology (ACC)/American Heart Association (AHA) guidelines give myocardial viability a class IIa (LOE "B") recommendation[16] and the European Society of Cardiology/European Association of Cardiothoracic Surgery (ESC/EACTS) guidelines give it a still lower class IIb (LOE "B") recommendation.[17] In clinical practice, certainly viability testing is useful and may help in predicting the response to revascularization or medical therapy, besides being a prognostic marker. However, it should be complemented by other astute observations like size and quality of the coronary artery, thickness of the ventricular myocardium of the subtended territory, regional wall motion abnormalities, and the risk assessment of the procedure.

PRACTICAL TIP

In patients having angina, myocardial revascularization is clearly indicated, but if they have only dyspnea, suggestive of HF, then one must be wary. Only if it is an angina equivalent, especially in diabetics; in critical coronary anatomy; or with significant viable myocardium, should myocardial revascularization be offered. However, in generic terms, these patients are less likely to do well after CABG. Cahill and Kharbanda suggest a simple algorithm for viability testing in ischemic cardiomyopathy (Fig. 1).[8]

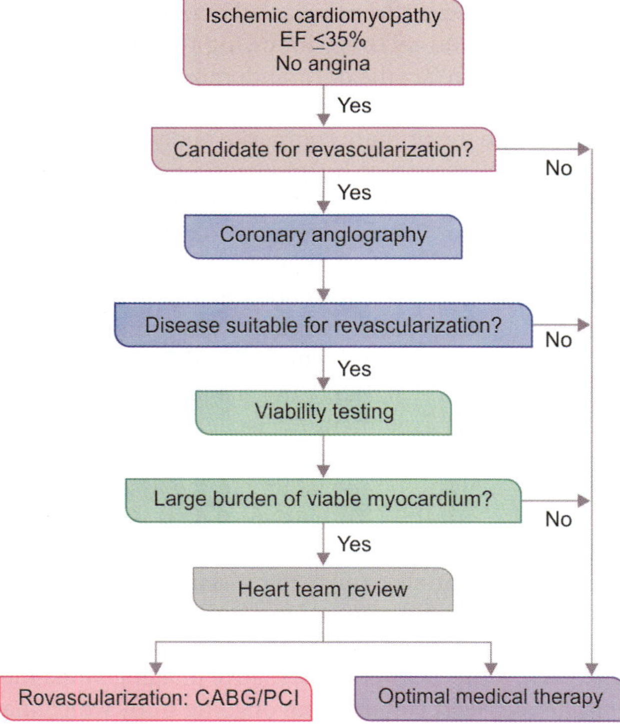

Fig. 1: Decision-making in ischemic cardiomyopathy.[9]
(CABG: coronary artery bypass graft; EF: ejection fraction; PCI: percutaneous coronary intervention)

CORONARY ARTERY BYPASS GRAFT IN LEFT VENTRICULAR DYSFUNCTION

There is a paucity of data of myocardial revascularization in HF with most studies including the MASS II (Medicine, Angioplasty or Surgery Study-II), COURAGE (Clinical Outcomes Utilizing Revascularization and Aggressive Drug Evaluation), ISCHEMIA (International Study of Comparative Health Effectiveness With Medical and Invasive Approaches), SYNTAX (Synergy Between Percutaneous Coronary Intervention With TAXUS and Cardiac Surgery), and FREEDOM (Future Revascularization Evaluation in Patients With Diabetes Mellitus: Optimal Management of Multivessel Disease) Trials, either excluding them or with less than 5% enrollment.

Left ventricular dysfunction in the cohort of patients undergoing CABG is much higher in India than in the Western world. In Cleveland Clinic experience, severe LV dysfunction was present in 8.5%[18] and in New York Heart Registry, it was present in approximately 15% of patients.[19] However, in India, it is present in up to 20% of patients.[18] Moreover, profile of patients too has changed with improved management of MI with thrombolysis and primary percutaneous coronary intervention (PCI). In San Donato experience, patients with classical dyskinetic remodeling of the apex decreased, with a corresponding increase in the patients demonstrating LV chamber distortment and a more global LV dilatation.[20] This has an impact on decision-making, as the former may be helped with surgical ventricular reconstruction (SVR), but not the latter. The goal of CABG in patients of HF is to get symptomatic relief, improve quality of life, prevent hospital readmissions, and most importantly, improve survival. Despite the advances all round, patients with severe LV dysfunction and HF, are a high-risk surgical group. In-hospital mortality ranges from 4.6% to 11%, which is much higher than a routine CABG.[21] However, despite higher morbidity and mortality associated with CABG in LV dysfunction, the mid- and long-term benefits of CABG over medical therapy alone are overwhelming (Fig. 2).[22] Therefore, patients with suitable anatomy, and more so if viability is demonstrated, should not be denied CABG (Fig. 1).[20]

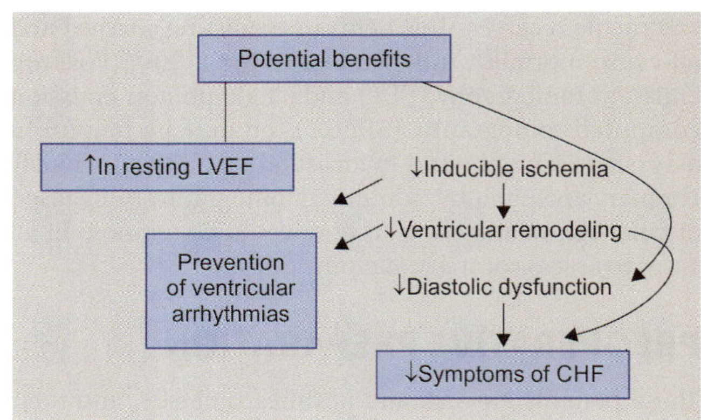

Fig. 2: Benefits of revascularization.[22]
(CHF: chronic heart failure; LVEF: left ventricular ejection fraction)

The STICH trial, the only RCT till date in this field, showed that at 5 years, the primary end point of all-cause mortality was no different (CABG 36% vs. OMT 41%; HR 0.86; p -0.12). Secondary endpoints of repeat revascularization plus mortality (CABG 39% vs. OMT 55%, p <0.001) and cardiovascular hospitalization plus mortality (CABG 58% vs. OMT 68%; p <0.001); however favored CABG (Fig. 3).[23] But, when the study was extended to 10 years, even the mortality benefit was demonstrated in favor of CABG (58.9% vs. 66.1%, HR 0.84; p -0.02) with a number needed to treat (NNT) to prevent 1 death of 14 (Fig. 4).[24] Even in a recent meta-analysis, revascularization was associated with a significant reduction in mortality compared to OMT (p <0.001) and there was a survival benefit (HR 0.82, p <0.001).[25]

Postoperatively antiplatelet drugs should be introduced at the earliest, preferably within the first 6 hours.[8] Beta-blockers and angiotensin converting enzyme (ACE) inhibitors and mineralocorticoid diuretics too have been shown to reduce morbidity and mortality. However, one should be cautious in introducing these in patients with

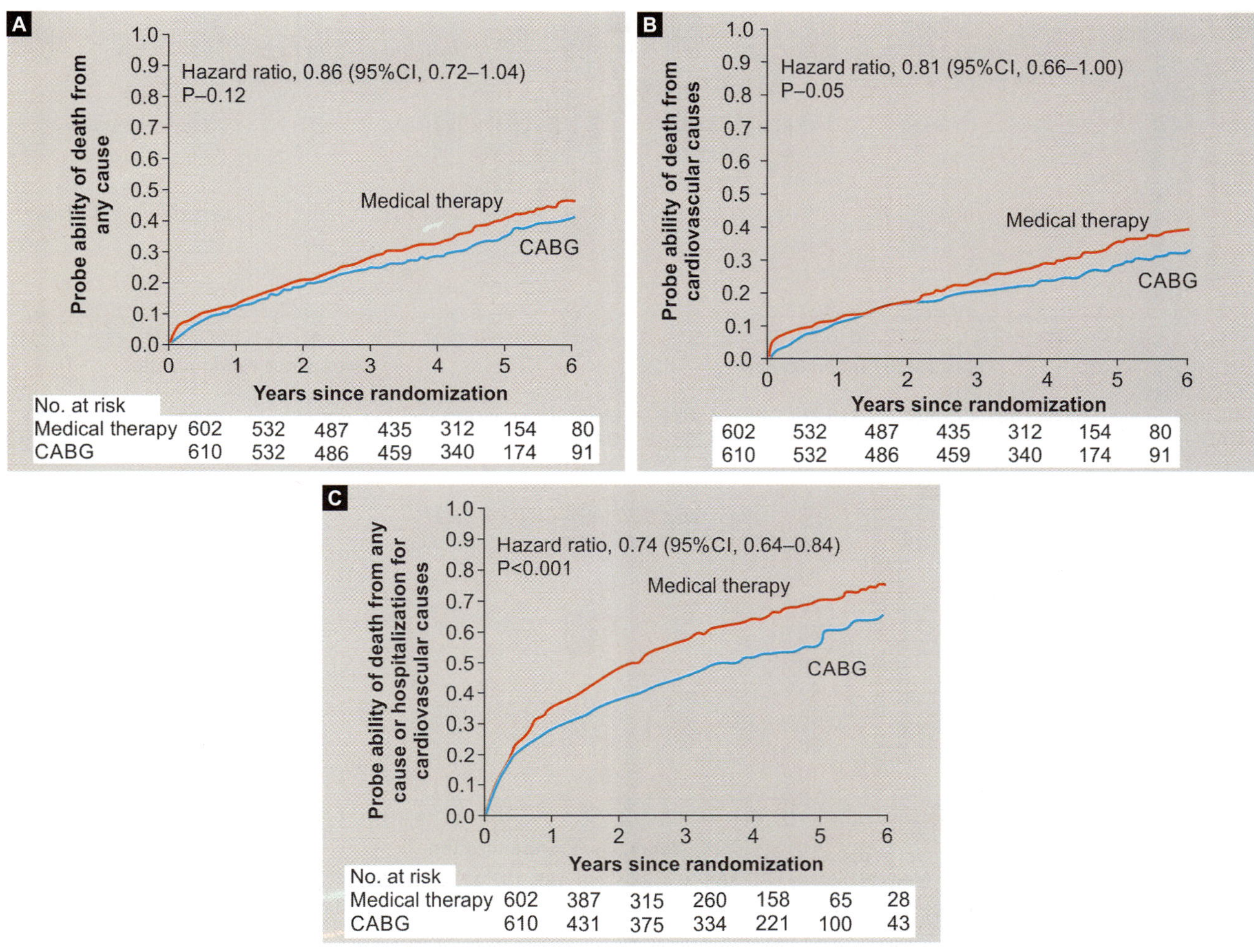

Figs. 3A to C: Intention to treat survival analysis—STICH trial.[23]

borderline hemodynamics and with pulmonary disease. One must also realize, that in STICH trial, the incidence of sudden cardiac death (SCD) at 5 years was 8.5% and it was maximum between 1 month and 3 months with patients with increased left ventricular end-systolic volume index (LVESVI)/raised BNP/atrial fibrillation having higher incidence.[26] Thus, risk stratification for SCD must occur early postoperatively as these patients may need anti-arrhythmic drugs, implantation of automatic internal cardiodefibrillator (AICD) or institution of cardiac resynchronization therapy (CRT).

Acute Cardiogenic Shock

Cardiogenic shock complicates 6–8% of patients with MI with a high mortality of 40–50%.[27] SHOCK (SHould we emergently revascularize Occluded Coronaries in cardiogenic shock) Trial conclusively showed that early revascularization improved long-term survival compared to medical therapy (6 months mortality 50.3% vs. 63.1% respectively, RR 0.80, p -0.03).[28] CABG thus is a class I recommendation for patients with cardiogenic shock not suitable for PCI.[17] The results are improving and mortality rates for CABG in acute cardiogenic shock, which were in the range of 20–50% earlier, have recently dropped to 18.7% in a large national registry.[29] Part of this reduction is because of increased utilization of mechanical circulatory support (MCS) in these patients. The choice of inotropes is contentious. However, a subgroup analysis of the SOAP II (Sepsis Occurrence in Acutely Ill Patients II) Trial suggests an advantage of noradrenaline over dopamine in patients with shock.[30]

Role of Surgical Ventricular Reconstruction

Role of SVR in LV dysfunction remains debatable. The STICH Trial was neutral in its addressing the question of benefits of SVR + CABG, compared with CABG alone.[31]

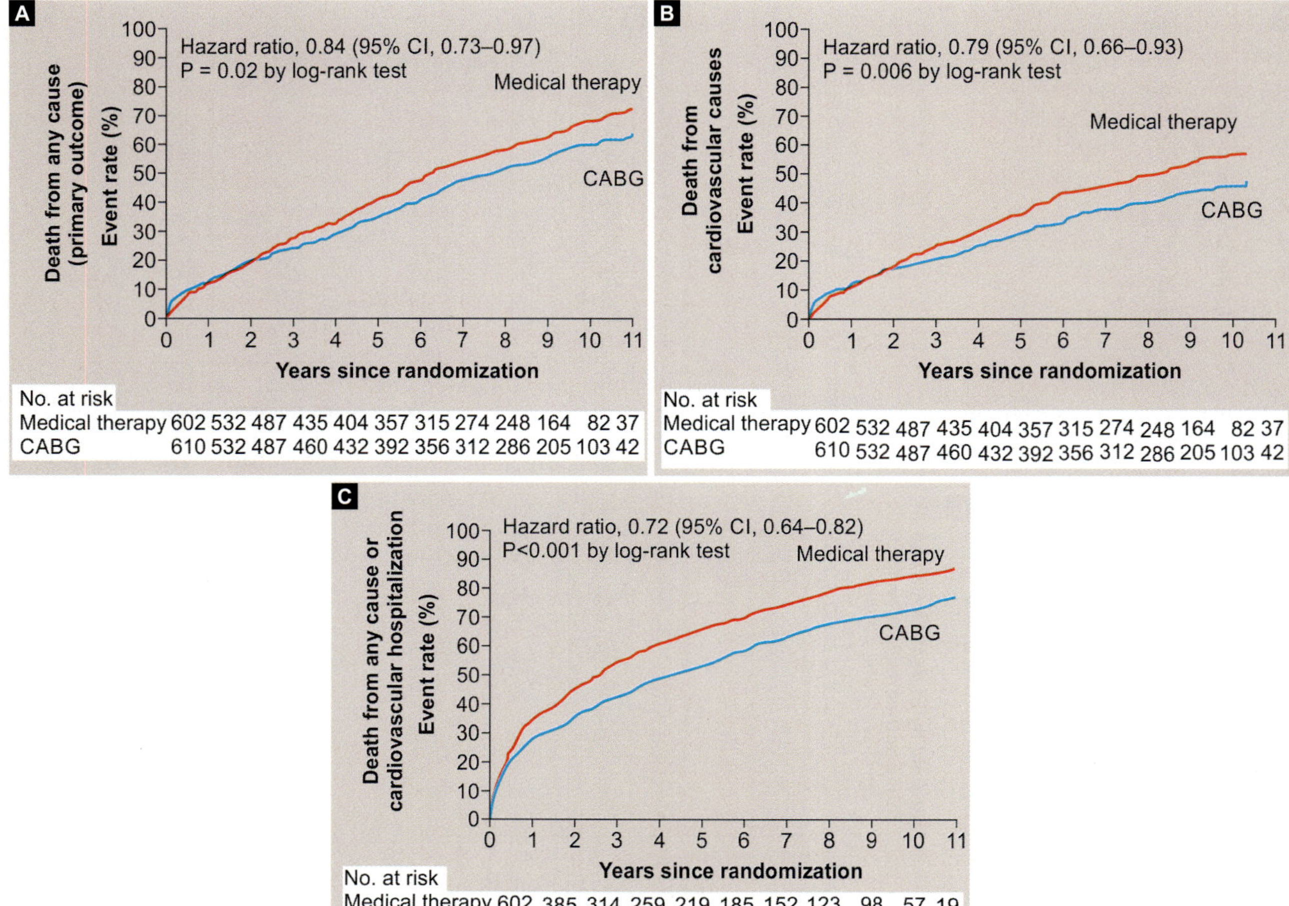

Figs. 4A to C: Kaplan–Meier estimates—STICH trial.[24]

Despite the controversies, SVR is an effective technique in patients with discrete scars and where postoperative LVESVI of <70 mL/m^2, along with maintenance of the elliptical shape of the LV, can be achieved.[20]

Off-pump Coronary Artery Bypass vs On-pump Surgery

Despite the equipoise between the Western and the Eastern World on the use of Off-Pump strategy, latter has been validated for high-risk cases as it reduces the operative mortality.[32,33] Ueki et al., in a propensity score matched analysis of the Japanese National Database, showed that the 30-day mortality was 1.7% with Off-Pump CABG vs. 3.7% with Pump-CABG (p-0.01) in patients with severe LV dysfunction.[34] This was corroborated by Keeling et al. looking at the Society of Thoracic Surgeons (STS) National database.[35] In fact, the reduced motion of the heart, and thus the reduced dp/dt, leads to better stabilization and makes the surgery technically less demanding. However, a meta-analysis comparing Off-Pump vs. Pump CABG found no significant mortality benefit of Off-Pump CABG (in-hospital mortality 4.4% vs. 5.4% respectively).[36] The debate of Off-Pump vs. Pump CABG thus remains unresolved and the surgeon's experience remains a major determining factor.

Use of Arterial Conduits

The use of internal mammary artery (IMA) to left anterior descending (LAD) coronary artery producing survival benefit is a well-established fact. However, evidence base for use of bilateral IMAs is lacking. Even the recent Arterial Revascularization Therapy (ART) trial has failed to demonstrate any benefit of bilateral IMAs, at least in intention to treat analysis.[37] Survival of patients with LV dysfunction is significantly worse than those with preserved LV function, and therefore they may not be surviving long enough to be able to exhibit the benefits of additional arterial grafting. Lytle et al.[38] and Galbut et al.,[39] demonstrated survival advantage for bilateral IMAs over single IMA, albeit only for those with ejection fraction (EF) ≥30%. However, Mohammadi et al.[40] failed to demonstrate any long-term survival advantage of bilateral IMAs. It is, therefore, recommended that an arterial graft to LAD should always be used. Additional arterial grafts should be used only after factoring in issues like age of the patient, presence of comorbidities, - especially DM, amount of myocardium in jeopardy, besides surgeon's comfort and experience with bilateral IMAs.

Elective Intra-aortic Balloon Pump Use

Perioperative use of Intra-aortic Balloon Pump (IABP) is commonplace. However, elective preoperative use in patients with severe LV dysfunction is a highly debatable issue. IABP SHOCK II Trial found no difference in either short-[41] or long-term[42] results with elective preoperative use of IABP in patients with acute coronary syndromes with cardiogenic shock, who were planned for myocardial revascularization. However, Zangrillo et al., in a meta-analysis of eight RCTs, found that elective preoperative IABP use was associated with a statistically significant reduction in perioperative mortality (3.5% vs. 11%).[43] In my personal and institutional ideology, if a patient has preoperative ongoing ischemia, IABP is an effective strategy. However, in a stable patient undergoing CABG, use of IABP is dictated by patient's hemodynamic profile while manipulating the heart during off-pump surgery and for those patients undergoing pump surgery, the call has to be taken at the first attempt to come off cardiopulmonary bypass (CPB). Certainly, if indicated, it should be used earlier than later, and multiple attempts to come off CPB and delaying institution of counterpulsation could actually be harmful.

Percutaneous Coronary Intervention vs. Coronary Artery Bypass Graft

Most studies comparing PCI vs. CABG like the Bypass Angioplasty Revascularization Investigation (BARI), Arterial Revascularization Therapy Study (ARTS), FREEDOM, and SYNTAX have excluded patients with LV dysfunction and HF, and therefore, there is very limited data on the optimum revascularization strategy for these patients. However, based on available data, the recent 2018 ESC/EACTS guidelines give CABG a class I recommendation, but PCI only a class IIa (C) recommendation.[17] The ACC/AHA guidelines, however, give CABG, only a class IIb recommendation and no recommendation at all for PCI,[8] thereby providing no guidance and in fact adding to the confusion. In a recent analysis of New York State Registry, PCI was validated in patients with LVEF ≤35% to be associated with a similar mortality to CABG (p-0.91), a lower risk of stroke, but an increased risk of MI and repeat revascularization.[44] To the contrary, Mamas et al. in an analysis of British Cardiovascular Intervention Society data from 2006 to 2011, showed that LV function was an independent predictor of 30-day mortality after PCI with LVEF <30% having an HR of 7.25 (p <0.0001).[45] Therefore, CABG has been advocated to be a better method of revascularization in these patients than PCI. Kang et al. in a meta-analysis of three real world registries showed that CABG reduced all-cause mortality (HR 0.43); cardiac mortality (HR 0.49), and need for repeat revascularization (HR 0.08; p <0.001), compared to PCI at a mid-term analysis.[46] Same findings were echoed in an independent meta-analysis by Cui et al.[47] Ngu et al. showed that there is greater improvement in ejection fraction with CABG.[48] Nagendran et al., in a propensity matched analysis, showed that these benefits get exaggerated in diabetics, with >60% relative risk reduction and 16% absolute risk reduction in 5-year mortality rate, with CABG as against PCI.[49] This may even have a substantial public health impact. Survival benefit of CABG over PCI was also demonstrated by Wolff et al. in a meta-analysis of 21 studies (HR 0.82; 95% CI 0.75–0.90; p <0.001).[25]

CONCLUSION

Despite paucity of data, CABG can be performed effectively and safely in patients with HF and LV dysfunction. Viability testing helps in prognostication, but must be viewed in light of clinical picture. Use of Off-Pump techniques and arterial conduits, in experienced hands, is not only desirable but beneficial for improved short- and long-term outcomes respectively. CABG trumps PCI because of its survival advantage and less major adverse cardiac and cerebrovascular events (MACCE), essentially driven by less MI and repeat revascularization, but countervailing increased stroke rates. However, more data is needed and RCTs should include patients with LV dysfunction.

REFERENCES

1. Huffman MD, Prabhakaran D. Heart failure: epidemiology and prevention in India. Natl Med J India. 2010;23(5):283-8.
2. Mishra S, Mohan JC, Nair T et al. Management protocols for chronic heart failure in India. Indian Heart J. 2018;70(1):105-27.
3. Velazquez EJ, Bonow RO. Revascularisation in severe left ventricular dysfunction. J Am Coll Cardiol. 2015;65(6):615-24.
4. Cheong BY, Muthupillai R, Wilson JM, et al. Prognostic significance of delayed-enhancement magnetic resonance imaging: survival of 857 patients with and without left ventricular dysfunction. Circulation. 2009;120(21):2069-76.
5. Roes SD, Kelle S, Kaandorp TA, et al. Comparison of myocardial infarct size assessed with contrast-enhanced magnetic resonance imaging and left ventricular function

and volumes to predict mortality in patients with healed myocardial infarction. Am J Cardiol. 2007;100(6):930-6.
6. Kwon DH, Halley CM, Carrigan TP, et al. Extent of left ventricular scar predicts outcomes in ischemic cardiomyopathy patients with significantly reduced systolic function: a delayed hyperenhancement cardiac magnetic resonance study. JACC Cardiovasc Imaging. 2009;2(1):34-44.
7. Aboul-Hassan SS, Stankowski T, Marczak J, et al. The use of preoperative aspirin in cardiac surgery: A systematic review and meta-analysis. J Card Surg. 2017;32(12):758-74.
8. Hillis LD, Smith PK, Anderson JL, et al. 2011 ACCF/AHA Guideline for Coronary Artery Bypass Graft Surgery: a report of the American College of Cardiology Foundation/American Heart Association Task Force on Practice Guidelines. Circulation. 2011;124(23):e652-735.
9. Cahill TJ, Kharbanda RK. Viability testing to guide myocardial revascularisation in patients with Heart Failure. Indian J Thorac Cardiovasc Surg. 2018;34(Suppl 3):S206-12.
10. Allman KC, Shaw LJ, Hachamovitch R, et al. Myocardial viability testing and impact of revascularization on prognosis in patients with coronary artery disease and left ventricular dysfunction: A meta-analysis. J Am Coll Cardiol. 2002;39:1151-8.
11. Ling LF, Marwick TH, Flores DR, et al. Identification of therapeutic benefit from revascularization in patients with left ventricular systolic dysfunction: Inducible ischemia versus hibernating myocardium. Circ Cardiovasc Imaging. 2013;6(3):363-72.
12. Beanlands RS, Nichol G, Huszti E, et al. PARR-2 Investigators. F-18-fluorodeoxyglucose positron emission tomography imaging-assisted management of patients with severe left ventricular dysfunction and suspected coronary disease. A randomized, controlled trial (PARR-2). J Am Coll Cardiol. 2007;50(20):2002-12.
13. Mc Ardle B, Shukla T, Nichol G, et al. PARR-2 Investigators. Long-term follow-up of outcomes with F-18-fluorodeoxyglucose positron emission tomography imaging-assisted management of patients with severe left ventricular dysfunction secondary to coronary disease. Circ Cardiovasc Imaging. 2016;9(9). pii:e004331.
14. Bonow RO, Maurer G, Lee KL, et al. STICH Trial Investigators. Myocardial viability and survival in ischemic left ventricular dysfunction. N Engl J Med. 2011;364(17):1617-25.
15. O'Meara E, Mielniczuk LM, Wells GA, et al. IMAGE HF investigators. Alternative imaging modalities in ischemic heart failure (AIMI-HF) IMAGE HF project I-A: Study protocol for a randomized controlled trial. Trials. 2013;14:218.
16. Yancy CW, Jessup M, Bozkurt B, et al. American College of Cardiology Foundation; American Heart Association Task Force on Practice Guidelines. 2013 ACCF/AHA guideline for the management of heart failure: a report of the American College of Cardiology Foundation/American Heart Association Task Force on practice guidelines. Circulation. 2013;128(16):e240-327.
17. Neumann FJ, Sousa-Uva M, Ahlsson A, et al. ESC Scientific Document Group. 2018 ESC/EACTS Guidelines on myocardial revascularization. Eur Heart J. 2019;40(2):87-165.
18. Kaul U, Bhatia V. Perspective on coronary interventions and cardiac surgeries in India. Ind J Med Res 2010;132:88-93.
19. Topkara VK, Cheema FH, Kesavaramanujam S, et al. Coronary artery bypass grafting in patients with low ejection fraction. Circulation. 2005;112(Suppl 9):I344-50.
20. Garatti A, Castelvecchio S, Canziani A, et al. CABG in patients with left ventricular dysfunction: indications, techniques and outcomes. Indian J Thorac Cardiovasc Surg. 2018;34(Suppl 3):S279-86.
21. Nagendran J, Norris CM, Graham MM, et al. APPROACH Investigators. Coronary revascularization for patients with severe left ventricular dysfunction. Ann Thorac Surg. 2013;96(6):2038-44.
22. Anavekar NS, Chareonthaitawee P, Narula J, et al. Revascularization in patients with severe left ventricular dysfunction: Is the assessment of viability still viable? J Am Coll Cardiol. 2016;67(24):2874-87.
23. Velazquez EJ, Lee KL, Deja MA, et al. STICH Investigators. Coronary-artery bypass surgery in patients with left ventricular dysfunction. N Engl J Med. 2011;364(17):1607-16.
24. Velazquez EJ, Lee KL, Jones RH, et al. STICHES Investigators. Coronary-artery bypass surgery in patients with ischemic cardiomyopathy. N Engl J Med. 2016;374(16):1511-20.
25. Wolff G, Dimitroulis D, Andreotti F, et al. Survival benefits of invasive versus conservative strategies in heart failure in patients with reduced ejection fraction and coronary artery disease: A meta-analysis. Circ Heart Fail. 2017;10(1). pii: e003255.
26. Rao MP, Al-Khatib SM, Pokorney SD, et al. STICH Trial Investigators. Sudden cardiac death in patients with ischaemic heart failure undergoing coronary artery bypass grafting: Results from the STICH randomised clinical trial (Surgical Treatment for Ischemic Heart Failure). Circulation. 2017;135(12):1136-44.
27. Katz JN, Stebbins AL, Alexander JH, et al. TRIUMPH Investigators. Predictors of 30-day mortality in patients with refractory cardiogenic shock following acute myocardial infarction despite a patent infarct artery. Am Heart J. 2009;158(4):680-7.
28. Hochman JS, Sleeper LA, Webb JG, et al. Early revascularization in acute myocardial infarction complicated by cardiogenic shock. SHOCK Investigators. Should we emergently revascularize occluded coronaries for cardiogenic shock. N Engl J Med. 1999;341(9):625-34.
29. Acharya D, Gulack BC, Loyaga-Rendon RY, et al. Clinical characteristics and outcomes of patients with myocardial infarction and cardiogenic shock undergoing coronary artery bypass surgery: Data from the Society of Thoracic Surgeons National Database. Ann Thorac Surg. 2016;101(2): 558-66.
30. De Backer D, Biston P, Devriendt J, et al. SOAP II Investigators. Comparison of Dopamine and norepinephrine in the treatment of shock. N Engl J Med. 2010;362(9):779-89.
31. Jones RH, Velazquez EJ, Michler RE, et al. STICH Hypothesis 2 Investigators. Coronary bypass surgery with or without surgical ventricular reconstruction. N Engl J Med. 2009;360(17):1705-17.

32. Kowalewski M, Pawliszak W, Malvindi PG, et al. Off-pump coronary artery bypass grafting improves short-term outcomes in high-risk patients compared with on-pump coronary artery bypass grafting: Meta-analysis. J Thorac Cardiovasc Surg. 2016;151(1):60-77.e1-58.
33. Lemma MG, Coscioni E, Tritto FP, et al. On-pump versus off-pump coronary artery bypass surgery in high-risk patients: Operative results of a prospective randomized trial (on-off study). J Thorac Cardiovasc Surg. 2012;143(3):625-31.
34. Ueki C, Miyata H, Motomura N, et al. Off-pump versus on-pump coronary artery bypass grafting in patients with left ventricular dysfunction. J Thorac Cardiovasc Surg. 2016;151(4):1092-98.
35. Keeling WB, Williams ML, Slaughter MS, et al. Off-pump and on-pump coronary revascularization in patients with low ejection fraction: A report from the society of thoracic surgeons national database. Ann Thorac Surg. 2013;96(1):83-9.
36. Kunadian V, Zaman A, Qiu W. Revascularization among patients with severe left ventricular dysfunction: a meta-analysis of observational studies. Eur J Heart Fail. 2011;13(7):773-84.
37. Taggart DP, Benedetto U, Gerry S, et al. Arterial Revascularization Trial Investigators. Bilateral versus single internal thoracic-artery grafts at 10 years. N Engl J Med. 2019;380(5):437-46.
38. Lytle BW, Blackstone EH, Sabik JF, et al. The effect of bilateral internal thoracic artery grafting on survival during 20 postoperative years. Ann Thorac Surg. 2004;78(6):2005-14.
39. Galbut DL, Kurlansky PA, Traad EA, et al. Bilateral internal thoracic artery grafting improves long-term survival in patients with reduced ejection fraction: a propensity-matched study with 30-year follow-up. J Thorac Cardiovasc Surg. 2012;143(4):844-53.e4.
40. Mohammadi S, Kalavrouziotis D, Cresce G, et al. Bilateral internal thoracic artery use in patients with low ejection fraction: Is there any additional long-term benefit? Eur J Cardiothorac Surg. 2014;46(3):425-31.
41. Thiele H, Zeymer U, Neumann FJ, et al. Intraaortic Balloon Pump in cardiogenic shock II (IABP-SHOCK II) trial investigators. Intra-aortic balloon counterpulsation in acute myocardial infarction complicated by cardiogenic shock (IABP-SHOCK II): Final 12 month results of a randomised, open-label trial. Lancet. 2013;382(9905):1638-45.
42. Thiele H, Zeymer U, Thelemann N, et al. IABPSHOCK II Trial (Intraaortic Balloon Pump in Cardiogenic Shock II) Investigators. Intraaortic Balloon Pump in cardiogenic shock complicating acute myocardial infarction: Long term 6-year outcome of the randomized IABP-Shock II Trial. Circulation. 2018. doi: 10.1161/CIRCULATIONAHA.118.038201.
43. Zangrillo A, Pappalardo F, Dossi R, et al. Preoperative intra-aortic balloon pump to reduce mortality in coronary artery bypass graft: A meta-analysis of randomized controlled trials. Crit Care. 2015;19:10.
44. Bangalore S, Guo Y, Samadashvili Z, et al. Revascularization in patients with multivessel coronary artery disease and severe left ventricular systolic dysfunction: Everolimus-eluting stents versus coronary artery bypass graft surgery. Circulation. 2016;133(22):2132-40.
45. Mamas MA, Anderson SG, O'Kane PD, et al. British Cardiovascular Intervention Society and the National Institute for Cardiovascular Outcomes Research. Impact of Left ventricular function in relation to procedural outcomes following percutaneous coronary intervention: Insights from the British Cardiovascular Intervention Society. Eur Heart J. 2014;35(43):3004-12a.
46. Kang SH, Lee CW, Baek S, et al. Comparison of outcomes of coronary artery bypass grafting versus drug-eluting stent implantation in patients with severe left ventricular dysfunction. Am J Cardiol. 2017;120(1):69-74.
47. Cui K, Zhang D, Lyu S, et al. Meta-analysis comparing percutaneous coronary revascularization using drug-eluting stent versus coronary artery bypass grafting in patients with left ventricular systolic dysfunction. Am J Cardiol. 2018;122(10):1670-76.
48. Ngu JM, Ruel M, Sun LY. Left ventricular function recovery after revascularization: Comparative effects of percutaneous coronary intervention and coronary artery bypass grafting. Curr Opin Cardiol. 2018;33(6):633-7.
49. Nagendran J, Bozso SJ, Norris CM, et al. Coronary artery bypass surgery improves outcomes in patients with diabetes and left ventricular dysfunction. J Am Coll Cardiol. 2018;71(8):819-27.

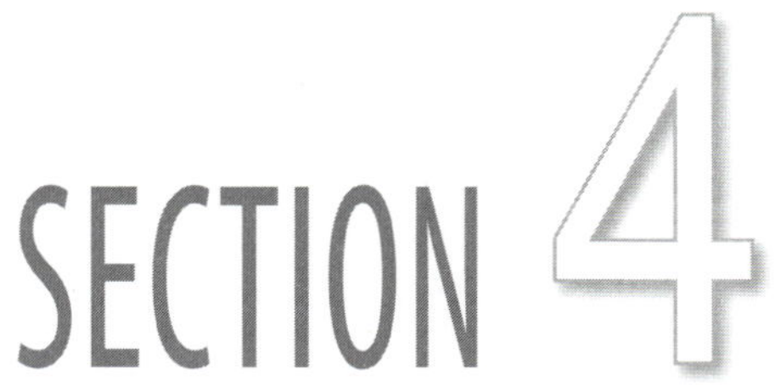

Stroke and Heart Failure

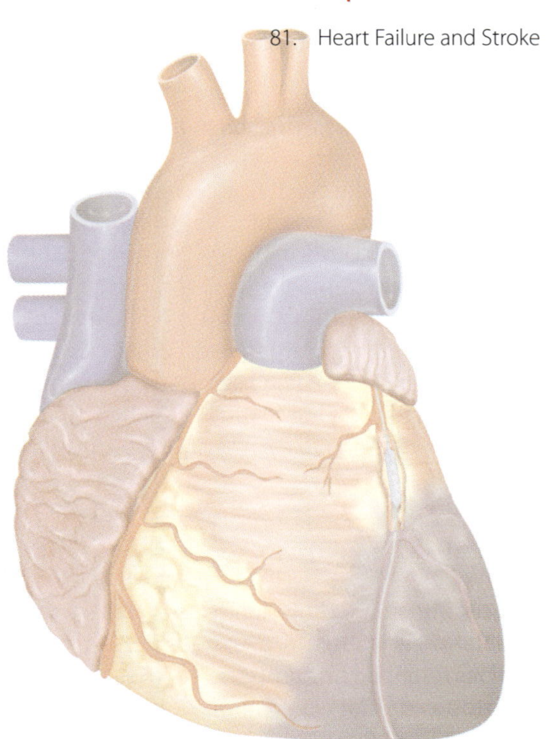

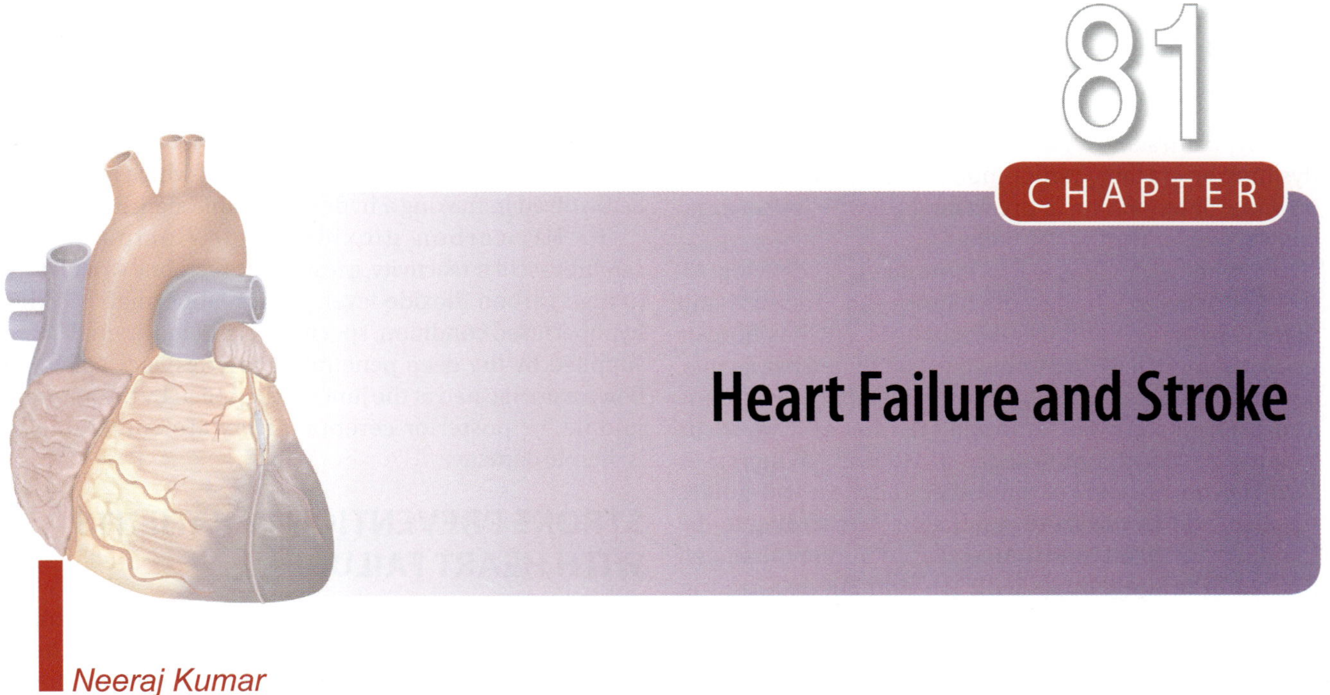

81 CHAPTER

Heart Failure and Stroke

Neeraj Kumar

INTRODUCTION

Heart failure (HF) is a global problem and a major cause of death and is a rapidly growing public health issue affecting approximately 40 million individuals worldwide.[1] HF is a clinical syndrome characterized by typical symptoms (e.g. breathlessness, ankle swelling, and fatigue) that may be accompanied by signs (e.g. elevated jugular venous pressure, pulmonary crackles, and peripheral edema) caused by a structural and/or functional cardiac abnormality, resulting in a reduced cardiac output and/or elevated intracardiac pressures at rest or during stress.[2] According to the guideline, HF with reduced ejection fraction (HFrEF) is defined as an ejection fraction of <40% (previously referred to as "systolic HF"), whereas HF with preserved ejection fraction (HFpEF) is defined as an ejection fraction of ≥50% (previously referred to as "diastolic HF"). Patients with an ejection fraction in the range of 40–49% are considered to have HF with mid-range ejection fraction (HFmrEF). HF typically develops as a result of several health problems related to congenital or acquired conditions and not a single illness. The major risk factors for HF are hypertension, coronary artery disease, valvular heart disease, diabetes, and atrial fibrillation (AF).[3]

Heart failure and stroke commonly coexist and share common risk factors, including AF. Heart failure was associated with a 17.4-fold increased risk for stroke compared with the general population in the first 30 days after HF diagnosis and remained elevated during 5 years of follow-up.[4] There is no doubt that the risk of stroke is increased in patients with HF. However, as HF is often accompanied by traditional risk factors for stroke, such as hypertension, coronary artery disease, (AF), diabetes mellitus, and obesity, it remains controversial that HF itself is an independent stroke risk factor

EPIDEMIOLOGY

It has been reported that 1–2% of the population has HF, and the prevalence increases with age.[5] The prevalence rate is <1% in individuals under 40 years of age, but is >10% in those over 80 years of age, and generally doubles in each decade of life.[6] Previous studies showed that approximately 10–24% of patients with stroke have HF,[7,8] and HF appears to be the cause of stroke in 9% of the patients.[9] According to the Framingham study,[10] the risk of ischemic stroke was two to three times higher in patients with HF than in those without HF, which was also supported by other community-based studies.[4] Recently, a population-based cohort study reported that patients with HF had a higher risk of all subtypes of stroke, as well as ischemic stroke, than the general population, it also demonstrated a significant relationship between HF and short-term and long-term risks of all stroke subtypes even after adjustment for a range of confounders, including AF or atrial flutter.[11]

PATHOPHYSIOLOGY OF STROKE IN CHF

Chronic heart failure (CHF) is a common cause of ischemic stroke, and several pathophysiologic mechanisms have been described. The most frequently recognized reasons for cardioembolic stroke in patients with CHF are thrombus formation due to atrial fibrillation or left ventricular (LV) hypokinesia.[12,13] Untreated AF can cause ventricular dysfunction via tachycardia-induced cardiomyopathy and promote deterioration in preexisting HF with loss of atrial contraction for ventricular filling.[14]

Patients with HF are also more likely to develop AF owing to changes in hemodynamics (i.e. pressure and volume overload) and cellular changes, such as fibrosis and/or automaticity, in association with shared risk factors, such as hypertension, age, diabetes, metabolic syndrome, and arteriosclerosis. Although HF and AF can occur independently, the prevalence of HF and AF increases further in the presence of each other, and these two entities often co-exist in the same population.[15] According to the Framingham Heart Study, AF occurred in more than half (57%) of the individuals with HF, and HF occurred in over one-third (37%) of the individuals with AF.[16] Patients with HF and AF are more prone to develop stroke and had a 5-fold increased risk than the control population.[17] Mogensen et al.[18] reported that the type of AF (paroxysmal, persistent or permanent, or new-onset) may be associated with the stroke risk in patients with HFrEF. In this study, persistent or permanent AF did not increase the stroke risk; however, paroxysmal [hazard ratio (HR), 1.34; 95% confidence interval (CI), 1.02–1.76] and new-onset (HR, 2.20; 95% CI, 1.25–3.88).

AF significantly increased the risk when compared to the absence of AF.

Akinetic ventricular segments and dilated left atrium or ventricle with stasis of the blood flow seen in HF may increase thrombus formation via a mechanism similar to that of AF patients, i.e. blood flow abnormalities.[19] Left ventricular wall motion abnormality (LVWMA) has been suggested as a low or an uncertain risk factor in terms of cerebral embolic risk.[20] LVWMA is associated with regional blood stasis and incomplete ventricular emptying, which may increase thrombogenicity and induce intraventricular thrombus formation.[21]

Heart failure patients are in the prothrombotic state. The prothrombotic state of HF was supported by the observation of platelet hyperactivity, increased thrombin generation, and impaired fibrinolysis.[22,23] This prothrombotic state was further enhanced by the activated sympathetic nervous system and renin-angiotensin-aldosterone system and by systemic inflammation, which are the characteristics of HF.

There are functional and/or structural damages in the blood vessels due to endothelial dysfunction or atherosclerosis in HF (vessel wall abnormalities).[24,25] In a defective endothelium, the release of endothelium-derived nitric oxide in response to stimuli is impaired, which, in turn, may promote monocyte and platelet adhesion to the endothelium, leading to thrombosis and thromboembolism.[26] In addition, the level of von Willebrand factor, a marker that reflects endothelial damage or dysfunction, is abnormally high in HF, which appears to be involved in making a hypercoagulable state in HF.

In HF, carbon dioxide levels fluctuate, and cerebrovascular reactivity, a response of cerebral vasculature to high carbon dioxide levels, is also abnormal.[27] In this hypoperfused condition, specific areas of the brain that are supplied by the deep penetrating arteries, lack collateral flow, or are located at the junction supplied by the anterior, middle, or posterior cerebral artery are vulnerable to ischemic damage.

STROKE PREVENTION IN PATIENTS WITH HEART FAILURE

The use of non-vitamin K antagonist oral anticoagulant (NOAC) as well as warfarin in patients with AF has been extensively studied. The current guidelines recommend assessing stroke risks in patients with AF using the CHA_2DS_2-VASc [congestive heart failure, hypertension, age≥75 years (double score), diabetes, prior stroke or transient ischemic attack (TIA; double score), vascular disease, age 65–74 years, sex class (female)] scoring system.[28,29] In both the American College of Cardiology/American Heart Association and European Society of Cardiology guidelines, oral anticoagulation is strongly recommended for patients with a CHA_2DS_2-VASc score of 2 or more.[28,29] In the case of a CHA_2DS_2-VASc score of 1, the American guideline permits all three options (no antithrombotic treatment, oral anticoagulant, or aspirin).[29] However, the more recently published European guideline recommends the use of oral anticoagulation as Class IIa with level of evidence B, as there is a growing evidence in which oral anticoagulants may be beneficial in men with a CHA_2DS_2-VASc score of 1 and in women with a CHA_2DS_2-VASc score of 2.[28] As the CHA_2DS_2-VASc score is at least 1 in patients with HF, an anticoagulation in those with HF and AF should be considered. In patients with contraindications to anticoagulants, such as high bleeding risks, left atrial appendage occlusion may be considered as Class IIb with level of evidence B.[28]

PREDICTORS OF STROKE IN PATIENTS WITHOUT ATRIAL FIBRILLATION

CHA2DS2-VASc Score

In a Danish cohort study,[30] CHA_2DS_2-VASc score was first used to predict ischemic stroke in patients with incident HF. In particular, the risk of ischemic stroke increased with a clear dose–response relationship as the score increased at high CHA_2DS_2-VASc scores (≥4), regardless of AF. Because of its modest predictive accuracy, the use of CHA_2DS_2-VASc score for stroke risk stratification may be limited in clinical practice. However, it was suggested that CHA_2DS_2-VASc score could be a useful tool for identifying "low-stroke risk" patients because CHA_2DS_2-VASc score yielded a high negative predictive value (92%; 95% CI, 91–93) for ischemic stroke at the 1-year follow-up. Identification of patients at a "truly low" risk would be important especially because they are less likely to benefit from anticoagulation. Due to the lack of a convenient and accurate model to predict stroke and the accompanied increased mortality in HF, Freudenberger et al. proposed a new scoring system for stroke prediction in patients with an ejection fraction of less than 35%, with a full model of their score, including 14 risk factors, and to provide better clinical practicability, a simpler, more practical score of only 8 of these components: age, blood oxygen urea, ejection fraction, hemoglobin, gender, diastolic blood pressure, diabetes mellitus, and prior stroke. In their study population (n = 2305), the new developed score performed modestly but was superior (statistically) to CHA_2DS_2-VASc score in stroke prediction [area under the curve (AUC) 0.660, 95% CI 0.58–0.74 vs. 0.52, 95% CI 0.398–0.63, p = 0.001].[31]

Compared with the data of the general population, data from a recent Danish nationwide registry indicated a 5-fold elevated 30-day ischemic stroke risk after first-time hospitalization for HF.[11]

In another community-based study, HF was associated with a 17-fold increased risk for ischemic stroke compared with that in the general population in the first 30 days after HF diagnosis. Taken together, anticoagulation for stroke prevention might be considered for patients with HF at a high risk based on several variables (e.g. age, diabetes, and prior stroke), especially within the first month after the diagnosis of HF. Further studies are needed to develop a clinical model to predict the stroke risk in patients with HF, including variables, such as time interval following the diagnosis of incident HF.

Stroke Prevention in Heart Failure

There are four randomized clinical trials investigating the effect of warfarin on stroke risk in patients with HF in comparison to aspirin: Warfarin/Aspirin Study in Heart Failure (WASH),[32] Heart Failure Long-Term Antithrombotic Study (HELAS),[33] Warfarin and Antiplatelet Therapy in Chronic Heart Failure (WATCH),[34] and Warfarin versus Aspirin in Reduced Cardiac Ejection Fraction (WARCEF).[35]

The WASH and HELAS trials were small studies, which were underpowered but showed no suggestion for the efficacy of anticoagulant therapy for HF patients in sinus rhythm.

The WATCH and WARCEF trials were larger studies (with WARCEF being a double-blind trial) and showed no significant benefit for the primary outcome that included mortality but a significant risk reduction for stroke (a secondary outcome) in patients treated with warfarin compared to aspirin; however, the positive effect was neutralized by an increased risk of major bleeding.

In WATCH, clopidogrel was superior neither to warfarin nor to aspirin. A meta-analysis of these four trials based on 3,665 patients showed that warfarin reduced the risk of cardiovascular events including stroke by 20% compared to antiplatelet therapy [risk ratio (RR) 0.79, 95% CI 0.63–1.00; I2 = 0%], but the risk of major bleeding was 2-fold higher (RR 2.00, 95% CI 1.44–2.78; I2 = 4%).

Consequently, the stroke risk reduction of warfarin was outweighed by the increased bleeding risk.[36]

NOACs, including dabigatran, rivaroxaban, apixaban, and edoxaban, have been approved by the Food and Drug Administration based on their respective clinical trials.[37-40] Subgroup analyses of these studies showed that NOACs were effective and safe in patients with HF and AF similar to warfarin. In general, compared with warfarin, NOACs have rapid onset and offset of action, yield more predictable anticoagulant responses, and can be administered at fixed doses without routine monitoring, thereby simplifying therapy.[41] In addition, dietary vitamin K intake does not affect NOACs; therefore, dietary restrictions are not required.[41] There are also few clinically important drug-to-drug interactions with NOACs. This profile of NOACs can be an advantage for patients with HF who often take polypharmacy[42] and have a high bleeding risk due to comorbidity.

CONCLUSION

Based on the current evidence, HF should be considered as an independent risk factor for stroke.

The CHA_2DS_2-VASc score might be useful to predict stroke risk in HF patients with or without AF in clinical routine. Thus far, there is only a recommendation for the oral anticoagulation use in patients with concomitant HF and AF, while in patients with HF and no AF, individualized risk stratification is preferred. Based on recent data, NOACs should be preferred over warfarin. Finally, the results of ongoing studies may clarify further aspects of anticoagulation in HF patients without AF.

REFERENCES

1. GBD 2015 Disease and Injury Incidence and Prevalence Collaborators. Global, regional, and national incidence, prevalence, and years lived with disability for 310 diseases and injuries, 1990-2015: A systematic analysis

for the Global Burden of Disease Study 2015. Lancet. 2016;388(10053):1545-602.
2. Dickstein K, Cohen-Solal A, Filippatos G, et al. ESC Committee for Practice Guidelines (CPG). ESC guidelines for the diagnosis and treatment of acute and chronic heart failure 2008: the Task Force for the Diagnosis and Treatment of Acute and Chronic Heart Failure 2008 of the European Society of Cardiology. Developed in collaboration with the Heart Failure Association of the ESC (HFA) and endorsed by the European Society of Intensive Care Medicine (ESICM). Eur Heart J. 2008;29(19):2388-442.
3. Writing Group Members, Lloyd-Jones D, Adams RJ, Brown TM, et al. American Heart Association Statistics Committee and Stroke Statistics Subcommittee. Heart disease and stroke statistics—2010 update. A report from the American Heart Association. Circulation. 2010;121(7):e46-215.
4. Witt BJ, Brown RD Jr, Jacobsen SJ, et al. Ischemic stroke after heart failure: A community-based study. Am Heart J. 2006;152(1):102-9.
5. Ponikowski P, Anker SD, AlHabib KF, et al. Heart failure: Preventing disease and death worldwide. ESC Heart Fail. 2014;1(1):4-25.
6. Writing Group Members, Mozaffarian D, Benjamin EJ, Go AS, et al. American Heart Association Statistics Committee; Stroke Statistics Subcommittee. Heart disease and stroke statistics--2016 update. A report from the American Heart Association. Circulation 2016;133(4):e38-360.
7. Divani AA, Vazquez G, Asadollahi M, et al. Nationwide frequency and association of heart failure on stroke outcomes in the United States. J Card Fail. 2009;15(1):11-6.
8. Ois A, Gomis M, Cuadrado-Godia E, et al. Heart failure in acute ischemic stroke. J Neurol. 2008;255(3):385-9.
9. Pullicino P, Homma S. Stroke in heart failure: Atrial fibrillation revisited? J Stroke Cerebrovasc Dis. 2010;19(1):1-2.
10. Kannel WB, Wolf PA, Verter J. Manifestations of coronary disease predisposing to stroke. The Framingham study. JAMA. 1983;250(21):2942-6.
11. Adelborg K, Szépligeti S, Sundbøll J, et al. Risk of stroke in patients with heart failure: A population-based 30-year cohort study. Stroke. 2017;48(5):1161-8.
12. Pullicino PM, Halperin JL, Thompson JL. Stroke in patients with heart failure and reduced left ventricular ejection fraction. Neurology. 2000;54(2):288-94.
13. Wolf PA, Abbott RD, Kannel WB. Atrial fibrillation is an independent risk factor for stroke: the Framingham Study. Stroke. 1991;22(8):983-8.
14. Anter E, Jessup M, Callans DJ. Atrial fibrillation and heart failure: treatment considerations for a dual epidemic. Circulation. 2009;119(18):2516-25.
15. Hohendanner F, Heinzel FR, Blaschke F, et al. Pathophysiological and therapeutic implications in patients with atrial fibrillation and heart failure. Heart Fail Rev. 2018;23(1):27-36.
16. Santhanakrishnan R, Wang N, Larson MG, et al. Atrial fibrillation begets heart failure and vice versa: temporal associations and differences in preserved versus reduced ejection fraction. Circulation. 2016;133(5):484-92.
17. Kang SH, Kim J, Park JJ, et al. Risk of stroke in congestive heart failure with and without atrial fibrillation. Int J Cardiol. 2017;248:182-7.
18. Mogensen UM, Jhund PS, Abraham WT, et al. PARADIGM-HF and ATMOSPHERE Investigators and Committees. Type of atrial fibrillation and outcomes in patients with heart failure and reduced ejection fraction. J Am Coll Cardiol. 2017;70(20):2490-500.
19. Falk RH, Foster E, Coats MH. Ventricular thrombi and thromboembolism in dilated cardiomyopathy: a prospective follow-up study. Am Heart J. 1992;123(1):136-42.
20. Ferro JM. Cardioembolic stroke: An update. Lancet Neurol. 2003;2(3):177-88.
21. Cusick DA, Bonow RO, Chaudhry FA. Left ventricular apical thrombus and myocardial viability: A dobutamine stress echocardiographic study. Echocardiography. 2000;17(6 Pt 1):547-54.
22. de Peuter OR, Kok WE, Torp-Pedersen C, et al. Systolic heart failure: A prothrombotic state. Semin Thromb Hemost. 2009;35(5):497-504.
23. Gibbs CR, Blann AD, Watson RD, et al. Abnormalities of hemorheological, endothelial, and platelet function in patients with chronic heart failure in sinus rhythm: Effects of angiotensin-converting enzyme inhibitor and beta-blocker therapy. Circulation. 2001;103(13):1746-51.
24. Sbarouni E, Bradshaw A, Andreotti F, et al. Relationship between hemostatic abnormalities and neuroendocrine activity in heart failure. Am Heart J. 1994;127(3):607-12.
25. Kubo SH, Rector TS, Bank AJ, et al. Endothelium-dependent vasodilation is attenuated in patients with heart failure. Circulation. 1991;84(4):1589-96.
26. Lip GY, Gibbs CR. Does heart failure confer a hypercoagulable state? Virchow's triad revisited. J Am Coll Cardiol. 1999;33(5):1424-6.
27. Georgiadis D, Sievert M, Cencetti S, et al. Cerebrovascular reactivity is impaired in patients with cardiac failure. Eur Heart J. 2000;21(5):407-13.
28. Kirchhof P, Benussi S, Kotecha D, et al. ESC Scientific Document Group. 2016 ESC guidelines for the management of atrial fibrillation developed in collaboration with EACTS. Eur Heart J. 2016;37(38):2893-962.
29. January CT, Wann LS, Alpert JS, et al. American College of Cardiology/American Heart Association Task Force on Practice Guidelines. 2014 AHA/ACC/HRS guideline for the management of patients with atrial fibrillation: A report of the American College of Cardiology/American Heart Association Task Force on Practice Guidelines and the Heart Rhythm Society. J Am Coll Cardiol. 2014;64(21):e1-76.
30. Melgaard L, Gorst-Rasmussen A, Lane DA, et al. Assessment of the CHA2DS2-VASc score in predicting ischemic stroke, thromboembolism, and death in patients with heart failure with and without atrial fibrillation. JAMA. 2015;314(10):1030-8.
31. Freudenberger RS, Cheng B, Mann DL, et al. WARCEF Investigators. The first prognostic model for stroke and death in patients with systolic heart failure. J Cardiol. 2016;68(2):100-3.

32. Cleland JG, Findlay I, Jafri S, et al. The Warfarin/Aspirin Study in Heart failure (WASH): A randomized trial comparing antithrombotic strategies for patients with heart failure. Am Heart J. 2004;148(1):157-64.
33. Cokkinos DV, Haralabopoulos GC, Kostis JB, et al. Efficacy of antithrombotic therapy in chronic heart failure: The HELAS study. Eur J Heart Fail. 2006;8(4):428-32.
34. Massie BM, Collins JF, Ammon SE, et al. WATCH Trial Investigators. Randomized trial of warfarin, aspirin, and clopidogrel in patients with chronic heart failure: The Warfarin and Antiplatelet Therapy in Chronic Heart Failure (WATCH) trial. Circulation. 2009;119(12):1616-24.
35. Homma S, Thompson JL, Pullicino PM, et al. WARCEF Investigators. Warfarin and aspirin in patients with heart failure and sinus rhythm. N Engl J Med. 2012;366(20):1859-69.
36. Shantsila E, Lip GY. Antiplatelet versus anticoagulation treatment for patients with heart failure in sinus rhythm. Cochrane Database Syst Rev. 2016;9:CD003333.
37. Giugliano RP, Ruff CT, Braunwald E, et al. ENGAGE AF-TIMI 48 Investigators. Edoxaban versus warfarin in patients with atrial fibrillation. N Engl J Med. 2013;369(22):2093-104.
38. Patel MR, Mahaffey KW, Garg J, et al. ROCKET AF Investigators. Rivaroxaban versus warfarin in nonvalvular atrial fibrillation. N Engl J Med. 2011;365(10):883-91.
39. Granger CB, Alexander JH, McMurray JJ, et al. ARISTOTLE Committees and Investigators. Apixaban versus warfarin in patients with atrial fibrillation. N Engl J Med. 2011;365(11):981-92.
40. Connolly SJ, Ezekowitz MD, Yusuf S, et al. RE-LY Steering Committee and Investigators. Dabigatran versus warfarin in patients with atrial fibrillation. N Engl J Med. 2009;361(12):1139-51.
41. Yeh CH, Hogg K, Weitz JI. Overview of the new oral anticoagulants: Opportunities and challenges. Arterioscler Thromb Vasc Biol. 2015;35(5):1056-65.
42. Lee SE, Cho HJ, Lee HY, et al. A multicenter cohort study of acute heart failure syndromes in Korea: Rationale, design, and interim observations of the Korean Acute Heart Failure (KorAHF) registry. Eur J Heart Fail. 2014;16(6):700-8.

SECTION 5

Arrhythmia and Heart Failure

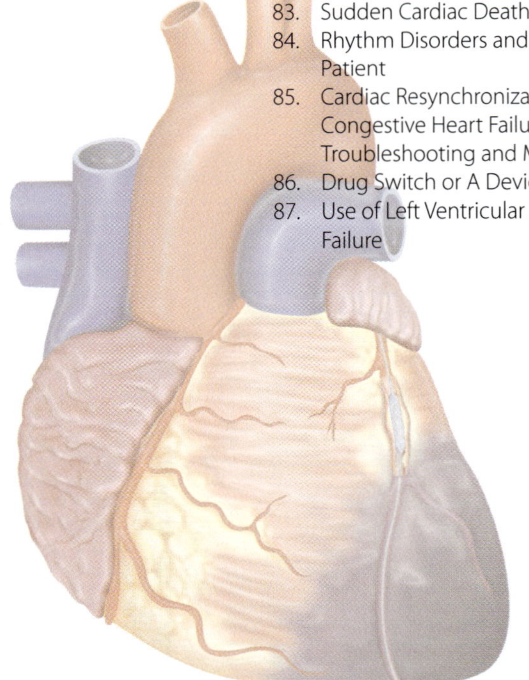

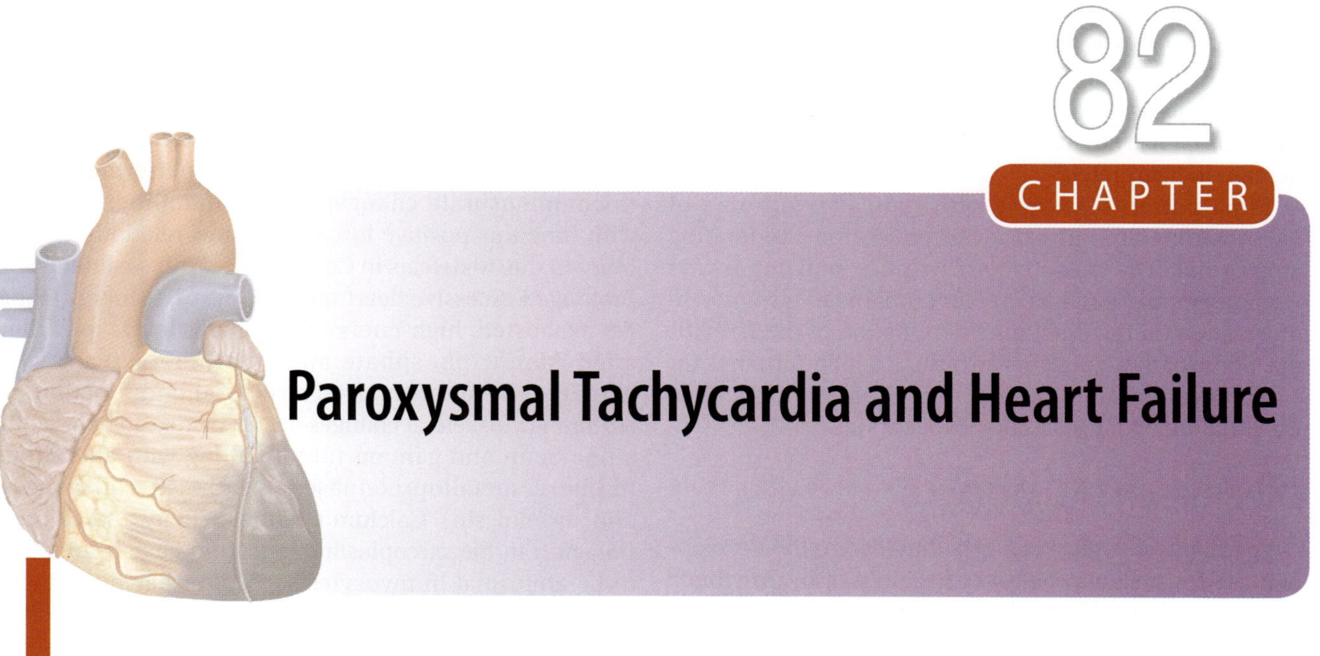

82

CHAPTER

Paroxysmal Tachycardia and Heart Failure

Danish H Kazmi, Aditya Kapoor

INTRODUCTION

Long-standing tachycardia is a well-recognized cause of heart failure (HF) and left ventricular (LV) dysfunction, and has led to the nomenclature, *tachycardia-induced cardiomyopathy (TIC) or tachycardiomyopathy (TCMP)*.[1,2] Unlike for most cardiomyopathies where precious little can be done to reverse the progression of the underlying disease, the often debilitating symptoms of patients with TCMP can be ameliorated if suspected and treated in time. Reversibility of ventricular function is common if the tachycardia can be treated effectively, either with drugs, catheter ablation or cardioversion. While the classic definition proposed by Gallagher refers to impairment of LV function secondary to chronic uncontrolled, sustained or incessant tachycardia, recurrent atrial and ventricular ectopy can also promote dyssynchrony. More contemporary definitions highlight the underlying etiology by specifying "atrial and/or ventricular dysfunction secondary to rapid and/or asynchronous/irregular myocardial contraction which is partially or completely reversed after treatment of the causative arrhythmia".[3,4] Therefore, the term "arrhythmia-induced cardiomyopathy" (AIC) is now emerging as an alternative to TIC/TCMP to describe the phenomenon of tachycardias/ectopic rhythms causing ventricular dysfunction and clinical HF. Although many patients with TIC have no previous structural heart disease, it can also manifest in patients with baseline left ventricular dysfunction from underlying structural heart disease that gets aggravated in the setting of prolonged tachycardia. The diagnosis is made after demonstrating recovery of left ventricular function with normalization of heart rate (by appropriate therapeutic measures) in the absence of other identifiable etiologies.

FACTORS GOVERNING DEVELOPMENT OF AIC

Sole existence of an arrhythmia does not mandate development of ventricular dysfunction in all patients. Predisposing factors include the heart rate, type and duration of tachycardia, existing heart disease, age, and other co-morbidities. An arrhythmia that is chronic, insidious, persistent, and well tolerated is more likely to result in AIC. Even though a heart rate limit above which TIC will appear is not well established, prolonged heart rate persistently >100 beats per minute deserves attention. The usual duration of onset of ventricular dysfunction after an underlying tachycardia is also difficult to ascertain but being a rate-dependent phenomenon, patients with higher tachycardia rates tend to develop AIC earlier. It is suggested that chronic tachycardia that occurs >10–15% of the day may result in AIC.[5] The presence of absence of underlying structural heart disease also dictates the time to onset, with deterioration of ventricular function developing earlier in those with baseline ventricular dysfunction. It has been described in patients of all ages including infants and children, in heart transplant patients, and even in utero.[6-8] A possible role of genetic influences has also been postulated with patients having homozygous deletion polymorphism in the angiotensin converting enzyme (DD) gene having a higher propensity to develop AIC, in the setting of chronic increase in heart rates.[9]

Most patients present with typical symptoms of HF, sometimes months or even years after the inciting tachycardia. The causative arrhythmia may not always be apparent and patients are often unable to give precise information on the exact time of initiation of the arrhythmia. Some of these patients are also at a long-term risk for sudden death, due to persistent and hitherto unknown ultrastructural changes in the myocardium.

EXPERIMENTAL MODELS

The pathophysiological changes that lead to the development of HF in patients who have a sustained tachyarrhythmia are not clearly understood. Experimental animal models initially pioneered by Whipple et al. have consistently shown that rapid atrial/ventricular pacing can lead to severe biventricular systolic dysfunction.[10] Hemodynamic abnormalities manifest as early as 24–48 hours with rise in filling pressures, increase in pulmonary artery pressures, and fall in systemic arterial pressures at 1 week. In the early remodeling phase, there may be no compromise in cardiac output or systemic perfusion pressures, but by second week, there is LV dilation and fall in LV ejection fraction (EF), and a sustained fall in cardiac output, EF, and clinical HF by approximately 3–5 weeks.[11-14] Cessation of pacing is known to cause improvement of left ventricular function within 24 hours and a return to normal within few weeks. The end-systolic and end-diastolic volumes may, however, continue to remain elevated 8–12 weeks after cessation of pacing and occasionally, EF may not normalize and some abnormalities in contractile function may persist.

PATHOPHYSIOLOGY AND STRUCTURAL CHANGES

Structural cardiac changes observed in TCMP may be primarily due to the tachyarrhythmia itself or the tachycardia may be secondary to the changes seen in cardiomyopathy. Various mechanisms have been proposed to explain the pathogenesis of ventricular dysfunction including myocardial energy depletion, reduced cellular energy stores, abnormal calcium handling, myocardial ischemia, altered subendocardial and subepicardial blood flow ratios and extracellular matrix remodeling.[5,15] Cellular changes also occur, e.g. loss of myocytes, myocellular elongation without an absolute increase in myocyte cross-sectional area, myofibril misalignment, disruption of basement membrane/sarcolemmal interfaces, loss of sarcomere register, changes in myocyte attachment to laminin, fibronectin, and the extracellular collagen matrix. Initially, increased contraction frequency causes an increase in myocardial contractile performance due to commensurate changes in Ca^{+2} handling; however, with time this positive force–frequency relationship gets blunted due to defects in Ca^{+2} cycling. With sustained and prolonged excessive heart rates, myocardial energy stores get exhausted, high-energy phosphates levels including adenosine triphosphate and creatine decrease with alteration in mitochondrial structural and function. In addition cytoskeletal changes occur: increased beta-actin, alpha-actin and gamma-tubulin along with alterations in matrix metalloproteinases (gelatinase, collagenase, and stromolysin). Calcium channel activity and calcium transport in the sarcoplasmic reticulum have been found to be abnormal in myocytes soon after pacing induced tachycardia, remaining upto 4–6 weeks after cessation of pacing. Models determining whether there is predisposition to sudden cardiac death have revealed increased dispersion in monophasic action potential duration, increased cesium chloride sensitivity in myocytes, and impaired potassium channel functioning, perhaps as a precursor to QT prolongation and malignant arrhythmias.[16] All these structural and cellular changes lead to chamber dilatation (usually without hypertrophy), mitral regurgitation, elevated ventricular filling pressures leading eventually to decreased contractility, reduction of cardiac output and HF. As part of the remodeling process, neurohormonal changes occur like rise in natriuretic peptide levels, activation of renin-angiotensin and endothelin pathways, impaired response to nitric oxide, and rise in norepinephrine levels, probably coupled to decreased sympathetic responsiveness and beta-1 receptor density.

UNDERLYING TACHYCARDIAS

Two categories of AIC can occur—either the arrhythmia may be the only reason for ventricular dysfunction (*arrhythmia-induced*), or the arrhythmia exacerbates preexisting ventricular dysfunction and/or worsens HF in a patient with concomitant structural heart disease (*arrhythmia-mediated*).[5,17] While both supraventricular (SVT) and ventricular arrhythmias can lead to AIC, the most common causes are long-standing atrial fibrillation (AF)/atrial flutter, incessant atrial tachycardia, and permanent junctional reciprocating tachycardia (PJRT) (Figs. 1 to 4).[18-23] In patients with AF, deterioration of myocardial function occurs not only due to the rapid ventricular rate but also because of the irregularity of ventricular response. Atrioventricular nodal reentry tachycardia (AVNRT) and atrioventricular tachycardia are relatively less frequently associated with AIC as these types of tachycardia are generally not incessant,

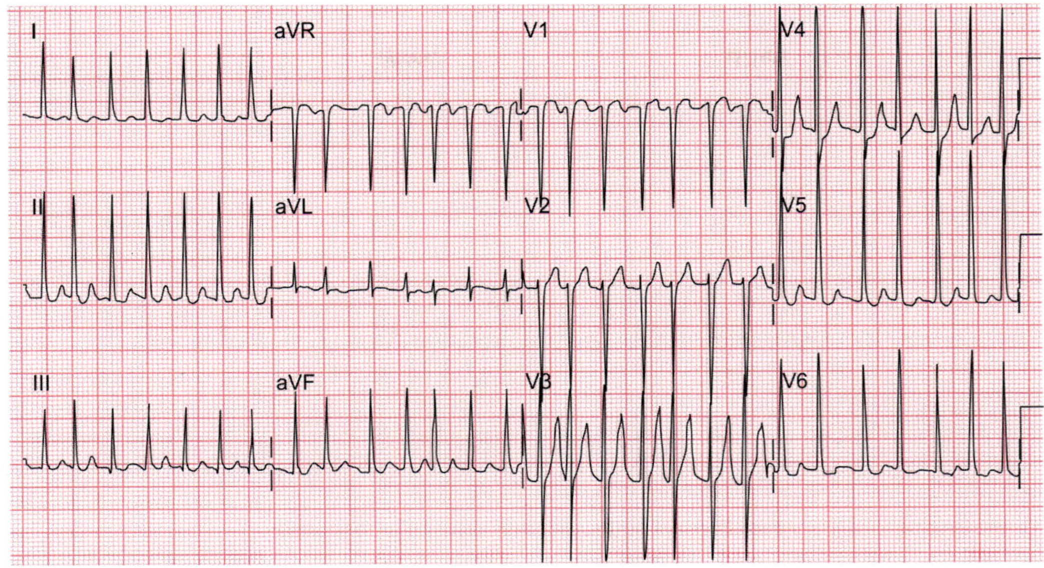

Fig. 1: Atrial fibrillation with fast ventricular response as a cause of tachycardiomyopathy.

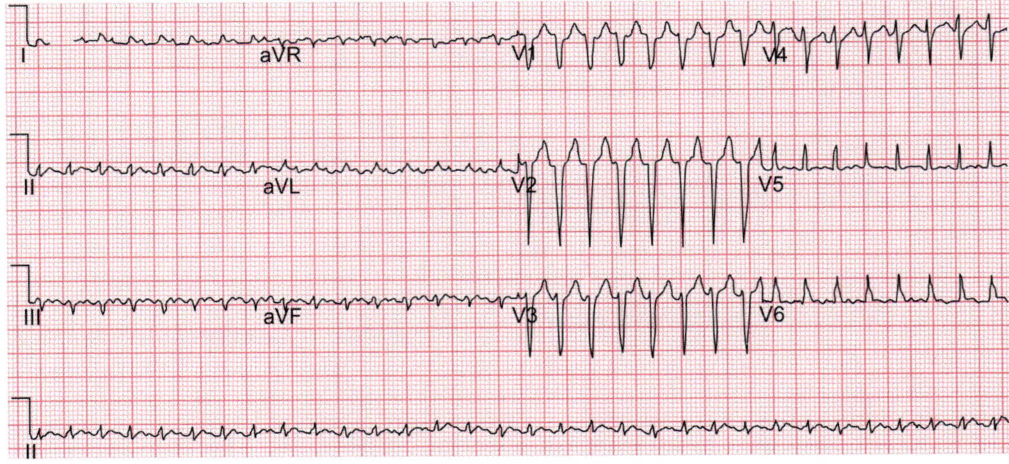

Fig. 2: Incessant atrial tachycardia in a 25-year-old male as a cause of heart failure.

except for PJRT which generally involves a slowly conducting posteroseptal accessory pathway.

Ventricular arrhythmias causing ventricular dysfunction are generally idiopathic in nature and sustained monomorphic VT is rarely a cause, being more often associated with preexisting structural heart disease. Idiopathic VT, if persistent, may result in reversible LV dysfunction, often arising from right ventricular outflow tachycardia (RVOT-VT) or the idiopathic left ventricular tachycardia (ILVT) type arising from the fascicles; rarely bundle-branch reentry VT (BBRT) can be the underlying mechanism.[24,25] Frequent premature ventricular contractions (PVCs) can cause asynergic and inefficient ventricular contraction resulting in abnormal left ventricular mechanics and torsional forces leading to development of regional ventricular wall motion abnormities and ventricular dysfunction. Different criteria for cutoffs for high ventricular premature complexes (VPC) burden have been reported with a high burden being variably defined as ranging from >10,000–25,000 PVCs/day and as >10–24% of total heartbeats/day.[26-28] PVCs of right ventricular (RV) origin (burden ≥10%), interpolated PVCs, asymptomatic PVCs, presence of retrograde P waves, and multiform VPC have a lower threshold of leading to AIC. A PVC QRS width >150 ms or epicardial origin is also a significant predictor probably because of the greater degree of dyssynchrony it promotes. An abnormal EF that improves by ≥15% or is normalized (becomes ≥50%) after an effective ablation procedure, is also considered as a criterion for PVC-induced cardiomyopathy.

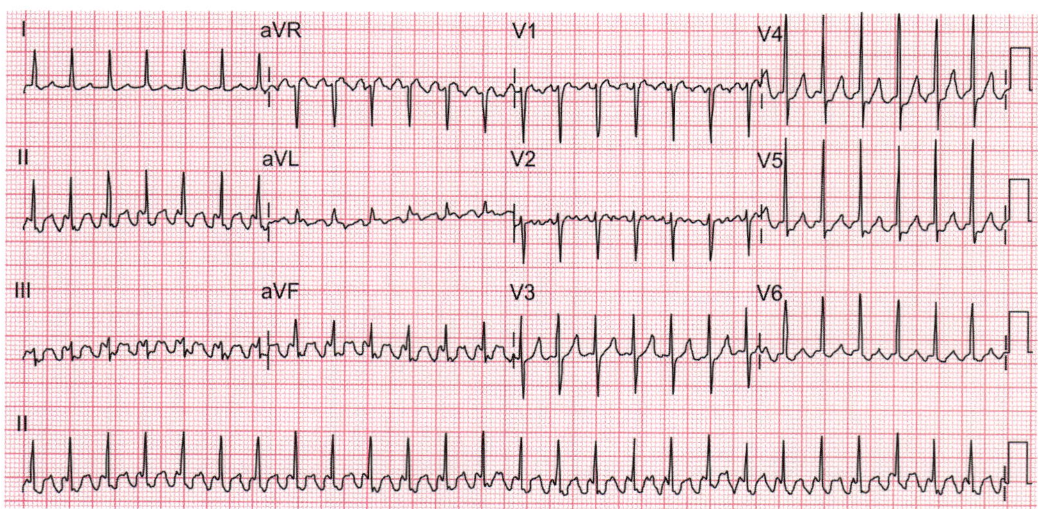

Fig. 3: Atrial flutter with fast ventricular response.

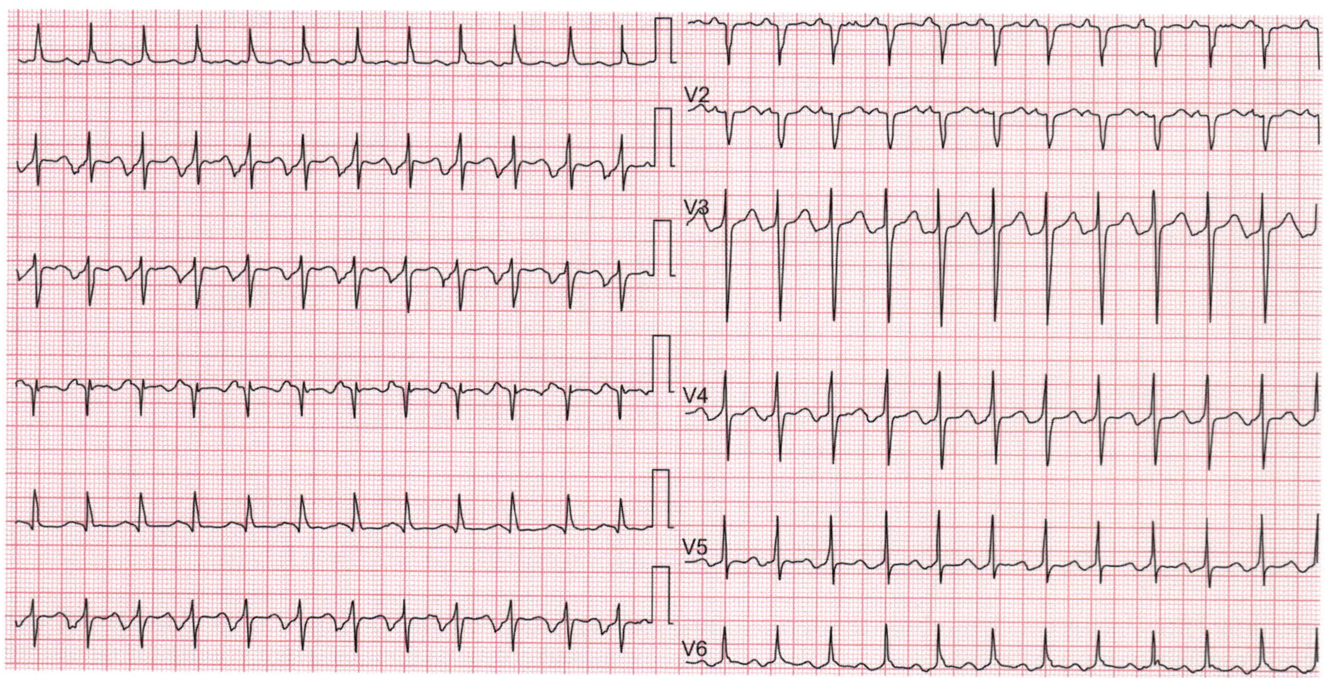

Fig. 4: Incessant permanent junctional reciprocating tachycardia is a relatively common cause of tachycardiomyopathy.

INCIDENCE

The incidence of AIC is difficult to ascertain, since the diagnosis is often of exclusion and is therefore likely to be under-recognized in clinical practice. Amongst patients with AF, up to 40–50% are prone to develop some degree of left ventricular dysfunction and TCMP while the reported incidence of patients with incessant or frequent paroxysmal atrial tachycardia (AT) developing cardiomyopathy is 5–10%, other series describe prevalence of 8–28% in focal/ectopic atrial tachycardias and 9–34% for ventricular ectopy and non-sustained VT.[18,29-32]

DIAGNOSIS

A diagnosis of TIC requires high index of suspicion since the underlying arrhythmia may not always be apparent and patients may not always present with symptoms of the arrhythmia and palpitations. Hence it should be suspected in all patients with unexplained or new onset ventricular dysfunction/HF especially in the setting of paroxysmal or incessant tachycardia. Even if an arrhythmia is identified at the time of ventricular dysfunction, the establishment of a cause–effect relationship is not always feasible and the diagnosis is generally established after restoration of cardiac function following heart rate control.

The exclusion of underlying structural heart disease is always a challenge as current imaging techniques including echocardiography and even MRI may not be easily able to differentiate focal/diffuse fibrosis which is either primary or secondary to the arrhythmia causing regional ventricular wall dysfunction or dyskinesis. In most cases, echocardiography reveals relatively normal LV dimensions (typically LV end-diastolic dimension below 5.5 cm) despite LV dysfunction and absence of significant LV hypertrophy. Patients generally have smaller LV dimensions and volumes adjusted for body surface area and LV mass compared with patients with idiopathic dilated cardiomyopathy. The lesser degree of LV enlargement is thought to be due to a relatively more rapid process in these patients as opposed to the chronic degenerative process seen in idiopathic dilated cardiomyopathies. Gadolinium late enhancement on MRI is an indicator of structural pathology indicating a scar and lesser likelihood of ventricular function response in the context of arrhythmia ablation. Studies have demonstrated that presence of wider and diffuse areas of low amplitude signals and reduced unipolar voltage area ≥one-third of LV endocardium indicate irreversible cardiomyopathy.[33] The resting HR may not give an indication of the mean HR (especially in case of underlying AF/VPCs). Hence ambulatory ECG monitoring is also important for diagnosis as well as identifying subclinical arrhythmias. Serial assessment of cardiac natriuretic peptides has also been reported to help differentiate AIC from irreversible dilated cardiomyopathy (rapid decline in levels following institution of rate control favoring the possibility of reversible cardiomyopathy).

TREATMENT

A timely diagnosis is important since reversal of ventricular function correlates with early institution of appropriate treatment, with the primary goals being:

- Improving symptoms
- Reversing LV dysfunction with appropriate heart rate control
- Preventing arrhythmia recurrence.

Case management differs according to the underlying tachyarrhythmia.

- In most patients with AF, both rate or rhythm control is comparable as far as long-term outcomes are concerned, and for those in permanent AF, lenient rate control (resting heart rate <110 beats/min) is sufficient and a strategy of more strict rate control (resting heart rate <80 beats/min and heart rate with moderate exercise <110 beats/min) is not superior.[34,35] However in many of these initial studies, AF and development of AIC was not specifically considered. Although the Atrial Fibrillation and Congestive Heart Failure (AF-CHF) trial which studied patients of AF with HF, reported that a rhythm control strategy did not improve all-cause mortality or worsening HF, nearly 40% of patients in the rate control arm were actually in sinus rhythm during follow-up.[36] In contrast, the CAFÉ-II (Controlled Study of Rate Versus Rhythm Control in Patients with Chronic AF and HF) study, a rhythm control strategy (amiodarone with cardioversion), was found to be superior to rate control in improving LV function, pro-BNP levels, and quality of life.[37]
  In patients of AF with HF, restoration and maintenance of sinus rhythm is known to be associated with more favorable results.[38,39]
  - If long-term adequate ventricular rate control cannot be achieved in patients with AF and AIC, rhythm control should be attempted using DC cardioversion, class Ic and III anti-arrhythmic drugs or catheter-based therapies. Catheter ablation offers an effective rhythm control strategy and avoids potentially toxic long-term anti-arrhythmic therapy. Patients most likely to do better with rhythm control approach are those with recent AF, no evidence of gross myocardial abnormalities on advanced imaging like MRI (absence of significant scar) and an otherwise normal ECG without significant conduction/repolarization abnormalities.
  - Atrioventricular junction ablation followed by pacemaker implantation is also an option for those patients in whom a definitive cure cannot be obtained by other means. However, this approach results in LV dysynchrony and is usually reserved as a last resort for elderly patients intolerant of rate/rhythm control medications.
- In patients with atrial flutter, good rate control is often difficult to achieve and given the high success rate and low risk of complications with catheter ablation, the latter is recommended when AIC secondary to persistent atrial flutter is suspected. For those in whom catheter ablation is not feasible, attempts at cardioversion with antiarrhythmic therapy or aggressive rate control should be used.

In other clinical situations, treatment should be directed toward termination of the responsible arrhythmia and to treating HF. This approach may include antiarrhythmic drug therapy, DC cardioversion, and catheter ablation whenever possible, and the position of ablation in the treatment algorithm differs according to the specific type of arrhythmia, degree of myocardial dysfunction, and symptom severity.

- In all cases of SVT-mediated cardiomyopathy, catheter ablation takes precedence over all strategies in most cases.[30,31,40,41] In cases of SVT, abolition of the culprit arrhythmia is achieved with RFA to a significantly higher extent than any other strategy and avoids the use of excessive anti-arrhythmic drugs which pose the risk of proarrhythmic effects.
- Therapy for PVC-mediated AIC also involves the use of either antiarrhythmic therapy or catheter ablation. Beta-blockers and nondihydropyridine calcium channel blockers may be used as the drugs of first choice and although without significant side effects, they have limited effectiveness. Other drugs like dofetilide, mexiletine, sotalol, or amiodarone may be more effective but have a more adverse side effect profile and are frequently reserved for patients who fail or are reluctant to undergo catheter ablation.
- The most optimal candidates for catheter ablation of recurrent PVCs who have a high likelihood of improvement of ventricular function following ablation, include young individuals without structural heart disease having >20,000 PVCs per day, ≤2 PVC morphologies, PVCs originating from outflow tracts or from the fascicles and with preserved myocardial wall thickness. An important target when complete elimination of all PVCs is not possible, especially in the context of multifocal PVCs, is reduction of PVC burden to <5,000/day. Elimination or significant reduction of PVC burden with ablation has been shown to improve functional status and left ventricular ejection fraction (LVEF).

PROGNOSIS

Although reversible, the extent of ventricular function recovery in patients with arrhythmia-induced cardiomyopathy following restoration to sinus rhythm is variable and depends on the duration as well as rate of the responsible arrhythmia and presence of absence of underlying structural heart disease. The greatest degree of left ventricular function recovery usually occurs within 4 weeks after elimination of the underlying arrhythmia. Early improvement (defined as ≥25% improvement of EF within a week) following catheter ablation has been reported to be predictive of complete normalization during long-term follow-up.[42] Complete normalization of EF may be a more gradual process, taking up to 6 months to 1 year (Figs. 5A and B). Occasionally, despite normalization of EF, persistent LV remodeling occurs, with elevated LV dimensions and volumes suggesting incomplete recovery at an ultrastructural level and the need for continued HF therapy for sometime. Experimental models suggest that left ventricular hypertrophy persisting after weeks of discontinuation of pacing is due to post-pacing response of myocytes to hypertrophic triggers, and is exaggerated by persistent LV dilatation.

Recurrent or new tachyarrhythmias impact LV function poorly with rapid decline in ventricular function, HF and a high incidence of adverse cardiac events and even sudden cardiac death, if the arrhythmia remains uncontrolled. This indicates that some structural cardiac abnormalities may persist even after an apparent recovery in ventricular function and abrupt discontinuation of HF treatment after normalization of EF should be avoided along with close monitoring for recurrence of the arrhythmia.

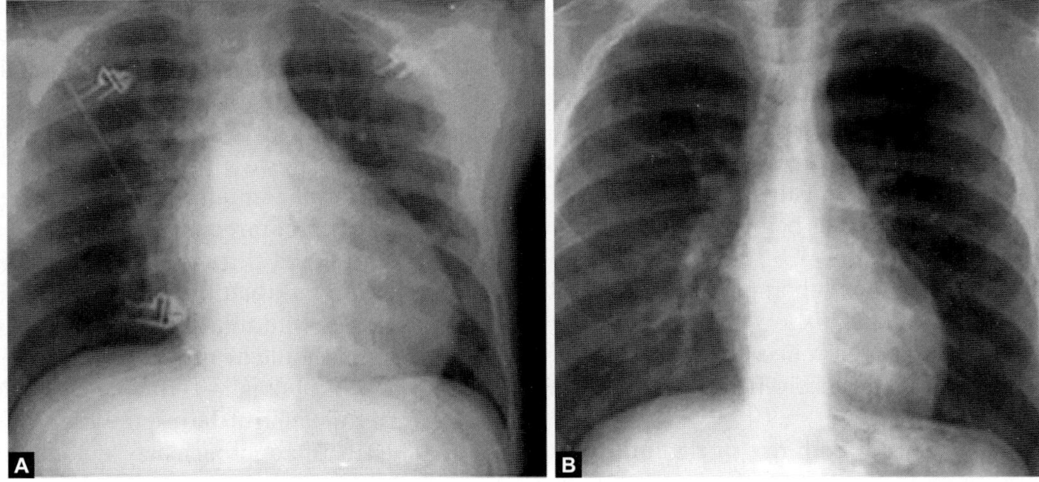

Figs. 5A and B: (A) X-ray chest in a patient with tachycardiomyopathy prior to ablation. (B) X-ray chest 6 months later following ablation.

CONCLUSION

Tachycardia-induced cardiomyopathy is classically defined as the reversible impairment of ventricular function induced by persistent arrhythmia and should be considered in all patients with a dilated cardiomyopathy of uncertain origin who have an underlying tachycardia. Abolishing the tachycardia with drugs or catheter ablation often results in clinical improvement and ventricular function recovery. Important pointers toward a diagnosis are as follows:

- Evidence of a previously normal EF and no other obvious cause of ventricular dysfunction, especially in the setting of a persistent elevation in heart rate
- Degree of LV dysfunction being out of proportion to other comorbidities
- Chronic incessant tachycardia occurring >10–15% of the day
- Recovery of LV function after control of tachycardia (by rate control, cardioversion or radiofrequency ablation within 1–6 months)
- Rapid decline in LVEF following recurrence of tachycardia in a patient with recovered LV function after previous control of tachycardia.

There is an initial adaptive/compensatory phase which manifests as cellular and extracellular remodeling, neurohormonal system activation with LV dilation, and can be identified by imaging modalities and biomarker estimation. This is followed by the second phase in which defects in excitation–contraction coupling lead to overt LV dysfunction and clinical HF.

It is often difficult to determine whether an arrhythmia is the initiator or consequence of cardiomyopathy in a patient with tachycardia and HF, raising the issue of a "chicken or egg" question. Early recognition of the relationship of culprit arrhythmia is important so that timely therapeutic measures can be instituted. Future research needs to focus on specific pathophysiological mechanisms, identifying clinical, genetic, and demographic characteristics that predispose a particular patient to develop AIC facilitating early detection and diagnosis, and finding optimal therapeutic strategies to prevent residual ultrastructural abnormalities and long-term adverse ventricular remodeling.

REFERENCES

1. Gallagher JJ. Tachycardia and cardiomyopathy: the chicken-egg dilemma revisited. J Am Coll Cardiol. 1985;6(5):1172-3.
2. Khasnis A, Jongnarangsin K, Abela G, et al. Tachycardia-induced cardiomyopathy: A review of literature. Pacing Clin Electrophysiol. 2005;28(7):710-21.
3. Chugh SS, Shen WK, Luria DM, et al. First evidence of premature ventricular complex-induced cardiomyopathy: A potentially reversible cause of heart failure. J Cardiovasc Electrophysiol. 2000;11(3):328-9.
4. Simantirakis EN, Koutalas EP, Vardas PE, et al. Arrhythmia-induced cardiomyopathies: The riddle of the chicken and the egg still unanswered? Europace. 2012;14(4):466-73.
5. Fenelon G, Wijns W, Andries E, et al. Tachycardiomyopathy: mechanisms and clinical implications. Pacing Clin Electrophysiol. 1996;19(1):95-106.
6. Ott P, Kelly PA, Mann DE, et al. Tachycardia-induced cardiomyopathy in a cardiac transplant recipient: Treatment with radiofrequency catheter ablation. J Cardiovasc Electrophysiol. 1995;6(5):391-5.
7. Sanchez C, Benito F, Moreno F, et al. Reversibility of tachycardia-induced cardiomyopathy after radiofrequency ablation of incessant supraventricular tachycardia in infants. Br Heart J. 1995;74(3):332-3.
8. Harrigan JT, Kangos JJ, Sikka A, et al. Successful treatment of fetal congestive heart failure secondary to tachycardia. N Engl J Med. 1981;304(25):1527-9.
9. Deshmukh PM, Krishnamani R, Romanyshyn M, et al. Association of angiotensin converting enzyme gene polymorphism with tachycardia cardiomyopathy. Int J Mol Med. 2004;13(3):455-8.
10. Whipple GH, Sheffield LT, Woodman EG. Reversible congestive heart failure due to chronic rapid stimulation of the normal heart. Pro N Engl Cardiovasc Soc. 1962;20:39-40.
11. Spinale FG, Hendrick DA, Crawford FA, et al. Chronic supraventricular tachycardia causes ventricular dysfunction and subendocardial injury in swine. Am J Physiol. 1990;259(1 Pt 2):H218-29.
12. Howard RJ, Moe GW, Armstrong PW. Sequential echocardiographic-Doppler assessment of left ventricular remodeling and mitral regurgitation during evolving experimental heart failure. Cardiovasc Res. 1991;25(6)468-74.
13. Moe GW, Angus C, Howard RJ, et al. Evaluation of indices of left ventricular contractility and relaxation in evolving canine experimental heart failure. Cardiovasc Res. 1992;26(4):362-6.
14. Armstrong PW, Stopps TP, Ford SE, et al. Rapid ventricular pacing in the dog: Pathophysiologic studies of heart failure. Circulation. 1986;74(5):1075-84.
15. Shinbane JS, Wood MA, Jensen DN, et al. Tachycardia-induced cardiomyopathy: A review of animal models and clinical studies. J Am Coll Cardiol. 1997;29(4):709-15.
16. Pak PH, Nuss HB, Tunin RS, et al. Repolarization abnormalities, arrhythmia and sudden death in canine tachycardia-induced cardiomyopathy. J Am Coll Cardiol. 1997;30(2):576-84.
17. Gopinathannair R, Etheridge SP, Marchlinski FE, et al. Arrhythmia-induced cardiomyopathies: Mechanisms, recognition, and management. J Am Coll Cardiol. 2015;66(15):1714-28.
18. Umana E, Solares CA, Alpert MA. Tachycardia-induced cardiomyopathy. Am J Med. 2003;114(1):51-5.
19. Grogan M, Smith HC, Gersh BJ, et al. Left ventricular dysfunction due to atrial fibrillation in patients believed to have idiopathic dilated cardiomyopathy. Am J Cardiol. 1992;69(19):1570-3.
20. Luchsinger JA, Steinberg JS. Resolution of cardiomyopathy after ablation of atrial flutter. J Am Coll Cardiol. 1998;32(1):205-10.

21. Gillette PC, Smith RT, Garson A Jr, et al. Chronic supraventricular tachycardia: A curable cause of congestive cardiomyopathy. JAMA. 1985;253(3):391-2.
22. Cruz FE, Cheriex EC, Smeets JL, et al. Reversibility of tachycardia-induced cardiomyopathy after cure of incessant supraventricular tachycardia. J Am Coll Cardiol. 1990;16(3):739-44.
23. Corey WA, Markel ML, Hoit BD, et al. Regression of a dilated cardiomyopathy after radiofrequency ablation of incessant supraventricular tachycardia. Am Heart J. 1993;126(6): 1469-73.
24. Anselme F, Boyle N, Josephson M. Incessant fascicular tachycardia: A cause of arrhythmia induced cardiomyopathy. Pacing Clin Electrophysiol. 1998;21(4 Pt 1):760-3.
25. Vijgen J, Hill P, Biblo LA, et al. Tachycardia-induced cardiomyopathy secondary to right ventricular outflow tract ventricular tachycardia: Improvement of left ventricular systolic function after radiofrequency catheter ablation of the arrhythmia. J Cardiovasc Electrophysiol. 1997;8(4):445-50.
26. Baman TS, Lange DC, Ilg KJ, et al. Relationship between burden of premature ventricular complexes and left ventricular function. Heart Rhythm. 2010;7(7):865-9.
27. Kanei Y, Friedman M, Ogawa N, et al. Frequent premature ventricular complexes originating from the right ventricular outflow tract are associated with left ventricular dysfunction. Ann Noninvasive Electrocardiol. 2008;13(1):81-5.
28. Niwano S, Wakisaka Y, Niwano H, et al. Prognostic significance of frequent premature ventricular contractions originating from the ventricular outflow tract in patients with normal left ventricular function. Heart. 2009;95(15):1230-7.
29. Roberst-Thomson KC, Kistle PM, Kalman JM. Atrial tachycardia: Mechanisms, diagnosis, and management. Curr Probl Cardiol. 2005;30(10):529-73.
30. Medi C, Kalman JM, Haqqani H, et al. Tachycardia-mediated cardiomyopathy secondary to focal atrial tachycardia: Long-term outcome after catheter ablation. J Am Coll Cardiol. 2009;53(19):1791-7.
31. Ju W, Yang B, Li M, et al. Tachycardiomyopathy complicated by focal atrial tachycardia: Incidence, risk factors, and long-term outcome. J Cardiovasc Electrophysiol. 2014;25(9):953-7.
32. Kawamura M, Badhwar N, Vedantham V, et al. Coupling interval dispersion and body mass index are independent predictors of idiopathic premature ventricular complex-induced cardiomyopathy. J Cardiovasc Electrophysiol. 2014;25(7):756-62.
33. Campos B, Jauregui ME, Park KM, et al. New unipolar electrogram criteria to identify irreversibility of nonischemic left ventricular cardiomyopathy. J Am Coll Cardiol. 2012;60(21)2194-204.
34. Olshansky B, Rosenfeld LE, Warner AL, et al.; AFFIRM Investigators. The Atrial Fibrillation Follow-up Investigation of Rhythm Management (AFFIRM) study: Approaches to control rate in atrial fibrillation. J Am Coll Cardiol. 2004;43(7):1201-8.
35. Van Gelder IC, Groenveld HF, Crijns HJ, et al.; RACE II Investigators. Lenient versus strict rate control in patients with atrial fibrillation. N Engl J Med. 2010;362(15):1363-73.
36. Roy D, Talajic M, Nattel S, et al.; Atrial Fibrillation and Congestive Heart Failure Investigators. Rhythm control versus rate control for atrial fibrillation and heart failure. N Engl J Med. 2008;358(25):2667-77.
37. Shelton RJ, Clark AL, Goode K, et al. A randomised, controlled study of rate versus rhythm control in patients with chronic atrial fibrillation and heart failure: (CAFE-II study). Heart. 2009;95(11):924-30.
38. Nerheim P, Birger-Botkin S, Piracha L, et al. Heart failure and sudden death in patients with tachycardia-induced cardiomyopathy and recurrent tachycardia. Circulation. 2004;110(3):247-52.
39. Nedios S, Sommer P, Dagres N, et al. Long-term follow-up after atrial fibrillation ablation in patients with impaired left ventricular systolic function: The importance of rhythm and rate control. Heart Rhythm. 2014;11(3):344-51.
40. Furushima H, Chinushi M, Sugiura H, et al. Radiofrequency catheter ablation for incessant atrioventricular nodal reentrant tachycardia normalized H-V block associated with tachycardia-induced cardiomyopathy. J Electrocardiol. 2004;37(4):315-9.
41. Bensler JM, Frank CM, Razavi M, et al. Tachycardia-mediated cardiomyopathy and the permanent form of junctional reciprocating tachycardia. Texas Heart Inst J. 2010;37(6): 695-8.
42. Hasdemir C, Kartal Y, Simsek E, et al. Time course of recovery of left ventricular systolic dysfunction in patients with premature ventricular contraction-induced cardiomyopathy. Pacing Clin Electrophysiol. 2013;36(5):612-7.

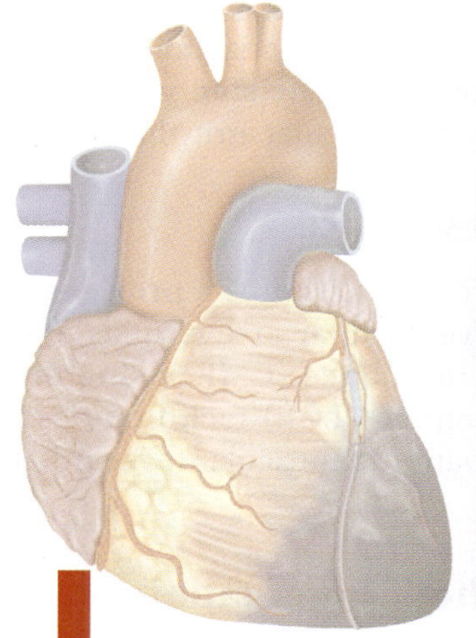

Sudden Cardiac Death in Heart Failure

Ravi Prakash, Kavita Tyagi, HK Chopra

INTRODUCTION

Heart failure (HF) is a complex clinical syndrome in which structural or functional myocardial abnormalities result in symptoms and signs of hypoperfusion and/or pulmonary or systemic congestion at rest or during exercise.[1] In spite of considerable advances in the treatment of HF in recent years, morbidity and mortality remain high with a 4-year survival of less than 50%.[1]

Sudden death is often defined as natural death, in which the time and mode of death is unexpected, and which occurs within 1 hour of the onset of symptoms.[2] Sudden cardiac death (SCD) can manifest as ventricular tachycardia (VT), ventricular fibrillation (VF), pulseless electric activity (PEA), or asystole.[2]

Sudden cardiac death accounts for about 40–45% of all deaths in HF reduced ejection fraction (HFrEF) patients, and the proportion of SCD is higher in patients with milder symptoms [New York Heart Association (NYHA) class II-III]. Indeed two-thirds of patients with NYHA functional class II experience SCD, compared with only one-third of those with NYHA functional class IV symptoms, who died preponderantly for advanced HF. Incidence of SCD in patients was higher than 20% per year before the era of disease modifying therapies, nevertheless with current pharmacologic and electrical therapy, incidence of SCD has decreased to about 3% per year.[2]

PATHOPHYSIOLOGY OF SUDDEN CARDIAC DEATH

Sudden cardiac death in patients with HFrEF requires the chance and complex interaction between a transient event (premature ectopics, electrolyte imbalance, ischemia) and underlying pathologic substrate (scar, fibrosis) that induces electrical instability.[3] In ischemic cardiomyopathy, origin of SCD is related to areas of the infarcted myocardium that are adjacent to thick scar formed over time. In patients with systolic dysfunction after a myocardial infarction, non-arrhythmic SCD frequently occurs during the first 4–6 weeks and is usually due to mechanical complications of myocardial infarction. Proportions of arrhythmic and non-arrhythmic SCD cases become equivalent approximately 1 month after the acute coronary syndrome.[4] These observations explain the guidelines' recommendation of delaying implantable cardioverter defibrillator (ICD) implantation for 40 days after myocardial infarction. In nonischemic cardiomyopathy, origin of SCD is related to multiple patchy areas of fibrosis without significantly visible scar found in ventricular myocardium. Reentry accounts for only 40% of the mechanisms of ventricular arrhythmias in patients with nonischemic cardiomyopathy, with the rest due to triggered activity.[5] The primary mechanism of SCD in patients with HF with preserved ejection fraction (HFpEF) seems related to myocardial fibrosis that alters regional conduction patterns and serves as islands of reentry. Ischemia is also likely to act as a contributor to ventricular arrhythmias in HFpEF.

RISK STRATIFICATION OF SCD IN HF

Risk stratification of SCD in patients with HF represents a clinical challenge. Risk stratification defines candidates for medical therapies and help selecting patients for ICD. Left ventricular ejection fraction (LVEF) is one of the most important determinants of risk of SCD in HF.[6] It is widely used to identify candidates for primary prevention therapy with ICD. Other modalities for risk stratification are also emerging; however, they are yet to be proved by properly designed studies.

Resting ECG

Prolonged QRS complex duration signifies ventricular arrhythmias through abnormal dispersion of depolarization and repolarization and resultant cardiac dyssynchrony. QRS duration of >120 msec (irrespective of morphology) predicts SCD in patients with dilated cardiomyopathy, independent of LVEF value.[6] However, well-designed prospective studies need to clarify the role of resting ECG in SCD risk stratification in HF.

Ambulatory Electrocardiogram

Twenty-four-hours Holter monitoring can be used to predict SCD in patients with HF with ischemic etiology. Patients with previous myocardial infarction and nonsustained ventricular tachycardia is said to have higher mortality.[7]

Microvolt T-wave Alternans

Microvolt T-wave alternans (MTWA) is a beat-to-beat fluctuation of T-wave amplitude and morphology, which has been associated with increased susceptibility for sustained ventricular arrhythmia.[7] Early studies showed that TWA was a powerful electrocardiographic tool in predicting SCD in patients, in ischemic and nonischemic cardiomyopathy. Despite considerable enthusiasm over TWA, subsequent large prospective trials failed to validate the role of TWA for risk stratification in patients with HF.

Signal-averaged Electrocardiography

Signal-averaged electrocardiography (SAECG) is a method to improve the signal-to-noise ratio of a surface electrocardiogram, thus facilitating the identification of low-amplitude signal at the end of QRS complex. This test was initially found to be a promising marker of SCD in patients with ischemic cardiomyopathy, and later in patients with nonischemic cardiomyopathy.[8] Nevertheless, subsequent studies have shown conflicting and less promising results.

However, SAECG has a high negative predictive value. For this reason, SAECG may be used as the first-line test to identify patients at low risk of SCD.

Speckle Echocardiography

Speckle-tracking echocardiography (STE) allows for the measurement of the different myocardial strains, providing an indirect evaluation of systolic function and presence of scar/fibrosis. In patients with ischemic dilated cardiomyopathy, a reduction of global longitudinal strain (GLS) has been independently associated with SCD, appropriate ICD therapy, and ventricular arrhythmias.[9]

Cardiac Magnetic Resonance

The presence of myocardial scar/fibrosis provides a substrate for malignant ventricular arrhythmias and SCD. Cardiac magnetic resonance (CMR) using the late gadolinium enhancement (LGE) technique can accurately identify and quantify ventricular myocardial scar/fibrosis.

Myocardial Sympathetic Innervation Imaging

Sustained activation of the sympathetic nervous system is thought to be a significant contributor to the progression of HF and adverse outcomes including SCD. Myocardial iodine-123 metaiodobenzylguanidine (123I-mIBG) imaging provides a noninvasive method to assess cardiac sympathetic function and risk stratify patients with HF.[10]

Autonomic Function Test

Heart rate variability (HRV) and heart rate turbulence (HRT) have been studied as markers of autonomic dysfunction that have a significant role in the development of ventricular arrhythmias in patients with HFrEF.

Heart rate variability is associated with increased ventricular arrhythmias and mortality. However, HRV does not appear to enhance prognostic stratification when directly compared to other markers of SCD. Moreover, in patients with nonischemic cardiomyopathy, HRV is related to left ventricular dysfunction but not to ventricular arrhythmias and SCD.[11]

Heart rate turbulence (i.e. the short-term fluctuation in sinus cycle length that follows a ventricular premature complex) is a noninvasive marker of electrical instability that has been shown to identify patients at high risk for SCD. However, in nonischemic population, HRT does not yield predictive power for SCD risk stratification.[11]

PREVENTION OF SUDDEN CARDIAC DEATH

The implantable cardioverter-defibrillator (ICD) has established itself as life-saving therapy in patients at risk for SCD. Over the last two decades, the indications have evolved from secondary prevention of sudden death to also include primary prevention in selected patients. For secondary prophylaxis, ICD placement is indicated as initial therapy in survivors of cardiac arrest due to ventricular fibrillation (VF) or hemodynamically unstable ventricular tachycardia (VT).

Currently, indications for primary prophylaxis account for most ICD implants. Class I indications for primary prophylaxis are as follows:

- Structural heart disease, sustained VT
- Syncope of undetermined origin, inducible VT or VF at electrophysiologic study (EPS)
- Left ventricular ejection fraction ≤35% due to prior myocardial infarction (MI), at least 40 days post-MI, NYHA class II or III
- Left ventricular ejection fraction ≤35%, NYHA class II or III
- Left ventricular ejection fraction ≤30% due to prior MI, at least 40 days post-MI
- Left ventricular ejection fraction ≤40% due to prior MI, inducible VT or VF at EPS.

CONCLUSION

Despite progress in pharmacological and electrical therapy, SCD remains the most frequent cause of mortality in patients with HFrEF. Early studies have identified LVEF and ischemic etiology as predictors of events. Most recently, imaging and advanced electrocardiographic techniques can enhance the identification of high-risk individuals who may benefit from a specific approach to prevent SCD. ICD can be of utmost advantage for SCD prevention in indicated group of HF patients, however, requiring proper patient selection and follow-up.

REFERENCES

1. Ziaeian B, Fonarow GC. Epidemiology and etiology of heart failure. Nat Rev Cardiol. 2016;13(6):368-78.
2. Hayashi M, Shimizu W, Albert CM. The spectrum of epidemiology underlying sudden cardiac death. Circ Res. 2015;116(12):1887-906.
3. Mendonca Costa C, Plank G, Rinaldi CA, et al. Modeling the electrophysiological properties of the infarct border zone. Front Physiol. 2018;9:356.
4. Zaman S, Kovoor P. Sudden cardiac death early after myocardial infarction: Pathogenesis, risk stratification, and primary prevention. Circulation. 2014;129(23):2426-35.
5. Goldberger JJ, Subačius H, Patel T, et al. Sudden cardiac death risk stratification in patients with nonischemic dilated cardiomyopathy. J Am Coll Cardiol. 2014;63(18):1879-89.
6. Wellens HJ, Schwartz PJ, Lindemans FW, et al. Risk stratification for sudden cardiac death: Current status and challenges for the future. Eur Heart J. 2014;35(25):1642-51.
7. Kusmirek SL, Gold MR. Sudden cardiac death: The role of risk stratification. Am Heart J. 2007;153(Suppl 4):25-33.
8. Jarrett JR, Flowers NC. Signal-averaged electrocardiography: History, techniques, and clinical applications. Clin Cardiol. 1991;14(12):984-94.
9. Ersbøll M, Valeur N, Andersen MJ, et al. Early echocardiographic deformation analysis for the prediction of sudden cardiac death and life-threatening arrhythmias after myocardial infarction. JACC Cardiovasc. Imaging. 2013;6(8):851-60.
10. Nakajima K, Nakata T, Doi T, et al. Validation of 2-year 123I-meta-iodobenzylguanidine-based cardiac mortality risk model in chronic heart failure. Eur Heart J Cardiovasc Imaging. 2018;19(7):749-56.
11. Kleiger RE, Miller JP, Bigger JT Jr, et al. Decreased heart rate variability and its association with increased mortality after acute myocardial infarction. Am J Cardiol. 1987;59(4):256-62.

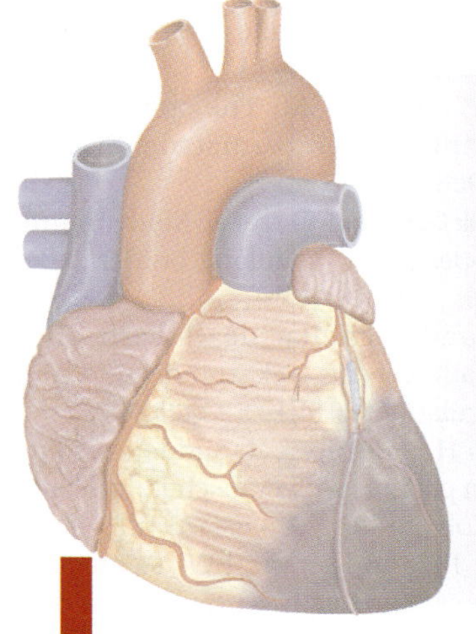

Rhythm Disorders and Cardiac Transplant Patient

Surendra K Chutani, Arun Chutani, Arti Shah, Bharat Kantharia

INTRODUCTION

Cardiac transplantation has significantly altered the treatment paradigm for end-stage heart disease. With current surgical techniques and postoperative immunosuppression of 1-year survival rate is more than 90%, 5-year survival rate is 70%, and median survival exceeds 10 years. Cardiac arrhythmias are common in orthotopic heart transplantation recipient, both in the early postoperative period and in late. There are several mechanisms for arrhythmogenesis in transplanted heart in early and late postoperative period.[1] In early postoperative surgical trauma to the sinoatrial and atrioventricular (AV) node, ischemia during preservation, surgical suture lines, and reading rejection over long-term associated with accelerated atherosclerosis contribute to the formation of arrhythmic substrate. In addition, the denervated donor heart has increased sensitivity to sympathetic activity including catecholamine and to parasympathetic activity involving adenosine and acetylcholine.

PATHOPHYSIOLOGICAL MECHANISMS

There are several mechanisms for arrhythmogenesis in the transplanted heart, with early postoperative arrhythmias resulting from different mechanisms than those occurring later.[2] Following factors are important:

- *Graft Ischemia Time:* Long cropped ischemia time can predispose to conduction system injury both in early and late postoperative. Ischemic and resulted into early mitochondrial damage and subsequent endocardial fibrosis. Prolonged graft ischemia more than 4 hours is classified as high-risk ischemia and carries a greater 30-day and 1-year mortality rates. When myocardial preservation is not adequate, risk of chronic rejection with endothelial damage is enhanced.[3]
- *Type of anastomosis: Bicaval versus Biatrial:* The most common technique used for donor to recipient anastomosis is bicaval method. It involves anastomosis at the level of two vena cava, the great vessels, and the left atrial cuff around the pulmonary veins. In bicaval suture method there less sinus node injury, tricuspid regurgitation and atrial dilatation. In biatrial method the recipient right and left atria are retained and sutured to the respective atria of the donor, hence the recipient sinuatrial (SA) node is preserved but it is not functional because of disruption of the blood supply and denervation. And there is complete conduction block across the suture line in the right atrium. When biatrial method is used there are the 2 P-waves on surface EKG, from recipient and donor atria respectively and might mimic atrial flutter; though on closer examination atrial revealed nonconductive atrial P-wave. Reestablishment of conduction across the atrial anastomosis site may produce tachycardia because of fibrillatory activity or flutter activity in the recipient atrium. Sinus activity from the recipient atrium may intermittently escape into donor atrium and manifest as frequent atrial ectopic or atrial parasystole. The scar in the atria can act as conduction barrier it is posing to atrial flutter, CT isthmus dependent atrial flutter or mitral annular atrial flutter. Therefore, the biatrial matted is more likely

associated with greater risk of a reentrant tachycardia and flutter.[4]

- *Denervation and renervation:* The donor heart is completely denervated during transplantation. The lack of parasympathetic activity has greater effects and most heart transplant patients have high resting heart rate and significantly reduced heart rate variability. Over time both sympathetic and parasympathetic innovation occurs, but the degree of reinnervation is incomplete, nonuniform and variable between patients and the heterogeneous within the same patient.
- *Cardiac allograft vasculopathy:* It is relatively common and has important prognostic significance. Ischemia resulting from vasculopathy or atherosclerosis is a likely precipitant for ventricular arrhythmias and sudden cardiac death (SCD). It can also result in ventricular dysfunction resulting in to increased risk of SCD.[5]
- *Nonspecific late graft failure:* Then progressive left ventricular dysfunction occurs without evidence of epicardial coronary artery narrowing by biopsy it is labeled as nonspecific graft failure. Such patients can ultimately develop severe left ventricular dysfunction and terminal arrhythmia manifested as pulseless electrical activity and asystole.[6]
- *Rejection:* The incidence of rejection is 20–30% in the first posttransplantation year. Atrial flutter and fibrillation have been attributed to acute rejection. Hence occurrence of atrial fibrillation (AF) or flutter should prompt evaluation for rejection. Repeated injection episodes can also lead to substrate for mechanism of atrial flutter because of scar formation. Myocardial injury due to infiltration of inflammatory cells, edema and subsequent scarring and ventricular dysfunction may predispose to ventricular arrhythmias. Patients with severe acute rejection can have SCD.[7]

MANAGEMENT OF POSTTRANSPLANT ARRHYTHMIA

Treatment of Sinus Bradycardia

Normalization of posttransplant sinus node dysfunction (SND) and bradyarrhythmias occurs spontaneously in up to 55% of patients during the first three postoperative months and a conservative strategy is reasonable in the early postoperative period. The administration of theophylline, terbutaline or albuterol has been advocated to increase the sinus rate and avoid implantation of a permanent pacemaker during the first three postoperative months. Atropine is not an effective treatment for bradycardia in the transplanted heart when vagal innervation is absent. Intravenous isoproterenol is suggested in the unlikely event that emergency treatment of bradycardia is needed in the heart transplant patient who does not have pacemaker wires in place.[8]

Patients with more severe bradycardia that persists for more than 2 weeks after transplantation usually require a permanent pacemaker; a rate-responsive dual chamber or atrial pacemaker implanted in the donor right atrium, if intact AV conduction is present, is recommended. The role of biventricular pacing is not known in cardiac transplant recipients who fulfill the criteria used for such therapy in non-transplant patients. Successful implementation of cardiac resynchronization therapy in heart transplant patients has been reported.[9]

Conduction Disturbances

The most common conduction abnormality following orthotopic heart transplant is a new right bundle branch delay not present on the donor electrocardiogram (ECG) prior to transplantation. This can occur in up to 70% of patients and is usually manifest as an incomplete right bundle branch block (RBBB) present immediately postoperatively. The incidence of RBBB is higher with biatrial versus bicaval anastomosis. Potential mechanisms for later RBBB include right ventricular hypertrophy from elevated pulmonary pressures or damage to the right bundle from endomyocardial biopsy sampling of the right ventricular septal wall.

Although the transplanted heart is denervated, AV nodal function is intact and the ability of the AV node to adapt to exercise with a shortening of the PR interval is retained since it remains sensitive to circulating catecholamine. High-grade AV block is uncommon, particularly in the early postoperative period. Although pacemaker implantation is performed in approximately 10–15% of cardiac transplant recipients, AV block accounts for less than 20% of these cases and median time to pacemaker implantation is later for AV block than for SND. The late development of heart block has been associated with an increase in mortality, often from transplant arteriopathy.

Indications for pacemaker placement are the same as for other patients with symptomatic bradyarrhythmias or chronotropic incompetence that are not expected to resolve. Patients who undergo bicaval cardiac transplants are less likely to require permanent cardiac pacing than those who undergo biatrial cardiac transplants.[10]

Supraventricular Arrhythmias

Atrial Premature Beats

Isolated atrial premature beats (APBs) and nonsustained atrial dysrhythmias are common in the early postoperative period, occurring in up to 76% of patients. The prevalence is lower at long-term follow-up, decreasing from 55% in the early postoperative period to 30% at mean of 24 months after transplantation in one report.[11]

Atrial Fibrillation or Flutter

Atrial fibrillation has been described in 10–24% of patients, while atrial flutter has been described in 12–15%. These arrhythmias often occur in even absence of significant rejection. Most episodes of AF occur within the first 30–60 days after transplantation with incidence ranging from 5% to 11%. This relatively low rate, compared to typical postpericardiectomy AF incidence is postulated to be due to surgical pulmonary vein isolation and cardiac denervation, which occurs with the heart transplantation surgery. Patients treated with long-term amiodarone therapy prior to heart transplantation have less early postoperative AF with no adverse impact on mortality. Late AF develops in 5–10% of patients and is associated with decrease in systolic function and increased overall mortality.[12]

Atrial flutter that occurs in the absence of rejection is a result of a macro reentrant circuit in a counterclockwise direction around the tricuspid ring, similar to that seen in typical atrial flutter in normal hearts. This circuit includes the isthmus between the tricuspid valve and the inferior vena cava, referred to as the cavotricuspid isthmus.

The cause of atrial dysrhythmias during rejection is not known. It is possible that the patchy nature of rejection results in heterogeneous impairment of atrial conduction and refractoriness, allowing for the formation of multiple micro reentrant circuits. Treatment of these arrhythmias includes control of the ventricular response rate and, if warranted, immunosuppressive therapy for rejection. Overdrive pacing can be performed at the time of myocardial biopsy with more than a 90% success in terminating atrial flutter.[13]

There are case reports and small series of successful radiofrequency ablation of atrial flutter in transplanted hearts. Interestingly, the usual suture line between the donor and recipient heart lies within the cavo-tricuspid isthmus, which, as noted above, is a critical component of the circuit of typical atrial flutter.

Supraventricular Tachycardia

A variety of supraventricular tachycardia (SVT) can occur in orthotopic heart transplant recipients, including AV reentrant tachycardia (AVRT) involving a concealed AV bypass tract, Wolff-Parkinson-White syndrome, and sustained atrial tachycardia. Radiofrequency catheter ablation has been performed in many of these patients with success and complication rates similar to nontransplant recipients.[14]

Interaction of diltiazem with immunosuppressive agents is important. Intravenous diltiazem is often used to control ventricular rates in patients with SVTs and/or AF. Diltiazem inhibits CYP3A and P glycoprotein that metabolize tacrolimus and cyclosporine. Consequently, heart transplant patients receiving diltiazem often have elevated tacrolimus or cyclosporine levels, which can result in renal dysfunction.[15]

Ventricular Arrhythmias

- Ventricular premature beats (VPBs) are common in the early posttransplant period, occurring in up to 100% of patients. The incidence of VPBs decreases after the early postoperative period and does not appear to be associated with rejection or other factors.[16]
- The frequency of nonsustained ventricular tachycardia (NSVT) also decreases over time.
- Sustained ventricular arrhythmias are uncommon in the donor heart; when they occur, they are usually associated with either severe transplant cardiac allograft vasculopathy or allograft rejection. Ventricular fibrillation has been reported in patients hospitalized for severe allograft rejection, while autopsy studies of patients with SCD have demonstrated a high prevalence of severe cardiac allograft vasculopathy or recent myocardial infarctions.[17]
- Limited outcome data exist for implantable cardioverter-defibrillator (ICD) therapy in heart transplant recipients. ICD therapy has been reported to effectively terminate ventricular arrhythmias in transplanted patients with severe left ventricular dysfunction, severe allograft vasculopathy, or history of cardiac arrest. The effect of ICD therapy on long-term survival and quality of life in this population is not known.[18]

CONCLUSION

While most arrhythmias after orthotopic heart transplantation are benign, there are several clinical associations. Early postoperative bradyarrhythmias due to SND are probably caused by surgical trauma to the sinoatrial node or its blood supply and can partly be avoided using a bicaval anastomosis technique. Atropine is not an effective treatment for bradycardia when vagal innervation is absent; intravenous isoproterenol is suggested in the unlikely event that emergency treatment of bradycardia is needed in the heart transplant patient without pacemaker wires in place. Sustained atrial flutter and fibrillation are commonly associated with allograft rejection. Thus, the presence of these arrhythmias should prompt a search for acute rejection by endomyocardial biopsy. Empiric steroid therapy should be considered in such patients prior to return of the biopsy results. Adenosine should not be used to try to elucidate the mechanism of supraventricular tachyarrhythmia since it can result in transient, but significant, bradyarrhythmias. Patients with frequent and symptomatic SVT may be treated with radiofrequency catheter ablation. Complex ventricular ectopy or AV block may be caused by either acute rejection or severe cardiac allograft vasculopathy. Affected patients should undergo endomyocardial biopsy followed, if rejection is not present, by coronary angiography to diagnose cardiac allograft vasculopathy. Insertion of a permanent pacemaker should be considered in patients with significant bradyarrhythmias, either from SND or high-grade AV block that are associated with decreased cardiac output and occur in the absence of acute rejection. Standard recommendations for ICD therapy apply to cardiac transplant recipients.

REFERENCES

1. Calzolari V, Angelini A, Basso C, et al. Histologic findings in the conduction system after cardiac transplantation and correlation with electrocardiographic findings. Am J Cardiol. 1999;84(6):756-9, A9.
2. Knight CS, Tallaj JA, Rayburn BK, et al. Bradycardia and syncope as a presentation of cardiac allograft rejection involving the conducting system. Cardiovasc Pathol. 2010;19(2):117-20.
3. Ellenbogen KA, Thames MD, DiMarco JP, et al. Electrophysiological effects of adenosine in the transplanted human heart. Evidence of supersensitivity. Circulation. 1990;81(3):821-8.
4. Flyer JN, Zuckerman WA, Richmond ME, et al. Prospective study of adenosine on atrioventricular nodal conduction in pediatric and young adult patients after heart transplantation. Circulation. 2017;135(25):2485-93.
5. Gallego-Page JC, Segovia J, Alonso-Pulpón L, et al. Re-innervation after heart transplantation: A multidisciplinary study. J Heart Lung Transplant. 2004;23(6):674-82.
6. Jacquet L, Ziady G, Stein K, et al. Cardiac rhythm disturbances early after orthotopic heart transplantation: Prevalence and clinical importance of the observed abnormalities. J Am Coll Cardiol. 1990;16(4):832-7.
7. Mackintosh AF, Carmichael DJ, Wren C, et al. Sinus node function in first three weeks after cardiac transplantation. Br Heart J. 1982;48(6):584-8.
8. Heinz G, Kratochwill C, Koller-Strametz J, et al. Benign prognosis of early sinus node dysfunction after orthotopic cardiac transplantation. Pacing Clin Electrophysiol. 1998;21(2):422-9.
9. Mason JW, Harrison DC. Electrophysiology and electropharmacology of the transplanted human heart. In: Narula OS (Ed). Cardiac Arrhythmias: Electrophysiology, Diagnosis and Management. Baltimore: Williams & Wilkins; 1979. p. 66.
10. DiBiase A, Tse TM, Schnittger I, et al. Frequency and mechanism of bradycardia in cardiac transplant recipients and need for pacemakers. Am J Cardiol. 1991;67(16): 1385-9.
11. Miyamoto Y, Curtiss EI, Kormos RL, et al. Bradyarrhythmia after heart transplantation. Incidence, time course, and outcome. Circulation. 1990;82(Suppl 5):IV313-7.
12. Melton IC, Gilligan DM, Wood MA, et al. Optimal cardiac pacing after heart transplantation. Pacing Clin Electrophysiol. 1999;22(10):1510-27.
13. Mariani JA, McDonald MA, Nanthakumar K, et al. Cardiac resynchronization therapy after atrioventricular node ablation for rapid atrial fibrillation in a heart transplant recipient with late allograft dysfunction. J Heart Lung Transplant. 2010;29(6):704-6.
14. Villa AE, de Marchena EJ, Myerburg RJ, et al. Comparisons of paired orthotopic cardiac transplant donor and recipient electrocardiograms. Am Heart J. 1994;127(1):70-4.
15. Li YG, Grönefeld G, Israel C, et al. Radiofrequency catheter ablation in patients with symptomatic atrial flutter/tachycardia after orthotopic heart transplantation. Chin Med J (Engl). 2006;119(24):2036-41.
16. Nof E, Stevenson WG, Epstein LM, et al. Catheter ablation of atrial arrhythmias after cardiac transplantation: Findings at EP study utility of 3-D mapping and outcomes. J Cardiovasc Electrophysiol. 2013;24(5):498-502.
17. Goy JJ, Kappenberger L, Turina M. Wolff-Parkinson-White syndrome after transplantation of the heart. Br Heart J. 1989;61(4):368-71.
18. Tsai VW, Cooper J, Garan H, et al. The efficacy of implantable cardioverter-defibrillators in heart transplant recipients: Results from a multicenter registry. Circ Heart Fail. 2009;2(3):197-201.

CHAPTER 85

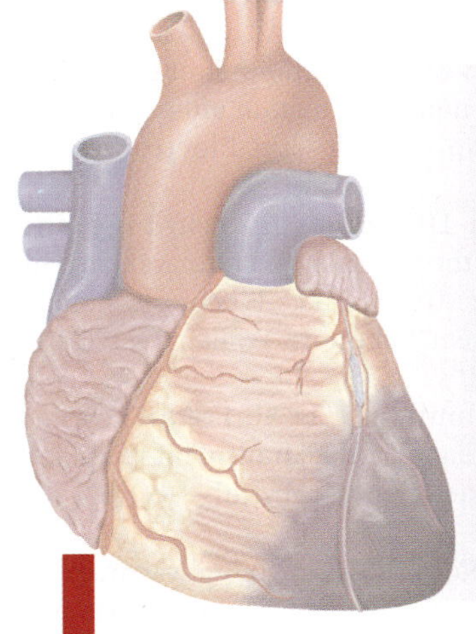

Cardiac Resynchronization Therapy in Congestive Heart Failure: State of Art, Troubleshooting and Management

Surendra K Chutani, Arun Chutani, Arti Shah, Bharat Kantharia

INTRODUCTION

The Role of Cardiac Resynchronization Therapy in Heart Failure Management

The purpose of cardiac resynchronization therapy (CRT) is to eliminate the dyssynchrony, which results from bundle branch block activation, and restore the mechano-energetic efficiency of the heart. Following CRT, both the left and right ventricles are stimulated in an attempt to recoordinate cardiac electrical activation and produce a synchronous and efficient contraction. Several large randomized controlled trials of biventricular (BiV) pacing have been conducted which have established the efficacy of this therapy, which yields both reductions in morbidity and mortality. As a result of landmark studies, class 1 indications exist for CRT in patients with symptomatic heart failure, a severely impaired LV [left ventricular ejection fraction (LVEF) <35%] and an echocardiography (ECG) demonstrating left bundle-branch block (LBBB) with significant electrical delay.[1]

CLINICAL RESPONSE TO CARDIAC RESYNCHRONIZATION THERAPY

Around 30–50% of patients fail to respond to transvenous, epicardial CRT. This group is classified as nonresponders although no unifying definition of response to CRT exists. Response can be measured in a variety of different clinical, functional and structural endpoints and patients can fail to respond for a variety of different reasons. The process of defining response to CRT is challenging as no universally accepted definition of CRT response exists. Response rates tend to be higher when clinical measures, such as subjective assessments of symptoms are used but are much lower when remodeling or outcome measurements are employed.

Symptomatic improvements do not always correlate with echocardiographic or functional classification improvements. There is also no consensus as to the optimal timeframe to reassess LV function when gauging remodeling. The most widely accepted definition of responder to CRT involves an assessment of left ventricular reverse remodeling (LVRR) 6 months after implantation, with reductions in LV end-systolic volume (LVESV) the most useful measure. Remodeling endpoints are typically associated with nonresponder rates between 30% and 50%.[1]

FACTORS ASSOCIATED WITH SUBOPTIMAL CRT RESPONSE/NON-RESPONSE TO EPICARDIAL CRT

The reasons why some patients fail to adequately respond to transvenous, epicardial CRT are multifactorial and involve several pre-, peri- and postimplant factors. Following are the possible factors:

- Suboptimal AV timing
- Arrhythmias

- Less than 90% BiV pacing
- Anemia
- Suboptimal LV lead position
- Suboptimal medical therapy
- Primary RV dysfunction
- Persistent mechanical dyssynchrony
- Underlying narrow QRS
- Compliance issues.

PREIMPLANT FACTORS ASSOCIATED WITH SUBOPTIMAL CRT RESPONSE/ NONRESPONSE TO EPICARDIAL CRT

Preimplant factors associated with nonresponse to CRT include inappropriate patient selection, baseline ECG morphology and QRS duration, gender, etiology, presence of myocardial scar, and disease severity.[2]

Patient Selection

Optimal patient selection is critical when looking to maximize response to CRT. It is indicated in patients with symptomatic heart failure with LBBB who exhibit impaired LV function and display evidence of ventricular dyssynchrony. Patients must have been established on optimal tolerated medical therapy and reversible causes of heart failure should have been excluded, including ischemia, arrhythmia, or valvular heart disease.

Electrocardiogram Morphology and QRS Duration

The presence of LBBB morphology is a strong predictor of response to CRT. Whilst no definitive data exists evaluating CRT response in patients with right bundle-branch block (RBBB), retrospective analysis suggests that this group of patients tends to do less well. Interestingly, when patients with heart failure and RBBB were analyzed using 3D noncontact mapping, they were found to exhibit significant LV activation delay in addition to the delay identified in the RV. In addition, LBBB activation is not exclusively associated with electrical conduction delay. In one analysis, up to a third of patients with LBBB who underwent electromechanical or noncontact mapping demonstrated normal transseptal activation time and a near-normal LV endocardial activation time.

The evidence for CRT in patients with nonspecific intraventricular conduction delay (NICD) who possess a wide QRS without the appearance of left or right bundle-branch block is also sparse. This ECG abnormality is present in between 3.8% and 5.8% of patients with impaired LV function. In addition, this can be caused by a variety of pathophysiological processes, which may independently influence response. Conflicting outcomes following the use of CRT in patients with NICD have been reported with some studies appearing to show benefits in quality of life, whilst others revealed no benefit in clinical composite score, remodeling or mortality. Morphology again appears to be the critical determinant with patients exhibiting an LBBB-like NICD morphology appearing to gain the most benefit. While reliably categorizing the activation pattern based on a 12-lead ECG alone can be challenging; this is possible using both invasive electroanatomical mapping and novel noninvasive body surface mapping technology.

Gender

Gender appears to play a key part in determining response to CRT. Female CRT recipients appear to achieve superior survival benefits when compared to male recipients, although lower rates of ischemic cardiomyopathy (ICM) confound this analysis. Interestingly, it appears that the degree of electrical dyssynchrony required predicting response to CRT differs between the sexes.

Etiology and Myocardial Scar

In approximately 50% of patients receiving CRT, the etiology of their heart failure would be ischemic in origin; however, ischemic etiology is an independent predictor of nonresponse to CRT. Studies have shown that patients with ICM experience have less improvement in LVEF than patients with nonischemic, dilated cardiomyopathy (DCM). The difference in remodeling has been attributed to a sequelae of the greater burden of scarred myocardium typically identified in ischemic patients, reducing the potential for LV remodeling.

Atrial Fibrillation

Approximately 25% of patients undergoing CRT implantation are in permanent atrial fibrillation (AF). Such patients with AF to concurrently exhibit older age, increased severity of heart failure and additional comorbidities than patients who present with sinus rhythm. Patients with AF are more likely to have a faster and more irregular heart than patients in sinus rhythm, and the etiology of their LV dysfunction may in some instances be a result of tachycardiomyopathy. When the presenting rhythm was analyzed in a randomized trial, CRT appeared to confer no benefit to patients with coexistent AF, whilst a 25% reduction in mortality was observed amongst those in sinus rhythm. One explanation for this discrepancy is that amongst the group with AF, only 50% of the patients experienced a BiV pacing burden in excess of 90%. In order to maximizing the percentage of

BiV pacing, it has been postulated that all patients with AF should undergo atrioventricular (AV) junctional ablation and this approach does appear to enhance the effects of CRT with the same magnitude as those seen in patients with sinus rhythm.

Upgrades to Cardiac Resynchronization Therapy

Patients with a bradycardia pacing system in situ who go on to develop heart failure symptoms account for around 23–28% of CRT implants. The deleterious effects of chronic RV pacing have been well established. As such, implantation of a BiV pacing system may be appropriate for patients with evidence of symptomatic heart failure and reduced ejection fraction who are expected to experience a high pacing burden. It is likely stricter adherence to professional practice guidelines identifying suitable patients to undergo an upgrade to a CRT system will improve the response rate to the therapy.

Peri-implant Factors

Peri-implant factors associated with nonresponse to CRT include utilizing appropriate LV lead technology and optimization of the LV lead stimulation site.

Left Ventricular Lead Technology

Transvenous, epicardial CRT was traditionally performed by implanting a bipolar pacing lead in a tributary of the coronary sinus, facilitating depolarization of the LV. Multisite pacing (MSP) where stimulation is delivered from two or more sites within the LV would intuitively appear preferable to single-site stimulation. In early pilot work, MSP was associated with greater reverse remodeling; however, in a larger, randomized study of prior nonresponders to CRT, no clinical or echocardiographic benefit was observed.

Multisite Pacing/Multipoint Pacing

Multisite pacing/multipoint pacing can also be delivered via multipoint pacing (MPP). This technique utilizes quadripolar LV pacing leads which have four integrated pacing cathodes along the course of the lead, allowing greater customization from any of the 10–17 MPP vectors available. The increased choice for the implanting physician means it is possible to program around frequently occurring issues including high pacing thresholds—potentially caused by areas of scar- or phrenic nerve stimulation (PNS), where LV depolarization causes diaphragmatic twitching. The use of MPP has been shown to yield greater improvements in acute hemodynamic response and in a small, randomized study, greater improvements in overall response.

Stimulation Site

The optimal LV pacing site displays large inter- and intrapatient variability amongst patients with both DCM and ICM. Delivering stimulation from a more apical position has largely been shown to yield less favorable outcomes, and this practice is not endorsed in current guidelines. In general, there is a consensus that the lateral free wall represents the most favorable target for LV lead deployment, typically within the lateral or posterolateral cardiac veins of the coronary sinus. Unfortunately, the constraints of the coronary sinus anatomy mean it is occasionally impossible to even implant an LV lead, let alone target a specific site, which displays desirable viability and latency.

Postimplant

Postimplant factors associated with nonresponse to CRT include remote monitoring, frequency of BiV pacing, device programming, and optimization.

Remote Monitoring

Almost all modern cardiac implanted electronic devices (CIEDs) have the capability to allow remote device follow-up. Large, randomized studies have consistently shown that remote device monitoring is both feasible and reduces the need for ambulatory outpatient clinic attendance. The use of remote monitoring has been shown to improve clinical outcomes for patients with heart failure as well as achieving a significant reduction in mortality.[3]

Biventricular Pacing Incidence

In order for a CRT system to function effectively, it is essential that it is able to deliver consistent BiV pacing. Frequent ventricular ectopic and atrial tachyarrhythmia can reduce the frequency of BiV pacing and were identified in up to a third of nonresponders to CRT.

There are several mechanisms by which atrial tachyarrhythmia reduce response to CRT. Rapid atrial rates can result in loss of ventricular stimulation, but of equal significance are the detrimental hemodynamic sequelae of the irregularity of the rhythm as well as the loss of intrinsic atrial function. A strategy of attempting to maintain sinus rhythm using pharmacological therapy in patients with heart failure conferred no benefit over a strategy of rate control. Other strategies to increase the frequency of BiV pacing include both catheter ablation. Recent work has suggested that this approach may even confer a survival benefit in patients with AF and heart failure. AV junction ablation is an alternative strategy in patients with AF and whilst rendering the patient-pacing dependent, appears highly effective when combined with BiV pacing. As such, this practice is endorsed in the most recent guidelines.

Ventricular extrasystolic beats (VPCs) can similarly disrupt the efficient function of a CRT system, reducing the frequency of effective BiV pacing and as such, contributing to non-response. Here the therapeutic target is to minimize the occurrence of such events with either pharmacological therapy or catheter ablation.[3]

Programming and Optimization

Appropriate programming can increase the frequency of BiV pacing but is also essential in order to ensure the optimal mechanical functioning of the heart, which facilitates greater response. The most important settings requiring optimization are the pacing mode, upper and lower rate limits, the LV capture voltage, the stimulation vector and A-V and V-V intervals. Programming a high upper tracking rate ensures BiV pacing is maintained during exercise. Similarly, the LV pacing output should include an adequate safety margin to ensure continual BiV pacing, although some modern devices can automatically adjust this parameter.

Iterative optimization of the A-V and V-V intervals using Doppler echocardiography is the established reference method of achieving optimal programming by ensuring optimal diastolic filling of the LV. Recent large multicenter studies evaluating this practice have shown it to be largely ineffective when compared to the use of empirical programming. A more promising technique, which optimizes the A-V and V-V intervals using an integrated hemodynamic sensor, is currently undergoing further assessment.[4]

BIVENTRICULAR ENDOCARDIAL PACING

The persistent rate of nonresponse to transvenous, epicardial CRT has led to the development of novel forms of undertaking CRT. Of these, BiV endocardial pacing (BiV ENDO), where LV stimulation occurs from within the LV cavity, holds a great deal of promise. This technique is associated with several advantages over epicardial activation. BiV ENDO pacing can be achieved using several different approaches including the use of novel, leadless pacing.

Benefits of Biventricular Endocardial Pacing

A large body of evidence exists highlighting the potential benefits of BiV ENDO CRT. Failure to implant an LV lead in a tributary of the coronary sinus during a transvenous, epicardial CRT procedure occurs in around 5–15% of cases. With improvements in delivery, kit in conjunction with greater operator experience and the widespread adoption of quadripolar pacing leads failure to implant an LV lead now occurs in under 5% of cases. This can occur due to difficulty cannulating the coronary sinus ostium or passing the LV lead into a CS branch, unsatisfactory pacing parameters or phrenic nerve stimulation (PNS) associated with LV pacing. Where LV lead implantation is feasible, it is confined to the available anatomy of the CS. Hence, the final lead position is dependent on the presence of a suitable target vein and when none exists, it may be necessary to accept a suboptimal position. In addition, around 26% of patients undergoing an upgrade procedure from a preexisting bradycardia pacing system may have central venous stenosis preventing the implantation of a transvenous LV lead. In this population, it can prove impossible to implant an LV lead in 20–50% of patients.

BiV ENDO pacing is not reliant on the CS anatomy and instead, operators can choose to deliver stimulation at any site within the LV cavity. This allows for customization of the stimulation site based on the patient's pathology and physiology. In addition, whilst lead-based pacing systems may still encounter issues such as central venous stenosis and occlusion, particularly in the upgrade population, newer wireless pacing systems, which can be delivered, via a retrograde aortic approach eliminate the need for central venous access.[5]

PHRENIC NERVE STIMULATION AND ACTIVATION THRESHOLD

Clinically PNS can complicate LV lead deployment during transvenous, epicardial CRT implantation and this complication is encountered in over 20% of patients at implant or at follow-up. Unfortunately, the likelihood of encountering PNS increases when the lead is deployed at sites most associated LV reverse remodeling. Reducing the LV pacing output is a recognized technique for overcoming PNS and it is important to note that endocardial capture thresholds appear lower than equivalent parameters observed during BiV EPI. Besides, if PNS is encountered during implantation of a BiV ENDO pacing system, the operator has the freedom of the entire LV cavity to select an alternative pacing site. Endocardial stimulation of the LV facilitates more rapid myocardial depolarization wave front propagation occurs along the shorter endocardial surface of the heart. This rapid activation is the earlier recruitment of fast conducting Purkinje fibers with the capability of quickly disseminating activation.[6]

ARRHYTHMOGENESIS

Cardiac resynchronization therapy delivers electrical stimulation to the epicardial surface of the LV wall. This pattern of activation is juxtaposed to the sequence exhibited during intrinsic myocardial activation, which follows an endocardial to epicardial course. Reversing the normal depolarization sequence is thought to promote repolarization heterogeneity, which can prolong the QTc interval in susceptible patients and result in malignant arrhythmias, BiV ENDO pacing was associated with reductions in both QT dispersion and T peak to end, two important markers of dispersion of repolarization.[7]

IMPROVING RESPONSE THROUGH ENDOCARDIAL PACING

BiV ENDO pacing has the capability to achieve greater electrical resynchronization and consequently, maximize response to CRT. Traditionally, BiV ENDO pacing has been performed in a relatively small number of patients, typically those with failure to achieve conventional CRT or those that have been nonresponders. The recently published ALternate Site Cardiac ResYNChronization (ALSYNC) study was the first multicenter study of LV endocardial pacing and demonstrated the feasibility and safety of LV endocardial CRT delivered through the atrial transseptal approach. The acute hemodynamic benefits of BiV ENDO appear superior to those achievable utilizing BiV EPI, even amongst a cohort of ischemic, nonresponders to conventional epicardial CRT. When a direct comparison between BiV ENDO and BiV EPI was performed, the optimal endocardial location appeared superior to the optimal epicardial pacing site.[8]

BIVENTRICULAR ENDOCARDIAL PACING SYSTEMS

Lead-Based Pacing Systems

Chronic BiV ENDO CRT has traditionally been delivered via a pacing lead delivered via either a transventricular-septal or atrial-septal puncture. Due to the risk of thrombus formation resulting in systemic embolization, lead-based LV endocardial pacing requires lifelong anticoagulation. Following a transseptal implant, the potential also exists for an adverse interaction between the mitral valve and an LV lead, which passes through it. The presence of a pacing lead can worsen valvular regurgitation and this phenomenon has been acknowledged with right-sided leads. Reassuringly in the largest series of transseptal LV endocardial pacing to date, no system-related valvular complications were recorded. Instead, echocardiography showed reductions in mitral regurgitation because of improved LV function. The other major concern is the increased risk of mitral valve endocarditis should the system become infected. Secondary infectious foci including both cerebral and renal abscess formation are associated with the systemic embolization of vegetation.[9]

Atrial Transseptal

Lead-based BiV ENDO is predominantly delivered via the atrial transseptal approach. Superior and inferior access is frequently required in order to puncture the atrial septum and successfully position the lead in the LV although several refinements of this procedure have been described.

Ventricular Transseptal

Ventricular transseptal techniques allow the deployment of the lead using only superior access, eliminating the need for femoral punctures. This approach may be associated with both a lower risk of stroke and disruption to mitral valve function by eliminating the presence of pacing leads in the left atrium crossing the mitral valve, although a target INR of 2.5–3 is still recommended.

Apical Transseptal

A hybrid surgical/percutaneous approach has also been described where the LV apex is accessed via a mini-thoracotomy facilitating the deployment of a lead at the LV apex, which is then tunneled up to a generator, implanted in the conventional subclavicular position. Whilst the results from this series of 20 patients appear promising, this is a more invasive option and a higher target international normalized ratio (INR) of 3–3.5 is recommended.

Leadless Pacing Systems

Whilst chronic BiV ENDO delivered via a pacing lead currently requires ongoing anticoagulants due to the risk of thrombus formation, newer wireless technology eliminated this risk. Formal anticoagulation is not required and this development increases the likelihood of endocardial pacing becoming more widespread.

TRANSARTERIAL LEADLESS LV ENDOCARDIAL PACING

A leadless BiV ENDO CRT pacing system has been developed, which eliminates the need for any form of pacing lead to be present within the left ventricle. Instead, stimulation is delivered to the endocardial surface of the heart acoustically from an ultrasound pulse generator, implanted subcutaneously in an intercostal space. The ultrasound waves stimulate a small receiver-electrode, which is deployed percutaneously via the femoral artery, into the LV cavity. Acoustic ultrasound energy is converted to an electronic pacing pulse by the receiver electrode. RV pacing, resulting in near simultaneous (within 3 ms) LV and RV endocardial activation triggers the pulse generator. Early clinical studies evaluating this system confirmed implantation was safe and capable of achieving consistent BiV capture whilst more recent work has shown the system to be highly efficacious and associated with a clinical response rate of 84.8%.

TRANSVENOUS LEADLESS LV ENDOCARDIAL PACING

The most commonly encountered complication associated with the use of the WiSE CRT system is femoral arterial access complications. In addition, not every patient has suitable anatomy to allow sufficient arterial access to allow the insertion of the electrode delivery catheter. Ischemic heart disease is common in this population and as such, concurrent peripheral vascular disease is frequently encountered. A method of transvenously accessing the LV cavity via an atrial transseptal puncture has been described to facilitate deployment of the pacing electrode.

CONCLUSION

Cardiac resynchronization therapy in congestive heart failure is very promising therapy. However, nonresponse to CRT is a multifactorial issue. Improving patient selection and postimplant device troubleshooting remains the cornerstone of optimizing patient outcomes. Whilst newer lead technology including multipoint pacing and a greater focus on the importance of site selection are likely to be beneficial, the limitations of transvenous, epicardial CRT are widely acknowledged. In patients where implanting a transvenous lead is not possible, consideration should be given to endocardial pacing. Newer leadless LV endocardial systems no longer mandate lifelong anticoagulation. In addition, endocardial pacing appears capable of yielding more effective electromechanical resynchronization. Given the ability to stimulate the LV from any location, this technique would appear to offer a significant benefit to patients where transvenous lead implantation is restricted to inferior sites.

REFERENCES

1. Tracy CM, Epstein AE, Darbar D, et al.; American College of Cardiology Foundation, American Heart Association Task Force on Practice Guidelines, Heart Rhythm Society. 2012 ACCF/AHA/HRS focused update of the 2008 guidelines for device-based therapy of cardiac rhythm abnormalities: a report of the American College of Cardiology Foundation/ American Heart Association Task Force on Practice Guidelines and the Heart Rhythm Society. [corrected]. Circulation. 2012;126(14):1784-800.
2. Birnie DH, Tang AS. The problem of non-response to cardiac resynchronization therapy. Curr Opin Cardiol. 2006;21(1):20-6.
3. Zareba W, Klein H, Cygankiewicz I, et al.; MADIT-CRT Investigators. Effectiveness of cardiac resynchronization therapy by QRS Morphology in the Multicenter Automatic Defibrillator Implantation Trial-Cardiac Resynchronization Therapy (MADIT-CRT). Circulation. 2011;123(10):1061-72.
4. Auricchio A, Fantoni C, Regoli F, et al. Characterization of left ventricular activation in patients with heart failure and left bundle-branch block. Circulation. 2004;109(9):1133-9.
5. Sweeney MO, Hellkamp AS, Ellenbogen KA, et al.; Mode Selection Trial Investigators. Adverse effect of ventricular pacing on heart failure and atrial fibrillation among patients with normal baseline QRS duration in a clinical trial of pacemaker therapy for sinus node dysfunction. Circulation. 2003;107(23):2932-7.
6. Zanon F, Baracca E, Pastore G, et al. Multipoint pacing by a left ventricular quadripolar lead improves the acute hemodynamic response to CRT compared with conventional biventricular pacing at any site. Heart Rhythm. 2015;12(5):975-81.
7. Reddy VY, Miller MA, Neuzil P, et al. Cardiac resynchronization therapy with wireless left ventricular endocardial pacing: The SELECT-LV Study. J Am Coll Cardiol. 2017;69(17):2119-29.
8. Sieniewicz BJ, Gould JS, Rimington HM, et al. Transseptal delivery of a leadless left ventricular endocardial pacing electrode. JACC Clin Electrophysiol. 2017;3(11):1333-5.
9. James SA, Rinaldi CA, Turley AJ, et al. First-in-man implantation of a leadless endocardial left ventricular pacing system (WISE-CRT) utilising a trans-septal approach. Hear. Rhythm. 2018;20(Suppl 4):iv16.

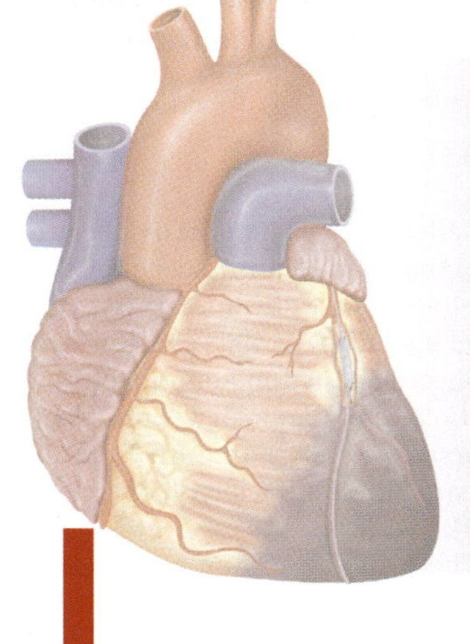

Drug Switch or A Device: How do I Decide?

Bagirath Raghuraman

INTRODUCTION

Better understanding of the mechanisms involved in heart failure (HF) coupled with giant strides in technology has led to exciting new innovations in the management of HF. These innovations are now revolutionizing the way HF is diagnosed and treated. Overall, this will translate into more accurate diagnosis and lead to better outcomes in the form of better quality of life and improved survival. Several high-level advances have been made in basic components including battery technology, the electronic components and materials which has enabled researchers to produce excellent new generation devices for HF that are cheaper, more efficacious, and can be individualized and customized according to each patient's requirement.

INNOVATIONS IN DIAGNOSTICS

Next-generation biomarkers which show promise are sST2, GDF-15, Gal-3, and miRNAs. These biomarkers are slowly adding value either alone in addition to established biomarkers or clinical variables in HF diagnosis and risk prediction. Multimarker approaches have definitely shown benefit over single biomarkers and soon research will bring up the best biomarker combination for HF management. At present, only brain natriuretic peptide (BNP), Nt-proBNP, and MR-proANP should be used in the context of HF diagnosis, prognosis and to monitor therapy.[1]

BREAKTHROUGHS IN MEDICINE

Ivabradine

Ivabradine, which is a sinus node inhibitor, was approved for the treatment of HF patients after the results and outcomes in chronic HF trial [SHIFT (Systolic Heart Failure Treatment with the IF Inhibitor Ivabradine Trial)].[2] The SHIFT study reported that a reduction in heart rate by 10 beats per minute over and above optimal therapy, was associated with an 18% relative risk reduction for cardiovascular death and hospitalization for worsening of HF ($p < 0.0001$), in patients with HF in sinus rhythm with a heart rate of ≥70 beats/min.

Angiotensin Receptor Neprilysin Inhibitor

As per the PARADIGM HF [Prospective Comparison of ARNI with Angiotensin-Converting Enzyme Inhibitor (ACEI) to Determine Impact on Global Mortality and Morbidity in Heart Failure] trial data, angiotensin receptor neprilysin inhibitor (ARNI) when compared with enalapril, reduced the risk of hospitalization for HF by 21% ($p < 0.001$) and decreased the symptoms and physical limitations of HF ($p = 0.001$). The ARNI group had higher proportions of patients with hypotension and nonserious angioedema but lower proportions with renal impairment, hyperkalemia, and cough than the enalapril group. The study concluded that ARNI was superior to enalapril in reducing the risks of death and of hospitalization for HF.[3]

Selective Antagonist of Mitofusin 1(Mfn1)-β2PKC Association[4]

We now know that β2PKC alters Mfn1 phosphorylation which damages the mitochondria. Of the six molecules that could block this β2PKC-Mfn1 interaction only selective antagonist of mitofusin 1-β2PKC association (SAMβA) did it in a way that did not affect β2PKC's other interactions. SAMβA treatment reestablishes mitochondrial morphology and function and improves cardiac contractility in rats with HF, suggesting that SAMβA may be a potential treatment for patients with HF. SAMβA also reduced a marker of oxidative stress in the heart cells which triggers cell death.

Riociguat

Riociguat is a member of the new class of compounds—soluble guanylate cyclase stimulators and has been found to be beneficial in the treatment of chronic thromboembolic pulmonary hypertension and right HF.[5]

Newer Inotropic Agents[6]

Conventionally dopamine, dobutamine, noradrenaline, adrenaline, milrinone, levosimendan and digoxin have been used since decades. Newer inotropes that have shown promise in recent clinical trials are listed in Table 1.

Further studies are required to establish the safety and efficacy of newer inotropic agents mentioned in Table 2.[7]

TABLE 2: Newer inotropic agents with mechanism.

Drugs	*Inotropic mechanism*
Nitroxyl donor, CXL-1020	SERCA activation plus vasodilation
Gene transfer	SERCA activation
Ryanodine receptor stabilizer; S44121	Ryanodine receptor stabilization
Etomoxir, Pyruvate	Energetic modulation

INNOVATIONS IN MONITORING SYSTEMS

Indwelling Monitoring Systems

CardioMEMS

The CardioMEMS system uses a miniaturized, wireless monitoring sensor that is implanted through femoral vein access into the pulmonary artery (PA) to directly measure pulmonary arterial pressure. Measuring PA pressure allows clinicians to proactively manage treatment with medication changes for patients with worsening HF before visible symptoms, such as weight gain and blood pressure changes occur. The system allows patients to transmit their PA pressure data from the comfort of their homes to their health-care providers, who then manage appropriate medication changes through phone or house visits. This reduces the likelihood of hospitalization. There is robust data from the CHAMPION (CardioMEMS Heart Sensor Allows Monitoring of Pressure to Improve Outcomes in NYHA Class III Heart Failure Patients) trial to support the benefit from the CardioMEMS device (Fig. 1).[8]

INNOVATIONS IN MEDICAL DEVICES

What's New in AICDs and CRT-D Space?

Within the past years, breakthroughs in sensor and nanotechnology have made automated implantable

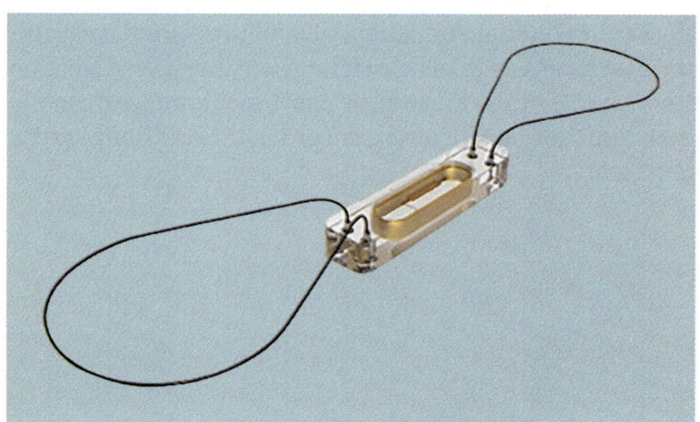

Fig. 1: CardioMEMS device.

TABLE 1: Newer inotropes with their action and class.

Inotrope	*Inotrope class*	*Action*	*Half life*	*Excretion*
Istaroxime	Na-K pump inhibitor and SERCA2a stimulator	Inhibits Na-K antiporter àincrease Ca intracellularly, stimulates SERCA2 on the sarcoplasmic reticulum, improves Ca management, Increases lusitropy	<1 hr	Systemic conversion to less active metabolite
Omecamtiv mecarbil	Myosin/Actin cross bridge enhancer	Interacts with ATPase on myosin, improving myosin/actin interaction	18.5 hrs	Renal and gastrointestinal excretion

cardioverter defibrillators (AICDs) and cardiac resynchronization therapy-defibrillators (CRT-Ds) safer and more reliable. Previously, the devices were imprecise at times and occasionally gave inappropriate shocks. Now, we can place multiple sensors more precisely in different chambers of the heart, allowing greater coordination. We can even convert nonresponders into good responders due to this fascinating leap of miniaturization technology. The newest pacemakers and defibrillators also contain sensors that can monitor other parameters like oxygen levels in the blood, physical activity, body temperature, adrenaline and hormone levels, and sync all that information to regulate the patient's heart rate more akin to what the heart does naturally.

CARDIAC CONTRACTILITY MODULATOR

Cardiac contractility modulation is a form of therapy using a cardiac contractility modulator which is intended for the treatment of patients with moderate to severe HF (NYHA class II–IV) who are symptomatic despite optimal medical therapy who can benefit from an improvement in cardiac output. The form of therapy enhances the strength of ventricular contraction and therefore the heart's pumping capacity by adjusting the myocardial contractility. The advantages of Chagas cardiomyopathy (CCM) over CRT-D is that it can be used in patients without left bundle branch block (LBBB), atrial fibrillation, CRT failures/nonresponders and in selected cases of heart failure with preserved ejection fraction (HFpEF). Further, it can be charged externally obviating the need for a surgical procedure to change pulse generators.[9]

AICD AND CRT-D BASED HOME MONITORING SYSTEMS

These devices can be used for home monitoring to detect arrhythmias and changes in the PA pressure. Most of these remote monitoring systems use a bedside base unit that collects and sends the patient information at night when the patient is sleeping. However, providers are starting to move toward interfacing the implantable devices to mobile devices or the patient's smartphones to enable constant monitoring (Table 3 and Figs. 2 and 3).

App based monitoring of HF patients is fast catching up as a way of keeping in touch with patients and picking them up early for more aggressive treatment in order to prevent hospitalization. "Dhadkan" from AIIMS and "Kaizala" from Narayana Health are front runners in using app based HF monitoring.

WEARABLES

Smart watch based monitoring keeps a tab on heart rate and blood pressure and alerts the healthcare provider if there is any abnormality. This has revolutionized patient monitoring by providing continuous data and constant alerts. Numerous devices are now available ranging from watches and bands to patches which can monitor heart rate

TABLE 3: Home monitoring system with company name.

Home monitoring system	*Company/Provider*
Merlin	Abbot
CardioMessenger Smart	Biotronic
MyCareLink—first app-based monitoring	Medtronic

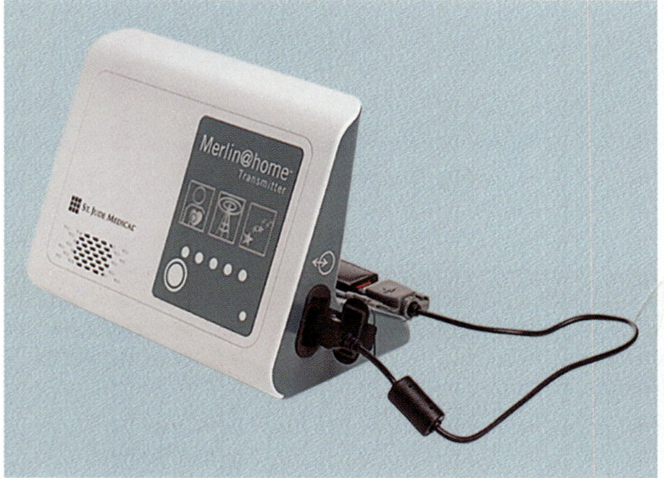

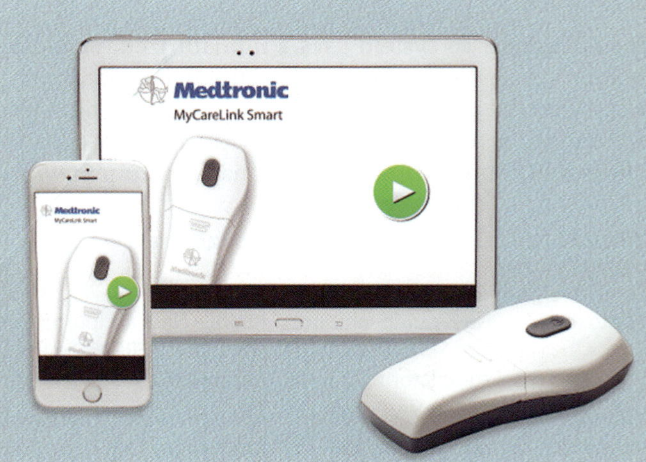

Fig. 2: Follow-up and feedback on smartphone: The world in your palm.

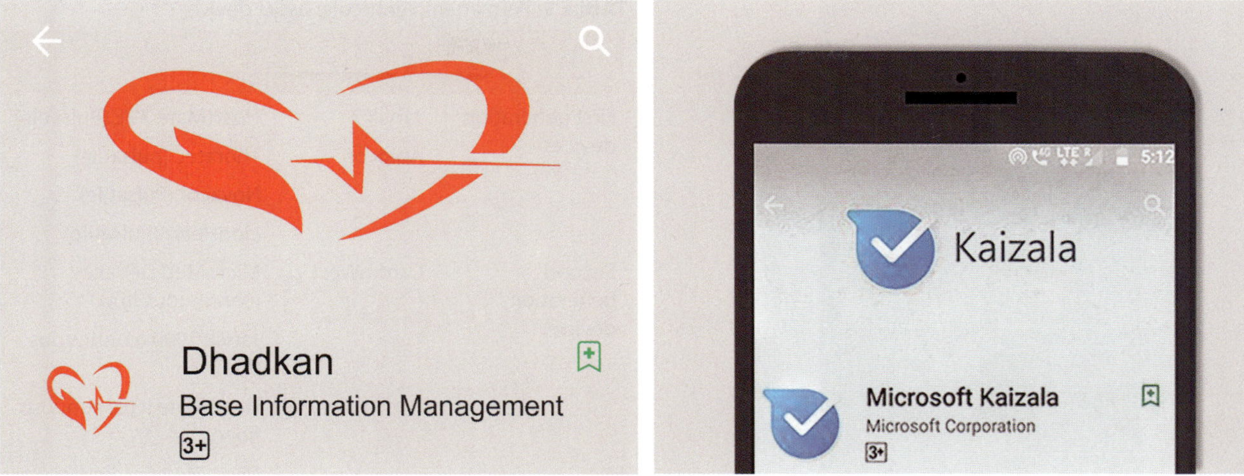

Fig. 3: App-based monitoring.

and record echocardiography (ECG) to detect arrhythmias (Fig. 4).

ULTRAFILTRATION

Aquapheresis therapy is extremely for treatment of patients with enormous volume overload. It can be done using AquadexFlexFlow System which uses a simplified approach to ultrafiltration for the removal of salt and water in patients with hypervolemia, or fluid overload. Compared to renal replacement devices used for ultrafiltration, the AquadexFlexFlow system is smaller and more portable. With this innovation, we can specify and adjust the exact amount and rate of fluid to be removed from each patient, resulting in a gradual reduction that has been shown to have no significant clinical impact on blood pressure, heart rate, or the balance of electrolytes (e.g. sodium, potassium, etc.) in the body. About 500 mL/hr of excess fluid can be removed without any clinically significant impact on the electrolyte balance (Fig. 5).[10,11]

TEMPORARY AND PERMANENT VENTRICULAR ASSIST DEVICES

Mechanical circulatory support for temporary or long-term support is increasingly used in the treatment of patients with severe HFrEF who have failed guideline-directed medical therapy (GDMT). Both American College of Cardiology (ACC) and European Society of Cardiology (ESC) guidelines also recommend that short-term mechanical support (nondurable systems) including extracorporeal life support and extracorporeal membrane oxygenation should be used in patients with acute profound HF as "bridge to decision" to gain time for heart transplantation or a permanent assist

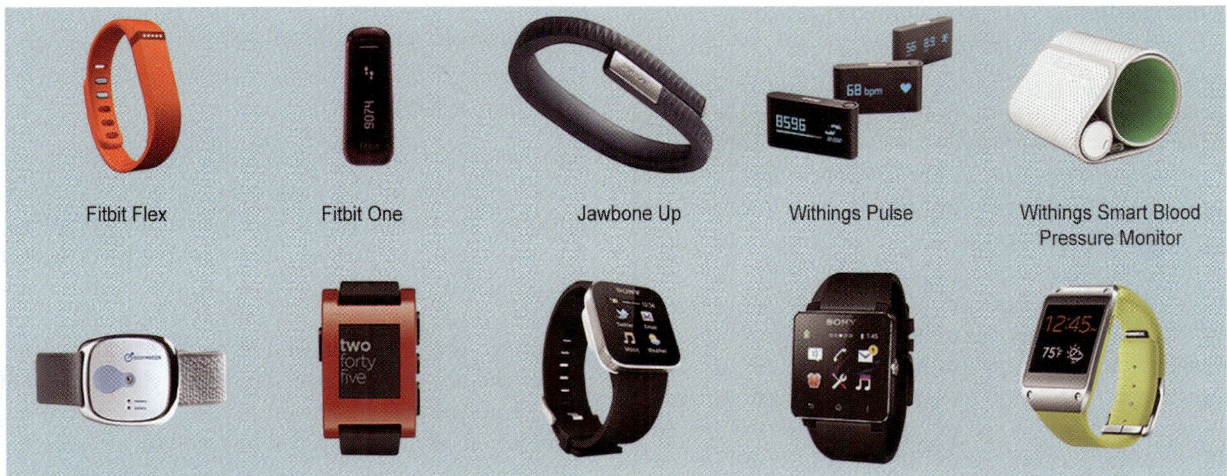

Fig. 4: Wearable devices.

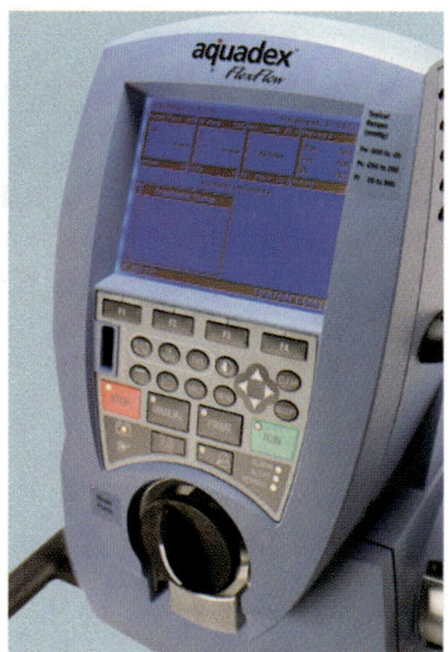

Fig. 5: AquadexFlexFlow system.

device evaluation. Both guidelines recommend that the implantation of a permanent left ventricular (LV) assist device should be considered in carefully selected patients with advanced HF (COR: IIa). The ESC Guidelines makes a distinction between LV assist device for bridge to transplant (COR: IIa LOE: C) and for patients who are not eligible for heart transplantation (COR: IIa, LOE: B) (Tables 4 and 5).[12]

Leviticus Cardio First in Human

The leviticus fully implanted ventricular assist device (FIVAD) system comprises internal and external components powered wirelessly. This is the first ventricular assist device (VAD) system that will allow patients to walk around without any physical impediments. With one charge, it can work for up to 8 hours. The FIVAD incorporates a heart pump produced by Jarvik Heart Inc. Leviticus Cardio's technology uses a receiver inductive coil implanted in the body alongside the VAD, coupled with a battery and an internal controller. An external coil, placed within a vest for easy carrying, charges the inner coil electromagnetically. The biggest limitation thus far in the journey of VADs has been the external cables, controller and battery case with batteries. This leap in technology achieved by Leviticus takes VAD engineering to the next level.

TABLE 4: Temporary assist devices available for use.

Device	Manufacturer
IABP	Maquet/Datascope
Impella	Abiomed
Tandem Heart (Cardiac Assist)	Cardiac Assist, Inc.; Pittsburgh
VA ECMO	Maquet
Centrimag	Abbot
Abiomed BVS 5000	ABIOMED Inc
PulseCath	Terumo
Procyrion	Aortix

(IABP: intra-aortic balloon pump; VA ECMO: venoarterial extracorporeal membrane oxygenation)

TABLE 5: Permanent ventricular assist devices.

Generation	*Total artificial heart*	*Ventricular assist device*
First generation devices	Jarvik 7	HeartMate XVE (Pulsatile)
	Abiocor	Thoratec (pulsatile)
		Novacor (Pulsatile)
		LionHeart (Pulsatile)
Second generation devices	CardioWest	MicroMed DeBakey (continuous flow)
		Jarvik 2000 (continuous flow)
		HeartMate II (continuous flow)
		MicroMed Cardiovascular
		HeartAssist 5 (continuous flow)
		CircuLite Synergy Micro-Pump (continuous flow)
Third generation devices		HeartMate III (Pulsatile)
		HeartMate X (continuous flow)
		HeartWare MVAD (continuous flow)
Fourth generation devices	SynCardia Total artificial heart	Magnevad

(MVAD: miniaturized ventricular assist device)

Heart in a Box

TransMedics' Organ Care System has come up with a concept known as "beating heart in a box"— works by pumping the donor heart with warm, oxygenated, and nutrient-enriched blood. The carbon fiber system is equipped with an oxygen tank, supply of donor blood, batteries, and special electric and mechanical equipment to monitor the organ, as well as a sterile plastic box that houses the donor organ during delivery, keeping it at the right temperature and humidity levels. This concept is extremely useful to keep the heart tissues viable during transport and shorten ischemic time which causes organ damage (Fig. 6).

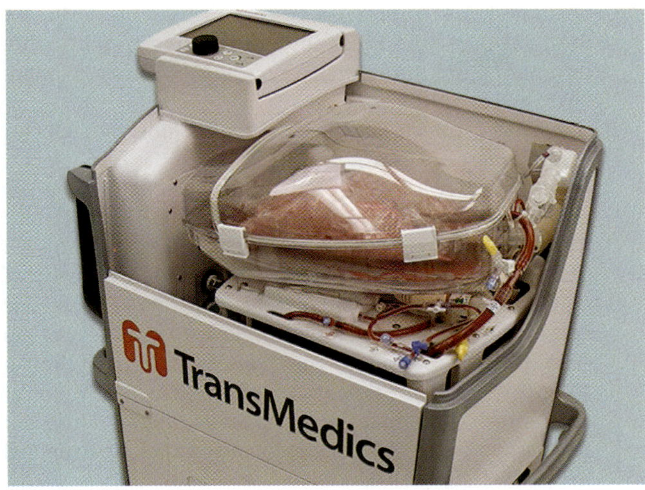

Fig. 6: TransMedics' organ care system.

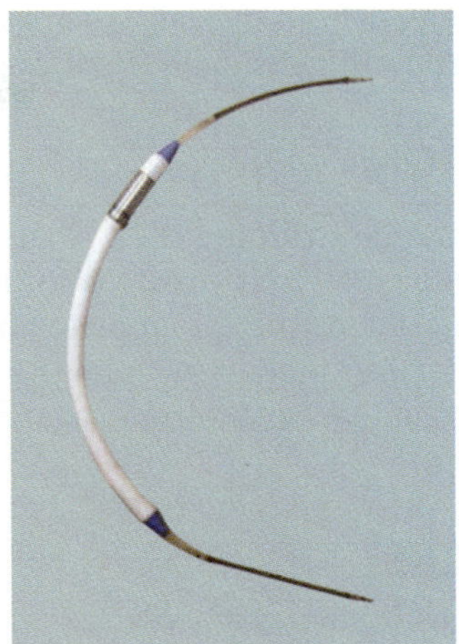

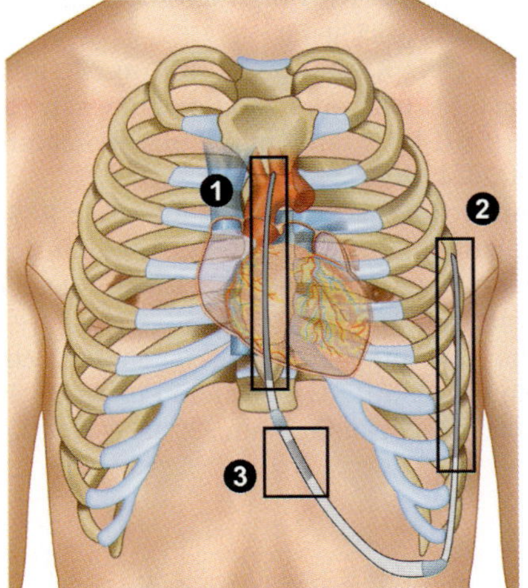

Fig. 7: Implantable defibrillator. 1. Position of the sternal coil, 2. Position of the side coil, 3. Active segment.

WHAT'S ON THE HORIZON

Here are some quick takes on what is coming up that can revolutionize HF management.

Stem Cell Therapy

After several attempts to harness the potential of stem cells, BioCardia which is a clinical-stage biotechnology-regenerative medicine company that is a front runner in innovative therapeutics for HF has come up with stem cells include CardiAMP™ Therapy and CardiALLO™ Therapy, which focus on HF resulting from heart attacks. The company was co-founded by Dr Simon Stertzer, who performed the first coronary balloon angioplasty in the US in 1978.

Implantable Defibrillators (Fig. 7)

This device was designed by Newpace. It involves using an implantable string subcutaneous defibrillator (ISSD) without a metal pulse generator. There are no leads within the heart. The implantation time is 20 minutes and extremely useful in sick HF patients who are unfit for longer procedure times. The device can be connected to a smartphone.

Robotic Sleeve

This device developed by Harvard University and Boston Children's Hospital researchers is useful for patients with thinned out heart muscle. The robot syncs with the heart through a thin silicone sleeve with soft pneumatic actuators that mimic the heart's outer muscle layers. It does so without any direct contact with the blood, as is the case with most currently available devices. This removes the need for potentially dangerous blood thinner medications.

3D Bioprinted Heart Tissue

Biolife4D has come up with a concept to bioprint a human cardiac muscle patch, which can be sutured over an area of dead heart muscle to speed up recovery from acute HF. The entire process involves reprograming a patient's blood cells into stem cells, which are then mutated to produce the specific types of cells suitable for the 3D bioengineering of a human heart.

Artificial Intelligence Algorithms

All devices and chips will be integrated with artificial intelligence (AI) systems and this will help to accurately monitor and alert physicians to treat patients better. It can even suggest ways to manage a crisis situation and help remote management from specialists across the globe. This is a fascinating new dimension in HF management.

CONCLUSION

Various biomarkers including sST2, GDF-15, Gal-3 and miRNAs besides BNP, Nt-proBNP and MR-proANP have important diagnostic, prognostic and therapeutic implications after drug therapy including ARNI, Ivabradine, SAMβA, Riociguat, Newer Inotropic agents, and various device therapies.

REFERENCES

1. Magnussen C, Blankenberg S. Biomarkers for heart failure: Small molecules with high clinical relevance. J Intern Med. 2018;283(6):530-43.
2. Swedberg K, Komajda M, Böhm M, et al.; SHIFT investigators. Ivabradine and outcomes in chronic heart failure (SHIFT): A randomised placebo-controlled study. Lancet. 2010;376(9744):875-85.
3. McMurray JJ, Packer M, Desai AS, et al.; PARADIGM-HF Investigators and Committees. Angiotensin-neprilysin inhibition versus enalapril in heart failure. N Engl J Med. 2014; 371(11):993-1004.
4. Ferreira JC, Campos JC, Qvit N, et al. A selective inhibitor of mitofusin 1-βIIPKC association improves heart failure outcome in rats. Nat Commun. 2019;10(1):329.
5. Ghofrani HA, D'Armini AM, Grimminger F, et al.; CHEST-1 Study Group. Riociguat for the treatment of chronic thromboembolic pulmonary hypertension. N Engl J Med. 2013;369(4):319-29.
6. Ginwalla M, Tofovic DS. Current status of inotropes in heart failure. Heart Fail Clin. 2018;14(4):601-16.
7. Hasenfuss G, Teerlink JR. Cardiac inotropes: Current agents and future directions. Eur Heart J. 2011;32(15):1838-45.
8. Abraham WT, Stevenson LW, Bourge RC, et al. CHAMPION Trial Study Group. Sustained efficacy of pulmonary artery pressure to guide adjustment of chronic heart failure therapy: Complete follow-up results from the CHAMPION randomised trial. Lancet. 2016; 387(10017): 453-61.
9. Abi-Samra F, Gutterman D. Cardiac contractility modulation: A novel approach for the treatment of heart failure. Heart Fail Rev. 2016;21(6):645-60.
10. Bart BA, Boyle A, Bank AJ, et al. Ultrafiltration versus usual care for hospitalized patients with heart failure: The relief for acutely fluid-overloaded patients with decompensated congestive heart failure (RAPID-CHF) trial. J Am Coll Cardiol. 2005;46(11):2043-6.
11. Jaski BE, Ha J, Denys BG, et al. Peripherally inserted veno-venous ultrafiltration for rapid treatment of volume overloaded patients. J Card Fail. 2003;9(3):227-31.
12. van der Meer P, Gaggin HK, Dec GW. ACC/AHA Versus ESC Guidelines on Heart Failure: JACC Guideline Comparison. J Am Coll Cardiol. 2019;73(21):2756-68.

CHAPTER 87

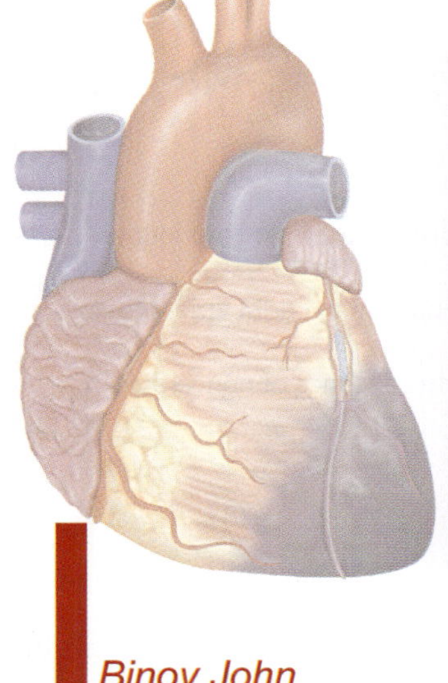

Use of Left Ventricular Assist Devices in Heart Failure

Binoy John

INTRODUCTION

Advances in coronary and cardiac care have facilitated prolonged survival and the life expectancy of the general population globally. However, this increased survival has come at the cost of more and more patients ending up with heart failure (HF) as they aged, due to various etiologies. HF is a global pandemic and world over, it is estimated that at least 26 million people suffer from HF and in Asia the prevalence of HF is found to be higher than that of the west, affecting 1.3–6.7% of the population. In India, it is estimated that 1.3–4.6 million people are affected by HF, with 0.5–1.8 million new cases of HF being diagnosed every year, which actually may be an underestimate. Though heart transplantation, which was performed first by Dr Christiaan Barnard in South Africa in 1967, more than five decades ago is considered the gold-standard in the treatment of advanced and refractory HF, the number of heart transplantations that happen globally is only 3,800–4,600 per year due to a stark shortage in donor hearts available for transplantation. It is this unmet need that has paved way for the rise of the machines, the mechanical circulatory support (MCS) devices or ventricular assist devices (VADs).

DEFINITION OF HEART FAILURE

Heart failure is a complex clinical syndrome that results from any structural or functional impairment of ventricular filling or ejection of blood. From a physiologic perspective, HF is defined as an inadequate cardiac output to meet metabolic demands or can be an adequate cardiac output secondary to compensatory neurohormonal activation, generally manifesting as increased left ventricular filling pressure. The American College of Cardiology (ACC)/ American Heart Association (AHA) have staged HF as Stages A, B, C, and D (Table 1).[1]

TABLE 1: ACC/AHA stages of heart failure.

Stages	Symptoms
A	At high risk for HF but without structural heart disease or symptoms of HF
B	Structural heart disease but without signs or symptoms of HF
C	Structural heart disease with prior or current symptoms of HF
D	Refractory HF requiring specialized interventions

(ACC: American College of Cardiology; AHA: American Heart Association; HF: heart failure)

The 5-year survival of stage A HF is 97%, stage B HF is 86%, stage C HF is 75%, and stage D is only 20%. The absolute mortality rate from HF is approximately 50% within 5 years of diagnosis of HF, despite advances in treatment. Once hospitalized and discharged, the need for repeated hospitalizations for these advanced HF patients becomes more frequent, with a 1 month hospital readmission rate as high as 25% (Table 2).[2]

Heart transplantation is the treatment of choice for advanced HF. But when donor hearts are not available or when the patient is not a heart transplant candidate, MCS devices are considered as an alternative and are used as appropriate to the clinical scenario.

TABLE 2: Definition of advanced heart failure.

1	Severe symptoms of heart failure with dyspnea or fatigue at rest, or with minimal exertion (New York Heart Association functional class III or IV)
2	Episodes of fluid retention (Pulmonary or systematic congestion, peripheral edema), or reduced cardiac output at rest (Peripheral hypoperfusion)
3	Objective evidence of severe cardiac dysfunction, shown by at least one of the following: a. Low left ventricular ejection fraction (30%) b. Severe abnormality of cardiac function on Doppler Echocardiography with a pseudonormal or restrictive mitral inflow pattern c. High left ventricular filling pressures (Mean pulmonary capillary wedge pressure >16 mm Hg, or mean right atrial pressure >12 mm Hg by pulmonary artery catheterization) d. High brain natriuretic peptide or N-terminal pro-brain natriuretic peptide plasma levels, in the absence of noncardiac causes
4	Severe impairment of functinoal capacity shown by one of the following: a. Inability to exercise b. 6-minute walk test distance <300 m or less in women or patients aged ≥75 years c. Peak oxygen consumption <12 to 14 mL/kg/min
5	History of at least one heart failure hospitalization in the past 6 months
6	Presence of all the previous features despite 'attempts to optimize therapy, including diuretics. Inhibitors of the rennin-angiotensin-aldosterone system, and β-blockers, unless these are poorly tolerated or contraindicated, and cardiac resynchronization therapy, when indicated

Mechanical circulatory support devices are essentially pumps which are designed either to assist or replace the function of the left or right ventricles of the heart or both and thereby assisting the systemic circulation to improve the perfusion of the organs and tissues.

The VADs are typically used in three clinical scenarios. First, as a bridge-to-transplant (BTT) indication, to stabilize a patient wait listed for cardiac transplantation until a donor heart is available; second, as a bridge-to-candidacy (BTC) indication, to stabilize a patient with the anticipation to enable possible future listing for heart transplant; and third, as a destination therapy (DT) indication, where the patient is given a VAD as a terminal treatment, as he is not a candidate for heart transplantation. But the patients who are placed on LVAD as DT are done so with the intention of BTT except for those patients who are contraindicated for cardiac transplant.

The salient features which categorize a MCS device comprise the ventricle or ventricles supported, the pump characteristics, the location of the pumping chamber, the mechanism of the pump, and the duration of support intended. VADs may be used on the left ventricle (LVAD), right ventricle (RVAD) or in both ventricles (BiVAD). Based on the pump characteristics the MCS devices may be pulsatile or nonpulsatile. The device pump can be extracorporeal (e.g. extracorporeal membrane oxygenation or ECMO, levitronix centrimag, impella) when located outside the body, paracorporeal (e.g. Berlin Heart Excor) when located outside the body, but adjacent to the body, intracorporeal (e.g. HeartMate IIP/VE, Novacor N100, HeartMate 3, HeartWare, HVAD, Jarvic 2000) when implanted within the body, or orthotopic in position as with the total artificial heart (TAH) (e.g. SynCardia, BiVacor). The earlier intracorporeal devices were all pulsatile devices and were very bulky and of poor durability with a propensity for malfunction and complications, which resulted in the patients being bedridden due to higher stroke rates and poor outcomes. These could only be used in larger patients. Thereafter, smaller versions were made and were implanted intra-abdominally, facilitating movement of these patients, but still suffered from high rates of device failure and lack of durability and higher rates of infections.[3]

HISTORY OF MECHANICAL CIRCULATORY SUPPORT

Mechanical circulation was initially introduced to facilitate open heart surgery and subsequently, the machines have evolved significantly since the development of the first cardiopulmonary bypass device, the Gibbon-IBM heart-lung machine. The Gibbon-IBM heart-lung machine was first used in 1953 for an atrial septal defect closure, by Dr Gibbon during an atrial septal defect closure in an 18-year-old lady.[4]

The first VAD however was implanted in 1963 by Dr DeBakey and Dr Liotta[5] in a patient named George

Washington, who went into a cardiac arrest after aortic valve replacement. The inflow of the VAD was attached to the left atrium and the outflow to the descending thoracic aorta achieving improvements in pump flows, and the patient improved until his death on the fourth postoperative day following brain damage, secondary to the cardiac arrest. The first TAH was performed in 1969, in a 47-year-old man, Haskell Karp with ischemic cardiomyopathy, who was awaiting cardiac transplantation at the St Luke's Episcopal Hospital, Houston as a BTT by Dr Cooley and Dr Liotta.[6] The patient underwent left ventricular aneurysmectomy after which the patient could not be weaned off the heart-lung machine and so a Liotta-TAH, a pneumatically powered pump with Dacron lined grafts and mechanical valves was implanted by Cooley and Liotta. The patient survived for 64 hours on TAH support, however, died of pseudomonas pneumonia, 32 hours postcardiac transplant. The continued development of the TAH resulted in the Akutsu III designed by Dr Tetsuzo Akutsu in 1970, which was thereafter implanted by Dr Cooley and colleagues as a BTT in 1981 in a patient with postcardiotomy shock after coronary artery bypass graft surgery.[7]

The first TAH as DT was performed by Dr DeVries in 1982 in the 61-year-old Dr Barney Clark who was diagnosed with nonischemic cardiomyopathy. He used the Jarvik 7 which was designed by Dr Jarvik. The patient however succumbed to death after 112 days following multiple complications like renal failure, pseudomembranous colitis, gastrointestinal bleeding, epistaxis, and aspiration pneumonia. The longest duration of usage of the Jarvik 7 was 620 days which was however complicated with infections and strokes.[8]

The first successful isolated LVAD implant was with the Novacor left ventricular assist system (LVAS) in 1984 as a BTT.[9] The Novacor LVAS was an electric, dual pusher-plate device that was constructed of a polyurethane pump sac with gelatin-sealed inflow and outflow grafts containing porcine bioprosthetic valves which facilitated unidirectional flow.[10] It was only in 1994, after three decades of work on MCS and the first announcement of the National Heart, Lung and Blood Institute (NHLBI) Artificial Heart program in 1964, that it was possible for the first patient with a pulsatile flow LVAD to be discharged from the hospital. The procedure was done by Dr OH Frazier.[11]

The first generation MCS devices which were introduced in 1980s were paracorporeal, pulsatile, and volume displacement pumps which were large in size, dependent on the preload and associated with poor durability (e.g. Thoratec PVAD, Abiomed BVS 5000, HeartMate XVE, and Novacor LVAS).

The second generation continuous flow nonpulsatile pumps were smaller in profile and capable of a similar degree of pumping support (10 L/min) and more durable and functionally dependent on both preload and afterload (e.g. HeartMate II, HeartWare and Jarvik, 2000). The second generation LVADs incorporated smaller continuous axial flow pumps, placement of which needed only less extensive surgery thereby decreasing surgical morbidity and mortality and could also be used in smaller sized patients. These were more durable, with lower thrombogenicity and thus lower stroke incidence. The better durability of these second generation pumps is because they have only a single moving part. The prototype of this second generation device is the HeartMate II. This is the LVAD which has been used maximally, with over 20,000 implants globally. This device conferred better survival rates and less organ failure in contrast to the first generation VADs. One-year survival with second generation devices are 81% for BTT and 73% for DT[12,13] though they still felt short vis-a-vis cardiac transplantation with 90% 1-year survival. Importantly, these modern devices enabled better self-care, gave better quality of life to the patients post-implant, facilitating ease of out-patient care and management.

The third generation LVADs are continuous flow devices which have been engineered to minimize contact between the pump and the axial rotor with the use of magnetic levitation technology, thereby also reducing the wear and tear of the device. The small size also enables implantation of the device under the pericardium and thus minimizing postoperative complications (e.g. HeartMate 3, DuraHeart, Incor, VentrAssist LVAD and HeartWare HVAD).

VENTRICULAR ASSIST DEVICES USAGE

The MCS device can be used for a short-term or temporarily for days to weeks, or long-term for months to years with the durable devices.

Temporary Mechanical Circulatory Support

Mechanical circulatory support can be used in temporary settings as in cardiogenic shock (CGS) refractory to medical therapy where a rapid augmentation of cardiac output and reduction in ventricular filling pressures are crucial for survival. Temporary MCS facilitates spontaneous recovery in scenarios as refractory myocarditis and Takotsubo cardiomyopathy. It also helps in aiding the decision time needed for advocating long-term MCS and cardiac transplantation in patients with chronic HF complicated by CGS. Temporary MCS is also useful in patients with severe HF to tide over immediate but reversible contraindications for a major operative procedure with a durable MCS, like coagulopathy from hepatic congestion, acute kidney injury from low cardiac output and high right atrial pressure, hypoalbuminemia resulting from bowel edema and cardiac cachexia, so that this temporary support would facilitate a candidacy for a durable MCS. However, it is important that the use of temporary MCS devices should be performed only when there is good expectation of a clinical improvement and as a rule should not be used if myocardial recovery is unlikely and the scope of a subsequent cardiac transplantation or the use of a long-term or durable VAD is not anticipated. But temporary MCS devices can be used rarely as a bridge to placement of a long-term durable VAD as a bridge-to-bridge (BTB) indication or a BTT, in clinical scenarios where there is difficulty in assessment of myocardial recovery, though not an approved indication. Temporary MCS includes the intra-aortic balloon pump (IABP), the extracorporeal life support (ECLS) or ECMO and percutaneous MCS devices as the Impella and Tandem heart.

Intra-aortic balloon pump is a mechanical device that increases myocardial oxygen perfusion and cardiac output by producing counterpulsations. It is a polyethylene balloon which is placed in the descending aorta approximately 2.0 cm below the left subclavian artery. It helps to improve the cardiac output by 0.5–1.0 L/min and is commonly used as the initial mechanical support to improve coronary perfusion in refractory CGS. The Intra-Aortic Balloon Counterpulsation in Acute Myocardial Infarction Complicated by Cardiogenic Shock II (IABP-Shock II) trial showed no significant improvement in 30 days survival outcomes.[14] Thereafter, most guidelines have shifted IABP from a Class I to Class IIa/III indication. However, many centers still use IABP as an easy-to-use support in cardiogenic shock scenarios when there is no access to higher therapies.

Extracorporeal life support/extracorporeal membrane oxygenation has been found to be useful as a temporary MCS. It is basically a form of cardiopulmonary bypass and the venoarterial ECMO (VA-ECMO) is a form of emergency biventricular support which is typically used as a last resort salvage therapy in CGS when implanting an IABP is or has not been helpful and placement of a VAD is not possible. The ECMO provides excellent hemodynamic support via a nonpulsatile centrifugal pump connected in-line with a membrane oxygenator which receives blood via inflow venous cannulas which are usually inserted into the femoral vein and returns oxygenated blood via an outflow arterial cannula which is inserted commonly into the femoral artery. Survival rates to discharge with ECMO in refractory CGS vary from 39% to 80% and is dependent on the basic clinical indication.[15] The key downside of ECMO is the lack of durability (mean of 4 days), inability to unload the left ventricle and potential hemorrhagic risk at the vascular access site. The patients who survive are often transitioned to a VAD or rarely a heart transplant.

Percutaneous Mechanical Circulatory Support

With the advances in MCS technology, new devices like the Impella have evolved. The Impella devices (ABIOMED) are essentially miniaturized percutaneous LVAD catheters. These are inserted via the femoral artery and placed retrograde across the aortic valve to provide adequate perfusion in hemodynamically unstable patients. However, these are not durable and are recommended for use only up to 7 days, though some centers have used them for up to 27 days via the right axillary artery approach. Left ventricular support by Impella devices can be with the Impella 2.5, the Impella cardiac power (Impella CP or Impella 3.5) and the Impella 5.0. These nonpulsatile micropumps propel blood from the left ventricle into the ascending aorta using the "Archimedes screw principle", which is the rotation of a small rotating screw-shaped surface inside a small hollow tube that crosses the aortic valve. The tip of the Impella is a pig tail that provides stabilization of the device in the left ventricle and is placed via the femoral artery so that the inlet resides in the left ventricle and the outlet rests in the ascending aorta. The pump which is connected to the console, allows for pressure monitoring and can be adjusted based on the desired degree of hemodynamic support. All the devices are preload dependent and are able to provide optimal left ventricular unloading. One benefit of the use of the Impella 5.0 is that it can be inserted via the axillary artery which allows the patient to be mobile and ambulant while on therapy. None of these peripheral devices can be placed or initiated at the patient bedside and must be inserted under fluoroscopic guidance.

Some of the advantages of the Impella devices are peripheral insertion, direct ventricular decompression, duration of support up to 21 days, and ability to support mobile patients with an axillary or central cannulation scenario. Disadvantages of this therapy are immobilization of the patient with femoral cannulation, high costs, concern of hemolysis, catheter migration with frequent need for reimaging and repositioning, and lack of pulmonary support.

The newest Impella device, the Impella RP (Abiomed)[16] offers right ventricle support in the setting of right ventricular dysfunction and failure. It is the first percutaneous pump designed for right heart support and can provide up to 14 days of support in both adult and pediatric patients with a body surface area ≥1.5 m^2 as per manufacture guidelines. The Impella RP is designed to provide up to 4 L/min of right heart support with the inlet resting in the right atrium and the outlet sitting in the main pulmonary artery. It is beneficial in providing right heart support in the setting of acute right HF and can be applied immediately after durable LVAD implant, post-heart-transplant or cardiac surgery.

The TandemHeart (Cardiac Assist Inc) is also a percutaneous LVAD which is placed via a trans-septal puncture.

VENTRICULAR ASSIST DEVICE SELECTION

The key contribution to the development and evolution of the MCS devices and therapy was the establishment of the Interagency Registry for Mechanically Assisted Circulatory Support (INTERMACS) national registry which was sponsored by the NHLBI and the information that was obtained from it. INTERMACS provides the largest data on the outcomes with durable MCS devices. It represents a collaborative effort of the NHLBI, Food and Drug Authority, device manufacturers and doctors and initiated patient enrollment and data collection in June 2006 and it was made mandatory in March 2009 that all hospitals in the USA entered the MCS data of all noninvestigative MCS devices approved for use by the Food and Drug Administration (FDA), into INTERMACS. Most important was the designing of the INTERMACS patient profile 1–7 based on the clinical status, hemodynamic profile, and degree of end-organ damage (Table 3).[17] Such a scale was designed for the purposes of perioperative risk prediction and stratification for future outcomes postimplant, including mortality and complications and also in correlating outcomes with the severity of the illness. The scale also aids in deciding the timing for use of the durable MCS devices.

The lower the number in the scale, the more gravely ill was the patient. Patients who underwent MCS device in INTERMACS patient profile 1 had the worst outcomes in contrast to more stable forms of advanced HF (INTERMACS Patient Profile 2 through 7).[18]

Ventricular assist device selection is typically a multidisciplinary one which is tailored to the patient's clinical status and needs. Patients who are INTERMACS Profile 3 and above are considered for BTT or DT with a durable long-term continuous flow MCS. However, the patients in INTERMACS Profile 1 or 2 who are by definition hemodynamically unstable should be immediately planned for a short-term MCS therapy. This acute and short-term support aids in improving the cardiac output and tissue perfusion and thus helps the patient to tide over impending mortality. However reports have shown that survival of patients undergoing as BTT is better when these devices are placed electively than on an emergency basis.[19]

The seventh INTERMACS annual report analyzed data of 15,745 patients who received MCS devices between the dates 23 June 2006 and 31 December 2014, of which 13,286 patients received LVADs. More than 90% (12,030) of them had received continuous flow LVAD, 955 of them pulsatile devices and 301 of them received TAH. The survival of patients with continuous flow devices had a 2-year survival of 70%.[20] Freedom from device exchange or mortality related to device malfunction was similar for both pulsatile and continuous flow devices in the initial 8 months at 96%. However, there was a linear decrease in freedom from device malfunction in the pulsatile device from 8 months to 24 months, being only 40% at 24 months in contrast to

TABLE 3: INTERMACS profiles.

Profile	*Definition*	*Description*
INTERMACS 1	Crash and burn	Hemodynamic instability in spite of increasing doses of catecholamines and/or mechanical circulatory support with critical hypoperfusion of target organs (Severe cardiogenic shock)
INTERMACS 2	Sliding on inotropes	Intravenous inotropic support with acceptable blood pressure but rapid deterioration of kidney function, nutritional state, or signs of congestion
INTERMACS 3	Dependent stability	Hemodynamic stability with low or Intermediate, but necessary due to hypotension, doses of inotropics, worsening of symptoms, or progressive kidney failure
INTERMACS 4	Frequent flyer	Temporary cessation of inotropic treatment is possible, but the patient presents frequent symptom recurrences and typically with fluid overload
INTERMACS 5	Housebound	Complete cessation of physical activity, stable at rest, but frequently with moderate water retention and some level of kidney dysfunction
INTERMACS 6	Walking wounded	Minor limitation on physical activity and absence of congestion while at rest. Easily fatigued by light activity
INTERMACS 7	Placeholder	Patient in NYHA functional class II or III with no current or recent unstable water balance

(INTERMACS: Interagency Registry for Mechanically Assisted Circulatory Support; NYHA: New York Heart Association)

the persistent freedom from malfunction of the continuous flow LVAD with 94% at 24 months.[18]

DURABLE OR LONG-TERM VENTRICULAR ASSIST DEVICES

The durable MCS or the long-term VADs include namely the Thoratec pVAD, Thoratec LVAD HeartMate II, HeartMate 3, HVAD, and CardioWest TAH. The HeartMate II is the most evaluated MCS device. It is a continuous flow rotary pump with an axial design and a bearing support for the impeller. An electric motor serves as the energy source for the pump, with power to the pump being delivered via a percutaneous lead with an external power source and a computerized controller. The pump is implanted in a pre-peritoneal pocket. It is used as both BTT and DT indications.

Bridge-to-transplant is an indication for MCS which includes patients in CGS or with advanced decompensated HF who are refractory to optimal medical therapy and in whom myocardial function is unlikely to recover, but are eligible candidates for cardiac transplantation. Durable devices are ideal for BTT as they facilitate long-term use and also allow untethered patient mobility and discharge of the patient from the hospital. These devices are indicated in patients with stable hemodynamics and preserved end-organ function, but have significant symptoms of HF and are on inotropic support or in patients who are not on inotropic support but who are symptomatic at rest.

The HeartMate II pivotal trial for a BTT indication was a prospective nonrandomized multicenter study in 133 patients with end-stage HF who were on a waiting list for a heart-transplant and received a HeartMate II device. The primary endpoint of the study was a composite of the proportion of patients who at 6 months had undergone cardiac transplantation or were explanted for cardiac recovery or had ongoing MCS with HeartMate II while remaining eligible for transplantation. Principal outcomes were seen in 100 patients (75%) who received HeartMate II.[21] At 3 months and 6 months there was significant improvement in NYHA functional class, 6-minute walk distance and in the quality of life based on the Minnesota Living with Heart Failure and Kansas City Cardiomyopathy questionnaires.[21] Major adverse events included postoperative bleeding, stroke, right heart failure, percutaneous lead infection, and device malfunction.

With the successful use in BTT indications and as experience with MCS device therapy provided support for longer durations, it evolved into the use of these devices as a permanent alternative to cardiac transplantation. DT uses durable MCS devices in patients with chronic refractory symptoms of advanced HF due to irreversible ischemic or nonischemic cardiomyopathy, who are otherwise stable hemodynamically without manifestations of significant organ injury, debilitation or cachexia and are not candidates for cardiac transplantation. The devices selected for use as DT are durable devices that allow for untethered hands-free mobility of the patient at home.

The HeartMate II DT pivotal trial for DT use of the device, randomly assigned 200 patients with NYHA class III B to IV symptoms and an LVEF ≤25% to receive a HeartMate II or HeartMate XVE.[22] Eligible patients also had to have either a maximal oxygen consumption not exceeding 14 mL/kg/min, required treatment with intravenous inotropic agents for 14 days or longer, or an intra-aortic balloon pump support for 7 days or more.[22] The primary endpoint was a composite of survival to 24 months without a disabling stroke or the need for an operation to repair or replace the device. A more than fourfold increase was observed in the percentage of HeartMate II patients who successfully attained the primary endpoint (46% versus 11%; $p < 0.001$).[23] All adverse events were less frequent among patients receiving HeartMate II with significant reductions in device related infections, sepsis, right heart failure, renal failure, and rehospitalizations. However, changes in functional capacity, 6-minute walk distance, and quality of life scores were similar between groups, suggesting that the improvements seen in these factors in VAD-supported patients are more closely linked to the favorable effects of the increase in cardiac output and reduction in left sided filling pressures rather than the characteristics of blood flow.

The benefits of MCS for DT in terms of survival, function, quality of life and for therapy in chronic advanced HF was established in the Randomized Evaluation of Mechanical Assistance in the Treatment of Congestive Heart Failure (REMATCH) trial which was a prospective randomized trial.[24] REMATCH compared the use of an LVAD with optimal medical therapy for patients with refractory chronic advanced HF. The results showed that mortality was halved in the LVAD group (relative risk 0.52; 95% confidence interval, 0.34–0.78) compared to the mortality seen in the control group treated with optimal medical therapy (92% at 2 years). Despite the serious adverse events associated with MCS like stroke, infection, bleeding, device, and malfunction, the LVAD group had a better quality of life than those treated medically.[24]

Criteria to be met by patients for DT are: (1) Ineligibility for heart transplant; (2) NYHA Class IIIB or IV symptoms for 45 of the preceding 60 days despite the use of maximally tolerated doses of drugs outlined in guidelines for heart-failure therapy; (3) LVEF < 25%; and (4) Peak exercise oxygen consumption (peak VO_2 of 14 mL/kg/min or less, unless the patient is dependent on intravenous inotropes for 14 days or IABP for 7 days.

After the approval of HeartMate II for DT in 2010, its usage increased with 46% being for DT, 30% as BTT and 26% as BTC as per 2014 statistics in contrast to 2008–2011 with 29% being DT, 32% being BTT and 38% being BTC. But survival by implant strategy has remained unchanged over the years though BTT patients fared significantly better after implant [BTT survival at 1 year: 86% and 3 years: 76% in contrast to DT (DT survival at 1 year: 76% and 3 years: 57%)].[20] With more and more delay in donor hearts being available for transplant it was seen that DT survival has improved over the years providing good quality of life, so much so that some patients may even remove themselves from the cardiac transplant waiting list.[20]

HeartMate III is the latest MCS device that has been approved by FDA for use for both BTT and DT indication. It is an implantable, continuous flow rotary pump with centrifugal design intended as a durable MCS device. The device is small facilitating intrapericardial placement, as the HVAD and uses a bearingless design with a complete magnetic levitation of the impeller. The HeartMate 3 device was studied vis-a-vis the HeartMate II which was an axial flow device, in the Multicenter Study of MagLev Technology in Patients Undergoing Mechanical circulatory Support Therapy with HeartMate 3 (MOMENTUM 3).[25] 1,028 patients with advanced HF were randomly assigned to receive either the HeartMate II (512 patients) or the HeartMate 3 (516 patients) irrespective of whether it was BTT or DT indication. The composite endpoints were survival at 2 years free of disabling stroke or reoperation to replace or remove a malfunctioning device. The principal secondary endpoint was pump replacement at 2 years. In the analysis of the primary endpoint, 397 patients (76.9%) in the centrifugal flow pump group in contrast to 332 patients (64.8%) in the axial flow pump group remained alive and free of disabling stroke or reoperation to replace or remove a malfunctioning device at 2 years [relative risk 0.84; 95% confidence interval (CI), 0.78–0.91; $p < 0.001$ for superiority]. Pump replacement was less common in the centrifugal flow pump group than in the axial flow pump group [12 patients (2.3%) vs. 57 patients (11.3%); relative risk, 0.21; 95% CI, 0.11–0.38; p,0.001]. Also, the number of events per patient year for stroke of any severity, major bleeding, and gastrointestinal hemorrhage were lower in the centrifugal flow pump group than in the axial flow pump group.[25]

COMPLICATIONS OF VENTRICULAR ASSIST DEVICES

The complications commonly associated with MCS devices are infection, bleeding, stroke, arrhythmias, renal dysfunction, and device malfunction, and it is the higher incidence of these complications which makes LVADs inferior to heart transplantation.

The rate of adverse events was significantly higher with pulsatile devices with a higher incidence of all complications especially bleeding, infection, and device malfunction. Infection was most commonly at the driveline site with Staphylococci being the most common organism.[26] Device malfunction occurs over time with wear and tear and is a measure of its durability and may be due to a mechanical issue as motor failure or biochemical causes like hemolysis or thrombus formation. Pump failure invariably results in a stroke, bleeding, or an infection of requiring a redo-surgery for pump exchange.

Though complication rates are much lower with the present day continuous flow pumps in contrast to the pulsatile pumps, the average rates of admissions still remain high with one of the studies showing an average of 1.64 ± 1.97 admissions per patient year follow-up.[27] The most common causes for readmission were gastrointestinal bleeds from anticoagulation and infection. It is notable that patients on LVAD as BTT have a significantly high wait-list mortality if and when a complication occurs. Also the patients who developed device-related complications pre-cardiac transplant had negative outcomes in the 1 year and 3 years post-cardiac transplant.[28] The major risk factors for mortality with continuous flow devices were INTERMACS Profiles 1 and 2, patients on hemodialysis, prior history of stroke, female sex, post-ICD implant, increased bilirubin and need for BiVAD as a single procedure.[20]

CONTRAINDICATIONS FOR VENTRICULAR ASSIST DEVICE INSERTION

Relative contraindications to LVAD include acute cardiogenic shock with uncertain neurologic status, active severe bleeding, active uncontrolled systemic infection, severe uncorrected aortic regurgitation, and a mechanical valve in aortic position which cannot be changed to a bioprosthetic valve. Also, patients who are physically unable to operate their pump and would not be able to respond to their device alarms are also considered unsuitable.[29]

CONCLUSION

Thus the concept of MCS which was initiated to facilitate open-heart surgery, has evolved over the decades and undergone refinement from the first generation to the new third generation devices. The percutaneous lead of the MCS device contributed to a lot of morbidity and also limitation of activities which affected the quality of life of the patient. The introduction of wireless energy transfer technology and the fully implantable VAD by Leviticus Cardio and others will eliminate the percutaneous lead and risk of drive-line infections and facilitate the MCS device to be charged transcutaneously allowing for much better movement and a significantly better quality of life and free movement.

REFERENCES

1. Writing Committee Members, Yancy CW, Jessup M, Bozkurt B, et al. American College of Cardiology Foundation/ American Heart Association Task Force on Practice Guidelines. ACCF/AHA guideline for the management of heart failure: A report of the American College of Cardiology Foundation/American Heart Association Task Force on practice guidelines. Circulation. 2013;128(16):e240-327.
2. Metra M, Ponikowski P, Dickstein K, et al. Heart Failure Association of the European Society of Cardiology. Advanced chronic heart-failure: A position statement from the study group on advanced heart failure of the Heart Failure Association of the European Society of Cardiology. Eur J Heart Fail. 2007;9(6-7):684-94.
3. Toeg HD, Al-Atassi T, Garcia JP, et al. An update on mechanical circulatory support for heart failure therapy. Curr Opin Cardiol. 2014;29(2):167-73.
4. Gibbon JH Jr. Application of a mechanical heart and lung apparatus to cardiac surgery. Minn Med. 1954;37(3):171-85.
5. DeBakey ME. Left ventricular bypass pump for cardiac assistance. Clinical experience. Am J Cardiol. 1971;27(1):3-11.
6. Cooley DA. The total artificial heart. Nat Med. 2003:9(1) 108-11.
7. Cooley DA, Akutsu T, Norman JC, et al. Total artificial heart in two-staged cardiac transplantation. Cardiovasc Dis. 1981;8(3):305-19.
8. DeVries WC. The permanent artificial heart. Four case reports. JAMA. 1988;259(6):849-59.
9. Portner PM, Oyer PE, Pennington DG, et al. Implantable electrical left ventricular assist system: Bridge to transplantation and the future. Ann Thorac Surg. 1989;47(1):142-50.
10. Oyer PE, Stinson EB, Portner PM, et al. Development of a totally implantable, electrically actuated left ventricular assist system. Am J Surg. 1980;140(1):17-25.
11. Frazier OH. First use of an untethered, vented electric left ventricular assist device for long-term support. Circulation. 1994;89(6):2908-14.
12. Lok SI, Martina JR, Hesselink T, et al. Single-center experience of 85 patients with a continuous-flow left ventricular assist device: Clinical practice and outcome after extended support. Eur J Cardiothorac Surg. 2013;44(3):e233-8.
13. Park SJ, Milano CA, Tatooles AJ, et al. HeartMate II Clinical Investigators. Outcomes in advanced heart failure patients with left ventricular assist devices for destination therapy. Circ Heart Fail. 2012;5(2):241-8.
14. Thiele H, Zeymer U, Neumann FJ, et al. Intraaortic Balloon Pump in cardiogenic shock II (IABP-SHOCK II) trial investigators. Intra-aortic balloon counterpulsation in acute myocardial infarction complicated by cardiogenic shock (IABP-SHOCK II): Final 12 month results of a randomised, open-label trial. Lancet. 2013;382(9905):1638-45.
15. Paden ML, Conrad SA, Rycus PT, et al. ELSO Registry. Extracorporeal Life Support Organization Registry Report 2012. ASAIOJ. 2013;59(3):202-10.
16. Anderson MB, Goldstein J, Milano C, et al. Benefits of a novel percutaneous ventricular assist device for right heart failure: The prospective RECOVER RIGHT study of the Impella RP device. J Heart Lung Transplant. 2015;34(12):1549-60.
17. Stevenson LW, Pagani FD, Young JB, et al. INTERMACS profiles of advanced heart failure: The current clinical picture. J Heart Lung Transplant. 2009;28(6):535-41.
18. Kirklin JK, Naftel DC, Kormos RL, et al. Fifth INTERMACS annual report: Risk factor analysis from more than 6,000 mechanical circulatory support patients. J Heart Lung Transplant. 2013;32(2):141-56.
19. Deng MC, Weynad M, Hammel D, et al. Selection and management of ventricular assist device patients: The Muenster experience. J Heart Lung Transplant. 2000;19(Suppl 8):S77-82.
20. Kirklin JK, Naftel DC, Pagani FD, et al. Seventh INTERMACS annual report: 15,000 patients and counting. J Heart Lung Transplant. 2015;34(12):1495-504.
21. Miller LW, Pagani FD, Russell SD, et al. HeartMate II Clinical Investigators. Use of a continuous-flow device in patients awaiting heart transplantation. N Engl J Med. 2007;357(9):885-96.
22. Slaughter MS, Rogers JG, Milano CA, et al. HeartMate II Investigators. Advanced heart failure treated with continuous-flow left ventricular assist device. N Engl J Med. 2009;361(23):2241-51.
23. Moazami N, Fukumachi K, Kobayashi M, et al. Axial and centrifugal continuous-flow rotary pumps: A translation from pump mechanics to clinical practice. J Heart Lung Transplant. 2013;32(1):1-11.
24. Rose EA, Gelijns AC, Moskowitz AJ, et al.; Randomized Evaluation of Mechanical Assistance for the Treatment of Congestive Heart Failure (REMATCH) Study Group. Long-term use of a left ventricular assist device for end-stage heart failure. N Engl J Med. 2001;345(20):1435-43.
25. Mehra MR, Uriel N, Naka Y, et al. MOMENTUM 3 Investigators: A fully magnetically levitated left ventricular assist device - Final report. N Engl J Med. 2019;380(17):1618-27.
26. Gordon RJ, Weinberg AD, Pagani FD, et al. Ventricular Assist Device Infection Study Group. Prospective, multicenter study of ventricular assist device infections. Circulation. 2013;127(6):691-702.
27. Hasin T, Marmor Y, Kremers W, et al. Readmissions after implantation of axial flow left ventricular assist device. J Am Coll Cardiol. 2013;61(2):153-63.
28. Quader MA, Wolfe LG, Kasirajan V. Heart transplantation outcomes in patients with continuous-flow left ventricular assist device-related complications. J Heart Lung Transplant. 2015;34(1):75-81.
29. Feldman D, Pamboukian SV, Teuteberg JJ, et al. The 2013 International Society for Heart and Lung Transplantation guidelines for mechanical circulatory support: Executive summary. J Heart Lung Transplant. 2013;32(2):157-87.

CHAPTER

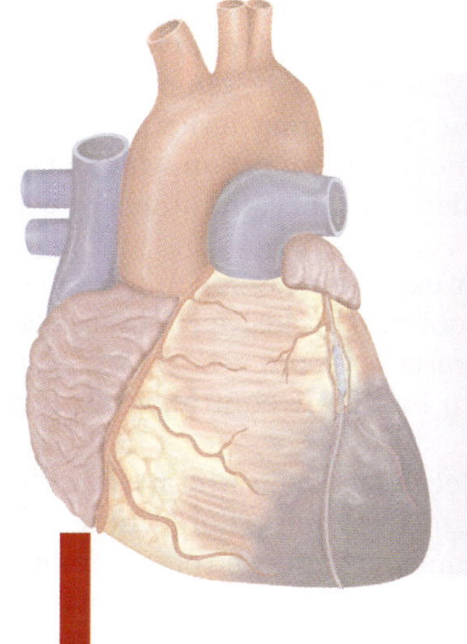

Minimally Invasive Left Ventricular Assist Devices

Yugal K Mishra, Sanket Garg

INTRODUCTION

Left ventricular assist devices (LVAD) have now become an established therapy for end-stage heart failure as bridge to transplant or as destination therapy. Over the years, the designs of implant have improved and evolved and so has the technical aspects in terms of preoperative and postoperative care as well as implantation techniques and this had vastly improved the results of implantation as well as decreased the postoperative morbidity. Full sternotomy and cardiopulmonary bypass (CPB) is the most widely used and accepted technique for LVAD implantation and is the standard of care but like in other cardiac surgery procedures, minimally invasive technique for LVAD implantation is becoming popular in suitable patients and many centers across world have published their experience with these techniques with successful results. Like any new technique some people might argue that it is not safe and there are many detractors who would say that patient is not here for cosmetic surgery but the advantage for minimally invasive techniques is not only cosmetic but others including less operative trauma, reduced blood requirements, avoidance of CPB and lot many others as shown in other minimally invasive cardiac surgery like valve surgery and minimally invasive direct coronary artery bypass (MIDCAB) and minimally invasive coronary artery bypass graft (CABG).

HISTORY

The concept of minimally invasive implantation was introduced by Hill et al. by using a combination of a right mini-thoracotomy and small left subcostal incision to implant the Thoratec paracorporeal LVAD. Subsequently, Gregory et al. described a less invasive approach for implanting LVAD via right mini-thoracotomy and a small subcostal incision. Nowadays, many more approaches have been described. These approaches can be classified as moving from on-pump techniques to off-pump techniques for LVAD implantation and alternate approaches to LVAD implantation. In this chapter, we will describe the various approaches and configurations of minimally invasive technique and sites of implantation and their pros and cons.

MINIMALLY INVASIVE STRATEGY

Typically the LVAD implantation is done on CPB by mid-sternotomy approach. However, institution of CPB in these borderline patients with failing hearts, multiorgan dysfunction, and multiple comorbidities is associated with many harmful side effects as has been well documented in the literature including release of inflammatory mediators, bleeding, renal and pulmonary dysfunction, and increased pulmonary vascular resistance. Most of these patients have preoperative evidence of renal insufficiency, pulmonary edema, and liver congestion and bleeding abnormalities. Institution of CPB in these patients often exacerbates these preexisting morbidities leading to postoperative bleeding, worsening renal and hepatic dysfunction, and right ventricular dysfunction. The use of off-pump strategy could help to minimize these potential harmful complications and this has been shown in a large randomized study in a select group of patients. The decreased use of blood products also avoids potential complications of blood transfusion as well as decrease the chances of recipient sensitization thus preserving the patient for future transplant. Though it is preferred if device implantation can be done by off-pump technique it is not mandatory to do it off-pump only and various sites have been used by many groups to do the minimally invasive LVAD implantation on CPB like femoral cannulation, ascending aorta, and two-stage RA cannulation by upper hemisternotomy, aorta and femoral vein, etc.

EVALUATION AND INVESTIGATIONS

The patient should be a candidate for LVAD implantation as per standard American College of Cardiology/American Heart Association (ACC/AHA) guidelines. Patients with preoperative right ventricular failure are better done with minimally invasive technique than with sternotomy. Inflow and outflow sites should be carefully marked preoperatively including the driveline site.

- *Transthoracic echo:* To evaluate for any intracardiac shunt, any intracardiac clot or any regurgitant lesion which may require fixation and to see for LV size and LV aneurysm. LV apex should be marked by transthoracic echo to mark the left thoracotomy inflow pump insertion site.
- *Computed tomography (CT) angiography and contrast-enhanced computed tomography (CECT) chest:* To look for any aortic calcification or any aortic abnormality. Also to rule out any pulmonary pathology or adhesions.
- *Carotid and peripheral Doppler:* Femoral vessel evaluation to look for flow and size of vessels in case of need for cardiopulmonary bypass or ECMO. Subclavian vessel should be looked for possible outflow graft landing and carotid vessel should be evaluated for any concomitant disease.
- *Pulmonary function test:* To evaluate for the lung functions.
- *Coronary angiography:* To rule out any concomitant coronary artery disease.

ANESTHESIA CONSIDERATIONS

General anesthesia is required. Double lumen endotracheal intubation is done to achieve lung collapse. The anesthetic management of rate and arrhythmias and blood pressure during LVAD placement is very important. This can be achieved by either rapid ventricular pacing or by transient bolus injection of intravenous adenosine.

The two most commonly used off-pump techniques for LVAD insertion are either to use rapid ventricular pacing or by the use of a bolus of intravenous adenosine to achieve a short bradycardiac arrest. The use of rapid ventricular pacing was reported by Centrofanti et al. in 2011 for Jarvik LVAD insertion.

The use of adenosine has the added advantage of reduced blood loss as it further reduces the volume of blood ejected during each cardiac cycle during device insertion. Adenosine mediates pulmonary vasodilation which may reduce pulmonary vascular resistance and thus protect the RV function.

There are some other experimental techniques like vacuum-assisted coring tool with occlusive endovascular balloon inserted via femoral artery, etc.

Blood pressure has to be tightly controlled during outflow graft placement.

But there are only a select few patients who are suitable for off-pump technique of LVAD insertion. There are patients who require concomitant correction of some other cardiac pathology like left ventricular/atrial clot removal, correction of aortic or mitral or tricuspid regurgitation or repair of any intracardiac shunt, etc. This is the subset of patients who are not suitable for off-pump techniques.

INSERTION TECHNIQUES

The LVAD insertion is divided into three steps:

1. Inflow cannula and pump insertion
2. Outflow graft insertion
3. Driveline insertion.

Inflow and Pump Insertion (Figs. 1A and B)

There are two insertion approaches for the minimally invasive techniques:

1. Left subcostal incision mainly used now for HeartMate II. The advantage is that it helps in making pocket for the device.

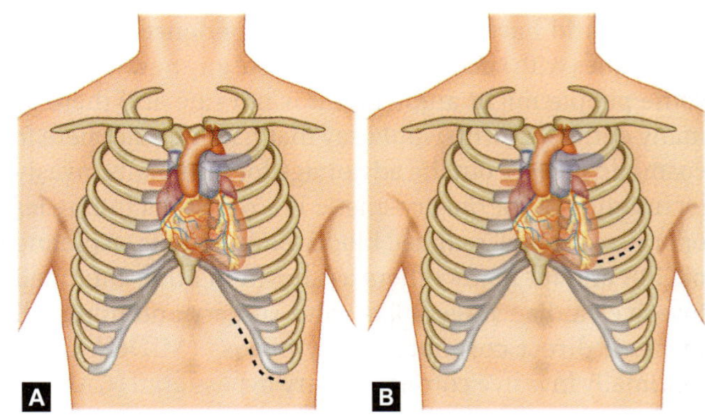

Figs. 1A and B: Inflow cannula sites. (A) Subdiaphragmatic; (B) Left thoracotomy.
Source: Makdisi G, Wang IW. Minimally invasive is the future of left ventricular assist device implantation. J Thorac Dis. 2015;7(9):E283-8.

2. Left anterior thoracotomy at 5th or 6th intercostal space. This is especially useful in cases of redo sternotomy or difficult sternal reentry patients. Also it has the advantage of single incision entry for complete procedure as the outflow graft can be placed in left axillary artery or descending thoracic aorta.

Outflow Graft Insertion (Figs. 2 and 3)

This could be done by multiple techniques and in different locations as per the surgeon preference, the patient profile, history of the patient like if it is a redo patient, porcelain aorta, flow in axillary artery, etc. The various locations approaches are right mini-thoracotomy, split upper hemisternotomy, axillary and subclavian arteries, supraceliac abdominal aorta, innominate artery, and descending aorta. But any outflow graft in any artery other than ascending aorta might cause flow turbulence and has to be placed very carefully.

Upper Hemisternotomy with Ascending Aortic Anastomosis for Outflow Graft

This is the most commonly used for on-pump minimally invasive strategy though should be avoided in case of planned heart transplant later in life as it will make second entry easier. The advantage is CPB can be initiated easily, can be associated with either inflow pump incisions or tunneling of the driveline to the right or left upper quadrant. For the majority of patients, the outflow graft is tunneled and passed within the pericardium and anastomosed to the proximal ascending aorta.

Right Mini-thoracotomy with Ascending Aortic Anastomosis for Outflow Graft

This technique is preferentially utilized in bridged patients to spare the sternal incision for heart transplantation. The outflow graft is inserted through a 4–6 cm right anterior mini-thoracotomy via 2nd or 3rd intercostal space. This allows direct access to the ascending aorta to initiate the CPB and/or to perform the outflow anastomosis.

Upper Hemisternotomy with Right Hemithoracotomy J Shape Incision

This is a combination of the previous two incisions. In this technique also the outflow graft is anastomosed to ascending aorta.

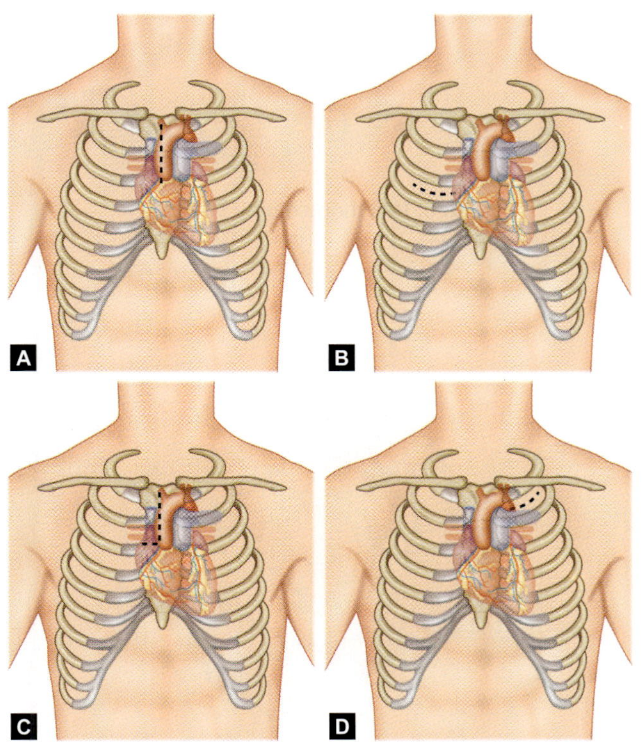

Figs. 2A to D: Outflow graft site insertion. (A) Upper hemisternotomy; (B) right minithoracotomy; (C) upper hemisternotomy and right hemithoracotomy J shape incision; (D) axillary.
Source: Makdisi G, Wang IW. Minimally invasive is the future of left ventricular assist device implantation. J Thorac Dis. 2015;7(9): E283-8.

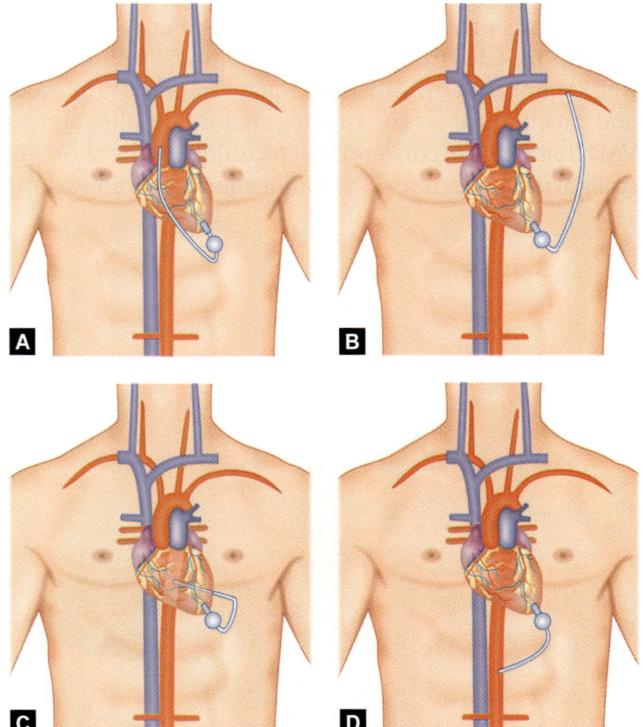

Figs. 3A to D: Minimally invasive LVAD insertion configurations. (A) OG to ascending aorta; (B) OG to axillary artery; (C) OG to descending aorta; (D) OG to supraceliac aorta.
(LVAD: left ventricular assist device; OG: outflow graft)
Source: Makdisi G, Wang IW. Minimally invasive is the future of left ventricular assist device implantation. J Thorac Dis. 2015;7(9):E283-8.

Left Thoracotomy with Left Axillary Artery

This is not the preferential site for outflow graft anastomosis and is used in case the ascending or descending aorta cannot be used for outflow graft anastomosis due to some reason like porcelain aorta. There are chances of flow turbulence with this anastomosis and pump flow should be carefully adjusted slowly over few days if this site is used for outflow graft. This site is especially useful in case of single left thoracotomy incision for outflow graft anastomosis.

Single Left Thoracotomy Incision with Descending Aorta Anastomosis (Figs. 4 to 6)

For this technique left ventricular apex is localized by on-table echocardiography and the surface marking is then used to enter the left pleural space and expose the LV apex. The LVAD positioning is mainly done by using transesophageal echocardiography and guidewire if needed. The outflow graft is anastomosed end-to-side to the descending aorta.

Left Thoracotomy with Supraceliac Abdominal Aorta

Driveline Insertion (Fig. 7)

The external driveline is the Achilles heel of assist devices and this remains true for both conventional techniques as well as minimally invasive techniques. It is prone to infection and mechanical stress, causing major complications in VAD therapy. The conventional technique is the short and straight driveline tunnel. A modification of this approach is a double subfascial tunneling. Some authors have described advantages in externalization of only the silicone portion of the driveline regarding infections.

POSTOPERATIVE MANAGEMENT

Patient has to be taught preoperatively and counseled about the pump management. The postoperative critical care management includes routine postoperative critical care as for any LVAD patient including antibiotic cover and anticoagulation and goal directed heart failure management.

Left ventricular assist device insertion by minimally invasive procedures is feasible and safe in a select group of patients as discussed and in this subset of patients

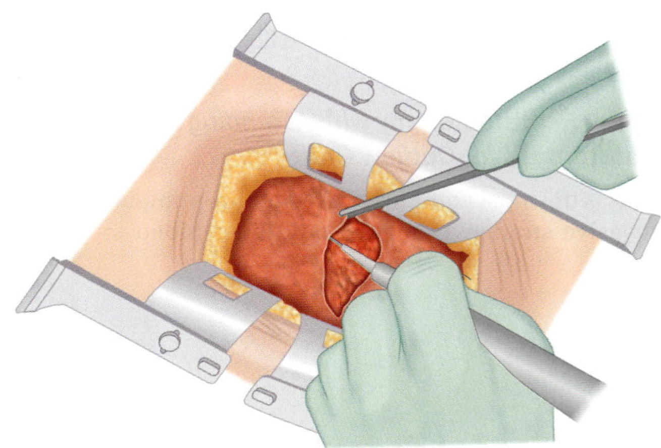

Fig. 5: Left thoracotomy incision.

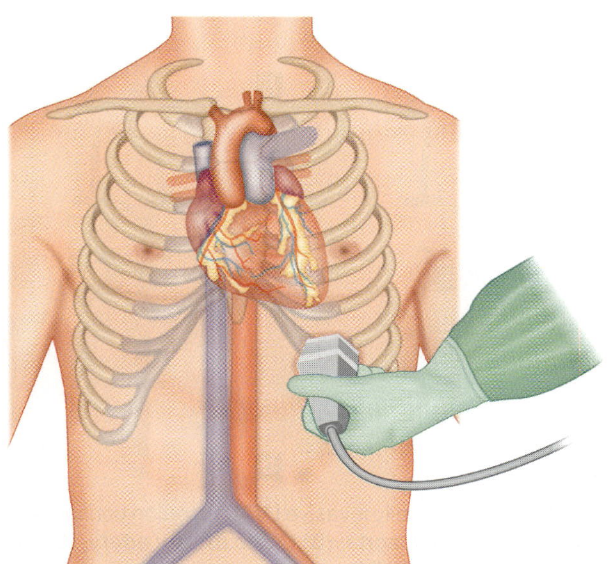

Fig. 4: Left ventricular apex localization.

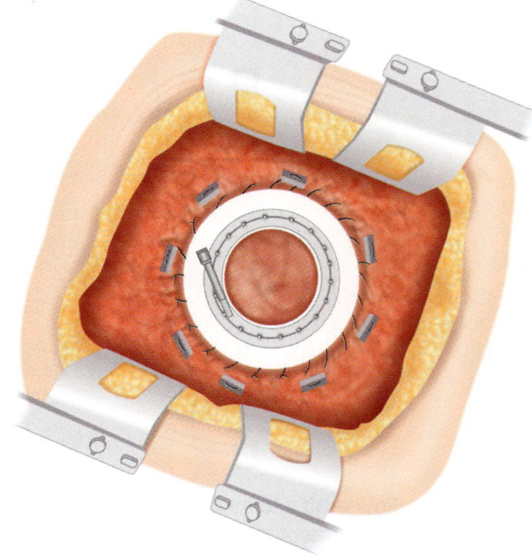

Fig. 6: Sewing ring insertion.

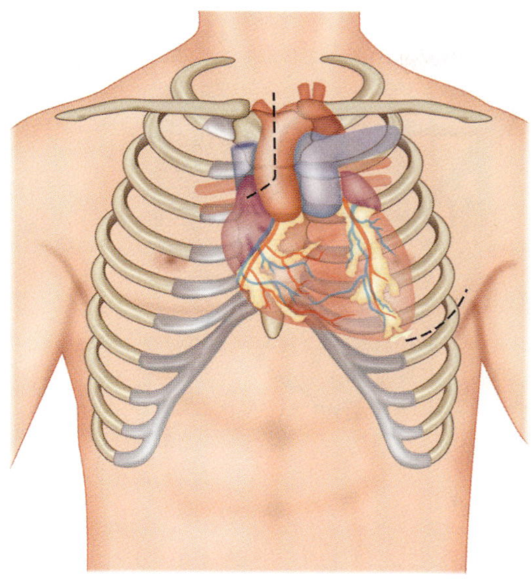

Fig. 7: Upper minimal J sternotomy with extension into the right second-to-third intercostal space.
Source: Schmitto JD, Denix E, Rojas SV, et al. Minimally invasive implantation: The procedure of choice! Operative Techniques in Thoracic and Cardiovascular Surgery. 2016;21:65-78.

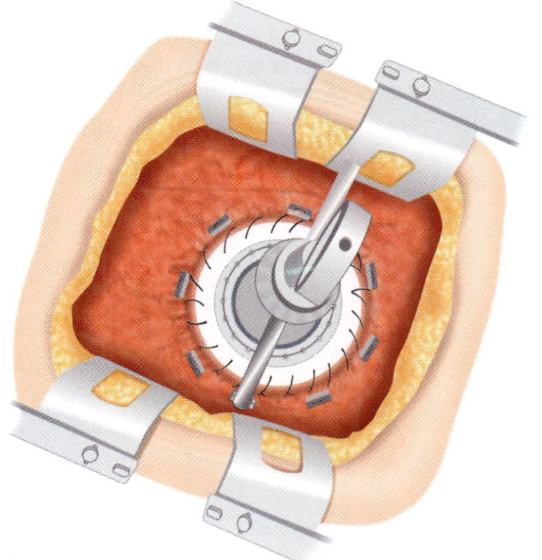

Fig. 8: Coring of left ventricular apex.
Source: Schmitto JD, Denix E, Rojas SV, et al. Minimally invasive implantation: The procedure of choice! Operative Techniques in Thoracic and Cardiovascular Surgery. 2016;21:65-78.

(Fig. 8), minimally invasive techniques may improve the survival and reduce mortality in LVAD insertion when compared to re-operative sternotomy (Fig. 9), LVAD implantation without the use of CPB has the potential to minimize postoperative complications such as excessive

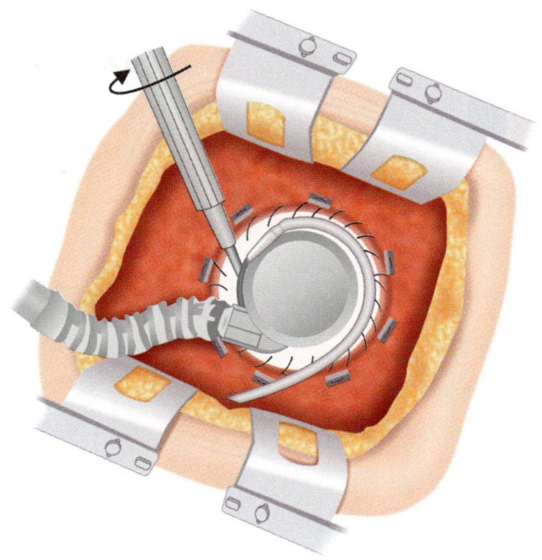

Fig. 9: Left ventricular cavity inspection and driveline.
Source: Schmitto JD, Denix E, Rojas SV, et al. Minimally invasive implantation: The procedure of choice! Operative Techniques in Thoracic and Cardiovascular Surgery. 2016;21:65-78.

bleeding during implantation without compromising hemodynamics. By minimizing the needs for blood transfusions, patients have decreased exposure to blood antigens which ultimately reduces the risk of sensitization in transplant candidates. Evidence for the safety of minimally invasive techniques of LVAD insertion are already in place and continue to grow with refinement in techniques and this technique is probably the future of LVAD insertion in selected patients as discussed (Figs. 10 and 11).

CONCLUSION

Left ventricular assist device insertion by minimally invasive procedures is feasible and safe; minimally invasive techniques improve the survival and reduce mortality in LVAD insertion and this has been proven by many authors as they share their experiences with these techniques and with refinements in techniques of minimally invasive LVAD insertion in select group of patients as discussed. LVAD implantation without the use of CPB has the potential to minimize postoperative complications such as excessive bleeding during implantation without compromising hemodynamics. By minimizing the needs for blood transfusions, patients have decreased exposure to blood antigens which ultimately reduces the risk of sensitization in transplant candidates. We believe that a combination of minimally invasive LVAD insertion with off-pump should be the ultimate goal of minimally invasive LVAD implantation.

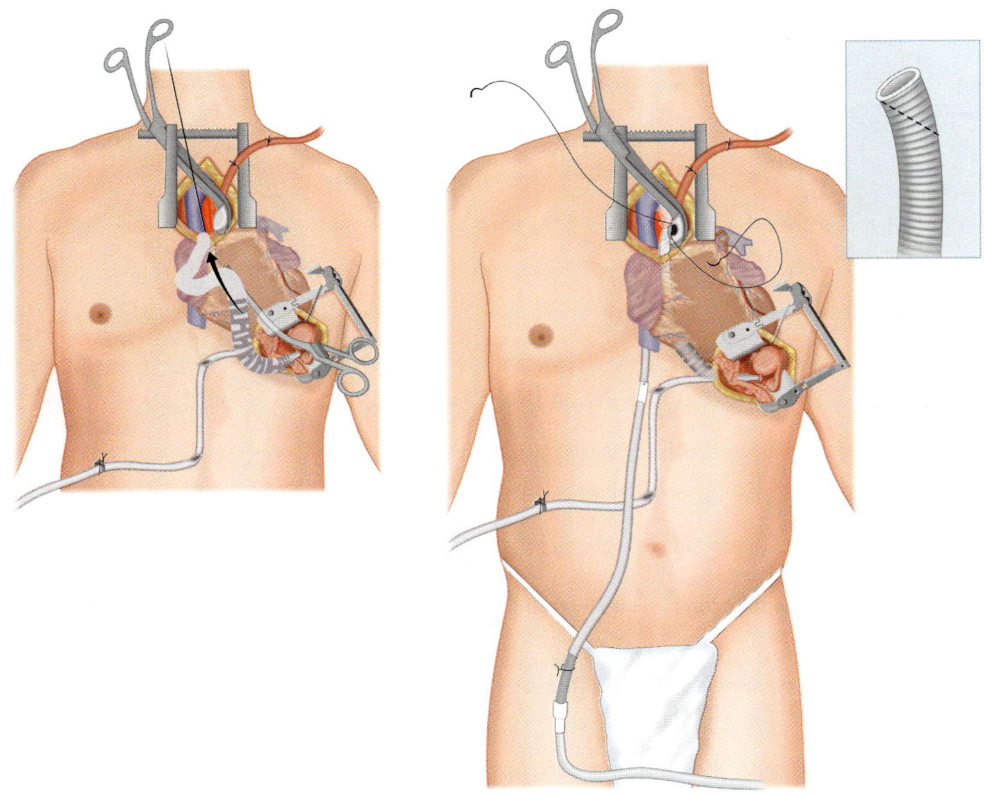

Fig. 10: Outflow graft tunneling via retrosternal space and anastomosis to ascending aorta along with driveline tunneling.
Source: Schmitto JD, Denix E, Rojas SV, et al. Minimally invasive implantation: The procedure of choice! Operative Techniques in Thoracic and Cardiovascular Surgery. 2016;21:65-78.

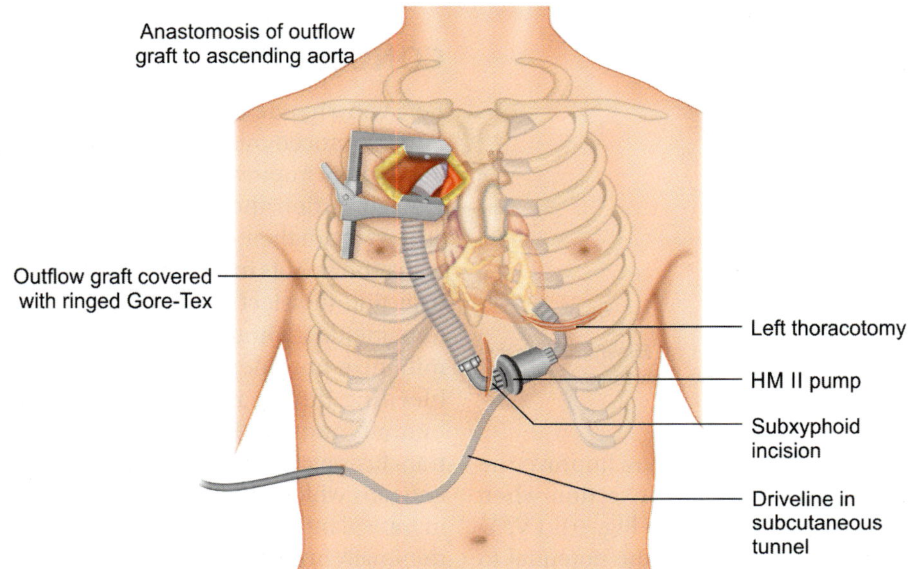

Fig. 11: Complete left ventricular assist device with outflow graft and driveline insertion.

BIBLIOGRAPHY

1. Anastasiadis K, Antonitsis P, Argiriadou H, et al. Use of minimal extracorporeal circulation circuit for left ventricular assist device implantation. ASAIO J. 2011;57(6):547-9.
2. Anyanwu AC, Itagaki S, Pinney S, et al. Initial experience with routine less invasive implantation of HeartMate II left ventricular assist device without median sternotomy. Eur J Cardiothorac Surg. 2014;46(6):985-90.
3. Anyanwu AC. Technique for less invasive implantation of Heartmate II left ventricular assist device without median sternotomy. Semin Thorac Cardiovasc Surg. 2011;23(3):241-4.
4. Awad H, Abd El Dayem M, Heard J, et al. Initial experience with off-pump left ventricular assist device implantation in single center: Retrospective analysis. J Cardiothorac Surg. 2010;5:123.
5. Belhaj A. Actual knowledge of systemic inflammation reaction during cardiopulmonary bypass. Recent Pat Cardiovasc Drug Discov. 2012;7(3):165-9.
6. Birks EJ, George RS, Hedger M, et al. Reversal of severe heart failure with a continuous-flow left ventricular assist device and pharmacological therapy: A prospective study. Circulation. 2011;123(4):381-90.
7. Centofanti P, La Torre M, Attisani M, et al. Rapid pacing for the off-pump insertion of the Jarvik left ventricular assist device. Ann Thorac Surg. 2011;92(4):1536-8.
8. Cheung A, Lamarche Y, Kaan A, et al. Off-pump implantation of the HeartWare HVAD left ventricular assist device through minimally invasive incisions. Ann Thorac Surg. 2011;91(4):1294-6.
9. Clive Landis R, Murkin JM, Stump DA, et al. Consensus statement: Minimal criteria for reporting the systemic inflammatory response to cardiopulmonary bypass. Heart Surg Forum. 2010;13(2):E116-23.
10. Cohn WE. New tools and techniques to facilitate off-pump left ventricular assist device implantation. Tex Heart Inst J. 2010;37(5):559-61.
11. El-Sayed Ahmed MM, Aftab M, Singh SK, et al. Left ventricular assist device outflow graft: Alternative sites. Ann Cardiothorac Surg. 2014;3(5):541-5.
12. Farrar DJ, Holman WR, McBride LR, et al. Long-term follow-up of Thoratec ventricular assist device bridge-to-recovery patients successfully removed from support after recovery of ventricular function. J Heart Lung Transplant. 2002;21(5):516-21.
13. Frazier OH, Myers TJ. Left ventricular assist system as a bridge to myocardial recovery. Ann Thorac Surg. 1999;68(2):734-41.
14. Frazier OH. Implantation of the Jarvik 2000 left ventricular assist device without the use of cardiopulmonary bypass. Ann Thorac Surg. 2003;75(3):1028-30.
15. Galiè N, Ussia G, Passarelli P, et al. Role of pharmacologic tests in the treatment of primary pulmonary hypertension. Am J Cardiol. 1995;75(3):55A-62A.
16. Gregoric ID, Cohn WE, Frazier OH. Diaphragmatic implantation of the HeartWare ventricular assist device. J Heart Lung Transplant. 2011;30(4):467-70.
17. Gregoric ID, La Francesca S, Myers T, et al. A less invasive approach to axial flow pump insertion. J Heart Lung Transplant. 2008;27(4):423-6.
18. Hill JD, Avery GJ, Egrie G, et al. Less invasive Thoratec LVAD insertion: A surgical technique. Heart Surg Forum. 2000;3(3):218-23.
19. Kirklin JK, Naftel DC, Kormos RL, et al. Fifth INTERMACS annual report: Risk factor analysis from more than 6,000 mechanical circulatory support patients. J Heart Lung Transplant. 2013;32(2):141-56.
20. Kirklin JK, Naftel DC, Kormos RL, et al. Second INTERMACS annual report: More than 1,000 primary left ventricular assist device implants. J Heart Lung Transplant. 2010;29(1):1-10.
21. Krabatsch T, Drews T, Potapov E, et al. Different surgical strategies for implantation of continuous-flow VADs-Experience from Deutsches Herzzentrum Berlin. Ann Cardiothorac Surg. 2014;3(5):472-4.
22. Lamy A, Devereaux PJ, Prabhakaran D, et al.; CORONARY Investigators. Off-pump or on-pump coronary-artery bypass grafting at 30 days. N Engl J Med. 2012;366(16):1489-97.
23. Makdisi G, Wang IW. Minimally invasive is the future of left ventricular assist device implantation. J Thorac Dis. 2015;7(9):E283-8.
24. Maltais S, Davis ME, Haglund N. Minimally invasive and alternative approaches for long-term LVAD placement: The Vanderbilt strategy. Ann Cardiothorac Surg. 2014;3(6):563-9.
25. Momeni M, Carlier C, Baele P, et al. Fibrinogen concentration significantly decreases after on-pump versus off-pump coronary artery bypass surgery: A systematic point-of-care ROTEM analysis. J Cardiothorac Vasc Anesth. 2013;27(1):5-11.
26. Ota T, Yerebakan H, Akashi H, et al. Continuous-flow left ventricular assist device exchange: Clinical outcomes. J Heart Lung Transplant. 2014;33(1):65-70.
27. Patil NP, Popov AF, Simon AR. Minimally invasive left ventricular assist device implantation: At the crossroads. J Thorac Dis. 2015;7(4):564-5.
28. Pintar T, Collard CD. The systemic inflammatory response to cardiopulmonary bypass. Anesthesiol Clin North Am. 2003;21(3):453-64.
29. Popov AF, Hosseini MT, Zych B, et al. HeartWare left ventricular assist device implantation through bilateral anterior thoracotomy. Ann Thorac Surg. 2012;93(2):674-6.
30. Popov AF, Mohite PN, Sabashnikov A, et al. Minimally invasive HeartWare LVAD implantation through single left thoracotomy. J Artif Organs. 2015;18(2):170-2.
31. Reeves JT, Groves BM, Weir EK. Adenosine and selective reduction of pulmonary vascular resistance in primary pulmonary hypertension. Circulation. 1991;84(3): 1437-9.
32. Riebandt J, Sandner S, Mahr S, et al. Minimally invasive thoratec Heartmate II implantation in the setting of severe thoracic aortic calcification. Ann Thorac Surg. 2013;96(3):1094-6.
33. Rojas SV, Avsar M, Hanke JS, et al. Minimally-invasive approach for left ventricular assist device implantation:

Lower mortality and improved early outcome in adult patients with severe heart failure. Thorac Cardiovasc Surg. 2013;61(S 01):OP52.
34. Sabashnikov A, Mohite PN, Simon AR, et al. HeartWare miniaturized intrapericardial ventricular assist device: Advantages and adverse events in comparison to contemporary devices. Expert Rev Med Devices. 2013;10(4):441-52.
35. Schechter MA, Patel CB, Blue LJ, et al. Improved early survival with a nonsternotomy approach for continuous-flow left ventricular assist device replacement. Ann Thorac Surg. 2015;99(2):561-6.
36. Schmitto JD, Molitoris U, Haverich A, et al. Implantation of a centrifugal pump as a left ventricular assist device through a novel, minimized approach: Upper hemisternotomy combined with anterolateral thoracotomy. J Thorac Cardiovasc Surg. 2012;143(2):511-3.
37. Selzman CH, Sheridan BC. Off-pump insertion of continuous flow left ventricular assist devices. J Card Surg. 2007;22(4):320-2.
38. Slaughter MS, Rogers JG, Milano CA, et al. HeartMate II Investigators. Advanced heart failure treated with continuous-flow left ventricular assist device. N Engl J Med. 2009;361(23):2241-51.
39. Sun BC, Firstenberg MS, Louis LB, et al. Placement of long-term implantable ventricular assist devices without the use of cardiopulmonary bypass. J Heart Lung Transplant. 2008;27(7):718-21.
40. Umakanthan R, Haglund NA, Stulak JM, et al. Left thoracotomy HeartWare implantation with outflow graft anastomosis to the descending aorta: A simplified bridge for patients with multiple previous sternotomies. ASAIO J. 2013;59(6):664-7.
41. Van Meter CH, Jr, Robbins RJ, Ochsner JL. Technique of right heart protection and deairing during heartmate vented electric LVAD implantation. Ann Thorac Surg. 1997;63(4):1191-2.
42. Wagner CE, Bick JS, Kennedy J, et al. Minimally invasive thoracic left ventricular assist device implantation; case series demonstrating an integrated multidisciplinary strategy. J Cardiothorac Vasc Anesth. 2015;29(2):271-4.
43. Wever-Pinzon O, Drakos SG, Kfoury AG, et al. Morbidity and mortality in heart transplant candidates supported with mechanical circulatory support: Is reappraisal of the current United network for organ sharing thoracic organ allocation policy justified? Circulation. 2013;127(4):452-62.

CHAPTER

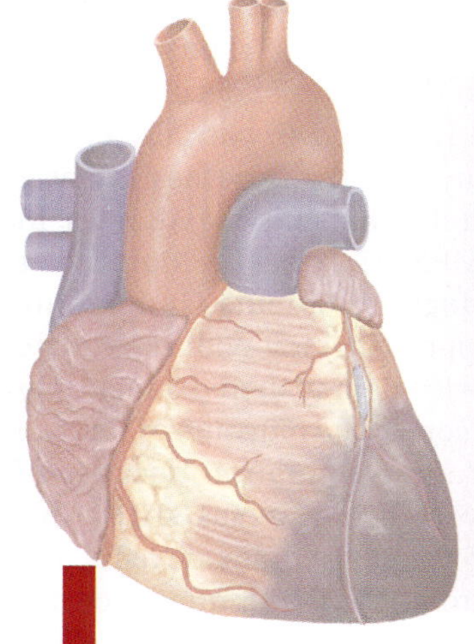

Newer Left Ventricular Assist Devices: Current Scenario

G Justin Paul, J Cecily Mary Majella

INTRODUCTION

Ventricular assist device has rapidly emerged as a durable and safe therapy for end-stage heart failure patients. Though originally conceived as bridge to transplant (BTT), significant advancements in medical management as well as technology with advent of newer generation devices have improved patient outcomes leading to increasing use as destination therapy (DT). Despite such improvement, however, the burden of adverse events remains significant and defines the most pressing issue in the current state of ventricular assist device (VAD) therapy. Eventual use of VAD technology as a comparable alternative to heart transplantation will ultimately rely on our ability to mitigate these risks. In this article, we will focus on new left VADs, ongoing investigations, and general trends that may have significant implications for future improvements in device-related outcomes, as the field continues to grow as the epitome of synergy between advancements in engineering and clinical medicine. Mechanical circulatory support (MCS) with VAD is a safe and efficacious treatment strategy for patients with end-stage heart failure (HF) that is refractory to medical therapy. Although these patients appreciate 81% and 70% survival at 1 year and 2 years, respectively,[1] they still experience high rates of VAD-related adverse events (AEs) which require our keen attention and understanding.

LEFT VENTRICULAR ASSIST DEVICE AS A BRIDGE-TO-TRANSPLANT/ DESTINATION THERAPY

Ventricular assist devices were originally conceived as temporary, BTT platforms. Initially, BTT was an effective strategy to rescue patients whose severity of HF precluded survival on medical therapy alone until a donor organ became available. However, it was recognized early on that utilizing VAD solely, as BTT was inadequate in addressing the growing prevalence of end-stage HF. This epidemiological challenge inspired the utilization of VADs as DT- potentially a durable and lifelong alternative to heart transplantation (HT).[2,3] The early-generation devices were pneumatically driven and pulsatile-flow which contributed to significant morbidity profiles including high incidence of device failure, and poor survival. Recognizing these limitations, subsequent clinical investigations began to focus on a new design in MCS that would come to actualize its potential as mainstream therapy for HF-continuous flow (CF) devices. Smaller and more durable, their early results demonstrated significantly improved survival and complication profiles, both for BTT and DT patients.[4-6] The Randomized Evaluation of Mechanical Assistance for the Treatment of Congestive Heart Failure (REMATCH) trial in 2001 by Rose et al.[2] first demonstrated the potential of using VADs as a durable DT platform with superior survival outcomes compared with conventional medical therapy alone. The trial was initially received with equal parts of excitement for the immense potential of this platform and legitimate trepidation over its alarmingly high rates of complications. Since then, the field has undergone several paradigm shifts with commensurate improvements in adverse effects profiles.

As the field transitioned toward CF-VADs, two distinct subclassification of CF design also emerged—axial and centrifugal mechanisms. Axial flow is generated by a propeller in a pipe, whereas centrifugal flow is generated by a bladed disk spinning in a cavity. During this era, two devices in particular, the axial-flow HeartMate II device and the centrifugal-flow HeartWare ventricular assist device (HVAD)[1] constituted the majority of devices implanted worldwide. Several key engineering differences between the two devices are that the HeartMate II rotor spins on blood-immersed ruby bearings, whereas the HVAD has a magnetically levitated, frictionless rotor. The HVADs smaller size is theoretically more conducive to biventricular or minimally invasive placement via thoracotomy. Some of the engineering differences between centrifugal and axial flow devices carry important physiological and management implications.[7] Although the effects of different flow-profiles are clinically harder to distinguish than laboratory, they point to important considerations for patient management. For instance, centrifugal output is exquisitely sensitive to loading conditions producing high pump-flow pulsatility in accordance with native ventricular activity. On the contrary, axial output is relatively inelastic across varied pressure gradients which during low LV volume states, can potentially lead to a higher incidence of suck-down event (a significant decrease in VAD output from contact between the VAD inflow cannula and the ventricular cavity or septum). It is multifactorial (e.g. inflow cannula position, high speed, and low ventricular volume), and may trigger ventricular tachyarrhythmia.[7] The most recent addition to the field of MCS is a new-generation centrifugal-flow device, the HeartMate III which has a fully magnetically levitated rotor, wider blood-flow paths, and artificial pulsatility. By programming the device to rhythmically decelerate and accelerate, the Heartmate III aimed to partially mimic and restore native pulsatility with the hypothesis, that it would reduce bleeding and thromboembolic AE rates. In the recently published MOMENTUM trial (the Multicenter Study of MagLev Technology in Patients Undergoing Mechanical Circulatory Support Therapy With HeartMate 3), the third-generation device demonstrated superiority over the HeartMate II in its composite outcome of survival without disabling stroke and reoperation because of malfunctioning device at 2 years (79.5% versus 60.2%). This difference was primarily driven by the dramatic reduction in the incidence of pump thrombosis (PT) requiring device exchange (1.6% versus 17.0%). Nonetheless, the excellent outcomes noted in both trials are emblematic of the exciting engineering potential and ongoing innovation that define this field (Table 1).

HEARTWARE VENTRICULAR ASSIST DEVICE ADVANTAGE (FIG. 1)

The HeartWare™ HVAD™ Pump is the smallest, full-support centrifugal VAD designed to be implanted completely within the pericardial space. The unique integrated inflow cannula design offers the flexibility to fit into smaller framed patients and treat more complex patients. It also allows for stable inflow—even with body habitus changes eliminating complication of malposition (Fig. 2).[4]

Easy to implant, the small size reduces the need for a pump pocket which may lead to decreased bleeding and decreased blood product use. It allows for less invasive exchange and explant.

A 10-mm outflow graft to the artery reduces the anastomotic size by approximately 50% compared to other devices, leading to flexibility of arterial landing sites (Table 2).

TABLE 1

Device type	*HeartWare HVAD*	*System HeartMate II*	*HeartMate III*
Speed range, rotations per minute	2,400–3,200	6,000–15,000	3,000–9,000
Rotor design	Centrifugal	Axial	Centrifugal
Pump position	Intrapericardial	Pump pocket	Intrapericardial
Blood flow gaps, mm	≈0.05	≈0.08	≈0.12
Food and Drug Administration–approved indication	Bridge to transplant (2012) Destination therapy (2017)	Bridge to transplant (2008) Destination therapy (2010)	Bridge to transplant (2017) Destination therapy (2017)
Magnetic levitation	Present		Present
Artificial pulsatility			Present
High inlet suction		Present	

(HVAD: heartware ventricular assist device)

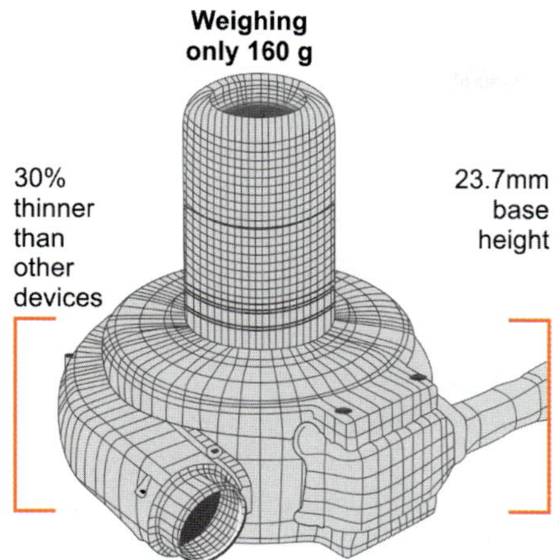

Fig. 1: Heartware ventricular assist device.

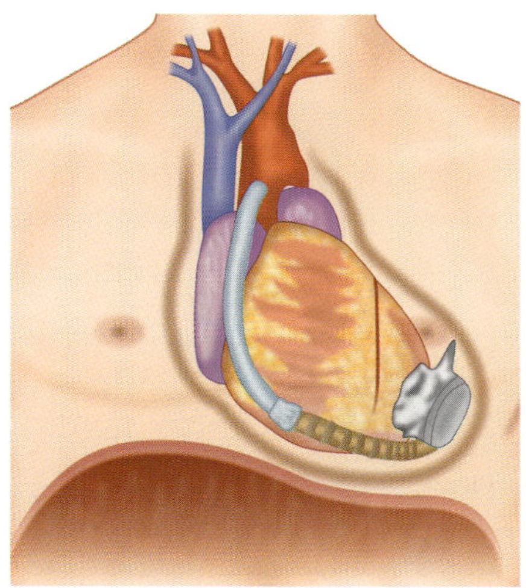

Fig. 2

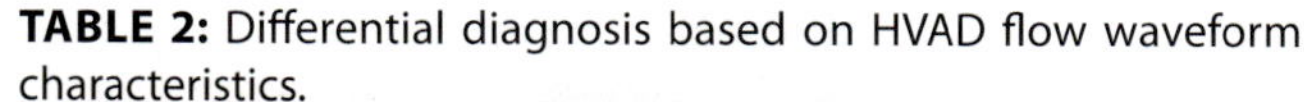

TABLE 2: Differential diagnosis based on HVAD flow waveform characteristics.

	Lower mean flow	*Higher mean flow*
Lower pulsatility	RVF, hypovolemia, tamponade, occlusion VFib/rapid VT	Hypotenstion/vasodilatation, aortic regurgitation, pump thrombosis (falsely elevated)
Higher pulsatility	HTN (with low trough), low RPMs, continuous suction (negatively deflected)	Hypervolemia, recovery?

(HTN: hypertension; HVAD: heartware continuous-flow ventricular assist device; RPM: revolutions per minute; RVF: right ventricular failure; VT: ventricular tachycardia; VF: ventricular fibrillation)

HeartMate II

The HeartMate II is a left ventricular assist device (LVAD) that is implanted alongside the patient's native heart with the purpose of pumping for the heart's left ventricle (Figs. 3 to 5).

The HeartMate II is surgically implanted just below the diaphragm in the abdomen. It acts as a conduit by attaching to the left ventricle and then to the aorta, leaving natural circulation in place. It assists in providing energy to propel blood throughout the body, as a healthy left ventricle would do. Food and Drug Administration (FDA) approved to use as a BTT or as destination therapy,[8,9] when the patient is not a transplant candidate (Fig. 6)

A new fully magnetically levitated centrifugal continuous-flow circulatory pump, HeartMate III has been engineered to reduce shear stress on blood elements and avert pump thrombosis. This pump has wide blood-flow passages and no mechanical bearings, is frictionless, and is programed to facilitate rapid changes in rotor speed to create an intrinsic artificial pulse. This fixed pulse which is asynchronous with the native heartbeat, reduces stasis in the pump.

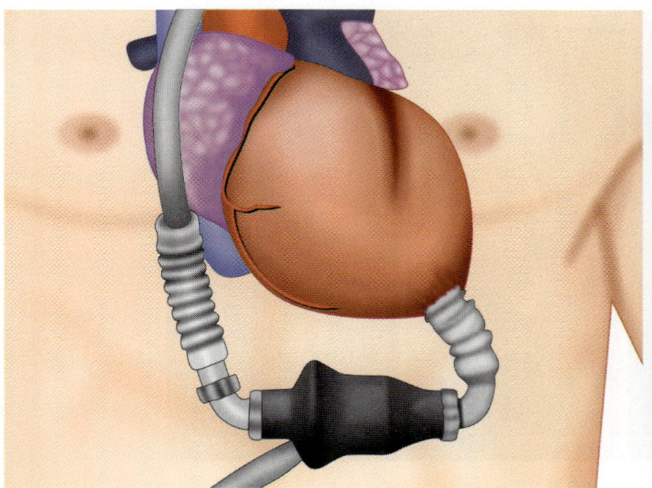

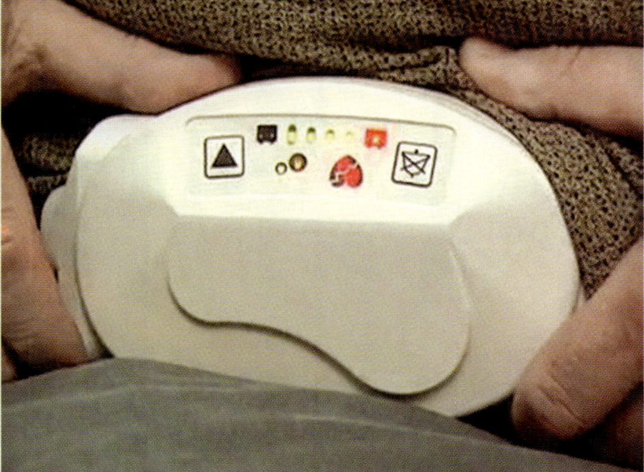

Fig. 3: Components of Heartmate II.

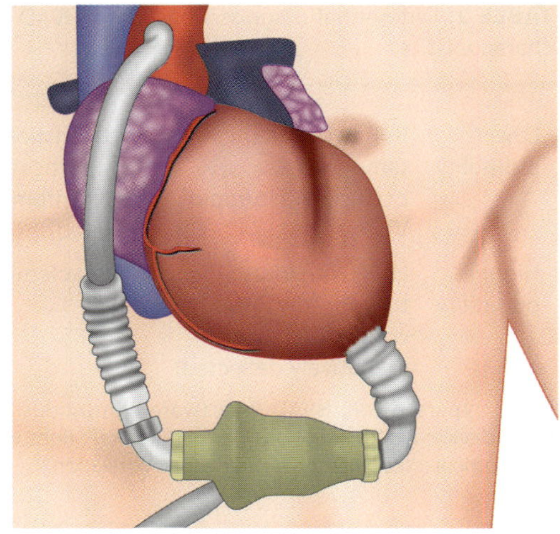

Implanted blood pump

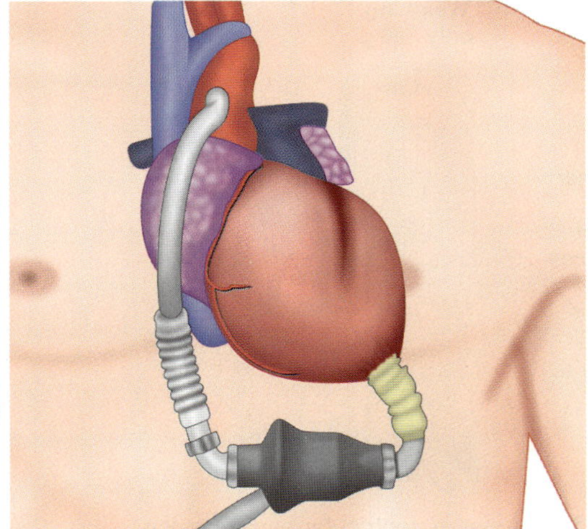

Inflow conduit

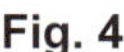

Fig. 4

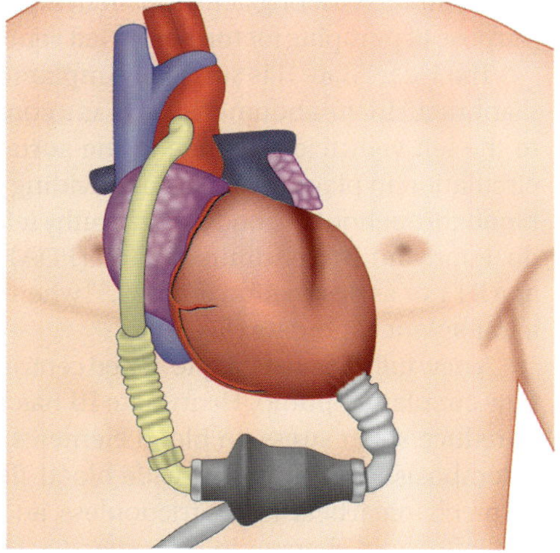

Outflow graft

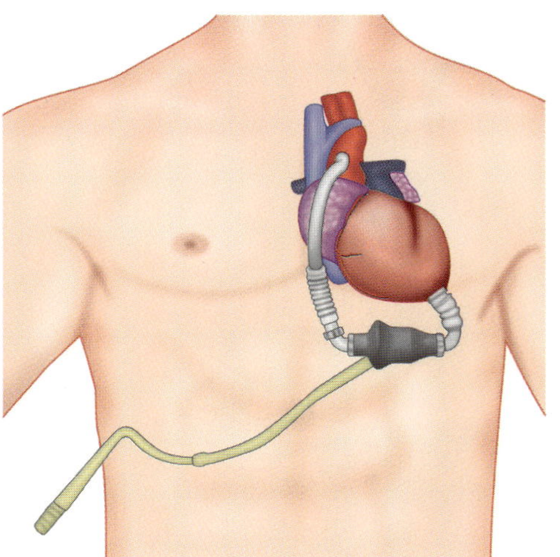

Percutaneous lead

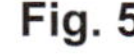

Fig. 5

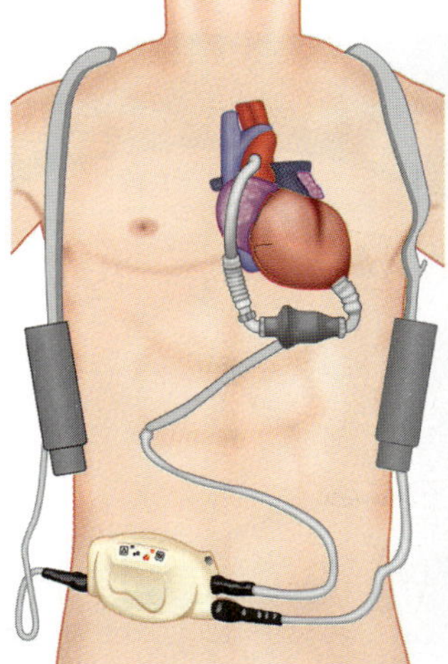

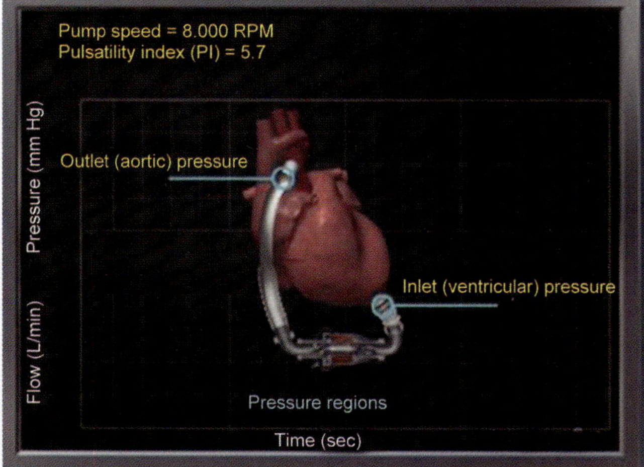

Fig. 6: HeartMate II.
(RPM: revolutions per minute)

HEARTMATE II AND HEARTMATE III-A COMPARITIVE ANALYSIS (FIG. 7)

Panel A shows a diagram of the axial-flow pump; blood enters at one end of the rotor and is driven along the axis of the rotor to the outflow of the pump.

Panel B shows a diagram of the fully magnetically levitated centrifugal-flow pump; blood enters at the central axis of the rotor and is driven outward centrifugally to the outflow of the pump. Both pumps are considered to be continuous-flow pumps (rather than pulsatile-flow pumps), because blood flow is continuous and not interrupted, although the centrifugal-flow pump incorporates rapid changes in rotor speed to create an intrinsic artificial pulse.

In the MOMENTUM 3 trial, implantation of the fully magnetically levitated centrifugal continuous-flow pump HeartMate III was associated with a higher rate of survival free of disabling stroke or survival free of reoperation to replace or remove the device at 6 months after implantation than was implantation of the mechanical-bearing axial continuous-flow pump HeartMate II among patients with advanced heart failure irrespective of their eligibility for transplantation. The incremental benefits associated with the centrifugal-flow pump observed in this 6-month analysis were due to the absence of suspected or confirmed pump thrombosis leading to surgical pump exchange or urgent transplantation.

Pump thrombosis which is manifested by elevations in hemolytic biomarkers, such as lactate dehydrogenase level or in sudden transient increases in pump power, is an important limitation to the use of currently available circulatory pumps. As the clinical syndrome progresses, worsening heart failure caused by the inability of the pump to unload the left ventricle becomes apparent and ultimately necessitates reoperation or urgent transplantation to replace or remove the pump. A recent analysis has also shown that the centrifugal-flow device does not cause loss of high-molecular-weight multimers of von Willebrand factor to the same degree that the axial-flow pump does.

There were no significant differences between the two pumps in the associated rates of other major complications including right heart failure (RHF), any stroke or disabling stroke, major infection including drive-line infections, or bleeding episodes, particularly gastrointestinal bleeding. A numerical, but not statistically significant, trend toward a higher rate of disabling strokes with the centrifugal-flow pump than with the axial-flow pump and a higher rate of RHF events managed with a right ventricular assist system with the axial-flow pump than with the centrifugal-flow

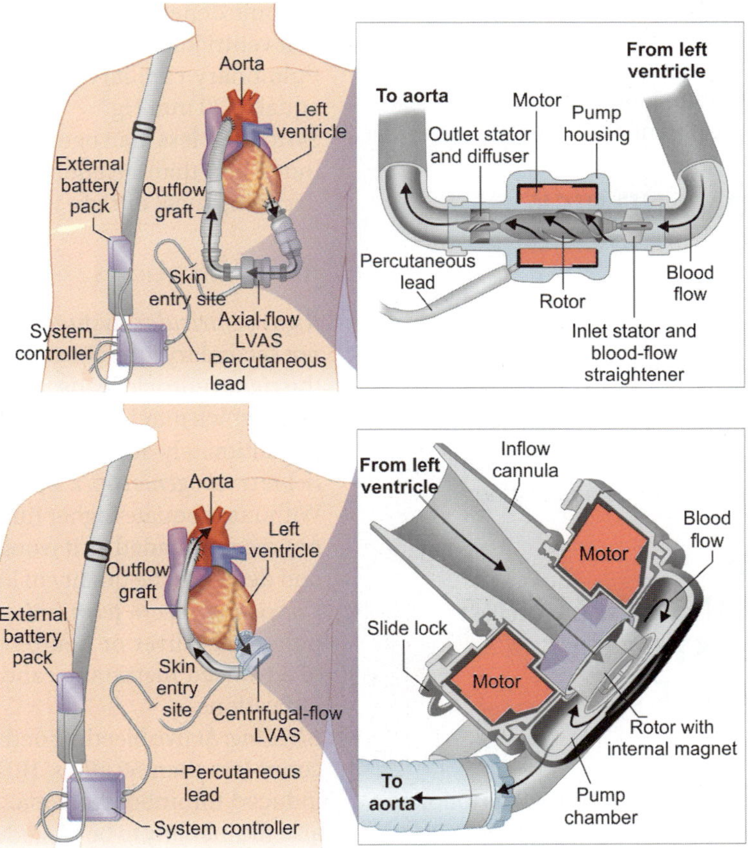

Fig. 7: Diagrams of the axial-flow pump and the centrifugal-flow pump.

pump. It is unclear whether pump thrombosis would remain infrequent, if anticoagulation doses were reduced in an effort to decrease rates of bleeding.

BIVENTRICULAR ASSIST DEVICE

This device is used for patients with either biventricular failure or right ventricular failure associated with left ventricular disease. The total artificial heart (TAH) has been a revolution. The SynCardia TAH is the most widely used TAH.

PULSATILITY INDEX

When the left ventricle contracts, the increase in ventricular pressure causes an increase in pump flow during cardiac systole. The magnitude of these flow pulses are measured and averaged over 15-second intervals to produce a "Pulsatility Index". The pulsatility index (PI) calculation represents cardiac pulsatility. PI values typically range from 1 to 10. In general, the magnitude of the PI value is related to the amount of assistance provided by the pump. Higher values indicate more ventricular filling and higher pulsatility (i.e. the pump is providing less support to the left ventricle). Lower values indicate less ventricular filling and lower pulsatility (i.e. the pump is providing greater support and further unloading the ventricle). PI values should be routinely monitored and should not vary significantly during resting conditions. Under otherwise stable conditions, a significant drop in value may indicate a decrease in circulating blood volume. PI values near or above 10 may indicate potential problems.

PATIENT SELECTION AND RISK STRATIFICATION

According to the most recent HF guidelines published by the American College of Cardiology and American Heart Association, VAD implantation is indicated for patients who have Stage D HF with reduced ejection fraction. However, although the demand is alarmingly high, VAD remains a highly invasive intervention that requires a careful, multidisciplinary evaluation of patients candidacy before implantation.

INDICATIONS AND CONTRAINDICATIONS REGARDING VENTRICULAR ASSIST DEVICE IMPLANTATION (TABLE 3)

Indications

Strong indications for either BTT, DT, or BTR are as follows.

- New York Heart Association (NYHA) class IV for 60–90 days

TABLE 3: Indications and contraindications regarding ventricular assist device implantation.

Indications	*Absolute contraindications*
Frequent hospitalizations for HF	Irreversible hepatic disease
Intolerance to neurochormonal antagonists	Irreversible renal disease
NYHA IIIb–IV functional limitations despite OMT	Irreversible neurological disease
End-organ dysfunction owing to low CO	Medical nonadherence
Increasing diuretic requirement	Severe psychosocial limitations
CRT nonresponder	
Inotrope dependence	
Low peak VO_2 (<14 mL/kg/min)	

(HF: heart failure; OMT: optimal medical therapy; NYHA: New York Heart Association; CO: cardiac output; CRT: cardiac resynchronization therapy)

Source: Adapted from Peura et al. and published with the permission of the American Heart Association.

- Maximal tolerated medical therapy and certified respiratory therapy/implantable cardioverter-defibrillator, if indicated
- Chronic dependence on inotropic agents
- Left ventricular ejection fraction (LVEF) less than 25%
- Pulmonary capillary wedge pressure greater than or equal to 20 mm Hg
- Systolic BP less than or equal to 80–90 mm Hg or cardiac index less than or equal to 2 L/min/m^2, evidence of declining renal or right ventricular function.

Contraindications

- *Right ventricular dysfunction:* Either primarily or RHF not secondary to left heart failure. Improper function of the right ventricle leads to insufficient filling of the left heart which may lead to inadequate inflow in the device and ultimately device malfunction.
- *Acute cardiogenic shock with a neurological compromise:* Without adequate higher functions, LVAD placement is not recommended as it would only increase morbidity and decrease the quality of life.
- *Coexisting severe terminal comorbidity:* Severe renal, pulmonary, liver or neurological disease or evidence of advanced metastatic cancer are considered contraindications.
- *Bleeding:* Active bleeding or thrombocytopenia (platelet count less than 50,000 × 10/L) or confirmed heparin-induced thrombocytopenia. Not just the bleeding but also the inability to be placed on anticoagulation makes this a contraindication.

- *Anatomical factors:* Hypertrophic cardiomyopathy or a large ventricular septal defect is a hindrance to devise placement and function.
- *Technical limitations:* Body surface area less than 1.2–1.5 m^2 or any other factor.
- *Social considerations:* LVAD management requires a high degree of patient compliance which necessitates adequate psychological function to comply with medications and device maintenance. It also requires family education in interpreting basic function and alarms. Thus, any difficulty posed by such factors could pose a contraindication to LVAD placement.

COMPLICATIONS (FIG. 8)

The vexing combination of existing RV dysfunction, pulmonary hypertension, and acute hemodynamic shifts often precipitates RHF early on post-VAD implantation in ≈15–25% of the patients with 4% requiring RVAD implantation within 2 weeks. Though its exact mechanism is unclear, it is believed to be driven by sudden increases in LV unloading and RV preload, which distorts RV geometry and unmasks underlying dysfunction.

TREATMENT SRATEGY FOR LVAD ASSOCIATED GI BLEED

Treatment srategy for LVAD associated gastrointestinal bleed in Flowchart 1.

CLINICAL PRESENTATION OF LVAD ASSOCIATED THROMBOSIS

Clinical presentation of LVAD associated thrombosis in Figure 9.

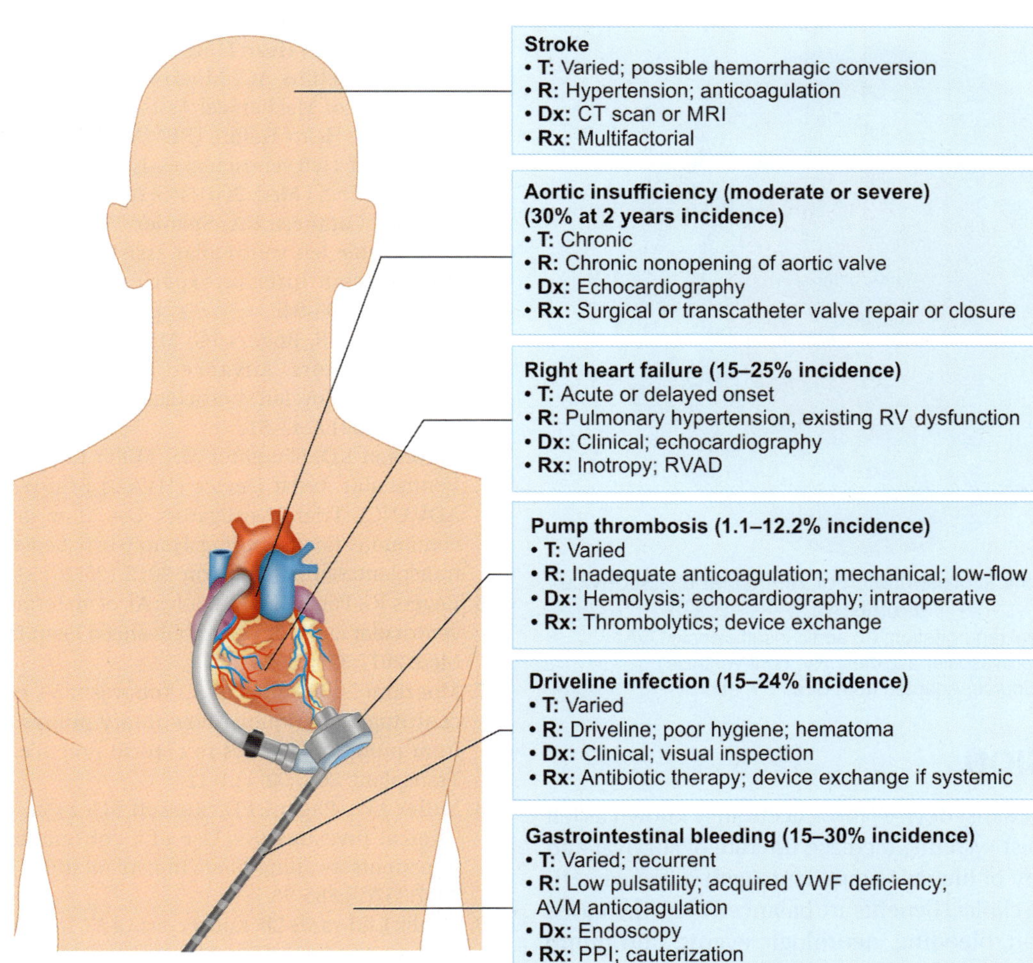

Fig. 8

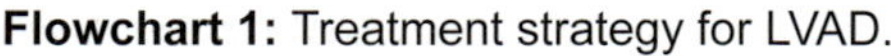

Flowchart 1: Treatment strategy for LVAD.

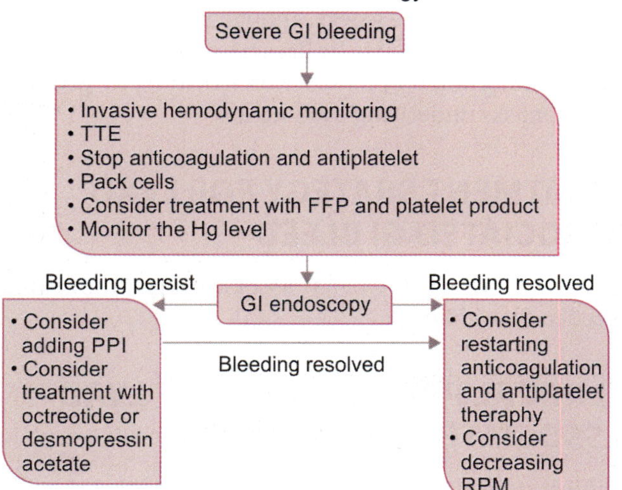

(GI: gastrointestinal; TTE: transesophageal echocardiogram; FFP: fresh frozen plasma; Hg: hemoglobin; PPI: proton pump inhibitor; RPM: remote patient monitoring)

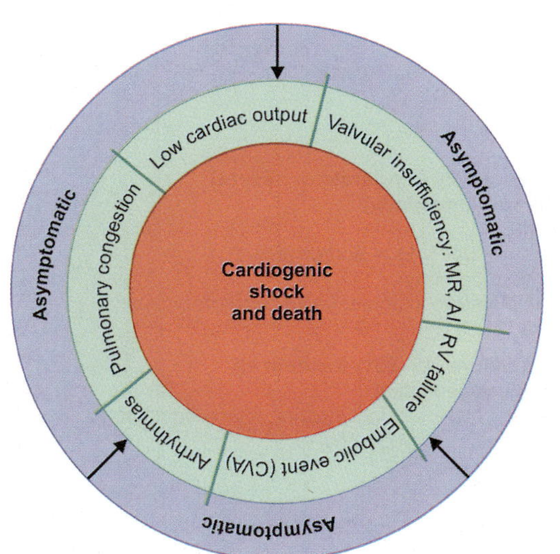

Fig. 9: The clinical presentation of ventricular assist device thrombosis.

(MR: mitral regurgitation; AI: aortic insufficiency; CVA: cerebrovascular accident; RV: right ventricle)

Source: Adapted from Birati EY, et al.

CONCLUSION

Left ventricular assist devices more accurately known as left ventricular assist systems, increase the rate of survival and improve quality of life among patients with advanced HF. However, these clinical benefits are balanced by an increased risk of infection, bleeding, neurologic events, and pump malfunction that is due principally to pump thrombosis. In conclusion, comparative analysis between the centrifugal-flow left ventricular assist system HeartMate III and the axial-flow left ventricular assist system HeartMate II in patients with advanced HF, there is evidence of incremental improvement in clinical outcomes with the centrifugal-flow pump that was attributable to a lower rate of reoperation for pump malfunction without an apparent between-group difference in the rate of other adverse events. In a remarkably short span of time, MCS using VAD has become a mainstream treatment option for end-stage HF, with a growing proportion of patients successfully undergoing VAD implantation as DT. Survival outcomes have and will continue to improve with the emergence of newer generations of CF-VADs. Although risks of various AEs are still significant, posing a predominant challenge for the coming decade, altogether, the synergy between medical management, and engineering innovations will continue to actualize the unlimited potential of MCS, marking one of the most exciting eras in the treatment of HF.

REFERENCES

1. Kirklin JK, Pagani FD, Kormos RL, et al. Eighth annual INTERMACS report: special focus on framing the impact of adverse events. J Heart Lung Transplant. 2017;36(10):1080-6.
2. Rose EA, Gelijns AC, Moskowitz AJ, et al. Randomized Evaluation of Mechanical Assistance for the Treatment of Congestive Heart Failure (REMATCH) Study Group. Long-term use of a left ventricular assist device or end-stage heart failure. N Engl J Med. 2001;345(20):1435-43.
3. Sun BC, Catanese KA, Spanier TB, et al. 100 long-term implantable left ventricular assist devices: the Columbia Presbyterian interim experience. Ann Thorac Surg. 1999;68(2):688-94.
4. Slaughter MS, Rogers JG, Milano CA, et al. HeartMate II Investigators. Advanced heart failure treated with continuous-flow left ventricular assist device. N Engl J Med. 2009;361(23):2241-51.
5. Aaronson KD, Slaughter MS, Miller LW, et al. HeartWare Ventricular Assist Device (HVAD) Bridge to Transplant ADVANCE Trial Investigators. Use of an intrapericardial, continuous-flow, centrifugal pump in patients awaiting heart transplantation. Circulation. 2012;125(25):3191-200.
6. Rogers JG, Pagani FD, Tatooles AJ, et al. Intrapericardial left ventricular assist device for advanced heart failure. N Engl J Med. 2017;376(5):451-60.
7. Moazami N, Fukamachi K, Kobayashi M, et al. Axial and centrifugal continuous-flow rotary pumps: A translation from pump mechanics to clinical practice. J Heart Lung Transplant. 2013;32(1):1-11.
8. Miller LW, Pagani FD, Russell SD, et al. HeartMate II Clinical Investigators. Use of a continuous-flow device in patients awaiting heart transplantation. N Engl J Med. 2007;357(9):885-96.
9. Stehlik J, Edwards LB, Kucheryavaya AY, International Society of Heart and Lung Transplantation, et al. The registry of the International Society for Heart and Lung Transplantation: 29th official adult heart transplant report-2012. J Heart Lung Transplant. 2012;31(10):1052-64.

CHAPTER

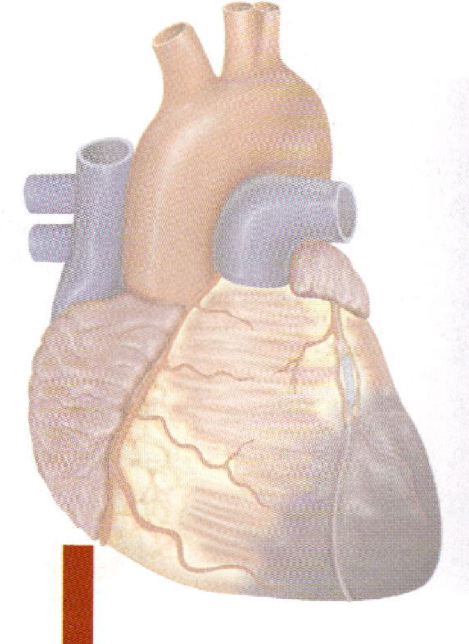

Device Therapy in Heart Failure

Ajay Naik, Aarya Naik

INTRODUCTION

Heart failure is the final frontier in cardiac disease management spectrum. When there is inexorable progression of disease despite lifestyle changes, guideline-directed optimal medical therapy, and interventions, devices become an important option to reduce morbidity and mortality. The device options may include cardiac implantable electronic devices (CIEDs) such as cardiac resynchronization therapy (CRT), implantable cardioverter defibrillator (ICD), or implantable hemodynamic monitors.

VENTRICULAR DYSSYNCHRONY AND CARDIAC RESYNCHRONIZATION THERAPY

- Progressive ventricular dilatation in heart failure (HF) results in conduction abnormalities.
- Bundle branch blocks, in particular left bundle branch block (LBBB) alter the timing and pattern of ventricular contraction. This worsens the mechanical function of the already failing ventricle.[1]
- The paradoxical septal motion and delayed activation of left ventricular (LV) free wall is well appreciated in LBBB and is termed as "Ventricular Dyssynchrony".
- Correction of the electrical conduction abnormality by biventricular (BiV) pacing, more generally referred to as CRT, results in improvement in mechanical function of the LV.
- Cardiac resynchronization therapy has proved to be one of the most important breakthroughs in the treatment of HF.[2]
- Cardiac resynchronization therapy is now established therapy in HF in indicated patients.

MECHANISM OF CARDIAC RESYNCHRONIZATION THERAPY

- Cardiac resynchronization therapy corrects the abnormal ventricular activation pattern seen in patients with LBBB conduction delay.
- Biventricular pacing results in the generation of two ventricular activation wavefronts, which result in a more normal pattern of ventricular activation.
- Left ventricular contraction is more efficient and stroke volume is improved, without an increase in myocardial oxygen consumption by the heart, and both mitral regurgitation and myocardial diastolic dysfunction are often decreased.[2]

LANDMARK CLINICAL TRIALS OF CARDIAC RESYNCHRONIZATION THERAPY

Cardiac resynchronization therapy has been clinically evaluated in 4,000 patients in landmark randomized controlled trials (Table 1). It has demonstrated benefit for patients with New York Heart Association (NYHA) class III

TABLE 1: Landmark randomized clinical trials of CRT.

Study	No. of patients	NYHA class	lVEF (%)	lVEDD (mm)	SR/AF	QRS (ms)	ICD
MUSTIC-SR	58	III	<35%	>60	SR	>150	No
MIRACLE	453	III, IV	<35%	>55	SR	>130	No
MUSTIC AF	43	III	<35%	>60	AF	>200	No
PATH CHF	41	III, IV	<35%	NA	SR	>120	No
MIRACLE ICD	369	III, IV	<35%	>55	SR	>130	Yes
CONTAK CO	227	II, IV	<35%	NA	SR	>120	Yes
MIRACLE ICD II	186	II	<35%	>55	SR	>130	Yes
PATH CHF II	89	III, IV	<35%	NA	SR	>120	Yes/no
COMPANION	1520	III, IV	<35%	NA	SR	>120	Yes/no
CARE HF	814	III, IV	<35%	>30 (indexed to height)	SR	>120	No
CARE HF extension 2006	813	III, IV	≤35%	>30 (indexed to height)	SR	>120	No
REVERSE 2008	610	I, II	<40%	>55	SR	>120	Yes/no
MADIT-CRT	1800	I, II	<30%	NA	SR	>130 ms	Yes
RAFT	1798 Canada	II, III	<30%	>60	SR/AF	>130 >200*	Yes

(AF: atriaL fibrillation; ICD: implantable cardioverter-defibrillator; lVEDD: Left ventricular end-diastolic diameter; lVEF: Left ventricular ejection fraction; NYHA: New York Heart Association; SR: sinus rhythm; CRT: cardiac resynchronization therapy)

*Patients in atrial fibrillation.

HF, in particular, and, to some degree, for those with class IV HF.[2]

BENEFITS OF CARDIAC RESYNCHRONIZATION THERAPY IN HEART FAILURE

- For Patients with moderate-to-severe HF (NYHA class III– IV), CRT has been shown in four of the landmark trials (MUSTIC SR, MIRACLE, CONTAK-CD, MIRACLE-ICD) to provide very consistent improvements in NYHA class, exercise capacity (6-minute hall walk distance) and peak oxygen consumption, and quality of life.
- CARE-HF study, a large trial, randomized patients to either CRT plus optimal medical therapy or CRT alone, provided the first demonstration that CRT without an ICD prolonged survival, and markedly reduced both morbidity and mortality, with the effect sustained over 37 months of follow-up.
- One of the most important mechanisms of action for the benefit of CRT was reverse remodeling, which evolved over the initial 18 months and had a sustained effect over time.[3]
- A meta-analysis of six randomized, controlled trials of CRT for more severe, chronic, and symptomatic LV systolic dysfunction found that CRT was associated with a 28% reduction in all-cause mortality and a 37% reduction in new hospitalizations for exacerbation of HF.[4]

INDICATIONS FOR CARDIAC RESYNCHRONIZATION THERAPY

A recent publication compared guidelines for CRT from major societies including American College of Cardiology Foundation (ACCF)/American Heart Association (AHA)/ Heart Rhythm Society (HRS), European Society of Cardiology (ESC) Heart Failure Association, ESC European Heart Rhythm Association (EHRA), Canadian Cardiac Society (CCS), National Heart Foundation of Australia and Cardiac Society of Australia and New Zealand, and National Institute of Health and Care Excellence (NICE) (Tables 1 and 2).[5]

- All cardiac societies' guidelines reviewed agree that patients with LBBB and a QRS duration >150 ms should be offered a CRT device provided they are in NYHA functional class III.
- There also appears to be general consensus among the international guidelines for CRT implantation in patients with LBBB and a QRS duration >150 ms in NYHA functional class II and ambulatory class IV.
- There are inconsistencies between recommendations for patients with LBBB and narrower QRS duration (129–149 ms) and non-LBBB patients (Tables 2 and 3).[5]

TABLE 2: Comparison of CRT recommendation for LBBB from various societies.

Guideline (Year)	QRS ≥150 ms		QRS 130–149 ms		QRS 110–129 1M	
	NYHA Functional Class III/IV	NYHA Functional Class II	NYHA Functional Class III/IV	NYHA Functional Class II	NYHA Functional Class III/IV	NYHA Functional CLass II
ESC HFA (2016)*	I, A	I, A	1,8	1,8	III, A	III, A
ESC EHRA (2013)	I, A	I, A	1, 8	1, 8	1, 8	1, 8
ACC/AHAIHRS (2013)	I, A	I, B	IIa, B	11a, B	IIa, B	IIa, B
CCS (2017)	I, High	I, High	I, High	I, High	III, Moderate	III, Moderate
Australian Guidelines (2011)	A		A		A	
NICE (2014)	CRT-P or CRT-D†	CRT-D	CRT-P or CRT-D†	CRT-D	CRT-P or CRT-D†	CRT-D

(ACC/AHA/HRS: American College of Cardiology/American Heart Association/Heart Rhythm Society; CCS: Canadian Cardiology Society; CRT-D: cardiac resynchronization therapy-defibrillator; CRT-P: cardiac resynchronization therapy-pacemaker; ESC EHRA: European Society of Cardiology European Hearth Rhythm Association; ESC HFA: European Society of Cardiology European Heart Rhythm Association; LBBB: left bundle branch block)

Values are class of recommendation, level of evidence, unless otherwise indicated. Australian guidelines provide only grade of recommendation A, not evidence level for these recommendations. NICE guidelines provide guidance on type of device rather than recommendation or evidence level.

*The ESC HFA guidelines do not specify NYHA functional class, rather they state that the guidelines refer to symptomatic patients with heart failure.

†Not for NYHA functional class IV.

TABLE 3: Comparison of CRT recommendation for non-LBBB from various societies.

Guideline (Year)	QRS ≥150 ms		QRS 130–149 ms		QRS 110–129 1M	
	NYHA Functional Class III/IV	NYHA Functional Class II	NYHA Functional Class III/IV	NYHA Functional Class II	NYHA Functional Class III/IV	NYHA Functional CLass II
ESC HFA (2016)*	IIa, B	IIa, B	IIb, B	IIb, B	III, A	III, A
ESC EHRA (2013)	IIa, B	IIa, B	IIb, B	IIb, B	IIb, B	IIb, B
ACC/AHAIHRS (2013)	IIa, A	IIb, B	IIb, B	III, B	IIb, B	III, B
CCS (2017)	IIb, Low	IIb, Low			III, Moderate	III, Moderate
Australian Guidelines (2011)	A		A		A	
NICE (2014)	CRT-P or CRT-D†	CRT-D	CRT-P‡		CRT-P‡	CRT-D

Values are class of recommendation, level of evidence, unless otherwise indicated. Australian guidelines provide only grade of recommendation A, not evidence level for these recommendations. NICE guidelines provide guidance on type of device rather than recommendation or evidence level.

*The ESC HFA guidelines do not specify NYHA functional class, rather they state that the guidelines refer to symptomatic patients with heart failure.

†Not for NYHA functional class IV.

‡Only for NYHA functional class IV.

PATIENTS WITH HF AND LESS CONVENTIONAL INDICATIONS FOR CRT[5]

Atrial Fibrillation

- Concomitant AF may be present in 10–50% of patients with moderate or severe HF.[5]
- Most randomized control trials of CRT excluded patients with AF, and those trials that did include patients with AF were small.
- Ventricular rate must be adequately controlled by pharmacologic intervention or atrioventricular nodal ablation in order to ensure a high degree of CRT pacing.

Conventional Pacemaker Indication and Heart Failure

- BLOCK-HF trial showed that biventricular pacing was superior to RV pacing in patients with HF and atrioventricular block (HFA guidelines provide a Class I recommendation for CRT after this trial).
- DAVID (Dual Chamber and VVI Implantable Defibrillator) trial, suggested a worse outcome in patients who were paced at >40% (ACC/AHA/HRS guidelines recommend CRT for patients with degree of anticipated RV pacing >40%).
- Although the complication rate is greater with an increasing number of leads implanted, a later upgrade

from a permanent pacemaker to a CRT is also associated with added risk.

Patients with HF and an ICD Indication

- The HFA guidelines state that if a patient is due to receive an ICD and has a QRS duration between 130 ms and 149 ms, a CRT-D should be considered, and if the QRS is >150 ms, a CRT-D is recommended.
- European Heart Rhythm Association guidelines favor CRT-P implantation in patients with advanced HF, severe renal insufficiency or dialysis, and other major comorbidities including frailty and cachexia. CRT-D, on the other hand, is recommended if the life expectancy is >1 year in patients with NYHA functional class II, ischemic heart disease, and no major comorbidities.
- No randomized study was powered to compare CRT-D versus CRT-P, COMPANION study compared these devices to optimal medical therapy. Most associations leave the choice of device to the implanting physician.

Upgrade from Conventional Pacing to Cardiac Resynchronization Therapy

- Patients who have received a conventional pacemaker or an ICD and develop worsening HF, and who have a high proportion of RV pacing may be considered for an upgrade to a CRT.
- Upgrades have become increasingly common in view of heightened awareness that RV pacing >40% may aggravate LV dysfunction and cause HF.

Patients in HF NYHA Functional Class I

- None of the ESC guidelines, CCS, or Australian guidelines provides recommendations for CRT for patients in NYHA functional class I.
- The ACC/AHA/HRS guidelines, on the other hand, provide a Class IIb recommendation, evidence level C, on condition that the patients have LBBB with a QRS >150 ms, HF caused by ischemia, and an LVEF <30% on guideline-directed medical therapy.

Heart Failure Patients with Narrow QRS

- There is increasing evidence that patients with a narrow QRS do not benefit from a CRT device.[5]
- Two meta-analyses have been published showing that CRT implantation in narrow QRS is associated with a poor prognosis.[6]

Nonresponders to Cardiac Resynchronization Therapy

- There is an approximately 30% non-responder rate across various clinical trials, when taking into account absence of LV remodeling or lack of symptom improvement.
- The main causes of non-response are suboptimal LV lead placement, suboptimal AV and VV timing, ventricular scar, and HF progression.
- The definition and treatment of these non-responders remain a major area of research, and efforts to convert these patients to responders remain an important goal.

Multisite and Multipoint Left Ventricular Pacing

- In order to overcome non-responder issues, newer algorithms are being utilized to stimulate the LV simultaneously or sequentially from multiple electrodes of the LV lead.
- Quadripolar LV lead has become the choice in most implants in the current era. (Fig. 1).

Epicardial Left Ventricular Lead

If the patient is undergoing surgery for revascularization/valvar indication an epicardial lead deployment by the surgeon at the optimal myocardial site can help overcome issues of absence or small calibre of veins at ideal target LV stimulation site.

Bundle of His Pacing for Heart Failure

- There has been considerable interest in bundle of His pacing for HF patients. This may be particularly attractive in patients who do not fulfill ideal criteria for conventional CRT such as RBBB, less wide QRS, AF with less wide QRS, IVCD, suboptimal target LV vein/pacing site, suboptimal LV pacing thresholds.
- Improvement in hardware and understanding of selective/nonselective His pacing mechanism may make this another option in HF device therapy.

Prevalence of HF and Target Population for CRT

- As per population studies, approximately 2% of adults aged 45 years have HF.[7] LV systolic dysfunction is prevalent in approximately half of these, of which, half are symptomatic. Of these symptomatic patients with reduced LVEF, approximately 40% have QRS >120 ms.

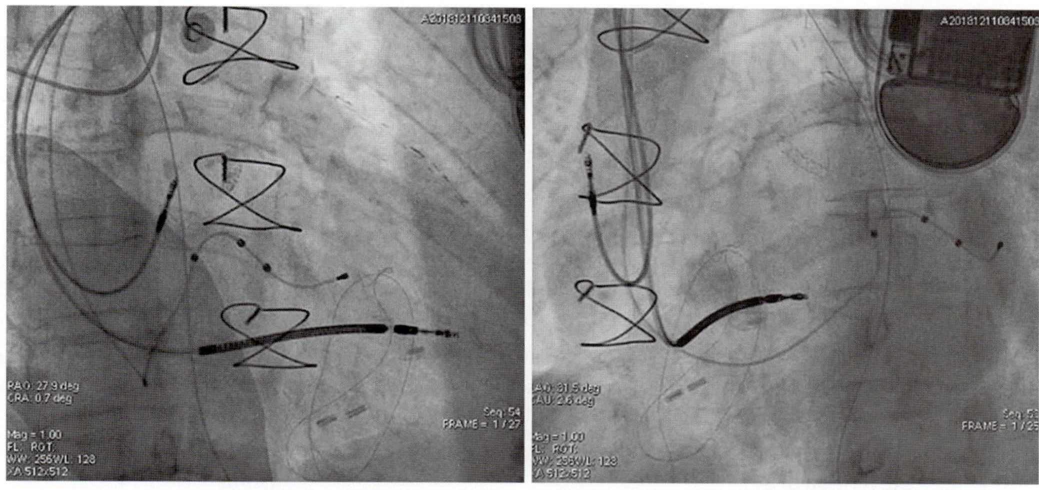

Fig. 1: Cardiac resynchronization therapy device with quadripolar LV lead, RAO, and LAO projections.
(LAO: left anterior oblique; LV: left ventricular; RAO: right anterior oblique)

- Approximately 25% of patients with reduced LVEF and prolonged QRS may have atrial fibrillation (AF). Some may have end-stage NYHA class IV HF symptoms or serious comorbidities foreshortening life expectancy (e.g. cancer). These are not currently considered ideal CIED patients.
- There would be a potential target population for CRT of approximately 0.1% of the adult population (or approximately 10 persons per 10,000). Current CRT or CRT-D implant rates are closer to 1:10,000.[5]

SUDDEN CARDIAC DEATH AND ICD THERAPY IN HF

Patients with HF and LV systolic dysfunction are at increased risk of sudden cardiac death (SCD). SCD is the leading cause of mortality in patients with HF and occurs at a rate 6–9 times seen in the general population.[1] ICD as both primary and secondary prophylactic therapy reduces total mortality by reducing the incidence of SCD.

Randomized Controlled Trials of ICD for HF

- The landmark trials establishing a role for ICDs as primary prevention of mortality in HF patients are the multicenter automatic defibrillator implantation II (MADIT II) and the sudden cardiac death-heart failure trial (SCD-HeFT) (Table 4).
- The Danish study to assess the efficacy of ICDs in patients with nonischemic systolic heart failure on mortality (DANISH) concluded that prophylactic ICD in patients with symptomatic systolic HF not caused by CAD was not associated with a significantly lower long-term rate of death from any cause than was usual clinical care.[1]
- A meta-analysis of 11 studies enrolling 8,657 participants with LV dysfunction including 3,128 patients without IHD and 5,439 patients with IHD has been recently published (Table 5).[8] In patients without IHD [nonischemic cardiomyopathy (NICM)] with HF, ICD therapy was found to reduce mortality by 24% (HR 0.76, 95% CI 0.64–0.90, p = 0.001). In patients with IHD, ICD implantation at a dedicated procedure also reduced mortality by 24% (HR 0.76, 95% CI 0.60–0.96, p = 0.02).
- With a significant 24% mortality reduction in both etiologies, it may no longer be necessary to distinguish between them when deciding on primary prevention ICD implantation. Thus, it is unlikely that current guideline recommendation for ICDs will change, despite the negative result of the DANISH trial.

Subcutaneous Implantable Cardioverter Defibrillator

- The subcutaneous ICD has emerged as a promising alternative to conventional ICD systems.[9] It avoids the potential periprocedural and long-term complications associated with the transvenous leads.
- It is an effective and safe modality with comparable defibrillation success rate and similar rates of inappropriate shock delivery to conventional ICDs.
- Subcutaneous implantable cardioverter defibrillator (S-ICD) is an option for patients without pacing requirements, particularly younger patients who would be exposed to a longer period of transvenous leads of conventional system and the attendant risk and complications.

TABLE 4: Major ICD trials and their outcomes.

Study	*Total population*	*Indication*	*% Women*	*Groups*	*Mortality*
MADIT I[2]	196	Primary prevention of SCD	8	Antiarrhythmic drug therapy versus ICD	54% relative reduction in mortality in ICD group; not stratified by sex
MADIT II[4]	1,232	Primary prevention of SCD	16	ICD versus medical therapy	Men: HR 0.66; p = 0.011 Women: HR 0.57; p = 0.132
SCD-HeFT[5]	2,521	Primary prevention of SCD	23	ICD versus medical therapy + amiodarone versus medical therapy alone	Men: HR 0.73; CI [0.57–0.93] Women: HR 0.96; CI [0.58–1.61]
MUSTT[3]	704	Primary prevention of SCD	10	Standard medical therapy versus medical therapy plus EP-guided therapy	Mortality in EP-guided therapy group— Men: 21% Women: 32% (p = 0.13)
DEFINITE[7]	458	Primary prevention of SCD	29	Medical therapy versus ICD	Men: HR 0.49; CI [0.27–0.90]; p = 0.019 Women: HR 1.14; CI [0.50–2.64]; p = 0.754
AVID[6]	1,885	Secondary prevention of SCD	22	Antiarrhythmic drug therapy versus ICD	Mortality in women: 15.5%, men: 14.4% compared with 24.5% in patients without ICD

(AVID: antiarrhythmics versus implantable defibrillators; DEFINITE: defibrillators in non-ischemic cardiomyopthy treatment evaluation; EP: electrophysiology; ICD: implantable cardioverter-defibrillator; MADIT: multicenter automatic defibrillator implantation trial; MUSTT: multicenter unsustained tachycardia trial; SCD: sudden cardiac death; SCD-HeFT: sudden cardiac death in heart failure trail)

TABLE 5: Impact of primary prevention ICD implanted during a dedicated procedure on all-cause mortality.[8]

	ICD (N)|No ICD (N)		*Weight*	*HR [95% CI]*
MADIT I 1996	95|101		12.85%	0.46 [0.26 , 0.82]
MADIT II 2002	742|490		27.83%	0.69 [0.51 , 0.93]
COMPANION 2004	325|331		26.28%	1.01 [0.74 , 1.40]
SCD-HeFT 2005	431|452		33.04%	0.79 [0.62 , 1.00]
Summary, random effects (p = 0.02)		0.25 0.50 1.00 2.00 ICD better Hazard ratio ICD worse	100.00%	0.76 [0.60 , 0.96]

(CI: confidence interval; HR: hazard ratio; ICD: implantable cardioverter defibrillator; SCD: sudden cardiac death)

Completely Leadless Cardiac Implantable Electronic Devices

There is ongoing research in the innovative field of complete leadless systems, wherein a subcutaneous ICD would be able to communicate with one or more leadless pacemakers to provide antitachycardia pacing or CRT function without the need for any transvenous leads.

Implantable Hemodynamic Monitors

- Sophisticated implantable hemodynamic monitors (IHMs) are being developed to allow continuous or intermittent assessment of hemodynamics, intracardiac, or pulmonary artery pressures.
- CardioMEMS heart sensor allows monitoring of pressure to improve outcomes in NYHA Class III HF Patients (CHAMPION) trial showed significantly fewer HF hospitalizations occurred in the treatment group compared to control group.[9] This led to approval of the first hemodynamic monitoring system for use in HF patients with NYHA Class III symptoms and a history of HF hospitalization within past 12 months.

CONCLUSION

Device therapy in HF is evolving rapidly over the past decades. CRT is an established therapy for reduction in mortality and morbidity in indicated patients with ventricular dyssynchrony and HF. CRT is safe, effective and patients demonstrate significant improvement in both clinical symptoms and multiple measures of functional status, exercise capacity, and outcomes. Prophylactic ICD implantation is also of proven benefit in HF patients. IHMs improve the clinician's ability to avoid episodes of HF decompensation and may improve the natural history of the disease. Ongoing research and innovations hold great promise for the future in the field of device therapy in HF.

REFERENCES

1. Abraham WT. Devices for monitoring and managing Heart Failure. In: Zipes DP, Libby P, Bonow RO, Mann DL, Tomaselli GF (Eds). Braunwald's Heart Disease: A Text book of Cardiovascular Medicine, 11th edition. Elsevier; 2019. pp. 543-52.
2. Linde C, Ellenbogen K, McAlister FA. Cardiac resynchronization therapy (CRT): Clinical trials, guidelines, and target populations. Heart Rhythm. 2012;9(Suppl 8):S3-13.
3. Ghio S, Freemantle N, Scelsi L, et al. Long-term left ventricular reverse remodelling with cardiac resynchronization therapy: results from the CARE-HF trial. Eur J Heart Fail. 2009;11(5):480-8.
4. Rossi A, Rossi G, Piacenti M, et al. The current role of cardiac resynchronization therapy in reducing mortality and hospitalization in heart failure patients: a meta-analysis from clinical trials. Heart Vessels. 2008;23(4):217-23.
5. Normand C, Linde C, Singh J, et al. Indications for Cardiac Resynchronization Therapy. A comparison of the major international guidelines. JACC Heart Fail. 2018;6(4):308-16.
6. Shah RM, Patel D, Molnar J, et al. Cardiac-resynchronization therapy in patients with systolic heart failure and QRS interval ≤130 ms: insights from a meta-analysis. Europace. 2015;17(2):267-73.
7. Redfield MM, Jacobsen SJ, Burnett JC Jr, et al. Burden of systolic and diastolic ventricular dysfunction in the community: appreciating the scope of the heart failure epidemic. JAMA. 2003;289(2):194-202.
8. Shun-Shin MJ, Zheng SL, Cole GD et al. Implantable cardioverter defibrillators for primary prevention of death in left ventricular dysfunction with and without ischemic heart disease: a meta-analysis of 8567 patients in the 11 trials. Eur Heart J. 2017;38(22):1738-46.
9. Sideris S, Archontakis S, Gatzoulis KA, et al. The subcutaneous ICD as an alternative to the conventional ICD system: Initial experience in Greece and a review of the literature. Hellenic J Cardiol. 2017;58(1):4-16.

CHAPTER

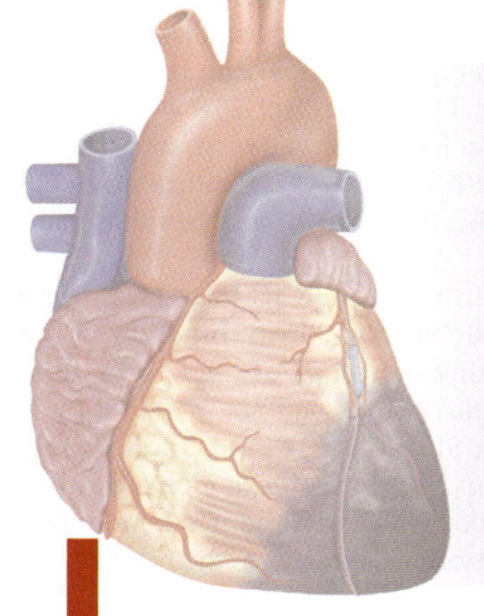

Durable Ventricular Assist Devices in Advanced Heart Failure

Nandini Nair, Santhosh KG Koshy

INTRODUCTION

The history of durable mechanical support dates back almost half a century. Early research on mechanical circulatory support systems in nonhuman systems led to the birth of mechanical circulatory support in humans. The first pump that was used to prolong life in a patient was pneumatic.[1] Novacor was the first pump placed in 1984 as a bridge-to-transplant (BTT).[2] Mechanical circulatory devices are now mainstream therapy with accelerated growth seen in the last decade.[3] Ventricular assist devices (VADs) have therefore evolved from being temporary support systems to life-long use now termed "destination therapy (DT)". Increasing utilization of left ventricular assist devices (LVADs) in the setting of donor organ shortage and higher incidence of end-stage heart failure, has led to further refinement of these devices to make them smaller and more portable. Such innovations have improved quality of life making VADs a more attractive option in life-threatening illness when organs are in shortage or the patients are not candidates for cardiac transplantation.

Increasing incidence and prevalence of heart failure has paved the way for LVAD therapy which has consequently evolved as an integral component of advanced heart failure care. VADs are now commonly used as a bridge-to-recovery/decision/transplant or as DT in end-stage heart failure.[4-7] Improvements through ongoing research in technology and pump design have made implantation easier with decreasing operative risks and related adverse events. The present-day axial and centrifugal pumps are more durable with fewer moving parts and are smaller in size. Patients with a smaller body habitus who were in the past not candidates for VAD therapy are now able to receive LVAD support in end-stage heart failure. The newer designs of continuous flow (CF) pumps as compared to earlier pulsatile pumps seem to prolong and improve quality of life.[8-10]

This chapter will address the evolution of durable VADs from the bulky, pulsatile devices in the past to the present day sleek, compact CF-VADs which have more long-term efficiency and highlight the major factors contributing to success of the CF-LVADs in today's advanced heart failure management.

Mechanical circulatory support involves two types of pumps—the "volume displacement pumps" and the "rotary pumps". The volume displacement devices constitute the first-generation pumps which provide pulsatility and the rotary pumps are the present day second and third generation continuous-flow pumps.

PULSATILE FLOW TO CONTINUOUS FLOW PUMPS

The pulsatile pumps (first generation) provide exemplary unloading of the ventricle and are engineered to provide a flow of 10 L/min. They have, however, fallen out of favor due to the fact that they are larger, exhibit more complexity, have a loud pulsatile sound, and are limited in durability due to several moving parts which are susceptible to wear and tear.[11,12] The evolution of technology has led to smaller sophisticated devices.

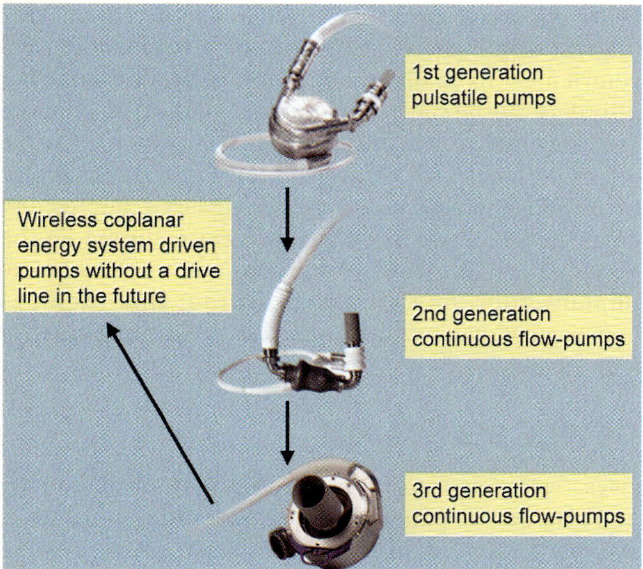

Fig. 1: Evolution of durable ventricular assist devices from the first generation to third generation and finally the wireless coplanar energy system which is a completely internalized pump lacking an external driveline.

The only current day pulsatile device in use is the SynCardia—total artificial heart (TAH) for biventricular failure.[13] All of the other current pumps in use are CF devices as described in Figure 1. The axial CF pumps have an internal rotor within the blood flow path that is suspended by contact bearings, which produces tangential velocity and kinetic energy resulting in a pressure gradient across the pump. The pump is powered by an external system driver via a percutaneous lead. Centrifugal CF pumps have an impeller or rotor suspended in the blood flow path using a noncontact bearing design, which uses either magnetic or hydrodynamic levitation. Since this system lacks mechanical contact, it reduces frictional wear and heat generation. These devices therefore have higher reliability and durability. Centrifugal CF pumps with magnetic levitation devices are larger because they require complex position sensing and control systems. The centrifugal CF pumps are typically placed in the pericardial space.

INDICATIONS FOR VENTRICULAR ASSIST DEVICES

The indications for durable VADs are BTT, bridge-to-recovery (BTR), and DT.

- *Bridge-to-transplant*: The landmark study that showed the benefit of VAD support on survival was the multicenter trial with the HeartMate VE. This was beginning of the era of durable mechanical support as BTT.[6]
- *Destination therapy*: It is a term used to denote use of VADs for advanced heart failure patients who are refractory to medical treatment and are not candidates for heart transplantation due to history of malignancy, older age, pulmonary hypertension, active smoking or advanced pulmonary/renal disease. The Randomized Evaluation of Mechanical Assistance for the Treatment of Congestive Heart Failure (REMATCH) trial was the landmark trial which showed significant improvement in survival and quality of life for DT patients.[4]
- *Bridge-to-recovery:* The BTR population is much smaller and rests on a number of important patient characteristics which depend on the stage/etiology of the disease process. The BTR concept is shown to work in conditions including myocarditis, postcardiotomy shock, myocardial infarction, and peripartum cardiomyopathy. The positive changes have been attributed to reverse remodeling and as well as improved response by the β-adrenergic system. Significant reduction in hypertrophy/fibrosis has been conceptual targets. Cellular calcium driven pathways improve after mechanical unloading of the ventricle leading to reduction in left ventricular end diastolic dimension and mass.[14,15] Such observations led to extension of this therapy to chronic heart failure. However, in the chronic heart failure patients the extent of recovery was not universally seen. In nonischemic patients with an acute inflammatory type of cardiomyopathy 10–11% recovery was observed.[15] The Harefield protocol used a selective beta 2 agonist, clenbuterol to increase the recovery in this population to 73%.[16] This protocol was not entirely reproducible in another study.[17] Left ventricular dysfunction did not improve in patients treated with high-dose clenbuterol but it increased skeletal muscle mass on LVAD support which could be advantageous.[17] Dandel et al. made an interesting observation in idiopathic dilated cardiomyopathy patients that heart failure recurred after LVAD explantation if the patients had a larger left ventricle and a lower ejection fraction when the LVAD was explanted.[18] More recently, the protocol used in two stages showed enough recovery for explantation of LVAD.[19] Studies on understanding the molecular mechanisms of LVAD-induced reverse remodeling are needed to develop consistent protocols for use in BTR.[20,21]

PATIENT SELECTION

The timing of LVAD placement drives the outcome.[22] Interagency for Mechanically Assisted Circulatory Support

(INTERMACS) registry developed by National Heart, Lung and Blood Institute[23] led to the establishment of the INTERMACS classification of disease acuity and its impact on outcomes. Table 1 summarizes the seven profiles starting from the sickest—life-threatening cardiogenic shock (profile 1) to the least sick—Advanced Heart Failure New York Heart Association (NYHA) class III (profile 7). The INTERMACS classification is used to drive the prognosis.

Summary of indication and contraindications for VAD placement is described in Table 2. No particular age cutoff has been postulated.[24] However, with age, renal dysfunction could affect prognosis in a big way. Increasing age especially >70 years needs attention when deducing LVAD risk, but increasing pre-LVAD creatinine, bilirubin, and an ischemic etiology predict higher mortality. Creatinine has been shown to be a very powerful predictor in post-LVAD survival. Elderly patients can undergo LVAD implantation and experience excellent survival if carefully selected.[25-27]

TABLE 1: INTERMACS (Interagency Registry for Mechanically Assisted Circulatory Support) profile for heart failure acuity.

Profile 1	Critically-ill cardiogenic shock
Profile 2	Progressive decline on inotropic support
Profile 3	Stable on inotropic support
Profile 4	Resting symptoms—at home on oral therapy
Profile 5	Intolerant to exertion
Profile 6	Exertion limited
Profile 7	Advanced NYHA class III symptoms

(NYHA: New York Heart Association)

TABLE 2: Indications and contraindications for ventricular assist device placement.

Indications	*Contraindications*
NYHA class IV	Severe RV failure
LVEF <25%	Uncorrected severe carotid artery disease
On IABP support for >7 days	End-stage renal disease on dialysis
On inotropic support >14 days	Irreversible cerebral injury
On optimal medical therapy >45 days	Sepsis/active infection
Peak oxygen consumption <14 mL/kg/min	Liver failure
	Disseminated intravascular injury
	Noncardiac illness limiting survival to <2 years

(NYHA: New York Heart Association; LVEF: left ventricular ejection fraction; IABP: intra-aortic balloon pump; RV: right ventricular)

Other important aspects in selection and timing of LVAD implantation is the severity of aortic regurgitation, right ventricular (RV) failure, active infection, and bleeding disorders. Aortic valve replacement is indicated in severe aortic regurgitation at the time of VAD implant to preserve organ perfusion. RV failure should be recognized and treated adequately before an LVAD is placed. If refractory RV failure exists, a biventricular device should be the option. Infections should be treated and resolved before implantation. Any bleeding disorder that excludes anticoagulation is a contraindication as CF pumps require anticoagulation.[28-34]

DEVICE SELECTION

Device selection depends on the availability in each country and also on the patient characteristics that make them suitable for a particular pump. Table 3 summarizes the landmark trials which led to the approval of present-day devices for BTT and/or DT.[4,6,8,13,35-38] The CF axial pump that is approved by the Food and Drug Administration (FDA) for both BTT and DT is the HeartMate II. The CF centrifugal pumps that are FDA approved for both BTT and DT are HVAD and HeartMate 3.

LIMITATIONS

Common complications are pump thrombosis, strokes, driveline infections, and gastrointestinal bleeding. Pump thrombosis is one of the dreaded complications seen more frequently in the second-generation CF-axial and CF-centrifugal pumps.[38-43] It is not noted significantly in the third generation CF-centrifugal pump (HeartMate 3), which has an intrinsically programed pulsatility every 2 seconds. This reduces stasis with periodic flush outs.[40] The second-generation CF-centrifugal pumps had a higher incidence of strokes which was found to be resolved when blood pressure was better controlled in addition to optimal anticoagulation.[44] Complications vary among pump types and predisposing factors of the patient. Driveline infections, gastrointestinal bleeding, and strokes were similar in the HeartMate 3 as compared to other contemporary pumps but pump thrombosis, hemolysis, and pump failure were not complications noted in a 1-year European study in this device.[45]

SUMMARY

A graphical summary of the evolution of devices is described in See Figure 1. The development of pumps is progressing in a fashion to make them smaller, more durable and completely internal with elimination of the driveline. The earliest of such a device was recently tested in patients.[46]

TABLE 3: Landmark studies in the evolution of durable ventricular assist devices.

Study	*Study type*	*Device type*	*Indication*	*Number of subjects*	*Conclusion*
Frazier et al.[6]	Multicenter clinical trial (nonrandomized)	HeartMate VE-LVAS Historical control IP HeartMate	BTT	280 48	Survival improved with Heartmate VE-LVAS
Rose et al.[4]	RCT	HeartMate XVE Control	DT	68 61	Significantly improved survival and quality of life at 1 year
Miller et al.[8]	Multicenter study without controls	HeartMate II-CF axial pump	BTT	133	Survival was 75% at 6 months and 68% at 12 months
Starling et al.[34]	Multicenter post-approval study	HeartMate II-CF axial pump Comparison group with 80% HeartMate XVE and 20% pVAD	BTT	169 169	Marked improvement in survival with HeartMate II versus control at 12 months
Aaronson et al.[35]	Multicenter prospective study	CF-centrifugal pump (HVAD) Control group received a contemporary pump	BTT	140	HVAD was non inferior to control group at 180 days
Rogers et al.[36]	Multicenter randomized trial	CF-centrifugal (HVAD) vs CF-axial pump	DT	297 148	CF—centrifugal pump (HVAD) was noninferior to CF-axial pump in terms of survival free from disabling stroke or device removal due to malfunction or failure
Milano et al.[37]	Multicenter Supplemental Trial	CF-centrifugal (HVAD) vs CF-axial pump	DT	308 157	Confirmed that blood pressure control would reduce the stroke rates in HVAD as HVAD had a higher stroke rate
Copeland et al.[13]	Nonrandomized prospective study in biventricular failure patients	TAH control	BTT	81 35	TAH improved survival to transplant and after transplant compared to controls with no device
Slaughter et al.[10]	Randomized study	CF-pump Pulsatile pump	DT	134 66	The CF pump improved survival from disablling stroke and device failure at 2 years as compared with pulsatile pump
Mehra et al.[38]	Randomized trial comparing CF-centrifugal and CF-axial pumps	CF-centrifugal pump (HeartMate 3) CF-axial pump (HeartMate II)	BTT or DT	152 142	CF pumps had a better disabling stroke—free survival at 6 months post implantation No pump thrombosis in CF—centrigual pump and 10.1% in CF—axial pump

(BTT: bridge-to-transplant; DT: destination therapy; TAH: total artificial heart; CF: continuous flow; RCT: randomized controlled trial; HVAD: HeartWare ventricular assist device; pVAD: percutaneous ventricular assist device)

CONCLUSION

The pulsatile biventricular support—TAH and nonpulsatile CF-VADs have become the mainstay of today's advanced heart failure management. The evolution of technology appears to be moving toward smaller, versatile pumps with safer implantation techniques with better long-term durability. The limitations of mechanical support devices include pump thrombosis, pump failure, strokes, driveline infections, and gastrointestinal bleeding. The newer CF centrifugal pumps have almost completely eliminated pump thrombosis and failure, but other complications still occur. As technology is refined in the years to come and as pumps become completely internalized driveline infections may disappear too. Therefore, the field of artificial organs is progressing rapidly in the setting of donor organ shortage.

REFERENCES

1. DeBakey ME. Left ventricular bypass pump for cardiac assistance. Clinical experience. Am J Cardiol. 1971;27(1):3-11.
2. Portner P, Oyer P, McGregor C. First human use of an electrically powered implantable ventricular assist system. Artif Organs. 1985;9:36.
3. Kirklin JK, Naftel DC. Mechanical circulatory support: Registering a therapy in evolution. Circ Heart Fail. 2008;1(3):200-5.
4. Rose EA, Gelijns AC, Moskowitz AJ, et al. Randomized Evaluation of Mechanical Assistance for the Treatment of Congestive Heart Failure (REMATCH) Study Group. Long-term use of a left ventricular assist device for end-stage heart failure. N Engl J Med. 2001;345(20):1435-43.
5. Park SJ, Tector A, Piccioni W, et al. Left ventricular assist devices as destination therapy: A new look at survival. J Thorac Cardiovasc Surg. 2005;129(1):9-17.
6. Frazier OH, Rose EA, Oz MC, et al. Multicenter clinical evaluation of the heartmate vented electric left ventricular assist system in patients awaiting heart transplantation. J Thorac Cardiovasc Surg. 2001;122(6):1186-95.
7. Frazier OH, Myers TJ, Westaby S, et al. Clinical experience with an implantable, intracardiac, continuous flow circulatory support device: Physiologic implications and their relationship to patient selection. Ann Thorac Surg. 2004;77(1):133-42.
8. Miller LW, Pagani FD, Russell SD, et al. HeartMate II Clinical Investigators. Use of a continuous-flow device in patients awaiting heart transplantation. N Engl J Med. 2007;357(9):885-96.
9. Pagani FD, Miller LW, Russell SD, et al. HeartMate II Investigators. Extended mechanical circulatory support with a continuous-flow rotary left ventricular assist device. J Am Coll Cardiol. 2009;54(4):312-21.
10. Slaughter MS, Rogers JG, Milano CA, et al. HeartMate II Investigators. Advanced heart failure treated with continuous-flow left ventricular assist device. N Engl J Med. 2009;361(23):2241-51.
11. Kirklin JK, Frazier OH. Developmental history of the mechanical circulatory support. In: Kirklin JK, Fraizer OH (Eds). ISHLT Monograph Series: Mechanical Circulatory Support, Volume 1. NY, USA: Elsevier; 2006. pp. 1-8.
12. Klotz S, Jan Danser AH, Burkhoff D. Impact of left ventricular assist device (LVAD) support on the cardiac reverse remodeling process. Prog Biophys Mol Biol. 2008;97(2-3):479-96.
13. Copeland JG, Smith RG, Arabia FA, et al. CardioWest Total Artificial Heart Investigators. Cardiac replacement with a total artificial heart as a bridge to transplantation. N Engl J Med. 2004;351(9):859-67.
14. Maybaum S, Mancini D, Xydas S, et al. LVAD Working Group. Cardiac improvement during mechanical circulatory support: A prospective multicenter study of the LVAD Working Group. Circulation. 2007;115(19):2497-505.
15. Simon MA, Kormos RL, Murali S, et al. Myocardial recovery using ventricular assist devices: Prevalence, clinical characteristics, and outcomes. Circulation. 2005;112(Suppl 9):I32-6.
16. Yacoub MH. A novel strategy to maximize the efficacy of left ventricular assist devices as a bridge to recovery. Eur Heart J. 2001;22(7):534-40.
17. George I, Xydas S, Mancini DM, et al. Effect of clenbuterol on cardiac and skeletal muscle function during left ventricular assist device support. J Heart Lung Transplant. 2006;25(9):1084-90.
18. Dandel M, Weng Y, Siniawski H, et al. Long-term results in patients with idiopathic dilated cardiomyopathy after weaning from left ventricular assist devices. Circulation. 2005;112(Suppl 9):I37-45.
19. Jakovljevic DG, Yacoub MH, Schueler S, et al. Left ventricular assist device as a bridge to recovery for patients with advanced heart failure. J Am Coll Cardiol. 2017;69(15):1924-33.
20. Ibrahim M, Yacoub MH. Bridge to recovery and weaning protocols. Heart Fail Clin. 2014;10(Suppl 1):S47-55.
21. Miyagawa S, Toda K, Nakamura T, et al. Building a bridge to recovery: The pathophysiology of LVAD-induced reverse modeling in heart failure. Surg Today. 2016;46(2):149-54.
22. Wozniak CJ, Stehlik J, Baird BC, et al. Ventricular assist devices or inotropic agents in status 1A patients? Survival analysis of the United Network of Organ Sharing database. Ann Thorac Surg. 2014;97(4):1364-71.
23. Stevenson LW, Pagani FD, Young JB, et al. INTERMACS Profiles of advanced heart failure: The current picture. J Heart Lung Transplant. 2009;28(6):535-41.
24. Feldman D, Pamboukian SV, Teuteberg JJ, et al. International Society for Heart and Lung Transplantation. The 2013 International Society for Heart and Lung Transplantation Guidelines for mechanical circulatory support: Executive summary. J Heart Lung Transplant. 2013;32(2):157-87.
25. Kirklin JK, Naftel DC, Pagani FD, et al. Seventh INTERMACS annual report: 15,000 patients and counting. J Heart Lung Transplant. 2015;34(12):1495-504.
26. Cotts WG, McGee EC Jr, Myers SL, et al. Predictors of hospital length of stay after implantation of a left ventricular assist device: An analysis of the INTERMACS registry. J Heart Lung Transplant. 2014;33(7):682-8.
27. Nair N, Gongora E. Reviewing the use of ventricular assist devices in the elderly: Where do we stand today? Expert Rev Cardiovasc Ther. 2018;16:11-20.
28. Holley CT, Fitzpatrick M, Roy SS, et al. Aortic insufficiency in continuous-flow left ventricular assist device support patients is common but does not impact long-term mortality. J Heart Lung Transplant. 2017;36(1):91-6.
29. Kormos RL, Teuteberg JJ, Pagani FD, et al. HeartMate II Clinical Investigators. Right ventricular failure in patients with the HeartMate II continuous-flow left ventricular assist

device: Incidence, risk factors, and effect on outcomes. J Thorac Cardiovasc Surg. 2010;139(5):1316-24.
30. Atluri P, Goldstone AB, Fairman AS, et al. Predicting right ventricular failure in the modern, continuous flow left ventricular assist device era. Ann Thorac Surg. 2013;96(3): 857-63.
31. Gustafsson F, Rogers JG. Left ventricular assist device therapy in advanced heart failure: Patient selection and outcomes. Eur J Heart Fail. 2017;19(5):595-602.
32. Klovaite J, Gustafsson F, Mortensen SA, et al. Severely impaired von Willebrand factor-dependent platelet aggregation in patients with a continuous-flow left ventricular assist device (HeartMate II). J Am Coll Cardiol. 2009;53(23):2162-7.
33. Demirozu ZT, Radovancevic R, Hochman LF, et al. Arteriovenous malformation and gastrointestinal bleeding in patients with the HeartMate II left ventricular assist device. J Heart Lung Transplant. 2011;30(8):849-53.
34. Starling RC, Naka Y, Boyle AJ, et al. Results of the post-US Food and Drug Administration-approval study with a continuous flow left ventricular assist device as a bridge to heart transplantation: A prospective study using the INTERMACS (Interagency Registry for Mechanically Assisted Circulatory Support). J Am Coll Cardiol. 2011;57(19):1890-8.
35. Aaronson KD, Slaughter MS, Miller LW, et al. HeartWare Ventricular Assist Device (HVAD) Bridge to Transplant ADVANCE Trial Investigators. Use of an intrapericardial, continuous-flow, centrifugal pump in patients awaiting heart transplantation. Circulation. 2012;125(25):3191-200.
36. Rogers JG, Pagani FD, Tatooles AJ, et al. Intrapericardial left ventricular assist device for advanced heart failure. N Engl J Med. 2017;376(5):451-60.
37. Milano CA, Rogers JG, Tatooles AJ, et al. ENDURANCE Investigators. HVAD: The ENDURANCE supplemental trial. JACC Heart Fail. 2018;6(9):792-802.
38. Mehra MR, Naka Y, Uriel N, et al. MOMENTUM 3 Investigators. A fully magnetically levitated circulatory pump for advanced heart failure. N Engl J Med. 2017;376(5):440-50.
39. Bourque K, Cotter C, Dague C, et al. Design rationale and preclinical evaluation of the HeartMate 3 left ventricular assist system for hemocompatibility. ASAIO J. 2016;62(4): 375-83.
40. Kirklin JK, Naftel DC, Kormos RL, et al. Interagency Registry for Mechanically Assisted Circulatory Support (INTERMACS) analysis of pump thrombosis in the HeartMate II left ventricular assist device. J Heart Lung Transplant. 2014;33(1):12-22.
41. Mehra MR, Stewart GC, Uber PA. The vexing problem of thrombosis in long-term mechanical circulatory support. J Heart Lung Transplant. 2014;33(1):1-11.
42. Mehra MR, Goldstein DJ, Uriel N, et al. MOMENTUM 3 Investigators. Two-Year outcomes with a magnetically levitated cardiac pump in heart failure. N Engl J Med. 2018;378:1386-95.
43. Uriel N, Colombo PC, Cleveland JC, et al. Hemocompatibility-related outcomes in the MOMENTUM 3 trial at 6 months: A randomized controlled study of a fully magnetically levitated pump in advanced heart failure. Circulation. 2017;135(21):2003-12.
44. Teuteberg JJ, Slaughter MS, Rogers JG, et al. ADVANCE Trial Investigators. The HVAD left ventricular assist device: Risk factors for neurological events and risk mitigation strategies. JACC Heart Fail. 2015;3(10):818-28.
45. Krabatsch T, Netuka I, Schmitto JD, et al. Heartmate 3 fully magnetically levitated left ventricular assist device for the treatment of advanced heart failure -1 year results from the Ce mark trial. J Cardiothorac Surg. 2017;12(1):23.
46. Pya Y, Maly J, Bekbossynova M, et al. First human use of a wireless coplanar energy transfer coupled with a continuous-flow left ventricular assist device. J Heart Lung Transplant. 2019;38(4):339-43.

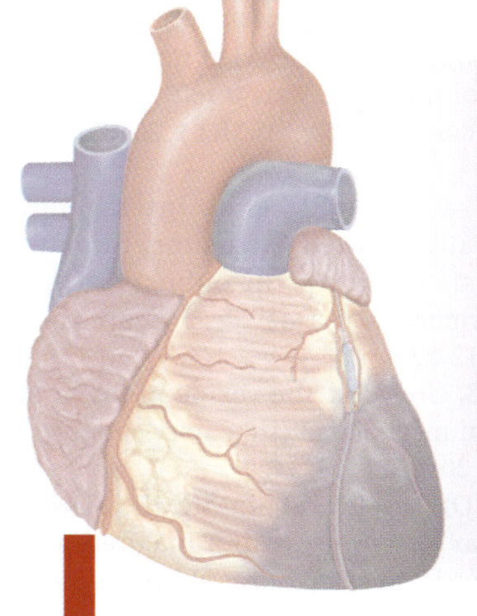

Review Outcomes of Recent Device Trials in Heart Failure

Aparna Jaswal, Wasim Rashid

INTRODUCTION

Heart failure (HF) is a complex clinical syndrome characterized by the reduced ability of the heart to pump and/or fill with blood. HF has been defined as global pandemic, since it affects around 26 million people worldwide.[1] In India, the estimates range between 1.3 million and 4.6 million, which translates to a prevalence of 0.12–0.44%, although this may be underestimated.[2]

The treatment of HF has evolved over the decades. Prior to 1980, treatments focused on lifestyle changes or limitations such as bed rest, inactivity, and fluid restrictions. Hemodynamic agents, digitalis, and diuretics comprised the mainstay of treatment. Heralded by the first Vasodilator Heart Failure Trial (V-Heft)[3] in 1980, vasodilators—particularly the combination of nitrates and hydralazine—were being prominently used along with positive inotropic agents. The decade of 1990s brought neurohormonal interventions to the forefront. Angiotensin-converting enzyme (ACE) inhibitors, beta-blockers, and spironolactone (for the treatment of advanced HF) were shown to alter the natural history of disease progression.[4-8] The year 2000 marked the beginning of the "Device Era". By then, the pharmacological era of HF therapy had almost drawn to a close till recently with the development of angiotensin-neprilysin inhibitor LCZ696.[9] Since the 2000s, we have witnessed the development of new devices [implantable cardioverter-defibrillators (ICDs), capillary refill times (CRTs), left ventricular assist devices (LVADs), etc.] for the treatment of HF.

Yet, despite major advances in therapies for HF with impaired left ventricular (LV) function over the past decades, HF is still among the leading causes for recurrent hospitalizations and mortality. There is a huge unmet demand for new devices in HF due to two main reasons. First, despite the careful selection criteria, approximately 30% of implanted patients fail to benefit from CRT highlighting the need for alternative device therapies in this population.[10] Second, two-thirds of patients with HF do not meet criteria for CRT due to normal or slightly prolonged QRS duration. Furthermore, HF with preserved ejection fraction, which accounts for 50% of HF patients with outcomes similar to those seen in heart failure with reduced ejection fraction (HFrEF), represents a wide therapeutic gap.[11] Hence, the purpose of this chapter is to summarize the latest innovations in device therapy of HF.

CARDIAC CONTRACTILITY MODULATION

Cardiac contractility modulation signals are nonexcitatory signals which are applied during the absolute refractory period (approximately 30 ms after detection of the QRS complex onset and consist of two biphasic +7 V pulses spanning a total duration of 20 ms). It has been shown to enhance the strength of LV contraction and improve exercise tolerance as well as quality of life (QoL) in patients with HF.[12,13] The signals influence cell function without any affecting activation sequence, the effects are independent of QRS duration, potentially filling a huge therapeutic gap.

Cardiac contractility modulation signals are provided by a pacemaker-like impulse generator (OPTIMIZER III, IMPULSE Dynamics) that connects to the heart via two standard active-fixation leads placed endocardially on the right ventricular (RV) septum. An additional right atrial lead is used to detect the timing of atrial activation which ensures appropriate timing of Chagas cardiomyopathy (CCM) signal delivery. A multicenter randomized, double-blind, and double crossover study examined its use in HF patients with ejection fraction (EF) ≤35% and New York Heart Association (NYHA) class II or III symptoms despite optimal medical therapy (OMT)—the FIX-HF-4 study.[14] The study met its primary endpoint, i.e. exercise tolerance, and QoL improved significantly during the on periods compared with the off periods. The second randomized study of CCM was a multicenter study involving 428 patients recruited from 50 sites in the US (FIX-HF-5 study).[15] Efficacy was assessed by ventilatory anaerobic threshold (VAT), peak VO_2 (pVO_2), and Minnesota Living with Heart Failure Questionnaire (MLWFQ) at 6 months. CCM did not improve VAT (the primary end point), but did improve pVO_2 and MLWHFQ and satisfied the noninferiority criteria for safety as well. A subgroup analysis demonstrated an improvement in the subgroup with left ventricular ejection fraction (LVEF) >25% and NYHA class III.[16] Subsequently, this led to the FIX-HF-5C study which was conducted to further evaluate the benefit of CCM in patients with LVEF ranging from 25% to 45%.[17] This study showed that CCM is safe, improves exercise tolerance, and QoL in the specified group of HF patients, and leads to fewer HF hospitalizations. The Food and Drug Administration (FDA) granted premarket approval application (PMA) for the OPTIMIZER Smart System in March 2019 for NYHA class III HF patients who remain symptomatic despite guideline directed medical therapy, who are in normal sinus rhythm, are not indicated for cardiac resynchronization therapy (CRT), and have an LVEF ranging from 25% to 45%.

NEUROMODULATION

The parasympathetic nervous system, which innervates the myocardium via the vagus nerve, modulates cardiac contractility and sinoatrial function. Both clinical and experimental evidence indicate that activation of the adrenergic nervous system and inhibition of the parasympathetic nervous system play a major role in the genesis of symptoms and disease progression in patients with HF and HFrEF.[18,19] This autonomic imbalance exerts adverse cardiac, vascular, and renal effects resulting in pathological myocardial remodeling, peripheral vasoconstriction, and salt and water retention. Both these pathophysiological observations and the success in treatment of HFrEF with adrenergic receptor blockade provide a rationale for therapies that inhibit adrenergic activity, enhance parasympathetic activity, or preferably, accomplish both.

Hence, therapeutic neurostimulation approaches have targeted either reflex activation of the parasympathetic tone and sympathetic inhibition via afferent fiber stimulation [spinal cord stimulation (SCS), carotid sinus nerve stimulation], or the efferent parasympathetic stimulation (cervical vagal and intracardiac vagal stimulation). A brief overview of these novel techniques is given below:

Spinal Cord Stimulation

Spinal cord stimulation showed promise in preclinical experiments to improve the systolic function of the LV and to decrease the ventricular arrhythmias associated with this condition. This therapy involves the placement of a stimulation electrode in the epidural space tunneled to a pulse generator in the paraspinal lumbar region. Thoracic Spinal Cord Stimulation for Heart Failure as a Restorative Treatment (SCS HEART study) was the first-in-man trial in patients with NYHA class III HF, LVEF 20–35%, and implanted defibrillator device carried out in 22 patients.[20] The results of this non-randomized trial were promising and suggested that high thoracic SCS is safe and feasible and potentially can improve symptoms, functional status, and LV function and remodeling in patients with severe symptomatic systolic HF. The DEFEAT-HF Study (Determining the Feasibility of Spinal Cord Neuromodulation for the Treatment of Chronic Systolic Heart Failure) was a prospective, multicenter randomized (3:2), parallel, single-blind, controlled study to investigate whether SCS was a feasible therapy for the treatment of systolic HF for patients with NYHA functional class III HF, LVEF ≤35%, QRS duration <120 ms, and LV end-diastolic dimension ≥55 mm. However, the study did not provide evidence to support a meaningful change in clinical outcomes for HF patients receiving SCS[21] highlighting the need of further larger, more cautiously designed studies with long-term follow-up.

Carotid Sinus Nerve Stimulation

Also known as baroreceptor activation therapy (BAT), this approach involves electrical stimulation of the carotid baroreceptors by an implanted device resembling a cardiac pacemaker resulting in centrally mediated reduction of sympathetic outflow and increased parasympathetic activity leading to reduced peripheral resistance and to increased arterial and venous compliance. Barostim HOPE-4HF was a prospective randomized study demonstrated that BAT is safe and efficient, and its effects are more pronounced in patients not treated with CRT at 6 months follow-up.[22,23] The next generation of BAT—the Neo system (CVRx Neo system) received CE mark in 2011. Attempts at stimulation of carotid sinus nerves via endovascular stimulation with a catheter in the internal jugular vein are also being investigated (ACES II study, Acute Carotid Sinus Endovascular Stimulation Study).[24]

CERVICAL VAGAL NERVE STIMULATION

The vagal nerve stimulation (VNS) system is an implantable neurostimulator system that delivers electrical impulses via an asymmetric bipolar multicontact cuff electrode around the vagus nerve in the neck. The stimulation electrode is tunneled to the intraclavicular region and attached to the pulse generator. Several studies in various chronic HF animal models have shown a reduction of the progression of HF and a survival benefit with cervical VNS.[25-27] Early phase II trials like CardioFit[28] and ANTHEM-HF[29] were promising with significant improvements in LVEF, NYHA class, improvements in NYHA, HF questionnaire scores, and 6-minute walk test. However, in the multicenter, randomized, double-blind, Phase II trial, Neural Cardiac Therapy for Heart Failure Study (NECTAR-HF) the primary efficacy end point, change in left ventricular end-systolic dimension (LVESD) from baseline to 6 months, was not significant.[30] The Increase of Vagal TonE in Congestive HF (INOVATE-CHF) trial was an international multi-center, randomized, and open-label Phase III trial designed to assess safety and efficacy of vagus nerve stimulation on cardiovascular outcome. About 707 patients with HFrEF were enrolled, in a 3:2 randomization ration to active VNS therapy vs. OMT (no implant). The primary endpoint of this study was a composite score of all-cause mortality and hospitalization due to worsening HF. The study was terminated sooner than expected, as there was no statistically significant improvement of the primary efficacy endpoint. QoL, NYHA functional class, and 6-minute walking distance were favorably affected, but LV end-systolic volume index was not different.[31]

INTRACARDIAC ATRIOVENTRICULAR NODAL VAGAL STIMULATION

Rapid ventricular rates during atrial fibrillation (AF) may further deteriorate HF or decrease the degree of LV resynchronization in patients with cardiac resynchronization devices or lead to inappropriate ICD shocks. Postganglionic cardiac vagal fibers, which preferentially supply the atrioventricular node, reside in an inferior right ganglionated plexus (IRGP) at the posteroinferior interatrial septum. This makes them amenable to stimulation from the endocardial surface, thus resulting in a graded response negative dromotropic effect.[32] The feasibility of such an approach was shown in a series of chronic human implants in HF patients with AF.[33] The Chronic Clinical Atrioventricular-Nodal Stimulation Download Study was a nonrandomized trial and demonstrated the feasibility of implementation of atrioventricular-nodal stimulation (AVNS) in a CRT and defibrillator system. AVNS increased ventricular interval >25% in 81% of patients. AVNS did not influence the safety profile of the CRT and defibrillator system.[34]

HIS BUNDLE PACING

The advent of His bundle pacing (HBP) as an alternative site of pacing holds tremendous promise, as it provides a more physiological, simultaneous activation of both the ventricles and can be used in selected patients as an alternative to CRT. In a feasibility study, it was shown that permanent HBP is feasible for patients with an indication for CRT using the LV port in lieu of a coronary sinus lead. In this initial experience, narrowing of QRS duration was achieved in 76% of patients with bundle branch block, and improvements in clinical and echocardiographic measures were observed with HBP.[35] In another study, HBP was attempted as a rescue strategy in patients with failed LV lead or nonresponse to biventricular pacing (BVP) (group I), or as a primary strategy in patients with AV block, blood brain barrier (BBB), or high ventricular pacing burden as an alternative to BVP (group II) in patients with indications for CRT. HBP was successful in 95–106 patients (90%)—30 in group I and 65 in group II. During mean follow-up of 14 months, both groups demonstrated significant narrowing of QRS, increase in LVEF, and improvement in NYHA functional class with HBP.[36] In a recent systematic review and meta-analysis permanent HBP resulted in narrow QRS duration of 116.3 ± 13.9 ms after implantation. LV functions, including echocardiographic parameters and clinical outcomes, significantly improved at follow-up (p <0.001).[37] The His Bundle Pacing vs. Coronary Sinus Pacing for Cardiac Resynchronization Therapy (His-SYNC) pilot trial was an investigator-initiated, prospective, and randomized controlled trial that aimed to assess the feasibility and efficacy of His-CRT as a first-line strategy compared to biventricular cardiac resynchronization therapy (BiV-CRT). The primary outcomes of the trial were change in QRS duration, improvement in LVEF at 6 months, and time to cardiovascular hospitalization or death at 12 months. In this first randomized pilot trial, His-CRT did not demonstrate significant improvements in electrocardiographic or echocardiographic parameters as compared to BiV-CRT.[38] This study was underpowered to detect differences less than 10% between groups, and a type II error is possible. Importantly, intention-to-treat (ITT) analysis in the presence of high crossover rates affected the ability to directly assess treatment efficacy. Improved patient selection may decrease crossover rates, and larger prospective studies may be useful to assess for smaller differences in effect size between CRT modalities.

CONCLUSION

There is a huge unmet need for new approaches in device therapy of HF as the current approaches cater to a small subgroup of patients with HF. Several innovative approaches hold tremendous promise as potentially path-breaking in catering to the needs of a larger proportion of these patients. However, more outcome studies are needed, and we may see a new era of second generation devices in the management of HF.

REFERENCES

1. Savarese G, Lund LH. Global public health burden of heart failure. Card Fail Rev. 2017;3(1):7-11.
2. Huffman MD, Prabhakaran D. Heart failure: Epidemiology and prevention in India. Natl Med J India. 2010;23(5):283-8.
3. Cohn JN, Archibald DG, Ziesche S, et al. Effect of vasodilator therapy on mortality in chronic congestive heart failure. Results of a Veterans Administration Cooperative Study. N Engl J Med. 1986;314(24):1547-52.
4. Swedberg K, Eneroth P, Kjekshus J, et al. Hormones regulating cardiovascular function in patients with severe congestive heart failure and their relation to mortality. CONSENSUS Trial Study Group. Circulation. 1990;82(5):1730-6.
5. Cohn JN, Johnson G, Ziesche S, et al. A comparison of enalapril with hydralazine-isosorbide dinitrate in the treatment of chronic congestive heart failure. N Engl J Med. 1991;325(5):303-10.
6. Yusuf S, Pitt B, Davis CE, et al. SOLVD Investigators. Effect of enalapril on survival in patients with reduced left ventricular ejection fractions and congestive heart failure. N Engl J Med. 1991;325(5):293-302.
7. Yusuf S, Pitt B, Davis CE, et al. SOLVD Investigators. Effect of enalapril on mortality and the development of heart failure in asymptomatic patients with reduced left ventricular ejection fractions. N Engl J Med. 1992;327(10):685-91.
8. Lechat P. The evolution of heart failure management over recent decades: From CONSENSUS to CIBIS. Eur Heart J Suppl. 2006;8(Suppl C):C5-C12.
9. McMurray JJV, Packer M, Desai AS, et al. PARADIGM-HF Investigators and Committees. Angiotensin-neprilysin inhibition versus enalapril in heart failure. N Engl J Med. 2014;371(11):993-1004.
10. Díaz-Infante E, Mont L, Leal J, et al. SCARS Investigators. Predictors of lack of response to resynchronization therapy. Am J Cardiol. 2005;95(12):1436-40.
11. Owan TE, Hodge DO, Herges RM, et al. Trends in prevalence and outcome of heart failure with preserved ejection fraction. N Engl J Med. 2006;355(3):251-9.
12. Burkhoff D, Ben-Haim SA. Nonexcitatory electrical signals for enhancing ventricular contractility: Rationale and initial investigations of an experimental treatment for heart failure. Am J Physiol Heart Circ Physiol. 2005;288(6):H2550-6.
13. Lawo T, Borggrefe M, Butter C, et al. Electrical signals applied during the absolute refractory period: An investigational treatment for advanced heart failure in patients with normal QRS duration. J Am Coll Cardiol. 2005;46(12):2229-36.
14. Borggrefe MM, Lawo T, Butter C, et al. Randomized, double blind study of non-excitatory, cardiac contractility modulation electrical impulses for symptomatic heart failure. Eur Heart J. 2008;29(8):1019-28.
15. Kadish A, Nademanee K, Volosin K, et al. A randomized controlled trial evaluating the safety and efficacy of cardiac contractility modulation in advanced heart failure. Am Heart J. 2011;161(2):329-37.e1-2.
16. Abraham WT, Nademanee K, Volosin K, et al. FIX-HF-5 Investigators and Coordinators. Subgroup analysis of a randomized controlled trial evaluating the safety and efficacy of cardiac contractility modulation in advanced heart failure. J Card Fail. 2011;17(9):710-7.
17. Abraham WT, Kuck KH, Goldsmith RL, et al. A randomized controlled trial to evaluate the safety and efficacy of cardiac contractility modulation. JACC Heart Fail. 2018;6(10):874-83.
18. Floras JS. Sympathetic nervous system activation in human heart failure: Clinical implications of an updated model. J Am Coll Cardiol. 2009;54(5):375-85.
19. Ponikowski P, Anker SD, Chua TP, et al. Depressed heart rate variability as an independent predictor of death in chronic congestive heart failure secondary to ischemic or idiopathic dilated cardiomyopathy. Am J Cardiol. 1997;79(12):1645-50.
20. Tse HF, Turner S, Sanders P, et al. Thoracic Spinal Cord Stimulation for Heart Failure as a Restorative Treatment (SCS HEART study): First-in-man experience. Heart Rhythm. 2015;12(3):588-95.
21. Zipes DP, Neuzil P, Theres H, et al. DEFEAT-HF Trial Investigators. Determining the feasibility of spinal cord neuromodulation for the treatment of chronic systolic heart failure: The DEFEAT-HF study. 2016;4(2):129-36.
22. Abraham WT, Zile MR, Weaver FA, et al. Baroreflex activation therapy for the treatment of heart failure with a reduced ejection fraction. JACC Heart Fail. 2015;3(6):487-96.
23. Halbach M, Abraham WT, Butter C, et al. Baroreflex activation therapy for the treatment of heart failure with reduced ejection fraction in patients with and without coronary artery disease. Int J Cardiol. 2018;266:187-92.
24. Tsioufis C, Iliakis P, Kasiakogias A, et al. Non-pharmacological modulation of the autonomic nervous system for heart failure treatment: WHERE do we stand? Curr Vasc Pharmacol. 2018;16(1):30-43.
25. Li M, Zheng C, Sato T, et al. Vagal nerve stimulation markedly improves long-term survival after chronic heart failure in rats. Circulation. 2004;109(1):120-4.

26. Zheng C, Li M, Inagaki M, et al. Vagal stimulation markedly suppresses arrhythmias in conscious rats with chronic heart failure after myocardial infarction. Conf Proc IEEE Eng Med Biol Soc. 2005;7:7072-5.
27. Zhang Y, Popovic ZB, Bibevski S, et al. Chronic vagus nerve stimulation improves autonomic control and attenuates systemic inflammation and heart failure progression in a canine high-rate pacing model. Circ Heart Fail. 2009;2(6):692-9.
28. De Ferrari GM, Crijns HJ, Borggrefe M, et al. CardioFit Multicenter Trial Investigators. Chronic vagus nerve stimulation: A new and promising therapeutic approach for chronic heart failure. Eur Heart J. 2010;32(7):847-55.
29. Premchand RK, Sharma K, Mittal S, et al. Autonomic regulation therapy via left or right cervical vagus nerve stimulation in patients with chronic heart failure: Results of the ANTHEM-HF trial. J Card Fail. 2014;20(11):808-16.
30. Zannad F, De Ferrari GM, Tuinenburg AE, et al. Chronic vagal stimulation for the treatment of low ejection fraction heart failure: Results of the NEural Cardiac TherApy foR Heart Failure (NECTAR-HF) randomized controlled trial. Eur Heart J. 2014;36(7):425-33.
31. Gold MR, Van Veldhuisen DJ, Hauptman PJ, et al. Vagus nerve stimulation for the treatment of heart failure: the INOVATE-HF trial. J Am Coll Cardiol. 2016;68(2):149-58.
32. Schauerte P, Mischke K, Plisiene J, et al. Catheter stimulation of cardiac parasympathetic nerves in humans: A novel approach to the cardiac autonomic nervous system. Circulation. 2001;104(20):2430-5.
33. Bianchi S, Rossi P, Della Scala A, et al. Atrioventricular (AV) node vagal stimulation by transvenous permanent lead implantation to modulate AV node function: Safety and feasibility in humans. Heart Rhythm. 2009;6(9):1282-6.
34. Bianchi S, Rossi P, Schauerte P, et al. Increase of ventricular interval during atrial fibrillation by atrioventricular node vagal stimulation: Chronic clinical atrioventricular-nodal stimulation download study. Circ Arrhythm Electrophysiol. 2015;8(3):562-8.
35. Ajijola OA, Upadhyay GA, Macias C, et al. Permanent His-bundle pacing for cardiac resynchronization therapy: Initial feasibility study in lieu of left ventricular lead. Heart Rhythm. 2017;14(9):1353-61.
36. Sharma PS, Dandamudi G, Herweg B, et al. Permanent His-bundle pacing as an alternative to biventricular pacing for cardiac resynchronization therapy: A multicenter experience. Heart Rhythm. 2018;15(3):413-20.
37. Qian Z, Zou F, Wang Y, et al. Permanent His bundle pacing in heart failure patients: A systematic review and meta-analysis. Pacing Clin Electrophysiol. 2019;42(2):139-45.
38. Upadhyay GA, Vijayaraman P, Nayak HM, et al. His-SYNC Investigators. His corrective pacing or biventricular pacing for cardiac resynchronization in heart failure. J Am Coll Cardiol. 2019;74(1):157-9.

SECTION 6

Hypertension

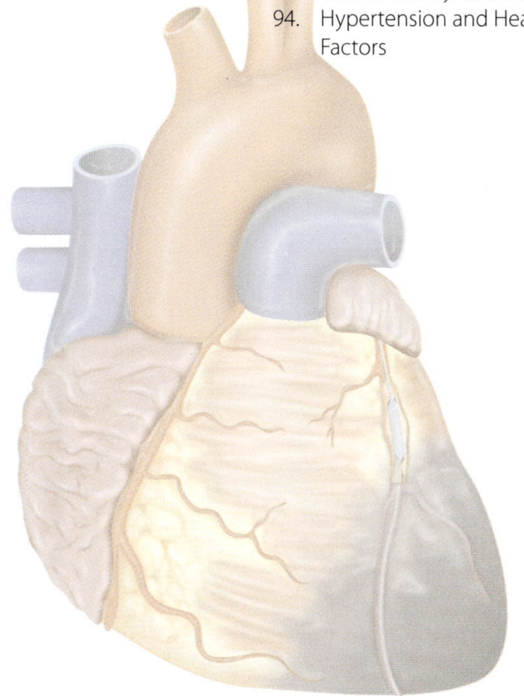

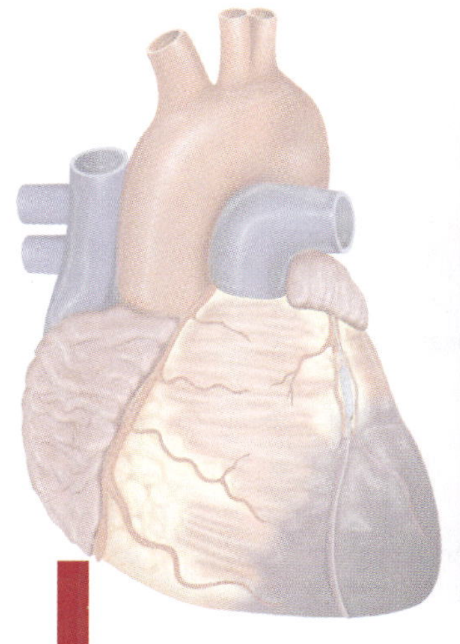

Cardiorenal Syndrome in Heart Failure

Sunil Prakash, Bhanu Mishra, Satender Yadav

INTRODUCTION

Cardiorenal Intersection

The kidney has a central role in total body water, electrolyte balance, and blood pressure regulation. It is therefore blessed with blood flows of 400 mL/min/100 g, which is approximately 20–25% of the cardiac output. Continuous communication between these two organs occurs at multiple levels, including the sympathetic nervous system, renin-angiotensin-aldosterone system (RAAS), antidiuretic hormone, endothelin, and natriuretic peptides (Fig. 1).

CHRONIC KIDNEY DISEASE

Chronic kidney disease (CKD) is defined as abnormalities of kidney structure and function, present for more than 3 months, with implications for health. With normative aging (age 20–80 years), the estimated glomerular filtration rate (eGFR) declines from about 130 mL/min/1.73 m^2 to 60 mL/min/1.73 m^2, a variety of pathobiologic processes appear to begin when the eGFR drops below 60 mL/min/1.73 m^2.[1]

HOW IS CKD DEFINED AS A CARDIOVASCULAR RISK STATE?

The association between cardiovascular disease (CVD) risk and CKD (reduced eGFR or presence of proteinuria >300 mg/day) has been confirmed by cohort studies in the general population[2] as well as in type 2 diabetes mellitus and preexisting high-risk coronary artery disease (CAD) patients.[3] The American College of Cardiology/American Heart Association task force and the National Kidney Foundation in 2003 recommended that CKD be considered a coronary heart disease (CHD) risk equivalent.[4,5] The results of the Alberta Kidney Disease Network in a population-based cohort of nearly 1.3 million adults were consistent with these recommendations and underlined the fact that all-cause mortality was higher in those with CKD than those with a previous myocardial infarction.[6,7] The Cardiovascular Health Study revealed that people with a serum creatinine >1.5 mg/dL had a 70% increase in risk for all-cause mortality after a 5-year follow-up.[8] More recently, a meta-analysis that includes 1,05,872 participants with urine albumin-to-creatinine ratio (ACR) measurements and 1,128,310 participants with urine protein dipstick measurements from 21 general population cohorts demonstrates that a reduced GFR < 60 mL/min/1.73 m^2 and presence of albuminuria were associated with high rates of all-cause and cardiovascular mortality independent of each other and traditional cardiovascular risk factors.[2]

CONTENTS AND DESCRIPTION

Renal Disease and Hypertension

Glomerular injury activates a variety of pathways that increase systemic blood pressure. Raised blood pressure sets up a vicious circle of more glomerular and tubule-interstitial

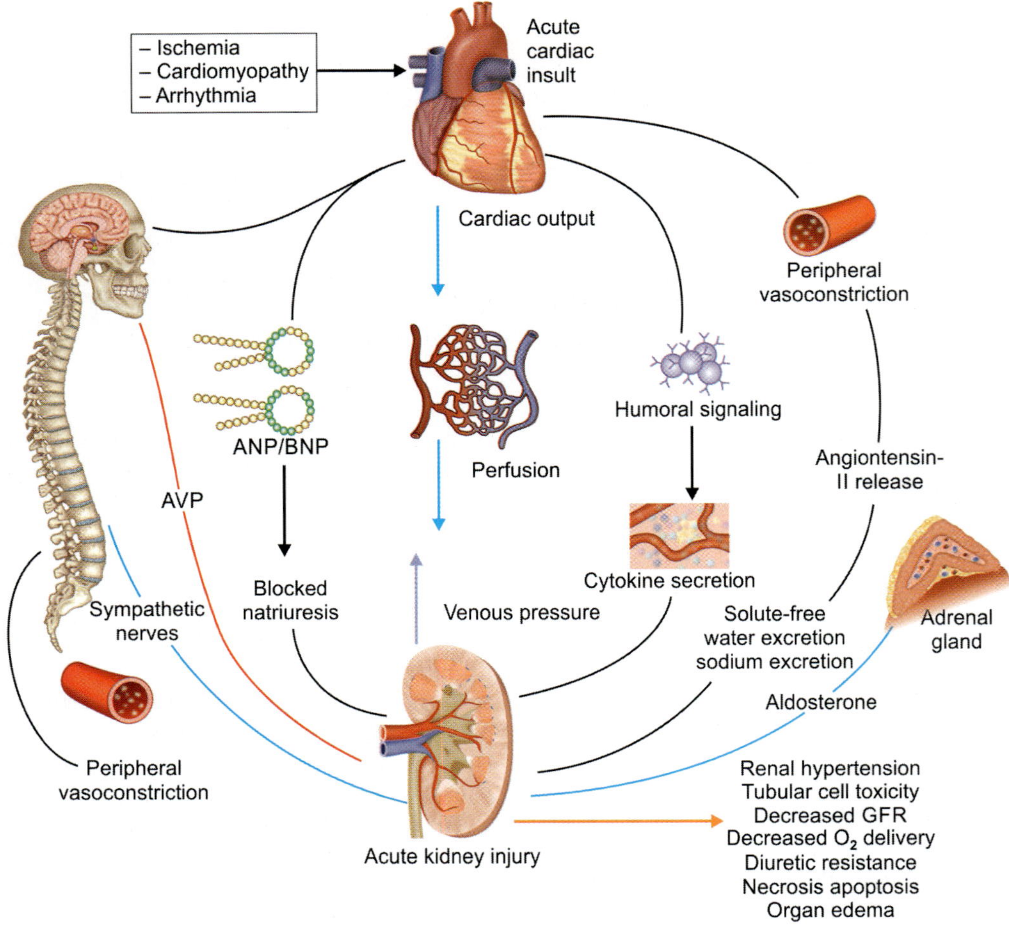

Fig. 1: Cardiorenal intersection.
(AVP: arginine vasopressin; ANP: atrial natriuretic peptide; BNP: B-type natriuretic peptide)

injury and worsening hypertension. Hypertension is the second leading cause of end-stage renal disease in the US, and has been reported in 85–95% of patients with CKD (stages 3–5). The relationship between hypertension and CKD is cyclic and reciprocal in nature. To date it remains the egg or hen story—which came first? Uncontrolled hypertension is a risk factor for developing CKD, and is associated with a more rapid progression of CKD, meanwhile, progressive CKD exacerbates hypertension due to volume expansion and increased systemic vascular resistance.[9] Tight blood pressure control remains the cornerstone in the management of CKD and CVD.[1]

Newer Diagnostic Tools of Cardiorenal Syndrome

The acute dialysis quality initiative classifies cardiorenal syndrome (CRS) into five types for ease of understanding and management (Table 1). Newer approach in diagnosis of CRS includes use of biomarkers of cardiac and kidney injury. These biomarkers have facilitated earlier diagnosis and comprehensive management of CKD and congestive cardiac failure (CCF).

Markers for glomerular filtration and integrity are serum creatinine, serum cystatin C, and albuminuria. Cystatin C, in serum, is associated with twice the risk of mortality and predicts-rehospitalization, and has prognostic value. Albuminuria has strong prognostic significance in all-cause mortality, cardiovascular death, and readmission, as brought about in CHARM, GISSI-HF, and Val-HeFT studies.[10]

Markers for renal tubular injury are neutrophil gelatinase-associated lipocalin (NGAL), tissue inhibitor of metalloproteinase-2 (TIMP-2), and insulin-like growth factor binding protein-7 (IGFBP-7). Urinary NGAL is produced in loop of Henle and PCT. NGAL is upregulated protein produced by the kidney in the setting of acute kidney injury (AKI), and has diagnostic and prognostic value in

TABLE 1: Cardiorenal syndrome classification.

Phenotype	*Nomenclature*	*Description*	*Clinical examples*
Type 1 CRS	Acute CRS	HF resulting in AKI	ACS/AHF resulting in cardiogenic shock and AKI
Type 2 CRS	Chronic CRS	Chronic HF resulting in CKD	Chronic HF
Type 3 CRS	Acute renocardiac syndrome	AKI resulting in AHF	HF in the setting of AKI from volume overload and metabolic disturbances in uremia
Type 4 CRS	Chronic renocardiac syndrome	CKD resulting in chronic HF	LVH and HF from CKD-associated cardiomyopathy
Type 5 CRS	Secondary CRS	Systemic process resulting in HF and kidney failure	Amyloidosis, sepsis, cirrhosis

(ACS: acute coronary syndrome; AHF: acute heart failure; AKI: acute kidney injury; CKD: chronic kidney disease; CRS: cardiorenal syndrome; HF: heart failure; LVH: left ventricular hypertrophy)

Flowchart 1

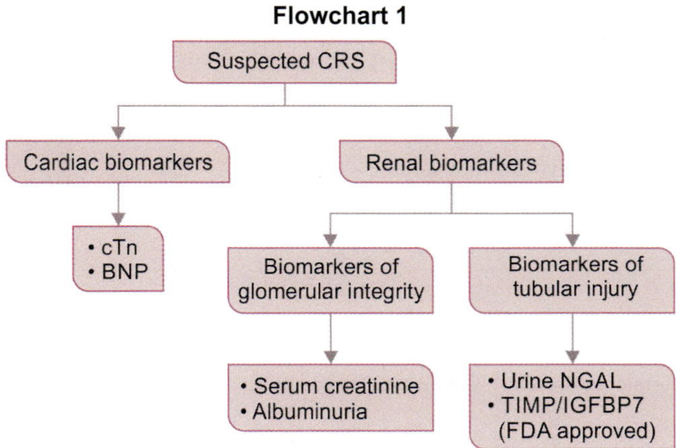

(BNP: B-type natriuretic peptide; CRS: cardiorenal syndrome; cTn: cardiac troponin; IGFBP7: insulin-like growth factor protein 7; NGAL: neutrophil gelatinase-associated lipocalin; TIMP: tissue inhibitor of metalloproteinase)

acute as well as chronic heart failure. It is handy tool in management of AKI and CRS. TIMP-2 and IFGBP-7 stood up in SAPPHIRE validation cohort as a biomarker which correlates better with AKI and CRS (Flowchart 1).[10]

Cardiac biomarkers like troponins and NT-proBNP are routinely used in bedside management of heart failure patients. Newer markers like suppressor of tumorogenecity-2 (ST2) and galectin-3 have now arrived on clinical horizon. ST2 is a decoy protein produced by endothelial cells in response to biomechanical strain, and its measurements offer incremental value in prognosticating heart failure outcomes. Galectin-3 is produced by cardiac macrophages and analysis of studies such as CORONA and COACH trials suggests that it is an independent marker of all-cause mortality (Table 2).[10]

Management of Hypertension, CCF and CKD

Previously guidelines suggested 140/90 mm Hg as starting point for pharmacological treatment.[11] Latest 2017 ACC/AHA hypertension guidelines now recommend office blood pressure target of <130/80 mm Hg for individuals with a 10-year cardiovascular risk >10%.

Management of fluid overload is central in the effective treatment of CRS. Assessment of volume status remains a vexatious issue. Newer methods to assess the same are bioimpedance vector analysis (BIVA), measurement of intraabdominal pressure (IAP), relative blood volume monitoring devices, and implantable and invasive hemodynamic monitoring devices. BIVA is a noninvasive bedside volume assessment technique based on the electric principle that the body is a circuit with a given resistance and reactance. BIVA has been combined with B-type natriuretic peptide (BNP) to guide management and prognosis.[10]

Diuretics, angiotensin-converting enzyme inhibitor (ACE-i)/angiotensin receptor blocker (ARB), beta-blockers, and aldosterone inhibitors are traditionally used in management of CRS. Newer drugs like neprilysin inhibitors combined with ARB (sacubitril/valsartan) have shown benefits as borne by PARADIGM-HF trial.[10]

CARESS-HF and UNLOAD trials have shown that intravenous diuretics should be tried first, preferably in infusion, to avoid braking phenomenon, which was found to be noninvasive and noninferior way with similar outcomes. Ultrafiltration, even though effective in removing fluids, did not improve mortality outcomes.[10]

Beta-blockers showed improved mortality benefits as evidenced in MERIT-HF (metoprolol) and Cardiac Insufficiency Bisoprolol Studies (CIBIS 2) (bisoprolol) study. However, evidence at lower levels of GFR is unsatisfactory.[10]

Mineralocorticoid receptor antagonist (MRA) has also been used as add-on therapy with ACE/ARB. Trials like Randomized Aldactone Evaluation Study (RALES) and Eplerenone in Mild Patients Hospitalization and Survival Study in Heart Failure (EMPHASIS-HF) have shown no significant improvement in patient outcomes, especially at lower GFRs. Conversely, hyperkalemia is a dreaded complication (Table 3).[10]

TABLE 2: Biomarkers for cardiac and renal injury.

Biomarkers	*Characteristics/site of origin*	*Diagnostic*	*Prognostic value*
Cardiac biomarkers			
cTn	Marker of myocardial injury	ACS	ACS, HF, CKD
BNP	Marker of myocardial stretch	HF, ACS, CRS	HF, CRS
sST2	Member of IL-1 family of receptors		HF, CRS
Galectin-3	Beta-galactoside binding lectin (intracellular and extracellular)		HF, CRS
Kidney biomarkers			
Biomarkers of glomerular integrity			
Serum creatinine	Skeletal muscle	AKI, CRS	HF, CRS
Cystatin C	All nucleated cells	CRS	CRS
Albuminuria	Marker of glomerular integrity/FCI disruption	CRS	CRS
Biomarkers of tubular injury			
TIMP/IGFBP7	Involved in G1 cell cycle arrest; may stimulate renal epithelium in an autocrine and paracrine fashion and sensitize for upcoming insults	AKI	AKI, recovery
Serum NGAL	25-kDa protein found in neutrophil granules; secreted by myocardium, renal tubules, activated immune cells, hepatocytes, lung, and colon	AKI	CRS
Urine NGAL	Loop of Henle, collecting ducts	AKI, CRS	CRS
NAG	PCT	CRS, AKI	CRS
KIM-1	Type 1 cell membrane glycoprotein expressed in regenerating PCT epithelium	AKI	CRS

(ACS: acute coronary syndrome; AKI: acute kidney injury; BNP: B-type natriuretic peptide; CKD: chronic kidney disease; CRS: cardiorenal syndrome; cTn: cardiac troponin; HF: heart failure; IGFBP7: insulin-like growth factor protien7; IL: interleukin; KIM-1: kidney injury molecule-1)

TABLE 3: Strength of evidence of various drugs in heart failure over stages of CKD.

CRT	Strong	Strong	Absent
ICD	Strong	Strong	Weak
H-ISDN	Weak	Weak	Absent
Digoxin	Weak	Weak	Weak
Ivabradine	Moderate	Moderate	Absent
Beta-blocker	Strong	Strong	Moderate
MRA	Strong	Strong	Absent
ARNi	Strong	Strong	Absent
ACE inhibitor/ARB	Strong	Strong	Weak
Diuretics	Absent	Absent	Absent
CKD stage	CKD 1 and 2	CKD 3	CKD 4 and 5

(ACE: angiotensin converting enzyme; ARB: angiotensin receptor blocker; ARNi: angiotensin receptor neprilysin inhibitor, CRT: cardiac resynchronization therapy; ICD: implantable cardiac defibrillator; H-ISDN: hydralazine-isosorbide dinitrate; MRA: mineralocorticoid receptor antagonist)

Refractory heart failure remains an unresolved issue in the elderly, and CKD aggravates it. Ultra-filtration therapies represent a potentially useful adjunctive treatment for frequently hospitalized patients with severe heart failure. Trials of extracorporeal UF therapies have failed to fulfill their early promise in treatment of diuretic-resistant heart failure. Chronic ambulatory peritoneal dialysis (CAPD) is a gentler domiciliary therapy that may reduce hospitalization, cost of treatment, and improve quality of life and survival in such patients. Patient selection and team effort by nephrology and cardiology service is key to successful use of CAPD in patients of refractory heart failure.[12] Incremental CAPD in addition to fluid removal by PD, correction of renal anemia, preservation of kidney function, and avoidance of high-dose diuretic therapy may play a role in maximizing clinical benefits.[13]

CONCLUSION

Better understandings of cardiac and renal cross-talk have laid the way for discovery of newer tools for early diagnosis of CRS. This has led to resurgence of interest in discovery of newer medications and applications in mitigating this common, difficult-to-treat, and potentially fatal syndrome.

The future should involve more multicentric clinical trials, discovery of newer drugs, and biomedical engineering partnerships to improve patient outcomes.

LIMITATIONS

Data regarding effective therapies for CRS in ESRD is sparse, and we need more focused trials evaluating the same. Even though biomarkers are helpful but in resource-poor countries their availability and cost-effectiveness is doubtful. The above view is from a nephrologist point of view, and a combined cardiologist perspective will facilitate better management of this dreaded clinical syndrome.

REFERENCES

1. Braunwald E, Bonow RO. Braunwald's Heart Disease: A Textbook of Cardiovascular Medicine, 9th edition. Philadelphia: Saunders; 2012. p. 1934–41.
2. Matsushita K, Van der Velde M, Astor BC, et al.; Chronic Kidney Disease Prognosis Consortium. Association of estimated glomerular filtration rate and albuminuria with all-cause and cardiovascular mortality in general population cohorts: a collaborative meta-analysis. Lancet. 2010;375(9731):2073-81.
3. Van Der Velde M, Matsushita K, Coresh J, et al.; Chronic Kidney Disease Prognosis Consortium. Lower estimated glomerular filtration rate and higher albuminuria are associated with all-cause and cardiovascular mortality. A collaborative meta-analysis of high-risk population cohorts. Kidney Int. 2011;79(12):1341-52.
4. Levey AS, Coresh J, Balk E, et al.; National Kidney Foundation. National Kidney Foundation practice guidelines for chronic kidney disease: evaluation, classification, and stratification. Ann Intern Med. 2003;139(2):137-47.
5. Sarnak MJ, Levey AS, Schoolwerth AC, et al.; American Heart Association Councils on Kidney in Cardiovascular Disease, High Blood Pressure Research, Clinical Cardiology, and Epidemiology and Prevention. Kidney disease as a risk factor for development of cardiovascular disease: A statement from the American Heart Association Councils on Kidney in Cardiovascular Disease, High Blood Pressure Research, Clinical Cardiology, and Epidemiology and Prevention. Circulation. 2003;108(17):2154-69.
6. Tonelli M, Muntner P, Lloyd A, et al.; Alberta Kidney Disease Network. Risk of coronary events in people with chronic kidney disease compared with those with diabetes: A population-level cohort study. Lancet. 2012;380(9844): 807-14.
7. Polonsky TS, Bakris GL. Chronic kidney disease: a coronary heart disease equivalent? Lancet. 2012;380(9844):783-5.
8. Fried LP, Kronmal RA, Newman AB, et al. Risk factors for 5-year mortality in older adults: The Cardiovascular Health Study. JAMA. 1998;279(8):585-92.
9. Rao MV, Qiu Y, Wang C, et al. Hypertension and CKD: Kidney Early Evaluation Program (KEEP) and National Health and Nutrition Examination Survey (NHANES), 1999-2004. Am J Kidney Dis. 2008;51(4 Suppl 2):S30-7.
10. Rangaswami J, Bhalla V, Blair JEA, et al.; American Heart Association Council on the Kidney in Cardiovascular Disease and Council on Clinical Cardiology. Cardiorenal Syndrome: Classification, Pathophysiology, Diagnosis, and Treatment Strategies: A Scientific Statement from the American Heart Association. Circulation. 2019;139(16):e840-78.
11. Whelton PK, Carey RM, Aronow WS, et al. 2017 ACC/AHA/AAPA/ABC/ACPM/AGS/APhA/ASH/ASPC/NMA/PCNA Guideline for the Prevention, Detection, Evaluation, and Management of High Blood Pressure in Adults: Executive summary: A report of the American College of Cardiology/American Heart Association Task Force on Clinical Practice Guidelines. J Am Soc Hypertens. 2018;12(8):579.e1-579.e73.
12. Puttagunta H, Holt SG. Peritoneal dialysis for heart failure. Perit Dial Int. 2015;35(6):645-9.
13. Nakayama M, Nakano H, Nakayama M. Novel therapeutic option for refractory heart failure in elderly patients with chronic kidney disease by incremental peritoneal dialysis. J Cardiol. 2010;55(1):49-54.

CHAPTER 94

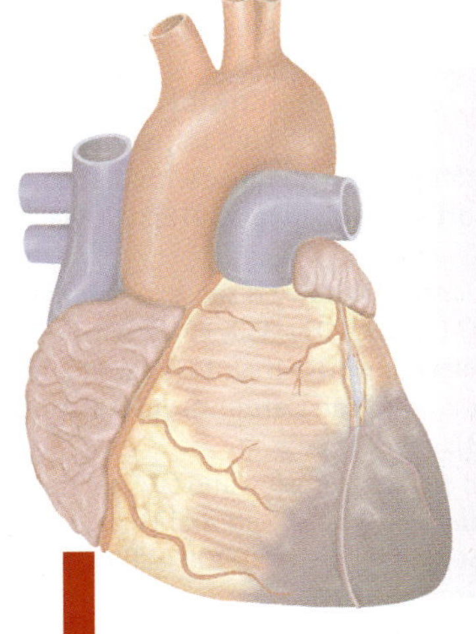

Hypertension and Heart Failure as Stroke Risk Factors

Pawan K Sharma, HK Chopra

INTRODUCTION

It is well known that long-standing hypertension is a prominent risk factor for developing heart failure. The Framingham Heart Study showed that during a follow-up of 20 years, about 91% patients developed hypertension before being diagnosed with new heart failure.[1] In the hypertensive people, history of myocardial infarction, diabetes, left ventricular hypertrophy, and valvular heart disease were associated with increased risk of developing heart failure irrespective of the gender. In the Framingham population, the lifetime risk of developing heart failure increased with age and was 20% at the age of 80 years. The risk of developing heart failure doubled with elevated blood pressure of 160/100 mm Hg compared to those with blood pressure of 140/90 mm Hg.[2] Heart failure is defined as a clinical syndrome with symptoms of dyspnea, ankle swelling, and fatigue that may be accompanied by signs such as elevated jugular venous pressure, pulmonary crackles, and peripheral edema, may be caused by structural and/or functional cardiac abnormality, resulting in a reduced cardiac output and/or elevated intracardiac pressures at rest or during stress.[3] Since the reduced heart function in heart failure cannot supply oxygenated blood to the brain, it may predispose to cerebral ischemia and lead to stroke. The prevalence rate of stroke doubles with each decade of life. In people younger than 40 years age it is <1% and increases up to >10% in age more than 80 years.[4]

It is estimated that approximately 40 million people have heart failure all over the world and this number may increase with improved survival due to advances in therapies and increasing age of the population.[5] Patients with heart failure and stroke have common risk factors such as atrial fibrillation. In fact, it is not uncommon to have both heart failure and stroke occurring together in the same patient. It has been noted that the risk of ischemic stroke is 2–3 times higher in patients with heart failure than in those without heart failure.[6-8] Major risk factors for heart failure are hypertension, coronary artery disease, valvular heart disease, diabetes, and atrial fibrillation.[9] It is still debated whether heart failure is an independent risk factor for increased incidence of stroke because most studies involving stroke in heart failure did not differentiate between patients who had atrial fibrillation and who did not have atrial fibrillation.

In Denmark, 2,89,353 patients with heart failure and 14,46,765 individuals from general population were followed from 1980 to 2012 and it was noted that heart failure was associated with increased risks of ischemic stroke, intracerebral hemorrhage, and subarachnoid hemorrhage over both the short- and long-term, and risks of all stroke subtypes remained positively associated with heart failure over 3 decades of follow-up.[10] A US cohort study involving 630 heart failure patients also demonstrated similar findings. The 30-day ischemic stroke risk was increased by 17-fold when compared with general population and it persisted for over 5 years.[8] Another study from UK reported that the risk of stroke in heart failure patients was 2–3-fold higher when compared with general population.[6] Several mechanisms have been proposed that increase the risk of ischemic stroke in heart failure patients. One possible mechanism is the formation of thrombi in the dilated, hypokinetic left ventricle because of wall-motion abnormalities and in the left atrium because of atrial fibrillation. Heart failure is also associated with increased activity of procoagulant factors, aggregation of thrombocytes, and endothelial dysfunction which may increase the risk of clot formation and thereby increasing the risk of ischemic stroke.[11] The increased risk of hemorrhagic stroke in heart failure may be a reflection of higher use of antithrombotic drugs.

HYPERTENSION AND HEART FAILURE

The hypertensive heart disease may progress through four different stages. Initially, there is: (1) isolated left ventricular diastolic dysfunction without left ventricular hypertrophy which may lead to (2) left ventricular diastolic dysfunction with concentric left ventricular hypertrophy which in turn leads to (3) clinical heart failure with preserved left ventricular function which can finally progress to (4) dilated cardiomyopathy with heart failure and reduced ejection fraction.[12]

This indicates that diastolic dysfunction and left ventricular hypertrophy leading to heart failure with preserved ejection fraction (HFpEF) is a much more common complication of long-standing hypertension. Some hypertensive patients develop normal blood pressure and then may have low BP as heart failure progresses and becomes more severe. This phenomenon is called "decapitated hypertension". Some patients with hypertension may have renal artery stenosis leading to heart failure. The clinical entity of flash pulmonary edema and bilateral atheromatous renal artery stenosis is known as Pickering syndrome.[13] It is obvious that both heart and kidney are target organs in hypertension and, therefore, hypertension may lead to heart failure and renal failure. This phenomenon of renal failure in heart failure is known as cardiorenal syndrome.[14]

Antihypertensive Therapy for Heart Failure Prevention

Beta-blockers are considered as standard of care in the treatment of heart failure. Patients with heart failure with reduced ejection fraction (HFrEF) in sinus rhythm should receive beta-blockers as they have been shown to reduce the mortality and admission to hospital.[15] Beta-blockers provide a risk reduction of 23% in heart failure patients ($p = 0.055$) but increase risk of stroke by 19% in the elderly.[16] Therefore, beta-blockers should not be considered as first-line therapy for prevention of heart failure. Calcium channel blockers have been shown to increase the risk of heart failure but decrease the risk of stroke when compared with angiotensin converting enzyme (ACE) inhibitors and angiotensin receptor blockers (ARBs).[17] Stroke remains the most devastating complication of hypertension. In the Antihypertensive and Lipid Lowering Treatment to Prevent Heart Attack Trial (ALLHAT) study, the alpha-blocker doxazosin was associated with a higher risk of stroke.[16] The thiazide diuretics, chlorthalidone and indapamide, provide significant heart failure risk reduction.[18] There is no outcome data for hydrochlorothiazide for heart failure or any other cardiovascular endpoint and, therefore, it should be avoided in hypertensive patients at risk of heart failure. The other thiazide diuretics such as chlorthalidone and indapamide can be used for treatment of hypertension and prevention of heart failure. The new agents like angiotensin II receptor neprilysin inhibitor and valsartan/sacubitril may become a useful antihypertensive drug in addition to its role in heart failure treatment.[19] Switching to vasodilating beta-blockers such as carvedilol or nebivolol may have additional antihypertensive benefit in patients at risk of developing heart failure.

HEART FAILURE AND STROKE

Globally, heart failure affects about 40 million people all over the world.[5] Heart failure and stroke are commonly seen in the same individual to coexist and share certain common risk factors, including atrial fibrillation. The risk of ischemic stroke is also 2–3 times higher in patients with heart failure than in those without heart failure.[6-8] In 2013, stroke was noted to be the second leading cause of death accounting for 11.8% of all deaths worldwide following ischemic heart disease which was responsible for 14.8% of all deaths.[20] Overall, the stroke burden has increased in both sexes of all ages worldwide.[20,21] To reduce the overall stroke burden, it is important to control the common modifiable lifestyle risk factors such as smoking, unhealthy diet, physical inactivity, and excessive use of alcohol. Control of other major risk factors, such as hypertension and atrial fibrillation (AF), appropriate treatment in the acute stage, and rehabilitation and long-term follow-up for secondary prevention should also be considered.

Stroke as a Consequence of Heart Failure

Heart failure is a common cause of ischemic stroke.[9] Many possible mechanisms have been proposed for increased incidence of cardioembolic stroke. Most frequent reason for cardioembolic stroke in heart failure patients is thrombus formation due to atrial fibrillation, left ventricular hypokinesis, or dilated cardiomyopathy.[22,23] Embolism to the brain could be of cardiac or aortic origin such as myocardial infarction, atrial fibrillation, valvular heart disease, complicated aortic plaque, or patent foramina ovale. Heart failure associated with hypertension, diabetes, and coronary artery disease are usually associated with atherosclerotic and lacunar stroke. In heart failure, there is activation of the sympathetic nervous system and of the renin-angiotensin-aldosterone system leading to a hypercoagulable state, increased aggregation of platelets, and reduced fibrinolysis.[24,25] Heart failure patients are also known to have endothelial dysfunction and malfunctioning of cerebral autoregulation.[26,27] Patients with heart failure are also at risk for stroke due to cerebral ischemia due to perfusion failure leading to large-artery atherosclerosis and small vessel occlusion. Hypotension in patients with heart failure may be an additional risk factor for stroke.[6]

Mechanism of stroke in heart failure has mostly been studied in patients with HFrEF. In patients with HFpEF, alterations in the cardiac structure, e.g. left ventricular hypertrophy or concentric remodeling and diffuse myocardial fibrosis may be responsible for myocardial stiffness along with left atrial enlargement which may lead to blood stasis, which in turn may contribute to stroke.[28,29] Previous studies have shown that 10–24% of patients with stroke have heart failure.[30-33] Heart failure appears to be the cause of stroke in 9% of patients.[11,34] Patients with stroke and heart failure have higher mortality rates, more severe neurologic deficits, and longer hospital stays than those without heart failure.[11] According to the Framingham study,[7] the risk of ischemic stroke was 2–3 times higher in patients with heart failure than in those without heart failure, which was also supported by other community-based studies.[6,8] A 30-year population-based cohort study has shown a significant relationship between heart failure and short-term and long-term risks of all stroke subtypes.[10]

Stroke Risk in Heart Failure with Atrial Fibrillation

Patients with heart failure are more likely to have risk factors, such as hypertension, advanced age, diabetes, metabolic syndrome, and arteriosclerosis. The heart failure may also lead to hemodynamic changes involving pressure and volume overload, cellular changes involving fibrosis and/or automaticity. This increases the risk of development of atrial fibrillation in heart failure patients.[35] Patients with heart failure and atrial fibrillation have 5-fold increased risk of stroke than the control population.[36] Untreated atrial fibrillation can cause tachycardia-induced cardiomyopathy which can lead to heart failure.[37] In a meta-analysis, it has been noted that although the all-cause mortality rate is significantly higher in the atrial fibrillation with HFrEF patients, there was no difference in the stroke risk between atrial fibrillation with HFrEF and HFpEF.[38]

Stroke Risk in Heart Failure with Sinus Rhythm

There are very few small, short-term follow-up studies which looked at if there is any relationship between stroke and heart failure with sinus rhythm. But there is consensus that the risk of ischemic stroke, thromboembolism, and death increases in patients with heart failure even with sinus rhythm.[10,36,39-41] A Korean study has shown that patients with heart failure but without atrial fibrillation had a 3.5-fold increased risk for stroke, while those with heart failure and atrial fibrillation demonstrated a >5-fold increased risk for stroke.[36] However, this study did not differentiate between heart failure types, HFrEF and HFpEF and the diagnosis were based on International Classification of Diseases (ICD) codes. Patients with HFrEF without atrial fibrillation have a lower stroke risk than those with atrial fibrillation (1.2% per year vs. 1.6% per year respectively).[41] Patients with HFpEF without atrial fibrillation showed a lower stroke risk than those with atrial fibrillation (1.0% per year vs. 1.8% per year, respectively).[40]

Silent Stroke in Heart Failure

Patients with heart failure have higher incidence of silent stroke. This silent stroke may be a precursor of a symptomatic stroke and likely contribute to cognitive impairment which is common in heart failure patients.[11] However, the clinical significance of a high prevalence of silent stroke in heart failure is unclear.[42] In addition to a clinical stroke, approximately 25–80% heart failure patients may have increased cognitive impairment including decreased attention, memory loss, and decreased concentration.[43-45] Several studies have reported changes such as gray matter atrophy and white matter hyperintensities in heart failure. Since there is rich vasculature in the cortical gray matter, the mechanism of gray matter loss is unknown but it has to be other than hypoperfusion.[45,46] Possible mechanisms for silent stroke or brain injury in heart failure could be due to diminished cerebral blood flow, neurohormonal changes involving cortisol and catecholamines, inflammatory responses associated with myocardial injury, and nutritional deficiency such as thiamine deficiency.[44]

Stroke Prevention in Heart Failure with Atrial Fibrillation

Stroke risk of a patient can be calculated by CHA_2DS_2-Vasc scoring system. The non-vitamin K antagonist oral anticoagulants (NOACs) and warfarin are usually recommended for CHA_2DS_2-Vasc score of 2 or more. In patients with contraindication to anticoagulants such as high bleeding risk, left atrial appendage occlusion may be considered.

Stroke Prevention in Heart Failure without Atrial Fibrillation

There have been four main trials of stroke prevention in patients with HFrEF who maintained sinus rhythm:

1. Warfarin versus Aspirin in Reduced Cardiac Ejection Fraction (WARCEF)
2. Warfarin and Antiplatelet Therapy in Chronic Heart Failure (WATCH)
3. Heart Failure Long-term Antithrombotic Study (HELAS)
4. Warfarin/Aspirin Study in Heart Failure (WASH).

In the WASH and HELAS trials, there was no significant difference between warfarin, aspirin, and placebo group at the composite end points of death, stroke or myocardial infarction.[47,48]

The WATCH trial showed that compared to aspirin or clopidogrel, warfarin reduced the incidence of ischemic stroke. However, the primary composite outcome of all-cause mortality, nonfatal myocardial infarction, and nonfatal stroke was neutral among the three antithrombotic groups.[49] The WARCEF trial was the largest study among the four trials. It showed that the incidence of ischemic stroke was lower with warfarin than with aspirin, however, the benefit was counteracted by an increase in major bleeding events.[50]

In a meta-analysis of these four trials, warfarin showed reduction in the stroke risk by 41% compared with that using aspirin. However, the risk of bleeding doubled, which offset the benefit of stroke prevention. Furthermore, there was no difference in the mortality rate, incidence rate of myocardial infarction, and hospitalization rate between the groups.[51] Based on these results, the use of warfarin for the prevention of stroke in patients with sinus rhythm seems to be beneficial at least in the HFrEF. However, the routine use of warfarin in patients with HFrEF but without atrial fibrillation appears to be limited as benefits are offset by the risk of bleeding. This suggests that anticoagulation may be beneficial only for certain patients with a higher stroke risk beyond the bleeding risk. It is also expected that NOACs may be better option for stroke prevention.

Is there a Time for Increased Risk of Stroke in Heart Failure?

Risk of stroke seems to be higher in the initial period following incident heart failure.[8,10,52,53] Nationwide Registry Data from Denmark demonstrated that the 30-day ischemic stroke risk increased 5-fold after first-time hospitalization for heart failure. It remained elevated for almost 30 years with 2-fold increase between 31 days and 365 days and 1.5-fold increase between 1 year and 30 years.[10] Similarly, in a Dutch cohort study, the risk of ischemic stroke increased by 4.6-fold in the first 30 days after heart failure diagnosis.[53] These studies have consistently demonstrated an increased risk of ischemic stroke in the first 30 days after the heart failure diagnosis. These results suggest that anticoagulation for stroke prevention might be considered for patients with heart failure at a high risk, especially within the first month after the diagnosis of heart failure. Further studies are needed to confirm this hypothesis and to develop a clinical model to predict the stroke risk in patients with heart failure.

CONCLUSION

Control of hypertension appears to be the best and simple strategy for preventing heart failure and stroke in majority of patients. Most antihypertensive drugs reduce the transition from hypertension to heart failure to some extent. However, the thiazide diuretics like chlorthalidone and indapamide seem to have an edge over other antihypertensive drugs in preventing heart failure. There is no outcome data on hydrochlorothiazide, therefore, it should be avoided in patients at risk for heart failure. Stroke and heart failure are frequently associated with high mortality and morbidity rates. Atrial fibrillation, which develops in more than half of patients with heart failure, is a major risk factor for stroke. The role of heart failure individually as a risk factor for stroke has been underestimated. There is a growing evidence that heart failure itself increases the risk of stroke regardless of atrial fibrillation through various mechanisms, mainly by thromboembolism. Previous studies showed benefit of warfarin in patients with heart failure without atrial fibrillation but this benefit was counteracted by the increased incidence of major bleeding. Recent studies have suggested that patients with heart failure at a higher risk of stroke may benefit from anticoagulation. Based on the stroke risk model, it may be possible to select the best strategy to prevent stroke in patients with heart failure. Moreover, NOACs, due to their favorable risk-benefit profile compared with warfarin are an attractive therapeutic option. Thus, NOACs may be effective for stroke prevention in patients with heart failure, especially those at high risk of stroke in the period of highest risk for developing stroke. This outlook needs to be proven in further studies.

REFERENCES

1. Levy D, Larson MG, Vasan RS, et al. The progression from hypertension to congestive heart failure. JAMA. 1996;275(20):1557-62.
2. Lloyd-Jones DM, Larson MG, Leip EP, et al. Framingham Heart Study. Lifetime risk for developing congestive heart failure: The Framingham Heart Study. Circulation. 2002;106(24):3068-72.

3. Ponikowski P, Voors AA, Anker SD, et al. ESC Scientific Document Group. 2016 ESC guidelines for the diagnosis and treatment of acute and chronic heart failure: The task force for the diagnosis and treatment of acute and chronic heart failure of the European Society of Cardiology (ESC) Developed with the special contribution of the Heart Failure Association (HFA) of the ESC. Eur Heart J. 2016;37(27):2129-200.
4. Mozaffarian D, Benjamin EJ, Go AS, et al. Writing Group Members, American Heart Association Statistics Committee, Stroke Statistics Subcommittee. Heart disease and stroke statistics-2016 update: A report from the American Heart Association. Circulation. 2016;133(4):e38-60.
5. GBD 2015 Disease and Injury Incidence and Prevalence Collaborators. Global, regional, and national incidence, prevalence, and years lived with disability for 310 diseases and injuries, 1990-2015: a systematic analysis for the Global Burden of Disease Study 2015. Lancet. 2016;388(10053): 1545-602.
6. Pullicino PM, McClure LA, Wadley VG, et al. Blood pressure and stroke in heart failure in the REasons for Geographic And Racial Differences in Stroke (REGARDS) study. Stroke. 2009;40(12):3706-10.
7. Kannel WB, Wolf PA, Verter J. Manifeststions of coronary disease predisposing to stroke. The Framingham Study. JAMA. 1983;250(21):2942-6.
8. Witt BJ, Brown RD Jr, Jacobsen SA, et al. Ischemic stroke after heart failure: a community-based study. Am Heart J. 2006;152(1):102-9.
9. Lloyd-Jones D, Adams RJ, Brown TM, et al. Writing Group Members, American Heart Association Statistics Committee and Stroke Statistics Subcommittee. Heart disease and stroke statistics–2010 update: A report from the American Heart Association. Circulation. 2010;121(7):e46-215.
10. Adelborg K, Szépligeti S, Sundbøll J, et al. Risks of stroke in patients with heart failure: A population-based 30-year cohort study. Stroke. 2017;48(5):1161-8.
11. Haeusler KG, Laufs U, Endres M. Chronic heart failure and ischemic stroke. Stroke. 2011;42(10):2977-82.
12. Iriarte M, Murga N, Sagastagoitia D, et al. Classification of hypertensive cardiomyopathy. Eur Heart J. 1993;14 Suppl J:95-101.
13. Masserli FH, Bangalore S, Makani H, et al. Flash pulmonary oedema and bilateral renal artery stenosis: the Pickering syndrome. Eur Heart J. 2011;32(18):2231-5.
14. Bock JS, Gottlieb SS. Cardiorenal syndrome: new perspectives. Circulation. 2010;121(23):2592-600.
15. Kotecha D, Manzano L, Krum H, et al. Beta-Blockers in Heart Failure Collaborative Group. Effect of age and sex on efficacy and tolerability of β blockers in patients with heart failure with reduced ejection fraction: individual patient data meta-analysis. BMJ. 2016;353:i1855.
16. Bangalore S, Wild D, Parkar S, et al. Beta-blockers for primary prevention of heart failure in patients with hypertension insights from a meta-analysis. J Am Coll Cardiol. 2008;52(13):1062-72.
17. Chen N, Zhou M, Yang M, et al. Calcium channel blockers versus other classes of drugs for hypertension. Cochrane Database Syst Rev. 2010;(8):CD003654.
18. Thomopoulos C, Parati G, Zanchetti A. Effects of blood pressure-lowering treatment. 6. Prevention of heart failure and new-onset heart failure–meta-analysis of randomized trials. J Hypertens. 2016;34(3):373-84.
19. Bavishi C, Masserli FH, Kadosh B, et al. Role of neprilysin inhibitor combinations in hypertension: insights from hypertension and heart failure trials. Eur Heart J. 2015;36(30):1967-73.
20. Feigin VL, Norrving B, Mensah GA. Global burden of stroke. Circ Res. 2017;120(3):439-48.
21. Feigin VL, Krishnamurthi RV, Parmar P, et al.; GBD 2013 Writing Group, GBD 2013 Stroke Panel Experts Group. Update on the global burden of ischemic and hemorrhagic stroke in 1990-2013: The GBD 2013 study. Neuroepidemiology. 2015;45(3):161-76.
22. Pullicino PM, Halperin JL, Thompson JL. Stroke in patients with heart failure and reduced left ventricular ejection fraction. Neurology. 2000;54(2):288-94.
23. Wolf PA, Abbott RD, Kannel WB. Atrial fibrillation as an independent risk factor for stroke: the Framingham Study. Stroke. 1991;22(8):983-8.
24. Caldwell JC, Mamas MA, Neyses L, et al. What are the thromboembolic risks of heart failure combined with chronic or paroxysmal AF? J Card Fail. 2010;16(4):340-7.
25. Jug B, Vene N, Salobir BG, et al. Procoagulant state in heart failure with preserved left ventricular ejection fraction. Int Heart J. 2009;50(5):591-600.
26. Georgiadis D, Sievert M, Cencetti S, et al. Cerebrovascular reactivity is impaired in patients with cardiac failure. Eur Heart J. 2000;21(5):407-13.
27. Lip GY, Gibbs CR. Does heart failure confer a hypercoagulable state? Virchow's triad revisited. J Am Coll Cardiol. 1999;33(5):1424-6.
28. Su MY, Lin LY, Tseng YH, et al. CMR-verified diffuse myocardial fibrosis is associated with diastolic dysfunction in HFpEF. JACC Cardiovasc Imaging. 2014;7(10):991-7.
29. Zile MR, Gottdiener JS, Hetzel SJ, et al. I-PRESERVE Investigators. Prevalence and significance of alterations in cardiac structure and function in patients with heart failure and a preserved ejection fraction. Circulation. 2011;124(23):2491-501.
30. Divani AA, Vasquez G, Asadollahi M, et al. Nationwide frequency and association of heart failure on stroke outcomes in the United States. J Card Fail. 2009;15(1):11-16.
31. Ois A, Gomis M, Cuadrado-Godia E, et al. Heart failure in acute ischemic stroke. J Neurol. 2008;255(3):385-9.
32. Hays AG, Sacco RL, Rundek T, et al. Left ventricular systolic dysfunction and the risk of ischemic stroke in a multiethnic population. Stroke. 2006;37(7):1715-9.
33. Appelros P, Nydevik I, Viitanen M. Poor outcome after first-ever stroke: Predictors for death, dependency, and recurrent stroke within the first year. Stroke. 2003;34(1):122-6.

34. Pullicino P, Homma S. Stroke in heart failure: Atrial fibrillation revisited? J Stroke Cerebrovasc Dis. 2010;19(1):1-2.
35. Hohendanner F, Heinzel FR, Blaschke F, et al. Pathophysiological and therapeutic implications in patients with atrial fibrillation and heart failure. Heart Fail Rev. 2018;23(1):27-36.
36. Kang SH, Kim J, Park JJ, et al. Risk of stroke in congestive heart failure with and without atrial fibrillation. Int J Cardiol. 2017;248:182-7.
37. Anter E, Jessup M, Callans DJ. Atrial fibrillation and heart failure: Treatment considerations for a dual epidemic. Circulation. 2009;119(18):2516-25.
38. Kotecha D, Chudasama R, Lane DA, et al. Atrial fibrillation and heart failure due to reduced versus preserved ejection fraction: A systematic review and meta-analysis of death and adverse outcomes. Int J Cardiol. 2016;203:660-6.
39. Lip GY, Piotrponikowski P, Andreotti F, et al. Heart Failure Association (EHFA) of the European Society of Cardiology (ESC) and the ESC Working Group on Thrombosis. Thromboembolism and antithrombotic therapy for heart failure in sinus rhythm: An executive summary of a joint consensus document from the ESC Heart Failure Association and the ESC Working Group on Thrombosis. Thromb Haemost. 2012;108(6):1009-22.
40. Abdul-Rahim AH, Perez AC, MacIsaac RL, et al.; Candesartan in Heart failure Assessment of Reduction in Mortality and Morbidity-Preserved (CHARM-Preserved) and the Irbesartan in Heart Failure with Preserved Systolic Function (I-Preserve) Steering Committees. Risk of stroke in chronic heart failure patients with preserved ejection fraction, but without atrial fibrillation: Analysis of the CHARM-Preserved and I-Preserve trials. Eur Heart J. 2017;38(10):742-50.
41. Abdul-Rahim AH, Perez AC, Fulton RL, et al. Investigators of the Controlled Rosuvastatin Multinational Study in Heart Failure (CORONA), GISSI-Heart Failure (GISSI-HF) Committees and Investigators. Risk of stroke in chronic heart failure patients without atrial fibrillation: Analysis of the Controlled Rosuvastatin in Multinational Trial Heart Failure (CORONA) and the Gruppo Italiano per lo Studio della Sopravvivenza nell'Insufficienza Cardiaca-Heart Failure (GISSI-HF) trials. Circulation. 2015;131(17):1486-94.
42. Hassell ME, Nijveldt R, Roos YB, et al. Silent cerebral infarcts associated with cardiac disease and procedures. Nat Rev Cardiol. 2013;10(12):696-706.
43. Pressler SJ. Cognitive functioning and chronic heart failure: A review of the literature (2002-July 2007). J Cardiovasc Nurs. 2008;23(3):239-49.
44. Havakuk O, King KS, Grazette L, et al. Heart failure-induced brain injury. J Am Coll Cardiol. 2017;69(12):1609-16.
45. Almeida OP, Garrido GJ, Beer C, et al. Cognitive and brain changes associated with ischaemic heart disease and heart failure. Eur Heart J. 2012;33(14):1769-76.
46. Vogels RL, van der Flier WM, van Harten B, et al. Brain magnetic resonance imaging abnormalities in patients with heart failure. Eur J Heart Fail. 2007;9(10):1003-9.
47. Cleland JG, Findlay I, Jafri S, et al. The Warfarin/Aspirin Study in Heart Failure (WASH): A randomized trial comparing antithrombotic strategies for patients with heart failure. Am Heart J. 2004;148(1):157-64.
48. Cokkinos DV, Haralabopoulos GC, Kostis JB, et al. HELAS Investigators. Efficacy of antithrombotic therapy in chronic heart failure: The HELAS study. Eur J Heart Fail. 2006;8(4):428-32.
49. Massie BM, Collins JF, Ammon SE, et al. WATCH Trial Investigators. Randomized trial of warfarin, aspirin and clopidogrel in patients with chronic heart failure: The Warfarin and Antiplatelet Therapy in Chronic Heart Failure (WATCH) trial. Circulation. 2009;119(12):1616-24.
50. Homma S, Thompson JL, Pullicino PM, et al. WARCEF Investigators. Warfarin and aspirin in patients with heart failure and sinus rhythm. N Engl J Med. 2012;366(20):1859-69.
51. Hopper I, Skiba M, Krum H. Updated meta-analysis on antithrombotic therapy in patients with heart failure and sinus rhythm. Eur J Heart Fail. 2013;15(1):69-78.
52. Lip GY, Rasmussen LH, Skjøth F, et al. Stroke and mortality in patients with incident heart failure: the Diet, Cancer and Health (DCH) cohort study. BMJ Open. 2012;2(4):pii:e000975.
53. Alberts VP, Bos MJ, Koudstaal P, et al. Heart failure and the risk of stroke: The Rotterdam Study. Eur J Epidemiol. 2010;25(11):807-12.

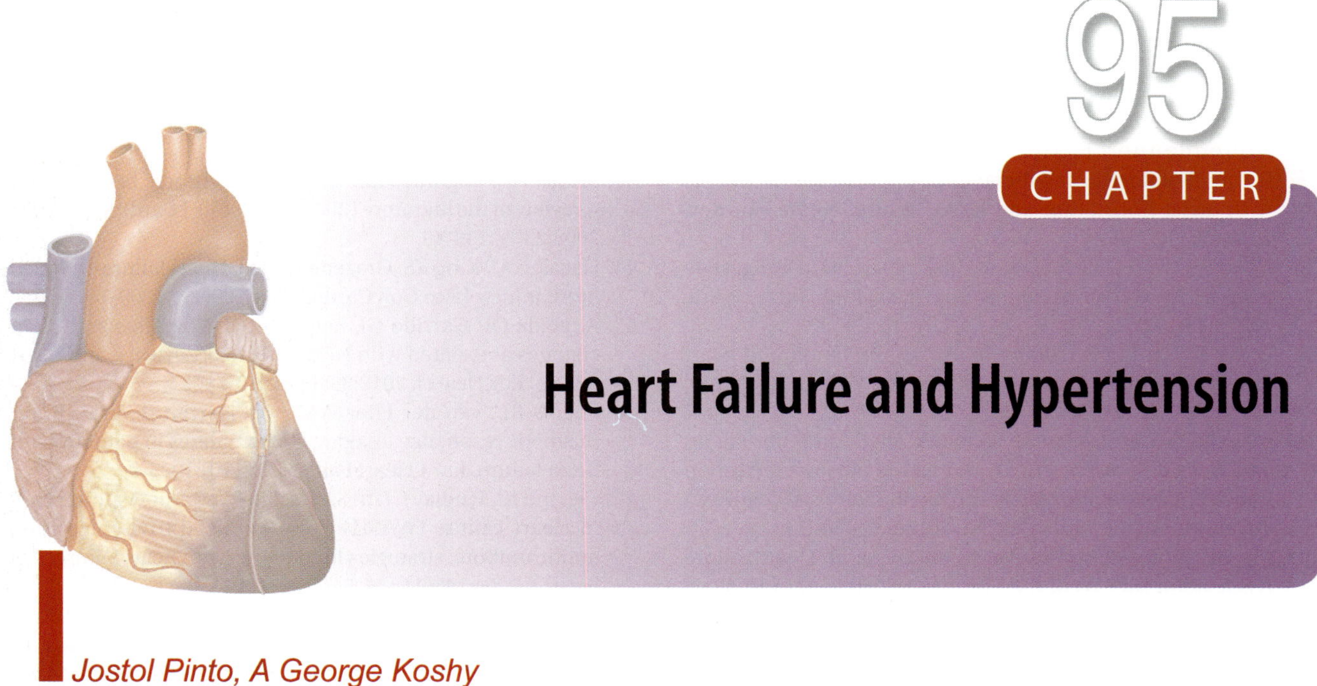

Heart Failure and Hypertension

Jostol Pinto, A George Koshy

INTRODUCTION

Heart failure (HF) is a common cause of significant morbidity, recurrent hospitalizations, potential mortality, and large financial burden in healthcare globally. HF has received mention in literature as early as 1500 BC in the Egyptian *Papyrus Ebers*. Over 40 million people (0.55% of the world's population) had HF in 2015.[1] Overall HF affects 2% of all adults;[2] this rises to about 8% for those over 65 years of age.[3] Hypertension is in no way less sinister. Complications of hypertension account for 9.4 million deaths worldwide every year. Hypertension is responsible for 45% of all cardiac deaths and 51% of all deaths due to stroke.[4] Worldwide, about 40% of adults above 25 years of age were hypertensive by 2008—that was a billion hypertensives already.[4] As of 2015, it affects between 16% and 37% of the global population.[5] In a recent study involving 1.3 million Indian adults, the crude prevalence of hypertension was 25.3% (age-standardized prevalence being 24.5% for men and 20.0% for women). Of note, the prevalence was 12.1% in the age group of 18–25 years. In terms of prevalence of hypertension, Kerala has the highest prevalence among South Indian states, and it figures among the top five states in our country (the other four being Punjab and Himachal Pradesh in the North, and Sikkim and Nagaland in the East).[6]

In recent medical literature, a lot has been elucidated about the relationship between systemic hypertension and its contribution to the progression of HF. It is well known that the most common causes of HF are coronary artery disease and hypertension; the less common causes include atrial fibrillation, valvular heart disease, cardiomyopathies, myocarditis, high output states, metabolic disorders, and obstructive sleep apnea.

Prior to understanding the complex but definite relationships between hypertension and HF, it is indeed pertinent that we first delve into the intricacies of HF per se.

PATHOGENESIS AND STAGES OF PROGRESSION

Definition

Heart failure is a progressive loss of functioning myocytes that prevents the heart from contracting normally—the inciting event could be abrupt or insidious in onset. It is a clinical syndrome that is characterized by typical symptoms and/or signs caused by structural and/or functional cardiac abnormalities that result in reduced cardiac output and/or elevated intracardiac pressures. While HF is often classified based on left ventricular ejection fraction (LVEF) as that with reduced [HF with reduced ejection fraction (HFrEF)], mid-range [HF with mid-range ejection fraction (HFmrEF)], or preserved [HF with preserved ejection fraction (HFpEF)] ejection fraction, in our review, it is better viewed as to whether it is of an acute or persistent nature.

Acute HF may occur in a normal heart or as a decompensation in an already failing heart. It is often precipitated by volume overload, inappropriate drug intake [missing essential drugs or intake of nonsteroidal anti-inflammatory drugs (NSAIDs) or pioglitazone], excessive salt in diet, myocardial infarction, arrhythmias, sepsis-myocarditis, or accelerated hypertension. Chronic HF is a progressive entity which may acutely decompensate due to insults or gradually worsen per se. Of note, hypertension can be responsible for either of the types of HF.

Pathology

Heart failure may occur due to a variety of causes. But the common mechanism underlying all these pathways is that dysfunction of part or all of myocytes increases the workload on the functional or partly functional myocytes. The resultant force of contraction now falls short of that expected by the Frank–Starling law due to decreased cross-linking between actin and myosin filaments.

The pathogenesis of HF occurs by progression of three interrelated pathways:

1. Neurohormonal (sympathetic, renin–angiotensin system, endothelin, natriuretic peptides, and cytokines)
2. Myocardial damage—myocyte and interstitial alterations [left ventricular (LV) remodeling, calcium leak, hypertrophy, apoptosis, fibrosis, reactive oxygen species, beta-adrenergic desensitization, and electrophysiology]
3. Endothelium/peripheral vasculature (constriction, nitric oxide, and cytokines).

Stages

According to the 2001 American College of Cardiology/ American Heart Association (ACC/AHA) working group, HF may be classified into four stages:

Stage A: Patients at high risk for developing HF, but no functional or structural heart disorder

Stage B: A structural heart disorder but no symptoms

Stage C: Previous or current symptoms of HF with structural heart disease

Stage D: Advanced disease requiring hospital-based support, a heart transplant, or palliative care.

The relationship between "New York and America":

- ACC Stage A has no corresponding New York Heart Association (NYHA) functional class
- ACC Stage B corresponds to NYHA I
- ACC Stage C corresponds to NYHA II and III
- ACC Stage D corresponds to NYHA III and IV.

CLINICAL FEATURES AND EVALUATION

Symptoms

Fatigue, dyspnea, paroxysmal nocturnal dyspnea, orthopnea, wheeze (cardiac asthma), and dizziness.

Signs

Cool extremities, crackles, cyanosis, laterally displaced apical impulse, third heart sound, murmurs pedal/sacral edema, ascites, hepatomegaly, raised jugular venous pressure, or a positive hepatojugular reflux.

Methods of Evaluation

Diagnosis of HF may be made clinically using the Framingham Criteria (two major or one major plus two minor criteria) which includes a list of nine major and seven minor criteria. It is 100% sensitive and 78% specific for this purpose.[7] Echocardiography and natriuretic peptide levels provide the necessary parameters to subclassify the diagnosis of HF into HFpEF, HFmrEF, or HFrEF.

Severity of HF may be graded based on the NYHA functional class, LVEF, and natriuretic peptide levels. Chest X-rays, electrocardiograms, levels of high-sensitivity troponins, renin, vasopressin, angiotensin II, and catecholamines provide corroborative information regarding the severity or progression of HF. For instance, coronary sinus plasma noradrenaline levels indeed predict mortality in HF. Coronary angiography or nuclear studies aid in determining if HF is associated with ischemia.

The 2017 ACC/AHA/HFSA Focused Update on Heart Failure Management recommends the following:[8]

- Measuring natriuretic peptides to diagnose or exclude HF in patients presenting with dyspnea (Class I, Level A)
- Measuring brain natriuretic peptide (BNP)/N-terminal proBNP (NT-proBNP) to prognosticate chronic HF (Class I, Level A)
- Measuring natriuretic peptides and/or troponin on admission to prognosticate acute decompensated heart failure (ADHF) (Class I, Level A)
- Measuring natriuretic peptides predischarge to establish postdischarge prognosis (Class IIa, Level B-R)
- Measuring natriuretic peptides to screen for those at risk of developing HF (Class IIa, Level B-R).

TREATMENT

Acute HF often presents as acute pulmonary edema and congestion. It is managed by administering oxygen, diuretics, nitrates, inotropic support, and ventilatory support and less often, by digoxin, cardioversion, or mechanical circulatory support. Novel approaches with debatable benefits include ultrafiltration, vasopressin antagonists, serelaxin, levosimendan, ularitide, aliskiren (direct renin inhibitor), cinaciguat, omecamtiv mecarbil, istaroxime, stresscopin, and rolofylline. Targets of treatment include blood pressure, volume status, renal function, and symptom relief.

In chronic HF, it depends on whether we are managing that with reduced or preserved EF. Treating HFpEF includes using diuretics, managing atrial fibrillation, valve surgery, or revascularization. Treatment of HFrEF employs angiotensin converting enzyme inhibitors/angiotensin receptor blockers (ACEIs/ARBs), beta-blockers, diuretics, aldosterone antagonists, revascularization, statins, capillary refill time (CRT), and/or implantable cardioverter defibrillator (ICD) in select cases. In both types, refractory HF may warrant the use of chronic inotropes, mechanical circulatory support, or even heart transplant.

The 2017 ACC/AHA/HFSA Focused Update on Heart Failure Management recommends the following:[8]

- *In Stage C HFpEF*:
    - To decrease hospitalizations, use aldosterone antagonists if EF >45%, BNP is elevated, HF admission within 1 year, creatinine <2.5 mg%, potassium <5 mEq/L (Class IIa, Level B-R)
    - No benefit from nitrates, PDE-5 inhibitors or nutritional supplements (Class III).
- *Treat anemia*:
    - IV iron replacement to improve QoL in NYHA class II and III if ferritin <100 ng/mL or if ferritin <100 ng/mL and transferrin saturation <20%
    - No benefit from erythropoietin (Class III).
- *Treat hypertension*:
    - Target BP <130/80 mm Hg in Stage A HF (Class I, Level B-R)
    - Target SBP <130 mm Hg in HFrEF (Class I, Level C-EO)
    - Target SBP <130 mm Hg in HFpEF after managing volume overload (Class I, Level C-LD).
- *Treat sleep-disordered breathing*: Use continuous positive airway pressure (CPAP) in patients with HF and obstructive sleep apnea (OSA) to improve sleep (Class IIb, Level B-R).

The comprehensive 2018 European Society of Cardiology/European Society of Hypertension (ESC/ESH) Guidelines for the management of arterial hypertension have outlined a convenient flowchart to initiate treatment at various stages of hypertension (Flowchart 1).[9]

RELATIONSHIP BETWEEN HYPERTENSION AND HEART FAILURE

As per the 2017 ACC/AHA classification, systemic hypertension in adults is now diagnosed with blood pressure over 130 mm Hg systolic or over 80 mm Hg diastolic. If systolic pressure is between 120 mm Hg and 129 mm Hg, it is now termed as "elevated BP".

Increased systolic blood pressure increases the afterload and lower diastolic pressure reduces the coronary perfusion pressure—both contribute to the vulnerability to HF.

While in younger patients, diastolic and mean pressures correlate better with the incidence of HF, in the elderly a better predictor of the same is pulse pressure.[10,11] Left ventricular hypertrophy (LVH) serves to play the role of an adaptation to systemic hypertension as well as a predecessor

Flowchart 1: Various stages of hypertension.

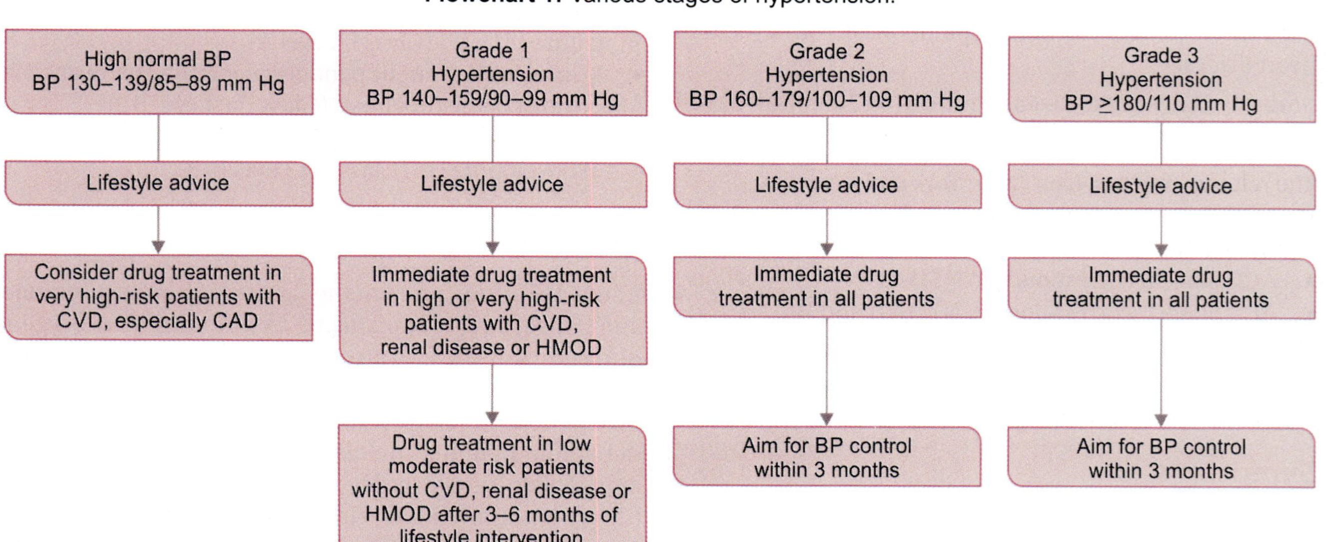

(CAD: coronary artery disease; CVD: cardiovascular disease; HMOD: hypertension-mediated organ damage)

of HF and hence, in a way, links the two pathologies. However, this relationship is in no way linear. Individuals have a varied hypertrophic response to a given level of hypertension, and not all cases of HF go through the stage of LVH. Nevertheless, the subcellular mechanisms underlying the development of hypertrophy due to hypertension share a platform in developing HF as well. The increased afterload of systemic hypertension causes wall stress on the LV. This releases intracellular calcium which activates calcineurin, which in turn activates genes like c-myc and c-jun which upregulate protein synthesis and increase levels of angiotensin II, norepinephrine, and insulin. The resulting hypertrophy of the LV due to an activated renin–angiotensin system disproportionately involves noncardiomyocytes. Thus, LVH caused by hypertension is an inhomogenous hypertrophy at the cellular level.

This strongly contrasts other cellularly homogenous forms of LVH like adaptive response in normotensive athletes, anemia, and even hyperthyroidism. The key difference is that in these conditions, there is no associated activation of the renin–angiotensin system.[12]

Myocardial damage is more evident when hypertension is the cause of hypertrophy. Fibrosis and increased deposition extracellular matrix decrease myocardial compliance and eventually contractility as well. This deposition is evidenced by elevated serum procollagen type I C-terminal propeptide, by delayed enhancement cardiac MRI, and by ^{111}In-labeled antimyosin antibodies. The resulting oxidative stress, hypoxia, and cytokines trigger apoptosis. It is fascinating how the signals (especially angiotensin), which mediate growth and hypertrophy, if persistent in terminally differentiated cells, paradoxically trigger apoptosis.[13]

Hypertension often but not necessarily passes through the stages of hypertrophy, diastolic dysfunction, or systolic dysfunction en route to the development of HF.

Acute HF may be brought about by transient sudden rise in systolic blood pressure more so in the presence of diastolic dysfunction, atrial fibrillation (loss of atrial contribution), coexistent coronary arterial disease, or mitral regurgitation. The normal ventricular compensation for an acute rise in afterload by increasing its end-diastolic volume is mitigated in diastolic dysfunction due to the reduced myocardial compliance of the inhomogeneously hypertrophied ventricle.

Hypertension as a Predictor of Heart Failure

In the Framingham Heart Study, hypertension preceded HF in 91% of the cases, and it imposed a two- to three-fold risk of developing HF after adjusting for age and other risk factors. In this cohort, HF was attributed to hypertension in 39% of men and 59% of women.[7] However, in a Swedish study of 7,500 patients followed up for 27 years, hypertension accounted as a cause for HF in 20.3% of patients.[14] Systemic hypertension is antecedent to HFpEF in over 85% of cases. About 75% of patients with HF and hypertension have a BP of >160/100 mm Hg.[15] HFpEF connotes a 5-year mortality of 60%, and over 50% of patients hospitalized with HF have HFpEF. These figures indeed make hypertension seem to have a significant role in the mortality caused by HF.

Challenges in the Association between Hypertension and Heart Failure

While this article focusses on the causation of HF by hypertension, common sense and evidence do, indeed, dictate that HF increases independently as age advances, renal disease progresses, with diabetes mellitus; these could be confounding factors in analyzing how strongly hypertension is associated with HF.

Further there is no definite threshold of blood pressure beyond which the occurrence of HF significantly increases.[15]

Hypertensive heart disease manifested as LVH is initially a compensatory mechanism in stalling HF in order to maintain cardiac output against the increased afterload, and indeed the EFs are supranormal in the early stages of LVH, but in itself is indeed a surrogate for HFpEF. Further, LVH accelerates atherosclerosis and potentiates arrhythmias, which in turn contribute to faster progression to HF. This weakens, in part, the association of hypertension with HF, as HF is also caused in part by the coexisting atherosclerotic vascular disease. If hypertension goes unchecked, this ultimately does result in HFrEF or at least exercise-induced systolic dysfunction.

Development of LVH itself is variable, for instance, for any given level of blood pressure, males are more likely to develop LVH earlier than females.

When we refer back to the stages of HF mentioned earlier, we understand that hypertension with or without diastolic dysfunction in itself qualifies as Stage A HF, while LVH qualifies as Stage B HF. So by definition, if hypertension itself constitutes an early stage of HF, then there is hardly any room for debate whether it causes the same.

A large proportion of patients with hypertensive LVH is having supranormal EF on echocardiography despite diastolic dysfunction. Supranormal function as a predecessor of failure is a concept challenging to fathom, and while partly defended as exercise-induced systolic dysfunction in a minority and diastolic HF by definition, it still does not completely clarify the concept of a supranormal EF coexisting with HFpEF.

Finally, there are certain drugs which successfully combat hypertension and yet do not mitigate HF, thus weakening the direct link between the two in therapeutic retrospect. Such drugs include calcium channel blockers (CCBs), alpha blockers, and combination of ACE inhibitors + ARBs.

Treatment of Both Hypertension and Heart Failure

The aim is not just to control blood pressure but to also slow down the adverse myocardial remodeling. These additional targets include neurohumoral mediators, fibrosis, diastolic dysfunction, and apoptosis.

These could be assisted by the use of appropriate agents—gene therapy (cellular signaling, neurohormonal modulation, and anti-apoptosis), ACEIs (anti-fibrotic and regress remodeling), losartan (antiapoptotic and regress remodeling), alpha-blockers, beta-blockers, MRAs, and endothelin antagonists.

Low Sodium, Rich Potassium Diet with Fluid Restriction

The WHO recommends that adults consume less than 2 g sodium or 5 g salt per day.[4] Popcorn, bacon, processed meat, and puffs contain about 1.5 g sodium per 100 g! Soy sauce contains 7 g sodium per 100 g.

The reduction of salt intake in Finland in the 1970s through mass media and legislation resulted in a decline of the national average of systolic and diastolic blood pressure by 10 mm Hg each. The WHO also recommends consuming at least 3.5 g of potassium per day. Every 100 g of beans/peas, nuts, bananas/dates/papaya provides about 1.3 g, 0.6 g, and 0.3 g of potassium, respectively.

Most drugs primarily employed for the treatment of HFrEF are antihypertensives—this cannot be plain coincidence. While their mechanisms of action are well studied as to how they reduce or reverse the progression of HF, or at least relieve symptoms of HF, it is equally true that they also control hypertension independently. Such drugs include ACEI/ARBs, beta-blockers, diuretics, nitrate-hydralazine, aldosterone antagonists, and even the latest in the list—angiotensin receptor-neprilysin inhibitor (ARNI).

Sacubitril–valsartan (angiotensin receptor neprilysin inhibitor) has been found to improve outcomes in HFpEF as evidenced by reduced NT-proBNP, left atrial size, improved myocardial circumferential strain, and a trend toward improved symptoms in the PARAMOUNT trial.[16] In an experimental model using Lewis rats with ischemic HF, ARNI was shown to reduce interstitial fibrosis and cardiomyocyte size, and increase vascular endothelial growth factor (VEGF-A) expression and angiogenesis with improved perfusion, thus improving global LV function.[17] These findings encourage the potential role of ARNI in reversing or reducing the pathologic changes of hypertension induced HFpEF as well.

In the ALLHAT study, amlodipine cohort had a 38% increased risk of HF when compared with the chlorthalidone cohort. In general, CCBs may be less preferred in treating hypertension in HF. Maximum data on regression of LVH are available with ACEIs and ARBs. CCBs, beta-blockers, and diuretics also produce modest reduction in LVH. But direct-acting vasodilators like hydralazine have no proven benefit in producing regression of LVH. However, sustained reduction of blood pressure indeed reduces the incidence of both LVH and HF.[18-20]

CONCLUSION

While the continuum of hypertension and HF is certainly gaining acceptance, corroborative and definitive links are still being sought. They share similarities in their risk factors and molecular bases, but more importantly in their treatment and prevention. With further neurohormonal therapeutics and gene therapy in the future, prevention of both may not be a very distant hope.

REFERENCES

1. GBD 2015 Disease and Injury Incidence and Prevalence Collaborators. Global, regional, and national incidence, prevalence, and years lived with disability for 310 diseases and injuries, 1990–2015: a systematic analysis for the Global Burden of Disease Study 2015. Lancet. 2016;388(10053):1545-602.
2. Metra M, Teerlink JR. Heart failure. Lancet. 2017;390(10106):1981-95.
3. McMurray JJ, Pfeffer MA. Heart failure. Lancet 2005;365(9474):1877-89.
4. WHO. (2013). A global brief on hypertension. WHO/DCO/WHD/2013.2. [online] Available from https://www.who.int/cardiovascular_diseases/publications/global_brief_hypertension/en/ [Last accessed November, 2019].
5. Poulter NR, Prabhakaran D, Caulfield M. Hypertension. Lancet. 2015;386(9995):801-12.
6. Geldsetzer P, Manne-Goehler J, Theilmann M, et al. Diabetes and Hypertension in India: A nationally representative study of 1.3 million adults. JAMA Intern Med. 2018;178(3):363-72.
7. McKee PA, Castelli WP, McNamara PM, et al. The natural history of congestive heart failure: the Framingham study. N Engl J Med. 1971;285(26):1441-6.
8. Yancy CW, Jessup M, Bozkurt B, et al. 2017 ACC/AHA/HFSA Focused Update of the 2013 ACCF/AHA Guideline for the Management of Heart Failure: A Report of the American College of Cardiology/American Heart Association Task Force on Clinical Practice Guidelines and the Heart Failure Society of America. Circulation. 2017;136(6):e137-61.
9. Williams B, Mancia G, Spiering W, et al.; ESC Scientific Document Group. 2018 ESC/ESH Guidelines for the

management of arterial hypertension. Eur Heart J. 2018;39(33):3021-104.

10. Kannel WB, Gordon T, Schwartz MJ. Systolic versus diastolic blood pressure and risk of coronary heart disease. The Framingham study. Am J Cardiol. 1971;27(4):335-46.
11. Vaccarino V, Holford TR, Krumholz HM. Pulse pressure and risk for myocardial infarction and heart failure in the elderly. J Am Coll Cardiol. 2000;36(1):130-8.
12. Weber KT, Brilla CG. Pathological hypertrophy and cardiac interstitium. Fibrosis and renin-angiotensin-aldosterone system. Circulation. 1991;83(6):1849-65.
13. Fortuño MA, Ravassa S, Fortuño A, et al. Cardiomyocyte apoptotic cell death in arterial hypertension: mechanisms and potential management. Hypertension. 2001;38(6):1406-12.
14. Wilhelmsen L, Rosengren A, Eriksson H, et al. Heart failure in the general population of men—morbidity, risk factors and prognosis. J Intern Med. 2001;249(3):253-61.
15. Levy D, Larson MG, Vasan RS, et al. The progression from hypertension to congestive heart failure. JAMA. 1996;275(20):1557-62.
16. Solomon SD, Zile M, Pieske B, et al. Prospective comparison of ARNI with ARB on Management Of heart failUre with preserved ejectioN fracTion (PARAMOUNT) Investigators. The Angiotensin Receptor Neprilysin Inhibitor LCZ696 in heart failure with preserved ejection fraction: A phase 2 double-blind randomised controlled trial. Lancet. 2012;380(9851):1387-95.
17. Pfau D, Thorn SL, Zhang J, et al. Angiotensin receptor neprilysin inhibitor attenuates myocardial remodelling and improves infarct perfusion in experimental heart failure. Sci Rep. 2019;9(1):5791.
18. Moser M, Hebert PR. Prevention of disease progression, left ventricular hypertrophy and congestive heart failure in hypertension treatment trials. J Am Coll Cardiol. 1996;27(5):1214-8.
19. Neal B, MacMohan S, Chapman N; Blood Pressure Lowering Treatment Trialists' Collaboration. Effects of ACE inhibitors, calcium antagonists, and other blood-pressure-lowering drugs: Results of prospectively designed overviews of randomised trials. Blood Pressure Lowering Treatment Trialists' Collaboration. Lancet. 2000;356(9246):1955-64.
20. ALLHAT officers and coordinators for the ALLHAT collaborative Research Group, The Antihypertensive and Lipid-Lowering Treatment to Prevent Heart Attack Trial. Major outcomes in high-risk hypertensive patients randomized to angiotensin-converting enzyme inhibitor or calcium channel blocker vs diuretic: The Antihypertensive and Lipid-Lowering Treatment to Prevent Heart Attack Trial (ALLHAT). JAMA. 2002;288(23):2981-97.

Bisoprolol in Heart Failure

AK Pancholia, HK Chopra

INTRODUCTION

Heart failure (HF) is a disease of epidemic proportions. Its prevalence ranges from 0.4% to 2% in the adult population of Western countries and increases 2- to 3-fold when patients with asymptomatic left ventricular (LV) dysfunction and with normal LV ejection fraction (EF) are included.[1-3] Despite recent advances, its prognosis remains poor. Half of the patients die within 3–5 years after their first diagnosis, and 1-year mortality rate may reach 50% in patients with severe HF.[4,5] Randomized controlled trials have allowed the selection of therapies able to improve quality of life and outcomes in patients with chronic HF. Hence, guidelines now recommend the administration of beta-blockers, angiotensin-converting enzyme inhibitors, angiotensin receptor blockers (ARBs), and, in New York Heart Association (NYHA) class III to IV patients, aldosterone antagonists, to improve prognosis of the patients with HF.[4,5] Diuretics are indicated for symptomatic treatment of fluid overload when present and manifest as pulmonary congestion or peripheral edema. Digoxin is also indicated to improve symptoms in patients with NYHA class III and IV HF.[5] Beta-blockers are therefore the mainstay of current medical treatment of HF. Bisoprolol was the first beta-blocker shown to have beneficial effects on outcomes in the Cardiac Insufficiency Bisoprolol Study II (CIBIS-II).[6]

ESSENTIAL CLINICAL PHARMACOLOGY

Beta-receptor Selectivity

Bisoprolol has high selectivity for beta-1 ARs with a beta-1 to beta-2 antagonist activity ratio of 119. Its selectivity for beta-1 ARs is higher compared with metoprolol, the other selective beta-blockers used in the treatment of HF (beta-1 to beta-2 ratio, 45).[7] This high selectivity might lead to better tolerability in patients with concomitant chronic obstructive pulmonary disease (COPD) as well as with peripheral vascular disease.[8-10]

Pharmacokinetics

Bisoprolol is almost completely absorbed in the intestine (90%) with very low liver first pass metabolism (10%). It has low plasma protein binding (30%) with a 1:1 ratio between hepatic metabolism and renal excretion. In normal subjects, its half-life is long (10–11 hours) and is further prolonged in patients with HF (17 ± 5 hours) and/or with severe renal failure allowing once-daily administrations.[11] Bisoprolol does not interfere with the metabolism of other drugs.

Modes of Administration

As with all beta-blockers in patients with HF, bisoprolol should be started with low doses with gradual (1- to 2-week intervals) uptitration to target doses. Treatment is generally started with 1.25 mg once daily with subsequent uptitration to 2.5 mg/daily, 3.75 mg/daily, 5 mg/daily, 7.5 mg/daily, and 10 mg/daily, if tolerated.[6] Target dose of bisoprolol was 5 mg in the first CIBIS trial, in which bisoprolol did not significantly reduce mortality, while it was 10 mg in CIBIS-II, in which bisoprolol reduced mortality.[6] Taking into account the differences in the initial as well as in the target doses (carvedilol, 3.125 mg bid to 25–50 mg bid, metoprolol succinate, 12–25 mg to 200 mg daily), similar protocols for initiation of therapy and uptitration must be used also for the other beta-blockers approved for HF treatment.[4,5]

EFFICACY STUDIES: CIBIS TRIALS

Bisoprolol fumarate has the advantage to have been studied largely in three major mortality trials in stable chronic heart failure (CHF) patients, demonstrating the important benefits of this beta-1 blocking agent and its good tolerability.

CIBIS Trial

Cardiac Insufficiency Bisoprolol Study (CIBIS) was the first randomized, double-blind, and placebo-controlled study with the primary objective to evaluate the impact of bisoprolol on mortality in patients with HF.[6] The inclusion criteria were ambulatory CHF patients in NYHA class III–IV, with a left ventricular ejection fraction (LVEF) <40%, receiving diuretics and vasodilator therapy and not registered on a waiting list for heart transplantation. At this time, the tolerability of a chronic beta-blocker therapy was unknown in a large population. An important prerequisite before inclusion was the need of a clinical phase of stability, without any episode of HF decompensation and the absence of major modification of HF therapy in the last 3 weeks before randomization. The initial dose of bisoprolol was 1.25 mg once daily, which could be increased 48 hours later to 2.5 mg/day and 1 month after to the maximal dose of 5 mg/day. CIBIS enrolled 641 patients with CHF, in NYHA class III in the vast majority (609, 95%). During a mean duration of follow-up of 1.9±0.1 years, there were 120 deaths, 67 (20.9%) in the placebo group and 53 (16.6%) in the bisoprolol group (Fig. 1).[12] This difference was not statistically significant with a risk reduction of 0.80 (0.56–1.15).

Despite this negative result, CIBIS was a very important study demonstrating the good tolerability of bisoprolol in a large CHF population, without evidence for any harmful effect of the beta-blocker therapy. Bisoprolol decreased the rate of hospitalization for worsening HF (17%) compared with 24% in the placebo group. Moreover, more patients in the bisoprolol group than in the placebo group improved their functional status. At the end of the trial, 21% of the patients receiving bisoprolol had an improvement of at least one class, compared with 15% in the placebo group. Deterioration of at least one NYHA class was similar in the two subgroups (13% vs. 11%).

CIBIS-II Trial

The CIBIS-II study was the first large randomized, double-blind, and placebo-controlled study demonstrating a dramatic reduction in mortality with a beta-blocking agent in CHF patients.[13] CIBIS-II enrolled 2,647 class III–IV stable CHF patients with a LVEF <35%, who were receiving diuretics and vasodilator therapy. In contrast to the CIBIS study, bisoprolol titration was forced to the maximal tolerated dose, with the highest possible dose of 10 mg/day. Bisoprolol induced a significant heart rate reduction (of 9.8±14.7 beats/min), with a limited effect on blood pressure (systolic blood pressure reduction of 4.1 ± 16.4 mm Hg with bisoprolol but of 2.3±16.4 mm Hg with placebo).[14] The study was prematurely stopped because of the significant mortality benefit associated with bisoprolol (Figs. 2 and 3).

After a mean follow-up period of 1.3 years, there were 384 deaths, with 228 (17.3%) deaths in the placebo arm and 156 (11.8%) in the bisoprolol arm [hazard ratio (HR) of 0.66 (0.54–0.81)]. Bisoprolol significantly reduced cardiovascular mortality, sudden cardiac death, and hospital admission

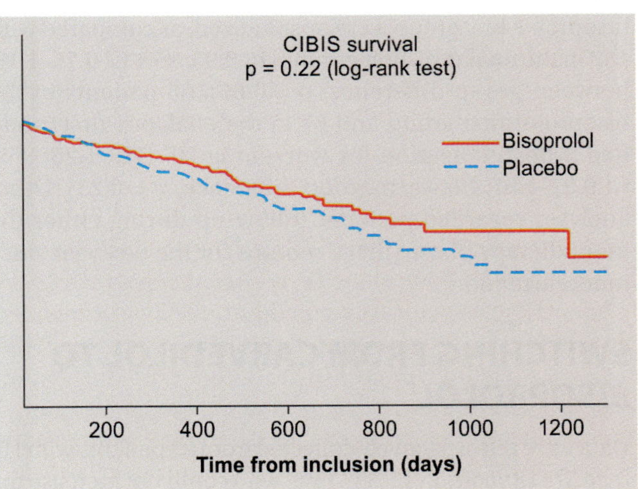

Fig. 1: Survival curve in Cardiac Insufficiency Bisoprolol Study patients.[12]

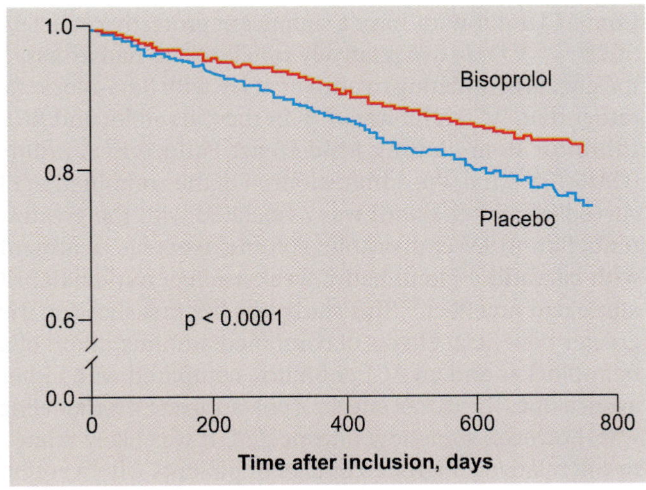

Fig. 2: Survival curve of Cardiac Insufficiency Bisoprolol Study II.[13]

In the bisoprolol-treated group of patients there was a **reduction** in	
• All-cause mortality (independent of etiology) by	**34%** (p<0.0001)
• Sudden death by	**44%** (p<0.0011)
• All-cause hospital admission by	**20%** (p<0.0006)
• Hospital admissions due to worsening heart failure by	**36%** (p<0.0001)

Fig. 3: Cardiac Insufficiency Bisoprolol Study II main results.[13]

(HR: 0.80 and hospital admission for worsening HF compared with placebo). The magnitude of the benefit was similar in NYHA subclasses, and independent of the etiology of HF. However, in patients with atrial fibrillation (20%), bisoprolol did not decrease total mortality when compared with placebo. In CIBIS, retrospective analysis suggested that patients with a LVEF of 20% benefit more from bisoprolol than other patients.[15] However, this was not confirmed in CIBIS-II, where the beneficial effect of bisoprolol was independent of the level of LV dysfunction.

CIBIS-III Trial

This study is to answer whether ACE inhibitor first or beta-blocker first in CHF. Despite the high significance of results obtained with beta-blocker therapy, all the data had been obtained with the administration of beta-blockers on top of standard therapy, including ACE inhibitors. However, there are reasons to believe that initiation of treatment with beta-blockers, rather than ACE inhibitors, may be beneficial as well. First, sympathetic activation may precede activation of the renin-angiotensin system in HF.[16] Second, beta-blockers may reduce renin-angiotensin activation to a greater extent than what achieved by ACE inhibitors with respect to sympathetic activation.[17] Third, sudden cardiac death (SCD) is the most important cause of death in the early course of HF[18] and beta-blockers, differently from ACE inhibitors, have a significant protective effect on SCD.[6,7, 18, 19] Only two relatively small studies had assessed the effects of initiating treatment of HF with beta-blockers, rather than ACE inhibitors.[20-22] In the Carvedilol and ACE Inhibitor Remodelling Mild Heart Failure EvaluatioN (CARMEN) trial, the administration of the combination of carvedilol and enalapril was associated with the greatest reduction in LV end-systolic volume, whereas treatment with carvedilol alone had a weaker effect and enalapril alone had no effect.[20] This study was the first showing the greater beneficial effects of combined administration of a beta-blocker and an ACE inhibitor, compared with either agent alone. The lack of effects of enalapril on LV remodeling was, however, somehow unexpected. It was likely related to the relatively high percentage of patients who were on enalapril before entry into the study and who might have developed tolerance to the effects of ACE inhibition. The study compared the effects of initiating HF treatment with a beta-blocker rather than an ACE inhibitor. Its design was therefore very similar to CIBIS-III. In the study, initiation of therapy with a beta-blocker was associated with a greater effect on LVEF and volumes. However, this study was not blinded. The hypothesis of the CIBIS-III trial was that initiation of treatment of HF with the beta-1-selective beta-blocker bisoprolol (to which enalapril is subsequently added) is as effective and safe as a treatment regimen based on the initiation with the ACE inhibitor enalapril (to which bisoprolol is subsequently added). Thus, the primary end point of the study was showing that initiation of therapy with bisoprolol, followed by combination therapy with enalapril after 6 months, was comparable (noninferior) to initiation of therapy with enalapril, followed by combination therapy with bisoprolol, after 6 months, with respect to the prevention of all-cause death and all-cause hospitalizations.[23] As already pointed out, CIBIS-III was designed as a noninferiority trial of bisoprolol first treatment vs. enalapril first treatment. The trial was successful with respect to its primary end point, i.e. bisoprolol-first was not inferior to enalapril first treatment (Fig. 4).

In the per-protocol sample, the primary end point was achieved in 163 patients in the bisoprolol-first group and 165 patients in enalapril-first group (absolute difference 0.7%, 95% CI 0.66–5.1%, HR 0.97%; 95% CI 0.78–1.21; noninferiority for bisoprolol-first vs. enalapril-first treatment, p = 0.046). There were 65 deaths in the bisoprolol-first group, as compared with 73 in the enalapril-first group (HR 0.88; 95% CI 0.63–1.22; between-group difference, p = 0.44), and cardiovascular deaths were not significantly different in the two groups [55 in bisoprolol-first treatment vs. 56 in enalapril-first treatment (HR 0.97; 95% CI 0.67–1.40; between-group difference, p = 0.86)]. 151 patients in the bisoprolol-first group were hospitalized, as compared with 157 in the enalapril-first group (HR 0.95; 95% CI 0.76–1.19; between-group difference, p = 0.66). 63 patients in the bisoprolol-first group and 51 in the enalapril-first group had a hospitalization for worsening HF (HR 1.25; 95% CI 0.87–1.81; between-group difference, p = 0.23). Other analyses regarded patients' follow-up during either the monotherapy phase (first 6 months) or the first year since randomization.[23]

SWITCHING FROM CARVEDILOL TO BISOPROLOL

Data were retrospectively collected from 23 patients with HF (age 57±18 years, LVEF 33±15%) who could not increase the dosage of carvedilol because of dizziness or hypotension,

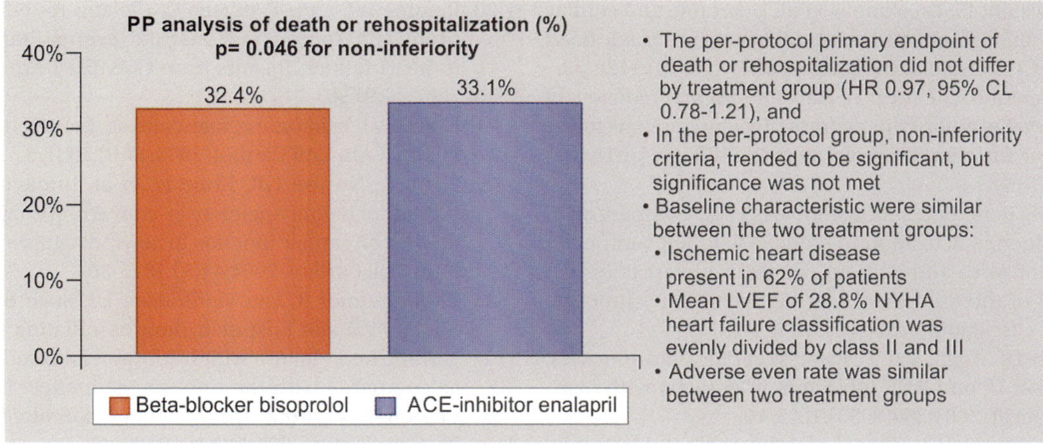

Fig. 4: Cardiac Insufficiency Bisoprolol Study IV: Primary end-points.
Source: www.clinical trial results.org

defined as systolic blood pressure <90 mm Hg. Before and immediately after, and 6 months after switching to bisoprolol ameliorates adverse effects in HF patients with dizziness or hypotension and help with continuation of beta-blocker treatment as well as dosage increase in HF patients with adverse symptoms or signs, allowing them to reach the target dose.[24]

CONCLUSION

Bisoprolol fumarate is a potent, highly selective beta-1 adrenergic blocker. Large mortality trials have clearly demonstrated the beneficial effects of bisoprolol on mortality and on morbidity compared with placebo. These favorable effects are associated with a reverse remodeling of the left ventricle and a significant improvement in LVEF. Finally, bisoprolol is well tolerated, with a limited number of side effects leading to its permanent withdrawal.

REFERENCES

1. Cowie MR, Mosterd A, Wood DA, et al. The epidemiology of heart failure. Eur Heart J. 1997;18(2):208-25.
2. Cleland JG, Khand A, Clark A. The heart failure epidemic: exactly how big is it? Eur Heart J. 2001;22(8):623-6.
3. Stewart S, MacIntyre K, Hole DJ, et al. More "malignant" than cancer? Five-year survival following a first admission for heart failure. Eur J Heart Fail. 2001;3(3):315-22.
4. Hunt SA, Abraham WT, Chin MH, et al. American College of Cardiology, American Heart Association Task Force on Practice Guidelines, American College of Chest Physicians, International Society for Heart and Lung Transplantation, Heart Rhythm Society. ACC/AHA 2005. Guideline Update for the Diagnosis and Management of Chronic Heart Failure in the Adult: a report of the American College of Cardiology/American Heart Association Task Force on Practice Guidelines (Writing Committee to Update the 2001 Guidelines for the Evaluation and Management of Heart Failure): developed in collaboration with the American College of Chest Physicians and the International Society for Heart and Lung Transplantation: endorsed by the Heart Rhythm Society. Circulation. 2005;112(12):e154-235.
5. Swedberg K, Cleland J, Dargie H, et al. Task Force for the Diagnosis and Treatment of Chronic Heart Failure of the European Society of Cardiology. Guidelines for the diagnosis and treatment of chronic heart failure: Executive summary (update 2005): The Task Force for the Diagnosis and Treatment of Chronic Heart Failure of the European Society of Cardiology. Eur Heart J. 2005;26(11):1115-40.
6. A randomized trial of beta-blockade in heart failure. The Cardiac Insufficiency Bisoprolol Study (CIBIS). CIBIS Investigators and Committees. Circulation. 1994;90(4):1765-73.
7. Bristow MR. Beta-adrenergic receptor blockade in chronic heart failure. Circulation. 2000;101(5):558-69.
8. Metra M, Nodari S, D'Aloia A, et al. Beta blockers in heart failure: Issues in the management of individual patients. Heart Fail Rev. 1999;4:65-77.
9. Sirak TE, Jelic S, Le Jemtel TH. Therapeutic update: Non-selective beta- and alpha-adrenergic blockade in patients with coexistent chronic obstructive pulmonary disease and chronic heart failure. J Am Coll Cardiol. 2004;44(3):497-502.
10. Le Jemtel TH, Padeletti M, Jelic S. Diagnostic and therapeutic challenges in patients with coexistent chronic obstructive pulmonary disease and chronic heart failure. J Am Coll Cardiol. 2007;49(2):171-80.
11. Leopold G, Kutz K. Bisoprolol: Pharmacokinetic profile. Rev Contemp Pharmacother. 1997;8:35-43.
12. de Groote P, Ennezat PV, Mouquet F. Bisoprolol in the treatment of chronic heart failure. Vasc Health Risk Manag. 2007;3(4):431-9.
13. The Cardiac Insufficiency Bisoprolol Study II (CIBIS-II): A randomised trial. Lancet. 1999;353(9146):9-13.

14. Lechat P, Hulot JS, Escolano S, et al. Heart rate and cardiac rhythm relationships with bisoprolol benefit in chronic heart failure in CIBIS II Trial. Circulation. 2001;103(10):1428-33.
15. Funck-Brentano C, Lancar R, Hansen S, et al. Predictors of medical events and of their competitive interactions in the Cardiac Insufficiency Bisoprolol Study 2 (CIBIS-2). Am Heart J. 2001;142(6):989-97.
16. Francis GS, Benedict C, Johnstone DE, et al. Comparison of neuroendocrine activation in patients with left ventricular dysfunction with and without congestive heart failure. A substudy of the Studies of Left Ventricular Dysfunction (SOLVD). Circulation. 1990;82(5):1724-9.
17. Campbell DJ, Aggarwal A, Esler M, et al. Beta-blockers, angiotensin II, and ACE inhibitors in patients with heart failure. Lancet. 2001;358(9293):1609-10.
18. Effect of metoprolol CR/XL in chronic heart failure: Metoprolol CR/XL Randomised Intervention Trial in Congestive heart failure (MERIT-HF). Lancet. 1999;353(9169):2001-7.
19. Packer M, Coats AJ, Fowler MB, et al. Effect of carvedilol on survival in severe chronic heart failure. N Engl J Med. 2001;344:1651-8.
20. Remme WJ, Torp-Pedersen C, Cleland JG, et al. Carvedilol protects better against vascular events than metoprolol in heart failure: Results from COMET. J Am Coll Cardiol. 2007;49(9):963-71.
21. Leier CV. Dismantling mandates in the treatment of heart failure. J Am Coll Cardiol. 2004;44(9):1831-3.
22. Sliwa K, Norton GR, Kone N, et al. Impact of initiating carvedilol before angiotensin-converting enzyme inhibitor therapy on cardiac function in newly diagnosed heart failure. J Am Coll Cardiol. 2004;44(9):1825-30.
23. Willenheimer R, van Veldhuisen DJ, Silke B, et al. Effect on survival and hospitalization of initiating treatment for chronic heart failure with bisoprolol followed by enalapril, as compared with the opposite sequence: Results of the randomized Cardiac Insufficiency Bisoprolol Study (CIBIS) III. Circulation. 2005;112(16):2426-35.
24. Taniguchi T, Ohtani T, Mizote I, et al. Switching from carvedilol to bisoprolol ameliorates adverse effects in heart failure patients with dizziness or hypotension. J Cardiol. 2013;61(6):417-22.

SECTION 7

Valvular

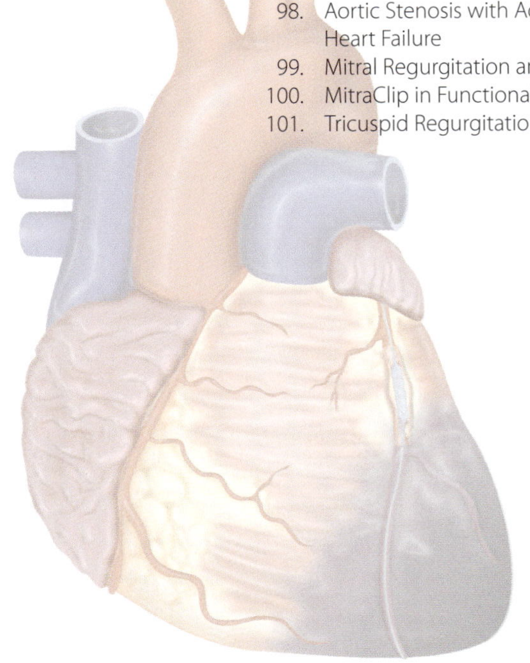

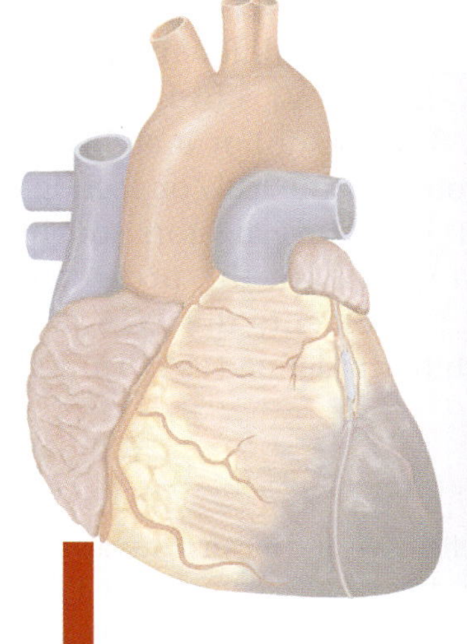

Echocardiographic Evaluation of Aortic Stenosis with Heart Failure

Adrian Chong, Sudhir Wahi

INTRODUCTION

Degenerative aortic stenosis (AS) is the most common native valvular heart disease in industrialized countries.[1,2] Untreated severe AS will result in left ventricular (LV) remodeling, systolic dysfunction with impaired left ventricular ejection fraction (LVEF), and ultimately congestive cardiac failure. Transthoracic echocardiography (TTE) remains the preferred diagnostic imaging modality in the assessment of valvular AS. Severe AS is defined by an AS jet peak flow velocity (AV V_{max}) >4.0 m/sec, mean transvalvular pressure gradient (MG) >40 mm Hg, and calculated aortic valve area (AVA) by the continuity equation of <1.0 cm^2 [or <0.6 cm^2/m^2 indexed for body surface area (AVAi)].[3-5] However, transvalvular velocities and gradients are flow-dependent parameters that decrease in parallel with a depressed LVEF and ensuing low stroke volume (SV) or flow state. As 5–10% of AS patients will present with severe AS and concomitant LV systolic dysfunction, this syndrome of low-flow low-gradient aortic stenosis (LFLGAS) with resultant discrepancies in the conventional hemodynamic criteria is not infrequently encountered. Correct evaluation of this high-risk subset of patients is critical as the mean survival is <1.5 years from symptom onset.[6,7]

CLASSICAL LOW-FLOW LOW-GRADIENT AORTIC STENOSIS (REDUCED LVEF)

Classical LFLGAS (CLFLGAS) with reduced LVEF is defined by the composite of an effective orifice area (EOA) or AVA <1.0 cm^2, LVEF <50%, mean gradient (MG) <40 mm Hg, and SV indexed (SVi) <35 mL/m^2.[4,5] Patients presenting with features of CLFLGAS consist of two pathophysiologically and prognostically different cohorts that must be differentiated in order to guide treatment decisions. Those with true severe aortic stenosis [TSAS; American College of Cardiology (ACC) stage D2] have progressive LV systolic dysfunction as a consequence of chronically elevated afterload and wall stress with resultant low transvalvular velocities, and gradients despite the persistently small EOA.[3] TSAS warrants intervention [European Society of Cardiology (ESC) class I level of evidence (LOE: B); ACC class I (LOE: A)] as LV functional recovery is expected following either surgical or transcatheter aortic valve replacement (SAVR or TAVR) depending on patient-specific procedural risks.[3,5,8] The alternative scenario is a patient with nonsevere valvular AS, but has a coexistent underlying cardiomyopathy responsible for the low-flow state. The apparent restricted leaflet mobility is due to the inability of the dysfunctional LV to generate sufficient energy or force to open the aortic cusps, hence resulting in "pseudo-severe" aortic stenosis (PSAS). The reported prevalence of PSAS is in the order of 5–35% of patients with LFLGAS.[9] Aortic valve replacement (AVR) is inappropriate and also carries a higher operative mortality, as the primary pathology is LV systolic dysfunction rather than true afterload mismatch from severe mechanical obstruction.[10] Data from the European Multicenter Registry of LFLGAS demonstrated that PSAS patients managed conservatively had a 5-year mortality rate of 43±11% which was significantly lower in comparison to those with TSAS (91±6%; P <0.001).[11] This was comparable to that of patients with isolated systolic heart failure and no valvular disease (52±11% for PSAS vs 44±10% for heart failure; P = 0.41) supporting the non-AVR medical approach as the treatment strategy for PSAS.

Low-dose dobutamine stress echocardiography (DSE) is the primary imaging tool to distinguish TSAS from PSAS in CLFLGAS.[3-5] The standard DSE protocol involves dobutamine infused at a starting dose of 2.5–5.0 mcg/kg/min, then increasing the rate at 3–5-minute intervals, to a maximum of 20 mcg/kg/min where maximal inotropic effect has been achieved. The optimal TTE imaging window must first be established at baseline, allowing subsequent reproducible pulsed and continuous wave Doppler interrogations of the left ventricular outflow tract (LVOT) and aortic valve (AV) at each stage, measuring the AV V_{max}, AV MG, LVOT/AV velocity time integrals, and AVA. Target endpoints include a heart rate increment by >10–20 bpm above baseline (or >100 bpm), or if a diagnostic threshold is achieved. Confirmation of TSAS requires a peak AV V_{max} velocity of >4.0 m/sec or MG of >40 mm Hg at any stage with the proviso that the AVA does not exceed 1.0 cm^2. PSAS is diagnosed by an increase in the AVA to >1.0 cm^2 (or >0.2 cm^2 increment from baseline) with augmented SV or flow rate paralleled by minimal change in the MG. This also allows assessment of LV contractile or flow reserve (CR/FR) defined as an increase in the SV or LVEF by >20%. The presence of CR/FR predicted lower operative mortality (CR present 5% vs. CR absent 32%; P = 0.0002), better functional improvement and increase in LVEF post-AVR, and increased survival.[12-14] However, the absence of CR/FR should not preclude consideration for SAVR or TAVR.[5,15] Similar data can be derived in the cardiac catheterization laboratory using dobutamine infusions and invasive hemodynamic measurements of gradients, cardiac output, and AVA.[16] Although the dobutamine challenge appears fundamentally simplistic, it should ideally be performed in specialized centers. Adverse effects (including arrhythmias and hypotension) are not uncommon and require premature termination of the test (~30%).[17] Increased susceptibility to hypotension from LV outflow obstruction and subendocardial hypoperfusion with resultant ischemia are likely contributors.[18,19] Experienced operators are also essential for accurate interpretation of the results.

A third subset of patients in this LFLGAS scenario exists where there is no significant augmentation in LVEF/SV, and neither diagnostic criteria for TSAS or PSAS are fulfilled, such that the true severity of AS remains "indeterminate". These patients have the worse overall prognosis as they remain undifferentiated, and consequently, "undertreated".[20,21] It has been recognized that individual patients will have variable SV or FR responses to dobutamine [different degrees of contractile reserve (inotropy), chronotropy, medication effects (e.g. β-blockade) or inability to tolerate the complete protocol]. The truly or pseudo-severe aortic stenosis (TOPAS) investigators sought to overcome this limitation with the projected AVA (EOA_{proj}).[17] EOA_{proj} represents the EOA at a standardized flow rate (arbitrarily defined as 250 mL/s) and is calculated as:

$$EOA_{proj} = EOA_{rest} + VC \times (250 - Q_{rest})$$

EOA_{rest} and Q_{rest} are the baseline AVA and mean transvalvular flow rate (Q = SV/ejection time). Valve compliance (VC) represents the rate of change in the EOA with increasing transvalvular flow (extrapolated from the regression slope of the EOA vs flow curve plotted during the incremental stages of the dobutamine infusion). In 23 patients with LFLGAS, who underwent low-dose DSE (15 TSAS and 8 PSAS) followed by surgical AVR, EOA_{proj} was superior to MG and EOA criteria in distinguishing TSAS from PSAS (TSAS: stress MG >30 mm Hg: sensitivity 80%, specificity 63%, correct classification 74%; stress EOA ≤1.0 cm^2: 67%, 63%, 65%; ΔEOA <0.3 cm^2: 87%, 13%, 61%; EOA_{proj} ≤1.0 cm^2: 93%, 63%, 83%). Indexed EOA_{proj} ≤0.55 cm^2/m^2 further enhanced the discriminatory value by improving sensitivity 100%, specificity 83%, and correct classification 95%. Surgical inspection and pathologic assessment of leaflet calcification was used as the reference standard. In CLFLGAS, EOA_{proj} at peak dose DSE has also been demonstrated to independently predict increased mortality.[22] However, the discriminatory value of EOA_{proj} is reduced, where the increase in FR is <15%, owing to less accurate VC estimations by this graphing approach. There is a simplified version of the EOA_{proj}, where VC is calculated (and substituted into the EOA_{proj} equation):[23]

$$VC_{simpl} = (AVA_{peak} - AVA_{rest})/(Q_{peak} - Q_{rest})$$

EOA_{proj} (simplified) correlated (r = 0.95, P <0.001) and agreed (0.004±0.07 cm^2) well with the conventional technique resulting in similar accuracy for differentiating TSAS from PSAS [ROC (AUC) 0.89 vs. 0.86 and correct classification 94% vs. 92%, respectively]. EOA_{proj} (simplified) can be easily incorporated into the "routine" low-dose DSE protocol to reduce the incidence of "indeterminate" CLFLGAS and/or increase diagnostic confidence to improve therapeutic decision-making (Fig. 1).

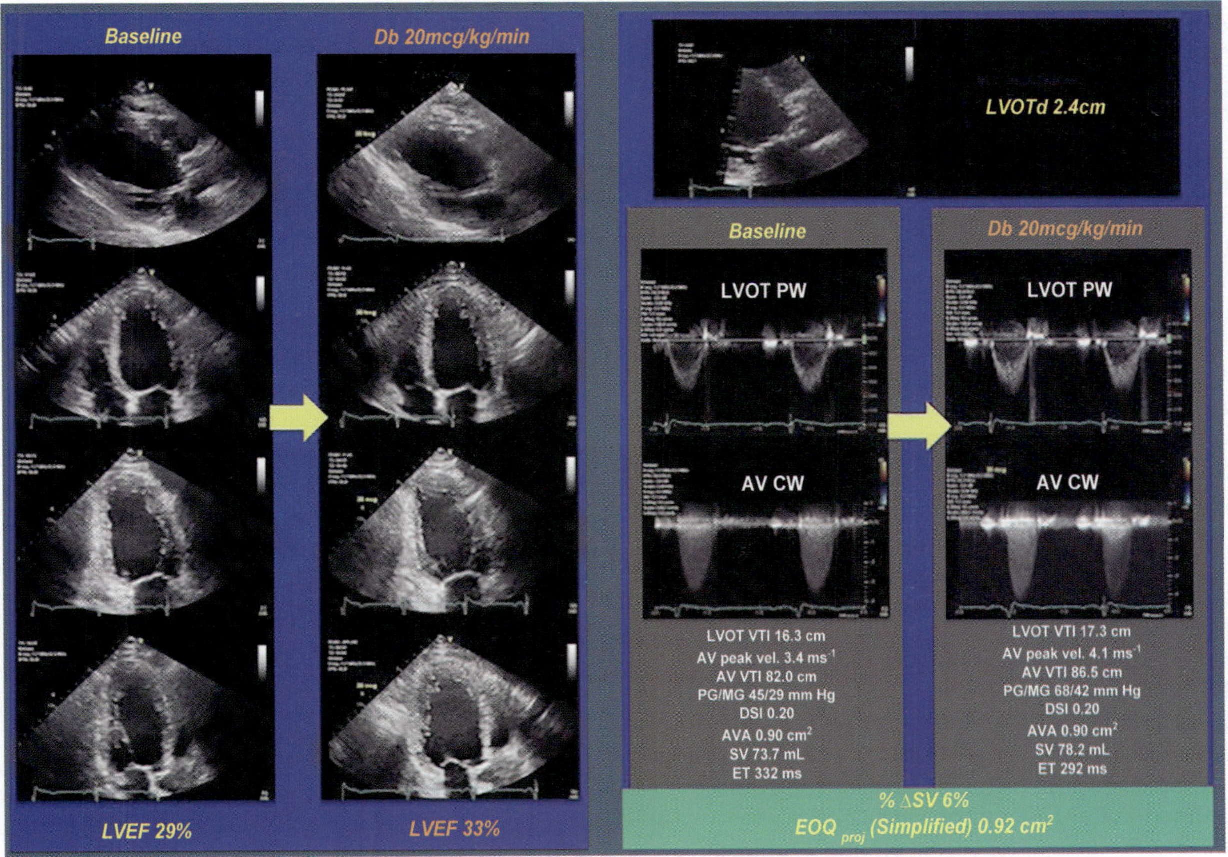

Fig. 1: Example of low-dose DSE performed for assessment of CLFLGAS and diagnosis of true severe AS [CR (-)].

(AS: aortic stenosis; AVA: aortic valve area; AV: aortic valve; VTI: velocity time integral; CLFLGAS: classical low-flow low-gradient aortic stenosis; CR: contractile reserve; CW: continuous wave; DSE: dobutamine stress echocardiography; DSI: delayed signal intensity; EOA: effective orifice area; ET: endotracheal tube; LVEF: left ventricular ejection fraction; LVOT: left ventricular outflow tract; MG: mean gradient; PG: proangiogenic growth; PW: pulse wave; SV: stroke volume)

PARADOXICAL LOW-FLOW LOW-GRADIENT AORTIC STENOSIS (PRESERVED LVEF)

Paradoxical low-flow low-gradient aortic stenosis (PLFLGAS) represents up to 30% of unselected AS cases and often present with heart failure symptoms despite a "preserved" LVEF.[24] PLFLGAS is hemodynamically defined by an AVA <1.0 cm^2, MG <40 mm Hg, LVEF ≥50%, and SVi <35 mL/m^2.[4,5] PLFLGAS is associated with a female preponderance, small concentrically hypertrophied LV cavities, higher LV global afterload, or valvuloarterial impedance [Z_{va} (mm Hg.mL^{-1}.m^{-2})] and lower survival.[25] PLFLGAS has been viewed as a more advanced disease stage, where chronic afterload excess has exceeded LV compensatory mechanisms, impaired myocardial function, reduced cardiac output, and pseudonormalized peripheral blood pressure. However, the severity of AS was originally based upon AVA, AVA corrected for pressure recovery (energy loss index), dimensionless velocity index, and VR, despite the proposed mechanisms for the low gradient being a low flow state, increased global afterload, and intrinsic myocardial dysfunction.[26] Consequently, as with CLFLGAS, PLFLGAS now represents a heterogeneous group comprised of patients with PSAS or TSAS (ACC stage D3, where AVR may be indicated [ESC class IIa (LOE: C), ACC class IIa (LOE: C)]. There is limited evidence supporting the use of low-dose DSE and/or EOA_{proj} as any attempt to augment flow would be intuitively difficult given the preexisting small LV cavities and low SV.[27] The echocardiographic differentiation between TSAS and PSAS remains the most challenging aspect of AS assessment faced by echocardiography laboratories today.

AORTIC VALVE CALCIUM SCORE BY MULTISLICE COMPUTED TOMOGRAPHY

An integrated approach to grade AS severity is often required when "indeterminate" cases are encountered. As leaflet calcification is the primary lesion in degenerative "calcific" AS, quantification using aortic valve calcium (AVC) scoring by multislice computed tomography (MSCT; Agatston method) may well be the final common pathway to determine anatomic severity, when hemodynamic assessments are inconclusive. Cueff et al. demonstrated that an AVC threshold of 1651AU was able to correctly classify TSAS and PSAS with a sensitivity 93%, specificity 75%, positive predictive value 93%, and negative predictive value 75% in the subset of patients with LFLGAS (AVA <1.0 cm^2, MG ≤40 mm Hg) and LVEF ≤40%.[28] Applying different AVC thresholds for severe AS [women: AVC ≥1274 AU, AVC density (AVCd; AVC indexed for aortic annulus area) ≥292 AU/cm^2; men: AVC ≥2065 AU, AVCd ≥476 AU/cm^2], Clavel et al. noted 45–66% of patients with LVEF 64 ± 7%, and discordant measurements (AVAi ≤0.6 cm^2, MG ≤40 mm Hg) had severe AS, independent of flow state.[29] These same AVC load cutoffs were also shown to incrementally predict excess mortality.[30] Current guidelines have predefined AVC thresholds of ≥3000/≥2000/<1600 AU and ≥1600/≥1200/<800 AU for very likely/likely/unlikely severe AS in men and women, respectively.[4]

CONCLUSION

Meticulous echocardiographic evaluation of TSAS, nonsevere valvular AS, and low pressure gradient AS, with or without comorbidities with multimodalities imaging may enhance the diagnostic, prognostic, and therapeutic implications which ultimately help in reducing cardiac morbidity and mortality.

REFERENCES

1. Carabello BA, Paulus WJ. Aortic stenosis. Lancet. 2009;373(9667):956-66.
2. Iung B, Vahanian A. Epidemiology of valvular heart disease in the adult. Nat Rev Cardiol. 2011;8(3):162-72.
3. Nishimura RA, Otto CM, Bonow RO, et al. American College of Cardiology/American Heart Association Task Force on Practice Guidelines. 2014 AHA/ACC guideline for the management of patients with valvular heart disease: A report of the American College of Cardiology/American Heart Association Task Force on Practice Guidelines. J Am Coll Cardiol. 2014;63(22):e57-185.
4. Baumgartner H Chair, Hung J Co-Chair, Bermejo J, et al. Recommendations on the echocardiographic assessment of aortic valve stenosis: A focused update from the European Association of Cardiovascular Imaging and the American Society of Echocardiography. Eur Heart J Cardiovasc Imaging. 2017;18(3):254-75.
5. Baumgartner H, Falk V, Bax JJ, et al. ESC Scientific Document Group. 2017 ESC/EACTS guidelines for the management of valvular heart disease. Eur Heart J. 2017;38(36):2739-91.
6. Horstkotte D, Loogen F. The natural history of aortic valve stenosis. Eur Heart J. 1988;(9 Suppl E):57-64.
7. Clavel MA, Magne J, Pibarot P. Low-gradient aortic stenosis. Eur Heart J. 2016;37(34):2645-57.
8. Nishimura RA, Otto CM, Bonow RO, et al. 2017 AHA/ACC focused update of the 2014 AHA/ACC guideline for the management of patients with valvular heart disease: A report of the American College of Cardiology/American Heart Association task force on clinical practice guidelines. J Am Coll Cardiol. 2017;70(2):252-89.
9. Burwash IG. Low-flow, low-gradient aortic stenosis: From evaluation to treatment. Curr Opin Cardiol. 2007;22(2):84-91.
10. Carabello BA, Green LH, Grossman W, et al. Hemodynamic determinants of prognosis of aortic valve replacement in critical aortic stenosis and advanced congestive heart failure. Circulation. 1980;62(1):42-8.
11. Fougères E, Tribouilloy C, Monchi M, et al. Outcomes of pseudo-severe aortic stenosis under conservative treatment. Eur Heart J. 2012;33(19):2426-33.
12. Schwammenthal E, Vered Z, Moshkowitz Y, et al. Dobutamine echocardiography in patients with aortic stenosi and left ventricular dysfunction: Predicting outcome as a function of management strategy. Chest. 2001;119(6):1766-77.
13. Monin JL, Quéré JP, Monchi M, et al. Low-gradient aortic stenosis: Operative risk stratification and predictors for long-term outcome: A multicenter study using dobutamine stress hemodynamics. Circulation. 2003;108(3):319-24.
14. Quere JP, Monin JL, Levy F, et al. Influence of preoperative left ventricular contractile reserve on postoperative ejection fraction in low-gradient aortic stenosis. Circulation. 2006;113(14):1738-44.
15. Tribouilloy C, Lévy F, Rusinaru D, et al. Outcome after aortic valve replacement for low-flow/low-gradient aortic stenosis without contractile reserve on dobutamine stress echocardiography. J Am Coll Cardiol. 2009;53(20):1865-73.
16. Nishimura RA, Grantham A, Connolly HM, et al. Low-output, low-gradient aortic stenosis in patients with depressed left ventricular systolic function: The clinical utility of the dobutamine challenge in the catheterization laboratory. Circulation. 2002;106(7):809-13.
17. Blais C, Burwash IG, Mundigler G, et al. Projected valve area at normal flow rate improves the assessment of stenosis severity in patients with low-flow, low-gradient aortic stenosis: The multicenter TOPAS (Truly or Pseudo-Severe Aortic Stenosis) study. Circulation. 2006;113(5):711-21.
18. Bountioukos M, Kertai MD, Schinkel AF, et al. Safety of dobutamine stress echocardiography in patients with aortic stenosis. J Heart Valve Dis. 2003;12(4):441-6.
19. Schinkel AF, Bountioukos M, Poldermans D, et al. Letter by Schinkel et al regarding article, "Projected valve area at

normal flow rate improves the assessment of stenosis severity in patients with low-flow, low-gradient aortic stenosis: The multicenter TOPAS (Truly or Pseudo-Severe Aortic Stenosis) study". Circulation. 2006;114(14):e526.
20. deFilippi CR, Willett DL, Brickner ME, et al. Usefulness of dobutamine echocardiography in distinguishing severe from nonsevere valvular aortic stenosis in patients with depressed left ventricular function and low transvalvular gradients. Am J Cardiol. 1995;75(2):191-4.
21. Grayburn PA, Eichhorn EJ. Dobutamine challenge for low-gradient aortic stenosis. Circulation. 2002;106(7):763-5.
22. Clavel MA, Fuchs C, Burwash IG, et al. Predictors of outcomes in low-flow, low-gradient aortic stenosis: Results of the multicenter TOPAS study. Circulation. 2008;118(14 Suppl):S234-42.
23. Clavel MA, Burwash IG, Mundigler G, et al. Validation of conventional and simplified methods to calculate projected valve area at normal flow rate in patients with low flow, low gradient aortic stenosis: The multicenter TOPAS (True or Pseudo Severe Aortic Stenosis) study. J Am Soc Echocardiogr. 2010;23(4):380-6.
24. Jander N, Minners J, Holme I, et al. Outcome of patients with low-gradient "severe" aortic stenosis and preserved ejection fraction. Circulation. 2011;123(8):887-95.
25. Hachicha Z, Dumesnil JG, Bogaty P, et al. Paradoxical low-flow, low-gradient severe aortic stenosis despite preserved ejection fraction is associated with higher afterload and reduced survival. Circulation. 2007;115(22):2856-64.
26. Dumesnil JG, Pibarot P, Carabello B. Paradoxical low flow and/or low gradient aortic stenosis despite preserved left ventricular ejection fraction: Implications for diagnosis and treatment. Eur Heart J. 2010;31(3):281-9.
27. Clavel MA, Ennezat PV, Maréchaux S, et al. Stress echocardiography to assess stenosis severity and predict outcome in patients with paradoxical low-flow, low-gradient aortic stenosis and preserved LVEF. JACC Cardiovasc Imaging. 2013;6(2):175-83.
28. Cueff C, Serfaty J, Cimadevilla C, et al. Measurement of aortic valve calcification using multislice computed tomography: Correlation with haemodynamic severity of aortic stenosis and clinical implication for patients with low ejection fraction. Heart. 2011;97(9):721-6.
29. Clavel MA, Messika-Zeitoun D, Pibarot P, et al. The complex nature of discordant severe calcified aortic valve disease grading: New insights from combined Doppler echocardiographic and computed tomographic study. J Am Coll Cardiol. 2013;62(24):2329-38.
30. Clavel MA, Pibarot P, Messika-Zeitoun D, et al. Impact of aortic valve calcification, as measured by MDCT, on survival in patients with aortic stenosis: Results of an international registry study. J Am Coll Cardiol. 2014;64(12):1202-13.

CHAPTER

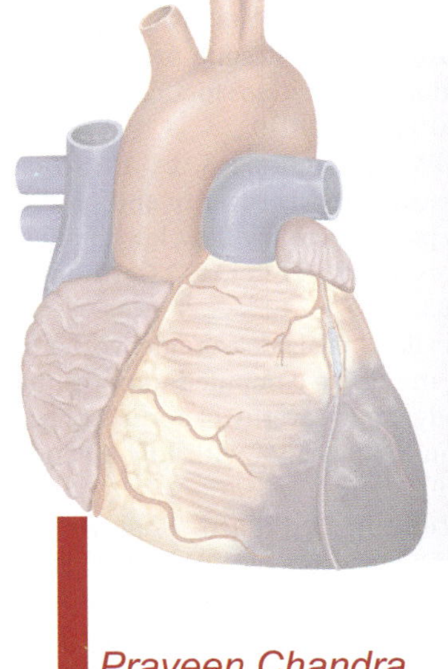

Aortic Stenosis with Aortic Regurgitation and Heart Failure

Praveen Chandra

INTRODUCTION

Heart failure (HF) has emerged as a major public health concern with an estimated prevalence of more than 26 million people worldwide.[1] Despite progressive improvements in health care, outcomes of patients with heart failure remains far from satisfactory. In the ESC-HF Pilot study, annual all-cause mortality rate in heart failure ranged from 7% to 17%.[2]

Valvular heart diseases (VHDs) rank among the leading causes of heart failure globally. Among patients with suspected heart failure, 14% had underlying significant VHD.[3] Among patients with moderate and severe native VHD included in the Euro Heart Survey, 69.8% presented with heart failure symptoms, and the most frequent valvular lesions were aortic stenosis (AS) and mitral regurgitation.[4]

The relationship between heart failure and valve pathology is complex. VHD may be the primary cause of heart failure or may develop as a consequence of congestive heart failure leading to clinical worsening. Patients with heart failure and VHD are at increased risk of adverse events including sudden cardiac death. Such patients require comprehensive evaluation and appropriate management strategy for improved outcomes.

Diseases of the aortic valve are the most common VHD seen in clinical practice with AS being the most common, accounting for 30% of patients referred to treatment, followed by aortic regurgitation (AR), which accounts for 10%.[5]

Isolated AS is characterized by pressure overload of the left ventricle (LV). In the presence of increased afterload as a result of fixed outflow tract obstruction, the LV undergoes concentric hypertrophy with increased LV mass index, thus maintaining a normal ejection fraction despite markedly elevated intraventricular pressures.

On the other hand, AR is a volume overload condition. In order to accommodate the abnormally large stroke volumes, LV undergoes chamber dilatation and eccentric hypertrophy. However, wall stress remains elevated according to law of Laplace (Stress = pressure × volume/ wall thickness).

However, when both AS and AR coexist, the combined pressure and volume overload result in a distinct form of myocardial stress. The LV has to simultaneously adjust for the increased stroke volume of AR and the increased afterload resulting from AS. This results in an intermediate phenotype characterized by LV end-diastolic dimensions lesser than that in pure AR but larger than that in pure AS. Hemodynamically, the concomitant volume and pressure overload imposes a double negative impact on LV mechanics and function (Fig. 1).

In a study by Popescu et al.[5] patients with mixed aortic valve disease (MAVD) were younger, more symptomatic, and had higher LV mass, pulmonary capillary wedge pressure, left ventricular end-diastolic pressure (LVEDP), and pulmonary artery pressure and a lower LV ejection fraction than those with isolated AS. Patients with severe AS who also have coexistent significant AR, have a significantly lower event-free survival than patients with pure AS.[6] Not only do such patients present with more severe LV hypertrophy and functional impairment at baseline, but they also have higher overall estimates of operative risk (higher EuroSCORE and STS-PROM).[7]

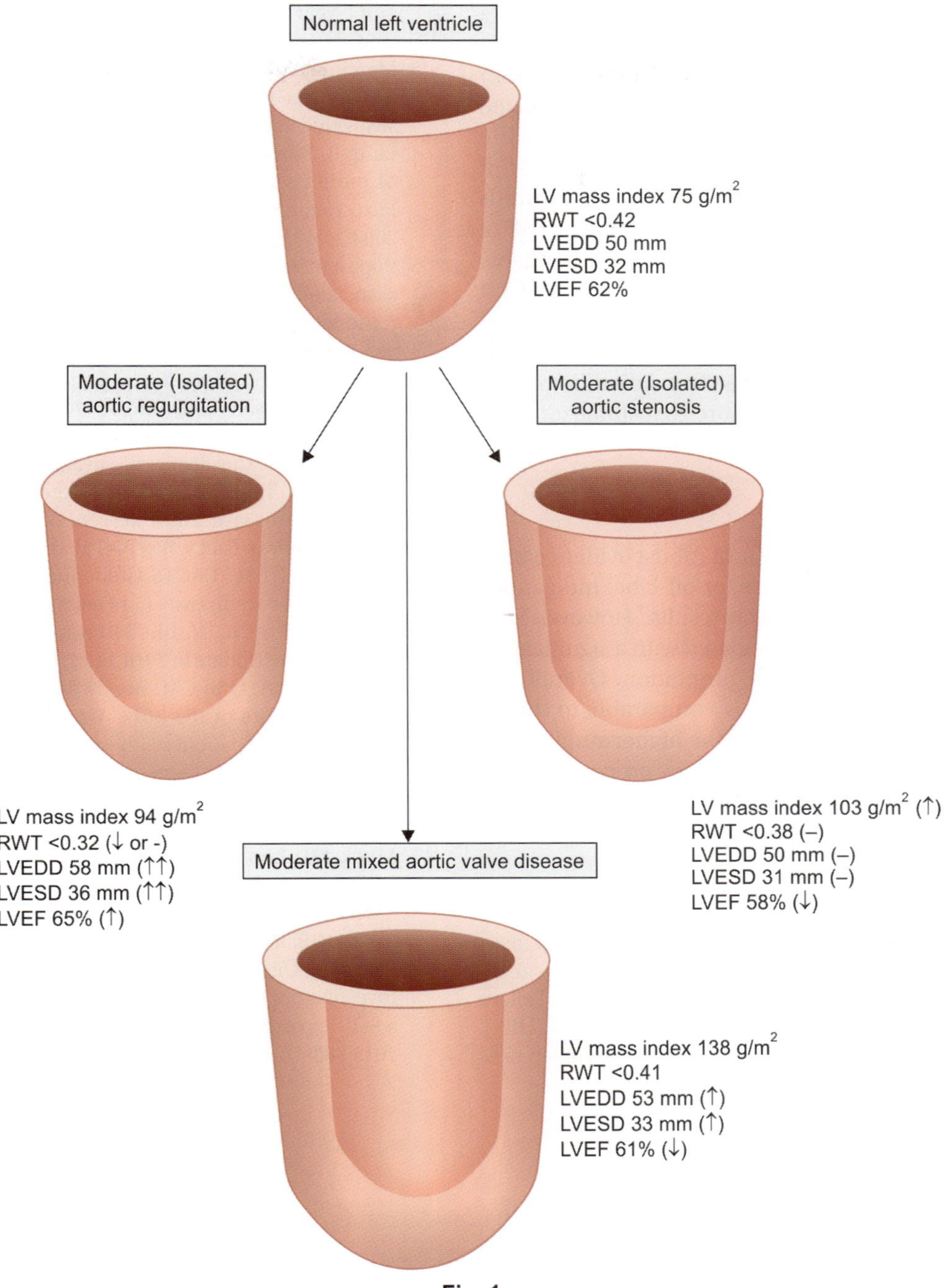

Fig. 1

(LV: left ventricle; LVEDD: left ventricular end-diastolic diameter; LVEF: left ventricular ejection fraction; LVESD: left ventricular end-systolic dimension; RWT: relative wall thickness)

In view of paucity of data regarding natural history of MAVD, evidence-based recommendations for the management of such patients is lacking. Current guidelines recommend basing decisions on the recommendation for the predominant lesion or in the case of balanced stenosis and regurgitation, indications for interventions should be based on symptoms and objective consequences.[8] As described above, MAVD represents a unique hemodynamic and pathophysiological entity and thus recommendations for isolated AS or AR may not be appropriate for this population.

During the past decade, transcatheter aortic valve implantation (TAVI) has revolutionized the management of aortic valve disease.[9] It has rapidly evolved from a treatment used on a compassionate basis for inoperable patients to being the standard of care in high-risk AS.[10] More recently, results from two additional randomized controlled trials (RCTs) have extended the available evidence to patients at low surgical risk. In the PARTNER 3 trial, TAVI with use of the balloon-expandable Edwards Sapien S3 prosthesis was associated with a lower risk of death, stroke, and rehospitalization at 1 year among low surgical risk patients.[11] In the EVOLUT Low Risk trial, TAVI with use of the self-expanding supra-annular CoreValve/Evolut prosthesis was shown to be noninferior to surgical valve replacement with respect to death and disabling stroke and superior in terms of heart failure rehospitalization at 2 years among patients at low surgical risk.[12]

CONCLUSION

The growing clinical experience and robust evidence base with TAVI has encouraged its use for off-label indications such as MAVD with mostly favorable results.[7] However, TAVI in this patient subgroup was associated with a significantly higher risk of prosthetic valve regurgitation. Overall, the outcome of patients with MAVD is comparable to that of patients with pure AS. Considering the higher surgical risk of MAVD patients and poorer outcomes on conservative management, TAVI may provide a favorable treatment option for this special population group.

REFERENCES

1. Savarese G, Lund LH. Global public health burden of heart failure. Card Fail Rev. 2017;3(1):7-11.
2. Maggioni AP, Dahlström U, Filippatos G, et al. Heart Failure Association of the European Society of Cardiology (HFA). EURObservational Research Programme: regional differences and 1-year follow-up results of the Heart Failure Pilot Survey (ESC-HF Pilot). Eur J Heart Fail. 2013;15(7):808-17.
3. Marciniak A, Glover K, Sharma R. Cohort profile: prevalence of valvular heart disease in community patients with suspected heart failure in UK. BMJ Open. 2017;**7**(1):e012240.
4. Lung B, Baron G, Butchart EG, et al. A prospective survey of patients with valvular heart disease in Europe: The Euro Heart Survey on Valvular Heart Disease. Eur Heart J. 2003;24(13):1231-43.
5. Popescu AC, Antonini-Canterin F, Enache R, et al. Impact of associated significant aortic regurgitation on left ventricular remodeling and hemodynamic impairment in severe aortic valve stenosis. Cardiology. 2013;124(3):174-81.
6. Honda S, Kitai T, Okada Y, et al. Impact of aortic regurgitation on the prognosis of severe aortic stenosis. Heart. 2012;98(21):1591-4.
7. Abdelghani M, Cavalcante R, Miyazaki Y, et al. Transcatheter aortic valve implantation for mixed versus pure stenotic aortic valve disease. EuroIntervention. 2017;13(10):1157-65.
8. Baumgartner H, Falk V, Bax JJ, et al. ESC Scientific Document Group. 2017 ESC/EACTS Guidelines for the management of valvular heart disease. Eur Heart J. 2017;38(36):2739-91.
9. Perrin N, Frei A, Noble S. Transcatheter aortic valve implantation: Update in 2018. Eur J Intern Med. 2018;55:12-9.
10. Nishimura RA, Otto CM, Bonow RO, et al. 2017 AHA/ACC focused update of the 2014 AHA/ACC Guideline for the management of patients with valvular heart disease: a report of the American College of Cardiology/American Heart Association Task Force on Clinical Practice Guidelines. J Am Coll Cardiol. 2017;70(2):252-89.
11. Mack MJ, Leon MB, Thourani VH, et al. PARTNER 3 Investigators. Transcatheter Aortic-Valve Replacement with a Balloon-Expandable Valve in Low-Risk Patients. N Engl J Med. 2019;380(18):1695-1705.
12. Pompa JJ, Deeb MG, Yakubov SJ, et al. Evolut Low Risk Trial Investigators. Transcatheter Aortic-Valve Replacement with a Self-Expanding Valve in Low-Risk Patients. N Engl J Med. 2019;380(18):1706-15.

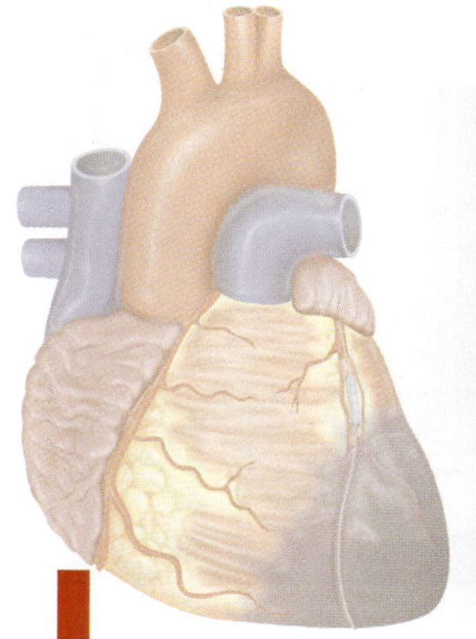

CHAPTER 99

Mitral Regurgitation and Heart Failure

Simmi Manocha, Kumar Hrishikesh, Prateek Bajaj

INTRODUCTION

Mitral regurgitation (MR) is among the most common valvular heart diseases. MR is classified as *primary (organic),* when caused principally due to structural or degenerative abnormality of mitral valve (leaflets, chordae, papillary muscles), e.g. mitral valve prolapse (myxomatous MV), infective endocarditis, rheumatic fever (RHD), cleft mitral leaflet (congenital abnormality). Secondary (functional) MR occurs in the absence of organic MV disease, usually due to LV dysfunction or mitral annular dilatation. Secondary MR is most commonly carpentier type IIIB and occasionally Type-I.[1] It is either ischemic resulting from LV remodeling after myocardial infarction (MI), resulting in papillary muscle dysfunction and systolic tenting and tethering of mitral leaflets, leading to eccentric regurgitation jet (predominantly). Nonischemic secondary MR is most commonly due to long standing hypertension or dilated cardiomyopathy (DCMP) resulting from global LV dilatation (mitral annular dilatation), leading to central regurgitant jet predominantly.[1]

MR is graded into mild, moderate and severe on the basis of various qualitative and quantitative indices by 2D, 3D echocardiography and transesophageal echocardiogram (Table 1 and Figures 1A to C).

PATHOPHYSIOLOGY OF MR CAUSING HEART FAILURE

Acute Phase

With abrupt onset of MR either by primary or secondary (ischemic) etiology, leads to sudden overloading of central circulation but a normal LV compliance resulting into elevated left atrial pressures and pulmonary venous hypertension. This leads to acute pulmonary edema and dyspnea (Fig. 2).

Chronic Compensated Phase

If the patient tolerates the acute phase, the LV myocardium shows adaptive changes to chronic volume overload (eccentric left ventricular hypertrophy and enlargement) but with normal systolic function of LV. In this phase patient remains asymptomatic.

TABLE 1: Quantitative echocardiographic criteria for severe MR in primary and secondary variants.

Quantitative Indices	*Primary (organic) MR*	*Secondary (Functional) MR*
EROA (Effective orifice area by PISA method)	≥0.4 cm^2	≥0.2 cm^2
Regurgitant volume (calculated by PISA method)	≥60 mL	≥30 mL
Regurgitant fraction	≥50%	≥50%
Vena contracta	≥7 mm	-
Jet area	Central jet covering >40% of LA area or holo systolic eccentric MR jet	

Source: Nishimma RA, OHO CM, Bonow RA, et. Al. AHA/ACC guided for the management of patient with valvular heart disease, a report of the ACC/AHA Task force on practice guidelines. J am Coll Cardiol. 2014;63:e57-187.

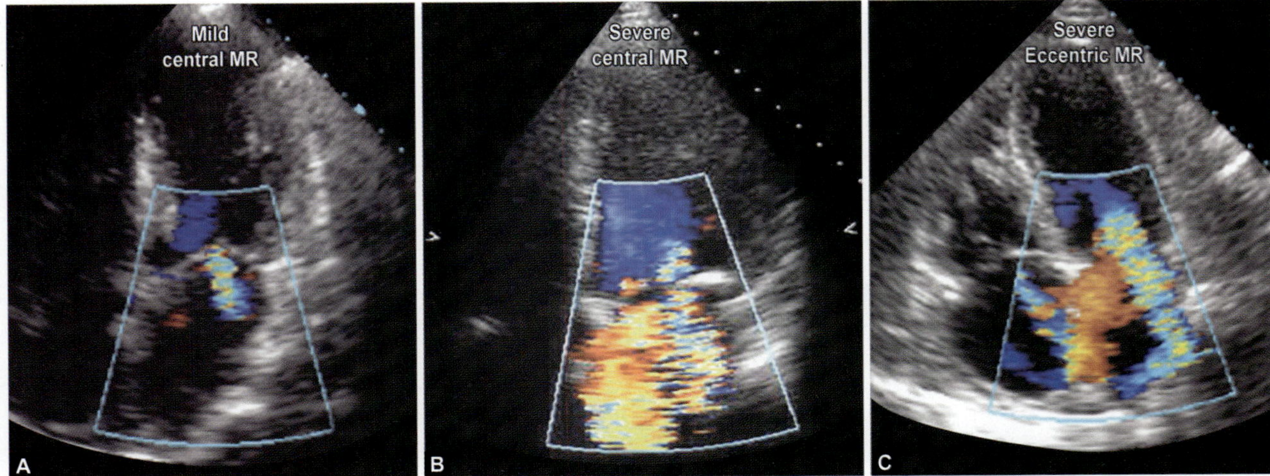

Figs. 1A to C: Showing severe MR.
Courtesy: European Association of Cardiovascular (ESC) Imaging[2]

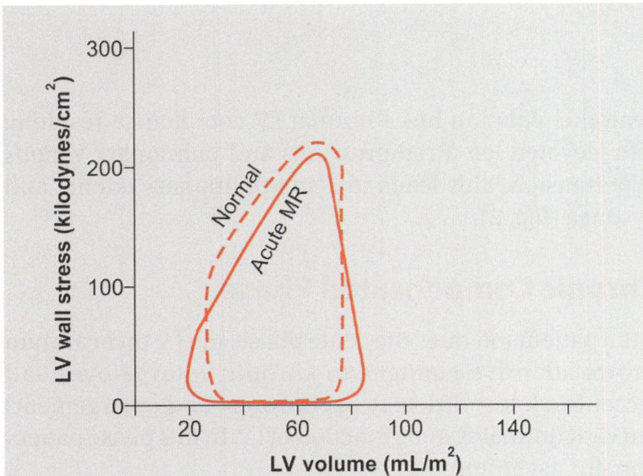

Fig. 2: LV stress-volume loop in acute MR. The early adaptation to acute MR consists of an increase in end-diastolic volume, a systolic unloading, that is characteristics of acute MR, and a decrease in end-systolic volume; as a result total stroke volume increases.[3]

This phase is very important as despite being asymptomatic phase of heart failure, early diagnosis and early intervention (medical/surgical) at this phase leads to very good prognosis.

Transition Phase with Mild LV Dysfunction

Eventually the compensatory adaptations of LV to increased volume overload, fails and mild LV dysfunction appears, which is reversible after intervention. In this phase symptoms like dyspnea on exertion (NYHA Class I/II) start but myocardium is in reversible state.

Decompensated Heart Failure

Ultimately in the absence of adequate medical or surgical intervention, progressive and irreversible structural and functional changes in LV take place resulting into moderate to severe LV dysfunction with increasing pulmonary artery pressure, which becomes irreversible later on. In this stage person is symptomatic (NYHA Class III/IV). Cardiac arrhythmia (AF) may develop in this stage.

This stage is delayed and neglected form of heart failure due to severe MR, as intervention at this stage does not yield good outcome. Myocardial remodeling is mostly irreversible at this stage (Fig. 3).

EARLY DIAGNOSIS OF HEART FAILURE

Advancement in management of heart failure is mostly dependent upon its early diagnosis at the stage of chronic compensated heart failure or transition stage, so that early medical or surgical intervention could reverse the myocardial remodeling.[4]

Strain echocardiography plays an important role is the diagnosis of these cases of heart failure with preserved ejection fraction (HFpEF), which represent almost 50% of overall cases of heart failure.[5] Longitudinal systolic strain (LS) measurement in HFpEF, by 2D speckle tracking strain echocardiography, has emerged as a more sensitive index of myocardial systolic performance than LVEF.[6] LS can detect subtle systolic dysfunction despite preserved global EF in HFpEF.[7] Also impaired LS, as defined by an absolute value less than 15.8%, is an independent prognostic marker in HFpEF patients and is associated with >2 fold increase in the composite end-point of cardiovascular death, heart

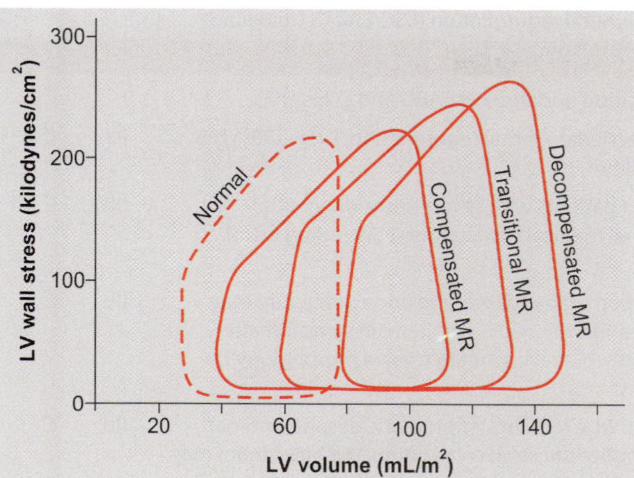

Fig. 3: LV stress-volume loops in three stages of chronic MR. As the ventricle adapts to the chronic hemodynamic burden, a progressive increase in LV end-diastolic volume and systolic wall strain occurs. LVEF progressively declines from 65% in compensated MR, to 55% during transitional stage, and finally to 45% or lower in Decompensated stage.[3]

failure hospitalization, or aborted cardiac arrest.[8] These large cohort studies implicate the need for routine use of strain imaging in prognosticating cases of heart failure specially HFpEF cases.

PARADOX: Heart Failure causing Secondary MR

Though, it is well known that severe MR (primary or secondary), causes heart failure in acute as well as chronic setting; long standing heart failure, as in cases of dilated cardiomyopathy (DCMP), causes remodeling of myocardium and retraction of papillary muscles and chordae as well as mitral annular dilatation leading to various grades of secondary MR.

It creates great confusion in deciding in patients of heart failure with severe secondary MR, that MR is the cause of HF or result of the same. Careful clinical history and secondary echocardiographic features resolves the mystery.

TREATMENT OF MR

Treatment of MR depends upon the etiology, whether it's a primary or secondary MR.

Optimal medical therapy in lines with the guidelines for the management of heart failure,[9] should be the first step in the management of all patient's with secondary MR. It improves symptoms, lessens MR and may delay the need for surgical intervention.

Beta-blockers and renin-angiotensin-aldosterone system inhibitors had the strongest supporting evidence for providing beneficial effects. Beta-blockers appear to lessen MR, prevent deterioration of LV function and improve survival in asymptomatic patient's with moderate - severe MR. ACE and ARB reduces MR especially in asymptomatic patients.

Urgent surgery is indicated in patients with acute severe MR. Surgery is obliviously indicated in symptomatic patients with severe primary MR.[10] In asymptomatic patients with LVEF-60%, LVESD ≥45 mm,[15] cardiac arrhythmia (AF)[13] and PASP ≥50 mm Hg,[14] becomes trigger for early surgery.

It is widely accepted that when feasible, *mitral valve repair* is the preferred treatment. When repair is not feasible,

TABLE 2: Indications for intervention in severe primary mitral regurgitation (ESC/EACTS Guidelines)

Recommendations	*Class*	*Level*
Mitral valve repair should be the preferred technique when the results are expected to be durable	I	C
Surgery is indicated in symptomatic patient with LVEF>30%[10–12]	I	B
Surgery is indicated is asymptomatic patients with LV dysfunction (LVESD ≥ 45% mm and/or LVEF>60%)	I	B
Surgery should be considered in asymptomatic patients with preserved LV function (LVESD < 45 mm and LVEF >60%) and atrial fibrillation secondary to mitral regurgitation or pulmonary hypertension (systolic pulmonary pressure at rest >50 mm Hg)[13,14]	IIa	B
Surgery should be considered in asymptomatic patients with preserved LVEF (>60%) and LVSED 40–44 mm when a durable repair is likely, surgical risk is low, the repair is performed in a heart valve center and at least one of the following findings is present: Flail leaflet or Presence of significant LA dilatation (volume index ≥60 mL/m² BSA) in sinus rhythm	IIa	C
Mitral valve repair should be considered in symptomatic patients with severe LV dysfunction (LVEF <30% and/or LVSED >55 mm) refractory to medical therapy when the likelihood of successful repair is high and comorbidity low	IIa	C
Mitral valve replacement may be considered in symptomatic patients with severe LV dysfunction (LVEF <30% and or LVSED >55 mm) refractory to medical therapy when the likelihood of successful repair is low and comorbidity low	IIb	C
Percutaneous edge to edge procedure may be considered in patients with symptomatic severe primary mitral regurgitation who fulfill the echocardiographic criteria of eligibility and are judged inoperable or at high surgical risk by the heart team, avoiding futility.	IIb	C

TABLE 3: Indications for mitral valve intervention in chronic secondary mitral regurgitation (ESC/EACTS Guidelines)

Recommendations	*Class*	*Level*
Surgery is indicated in patients with severe secondary mitral regurgitation undergoing CABG and LVEF>30%	I	C
Surgery should be considered in symptomatic patients with severe secondary mitral regurgitation, LVEF <30% but with an option for revascularization and evidence of myocardial viability	IIa	C
When revascularization is not indicated, surgery may be considered in patients with severe secondary mitral regurgitation and LVEF>30% who remain symptomatic despite optimal medical management (including CRT if indicated) and have a low surgical risk	IIb	C
When revascularization is not indicated and surgical risk is not low, a percutaneous edge to edge procedure may be considered in patients with severe secondary mitral regurgitation and LVEF >30% who remain symptomatic despite optimal medical management (including CRT if indicated) and who have a suitable valve morphology by echocardiography, avoiding futility	IIb	C
In patients with severe secondary mitral regurgitation and LVEF <30% who remain symptomatic despite optimal medical management (including CRT if indicated) and who have no option for revascularization, the heart team may consider a percutaneous edge to edge procedure or valve surgery after careful evaluation for a ventricular assist device or heart transplant according to individual patient characteristics.	IIb	C

mitral valve replacement (MVR) with preservation of subvalvular apparatus, is favored (Table 2).

Transcatheter MV interventions have been developed to correct primary MR either through a transeptal or a transapical approach. Among the transcatheter procedures, currently only the edge to edge mitral repair is widely adopted.[16]

Experience with transcatheter annuloplasty, transapical chordal implantation or valve replacement is still limited and general recommendations cannot be made. Transcatheter mitral valve treatment should be discussed by heart team in symptomatic patients who are at high surgical risk or are inoperable. *Percutaneous edge to edge repair* is generally safe and can improve symptoms and provide reverse remodeling. However rate of residual MR up to 5 years is higher than with surgical repair.[17]

In contrast to primary MR, there is currently no evidence that a reduction of secondary MR improves survival. In patients with CAD undergoing revascularization the optimal surgical approach remains controversial.[18] While MV repair with an undersized complete ring to restore leaflet coaptation and valve competence is preferred technique, valve replacement should be considered in patients with risk factors for residual or recurrent MR.[19] Indications for surgery in secondary MR are particularly restrictive, when concomitant revascularization is not an option owing to significant operative mortality, high rates of recurrent MR and absence of proven survival benefit.[20,21]

Percutaneous edge to edge repair for secondary MR is a low risk option, but its efficacy to reduced MR remains inferior to surgery.[22] It can improve symptoms functional capacity and quality of life and may induce reverse LV remodeling (Table 3).[23]

Similar to surgery, a survival benefit compared with optimal medical therapy according to current guidelines[9] has not been proven yet.

REFERENCES

1. Anita WA, Michael JM, Gregg WS. secondary mitral regurgitation in heart failure: JACC. 2015;65(12).
2. European Journal of Echocardiography, 2003;4(4) 237–61. https://doi.org/10.1016/j.euje.2003.07.001
3. Collham H, Gaosch WH, Meyer TE. Left ventricular response to mitral regurgitation. Circulation AHA. 2008;118:2298-303.
4. Robert JM, Michel GK. Longitudinal stream in heart failure with preserved ejection fraction circulation. 2014;5:132: 368-70.
5. Sulan TE, Hadge DO, Herges RM, et al. Trends in presence and outcome of heart failure with preserved ejection fraction. M Engl J Med. 2006;355:251-9.
6. Gorscan J III, Tanaka H. Echocardiographic assessment of myocardial strain. J Am Coll Cordial. 2011;58:1401-13.
7. Kraigher-Krainer E, Shah AM, Gupta DK, et al. Paramount investigations, impaired systolic function by strain imaging in HFpEF. J AM Coll Cardiol. 2014;63:447-56.
8. Shah AM, Claget B, Sweitzer MJ, et al. The prognostic importance of impaired systolic function in HFpEF and the impact of spiromolartome. Circulation. 2015;132-402-414.
9. Ponikowski P, Voors AA, Anker SD, et al. 2016 ESC Guidelines for the diagnosis and treatment of acute and chronic heart failure: Developed with the special contribution of the Heart Failure Association (HFA) of the ESC. Eur Heart J. 2016;37:2129-200.
10. Tribouillory CM, Enriquez-Sarano M, Schaff HV, et al. Impact of preoperative symptoms on survival after surgical correction of organic mitral regurgitation: rationale for optimizing surgical indications. Circulation. 1999;99: 400-5.

11. Enriquez-Sarano M, Tajik AJ, Schaff HV, et al. Echocardiographic prediction of left ventricular function after correction of mitral regurgitation: results and clinical implications. J Am Coll Cardiol. 1994:24:1536-43.
12. Haan CK, Cabral CI, Conetta DA, et al. Selecting patients with mitral regurgitation and left ventricular dysfunction for isolated mitral valve surgery. Ann Thorac Surg. 2004;78:820-5.
13. Badhwar V, Peterson ED, Jacobs JP, et al. Longitudinal outcome of isolated mitral repair in older patients: results from 14,604 procedures performed from 1991 to 2007. Ann Thorac Surg. 2012;94:1870-7.
14. Le Tourneau T, Richardson M, Juthier F, et al. Echocardiography predictors and prognostic value of pulmonary artery systolic pressure in chronic organic mitral regurgitation. Heart. 2010;96-1311-7.
15. Erriquez-Sarano M, Tajik AJ. Schaff HV, et al. Echocardiographic prediction of survival after surgical correction of organic mitral regurgitation. Circulation. 1994;90:830-7.
16. Feldmen T, Foster E, Glower DD, et al. Everest II investigators. Percutaneous repair or surgery for mitral regurgitation. N Engl J Med. 2011;364:1395-406.
17. Feldmen T, Kar S, Elmariah S, et al. Everest-II investigators. Randomized comparison of percutaneous repair and surgery for mitral regurgitation; 5-year results of Everest II. J Am Coll Cardiol. 2015;66:2844-54.
18. Acker MA, Parides MK, Perrault LP, et al. Mitral valve repair versus replacement for severe ischemic mitral regurgitation. N Engl J Med. 2014;370:23-32.
19. Nishimma RA, OHO CM, Bonow RA, et al. AHA/ACC guided for the management of patient with valvular heart disease, a report of the ACC (AHA Task force on practice guidelines. J Am Coll Cardiol. 2014;63:e57-187.
20. Mihaljevic T, Lam BK, Rajeswaran J, et al. Impact of mitral valve annuloplasty combined with revascularization in patients with functional ischemic mitral regurgitation. J Am Coll Cardiol. 2007;49:2191-201.
21. Wu AH, Aaronson KD, Bolling SF, et al. Impact of mitral valve annuloplasty or mortality risk in patients with mitral regurgitation and left ventricular systolic dysfunction. J Am Coll Cardiol. 2005;45:381-7.
22. Mauri L, Foster E, Glower DD, et al. Everest II investigator. 4 years results of a randomized controlled trial of percutaneous repair versus surgery for mitral regurgitation. J An Coll Cardiol. 2013;62:317-28.
23. Maisano F, Franzen O, Baldus S, et al. Percutaneous mitral valve interventions in the read world: early and 1 year results from the ACCESS-EU a prospective, multicenter, nonrandomized post-approval study if the MitraClip therapy in Europe. J Am Coll Cardiol. 2013;62:1052-61.

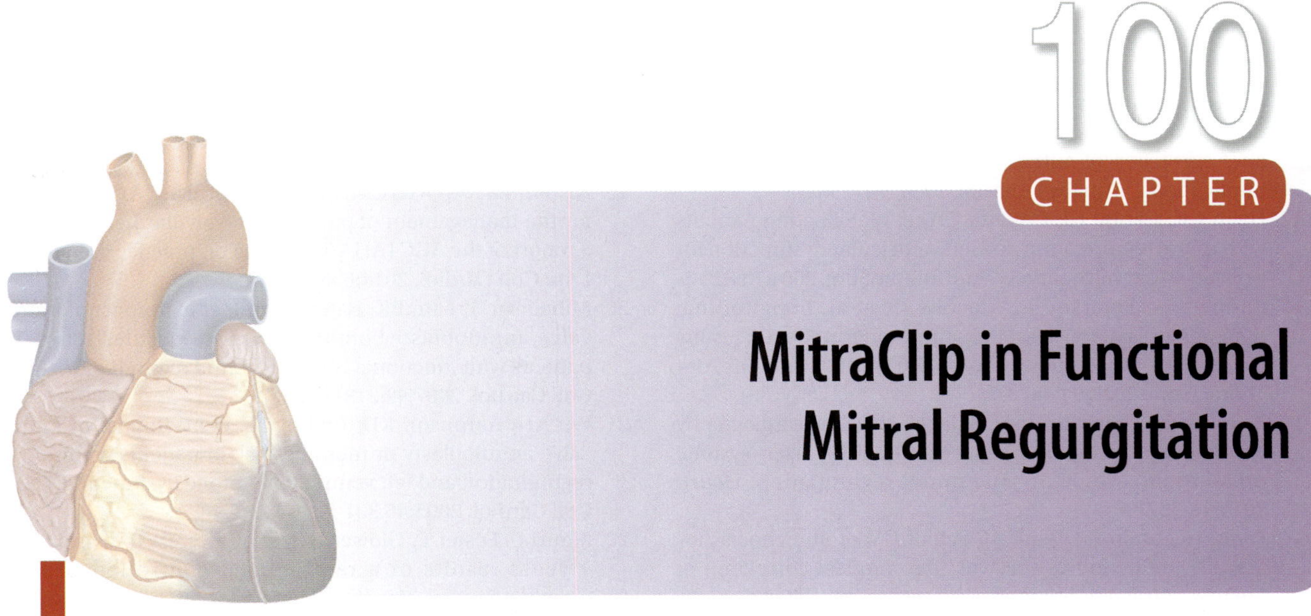

MitraClip in Functional Mitral Regurgitation

Aslaniff Roslan, Jayakhanthan Kolathaivelu, NN Khanna

INTRODUCTION

Mitral valve disease is the second most common valve problem after aortic stenosis.[1] The most common mitral valve disease is mitral regurgitation (MR). MR can be divided into two groups and is classified by leaflet movements, the Carpentier classification (Fig. 1). The first group is primary MR, in which there are abnormalities of the mitral valve leaflets and/or subvalvular apparatus, most commonly degenerative mitral regurgitation (DMR) due to fibroelastin deficiency or myxomatous degeneration (Carpentier 2) and rheumatic mitral valve disease with restricted closure in both systole and diastole (Carpentier 3a). In the initial MitraClip studies, EVEREST (Endovascular Valve Edge-to-Edge Repair Study) and EVEREST 2 trials, most of the patients had DMR.[2] For DMR however, the gold standard treatment is mitral valve repair in which appropriate timing give same survival as age-matched control.[3]

The second group, which is of the majority, is functional mitral regurgitation (FMR) in which the leaflets and subvalvular apparatus is normal. In this group, the most common pathophysiology is dilated left ventricle or regional wall motion abnormalities in which the mitral valve leaflets is tethered and tented due to distortion of papillary muscles placements (Carpentier 3b). This is compounded over time by dilated mitral valve annulus, especially in the posterior direction (Carpentier 1). Usually, however the Carpentier 3b mechanism predominates. The other situation where one can see pure mitral annulus dilatation is in chronic atrial fibrillation, where the left ventricle size and function are normal. This is called atriogenic functional mitral regurgitation (AFMR) and at the moment little is known on how best to approach this entity.[4]

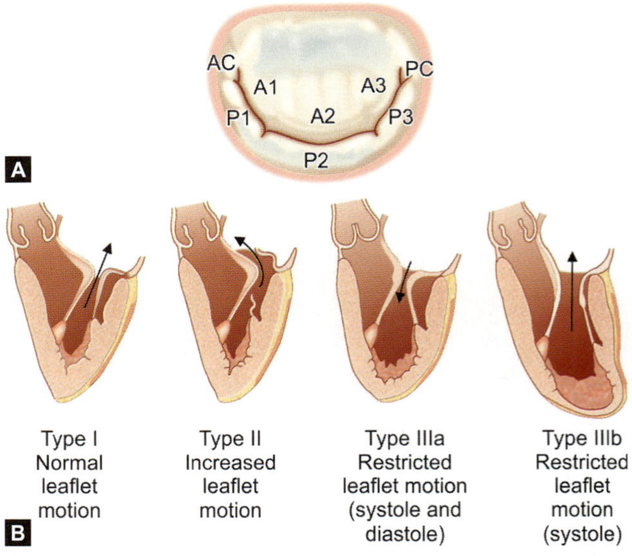

Fig. 1: (A) The middle scallop of the posterior leaflet is designated as P2 and the adjacent lateral and medial segments are P1 and P3. The opposing segments of the anterior leaflet are designated as A1, A2, and A3. AC and PC represent the anterolateral and posteromedial commissures; (B) Leaflet dysfunction (Carpentier type I, type II, and type III) is classified on the basis of motion of the free margin of the leaflet in relation to the annular plane.[5]
(Modified from Carpentier et al., 2010)

Most of FMR is the combination of Type 1 and Type 3b in the Carpentier classification

(Clinical trial design principles and end-point definitions for transcatheter mitral valve repair and replacement: *Part 1: clinical trial design principles: A consensus document from the mitral valve academic research consortium).*

FUNCTIONAL MITRAL REGURGITATION

In FMR, irrespective it is ischemic or nonischemic in etiology, the management is controversial. For those whom revascularization is an option, the best strategy is to attempt revascularization in whichever way deemed more beneficial for the ventricle. If the patient is a surgical candidate, the latest study has shown that the intervention is only indicated for severe MR and replacement is favorable if the patients have predominant tenting and tethering of leaflets as this approach have lower recurrence of MR, better left ventricle remodeling, although there is no overall mortality benefit.[6] This dilemma and the uncertainty of outcomes with surgical correction put MitraClip under a spotlight. The hope of solving this problem for patient with severe MR without any revascularization options.

The MitraClip

The MitraClip procedure (Abbott Vascular, Santa Clara, CA) was introduced in 2003. As of July 2017, more than 50,000 patients have been treated worldwide.[7] MitraClip is a percutaneous procedure done via femoral vein access and transseptal punctures. The MitraClip system consists of a steerable guide catheter and a clip delivery system (CDS), which includes the clip attached at the end of the CDS. The guide catheter is 24 French proximally, and tapers to 22 French at the point where it crosses the interatrial septum. Leaflet tissue is secured between the clip arms and opposing grippers. The clip arms are then closed to 0°, then locked to effect and maintain coaptation of the two leaflets (Fig. 2).[1]

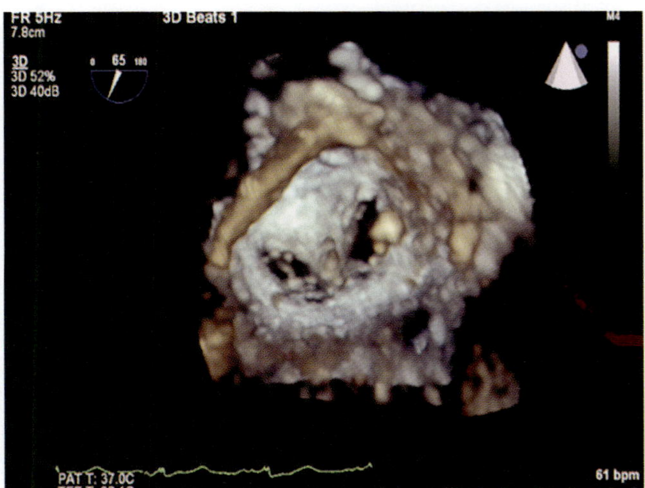

Fig. 2: 3D-echocardiogram shows en face view of the mitral valve with MitraClip positioned at A2-P2 segment.
Source: Image from Roslan et al. Butterfly in the heart, infective endocarditis after MitraClip procedure.[8]

Study has shown that the degree of FMR correlates directly with survival.[9] MitraClip mimics the surgical Alfieri procedure in which the clip mimic the stitching bringing together part of the anterior and posterior mitral valve leaflet, leaving two orifices if only single clip is used.

Outcome of MitraClip in Functional Mitral Regurgitation

In 2018, two landmark trials with opposing results were presented a month apart. The first; Percutaneous Repair or Medical Treatment for Secondary Mitral Regurgitation (MITRA-FR) was a negative study. The primary end-points in MITRA-FR which is rehospitalization from heart failure and all-cause mortality in 1 year were not achieved. There were numerically greater hospitalization and all-cause mortality in the intervention group even though this was statistically not significant.[10] The second; transcatheter Mitral-Valve Repair in Patients with Heart Failure (COAPT) trial however showed significantly positive results in the primary end-points; hospitalization for heart failure at 2 years and even more interestingly all-cause mortality benefit at the end of 2 years.[12] The question was how come two trials with the same intervention have very different outcomes?

When we looks at the detail of these trials, the two most important differences are the degree of MR and how dilated the left ventricle was. In the MITRA-FR study, the average effective regurgitant orifice area (EROA) is 0.30 cm^2 and in COAPT trial the average EROA is 0.4 cm^2. This means that the MR severity is more in COAPT trial. Second, the left ventricle in the MITRA-FR study is bigger [left ventricular (LV) end diastolic volume index, average 135 mL/m^2 for MITRA-FR and average of 101 mL/m^2 for COAPT] suggesting more advance left ventricle disease.[11] In essence, patients in COAPT trial have more severe MR and less sick left ventricle compare to those in MITRA-FR trial (Fig. 3). The other way to look at this is that patients in MITRA-FR trial have sicker ventricles and the MR is likely a bystander; not contributing to the LV dysfunction. On the other hand, patients in COAPT trial the LV dysfunction contributed to the MR which worsened the LV function. That means there is more contribution from the MR to the LV dysfunction. Hence, these population of patients fair better with MitraClip.[11] The other important difference is the fact that all patients in COAPT trial is already on maximally tolerated heart failure medications including

	MITRA-FR	COAPT
Baseline clinical characteristics		
Age, year	70±10	72±11
NYHA class, %		
I	0	0.2
II	32.9	39.0
III	58.5	52.5
IV	8.6	8.3
Surgical risk		
STS score ≥8%		42.7%
EuroSCORE II, median and IQR		6.2 (3.5–11.0)
Baseline echocardiographic characteristics		
MR severity, %		
Moderate (EROA 20–29 mm^2)	52	14
Moderate-to-severe (EROA 30–39 mm^2)	32	46
Severe (EORA ≥ 40 mm^2)	16	41
EROA, mm^2	31 ± 10	41 ± 15
LV end-diastolic volume index, mL/m^2	135 ± 35	101 ± 34
LV ejection fraction, %	33 ± 7	31 ± 9

Fig. 3: Similarities and differences between MITRA-FR and COAPT with respect to baseline characteristics of the study population.[11]

(MITRA-FR: percutaneous repair or medical treatment for secondary mitral regurgitation; COAPT: mitral-valve repair in patients with heart failure; NYHA: New York heart association; STS: Society of Thoracic Surgeons; MR: mitral regurgitation; EROA: effective regurgitant orifice area; LV: left ventricular; IQR: interquartile range)

cardiac resynchronization therapy if needed, and there were much less changes in medications during and after the intervention. The COAPT trial also had double the number of patients of MITRA-FR with longer follow-up looking at 2 years outcome and much closer involvement of heart failure consultants.[13]

So what does these trials mean for our patient selection? The most suitable candidates from these two trials at least are those with severe MR, LV end systolic dimension that is less than 7 cm and patients who are still symptomatic despite maximal tolerated goal-directed medical therapy. These patients must be carefully selected with the involvement of Heart team discussion (Fig. 4).[11,13]

CONCLUSION

The explosion of percutaneous transcatheter valve intervention, led by the immense success of transcatheter aortic valve implantation (TAVI) herald the new era of valvular intervention. Surprisingly mitral valve intervention has lagged behind aortic valve intervention due to the complexity of the leaflets, the dynamic saddle-shaped annulus, and the difficulty of delivering bulky device trans-septally. However, with the MitraClip we have a new armamentarium in dealing with the complex FMR. The COAPT trial has brought optimism for this approach and we wait with bated breath for the outcome of RESHAPE-HF2 trial.

REFERENCES

1. Alegria-Barrero E, Franzen OW. Mitral regurgitation-A multidisciplinary challenge. ECR Cardiol. 2014;9(1):49-53.
2. Feldman T, Kar S, Rinaldi M, et al. Percutaneous mitral repair with the MitraClip system: safety and midterm durability in the initial EVEREST (Endovascular Valve Edge-to-Edge REpair Study) cohort. J Am Coll Cardiol. 2009;54(8):686-94.
3. McNeely CA, Vassileva CM. Long-term outcomes of mitral valve repair versus replacement for degenerative disease: A systematic review. Curr Cardiol Rev. 2015;11(2): 157-62.

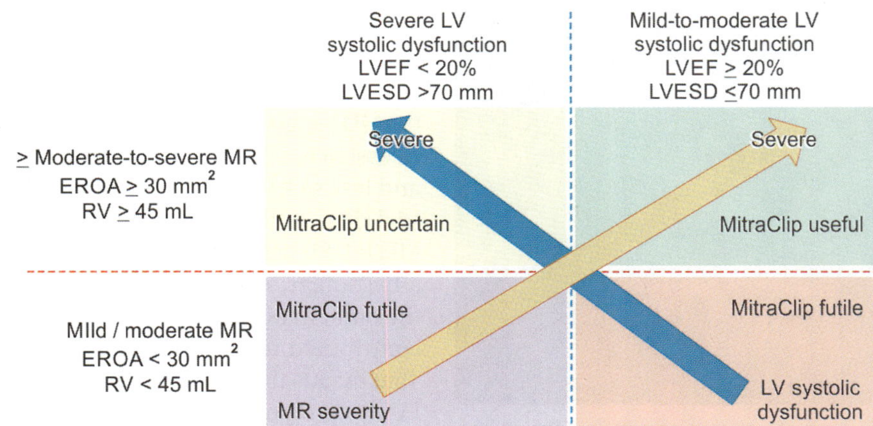

Fig. 4: Utility vs futility of MitraClip procedure according to severity of MR and LV systolic dysfunction.[11]

(LV: left ventricular; MR: mitral regurgitation; LVEF: left ventricular ejection fraction; LVESD: left ventricular end-systolic dimension; EROA: effective regurgitant orifice area)

4. Deferm S, Bertrand PB, Verbrugge FH, et al. Atrial Functional Mitral Regurgitation JACC Review Topic of the Week. J Am Coll Cardiol. 2019;73(19):2465-76.
5. Carpentier A, Adams DH, Filsoufi F. Carpentier's reconstructive valve surgery. From valve analysis to valve reconstruction. Philadelphia, US: Saunders, Elsevier, 2010.
6. Acker MA, Parides MK, Perrault LP, et al. Mitral-valve repair versus replacement for severe ischemic mitral regurgitation. N Engl J Med. 2014;370:23-32.
7. Abbott Vascular. TMVr with MitraClip therapy: clinical experience. [online] Available from: http://mitraclip.com/hcp/tmvr_mitraclip_therapy/clinical_experience. [Last accessed November, 2019]
8. Roslan A, Kamsani SH, Aktifanus ATJ, et al. Butterfly in the heart, Infective Endocarditis after MitraClip procedure. CASE. 2018;2(2):63-5.
9. Ciarka A, Van de Veire N. Secondary mitral regurgitation: pathophysiology, diagnosis, and treatment. BMJ Heart. 2011;97(12):1012-23.
10. Obadia JF, Messika-Zeitoun D, Leurent G, et al. Percutaneous Repair or Medical Treatment for Secondary Mitral Regurgitation. N Engl J Med. 2018;379(24):2297-306.
11. Pibarot P, Delgado V, Bax JJ. MITRA-FR vs. COAPT: lessons from two trials with diametrically opposed results. European Heart J Cardiovasc Imaging. 2019;20(6):620-4.
12. Stone GW, Lindenfeld J, Abraham WT, et al. Transcatheter mitral-valve repair in patients with heart failure. N Engl J Med. 2018;379(24):2307-18.
13. Atianzar K, Zhang M, Newhart Z, et al. Why Did COAPT Win While MITRA-FR Failed? Defining the Appropriate Patient Population for MitraClip. Interv Cardiol. 2019;14(1):45-7.

Tricuspid Regurgitation and Heart Failure

Aniruddha De

INTRODUCTION

About 1.6 million Americans have moderate to severe tricuspid regurgitation (TR), but less than 8,000 tricuspid valve (TV) operations are performed annually in the USA. The etiology of TR is due to either primary or secondary causes. Primary TR was usually observed in patients with congenital heart disease and seldom found in adults. Secondary TR is mainly associated with left-sided valvular or myocardial disease and pulmonary hypertension (PH). However, there is a subgroup of adult patients without any congenital anomalies, PH or left-sided heart disease who develop symptomatic isolated TR. High mortality and morbidity are often associated with heart failure throughout the world.[1] Moderate to severe TR is always associated with high mortality when compared to trivial or mild TR.[2] Higher incidence of heart failure and worst survival was often observed in patients with more than moderate TR.[3] It has been observed that TR severity is considered as an independent factor for long-term survival.[4] Even, isolated TR is found to be associated with increased mortality and morbidity.[5] Moderate to severe TR was found to be associated with high mortality which is independent of systolic pulmonary artery pressure (sPAP) and left ventricular (LV) ejection fraction though sPAP is considered as an indicator of TR severity by echocardiographic parameter.[4,6-8] Hence, severity of TR, may play crucial roles in predicting outcome of patients with heart failure and significant TR.

ECHOCARDIOGRAPHIC EXAMINATION

The following echocardiographic examination is essential for evaluating the association between TR and heart failure:

- Evaluation of left atrial (LA) size
- Left ventricular geometry and function.
- Right heart dimensions:
  - Right ventricular (RV) basal and mid-diameter at end diastole
  - Right atrial (RA) area at end systole and diastole
  - Right atrial volume (minimum and maximum) from RV focused view
  - Right ventricular free wall thickness at end-diastole from the subcostal view.
- Right ventricular function:
  - Tricuspid annular plane systolic excursion (TAPSE)
  - Right ventricular fractional area change (FAC).
- Right atrial function:
  - Right atrial emptying volume
  - Right atrial emptying fraction.
- Systolic pulmonary artery pressure and right atrial pressure (RAP):
  - Systolic pulmonary artery pressure was obtained from peak TR jet velocity with an estimated RAP
  - Right atrial pressure was estimated from diameter of inferior vena cava (IVC) and inspiratory collapsibility.
- Tricuspid regurgitation was measured by vena contracta which is the narrowest portion of the TR jet from the apical four-chamber view.
- Right ventricular free wall longitudinal strain (LS).

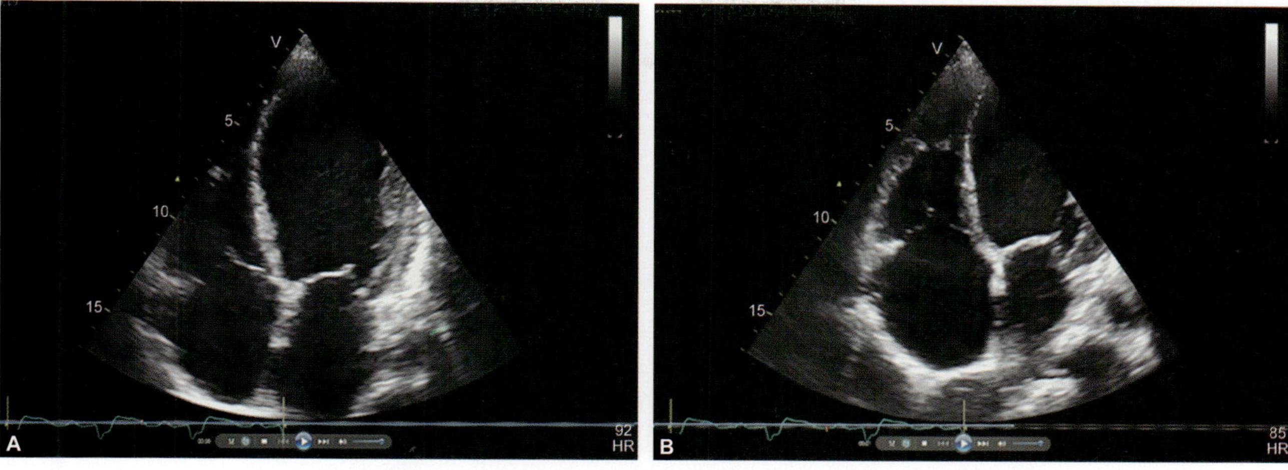

Figs. 1A and B: Left ventricular dysfunction and enlarged right atrium.

OBSERVATION

The following observations were found from different studies where heart failure is associated with TR:

- Increased mortality was observed in patients with heart failure and moderate to severe TR with large atrial size.
- Right ventricular dysfunction and failure often correlated well with the survival for any cardiovascular disease, whereas RA size reflects the magnitude of RV dysfunction.[9,10]
- Prognosis in patients with PH, heart failure with both preserved and reduced ejection fraction can be predicted by the TAPSE which reflects RV function.[11-13]
- Functional TR is the most common cause of TR and is often secondary to left-sided heart diseases. Significant late morbidity and mortality are often observed if simultaneous repair of TR is not done while correcting the left-sided lesion. As a result, these patients develop progressive RV dysfunction and need for second operation with high mortality.[14]
- Right ventricular longitudinal function can also be assessed by RV LS and speckle tracking echocardiography and provide valuable information in patients with heart failure.[15,16]
- Advanced LV dysfunction, chronic obstructive pulmonary disease (COPD), and pulmonary emboli can lead to increased RV pressures in heart failure patients (Figs. 1A and B).[17]
- Increased RV systolic pressures will cause more TR and maintaining a vicious circle. As a result, RV failure will develop due to increased pressure and volume overload and worsening RV performance.
- Severe TR may develop in any valvular or myocardial disease (Figs. 2A and B). The severe regurgitation

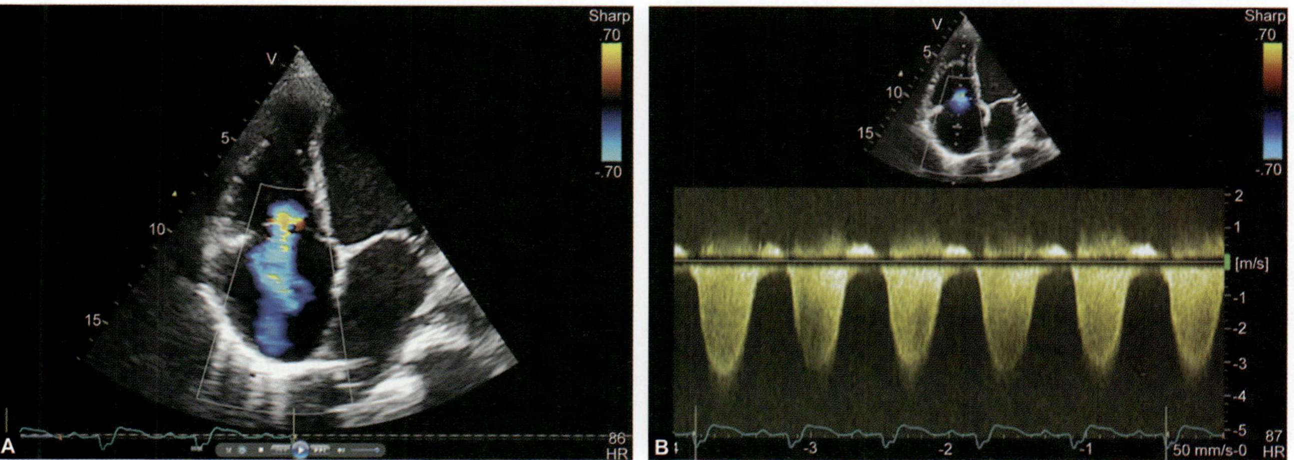

Figs. 2A and B: Moderate to severe tricuspid regurgitation pulmonary hypertension.

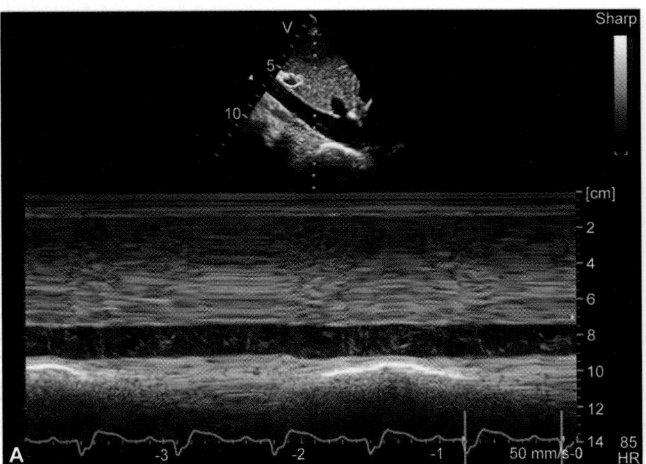

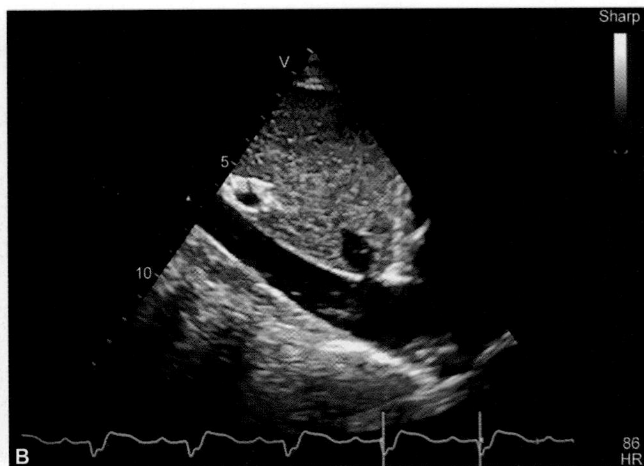

Figs. 3A and B: Dilated inferior vena cava with little respiratory variation.

toward the RA due to incompetent valve can lead to RA dilatation. As a result, RV volume overload increased by the large regurgitant volume and venous return flow. However, mild or moderate TR may not lead to significant hemodynamic disturbances as the right atrium is much compliant. But RA and RV end-diastolic pressure rise due to high volume overload associated with severe TR and often leads to right-sided heart failure.[18] This suggests that progressive TR volume plays a key role in the disease progression in heart failure patients complicated by significant TR.

- A significantly reduced pulmonary artery systolic pressure should be treated as an ominous sign of worsening RV performance which in turn increased mortality in heart failure patients with severe TR.
- Echocardiographic TR predicted event-free survival in patients with severe heart failure referred for cardiac transplant evaluation. Echocardiographic TR is a reliable marker of RV systolic dysfunction and strongly associated with features of RV dysfunction, namely, RV dilation, RV hypokinesia, and lower percentage of RV systolic area change.[19]
- Patients with severe MR or TR represent high-risk subsets of patients with left ventricular systolic dysfunction (LVSD). Future study is warranted to determine whether pharmaceutical or surgical strategies to relieve MR and TR have a favorable impact on survival.[20]
- Tricuspid regurgitation severity is associated with worse survival in patients regardless of left ventricular ejection fraction (LVEF) or pulmonary artery pressure. Severe TR is associated with a poor prognosis, independent of age, biventricular systolic function, RV size, and IVC dilation.[21]

PRESENTATION

The presentation of isolated TR is as follows:

- Elevated central venous pressure with systolic pulsation indicating a high RA pressure and large C-V wave.
- Features of right heart failure (neck fullness, hepatomegaly, edema, and ascites).
- Low cardiac output (fatigue).
- Exertional dyspnea due to increased ventricular interaction with the dilated RV causing reduced compliance of the left ventricle.
- Hepatic and renal failure may develop due to venous congestion and persistent low perfusion pressure.
- Isolated severe TR may present with features of right heart failure despite normal LV function, normal left-sided cardiac valves, and normal pulmonary arterial pressures.

Similar findings may be seen in constrictive pericarditis and restrictive cardiomyopathy and should be considered in the differential diagnosis.

CLINICAL UTILITY

Left ventricular morphology and function by echocardiography was always the focus of attention in heart failure patients. Systolic and diastolic LV function are routinely assessed for any clinical decisions and prognosis for heart failure patients. Whereas, routine use of RA/RV morphology and function estimation are not done in all patients with heart failure.

A RA area ≥27 cm^2 at baseline, a dynamic increase in TR volume ≥15 mL, a dynamic increase of RV dilatation ≥10 mm, and a dynamic reduction in sPAP ≥10 mm Hg are indicators of worse outcome for heart failure patients with moderate/severe functional TR. A particularly dramatic impairment of short-term survival is related to the accumulation of two or more of these echocardiographic parameters.[14]

Management of majority of patients with symptomatic TR can be done by diuretics and treatment of underlying disease process by reducing volume overload. It is still not known whether diuretics alter the disease progression or temporary giving symptomatic relief in patients with primary valvular heart disease. Hence, TV surgery is considered as definitive therapy for severe symptomatic TR.

Tricuspid valve replacement for severe TR can be performed with an acceptable operative mortality if patients undergo surgery before the onset of advanced heart failure symptoms. Late mortality is associated with a high preoperative Charlson index, short right index of myocardial performance ratio, and advanced New York Heart Association class.[22]

Tricuspid regurgitation due to primary abnormalities of the tricuspid leaflets is extremely rare. In majority of cases it is "functional" in nature and is due to geometric alterations caused by dilatation of right ventricle.[23,24] Significant functional TR usually found in association with left-sided heart disease, which often dominates the clinical symptoms. As a result, a vicious cycle is established which causes further RV dilatation and dysfunction. Hence, worsening of TR is due to more annular dilatation, displacement of papillary muscles, and leaflet tethering of TV.

Important parameters for the persistence of TR after mitral valve repair are severity of leaflet tethering and the diameter of tricuspid annulus. Geometry, size, function of both ventricle, and pulmonary artery pressures are other important parameters should be considered carefully in evaluating patients who should undergo tricuspid valve surgery. Three-dimensional (3D) echocardiography can give valuable information of TV apparatus before undertaking surgery of a leaking TV whether it can be successfully repaired or not. However, long-term prospective studies are required to confirm the predictive value of such parameters.

As per current guidelines,[25,26] surgical correction of functional severe TR should be considered in symptomatic patients during left-sided valve surgery. Surgery of TV can be done in mild or moderate TR if it is associated with annular dilatation. However, high incidence of perioperative mortality, residual and recurrent TR after surgical correction is observed in several studies.[27-29]

It has also been observed that the incidence of isolated TR is increased with the rising prevalence of atrial fibrillation (AF) and intracardiac devices.[30-32] However, existing guidelines fail to address the correct management and definite therapies. Intracardiac leads can entangle the subvulvar apparatus, adhere, impinge, and even perforate the leaflets (Flowcharts 1 and 2).

CONCLUSION

Echocardiographic evaluation of severity of TR has prognostic and therapeutic implications in heart failure with preserved ejection fraction (HFpEF) and heart failure with reduced ejection fraction (HFrEF). Echo-guided therapeutic intervention is therefore need of the hour to stratify the clinical implications in reducing the cardiac mortality.

Flowchart 1: The etiology of tricuspid regurgitation can be divided according to the presence or absence of organic valvular disease. Patients with isolated primary or secondary tricuspid regurgitation (highlighted in the yellow boxes) represent an emerging patient population about whom little is known.[33]

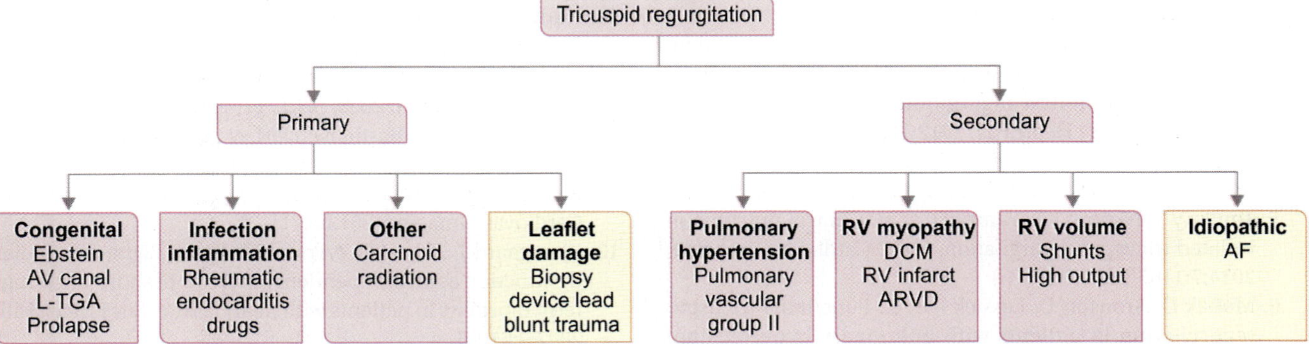

(AF: atrial fibrillation; ARVD: arrhythmogenic right ventricular dysplasia; AV: aortic valve; DCM: dilated cardiomyopathy; L–TGA: L-transposition of the great arteries; RV: right ventricle)

Flowchart 2: Algorithm for the management of severe isolated tricuspid regurgitation.[33]

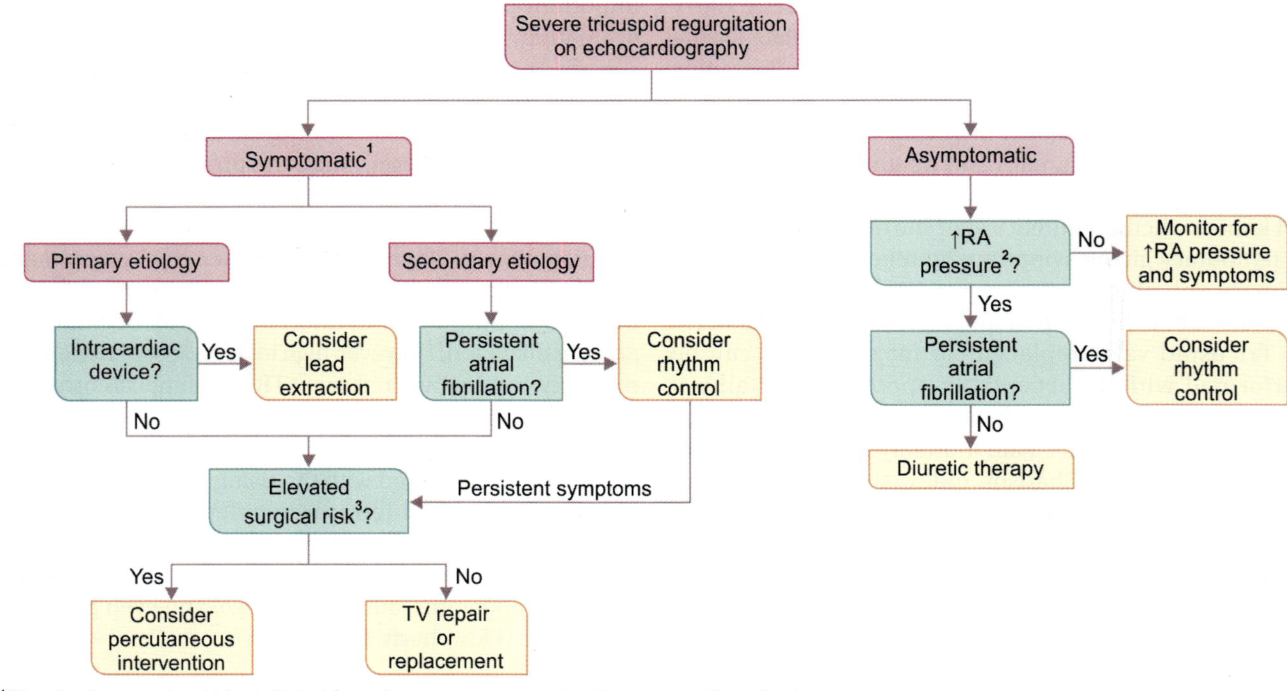

[1]Diuretic therapy should be initiated for volume management in all symptomatic patients.
[2]Right atrial pressure assessed by physical examination (markedly elevated and pulsatile venous pressure), echocardiogram, or hemodynamic catheterization.
[3]Surgical risk determined by degree of right ventricular dysfunction and comorbidities.
(RA: right atrium; TV: tricuspid valve)

REFERENCES

1. Hobbs FD, Roalfe AK, Davis RC, et al. Prognosis of all-cause heart failure and borderline left ventricular systolic dysfunction: 5 year mortality follow-up of the Echocardiographic Heart of England Screening Study (ECHOES). Eur Heart J. 2007;28:1128-34.
2. Agricola E, Marini C, Stella S, et al. Effects of functional tricuspid regurgitation on renal function and long-term prognosis in patients with heart failure. J Cardiovasc Med (Hagerstown). 2017;18(2):60-8.
3. Agricola E, Stella S, Gullace M, et al. Impact of functional tricuspid regurgitation on heart failure and death in patients with functional mitral regurgitation and left ventricular dysfunction. Eur J Heart Fail. 2012;14:902-8.
4. Nath J, Foster E, Heidenreich PA. Impact of tricuspid regurgitation on long-term survival. J Am Coll Cardiol. 2004;43:405-9.
5. Topilsky Y, Nkomo VT, Vatury O, et al. Clinical outcome of isolated tricuspid regurgitation. JACC Cardiovasc Imaging. 2014;7:1185-94.
6. Mutlak D, Aronson D, Lessick J, et al. Functional tricuspid regurgitation in patients with pulmonary hypertension: is pulmonary artery pressure the only determinant of regurgitation severity? Chest. 2009;135:115-21.
7. Berger M, Haimowitz A, Van Tosh A, et al. Quantitative assessment of pulmonary hypertension in patients with tricuspid regurgitation using continuous wave Doppler ultrasound. J Am Coll Cardiol. 1985;6:359-65.
8. Ghio S, Gavazzi A, Campana C, et al. Independent and additive prognostic value of right ventricular systolic function and pulmonary artery pressure in patients with chronic heart failure. J Am Coll Cardiol. 2001;37:183-8.
9. Raymond RJ, Hinderliter AL, Willis PW, et al. Echocardiographic predictors of adverse outcomes in primary pulmonary hypertension. J Am Coll Cardiol. 2002;39:1214-9.
10. Haddad F, Doyle R, Murphy DJ, et al. Right ventricular function in cardiovascular disease, part II: pathophysiology, clinical importance, and management of right ventricular failure. Circulation. 2008;117:1717-31.
11. Fine NM, Chen L, Bastiansen PM, et al. Outcome prediction by quantitative right ventricular function assessment in 575 subjects evaluated for pulmonary hypertension. Circ Cardiovasc Imaging. 2013;6:711-21.
12. Kjaergaard J, Akkan D, Iversen KK, et al. Right ventricular dysfunction as an independent predictor of short- and long-term mortality in patients with heart failure. Eur J Heart Fail. 2007;9:610-6.
13. Mohammed SF, Hussain I, AbouEzzeddine OF, et al. Right ventricular function in heart failure with preserved ejection fraction: a community-based study. Circulation. 2014;130:2310-20.

14. Wang N, Fulcher J, Abeysuriya N, et al. Tricuspid regurgitation is associated with increased mortality independent of pulmonary pressures and right heart failure: a systematic review and meta-analysis. Eur Heart J. 2019;40(5):485-7.
15. Cameli M, Lisi M, Righini FM, et al. Right ventricular longitudinal strain correlates well with right ventricular stroke work index in patients with advanced heart failure referred for heart transplantation. J Card Fail. 2012;18:208-15.
16. Motoki H, Borowski AG, Shrestha K, et al. Right ventricular global longitudinal strain provides prognostic value incremental to left ventricular ejection fraction in patients with heart failure. J Am Soc Echocardiogr. 2014;27:726-32.
17. Oakley C. Importance of right ventricular function in congestive heart failure. Am J Cardiol. 1988;62:14A-9A.
18. Rao S, Tate DA, Stouffer GA. Hemodynamic findings in severe tricuspid regurgitation. Catheter Cardiovasc Interv. 2012;81:162-9.
19. Hung J, Koelling T, Semigran MJ, et al. Usefulness of echocardiographic determined tricuspid regurgitation in predicting event-free survival in severe heart failure secondary to idiopathic-dilated cardiomyopathy or to ischemic cardiomyopathy. Am J Cardiol. 1998;82(10): 1301-3, A10.
20. Koelling TM, Aaronson KD, Cody RJ, et al. Prognostic significance of mitral regurgitation and tricuspid regurgitation in patients with left ventricular systolic dysfunction. Am Heart J. 2002;144(3):524-9.
21. Nath J, Foster E, Heidenreich PA. Impact of tricuspid regurgitation on long-term survival. J Am Coll Cardiol. 2004; 43(3):405-9.
22. Topilsky Y, Khanna AD, Oh JK, et al. Preoperative Factors Associated With Adverse Outcome After Tricuspid Valve Replacement. Circulation. 2011;123:1929-39.
23. Kim H-K, Kim Y-J, Park J-S, et al. Determinants of the severity of functional ricuspid regurgitation. Am J Cardiol. 2006;98:236–242.
24. Fukuda S, Gillinov AM, Song J-M, et al. Echocardiographic insights into atrial and ventricular mechanisms of functional tricuspid regurgitation. Am Heart J. 2006;152:1208-14.
25. Vahanian A, Alfieri O, Andreotti F, et al.; Joint Task Force on the Management of Valvular Heart Disease of the European Society of Cardiology (ESC); European Association for Cardio-Thoracic Surgery (EACTS). Eur Heart J. 2012;33: 2451-96.
26. Bonow RO, Carabello BA, Chatterjee K, et al. 2008 Focused update incorporated into the ACC/AHA 2006 guidelines for the management of patients with valvular heart disease: a report of the American College of Cardiology/American Heart Association Task Force on Practice Guidelines (Writing Committee to Revise the 1998 Guidelines for the Management of Patients With Valvular Heart Disease): endorsed by the Society of Cardiovascular Anesthesiologists, Society for Cardiovascular Angiography and Interventions, and Society of Thoracic Surgeons. Circulation. 2008;118: e523-661.
27. Topilsky Y, Khanna AD, Oh JK, et al. Preoperative factors associated with adverse outcome after tricuspid valve replacement/clinical perspective. Circulation. 2011;123: 1929-39.
28. McCarthy PM, Bhudia SK, Rajeswaran J, et al. Tricuspid valve repair: durability and risk factors for failure. J Thorac Cardiovasc Surg. 2004;127:674-85.
29. Raja SG, Dreyfus GD. Surgery for functional tricuspid regurgitation: current techniques, outcomes and emerging concepts. Expert Rev Cardiovasc Ther. 2009;7:73-84
30. Nath J, Foster E, Heidenreich PA. Impact of tricuspid regurgitation on long-term survival. J Am Coll Cardiol. 2004;43:405-9.
31. Topilsky Y, Nkomo VT, Vatury O, et al. Clinical outcome of isolated tricuspid regurgitation. JACC Cardiovasc Imaging. 2014;7:1185-94.
32. Paniagua D, Aldrich HR, Lieberman EH, et al. Increased prevalence of significant tricuspid regurgitation in patients with transvenous pacemakers leads. Am J Cardiol. 1998;82:1130-2.
33. Fender EA, Zack CJ, Nishimura RA. Isolated tricuspid regurgitation: outcomes and therapeutic interventions. Heart. 2017;104(10):heartjnl-2017-311586.

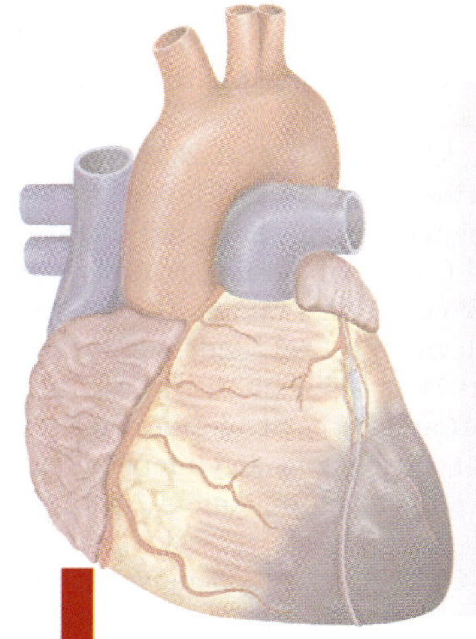

Pulmonary Hypertension and Heart Failure

Ashish Jaikishan, Amit K Gupta, Sameer Srivastava

INTRODUCTION

Pulmonary hypertension (PH) defines a group of clinical conditions presenting with abnormal elevation in the pulmonary circulation pressure.[1,2] The normal mean pulmonary artery pressure (mPAP) at rest is 143.3 mm Hg, and the upper limit of normal is 20.6 mm Hg.[3] Nevertheless, PH is defined as an increase of mPAP ≥25 mm Hg at rest, as assessed by right heart catheterization (RHC). PH was previously classified into two categories: (1) primary PH; or (2) secondary PH according to presence of identified causes or risk factors. Since second World Symposium on PH held in Evian, in 1998, a clinical classification was established in order to individualize different categories of PH sharing similar pathological findings, similar hemodynamic characteristics, and similar management. Five groups of disorders that cause PH were identified: pulmonary arterial hypertension (PAH) (Group 1); PH due to left heart disease (Group 2); PH due to chronic lung disease and/or hypoxia (Group 3); chronic thromboembolic PH (Group 4); and PH due to unclear multifactorial mechanisms (Group 5).

PULMONARY HYPERTENSION DUE TO LEFT HEART FAILURE

This group belongs to group 2 of PAH classification. Among the various PH groups, PH associated with left heart failure (HF) represents the most common form of PH, accounting for 65–80% of all PH cases.[4] In comparison to PAH, patients with pulmonary hypertension due to left heart disease (PH-LHD) are more often older, female, having systemic hypertension and most, if not all, of the features of the metabolic syndrome. PH is due to elevated filling pressures of the left heart chambers which are transmitted backward to the pulmonary circulation. Pulmonary vascular resistance (PVR) is usually normal (<3 woods unit), along with the gradient between mPAP and pulmonary capillary wedge pressure (PCWP) (transpulmonary gradient; <12 mm Hg) and the gradient between diastolic PAP and PCWP [diastolic pressure gradient (DPG); <5–7 mm Hg]. However, with chronic elevation of left-sided filling pressure, there is activation of neurohormonal mediators as well as neurogenic effects, which may cause excess vasoconstriction with/without vascular remodeling, resulting in "disproportionate" increase of PAP, and thereby elevating transpulmonary pressure gradient (TPG) and PVR, which has been described as "reactive", "out-of-proportion", or "mixed" PH (Fig. 1).

Based on the levels of DPG, there are two types of PH-LHD: "isolated postcapillary PH" [pulmonary arterial wedge pressure (PAWP) >15 mm Hg and diastolic pressure difference (DPD) <7 mm Hg] and "combined postcapillary PH and precapillary PH" (PAWP >15 mm Hg and DPG ≥7 mm Hg). DPD is less dependent of stroke volume and loading conditions, and correlates with pulmonary vascular remodeling in PH-LHD, better than TPG.

In heart failure with reduced ejection fraction (HFrEF), the prevalence of PH as assessed by RHC was reported to be between 40% and 75%, while in heart failure with preserved ejection fraction (HFpEF), recent studies utilizing either

TABLE 1: Prevalence of PH in HF (selected studies).

First author (Ref. #)	*N*	*Type*	*Definition of PH*	*Population*	*EF*	*Percentage of measurable TRV*	*Prevalence of PH*	*Corrected prevalence of PH*
Bursi[7]	1,049	Echo	TTG + RAP ≥35 mm Hg	Epidemiological		91%	79%	72%
Damy[8]	1,380	Echo	TTG ≥35 mm Hg	Hull HF clinic	26% preserved	26%	25%	7%
Lam[6]	244	Echo	TTG + RAP ≥35 mm Hg	Olmsted County HF survey	Only EF ≥50%	83%	83%	69%
Leung[9]	455	Invasive	mPAP ≥25 LVEF 15%	Catheterization laboratory			52%	
Robbins[5]	122	Invasive	mPAP ≥25 PAWP >15	PH reference center	Mixed	NA	23%	20%

(PH: pulmonary hypertension; EF: ejection fraction; TRV: tricuspid valve replacement; TTG: tissue transglutaminase; RAP: right atrial pressure; mPAP: mean pulmonary artery pressure; HF: heart failure; LVEF: left ventricular ejection fraction; PAWP: pulmonary artery wedge pressure)

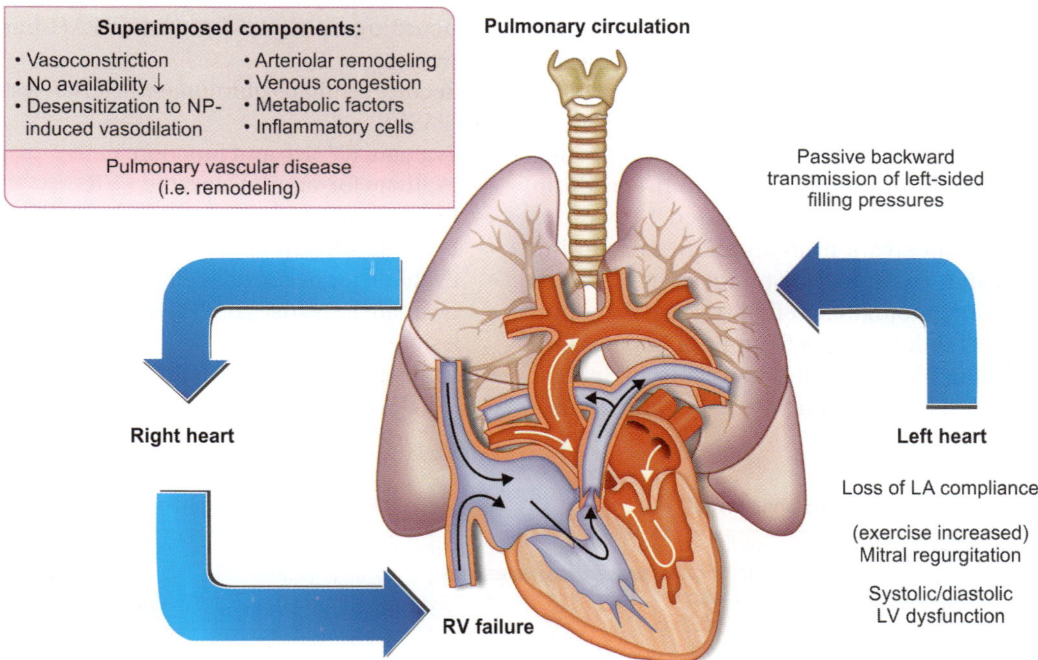

Fig. 1: Pathobiology of PH related to left heart disease.
(PH: pulmonary hypertension; RV: right ventricular; LA: left atrium; LV: left ventricular)

echocardiography or RHC indicated PH prevalence in range between 36% and 83%. Lam et al. in a community-based study found that presence of PAH in patients of HF was strongly associated with mortality. Increased PAWP, mean PAP, and PVR, and a reduced PA compliance/capacitance are predictors of poor survival in HF.

Elevations of pulmonary pressures and PVR represents an increase of both resistive and pulsatile right ventricular (RV) afterload, this in turn causes functional tricuspid regurgitation, dilatation, and maladaptive remodeling of right heart chambers and ultimately results in RV dysfunction and failure.

RIGHT HEART FAILURE DUE TO PULMONARY ARTERIAL HYPERTENSION

When RV afterload is elevated, RV function becomes a major determinant of functional capacity and prognosis, as in WHO group 1 PH (PAH) or congenital heart diseases, such as pulmonic stenosis.[10] Right heart failure (RHF) in presence of left-sided failure is the most common scenario. Right ventricular failure (RVF) in PAH differs from left ventricular failure (LVF) in etiology, prognosis, and therapy. Compared with LVF, PAH-associated RVF:

- Enlarged RV compressing LV—reflecting ventricular interdependence
- Reduced RV perfusion due to microvascular ischemia or decreased coronary artery perfusion pressure
- High and fixed transpulmonary gradient.

In adult PAH patients, there is a high inpatient mortality when there is RV failure requiring inotropic support (≥40%) compared to patients with LVF requiring inotropes (13–14%). Chronic pressure overload that occurs in all categories of PH, stimulates RVH. RVH compensates for increased afterload and maintains cardiac output. However, as time progressed, RV ischemia develops and may result in RV decompensation due to persistently elevated wall stress, thereby leading to RV dysfunction and failure (Fig. 2).

Right ventricular failure reflects inability of the RV to perfuse lung circulation adequately to maintain LV filling at low venous/diastolic pressures. It is characterized by reduced cardiac index (<2.5 L/min per square meter) and increased RV filling pressures [right atrial pressure (RAP) ≥8 mm Hg]. On physical examination, manifest as an elevation in jugular venous pressure (JVP), reflecting elevated RAP, RV lift on palpation of the precordium indicates RV enlargement. A right-sided S-3 sound on auscultation indicates a noncompliant and failing RV. Kussmaul's sign (paradoxical increase in JVP with inspiration) and hepatojugular reflux (rise in JVP upon pressure over liver/abdomen) are features of impaired RV reserve. In addition, RVF frequently results in peripheral edema and hepatic congestion on physical examination.

Due to pulmonary vascular disease, there is elevated afterload which initiates RVH in PAH, it is the decline in RV function [manifested as reduced right ventricular ejection fraction (RVEF) and RV dilatation] that predicts adverse prognosis (Fig. 3). Consistent with this, impaired RVEF predicts clinical worsening in PAH more accurately than elevated PVR.

DIAGNOSTIC EVALUATION OF THE PATIENT WITH SUSPECTED PULMONARY HYPERTENSION

Echocardiography

It can evaluate for the cause of PAH. Checklist for echocardiographic evaluation of PAH has been given below:

- Record estimate pulmonary arterial systolic pressure (PASP)
- Evaluate RV size and function
- Evaluate for signs of elevated PVR
- Estimate volume status
- Evaluate severity of TR
- Evaluate for pericardial effusion
- Evaluate for causes of PH (left heart disease and shunt lesions)
- Differentiate PAH from pulmonary venous hypertension (PVH) (Fig. 4).

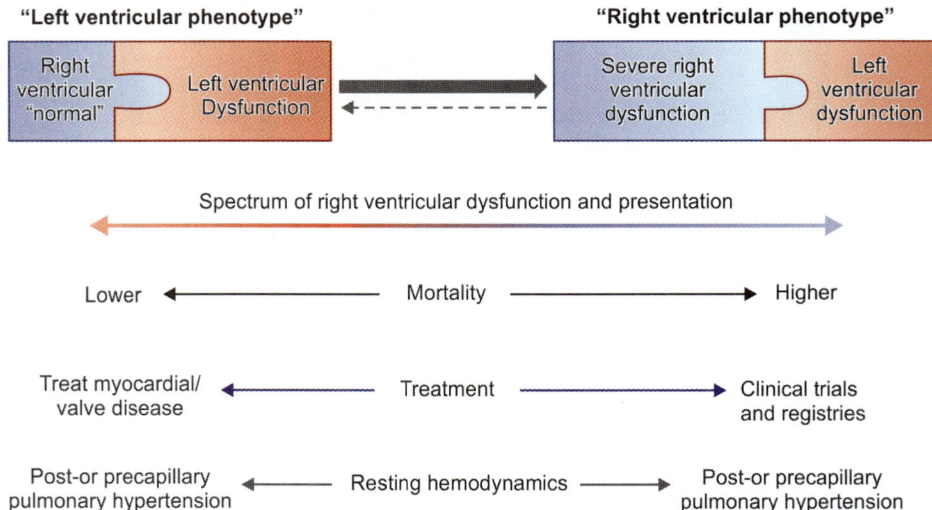

Fig. 2: Left ventricular phenotype versus right ventricular phenotype in pulmonary hypertension associated with left heart disease. Spectrum shows right ventricular dysfunction and presentation, the impact on mortality, therapeutic implications, and resting pulmonary hemodynamics.

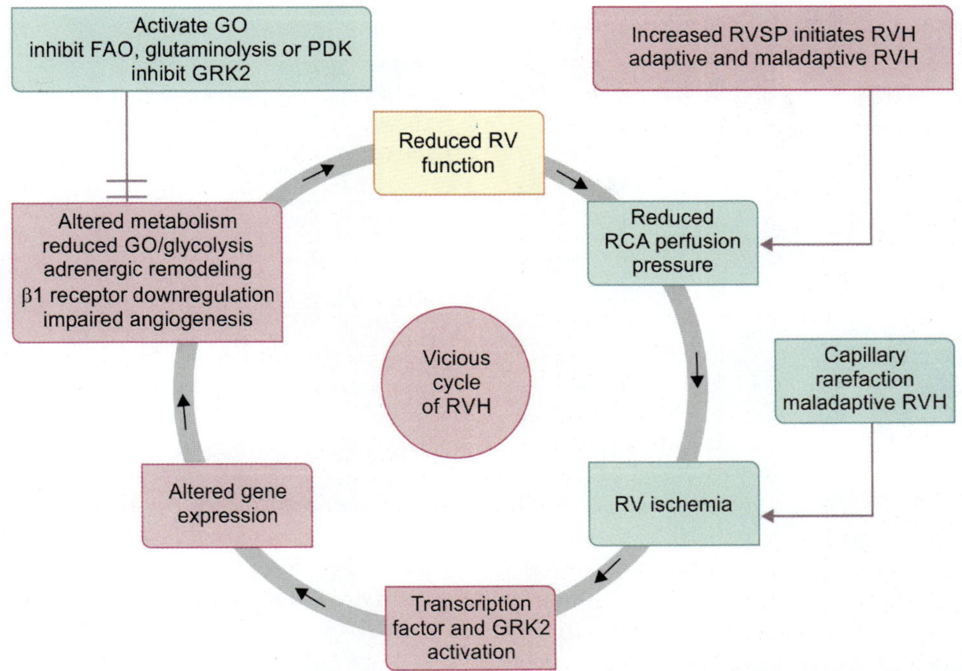

Fig. 3: Pathobiology of right ventricular (RV) failure in pulmonary arterial hypertension. Vicious cycle of RV failure including metabolic changes and RV ischemia.

(FAO: fatty acid oxidation; GO: glucose oxidation; GRK2: G-protein receptor kinase 2; PDK: pyruvate dehydrogenase kinase; RCA: right coronary artery; RVH: right ventricular hypertrophy; RVSP: right ventricular systolic pressure)

Invasive Hemodynamic Testing

Cardiac catheterization is an essential step in the diagnosis of PH, especially PAH, and should be performed prior to the initiation of PAH-specific therapy.

Dynamic Testing During Invasive Hemodynamic Studies

In PAH patients with idiopathic, heritable, or anorexigen-induced PAH, acute pulmonary vasodilator testing is indicated. Most commonly used vasodilator used is inhaled nitric oxide (iNO).

Test is considered to be positive when it includes all of the following: (1) decrease in mPAP to ≤40 mm Hg; (2) decrease of at least 10 mm Hg in mPAP; and (3) unchanged or increased cardiac output.

Calcium channel blocker therapy can be given to patient with positive vasodilator response.[11]

Cardiac Magnetic Resonance Imaging

It provides most accurate noninvasive measurement of RV volumes, mass, and ejection fraction. Gadolinium contrast injection during cardiovascular magnetic resonance (CMR) can be used to evaluate for focal RV fibrosis; patients with PAH often exhibit late gadolinium enhancement at the RV insertion points.

TREATMENT

General Measures

Basic counseling and disease state education is very essential.[12] Low-level graded aerobic exercise such as walking, oxygen supplementation to keep saturation above 90% at rest and with exertion, sleep, or altitude is advisable. Heavy physical exertion and isometric exercise are to be avoided, as this may evoke exertional syncope. A sodium restricted diet is advised and is particularly important to manage volume status in those with RVF. Routine immunizations, such as those against influenza and pneumococcal pneumonia, are advised.

Medical Therapy

Calcium-Channel Blockers

Calcium-channel blockers can be a very effective treatment for those few patients with an acute response to vasodilator testing.

Prostacyclins

Prostacyclin synthase expression is reduced in endothelial cells from PAH patients, resulting in inadequate production of prostaglandin I2 (i.e. prostacyclin), a vasodilator with antiproliferative effects. Commercially available:

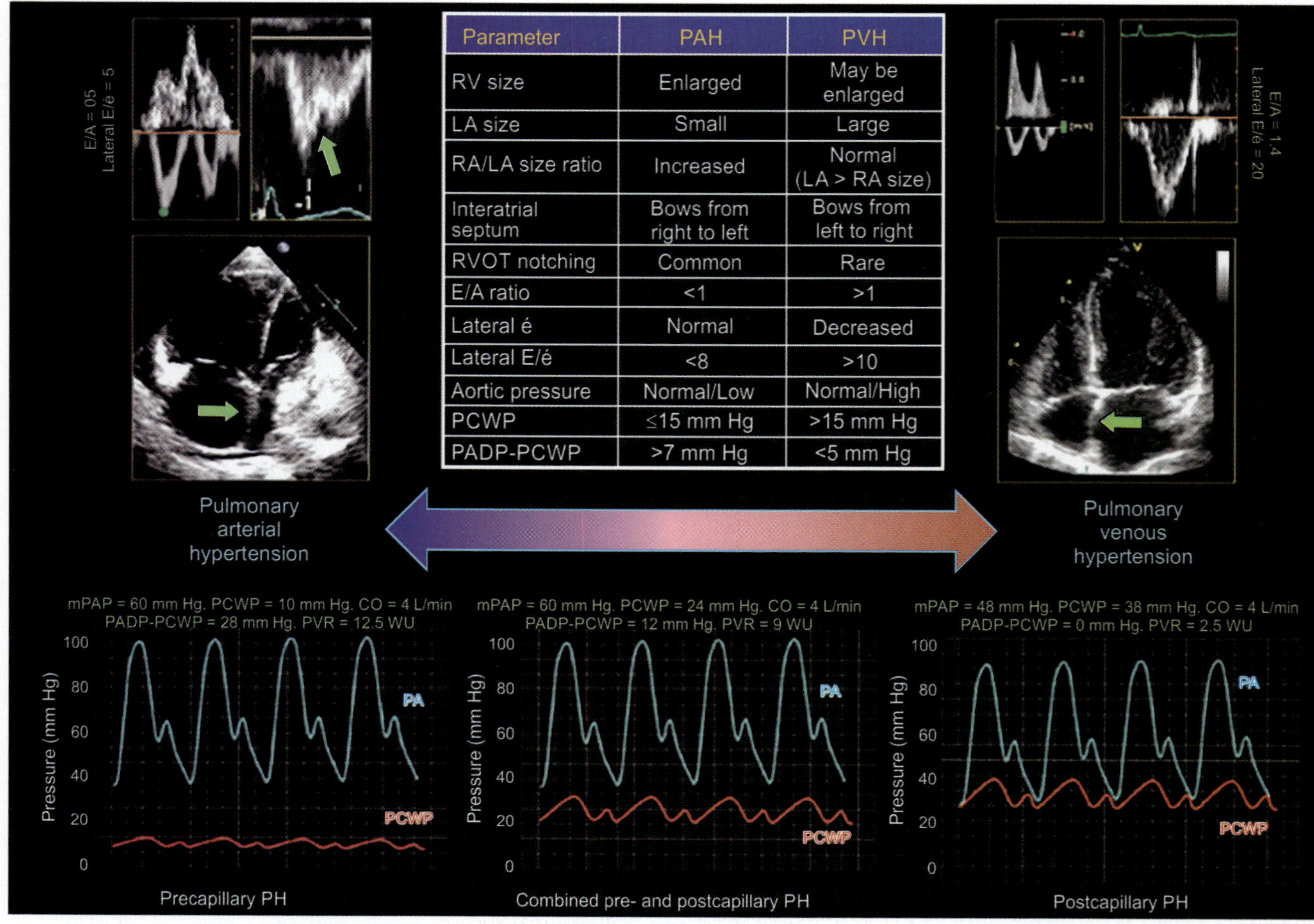

Parameter	PAH	PVH
RV size	Enlarged	May be enlarged
LA size	Small	Large
RA/LA size ratio	Increased	Normal (LA > RA size)
Interatrial septum	Bows from right to left	Bows from left to right
RVOT notching	Common	Rare
E/A ratio	<1	>1
Lateral é	Normal	Decreased
Lateral E/é	<8	>10
Aortic pressure	Normal/Low	Normal/High
PCWP	≤15 mm Hg	>15 mm Hg
PADP-PCWP	>7 mm Hg	<5 mm Hg

Fig. 4: Pulmonary arterial hypertension versus pulmonary venous hypertension: (Echocardiographic and invasive hemodynamic differentiation.)

epoprostenol (continuous IV), treprostinil (continuous subcutaneous, continuous IV, intermittent inhaled, and oral) and iloprost (intermittent inhaled).[13]

Endothelin Receptor Antagonist

Increased tissue expression and increased plasma levels of endothelin-1, a potent vasoconstrictor and stimulator of cell proliferation, have been described in PAH.

Endothelin receptor antagonists are the first class of drugs which are orally administered in PAH. They selectively blocking endothelin-A receptors or by dual blockage of endothelin-A and -B receptors. Bosentan, ambrisentan, and macitentan are commercially available Endothelin antagonists.

Phosphodiesterase Type 5 Inhibitors

Nitric oxide is a potent vasodilator of the pulmonary circulation, acting through the increase in cyclic guanosine monophosphate (cGMP), and cleared mainly as a result of degradation by phosphodiesterase-5 (PDE-5).

Phosphodiesterase-5 inhibitors, which decrease cGMP degradation, and soluble guanylate cyclase stimulators, which increase cGMP and NO production, e.g. sildenafil and tadalafil.

Soluble guanylate cyclase stimulators. Riociguat is a first-in-class soluble guanylate cyclase stimulator. It directly stimulates soluble guanylate cyclase independent of NO, and increases the cGMP levels.

Lung Transplantation and Bridge to Transplantation with Extracorporeal Life Support

Patient refractory to drug therapy can be referred for lung transplant. Transplant referral should occur before the patient develops severe RV failure and that eligible patients should be counseled about lung transplant early in their diagnosis. Lung transplantation is a life-saving procedure in severe PAH with survival rates after 1, 5, 10, and 15 years of 70%, 50%, 39%, and 26% (heart-lung transplantation) and 79%, 52%, 43%, and 30% (double-lung transplantation), respectively.[14-16]

Atrial Septostomy

Balloon atrial septostomy (artificial creation of a right-to-left shunt to decompress the right heart) can be performed percutaneously with careful graded balloon dilation but high periprocedural mortality in patients with markedly elevated RAP and should only be considered as a palliative therapy or bridge to transplantation in centers with experience in this procedure.[17]

REFERENCES

1. McLaughlin VV, Archer SL, Badesch DB, et al. ACCF/AHA 2009 expert consensus document on pulmonary hypertension: a report of the American College of Cardiology Foundation Task Force on Expert Consensus Documents and the American Heart Association. J Am Coll Cardiol. 2009;53:1573-619.
2. McLaughlin VV, Shah SJ, Souza R, et al. Management of Pulmonary Arterial Hypertension. JACC. 2015;65(18):1976-97.
3. Kovacs G, Berghold A, Scheidl S, et al. Pulmonary arterial pressure during rest and exercise in healthy subjects: a systematic review. Eur Respir J. 2009;34:888-94.
4. Rosenkranz S, Gibbs JS, Wachter R, et al. Left ventricular heart failure and pulmonary Hypertension. Eur Heart J. 2016;37:942-54.
5. Robbins IM, Newman JH, Johnson RF, et al. Association of the metabolic syndrome with pulmonary venous hypertension. Chest. 2009;136:31-6.
6. Lam CS, Roger VL, Rodeheffer RJ, et al. Pulmonary hypertension in heart failure with preserved ejection fraction: a community-based study. J Am Coll Cardiol. 2009;53:1119-26.
7. Bursi F, McNallan SM, Redfield MM, et al. Pulmonary pressures and death in heart failure: a community study. J Am Coll Cardiol. 2012;17:222-31.
8. Damy T, Goode KM, Kallvikbacka-Bennett A, et al. Determinants and prognostic value of pulmonary arterial pressure in patients with chronic heart failure. Eur Heart J. 2010;31:2280-90.
9. Leung CC, Moondra V, Catherwood E, et al. Prevalence and risk factors of pulmonary hypertension in patients with elevated pulmonary venous pressure and preserved ejection fraction. Am J Cardiol. 2010;106:284-6.
10. Brickner ME, Hillis LD, Lange RA. Congenital heart disease in adults. First of two parts. N Engl J Med. 2000;342:256-63.
11. Sitbon O, Humbert M, Jais X, et al. Long-term response to calcium channel blockers in idiopathic pulmonary arterial hypertension. Circulation. 2005;111:3105-11.
12. Mereles D, Ehlken N, Kreuscher S, et al. Exercise and respiratory training improve exercise capacity and quality of life in patients with severe chronic pulmonary hypertension. Circulation. 2006;114:1482-9.
13. Tuder RM, Cool CD, Geraci MW, et al. Prostacyclin synthase expression is decreased in lungs from patients with severe pulmonary hypertension. Am J Respir Crit Care Med. 1999;159:1925-32.
14. Fadel E, Mercier O, Mussot S, et al. Long-term outcome of double-lung and heart-lung transplantation for pulmonary hypertension: a comparative retrospective study of 219 patients. Eur J Cardiothorac Surg. 2010;38:277-84.
15. Granton J, Mercier O, De Perrot M. Management of severe pulmonary arterial hypertension. Semin Respir Crit Care Med. 2013;34:700-13.
16. Humbert M, Lau EM, Montani D, et al. Advances in therapeutic interventions for patients with pulmonary arterial hypertension. Circulation. 2014;130:2189-208.
17. Sandoval J, Gaspar J, Pena H, et al. Effect of atrial septostomy on the survival of patients with severe pulmonary arterial hypertension. Eur Respir J. 2011;38:1343-8.

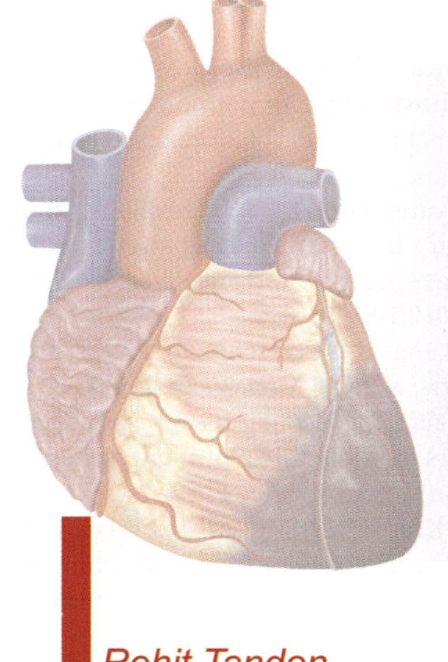

Pulmonary Stenosis, Pulmonary Regurgitation and Heart Failure: Diagnosis and Management Strategies

Rohit Tandon

INTRODUCTION

Historically, right-sided valvular disease has received less attention from clinicians and researchers than left-sided valve disease, in part because of a protracted latent asymptomatic period. It is increasingly recognized that pulmonary valve (PV) disease is not benign and has a significant and independent impact on morbidity and mortality. In this era of increasing awareness and improved treatment options for patients with valve disease, it is important that clinicians consider the diagnosis of PV disease, understand its pathophysiology, choose appropriate confirmatory testing, and refer patients for timely intervention to prevent clinical deterioration with associated adverse consequences.

PULMONARY VALVE STENOSIS

The majority (95%) of pulmonary stenosis (PS) cases are related to congenital or genetic disorders. Noonan syndrome, an autosomal dominant disorder, is commonly associated with PS. The abnormal PV may be classified as acommisural, unicommissural, bicuspid, or dysplastic. Carcinoid syndrome and rheumatic valve disease may cause PS but essentially always occur in conjunction with other valve disease. Most patients with mild to moderate PS are asymptomatic. Severe PS may cause fatigue and dyspnea. Systemic or suprasystemic right ventricular (RV) pressures can cause exertional light headedness, syncope, and eventually right-sided heart failure.

Clinical Examination

In mild PS, pulmonary ejection sound that decreases in intensity with inspiration and a pulmonary ejection murmur that increases with inspiration may be heard and thus mimics a functional murmur. In severe PS, a wave and RV lift are common. A pulmonary ejection systolic murmur is audible and may be palpable at the upper left sternal border with radiation to the neck. With increasing PS severity, the ejection click moves closer to the first heart sound and eventually disappears; the second heart sound becomes widely split. A right-sided fourth heart sound may be heard.

Electrocardiogram (ECG) in severe PS is characterized by right atrial (RA) enlargement, right-axis deviation, RV hypertrophy, and RV strain pattern.

On chest radiograph, right-sided heart enlargement, dilatation of the pulmonary artery, and diminished vascular lung markings may be noted.[1]

Two-dimensional echocardiography demonstrates thickened PV cusps with systolic doming dilated pulmonary artery with/without subvalvular or supravalvular obstruction. The severity of PS is determined peak transpulmonic velocity using continuous wave Doppler. Severe PS is defined as a peak gradient 60 mm Hg, moderate PS peak gradient of 36–60 mm Hg, and mild PS peak gradient 36 mm Hg.[1] Cardiac catheterization should be considered when clinically discordant data is present or to facilitate intervention. The long-term follow-up of 592 patients with PS in the Second Natural History Study

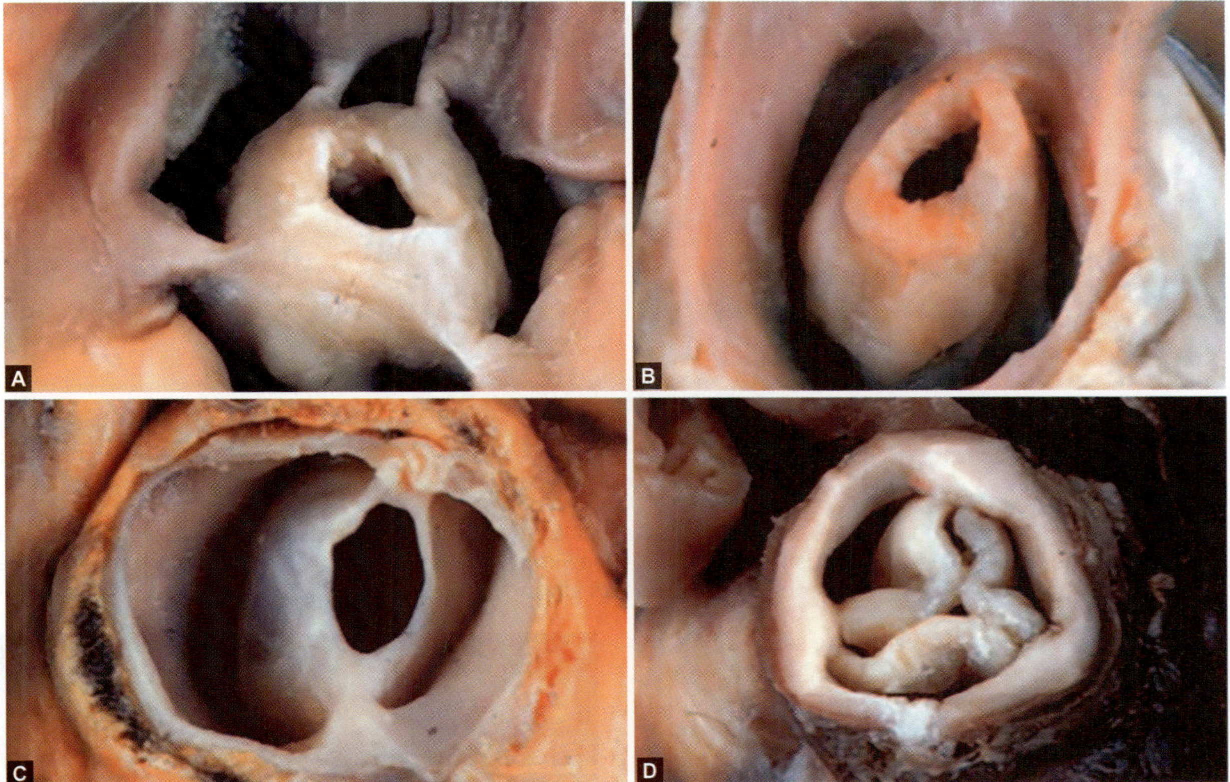

Figs. 1A to D: The abnormal pulmonary valve may be classified as acommisural (A) with prominent systolic doming of the valve cusps and an eccentric orifice, unicommissural (B), bicuspid with fused commissures (C), or dysplastic (D) with severely thickened and deformed valve cusps.

reported an overall survival at 25 years of 96%. Event-free survival was closely related to pressure gradient. On the basis of these surgical data, relief of PS is recommended for all patients with a peak gradient ≥50 mm Hg.[1] Percutaneous pulmonary balloon valvuloplasty (PBV) is the treatment of choice for most patients. In patients with mild PS, symptoms are uncommon, progression is minimal, and outcome is excellent only periodic follow-up is recommended. Approximately 25% of patients with moderate PS eventually require intervention. Predictors of the need for intervention include higher peak systolic gradient and reduced cardiac output.[2] Intervention in the Second Natural History Study involved surgical valvotomy. Reoperation was reported in only 4% of patients during a 10-year follow-up.[2]

In a subsequent longitudinal study of 90 consecutive patients with PS treated with operation, reoperation was required in 15%, primarily for pulmonary regurgitation (PR) (9%). At last follow-up, moderate to severe PR was present in 37%, emphasizing the importance of follow-up after PS intervention.[3]

Asymptomatic athletes with a peak PS gradient <40 mm Hg and normal RV function can participate in all competitive sports with annual reevaluation. Athletes with a peak PS gradient >40 mm Hg can participate in low-intensity competitive sports or can be referred for intervention. 2–4 weeks after PBV, asymptomatic athletes with mild residual PS and normal ventricular function can participate in all competitive sports. After operation, an interval of 3 months is suggested before sports participation is resumed.[4]

Pregnancy is generally well tolerated in PS patients. Severe PS may be associated with an increased risk during labor and delivery and postpartum. PBV can be performed with low risk during pregnancy for symptomatic severe PS. These patients are at increased risk of having an infant with congenital heart disease, particularly those with Noonan's syndrome.[5]

Pulmonary balloon valvuloplasty is the procedure of choice for children and adults with severe or symptomatic PS and carries a low risk of morbidity, mortality, and restenosis.[1,6-9]

However, a high frequency of PR has been reported; after PBV, 57% of children had moderate or severe PR at the last follow-up.[10]

These data emphasize the need for lifelong follow-up after PBV. PBV is performed most often with a circular oversized balloon that reportedly separates congenitally

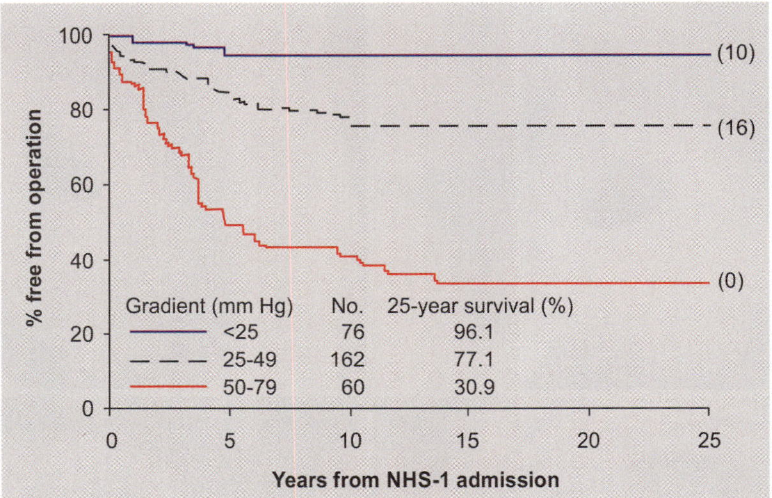

Fig. 2: Survival curve from Second Natural History Study. Kaplan–Meier curves of percentage free from surgery for 300 PS patients managed medically, grouped by gradient at admission to the First Natural History Study (NHS-1). Numbers in parentheses indicate number of patients remaining under observation 25 years after admission.

fused commissures. Thus, best results are seen in patients with congenital stenosis with fused, but thin, leaflets and a normal annulus size. After PBV, the transpulmonic gradient usually decreases by two-thirds of its baseline value.[11,12]

The procedure is not recommended in patients with acquired PS related to carcinoid or rheumatic disease because of the nature of valve involvement, commonly associated PR, and concomitant other valve involvement. PS often is associated with some degree of subvalvular muscular obstruction resulting from hypertrophy of the RV myocardium. After relief of PS, infundibular obstruction may worsen transiently but then tends to regress over months with eventual resolution.[13,14]

Acute severe obstruction can cause "suicidal" RV, which results in suprasystemic RV pressure with resultant cyanosis and hemodynamic instability. Beta-Blocker therapy is recommended before PBV to prevent or reduce the severity of this complication; therapy generally is discontinued after 3–6 months. In patients who have a poor result with PBV, unfavorable valve morphology, hypoplastic pulmonary annulus, fixed subvalvar or supravalvar PS, or severe PR, surgical valvotomy or valve replacement may be preferred. The choice of PV prosthesis type must be individualized. Bioprostheses are preferred for PV replacement. Homografts demonstrate unpredictable durability and may degenerate prematurely, with obstruction, regurgitation, or both, especially in the setting of pressure half-time (PHT). Mechanical valves are thrombogenic and generally not used in the low-pressure right side of the heart unless the patient requires lifelong warfarin for another reason.[15]

Percutaneous PV implantation facilitates significant reduction in RV systolic pressure and RV outflow tract gradient; freedom from reoperation was 70% at 70 months. This procedure might reduce the number of operations needed over the total lifetime of patients with RV to pulmonary artery conduits.[16]

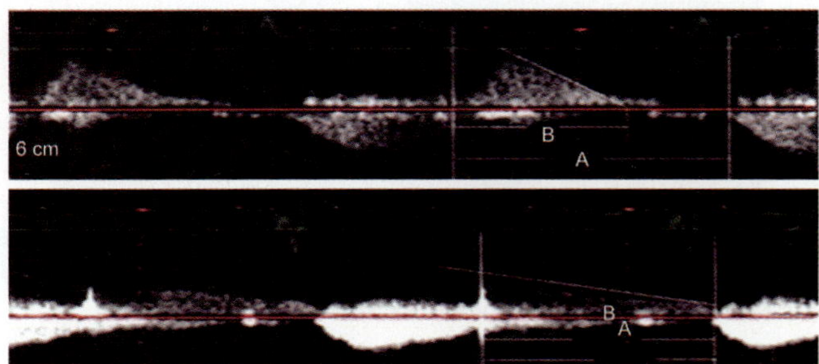

Fig. 3: Continuous wave Doppler echocardiographic recordings of pulmonary flow from a patient with severe (top) and mild (bottom) pulmonary regurgitation (PR). The duration of regurgitant flow (B) with respect to total diastole (A) is shorter in the patient with severe PR.

PULMONARY VALVE REGURGITATION

In adults, pathological PR most often is the consequence of prior interventions for congenital heart disease such as tetralogy of Fallot repair with placement of an outflow tract patch or surgical valvotomy for isolated congenital PS.[3]

Additional causes of PR include rheumatic or carcinoid heart disease, trauma, endocarditis, and pulmonary artery and annular dilation; PR also can occur secondary to PHT. Patients with long-standing severe PR develop progressive RV dilation and reduced RV function. This can lead to the inability to augment cardiac output with exercise and to congestive heart failure. In addition, the dilated and dysfunctional RV is associated with QRS prolongation, ventricular arrhythmias, and sudden death. This mechanical-electric association has been well documented in patients with transannular patch repair of tetralogy of Fallot.[17]

Pathophysiology of Pulmonary Regurgitation

Functionally severe PR is different from severe AR for two reasons. First, forward pulmonary blood flow can be maintained indirectly by the work of the left heart via the systemic venous return and by RA contraction. The second difference is that the pulmonary microvascular bed, is of low resistance. Flow that passes forward through alveolar capillaries in systole is unlikely to pass back again in diastole, there being no significant reversal of gradient. The pulmonary microvascular bed, therefore, has a valve-like effect in the setting of severe PR. That is why severe PR has regurgitant fraction of only about 40%,[5,18] which is generally well tolerated for a long period of time. However, conditions that lead to elevated pulmonary artery pressure, e.g. branch pulmonary arterial stenosis, acquired bronchopulmonary disease, left ventricular dysfunction, or pulmonary vascular disease can lead to increase in its severity.

Clinical Examination

Pulmonary regurgitation patients may demonstrate a parasternal lift when the RV is enlarged. The murmur of PR is typically a soft, diastolic, decrescendo murmur best heard in the left upper sternal region in patients with normal pulmonary pressures. It begins after the pulmonic closure sound and may be accompanied by a pulmonic systolic ejection murmur. An increase in intensity of the murmur may be noted during inspiration. The murmur is easily audible and occasionally palpable in patients with pulmonary hypertension.

Investigations

Nonspecific ECG findings are noted in patients with PR. The total QRS duration and the rate of QRS increase reflect the impact of PR on the RV in patients with tetralogy of Fallot. QRS prolongation, with rSr morphology in the right precordial leads, reflecting volume overload of the RV is usually seen. QRS duration increases with time, reflecting progressive RV enlargement. QRS duration and QRS change have prognostic implications for malignant arrhythmia and sudden cardiac death (SCD). RV dilatation and stretch slows interventricular conduction and creates a mechanoelectrical substrate for reentry circuits, predisposing to sustained ventricular tachycardia. QRS duration of 180 ms or more is shown to be a highly sensitive predictor of sustained ventricular tachycardia and SCD in patients with previous tetralogy repair.[19] While QRS lengthening, seen immediately after repair, reflects surgical injury to the myocardium and on the right bundle branch, late QRS prolongation almost universally reflects RV dilatation, mostly due to PR. Interval change in QRS duration, thus, may have a greater prognostic value for sustained ventricular tachycardia and SCD than absolute QRS measurements at any point in time.[5] This is particularly relevant to contemporary cohorts undergoing tetralogy repair via a transatrial/transpulmonary approach, where direct myocardial damage is limited, thus initial

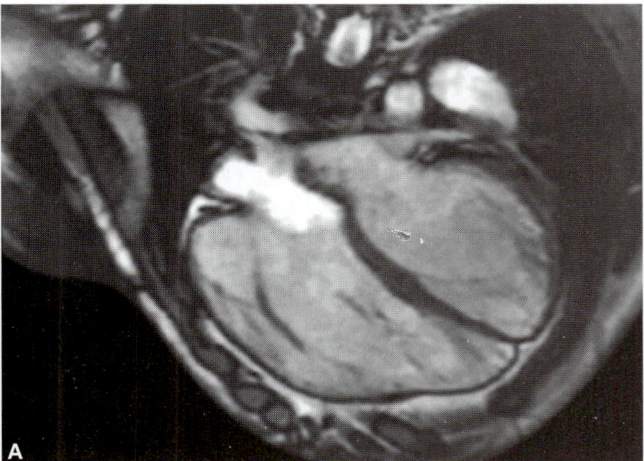

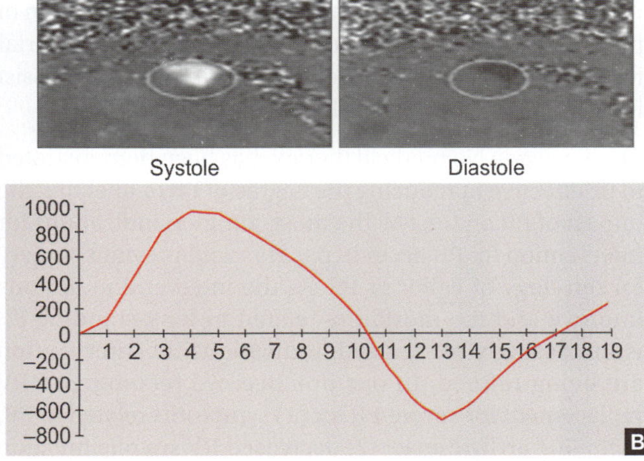

Figs. 4A and B: Cardiovascular magnetic resonance for assessment of biventricular function and pulmonary regurgitation (PR) in a patient following repair of tetralogy of Fallot. (A) Four chamber view shows right ventricular dilatation and hypertrophy in a patient with severe PR. (B) Phase velocity mapping measuring the flow across the pulmonary artery in systole and diastole (below the curve) in the same patient.

postoperative QRS prolongation is less compared with older cohorts who underwent tetralogy repair via a right ventriculotomy.[20]

Chest radiography may demonstrate cardiomegaly, involving the right-sided chambers and pulmonary artery enlargement. Patients with severe PR characteristically have dilatation of the pulmonary trunk and central pulmonary arteries. There is also RV enlargement, evident as filling of the retrosternal space on lateral projections.

Echocardiography

The diagnosis of PR is usually made by echocardiography and graded on a 1–4 scale with color Doppler imaging. A trivial or mild degree of PR is detectable in most normal individuals.[19]

Pathological PR is typically a wide holodiastolic jet. The density of the continuous-wave Doppler signal and deceleration PHT correspond to the degree of regurgitation and the RV pressures. When PR is unrestricted and the pulmonary pressures are low, the Doppler color-flow map may be laminar, leading to underappreciation of the PR severity.[20,21]

Cardiac magnetic resonance imaging (MRI) is commonly used to assess right-sided heart size and function in asymptomatic patients with severe PR to determine the optimum time of valve replacement. Cardiac catheterization is rarely performed to assess PR. Most patients with mild degrees of PR have a benign clinical course. Chronic severe PR often is well tolerated for many years. However, the RV may dilate and develop systolic dysfunction, analogous to the effect of chronic aortic regurgitation on the left ventricle. Severe RV dilation is associated with an increased risk of sudden death related primarily to arrhythmias.[17]

Exercise testing is a useful adjunct for the evaluation of functional class. Changes in exercise capacity with serial testing may precede the onset of overt symptoms and assist in deciding on timing of PVR in these patients.

Management: No medical therapy has been demonstrated to be effective in reducing the degree of PR or affecting the impact of PR on the RV. The most common indications for intervention for PR occur in patients with previous surgery for tetralogy of Fallot or PS. As the intervention options improve and the morbidity related to long-standing PR is increasingly recognized, indications for intervention are being refined. In our practice, we recommend PV replacement for severe PR for (1) symptoms related to PR, including arrhythmias; (2) decreased RV systolic function (ejection fraction <40% by cardiac MRI); (3) progressive RV dilation (cardiac MRI RV end-diastolic volume 160 mL/m^2 or 82 mL/m^2 for RV end-systolic volume; (4) decline in functional aerobic capacity; (5) moderate or worse tricuspid regurgitation (TR) related to progressive annular dilatation; (6) severe PR in a patient requiring another cardiac operation; and (7) concern about risk of arrhythmia in patients with prolonged or increasing QRS duration (total QRS duration >180 milliseconds or QRS duration increase 3.5 ms/year.[17]

Right ventricular size tends to normalize and functional status improves after PV replacement for PR late after tetralogy of Fallot surgery.[22] However, RV function may not fully recover once marked enlargement (>170 mL/m^2) and systolic dysfunction are evident.[23,24]

Most patients (even those who consider themselves asymptomatic) improve their functional class after PVR. There are conflicting reports, however, regarding recovery of RV function following PVR. When timely PVR is performed, there is almost universally, reduction of RV size and improvement of RV ejection fraction. In contrast, when PVR is performed late, RV recovery is incomplete.

So to preserve RV function, PVR in adults should be considered before RV dysfunction and overt symptoms of RV failure ensue. Surveillance should be directed at monitoring RV dilatation and its sequelae, rather than PR per se. Clinical findings accompanying ventricular dilatation are decreased exercise tolerance and other signs and symptoms of heart failure. It is important to obtain an estimate of RV pressure—for example, from a TR jet by Doppler echocardiography. Evidence of elevated RV pressure should initiate a search for RV outflow tract obstruction or pulmonary artery stenosis with help of cardiac computed tomography (CT) or MRI.

CONCLUSION

Meticulous echocardiographic evaluation PS, PR in heart failure with multimodality imaging with enhance the diagnostic, prognostic, and therapeutic implications thereby help in reducing the cardiac morbidity and mortality.

REFERENCES

1. Bonow R, Carabello B, Kanu C, et al. American College of Cardiology/American Heart Association Task Force on Practice Guidelines; Society of Cardiovascular Anesthesiologists; Society for Cardiovascular Angiography and Interventions; Society of Thoracic Surgeons. ACC/AHA 2006 guidelines for the management of patients with valvular heart disease: a report of the American College of Cardiology/American Heart Association Task Force on Practice Guidelines (Writing Committee to Revise the 1998 Guidelines for the Management of Patients With Valvular Heart Disease): developed in collaboration with the Society of Cardiovascular Anesthesiologists: endorsed by the Society for Cardiovascular Angiography and Interventions and the Society of Thoracic Surgeons. Circulation. 2006;114:e84-231.

2. Hayes C, Gersony W, Driscoll D, et al. Second natural history study of congenital heart defects: results of treatment of patients with pulmonary valvar stenosis. Circulation. 1993;87(Suppl 2):I28-37.
3. Roos-Hesselink JW, Meijboom FJ, Spitaels SE, et al. Long-term outcome after surgery for pulmonary stenosis (a longitudinal study of 22-33 years). Eur Heart J. 2006;27: 482-8.
4. Graham T Jr, Driscoll D, Gersony W, et al. Task Force 2: congenital heart disease. J Am Coll Cardiol. 2005;45:1326-33.
5. Drenthen W, Pieper P, Roos-Hesselink J, et al. ZAHARA Investigators. Outcome of pregnancy in women with congenital heart disease: a literature review. J Am Coll Cardiol. 2007;49:2303-11.
6. David S, Goussous Y, Harbi N, et al. Management of typical and dysplastic pulmonic stenosis, uncomplicated or associated with complex intracardiac defects, in juveniles and adults: use of percutaneous balloon pulmonary valvuloplasty with eight-month hemodynamic follow-up. Cathet Cardiovasc Diagn. 1993;29:105-12.
7. Kaul U, Singh B, Tyagi S, et al. Long-term results after balloon pulmonary valvuloplasty in adults. Am Heart J. 1993;126:1152-5.
8. Lau K, Hung J. Controversies in percutaneous balloon pulmonary valvuloplasty: timing, patient selection and technique. J Heart Valve Dis. 1993;2:321-5.
9. Sievert H, Kober G, Bussman W, et al. Long-term results of percutaneous pulmonary valvuloplasty in adults. Eur Heart J. 1989;10:712-7.
10. Garty Y, Veldtman G, Lee K, et al. Late outcomes after pulmonary valve balloon dilatation in neonates, infants and children. J Invasive Cardiol. 2005;17:18-22.
11. Chen C, Cheng T, Huang T, et al. Percutaneous balloon valvuloplasty for pulmonic stenosis in adolescents and adults. N Engl J Med. 1996;335:21-5.
12. Fawzy M, Awad M, Galal O, et al. Long-term results of pulmonary balloon valvulotomy in adult patients. J Heart Valve Dis. 2001;10:812-8.
13. Fawzy M, Galal O, Dunn B, et al. Regression of infundibular pulmonary stenosis after successful balloon pulmonary valvuloplasty in adults. Cathet Cardiovasc Diagn. 1990;21: 77-81.
14. Teupe C, Burger W, Schrader R, et al. Late (five to nine years) follow-up after balloon dilation of valvular pulmonary stenosis in adults. Am J Cardiol. 1997;80:240-2.
15. Waterbolk T, Hoendermis E, den Hamer I, et al. Pulmonary valve replacement with a mechanical prosthesis: promising results of 28 procedures in patients with congenital heart disease. Eur J Cardiothorac Surg. 2006;30:28-32.
16. Lurz P, Coats L, Khambadkone S, et al. Percutaneous pulmonary valve implantation: impact of evolving technology and learning curve on clinical outcome. Circulation. 2008;117:1964-72.
17. Therrien J, Siu S, Harris L, et al. Impact of pulmonary valve replacement on arrhythmia propensity late after repair of tetralogy of Fallot. Circulation. 2001;103:2489-94.
18. Brown J, Ruzmetov M, Rodefeld M, et al. Right ventricular outflow tract reconstruction with an allograft conduit in non-Ross patients: risk factors for allograft dysfunction and failure. Ann Thorac Surg. 2005;80:655-63.
19. Klein A, Burstow D, Tajik A, et al. Age-related prevalence of valvular regurgitation in normal subjects: a comprehensive color flow examination of 118 volunteers. J Am Soc Echocardiogr. 1990;3:54-63.
20. Zoghbi WA, Enriquez-Sarano M, Foster E, et al. Recommendations for evaluation of the severity of native valvular regurgitation with twodimensional and Doppler echocardiography. J Am Soc Echocardiogr. 2003;16:777-802.
21. Silversides C, Veldtman G, Crossin J, et al. Pressure half-time predicts hemodynamically significant pulmonary regurgitation in adult patients with repaired tetralogy of Fallot. J Am Soc Echocardiogr. 2003;16:1057-62.
22. Oosterhof T, van Straten A, Vliegen H, et al. Preoperative thresholds for pulmonary valve replacement in patients with corrected tetralogy of Fallot using cardiovascular magnetic resonance. Circulation. 2007;116:545-51.
23. Buechel E, Dave H, Kellenberger C, et al. Remodelling of the right ventricle after early pulmonary valve replacement in children with repaired tetralogy of Fallot: assessment by cardiovascular magnetic resonance. Eur Heart J. 2005;26:2721-7.
24. Therrien J, Siu S, McLaughlin P, et al. Pulmonary valve replacement in adults late after repair of tetralogy of Fallot: are we operating too late? J Am Coll Cardiol. 2000;36:1670-5.

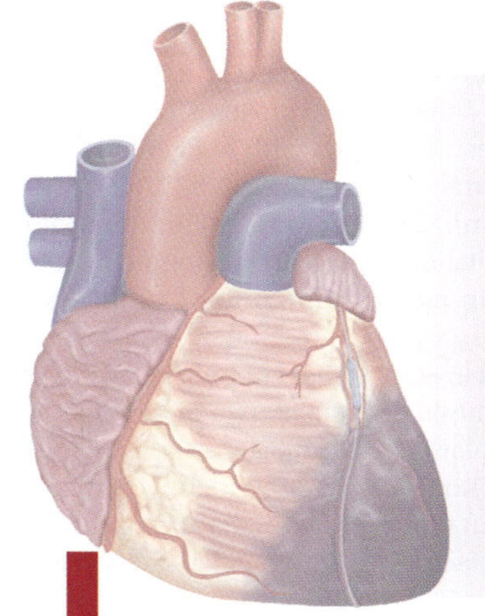

Riociguat in CTEPH with Heart Failure

Arnab Banerjee, Debabrata Roy

INTRODUCTION

Chronic thromboembolic pulmonary hypertension (CTEPH) is one of the many causes of pulmonary hypertension (PH) that results from the gradual and progressive obstruction of the pulmonary vasculature by residual and organized thrombi. This fault in the pulmonary vasculature results in gradual increase in pulmonary vascular resistance (PVR), PH, and premature death due to right ventricular failure.[1-3] Pulmonary endarterectomy (PEA) has long been the gold standard of treatment of CTEPH, and can potentially cure the disease if it is successful.[4] However, in about 30–40% of the patients, the disease is inoperable, and about 50% of the patients with develop recurrent or persistent disease after the operation.[5]

Riociguat is a soluble guanylate cyclase (sGC) stimulator that has been approved for the treatment of inoperable and recurrent or persistent CTEPH.[6] Nitric oxide (NO) is produced from arginine by the action of the enzyme, nitric oxide synthase (NOS), giving birth to citrulline as a by-product. NOS is of three types: (1) inducible NOS (iNOS), (2) neuronal NOS (nNOS), and (3) endothelial NOS (eNOS). NO then binds to the heme group of the sGC, and potentiates the enzyme, resulting in increased production of cyclic guanosine monophosphate (cGMP) from guanosine triphosphate (GTP). cGMP acts as a second messenger and leads to the formation and activation substances like cGMP-dependent protein kinases [(e.g. protein kinase G (PKG)], phosphodiesterases (PDEs), etc. Protein kinase G leads to the activation of myosin phosphatase which in turn accentuates the release of calcium from the intracellular stores of the smooth muscle cells resulting in subsequent relaxation of the muscles concerned, and vasodilation. cGMP also leads to the activation of the PDEs which converts cGMP to GTP, thus resulting in a negative feedback cycle. This is stopped by PDE inhibitors like sildenafil, tadalafil. However, detailed discussion of all these pathways is beyond the scope of the current article. For the time being, we will concentrate on riociguat and its action in CTEPH.

Riociguat has a dual mode of action, sensitizing sGC to endogenous NO by stabilizing the bond between NO and sGC, and directly stimulating sGC via a different binding site, independently of the action of NO. This dual potentiation facilitates the NO–sGC–cGMP pathway and increases generation of cGMP, thereby augmenting smooth muscular relaxation and vasodilation (Fig. 1).

CHRONIC THROMBOEMBOLIC PULMONARY HYPERTENSION

Definitions and Description

Pulmonary hypertension is defined as a resting mean pulmonary arterial pressure (mPAP) of ≥25 mm Hg measured by invasive right heart catheterization. There are different types of PH, which are differentiated according to their etiological factors and clinical and diagnostic characteristics. This mode of classification of PH has been modified and amended several times, the most recent being in 2013 at the Fifth World Symposium on PH held in Nice, France. In this system of 5 groups, group 2 is postcapillary PH (venous), primarily due to left ventricular failure,

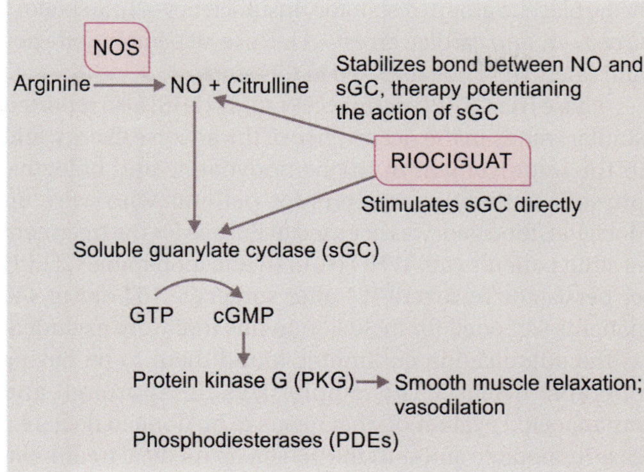

Fig. 1: NO–sGC–cGMP pathway.
(cGMP: cyclic guanosine monophosphate; GTP: guanosine triphosphate; NO: nitric oxide; NOS: nitric oxide synthases)

whereas all the other groups comprise one or the other varieties of precapillary PH, or more precisely, pulmonary arterial hypertension (PAH). CTEPH represents group 4 and is different from all other forms of PH, including group 1 PAH, which can masquerade as CTEPH as far as clinical symptoms and signs are concerned.

Chronic thromboembolic pulmonary hypertension is diagnosed if, after effective therapeutic anticoagulation of at least 3 months duration, the patient's mPAP is found to be ≥25 mm Hg and the corresponding pulmonary capillary wedge pressure (PCWP) is ≥15 mm Hg, along with at least one mismatched segmental perfusion defect showed by ventilation/perfusion (V/Q) scintigraphy, multidetector-computed tomography angiography (MD-CTA) or pulmonary angiography.[7] Of all these modalities, V/Q scintigraphy is the cheapest, readily available, preferred and most recommended screening test for CTEPH, with segmental perfusion defects being the major difference between CTEPH and PAH.[8] Segmental defects are usually absent in PAH, or if present, are noticed in the peripheral small regions, and the magnitude of the defects are usually quite small or insignificant.

Etiology

The only known and confirmed etiological factor for CTEPH is an unresolved episode of acute pulmonary embolism (PE), resulting de novo or from an episode of venous thromboembolism (VTE).[9] These unresolved embolic and thrombotic materials in the pulmonary vasculature give birth to an abnormal proliferation of the endothelium and smooth muscle in vessel walls, ultimately leading to the fibrotic and proliferative changes in the vasculature. The result is permanent vascular remodeling and arteriopathy of distal resistance vessels that the world acknowledges as CTEPH. Incomplete resolution of the thrombus may be due to the inherent quality of the thrombus *per se*, or due to an imbalance between the procoagulant and anticoagulant cascades, with the scales tipping in favor of a procoagulant state due to any cause, be it genetic or acquired. Small vessel thrombi are also responsible for these changes, as is an inadequate level of angiogenesis in the diseased segment, potentiating the process of fibrosis. In the absence of PE, the etiopathogenesis is unknown. Previous PE/VTE and recurrent VTE, infected pacemaker, ventriculoatrial shunt, splenectomy, antiphospholipid antibodies, and lupus anticoagulant are the risk factors which are increasingly associated with CTEPH.[10]

Diagnosis

Rapid and accurate diagnosis is essential for the successful treatment. Clinical signs and symptoms are nonspecific and risk factors, such as history of VTE or PE may be absent. The recommended preliminary step in diagnosis is 2D-echocardiography. Cardiopulmonary exercise testing (CPET) is a supplementary tool that can help in diagnosing early physical difficulties and point to a definitive assessment. Ventilation/perfusion scintigraphy is the imaging modality of choice to exclude CTEPH.[11] Single photon emission computed tomography (SPECT) is gaining popularity in this segment. Invasive pulmonary hemodynamic assessment by right heart catheterization is essential before taking decisions regarding treatment, although there is much buzz in recent times about noninvasive hemodynamic monitoring. Though digital subtraction angiography (DSA) is the gold standard test to diagnose and delineate the extent of the thrombus and the status of operability, newer techniques, such as computed tomography (CT) and magnetic resonance (MR) angiography are increasingly being used with a good degree of sensitivity and specificity for segmental disease. DSA is still superior in subsegmental and distal disease. Promising new models include dual-energy CT,[12] combination of rotational angiography and cone beam CT, and positron emission tomography (PET). PET-guided metabolic imaging is very effective in differentiating CTEPH from malignant lesions like mediastinal or pulmonary artery sarcoma (PAS).[13] These techniques reduce the margin of error, apart from proving valuable information regarding planning of treatment. Further reliability and validation studies are needed for these tests to be implemented in routine clinical use, let alone the prospect of reduction in costs of these newer tools.[14]

Treatment

The traditional treatment of CTEPH has long been pulmonary endarterectomy which is potentially curable. The perioperative mortality in most experienced centers is less than 5%, and the surgery in most cases result in near normalization of the pulmonary and right ventricular hemodynamic parameters.[15] Lesions that are located too distally in the pulmonary arterial tree may not be amenable or accessible to surgical treatment. Balloon pulmonary angioplasty may be a viable option in these cases for segmental/subsegmental disease. Drug eluting balloons for these cases are being tried. About half of the patients will face recurrent disease after successful surgery.Medical treatment targeting various pathways of the endothelial milieu is the new fad in the pharmacological armamentarium of this disease.[16]

Of the various drugs available for the treatment of CTEPH, riociguat is a promising option. Other classes of drugs that are available for the treatment of CTEPH are prostanoids (epoprostenol, treprostinil, and iloprost), endothelin receptor antagonists (bosentan, ambrisentan, macitentan) and PDE-5 inhibitors (sildenafil, tadalafil, vardenafil).

TRIALS OF RIOCIGUAT

CHEST-1

The efficacy and safety of riociguat were assessed in CHEST-1, a multicenter, phase III, randomized, double-blind, placebo-controlled study. 261 patients were enrolled, all of whom had either inoperable disease as assessed by an adjudication committee consisting of experienced CTEPH operators, or recurrent or persistent disease after operation. They had a mean 6-min walk distance (6MWD) of 150–450 m, PVR > 300 dynes/cm^{-5} and mPAP ≥ 25 mm Hg. Randomization was done to administer the patients placebo or riociguat at an initial dose of 1 mg three times daily. The dose was adjusted in the first 8 weeks of the study on the basis of tolerability, and side effects, and in the patients who did not have hypotension, the dose was optimized to 2.5 mg TDS. That individualized dose was given for the next 8 weeks. At the end of the 16th week, 77% of patients taking the maximal riociguat dose of 2.5 mg TDS. The dose of the study drug was decreased in 18 patients (10%) in the riociguat group compared to three (3%) in the placebo group. At the end of week 16, there was an increase in the 6MWD (the primary end-point) 39 m in the patient group getting riociguat compared to a 6 m decrease in the placebo arm (95% confidence interval (CI) 25–67 m; p < 0.001). Apart from that, there was a significant betterment in the World Health Organization (WHO) functional class in the riociguat arm (33%) compared to the placebo arm (15%; p = 0.003). However, there was no statistically significant difference in the rate of worsening between the two groups. Headache, dizziness, dyspepsia, peripheral edema and nasopharyngitis were the most common side effects noted. Right ventricular failure, syncope and hemoptysis were the most fearsome adverse events. Deaths potentially related to the side effects occurred in two patients (1%) in the riociguat group (heart failure—1 and acute renal failure-1) and in three patients (3%) in the placebo group (respiratory insufficiency—1, circulatory arrest—1, and cardiac arrest—1). Dose-dependent efficacy and safety were not analyzed in this study.

Phase IIIb CTEPH early access study (EAS) also reported similar trends in the occurrence of the adverse events, and in the improvement in the hemodynamic and objective physical activity parameters for patients who were on riociguat. Riociguat was licensed in Europe for the treatment of adult patients with WHO FC II/III and inoperable CTEPH or persistent/recurrent PH after surgery.[17] 164 out of 446 patients screened for inclusion in this trial were excluded, as the adjudication committee found them to be having operable disease. This emphasizes the thorough and multifaceted evaluation that needs to be done to declare a case inoperable and start the person on medical treatment, as PEA still is the treatment of choice in CTEPH.

Increased proportion of the patients who were on riociguat achieved a 6MWD ≥ 380 m, WHO FC I/II and PVR < 500 dynes/cm^{-5}. Little change was observed in placebo-treated patients. Similar trends in improvement were noted in thresholds for cardiac index, SvO_2, N-terminal-pro B-type natriuretic peptide (NT-proBNP) level and right atrial pressure. Apart from all these fantastic effects, riociguat treated patients achieved a combination of response criteria for 6MWD, WHO FC, cardiac index, SvO_2, and NT-proBNP level more frequently. All these data show the magnitude of positive effect that riociguat promises.

PATENT-1

The PATENT-1 study was published almost simultaneously with the CHEST-1 trial. It was a 12-week, double-blind, placebo-controlled trial conducted in patients with PAH. In this study, 443 patients with symptomatic PAH were randomized in a 2:4:1 fashion to placebo, dose-adjusted riociguat with a maximum dosage of 2.5 mg three times daily, or dose-adjusted riociguat with a maximum dosage of 1.5 mg three times daily. There was an increment in the 6MWD by a mean of 30 m in the 2.5 mg maximum-dose group and decrement by 6 m in the placebo group (95% CI, 20–52 m; $p < 0.001$). This result was maintained irrespective of the baseline PAH therapy. Patients in WHO functional class III or IV PAH (95% CI, 37–81 m) at baseline had a significantly better response than those in WHO functional class I or II PAH (95% CI, –9 to 36 m). Patients in the riociguat 2.5 mg maximum-dose group had significant improvement in PVR (–226 dyn·s·cm^{-5}; 95% CI, –281 to –170 dyn·s·cm^{-5}; $p < 0.001$) and WHO functional class ($p = 0.003$) compared to the placebo group along with a decreased incidence of clinical worsening when compared to the placebo group.

Riociguat Long-term Data: CHEST-2

Long-term safety of riociguat was assessed in CHEST-2 trial, an extension of the CHEST-1 trial. 237 patients (98%)

enrolled in CHEST-2. Patients who received placebo in CHEST-1 were initially started on a dose of 1 mg TDS and the dose was individualized as in the CHEST-1 study). The primary objective was to assess the safety of riociguat in the long-term (mean treatment duration—83 weeks, median—75 weeks). Nasopharyngitis (23%), dizziness (19%), peripheral edema (18%), and diarrhea (14%) were most common. Hypotension was seen in 6% and syncope in 7%, but they resolved in all these cases with continued use. The mean±SD change observed from baseline in 6MWD was +52 ± 66 m at 1 year (n = 209) and +50 ± 68 m at 2 years (n = 162). All the positive effects that were noticed in the CHEST-1 trial were retained in the CHEST-2 trial. The estimated overall survival rate was 93% (95% CI 89–96%) at 2 years,[18] and no new kind of adverse effects were observed.

CONCLUSION

Chronic thromboembolic pulmonary hypertension is a devastating condition which can lead to rapid deterioration of functional capacity and even death. Till date pulmonary endarterectomy has been the only potentially curable treatment available. However, recent advances in medicine and insight into the causative and etiopathogenetic pathways have led to the introduction of a number of drugs that can lead to improvement in the disease. Recently, riociguat has been approved for the treatment of this condition, and it has been shown that it leads to considerable improvement in functional capacity of the patients. Side effect profile of the drug is quite favorable. It has been used as primary treatment for inoperable disease as well as a bridge to surgery for these patients. Considering all the options available for the treatment of CTEPH, riociguat is a promising option. However more research is needed in this field, for the development of more definitive therapy, as well as refinement of the existing ones.

REFERENCES

1. Lang IM, Klepetko W. Chronic thromboembolic pulmonary hypertension: an updated review. Curr Opin Cardiol. 2008;23:555-9.
2. Peacock A, Simonneau G, Rubin L. Controversies, uncertainties and future research on the treatment of chronic thromboembolic pulmonary hypertension. Proc Am Thorac Soc. 2006;3:608-14.
3. Simonneau G, Robbins IM, Beghetti M, et al. Updated clinical classification of pulmonary hypertension. J Am Coll Cardiol. 2009;54:S43-54.
4. Kim NH, Delcroix M, Jenkins DP, et al. Chronic thromboembolic pulmonary hypertension. J Am Coll Cardiol. 2013;62:D92-9.
5. Mayer E, Jenkins D, Lindner J, et al. Surgical management and outcome of patients with chronic thromboembolic pulmonary hypertension: results from an international prospective registry. J Thorac Cardiovasc Surg. 2011;141:702-10.
6. Grimminger F, Weimann G, Frey R, et al. First acute haemodynamic study of soluble guanylate cyclase stimulator Riociguat in pulmonary hypertension. Eur Respir J. 2009;33:785-92.
7. Lang IM, Pesavento R, Bonderman D, et al. Risk factors and basic mechanisms of chronic thromboembolic pulmonary hypertension: a current understanding. Eur Respir J. 2013;41:462-8.
8. Galiè N, Hoeper MM, Humbert M, et al. Guidelines for the diagnosis and treatment of pulmonary hypertension Eur Respir J. 2009;34:1219-63.
9. Bonderman D, Wilkens H, Wakounig S, et al. Risk factors for chronic thromboembolic pulmonary hypertension. Eur Respir J. 2009;33:325-31.
10. Lang IM, Madani M. Update on chronic thromboembolic pulmonary hypertension. Circulation. 2014;130:508-18.
11. He J, Fang W, Lv B, et al. Diagnosis of chronic thromboembolic pulmonary hypertension: comparison of ventilation/perfusion scanning and multidetector computed tomography pulmonary angiography with pulmonary angiography. Nucl Med Commun. 2012;33:459-63.
12. Takagi H, Ota H, Sugimura K, et al. Dual-energy CT to estimate clinical severity of chronic thromboembolic pulmonary hypertension: comparison with invasive right heart catheterization. Eur J Radiol. 2016;85:1574-80.
13. Ito K, Kubota K, Morooka M, et al. Diagnostic usefulness of 18F-FDG PET/CT in the differentiation of pulmonary artery sarcoma and pulmonary embolism. Ann Nucl Med. 2009;23:671-6.
14. Gopalan D, Delcroix M, Held M. Diagnosis of chronic thromboembolic pulmonary hypertension. Eur Respir Rev. 2017;26:(143). pii: 160108.
15. Taboada D, Pepke-Zaba J, Jenkins DP, et al. Outcome of pulmonary endarterectomy in symptomatic chronic thromboembolic disease. Eur Respir J. 2014;44:1635-45.
16. Pepke-Zaba J, Ghofrani HA, Hoeper MM. Medical management of chronic thromboembolic pulmonary hypertension. Eur Respir Rev. 2017;26:(143). pii: 160107.
17. Bayer AG. (2014). Adempas (riociguat): EU Summary of Product Characteristics. [online] Available from https://www.ema.europa.eu/en/documents/product-information/adempas-epar-product-information_en.pdf [Last accessed November, 2019].
18. Simonneau G, D'Armini AM, Ghofrani HA, et al. Predictors of long-term outcomes in patients treated with Riociguat for chronic thromboembolic pulmonary hypertension: data from the CHEST-2 open-label, randomised, long-term extension trial. Lancet Respir Med. 2016;4:372-80.

105

CHAPTER

Rheumatic Heart Disease and Heart Failure

IB Vijayalakshmi

INTRODUCTION

The heart failure (HF) is a complex clinical syndrome, with multiple etiologies and diverse clinical manifestations, as it can result from many structural or functional cardiac disorders including acute rheumatic fever (ARF) and its long-term sequel chronic rheumatic heart disease (RHD). The ARF with carditis leads to acute mitral/aortic/tricuspid regurgitation (TR) causing HF or chronic RHD in which permanent damage to heart valves is caused, leading to leaking or stenosis of valves or combination of both. Unfortunately "carditis" is the only presentation of ARF that causes HF and death during acute stage, or leads to permanent damage with long-term morbidity and mortality due to RHD and HF. In developing country like Bharat (India), the ARF and chronic RHD are very important causes of HF. There are now well established guidelines for the management of HF in ischemic heart disease (IHD) in adults[1,2] but no equivalent consensus for children with HF caused by ARF and RHD.

EPIDEMIOLOGY

Rheumatic heart disease is highly prevalent in developing nations, where it is the leading cause of cardiovascular morbidity including HF.[3-8] It is estimated that 15.6 million people are affected worldwide by ARF. In India, 300,000 out of 500,000 individuals that acquire ARF every year go on to develop chronic RHD.[9] As many as 39% of persons with ARF may develop varying degrees of carditis associated with valve insufficiency, congestive heart failure (CHF) and even death. About 60% of the approximately 470,000 patients diagnosed with ARF annually eventually develop RHD, joining the approximately 33 million worldwide with RHD.[10] Chronic manifestations due to residual and progressive valve deformity occur in 9–39% of adults with previous ARF. Fusion of the valve apparatus resulting in stenosis or combination of stenosis and insufficiency develops 2–10 years after an episode of ARF, and recurrent episodes may cause progressive damage to the valves. About 3 million people have chronic HF requiring repeated hospitalization.[9,10] In developing nations, it has been reported that RHD is the cause of HF in 20.1% of all HF patients. Rheumatic heart disease remains a major public health problem in many parts of the world.[11,12] Globally, India contributes nearly 25–50% of newly diagnosed cases, deaths, hospitalizations due to RHD. As per WHO estimates, nearly 133 million deaths annually were attributable to RF/RHD in the Southeast Asia region which includes Indian subcontinent.[11]

Out of 212 patients admitted to ICU, at Sri Jayadeva Institute of Cardiovascular Sciences and Research (SJICSR), in just 3 months of study period, majority of them (166 patients—78%) were with HF, 27 patients with infection, 10 with anemia, 8 patients with cerebrovascular accident (CVA) peripheral embolism in 4 patients with acute coronary syndrome, 3 patients with pericardial effusion, 3 patients with prosthetic valve thrombosis and 1 patient with complete heart block. Out of these 212 patients admitted to ICU, 37 patients (17.45%) expired despite the best treatment.[13]

PATHOPHYSIOLOGY OF HEART FAILURE

In a healthy heart, increased filling of the ventricle results in increased contraction force (by the Frank–Starling law of the heart) and hence increase in cardiac output (CO). But in failing heart, this mechanism fails, as the ventricle is loaded with excessive blood, which the myocardium fails to pump, leading to decreased CO. At this stage venous pressures increase and is accompanied by molecular abnormalities that cause progressive deterioration of the failing heart and premature death of myocardial cells.[14] At the onset of HF various compensatory mechanisms come into action. But these compensatory mechanisms meant for short time are not sustained for a long time, eventually HF occurs. The compensatory increase in sympathetic tone increases the heart rate causing tachycardia, augments myocardial contractility that leads to systemic vasoconstriction which helps to maintain tissue perfusion pressure temporarily at the cost of worsening the load on the heart. But when sympathetic action is undeterred, tachycardia and peripheral vasoconstriction (increased afterload) for a long time leads to substantial increase in cardiac work and myocardial oxygen consumption and demand also increases. The compensatory stimulation of renin-angiotensin-aldosterone system (RAAS) causes vasoconstriction and renal retention of salt and water which increases diastolic filling pressure and increase myocardial contractility through Frank-Starling mechanism.[15] But when these effects are excessive, it causes systemic and pulmonary venous congestion and increases after load. In addition, RAAS, is responsible in mediating renal hyporesponsiveness to the natriuretic peptides, which also facilitates progression of HF.[16] The compensatory ventricular hypertrophy initiated and regulated by many of the signaling molecules that mediate the neurohormonal responses in the failing heart provides more contractile elements. However, abnormal maladaptive hypertrophy ultimately results in myocardial cell death and fibrosis which makes the HF worse. The compliance is the relationship between ventricular end-diastolic pressure and ventricular end-diastolic volume. Compliance is not constant; it is altered by acute and chronic processes such as changes in heart rate or contractility, which are both changed in RHD. This alteration in heart rate due to tachycardia/atrial fibrillation with fast ventricular rate and decreased CO leads to HF.

MECHANISM OF HEART FAILURE IN MITRAL STENOSIS

Mitral stenosis (MS) is the most common lesion in RHD. The MS leads to hypertrophy of left atrium (LA) and its dilatation due to increased pressure, causing atrial fibrillation and mural thrombosis. Left ventricle (LV) is under filled and "protected" by stenosis of mitral valve. LV is usually small or normal in size and contour. Pulmonary arterial pressure increases leading to intimal and medial hypertrophy of pulmonary arteries and increase in pulmonary vascular resistance (PVR). As a result there is right ventricular (RV) dilatation from pressure overload. There is a main pulmonary artery (MPA) dilatation, leading to functional pulmonary valve regurgitation (Graham Steel murmur). Chronic edema of alveolar walls and interstitial edema leading to fibrosis and pulmonary hemosiderosis, leading to breathlessness.

The MS causes:

- Dyspnea on exertion or even at rest (orthopnea), paroxysmal nocturnal dyspnea (PND), pulmonary edema—all due to the high pulmonary capillary pressures.
- Hemoptysis, frequent "bronchitis" can also occur at least in part from high pulmonary pressures. Bronchitis is due to a bronchial hyperemia that leads to increased mucous secretion (passive congestion leads to hyperemia).
- Fatigue—occurs in severe MS and suggests a chronically low CO, often accompanied by RV failure.
- Initial symptom may be of HF from new onset of atrial fibrillation.

In other words, narrowed mitral valve orifice area in severe MS, interferes with blood flow from LA to LV. This leads to build up of pressure in LA and the pulmonary veins (PV), leading to fluid accumulation and causing interstitial edema of the lungs. The increased pressure in pulmonary veins and capillaries is transmitted to pulmonary arteries leading to pulmonary artery hypertension (PAH). This strains the right ventricle (RV), leading to TR and right HF. The elevated pulmonary pressure is a passive phenomenon in most patients, hence PVR is normal. However, a subset (15%) of patients with MS also develop increased PVR so that pulmonary artery (PA) pressure becomes further elevated and frequently causes RV failure because the geometry of the RV is not designed to handle very high PA pressure. RV failure and LV failure have the common characteristics of a low resting CO and high sympathetic tone (Fig. 1). In RV failure, central venous pressure (CVP) rises to utilize the Frank-Starling mechanism but the elevated CVP also leads to jugular vein distension, hepatomegaly, peripheral edema, ascites and possibly defects in coagulation secondary to liver dysfunction.[16]

Electrocardiogram in Mitral Stenosis

If patient of MS is in normal sinus rhythm (NSR), then ECG shows right axis deviation, right ventricular hypertrophy with left atrial enlargement (P-wave duration in lead II

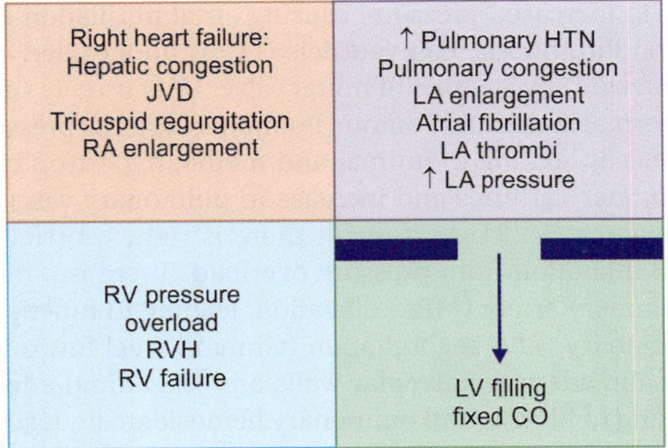

Fig. 1: Pathophysiology in mitral stenosis.

≥0.12 s and/or a P-wave axis between +45 and –30) widened notched P-wave in lead II and mid chest leads as the most common ECG finding called "P-mitrale" (Fig. 2). In severe MS patients with significant PAH, the ECG shows peaked P wave > 2.5 called as P-pulmonale due to RA enlargement. Atrial fibrillation is seen in nearly half of the patients with MS with HF. The most dreaded complication of atrial fibrillation in RHD may cause HF and stroke/thromboembolic events.

Chest X-ray in Mitral Stenosis

The following features are seen in plane CXR in posteroanterior (PA) view:

- Straightening of left heart border of cardiac silhouette is seen due to under, filled LV, convexity along left heart border due to enlarged left atrial appendage and full pulmonary bay due to dilated MPA caused by PAH (Fig. 3).
- Left atrial enlargement causing double shadow along the right border. Extreme enlargement of left atria and appendage cause double density on the PA with posterior displacement of the esophagus laterally and

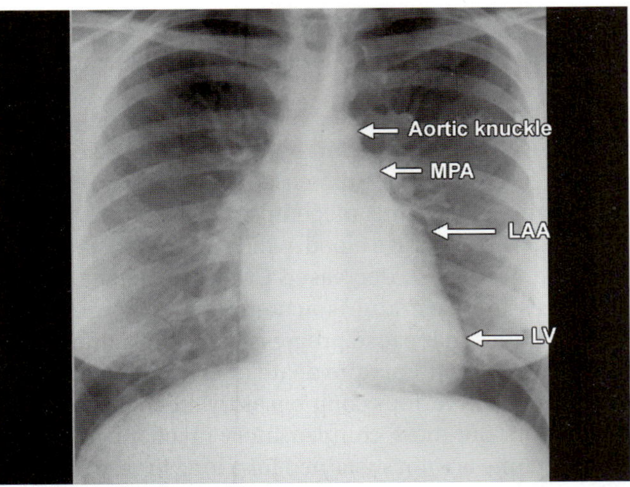

Fig. 3: Plain X-ray chest in posteroanterior (PA) view shows straightening of left border formed by aortic knuckle, main pulmonary artery (MPA), left atrial appendage (LAA) and left ventricle (LV) and apex is lifted up due to RVH in a 23-year-old lady with severe mitral stenosis with pulmonary artery hypertension (PAH).

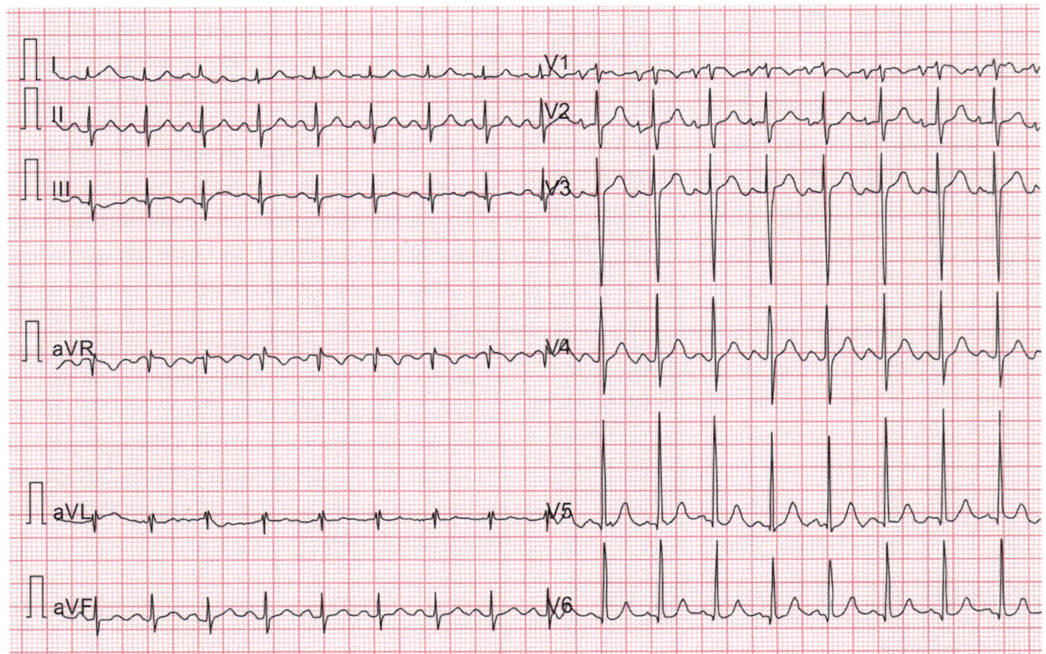

Fig. 2: The 12-lead ECG shows left atrial enlargement [P-wave duration in lead II ≥0.12 s and widened notched P-wave in lead II and mid-chest leads ("P-mitrale") in a 16-year-old girl of rheumatic heart disease (RHD) with mitral stenosis (MS)].

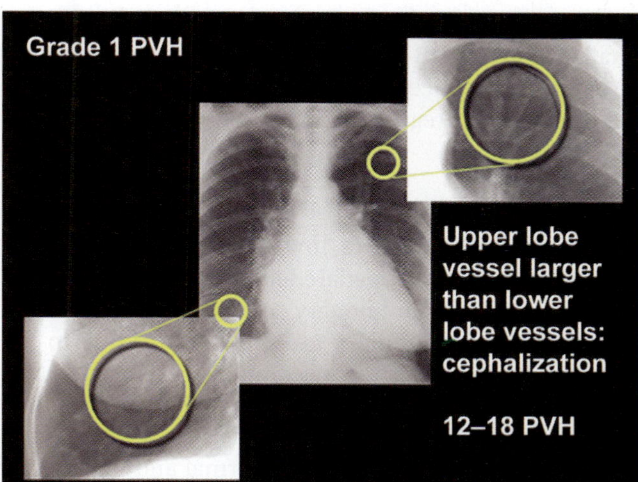

Fig. 4: Chest X-ray (CXR) in posteroanterior (PA) view shows cephalization. Zoomed picture (yellow circles) shows the upper lobe vessels larger than lower lobe vessels indicate mild grade I pulmonary venous hypertension.[12-18]

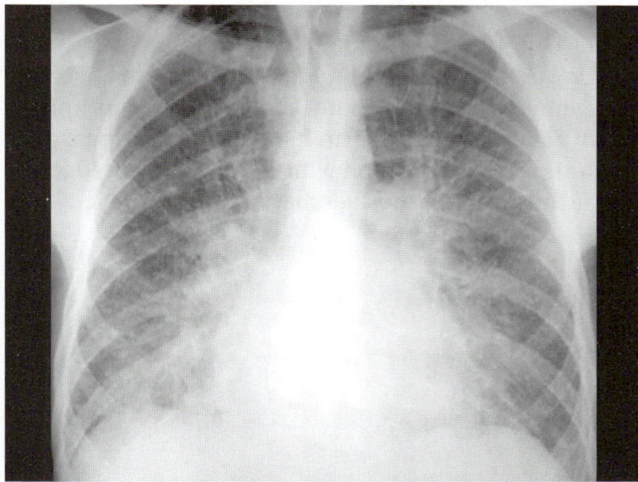

Fig. 5: X-ray chest posteroanterior (PA) view in a 16-year-old boy with rheumatic heart disease (RHD) with mitral stenosis (MS) shows along with cephalization there is prominent hilar bronchovascular markings indicating moderate or grade II pulmonary venous hypertension.[19-23]

left mainstem bronchus elevation causing the widening angle of carina.

- Increased cephalic pulmonary blood flow indicating increased pulmonary pressure. Depending on pulmonary vasculature on CXR, one can assess the possible pressure (Figs. 4 to 6).[12-23]
- Calcified mitral valve. (*Note:* Calcification of the annulus but not the leaflets may lead to regurgitation but not stenosis).
- Kerley B lines.
- PA and RV enlargement.

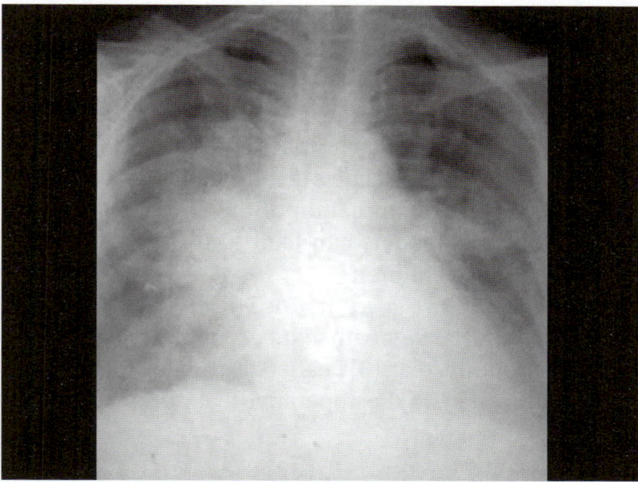

Fig. 6: X-ray chest in posteroanterior (PA) view shows "bat wing appearance" indicating severe or grade 3 pulmonary venous hypertension (PVH) due to alveolar edema (>25 PVH).

Echocardiography

The transthoracic echocardiography (TTE) is the primary imaging tool and should be performed in all women suspected of MS for assessment of hemodynamic severity (mean gradient, mitral valve area and PA pressure), assessment of concomitant valvular lesions and assessment of valve morphology to determine suitability for balloon mitral valvotomy (BMV).

Mechanism of Heart Failure in Mitral Regurgitation

Pathophysiology and symptoms of MR are due to the regurgitation of blood into the LA which forces both the LA and LV to enlarge in order to accommodate not only normal forward blood flow from pulmonary veins, but also the regurgitant volume from LV. The dilated LA accommodates the large regurgitant volume and thus minimizes the rise in LA pressures. Consequently, the pulmonary vasculature is not subjected to high pressures in initial stages. So patient with MR is asymptomatic for many years. LV dilatation, plus modest muscle hypertrophy, maintains a normal forward output. But the LV cannot enlarge indefinitely. Hence eventually forward output suffers and the patient develops early easy fatigability as opposed to shortness of breath. Dyspnea on exertion is a common symptom as the LV myocardium deteriorates as LV end-diastolic pressure (LVEDP) rises[11] and congestive symptoms (PND, orthopnea, dyspnea) appear as the pulmonary capillary pressures rise with LVEDP. Such symptoms suggest at least some, if not severe, LV failure.

ACUTE MITRAL REGURGITATION WITH HEART FAILURE

There is severe inflammatory process in mitral valve apparatus, especially the chordae tendineae and anterior and/or posterior mitral leaflets in the patients with ARF with carditis.[17] Severe inflammation of the chordal structures and mitral valve leaflets can lead to isolated MR, seen predominantly in children.

The various causes for acute MR are: (1) Valvulitis, thickened mitral leaflets with reduced mobility. (2) Chordae tendineae rupture/tear. (3) Leaflet destruction/perforation (e.g. endocarditis). (4) Postoperative leaky prosthetic valve (usually paravalvular).

Pathophysiology

In acute regurgitation LA is small as time is not there for it to dilate. Hence LA is not compliant; in consequence the "V" wave is large and LA pressures become more elevated than in chronic MR. RV failure is common in acute MR. High PAH may lead to RV failure via increased MR causing increased left atrial pressure (LAP) leading to increased PA pressure causing RV decompensation. The systemic vasodilation leads to a decreased regurgitant fraction by shrinking the LV and allowing closer apposition of the mitral valve apparatus. 50% regurgitation in acute MR is much more serious than 50% regurgitation on a chronic basis because the LV is smaller in acute MR and forward stroke volume and CO is remarkably reduced in acute MR more than in chronic MR. The degree of regurgitation worsens with LV dilatation.

Symptoms

Easy fatigability (due to low CO), dyspnea (due to pulmonary congestion), pedal edema (RV decompensation) are common. Frank pulmonary edema occurs with severe dysfunction (e.g. papillary muscle rupture) due to the very high LA pressures that accompany severe acute MR. Cardiogenic shock may be the consequence of an impaired forward CO, leading to acute severe dyspnea, CHF and hypotension. The LV size may be normal and may not be hyperdynamic. Loud S1 systolic murmur may or may not be pansystolic inflow/rumble is heard and S3 may be the only abnormality.

ECG in Mitral Regurgitation

The ECG in mitral regurgitation shows LA enlargement and LVH (50% of patients with severe MR), both LA and LV enlargement with AF in about 33% and RV hypertrophy in 15% of patients RVH is seen in 15%, combined hypertrophy in 5% and atrial fibrillation with course see-saw edge like course flutter fibrillary waves may be seen (Fig. 7).

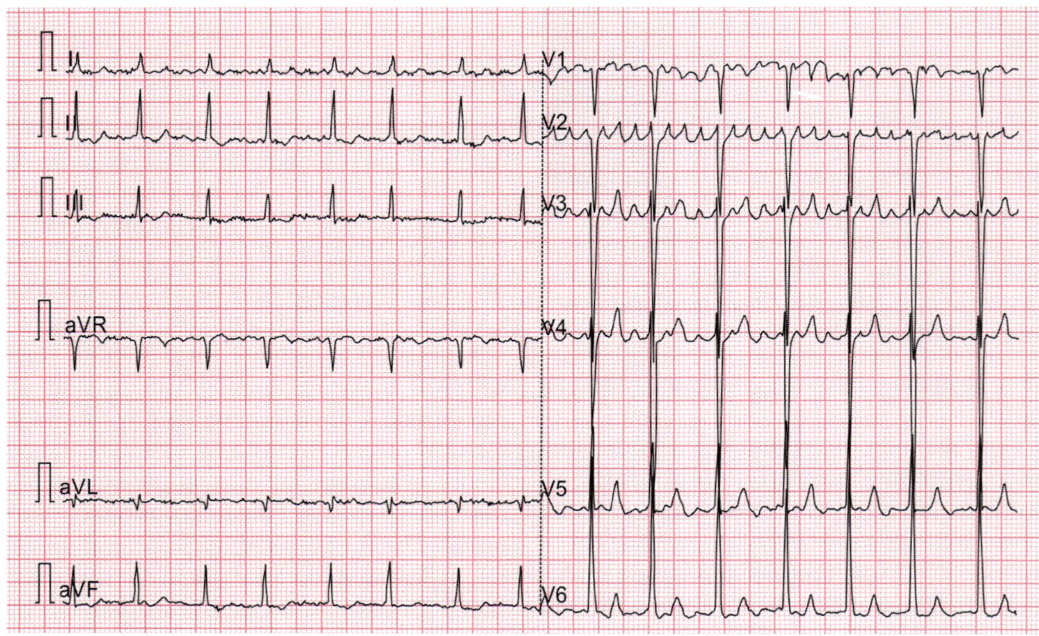

Fig. 7: ECG shows course flutter fibrillary waves with varying R-R intervals in a 26-year-old lady with rheumatic heart disease (RHD) with mitral regurgitation (MR).

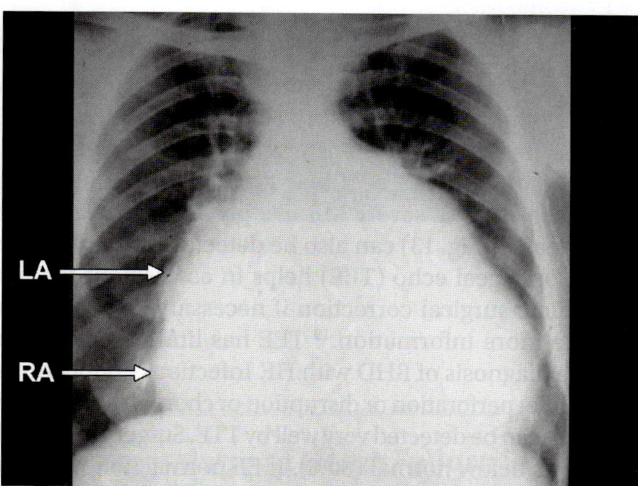

Fig. 8: Chest X-ray shows cardiomegaly, left atrial (LA) border extending beyond the right atrial (RA) border, prominent upper pulmonary veins illustrating staghorn appearance in a 32-year-old woman with rheumatic heart disease (RHD) with severe mitral regurgitation.

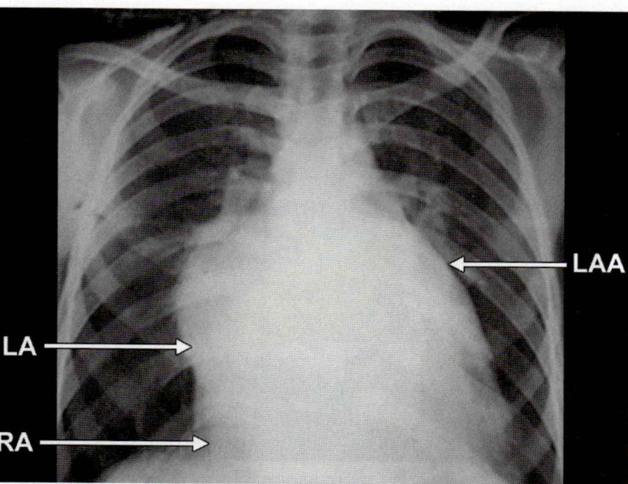

Fig. 9: Chest X-ray (CXR) in posteroanterior (PA) view shows giant left atrium (LA), the border of LA is seen much beyond the right atrium (RA) with a prominent left atrial appendage (LAA).

Chest X-ray in Mitral Regurgitation

Chest X-ray in PA view shows cardiomegaly due to dilatation of both left ventricle (LV) and LA. The double shadow on the right border due to enlargement of LA, prominent cephalic vessels (staghorn appearance) are seen due to increased pulmonary venous pressure (Fig. 8). Cephalization of pulmonary veins is called as "staghorn appearance" or "inverted moustache" is seen in the upper zone. The giant LA is seen even beyond RA border (Fig. 9) CXR is also very useful after mitral valve repair and reduction in size of LA after surgical plication of giant LA the X-ray see the difference before and after surgery (Figs. 10A and B).

Two-dimensional Echocardiography

In patients with MR, TTE is the commonly used to assess the mechanisms, severity, reparability, and consequences of MR.[19] The size and function of the left and right ventricle, the size of the LA, the degree of PAH and the presence of other associated valve lesions need to be evaluated. The severity of MR can be assessed more accurately by measurement of the width of the "vena contracta" (Fig. 11). One can provide precise anatomical delineation of the different lesions,

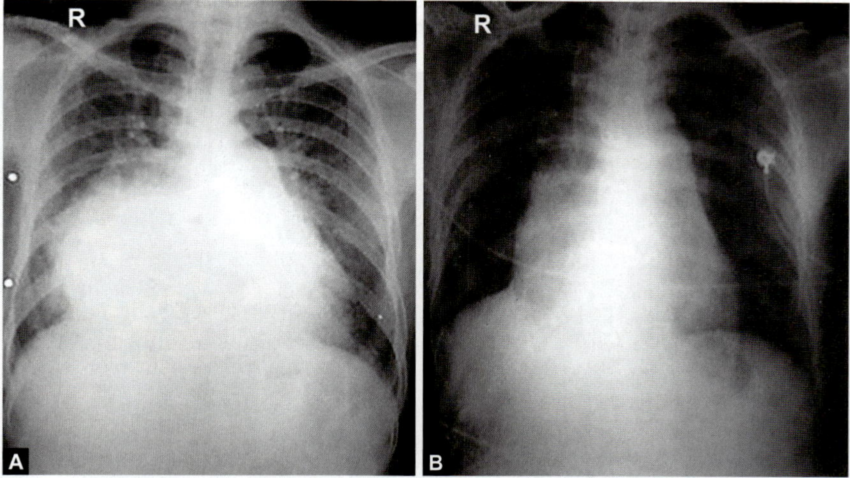

Figs. 10A and B: (A) X-ray in posterioranterior (PA) view shows cardiomegaly with gross dilatation of left atrium (LA) extending beyond the right atrium (RA), cephalization of pulmonary veins in upper zone; (B) Post-operation after mitral valve repair and plication of LA chest X-ray (CXR) shows no cardiomegaly and no LA enlargement and no venous congestion.

Inadequate aortic valve closure allows blood to enter the LV from the aorta during diastole. With aortic regurgitation, leads to rapid fall in pressure and aortic diastolic pressure becomes very low. LVEDP is elevated because of the regurgitant flow that tries to equilibrate LVEDP with diastolic aortic pressure, but a short diastolic time period and a large, compliant LV may prevent the equalization of pressures from occurring. LA pressures and pulmonary artery wedge (PAW) may not be very elevated. Forward

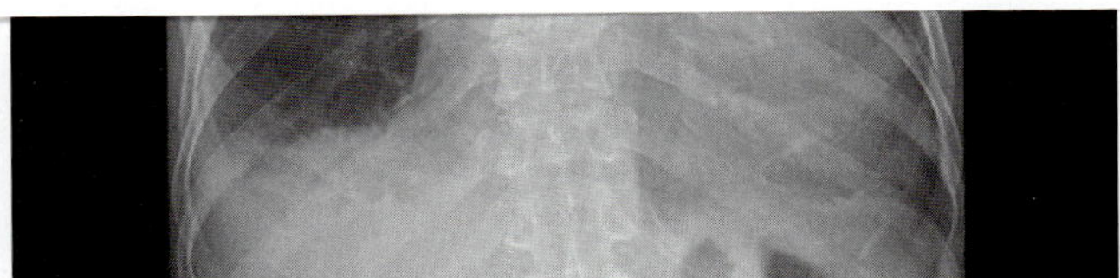

Fig. 14: Chest X-ray (CXR) in posteroanterior (PA) view shows gross cardiomegaly due to large left ventricle in a 43-year-old man with rheumatic heart disease (RHD) with mitral stenosis (MS) and mitral regurgitation (MR) with severe aortic regurgitation.

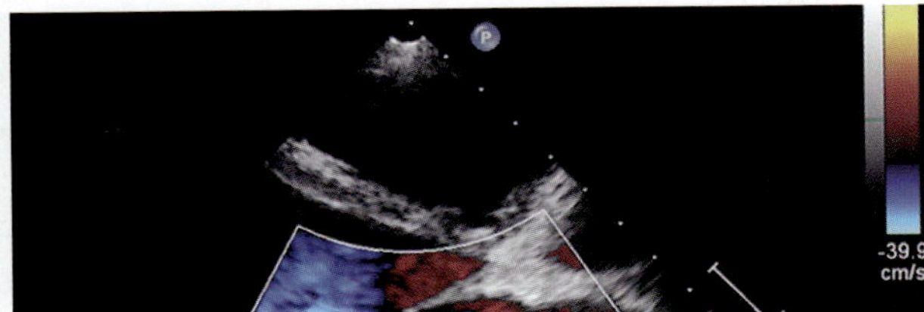

which must be related to the segmental and functional anatomy according to the Carpentier classification in order to assess the feasibility of repair. One can also assesses mitral annular dimensions by echocardiography.[18] TTE can also detect the cause for severe MR, e.g. chordal tear can be detected in apical four chamber view (Fig. 12). The other cases of severe MR like perforation of anterior

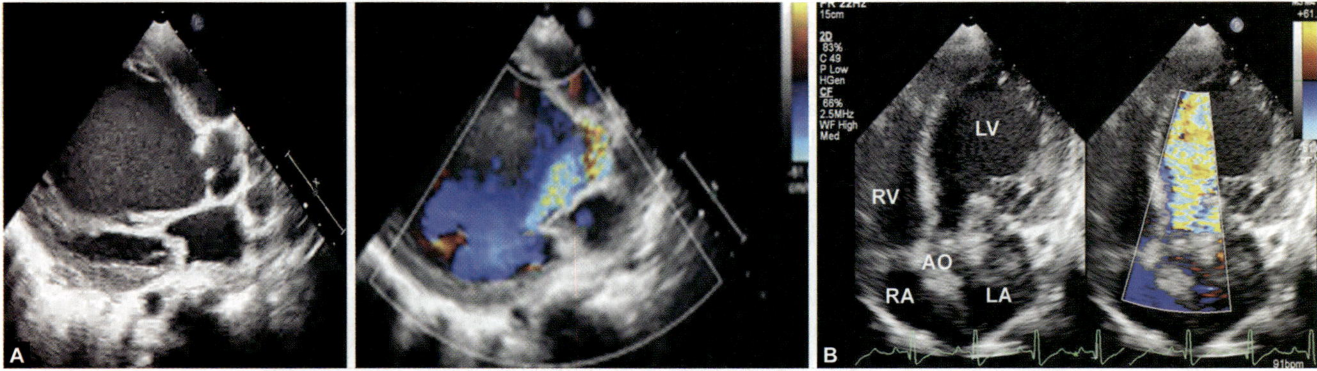

Figs. 15A and B: (A) Transthoracic echocardiography (TTE) in parasternal long-axis view showed dilated LV with reduced contraction, thickened, beaded AV, and MV with reduced mobility; colored Doppler showed severe AR and mild MR; (B) Apical five chamber view with color Doppler shows severe AR in a 12-year-old boy who presented with history of breathlessness NYHA IV symptoms in cardiogenic shock and treated as dilated cardiomyopathy (DCM) elsewhere as the diagnosis of rheumatic heart disease (RHD) was missed.

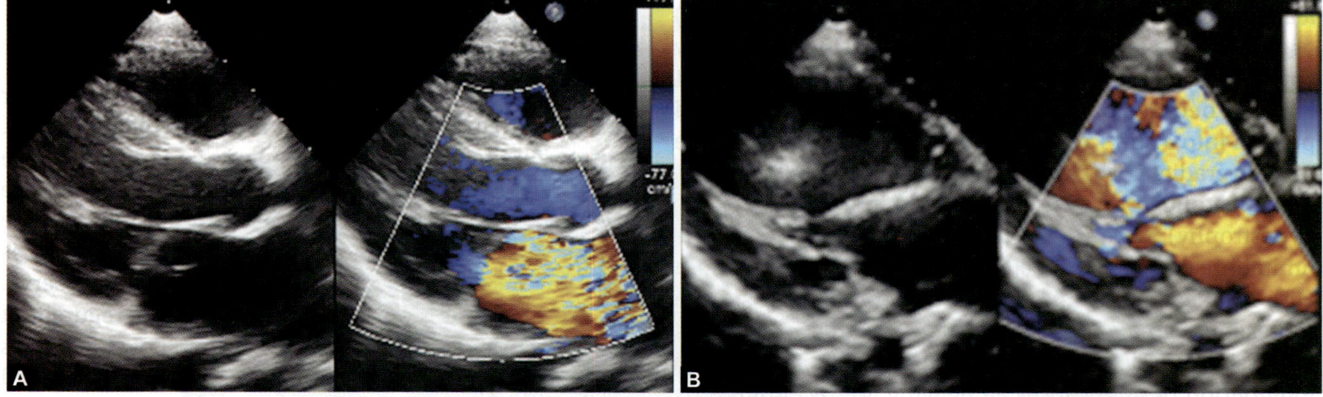

Figs. 16A and B: (A) Transthoracic echocardiography (TTE) in parasternal long-axis view with color Doppler in systole shows severe MR; (B) Diastole shows severe AR in a13-year-old boy with history of fever, easy fatigability for 7 days with multiple migratory joint pains involving large joints, restriction of movements. ASLO-480 and CRP-positive.

flow may raise LV diastolic pressure so quickly as to cause premature closure of the mitral valve. Premature closure prevents the LAP from becoming equal to the high LVEDP, but it also prematurely stops filling of the LV from the LA. Note that this means that PAW pressure will be less than LVEDP. If the patient has associated MR then, this protection is lost (Figs. 16A and B). Some acute compensation is achieved by high sympathetic tone and tachycardia, the former preserves BP while the latter improves total CO and limits diastolic pressure fall off.[20]

Mechanism of Heart Failure in Tricuspid Stenosis

Tricuspid stenosis (TS), which is mostly of rheumatic origin, is rarely observed in developed countries although it is still seen in developing countries.[20] Detection requires careful clinical and TTE evaluation, as it is almost always associated with mitral/aortic valve lesions that dominate the presentation.[11] Evaluation and clinical signs are often masked by those of the associated other valvular lesions, especially MS.[14]

Echocardiography

Echocardiography provides the most useful information. Tricuspid stenosis is often overlooked and requires careful evaluation (Fig. 17). The pressure half-time method is less valid for the assessment of the severity of TS than of MS and the continuity equation is rarely applicable because of the frequency with which associated regurgitation is present. Planimetry of the valve area is usually impossible unless 3D echocardiography is used. Generally no accepted grading of severity TS exists. A mean gradient ≥5 mm Hg at normal heart rate is considered indicative of clinically

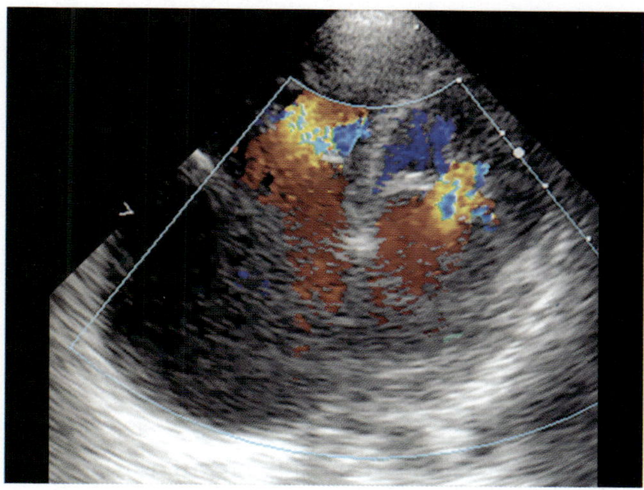

Fig. 17: Transthoracic echocardiography (TTE) in apical 4-chamber view with color Doppler shows MS and TS in a 8-year-old boy of rheumatic heart disease (RHD) with juvenile MS.

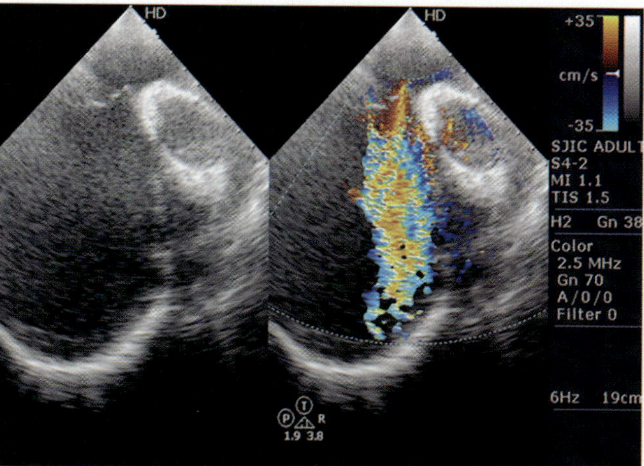

Fig. 18: Transthoracic echocardiography (TTE) in apical 4-chamber view shows giant RA with severe TR in a 34-year-old lady with HF who had under gone balloon mitral valvuloplasty (BMV) earlier and developed restenosis with severe pulmonary artery hypertension. She also had moderate AS and AR.

significant TS.[16] Echocardiography should also examine the presence of commissural fusion, the anatomy of the valve and its subvalvular apparatus, which are the most important determinants of reparability and the degree of concomitant TR.

Mechanism of Heart Failure in Tricuspid Regurgitation

Tricuspid regurgitation (TR) develops either primarily due to ARF or secondary to severe pulmonary hypertension due to chronic RHD with MS/MR. The right atrium (RA) and right ventricle dilate secondary to volume overload by TR. Right HF secondary TR is due to annular dilatation and RV pressure and/or volume overload (Fig. 18). Pressure overload is most often caused by pulmonary hypertension resulting from left-sided heart failure.[20,21]

Pregnancy and Rheumatic Heart Disease[18,22,23]

The RHD may increase the maternal and fetal risks during pregnancy. Patients with RHD respond differently to the hemodynamics of pregnancy depending on the type and severity of maternal valvular disease, the resulting abnormalities of functional capacity, LV function and pulmonary pressure. The pregnancy increases the heart rate, blood volume and CO and this is poorly tolerated by women with left-sided obstructive lesions. On the other hand, the decrease in systemic vascular resistance often benefits women with regurgitant lesions until delivery, when the abrupt increase in vascular resistance may precipitate pulmonary edema. The women with pulmonary hypertension are particularly intolerant of the hemodynamic changes of pregnancy and represent an exceptionally high-risk group.

In pregnant women with moderate or severe MS (valve area < 1.5 cm^2), HF is progressive and eventually pulmonary edema can occur, particularly during the second and third trimesters.[18,21,22] An increase in LA and pulmonary pressures contributes to atrial wall stress and the development of atrial fibrillation (AF). Also even in previously asymptomatic women, AF, fever, anemia can cause hemodynamic decompensation. The maternal and fetal outcomes are directly related to the severity of MS and the prepregnancy NYHA functional class. Though AF is (<15%), it carries the additional risk of thromboembolic events. The mortality is between 0 and 3%.[18,22,23] The prematurity rates are 20–30%, intrauterine growth retardation 5–20% and stillbirth 1–3%.[18,22] The fetal morbidity has been estimated at approximately 33% in patients with severe MS with HF, compared to 28% in patients with moderate MS and 14% in patients with mild MS.[22] The absolute mortality appears to be low, despite reported high morbidity.[18]

Why does pregnancy aggravate heart failure in mitral stenosis?

Increase in blood volume by 30–50% leads to increase in capillary hydrostatic pressure that causes pulmonary edema. Decrease in SVR and increase in HR 10–20 beats/min causing reduced diastolic filling time of LV. Increase in CO by 30–50% leads to increase in transmitral valvular gradient. The rise in LA pressure during labor and delivery leads to sympathetic stimulation causing rise in heart rate

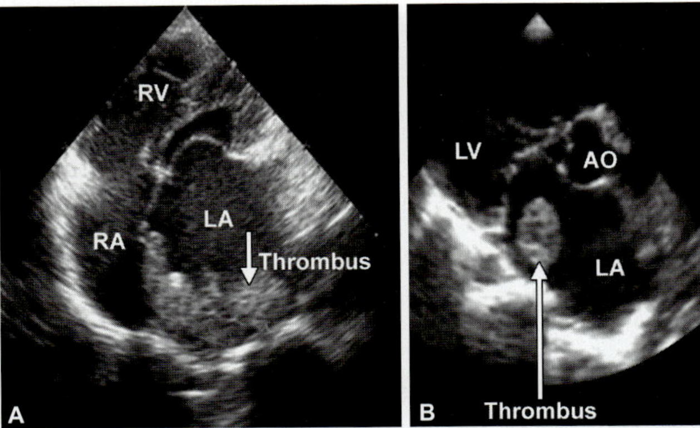

Figs. 19A and B: (A) Transthoracic echocardiography (TTE) in rheumatic heart disease (RHD) with MS shows mural thrombus attached to the roof of LA; (B) TTE shows ball wall mobile thrombus in LA in a 24-year-old lady with RHD, severe MS.

(HR) and CO. The sudden increase in venous return as compression on inferior vena cava (IVC) by the fetus is no more there after delivery and also autotransfusion blood occurs from placental bed increases the preload and makes the symptoms of MS worse. Atrial enlargement in pregnancy causes atrial fibrillation precipitating HF. To compound the problem hypercoagulability during labor increases risk of thromboembolic episodes especially if mural thrombus is detected on TTE (Figs. 19A and B).

Manifestations of Heart Failure in Rheumatic Heart Disease

Irrespective of which valve is involved, the first manifestation of CHF is usually tachycardia. An obvious exception to this finding occurs in CHF due to a primary bradyarrhythmias or complete heart block. As the severity of CHF increases, signs of venous congestion usually ensue. Left-sided HF is generally associated with signs of pulmonary venous congestion, whereas right-sided HF is associated with signs of systemic venous congestion. Marked failure of either ventricle, however, can affect the function of the other, leading to systemic and pulmonary venous congestion. Later stages of CHF are characterized by signs and symptoms of low CO. Generally, CHF with normal CO is called compensated CHF, and CHF with inadequate CO is considered decompensated.

Diagnosis

Early diagnosis of HF in RHD is very important to initiate appropriate treatment to reduce morbidity, mortality, and cost of repeated hospitalizations. However, the diagnosis can be challenging at times as not all HF patients exhibit typical symptoms and neither do all patients who have seemingly typical symptoms have HF.[23] Hence, clinical evaluation and diagnostic tools are the two key aspects for the accurate diagnosis. Clinical evaluation involves a detailed history (individual and family) and thorough physical examination.[24,25] Observation of various signs and symptoms elucidated during the clinical evaluation aid in the process of diagnosis.[24,25] It may be specifically difficult to recognize and interpret the signs and symptoms of HF in patients who are obese or elderly or have comorbid chronic lung disease.[24]

TREATMENT OF HEART FAILURE IN RHEUMATIC HEART DISEASE

The goals of therapy for HF in ARF and RHD can largely be divided into supportive care and correction of underlying causes. Supportive care is focused on optimizing CO and is achieved by reducing preload, modulating HR, increasing contractility, and reducing afterload (except in the presence of obstructive lesions). The use of mechanical assistance in fulminant or end-stage HF is increasing, with extracorporeal membrane oxygenation (ECMO) or mechanical assist devices. Acutely the goal is to maintain CO and organ perfusion, chronically to allow for normal growth and development. Correction of the underlying cause mainly applies to surgical correction or palliation of structural lesions, but will also include treatment of underlying diseases, such as correction of thyroid dysfunction or anemia, and treatment of renal failure. Prevention of complications is an important consideration particularly in tight MS, as they are at significant risk of mural thrombus. Anticoagulation with warfarin or low molecular weight heparin should be used.

Management

Even if patient needs surgery, medical stabilization with vasodilator therapy will help. Some patients will also need inotropic support and/or intra-aortic balloon pump (IABP). Treatment for acute MR is similar to chronic MR—except that contractility may need more active support. Vasodilator therapy may have limited effectiveness because the total CO of a normal-sized ventricle is smaller than that of a chronically enlarged ventricle. Vasodilation may lead to hypotension if the rise in CO fails to match the drop in SVR. Induction of anesthesia must proceed slowly and drugs must be given in small increments. Loss of sympathetic tone may rapidly lead to a fall in SVR and BP. Operative mortality for emergent valve replacement correlates with the end-systolic volume (ESV). If the ESV is normal (30–90 cc/m^2), MVR is well tolerated. If ESV is more than 90 cc/m^2, then high operative mortality is seen. Diuretics are useful in the presence of HF, but of limited efficacy unless the lesion is taken care of.

Nondrug Therapy

A major focus of pediatric medicine is growth and nutrition. Children with HF are no exception to this. Lethargy and gut congestion may lead to decreased oral intake and assimilation, while energy expenditure is often more due to increased catabolism. Underlying metabolic conditions may require specific dietary therapy. The most crucial of these is nutrition; it is essential that adequate nutrition be supplied to the child in HF, but excess sodium should be avoided. In the case of infants, reduced-volume, high energy feeds, 120–150 kcal/kg/day may be required in order to supply the body with the increased energy demands of HF, without overburdening the circulation with excess fluid.

Treatment of the Precipitating Events

Most of the important variables subject to manipulation in the management of rheumatic heart disease can be organized into four categories: (1) Rate and rhythm, (2) Preload, (3) Afterload, and (4) Contractility. If one can remember these four items and the pathophysiology of the lesion, the management of each item should become apparent. Almost always, the worsening in clinical state of apatient with CHF can be traced to a precipitating event, the treatment of which leads to significant improvement. The checklist includes rheumatic activity, infective endocarditis, intercurrent infections, anemia, electrolyte imbalances, arrhythmia, pulmonary embolism, drug interactions, drug toxicity or noncompliance, and other system disturbances.

Treatment of Congested State

This deals with the conventional medical management of CHF. The therapy is often resorted to before a definitive diagnosis is made, and is chronically used. It is aimed at reducing the pulmonary or systemic congestion (diuretics), reducing the disproportionately elevated afterload (vasodilators including ACE inhibitors), increasing contractility (inotropes), and other measures.

OTHER OPTIONS

Extracorporeal membrane oxygenation has evolved into an excellent method of preoperative and postoperative support in the treatment of HF. Along with ECMO, the left ventricular assist device (LVAD) and the IABP have also found a place in the management of RHD patients with HF. There is a 74% survival rate and the long-term outcome has been excellent in most cases.[26,27]

Ventricular Assist Devices

The use of mechanical assist devices for the treatment of end-stage HF in children awaiting transplant has been increasing as the device design has allowed for lower pump volumes. In the older child and adolescent, use of a mechanical assist device results in successful bridge to transplantation in 80% of cases.[28,29]

Heart Transplantation

Heart transplantation remains the therapy of choice for end-stage HF in RHD refractory to surgical and medical therapy. Current 1-year survival after heart transplantation in children is 85%; overall survival 20 years after transplantation is 40%.

CONCLUSION

The cardiac involvement is the most serious complication of ARF and causes significant morbidity and mortality. Heart failure in ARF and RHD patients continues to be a challenge to the treating clinicians. The number of patients with RHD and HF increases if timely interventions and surgery are not performed. Although guidelines have been developed for the management of decompensated HF in other conditions, they are limited in RHD with HF because of the paucity of proper studies. Recent advances in our understanding of the pathophysiologic mechanisms involved in the HF have led to changes in our approach to the treatment of RHD with HF. The management of HF in ARF and RHD poses many challenges and requires a comprehensive and integrative approach by cardiologists and cardiac surgeons. The goals of RHD therapy have shifted from treating HF to prevention of ARF, RHD and HF.

REFERENCES

1. WHO. The World Health Report 2000—Health System: improving performance. Geneva: WHO; 2000.
2. Medscape. (2019). Rheumatic Fever Clinical Presentation. [online] Available from https://emedicine.medscape.com/article/236582-clinical [Last accessed, 2019].
3. Eisenberg MJ. Rheumatic heart disease in the developing world: prevalence, prevention, and control. Eur Heart J. 1993;14:122-8.
4. Marijon E, Ou P, Celermajer DS, et al. Prevalence of rheumatic heart disease detected by echocardiographic screening. N Engl J Med. 2007;357:470-6.
5. Padmavati S. Rheumatic heart disease: prevalence and preventive measures in the Indian subcontinent. Keywords: rheumatic heart disease; rheumatic fever. Heart. 2001;86:127.
6. Carapetis JR, Steer AC, Mulholland EK, et al. The global burden of group A streptococcal diseases. Lancet Infect Dis. 2005;5:685-94.

7. Damasceno A, Cotter G, Dzudie A, et al. Heart failure in sub-saharan Africa: time for action. J Am Coll Cardiol. 2007;50:1688-93.
8. WHO. The World Health Report 2004—changing history. Geneva: WHO; 2004.
9. World Health Organization. Rheumatic fever and rheumatic heart disease. Report of a WHO Study Group. Technical Report Series No. 764. World Health Organization: Geneva; 1988.
10. Nieminen MS, Böhm M, Cowie MR, et al. Executive summary of the guidelines on the diagnosis and treatment of acute heart failure: the Task Force on Acute Heart Failure of the European Society of Cardiology. Eur Heart J. 2005;26: 384-416.
11. Amoah AG, Kallen C. Aetiology of heart failure as seen from a National Cardiac Referral Centre in Africa. Cardiology. 2000;93:11-8.
12. World Health Organization. Rheumatic fever and rheumatic heart disease. World Health Organ Tech Rep Ser. 2004;923: 1-122.
13. Vijayalakshmi IB. Rheumatic heart disease—A neglected giant. In: PK Deb (Ed). Cardiology Update 2012. Kolkata: CSI; 2012. pp.15-22.
14. Sipido KR, Eisner D. Something old, something new: changing views on the cellular mechanism of heart failure. Cardiovasc Res. 2005;68:167-74.
15. Mehra MR, Uber PA, Potluri S. Renin angiotensin aldosterone and adrenergic modulation in chronic heart failure: contemporary concepts. Am J Med Sci. 2002;20:1465-8.
16. Otto CM, Bonow RO. Valvular heart disease. In: Libby P, Bonow RO, Mann DL, Zipes DP (Eds). Braunwald's Heart Disease: A Textbook of Cardiovascular Medicine, 8th edition. Philadelphia, PA: WB Saunders; 2007. pp.1625-712.
17. Vijayalakshmi IB. The efficacy of echocardiographic criterions for the diagnosis of carditis in acute rheumatic fever. Cardiol Young. 2008;18:586-92.
18. Lancellotti P, Moura L, Pierard LA, et al. European Association of Echocardiography recommendations for the assessment of valvular regurgitation. Part 2: mitral and tricuspid regurgitation (native valve disease). Eur J Echocardiogr. 2010;11:307-32.
19. Salcedo EE, Quaife RA, Seres T, et al. A framework for systematic characterization of the mitral valve by real-time three-dimensional transesophageal echocardiography. J Am Soc Echocardiogr. 2009;22:1087-99.
20. Le Tourneau T, Messika-Zeitoun D, Russo A, et al. Impact of left atrial volume on clinical outcome in organic mitral regurgitation. J Am Coll Cardiol. 2010;56:570-8.
21. Vahanian A, Alfieri O, Andreotti F, et al. Guidelines on the management of valvular heart disease (version 2012). Joint Task Force on the Management of Valvular Heart Disease of the European Society of Cardiology (ESC); European Association for Cardio-Thoracic Surgery (EACTS). Eur Heart J. 2012;33:2451-96.
22. Elkayam U, Bitar F. Valvular heart disease and pregnancy part I: native valves. J Am Coll Cardiol. 2005;46:223-30.
23. Lesniak-Sobelga A, Tracz W, KostKiewicz M, et al. Clinical and echocardiographic assessment of pregnant women with valvular heart diseases—maternal and fetal outcome. Int J Cardiol. 2004;94:15-23.
24. Hameed A, Karaalp IS, Tummala PP, et al. The effect of valvular heart disease on maternal and fetal outcome of pregnancy. J Am Coll Cardiol. 2001;37:893-9.
25. Silversides CK, Colman JM, Sermer M, et al. Cardiac risk in pregnant women with rheumatic mitral stenosis. Am J Cardiol. 2003;91:1382-5.
26. Zelop C, Heffner LF. The downside of cesarean delivery: short- and long-term complications. Clin Obstet Gynecol. 2004:47;386-93.
27. Burch M, Aurora P. Current status of paediatric heart, lung, and heart-lung transplantation. Arch Dis Child. 2004;89:386-9.
28. Blume ED, Naftel DC, Bastardi HJ, et al. Outcomes of children bridged to heart transplantation with ventricular assist devices: a multi-institutional study. Circulation. 2006;113:2313-9.
29. Khan A, Gazzaniga AB. Mechanical circulatory assistance in paediatric patients with cardiac failure. Cardiovasc Surg. 1996;4:43-9.

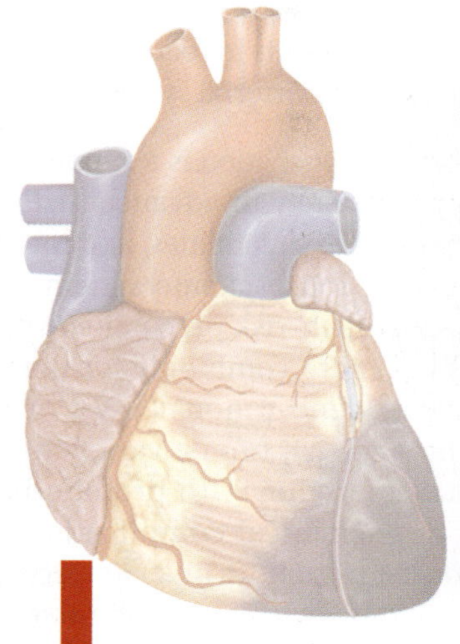

CHAPTER

Heart Support Devices in Heart Failure

Vivudh P Singh, Vishal Rastogi, Vijay Kumar, Ashok Seth

INTRODUCTION

Remarkable advances in surgical approaches for the management of heart failure (HF) have occurred over the past decade. Mechanical circulatory support (MCS) devices are the new paradigm shift in treatment armamentarium for patients with advanced HF refractory to optimal medical therapy. In patients with acute decompensated HF or cardiogenic shock, temporary percutaneous MCS devices, including intra-aortic balloon pump (IABP), extracorporeal membrane oxygenation (ECMO), and the axial flow Impella device, can be employed to support end-organ perfusion while awaiting myocardial recovery, hemodynamic stability, or in irreversible cases, facilitate additional time to consider candidacy for more durable therapeutic options such as long-term MCS or cardiac transplantation.[1,2] Although heart transplantation remains the gold standard therapeutic intervention for end-stage chronic HF, with over 50% of patients now surviving beyond 10 years,[3] this therapy remains limited by a chronic shortage of donor organs. Durable left ventricular assist device (LVAD) therapy, whether as interim stabilization and/or optimization while awaiting heart transplantation or as lifetime support for patients deemed ineligible for transplantation, has significantly improved survival, functional capacity, and quality of life for advanced HF patients.[3-8]

Device options: Mechanical circulatory support can be classified in number of ways. Four factors determine classification: duration of support (short-term vs long-term), configuration of ventricular assist (biventricular vs univentricular), pump flow pattern (pulsatile vs continuous-flow), and location of implantation (extracorporeal vs extracorporeal).

Short-term device options: Mechanical circulatory support is considered short-term when the duration of support is from days to weeks.

IABP: The intra-aortic balloon pump has been the most widely used MCS device in the world over the past 50 years. The device is intuitive to most cardiovascular specialists and can be inserted in a variety of clinical settings including the catheterization laboratory and cardiac care unit. The IABP consists of a 7.5–9.5 Fr catheter inserted in the femoral artery. The device consists of a variably sized balloon that inflates during ventricular diastole and deflates during ventricular systole. The balloon is positioned distal to the left subclavian artery and above the renal arteries.

Impella: The Impella series of devices is capable of providing partial or full support of both left and right ventricular function. The principles of the Impella heart pump design allow for direct unloading of the ventricle from the inflow, and increased MAP and flow in the aorta from the outflow of the device. The ability to unload the ventricle by reducing ventricular end-diastolic pressures and volumes reduce wall tension, microvascular resistance, and increasing coronary perfusion. This results in overall improvement in oxygen supply while simultaneously reducing oxygen demand. The 9 Fr catheter-based system can be inserted peripherally using an over the wire technique or centrally into the aorta. The left ventricular devices are shaped like a

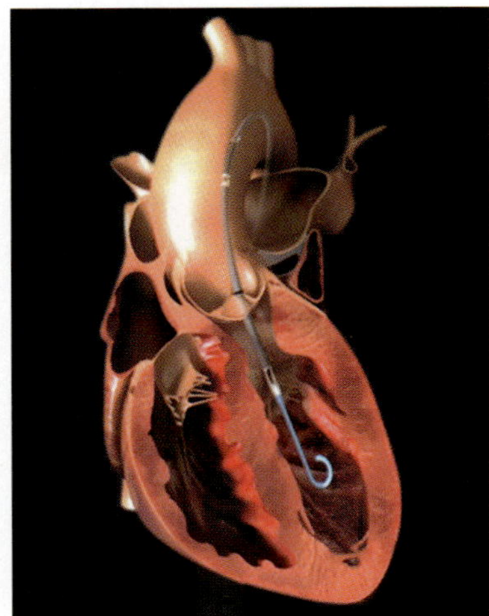

Fig. 1: Impella device.

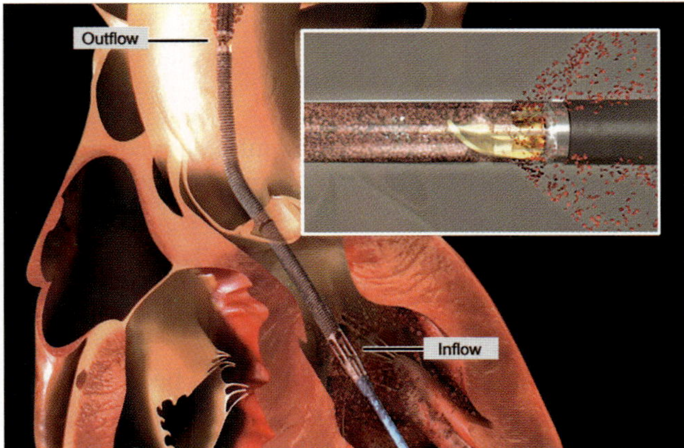

Fig. 2: TandemHeart.

pigtail catheter with an incorporated microaxial pump that draws blood from the ventricle and ejects it into the aorta. The smallest version of the device provide up to 2.5 L/min of output while the larger devices can deliver up to 5 L/min. The right-sided Impella (Impella RP) is inserted via the femoral vein and positioned such that the inflow sits at the inferior vena cava-right atrial junction and the outflow is in the pulmonary artery just above the pulmonic valve (Fig. 1).

The Impella products were designed for short-term support and have approval for use up to 6 hour. In practice, many centers extend the support duration and tailor it to patient need and effective circulatory support.

TandemHeart: The TandemHeart (Fig. 2) ventricular assist device (VAD) is an extracorporeal, centrifugal flow device that is capable of 5 L/min output. Left atrial access is obtained by venous cannulation that traverses the intra-atrial septum. The blood is returned to the arterial circulation via a catheter placed in the contralateral femoral artery. The relative instability of the system necessitates the patient be bed- bound during support as retraction of the inflow cannula into the right atrium results in recirculation of deoxygenated blood in the systemic arterial system.

ECMO: Extracorporeal membrane oxygenation is a support strategy used with increasing frequency in advanced HF centers based upon rapid deployment capabilities, and the ability to support both the circulatory and respiratory systems. ECMO has been used to support high-risk percutaneous coronary intervention (PCI) but more commonly for the treatment of respiratory failure [veno-venous (V-V)] or cardiogenic shock [veno-arterial (V-A)] from a variety of causes including myocardial infarction with profound ventricular dysfunction or a mechanical complication such as a ventricular septal defect or rupture of a papillary muscle, refractory ventricular tachycardia, and cardiac arrest. The ECMO circuit consists of cannula inserted either percutaneously via the femoral vasculature or centrally. Veno-venous ECMO is used for respiratory failure—blood is drawn from the right atrium and circulated through an oxygenator where there is passive exchange of O_2 and CO_2 prior to return of oxygenated blood to the right atrium. Success of V-V ECMO depends upon adequate function of the right ventricle. In V-A ECMO, blood is drawn from the right atrium and passed through the oxygenator prior to return to the arterial circulation. In the V-A configuration, the ECMO circuit is essentially functioning as a biventricular support device.

There are several important clinical considerations when using peripheral ECMO. First, return of oxygenated blood to the iliofemoral system may be insufficient to ensure adequate oxygenation of the head vessels and heart. The oxygen saturation in the right arm is a good indicator of adequacy of central and cerebral oxygenation. Second, peripherally cannulated patients with profound left ventricular dysfunction may develop pulmonary edema resulting an elevated left ventricular pressure. Despite cannulation of the right heart, residual pulmonary circulation, Thebesian vein drainage and aortic insufficiency all may contribute to LV volume loading. Daily chest radiographs should be performed to monitor the pulmonary volume status. If pulmonary edema is noted, additional venting of the LV is required to avoid permanent lung injury. Venting techniques include surgical placement of an LV apical drain, or further support with a percutaneous device such as IABP or Impella. Additional ECMO complications include insertion site bleeding, infections and vascular occlusion. In the case of peripheral ECMO, arterial occlusion from the large arterial cannula may result in lower extremity arterial insufficiency. An antegrade perfusion catheter may be prophylactically placed that provides oxygenated blood distally in the leg with arterial cannulation (Fig. 3).

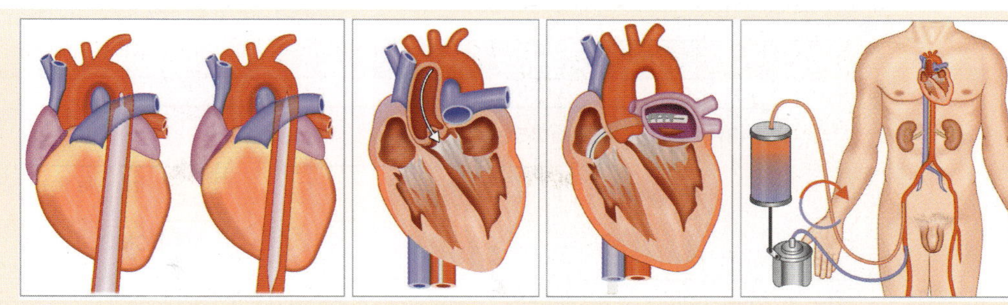

	IABP	Impella	TandemHeart	VA-ECMO
Cardiac flow	0.3–0.5 L/min	1.5 L/min (Impella 2.5, Impella CP, Impella 5)	2.5–5 L/min	3–7 L/min
Mechanism	Aorta	LV → AO	LA → AO	RA → AO
Maximum implant days	Weeks	7 days	14 days	Weeks
Sheath size	7.8 Fr	13–14 Fr Impella 5.0–21 Fr	15–17 Fr arterial 21 Fr venous	14–16 Fr arterial 18–21 Fr venous
Femoral artery size	>4 mm	Impella 2.5 and CP-5–5.5 mm Impella 5–8 mm	8 mm	8 mm
Cardiac synchrony or stable rhythm	Yes	No	No	No
Afterload	↓	↓	↑	↑↑↑
MAP	↑	↑↑	↑↑	↑↑
Cardiac flow	↑	↑↑	↑↑	↑↑
Cardiac power	↑	↑↑	↑↑	↑↑
LVEDP	↓	↓↓	↓↓	↔
PCWP	↓	↓↓	↓↓	↔
LV preload	—	↓↓	↓↓	↓
Coronary perfusion	↑	↑	—	—
Myocardial oxygen demand	↓	↓↓	↔↓	↔

Fig. 3: Comparison of mechanical circulatory support (MCS) devices.
(IABP: intra-aortic ballon pump; MAP: mean arterial pressure; LA: left atrial; LV: left ventricular; LVEDP: left ventricular end-diastolic pressure; PCWP: pulmonary capillary wedge pressure; RA: right atrial; VA-ECMO: venoarterial extracorporeal membrane oxygenation)

LONG-TERM SUPPORT

Durable LVAD therapy, whether as interim stabilization and/or optimization while awaiting heart transplantation or as lifetime support for patients deemed ineligible for transplantation, has significantly improved survival, functional capacity, and quality of life for advanced HF patients.

The early design of long-term devices featured pulsatile pump technology because pulsatility was believed to be necessary for organ perfusion and recovery. These early devices contained valves which were able to produce stroke volume of 65–85 mL. Device durability was a major issue in view of physical wear and tear. Subsequent generations of these devices featured continuous flow pumps with fewer moving parts and improved durability. Studies demonstrated that continuous flow devices provided improved outcomes with regards to survival, quality of life, functional capacity, and adverse events.

Long-term Device Options

HeartMate II (Abbott Medical, Lake Bluff, IL): The HeartMate II is an axial flow pump that was the first continuous flow device approved in the US for bridge to transplant and destination therapy. The functional aspect of the device is an elongated impeller that is suspended in the bloodstream by synthetic ruby bearings. Clinically, the device operates

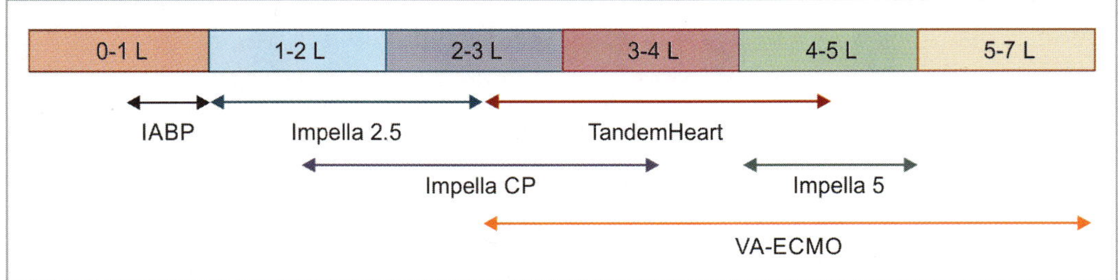

Fig. 4: Comparison of mechanical circulatory support (MCS) devices impact on cardiac flow.
(VA-ECMO: Venoarterial extracorporeal membrane oxygenation; IABP: intra-aortic balloon pump)

between 8000 and 12,000 RPM and is capable of providing up to 10 L/min of output under optimized conditions. ROADMAP trial enrolled 200 patient's ineligible for transplant. But whose HF had not yet progressed to the need for inotropic support to test the hypothesis that an earlier implant strategy may improve outcomes. The trial was not randomized and patients were allowed to select the most desired treatment at enrollment. Of the 103 patients who opted for medical therapy as an initial treatment, 18 crossed over to VAD by 12 months. Importantly, the crossover cohort did not have a higher postimplant mortality. The primary endpoint of ROADMAP was also survival with increased 6-min walk distance of ≥75 m, an endpoint successfully achieved by 2.4x more LVAD patients than those staying on medical therapy.

HeartMate III (Abbott Medical, Lake Bluff, IL): HeartMate III is a centrifugal flow device implanted in the pericardium that has a rotor suspended by an electromagnet. The device has no bearings and wider gaps between the rotor and the pump casing, design features anticipated to reduce the risks of pump thrombosis. The HeartMate III has completed analysis in Europe and the US. The US clinical trial was designed to test short- (6 months) and long-term (24 months) support. The short-term trial randomized to HMII (n = 142) versus HMIII (n = 152). The primary endpoint of survival without stroke or device failure met the primary non-inferiority endpoint for HeartMate III. In a pre-specified analysis in the case of non-inferiority, the HeartMate III was found to be statistically superior (86.2% vs 76.8%, p = 0.04) for the composite primary endpoint, a finding driven mostly by a reduction in device failure.

HVAD (Medtronic, Minneapolis, MN): The HeartWare Ventricular Assist System (HVAD) is an intrapericardial centrifugal flow pump capable of providing up to 10 L/min of flow under optimized physiological conditions but typically has flows of 4–5 L/min clinically. The output of centrifugal flow devices is more sensitive to afterload than the axial flow pumps highlighting the importance of blood pressure control.

JARVIK 2000: The Jarvik 2000 is a small axial flow device implanted entirely in the left ventricle. This pump has several unique features including the ability to anastomose the outflow graft to the descending aorta, a driveline that can be tunneled to the posterior auricular area that may lower the risk of infection and a variable speed controller.

Total Artificial Heart

The quest for a total artificial heart (TAH) began with the advent of MCS devices. Conceptually, the TAH is quite attractive as it offers the ability to replace the entire failing heart. The successful design and implementation of a TAH in clinical practice, however, has been much more elusive (Fig. 4). Furthermore, the rapid expansion of VAD technology has overshadowed TAH development. As a result, the majority of patients with advanced HF can be successfully managed with an LVAD or biventricular assist device (BIVAD) and the necessity of a TAH is debatable. The current indications for a TAH are limited and include severe biventricular failure, myocardial rupture, post-transplant rejection, LV thrombus, restrictive cardiomyopathy (amyloidosis and hypertrophic cardiomyopathy), and refractory ventricular dysrhythmia.

At present, the only TAH that is Food and Drug Administration (FDA) approved is the *CardioWest TAH* (Syncardia Systems Inc, Tucson, AZ, USA), a pneumatically powered pulsatile dual chamber device. Two percutaneous drivelines connect the TAH to an external power source. The patient must remain in hospital, although the recent development of a portable wearable power source, the Freedom driver, may ultimately permit discharge to home. There have been nearly 1,000 implants worldwide. A multicenter trial compared 81 critically ill patients with biventricular failure who received the CardioWest TAH to a 35-patient historical control group who received medical therapy alone. Survival to transplantation was 79% in the CardioWest TAH cohort and 46% in the control group. Post-transplantation survival was also superior in the TAH group, with 86% at 1 year and 64% at 5 years versus 69%

and 34% in the control patients. The CardioWest patients also showed substantial improvement in hepatic and renal function parameters within weeks of TAH implantation. Adverse events included significant bleeding (28%), driveline infection (DLI) (21%), stroke with residual neurologic deficit (0.07%), and device malfunction (0.01%).

COMPLICATIONS

Despite decades of development most VAD therapies are limited due to three longstanding complications. One is bacterial infection from percutaneous drivelines, which is the most frequent LVAD-associated problem. Another is thromboembolic events associated with blood-contacting surfaces, which includes both pump thrombus formation and blood clotting in the circulatory system. And the third is bleeding, mainly at the surgical site during the early postoperative period and gastrointestinal bleeding that usually begins three months after continuous flow LVAD implantation.

Driveline Infections

This risk factor has proven difficult to avoid in these pumps as drivelines that provide power, control, and communication are percutaneously sutured to remain secure, and this driveline exit site creates a conduit for bacterial entry that often leads to DLI. The prevalence and seriousness of DLI, which often leads to erythema, hyperthermia, purulent drainage, and significantly lower survival rate, increased as LVAD therapy expanded from short-term to long-term use. Although approximately 70% of infected patients require rehospitalization in the first year decrease DLI incidents include optimization of driveline implantation techniques and minimization of pump profile and operational invasiveness, which has resulted in smaller and more efficient devices such as the entirely intrapericardial HVAD (HeartWare) and completely intrathoracic HeartMate III.

Pump thrombosis: Another significant cause of LVAD complications is thromboembolism associated with blood-contacting surfaces. Pump thrombosis, where blood clots form at the blood-device interface, is a multifactorial process caused by misuse of anticoagulants, abnormal angulation of cannulas, and surface mediation of blood-contacting devices. The annual incidence of pump thrombosis in LVAD patients exceeds 10%, of which nearly one-third lead to serious complications including aortic insufficiency, hemolysis, neurologic events, and cardiogenic shock. In order to minimize the rate of chronic pump thrombosis, innumerable changes in VAD designs have been made over the years. Modern LVAD surface area has been scaled down, impeller profiles have been adjusted, implantation invasiveness has been minimized, and less reactive surface materials have been chosen.

Gastrointestinal Bleeding

The reported incidence of gastrointestinal bleeding (GIB) after continuous flow LVAD implantation is alarmingly high, as much as 61% by one account. There are several factors leading to GIB syndrome, but with third-generation continuous flow pumps the low pulsatility flow profile combined with increased oxidative and shear stresses seem to cause hematological abnormalities such as platelet dysfunction and von Willebrand factor (vWF) degradation (Figs. 5A to C).[9-12]

INNOVATIONS FOR EFFECTIVE LONG-TERM CARDIAC SUPPORT

Transcutaneous energy transmission (TET) technology that transfers power across intact skin makes devices completely implantable and therefore free of the risk of device-related infection. Different methods of transmitting energy across skin such as ultrasonic energy transfer and acoustic energy transfer have been previously developed, but because inductive coupling TET outperforms the others by more than double in terms of efficiency, the latter has been used in devices like AbioCor TAH (AbioMed), and the LionHeart LVAD (Arrow International, Reading, PA, USA) (Table 1). This system required transmit and receive coils must remain very close. So the receiver coil should be implanted just under skin and external coil secured over adhesive dressing.

This proximity restriction requires the receive coil to be implanted just under the skin and the external transmit coil to be secured in a single position on the skin surface with an adhesive dressing. Brief separation period of 30 minutes can be sustained. Another limitation is its lower energy efficiency, it consumes approximately 20% of the generated power during operation. Other drawbacks like fatal component failure, bleeding, and pain due to the large cumulative volume of all implanted parts also play a big role in preventing TET technology from being the main VAD powering method today (Figs. 6A and B).

Muscle-powered VAD: The use of electrically stimulated skeletal muscle as an endogenous power source to drive circulatory support systems is another alternative that is currently under study. It is basically an energy converter which converts contractile energy of muscle into energy. Large muscle such as latissimus dorsi muscle due to its

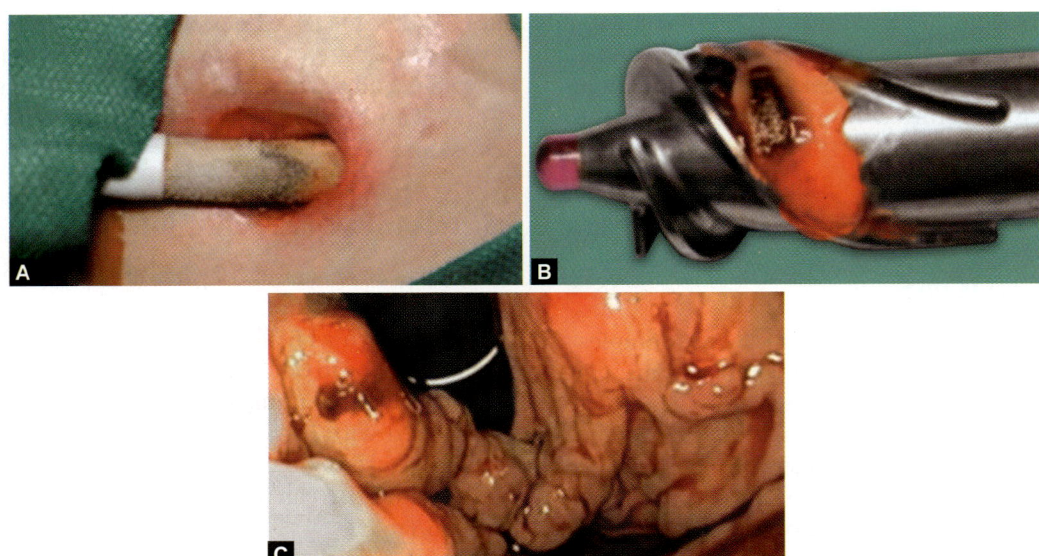

Figs. 5A to C: Longstanding complications after left ventricular assist device (LVAD) implantations are driveline infections (A), pump thrombosis (B), and gastrointestinal bleeding (C).

TABLE 1: Commonly used cardiac assist devices and their key characteristics.

Category	*Product*	*Type of support*	*Duration of support*	*Advantages*	*Limitations*
Early methods of cardiac support	ECMO	BiVAD	Short-term	Extracorporeal artificial heart-lung bypass for acute support	Upper body hypoxia, LV dilatation, thrombosis
	IABP	Descending aorta	Short-term	Increases myocardial oxygen perfusion and cardiac output	Thrombosis, aortic rupture, arterial flow obstruction
Ist generation–pulsatile flow	HeartMate XVE	LVAD	Long-term	Improved enough to receive FDA approval for DT in 2003 and CE mark in 2004	Bulky and heavy
	Berlin heart EXCOR	BiVAD	BTT	Pediatric uses with various pump sizes	Not completely implanted
	Novacor LVAS	LVAD	BTT	Longer durability and higher reliability at the time	Still large and bulky with three extracorporeal hardware
	HeartMate I	LVAD	BTT/BTR	Introduced textured blood contacting surface to reduce thrombosis	Large size and complications like bleeding and driveline infection
	Thoratec PVAD	Uni or BiVAD	Short-term	Weeks to months support for patient's home discharge postcardiotomy	Common side effects from pneumatic driveline
	ABioMed BVS 5000	Uni or BiVAD	Short-term	Resuscitate critically ill patients for acute stabilization	Risks of bleeding, coagulopathy, and end-organ damage
	Jarvik 7	TAH	Long-term	World's first permanent total artificial heart; more used as a BTT now	Thrombotic deposition and cerebral embolic events

Contd...

Contd...

Category	*Product*	*Type of support*	*Duration of support*	*Advantages*	*Limitations*
	AbioCor TAH	TAH	Long-term	Uses TET technology without aid of wires	Discomfort with TET system, bulkiness, clotting at device surfaces
	ABioMed Impella RP	IVC-to-PA	Short-term	First and only FDA approved percutaneous heart pump for RV support	Thrombotic vascular complications and hemolysis
	TandemHeart	LA-to-FA	Short-term	Significantly reduces preload and augments cardiac output	Risks of cannula migration, thromboembolism, and cardiac tamponade
2nd generation—continuous axial Flow	HeartMate II	LVAD	Long-term	FDA approval for DT, Improved survival rate and patient quality of life. Most commonly installed LVAD in 2000s	Bleeding, cardiac arrhythmia, infection, sepsis
	Heart Assist 5	LVAD	Long-term	Small size and weight, CE mark approved remote monitoring system in 2012	Bleeding, thrombosis, infections
	Jarvik 2000	LVAD	Long-term	Pediatric uses, FDA approval for trial using as a DT in 2012	Class 2 device recall for a potential external cable damage in 2018
	ABioMed Impella	FA-to-LV	Short-term	Minimally invasive, varying sizes	Hemolysis, aortic valve injury, infection
3rd generation—continuous centrifugal flow	HeartWare HVAD	LVAD	Long-term	Small size, magnetically levitated rotor, FDA approval for DT in 2017	Risks of infection, bleeding, arrhythmia, stroke
	HeartMate III	LVAD	Long-term	Magnetically levitated rotor, FDA approval for DT in 2018	Risks of infection, bleeding, arrhythmia, stroke
	DuraHeart	LVAD	Long-term	Favorable clinical outcomes as BTT in Japan and Europe	Hemolysis, thromboembolism, bleeding
	HeartWare MVAD	LVAD	Long-term	Miniature size for pediatric uses	Risks of infection, bleeding and thrombosis
	CentriMag	Uni-VAD	Short-term	Magnetically suspended rotor for acute therapy. Minimal shear force on RBCs and hemolysis	Bleeding, infection, respiratory failure, hemolysis, neurologic dysfunction
Non-blood-contacting VADs	CorInnova	Ventricular epicardium	Potentially long-term	Minimally invasive, non-blood-contacting, soft material	Studies done on large animals only
	Biomimetic DCCS	Ventricular epicardium	Potentially long-term	Soft material, non-blood-contacting, compression and torsion applications	Still under development
	Muscled-powered DCCS	Ventricular epicardium	Potentially long-term	Tether-free, non-blood-contacting, Biocompatible soft material	Still under development
	C-pulse Device	Ascending aorta	Short-term	Non-blood-contacting	No longer commercially available

(IVC: inferior vena cava; FA: femoral artery, LA: left atrial, PA: pulmonary artery)

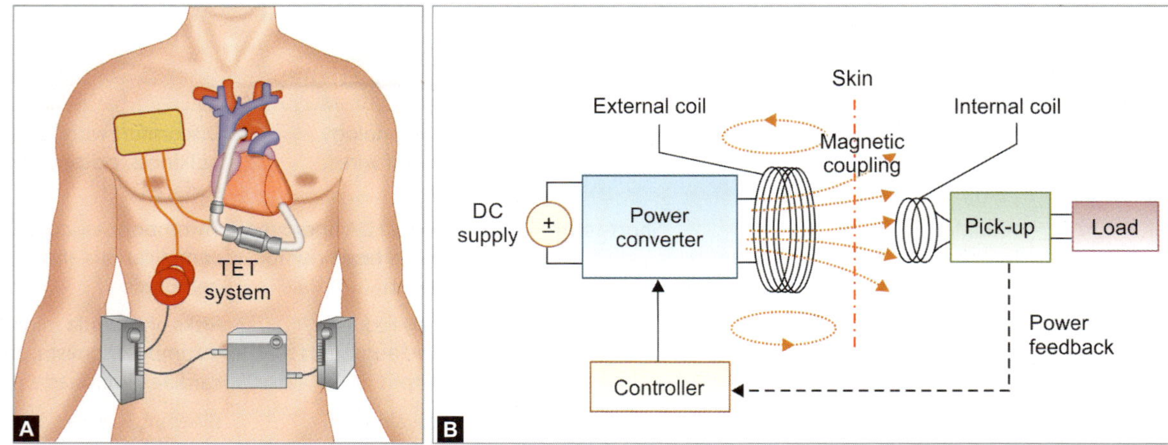

Figs. 6A and B: Schematics of the transcutaneous energy transmission (TET) system (A) in patient use and (B) with an electromagnetic coupling between the internal and external coils located inside and outside of patient skin.

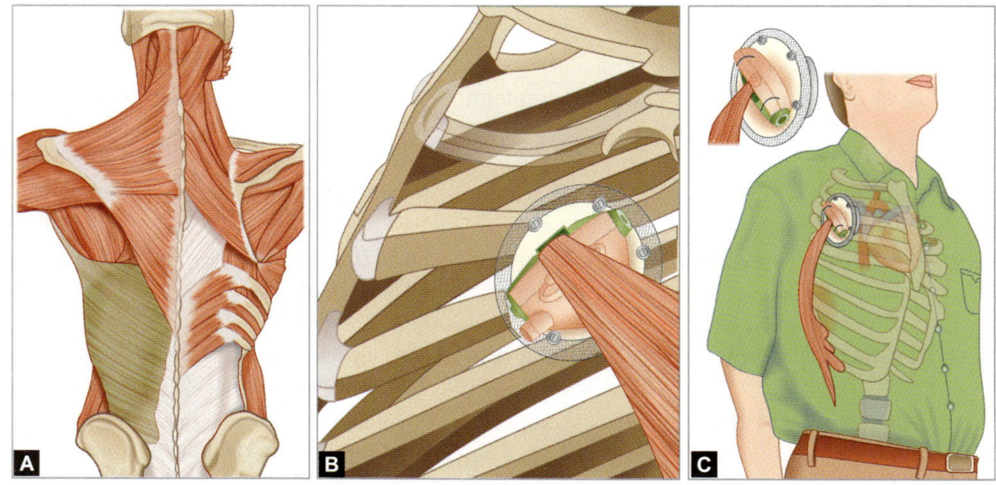

Figs. 7A to C: Muscle-powered ventricular assist devices (VADs) could use the latissimus dorsi (A) as its power source and convert this endogenous muscular power into hydraulic energy via a completely implantable muscle energy converter (B) that can potentially power pulsatile VADs for long-term use (C).

large size, surgical accessibility, proximity to the thoracic cavity, and steady-state work capacity are prime target (Figs. 7A to C).

Non-blood Contacting Cardiac Assist Devices

These devices can be applied externally without getting in contact with bloodstream and programmed to deliver compression during systole (copulsation) and diastole (counterpulsation). Thus increasing arterial pressure and reducing aortic pressure by lowering cardiac afterload. *Counterpulsation extraaortic balloon pump (EABP)* that wraps and compresses the external surface of the ascending aorta like the C-pulse device and shown to improve diastolic pressure, coronary blood flow and cardiac output.

CONCLUSION

As India progress toward a developed economy we will have loads of patient with advanced HF refractory to standard therapies and shortage of donor organ. VAD therapy will be a mainstay of providing a bridge to life. Limitation of cost, adverse event and availability will be key determinant to this era. Advance in technology with fully implantable VAD reduced cost and low adverse event will lead to wider use of therapy.

REFERENCES

1. National Heart, Lung, and Blood Institute (NHLBI). (2018). Heart Failure. [online] Available from https://www.nhlbi. nih. gov/health-topics/heart-failure [Last accessed November, 2019].
2. Ambrosy AP, Fonarow GC, Butler J, et al. The global health and economic burden of hospitalizations for heart failure: lessons learned from hospitalized heart failure registries. J Am Coll Cardiol. 2014;63:1123-33.
3. Mancini D, Colombo PC. Left Ventricular Assist Devices: A Rapidly Evolving Alternative to Transplant. J Am Coll Cardiol. 2015;65:2542-55.
4. Mandras SA, Crespo J, Patel HM. Innovative application of immunologic principles in heart transplantation. Ochsner J. 2010;10:231-5.
5. Lahpor JR. State of the art: implantable ventricular assist devices. Curr Opin Organ Transplant. 2009;14:554-59.
6. Boyle A. Current status of cardiac transplantation and mechanical circulatory support. Curr Heart Fail Rep. 2009;6:28-33.
7. Birks EJ. A changing trend toward destination therapy. Tex Heart Inst J. 2011;38:552-4.
8. Rose EA, Gelijns AC, Moskowitz AJ, et al. Long-term use of a left ventricular assist device for end-stage heart failure. N Engl J Med. 2001;345:1435-43.
9. Slaughter MS, Rogers JG, Milano CA, et al. Advanced heart failure treated with continuous flow left ventricular assist device. N Engl J Med. 2009;361:2241-51.
10. Miller LW, Pagani FD, Russell SD, et al. Use of a continuous-flow device in patients awaiting heart transplantation. N Engl J Med. 2007;357:885-96.
11. Aaronson KD, Slaughter MS, Miller LW, et al. Use of an intrapericardial, continuous-flow, centrifugal pump in patients awaiting heart transplantation. Circulation. 2012;125:3191-200.
12. Mehra MR, Naka Y, Uriel N, et al. A fully magnetically levitated circulatory pump for advanced heart failure. N Engl J Med. 2017;376:440-50.

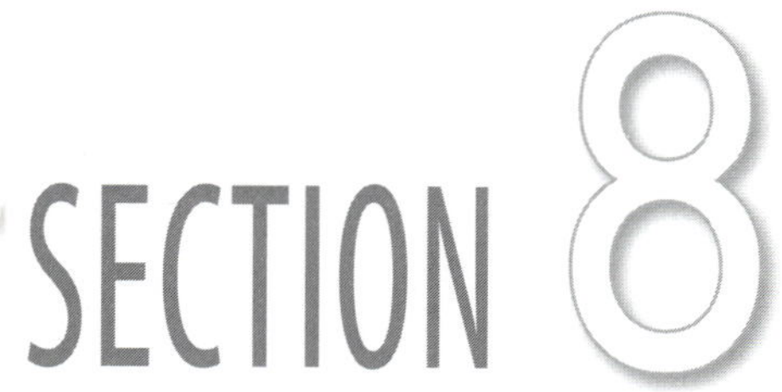

Congenital Heart Disease and Heart Failure

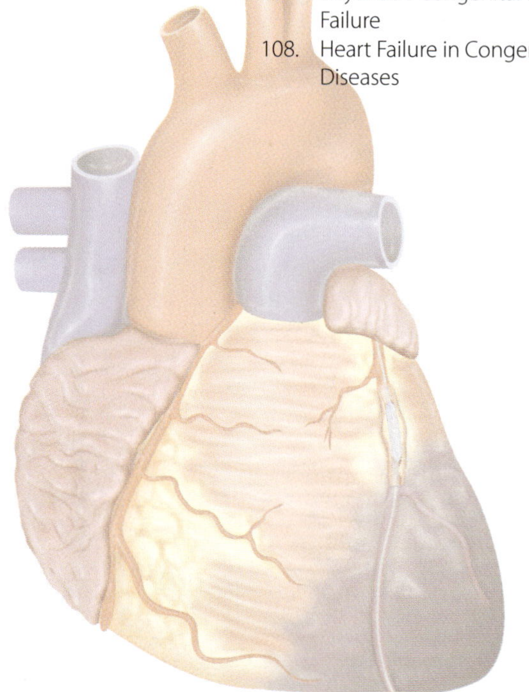

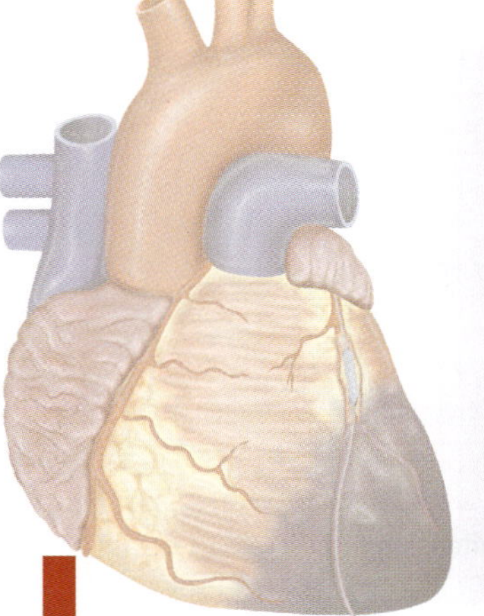

Acyanotic Congenital Heart Disease and Heart Failure

Arvind Balaji, Sivasubramanian Ramakrishnan

INTRODUCTION

Heart failure (HF) is defined as a complex clinical syndrome that can result from any structural or functional cardiac disorder that impairs the ventricular filling or ejection resulting in failure of heart to supply blood to either systemic or pulmonary circulation at appropriate flow.[1] Acyanotic congenital heart diseases (ACHDs) are the most common forms of congenital heart disease (CHD). They comprise lesions with left to right shunt at atrial, ventricular or great artery level, regurgitant lesions of either of the atrioventricular (AV) valves, resulting in volume overload of a cardiac chamber, or those due to obstruction of semilunar valves, which in turn result in pressure overload of either ventricles. Ultimately most of these lesions result in heart failure, at various ages depending on the location and severity of the lesion. With improvements in cardiac surgery, a growing population of corrected or palliated (Fontan pathway) CHDs enjoy increased longevity, albeit their risk of developing HF. Understanding the pathophysiology of these lesions help in prevention and management of HF symptoms in these patients and plan definitive interventions.

EPIDEMIOLOGY

The prevalence of HF in CHD varies among various regions of the world. A retrospective study from Nepal reported a HF prevalence of 54.8% among individuals with CHD aged up to 15 years.[2] Another prospective study from India, reported a 40.8% prevalence of HF among under 5 years children with CHDs who were also malnourished, whereas a study from Norway had reported that 8% of CHD patients between 2 weeks and 11 years presented with decompensated HF, subsequent to discharge from hospital after birth.[3,4] Exclusive data for acyanotic CHD are however not available.

PATHWAYS OF HEART FAILURE IN ACYANOTIC CONGENITAL HEART DISEASE

Lesions with left to right shunts result in pulmonary overcirculation, and is traditionally considered the most common cause of clinical HF. Abnormal loading conditions of ventricles (e.g. left ventricular volume overload as in case of post-tricuspid shunts, left ventricular pressure overload in case of severe aortic stenosis) are hypothesized to cause neurohormonal activation which results in myocardial remodeling and initiates the HF pathways. Hypertension and arrhythmias are often overlooked causes of HF in patients with ACHD (Flowchart 1).

Genetic pathways unrelated to the hemodynamic stressors, have also been shown to result in HF like presentation. Many pathways involved in the cardiac embryogenesis also play a role in myocardial structure and integrity. Hence, aberrations in these pathways can cause both CHD and cardiomyopathy (e.g. Noonan syndrome).[3] Left ventricular noncompaction (LVNC) is another such disorder, more often than not associated with CHD and heart failure. Monogenic causes of CHD are predominantly associated with syndromic CHD (e.g. *TBX5*

Flowchart 1: Causes of heart failure in acyanotic congenital heart disease.

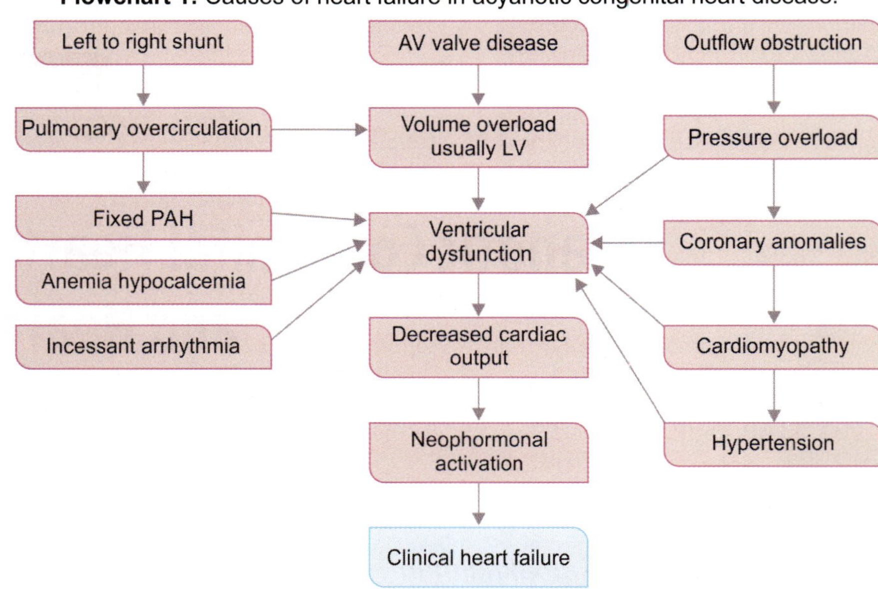

(AV: atrioventricular; LV: left ventricle; PAH: pulmonary arterial hypertension)

gene mutation in Holt–Oram syndrome, *JAG1* or *NOTCH2* gene mutations in Alagille syndrome), whereas the role of genetics in nonsyndromic CHD is still incompletely understood.[5] Another hypothesis is the presence of overlapping pathways in which there are aberrations at [e.g. deoxyribonucleic acid (DNA) methylation] or genetic level (e.g. calcium signaling, extracellular matrix protein expression) coexisting in patients with CHD, or might be triggered by the hemodynamic load which make them prone to development of heart failure.[6,7]

PATHOPHYSIOLOGY

The low cardiac output and compromised perfusion activate compensatory mechanisms, such as activation of renin-angiotensin-aldosterone system (RAAS) and the sympathetic nervous system. The downstream events occur explained in Flowchart 2, and when undeterred, set the stage for a state of chronic heart failure.[8] At the cellular level, there is depletion of intracellular calcium, secondary to sustained leak from sarcoplasmic reticulum induced by sympathetic activation, ultimately reducing cardiac contractility. The natriuretic peptides, ameliorate much of the harmful effects of these SNS and RAAS. However, in HF states, the levels of neprilysin, an enzyme which inactivates the NPs, is upregulated, limiting their beneficial effects.[9]

CLINICAL FEATURES

The diagnosis of HF is largely clinical. Various clinical classification systems are available to grade severity of HF across age groups. The presentation also depends on right of left heart failure. Right HF presents as elevated JVP, ascites, pedal edema and hepatomegaly, whereas, left HF manifests as dyspnea, orthopnea and pulmonary edema (Table 1).

Classification based on perfusion (warm vs cold) and congestion or filling pressure (dry vs wet) status provides a better management perspective, the ultimate goal being to achieve a warm and dry state, i.e. with adequate perfusion and normal filling pressures. Patients with congestion and hypoperfusion (wet and cold) are the worst subsets with highest risk of mortality.[10]

ETIOLOGY OF HEART FAILURE IN CHILDREN

Age of presentation also may give clue regarding the underlying etiology as shown in Table 2.

DIAGNOSTIC APPROACH

Detailed history and physical examination along with chest roentgenogram, 12-lead electrocardiogram and basic laboratory parameters including hemoglobin, electrolytes, renal and hepatic function are performed in all patients. Anatomic and hemodynamic evaluation [echocardiography, cardiac catheterization, computed tomography or cardiac magnetic resonance imaging (MRI)], with an aim to search for relievable or repairable (surgical or transcatheter) structural abnormality remains the key. CHD patients may develop pulmonary hypertension and

Flowchart 2: Clinical approach to pediatric heart failure.

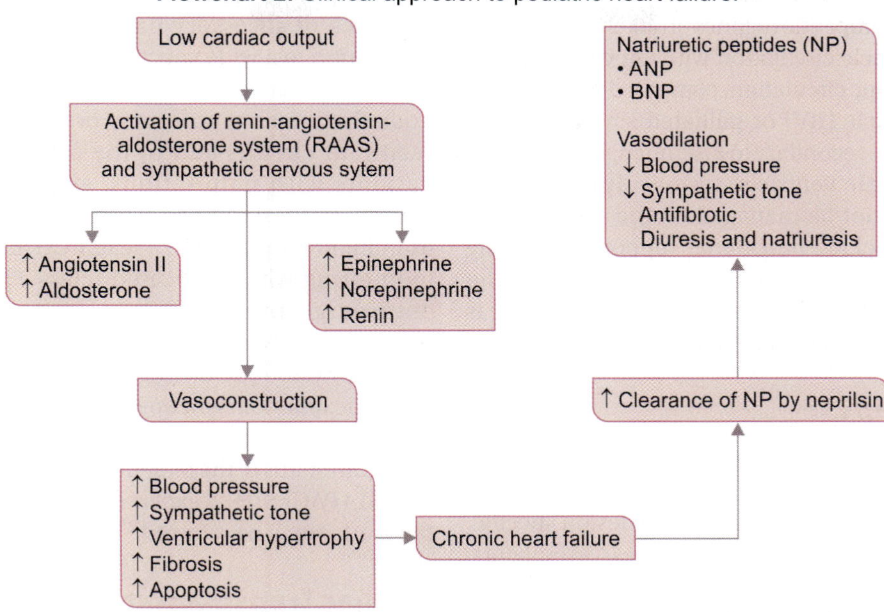

(ANP: atrial natriuretic peptide; BNP: B-type natriuretic peptide)

TABLE 1: Heart failure classification for children.

NYHA classification (for children > 6 years age)	Modified Ross classification (for children <6 years age)
Asymptomatic	Asymptomatic
Moderate limitation of physical activity	Mild tachypnea or feeding diaphoresis in infants, dyspnea on exertion in older children
Marked limitation of physical activity	Marked tachypnea or feeding diaphoresis, dyspnea on exertion, prolonged feeding times with growth failure
Symptoms at rest	Tachypnea, retractions, grunting or diaphoresis at rest

(NYHA: New York Heart Association)

they should be evaluated for and its severity and eligibility for PAH targeted therapies.

MANAGEMENT

It generally involves correction of the underlying defect either surgically or percutaneously. The role of medical care, though mostly supportive, cannot be overstated. Most of the management strategies have been extrapolated from standard adult HF therapy guidelines.[11,12] It is important to recognize that the benefits are not proven, and rarely there may be adverse events to treatment which may be unique to a particular CHD (e.g. aggressive diuresis in a patient with severe pulmonary stenosis and HF). The heterogeneity of

TABLE 2: Causes of heart failure as per age in children.

Age	*Possible etiologies*
Day 1/fetal	Birth asphyxia related, metabolic (hypocalcemia, hypomagnesemia), myocarditis, anemia, sepsis, severe tricuspid regurgitation (Ebstein's, birth trauma), severe congenital mitral regurgitation, rate related (SVT or CHB)
1st week of life	Critical aortic stenosis, critical pulmonary stenosis, coarctation of aorta, hypoplastic left heart syndrome, (mostly the ductus dependent cardiac lesions), obstructed total anomalous pulmonary venous connection (TAPVC). Adrenal insufficiency, renal failure, systemic hypertension
2nd week of life	Atrioventricular septal defects (AVSDs), persistent truncus arteriosus, TAPVC (unobstructed type), large ventricular septal defects (VSDs), single ventricle, large persistent ductus arteriosus
1st–2nd month of life	VSD, PDA, AVSD, aortopulmonary window, anomalous left coronary artery from pulmonary artery
Older children	Acute rheumatic fever, rheumatic heart disease, infective endocarditis, nonspecific aortoarteritis, cardiomyopathies, tachycardiomyopathies

(SVT: supraventricular tachycardia; CHB: complete heart block; PDA: patent ductus arteriosus)

CHD population adds to more complexity. The benefits of these extrapolated therapeutic regimes are likely to be higher in those with biventricle circulation with left ventricle (LV) supporting the systemic circulation, compared to those with systemic right ventricle (RV) or palliated single ventricle (Fontan). Heart failure secondary to Eisenmenger syndrome, failure of subpulmonic ventricle, systolic dysfunction of systemic RV should not be managed on the same lines.[13] General measures include nutritional support in growing children, targeting an intake of 30–50% more than the recommended daily allowance. Reduction of fluid intake is recommended only in patients with refractory edema.

Pharmacotherapy

The main focus of medical therapy is to reduce pulmonary wedge pressure, while increasing cardiac output and to prevent progression. The strategy should be lesion specific. In the acute stages, stabilization with inotropes/vasodilators, diuretics, mechanical ventilation are desirable. Potential precipitating factors, such as anemia, arrhythmias, and hypertension should be actively looked for and addressed.

Diuretics: These drugs act by reducing systemic and venous congestion. Loop diuretics (e.g. furosemide) are the more potent and preferred agents. Aldosterone antagonists (e.g. spironolactone) possess additional beneficial effects of attenuating myocardial remodeling and catecholamine release. Dyselectrolytemias (hyponatremia, hypo- or hyperkalemia) need to be monitored for, which can lead to life-threatening complications occasionally.

Angiotensin-converting enzyme (ACE) inhibitors remain the mainstay of treatment of chronic heart failure. They exert beneficial effects by reducing the afterload and reversing myocardial remodeling.[14] Beta-blockers have been widely used in young children with ventricular dysfunction, despite inconclusive evidence.[15,16] Carvedilol and metoprolol are the most commonly used drugs. They are usually started at small doses and gradually uptitrated. Beta-blockers are usually contraindicated in acute decompensated HF.

Digoxin: Digoxin has been shown to reduce hospitalization rates in adult HF, though it did not show survival benefit.[17] Though benefits in ACHD also is not demonstrated, it continues to be widely prescribed. One should be aware of the narrow therapeutic range and its potential harmful effects in acute myocarditis, and in presence of hypokalemia, hypomagnesemia, and renal failure.

Arrhythmias

Progressive HF and arrhythmias are the predominant modes of death in patients with CHD.[18] There are multiple abnormalities in the conduction pathway including presence of accessory pathway which predispose this population to a wide spectrum of rhythm disturbances. In the postoperative state, additional factors, such as sinus node dysfunction, atriotomy or ventriculotomy induced reentrant circuits add to the causes of arrhythmias.[19] Patients with palpitations, syncope or presyncope, worsening HF should have a detailed history and physical examination including 12-lead ECG and ambulatory ECG monitoring when indicated (class 1).[20] Workup to rule out regurgitant or obstructive lesions which potentially contribute to arrhythmias to be performed (class 1). Electrophysiologic testing is indicated in adult patients with unexplained syncope and "high-risk" postoperative CHD substrates. Subsequent management depends on the symptom status of the patient which is addressed in detail in the 2014 PACES/HRS expert consensus statement, to which the reader may be referred.[20]

Cardiac Transplantation

Mostly getting an appropriate donor is a challenge especially in infants and younger patients. Transplantation is reserved for children with corrected or uncorrectable lesions with severe ventricular dysfunction with failed pharmacological management. Early survival after transplant is overall poorer for CHD, whereas in the long-term, the median survival was better for CHD patients, compared to other pretransplant diagnosis.[21]

CONCLUSION

Acyanotic congenital heart disease is an important cause of HF in children and understanding the mechanisms involved helps in rationale management of the symptoms. Since there are only limited data available regarding the management of these patients, most of the pharmacologic strategies are extrapolations from adult HF guidelines. This may not be appropriate in few CHDs and it is important to personalize therapy to each patients' hemodynamics. The ultimate goal is to correct anatomic abnormalities, preserve myocardial function and stall the progression to end-stage HF. With accumulating evidence, and a multidisciplinary approach the outcomes of HF in this patient population are likely to improve.

REFERENCES

1. Hunt SA, Abraham WT, Chin MH, et al. 2009 Focused update incorporated into the ACC/AHA 2005 Guidelines for the Diagnosis and Management of Heart Failure in Adults A Report of the American College of Cardiology Foundation/American Heart Association Task Force on

Practice Guidelines Developed in Collaboration With the International Society for Heart and Lung Transplantation. J Am Coll Cardiol. 2009;53(15):e1-90.

2. Shah GS, Singh MK, Pandey TR, et al. Incidence of congenital heart disease in tertiary care hospital. Kathmandu Univ Med J (KUMJ). 2008;6(1):33-6.
3. Wessels MW, De Graaf BM, Cohen-Overbeek TE, et al. A new syndrome with noncompaction cardiomyopathy, bradycardia, pulmonary stenosis, atrial septal defect and heterotaxy with suggestive linkage to chromosome 6p. Hum Genet. 2008;122(6):595-603.
4. Vaidyanathan B, Nair SB, Sundaram KR, et al. Malnutrition in children with congenital heart disease (CHD) determinants and short term impact of corrective intervention. Indian Pediatr. 2008;45(7):541-6.
5. Fahed AC, Gelb BD, Seidman JG, et al. Genetics of congenital heart disease: the glass half empty. Circ Res. 2013;112(4):707-20.
6. Zaidi S, Choi M, Wakimoto H, et al. De novo mutations in histone-modifying genes in congenital heart disease. Nature. 2013;498(7453):220-3.
7. Creemers EE, Wilde AA, Pinto YM. Heart failure: advances through genomics. Nat Rev Genet. 2011;12(5):357-62.
8. Goldsmith SR. Interactions between the sympathetic nervous system and the RAAS in heart failure. Curr Heart Fail Rep. 2004;1(2):45-50.
9. Knecht M, Pagel I, Langenickel T, et al. Increased expression of renal neutral endopeptidase in severe heart failure. Life Sciences. 2002;71(23):2701-12.
10. Kantor PF, Lougheed J, Dancea A, et al. Presentation, diagnosis, and medical management of heart failure in children: Canadian Cardiovascular Society guidelines. Can J Cardiol. 2013;29(12):1535-52.
11. Ponikowski P, Voors AA, Anker SD, et al. 2016 ESC Guidelines for the diagnosis and treatment of acute and chronic heart failure: The Task Force for the diagnosis and treatment of acute and chronic heart failure of the European Society of Cardiology (ESC) Developed with the special contribution of the Heart Failure Association (HFA) of the ESC. Eur Heart J. 2016;37(27):2129-200.
12. Yancy CW, Jessup M, Bozkurt B, et al. 2013 ACCF/AHA Guideline for the Management of Heart Failure. Circulation. 2013;128(16):e240-327.
13. Stout KK, Broberg CS, Book WM, et al. Chronic Heart Failure in Congenital Heart Disease: A Scientific Statement from the American Heart Association. Circulation. 2016;133(8):770-801.
14. Momma K. ACE inhibitors in pediatric patients with heart failure. Paediatr Drugs. 2006;8(1):55-69.
15. Shaddy RE, Boucek MM, Hsu DT, et al. Carvedilol for children and adolescents with heart failure: a randomized controlled trial. JAMA. 2007;298(10):1171-9.
16. Blume ED, Canter CE, Spicer R, et al. Prospective single-arm protocol of carvedilol in children with ventricular dysfunction. Pediatr Cardiol. 2006;27(3):336-42.
17. Digitalis Investigation Group. The effect of digoxin on mortality and morbidity in patients with heart failure. N Engl J Med. 1997;336(8):525-33.
18. Oechslin EN, Harrison DA, Connelly MS, et al. Mode of death in adults with congenital heart disease. Am J Cardiol. 2000;86(10):1111-6.
19. Escudero C, Khairy P, Sanatani S. Electrophysiologic Considerations in Congenital Heart Disease and their Relationship to Heart Failure. Can J Cardiol. 20131;29(7):821-9.
20. Khairy P, Van Hare GF, Balaji S, et al. PACES/HRS Expert Consensus Statement on the Recognition and Management of Arrhythmias in Adult Congenital Heart Disease: Developed in Partnership Between the Pediatric and Congenital Electrophysiology Society (PACES) and the Heart Rhythm Society (HRS). Endorsed by the Governing Bodies of PACES, HRS, the American College of Cardiology (ACC), the American Heart Association (AHA), the European Heart Rhythm Association (EHRA), the Canadian Heart Rhythm Society (CHRS), and the International Society for Adult Congenital Heart Disease (ISACHD). Can J Cardiol. 2014;30(10):e1-63.
21. Kirk R, Dipchand AI, Edwards LB, et al. The Registry of the International Society for Heart and Lung Transplantation: Fifteenth Pediatric Heart Transplantation Report—2012. J Heart Lung Transplant. 2012;31(10):1065-72.

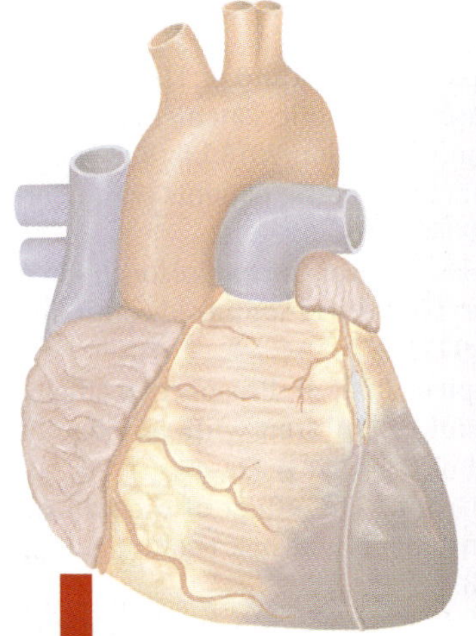

Heart Failure in Congenital Cyanotic Heart Diseases

Sonia A El-Saiedi, Gaser A Abdelmohsen, Ahmed M Dohain

INCIDENCE AND DISEASE BURDEN

Approximately 8–12 per 1,000 live births are born with congenital heart disease (CHD) and about 28% of major congenital defects have congenital heart lesions, moreover approximately one-third of infant deaths secondary to congenital anomalies are related to congenital heart lesions. Congenital heart diseases may be cyanotic or acyanotic, congenital cyanotic heart disease (CCHD) represents about 25–31% of CHD.[1-6]

ETIOLOGY

The genetic background of CHD is incompletely understood, it was thought that the cause of CHD is multifactorial due to interaction between genetic predisposition and environmental riskfactors, CHD may be isolated or associated with chromosomal abnormalities (trisomy 21, trisomy 13 or 18), genetic syndromes (DiGeorge, Noonan, Alagille, Heterotaxy) or associated with maternal diseases like diabetes, maternal exposure to teratogens like drugs (e.g. Ebstein anomaly with lithium), infections (e.g. rubella) or radiations.[7,8]

CLASSIFICATIONS OF CONGENITAL CYANOTIC HEART DISEASE

There are many classifications of CCHD described here.

Anatomical Classification[6]

Congenital cyanotic heart disease with right heart obstruction:
- Tricuspid atresia
- Pulmonary atresia with ventricular septal defect (PA-VSD)
- Pulmonary atresia with intact ventricular septum (PA-IVS)
- Critical pulmonary stenosis (PS)
- Fallot tetralogy.

Congenital cyanotic heart disease with left heart obstruction:
- Hypoplastic left heart syndrome (HLHS)
- Interrupted aortic arch (IAA)
- Critical aortic stenosis (AS) with right to left patent ductus arteriosus (PDA)
- Severe coarctation of aorta (COA) with right to left PDA.

Others lesions:
- Transposition of the great arteries (TGAs)
- Double outlet right ventricle (DORV)
- Truncus arteriosus (TA)
- Total anomalous pulmonary venous return (TAPVR)
- Ebstein anomaly
- Single ventricle associated with decreased pulmonary blood flow
- Eisenmenger's syndrome.

Functional Classification[9,10]

Congenital cyanotic heart disease could be classified functionally into:
- Congenital cyanotic heart disease with decreased pulmonary blood flow:
  - Critical/severe PS with right to left shunt across atrial septal defect (ASD)
  - Fallot tetralogy/PA-VSD
  - Tricuspid atresia with severe PS or restrictive VSD and normally related great vessels

- Ebstein anomaly with right to left ASD
- Single/double inlet ventricle with pulmonary stenosis.
- Congenital cyanotic heart disease with increased pulmonary flow:
  - Double outlet right ventricle
  - Truncus arteriosus
- Congenital cyanotic heart disease compatible with prenatal but incompatible with postnatal period:
  - Transposition of the great artery
  - Pulmonary atresia either with intact IVS or with VSD
  - Hypoplastic left heart syndrome/interrupted aortic arch
  - Total anomalous pulmonary venous return.

PATHOPHYSIOLOGY OF CYANOSIS AND HEART FAILURE IN CCHD

Normally the right side of the heart receives deoxygenated blood from systemic veins, this deoxygenated blood is then pumped to the lungs where oxygenation takes place, the oxygenated blood then returns to left side of the heart where it is pumped into the aorta and then to the whole body. In normal conditions the deoxygenated blood in the right side of the heart does not mix with the oxygenated blood in left side of the heart. Cyanosis usually occurs in two conditions: (1) Lung issues: When the deoxygenated blue blood returned from the lung to the heart without oxygenation due to lung pathology (pneumonia, lung collapse or pulmonary edema) or intrapulmonary shunts (pulmonary arteriovenous fistula) and cyanosis in this case is due to pulmonary causes. (2) Intracardiac right-to-left shunt: In CCHD, cyanosis is due to intracardiac right-to-left shunt across either patent foramen ovale (PFO), VSD or PDA. In these conditions the deoxygenated blue blood shunts to the left side of the heart bypassing the lungs and mixes with the oxygenated blood causing cyanosis, the degree of cyanosis usually depends on the magnitude of right-to-left shunt (the more the right-to-left shunt the more the cyanosis) and the pulmonary blood flow as it is the only source of oxygenated blood (the less the pulmonary blood flow the more the cyanosis).[11-14]

Congenital cyanotic heart disease could be associated with heart failure due to several mechanisms: (1) Increased pulmonary blood flow and lung plethora: Normally during fetal life, the pulmonary vascular resistance (PVR) is very high and usually starts to drop gradually after birth, with physiological decrease of PVR, some patients with CCHD may develop marked increase of pulmonary blood flow, this will lead to significant lung plethora with transudation of fluids around and inside the alveoli, and patients will present clinically by tachypnea and recessions. (2) Pulmonary venous congestion: Pulmonary venous congestion can happen in cases with impaired pulmonary venous drainage. Impaired pulmonary venous drainage can occur in cases with significant left ventricular dysfunction (e.g. critical COA, critical AS) as in these cases the left ventricular end diastolic pressure (LVEDP) is elevated and impairing drainage of blood from left atrium to the left ventricle. Pulmonary venous congestion can also occur in cases of compression of pulmonary veins impairing pulmonary venous drainage to the left atrium, like in cases with obstructed TAPVR (due to compression/stenosis of vertical vein) or in cases with HLHS or mitral atresia with restrictive ASD. Pulmonary venous congestion which leads to transudation of fluids around and inside the alveoli causing tachypnea and recessions. (3) Right side heart failure: CCHD could be associated with right-sided heart failure and hepatic congestion. Right-sided heart failure can occur either due to right ventricular dysfunction secondary to increased RV afterload associated with severe outlet obstruction (PA-IVS, critical PS). Right heart failure can also develop secondary to RV volume overload associated with severe tricuspid regurgitation (Ebstein anomaly) or severe pulmonary regurgitation after catheter or surgical intervention (PA-IVS, critical PS or Fallot tetralogy after surgical repair with transannular patch) or inadequate mixing as in cases of tricuspid atresia and restrictive ASD.[11-16]

CLINICAL PICTURE OF CONGENITAL CYANOTIC HEART DISEASE

Careful history and examination is crucial for evaluation of patients with CCHD.

History

- Cyanosis: Bluish discoloration of mucous membranes and skin
- Rapid breathing
- Decrease oral feeding: Decrease amount in each feed and baby takes more time in each feed with significant dyspnea and sweating.
- Interrupted feeding
- Failure to thrive
- Recurrent chest infections that may need hospital admissions.
- Palpitation and exercise intolerance in older kids.

Signs

- Tachycardia
- Tachypnea with intercostal and subcostal recessions
- Enlarged tender liver
- Hyperdynamic pericardium in cases of increased pulmonary blood flow or with significant valvular regurgitation

- Sternal heave in cases with significant RV hypertrophy
- Heart murmur
- Weak femoral pulsations as in cases with COA
- Blood pressure difference between upper and lower extremities (higher in upper) in cases with COA
- Shock/hypoperfusion and decreased capillary refill as in sever left-sided obstructive lesions when the PDA starts to close
- Fine crackles in cases with pulmonary edema
- Differential cyanosis: Oxygen saturation is higher in upper extremities than lower extremities as in cases with PPHN, IAA, and critical COA
- Reversed differential cyanosis: Oxygen saturation is lower in upper extremities than lower extremities as in cases with TGA with severe PHTN.

SCREENING OF CONGENITAL CYANOTIC HEART DISEASE

Prenatal screening: Fetal echocardiography plays an important role in identification of CCHD; it must be done if obstetric ultrasound revealed suspicion of CHD. The main limitations for its accuracy are: it depends on operator experience moreover maternal overweight and fetal position may affect the quality of the study.[17-19]

Pulse oximetry: Pulse oximetry plays an important role in screening of newborn with CCHD; it should be done at least after 24 hours of life, or just before discharge from the nursery. Pulse oximetry should be done in the right hand (preductal) and in any foot (postductal), three readings separated by 1 hour are required. If oxygen sat <90–95 or the difference between right hand and any foot >3% consultation of pediatric cardiologist should be done to exclude CCHD.[20-23]

Hyperoxia test: This test could be used to distinguish between cyanosis due to lung issues and cyanosis due to CCHD. Arterial blood gas should be done while patient is breathing room air and after 100% oxygen for 10 minutes through hood, mask or endotracheal tube. If PO_2 after 100% oxygen is ≥100 mm Hg, the cause of cyanosis most probably is due to lung issues, and if PO_2 < 100 mm Hg, most probably CCHD is the cause of cyanosis.[24]

Electrocardiogram: ECG can show axis, chamber enlargement, sinus tachycardia associated with heart failure.

Chest X-ray (CXR): It should be done routinely for patients with CCHD; CXR can show pulmonary edema, cardiomegaly, and increased bronchovascular markings as in cases with increased pulmonary blood flow or decreased pulmonary venous drainage. It can help in diagnosis if specific cardiac shapes are identified (egg on side as in TGA, boot shaped as in Fallot tetralogy).[11]

Echocardiography: Echocardiography is a noninvasive accurate modality for diagnosis of CHD; it can delineate anatomy, direction of shunts, and gradient across lesions, chambers size and cardiac function. The main limitations of echocardiography are: it cannot evaluate peripheral pulmonary arteries or veins and limited field of view if the patient has hyper inflated lungs.[25]

Multidetector computed tomography/cardiac MRI: It is complementary to echocardiography, it can evaluate both intra- and extracardiac anatomy, and it is superior to echocardiography in evaluation of peripheral pulmonary arteries or veins, coronary arteries and other vascular structures.[26,27]

MANAGEMENT OF HEART FAILURE IN CHILDREN WITH CYANOTIC HEART DISEASES

Cyanotic congenital heart defects include ductal-dependent pulmonary circulation (e.g. pulmonary atresia with or without VSD, tricuspid atresia) and ductal-dependent systemic circulation (IAA, HLHS). If ductal-dependent lesion is suspected or confirmed, prostaglandin (PGE1) infusion should be started. The dose starts from 0.05 µg/kg/min to 0.1 µg/kg/min.

When the desired response (i.e. increase in oxygen saturation, pH improvement or increase in systemic blood pressure) is achieved, the dose should gradually be reduced to 0.01 µg/kg/min. If there is no effect after starting PGE1, then the dose can be increased up to 0.4 µg/kg/min. The most common side effects of PGE1 intravenous (IV) infusion include apnea, bradycardia, fever, flushing, hypotension and edema.[28]

Interventional Cardiac Catheterization

- *Atrial septostomy*: It is indicated for infants who need mixing of blood for maintaining saturation and cardiac output. The most common indication is TGA with intact interventricular septum (IVS). Other less common indications include total anomalous pulmonary venous connection (TAPVC) with restrictive ASD, tricuspid atresia, pulmonary atresia and mitral atresia. Infants older than 6–8 weeks may require a septostomy with a blade as the septum becomes thicker.[29]
- *PDA stenting*: It is occasionally performed in infants with duct dependent systemic circulation such as HLHS, especially in centers offering transplantation as an alternative to staged palliative surgery. It maintains

duct patency as a bridge to transplantation. Stenting for duct-dependent pulmonary circulation is no longer performed in most centers and the majority of patients undergo a surgical aortopulmonary shunt instead.[30]

- *Radiofrequency perforation*: It can be performed for infants born with pulmonary atresia and intact IVS. If the atresia is membranous, it is possible to burn a hole in the valve with a radiofrequency wire. A balloon can be used to enlarge the hole afterward to secure antegrade flow to the lungs.[30]
- *RVOT stenting*: In the era of primary TOF repair, some young infants have significant risk factors such as small pulmonary arteries, major aortopulmonary collateral arteries (MAPCAs), small body weight and other comorbidities. In such cases, right ventricular outflow tract (RVOT) stenting could be a bridging procedure. It will relieve the cyanosis and allow for both somatic and pulmonary artery growth.[31]
- *Balloon valvuloplasty and angioplasty*: The use of balloons to treat both AS and PS is well established. Treatment of coarctation or branch PS includes ballooning and sometimes stenting of the stenotic segment is needed.[32]

Extracorporeal Membrane Oxygenation

- Preoperative support: Some patient may present initially with cardiogenic shock. Not stable to undergo any kind of surgical repair, they can benefit from preoperative ECMO support when conventional resuscitation measures are unsuccessful at stabilization. For example, a patient with D-TGA and an intact IVS may present with severe hypoxic shock. With not enough time to allow for opening up the ductus arteriosus via PGE1 infusion, these patients can be supported with ECMO until the metabolic acidosis resolves and organ function returns back to normal (thus allowing for the surgery to be done in much better circumstances). Another example can be patients with obstructed TAPVC (often infracardiac as they are more liable). They may present with profound cardiogenic shock that might necessitate ECMO support before going to surgery. Preoperative ECMO support allows resuscitation and stabilization of patients before the additional insult of cardiopulmonary bypass (CPB) and potential deep hypothermic circulation arrest. In addition, it decreases mortality and hypoperfusion associated morbidities such as renal failure.[29]
- Postoperative support: The most common use of ECMO in patients with cyanotic heart disease is postoperative support for low cardiac output, extracorporeal cardiopulmonary resuscitation (ECPR) and failure to come off of CPB.
- Bridge to transplant: Patients with uncorrectable congenital cardiac defects or irreversible cardiomyopathies presenting with profound shock or cardiac arrest can be supported by ECMO and listed for transplantation. If body size is sufficient, it can even be converted into a ventricular assist device (VAD), providing longer periods of support than ECMO as a bridge to transplantation.[29]

Ventricular-assisted Devices

Despite modern advances in medical and surgical therapies for CHDs, some children are not adequately treated enough or undergo palliative procedures which can eventually lead to progressive heart failure. These patients progress to end-stage heart failure for which heart transplant remains the standard of care.

Ventricular-assisted devices used in pediatric patients has become an acceptable therapy for heart failure and bridge to transplant. However, application of VADs in heart failure patients with single ventricle remains uncommon and the published date is limited. VADs offer the advantage of longer duration of support, possibility of hospital discharge, and rehabilitation of the patients' medical, psychological and nutritional conditions.[33]

Heart Transplantation

Currently, it is the best long-term treatment for children with end-stage heart failure. Survival rates vary significantly according to different indications of heart transplant and age groups, with a higher survival rate among younger transplant recipients. The current expected survival for infants receiving a heart transplant is almost 20 years.[34] Congenital heart disease is the indication for more than 50% of pediatric heart transplantations; a substantial portion of which have single ventricle physiology.[35] Patient with CHD have a lower survival rate after heart transplantation, most of the mortalities occurring within the perioperative period.[36]

In a multicenter study, the 5-year survival rate of a large group of patients with CHD (that had undergone heart transplantation) was 80%. All patients in that study were greater than 6 months of age.

The main indications for heart transplantation in cyanotic CHD include:[36]

- Primary heart transplantation for HLHS or Ebstein's anomaly.
- Tetralogy of Fallot (repaired or palliated) and other complex cyanotic heart diseases
- Single ventricle with or without Fontan circulation
- Systemic right ventricle (CC-TGA or TGA after atrial switch operation).

Fetal Intervention

Cardiac lesions that are amenable to fetal intervention are characterized by their rapid progress from mild to severe forms during gestation. This can result in irreversible myocardial damage and chamber, valve, or vessel hypoplasias at birth. There is a time limited window of opportunity to intervene in such unique groups of cardiac defects. The main objective of fetal cardiac intervention is to alter the natural history of an anomaly which, in turn, could be lifesaving to the fetus or improve the state at birth further reducing morbidity and/or mortality.

Currently, fetal cardiac intervention is not yet an alternative to neonatal surgical repair. However, there have been some reported successes in techniques for in utero cardiac approaches.[37]

Fetal catheter intervention may be considered for fetuses with:

- Aortic stenosis with antegrade flow and evolving HLHS (particularly fetuses with a severely restrictive ASD or intact atrial septum)
- Pulmonary atresia and intact interatrial septum with evolving hypoplastic right heart syndrome.

These considerations are classified as per class IIB, level of evidence B/C.[38]

In addition, fetuses with hypoplastic tricuspid valve annulus seem to be good candidates for pulmonary valve in utero intervention allowing for sufficient and significant heart growth.[39]

Cell-based Therapies

Over the last decade, there was development in multiple types of cell-based products that could mitigate the damage effect of acquired cardiac diseases in adults. Recently, there are pediatric CHD clinical trials in place of cell-based therapies focusing on single ventricle physiology. New innovations, such as bioengineered cells and scaffolds, may result in development of bioengineered patches, valves, conduits and even whole organs.[28]

REFERENCES

1. Mason CA, Kirby RS, Sever LE, et al. Prevalence is the preferred measure of frequency of birth defects. Birth Defects Res A Clin Mol Teratol. 2005 Oct;73(10):690-2.
2. Dolk H, Loane M, Garne E, et al. Congenital heart defects in Europe: prevalence and perinatal mortality, 2000 to 2005. Circulation. 2011;123:841-9.
3. van der Linde D, Konings EE, Slager MA, et al. Birth prevalence of congenital heart disease worldwide: a systematic review and meta-analysis. J Am Coll Cardiol. 2011;58:2241-7.
4. Bernier PL, Stefanescu A, Samoukovic G, et al. The challenge of congenital heart disease worldwide: epidemiologic and demographic facts. Semin Thorac Cardiovasc Surg Pediatr Card Surg Annu. 2010;13:26-34.
5. Shah GS, Singh MK, Pandey TR, et al. Incidence of congenital heart disease in tertiary care hospital. Kathmandu Univ Med J (KUMJ). 2008;6:33-6.
6. Hoffman JIE, Kaplan S. The incidence of congenital heart disease. J Am Coll Cardiol. 2002;39:1890-900.
7. Gelb BD, Chung WK. Complex genetics and the etiology of human congenital heart disease. Cold Spring Harb Perspect Med. 2014;4:a013953.
8. Blue GM, Kirk EP, Sholler GF, et al. Congenital heart disease: Current knowledge about causes and inheritance. Med J Aust. 2012;197:155-9.
9. Kashyap S. Approach and management of cyanotic newborn: Guidance for primary caretakers. Gujarat Med J. 2010;65: 94-6.
10. Thiene G, Frescura C. Anatomical and pathophysiological classification of congenital heart disease. Cardiovasc Pathol. 2010;19:259-74.
11. Masarone D, Valente F, Rubino M, et al. Pediatric heart failure: A practical guide to diagnosis and management. Pediatr Neonatol. 2017;58:303-12.
12. Knudson JD, Cabrera AG. The pathophysiology of heart failure in children: The basics. Curr Cardiol Rev. 2016;12: 99-103.
13. Chowdhury D. Pathophysiology of congenital heart diseases. Ann Card Anaesth. 2007;10:19-26.
14. Kyavar M, Sadeghpour A. Cyanosis. In: Sadeghpour A, Kyavar M, Alizadehasl A (Eds). Comprehensive Approach to Adult Congenital Heart Disease. London: Springer-Verlag; 2014. pp. 37-43.
15. Sharma M, Nair MN, Jatana SK, et al. Congestive heart failure in infants and children. Med J Armed Forces India. 2003;59:228-33.
16. Rao PS. Diagnosis and management of cyanotic congenital heart disease: part I. Indian J Pediatr. 2009;76:57-70.
17. Allan L. Technique of fetal echocardiography. Pediatr Cardiol. 2004;25:223-33.
18. SMGroup, Iliescu DG. (2016). Introduction to Fetal Echocardiography. [online] Available from https://smjournals.com/ebooks/echocardiography/chapters/ECHO-16-05.pdf [Last accessed November, 2019].
19. Hutchinson D, McBrien A, Howley L, et al. First-trimester fetal echocardiography: Identification of cardiac Structures for screening from 6 to 13 weeks' gestational age. J Am Soc Echocardiogr. 2017;30:763-72.
20. Mathur NB, Gupta A, Kurien S. Pulse oximetry screening to detect cyanotic congenital heart disease in sick neonates in a neonatal intensive care unit. Indian Pediatr. 2015;52:769-72.
21. Movahedian AH, Mosayebi Z, Sagheb S. Evaluation of pulse oximetry in the early detection of cyanotic congenital heart disease in newborns. J Tehran Univ Hear Cent. 2016;11:73-8.
22. MN P, Zamora J, Suresh G, et al. Pulse oximetry screening for critical congenital heart defects. Cochrane Database Syst Rev. 2018;3:CD011912.

23. Hu X, Ma X, Zhao Q, et al. Pulse oximetry and auscultation for congenital heart disease detection. Pediatrics. 2017;140:(4). pii: e20171154.
24. Singh Y, Chee YH, Gahlaut R. Evaluation of suspected congenital heart disease. Paediatr Child Heal (United Kingdom). 2015;25:7-12.
25. Lai WW, Geva T, Shirali GS, et al. Guidelines and standards for performance of a pediatric echocardiogram: A report from the Task Force of the Pediatric Council of the American Society of Echocardiography. J Am Soc Echocardiogr. 2006;19:1413-30.
26. Crean A. Cardiovascular MR and CT in congenital heart disease. Heart. 2007;93:1637-47.
27. Siripornpitak S, Pornkul R, Khowsathit P, et al. Cardiac CT angiography in children with congenital heart disease. Eur J Radiol. 2013;82:1067-82.
28. Holst KA, Said SM, Nelson TJ, et al. Current interventional and surgical management of congenital heart disease: Specific focus on valvular disease and cardiac arrhythmias. Circ Res. 2017;120:1027-44.
29. Hines MH. ECMO and congenital heart disease. Semin Perinatol. 2005;29:34-39.
30. Andrews RE, Tulloh RM. Interventional cardiac catheterisation in congenital heart disease. Arch Dis Child. 2004;89:1168-73.
31. Sandoval JP, Chaturvedi RR, Benson L, et al. Right ventricular outflow tract stenting in tetralogy of Fallot infants with risk factors for early primary repair. Circ Cardiovasc Interv. 2016;9:1-10.
32. El-saiedi SA, Attia WA, Sobhy R. Transcatheter repair of congenital heart defects in the young. EMJ. 2017;36-44.
33. Carlo WF, Villa CR, Lal AK, et al. Ventricular assist device use in single ventricle congenital heart disease. Pediatr Transplant. 2017;21:1-8.
34. Dipchand AI, Kirk R, Edwards LB, et al. The Registry of the International Society for Heart and Lung Transplantation: Sixteenth Official Pediatric Heart Transplantation Report—2013; focus theme: age. J Heart Lung Transplant. 2013;32:979-88.
35. Voeller RK, Epstein DJ, Guthrie TJ, et al. Trends in the indications and survival in pediatric heart transplants : a 24-year single-center experience in 307 Patients. Ann Thorac Surg. 2012;94(3):807-15; discussion 815-6.A
36. Lamour JM, Kanter KR, Naftel DC, et al. The effect of age, diagnosis, and previous surgery in children and adults undergoing heart transplantation for congenital heart disease. J Am Coll Cardiol. 2009;54:160-5.
37. Lee K, Khoshnood B, Chen L, et al. Infant mortality from congenital malformations in the United States, 1970-1997. Obstet Gynecol. 2001;98:620-7.
38. Yuan SM. Fetal cardiac interventions: an update of therapeutic options. Rev Bras Cir Cardiovasc. 2014;29:388-95.
39. Van Aerschot I, Rosenblatt J, Boudjemline Y. Fetal cardiac interventions: myths and facts. Arch Cardiovasc Dis. 2012;105:366-72.

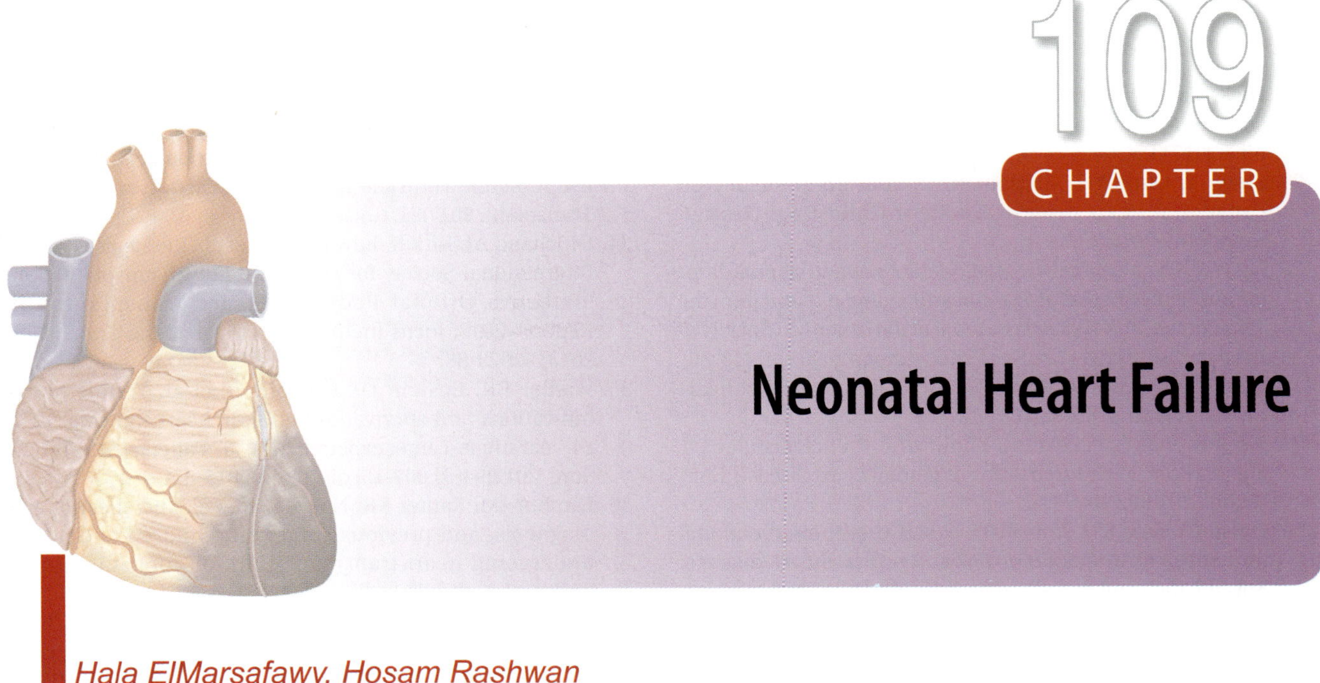

Neonatal Heart Failure

Hala ElMarsafawy, Hosam Rashwan

INTRODUCTION

Neonatal heart failure (HF) is a progressive clinical and pathophysiological disease caused by cardiovascular and noncardiovascular abnormalities that results from impairment of the ventricle to fill with or eject blood properly.[1] The most common cause of neonatal HF is structural congenital heart disease.[2] The causes of HF can be divided into several diverse overlapping categories:

- Cardiovascular versus noncardiovascular
- *Pathophysiologic*: Ventricular pump dysfunction with decreased contractility, or altered preload or afterload with preserved contractility
- Congenital cardiac malformation versus structurally normal heart (cardiomyopathy).[2]

CONGENITAL HEART DISEASES

Neonate with septal defects usually presents between 2 weeks and 8 weeks of age with congestive heart failure (CHF) as there is fall in pulmonary vascular resistance causing increase in pulmonary blood flow, rarely there can be an early presentation as in preterm child where precipitous fall in pulmonary vascular resistance (PVR) occurs causing large left to right shunt. In any newborn presenting with CHF, one should always look for other causes contributing to heart failure in addition to septal defects as:

- Associated obstructive lesion, especially coarctation of aorta, interrupted aortic arch or rarely aortic stenosis.
- Multiple levels of shunts, e.g. at atrial, ventricular and great artery.[1]

Ventricular dilation is initially adaptive to increase stroke volume, but eventually reaches an unfavorable point on the Frank–Starling curve, and decreases in cardiac contractility ensue. Congenital heart disease may induce low cardiac output via obstructive lesions of left-sided heart structures (e.g. critical aortic stenosis, hypoplastic left heart syndrome, critical coarctation), regurgitant lesions (e.g. severe mitral or aortic regurgitation), or lesions with obstruction to pulmonary venous return and inadequate atrial level shunting.[3]

Arteriovenous malformations (AVMs) also cause heart failure like anomalous origin of pulmonary artery from ascending aorta and Tetralogy of Fallot with absent pulmonary valve syndrome.[1] Anomalous origin of the left coronary artery from the pulmonary artery (ALCAPA) is an important but rare cause of ischemic cardiomyopathy in young infants. Correct establishment of this diagnosis in an infant with a dilated, dysfunctional left ventricle (LV) is critical because corrective surgery is available with excellent short- and long-term results. The onset of symptoms typically occurs within the first 1–3 months of life, when the pulmonary vascular resistance drops and is manifested by irritability, poor feeding, and tachypnea. However, in some patients, sufficient collateralization may occur to mitigate or prevent early symptoms. The electrocardiography (ECG) will show ST segment abnormalities and prominent Q waves; the echocardiogram shows a dilated, dysfunctional LV, frequently with mitral regurgitation. Reimplantation of the left main coronary artery is the surgical treatment of choice, with excellent long-term results.[4]

INHERITED CARDIOMYOPATHY

Neonatal cardiomyopathy is a diverse group of diseases with various morphological and functional phenotypes that affect the heart muscle and alter cardiac performance in neonates.[5] Cardiomyopathy can be segregated by gross cardiac phenotype into five general classifications: (1) dilated cardiomyopathy (DCM), (2) hypertrophic cardiomyopathy (HCM), (3) restrictive cardiomyopathy, (4) arrhythmogenic ventricular cardiomyopathy, and (5) left ventricular noncompaction cardiomyopathy (LVNC). The overall incidence of discovered cardiomyopathy (with or without heart failure symptoms) was 1.13/100,000 in the Pediatric Cardiomyopathy Registry (PCMR) in the United States and 1.24/100,000 in the National Australian Childhood Cardiomyopathy Study. These numbers were significantly higher for the neonatal group, at 8.34/100,000 and 7.84/100,000, respectively.[6,7] Neonatal DCM was 1.5 higher in neonates in PCMR.[8] DCM means the presence of a dilated LV chamber with decreased LV wall thickness, and systolic and/or diastolic dysfunction. It usually presents before the age of 1 year (41 %) with myocarditis being the most common cause according to PCMR.[6] However, the diagnosis of myocarditis remains challenging especially in infants where biopsy would be difficult to do. DCM have genetic background in almost 20% of cases[9] and familial DCM in fact represents about 40% of cases and mostly are autosomal dominant.[10]

Hypertrophic cardiomyopathy is characterized by hypertrophy of the left (and occasionally right) ventricle with histologic features of myocyte hypertrophy, myofibrillar disarray, and interstitial fibrosis. The survival for patients that present in the first year is low according to PCMR.[11] The genetic element plays a major role in half of the sporadic cases and two-thirds of familial ones.[12] Abnormalities in proteins of sarcomere contributes to the disease in adults, but this is not the case in children where genetic and metabolic causes are more common like glycogen storage disorders (GSD) (e.g. Pompe disease), lysosomal storage disease (e.g., sialidosis and Fabry disease), and mitochondrial disorders.[9]

Left ventricular noncompaction is characterized by the presence of prominent trabeculae, intertrabecular recesses, and thickening of the myocardium in two distinct layers composed of compacted and noncompacted tissue. The median age of presentation is 90 days and is usually in the form of low cardiac output or congestive heart failure.[13] The first gene described as causative of isolated LVNC was *TAZ*, which is responsible for Barth syndrome.[14]

METABOLIC AND TOXIC CARDIOMYOPATHIES

Fatty acid oxidation defects present with hypoketotic hypoglycemia with heart energy utilization is disrupted.[15] Carnitine is needed for transport of fatty acids across the inner mitochondrial membrane and its deficiency causes cardiomyopathy. It may be advised to give carnitine to neonates and infants with a suspected cardiomyopathy till establishing the diagnosis.[16]

Disorders of mitochondrial metabolism can present with cardiomyopathy with HCM is most common. Barth syndrome (X-linked DCM/LVNC with cyclic neutropenia and skeletal myopathy) is a classic example.[17] The infantile form of Pompe disease is the prototypical GSD with symptoms occurring in neonatal life. It results from decreased activity of α-1,4-glucosidase and presents as HCM, macroglossia, and hypotonia.[18] Cardiomyopathy in infants of diabetic mothers (IDM) includes biventricular hypertrophy proportional to the degree of maternal hyperglycemia in pregnancy. Regression is the role and use of beta-blockade may help reverse remodeling.[19]

Neonatal myocardium is particularly sensitive to perturbations in calcium transport, administration of calcium-channel blockers, particularly non-dihydropyridine class (e.g. verapamil) should be done with extreme caution.

INFLAMMATORY AND INFECTIOUS CARDIOMYOPATHIES

Myocarditis usually has a fulminant course and mimic overwhelming sepsis and necessitate mechanical ventilator and/or circulatory support. It is acquired or transplacental in 3rd trimester.[20] Kawasaki disease (KD) is a systemic inflammatory process manifesting as prolonged fever, rash, conjunctivitis, lymphadenopathy, and mucosal erythema. It is more common in first 5 years of life but when presents in first 6 months, it is usually atypical with high incidence of coronary aneurysms. KD may also cause myocarditis and affect systolic and diastolic functions of the heart.[21] Endocarditis is a cardiac infection of the heart lining and/or cardiac valves. It usually happens in neonates with indwelling central catheters. It manifests as rapidly progressive valve disease or a sepsis syndrome.[22]

ARRHYTHMIA

Arrhythmias, though rare, are not uncommon in full-term and preterm newborns. Maternal diabetes, toxemia and other postnatal conditions, e.g. asphyxia, hypothermia, metabolic and electrolyte imbalances, all contribute to rhythm disturbances. High index of suspicion in all neonates with left ventricular dysfunction is necessary to diagnose this condition. A critical evaluation of ECG is essential especially because many of these ECGs may casually be interpreted as sinus tachycardia, which is commonly associated with LV dysfunction. It is not necessary to have very fast heart rate to diagnose this condition. Suspicion is aroused when—

- The heart rate shows no variability and is fixed between 150 beats/min to 180 beats/min
- Abnormal P wave axis
- Atrioventricular (AV) dissociation.

Disruption of AV synchrony and loss of heart rate variability are responsible for development of heart failure.[23]

TACHYARRHYTHMIA

Classified into two groups: (1) Narrow QRS tachycardia, and (2) wide QRS tachycardia.

- *Narrow QRS tachycardia:* Ectopic atrial tachycardias, orthodromic, or antidromic AV reentrant tachycardias, the permanent form of reciprocating junctional tachycardia and atrial flutter are the most commonly described neonatal arrhythmias associated with cardiac dilation and systolic dysfunction. When starts in utero, incessant tachycardia can induce hydrops fetalis. Although paroxysmal supraventricular tachycardia (SVT) caused by accessory pathway [Wolff-Parkinson-White (WPW syndrome)] is the commonest mechanism in the neonatal period, this condition rarely causes heart failure because it is rarely sustained. The much rarer varieties of sustained supraventricular tachycardia (called junctional ectopic tachycardia) is more often responsible for heart failure because of its sustained nature. Atrial arrhythmias, like atrial flutter or atrial fibrillation are very rarely seen in pediatric practice, more so in neonate. Structural heart defects are not common in this group. Termination of the dysrhythmia will mostly cause return of ventricular function over a period of weeks to months.[24]
- *Wide QRS tachycardia:* It is relatively rare in neonatal period and is usually associated with some structural cardiac damage as in myocarditis or cardiac tumor.

Management

Early Management

- Circulatory collapse with a tachycardia whether broad or narrow complex requires direct current cardioversion, which should be synchronized
- If the compromise is not critical, try adenosine first
- In the infant with a narrow complex tachycardia who is not compromised, facial immersion can be tried. With the infant wrapped in a towel and connected to an ECG, the face is immersed for approximately five seconds into a bowl of cold water. It is safe and effective.[25] Ocular pressure is not recommended at any age, and carotid massage does not work and compresses the airway.

Adenosine at an initial dose of 200 mcg/kg can be given rapidly intravenously into a large vein (such as the antecubital fossa). Up to 500 mcg/kg is occasionally required.[26] Failure of adenosine to terminate the tachycardia may be due to:

- Inadequate dosage or too slow administration of the drug.
- The mechanism being atrial tachycardia as adenosine blocks the AV node, it may reveal atrial flutter or atrial tachycardia as the cause of the problem.
- The mechanism being ventricular tachycardia (VT).

Transient termination of a conduction system dependent tachycardia, with a few beats of sinus rhythm before restarting, is not uncommon. In this case, additional antiarrhythmic treatment is required. Intravenous amiodarone is increasingly used. Reasons being:

- It will work if the diagnosis is SVT or VT.
- It has little negative inotropic effect, so it is relatively safe when myocardial function may be compromised.
- It is effective with atrial flutter and safer than intravenous flecainide because it slows AV nodal conduction as well as slowing and eventually interrupting the flutter circuit.

Maintenance Therapy

Various pharmaceutical agents are used in the management of neonatal tachycardias. The standard classification of commonly used drugs is the Vaughan Williams' classification of antiarrhythmics.

Commonly used medications are beta-blocker, amiodarone, flecainide, and sotalol. Digoxin is sometimes used as adjunctive treatment to provide some AV block in combination with another agent, particularly flecainide, but also sotalol and amiodarone. The natural history of SVT presenting in the neonate suggests that spontaneous resolution usually occurs in the first year of life.[26,27]

BRADYARRHYTHMIAS

Depending on the heart rate, bradyarrhythmias (commonest being complete heart block) can cause heart failure even in fetal life. Careful and regular heart evaluation of these neonates is essential in order to advise pacemaker. Congenital complete heart block is often present as sequelae of transplacental passage of maternal anti-SSA (Sjögren's syndrome-related antigen A) or anti-SSB (Sjögren's-syndrome-related antigen B) antibodies, or as an associated feature of certain complex congenital heart defects such as heterotaxy syndrome. Persistent heart block can induce ventricular dilation and dysfunction.[28]

The current recommendations for permanent pacemaker in neonates are:

- *Symptoms*: Most commonly heart failure
- Heart rate less than 55 beats per minute and 70 beats per minute with structural heart defect
- Left ventricular dysfunction on echocardiography.

NONCARDIAC HEART FAILURE

- *Twin-twin transfusion syndrome (TTTS):* The recipient twin will often have ventricular hypertrophy in variable degrees. However, regression mostly occurs after birth. Fetal therapy with laser photocoagulation of the interplacental connections has shown success in resolving these cardiac abnormalities.[29] Moreover, monochorionic twin pregnancies especially those complicated by TTTS are at high risk for coronary heart disease (CHD), a detailed prenatal and postnatal echocardiography may be an advantage for early detection of CHD and might improve perinatal management, which should be evaluated in further studies.[30]
- *Pulmonary hypertension:* Outside of its association with congenital diaphragmatic hernia, pulmonary hypertension in neonates and infants may be seen in two categories: (1) persistent pulmonary hypertension of the newborn, and (2) pulmonary hypertension of chronic lung disease, which is a disease of premature infants.[31]
- **Vein of Galen malformation:**
  - Arteriovenous malformations are abnormal connections between an artery and a vein whereby the interconnecting capillary network is missed.[32] They frequently occur in midline regions of the brain.[33] The incidence of cerebral AVMs amounts to 1.21 per 100,000 persons per year.[34]
  - Vein of Galen is a short midline venous structure formed by the confluence of the two internal cerebral veins and the basal veins of Rosenthal. It is the caudal remnant of the median prosencephalic vein, which is a centrally located vessel that drains the choroid plexus. The Galenic vein is believed to be formed from the cerebral vasculature between 6 weeks and 11 weeks of gestation.[35]
  - The aneurysmal malformation of the Galenic vein is a rare congenital cerebral arteriovenous anomaly with an incidence of 1:25,000 that comprises 30% of the pediatric vascular and 1% of all pediatric congenital anomalies.[36]
  - Its pathogenesis is unknown but findings suggest that an endoglin mutation might be linked with vein of Galen aneurysmal malformation.[37]
  - Vein of Galen aneurysmal malformation is developed between 6 weeks and 11 weeks of gestation and can be diagnosed in the prenatal period by ultrasonography. Moreover, it is accompanied by high output heart failure and sometimes it can present with an audible cranial bruit.[38]
  - The main presentations of these patients are accompanied with CHF. It is important to highlight the fact that not all cases of cardiac failure may be due to a primary cardiac cause. An early diagnosis with a prompt referral is crucial in the management of this life-threatening condition.
  - A systolic murmur, as the first clinical manifestation of high cardiac output failure induced by cerebral arteriovenous malformations (CAVMs) after birth, has been reported by Barajas-Gamboa et al. in Mexico.[39]
- **Myocardial ischemia:**
  - The influence of hypoxemia related myocardial dysfunction in the newborn occurs in 30% of asphyxiated neonates[40] and is thought to be secondary to direct effect of ischemia on cardiac myocytes. Enzymatic indicators of myocardial injury in the asphyxiated newborns are elevated and often associated with electrocardiographic changes. The measurement of cardiac troponin may have a role in the early identification of neonates with myocardial damage secondary to ischemia. However, cardiac abnormalities often are underdiagnosed and require a high index of suspicion.
  - Hypoxia is responsible for multiorgan dysfunction causing deaths, but particularly results in myocardial damage despite "preferential'" myocardial perfusion.[41]
  - Myocardial dysfunction secondary to perinatal asphyxia is more frequent than thought, for which it will be useful to submit asphyxiated neonates to ECG monitoring and assay of cardiac enzyme markers complemented with clinical findings.[42]
- *Anemia*: The diagnosis of heart failure is based on a combination of characteristic signs and physical findings of impaired cardiac output, respiratory distress, and poor growth. Imaging studies generally are used to confirm the diagnosis of heart failure when there is a clinical uncertainty. Jaundice, feeding intolerance, tachypnea, tachycardia, hepatomegaly and delayed capillary refill are usually detected. Echocardiography was almost normal with minimally affected left ventricular function.[43]
- Other causes of heart failure are sacrococcygeal teratoma, perinatal hypoxic-ischemic injury and coronary thrombosis.

Diagnosis

Detailed History

- The mother's prenatal history specially any illnesses or toxic exposures
- A family history, extending at least three generations, if possible
- Deaths that are sudden or unexplained.

Examination

- Baby's weight
- Blood pressure and saturations in the right upper and a lower extremity is critical to exclude coarctation and assess for hypertension

- Abnormal murmurs, a gallop rhythm, thrills, and the intensity of the heart sounds.

Laboratory

- Serum chemistry panel, hepatic function panel, complete blood count with differential, thyroid function studies, a B-type natriuretic peptide, and serum troponin level
- Blood polymerase chain reaction (PCR) for adenovirus, parvovirus B19, human herpes virus 6, enterovirus, cytomegalovirus, and human immunodeficiency virus, if myocarditis was suspected
- Metabolic consultation and basic metabolic laboratories, including urine organic acids, serum amino acids, and a serum carnitine level.

Genetic Studies

- Commercially available testing for gene mutations associated with cardiomyopathy
- Whole exome sequencing.

Echocardiography

- A full anatomic study to evaluate for congenital and acquired conditions
- Assessments of LV systolic function including shortening fraction and ejection fraction
- Assessment of right ventricular systolic function is more limited
- Quantification of AV and semilunar valve regurgitation
- Assessment of diastolic function via tissue Doppler imaging by measuring myocardial velocities at the mitral valve annulus
- Strain rate imaging and 3D volumetric measures of right and left ventricular systolic function are currently under investigation but have not gained wide use in the evaluation of children and infants due to technical challenges and lack of easy reproducibility.

Cardiac Magnetic Resonance Imaging

- Is challenged by the need for sedation and/or general anesthesia
- Higher heart rates in children (especially neonates) further hamper ECG gating
- Cardiac magnetic resonance imaging (MRI) is superior to echocardiography in image quality of both the LV and right ventricle and allows for accurate volumetric calculation of ejection fraction of both ventricles
- Assessment for myocardial scarring via the presence of late gadolinium enhancement and T1 mapping.

Cardiac Catheterization

- Confirmation of coronary anatomy is best accomplished with selective coronary injection or aortic root angiography and should be considered if there is persistent suspicion of ALCAPA following other imaging evaluation
- When severe valvar congenital heart disease (e.g. critical aortic stenosis) is the etiology for acute heart failure catheterization can offer an interventional modality, in addition to its diagnostic utility
- In cases of refractory arrhythmias, invasive intracardiac electrophysiologic procedures can be considered for diagnosis confirmation or very rarely for intervention.

Management

Stabilization

- *Diuretics*: In stable infants, diuretics may be all what is needed. Furosemide should be started without delay. Diuretics are safe; however, anticipation for hypotension, renal insufficiency and electrolyte imbalances is needed.
- Inotropes should be used if there is a drop in systemic perfusion or resistance.
  - Milrinone is a phosphodiesterase inhibitor that increases cyclic adenosine monophosphate (cAMP). As calcium reuptake in the myocyte is dependent on cAMP, milrinone is also thought to enhance cardiac relaxation, so-called lusitropy. It is inodilator causing inotropy, afterload reduction and pulmonary vasodilatation without sustained rise in heart rate. It is safe in neonates and PRIMACORP study showed that milrinone decreases the risk of low cardiac output syndrome in neonates postoperative. Infusions start at low dose (0.1–0.3 mcg/kg/min) and up-titrated to a maximum of approximately 0.75 mcg/kg/min.[44]
  - Sympathomimetics as dopamine and dobutamine are used in cases of hypotension. Dobutamine is inodilator that increases contractility and reduces afterload by acting on adrenergic receptors, however. The net effect in children has been shown to be improved myocardial function, increased cardiac index, and stroke volume with less dramatic increase in heart rate. Dopamine acts on dopaminergic and adrenergic receptors, hence increases contractility by stimulating B adrenergic receptors and increases afterload by acting on alpha-1 adrenergic receptor. It causes tachycardia and is proarrhythmic. Epinephrine may be used in cardiogenic shock. It sustains blood pressure but causes tachycardia, myocardial ischemia, and arrhythmia.
- *Calcium chloride*: In neonates, the myocardial calcium stores are generally inadequate for the stresses induced by acute heart failure. So, neonates can be particularly sensitive to increased calcium concentrations with

significant improvements in cardiac contractility being directly tied to serum calcium levels. Calcium additionally has the benefit of not increasing heart rate or cardiac oxygen demand, in contrast to the effects of catecholamine medications.

- *Vasodilators*: They are helpful in patients with low cardiac output accompanied by high systemic vascular resistance.
  - Nitroprusside is a commonly used vasodilator with rapid onset and effect that can be used in neonates although utility is limited by cyanide toxicity.
  - Nicardipine is a dihydropyridine calcium channel blocker that has vasodilator effects on the vascular system without intrinsic myocardial inhibition. However, caution has been recommended in its use in neonates due to their low calcium stores.
  - Nesiritide, the recombinant form of brain natriuretic peptide, has been used in adults and children as an infusion for patients with acute decompensated heart failure and in adults was shown to improve outcomes although not clearly better than other vasodilators.[45]

Maintenance Therapy

Afterload reduction in chronic heart failure is mainly achieved by blockade of the conversion of angiotensin I to angiotensin II via angiotensin-converting enzyme inhibitors (ACEIs). Decreased angiotensin II yields less vasoconstriction and aldosterone production, as well as inhibiting the reuptake of sodium, potassium, and water in the tubules and collecting duct.

Adrenergic blockade with beta antagonists has been shown to provide additive survival benefits. Carvedilol, a nonselective beta-blocker with additional alpha-1 antagonism and antioxidative properties, has shown mild morbidity and mortality improvements in adult studies.

Use of digoxin, a cardiac glycoside that increases sarcoplasmic calcium concentrations via inhibition of the Na/KATPase continues to be common in some pediatric centers in part because of use in dysrhythmias, but it is no longer considered frontline for management of heart failure.[46]

Extracorporeal Membrane Oxygenation

Extracorporeal membrane oxygenation (ECMO) is now a readily available and often-successful means of short-term support in children of all ages. Limitations of ECMO include the need for systemic anticoagulation, the need for large-bore cannulae often with central placement through the chest in infants, and risk of both embolic and hemorrhagic complications.

Heart Transplantation

The primary indication for heart transplantation in infants remains congenital heart disease; however, in the last 3 decades, the number of cardiomyopathy cases has increased so that now only 55% of recipients have congenital disease to 41% cardiomyopathy, compared to approximately 75% congenital heart disease in the 1980s. Current data show a median survival of approximately 20 years, which has been steadily improving over time. For those patients who survive the first year the median survival stretches out to greater than 25 years. For those patients surviving 5 years posttransplant, greater than 60% will survive to 25 years.[47]

REFERENCES

1. Levy PT, Tissot C, Eriksen BH, et al. Application of neonatologist performed echocardiography in the assessment and management of neonatal heart failure unrelated to congenital Heart Disease. Pediatr Res. 2018;84(Suppl 1):78-88.
2. Hsu DT, Pearson GD. Heart failure in children: part I: history, etiology, and pathophysiology. Circulation: Heart Fail. 2009;2(1):63-70.
3. Kemper AR, Mahle WT, Martin GR, et al. Strategies for implementing screening for critical congenital heart disease. Pediatrics. 2011;128(5):e1259-67.
4. Ma K, Wang L, Hua Z, et al. Outcomes of coronary transfer for anomalous origin of the left coronary artery from the pulmonary artery. Eur J Cardiothorac Surg. 2015;47(4):659-64.
5. Nugent AW, Daubeney PE, Chondros P, et al. The epidemiology of childhood cardiomyopathy in Australia. N Engl J Med. 2003;348(17):1639-46.
6. Wilkinson JD, Landy DC, Colan SD, et al. The pediatric cardiomyopathy registry and heart failure: key results from the first 15 years. Heart Fail Clin. 2010;6(4):401-13.
7. Nugent AW, Daubeney PE, Chondros P, et al. The epidemiology of childhood cardiomyopathy in Australia. N Engl J Med. 2003;348(17):1639-46.
8. Towbin JA, Lowe AM, Colan SD, et al. Incidence, causes, and outcomes of dilated cardiomyopathy in children. JAMA. 2006;296(15):1867-76.
9. Kindel SJ, Miller EM, Gupta R, et al. Pediatric cardiomyopathy: importance of genetic and metabolic evaluation. J Card Fail. 2012;18(5):396-403.
10. Towbin J, Bowles N. The failing heart. Nature. 2002;415(6868):227-33.
11. Colan SD, Lipshultz SE, Lowe AM, et al. Epidemiology and cause-specific outcome of hypertrophic cardiomyopathy in children: findings from the Pediatric Cardiomyopathy Registry. Circulation. 2007;115(6):773-81.
12. Morita H, Rehm HL, Menesses A, et al. Shared genetic causes of cardiac hypertrophy in children and adults. N Engl J Med. 2008;358(18):1899-908.
13. Pignatelli RH, McMahon CJ, Dreyer WJ, et al. Clinical characterization of left ventricular noncompaction in

children: a relatively common form of cardiomyopathy. Circulation. 2003;108(21):2672-8.
14. Bleyl SB, Mumford BR, Brown-Harrison MC, et al. Xq28-linked noncompaction of the left ventricular myocardium: prenatal diagnosis and pathologic analysis of affected individuals. Am J Med Genet. 1997;72(3):257-65.
15. Baruteau J, Sachs P, Broue P, et al. Clinical and biological features at diagnosis in mitochondrial fatty acid beta-oxidation defects: a French pediatric study of 187 patients. J Inherit Metab Dis. 2013;36(5):795-803.
16. Helton E, Darragh R, Francis P, et al. Metabolic aspects of myocardial disease and a role for L-carnitine in the treatment of childhood cardiomyopathy. Pediatrics. 2000;105(6):1260-70.
17. Scaglia F, Towbin JA, Craigen WJ, et al. Clinical spectrum, morbidity, and mortality in 113 pediatric patients with mitochondrial disease. Pediatrics. 2004;114(4):925-31.
18. Kishnani PS, Amartino HM, Lindberg C, et al. Timing of diagnosis of patients with Pompe disease: data from the Pompe registry. Am J Med Genet A. 2013;161A(10):2431-43.
19. Huang T, Kelly A, Becker SA, et al. Hypertrophic cardiomyopathy in neonates with congenital hyperinsulinism. Arch Dis Child Fetal Neonatal Ed. 2013;98(4):F351-4.
20. Teele SA, Allan CK, Laussen PC, et al. Management and outcomes in pediatric patients presenting with acute fulminant myocarditis. J Pediatr. 2011;158(4):638-43 e1.
21. Hangai M, Kubota Y, Kagawa J, et al. Neonatal Kawasaki disease: case report and data from nationwide survey in Japan. Eur J Pediatr. 2014;173(11):1533-6.
22. Lin YT, Hsieh KS, Chen YS, et al. Infective endocarditis in children without underlying heart disease. J Microbiol Immunol Infect. 2013;46(2):121-8.
23. Lipshultz SE, Adams MJ, Colan SD, et al. Long-term cardiovascular toxicity in children, adolescents, and young adults who receive cancer therapy: pathophysiology, course, monitoring, management, prevention, and research directions: a scientific statement from the American Heart Association. Circulation. 2013;128(17):1927-95.
24. Moore JP, Patel PA, Shannon KM, et al. Predictors of myocardial recovery in pediatric tachycardia-induced cardiomyopathy. Heart Rhythm. 2014;11(7):1163-9.
25. Sreeram N, Wren C. Supraventricular tachycardia in infants: response to initial treatment. Arch Dis Child. 1990;65(1):127-9.
26. Dixon J, Foster K, Wyllie J, et al. Guidelines and adenosine dosing in supraventricular tachycardia. Arch Dis Child. 2005;90(11):1190.
27. van Engelen AD, Weijtens O, Brenner JI, et al. Management outcome and follow-up of fetal tachycardia. J Am Coll Cardiol. 1994;24(5):1371-5.
28. Silvetti MS, Drago F, Rava L. Determinants of early dilated cardiomyopathy in neonates with congenital complete atrioventricular block. Europace. 2010;12(9):1316-21.
29. Roberts D, Neilson JP, Kilby MD, et al. Interventions for the treatment of twin-twin transfusion syndrome. Cochrane Database Syst Rev. 2014;30(1):CD002073.
30. Springer S, Mlczoch E, Krampl-Bettelheim E, et al. Congenital heart disease in monochorionic twins with and without twin-to-twin transfusion syndrome. Prenat Diagn. 2014;34(10):994-9.
31. Hansmann G. Pulmonary hypertension in infants, children, and young adults. J Am Coll Cardiol. 2017;69(20):2551-69.
32. Riasi HR, Salehi F, Sanati AR. Fluctuating neurologic symptoms in a patient with brain lesion. J Med Cases. 2017;8(2):67-9.
33. Hortobágyi T, Szüts A, Csenki M, et al. Vein of Galen malformation combined with atrial septal defect in a neonate. Clin Neuropathol. 2003;22(4):193-8.
34. Daroff RB, Jankovic J, Mazziotta JC, Pomeroy S (Eds). Bradley's Neurology in Clinical Practice. Philadelphia: Elsevier Health Sciences; 2015.
35. Fayyaz A, Qureshi IA. Vein of Galen aneurysm: antenatal diagnosis: a case report. J Pak Med Assoc. 2005;55(10):455.
36. Wagner MW, Vaught AJ, Poretti A, et al. Vein of Galen aneurysmal malformation: Prognostic markers depicted on fetal MRI. Neuroradiol J. 2015;28(1):71-5.
37. Tsutsumi Y, Kosaki R, Itoh Y, et al. Vein of Galen aneurysmal malformation associated with an endoglin gene mutation. Pediatrics. 2011;128(5):e1307-10.
38. De Beritto T, Khan OA, Hageman JR, et al. Vein of Galen arteriovenous malformation in a neonate. Pediatr Ann. 2015;44(10):e243-6.
39. Barajas-Gamboa JS, Diaz-Perez JA, Leon-Camargo Y, et al. Systolic heart murmur as first manifestation of high output heart failure due to the vein of galen malformation. Arch Cardiol Mex. 2012;82(3):214-7.
40. Martín-Ancel A, García-Alix A, Cabañas FGF, et al. Multiple organ involvement in perinatal asphyxia. J Pediatr. 1995;127(5):786-93.
41. Legido A, Katsetos C, Mishra O, et al. Perinatal hypoxic ischemic encephalopathy: current and future treatments. Internat Pediatr. 2000;15(3):138-46.
42. Agrawal J, Shah GS, Poudel P, et al. Electrocardiographic and enzymatic correlations with outcome in neonates with hypoxic-ischemic encephalopathy. Ital J Pediatr. 2012;38(1):33.
43. Bilgin H, Eren A, Kara S. Hemolytic anemia and heart failure caused by anti-C and anti-E immunization. J Coll Physicians Surg Pak. 2016;26(6):539-40.
44. Abraham WT, Adams KF, Fonarow GC, et al. In-hospital mortality in patients with acute decompensated heart failure requiring intravenous vasoactive medications: an analysis from the Acute Decompensated Heart Failure National Registry (ADHERE). J Am Coll Cardiol. 2005;46(1):57-64.
45. Jefferies JL, Price JF, Denfield SW, et al. Safety and efficacy of nesiritide in pediatric heart failure. J Card Fail. 2007;13(7):541-8.
46. O'Connor MJ, Rosenthal DN, Shaddy RE. Outpatient management of pediatric heart failure. Heart Fail Clin. 2010;6(4):515-29.
47. Benden C, Goldfarb SB, Edwards LB, et al. The registry of the International Society for Heart and Lung Transplantation: seventeenth official pediatric lung and heart-lung transplantation report--2014; focus theme: retransplantation. J Heart Lung Transplant.f 2014;33(10):1025-33.

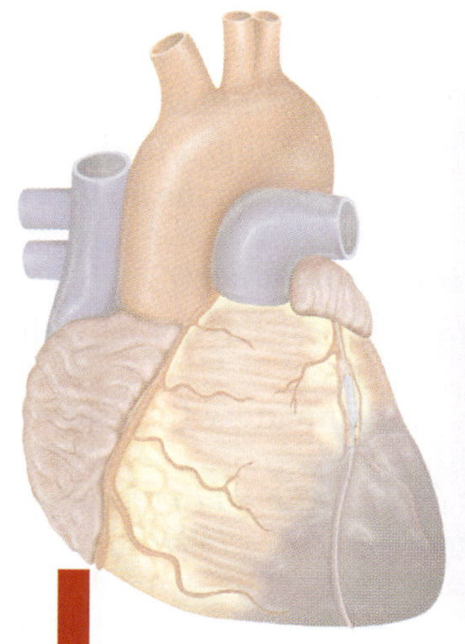

Prevention of Heart Failure in Children

Smita Mishra, Shariq Hoda

INTRODUCTION

Heart failure (HF) is a clinical syndrome characterized by the inability of the heart to supply cardiac output at a pace necessary to meet the metabolic demands of the body at the normal filling pressure/ventricular diastolic pressure.[1-3] The presentation of pediatric HF is diverse because of numerous underlying etiologies. Consequently, traditional preventive strategies adapted for adult HF cannot be imitated for HF in children. This chapter is a brief review of level of prevention of HF in young population.

LEVELS OF PREVENTION IN PEDIATRIC HEART FAILURE

- *Primary prevention*: It includes preventing exposures or increasing resistance to the cause of disease by identifying multiple "upstream factors" in the form of social determinants of early onset of adult cardiovascular diseases (CVDs). In congenital heart diseases (CHDs) there are scarcely any modifiable factors.
- *Secondary prevention*: This includes early detection, treatment, prevention of recurrence, and rehabilitation of a heart disease.
- *Tertiary prevention*: The tertiary prevention includes management of long-term issues (e.g. chronic HF) by drug, devices or palliation so to maximize functional abilities, quality of life, and life expectancy in those cases where primary or secondary prevention do not have a role.

TARGETING THE ANTENATAL FACTORS FOR PREVENTION OF HEART DISEASES[3-6]

- *Fetotoxic and teratogenic effects of drug or metabolic factors* (antiepileptic drugs like eptoin, or anticoagulants like warfarin—daily dose of >5 mg, contraceptives, lithium, coffee, alcohol, cocaine, and high HbA1c), *infections, malnutrition and hyperglycemia, and radiation during the period of organogenesis.*[4-6]
- *Role of hyperhomocysteinemia and vitamin deficiencies (B2, B6, B12, and folic acid) as the possible candidate for preconception screening.*[6]
- *Maternal overnutrition and obesity as the cause of* programed cardiac dysfunction and up-regulation of fetal genes.[6]
- *CHD and consanguinity*[3-6]: The parental consanguinity may have a higher chance of CHD in babies of consanguineous parents.

APPROPRIATE INVESTIGATIONS

The investigations are required to make the diagnosis of cardiac ailment as well as malfunctioning of other systems (X-ray chest, electrocardiogram, hematology, lipid profile, renal function test, liver function test, lipid profile, ultrasound abdomen, arterial blood gas analysis, etc.). Besides the echocardiography, several other imaging modalities (CT-MR angio, conventional angiograms and electrophysiological studies) may be needed on several occasions.

HEART FAILURE IN DIFFERENT TYPE OF CARDIAC DISEASES

Congenital Heart Diseases[7,8]

Saxena et al. reported prevalence of CHD is 8.07/1,000 live birth in a single institution study. Due to the increasing number of successful interventions for CHD per year, the size of the population of patients with grown-up congenital heart disease (GUCH) is expanding. The fetal diagnosis of complex CHD and subsequent termination of pregnancy may be a secondary prevention strategy.

Acyanotic Heart Diseases

Atrial septal defect (ASD) is a pretricuspid shunt lesion which often presents with arrhythmia, HF in adulthood or infrequently as the Eisenmenger syndrome. Large post-tricuspid shunt lesions, like ventricular septal defect, patent ductus arteriosus, aortopulmonary window, present with high output heart failure with preserved ejection function (HFpEF) in first few months of life. The valvular or vascular obstructive lesions [pulmonary stenosis (PS), aortic stenosis (AS), coarctation of aorta (COA)] are also acyanotic heart defect (HD) and may present with cardiocirculatory failure but can be managed well to interventions. The interventions in acyanotic CHDs are usually one time and expected to have a good long-term outcome in terms of quality or quantity of life.

Cyanotic Congenital Heart Disease

The babies with cyanotic congenital heart disease (CCHD) have central cyanosis and hypoxia. They are classified as tetralogy of Fallot (TOF), transposition of great arteries (TGA) (transposition physiology and admixture) (total anomalous pulmonary venous drainage, truncus, etc.) and need early intervention. Many of them are duct dependent and would present as cardiac emergencies [cyanotic spell or congestive heart failure (CHF)].

Early detection and intervention (secondary prevention) are the best opportunities for a baby with CHD to escape long-term complications like Eisenmenger syndrome, severe hypoxia, ventricular dysfunction, and terminal arrhythmia. Palliative interventions like prostaglandin infusing balloon atrial septostomy or shunt surgery may save the life till a definitive intervention is done. Fontan or univentricular cardiac surgery is a palliative surgery which improves the quality of life by complete physiological correction when anatomical correction is unachievable due to the complexity of HD.

Acute Rheumatic Fever and Rheumatic Heart Disease[1,2,9,10]

Acute rheumatic fever (ARF) and rheumatic heart disease (RHD) start in childhood and extend upto adulthood. It has been dealt with details elsewhere in the book.

Strategy to Control of Acute Rheumatic Fever

- Prompt treatment of streptococcal sore throat with appropriate antibiotics.
- Appropriate use of anti-inflammatory (aspirin or steroids) treatment of ARF.
- *Secondary prophylaxis (SP) of ARF and prevention of chronic valvular heart diseases (VHDs)* with intramuscular injection of long-acting penicillin at monthly or 3 weekly interval in an individual who does not have an allergy to penicillin, is the best method to prevent the recurrence of ARF and progression of VHD.

Cardiomyopathies[11–13]

In brief, cardiomyopathies (CMPs) are the heterogeneous group of myocardial diseases causing significant mortality and morbidity due to HF. The CMPs can present as:
- Heart failure with reduced ejection fraction (HFrEF)
- Heart failure with preserved ejection fraction.

Heart Failure with Reduced Ejection Fraction

Dilated CMP (DCMP) always presents with reduced ejection fraction.

Etiology: The etiological factors of DCMP are as follows:
- (1) Genetic (cardiac phenotype, neuromuscular); (2) Infection [postmyocarditis, human immunodeficiency virus (HIV), and Chagas]; (3) Systemic immune-mediated diseases (autoimmune and autoinflammatory); (4) Toxic (alcohol, cobalt, and anabolic steroids)/infiltrative (hemochromatosis and amyloidosis); (5) Drugs (chemotherapeutic agents and others like clozapine); (6) Endocrine (thyroid dysfunction, diabetes mellitus, pheochromocytoma, and acromegaly).
- Viral infection, HIV infection, and Chagas disease (trypanosoma cruzi infection) may also cause DCMP by acute direct myocardial damage leading to cell necrosis, stimulation of natural killer cells, macrophages, and T lymphocytes, cascading a subacute autoimmunity response for a prolonged period. DCMP may also be caused by cardiotoxicity because of drugs (described here).

Heart failure prevention in DCMP is difficult and the goals and objectives of GDMT (guideline-directed medical therapy) include to minimize ventricular volume overload, oxidative stress, adverse ventricular remodeling and yielding a complete structural and functional recovery. Withdrawal of a culprit drug or vitamin D therapy may reverse the course of DCMP in affected children. On the other hand, management with immunoglobulins, cytotoxic drugs, pulmonary artery banding, and cardiac transplant may also be successful in selected group of patients.

HF with Preserved Ejection Fraction

Hypertrophic cardiomyopathy (HCMP): In children, HCMP is defined as "left ventricular (LV) wall thickness more than two standard deviations greater than the predicted mean" (z score >2). It is the most common cause of sudden cardiac death (SCD—0.5–1%/year) in the younger population. Genetically, nine responsible genes have been identified to be associated with the HCM. Up to two-thirds of cases may be due to the genes responsible for the cardiac myosin-binding protein and β cardiac myosin heavy chain.

Hypertrophic cardiomyopathy-related cardiac events are intractable arrhythmia (atrial fibrillation, ventricular arrhythmia), myocardial ischemia, HF, and SCD.

Therapy: HCMP is managed by reducing the LV outflow tract (LVOT) gradient either medically (nonvasodilating beta-blockers, e.g. bisoprolol, nondihydropyridine calcium channel blockers like verapamil or diltiazem with or without disopyramide, newer molecule MYK-461) or by invasive *(surgical myomectomy or alcohol ablation) methods.*

Implantable convertor Defibrillator (ICD) in children: See below.

Restrictive cardiomyopathy (RCM): RCM presents with HFpEF initially, but later ventricular dysfunction (HFrEF) settles in RCM. It is broadly classified as infiltrative, storage disease, noninfiltrative, and endomyocardial disease. The treatment includes early detection by family screening, management of underlying conditions like amyloidosis or hemosiderosis, management of symptoms, arrhythmia, and if required, cardiac transplant may be recommended.

Infective Endocarditis[14]

The annual incidence rate of infective endocarditis (IE) is 0.05 and 0.12 cases per 1,000 pediatric admissions. IE usually affects the structurally abnormal heart and can be caused by a wide spectrum of organism which includes virulent and nonvirulent bacteria, fungus, etc. IE may change the natural history of hemodynamically insignificant CHD.

Arrhythmia[15]

Isolated cardiac arrhythmias may cause HF in infants and children and can affect the quality of life. Arrhythmia with cardiac conditions may be kept in three groups—(1) Unoperated heart diseases like—Ebstein's anomaly or corrected transposition of great arteries presenting with WPW syndrome; (2) Arrhythmia in postoperative patients (atrial/junctional tachycardia, heart blocks); and (3) Intractable arrhythmia end-stage cardiac disease; arrhythmias may cause the secondary CMP if remained undetected.

Just like in adult arrhythmia, the combination of pharmacotherapy, electrical therapies, antitachycardic pacing, antiarrhythmic devices, and surgical or interventional catheterization, in accordance to recently published guidelines for rhythm disorders in pediatric and adolescent age group to be followed for both, the short-term and long-term management. Drugs like verapamil may cause life-threatening bradycardia in infants. Radiofrequency ablation is usually avoided in young children who are amenable to pharmacotherapy. Bradyarrhythmia or congenital heart block is treated with pacemaker implantation (epicardial or endocardial leads). Long QT syndrome needs to be treated under same protocol as for the adults. Ventricular arrhythmia is uncommon in pediatrics and can be managed according to the guidelines.[15]

Coronary Artery Disease in Pediatrics

Risk stratification [American Heart association (AHA)] of groups of cardiac conditions which may be responsible for premature onset of coronary artery disease (CAD), is as follows:[16]

- *High risk group*: Homozygous familial hypercholesterolemia, diabetes mellitus type 1 and 2, chronic renal failure, Kawasaki disease (KD) with coronary aneurysm, etc.
- *Moderate risk*: Severe obesity, heterozygous familial hypercholesterolemia, hypertension, coarctation, LP (a), chronic renal disease, aortic stenosis, and postradiation therapy for childhood cancer.
- *At risk group*: Obesity, insulin resistance with comorbidities (dyslipidemia, nonalcoholic fatty liver, and polycystic ovary), hypertension (white coat), HCM and other CMPs, pulmonary hypertension, chronic inflammatory conditions, s/p coronary artery translocation for anomalous coronary arteries or transposition of the great arteries, childhood cancer (cardiotoxic chemotherapy only), and KD with regressed aneurysms (z score ≥5).

EVOLUTION OF HEART FAILURE

Recent guidelines [AHA/American College of Cardiology (ACC)] divide HF in stages A to D as follows: Stage A [patient has risk factors like metabolic syndrome (MS) but no HF]; Stage B (no HF but pre-existing heart disease present with microcellular changes); Stage C (compensated HF); and D (decompensated HF).

Congenital heart diseases: *(See Risk group 3 AHA/ACC classification).*

Childhood Cancer and Cardiovascular Diseases (Risk Group 2 and 3)

Exposure to radiation (>1,500 centigray of radiation), *anthracycline treatment,* and *hematopoietic stem cell transplantation* have been found to be associated with increased CVD mortality.[16]

Kawasaki Diseases[17]

Kawasaki diseases or mucocutaneous lymph node syndrome is a multisystem autoimmune disease. Diagnosis of KD is based on clinical parameters. Coronary artery abnormalities (ectasia, aneurysm, and stenosis) are the hallmark of KD and may be found in 25–40% of cases, usually after the 10th day of illness. KD is uniquely responsible for myocardial infarction in small children born with otherwise healthy heart.

Intravenous immunoglobulin (2 g/kg infusion over the 12–18 hours as the single dose) along with anti-inflammatory doses of aspirin (30–50 mg/kg/day) within 10 days of fever is cardioprotective for 95% of cases. During the viral infection, use of aspirin may not be safe in children and other antiplatelet agents may be tried. Many other drugs like methylprednisolone pulse therapy and infliximab have been used successfully to control the acute inflammation in resistant cases.

Long-term monitoring of patients with coronary anomalies, includes at least yearly ECG/echo/stress test/CT Angio/MRI/conventional Angio, etc.

Atherosclerosis in Children, Adolescents, and Young Adults[18,19]

As discussed above environmental factors, like intrauterine growth restriction (IUGR) or maternal diabetes mellitus, start functioning from the fetal life. With an unhealthy lifestyle and genetic predisposition, the process of AS accelerates.

Metabolic Syndrome in Children[18]

Obesity clustering with insulin resistance, dyslipidemia or hypertension is the hallmark of metabolic syndrome.

Obesity, Diabetes Type 2 in Children Adolescent and Young Adults[1–3,16,18,19]

The set of recommendations (WHO) have been established to promote intake of healthy food, physical activity of school-age children, preconception, and pregnancy care. In high-income countries, such as the United States and Australia, rates of combined childhood overweight and obesity ranged between 20–35%, while in India, reported occurrence is also significantly higher (18.5% overweight and 5.3% obese) amongst the 8–18 years age group.[20]

Hypertension

The hypertension in childhood causes aortic stiffness, increased coronary artery calcium score, carotid intima media thickness (cIMT), abnormal epithelial function as well as ventricular hypertrophy. Hypertension may damage many other target organs (kidney, brain, and eyes). A secondary cause cannot be ruled out unless meticulous investigations are done to exclude systemic inflammatory disorders, renal/endocrinal diseases or coarctation of the aorta.

Therapeutics for Hypertension[21]

Current guidelines recommend lifestyle changes, including maintaining a normal body mass index (18.5–24.9 kg/m^2), adopting the DASH (Dietary Approaches to Stop Hypertension), and reducing dietary sodium to 2.4 g. To avoid end-organ damage BP must be kept <95th percentile if no renal pathology detected or <90th percentile if a renal pathology has been identified.

PREVENTION OF CARDIOVASCULAR DISEASES IN PEDIATRIC AGE GROUP[1–3,16,18,22]

It is logical to screen children and adolescent, across the board for evidence of metabolic syndrome and hyperlipidemia. Ideal age of screening for lipid disorder is 2–10 years or preadolescent age group. Abnormal cardiac biomarkers like brain natriuretic peptides (NT-proBNP, BNP), cardiac troponin levels, and others [arginine vasopressin, epinephrine, and norepinephrine, interleukins, C-reactive protein, microalbuminuria, gut peptides glucagon-like peptide-1 (GLP-1) and GLP-2, adipocytokines, lipoproteins, and apolipoproteins] may play important role in future management of HF. Left ventricular hypertrophy and left bundle branch block are two important risk phenotypes requiring the close follow-up of a patient.

PREVENTION AND MANAGEMENT OF HEART FAILURE IN CHILDREN AND ADOLESCENTS PRESENTING WITH HIGH RISK OF CVD[1–3,16,18–22]

Diet and Exercise

Diet

The National Cholesterol Education Program experts recommend dietary treatment in children above 2 years of age. Adequate calories should be provided to maintain the normal development and growth.

Type 1 diet: Calories from fat <30%; saturated fat: 8–10% of daily kcal/estimated energy requirements; cholesterol: <300 mg/day; no trans fat; fibers: 14 g/1,000 kcal; no added sugar in juice, limit sodium intake.

Type 2 diet: Calories from fat <30%; saturated fat: <7% of daily kcal/estimated energy requirements; cholesterol: <150 mg/day; no trans fat. Plant stanol, sterol esters up to 2 g/day; water soluble fibers: 6 g/day for age group 2–12 years and >12 years 12 g/day; no added sugar in juice, instead of simple consume a complex carbohydrate. Increase intake of omega 3 fatty acids (increase dietary fishes or take supplements).

Role of fibers: Fibers are protective of intestinal epithelium as it is metabolized by intestinal bacteria into short-chain fatty acids which in turn perform important immunoregulatory functions.

Exercise[2,22]

Duration of exercise:

- Moderate-intensity aerobic exercise at least 2 hours and 30 minutes per week.
- Participation in aerobic exercise, such as brisk walking so that heart beat rises above the basal value, for at least 10 minutes at a time spread throughout the week.

Yoga: The yoga provides the benefits of exercise-induced burning of calories and fat. Exercise also improves functional capacity and quality of life in patients with HF.

Heart Failure in Children: Therapeutic Aspects

The basic requirements for rational drug therapy are: (1) Complete correct diagnosis (anatomical and pathophysiological cause of CHF)—it is important to have timely diagnosis and intervention for all significant CVDs like critical stenotic lesions, shunt lesions, ALCAPA, hypocalcemia-induced DCMP. (2) Clear understanding of pharmacology of various drugs (includes pharmacokinetics, drug dosages, potential efficacy, and side effects). (3) Meticulous monitoring of patient for therapeutic end points and side. (4) Readiness to modify or change the drug therapy if ongoing treatment is not effective or unacceptably toxic.

Pharmacological Intervention: Timely and Adequate Drug Therapy (Tables 1 and 2)

Guideline-directed Medical Therapy[2]

Guideline-directed medical therapy is a protocolized targeted drug therapy, by a group of drugs [diuretics, beta blockers, angiotensinogen-converting enzyme (ACE) inhibitors or receptor blockers] to counter the harmful compensatory mechanism induced by the process of HF itself.

Conventional Drugs[2,8,9,12,14,22]

- *Digoxin*: Though the digitalis glycoside has been shown to improve symptoms in patients with HF with reduced systolic function, but they fail to provide survival benefit in adults or in children.

TABLE 1: Pharmacotherapy of heart failure.

	Preserved systolic function *Left–right shunt*	*MR/AR*	*Ventricular dysfunction*	*Pressure overload*	*RV dysfunction*
Diuretics	I	I	I	IIa	I
Digoxin	IIa	IIa	I (for symptoms)	III	IIa
ACEi	IIa	I	I	III	I
Beta blockers	III	III	IIa	III	IIb
Digoxin	IIa	IIa	I (for symptoms)	III	IIa
Anticoagulant	III	III	IIa	Urgent intervention to relieve obstruction	

(ACEi: angiotensin-converting enzyme inhibitor; AR: aortic regurgitation; MR: mitral regurgitation; RV: right ventricle)

TABLE 2: Medical therapy according to the functional class of HF.

Functional class	*Therapeutics*
NYHA/Ross class 1	Pulse diuretics/ACE inhibitors can be started safely.
NYHA/Ross class II	Diuretics/ACE inhibitor/beta blocker/aldosterone (can be started safely at outpatient basis)
NYHA/Ross class III	All of above drugs but to be started with caution and monitoring. The patient may need admission
NYHA/Ross class IV	All of above with monitoring because they may not be tolerated in the presence of overtly unstable hemodynamics. Even if tolerated well, a suboptimal response is expected. Hospitalization and inotropes and vasodilators are recommended
Intractable symptom	Additionally, mechanical devices can be considered.

(ACE: angiotensinogen-converting enzyme; HF: heart failure; NYHA: New York Heart Association)

- *Diuretics*: Diuretics are currently recommended for all patients with HF who have volume overload of the ventricle. Diuretics from different groups (A–C) can be combined for greater efficacy: (*A*) *Loop diuretics*: e.g. furosemide and torsemide. (*B*) *Thiazides*: e.g. hydrochlorothiazide and metolazone. (*C*) *Aldosterone antagonists*: e.g. spironolactone and eplerenone.
  - *Furosemide*: It is a diuretic as well as a venodilator.
  - *Torsemide:* It is a loop diuretic, more potent than furosemide, (10 mg of torsemide is equivalent to 40 mg of furosemide).
  - *Thiazides*: These are relatively milder diuretics (except for metolazone) primarily used in mild hypertension and edema. Metolazone is 10 times more potent than hydrochlorothiazide.
  - *Aldosterone antagonists*: Spironolactone (doses 1 mg/kg/day) aldosterone is one of the local hormones responsible for the adverse remodeling of a failing heart and due to its potassium sparing effect, it has been used as the adjunct therapy with the loop diuretics.
- *Vasodilators: Angiotensin-converting enzyme inhibitors (ACEi)*: ACEi decreases the adrenergic drive and block activation of renin-angiotensin-aldosterone system. ACEi therapy is recommended as the first-line treatment for HF, when it is not secondary to an obstructive lesion. Improvement in symptoms and survival has been shown in adults with symptomatic HF on ACEi.
- *Angiotensin receptor blockers (ARBs)*: ARBs are competitive antagonists of the angiotensin II receptors. ARBs block angiotensin II receptors present in muscles adjacent to blood vessels (BV) and allow vasodilatation. In the process, they reduce systemic vascular resistance and bring down the ventricular afterload.
- *Beta blockers*: Several studies have shown the benefits of beta blocker therapy in adult patients with HF. Carvedilol has been shown to decrease mortality and risk of clinical progression of HF. It improves functional class and fractional shortening in children with ventricular dysfunction.
- *Ivabradine*: Basal tachycardia has been found to be associated with HF-related mortality in adults. Ivabradine is a relatively new drug with an overall favorable safety profile to reduce the tachycardia.
- *Vasodilators*: Older patients intolerant to ACE inhibitor can be put on other vasodilators (hydralazine, nitrates, calcium antagonists, nesiritide, etc.)
- *Antiplatelet/anticoagulation in HF*:[1-3,20] Patients with severe LV dysfunction, atrial fibrillation, and those with prosthetic implants need to be put on anticoagulation/antiplatelet therapy to avoid thrombosis and cerebrovascular accidents.
- *Micronutrients in HF*:[23] A normal heart consumes over 6 kg of adenosine triphosphate (ATP) for its pumping action, daily. During the life, the heart needs to maintain the essential level of efficiency by inexhaustibly replenishing the enzymes, membranes, and other substrates daily. Therefore, it needs a relentless supply of macronutrients (amino acids, lipids, and carbohydrates) as well as micronutrients. Micronutrients have the subtle presence in food and if deficient, they can negatively affect cardiac function. *Amino acids* are structural edifice of proteins and also participate in energy substrate metabolism.

CoQ10 (ubiquinone) helps in ATP formation in various tissues including heart.

Vitamin D is essential for calcium-homeostasis and hence become a moderator for cardiac contractility.

Ribose, a naturally occurring pentose sugar, enhances ATP levels and thus, augment ventricular diastolic compliance in CAD.

Magnesium: *Magnesium* deficiency may lead to ventricular arrhythmia and SCD.

Deficiencies of the B group vitamins, L-carnitine, Zn, selenium and vitamin C, are prevalent and may also contribute to the downhill course of failing hearts.

MANAGEMENT OF HYPERLIPIDEMIA: PHARMACOTHERAPY[3-24]

- *Statins*: The statins are 3-hydroxy-3-methyl-glutaryl-coenzyme A (HMG-CoA) reductase inhibitors.[24] The HMG-CoA reductase is the first enzyme of the HMG-CoA reductase pathway. By blocking it competitively, they inhibit cholesterol synthesis in the liver. In 0.1–1% of patients using statins, onset of myopathy may increase serum creatine kinase >10 times the upper limit of normal.
- *Bile acid sequestrants (cholestyramine and colestipol)*: This medication can prevent the uptake of bile salts by binding them in the gastrointestinal tract.
- *Other drugs*: Drugs like ezetimibe (a cholesterol absorption inhibitor), niacin (nicotinic acid), fibric acid derivatives, omega-3 fatty acids, and orlistat have been found effective in adults and they are also expected to be useful in pediatric cases.

Cardiac Resynchronization Therapy (CRT)

Asynchronous contraction of the LV in patients with HFrEF leads to mechanical inefficiency and aggravates the mitral regurgitation. The cardiac resynchronization therapy (CRT) involves pacing of the LV or both ventricles or both ventricles and the right atrium to achieve synchrony.[2,25]

Cardiac Transplantation for Heart Failure in Children[1-3,26]

Cardiac transplantation is done for end-stage HF or for complex CHD (HLHS, failed Fontan surgery, and CMPs). This surgery is contraindicated in patients with primary or secondary postpartum hemorrhage (PPH) (PVRI >6 Woods unit), chronic liver and kidney diseases, recent or recurrent malignancy, serious active or recurrent infection, HIV infection, genetic or metabolic diseases with poor long-term prognosis, and pharmacologically irreversible pulmonary hypertension (pulmonary vascular resistance >6 μm^2). The pediatric survival rate is 80% after 1 year, about 70% after 5 years.

Genetic Approach: Promising Approach Still Awaited[27]

Gene therapy for CVD, though a promising therapeutic modality, is still in preclinical stage. Few interesting advances in this direction include the successful use of angiogenic in experiments, possibility of modification of β-adrenergic pathways, and modification in molecules involved in cardiomyocyte Ca2+ cycling. Stem cell therapy is expected to reverse the underlying pathological changes in cardiac myocytes.

SUMMARY

In the present era of technical evolution and lifestyle modifications, pediatric age-group stands vulnerable to both childhood heart diseases and early onset of adult heart issues. It is now well established that atherosclerosis (AS) may start as early as perinatal period. Moreover, patients with KD, survivors of CHDs, metabolic disorders, inflammatory disorders, and malignancies are new entries in the spectrum. In the presence of modified sedentary lifestyle, lack of exercise, unhealthy dietary habits, and obesity lead to premature AS and CAD. Obesity is a proinflammatory state and predecessor of type 2 DM. All aforesaid conditions target vital organs like kidney, heart, brain, liver, and eyes. Timely risk stratification, appropriate interventions, dietary modifications, introduction of exercise, and whenever required use of appropriate pharmacotherapy as well as arrhythmia management are desired for a successful preventive pediatric HF program.

BIBLIOGRAPHY

1. Kay MA. State-of-the-art gene-based therapies: The road ahead. Nat Rev Genet. 2011;12:316-28.
2. Nordestgaard BG, Langsted A, Mora S, et al. Fasting Is Not Routinely Required for Determination of a Lipid Profile: Clinical and Laboratory Implications Including Flagging at Desirable Concentration Cutpoints-A Joint Consensus Statement from the European Atherosclerosis Society and European Federation of Clinical Chemistry and Laboratory Medicine. European Atherosclerosis Society (EAS) and the European Federation of Clinical Chemistry and Laboratory Medicine (EFLM) Joint Consensus Initiative. Clin Chem. 2016;62(7):930-46.

REFERENCES

1. Dickstein K, Cohen-Solal A, Filippatos G, et al. ESC Guidelines for the diagnosis and treatment of acute and chronic heart failure 2008: the Task Force for the Diagnosis and Treatment of Acute and Chronic Heart Failure 2008 of the European Society of Cardiology. Developed in collaboration with the Heart Failure Association of the ESC (HFA) and endorsed by the European Society of Intensive Care Medicine (ESICM). Eur Heart J. 2008;29:2388-442.
2. Swedberg K, Cleland J, Dargie H, et al. Guidelines for the diagnosis and treatment of chronic heart failure: The Task Force for the Diagnosis and Treatment of Chronic Heart Failure of the European Society of Cardiology. Eur Heart J. 2005;26(11):1115-40.
3. Romdhane HB, Damasceno A, Ebrahim S, et al. Prevention of Cardiovascular Disease Guidelines for assessment and

management of cardiovascular risk. [online] Available from https://www.who.int/cardiovascular_diseases/guidelines/Full%20text.pdf [Last accessed November, 2019].
4. Fall CH. Fetal malnutrition and long-term outcomes. Nestle Nutr Inst Workshop Ser. 2013;74:11-25.
5. Tikkanen J, Heinonen OP. Maternal exposure to chemical and physical factors during pregnancy and cardiovascular malformations in the offspring. Teratology. 1991;43(6):591-600.
6. Kapusta L, Haagmans ML, Steegers EA, et al. Congenital heart defects and maternal derangement of homocysteine metabolism. J Pediatr. 1999;135(6):773-4.
7. Saxena A, Mehta A, Sharma M, et al. A cross-sectional observational study from North India. Ann Pediatr Cardiol. 2016;9(3):205-9.
8. Mishra S. Congestive heart failure—Current concept in Management. IJPP. 2017;19(3):231-44.
9. RHD action. RHD Global Status Report 2015-2017. [online] Available from http://rhdaction.org/sites/default/files/RHD%20Global%20Status%20Report%202015-17.pdf [Last accessed November, 2019].
10. Mishra S, Saxena A, Mishra Y, et al. Working Group on Pediatric Acute Rheumatic Fever and Cardiology Chapter of Indian Academy of Pediatrics. Consensus guidelines on pediatric acute rheumatic fever and rheumatic heart disease. Indian Pediatr. 2008;45(7):565-73.
11. Richardson P, McKenna W, Bristow M, et al. Report of the 1995 World Health Organization/International Society and Federation of Cardiology Task Force on the definition and classification of cardiomyopathies. Circulation. 1996;93:841-2.
12. McNamara DM, Starling RC, Cooper LT, et al. Clinical and demographic predictors of outcomes in recent onset dilated cardiomyopathy: results of the IMAC (Intervention in Myocarditis and Acute Cardiomyopathy)-2 study. J Am Coll Cardiol. 2011;58:1112-8.
13. Howlett JG, Chan M, Ezekowitz JA, et al. The Canadian Cardiovascular Society Heart Failure Companion: Bridging Guidelines to Your Practice. Can J Cardiol. 2016;32(3):296-310.
14. Habib G, Lancellotti P, Antunes MJ, et al. 2015 ESC guidelines for the management of infective endocarditis: The Task Force for the Management of Infective Endocarditis of the European Society of Cardiology (ESC). Eur Heart J. 2015;36:3075-128.
15. Hernández-Madrid A, Paul T, Abrams D, et al. ESC Scientific Document Group. Arrhythmias in congenital heart disease: a position paper of the European Heart Rhythm Association (EHRA), Association for European Paediatric and Congenital Cardiology (AEPC), and the European Society of Cardiology (ESC) Working Group on Grown-up Congenital heart disease, endorsed by HRS, PACES, APHRS, and SOLAECE. Europace. 2018;20(11):1719-53.
16. de Ferranti SD, Steinberger J, Ameduri R, et al. Cardiovascular Risk Reduction in High-Risk Pediatric Patients: A Scientific Statement from the American Heart Association. Circular. 2019;139(13):e603-e634.
17. Lin YT, Manlhiot C, Ching JC, et al. Repeated systematic surveillance of Kawasaki disease in Ontario from 1995 to 2006. Pediatr Int. 2010;52(5):699-706.
18. Huang PL. A comprehensive definition for metabolic syndrome. Dis Model Mech. 2009;2(5-6):231-7.
19. Skilton MR. Intrauterine risk factors for precocious atherosclerosis. Pediatrics. 2008;121(3):570-4.
20. Misra A, Shah P, Goel K, et al. The high burden of obesity and abdominal obesity in urban Indian schoolchildren: a multicentric study of 38,296 children. Ann Nutr Metab. 2011;58(3):203-11.
21. Flynn JT, Kaelber DC, Baker-Smith CM, et al. Clinical Practice Guideline for Screening and Management of High Blood Pressure in Children and Adolescents. Pediatrics. 2017;140(3). pii: e20171904.
22. Expert Panel on Integrated Guidelines for Cardiovascular Health and Risk Reduction in Children and Adolescents, National Heart, Lung, and Blood Institute. Expert Panel on Integrated Guidelines for Cardiovascular Health and Risk Reduction in Children and Adolescents: summary report. Pediatrics. 2011;128(suppl 5):S213-56.
23. Soukoulis V, Dihu JB, Sole M, et al. Micronutrient deficiencies an unmet need in heart failure. J Am Coll Cardiol. 2009;54:1660-73.
24. Avis HJ, Vissers MN, Stein EA, et al. A systematic review and meta-analysis of statin therapy in children with familial hypercholesterolemia. Arterioscler Thromb Vasc Biol. 2007;27:1803-10.
25. Motonaga KS, Dubin AM. Cardiac Resynchronization Therapy for Pediatric Patients With Heart Failure and Congenital Heart Disease A Reappraisal of Results Circulation. 2014;129(18):1879-91.
26. Dipchand AI. Current state of pediatric cardiac transplantation. Ann Cardiothorac Surg. 2018;7(1):31-55.
27. Curfman G. Stem cell therapy for heart failure: An unfulfilled promise? JAMA. 2019;321(12):1186-7.

Pediatric Stroke and Heart Failure

Chandril Chugh, Himanshu Agarwal

INTRODUCTION

Stroke is defined by the World Health Organization (WHO) as a clinical syndrome consisting of rapidly developing clinical signs of focal (or global in case of coma) disturbance of cerebral function lasting more than 24 hours or leading to death with no apparent cause other than a vascular origin.[1] Stroke is classified broadly into three categories; ischemic stroke, hemorrhagic stroke, and subarachnoid hemorrhage. Ischemic stroke occurs due to blockage of blood vessel which limits the blood supply to the brain whereas hemorrhagic stroke occurs due to rupture of blood vessel leading spillage of blood in the intracranial cavity.[2] Depending on the site of blood spillage the hemorrhagic stroke could be classified as intracerebral hemorrhage or subarachnoid hemorrhage.

Stroke is common in the pediatric age group. The incidence ranges from 1 in 1,600 to 4,000 neonates at birth and 2.3 to 13 per 100,000 older children per year.[3,4] Although the pediatric brain is much more forgiving than an adult brain, stroke can still cause irreversible brain damage and cognitive decline. Stroke can cause death in up to 25% of cases and permanent disability in 66% patients.[5,6] About 80% of all pediatric strokes are ischemic.[7] Stroke is more common amongst boys as compared to girls. Pediatric strokes are frequently missed or misdiagnosed due to the prevalent notion that stroke is less common amongst the pediatric age group. Lack of awareness in the general population as well as the medical specialists are the two main reasons which delay diagnosis and treatment of stroke. In one study it was shown that pediatric stroke patients presented more than 24 hours after their symptoms started and the time taken to image the brain after presentation could be as long as 7 hours.[8] Early diagnosis of stroke and its timely treatment is paramount in providing good care and ensuring good outcome.

ISCHEMIC STROKE CLASSIFICATION

According to the multicenter Trial of Acute Stroke Treatment (TOAST) there are three kinds of ischemic stroke:[9]

1. Large vessel stroke
2. Small vessel stroke or lacunar stroke
3. Cardioembolic stroke.

Large artery strokes could be due to thrombotic or embolic occlusion of the major arteries of the brain like the internal carotid artery, middle cerebral artery, anterior cerebral artery or the vertebrobasilar system. Lacunar strokes are more often due to involvement of smaller or perforating blood vessels supplying the deeper structures of the brain.

CLINICAL PRESENTATION

Hallmark of stroke symptoms is that they begin suddenly; however, only 85% of pediatric strokes present with sudden onset of symptoms. Stroke symptoms are dependent on the area of the brain which is affected. A child may present with weakness on one side of the body, slurring of speech, inability to speak properly or altered mental status. Strokes involving the posterior circulation present with dizziness, ataxia, headaches or altered sensorium. Approximately 50% of pediatric patients can present with altered mental status. Headache has been observed in 40% of children with ischemic stroke, 46% with hemorrhagic stroke, and 51% with transient ischemic attack. Hemiplegia is by far the most common focal neurological symptom at presentation.[10,11] As compared to adult strokes, seizures at the stroke onset may account for about 30–50% of pediatric cases.[12]

In perinatal strokes, seizures and lethargy are far more common a few days after birth. Focal neurological signs may not develop at the onset and may take months to show up. Lethargy, apnea spells, or hypotonia are the most common symptoms in this age group.[8,13] Toddlers, often present with irritability, sleepiness, decreased feeding, hypothermia, and cold extremities.[14] Certain specific conditions such as cerebral venous sinus thrombosis and subarachnoid hemorrhage may present with characteristic signs on physical examination that are helpful in diagnosis. Apart from altered mental status and seizures, a child may exhibit signs of increased intracranial pressure such as downward gaze, bulging anterior fontanelle and dilated scalp veins. Frequent vomiting, headaches, neck rigidity, and meningismus also point towards subarachnoid hemorrhage. Depending on the arterial territory involved, focal neurological signs may develop. Involvement of middle cerebral artery can cause hemiparesis, gaze deviation with or without aphasia. Anterior cerebral artery involvement may cause weakness in the contralateral lower extremity. Vertigo, ataxia, nystagmus, and difficulty swallowing are consistent with an ischemic event in the posterior circulation.[11]

RISK FACTORS: ISCHEMIC STROKE

- Sickle cell disease
- Moyamoya syndrome
- Alagille syndrome
- Radiation vasculopathy
- Arterial dissection
- Collagen vascular disorders:
  - Ehlers-Danlos type IV
  - Marfan syndrome
  - COL4A1 mutations
  - Fibromuscular dysplasia
  - Focal cerebral arteriopathy
  - Primary angiitis of the central nervous system.
- Systemic vasculitides and autoimmune disorders:
  - Wegener granulomatosis
  - Microscopic polyangiitis
  - Polyarteritis nodosa
  - Takayasu arteritis
  - Systemic lupus erythematosus
  - Mixed connective tissue disease
  - Henoch-Schönlein purpura
  - Hemophagocytic lymphohistiocytosis
  - Kawasaki disease
  - Inflammatory bowel disease
  - Human immunodeficiency virus.
- Vasospasm:
  - Reversible cerebral vasoconstriction syndrome
  - Subarachnoid hemorrhage
  - Cocaine use.
- Prothrombotic conditions:
  - Polycythemia
  - Deficiency of protein C, protein S, and antithrombin III
  - Factor V Leiden mutation/activated protein C resistance
  - Prothrombin 20210 gene mutation
  - Elevated factor VIII
  - Elevated von Willebrand factor antigen
  - Hyperhomocysteinemia
  - Elevated lipoprotein(a)
  - Antiphospholipid antibodies.
- Migraine with aura
- Estrogen-containing oral contraceptive use
- Pregnancy and postpartum
- Malignancy
- L-Asparaginase and other chemotherapeutics
- Cardiac disorders:
  - Congenital heart disease, especially with right-to-left shunt
  - Cardiac catheterization or surgery
  - Extracorporeal membrane oxygenation
  - Left ventricular assist devices
  - Endocarditis
  - Valvular abnormalities
  - Cardiomyopathy.
- Genetic/metabolic disorders:
  - Mitochondrial encephalomyopathy, lactic acidosis, and stroke-like episodes (MELAS)
  - Cerebral autosomal dominant arteriopathy with subcortical infarcts and leukoencephalopathy (CADASIL)
  - Homocystinuria
  - Fabry disease.
- Organic acidemias:
  - Glutaric aciduria type II
  - Methylmalonic acidemia
  - Propionic acidemia
  - Isovaleric acidemia
  - Congenital disorders of glycosylation
  - Adenosine deaminase 2 deficiency.
  - Sulfite oxidase deficiency
- Infection:
  - Meningitis
  - *Streptococcus pneumoniae*

  - Tuberculosis
  - *Aspergillus* species
  - Varicella vasculopathy
  - Sinusitis
  - Mastoiditis
  - Sepsis.
- **Drugs:** Cocaine, amphetamines, lysergic acid diethylamide (LSD), glue, heroin, and ergot alkaloids.

RISK FACTORS FOR HEMORRHAGIC STROKE

- Arteriovenous malformation
- Arteriovenous fistula
- Aneurysm
- Cavernous malformation
- Capillary telangiectasia
- Venous angioma
- Vasculopathy:
  - Sickle cell disease
  - Moyamoya syndrome.
- Coagulation disorders:
  - Thrombocytopenia
  - Hemophilia
  - Hepatic failure
  - Vitamin K deficiency
  - Anticoagulant therapy.
- Other: Brain tumor
- Hemorrhage due to cerebral sinovenous thrombosis
- Hemorrhagic transformation of ischemic infarction.

CARDIAC DISEASES

Cardiac diseases are the most common cause of stroke in pediatric age group. Most of the strokes due to cardiac diseases are embolic. Congenital heart diseases predispose to stroke due to polycythemia or anemia. Diseases which cause structural damage like rheumatic heart disease or patients with prosthetic heart valve are at high risk of embolic stroke.[15] Patent foramen ovale has been widely discussed as one of the causes of embolic stroke as well.[16]

SICKLE CELL DISEASE

Sickle cell disease is another common cause of stroke in children. Abnormal erythrocytes are more likely to cause microcirculation thrombi leading to vascular occlusion. Sickle cells are also more likely to be sequestered in the spleen leading to anemia and decreased oxygen carrying capacity. Sickle cell disease predisposes to arteriopathy due to chronic inflammation leading to damage to vessel wall and impaired blood flow. Ischemic strokes are more common in younger age group whereas the older patients present with hemorrhage. There is a 70% chance of recurrence of neurological symptoms in patients with sickle cell disease.[17,18]

PROTHROMBOTIC STATES

About 13% of children with arterial stroke and up to 67% with venous stroke are found to have a hereditary thrombophilia. Children with prothrombotic states may have a family history of stroke or myocardial infarction (MI) in previous three generations, deep vein thrombosis (DVT), pulmonary embolism or multiple miscarriages. In adolescent females; oral contraceptives pills, uterine implants, depot injections, and other hormonal therapies can increase the risk of thrombosis.

Malignancy and chemotherapeutic agents increase the risk of thrombotic complications. Malignancy is known to produce a hypercoagulable state. Radiation therapy is an independent risk factor for development of vasculopathy which can increase stroke risk. Chemotherapeutic agents, particularly L-Asparaginase, predispose to venous thrombosis. Foreign bodies such as arterial or venous catheters in children with malignancy or other major medical conditions can act as a nidus for formation of thrombi that may then embolize.

INFECTION

Bacterial infections like otitis media, meningitis, and mastoiditis are frequently associated with cerebral venous thrombosis. Up to 25% patients with meningitis can have stroke during the course of illness. Mycoplasma, chlamydiae, tuberculosis, and neurobrucellosis are other examples of infection which can cause stroke due to local vasculitis and thrombus formation. Viruses like varicella, human immunodeficiency virus (HIV), *Enterovirus*, *Parvovirus*, and coxsackie have been associated with strokes as well.[19-22]

TRAUMA

Traumatic injury to the blood vessels of the neck also known as cervical neck dissection is a very common cause of stroke in the young. Some people may be predisposed to vascular dissection due to genetic collagen vascular disorders. In such cases, trivial trauma or activities like sneezing, coughing or neck manipulation may cause vascular dissection. In others, hyperextension or rotational injuries experienced during minor head trauma, motor vehicle collisions, sports such as wrestling, or even chiropractic manipulation can also result in strokes.[23-25]

MANAGEMENT OF ACUTE STROKE

The most important factor in the management of acute ischemic stroke is time. Patient with ischemic stroke loses 190,0000 brain cells every minute, about 14,000,000,000 nerve connections are destroyed every minute, and 12 km (7.5 miles) of nerve fibers are lost every minute. The brain ages 3.6 years for every hour, it is deprived of blood supply.[26]

Once the clinical diagnosis of an acute stroke is made the following steps need to be followed:
- Ensure that the patient is medically stable.
- Evaluate for reversible causes of neurological symptoms.
- Determine the nature of stroke (ischemic vs. hemorrhagic).
- Treatment of stroke.
- Determine the causes of stroke (investigations).

Ensure the Patient is Medically Stable: Never Forget the Airway, Breathing, and Circulation

In the treatment of acute stroke, time is of the essence. Medical stability of the patient should be established as soon as possible so that stroke management can proceed. Airway, breathing and circulation need to be assessed like in every medical emergency. Large strokes, intracranial hemorrhage (ICH), strokes affecting posterior circulation present with loss of consciousness, bulbar dysfunction, and sometimes respiratory distress. Hypoxia should be avoided at all costs and intubation should be considered if the airway is not protected or the patient needs ventilator support.

Evaluation of Reversible causes of Neurological Symptoms

In pediatric population, number of neurological ailments can present with focal neurological symptoms and need to be ruled out. Stroke differential diagnosis includes a wide array of diseases:
- Complicated migraine
- Seizure/postictal symptoms not due to stroke
- Hemorrhage (hemorrhagic stroke and traumatic hemorrhage)
- Intracranial infection (meningitis and abscess)
- Trauma
- Tumor
- Demyelinating disease (multiple sclerosis and acute disseminated encephalomyelitis)
- Posterior reversible encephalopathy syndrome (PRES)
- Toxic exposure
- Metabolic derangement
- Idiopathic intracranial hypertension (pseudotumor cerebri)
- Postinfectious process (cerebellitis and acute cerebellar ataxia)
- Musculoskeletal cause of weakness
- Somatoform disorder.

Determine the Nature of Stroke (Ischemic vs. Hemorrhagic)

Plain head computed tomography (CT) scan is sufficient to rule out ICH and it may also show mass effect, evidence of a mass lesion or other inflammatory processes. Head CT may not show the evidence of an ischemic stroke in the acute phase.[27]

Magnetic resonance imaging (MRI) with diffusion-weighted imaging remains the "gold standard" for the investigation of arterial ischemic stroke in infants and children, due to its greater sensitivity and specificity.[28] Vascular imaging which includes a CT angiogram, MR angiogram or a diagnostic angiogram may be considered if involvement of a large blood vessel like the internal carotid artery, middle cerebral artery or the vertebrobasilar system is suspected. MR venogram is helpful in diagnosing cerebral venous sinus thrombosis and a transcranial Doppler may be helpful in managing patients with sickle cell disease as well as vasoconstriction syndromes.

Laboratory Investigations

Following tests may be considered depending upon the patient history in the diagnostic workup:[12,29]
- Antithrombin III
- Prothrombin gene mutation
- Homocysteine level
- Methylenetetrahydrofolate reductase (MTHFR) allele
- Fibrinogen disorder
- Plasminogen activator inhibitor disorder
- Factor VII/VIII elevation
- Factor XII deficiency
- Plasma amino acids/urine amino and organic acids
- Serum and cerebrospinal fluid (CSF) lactate/pyruvate
- Hemoglobin electrophoresis
- Triglycerides/cholesterol
- Lipoprotein(a)
- Miscellaneous bacterial, fungal, spirochetal, and parasitic
- Viral and rickettsial tests [i.e. Lyme, purified protein derivative (PPD), venereal disease research laboratory (VDRL)
- Serum and CSF varicella titers
- Human immunodeficiency virus titers
- Contrast transesophageal echo (TEE)
- Electroencephalogram (EEG)
- Lumbar puncture

- Holter monitoring
- Transcranial Doppler.

TREATMENT: ISCHEMIC STROKE

Guidelines for the treatment of pediatric stroke recommend anticoagulation with heparin or low molecular weight heparin in cases of arterial dissection or cardioembolic causes. Aspirin has also been recommended in cases where an embolic cause is not certain. Guidelines do not recommend the use of both thrombolysis by tissue plasminogen activator (t-PA, Alteplase) and mechanical thrombectomy in children outside specific research protocols. However, pediatric cases have been treated with intravenous thrombolysis and intra-arterial thrombolysis on cases by case basis all over the world.[30-32]

Endovascular mechanical thrombectomy has also been used in children despite, as already explained, guidelines advise against its exportation in the pediatric population. The potential candidates for this approach may be pediatric patients with a large intracranial artery occlusion. Safety guidelines are needed considering the risks associated with the treatment of children as small adults and the inappropriateness of devices often designed for adult use.[33]

CEREBRAL SINUS VENOUS THROMBOSIS

Patients with cerebral venous sinus thrombosis are treated with full anticoagulation based on weight of the patient. Cerebral sinus venous thrombosis (CSVT) has a high mortality rate without anticoagulation.

INTRACRANIAL HEMORRHAGE

Management of ICH primarily involves supportive care and discontinuation of offending agents if any. Fresh frozen plasma, prothrombin complex concentrate or recombinant factor VII, have all been used in pediatric age group with variable results.[34] Surgical management of hemorrhagic stroke is controversial. There may be benefit of early surgical evacuation in patients with clinical deterioration due to mass effect. Children may warrant more aggressive intervention given their lack of cerebral atrophy which, in older adults, could potentially accommodate some degree of hematoma expansion. Although a recent prospective, multicenter trial suggested that surgical evacuation of a supratentorial intraparenchymal hemorrhage does not improve chances of good recovery or moderate disability beyond best medical management, a recent meta-analysis does suggest that surgical evacuation is associated with a reduction in the odds of being dead or dependent.[35]

CONCLUSION

Pediatric strokes are not uncommon and carry high morbidity and mortality. Timely diagnosis and treatment of stroke can save lives and enable the patient to have a good life. With the advent of newer ways to treat stroke through mechanical thrombectomy for up to 24 hours in adults, more and more patients are being benefited. Pediatric stroke; however, faces the biggest challenge of being difficult to diagnose and difficult to treat mechanically due to small caliber of blood vessels. There is a great need for pediatric stroke specialists and well-trained interventional neurologists who can diagnose stroke and treat it safely.

REFERENCES

1. Hatano S. Experience from a multicentre stroke register: a preliminary report. Bull World Health Organ. 1976;54(5):541-53.
2. Caplan LR. Basic pathology, anatomy, and pathophysiology of stroke. Caplan's Stroke: A Clinical Approach, 4th edition. Philadelphia: Saunders Elsevier; 2009. p. 22.
3. Chung B, Wong V. Pediatric stroke among Hong Kong Chinese subjects. Pediatrics. 2004;114(2):e206-12.
4. Schoenberg BS, Mellinger JF, Schoenberg DG. Cerebrovascular disease in infants and children: a study of incidence, clinical features, and survival. Neurology. 1978;28(8):763-8.
5. Lanthier S, Carmant L, David M, et al. Stroke in children: the coexistence of multiple risk factors predicts poor outcome. Neurology. 2000;54(2):371-8.
6. Riela AR, Roach ES. Etiology of stroke in children. J Child Neurol. 1993;8(3):201-20.
7. Carvalho KS, Garg BP. Arterial strokes in children. Neurol Clin. 2002;20(4):1079-100.
8. Gabis LV, Yangala R, Lenn NJ. Time lag to diagnosis of stroke in children. Pediatrics. 2002;110(5):924-8.
9. Adams HP Jr, Davis PH, Leira EC, et al. Baseline NIH Stroke Scale score strongly predicts outcome after stroke: A report of the Trial of Org 10172 in Acute Stroke Treatment (TOAST). Neurology. 1999;53(1):126-31.
10. Eeg-Olofsson O, Ringheim Y. Stroke in children. Clinical characteristics and prognosis. Acta Paediatrica Scandinavica. 1983;72(3):391-5.
11. Satoh S, Shirane R, Yoshimoto T. Clinical survey of ischemic cerebrovascular disease in children in a district of Japan. Stroke. 1991;22(5):586-9.
12. Younkin DP. Diagnosis and treatment of ischemic pediatric stroke. Curr Neurol Neurosci Rep. 2002;2(1):18-24.
13. Bouza H, Rutherford M, Acolet D, et al. Evolution of early hemiplegic signs in full-term infants with unilateral brain lesions in the neonatal period: a prospective study. Neuropediatrics. 1994;25(4):201-7.
14. Meyer-Heim AD, Boltshauser E. Spontaneous intracranial haemorrhage in children: aetiology, presentation and outcome. Brain Dev. 2003;25(6):416-21.
15. Ganesan V, Prengler M, McShane MA, et al. Investigation of risk factors in children with arterial ischemic stroke. Ann Neurol. 2003;53(2):167-73.

16. Webster MWI, Smith HJ, Sharpe DN, et al. Patent foramen ovale in young stroke patients. Lancet. 1988;2(8601):11-2.
17. Balkaran B, Ghar G, Morris JS, et al. Stroke in a cohort of patients with homozygous sickle cell disease. J Pediatr. 1992;120(3):360-6.
18. Kato GJ, Hebbel RP, Steinberg MH, et al. Vasculopathy in sickle cell disease: biology, pathophysiology, genetics, translational medicine, and new research directions. Am J Hematol. 2009;84(9):618-25.
19. Park YD, Belman AL, Kim TS, et al. Stroke in pediatric acquired immunodeficiency syndrome. Ann Neurol. 1990;28(3):303-11.
20. Moriarty DM, Haller JO, Loh JP, et al. Cerebral infarction in pediatric acquired immunodeficiency syndrome. Pediatr Radiol. 1994;24(8):611-2.
21. Hutchison JS, Ichord R, Guerguerian AM, et al. Cerebrovascular disorders. Semin Pediatr Neurol. 2004;11(2):139-46.
22. Salih MA, Abdel-Gader AG, Al-Jarallah AA, et al. Infectious and inflammatory disorders of the circulatory system as risk factors for stroke in Saudi children. Saudi Med J. 2006;27 Suppl:S41-52.
23. Fullerton HJ, Johnston SC, Smith WS. Arterial dissection and stroke in children. Neurology. 2001;57(7):1155-60.
24. Graham CJ, Schwartz JE, Stacy T. Stroke following oral trauma in children. Ann Emerg Med. 1991;20(9):1029-31.
25. Kim SH, Kosnik E, Madden C, et al. Cerebellar infarction from a traumatic vertebral artery dissection in a child. Pediatr Neurosurg. 1997;27(2):71-7.
26. Saver JL. Time is brain—quantified. Stroke. 2006;37:263-6.
27. Fleisher GR, Ludwig S. Textbook of Paediatric Emergency Medicine. Philadelphia: Wolters Kluwer/Lippincott Williams & Wilkins Health; 2010.
28. Gadian G, Calamante F, Kirkham FJ, et al. Diffusion and perfusion magnetic resonance imaging in childhood stroke. Child Neurology. 2000;15(5):279-83.
29. deVeber G. Arterial ischemic strokes in infants and children: an overview of current approaches. Semin Thromb Hemost. 2003;29(6):567-73.
30. Amlie-Lefond C, deVeber G, Chan AK, et al. Use of alteplase in childhood arterial ischaemic stroke: a multicentre, observational, cohort study. Lancet Neurol. 2009;8(6):530-6.
31. Poisson SN, Schardt TQ, Dingman A, et al. Etiology and Treatment of Arterial Ischemic Stroke in Children and Young Adults. Curr Treat Options Neurol. 2014;16:315.
32. Bernard TJ, Goldenberg NA, Armstrong-Wells J, et al. Treatment of Childhood Arterial Ischemic Stroke. Ann Neurol. 2008;63:679-96.
33. Ellis MJ, Amlie-Lefond C, Orbach DB. Endovascular therapy in children with acute ischemic stroke: review and recommendations. Neurology. 2012;79(13 Suppl 1):S158-64.
34. Mayer SA, Brun NC, Begtrup K, et al. Efficacy and safety of recombinant activated factor VII for acute intracerebral hemorrhage. N Engl J Med. 2008;358(20):2127-37.
35. Prasad K, Mendelow AD, Gregson B. Surgery for primary supratentorial intracerebral hematoma: a meta-analysis of 10 randomized controlled trials. Stroke. 2009;40(11):e624-6.

SECTION 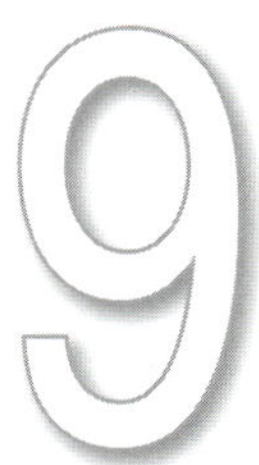

Metabolic

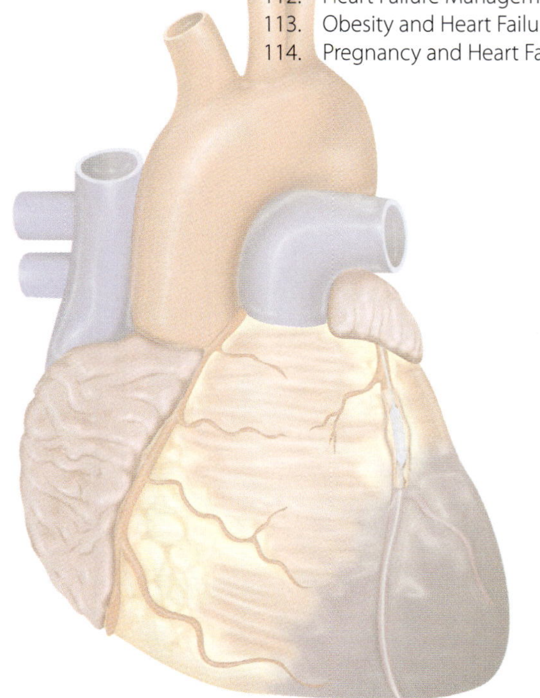

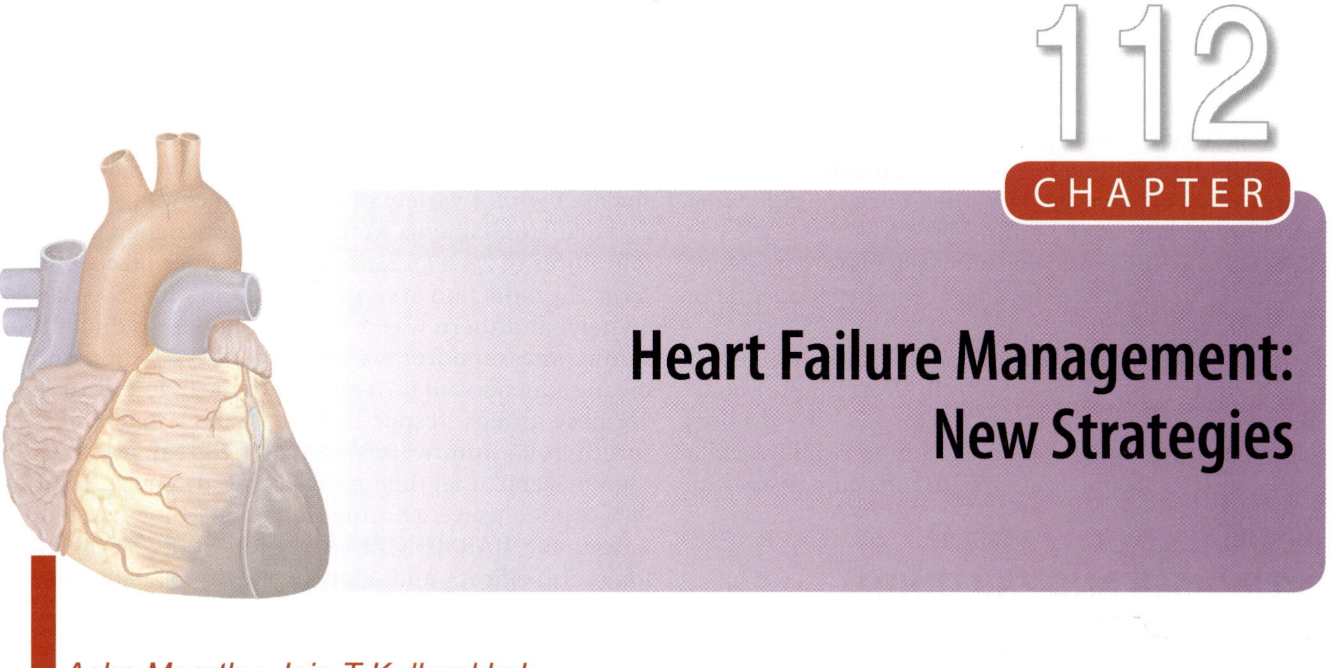

Heart Failure Management: New Strategies

Asha Moorthy, Jain T Kallarakkal

INTRODUCTION

Heart failure (HF), in the past three decades, has shown significant improvement in survival rates, but the 5-year mortality rate remains as high as 50% with significant morbidity. In the past decade, there was no significant change in the treatment modalities of HF. Hence, there is an overwhelming need for new therapies which can improve community-based outcome for patients with HF which is still suboptimal.

LCZ696 (SACUBITRIL/VALSARTAN)

Angiotensin receptor neprilysin inhibitor has shown beneficial outcomes in HF and is approved by Food and Drug Administration (FDA) for the treatment of chronic HF patients since 2015. Sacubitril is the prodrug for active LBQ657. In HF patients with reduced ejection fraction, the PARADIGM-HF (Prospective comparison of ARNI with ACEI to Determine Impact on Global Mortality and morbidity in Heart Failure)[1] trial has shown significant improvement. The trial was stopped early due to significant clinical benefit during a mean follow-up of 27 months. Management of heart failure with preserved ejection fraction [PARAMOUNT (Prospective Comparison of ARNI with ARB on Management of Heart Failure with Preserved Ejection Fraction)] trial[2] has studied prospectively HF patients with preserved ejection fraction. It compared LCZ696 with valsartan. The study showed significant decrease in N-terminal pro-brain natriuretic peptide (NT-proBNP) levels in the LCZ696 group at 12 weeks but no longer significant at 36 weeks. Although the investigators found a significant reduction in systolic blood pressure (SBP), there was no change in left ventricular (LV) size, function, or mass and diastolic function, New York Heart Association (NYHA) functional class, or quality of life scores at 12 weeks. At 36 weeks, there was a reduction in left atrial volume and improvement in NYHA functional class in the LCZ696 group compared with the valsartan group. There were similar adverse event rates among patients receiving LCZ696 compared with valsartan (15% vs. 20%). The trial was not designed or powered to detect clinical outcomes, but it has provided the rationale for larger ongoing clinical outcomes studies.

EPLERENONE

Inhibition of renin-angiotensin-aldosterone system (RAAS) by mineralocorticoid receptor antagonist (MRA) has become a milestone in the current HF treatment in symptomatic (NYHA class III and IV) patients with heart failure with reduced ejection fraction (HFrEF). Aldosterone promotes the retention of sodium, the loss of magnesium and potassium, sympathetic activation, parasympathetic inhibition, myocardial and vascular fibrosis, baroreceptor dysfunction, and vascular damage and impairs arterial compliance. The pathophysiological findings made MRA a cornerstone in the treatment of HF.

Spironolactone and eplerenone belong to this group. Side effects like painful gynecomastia are less seen with eplerenone when compared with spironolactone. Incidence of renal dysfunction and hyperkalemia are same in patients on eplerenone and spironolactone. Based on the results of RALES[3] (Randomized Aldactone Evaluation Study) and EPHESUS[4] (Eplerenone Post-Acute Myocardial Infarction Heart Failure Efficacy and Survival Study), the guidelines recommended that the addition of low-dose MRA to optimal therapy be considered in all patients with moderate to severe chronic HF in the absence of hyperkalemia or significant renal dysfunction.

In the EMPHASIS-HF[5] (Eplerenone in Mild Patients Hospitalization and Survival Study in Heart Failure) study, eplerenone reduced significantly (by 37%) the primary composite outcome of risk of death from cardiovascular causes and first hospitalization for HF in comparison with placebo.

PATIROMER AND ZIRCONIUM CYCLOSILICATE

Two novel potassium absorbents, patiromer calcium and sodium zirconium cyclosilicate (ZS-9), are designed to increase potassium loss via the gastrointestinal tract. Although they have not yet been approved by the FDA, both have demonstrated efficacy and safety in recent trials. As MRA is indicated in HF and hyperkalemia is its major side effect especially with concomitant renal dysfunction, role of these drugs were evaluated. Patiromer is a nonabsorbable polymer that binds potassium in exchange for calcium throughout the gastrointestinal tract. This agent, increases fecal excretion of potassium and consequently decreases plasma potassium levels. The PEARL-HF[6] study tested the combined use of patiromer with spironolactone in 105 HF patients receiving standard care but with previous documented hyperkalemia or chronic kidney disease (CKD). Patiromer significantly lowered serum potassium levels from baseline relative to placebo and prevented the development of hyperkalemia for more than 4 weeks in normokalemic patients with HF. The OPAL-HK[7] (A Two-Part, Single-Blind, Phase 3 Study Evaluating the Efficacy and Safety of Patiromer for the Treatment of Hyperkalemia) assessed the efficacy and safety of patiromer in 243 patients with CKD on RAAS inhibitors with high levels of serum potassium. In this study, a mean reduction in plasma potassium levels was 1.0 mEq/L after the initial 4 weeks of active treatment. When patiromer treatment was stopped at the end of the active treatment period, hyperkalemia rapidly recurred over 8 weeks. The recurrence of hyperkalemia during this period was significantly higher in the placebo group than in the patiromer group (60% vs. 15%, $p < 0.001$), indicating the need for persistent treatment to maintain normokalemia.

Sodium zirconium cyclosilicate is a high-specificity inorganic crystal that entraps potassium in the intestinal tract. Instead of exchanging calcium, ZS-9 exchanges sodium and hydrogen ions for potassium. The efficacy of ZS-9 was assessed in a multicenter randomized controlled trial (RCT) including 753 patients with hyperkalemia associated with a variety of diseases, including CKD, HF, and diabetes. Patients were randomly assigned to one of four doses of ZS-9 (1.25, 2.5, 5, or 10 g) or placebo for 2 days. The reduction of serum potassium with ZS-9 started acutely, and there was a dose-dependent reduction in serum potassium from baseline to 2 days, with absolute mean reductions of 0.73 and 0.53 mEq/L in the 10- and 5-g dose groups, respectively ($p < 0.001$). Reductions in serum potassium were significantly greater with ZS-9 than placebo at all time points on study day 2. Notably, 98% of patients were normalized on the 10-g dose within 2 days. The HARMONIZE[8] study was an RCT evaluating long-term efficacy and safety of ZS-9 in 258 patients with hyperkalemia. Patients achieving normokalemia (3.5–5.0 mEq/L) were randomly assigned to different doses of ZS-9 (5, 10, or 15 g) or placebo for 28 days in the maintenance phase. Mean baseline potassium was 5.6 mEq/L and declined to 4.5 mEq/L after 48 hours of 10-g ZS-9 treatment in the acute phase. Significant reduction in potassium was observed within 1 hour of ZS-9 administration, and 84% of patients achieved normokalemia at 24 hours and 98% at 48 hours. Furthermore, studies assessing the long-term efficacy and safety profile of this novel drug are ongoing (ClinicalTrials.gov identifier: NCT02163499). These recent trials of patiromer and ZS-9 represented short-term safety and efficacy of these attractive therapeutic strategies in patients who develop hyperkalemia during RAAS inhibition. However, the durability of the beneficial effects and the long-term safety of these agents still have to be elucidated. In addition, there are no prospective data answering whether intensive RAAS inhibition with the use of patiromer or ZS-9 would improve the efficacy of RAAS inhibition and cardiovascular outcomes. Further study is needed to address these issues.

IVABRADINE

The detrimental effects of elevated heart rates (HRs) in patients with HF (with reduced ejection fraction and preserved ejection fraction) are well appreciated. Ivabradine works by inhibiting an important pacemaker current (I_f) in the sinoatrial node. It was well documented that single intravenous administration of ivabradine produced pronounced reductions in HR in patients with LV dysfunction, without altering echocardiographic indicators of LV function. The Systolic Heart failure treatment with the IF Inhibitor Ivabradine Trial (SHIFT)[9] evaluated the effect of HR reduction by ivabradine in addition to guideline-based treatment on cardiovascular outcomes, symptoms, and quality of life in patients with HFrEF. SHIFT has shown that HR is a modifiable risk factor, because through the modification of HR without any other known cardiovascular effects risk was reduced.

RELAXIN

Relaxin is a naturally occurring hormone that is produced by the corpus luteum and placenta in pregnancy. Recent studies have shown that relaxin is also produced by the vasculature and failing myocardium. Relaxin interacts with a G protein-coupled receptor, leading to increased cyclic adenosine monophosphate (cAMP). As a result, nitric oxide production is increased by the increased activity of inducible nitric oxide synthase (iNOS) and endothelial nitric oxide synthase (eNOS) expression. Additionally, relaxin upregulates the activity of vascular matrix metalloproteinase-2 (MMP-2) which can activate endothelin-1, leading to endothelin-B receptor activation and subsequent nitric oxide production. Activation of the endothelin-B receptor is likely involved in the relaxin-mediated increases in renal blood flow. Thus, relaxin increases cardiac output, arterial compliance, and renal blood flow, supporting important physiological changes during pregnancy. Given its potent vasodilator properties as well as its ability to increase renal perfusion, relaxin became of interest as a potential therapy for acute HF. The Pre-RELAX-AHF[10] (Relaxin in Acute Heart Failure) study evaluated the effects of relaxin in 234 patients with acute decompensated heart failure (ADHF) within 16 hours from presentation. Patients were randomly assigned to receive four doses of relaxin or placebo for 48 hours. The key findings were that dyspnea relief and safety were optimal at 30 μg/kg per day and sustained results for dyspnea improvement. This dose also led to a substantial reduction in the composite endpoint of cardiovascular mortality or readmission due to HF or renal failure as well as a decrease in cardiovascular mortality at 180 days. However, several subjects (14%) had to discontinue relaxin therapy because of the significant fall in blood pressure. The RELAX-AHF[11] was an RCT enrolling 1,161 ADHF patients who have a SBP of more than 125 mm Hg and renal dysfunction. Patients were randomly assigned to receive serelaxin 30 μg/kg per day or placebo as a continuous 48-hour infusion within 16 hours from presentation. In this study, serelaxin significantly improved dyspnea, shortened the length of hospital stay, and decreased the incidence of worsening HF as compared with placebo. There was also an improvement in the 6-month mortality outcomes and no evidence of adverse effects of this agent on kidney function. Although relaxin has shown success in improving the clinical course of patients with ADHF during the initial hospitalization with an acceptable safety profile, a larger trial (RELAX-AHF-2, $n = 2{,}685$) is ongoing to hopefully validate whether this drug could indeed provide long-term mortality benefit.

ULARITIDE

Ularitide is a chemically synthesized form of urodilatin, a human natriuretic peptide (NP), produced by differential processing of pro-atrial natriuretic peptide (ANP) in distal renal tubule cells. It is a 32-amino acid-containing peptide with the same structure as the 28-amino acid-containing ANP, except for the addition of four amino acids at the N-terminal extension. In Phase I–II clinical HF studies, ularitide demonstrated beneficial effects such as vasodilation and preserved renal function for up to 3 days. In a randomized, double-blind, placebo-controlled Phase IIa and IIb study of 245 patients with ADHF, 24-hour infusions of ularitide lowered cardiac filling pressures, improved dyspnea, and preserved short-term renal function. In addition, troponin assessments did not indicate short-term myocardial damage, while the potent vasoconstrictor endothelin was significantly decreased.

The Prospective Double-blind Study in Patients with Symptomatic, Decompensated Chronic Heart Failure (SIRIUS) II[12] study was aimed to assess the clinical effects of ularitide in 221 patients with ADHF. The primary endpoint was a significant decrease in pulmonary capillary wedge pressure (PCWP) as well as improvement in dyspnea at 6 hours after completion of the 24-hour infusion. Ularitide demonstrated a significant reduction of PCWP for all three dosage groups (7.5, 15, and 30 ng/kg per minute). At higher doses, the agent reduced systemic vascular resistance and increased cardiac index. Besides the beneficial hemodynamic effects, improvement in dyspnea was reported. The most frequently reported drug-related adverse events were dose-dependent blood pressure decrease. Currently, a randomized, placebo-controlled, phase 3 study—Efficacy and Safety of Ularitide for the Treatment of Acute Decompensated Heart Failure (TRUE-AHF), $n = 2{,}152$—is ongoing to measure the effect of 48-hour infusion of ularitide. NPs offer us a unique and attractive strategy for HF treatment, acting as diuretic, natriuretic, vasoactive agents without any inotropic or chronotropic effects. However, the future role of NPs in ADHF therapy is still not yet clear, especially following the rise and fall of nesiritide use. Initial trials with ularitide, a synthetically produced urodilatin, showed hemodynamic and clinical benefits in patients with ADHF. Although ularitide has potential to be an alternative to nesiritide or carperitide, much more evidence is needed to evaluate the role of this agent in HF therapy.

CONCLUSION

Newer drugs are promising in the management of chronic HF. The unambiguous superiority of clinical outcomes with various drugs in patients with HFrEF trial represents a significant achievement with important clinical implications.

REFERENCES

1. McMurray JJ, Packer M, Desai AS, et al. Angiotensin-neprilysin inhibition versus enalapril in heart failure. N Engl J Med. 2014;371:993-1004.
2. Ruilope LM, Dukat A, Bohm M, et al. Blood-pressure reduction with LCZ696, a novel dual-acting inhibitor of the angiotensin II receptor and neprilysin: a randomised, double-blind, placebo controlled, active comparator study. Lancet. 2010;375:1255-66.
3. Pitt B, Zannad F, Remme WJ, et al. The effect of spironolactone on morbidity and mortality in patients with severe heart failure. Randomized Aldactone Evaluation Study Investigators. N Engl J Med. 1999;341(10):709-17.
4. Pitt B, Remme W, Zannad F, et al. Eplerenone, a selective aldosterone blocker, in patients with left ventricular dysfunction after myocardial infarction. N Engl J Med. 2003;348(14):1309-21.
5. Zannad F, McMurray JJ, Krum H, et al. Eplerenone in patients with systolic heart failure and mild symptoms. N Engl J Med. 2011;364(1):11-21.
6. Pitt B, Anker SD, Bushinsky DA, et al. Evaluation of the efficacy and safety of RLY5016, a polymeric potassium binder, in a double-blind, placebo-controlled study in patients with chronic heart failure (the PEARL-HF) trial. Eur Heart J. 2011;32(7):820-8.
7. Weir MR, Bakris GL, Bushinsky DA, et al. Patiromer in patients with kidney disease and hyperkalemia receiving RAAS inhibitors. N Engl J Med. 2015;372(3):211-21.
8. Kosiborod M, Rasmussen HS, Lavin P, et al. Effect of sodium zirconium cyclosilicate on potassium lowering for 28 days among outpatients with hyperkalemia: the HARMONIZE randomized clinical trial. JAMA. 2014;312(21):2223-33.
9. Swedberg K, Komajda M, Böhm M, et al. Ivabradine and outcomes in chronic heart failure (SHIFT): a randomised placebo-controlled study. Lancet. 2010;376(9744): 875-85.
10. Teerlink JR, Metra M, Felker GM, et al. Relaxin for the treatment of patients with acute heart failure (Pre-RELAX-AHF): a multicentre, randomised, placebo-controlled, parallel-group, dose-finding phase IIb study. Lancet. 2009;373(9673):1429-39.
11. Teerlink JR, Cotter G, Davison BA, et al. Serelaxin, recombinant human relaxin-2, for treatment of acute heart failure (RELAX-AHF): a randomised, placebo-controlled trial. Lancet. 2013;381(9860):29-39.
12. Mitrovic V, Seferovic PM, Simeunovic D, et al. Haemodynamic and clinical effects of ularitide in decompensated heart failure. Eur Heart J. 2006;27(33):2823-32.

Obesity and Heart Failure

SS Iyengar

"The impact of obesity in cardiovascular and metabolic diseases is more than just skin deep, and we as scientific community have only scratched the surface."[1]

INTRODUCTION

Obesity is defined as an abnormal accumulation of fat in the body, resulting in ≥20% excess body weight as compared to ideal body weight. This excess baggage carries with it an increased risk of morbidity and mortality due to its adverse effects on various systems of the body through various mechanisms, cardiovascular system being no exception. Heart failure (HF) has been defined as a clinical syndrome characterized by typical symptoms and signs due to a structural and/or functional cardiac abnormality, resulting in a reduced cardiac output and/or elevated intracardiac pressures at rest or during stress.[2]

Very rightly and thoughtfully, obesity is featured in as "Stage A Heart Failure".[3] Stage A of HF includes patients at high risk of developing HF because of the presence of conditions that are strongly associated with the development of HF. Such patients have no identifiable structural or functional abnormalities of the pericardium, myocardium, or cardiac valves and have no signs or symptoms of HF. The conditions in stage A HF are hypertension, atherosclerotic disease, diabetes, obesity, metabolic syndrome, patients using cardiotoxic drugs, and individuals with a family history of cardiomyopathy.[3] Recent global obesity reports estimated that at least 30% of men and 35% of women are obese in many countries worldwide that includes Asian countries.[4,5] Obesity-related cardiomyopathy is estimated to cause 11% of HF cases in males and up to 14% in women.[6]

OBESITY ASSESSMENT

Body mass index (BMI) is the most commonly used and a simple quantifier of obesity despite few flaws associated with it. World Health Organization (WHO) classifies obesity into different categories based on BMI (Table 1).[7]

There are other quantifiers, centered around central obesity. Central obesity is deemed to be present with the threshold values mentioned below.

- Waist circumference: >102 cm for men and >88 cm for women
- Waist to hip ratio: >0.9 in men and >0.85 in women
- Waist to height ratio: 0.5 or more for men and women.

These threshold values differ based on ethnicities.

TABLE 1: WHO classification of body mass index (BMI).

BMI (kg/m²)	*Class*
<18.5	Underweight
18.5–24.9	Normal range
25–29.9	Overweight
30–34.9	Class I obesity
35–39.9	Class II obesity
40 or more	Class III or morbid obesity

A consensus statement from India[8] classified BMI as follows:

- Normal: 18–22.9 kg/m^2
- Overweight: 23–24.9 kg/m^2
- Obese: >25 kg/m^2.

Cutoff values for waist circumference as a measure of central obesity for different ethnicities are shown in Table 2.[9]

HOW DOES OBESITY CAUSE HEART FAILURE?

An interesting term has been coined to name a new concept—"adiposopathy" (or sick fat). In this condition, there is an abnormal adverse response by the fat tissue organ to a stimulus.[10]

It is an outdated understanding for long now that the fat tissue in the body or the "adipose organ" is merely a storage house of energy in the form of lipids, which is built up or broken down according to the needs of the body. Now it has been recognized that adipose tissue is an exquisitely active metabolic and endocrine organ, in cross talk with various systems of the body, secreting active peptides, and nonpeptide substances.

ASSOCIATED FACTORS WITH VISCERAL ADIPOSITY

The characteristic pathologic feature of adiposopathy is the accumulation of fat in the abdominal cavity in the form of visceral adipose tissue (VAT). There are several factors which are associated with excess of VAT (Fig. 1).[11]

Gender-based differences in VAT are related to hormonal factors and VAT mass increases after menopause. VAT has ethnicity variations, South Asians manifesting diabetes at a lower BMI than whites and blacks being less prone for visceral obesity.[12,13]

Studies have shown association between visceral adiposity and hypertension, atherosclerotic cardiovascular disease (ASCVD), and HF.[14,15] Excess of VAT, when present in patients with diabetes mellitus, has also been shown to be associated with lower systolic and diastolic strain rates,

TABLE 2: Ethnicity and waist circumference for central obesity.

Ethnic group	Waist circumference (cm) (central obesity)	
	Male	Female
Europeans	94 cm or more	80 cm or more
South Asians	90 cm or more	80 cm or more
Chinese	90 cm or more	80 cm or more
Japanese	85 cm or more	90 cm or more

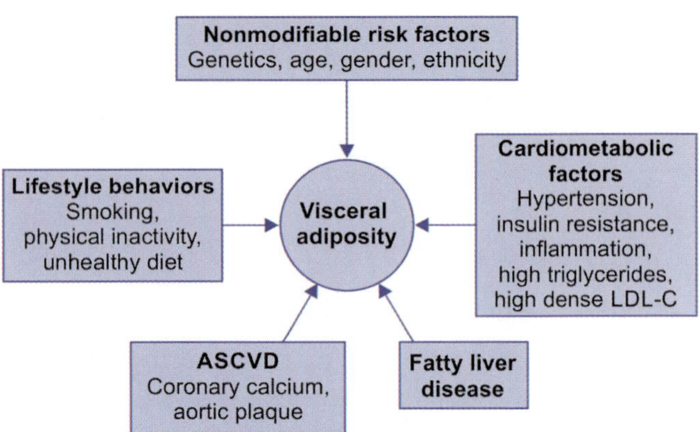

Fig. 1: Factors associated with increased visceral adiposity.[1] (ASCVD: arteriosclerotic cardiovascular disease; LDL-C: low-density lipoprotein cholesterol)

excess of triglyceride intramyocardially, and prolonged myocardial T1 by magnetic resonance imaging (MRI) (a measure of relaxation time).[16] Pericardial and epicardial fat deposits have also been shown to be associated with ASCVD coronary events in the general population independent of traditional risk factors. Genetic association has been shown between central obesity, coronary heart disease, and type 2 diabetes mellitus.[17]

Obstructive sleep apnea (OSA) has been referred to as "A Sleeping Beast" by McKee and Auckley.[18] The Sleep Heart Health Study of 6,424 adults with cardiovascular disease found that OSA was associated with a 2.38 relative odds of having HF.[19] OSA has adverse effects on cardiovascular system through mechanical, neurohumoral, and inflammatory mechanisms consequent to hypoxia, arousal, and intrathoracic pressure changes.[19]

PATHOGENIC MECHANISMS (FLOWCHART 1)

Adipose tissue has important interactions with other systems of the body, including cardiovascular system that helps in understanding the pathogenic mechanisms of HF in obesity. VAT, an active metabolic and endocrine organ, through direct and indirect mechanisms paves the path for HF, the mechanisms exhibiting overlapping as well as integrated effects. Visceral obesity has local effects on the myocardium, producing hypertrophy, fibrosis, and activation of inflammatory pathways. Hypervolumia and direct lipotoxicity add to the insult.

In a population-based cohort of obese adults, visceral fat, and subcutaneous fat were assessed by MRI and their association with various biomarkers was studied. After adjusting for age, sex, race, menopause, and BMI, it was found that VAT showed significant association with insulin

Flowchart 1: Obesity and heart failure—possible mechanisms.

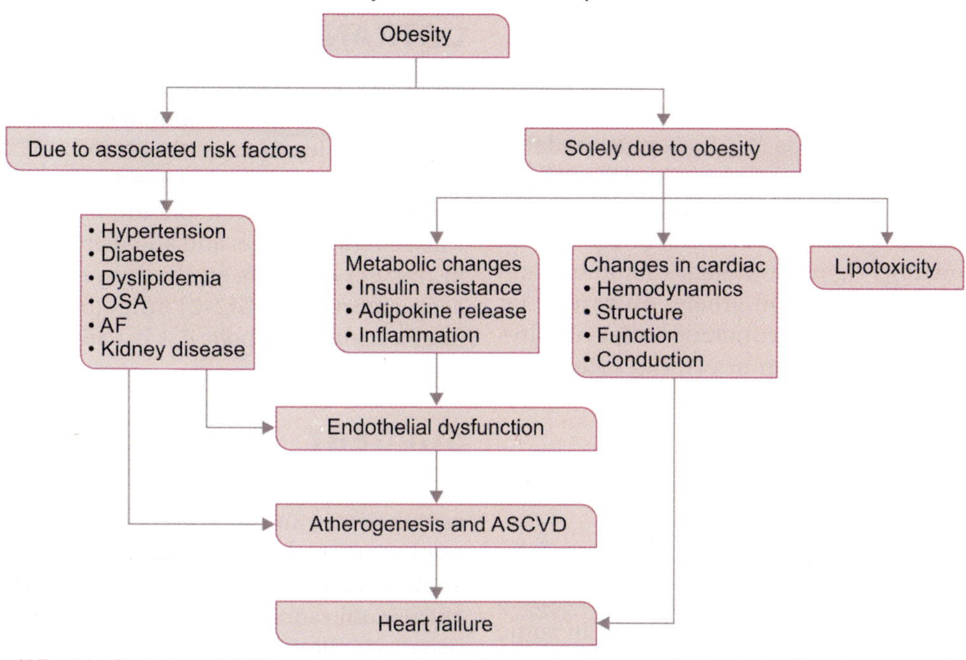

(AF: atrial fibrillation; ASCVD: arteriosclerotic cardiovascular disease; OSA: obstructive sleep apnea)

resistance, lower levels of adiponectin, raised small dense low-density lipoprotein (LDL) cholesterol, and increased LDL and very-low-density lipoprotein (VLDL) particle number. Visceral adiposity was also associated with prevalent diabetes, metabolic syndrome, hepatic steatosis, aortic plaque, and with C-reactive protein.[20]

NATRIURETIC PEPTIDES AND OBESITY

Observational studies have shown that visceral obesity is associated with lower natriuretic peptide levels in asymptomatic individuals, which has been referred to as "natriuretic peptide deficiency" and, "lower body adipose tissue" is associated with higher natriuretic peptide levels. Natriuretic peptides stimulate lipolysis, promote browning of adipocytes and stimulate adiponectin secretion from adipocytes. The natriuretic peptides have "lipomobilizing" effects and have a favorable influence on body fat metabolism and distribution.[21,22] Recently, leptin-aldosterone-neprilysin axis has been proposed to contribute to the evolution and progression of HF in people with obesity.[23] Visceral adiposity has been found to be associated with the three types of HF—heart failure with reduced ejection fraction (HFrEF), heart failure with preserved ejection fraction (HFpEF), and high output HF and all of them are associated with elevated levels of aldosterone and leptin. Leptin activates sympathetic nervous system and renin-angiotensin system and also directly facilitates secretion of aldosterone. Adiposity and renal sympathetic nerves enhance neprilysin activity. This interplay is ominous and deleterious for the heart.

CLINICAL IMPLICATIONS

Diagnosis

Obesity may complicate diagnosis of HF, since obesity by itself can cause dyspnea, exercise intolerance, and ankle swelling. Moreover, in obese subjects with poor echocardiographic window, echocardiographic imaging would be difficult.

Natriuretic Peptides

Obese individuals have low levels of natriuretic peptides.[24] Does this pose a problem in diagnosis and prognosis based on brain natriuretic peptide (BNP) levels? 12,230 participants who were free of HF at baseline and had a BMI ≥18.5 kg/m^2 in Atherosclerosis Risk in Communities (ARIC) study were followed up for a median of 20.6 years. There was an inverse association between baseline BMI and N-terminal pro-BNP (NT-proBNP) levels. But higher baseline NT-proBNP level was associated with increased risk of HF in all BMI categories, and it predicted risk even in subjects with severe obesity (BMI >35 kg/m^2). The study concluded that serum NT-proBNP estimation has significant prognostic value even among individuals with obesity.[25]

Heart Failure with Preserved Ejection Fraction

Obese HFpEF phenotype is probably a distinct entity. In United States, it is reported that 80% of patients with HFpEF are overweight or obese.[26,27] In a multimodality study of obese and nonobese patients with HFpEF and controls, obese group compared with other two groups, had increased plasma volume and more concentric left ventricular remodeling, right ventricular dilatation, and right ventricular dysfunction had greater epicardial fat thickness.[28] The study authors concluded that obesity-related HFpEF is a genuine form of cardiac failure and a clinically relevant phenotype demanding specific therapeutics.

OBESITY PARADOX

Obesity is a well-entrenched risk factor for developing HF. But once HF is diagnosed and well established, an interesting paradox may be witnessed. As seen in some other chronic illnesses, obesity is associated with lower mortality across a wide range of BMIs, which is referred to as the "obesity paradox". The risk of developing HF is higher in patients who are obese, but being obese or overweight provides survival advantage compared with normal weight or low weight patients. It was first described by Horwich et al.[29] in 2001. A large meta-analysis showed that HF patients who were overweight or obese had a favorable outcome in all cause and cardiovascular mortality.[30] The "obesity paradox" has been reported in patients whether they have HFrEF or HFpEF, ischemic or nonischemic cardiomyopathy.[31] A "U-shaped" relationship has been described in some studies, i.e. a BMI between 36 kg/m^2 and 40 kg/m^2 showing the lowest 1-year mortality, patients with BMI <20 kg/m^2 having the highest mortality, followed by patients with BMI >45 kg/m^2.[32,33] The clear mechanism to explain "obesity paradox" remains elusive. The studies reporting obesity paradox have been mostly retrospective. Obese patients probably get clinician's attention early. The renin-angiotensin system may be less active in obese and they tolerate drug therapy better.[34,35]

Recommendations regarding intentional weight loss remain unclear. European Society of Cardiology guidelines on HF[2] state the following:

- In patients with HF with moderate degrees of obesity (BMI, 35 kg/m^2), weight loss cannot be recommended.
- In more advanced obesity (BMI 35–45 kg/m^2), weight loss may be considered to manage symptoms and exercise capacity.

SODIUM-GLUCOSE COTRANSPORTER-2 INHIBITORS

In a study, 3,300 patients underwent estimation of body fat content and distribution in the form of estimated total body fat, index of central obesity, and visceral adiposity index.[36] These are the indices which closely correlate with cardiometabolic risk factors. Empagliflozin reduced weight, waist circumference, and adiposity indices versus placebo in this cohort. This study showed that sodium-glucose cotransporter-2 (SGLT-2) inhibitors have the potential to reduce cardiometabolic risk in patients with type 2 diabetes mellitus.

SURGERY

Surgical therapies for weight loss such as gastric bypass, gastric sleeve, and laparoscopic gastric banding have been used to treat severe obesity and type 2 diabetes mellitus. They have been shown to reduce visceral fat and improve glucose utilization. Observational studies suggest long-term benefits for both HFrEF and HFpEF after bariatric surgery.[37]

INTERVENTIONS FOR ADVANCED HEART FAILURE

In obese patients with advanced HF, increased BMI was strongly associated with a decreased likelihood of receiving a cardiac transplant once placed on the waiting list.[38]

There is limited data on use of mechanical left ventricular-assisted devices (LVADs) for obese HF patients. In a recent study of 3,856 patients who received continuous flow, LVAD between 2004 and 2014, the risk of death or delisting from transplant list while on LVAD was not significantly different between patients with different BMI. However, complications of thrombosis and device infection were significantly more in patients with BMI above 35 kg/m^2. There was an increased risk of mortality after transplant for obese patients compared with those with normal BMI.[39]

CONCLUSION

Obesity is a heavy and growing health problem, as is HF. Obesity is a risk factor for HF and has implications in diagnosis, prognosis, and therapeutics. Preventive measures have a great potential in facing this dual challenge.

REFERENCES

1. Neeland IJ, Poirier P, Després JP. Cardiovascular and metabolic heterogeneity of obesity: clinical challenges and implications for management. Circulation. 2018;137:1391-406.

2. Ponikowski P, Voors AA, Anker SD, et al. 2016 ESC Guidelines for the diagnosis and treatment of acute and chronic heart failure: The Task Force for the diagnosis and treatment of acute and chronic heart failure of the European Society of Cardiology (ESC) Developed with the special contribution of the Heart Failure Association (HFA) of the ESC. Eur Heart J. 2016;37:2129-200.
3. Jessup M, Abraham WT, Casey DE, et al. 2009 focused update: ACCF/AHA Guidelines for the Diagnosis and Management of Heart Failure in Adults: a report of the American College of Cardiology Foundation/American Heart Association Task Force on Practice Guidelines: developed in collaboration with the International Society for Heart and Lung Transplantation. Circulation. 2009;119:1977-2016.
4. Afshin A, Forouzanfar MH, Reitsma MB, et al. Health effects of overweight and obesity in 195 countries over 25 years. N Engl J Med. 2017;377:13-27.
5. Ng M, Fleming T, Robinson M, et al. Global, regional, and national prevalence of overweight and obesity in children and adults during 1980-2013: a systematic analysis for the Global Burden of Disease Study 2013. Lancet. 2014;384:766-81.
6. Glenn DJ, Wang F, Nishimoto M, et al. A murine model of isolated cardiac steatosis leads to cardiomyopathy. Hypertension. 2011;57(2):216-22.
7. World Health Organization. (2000) Obesity: Preventing and managing the global epidemic. Report of a WHO Consultation (WHO Technical Report Series 894). [online] Available from https://www.who.int/nutrition/publications/obesity/WHO_TRS_894/en/ [Last accessed November, 2019].
8. Misra A, Chowbey A, Makkar BM, et al. Consensus statement for diagnosis of obesity, abdominal obesity and metabolic syndrome for Asian Indians and recommendations for physical activity, medical and surgical management. J Assoc Physic India. 2009;57:163-70.
9. Alberti KG, Zimmet P, Shaw J, et al. The metabolic syndrome: a new worldwide definition. Lancet. 2005;366:1059-62.
10. Bays HE. Adiposopathy: is "sick fat" a cardiovascular disease? J Am Coll Cardiol. 2011;57:2461-73.
11. Neeland IJ, Ayers CR, Rohatgi AK, et al. Associations of visceral and abdominal subcutaneous adipose tissue with markers of cardiac and metabolic risk in obese adults. Obesity. 2013;21:e439-47.
12. Araneta MR, Kanaya AM, Hsu WC, et al. Optimum BMI cut points to screen Asian Americans for type 2 diabetes. Diabetes Care. 2015;38:814-20.
13. Després JP, Couillard C, Gagnon J, et al. Race, visceral adipose tissue, plasma lipids, and lipoprotein lipase activity in men and women: the Health, Risk Factors, Exercise Training, and Genetics (HERITAGE) family study. Arterioscler Thromb Vasc Biol. 2000;20:1932-8.
14. Chandra A, Neeland IJ, Berry JD, et al. The relationship of body mass and fat distribution with incident hypertension: observations from the Dallas Heart Study. J Am Coll Cardiol. 2014;64:997-1002.
15. Neeland IJ, Turer AT, Ayers CR, et al. Body fat distribution and incident cardiovascular disease in obese adults. J Am Coll Cardiol. 2015;65:2150-1.
16. Levelt E, Pavlides M, Banerjee R, et al. Ectopic and visceral fat deposition in lean and obese patients with type 2 diabetes. J Am Coll Cardiol. 2016;68:53-63.
17. Emdin CA, Khera AV, Natarajan P, et al. Genetic association of waist-to-hip ratio with cardiometabolic traits, type 2 diabetes, and coronary heart disease. JAMA. 2017;317:626-34.
18. McKee Z, Auckley DH. A sleeping beast: Obstructive sleep apnea and stroke. Ccleveland Clinic J Med. 2019;86:407-15.
19. Shahar E, Whitney CW, Redline S, et al. Sleep-disordered breathing and cardiovascular disease: cross-sectional results of the Sleep Health Study. Am J Respir Crit Care Med. 2001;163(1):19-25.
20. Neeland IJ, Ayers CR, Rohatgi A, et al. Association of visceral and subcutaneous adipose tissue mass with markers of cardiometabolic risk in obese adults: Observations from the Dallas heart study. J Am Coll Cardiol. 2018;59:e1786.
21. Neeland IJ, Winders BR, Ayers CR, et al. Higher natriuretic peptide levels associate with a favorable adipose tissue distribution pro le. J Am Coll Cardiol. 2013;62:752-60.
22. Tsukamoto O, Fujita M, Kato M, et al. Natriuretic peptides enhance the production of adiponectin in human adipocytes and in patients with chronic heart failure. J Am Coll Cardiol. 2009;53:2070-7.
23. Packer M. Leptin-aldosterone-neprilysin axis: identification of its distinctive role in the pathogenesis of the three phenotypes of heart failure in people with obesity. Circulation. 2018;137(15):1614-31.
24. Madamanchi C, Alhosaini H, Sumida A, et al. Obesity and natriuretic peptides, BNP and NT-proBNP: Mechanisms and diagnostic implications for heart failure. Int J Cardiol. 2014;176:6117.
25. Ndumele CE, Matsushita, K, Sang Y, et al. N-Terminal Pro-Brain Natriuretic Peptide and Heart Failure Risk Among Individuals with and without Obesity. The Atherosclerosis Risk in Communities (ARIC) Study. Circulation. 2016;133:631-8.
26. Upadhya B, Haykowsky MJ, Eggebeen J, et al. Sarcopenic obesity and the pathogenesis of exercise intolerance in heart failure with preserved ejection fraction. Curr Heart Fail Rep. 2015;12:20514.
27. Kitzman DW, Brubaker P, Morgan T, et al. Effect of caloric restriction or aerobic exercise training on peak oxygen consumption and quality of life in obese older patients with heart failure with preserved ejection fraction: a randomized clinical trial. JAMA. 2016;315:36-44.
28. Obokata M, Reddy YNV, Pislaru SV, et al. Evidence supporting the existence of a distinct obese phenotype of heart failure with preserved ejection fraction. Circulation. 2017;136:6-19.
29. Horwich TB, Fonarow GC, Hamilton MA, et al. The relationship between obesity and mortality in patients with heart failure. J Am Coll Cardiol. 2001;38:789-95.
30. Oreopoulos A, Padwal R, Kalantar-Zadeh K, et al. Body mass index and mortality in heart failure: a meta-analysis. Am Heart J. 2008;156:13-22.
31. Nagarajan V, Kohan L, Holland E, et al. Obesity paradox in heart failure: a heavy matter. ESC Heart Fail. 2016;3:227-34.

32. Nagarajan V, Cauthen CA, Starling RC, et al. Prognosis of morbid obesity patients with advanced heart failure. Congest Heart Fail. 2013;19:160-4.
33. Kapoor JR, Heidenreich PA. Obesity and survival in patients with heart failure and preserved systolic function: a U-shaped relationship. Am Heart J. 2010;159:75-80.
34. Fonarow GC, Srikanthan P, Costanzo MR, et al. An obesity paradox in acute heart failure: analysis of body mass index and inhospital mortality for 108,927 patients in the Acute Decompensated Heart Failure National Registry. Am Heart J. 2007;153:74-81.
35. Lavie CJ, Milani RV, Ventura HO. Obesity and cardiovascular disease: risk factor, paradox, and impact of weight loss. J Am Coll Cardiol. 2009;53:1925-32.
36. Neeland IJ, McGuire DK, Chilton R, et al. Empagliflozin reduces body weight and indices of adipose distribution in patients with type 2 diabetes mellitus. Diab Vasc Dis Res. 2016;13(2):119-26.
37. Rodriguez Flores M, Aguilar Salinas C, Piché ME, et al. Effect of bariatric surgery on heart failure. Expert Rev Cardiovasc Ther. 2017;15:567-79.
38. Weiss ES, Allen JG, Russell SD, et al. Impact of recipient body mass index on organ allocation and mortality in orthotopic heart transplantation. J Heart Lung Transplant. 2009;28:1150-7.
39. Clerkin KJ, Naka Y, Mancini DM, et al. The impact of obesity on patients bridged to transplantation with continuous-flow left ventricular assist devices. JACC Heart Fail. 2016;4:761-8.

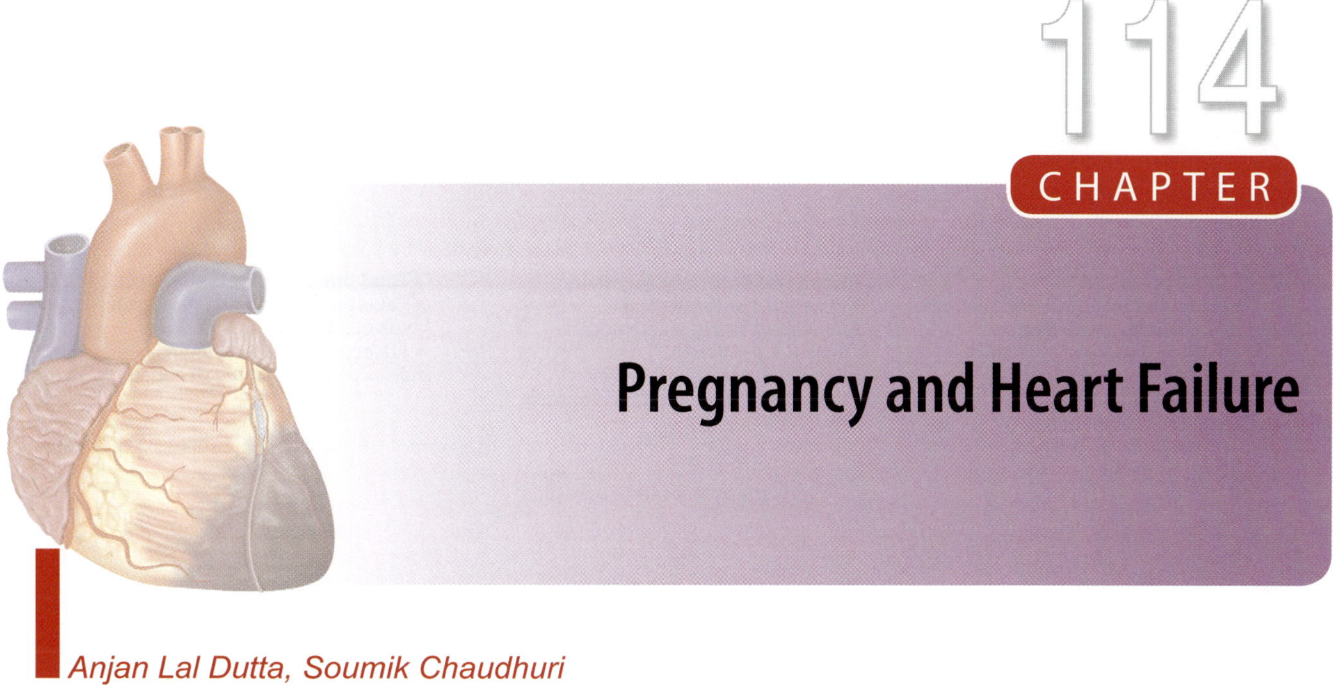

114

CHAPTER

Pregnancy and Heart Failure

Anjan Lal Dutta, Soumik Chaudhuri

INTRODUCTION

Cardiovascular diseases are important and established causes of increased maternal mortality accounting for almost 36.5% of mortality reported in Southern Asia.[1] UK data attributes cardiac disease as the cause of 20% of total mortality and is regarded as the most common overall cause of indirect maternal death.[2] The preponderance of deaths is due to some form of ventricular failure and can occur even in late postpartum period. Thus, the common occurrence and high mortality of cardiac disease in pregnant woman makes it imperative for us to identify risk factors for heart failure early in pregnancy, as well as identify signs of impending failure and manage the same with due care for both maternal and fetal well-being.

CARDIOVASCULAR CHANGES DURING PREGNANCY

During pregnancy, the changes in the cardiovascular system begin early and persist till labor and beyond. There is an endothelium-dependent, peripheral vasodilatation that starts by the end of the second month, increasing cardiac output by almost 20%, and is primarily regulated by prostaglandin I2 (PGI2) and estradiol. Systemic vascular resistance (SVR) falls by a fourth (25%) and the cardiac output is maximally increased by around 40% during pregnancy, at about 20–28 weeks of gestation. The primary hemodynamic variation is an increased stroke volume aided by a minor rise in heart rate. The heart undergoes a physiological dilation due to early increases in end-diastolic volume and ventricular wall muscle mass. Myocardial contractility is increased. The stroke volume starts decreasing near term, but the cardiac output is preserved due to an increase in maternal heart rate by about 10–20 bpm. Blood pressure shows a slight fall in the first two trimesters but returns to previous levels by the third.[3] The pulmonary capillary wedge pressure (PCWP) generally does not increase substantially and, coupled with a decrease in pulmonary vascular resistance (PVR) as well as serum colloid osmotic pressure, this leads to the osmotic pressure/PCWP gradient decreasing by almost 30% during pregnancy. This makes pregnant women particularly prone to pulmonary edema, either by increase in preload (fluid infusion) or increased pulmonary capillary permeability (pre-eclampsia) or both.

The process of labor leads to significant rise in cardiac output (15% in the initial stages leading to almost 50% by second stage of labor). The contracting uterus autotransfuses up to 300–500 mL of blood back into the circulation and attendant pain and anxiety further increase blood pressure and heart rate, due to sympathetic stimulation. Immediately after delivery, there is a rapid rise in cardiac output due to relief of the vena caval obstruction and the contracting uterus keeps emptying blood into the systemic circulation. Cardiac output precipitously increases by 60–70%, followed by an even faster decline to prelabor levels within an hour of delivery. Thus, women with cardiovascular disease are at the highest risk of pulmonary edema during the second stage of labor and the immediate postpartum period. Cardiac output tends to return to prepregnancy levels by 2 weeks postpartum, although it may persist longer in some patients of pre-eclampsia.[3] These pathophysiological changes are summarized in Flowchart 1.

Flowchart 1: Hemodynamic changes in pregnancy that act as precipitating factors for heart failure.

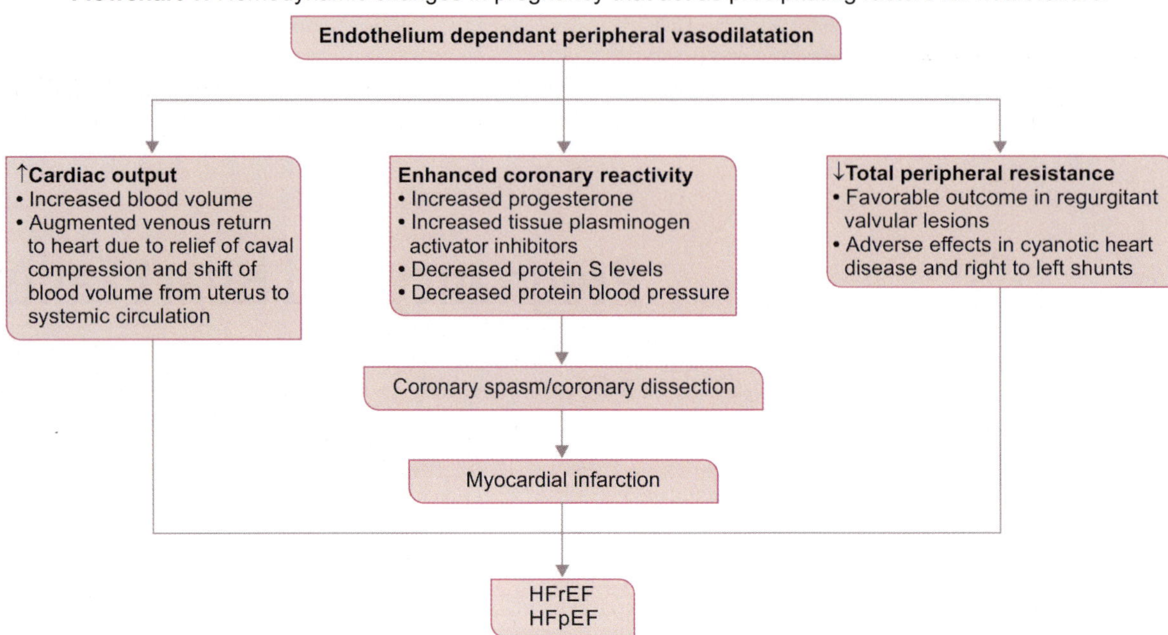

(HFpEF: heart failure with preserved ejection fraction; HFrEF: heart failure with reduced ejection fraction)

ETIOLOGY OF HEART FAILURE IN PREGNANCY (BOX 1)

Among these, peripartum cardiomyopathy, amniotic fluid embolism, and pre-eclampsia are specific pregnancy-related causes of heart failure whereas the others are comorbid conditions complicating pregnancy. We shall now discuss a few of the important etiologies in more detail

BOX 1: Causes of heart failure in pregnancy.

- Increased vascular resistance:
  - Pre-eclampsia
  - Hypertensive cardiomyopathy
  - Pulmonary hypertension and right heart failure
- Diseases affecting the aortic root:
  - Takayasu's arteritis
  - Marfan's syndrome
  - Atherosclerotic disease
- Ventricular failure:
  - Peripartum cardiomyopathy
  - Hereditary cardiomyopathies
  - Autoimmune and viral cardiomyopathies
  - Drug-induced cardiomyopathy
- Amniotic fluid embolism
- Valvular heart disease:
  - Stenotic lesions
  - Regurgitant lesions
- Congenital heart diseases:
  - Eisenmenger's syndrome
  - Marfan's with dilated aortic root
  - Post-Fontan procedure
  - Congenitally stenosed valves
  - Coarctation of aorta

Pre-eclampsia

Pregnancy-induced hypertension and pre-eclampsia are characterized by a hyperdynamic circulation leading to an increase in contractility of the left ventricle. This, coupled with an increase in SVR and administration of intravenous fluids, causes rapid increase in the left atrial filling pressures and consequent pulmonary edema. It is one of the predominant causes of hypertensive maternal mortality. Severe pre-eclampsia may present with transient impairment of systolic function, but the primary cardiac derangement is due to diastolic dysfunction.[4] Right heart filling pressures are usually normal.[5]

Hypertension

Chronic, pre-existent hypertension is rapidly increasing in frequency worldwide and is prevalent in up to 3% of all pregnant women. It leads to an increased risk of abruptio placentae, pre-eclampsia, and preterm births.[6] In the absence of superimposed pre-eclampsia, it generally leads to a mild pulmonary edema at 32–34 weeks of gestation due to an increased plasma volume and diastolic dysfunction.[7]

Pulmonary Hypertension

These may be idiopathic in nature (primary) or be secondary to other causes, further subdivided into pre- and postcapillary types. The secondary ones are usually cardiac diseases causing increased left-sided filling pressures or pulmonary parenchymal disease. Pregnant women with primary pulmonary hypertension are prone to acute right-sided heart failure immediately after delivery and the initial presentation may be sudden cardiac death. The mechanism for this acute deterioration is still not clear.[8]

Aortic Root Diseases

The most common diseases include Takayasu's arteritis and Marfan's syndromes. Heart failure; however, is a relatively rare presentation and they predominantly present with hypertension, or even acute aortic dissection especially with a dilated aortic root.[9]

Peripartum Cardiomyopathy

The most common cause of cardiac mortality during pregnancy.[10] This is a defined as the development of left ventricular systolic dysfunction with an ejection fraction <45% in the last month of pregnancy or 6 months postdelivery, in previously normal women. The main pathology is a possible induction of myocyte apoptosis due to a 16 kDa cathepsin cleavage product of prolactin.[11] Oxidative stress and inflammatory changes due to development of autoimmunity, may also play a role.[12] More often than not, it is a dilated cardiomyopathy due to no identifiable etiology. Imbalances in antiangiogenic versus angiogenic may also lead to development of cardiomyopathy.[13]

Hereditary Cardiomyopathies

These include dilated cardiomyopathy (DCMO-myocyte mutations), hypertrophic cardiomyopathy (HOCM-sarcomere mutation), and arrhythmogenic right ventricular cardiomyopathy (ARVC-desmosome mutation).[14] HOCM is generally well tolerated in pregnancy and depends on prepregnancy symptoms.[15] In DCMO patients, risk of heart failure during pregnancy is predicted by the magnitude of prepregnancy signs. The risk of sudden cardiac death in ARVC is unrelated to occurrence of pregnancy.[16]

Other Forms of Cardiomyopathy

Drugs known to cause cardiomyopathy are a vast list, with important ones including cocaine abuse, alcohol, methamphetamine, cyclophosphamide, and zidovudine among others. They rarely cause acute heart failure. Viral/autoimmune myocarditis may also lead to dilated cardiomyopathy and consequent heart failure.[17]

Amniotic Fluid Embolism

An uncommon but potentially fatal complication of labor, this presents with acute onset pulmonary edema, bleeding diathesis, seizure, and ultimately cardiovascular collapse.[18] The release of fetal squames and amniotic fluid into the maternal circulation leads to acute pulmonary hypertension, setting off left ventricular failure which requires prolonged inotropic support.

Ischemic Heart Disease

This is an unlikely cause of heart failure in pregnancy, with mortality stemming from an acute myocardial infarction.[19] Apart from conventional causes of coronary artery disease, anomalous coronary artery origin and coronary artery dissection may also present with similar symptoms and is related to the excess progesterone levels, leading to structural changes in vessel walls viz. loss of normal corrugation in elastic fibers, breaking up of reticular fibers, and decrease in the amount of acid mucopolysaccharides.[19] Deaths are rare.

Valvular Lesions

Increased plasma volume and a hyperdynamic circulation of pregnancy (maximal at 34 weeks and an acute rise immediately postpartum) may precipitate pulmonary edema in rheumatic valvular heart disease. Increases in pulse rate, accentuated by labor pains, diminish left ventricular filling times, thus increasing the risk of heart failure in women with mitral stenosis. Regurgitant lesions are generally better tolerated in pregnancy due to a decrease in SVR.[20] The immediate postdelivery period remains at high alert due to the sudden rise in blood volume. Anemia, arrhythmias and hyperthyroidism amplify the risk of pulmonary edema in valve disease and many patients may be diagnosed for the first time during pregnancy.[19]

Congenital Abnormalities

Corrected congenital heart disease women usually have uncomplicated pregnancies if their prepregnancy exercise tolerance was good.[21] Among uncorrected lesions, Eisenmenger syndrome and Marfan's with a dilated aortic root have the worst prognosis. Congenital stenosis, cyanotic disease without pulmonary hypertension, and a Fontan circulation have a moderate risk of heart failure whereas the septal defects (without pulmonary hypertension) are at low-risks.[21]

CLINICAL PRESENTATION

Acute heart failure in pregnancy may present as either left or right or biventricular heart failure. The most common symptom is dyspnea (or tiredness as usually perceived by pregnant women). Progesterone produces a physiological, increased respiratory drive to offload carbon dioxide from the fetus to the mother, and may cause a perceived dyspnea, not associated with cardiac disease. Presence of associated symptoms like paroxysmal nocturnal dyspnea, palpitations, and orthopnea need further evaluation.[22] Clinical signs of pregnancy like a mildly raised jugular venous pressure and a bounding pulse may confound diagnosis of cardiac failure. Peripheral edema tends to peak near time of delivery. Sinus arrhythmia may be physiologically present at this time.[23] Flow murmurs and a downwardly displaced apex are commonly seen as is a third heart sound.[23] The significant cardiac findings would include a diastolic or pansystolic murmur, arrhythmias, hypotension, a collapsing pulse, cyanosis, clubbing or an unexplained tachypnea or acute respiratory distress.

INVESTIGATIONS

The basic investigations must include an electrocardiogram (ECG) and chest X-ray (CXR). Increased pulmonary vascular markings are normal in advanced pregnancy and the ECG may show nonspecific ST segment abnormalities and/or supraventricular tachycardias as a normal finding.[22] Echocardiography should be routinely employed in pregnant women with symptoms suggestive of cardiac disease. Other investigations, as necessary in a cardiological evaluation, are also indicated.

TABLE 1: WHO classification for adverse outcomes in pregnant women with cardiac disease.

Class	Conditions
Class I: No increased risk of adverse outcomes	Repaired septal defects or patent ductus arteriosus, mitral valve prolapse, mild pulmonary stenosis, isolated ventricular ectopics
Class II: Mild increase of risk of adverse outcomes	All other arrhythmias, unrepaired tetralogy of Fallot, unrepaired septal defects
Class III: Approach to risk is individualized	Mild left ventricular (LV) systolic impairment, mild native valvular heart disease, bicuspid aortic valve with aorta <45 mm, Marfan's syndrome without aortic dilation
Class IV: Significant risk of adverse outcomes	Complex/unrepaired cyanotic heart diseases, mechanical valves, Fontan circulation, bicuspid aortic valve with aorta = 45–50 mm, Marfan's syndrome with aortic dilation = 40–45 mm
Class V: Pregnancy is contraindicated	Severe pulmonary hypertension, bicuspid aortic valve with aorta >50 mm, Marfan's syndrome with aortic dilation >45 mm, severe mitral/aortic stenosis, severe LV systolic dysfunction

RISK STRATIFICATION OF CARDIAC DISEASE IN PREGNANCY

The most widely accepted risk scoring system in pregnancy, for outcome of cardiac disease, is the WHO risk profile (Table 1).[10] Others include the CARPREG and ZAHARA risk profiles.

DIFFERENTIAL DIAGNOSIS

The differential diagnosis for heart failure in pregnancy includes the following, among others:[24]

- Adult respiratory distress syndrome (ARDS)
- Parenchymal pulmonary diseases
- Interstitial lung diseases
- Pulmonary thromboembolism
- Diabetic ketoacidosis
- Lactic acidosis
- HELLP syndrome (**H**emolysis, **E**levated **L**iver enzymes, and **L**ow **P**latelets)

PRINCIPLES OF MANAGEMENT

Drug Therapy

Diuretics: Diuretics are the preferred primary line of treatment for most pregnant women presenting with heart failure.[25] Reducing preload decreases left-sided filling pressures allowing the reabsorption of interstitial fluid in the lung. Theoretically, this may also decrease placental perfusion and adversely affect fetal growth, but there is no evidence that diuretics are an independent risk factor for fetal growth restriction and their use in symptomatic mothers is justified, especially when left ventricular function is compromised.[26] However, in conditions such as pre-eclampsia, the primary pathology is an increased vascular resistance with a concomitant left ventricular diastolic dysfunction. Parenteral vasodilators for afterload reduction allow for a rise in stroke volume and cardiac output and are the preferred treatment. Diuretic therapy may actually worsen such patients by depleting an already contracted intravascular volume. Bedside echocardiography or, if available, invasive hemodynamic monitoring help in managing such similar phenotypic presentations.[27] Nitroglycerine, used as a mixed venous and arterial vasodilator, has an important role in sick women with hypertension (due to pre-eclampsia), accentuated by left ventricular systolic failure, and coincident renal failure, by increasing venous capacitance.

Angiotensin-converting enzyme inhibitors (ACEIs): ACEI and angiotensin receptor blockers (ARBs) are accepted forms of therapy in nonpregnant individuals with heart failure, but are contraindicated in pregnancy due to a number of reasons. There is a primary hyperreninism in pregnancy precluding their use. Furthermore, they may affect perfusion of specific organs, especially the uterus.[28] Mothers receiving ACEI during pregnancy have increased risk of neonatal renal failure in the fetus as well. Current data; however, allows for their safe use during breastfeeding.[29]

Beta-blockers: Beta-adrenergic blockade decreases the heart rate and allowing for greater diastolic filling. They are associated with improved mortality and morbidity in patients with systolic dysfunction <40%. The use of beta-blockers in women with hypertension has shown an increased propensity towards intrauterine growth restriction and increased perinatal mortality.[30] However, it still remains a relative contraindication and is recommended in conditions where the mother's life is at risk and both the maternal disease and its treatment can cause adverse perinatal outcome.

Spironolactone: Being a potassium-sparing aldosterone antagonist, it causes a mild diuresis and works synergistically with other diuretics, significantly reducing mortality in heart failure.[31] Its antiandrogen effects, and possible teratogenesis (in animal models), make it a relative contraindication in pregnancy. In the puerperium, treatment proceeds according to need of the. Use during breastfeeding is relatively safe.

Bromocriptine: This drug may play a role in peripartum cardiomyopathy by suppressing prolactin secretion, as the cathepsin-cleavage product of prolactin has apoptotic effects on the myocardium. However, data is limited and consensus is still lacking. A multicenter randomized study is currently underway for this very purpose.[32]

Treatment of Arrhythmias

The most common arrhythmia is usually atrial fibrillation treated with beta-blockers and/or digoxin. Sustained ventricular tachyarrhythmias need continuous monitoring and use of amiodarone and implantable cardioverter defibrillators.[33] Sudden cardiac death causes almost 50% of deaths associated with heart failure.

Assist Devices

There is limited data on assist devices as adjunct bridge therapy till cardiac transplantation and is directed by clinical assessment of such needs. Inotropic support is indicated in severely impaired ventricular function with persistent hypotension due to refractory heart failure. Randomized data is lacking regarding characterization of specific subsets.[33]

Supportive Measures

These include treatment of aggravating factors like anemia, infection, and hyperthyroidism (both subclinical and overt).[34] Urinary sepsis is often overlooked and needs to be recognized in good time. Regular monitoring of vital signs and maintenance of oxygenation is of paramount importance. Thromboprophylaxis with subcutaneous low molecular weight heparin as a daily dose of 40 mg of enoxaparin should be considered in all pregnant women.[35]

Obstetric Management

The obstetric management of decompensated heart failure should be a weighted risk between maternal risk in continuing pregnancy versus the consequence of preterm birth for the baby. Most cardiac causes are usually pretrialled with medical therapy before considering termination of the pregnancy. Pre-eclampsia; however, is always an indication for ending the pregnancy because of high fatality rate. Labor causes an increase in left ventricular workload, a sympathetic rise in pain-induced catecholamines and an acute increase in intravascular blood volume at the point of delivery. The second stage of labor is usually cut short by assisted methods such as vacuum extractor or forceps. Cesarean delivery itself is associated with risks of anesthesia and postoperative complications, apart from hemorrhage and the choice of vaginal or cesarean delivery must be individualized to each case with a close eye on other obstetric comorbidities and the severity of the cardiac lesion. There is absolutely no justification for routine cesarean delivery in heart failure during pregnancy, unless obstetrically indicated in the patient.[36]

The Puerperium and Long-term Management

Placental delivery leads to vigorous uterine contractions and expulsion of blood into the systemic circulation, leading to a fluid overload state. Stenosed valves and failing ventricles will benefit from diuretic therapy at this time. Oxytocic drugs used in the active management of the third stage of labor lead to vasodilatation and low doses are generally recommended whereas ergometrine preparations are vasoconstrictive and best avoided.[37] Prophylactic antibiotics are advised to limit the risk of endocarditis.[38] The presence of peripartum cardiomyopathy may preclude breastfeeding.

CONCLUSION

The presence of cardiac disease significantly increases the maternal morbidity and mortality. Heart failure may appear de novo in pregnancy or previously well-controlled diseases may worsen due to the hemodynamic changes. A low index of suspicion, along with adequate knowledge of precipitating factors, will help us improve diagnosis and management of heart failure in pregnancy.

REFERENCES

1. Say L, Chou D, Gemmill A, et al. Global causes of maternal death: a WHO systematic analysis. Lancet Glob Health. 2014;2:e323-33.
2. Knight M, Kenyon S, Brocklehurst P, et al. Saving Lives, Improving Mothers' Care—Lessons learned to inform

future maternity care from the UK and Ireland Confidential Enquiries into Maternal Deaths and Morbidity 2009-2012, Oxford, UK: Healthcare Quality Improvement Partnership; 2014.
3. Wilson M, Morganti AA, Zervoudakis I, et al. Blood pressure, the renin-aldosterone system and sex steroids throughout normal pregnancy. Am J Med. 1980;68(1):97-104.
4. Young P, Johanson R. Haemodynamic, invasive and echocardiographic monitoring in the hypertensive parturient. Best Pract Res Clin Obstet Gynaecol. 2001;15:605-22.
5. Belfort M, Anthony J, Kirshon B. Respiratory function in severe gestational proteinuric hypertension: the effects of rapid volume expansion and subsequent vasodilatation with verapamil. BJOG. 1991;98:964-72.
6. Seely EW, Ecker J. Chronic hypertension in pregnancy. N Engl J Med. 2011;365:439-46.
7. Lindheimer MD, Taler SJ, Cunningham FG. ASH position paper: hypertension in pregnancy. J Clin Hypertens (Greenwich). 2009;11:214-25.
8. Weiss BM, Zemp L, Seifert B, et al. Outcome of pulmonary vascular disease in pregnancy: a systematic overview from 1978 through 1996. J Am Coll Cardiol. 1998;31:1650-7.
9. Milewicz DM, Dietz HC, Miller DC. Treatment of aortic disease in patients with Marfan syndrome. Circulation. 2005;111:e150-7.
10. Sliwa K, Libhaber E, Elliott C, et al. Spectrum of cardiac disease in maternity in a low-resource cohort in South Africa. Heart. 2014;100:1967-74.
11. Hilfiker-Kleiner D, Sliwa K. Pathophysiology and epidemiology of peripartum cardiomyopathy. Nat Rev Cardiol. 2014;11:364-70.
12. Ansari AA, Fett JD, Carraway RE, et al. Autoimmune mechanisms as the basis for human peripartum cardiomyopathy. Clin Rev Allergy Immunol. 2002;23:301-24.
13. Patten IS, Rana S, Shahul S, et al. Cardiac angiogenic imbalance leads to peripartum cardiomyopathy. Nature. 2012;485:333-8.
14. Watkins H, Ashrafian H, Redwood C. Inherited cardiomyopathies. N Engl J Med. 2011;364:1643-56.
15. Autore C, Conte MR, Piccininno M, et al. Risk associated with pregnancy in hypertrophic cardiomyopathy. J Am Coll Cardiol. 2002;40:1864-9.
16. Basso C, Corrado D, Marcus FI, et al. Arrhythmogenic right ventricular cardiomyopathy. Lancet. 2009;373:1289-300.
17. Kallwellis-Opara A, Staudt A, Trimpert C, et al. Autoimmunological features in inflammatory cardiomyopathy. Clin Res Cardiol. 2007;96:469-80.
18. Moore J, Baldisseri MR. Amniotic fluid embolism. Crit Care Med. 2005;33:S279-85.
19. Roos-Hesselink JW, Ruys TP, Stein JI, et al. Outcome of pregnancy in patients with structural or ischaemic heart disease: results of a registry of the European Society of Cardiology. Eur Heart J. 2013;34:657-65.
20. Sliwa K, Johnson MR, Zilla P, et al. Management of valvular disease in pregnancy: a global perspective. Eur Heart J. 2015;36:1078-89.
21. Engelfriet P, Boersma E, Oechslin E, et al. The spectrum of adult congenital heart disease in Europe: morbidity and mortality in a 5-year follow-up period. Eur Heart J. 2005;26:2325-33.
22. Hytten F, Chamberlain G. Clinical Physiology in Obstetrics. Boston, MA: Blackwell Scientific Publications; 1980.
23. Nelson-Piercy C, Chakravarti S. Cardiac disease and pregnancy. Anaesthes Intensive Care. 2007;8:312-6.
24. Soubra SH, Guntupalli KK. Critical illness in pregnancy: an overview. Crit Care Med. 2005;33:S248-55.
25. terMaaten JM, Dunning AM, Valente MA, et al. Diuretic response in acute heart failure—an analysis from ASCEND-HF. Am Heart J. 2015;170:313-21.
26. Belfort M, Akovic K, Anthony J, et al. The effect of acute volume expansion and vasodilatation with verapamil on uterine and umbilical artery Doppler indices in severe preeclampsia. J Clin Ultrasound. 1994;22:317-25.
27. Clark SL, Greenspoon JS, Aldahl D, et al. Severe preeclampsia with persistent oliguria: management of hemodynamic subsets. Am J Obstet Gynecol. 1986;154:490-4.
28. Irani RA, Xia Y. The functional role of the renin–angiotensin system in pregnancy and preeclampsia. Placenta. 2008;29:763-71.
29. Shotan A, Widerhorn J, Hurst A, et al. Risks of angiotensin-converting enzyme inhibition during pregnancy: experimental and clinical evidence, potential mechanisms, and recommendations for use. Am J Med. 1994;96:451-6.
30. Swan L, Lupton M, Anthony J, et al. Controversies in pregnancy and congenital heart disease. Congenit Heart Dis. 2006;1:27-34.
31. Pitt B, Zannad F, Remme WJ, et al. The effect of spironolactone on morbidity and mortality in patients with severe heart failure. N Engl J Med. 1999;341:709-17.
32. Haghikia A, Podewski E, Berliner D, et al. Rationale and design of a randomized, controlled multicentre clinical trial to evaluate the effect of bromocriptine on left ventricular function in women with peripartum cardiomyopathy. Clin Res Cardiol. 2015;104:911-7.
33. Dickstein K, Cohen-Solal A, Filippatos G, et al. ESC Guidelines for the diagnosis and treatment of acute and chronic heart failure 2008. Eur J Heart Fail. 2008;10:933-89.
34. Learoyd DL, Fung HY, McGregor AM. Postpartum thyroid dysfunction. Thyroid. 1992;2:73-80.
35. Ageno W, Squizzato A, Garcia D, et al. Epidemiology and risk factors of venous thromboembolism. Semin Thromb Hemost. 2006;32:651-8.
36. European Society of Gynecology (ESG), Association for European Paediatric Cardiology (AEPC), German Society for Gender Medicine (DGesGM), et al. ESC Guidelines on the management of cardiovascular diseases during pregnancy: the Task Force on the Management of Cardiovascular Diseases during Pregnancy of the European Society of Cardiology (ESC). Eur Heart J. 2011;32:3147-97.
37. Bohlmann MK, Rath W. Medical prevention and treatment of postpartum hemorrhage: a comparison of different guidelines. Arch Gynecol Obstet. 2014;289:555-67.
38. Dayer MJ, Jones S, Prendergast B, et al. Incidence of infective endocarditis in England, 2000–13: a secular trend, interrupted time-series analysis. Lancet. 2015;385:1219-28.

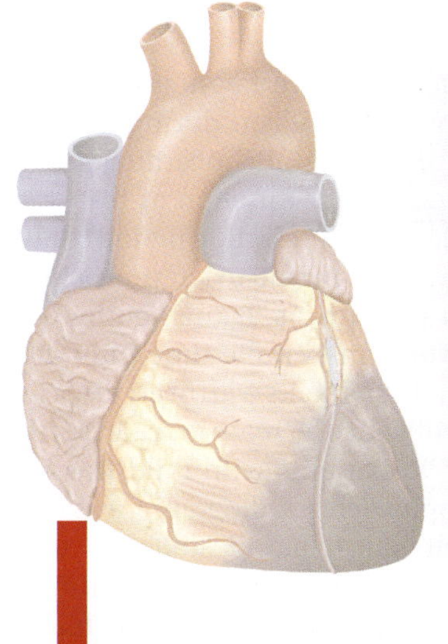

Hypothyroidism and Heart Failure

Vidyut Jain, Mayank Jain

INTRODUCTION

Hypothyroidism affects between 4% and 10% of the population, and the prevalence of subclinical hypothyroidism is reported to be as high as 10% in various studies.[1-3] The renewed interest in the role of the thyroid gland in heart failure (HF) is evident by changes in thyroid hormones (TH) in patients with chronic HF.[1] In addition, recent studies have demonstrated that a reduced serum T3 concentration has a strong predictive power for cardiovascular mortality in various categories of cardiac patients,[4] thus opening the prospect of additional approach for the treatment of HF based on thyroid hormone replacement.

REVIEW OF LITERATURE

The inclusion of thyroid hormone in the plethora of hormones already involved in the pathogenesis and treatment of HF further enhances the "systemic disease" characterization of HF. However, this should not come as a surprise when one remembers the numerous direct and indirect effects of TH on the cardiovascular system and the significant similarities that can be found between the hypothyroid phenotype and the HF phenotype.[5] In addition to the classical "cardiovascular side effects" of primary thyroid dysfunction, such as those on peripheral vascular resistance, heart rate, and myocardial contractility and relaxation, more recent research has identified novel cellular and molecular mechanisms by which thyroid hormone might exert its action in HF. These changes results into low level of serum T3 levels which affect both genomic and nongenomic mechanisms in the heart and in the vasculature in the setting of congestive HF.[6] In brief, these include erythropoietin synthesis,[7] endothelial nitric oxide synthesis,[8,9] protein kinase Akt pathway,[10] angiogenesis,[8] renin substrate synthesis in the liver,[11] and gene expression of natriuretic hormones.[12] Thus, TH interact with the other hormones involved in HF and disturb cardiac hemodynamics. This review attempts to highlight the effects of overt and subclinical hypothyroidism on the heart failure.

Cellular and Molecular Mechanisms Underlying the Effects of Thyroid Hormones on the Cardiovascular System

Thyroid hormones have a variety of effects on the cardiovascular system that can greatly impact cardiac function. Genomic effects of TH are mediated by TH nuclear receptors located in the intracellular compartment. The protein receptors bind T3 with greater (>10) affinity than T4.[13] Thyroid hormone plays important cardioprotective role through multiple pathways directly or indirectly by acting at the level of the myocytes, the interstitium, and the vasculature.[14] THs have an antiapoptotic effect on myocytes via activation of the phosphatidylinositol 3-kinase/serine/threonine protein kinase and protein kinase C signaling cascades, the expression, phosphorylation, and translocation of heat shock proteins 70 and 27, and the suppression of p38 mitogen-activated protein kinase signaling.[15] In addition, TH replacement reduces interstitial fibrosis in animal models of ischemic and nonischemic HF, and this effect can be up to some extent influence of TH on the activity of metalloproteinases and their inhibitors.[16] Furthermore, the antifibrotic effect of TH is also linked to the T3-induced inhibition of profibrotic pathways,[17] and is supported by the association of low serum T3 levels with the presence of cardiac fibrosis in patients with idiopathic dilated cardiomyopathy.[18] Hypothyroidism leads to decreased cardiac output due to impaired filling of ventricle on one hand and increased systemic vascular resistance on the other side. In addition, there is a decreased availability of vasodilating endothelial nitric oxide, thus increasing arterial stiffness. On a molecular level, these alterations result from reduced expression of sarcoplasmic reticulum Ca^{2+}-ATPase and increased expression of phospholamban, which inhibits ATPase. TH also impacts the renin-angiotensin-aldosterone system. Renin substrates are synthesized in the liver under the stimulus of T3. Thus, in a hypothyroid state, diastolic blood pressure increases, pulse pressure narrows, and renin levels decrease. This results in diastolic hypertension that is often sodium sensitive.[1] Erythropoietin secretion is increased by T3, which can explain the normochromic, normocytic anemia often found in hypothyroidism. Proposed theory also implicates that TH also regulate chronotropic genes through transcription as well as the beta-adrenergic system in cardiomyocytes. As a result of these mechanisms, heart rate decreases in hypothyroidism. Varied alterations in lipid parameters are noted in both overt and subclinical hypothyroidism, including elevated total cholesterol, low-density lipoprotein (LDL) cholesterol, and apolipoprotein B. A hypothyroid state results in decreased expression of hepatic LDL receptors and reduced activity of cholesterol-α-monooxygenase, which breaks down cholesterol, resulting in decreased LDL clearance.[14] Also noted are elevations in both C-reactive protein and homocysteine.[1,19] TH affect endothelial functions mediated by thyroid hormone receptor (THR)-α1 and THR-β. Activation of THR-α1 increases coronary blood flow, decreases coronary resistance in mouse models, and increases production of nitric oxide in endothelial and vascular smooth muscle cells. TH activation of THR-β induces angiogenesis by initiating the mitogen-activated protein kinase pathway.[14] Severe hypothyroidism can also cause pericardial effusion. Though the mechanism is unclear, increased capillary permeability and reduced lymphatic drainage from the pericardial space have been suggested.[14] Hypothyroidism can also be associated with a decrease in insulin sensitivity due to downregulation of glucose transporters and direct effects on insulin secretion and clearance.[20]

Cardiac Morphology and Function in Subclinical Hypothyroidism

Systolic and diastolic functions have been assessed in patients with subclinical hypothyroidism during the last 10–15 years by a variety of techniques. Echocardiographic studies showed that left ventricular function at rest was impaired, as indicated by a longer pre-ejection period (PEP) and increased ratio of pre-ejection period to left ventricular ejection time (PEP/ET) in patients as against euthyroid subjects.[21-23] These alterations in systolic time intervals were similar to those reported in patients with overt disease. Moreover, a mild (albeit significant) decrease in mean aortic acceleration was reported in patients with mild thyroid hormone deficiency.[24] Doppler echocardiography was first used in 1999 to evaluate left ventricular diastolic function in subjects with mild thyroid hormone deficiency.[24] Doppler-derived indices of left ventricular diastolic filling revealed abnormalities of myocardial relaxation. Impaired left ventricular diastolic function, characterized by slowed myocardial relaxation and impaired early ventricular filling, was the most consistent cardiac abnormality identified in young and middle-aged patients with Hashimoto thyroiditis and a mild but persistent increase in TSH compared to controls.[24] Isovolumic relaxation time (IRT) was significantly prolonged in all studies performed in patients with mild hypothyroidism.[21-25] Moreover, the ratio of early to late diastolic mitral flow velocity (E/A ratio) was significantly reduced, mainly because of an increased A wave.[23-25] Interestingly, diastolic function improved in all studies in which patients were evaluated after replacement therapy;[22-24] two such studies were double-blind placebo-controlled investigations.[22,23] Impaired left ventricular diastolic function at rest may be an important cause of systolic dysfunction on effort in patients with thyroid hormone deficiency.[26] The slowed rate of left ventricular relaxation could critically impair ventricular filling during exercise, leading to left ventricular systolic dysfunction. Impaired left ventricular systolic[27] and diastolic[28] function on effort were documented by Doppler echocardiography and cardiopulmonary exercise testing in patients with subclinical hypothyroidism compared with euthyroid controls. Moreover, systolic and diastolic function on effort improved after L-T4 replacement therapy in patients with subclinical hypothyroidism in studies performed with radionuclide ventriculography, Doppler echocardiography, and cardiopulmonary exercise testing.[27-30] Ultrasonic video densitometry was used to evaluate young and middle-aged patients affected by Hashimoto thyroiditis and subclinical hypothyroidism.[31] Video densitometric analysis revealed a lower cyclic variation index (CVI) in these patients than in controls at both the septum and posterior wall, resulting in an inverse relationship between CVI and the PEP/ET ratio.[31] Pulsed tissue Doppler imaging, which is minimally affected by alterations of afterload and heart rate, was used to provide, for the first time, information about myocardial systolic and diastolic properties in the various regional segments of the left ventricle, thereby permitting quantitative analysis of myocardial wall motion in subclinical hypothyroidism.[21] Tissue Doppler imaging analysis revealed that patients with mild hypothyroidism had similar changes in myocardial time intervals in several left ventricular segments as reported in overt disease.[21,25] Myocardial time intervals, evaluated as precontraction time (PTCm), the PTCm/myocardial contraction time ratio, and myocardial relaxation time (RTm), were prolonged at the level of both the posterior septum and the mitral annulus in patients with autoimmune subclinical hypothyroidism compared to controls.[21] More sophisticated techniques have recently been used to assess systolic and diastolic function in patients with subclinical hypothyroidism. Cardiac magnetic resonance imaging is currently the most accurate and reproducible noninvasive technique, providing an excellent evaluation of cardiac volumes and function. Cardiac volumes and systolic performance were significantly altered in patients with subclinical hypothyroidism. Moreover, preload (end-diastolic volume) was significantly decreased and afterload (systemic vascular resistance, SVR) significantly increased, leading to impaired cardiac performance in patients with mild thyroid failure.[32] The end-diastolic volume, stroke volume, ejection fraction, and cardiac index increased and SVR decreased after L-T4 therapy.[32] All these studies, performed in young and middle-aged subjects with mild thyroid hormone deficiency, support the hypothesis that long-term subclinical hypothyroidism can affect cardiac morphology and function, depressing systolic function at rest, inducing left ventricular diastolic dysfunction at rest and during exercise, and impairing left ventricular systolic function on exercise (Box 1).

BOX 1: Long-term cardiovascular consequences of persistent mild thyroid hormone deficiency.

- Cardiac morphology and function:
  - Depressed systolic function at rest
  - Left ventricular diastolic dysfunction at rest and during exercise
  - Impaired left ventricular systolic function on exercise
- Vascular abnormalities:
  - Increased systemic vascular resistance
  - Increased prevalence of diastolic hypertension
  - Increased arterial stiffness
  - Endothelial dysfunction
  - Increased carotid artery intima–media thickness

All the cardiovascular alterations reported in patients with subclinical hypothyroidism are similar to those observed in patients with overt hypothyroidism, suggesting that there is a continuum in the cardiac changes that occur through mild, subclinical disease into overt hypothyroidism.[33,34] Only one study was performed in elderly subjects (mean age 61 years) with a mean serum TSH level of 5.4 mIU/L.[35] In that study, using tissue Doppler imaging, subclinical hypothyroidism was not associated with significant differences in diastolic or systolic function compared with euthyroid controls. However, these elderly subjects were recruited from an epidemiological study and not from clinical practice;[36] thus, it is not possible to rule out that these patients were affected by transient subclinical hypothyroidism. Many patients with subclinical hypothyroidism are elderly, and the onset or progression of the disease in these vulnerable subjects may precipitate cardiac decompensation and promote congestive heart failure.[33] Only one study evaluated the risk of heart failure in patients with subclinical hypothyroidism and stratified the risk according to TSH levels (4.5–6.9, 7.0–9.9, and ≥ 10 mIU/L).[37] This study reported an increased risk of congestive heart failure among adults aged 70–79 years with a TSH level of 7.0 mIU/L or greater.[37]

Subclinical Hypothyroidism and the Risk of Heart Failure Events

Subclinical hypothyroidism (SHypo) seems to be associated with diastolic and systolic cardiac dysfunction, and thyroxine replacement improves cardiac function in patients with SHypo.[26] However, only a few studies have directly addressed the relationship between SHypo and HF. The Health, Aging, and Body Composition study is a population-based study of a cohort of elderly men and women (age 70–79) that began in 1997 in the areas surrounding Pittsburgh, Pennsylvania, and Memphis, Tennessee, USA. Among the 2,730 black and white adults who were followed for 4 years,[37] participants with a TSH level greater than 0.1 mU/L but less than 4.5 mU/L were considered euthyroid. Free T4 was measured in all participants with a TSH level of 7.0 mU/L or greater. Hypothyroidism was further classified according to TSH levels: Mild elevation (4.5–6.9 mU/L), moderate elevation (7.0–9.9 mU/L), and marked elevation (10.0 mU/L or greater). Participants with overt thyroid disease under amiodarone or thyroid hormone therapy were excluded. Rodondi et al. found that participants with a TSH of 7.0 mU/L or greater had a higher rate of HF events than euthyroid subjects (35.0 vs. 16.5/1,000 person-years, p = 0.006.[37] In multivariate analysis, including adjustment for prevalent cardiovascular disease and HF, the risk of HF was about three times as high among those with high TSH levels.

In those with a TSH level of 7.0–9.9 mU/L, the hazard ratio (HR) was 2.58 (95% CI 1.19–5.60), and it was 3.26 (95% CI 1.37–7.77) for those with a TSH of 10.0 mU/L or greater. After exclusion of 175 participants with prevalent HF, there were 127 who had incident HF events. The adjusted HR for incident HF events was 2.33 (95% CI 1.10–4.96; $p = 0.03$) in those with a TSH level of 7.0 mU/L or greater. Among the participants with prevalent HF, 51 had recurrent HF events; the adjusted HR was 7.62 (95% CI 2.25–25.77; $p = 0.001$) in those with a TSH level of 7.0 mU/L or greater. Results were similar after excluding thyroid hormone users, and there was no interaction with race or sex ($p > 0.20$ for each interaction). However, these results were limited by the lack of routine echocardiography, which limited the identification of HF and the type of cardiac dysfunction involved. This issue was also examined among 3,065 adults over 65 years of age in the Cardiovascular Health Study, who underwent echocardiography at baseline and at follow-up.[38] The definition of SHypo was the same as in the study described above. The authors compared adjudicated incident HF events over 12 years of follow-up and changes in cardiac function over 6 years between participants with SHypo, SHyper, and euthyroidism. They found a greater incidence of HF events among participants with a TSH level above 10 mU/L than among euthyroid participants (45.2 vs. 22.2/100 person-years, $p = 0.003$), but not among those with TSH between 4.5 and 9.9 mU/L or among those with SHyper. Compared to euthyroid participants, most baseline echocardiographic parameters did not differ by thyroid status; participants with TSH of 10.0 mU/L or greater had a higher peak E velocity (0.80 vs. 0.72 m/s, $p = 0.002$), and this difference persisted after adjustment for age, gender, heart rate, and systolic blood pressure. Peak E velocity, a sign of decreased left ventricular compliance, was associated with incident HF in the overall study sample (HR 1.14 for each 0.1 m/s increment, 95% CI 1.09–1.18, $p < 0.001$) and in those with TSH of 10.0 mU/L or greater (HR 1.45, 95% CI 1.20–1.76, $p < 0.001$) after adjustment for age, gender, and systolic blood pressure. Over 5 years, most changes in echocardiographic parameters did not significantly differ by thyroid status, except that participants with TSH of 10.0 mU/L or greater had a larger increase in left ventricular mass (+21 vs. +4 g, $p = 0.04$) and a greater proportion of HF events associated with low ejection fraction than did euthyroid participants (80% vs. 45%, $p = 0.08$). Two small cross-sectional studies also evaluated the association between TH and HF. One small cross-sectional study found that 8 of 31 patients (26%) with HF had a TSH level greater than 3.6 mU/L, with normal T4 levels.[39] Fruhwald et al. found either functional or morphological thyroid disorder in 59 of 61 patients with invasively diagnosed idiopathic dilated cardiomyopathy.[40] However, neither study was prospective or included a control group without HF. In conclusion, SHypo is associated with a moderately elevated risk of HF among older adults with a TSH greater than 10 mU/L. This issue has not been examined in cohorts of younger adults. To date, there is no evidence that SHyper is associated with clinical HF events, but only one study has examined this issue.[38]

Impact of Hypothyroidism on Heart Failure

In hypothyroid state, cardiovascular effects are opposite of hyperthyroidism and cardiac output falls by 30–50%.[41] Hypothyroidism is often associated with bradycardia, low pulse pressure, cold intolerance, increased diastolic blood pressure, and fatigue. Structural and functional changes in cardiovascular system have been reported in patients with hypothyroidism, with a severity that depends on the degree and duration of exposure to hypothyroid state.[1,28,32,33,42–44] Overt hypothyroidism is seen in about 3% of the adult female population. Overt and subclinical hypothyroidism results in an increased SVR with a reduced cardiac output, bradyarrhythmias, a higher prevalence of hypertension, imbalance in cardiac natriuretic hormone, changes in lipid profile, accelerated atherosclerosis, damage of the physical and intellectual capacities, and an impaired quality of life. Hypothyroidism is a risk factor of HF in the general population. Acute hypothyroidism and HF, often simulates as there is decreased cardiac output; decreased cardiac contractility and an altered gene expression profile (alteration in myosin heavy chain isoform expression and alterations in the activity of the sarcoplasmic reticulum Ca^{2+} pump that are induced by its interactions with phospholamban, a reversible inhibitor). In most cases, these changes are the result of reduced T3 level (<3.1 pmol/L), the physiological T3 therapy improving cardiac function. A systematic review and meta-analysis to clarify the association of hypothyroidism and all-cause mortality, as well as cardiac death and/or hospitalization in patients with HF, was conducted by Ning et al.[45] They included 13 articles that reported relative risks estimates and 95% confidence intervals for hypothyroidism with outcomes in patients with HF. It was also observed that hypothyroidism also leads to increased all-cause mortality as well as cardiac death and/or hospitalization in patients with HF. Overt hypothyroidism is usually associated with grade I diastolic dysfunction, but grade II diastolic dysfunction, called "pseudonormal filling dynamics", can also be found.[46] There are also data showing that hypothyroidism results in an increased AF susceptibility (HR = 1.23; 95% CI: 0.77–1.97),[47] quite similar to hyperthyroidism, but affecting other atrial electrophysiological parameters than hyperthyroidism.

Hypothyroidism also significantly alters ionic channel expression and function, thus decreasing heart rate, and prolonging sinus node recovery time and atrial ERP. In hypothyroid patients, increased atrial interstitial collagen and fibrosis may lead to longer atrial ERP and lead to increased conduction heterogeneity, thus favoring reentry formation and AF vulnerability. On the other hand, ion channel remodeling and dispersion may enhance AF arrhythmogenesis.

CONCLUSION

Heart failure in hypothyroidism is fairly common. Timely recognition is proved to be of great value in management of heart failure. L-T4 replacement therapy reduces myocyte apoptosis and is able to improve cardiovascular performance and ventricular remodeling in hypothyroidism.[48,49] It is noteworthy to recognize that normal cardiovascular hemodynamic restoration can take place without a significant increase in resting heart rate in the treatment of hypothyroidism. Treatment and management of subclinical and overt hypothyroidism should be tailored to each patient. L-T4 dose varies according to age, weight, severity, and duration of hypothyroidism and cardiac condition of the patient. Treatment of subclinical and overt hypothyroidism with appropriate doses of L-T4 is associated with benefits in restoring of normal TSH values (after 6–12 months of substitution therapy). In hypothyroidism, systolic and diastolic functions (left ventricular predominantly) are affected. For patients with systolic and diastolic HF and in the elderly (>70 years), a small dose of L-T4 should be started, 25 or 50 µg daily. The dose of L-T4 should be increased by 25 µg/day every 3–4 weeks until a full replacement dosage is reached. This treatment should be individualized and permanently monitored, the aim being to reach a stable serum TSH around 1–5 mIU/L. One needs to be careful in treating very elderly hypothyroid patients (>80–85 years) with elevated serum up to TSH ≤10 mIU/L in whom avoiding hormonal treatment unless they are very symptomatic.[20]

REFERENCES

1. Klein I, Danzi S. Thyroid disease and the heart. Circulation. 2007;116(15):1725-35.
2. Ochs N, Auer R, Bauer DC, et al. Meta-analysis: subclinical thyroid dysfunction and the risk for coronary heart disease and mortality. Ann Intern Med. 2008;148(11):832-45.
3. Razvi S, Shakoor A, Vanderpump M, et al. The influence of age on the relationship between subclinical hypothyroidism and ischemic heart disease: a meta-analysis. J Clin Endocrinol Metab. 2008;93(8):2998-3007.
4. Pingitore A, Landi P, Taddei MC, et al. Triiodothyronine levels for risk stratification of patients with chronic heart failure. Am J Med. 2005;118(2):132-6.
5. Lowes BD, Minobe W, Abraham WT, et al. Changes in gene expression in the intact human heart. Downregulation of alpha-myosin heavy chain in hypertrophied, failing ventricular myocardium. J Clin Invest. 1997;100(9):2315-24.
6. Davis PJ, Davis FB. Nongenomic actions of thyroid hormone on the heart. Thyroid. 2002;12:459-66.
7. Fish SA, Mandel SJ. The blood in thyrotoxicosis. In: Bravermann L, Utiger R (Eds) Werner and Ingbar's The Thyroid. Philadelphia: Lippincott Williams and Wilkins; 2005. pp. 595-98.
8. Vargas F, Moreno JM, Rodríguez-Gómez I, et al. Vascular and renal function in experimental thyroid disorders. Eur J Endocrinol. 2006;154(2):197-212.
9. Napoli R, Biondi B, Guardasole V, et al. Impact of hyperthyroidism and its correction on vascular reactivity in humans. Circulation. 2001;104(25):3076-80.
10. Kuzman JA, Gerdes AM, Kobayashi S, et al. Thyroid hormone activates Akt and prevents serum starvation induced cell death in neonatal rat cardiomyocytes. J Mol Cell Cardiol. 2005;39(5):841-4.
11. Laragh JH, Sealey JE. Relevance of the plasma renin hormonal control system that regulates blood pressure and sodium balance for correctly treating hypertension and for evaluating ALLHAT. Am J Hypertens. 2003;16(5 Pt 1):407-15.
12. Lewicki JA, Protter AA. Physiological studies of the natriuretic peptide family. In: Laragh JH, Brenner BM (Eds). Hypertension: pathophysiology, diagnosis and management. New York: Raven Press; 1995. 1029-53.
13. Sandler B, Webb P, Apriletti JW, et al. Thyroxine-thyroid hormone receptor interactions. J Biol Chem. 2004;279(53):55801-8.
14. Jabbar A, Pingitore A, Pearce SH, et al. Thyroid hormones and cardiovascular disease. Nat Rev Cardiol. 2017;14(1):39-55.
15. Pantos C, Mourouzis I, Saranteas T, et al. Thyroid hormone improves post ischaemic recovery of function while limiting apoptosis: a new therapeutic approach to support hemodynamics in the setting of ischaemia-reperfusion? Basic Res Cardiol. 2009;104(1):69-77.
16. Kinugawa K, Jeong MY, Bristow MR, et al. Thyroid hormone induces cardiac myocyte hypertrophy in a thyroid hormone receptor a1-specific manner that requires TAK1 and p38 mitogen activated protein kinase. Mol Endocrinol. 2005;19(6):1618-28.
17. van Rooij E, Quiat D, Johnson BA, et al. A family of microRNAs encoded by myosin genes governs myosin expression and muscle performance. Dev Cell. 2009;17(5):662-73.
18. Wang W, Guan H, Fang W, et al. Free triiodothyronine level correlates with myocardial injury and prognosis in idiopathic dilated cardiomyopathy: evidence from cardiac MRI and SPECT/PET imaging. Sci Rep. 2016;6:39811.
19. Vargas-Uricoechea H, Bonelo-Perdomo A, Sierra-Torres CH. Effects of thyroid hormones on the heart. Clin Investig Arterioscler. 2014;26(6):296-309.

20. Pearce SH, Brabant G, Duntas L, et al. 2013 ETA Guideline: Management of subclinical hypothyroidism. Eur Thyroid J. 2013;2(4):215-28.
21. Vitale G, Galderisi M, Lupoli GA, et al. Left ventricular myocardial impairment in subclinical hypothyroidism assessed by a new ultrasound tool: pulsed tissue Doppler. J Clin Endocrinol Metab. 2002;87(9):4350-5.
22. Monzani F, Di Bello V, Caraccio N, et al. Effect of levothyroxine on cardiac function and structure in subclinical hypothyroidism: a double blind, placebo-controlled study. J Clin Endocrinol Metab. 2001;86(3):1110-5.
23. Yazici M, Gorgulu S, Sertbas Y, et al. Effects of thyroxin therapy on cardiac function in patients with subclinical hypothyroidism: index of myocardial performance in the evaluation of left ventricular function. Int J Cardiol. 2004;95(2-3):135-43.
24. Biondi B, Fazio S, Palmieri EA, et al. Left ventricular diastolic dysfunction in patients with subclinical hypothyroidism. J Clin Endocrinol Metab. 1999;84(6):2064-7.
25. Aghini-Lombardi F, Di Bello V, Talini E, et al. Early textural and functional alterations of left ventricular myocardium in mild hypothyroidism. Eur J Endocrinol. 2006;155(1):3-9.
26. Biondi B, Palmieri EA, Lombardi G, et al. Effects of subclinical thyroid dysfunction on the heart. Ann Intern Med. 2002;137(11):904-14.
27. Kahaly GJ. Cardiovascular and atherogenic aspects of subclinical hypothyroidism. Thyroid. 2000;10(8):665-79.
28. Brenta G, Mutti LA, Schnitman M, et al. Assessment of left ventricular diastolic function by radionuclide ventriculography at rest and exercise in subclinical hypothyroidism, and its response to L-thyroxine therapy. Am J Cardiol. 2003;91(11):1327-30.
29. Bell GM, Todd WT, Forfar JC, et al. End-organ responses to thyroxine therapy in subclinical hypothyroidism. Clin Endocrinol. 1985;22(1):83-9.
30. Forfar JC, Wathen CG, Todd WT, et al. Left ventricular performance in subclinical hypothyroidism. Q J Med. 1985;57(224):857-65.
31. Di Bello V, Monzani F, Giorgi D, et al. Ultrasonic myocardial textural analysis in subclinical hypothyroidism. J Am Soc Echocardiogr. 2000;13(9):832-40.
32. Ripoli A, Pingitore A, Favilli B, et al. Does subclinical hypothyroidism affect cardiac pump performance? Evidence from a magnetic resonance imaging study. J Am Coll Cardiol. 2005;45(3):439-45.
33. Biondi B, Klein I, Hypothyroidism as a risk factor for cardiovascular disease. Endocrine. 2004;24(1):1-13.
34. Galderisi M, Vitale G, D'Errico A, et al. Usefulness of pulsed tissue Doppler for the assessment of left ventricular myocardial function in overt hypothyroidism. Ital Heart J. 2004;5(4):257-64.
35. Iqbal A, Schirmer H, Lunde P, et al. Thyroid stimulating hormone and left ventricular function. J Clin Endocrinol Metab. 2007;92(9):3504-10.
36. Cappola AR. Subclinical thyroid dysfunction and the heart. J Clin Endocrinol Metab. 2007;92:3404-5.
37. Rodondi N, Newman AB, Vittinghoff E, et al. Subclinical hypothyroidism and the risk of heart failure, other cardiovascular events, and death. Arch Intern Med. 2005;165(21):2460-6.
38. Rodondi N, Bauer D, Cappola A, et al. Subclinical thyroid dysfunction, cardiac function and the risk of heart failure: The Cardiovascular Health Study. J Am Coll Cardiol. 2008;52(14):1152-9.
39. Manowitz NR, Mayor GH, Klepper MJ, et al. Subclinical hypothyroidism and euthyroid sick syndrome in patients with moderate-to-severe congestive heart failure. Am J Ther. 1996;3(12):797-801.
40. Fruhwald FM, Ramschak-Schwarzer S, Pichler B, et al. Subclinical thyroid disorders in patients with dilated cardiomyopathy. Cardiology. 1997;88(2):156-9.
41. Danzi S, Klein I. Thyroid hormone and the cardiovascular system. Minerva Endocrinol. 2004;29(3):139-50.
42. Biondi B, Palmieri EA, Lombardi G, et al. Subclinical hypothyroidism and cardiac function. Thyroid. 2002;12(6):505-10.
43. Biondi B. Cardiovascular effects of mild hypothyroidism. Thyroid. 2007;17(7):625-30.
44. Chaker L, Baumgartner C, den Elzen WP, et al. Thyroid studies collaboration. Subclinical hypothyroidism and the risk of stroke events and fatal stroke: An individual participant data analysis. J Clin Endocrinol Metab. 2015;100(6):2181-91.
45. Ning N, Gao D, Triggiani V, et al. Prognostic role of hypothyroidism in heart failure: a meta-analysis. Medicine (Baltimore). 2015;94(30):e1159.
46. Tiryakioglu SK, Tiryakioglu O, Ari H, et al. Left ventricular longitudinal myocardial function in overt hypothyroidism: a tissue Doppler echocardiographic study. Echocardiography. 2010;27(5):505-11.
47. Kirchhof P, Benussi S, Kotecha D, et al. ESC Scientific Document Group.. 2016 ESC Guidelines for the management of atrial fibrillation developed in collaboration with EACTS. Eur Heart J. 2016;37(38):2893-962.
48. Cooper DS, Biondi B. Subclinical thyroid disease. Lancet. 2012;379(9821):1142-54.
49. Ravzi S, Ingoe L, Keeka G, et al. The beneficial effect of Lthyroxine on cardiovascular risk factors, endothelial function and quality of life in subclinical hypothyroidism: randomized, crossover trial. J Clin Endocrinol Metab. 2007;92(5):1715-23.

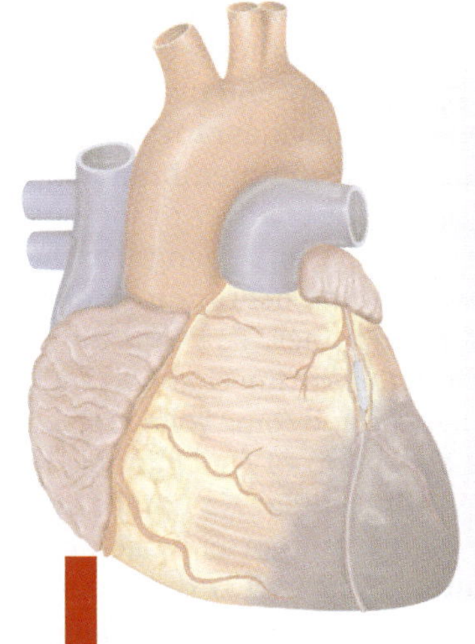

Hyperthyroidism and Heart Failure

Jabir A, Musna PJ, Jimmy George

INTRODUCTION

Heart failure is a major health problem representing a substantial number of emergency department presentations and admissions and is a leading cause of hospitalization globally.[1] Approximately 26 million people worldwide are living with heart failure.[2] Thyroid disease is quite common and perhaps after diabetes mellitus, it is the most common endocrine disorder which affects the cardiovascular system. It is present in 5–10% of the population. In the younger age group, thyroid dysfunction affects more of adult female to the tune of 9–15% of the population and smaller percentage of adult males. The incidence of thyroid dysfunction in males catches up with the females as the age advances. It is estimated that and some of the most characteristic signs and symptoms of thyroid disorders are result from the effects of thyroid hormone on cardiovascular system.[3-5] There is an intimate relationship between the heart and thyroid gland linked by their embryological relationship. Both hyperthyroidism and hypothyroidism produce changes in cardiac contractility, myocardial oxygen consumption, cardiac output, blood pressure, and systemic vascular resistance (SVR) and may induce arrhythmias.[6,7] These cardiovascular changes are almost always reversible with the achievement of euthyroid status.

PHYSIOLOGY OF THYROID HORMONE AND ITS EFFECT ON CARDIOVASCULAR SYSTEM

The thyroid gland produces two hormones, (1) thyroxine (T4) and (2) triiodothyronine (T3). T4 and T3 are synthesized by the thyroid gland in response to thyroid-stimulating hormone (TSH). The major form of thyroid hormone is thyroxine (85%), which acts mostly as a prohormone. Most of T4 is converted to biologically active T3 through the removal of an iodide by 5-monodeiodination in the liver, kidney, and skeletal muscle.[8,9] T3 is the biologically active hormone and it accounts for most of the biologic effects, including stimulation of tissue thermogenesis, alterations in the expression of various cellular proteins, and actions on the heart and vascular smooth muscle cells. Thyroid gland secretion is predominantly T4 and it secretes only less than 20% of circulating T3. The major part of circulating T3 is produced by conversion of T4 to T3 utilizing the deiodinase enzyme in the extrathyroidal tissue. There is no significant intracellular deiodinase activity in cardiac cells; therefore, in the heart, T3 hormone which is transported into the myocyte acts directly.[10] Both T4 and T3 circulate in the blood almost entirely (>95%) protein bound. The remaining unbound T3 is transported through a variety of membrane transport proteins to the cell nucleus to regulate expression of selected genes.[11] Thyroid hormones have a broad range of effect on cardiovascular system, particularly on the heart. They have direct genomic actions on cardiomyocytes by binding to nuclear receptors as well as extranuclear nongenomic actions on the ion channels in the cardiomyocyte cell membrane. The T3 and T4 have also effects on the peripheral circulation.[12]

Thyroid hormone upregulates expression of the sarcoplasmic reticulum calcium-activated ATPase (SERCA) and downregulates phospholamban expression, thereby enhancing myocardial relaxation. SERCA is an important ion channel that regulates myocyte calcium cycling. Reuptake of calcium into the sarcoplasmic reticulum early in diastole in part determines the rate at which the left ventricle relaxes (isovolumic relaxation time). The polymeric protein phospholamban regulates the activity of SERCA. Inotropic agents that enhance cardiac contractility through increases in myocyte cyclic adenosine monophosphate (cAMP) act by stimulating the phosphorylation of phospholamban. Thyroid hormone enhances phosphorylation of phospholamban, and even milder degree of hypothyroidism can contribute to diastolic dysfunction and heart failure.[13-15] They also increase expression of the more rapid contractile isoforms of the myosin heavy chain (α isoforms), which contributes to enhanced systolic function (Table 1).[16]

TABLE 1: Effect of thyroid hormone on cardiac gene expression.[16-18]

Positively regulated	*Negatively regulated*
α-myosin heavy chain	β-myosin heavy chain
Sarcoplasmic reticulum Ca2_-ATPase	Phospholamban
Na_/K_-ATPase	Adenylyl cyclase catalytic subunits
β1-Adrenergic receptor	Thyroid hormone receptor _1
Atrial natriuretic hormone	Na_/Ca2_ exchanger
Voltage-gated potassium channels (Kv1.5, Kv4.2, and Kv4.3)	

Since thyroid hormone-regulated genes are involved in structural and regulatory proteins, long-term exposure to high T3 levels can increase the synthesis of cardiac proteins, leading to cardiac hypertrophy and dysfunction. However, extranuclear nongenomic activities provoke rapid changes in the cardiac myocyte plasma membrane and cytoplasmic organelles. These include changes in sodium, potassium, and calcium ion channels; and changes to the intracellular signaling pathways in the heart and smooth muscle cells. On the plasma membranes, T3 exerts direct extragenomic actions on the functions of ion channels such as Na/K ATPase, Na/Ca^{++} exchanger, and some voltage gated K channels. It prolongs the activation of Na channels in myocardial cells and induces intracellular Na uptake and secondary activation of the Na-Ca antiporter, which can partly explain the positive inotropic effect.[19] T3 exerts a direct effect on L-type calcium channels, resulting in abbreviation of action potential duration. The strong inotropic activity of thyroid hormones is also demonstrated to be due to an increased number of β-adrenergic receptors.[20] However, a carefully controlled study of subhuman primates found no increase in sensitivity of the heart or cardiovascular system to catecholamines in experimental hyperthyroidism.[21] The heart rate increases due to increased sinoatrial activity (direct action), lower threshold for atrial activity, and shortened atrial repolarization (Fig. 1).[22,23]

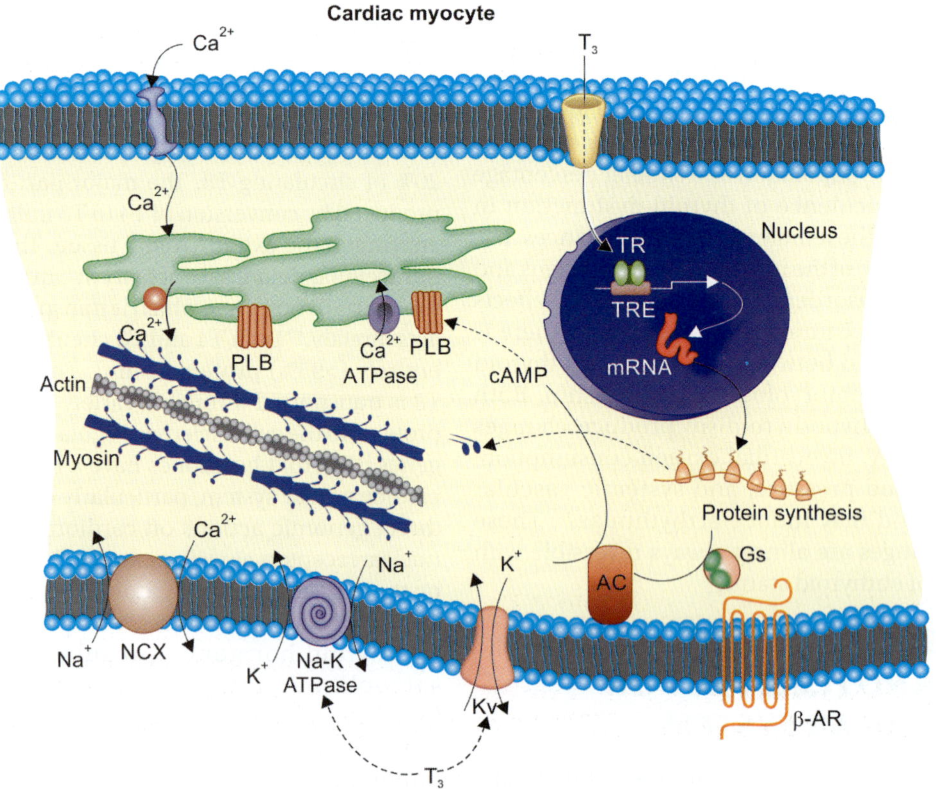

Fig. 1: Effects of thyroid hormone on cardiac myocytes.[24]

HEMODYNAMIC EFFECTS OF THYROID HORMONES

Hemodynamic effects of thyroid hormones are nongenomic and faster. In the peripheral vascular system, increased metabolic demand with increased oxygen utilization, increased production of metabolic end products, and relaxation of arterial smooth muscle fibers by thyroid hormone cause significant vasodilatation.[25] This fall in SVR plays the central role in all hemodynamic changes.[26] Decreased SVR causes an increase in heart rate. Selective increase in blood flow to skin, skeletal muscles and heart, leads to a fall in diastolic pressure and widening of pulse pressure. Vasodilatation causes reduction in renal perfusion and activation of the renin-angiotensin system that causes sodium retention and increased blood volume.[27] Thyroid hormones regulate erythropoietin secretion and increased red cell mass, may also contribute to increase in blood volume.[24] Improved diastolic relaxation and increased blood volume increased left ventricular end-diastolic volume (LVEDV). Reduced SVR and increased LVEDV means increased preload and decreased after load; thus the stroke volume increases. Increased stroke volume and increased heart rate lead to doubling or tripling of cardiac output, which cannot be explained by an increased metabolic rate alone. However, the pulmonary vascular resistance does not fall and because of the greater output to the pulmonary circulation, the pulmonary artery pressure increases. This leads to a rise in mean venous pressure, hepatic congestion, and peripheral edema associated with right-sided heart failure.[28]Administration of arterial vasoconstrictors decreased the peripheral blood flow and cardiac output by 34% in patients with hyperthyroidism but not in normal subjects.[29,30]

Together with hemodynamic changes, and increased contractility due to increased metabolic demand and the direct effect of the thyroid hormone on heart muscle, there is a dramatic increase in cardiac output.[31,32] In hyperthyroidism, these combined effects increase cardiac output 50–300% higher than in normal individuals.[3-8] In hypothyroidism, the cardiovascular effects are diametrically opposite and cardiac output may decrease by 30–50%. Local iodothyronine deiodinase upregulation may also be involved in cardiac remodeling via activation of thyroid hormone signaling pathways involving Akt and p38 mitogen-activated protein kinase (MAPK) in thyrotoxic-dilated cardiomyopathy.[33] Preclinical studies in which Akt was blocked by an angiotensin-II type 2 receptor blocker showed that this blockage might prevent thyroxine-mediated cardiac hypertrophy. Hypertrophied myocytes may be susceptible to apoptotic stimulation by angiotensin II in hyperthyroidism.[34]

In hyperthyroidism, SVR decreases, and blood volume and perfusion in peripheral tissues increase. The observation that hyperthyroidism is associated with increased vascularity suggests that T3 may increase capillary density via increased angiogenesis.[35] Hyperthyroidism has been documented as a secondary cause of isolated systolic hypertension. A widened pulse pressure is characteristic of hyperthyroidism. Recent reports have shown that arterial stiffness is increased in hyperthyroidism despite the low SVR.[36] Thus excess thyroid hormone typically causes systolic blood pressure to rise, and the increase can be quite dramatic in older patients with impaired arterial compliance as a result of atherosclerotic disease.[37] In hypothyroidism, endothelial dysfunction and impaired VSM relaxation vasodilatation as a result of a reduction in nitric oxide availability lead to reduced arterial compliance, which leads to increased SVR.[38]These effects lead to diastolic hypertension in around 30% of patients, and thyroid hormone replacement therapy restores endothelial-derived vasorelaxation and blood pressure to normal in most.

Thyroid Disease and Pulmonary Hypertension

Approximately 20% of patients with pulmonary hypertension have thyroid disease as a comorbidity, which is more frequent than the general population,[39] but primarily with hyperthyroidism. It has been suggested that the effect of thyroid hormone to decrease SVR may not occur in the pulmonary vasculature. Higher pressure in the left atrium increases pressure in the pulmonary veins, which stimulates baroreceptors and causes a reflex contraction in the arterioles, ultimately leading to increased pulmonary resistance and pulmonary artery hypertension. The resulting increase in pulmonary artery pressure increases the load on the right ventricle. Several case reports have documented that hyperthyroidism may present as right heart failure and tricuspid regurgitation which normalizes with treatment of hyperthyroidism (Fig. 2).[40-43]

Hyperthyroidism and Heart

Hyperthyroidism affects 2–5% of the population[44,45] and mortality is increased by 20% and the major causes of death are cardiac.[46] The major etiologies of thyrotoxicosis are hyperthyroidism caused by Graves' disease, toxic multinodular goiter (MNG), and toxic adenomas. Meanwhile, the cause of hyperthyroidism may also change the cardiovascular risk; patients with toxic multinodular

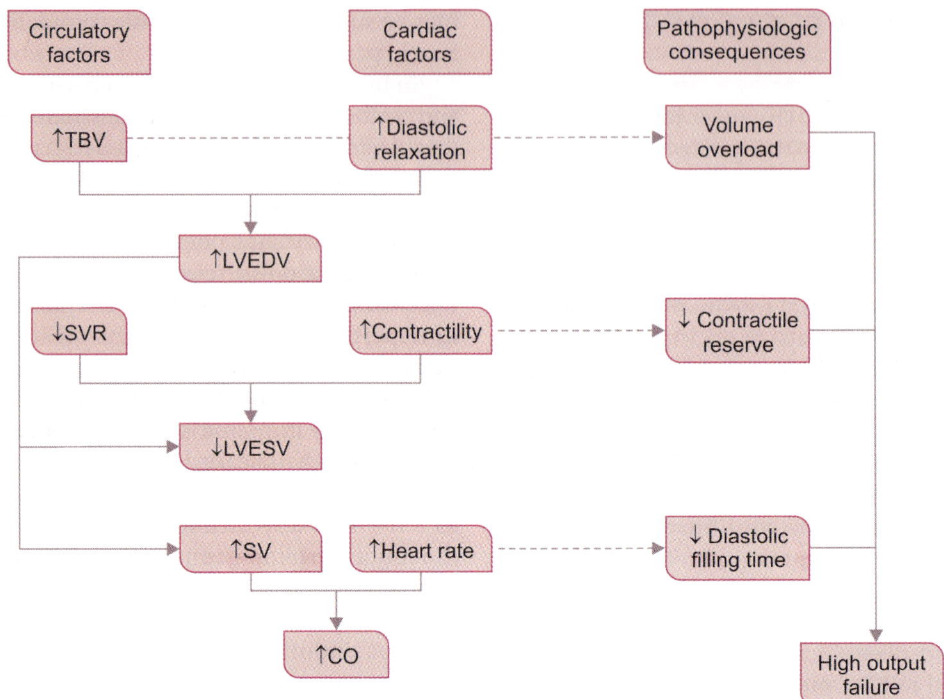

Fig 2: Effects of thyroid hormone on cardiovascular hemodynamics.[43]
(LVEDV: left ventricular end-diastolic volume; LVESV: left ventricular end-systolic volume;SVR: systemic vascular resistance; TBV: total blood volume)

goiter have higher cardiovascular risk than patients with Graves' disease, probably because of older age, and patients with Graves' disease may have autoimmune complications, such as valvular involvement, cardiomyopathy and pulmonary arterial hypertension (PAH).[47]

HYPERTHYROIDISM AND HEART FAILURE

Most patients with hyperthyroidism complain of palpitations and breathlessness on exertion, although symptoms such as weight loss in the presence of a normal or increased appetite, heat intolerance, and irritability tend to predominate. Characteristically there is a sinus tachycardia with high volume and often collapsing pulse, and a wide pulse pressure. The apex beat is forceful, flow murmurs are common. Mild ankle edema is common but is rarely caused by cardiac failure and usually a manifestation of the reduced of urinary sodium excretion by the kidneys (Table 2).[24]

Overt cardiac failure is uncommon in hyperthyroidism and usually occurs in the context of rapid atrial fibrillation (AF) in older patient with preexisting ischemic or valvular heart disease. Most of the hyperthyroid patients experience exercise intolerance and exertional dyspnea, in part because of weakness in the skeletal and respiratory muscle, however, it is mainly due to the inability to increase heart rate or lower vascular resistance further, as normally occurs in exercise.[48,3]

TABLE 3: Cardiovascular manifestations of hyperthyroidism.

Palpitations	Systolic hypertension
Exercise intolerance	Atrial fibrillation
Exertional dyspnea	Cardiac hypertrophy
Anginal chest pain	Hyperdynamic precordium
Peripheral edema	Congestive heart failure

Hyperthyroidism is characterized by a high left ventricular ejection fraction (LVEF) at rest and there is failure of LVEF to increase further on exercise. The heart in hyperthyroidism is performing at its peak capacity and further increase in cardiac function in response to increased demand is still possible. Hence, the term "high output heart failure" has not been used now, because the heart is still able to increase cardiac output at rest and with exercise to an extent. In the setting of low SVR and decreased preload, cardiac functional reserve is maximally utilized and cannot rise further to accommodate the demands of maximal exercise. This loss of cardiac functional reserve which contributes to the effort intolerance.[3,49] The exercise intolerance also appears to result from associated pulmonary hypertension as the pulmonary vascular resistance does not fall and the greater output to the pulmonary circulation, causes an increase in pulmonary artery pressure.[28]

About 6% of thyrotoxic patients develop heart failure and less than 1% develops dilated cardiomyopathy with impaired left ventricular systolic dysfunction, due to a tachycardia-mediated mechanism leading to an increased level of cytosolic calcium during diastole with reduced contractility of the ventricle and diastolic dysfunction.[50] More specifically, thyrotoxic cardiomyopathy is defined as myocardial damage caused by toxic effects of excessive thyroid hormone, resulting in altered myocyte energy production, intracellular metabolism, and myofibril contractile function. In the recent study of Yue et al., diastolic dysfunction was more prominent in thyrotoxic patients older than 40 years of age, whereas in younger ones a marked reduction in peripheral vascular resistance and increased cardiac output were prominent. Main manifestations are left ventricular hypertrophy, heart rhythm disturbances, primary AF, dilation of the heart chambers, heart failure, PAH, and diastolic dysfunction.[51]

In a group of patients with severe and chronic hyperthyroidism, sinus tachycardia or AF can produce tachycardiomyopathy and heart failure. This explains the subset of patients with hyperthyroidism, low cardiac output, and impaired left ventricular function, who are in AF at the time of diagnosis.[3] Preexistent ischemic or hypertensive heart disease may also predispose the hyperthyroid patient to the development of heart failure.[6] Both Graves' and Hashimoto's diseases are reported to be associated with an increased prevalence of mitral valve prolapse and it will predispose to left atrial enlargement and AF.[52] Among people >60 years of age, subclinical hyperthyroidism is associated with increased risk for AF, which in turn could lead to congestive heart failure.[53,54]

Atrial Fibrillation in Hyperthyroidism

The most common rhythm disturbance in hyperthyroidism is resting sinus tachycardia. However, the most common arrhythmia is AF and prevalence of AF ranges from 2% to 20%, peaking at up to 15% in patients older than 70 years of age.[23,55,56] Arial fibrillation is generally accompanied by a rapid ventricular response. The prevalence increases with age and is higher in men and rare in patients under 40 years of age unless there is longstanding severe thyrotoxicosis or coexistent structural heart disease. Prevalence of AF is now falling because of early diagnosis of hyperthyroidism in its natural history. The data from Danish National Registry showed in a cohort of 40,628 hyperthyroid patients, 8.3% of patients developed AF; male gender, ischemic heart disease, valvular heart disease, and congestive heart failures were associated with the highest risk for AF. Subclinical hyperthyroidism has the same relative risk for AF similar to overt hyperthyroidism.[53]

DIAGNOSIS OF THYROID FUNCTION DISORDERS

The serum TSH level is the most sensitive measure for the diagnosis of thyroid dysfunction. Serum TSH level increases in patients with primary hypothyroidism to >4.5 mU/L, and they are low (<0.1 mU/L) in hyperthyroidism due to the feedback inhibition of pituitary synthesis of thyrotropin. In the presence of abnormal TSH levels, measurement of free thyroxine (FT4) and total T3 (TT3) or free T3 (FT3) can distinguish subclinical from overt thyroid dysfunction. Subclinical hypothyroidism is diagnosed when the serum TSH is above the upper limit of the normal reference range and free thyroid hormones are within their respective reference range. It occurs in up to 4–20% of the adult population, and its prevalence increases with advancing age.[57,58] In 2–5% of patients (and more in areas of borderline iodine intake), only T3 is increased (T3 toxicosis). The converse state of T4 toxicosis, with elevated total and unbound T4 and normal T3 levels, is occasionally seen when hyperthyroidism is induced by excess iodine. Measurement of thyroperoxidase (TPO) antibodies or TSH receptor antibody (TRAb) may be useful, if the diagnosis is unclear clinically but is not needed routinely.[58]

MANAGEMENT

An untreated high-output state with hyperthyroidism can lead to ventricular dilation, persistent tachycardia, and eventual chronic heart failure which can be fatal.[59] In a study by Mitchell et al., patients with abnormal thyroid function and heart failure had 60% increased mortality compared to euthyroid patients with heart failure.[60] Apart from treatment to achieve euthyroid state, β-adrenergic blockade to reduce heart rate to less than 10–15% of baseline and diuretics to improve congestive symptoms are the treatment options for hyperthyroid patients with heart failure. Propranolol (10–40 mg, three to four times a day) has the advantage of blocking the conversion of T4 to T3 in peripheral tissues, but other cardioselective β-blockers have a longer half-life and are equally effective with improved compliance.[28,61] Digoxin is less beneficial due to greater blood volume distribution, increased rate of digitalis clearance and the need to block more Na-K-ATPase in the myocardium.[62] Vasodilators are contraindicated heart failure with hyperthyroidism. The direct inotropic effects of thyroid hormone will persist, so definitive therapy should be accomplished early.[28]

Atrial fibrillation usually reverts to sinus rhythm by achievement of a euthyroid status and β-adrenergic blockade is effective to control the ventricular rate. Increased plasma clearance of β-blockers usually necessitates higher doses.[63] In cardiac arrhythmias, intravascular infusion of calcium blockers should be avoided due to the risk of a further fall in SVR.[64] Digitalis in hyperthyroidism-associated AF is less effective with less predictable response. Successful treatment with either radioiodine or thiouracil is associated with conversion to sinus rhythm in a majority of patients within 2–3 months. Older patients (>60 years old) with AF of longer duration are less likely to spontaneously revert to sinus rhythm. Therefore, after the patient has been rendered chemically euthyroid, if AF persists, electrical or pharmacological cardioversion should be attempted. In the patients with AF the maintenance of sinus rhythm is not possible until the euthyroid state is restored, so electrical cardioversion is not recommended without euthyroid status,[65] when treated, the majority of patients can be restored to sinus rhythm and will remain so for prolonged periods of time. It is advised to evaluate each patient about the need for anticoagulation on a case-by-case basis. When oral anticoagulants are used, hyperthyroid patients will need smaller doses than euthyroid ones, due to faster elimination of vitamin-K dependent clotting factors.[28]

Heart failure secondary to hyperthyroidism has been considered a reversible cause of cardiomyopathy. There are several reports of patients with symptomatic heart failure who demonstrated reversal of echocardiographic measurements and clinical symptoms after achieving a euthyroid state.[66,67] Correction of the thyroid dysfunction is crucial. However, some studies have suggested that cardiovascular symptoms and signs, abnormal hemodynamics, and cardiac dysrhythmias can be persistent.[68] It is probable that individual patient characteristics such as age, comorbidities, and underlying risk factors for cardiac dysfunction significantly influence how one responds to treatment of thyrotoxic cardiomyopathy. Radioiodine (iodine131) is the preferred treatment in patients who desires definitive control of hyperthyroidism, the avoidance of surgery, and the potential side effects of antithyroid drugs (ATDs). 12–18 month course of carbimazole with noticeable clinical improvement within 10–14 days is recommended as treatment options in patients with high likelihood of remission with small goiters, and negative or low-titer TRAb; pregnancy; patients with moderate-to-severe active GO; and patients who need more rapid biochemical disease control. Most patients will be biochemically euthyroid within 4–6 weeks with ATDs. There may be an exacerbation of hyperthyroidism a few days after treatment with radioiodine because of a transient increase in serum thyroid hormone concentrations and hence patients with AF and cardiac failure should achieve euthyroid status with an ATD before giving radioiodine. Pretreatment with β-adrenergic blockade is recommended in all thyrotoxic patients with resting heart rate more than 90 beats per minute or associated cardiovascular disease.[61]

Hyperthyroidism is associated with an increase in cardiovascular and cerebrovascular mortality, which is most evident in the first year following treatment with radioiodine. A large series from a single center, based on more than 100,000 patient years of follow-up, showed that the standardized mortality ratio, in the year after ablative radioiodine, was 1.8:1[95% confidence interval (CI) 1.6–2:1].[69] At least some of this excess mortality could probably be avoided by earlier diagnosis and more aggressive treatment of the hyperthyroidism and its cardiovascular complications. The most recent data indicate that SH subjects appear to be at particular risk for the development of heart failure, especially older subjects and those with lower TSH levels. [70-72] Hence, American Thyroid Association recommends treatment of subclinical hypothyroidism, when TSH is persistently <0.1 mU/L, in all individuals 65 years of age; in patients with cardiac risk factors or heart disease, and in individuals with hyperthyroid symptoms.[61]

AMIODARONE AND THYROID

Amiodarone is a benzofuran derivative with 37% molecular weight of iodine and various effects on thyroid dysfunction are due to its high iodine content.[73] Amiodarone metabolism causes release of large amount of iodine that blocks thyroid hormone synthesis—the so-called Wolff–Chaikoff effect. This may be noticed in first few weeks but usually followed by normal thyroid hormone functioning. Amiodarone-induced hypothyroidism (AIH) is mostly due to this effect. AIH is mostly seen in females and elderly in the first few weeks of starting amiodarone. The overall prevalence of AIH is 15–30%. Treatment is usually by either thyroid hormone replacement or stopping of amiodarone.[11]

Amiodarone-induced thyrotoxicosis (AIT) is less common and mostly seen with chronic intake of amiodarone. There are mainly two types. AIT I is usually seen in areas of iodine deficiency with preexisting thyroid disease and MNG. It is mainly due to the high iodine content of amiodarone and iodine-induced excess thyroid hormone synthesis. AIT II is seen in normal thyroid tissue with glandular injury and preformed thyroid hormones leaks from damaged follicular cells. This is usually associated with elevated IL-6. Color-flow Doppler ultrasound shows decreased vascularity in type 2 AIT and increased vascularity in type 1 AIT. Radioactive iodine uptake, is usually low in type 2 AIT due to destruction of thyroid tissue and in type 1 AIT, iodine uptake may be high.[11,24,73]

Because of high thyroidal and total-body iodine content, use of radio iodine ablation is always ineffective. Treatment with ATDs has inconsistent effectiveness and it may be useful in type I AIT. Corticosteroid is beneficial, mainly in patients with type II AIT. However, corticosteroids can be given in all patients and response to treatment occurs within 2–4 weeks. If unresponsive to glucocorticoids, total thyroidectomy can be performed safely after preoperative treatment with beta-blockers and can rapidly reverse the hyperthyroidism without inducing thyroid storm.[74] Whether discontinuation of amiodarone is mandatory or not is controversial. No evidence supports that stopping amiodarone hastens the recovery from hyperthyroidism. The effect on thyroid does not depend on the dose and can occur at any time during treatment and this effect can persist up to 1 year after discontinuing therapy. Baseline thyroid function should be monitored in the beginning of amiodarone therapy and follow-up is needed every 3 months.[73]

CONCLUSION

Both hyperthyroidism and hypothyroidism produce changes in cardiac contractility, myocardial oxygen consumption, cardiac output, blood pressure, and SVR and may induce arrhythmias.[6,7] These cardiovascular changes are almost always reversible with the achievement of euthyroid status in heart failure. The severity and prognosis of heart failure with hyperthyroidism significantly change from hyperthyroid euthyroid state, thereby help in reducing morbidity and mortality.

REFERENCES

1. Donze J, Lipsitz S, Bates DW, et al. Causes and patterns of readmissions in patients with common comorbidities: retrospective cohort study. BMJ. 2013;347:f7171.
2. Ponikowski P, Anker SD, AlHabib KF, et al. Heart failure: preventing disease and death worldwide. ESC Heart Failure. 2015;1:4-25.
3. Klein I, Ojamaa K. Thyroid hormone and the cardiovascular system. N Engl J Med. 2001;344:501-9.
4. Dillmann WH. Cellular action of thyroid hormone on the heart. Thyroid. 2002;12:447-52.
5. Danzi S, Klein I. Thyroid hormone and the cardiovascular system. Minerva Endocrinologica. 2004;29:139-50.
6. Kahaly GJ, Dillmann WH. Thyroid hormone action in the heart. Endocrine Rev. 2005;26:704-28.
7. Biondi B, Palmieri EA, Lombardi G, et al. Effects of thyroid hormone on cardiac function: the relative importance of heart rate, loading conditions, and myocardial contractility in the regulation of cardiac performance in human hyperthyroidism. J Clin EndocrinolMetab. 2002;87:968-74.
8. Maia AL, Kim BW, Huang SA, et al. Type 2 iodothyronine deiodinase is the major source of plasma T3 in euthyroid humans. J Clin Invest. 2005;115:2524-33.
9. Bianco AC, Salvatore D, Gereben B, et al. Biochemistry, cellular and molecular biology, and physiological roles of the iodothyronine selenodeiodinases. Endocrine Rev. 2002;23:38-89.
10. Everts ME, Verhoeven FA, Bezstarosti K, et al. Uptake of thyroid hormones in neonatal rat cardiac myocytes. Endocrinology. 1996;137:4235-42.
11. Klein I, Danzi S. Thyroid disease and the heart. Curr Probl Cardiol. 2016;41(2):65-92.
12. Jabbar A, Pingitore A, Pierce SHS, et al. Thyroid harmones and Cardiovascular disease. Nature Reviews Cardiology. 2017;14:41.
13. Hartong R, Wang N, Kurokawa R, et al. Delineation of three different thyroid hormone-response elements in promoter of rat sarcoplasmic reticulum Ca^{2+} ATPase gene. J Biol Chem. 1994;269:13021-9.
14. Mintz G, Pizzarello R, Klein I. Enhanced left ventricular diastolic function in hyperthyroidism: noninvasive assessment and response to treatment. J Clin Endocrinol Metab. 1991;73:146-50.
15. Kiss E, Jakab G, Kranias EG, et al. Thyroid hormone-induced alterations in phospholamban protein expression: regulatory effects on sarcoplasmic reticulum Ca^{2+} transport and myocardial relaxation. Circ Res. 1994;75:245-51.
16. Danzi S, Dubon P, Klein I. Effect of serum T3 on the regulation of cardiac gene expression: role of histone acetylation. Am J Physiol Heart Circ Physiol. 2005;289:1506-11.
17. Haddad F, Bodell PW, Qin AX, et al. Role of antisense RNA in coordinating cardiac myosin heavy chain gene switching. J Biol Chem. 2003;278:37132-8.
18. Hu X, Lazar MA. Transcriptional repression by nuclear hormone receptors. Trends Endocrinol Metab. 2000;11:6-10.
19. Dudley SC Jr, Baumgarten CM. Bursting of cardiac sodium channels after acute exposure to 3,5,3'-triiodo-L-thyronine. Circ Res. 1993;73:301-13.
20. Hammond HK, White FC, Buxton IL, et al. Increased myocardial beta-receptors and adrenergic responses in hyperthyroid pigs. Am J Physiol. 1987;252:H283-90.
21. Hoit BD, Khoury SF, Shao Y, et al. Effects of thyroid hormone on cardiac b-adrenergic responsiveness in conscious baboons. Circulation. 1997;96:592-8.
22. Cacciatori V, Bellavere F, Pezzarossa A, et al. Power spectral analysis of heart rate in hyperthyroidism. J Clin Endocrinol Metab. 1996;81:2828-35.
23. Bielecka-Dabrowa A, Mikhailidis DP, Rysz J, et al. The mechanisms of atrial fibrillation in hyperthyroidism. Thyroid Res. 2009;2:4.
24. Klein I, Danzy S. Thyroid disease and the heart. Circulation. 2007;116:1725-35.
25. Panagoulis C, Halapas A, Chariatis E, et al. Hyperthyroidism and heart. Hellenic J Cardiol. 2008;49:169-75.
26. Park KW, Dai HB, Ojamaa K, et al. The direct vasomotor effect of thyroid hormones on rat skeletal muscle resistance arteries. Anesth Analog. 1997;85:734-8.
27. Resnick LM, Laragh JH. Plasma renin activity in syndromes of thyroid hormone excess and deficiency. Life Sci. 1982;30:585-6.

28. Klein I, Levey GS. Unusual manifestations of hypo thy roidism. Arch Intern Med. 1984;144:123-8.
29. Fadel BM, Ellahham S, Ringel MD, et al. Hyperthyroid heart disease. Clin Cardiol. 2000;23:402-8.
30. Kontos HA, Shapiro W, Mauck HP Jr, et al. Mechanism of certain abnormalities of the circulation to the limbs in thyrotoxicosis. J Clin Invest. 1965;44:947-56.
31. Theilen EO, Wilson WR. Hemodynamic effects of peripheral vasoconstriction in normal and thyrotoxic subjects. J Appl Physiol. 1967;22:207-10.
32. Danzi S, Klein I. Thyroid hormone and blood pressure regulation. Curr Hypertens Rep. 2003;5:513-20.
33. Walsh JP, Bremner AP, Bulsara MK, et al. Subclinical thyroid dysfunction and blood pressure: a community-based study. Clin Endocrinol. 2006;65:486-91.
34. Prisant LM, Gujral JS, Mulloy AL. Hyperthyroidism: a secondary cause of isolated systolic hypertension. J Clin Hypertens. 2006;8:596-9.
35. Merce J, Ferras S, Oltra C, et al. Cardiovascular abnormalities in hyperthyroidism: a prospective Doppler echocardiographic study. Am J Med. 2005;118:126-33.
36. Vargas F, Moreno JM, Rodriguez-Gomez I, et al. Vascular and renal function in experimental thyroid disorders. Eur J Endocrinol. 2006;154:197-212.
37. Palmieri EA, Fazio S, Palmieri V, et al. Myocardial contractility and total arterial stiffness in patients with overt hyperthyroidism: acute effects of beta1-adrenergic blockade. Eur J Endocrinol. 2004;150:757-62.
38. Taddei S, Caraccio N, Virdis A, et al. Impaired endothelium-dependent vasodilatation in subclinical hypothyroidism: beneficial effect of levothyroxine therapy. J Clin Endocrinol Metab. 2003;88:3731-7.
39. Vallabhajosula S, Radhi S, Cevik C, et al. Hyperthyroidism and pulmonary hypertension: an important association. Am J Med Sci. 2011;342(6):507-12.
40. Siu CW, Zhang XH, Yung C, et al. Hemodynamic changes in hyperthyroidism-related pulmonary hypertension: a prospective echocardiographic study. J Clin Endocrinol Metab. 2007;92(5):1736-42.
41. Sugiura T, Yamanaka S, Takeuchi H, et al. Autoimmunity and pulmonary hypertension in patients with Graves' disease. Heart Vessels. 2015;30(5):642-6.
42. Marvisi M, Zambrelli P, Brianti M, et al. Pulmonary hypertension is frequent in hyperthyroidism and normalizes after therapy. Eur J Intern Med. 2006;17:267-71.
43. Woeber KA. Thyrotoxicosis and the Heart. N Engl J Med. 1992;327:94-8.
44. Wang C, Crapo LM. The epidemiology of thyroid disease and implications for screening. Endocrinol Metabol Clin North Am. 1997;26:189-218.
45. Bulow PI, Laurberg P, Knudsen N, et al. Increase in incidence of hyprthyroidism predominantly occurs in young people after iodine fortification of salt in Denmark. J Clin Endocrinol Metab. 2006;91:3830-4.
46. Brandt F, Green A, Hegedüs L, et al. A critical review and meta-analysis of the association between over thyperthyroidism and mortality. Eur J Endocrinol. 2011;165:491-7.
47. Biondi B, Kahaly GJ. Cardiovascular involvement in patients with different causes of hyperthyroidism. Nat Rev Endocrinol. 2010;8:431-43.
48. Klein I, Levey GS. The cardiovascular system in thyro-toxicosis. In: Braverman LE, Utiger RD (Eds). Werner and Ingbar's the thyroid: a fundamental and clinical text. Philadelphia: Lippincott and Williams & Wilkins; 2000. pp. 596-604.
49. Kahaly GJ, Kampmann C, Mohr-Kahaly S. Cardiovascular hemodynamics and exercise tolerance in thyroid disease. Thyroid. 2002;12:473.
50. Dahl P, Danzi S, Klein I. Thyrotoxic cardiac disease. Curr Heart Fail Re. 2008;5:170-6.
51. Yue WS, Chong BH, Zhang XH, et al. Hyperthyroidism induced left ventricular diastolic dysfunction: implication in hyperthyroidism-related heart failure. Clin Endocrinol (Oxf). 2011;74:636-43.
52. Evangelopoulou ME, Alevizaki M, Toumanidis S, et al. Mitral valve prolapse in autoimmune thyroid disease: an index of systemic autoimmunity? Thyroid. 1999;9:973-7.
53. Frost L, Vestergaard P, Mosekilde L. Hyperthyroidism and risk of atrial fibrillation or flutter: a population-based study. Arch Intern Med. 2004;164:1675-8.
54. Sawin CT, Geller A, Wolf PA, et al. Low serum thyrotrop in concentrations as a risk factor for atrial fibrillation in older persons. N Engl J Med. 1994;331:1249-52.
55. Auer J, Scheibner P, Mische T, et al. Subclinical hyperthyroidism as a risk factor for atrial fibrillation. Am Heart J. 2001;142:838.
56. Vardas PE, Mavrakis HE. Atrial fibrillation: a symptom treated as a disease? Hellenic J Cardiol. 2006;47:191-3.
57. Biondi B. The normal TSH reference range: what has changed in the last decade? J Clin Endocrinol Metab. 2013;98: 3584.
58. Biondi B, Wartofsky L. Treatment with thyroid hormone. Endocr Rev. 2014;35:433.
59. Biondi B. Mechanisms in endocrinology: Heart failure and thyroid dysfunction. Eur J Endocrinol. 2012;167(5): 609-18.
60. Mitchell JE, Hellkamp AS, Mark DB, et al. Thyroid function in heart failure and impact on mortality. JACC Heart Fail. 2013;1(1):48-55.
61. Ross DS, Burch HB, Cooper DS, et al. 2016 American Thyroid Association Guidelines for diagnosis and management of hyperthyroidism and other causes of thyrotoxicosis. Thyroid. 2016;26(10):1343-421.
62. Chaudhury S, Ismail-Beigi F, Gick GG, et al. Effect of thyroid hormone on the abundance of Na, K, ATPase alpha subunit messenger ribonucleic acid. Mol Endocrinol. 1987;1:83-9.
63. Shenfield GM. Influence of thyroid dysfunction on drug pharmacokinetics. Clin Pharmacokinet. 1981;6:275-97.
64. Nakazawa HK, Sakurai K, Hamada N, et al. Management of atrial fibrillation in the post-thyrotoxic state. Am J Med. 1982;72:903-6.
65. Nakazawa H, Lythall DA, Noh J, Ishikawa N, et al. Is there a place for the late cardioversion of atrial fibrillation? A long-term follow-up study of patients with post-thyrotoxic atrial fibrillation. Eur Heart J. 2000;21:327-33.

66. Al-Ghamdi AS, Aljohani N. Graves' thyrotoxicosis-induced reversible cardiomyopathy: a case report. Clin Med Insights Case Rep. 2013;6:47-50.
67. Choudhury RP, MacDermot J. Heart failure in thyrotoxicosis, an approach to management. Br J Clin Pharmacol. 1998;46(5):421-4.
68. Osman F, Franklyn JA, Holder RL, et al. Cardiovascular manifestations of hyperthyroidism before and after antithyroid therapy: a matched case-control study. J Am Coll Cardiol. 2007;49(1):71-81.
69. Franklyn JA, Maisonneuve P, Sheppard MC, et al. Mortality after the treatment of hyperthyroidism with radioactive iodine. N Engl J Med. 1998;338:712-8.
70. Selmer C, Olesen JB, Hansen ML, et al. Subclinical and overt thyroid dysfunction and risk of all-cause mortality and cardiovascular events: a large population study. J Clin Endocrinol Metab. 2014;99:2372-82.
71. Collet TH, Gussekloo J, Bauer DC, et al. Thyroid Studies Collaboration 2012 Subclinical hyperthyroidism and the risk of coronary heart disease and mortality. Arch Intern Med. 172:799-809.
72. Gencer B, Collet TH, Virgini V, et al. Thyroid Studies Collaboration 2012 Subclinical thyroid dysfunction and the risk of heart failure events: an individual participant data analysis from 6 prospective cohorts. Circulation. 2012;126:1040-9.
73. Bogazzi F, Bartalena L, Martino E. Approach to the patient with amiodarone-induced thyrotoxicosis. J Clin Endocrinol Metab. 2010;95(6):2529-35.
74. Tomisti L, Materazzi G, Bartalena L, et al. Total thyroidectomy in patients with amiodarone-induced thyrotoxicosis and severe left ventricular systolic dysfunction. J Clin Endocrinol Metab. 2012;97(10):3515-21.

SECTION 10

Nutritional

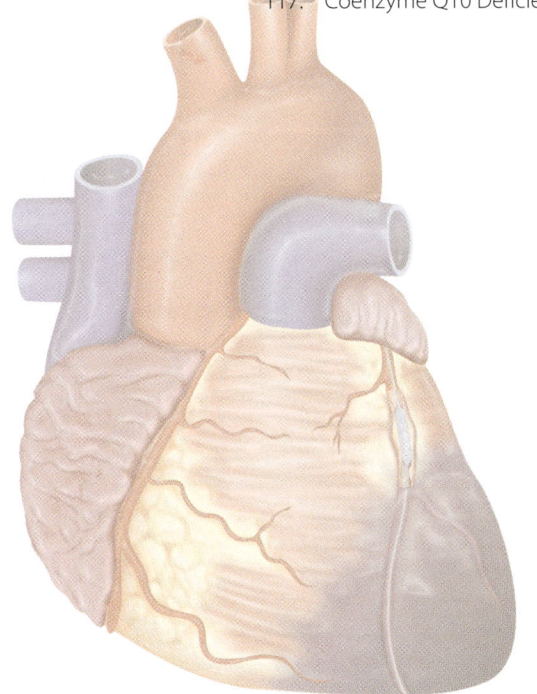

117 CHAPTER

Coenzyme Q10 Deficiency and Heart Failure

Pawan K Sharma, HK Chopra

INTRODUCTION

Coenzyme Q10 (CoQ10) is structurally similar to vitamin K and was first isolated from beef heart mitochondria in 1957.[1] CoQ10 occurs in organ meats, such as heart, liver, kidney, beef, and other food sources, such as soy oil, sardines, and peanuts.[2] Natural production of CoQ10 decreases with increasing age especially in the heart.[3] CoQ10 is insoluble in water and should be protected from light.[4] The CoQ10 is fat soluble and its absorption is significantly improved when taken with a fatty meal, such as soy or vegetable oil.[5] It is slowly absorbed with peak blood levels occurring 5–10 hours after oral administration. Normal blood levels of CoQ10 are 0.7–1.0 mcg/mL.[4] CoQ10 is the coenzyme for three mitochondrial enzymes (complexes I, II, and III). It accepts electrons from complexes I and II and transports them to complex III. It plays an important role in the production of adenosine triphosphate (ATP) by participating in reactions within the electron transport chain in the mitochondria.[6] CoQ10 also functions as a strong antioxidant by inhibiting the function of free radicals which have damaging effects on the body.[7,8] CoQ10 also improves endothelial function and increases nitric oxide bioavailability.[9] The CoQ10 also has effects on stabilization of Ca-dependent slow channels, inhibition of intracellular phospholipases, prostaglandin metabolism, free-radical scavenging, and direct membrane stabilization.[5] CoQ10 exists in three different oxidation states which include the fully reduced ubiquinol form (CoQ10H2), the radical semiquinone intermediate (CoQ10H), and fully oxidized ubiquinone form (CoQ10).

Coenzyme Q10 helps maintaining the optimal pH by transporting the protons across lysosomal membranes.[9,10] In the mitochondria, CoQ10 continually transports protons and electrons from one bioenergy enzyme to another. In isolated mitochondria, CoQ10 can protect membrane proteins and DNA from the oxidative damage which may occur during lipid peroxidation.[11] Sufficient concentrations of CoQ10 are required in the body cells to continuously generate energy and support their functions.[9,12] Pathophysiology of heart failure (HF) suggests that it is an energy-depleted state associated with low myocardial ATP production, mitochondrial dysfunction, abnormal calcium handling, increased reactive oxygen species generation, and endothelial dysfunction. It has also been shown that patients with lower ejection fraction and advanced HF have low levels of CoQ10. The CoQ10 has an important role in production of ATP, has potent anti-inflammatory action and may improve endothelial function. These actions suggest that CoQ10 may be an important therapeutic option in the treatment of congestive heart failure (CHF).

PHARMACOLOGY OF COENZYME Q10

Coenzyme Q10 is available in capsules, gel, and toothpaste forms. It is fat soluble and lipid vehicles, such as vegetable oil and vitamin E improve its absorption rate. The half-life is about 34 hours. It is eliminated primarily via the biliary tract, and up to 60% of oral dose can be recovered in the feces.[13] The recommended dose for health maintenance is 30 mg. A dose of 30–60 mg per has been used to prevent deficiency. Therapeutic dose of CoQ10 ranges from 200 mg to 400 mg daily. Treatment of cardiovascular disease requires elevated blood levels of 2–3 mcg/mL or even higher.[14]

ROLE OF COENZYME Q10 IN CONGESTIVE HEART FAILURE

Higher concentrations of CoQ10 are found in the heart muscle cells probably because myocardial cells require high energy for their function. CoQ10 has been shown to play an important role in the treatment of chronic HF and improving stress-induced cardiac dysfunction.[15,16] About 23 million people suffer from HF worldwide.[17] Despite significant advancements in the management of heart failure, mortality rates remain higher than 10% per year and can range between 20% and 50% in severe cases.[18] Folkers et al. demonstrated that myocardial CoQ10 level was linked with symptomatic severity of CHF because lowest levels are seen in patients with New York Heart Association (NYHA) class IV and the higher levels in patients in NYHA class I.[19] This may suggest that by replenishing CoQ10 deficiency, there may be improvement in ATP synthesis and thereby it may be useful in the treatment of heart failure.

From 1985 to 1993, Langsjoen and his group added CoQ10 to the medical regimens of 424 patients with various cardiovascular disease including ischemic cardiomyopathy, dilated cardiomyopathy, primary diastolic dysfunction, hypertension, mitral valve prolapse, and valvular heart disease. Of the 424 patients, 58% showed improvement by one NYHA class, 28% by two classes and 1.2% by three classes. The echocardiogram showed significant improvement in left ventricular function. Most patients were taking from one to five cardiac medications which dropped significantly after CoQ10 was added to the treatment: 43% of patients were able to stop taking between one to three cardiovascular drugs with the addition of CoQ10 therapy. Only 6% of the patients required the addition of one drug.[20] It was believed that the improvement in diastolic function led to blood pressure lowering and decreased catecholamine state.[20] There has been significant improvement in left ventricular ejection fraction (LVEF) by 3.7% when CoQ10 100–300 mg/day was supplemented for 1–6 months in the treatment of heart failure. This effect was more prominent in patients who were not taking angiotensin-converting enzyme inhibitor (ACEI).[21] The ejection fraction improved by 6.74% in patients not taking any ACEI therapy as compared to only 1.16% change with use of ACEI.[21] It has also been shown that in patients with heart failure, lower plasma CoQ10 levels are associated with higher mortality[22] and reflects severe advanced heart failure.[23]

A large randomized trial involving 641 patients has shown that CoQ10 supplementation, when compared with placebo, reduces the risk of hospitalization due to HF (73 vs 118, $p < 0.001$) and other complications of heart failure, such as pulmonary edema and cardiac asthma (20 vs 51 and 97 vs 198, $p < 0.001$).[24] The Q-SYMBIO trial showed that long-term CoQ10 treatment of patients with chronic HF is safe, improves symptoms, and reduces major adverse cardiovascular events (MACEs).[25] The Q-SYMBIO trial was a prospective, randomized, double-blind, placebo controlled, multicenter trial, enrolling 420 patients with moderate-to-severe CHF. Compared to placebo (n-218), CoQ10 was given at 100 mg orally three times a day for 2 years. The primary short-term endpoints at 16 weeks were changes in NYHA functional class, 6-minute walk test, and levels of N-terminal pro-B type natriuretic peptide. The primary long-term end-point at 2 years was composite major adverse cardiovascular events (MACEs). It was noted that there were no significant changes in short-term endpoints. The primary long-term end-point was reached in 15% of patients in the CoQ10 group compared to 26% in the placebo group.

The secondary endpoints were significantly lower in the CoQ10 group compared to the placebo group. The cardiovascular mortality was 9% versus 16%, $p = 0.026$; all-cause mortality was 10% versus 18%, $p = 0.018$ and incidence of hospital stay for HF was lower in the CoQ10 group versus the placebo group (8% vs 14%, $p = 0.033$). A significant improvement of NYHA class was seen in the CoQ10 group after 2 years (58% vs 45%, $p = 0.028$). Compared to placebo group, the CoQ10 group showed significant serum N-terminal pro-B type natriuretic peptide (NT-proBNP) reduction (60%, 1137 pg/mL vs 52% 881 pg/mL, $p > 0.05$). Although, the Q-SYMBIO study suggested potential benefits of CoQ10 therapy in the treatment of heart failure, but this study had significant limitation that despite being conducted in >17 centers in 9 countries, it took about 8 years to complete the enrollment. The Q-SYMBIO trial also suggested that there was trend towards benefit in elderly patients, male patients, NYHA functional class III, patients with dilated cardiomyopathy, patients with N-terminal prohormone of brain natriuretic peptide >300 pg/mL, patients with LVEF >30% ($p = 0.065$). Current HF guidelines do not recommend initiation of nutritional supplementation for the treatment of heart failure. But the long-term supplementation of CoQ10 in patients with HF seems safe, appears to produce symptomatic improvements, and more importantly has been found to significantly reduce MACEs and mortality. If future large randomized studies confirm the results of the Q-SYMBIO trial, CoQ10 may become a part of standard guidelines in patients with heart failure.

CoQ10 AND HEART FAILURE WITH PRESERVED EJECTION FRACTION

Heart failure with preserved ejection fraction (HFpEF) occurs when left ventricular systolic function is preserved and there is reduced ventricular compliance in diastole, resulting in increased left ventricular end-diastolic pressure. HFpEF is also believed to be due to abnormal energetics.[26] HFpEF patients may also have increased inflammatory mediators (such as tumor necrosis factor, factor—alpha, interleukin-6, soluble ST2, and pentraxin-3) which may result in endothelial dysfunction.[27] These may result in abnormal cardiac remodeling and ventricular relaxation. Since the CoQ10 plays a positive role in energetics, ameliorates proinflammatory mediators, and improves endothelial dysfunction, it may have a potential role in the treatment of HFpEF. Since there are no randomized trials evaluating the role of CoQ10 supplementation in the treatment of HFpEF, future trials of CoQ10 in HFpEF patients should be considered.

CoQ10 AND OTHER CARDIOVASCULAR CONDITIONS

Hypertension

In a small, crossover, placebo-controlled, randomized study evaluating antihypertensive effect of CoQ in patients with essential hypertension, treatment with CoQ10 demonstrated a statistically significant decrease in both systolic and diastolic blood pressure ($p < 0.001$) suggesting the antihypertensive effect of CoQ10.[14] In a study, involving 109 patients with essential hypertension CoQ10 was added at an average oral dose of 225 mg per day to their existing antihypertensive regimen. Within 1–6 months, there was a gradual improvement in functional status and a decrease in antihypertensive drug therapy. The NYHA functional class improved from a mean of 2.40–1.36 ($p < 0.001$) , and 51% of patients stopped using one to three antihypertensive drugs at an average of 4.4 months after starting CoQ10.[28] In another trial, addition of 120 mg per day of CoQ10 to conventional medical therapy for 8 weeks in patients with hypertension and coronary artery disease decreased systolic blood pressure by an average of 12 mm Hg and diastolic blood pressure by an average of 6 mm Hg, in comparison to a placebo containing B-complex vitamins.[29] In patients with isolated systolic hypertension, supplementation with both CoQ10 (120 mg/day) and vitamin E (300 IU/day) for 12 weeks resulted in an average decrease of 17 mm Hg in systolic blood pressure compared with 300 IU/day of vitamin E alone.[30] A meta-analysis of clinical trials in hypertensive patients using 100–120 mg per day of CoQ10, showed that the systolic blood pressure reduced by 11–17 mm Hg and diastolic blood pressure by 8–10 mm Hg.[31]

Myocardial Infarction and Cardiac Surgery

Pretreatment of animals with CoQ10 has been found to decrease myocardial damage due to ischemia-reperfusion.[32] Three placebo-controlled trials found that CoQ10 pretreatment with 100–300 mg/day for 7–14 days prior to surgery provided some benefit in short-term outcome measures after CABG surgery.[33,34]

Angina Pectoris

Five small placebo-controlled studies when compared to placebo, the addition of CoQ10 to conventional medical therapy in patients with chronic stable angina improved exercise tolerance and reduced or delayed electrocardiographic changes associated with myocardial ischemia. However, only two of the studies found significant decrease in symptom frequency and nitroglycerine consumption with CoQ10 supplementation. Presently, there is only limited evidence suggesting that CoQ10 supplementation would be a useful adjunct to conventional angina therapy.[35]

POTENTIAL ROLE IN NONCARDIAC DISEASES

Diabetes Mellitus

Diabetic patients have lower levels of CoQ10 compared to healthy controls. But there is no improvement in control of glycemia in both type 1 or 2 diabetics despite CoQ10 supplementation.[36,37] It has, therefore, been suggested that CoQ10 can be safely used in diabetic patients with cardiovascular disease.

Use with Doxorubicin and Cancer

In a placebo-controlled trial involving mice, 100 mg per day of CoQ10 given for 3–5 days prior to doxorubicin treatment showed statistically significantly improved survival ($p < 0.05$).[38] But, large-controlled clinical trials may prove this the effects of CoQ10 supplementation in patients taking doxorubicin.

Acquired Immune Deficiency Syndrome

Small clinical experience in AIDS-related complex (ARC) patients has suggested improved survival after CoQ10 supplementation. CoQ10 treatment has also shown increase in T4/T8 ratios and CoQ10 blood levels.[39]

Muscular Dystrophy

In a double-blind, placebo-controlled trial, treatment with CoQ10 has shown improved physical performance in patients with muscle dystrophy.[40]

Pregnancy

Normally, the plasma CoQ10 levels increase during each trimester of pregnancy. However, low CoQ10 levels have direct relationship with spontaneous abortion and spontaneous contractile activity in the third trimester. An increase in plasma CoQ10 level can decrease contractile activity of the uterine muscle and may help reducing the chances of spontaneous abortion.[41]

Periodontal Disease

It has been seen that gingival disease is related to lower levels of CoQ10. When given orally, CoQ10 seems to help reducing the periodontal disease by reducing the gingival inflammation. Topical application of CoQ10 dissolved in soya oil to the periodontal pockets also reduces bleeding and depth of pockets.[42]

SIDE EFFECTS OF CoQ10

Coenzyme Q10 is very safe and does not seem to have any significant side effects. Less than 1% patients report epigastric discomfort, diarrhea, nausea, or appetite suppression. Side effects can be minimized by decreasing the dosage or if daily doses higher than 100 mg are divided into two or three daily doses.[5] Dose >100 mg in the evening may cause mild insomnia in some individuals. Mild increase in serum transaminases has been seen in patients taking 300 mg/day for extended periods but no significant hepatic toxicity is seen otherwise.[5] In a study of 2,664 patients with HF, 36 patients (1.5% of all patients) reported 38 adverse events with nausea being the most common symptom (n = 30) followed by allergic maculopapular rash (n = 3). Seven patients with nausea and two with allergic maculopapular rash discontinued the drug, whereas the remaining patients tolerated a reduced dose of CoQ10.[43]

DRUG INTERACTIONS

Warfarin

Concomitant use of warfarin and CoQ10 supplementation can decrease the anticoagulant effect of warfarin because CoQ10 has some structural similarity to vitamin K.[44] Prothrombin time/international normalized ratio (PT/INR) should be monitored closely in patients taking warfarin and CoQ10 concomitantly.

HMG-CoA Reductase Inhibitors (Statins)

HMG-CoA reductase inhibitors which reduce the biosynthesis of cholesterol also lower the blood levels of CoQ10 by 20–30% by blocking its biosynthesis. This occurs because HMG-CoA reductase inhibitors partially share the biosynthetic pathway of CoQ10 and cholesterol.[45] Large studies are needed to examine the content of CoQ10 in target organs. Therefore, it is unclear whether statin therapy affects CoQ10 concentration in body tissues and target organs.[46-48] It is still unclear whether CoQ10 supplementation is beneficial for those taking statins.

Gemfibrozil

Gemfibrozil lowers endogenous levels of CoQ10.[49] Large clinical trial may help to elucidate the role of CoQ10 supplementation in patients taking gemfibrozil.

Other Drugs

Beta-blockers can inhibit CoQ10-dependent enzymes. CoQ10 may also protect against the adverse effects of clonidine, diazoxide, hydralazine, hydrochlorothiazide, and methyldopa.[50] Larger studies are needed to see, if CoQ10 supplementation has any beneficial effect in patients taking these drugs.

CONCLUSION

Coenzyme Q10 is widely available, relatively inexpensive, and is well tolerated by most patients. Based on the results of large clinical studies, there is enough evidence of potential benefit of CoQ10 in the treatment of CHF. Numerous small studies on CoQ10 have also shown potential benefits in various other diseases, but large, randomized trials are needed to evaluate the role of CoQ10 in these conditions. Lower myocardial levels of CoQ10 have been seen in patients with increasing severity of heart failure. This decline may be exacerbated by concurrent treatment with statins and beta-blockers, which can suppress endogenous CoQ10 synthesis. Some trials on CoQ10 supplementation in HF patients have reported improvements in functional parameters, such as ejection fraction, stroke volume, and cardiac output, with very favorable safety profile. Some trials have also shown that benefits tended to be greater in patients not treated with ACEIs. It has also been shown that lower plasma CoQ10 levels in HF patients correlate with higher mortality. The landmark Q-SYMBIO trial, a multicenter randomized, placebo-controlled trial highlighted the beneficial effects of supplemental CoQ10 in heart failure. Thus, the evidence suggests that CoQ10 supplementation may be a useful option for effective management of heart failure with the advantage of excellent clinical tolerance at a lower cost. Since CoQ10 has been shown to have no effect on glycemic control in diabetics, it can be safely used in a large number of HF patients suffering with diabetes.

REFERENCES

1. Crane FL, Hatefi Y, Lester EI, et al. Isolation of a quinone from beef heart mitochondria. Biochim Biophys Acta. 1957;25:220-1.
2. Challem J. Coenzyme Q10: It may just be the miracle vitamin of the 1990s. The Nutrition Reporter. 1996.
3. Marincola R. Neurobiology and quantified pharmaco EEG of coenzyme Q10. J Orthomolecular Med. 1997;12(2):87-95.
4. Allen LV. Coenzyme Q10 high strength capsules. US Pharm. 1999;24(5):96-9.
5. Pepping J. Alternative therapies: Coenzyme Q10. Am J Health Syst Pharm. 1999;56(6):519-21.
6. Silverman H, Romano J, Elmer G. The Vitamin Book. New York, NY: Bantam Books; 1993.
7. Weber C, Jakobsen TS, Mortensen SA, et al. Antioxidative effect of dietary coenzyme Q10 in human blood plasma. Internat J Vit Nutr Res. 1994;64:311-5.
8. Folkers K, Osterborg A, Nylander M, et al. Activities of vitamin Q10 in animal models and a serious deficiency in patients with cancer. Biochem Biophys Res Commu. 1997;234(2):296-9.
9. Crane FL. Biochemical functions of coenzyme Q10. J Am Coll Nutr. 2001;20(6):591-98.
10. Nohl H, Gille L. The role of coenzyme Q in lysosomes. In: Kagan VEQ PJ (Ed). Coenzyme Q: Molecular Mechanisms in Health and Disease. Boca Raton: CRC Press; 2001. pp. 99-106.
11. Ernster L, Dallner G. Biochemical, physiological and medical aspects of ubiquinone function. Biochim Biophys Acta. 1995;1271(1):195-204.
12. Bliznakov EG. From sharks to coenzyme Q10. Adv Exp Med Biol. 1976;73:441-50.
13. Ubidecarenone drug monograph (online monograph). Englewood, CO: Micromedex; 1995.
14. Digiesi V, Cantini F, Brodeck B. Effect of coenzyme Q10 on essential arterial hypertension. Curr Ther Res. 1990;47:841-5.
15. Langsjoen P, Vadhanavikit S, Folker K. Response of patients in class III and IV of cardiomyopathy to therapy in a blind and crossover trial with coenzyme Q10. Proc Natl Acad Sci. 1985;82:4240-4.
16. Judy W, Hall J, Toth P, et al. Double blind- double crossover study of coenzyme CoQ10 in heart failure. In: Folkers K, Yamamura Y, eds. Biomedical and Clinical Aspects of Coenzyme Q. Amsterdam, Netherlands: Elsevier Science; 1986.
17. McMurray JJ, Petrie MC, Murdoch DR, et al. Clinical epidemiology of heart failure: public and private health burden. Eur Heart J. 1998;19 (suppl P):P9-16.
18. Ho KK, Pinsky JL, Kannel WB, et al. The epidemiology of heart failure: the Farmington Study. J Am Coll Cardiol. 1993;22 (4 suppl A):6a-13a.
19. Folkers K, Vadhanavikit S, Mortensen SA. Biochemical rationale and myocardial tissue data on the effective therapy of cardiomyopathy with coenzyme Q10. Proc Natl Acad Sci USA. 1985;82:901-4.
20. Langsjoen H, Langsjoen P, Willis R, et al. Usefulness of coenzyme Q10 in clinical cardiology: A long-term study. Mol Aspects Med. 1994;15(suppl):S2165-75.
21. Sander S, Coleman CI, Patel AA, et al. The impact of coenzyme Q10 on systolic function in patients with chronic heart failure. J Card Fail. 2006;12:464-72.
22. Molyneux SL, Florkowski CM, George PM, et al. Coenzyme Q10: an independent predictor of mortality in chronic heart failure. J Am Coll Cardiol. 2008;52:1435-41.
23. McMurray JJ, Dunselman P, Wedel H, et al. Coenzyme Q10, rosuvastatin, and clinical outcomes in heart failure: a pre-specified substudy of CORONA (controlled rosuvastatin multinational study in heart failure). J Am Coll Cardiol. 2010;56:1196-204.
24. Morisco C, Trimarco B, Condorelli M. Effect of coenzyme Q10 therapy in patients with congestive heart failure: a long-term multicenter randomized study. Clin Investig. 1993;71(8 suppl): S134-6.
25. Mortensen SA, Rosenfeldt F, Kumar A, et al. The effect of coenzyme Q10 on morbidity and mortality in chronic heart failure. Results from Q-SYMBIO: A Randomized Double-Blind Trial. J Am Coll Cardiol HF. 2014;2:641-9.
26. Zile MR, Brutsaert DL. New concepts in diastolic dysfunction and diastolic heart failure: part II. Causal mechanisms and treatment. Circulation. 2002;105:1503-8.
27. Paulus WJ, Tschope C. A novel paradigm for heart failure with preserved ejection fraction: comorbidities drive myocardial dysfunction and remodeling through coronary microvascular endothelial inflammation. J Am Coll Cardiol. 2013;62:263-71.
28. Langsjoen P, Willis R, Folkers K. Treatment of essential hypertension with coenzyme Q10. Mol Aspects Med. 1994;15(suppl):S265-72.
29. Singh RB, Niaz MA, Rastogi SS, et al. Effect of hydrosoluble coenzyme Q10 on blood pressure and insulin resistance in hypertensive patients with coronary artery disease. J Hum Hypertens, 1999;13(3):203-8.
30. Burke BE, Neuenschwander R, Olson RD. Randomized, double-blind, placebo-controlled trial of coenzyme Q10 in isolated systolic hypertension. South Med J. 2001;94(11): 1112-7.
31. Rosenfeldt FL, Haas SJ, Krum H, et al. Coenzyme Q10 in the treatment of hypertension: a meta-analysis of the clinical trials. J Hum Hypertens. 2007;21:297-306.
32. Lonnrot K, Tolvanen JP, Porsti I, et al. Coenzyme Q10 supplementation and recovery from ischemia in senescent rat myocardium. Life Sci. 1999;64(5):315-23.
33. Rosenfeldt FL, Pepe S, Linnane A, et al. The effects of ageing on the response to cardiac surgery: protective strategies for the ageing myocardium. Biogerontology. 2002;3(1-2):37-40.

34. Langsjoen PH, Langsjoen AM. Overview of the use of CoQ10 in cardiovascular disease. Biofactors. 1999;9(2-4):273-84.
35. Tran MT, Mitchell TM, Kennedy DT, et al. Role of coenzyme Q10 in chronic heart failure, angina and hypertension. Pharmacotherapy. 2001;21(7):797-806.
36. Lim SC, Lekshminarayanan R, Goh SK, et al. The effect of coenzyme Q10 on microcirculatory endothelial function of subjects with type 2 diabetes mellitus. Atherosclerosis. 2008;196:966-9.
37. Eriksson JG, Forsen TJ, Mortensen SA, et al. The effect of coenzyme Q10 administration on metabolic control in patients with type 2 diabetes mellitus. Biofactors. 1999;9(2-4):315-8.
38. Combs A, Choe J, Truong D, et al. Reduction by coenzyme Q10 of the acute toxicity of Adriamycin in mice. Res Commun Chem Pathol Pharmacol. 1977;18:565-8.
39. Folkers K, Hanioka T, Xia LJ, et al. Coenzyme Q10 increases T4/T8 ratios of lymphocytes in ordinary subjects and relevance to patients having the AIDS related complex. Biochem Biophys Res Commun. 1991;176(2):786-91.
40. Folkers K, Simonsen R. Two successful double blind trials with coenzyme Q10 (vitamin Q10) on muscular dystrophies and neurogenic atrophies. Biochem Biophys Acta. 1995;1271 (1):281-6.
41. Nola G, Littarru G, De Santis M, et al. Coenzyme Q10 in pregnancy. Fetal Diagn Ther. 1996;11(4):264-70.
42. Wilkinson E, Arnold R, Folkers K. Treatment of periodontal and other soft tissue diseases of the oral cavity with coenzyme Q. In: Folkers K, Yamamura Y (Eds). Biomedical and Clinical Aspects of Coenzyme Q, Vol 1. Amsterdam, Netherlands: Elsevier/ North Holland Biomedical; 1977.
43. Baggio E, Gandini R, Plancher AC, et al. Italian multicenter study on the safety and efficacy of coenzyme Q10 as adjunctive therapy in heart failure. CoQ10 Drug Surveillance Investigators. Mol Aspects Med. 1994;15(suppl): S287-94.
44. Heck AM, DeWitt BA, Lukes AL. Potential interactions between alternative therapies and warfarin. Am J Health Syst Pharm. 2000;57(13):1221-7.
45. Mortensen S, Leh A, Agner E, et al. Dose-related decrease of serum coenzyme Q10 during treatment with HMG-CoA reductase inhibitors. Mol Aspects Med. 1997;18(suppl): S137-44.
46. Laaksonen R, Jokelainen K, Laakso J, et al. The effect of simvastatin treatment on natural antioxidants in low-density lipoproteins and high-energy phosphates and ubiquinone in skeletal muscle. Am J Cardiol. 1996;77(10);851-4.
47. Laaksonen R, Jokelainen K, Sahi T, et al. Decreases in serum ubiquinone concentrations do not result in reduced levels in muscle tissue during short-term simvastatin treatment in humans. Clin Pharmacol Ther. 1995;57(1):62-6.
48. Elmberger PG, Kalen A, Lund E, et al. Effects of pravastatin and cholestyramine on products of the mevalonate pathway in familial hypercholesterolemia. J Lipid Res. 1991;32(6):935-40.
49. Aberg F, Appelkvist E, Broijersen A, et al. Gemfibrozil-induced decrease in serum ubiquinone and alpha- and gamma-tocopherol levels in men with combined hyperlipidemia. Eur J Clin Invest. 1998;28:235-42.
50. Kishi T, Watanabe T, Folkers K. Bioenergetics in clinical medicine XV. Inhibition of coenzyme Q10-enzymes by clinically used adrenergic blockers of beta-receptors. Res Commun Chem Pathol Pharmacol. 1977;17(1):157-64.

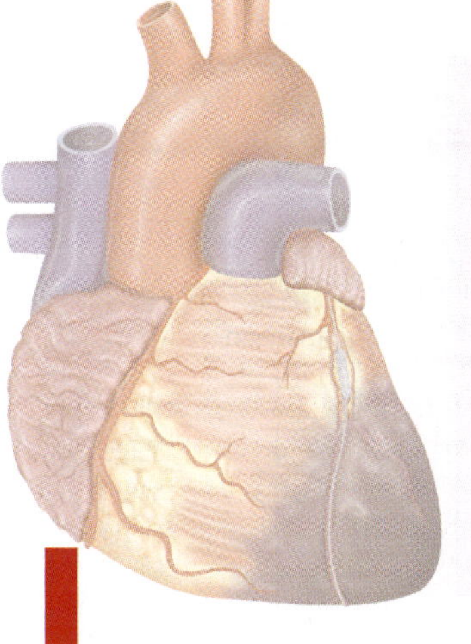

Iron Deficiency and Heart Failure

Mohan Bhargava, Mohit M Bhagwati

INTRODUCTION

Anemia is a common comorbidity associated with heart failure (HF) in general and heart failure with reduced ejection fraction (HFrEF) in particular across different studies.[1] The prevalence of anemia varies differently as per the population studied. For instance, it was 22% in SOLVD database and around 19% in COPERNICUS trial.[2,3] A meta-analysis done by Groenveld HF et al. reported the prevalence of anemia as 37.2% in HF patients.[4] It has also been seen that the severity of anemia is related to the New York Heart Association (NYHA) class and increases in severity as the NYHA class worsens.[5] Anemia in HF is multifactorial and can be due to iron deficiency (ID), associated chronic kidney disease (CKD) or chronic inflammation, blood loss through gastrointestinal tract, or too many blood tests. Anemia can be due to functional ID in presence of various inflammatory mediators in HF or it can be due to decreased erythropoiesis secondary to decreased renal blood flow or increased angiotensin II. Anemia can also be due to absolute ID secondary to malabsorption, bleeding or anorexia or in some cases there is "dilutional anemia" due to fluid retention.[6] The pathogenesis of anemia in HF is depicted in Flowchart 1. The patients with HF usually have reduced quality of life (QoL) and restricted exercise capacity, therefore treating anemia to improve QoL and exercise capacity was the initial notion behind treating anemia in HF.

FAILURE OF ERYTHROPOIETIN

The initial attempt to correct anemia in HF was undertaken in Tel Aviv in 1990, where patients were treated with a combination of subcutaneous erythropoietin and intravenous (IV) iron.[7] Patients showed significant improvements in left ventricular ejection fraction (LVEF), NYHA class and mean hemoglobin (Hb) concentration over 6 months. This led to plethora of research into treatment of anemia in HF. The initial notion of the researchers was that erythropoietin should be the weapon to fight anemia in HF like in other chronic diseases. There were several small studies which showed benefits of erythropoietin including a meta-analysis of 11 such randomized trials by Kotecha et al.[8] However, the proposed pathway to treat anemia in HF could not see the light of day after the results of a landmark negative trial, RED-HF.[9] It was a randomized, double-blind, placebo-controlled trial in 2,278 patients with HF and mild-to-moderate anemia. In this trial, treatment with an erythropoietin derivative, darbepoetin alfa did not show any improvement in the primary end-point of death from any cause or hospitalization for worsening HF. On the downside, there was a significant increased rate of thromboembolic events (13.5% vs 10.0%, respectively; $p = 0.009$) and an increased risk of ischemic stroke (4.5% vs 2.8%, respectively; $p = 0.03$). This trial concluded that the approach to treat anemia using erythropoietin in HF is counterproductive. During the same time period, there were multiple small

Flowchart 1: Pathogenesis of Iron deficiency in HF.[6]

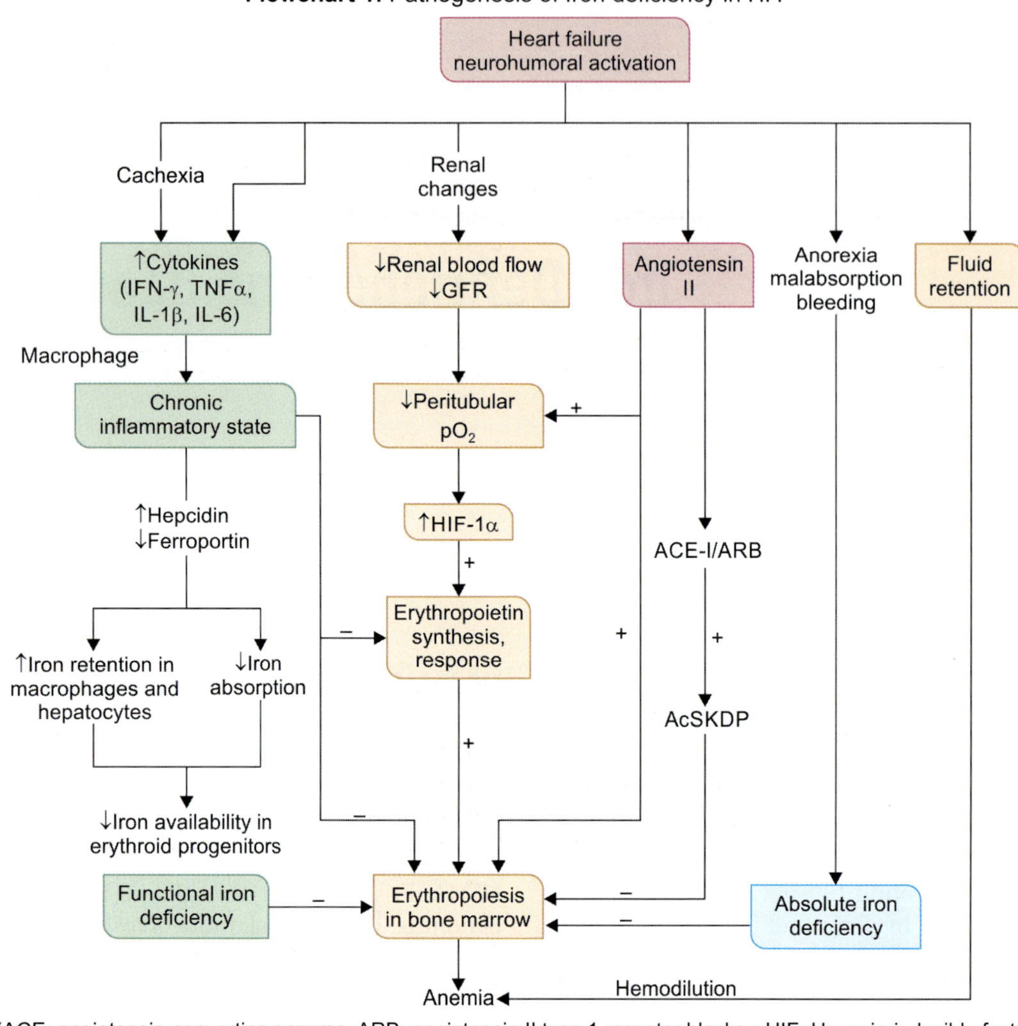

(ACE: angiotensin-converting enzyme; ARB; angiotensin II type 1 receptor blocker; HIF: Hypoxia-inducible factor; IFN: interferon; TNF: tumor necrosis factor)

studies where treatment with IV iron without erythropoietin improved clinical status, exercise capacity and QoL without any major adverse effects. This led to the era of belief that treating ID with or without anemia should be the further area of research in HF patients.[10,11]

IRON DEFICIENCY IN HEART FAILURE

Iron is one of the most essential trace element in human body. It is crucial in maintaining the oxygen-carrying capacity of the blood through erythropoiesis, oxygen transport, delivery, and its utilization. It is a key component of hemoglobin, myoglobin, and diverse enzymes involved in cellular respiration, oxidative phosphorylation, citric acid cycle, oxygen radical production, nitric oxide generation, and several other functions.[12] ID is very common in HF with as many as 50% of HF have low levels of available iron with or without anemia. ID can be absolute or functional. Absolute ID is present when total body iron is decreased due to decreased intake, decreased absorption or increased loss. Functional ID is present when total body iron is normal or increased but it is inadequate to meet the needs of target tissues because of sequestration in the storage pool. Functional ID is mainly due increase in the levels of a peptide called hepcidin secreted by hepatocytes. Hepcidin is the chief regulator of iron storage and release by controlling the activity of ferroportin, a transmembrane iron exporter, both at the site of iron absorption (gut mucosa cells in the duodenum) as well as at the site of iron storage (macrophages and hepatocytes). The ferroportin is destroyed by lysosome once it is bound by hepcidin which leads to reduced iron release and thus, functional ID.[13] The levels of hepcidin increase in chronic HF like other chronic diseases, such as chronic kidney disease or cancer.

Iron deficiency results in impaired oxidative metabolism and cellular energetics which decreases oxygen storage in myoglobin and reduces tissue oxidative capacity leading to mitochondrial and LV dysfunction. Reduced myocardial iron is associated with lower activity of citric acid cycle enzymes (aconitase and citrate synthase); diminished reactive oxygen species (ROS) protecting enzymes and reduced mitochondrial oxygen consumption.[14,15] Moreover, reduced myocardial iron in HF might therefore further promote impaired protection against ROS in combination with utilization of glucose rather than fatty acid and hence, might contribute to myocardial dysfunction and adverse remodeling.[16]

Clinically, it has been shown that ID in patients with HF is associated with impaired QoL, reduced exercise capacity, and overall poor prognosis independently of anemia and LVEF. In a prospective study done by Jankowska EA et al. on 443 patients with HF [(mean LVEF 26%), ID (serum ferritin <100 µg/L or 100–300 µg/L with transferrin saturation (TSAT) <20%] was present in 35%. Peak VO_2 was significantly lower in those with ID compared with those without ID (peak VO_2, 13.3 ± 4.0 versus 15.3 ± 4.5 $mL \cdot min^{-1} \cdot kg^{-1}$). This association was independent of clinical variables including anemia.[17] In one more study of 546 Polish patients with HF, ID (ferritin <100 µg/L or 100–300 µg/L with TSAT <20%) was present in 37% of patients of which, 57% were anemic and 32% were not anemic. On multivariable analysis, it was found that ID but not anemia was associated with a higher risk of death or heart transplantation [hazard ratio (HR), 1.58; 95% confidence interval (CI), 1.14–2.17; $P < 0.01$].[18] There are other Asian and international cohorts of HF patients where it has been seen that ID and not anemia is associated with mortality in HF patients.[19,20] Therefore ID needs to be addressed in HF patients irrespective of their anemic status.

Diagnosis of ID in HF

Diagnosing ID in a cardiac patient has been a challenge since inception. The gold standard technique remains a bone marrow aspiration and study with Prussian blue stain for absence of iron granules. However, it is invasive and impractical for physicians to do it on routine basis. Reliable cutoff values for lab markers were available for kidney disease and cancer but not HF. Early studies of ID in HF, used a ferritin concentration of <400 mg/L as a marker of ID and some studies used ferritin concentration of <100 mg/L or a combination of ferritin concentrations ranging between 100 mg/L and 299 mg/L together with a TSAT level of <20% as identifying ID. As the latter cutoff values were validated in a double-blind trial, European Society of Cardiology (ESC) guidelines accepted the said criteria for diagnosis of ID in HF (Table 1).[21]

TABLE 1: Diagnostic criteria of iron deficiency in heart failure.

Iron deficiency in heart failure (irrespective of anemia)	Serum ferritin <100 µg/dL OR Serum ferritin of 100–299 µg/dL with a transferrin saturation (TSAT) <20%

After diagnosing ID, the next step is to estimate the iron deficit and the required dose of IV iron for the correction of ID. Conventionally, Ganzoni's formula published in 1970 has been used to estimate ID in chronic diseases and the same is true for HF.[22] This equation assumes a target hemoglobin value of 15.0 g/dL (bodyweight of >35 kg) or 13.0 g/dL (lower body weight). An extra depot dose of 500 mg is usually added to the calculated deficit as the said equation does not take into account the iron stores. The equation is as follows:

Iron deficit (mg) = [2.4 × Body weight (kg) × Hb deficit (Target Hb-Patient's Hb)] + 500 mg for stores.

The calculated result is usually higher than 1,000 mg in most cases. IV iron is then administered as per the dosage guidelines in one or two sittings based on the iron deficit. The choice of the iron preparation and its route of administration are discussed later in the chapter.

Oral Iron Therapy in HF

The most common form of iron used in our country to treat ID anemia is the oral iron tablets which contain ferrous salts of iron. This oral iron tablets are readily available and inexpensive to buy and convenient to prescribe. However, in HF patients, oral iron is not absorbed well due to gut edema in HF and due to effects of hepcidin as discussed earlier. Oral iron has many adverse events particularly gastrointestinal. It needs to be taken empty stomach with multiple do's and don'ts regarding food and dairy products which hampers its compliance. The normal dosage is 100–200 mg per day. The response usually takes 1 or 3 weeks, shown by an increase in reticulocytes or hemoglobin. It is a slow acting process and it usually takes 2–6 months to replenish iron stores. Two clinical studies evaluated the use of oral iron preparations in patients with HF. IRON 5-(Short Term Oral Iron Supplementation in Systolic Heart Failure Patients Suffering From Iron Deficiency Anemia) HF trial and IRONOUT HF (Oral Iron Repletion Effects On Oxygen Uptake in Heart Failure) trial.[23,24] The first trial was prematurely terminated and the second trial failed to show any improvement in HF patients. The primary end-point of the IRONOUT HF trial was a change in peak oxygen uptake from baseline to 16 weeks and secondary end-points were 6-minute walk test (6MWT) and change in N- terminal-pro-brain natriuretic peptide (NT-proBNP) levels. None of these were statistically significant.[24] Therefore, it concluded that oral iron therapy has no role in HF patients.

Intravenous Iron Therapy in HF

As discussed above, oral iron therapy never appeared a practical solution in treating ID in HF. Therefore, significant research was done using IV iron for correction of ID in HF. There are many IV preparations available in the market; however, most studies in patients with HF and ID have used either iron sucrose or ferric carboxymaltose (FCM). The old IV preparation of iron dextran is not used in routine. Multiple studies have been done to study effects of IV iron in HF so far and the primary objective of these studies has been to look for the safety and efficacy of IV iron on exercise capacity, NYHA class, and QoL.

The first landmark study of IV iron in HF was FAIR HF trial done with ferric carboxymaltose. 459 patients of HF in NYHA class II or class III having ID were randomized to FCM or placebo. The primary outcome, Patient Global Assessment (PGA) at 24 weeks was reported as much or moderately improved in 50% of the IV iron group versus 28% of the placebo group ($p < 0.001$). NYHA class I or II at 24 weeks was 47% versus 30% ($p < 0.001$), respectively. Results were the same irrespective of the presence of anemia. Significant improvement was seen in the distance on a 6MWT ($p < 0.001$). Deaths and repeat hospitalization were lesser in FCM group. At follow-up, mean hemoglobin was 13.0 g/dL versus 12.5 g/dL ($p < 0.001$), respectively.[25] CONFIRM-HF was a multicenter, double-blind, placebo-controlled trial that enrolled 304 ambulatory symptomatic HF patients with LVEF ≤45%, elevated natriuretic peptides, and ID (ferritin <100 ng/mL or 100–300 ng/mL if TSAT <20%). Patients were randomized 1:1 to treatment with FCM or placebo. Treatment with FCM significantly prolonged 6MWT distance at week 24 (difference FCM vs placebo, 33 ± 11 m; $p = 0.002$). The treatment effect of FCM was consistent in all subgroups and was sustained to week 52 (difference FCM vs placebo, 36 ± 11 m; $p < 0.001$). Throughout the study, an improvement in NYHA class, PGA, QoL, and fatigue score in patients treated with FCM was detected with statistical significance observed from week 24 onward. Treatment with FCM was associated with a significant reduction in the risk of hospitalizations for worsening HF (HR, 0.39; 95% CI, 0.19–0.82; $p = 0.009$). Incidence of deaths and adverse events were comparable between both groups.[26] EFFECT-HF trial was a prospective randomized, controlled, multicenter, open-label trial of 172 patients with blinded end-point evaluation that examined the effect of treatment with IV ferric carboxymaltose compared with standard of care on exercise capacity in patients with symptomatic chronic HF and ID. There were no differences between study and control group on peak VO_2 ($p = 0.93$). Patients with anemia did not benefit more than patients without anemia (p for interaction = 0.758), and in patients treated with FCM, there was no association between the change in hemoglobin and the change in peak VO_2 (for FCM, $r = 0.0758$, $p = 0.51$). Patients in the FCM had improved NYHA class compared with the control group ($p < 0.05$). PGA was favorably affected in FCM group at 12 and 24 weeks post-treatment ($p < 0.05$). B-type natriuretic peptide and NT-proBNP were similar at baseline in both groups, but there was no statistical change in values between the two groups. No hypersensitivity reactions to FCM or hypophosphatemia were reported.[27] There were two meta-analysis published in 2016 and 2017 which indicate that IV iron therapy has beneficial effects in reducing mortality and rehospitalization in HF patients apart from its effects on QoL, NYHA class, and exercise capacity.[28,29] With this proof of principle, there are ongoing trials like FAIR-HF2 and HEART-FID which will evaluate effect of FCM in reducing hard end-points like mortality and rehospitalization in HF. We have sufficient data of utility of IV iron in HFrEF, however, the situation in HF with preserved ejection fraction (HFpEF) is less clear, and another prospective trial, the FAIR-HFpEF trial. Then, AFFIRM-AHF (Study to Compare FCM With Placebo in Patients With Acute Heart Failure and Iron Deficiency) trial, a randomized, double-blind placebo-controlled trial is comparing the effect of IV FCM in patients with ID who are hospitalized for acute HF.

GUIDELINE DIRECTED TREATMENT OF IRON DEFICIENCY IN HF

Diagnostic algorithm for the treatment of ID in HF in accordance ESC guidelines has been depicted in Flowchart 2.[30] ESC recommends that that all patients with HF should be tested for ID by using serum assessment of ferritin and TSAT. Anemia should be ruled out by using complete blood count assessment both are class I, level of evidence: C recommendations. IV ferric carboxymaltose should be considered in symptomatic patients (serum ferritin <100 mg/L, or ferritin between 100 mg/L and 299 mg/L and TSAT <20%) in order to alleviate HF symptoms and improve exercise capacity and QoL with class IIa, level of evidence: A recommendations.[21] The American Heart Association (AHA)/American College of Cardiology (ACC) guidelines of 2017 recommend that in patients with NYHA functional class II and III HF and ID (ferritin <100 mg/L or 100–300 mg/L if TSAT is < 20%), IV iron replacement might be reasonable to improve functional status and QoL (class

Flowchart 2: Diagnostic algorithm for treatment of iron deficiency in patients with HF according to ESC guidelines and expert consensus recommendations.[30]

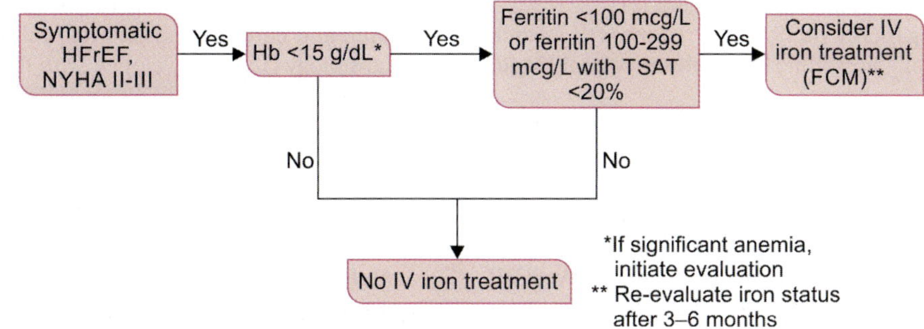

(FCM: ferric carboxymaltose; HFrEF: heart failure with reduced ejection fraction; HF; heart failure; IV: intravenous; NYHA: New York Heart Association; TSAT: transferrin saturation)

TABLE 2: Guidelines for the treatment of ID in heart failure.

	Guidelines description	*Class of recommendation*
American Heart Association	In patients with HFrEF with NYHA class II or III and ID, IV iron replacement might be reasonable to improve functional status and quality of life	IIb
European Society of Cardiology	IV FCM should be considered in symptomatic patients with HFrEF and ID to alleviate symptoms and improve exercise capacity and quality of life	IIa

(FCM: ferric carboxymaltose; HFrEF: heart failure with reduced ejection fraction; ID: iron deficiency; IV: intravenous; NYHA: New York Heart Association)

IIb level of evidence) (Table 2).[31] ESC recommends use of FCM, however, ACC/AHA does not mention any specific iron preparation. There are certain small studies with iron sucrose in HF, however, as the major randomized data is with FCM, the authors believe that FCM should be the iron preparation of choice. Regarding erythropoietin stimulating agents (ESA), ACC/AHA gives class III recommendation (contraindication) for use of ESA in patients with HF. The maximum dose of FCM is 1,000 mg or 1 g in one sitting and if the estimated deficit is more than 1 g, repeat infusion can be given after 2 weeks of initial dose.

CONCLUSION

Iron deficiency is widely present in patients with HFrEF (almost 50%) and is independent predictor of worse functional capacity and survival with or without the presence of anemia. It is defined as—ferritin <100 µg/dL or ferritin of 100–299 µg/dL with a TSAT <20%. All HFrEF patients should be screened for ID and an iron deficit should be calculated using Ganzoni's formula. IV iron therapy using iron FCM should be used to treat ID as oral iron therapy not beneficial in HFrEF. There is fair amount of evidence showing improvement in patient-reported outcomes and functional capacity and there is ongoing research to study mortality and rehospitalization benefit.

REFERENCES

1. Felker GM, Adams KF Jr, Gattis WA, et al. Anemia as a risk factor and therapeutic target in heart failure. J Am Coll Cardiol. 2004;44(5):959-66.
2. Al-Ahmad A, Rand WM, Manjunath G, et al. Reduced kidney function and anemia as risk factors for mortality in patients with left ventricular dysfunction. J Am Coll Cardiol. 2001;38(4):955-62.
3. Anker S, Coats AJS, Roecker EB, et al. Hemoglobin level is associated with mortality and hospitalization in patients with severe chronic heart failure: results from the COPERNICUS study. J Am Coll Cardiol. 2004;43(suppl A).
4. Groenveld HF, Januzzi JL, Damman K, et al. Anemia and mortality in heart failure patients a systematic review and meta-analysis. J Am Coll Cardiol. 2008;52(10):818-27.
5. Adams KF Jr, Patterson JH, Oren RM, et al. Prospective assessment of the occurrence of anemia in patients with heart failure: results from the Study of Anemia in a Heart Failure Population (STAMINA-HFP) Registry. Am Heart J. 2009;157(5):926-32.
6. Anand IS, Gupta P. Anemia and iron deficiency in heart failure: Current concepts and emerging therapies. Circulation. 2018;138(1):80-98.
7. Silverberg DS, Wexler D, Blum M, et al. The use of subcutaneous erythropoietin and intravenous iron for the treatment of the anemia of severe, resistant congestive heart failure improves cardiac and renal function and functional cardiac class, and markedly reduces hospitalizations. J Am Coll Cardiol. 2000;35:1737-44.

8. Kotecha D, Ngo K, Walters JA, et al. Erythropoietin as a treatment of anemia in heart failure: systematic review of randomized trials. Am Heart J. 2011;161:822-31.
9. Swedberg K, Young JB, Anand IS, et al. Treatment of anemia with darbepoetin alfa in systolic heart failure. N Engl J Med. 2013;368:1210-9.
10. Bolger AP, Bartlett FR, Penston HS, et al. Intravenous iron alone for the treatment of anemia in patients with chronic heart failure. J Am Coll Cardiol. 2006;48:1225-7.
11. Toblli JE, Lombraña A, Duarte P, et al. Intravenous iron reduces NT-pro-brain natriuretic peptide in anemic patients with chronic heart failure and renal insufficiency. J Am Coll Cardiol. 2007;50:1657-65.
12. Dunn LL, Suryo Rahmanto Y, Richardson DR. Iron uptake and metabolism in the new millennium. Trends Cell Biol. 2007;17:93-100.
13. Andrews NC. Closing the iron gate. N Engl J Med. 2012;366:376-7.
14. Brownlie T 4th, Utermohlen V, Hinton PS, et al. Tissue iron deficiency without anemia impairs adaptation in endurance capacity after aerobic training in previously untrained women. Am J Clin Nutr. 2004;79:437-43.
15. Dong F, Zhang X, Culver B, et al. Dietary iron deficiency induces ventricular dilation, mitochondrial ultrastructural aberrations and cytochrome c release: involvement of nitric oxide synthase and protein tyrosine nitration. Clin Sci (Lond). 2005;109:277-86.
16. Maeder MT, Khammy O, dos Remedios C, et al. Myocardial and systemic iron depletion in heart failure implications for anemia accompanying heart failure. J Am Coll Cardiol. 2011;58:474-80.
17. Jankowska EA, Rozentryt P, Witkowska A, et al. Iron deficiency predicts impaired exercise capacity in patients with systolic chronic heart failure. J Card Fail. 2011;17:899-906.
18. Jankowska EA, Rozentryt P, Witkowska A, et al. Iron deficiency: an ominous sign in patients with systolic chronic heart failure. Eur Heart J. 2010;31:1872-80.
19. Yeo TJ, Yeo PS, Ching-Chiew Wong R, et al. Iron deficiency in a multi-ethnic Asian population with and without heart failure: prevalence, clinical correlates, functional significance and prognosis. Eur J Heart Fail. 2014;16: 1125-32.
20. Klip IT, Comin-Colet J, Voors AA, et al. Iron deficiency in chronic heart failure: an international pooled analysis. Am Heart J. 2013;165:575-82.
21. Ponikowski P, Voors AA, Anker SD, et al. 2016 ESC Guidelines for the diagnosis and treatment of acute and chronic heart failure: The task force for the diagnosis and treatment of acute and chronic heart failure of the European Society of Cardiology (ESC). Developed with the special contribution of the Heart Failure Association (HFA) of the ESC. Eur J Heart Fail. 2016;18:891-975.
22. Ganzoni AM. Intravenous iron-dextran: therapeutic and experimental possibilities. Schweiz Med Wochenschr. 1970;100:301-3.
23. Beck-da-Silva L, Piardi D, Soder S, et al. IRONHF study: a randomized trial to assess the effects of iron in heart failure patients with anemia. Int J Cardiol. 2013;168:3439-42.
24. Lewis GD, Malhotra R, Hernandez AF, et al. Effect of oral iron repletion on exercise capacity in patients with heart failure with reduced ejection fraction and iron deficiency: the IRONOUTHF randomized clinical trial. JAMA. 2017;317:1958-66.
25. Anker SD, Comin Colet J, Filippatos G, et al. Ferric carboxymaltose in patients with heart failure and iron deficiency. N Engl J Med. 2009;361:2436-48.
26. Ponikowski P, van Veldhuisen DJ, Comin-Colet J, et al. Beneficial effects of long-term intravenous iron therapy with ferric carboxymaltose in patients with symptomatic heart failure and iron deficiency. Eur Heart J. 2015;36(11):657-68.
27. van Veldhuisen DJ, Ponikowski P, van derMeer P, et al. Effect of ferric carboxymaltose on exercise capacity in patients with chronic heart failure and iron deficiency. Circulation. 2017;136:1374-83.
28. Jankowska EA, Tkaczyszyn M, Suchocki T, et al. Effects of intravenous iron therapy in iron deficient patients with systolic heart failure: A meta-analysis of randomized controlled trials. Eur J Heart Fail. 2016;18:786-95.
29. Anker SD, Kirwan BA, van Veldhuisen DJ, et al. Effects of ferric carboxymaltose on hospitalisations and mortality rates in iron-deficient heart failure patients: an individual patient data meta-analysis. Eur J Heart Fail. 2018;20:125-33.
30. vonHaehling S, Ebner N, Evertz R, et al. Iron Deficiency in Heart Failure: An Overview. JACC Heart Fail. 2019;7(1):36-46.
31. Yancy CW, Jessup M, Bozkurt B, et al. 2017 ACC/AHA/ HFSA focused update of the 2013 ACCF/AHA guideline for the management of heart failure: a report of the American College of Cardiology/American Heart Association Task Force on Clinical Practice Guidelines and the Heart Failure Society of America. Circulation. 2017;36(6):e137-161.

SECTION 11

Heart Failure and Cardio-oncology

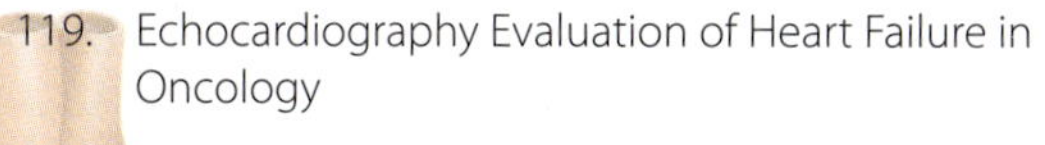

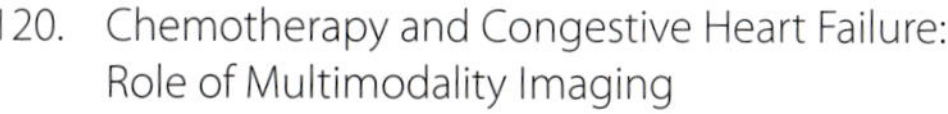

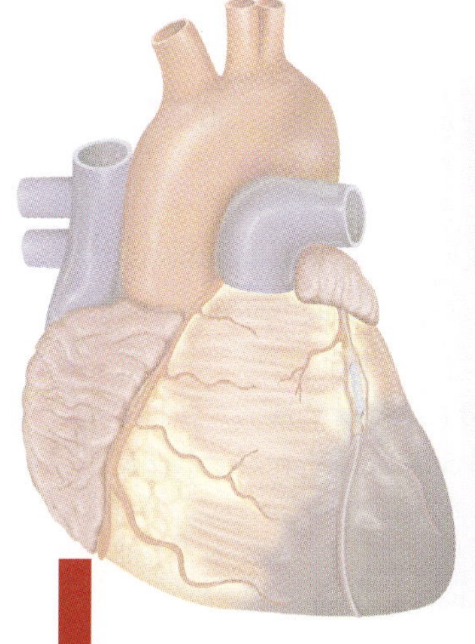

Echocardiography Evaluation of Heart Failure in Oncology

Madhu Mary Minz, Manish Bansal, Ravi R Kasliwal, HK Chopra

INTRODUCTION

According to the World Health Organization, cancer is the second largest cause of death globally and has accounted for about 9.6 million deaths in 2018.[1] India recorded about 3.9 million cancer cases in 2016 according to National Cancer Program of the Indian council of Medical Research. The medical science has made great advancements in combating cancer with significant improvements in survival rates. However, these achievements have come at the expense of cancer therapy related complications, most notably, those affecting the cardiovascular system. Indeed, cardiovascular complications are amongst the leading causes of death in patients who have been successfully cured of their cancers. Therefore, prevention, prompt recognition, and effective management of cardiac complications assume great significance in the overall management of the cancer patients.

WHAT IS CARDIOTOXICITY

Cancer-related cardiotoxicity is defined as any cardiac injury (functional or structural) due to the cancer itself, or cancer treatment—be it chemotherapy, radiation or both. The conventional chemotherapeutics, some of the newer anticancer signaling inhibitors and radiation therapy carry a substantial risk of premature cardiovascular complications, which may include:

- Myocardial dysfunction and heart failure
- Myocardial ischemia
- Arterial hypertension
- Arrhythmia/QT prolongation
- Valvular heart disease
- Thromboembolic disease
- Pericardial disease
- Peripheral vascular disease.

Table 1 summarizes mechanisms of common cardiac complications related to various cancer chemotherapeutic drugs.[2]

Myocardial dysfunction is the most commonly recognized and the most dreadful cardiac complication of cancer drugs. This chapter provides an overview of recognition and management of cancer therapy-related myocardial dysfunction, with emphasis on the role of echocardiography.

Several definitions have been proposed for cancer therapy-related cardiac dysfunction (CTRCD). The Cardiac Review and Evaluation Committee supervising trastuzumab trials defined CTRCD as one or more of the following:[3]

- Cardiomyopathy with decrease in left ventricular ejection fraction (LVEF) globally or due to regional changes in interventricular septum contraction
- Symptoms associated with heart failure
- Signs of heart failure like S3 gallop, tachycardia or both
- Decline in LVEF of at least 5–<55% with signs and symptoms of heart failure or asymptomatic decrease in LVEF of at least 10–<55%.

More recently, the American Society of Echocardiography (ASE) and the European Association of Cardiovascular Imaging (EACVI) have jointly proposed that >10% decline in LVEF to <53% confirmed on two examinations at least 2–3 weeks apart should be taken as CTRCD.[4]

TABLE 1: Mechanisms of common cardiac complications related to cancer chemotherapeutic drugs.

Drug	*Cancers for which used*	*Cardiac toxicity*
Anthracyclines		
Doxorubicin and epirubicin	Breast, lymphoma, lung, and leukemia	Myocardial injury due to oxidative stress and irreversible damage to cardiomyocytes membrane
Antimetabolites		
Capecitabine	Breast, colon	Myocardial ischemia, endothelial cell injury, and thrombosis
5-Fluorouracil	Breast, gastric	Endothelial cell injury, arterial vasospasm, and myocardial ischemia
Monoclonal antibodies		
Trastuzumab	Breast, gastric	Changes in contractile protein and mitochondria
Bevacizumab	Breast, colon, lung	Arterial hypertension, endothelial cell injury, venous/ arterial thrombosis
Alkylating agents		
Cyclophosphamide	Lymphoma, leukemia, and myeloma	Myocardial ischemia and endothelial cell injury
Cisplatin	Testicular, ovary	Arterial hypertension
Antimicrotubule agents		
Vinca alkaloids (vincristine, vinblastine)	Breast, lymphoma	Myocardial ischemia, arterial hypertension
Taxanes (paclitaxel and docetaxel)	Breast, lung	Myocardial ischemia
Tyrosine kinase inhibitors		
Lapatinib and sunitinib	Breast, lung, gastric	Arterial hypertension, thrombosis
Proteasome inhibitors		
Bortezomib, carfilzomib, and ixazomib	Myeloma	Proteasome injury

Myocardial injury occurs due to direct or indirect action of chemotherapy and depends on drug accumulative dose, preparation, route of administration, and sequential/ concomitant use of other drugs. Additionally, certain cardiovascular peptides like copeptin have been implicated in myocardial injury independent of the treatment in cases of breast cancer.[5] Finally, the recently published CANTOS (Canakinumab Anti-inflammatory Thrombosis Outcomes Study) trial has also suggested the role of interleukein-1β signaling pathway and inflammation in the pathogenesis of cancers.[6]

Myocardial injury due to cancer chemotherapy can be broadly categorized into two types:[7]

1. Type 1—irreversible injury or structural injury as with anthracyclines, and
2. Type 2—reversible injury and no structural abnormality as in case of trastuzumab.

This distinction is important for defining monitoring protocols for various cancer drugs.

Apart from chemotherapy, radiation therapy is also known to result in cardiac complications. Supradiaphragmatic radiation can lead to accelerated atherosclerosis, myocardial injury, plaque rupture, thrombosis, valve disease, and pericardial involvement. These can present as acute coronary syndrome or arrhythmias immediately after irradiation, or several years later as valvular, pericardial, or myocardial fibrosis.[8]The total dose of radiation therapy (>30–35 Gy), division into frequent fractions (>2 Gy), use of concomitant or sequential cardiotoxic chemotherapy, and certain irradiation techniques predispose the patients to the risk of developing cardiac toxicity postradiation.[9]

DIAGNOSIS OF CANCER THERAPY-RELATED CARDIOTOXICITY

The diagnosis of cancer therapy-related cardiotoxicity requires high index of clinical suspicion and regular monitoring and evaluation, which includes careful clinical examination, electrocardiogram (ECG), use of biomarkers, and cardiac imaging. The patients undergoing cancer treatment should be assessed at baseline for their risk of

TABLE 2: Risk factors for the development of cancer therapy related cardiac dysfunction.

Demographic and traditional risk factors	• Age(<18 years, >50 years) • Diabetes mellitus • Hypertension • Dyslipidemia • Family h/o premature coronary artery disease
Lifestyle risk factors	• Smoking/tobacco consumption • High alcohol intake • Obesity • Sedentary lifestyle
Current heart disease	• Coronary artery disease (previous myocardial infarction, angina, previous coronary revascularization) • Asymptomatic LV systolic dysfunction (LVEF < 50% or high BNP) • Heart failure (with normal/reduced LVEF) • Moderate to severe valvular heart disease with LVH or LV dysfunction • Hypertrophic cardiomyopathy • Dilated cardiomyopathy • Restrictive cardiomyopathy • Cardiac sarcoidosis • Significant cardiac arrhythmias (e.g. atrial fibrillation, ventricular tachyarrhythmias, etc.)
Previous use of cardiotoxic cancer drugs	• Previous anthracycline use • Prior radiotherapy to chest or mediastinum

Based on recommendations from the European Society of Cardiology.[2]

(BNP: brain natriuretic peptide; LV: left ventricular; LVEF: left ventricular ejection fraction; LVH: left ventricular hypertrophy)

developing cardiotoxicity (Table 2). The frequency and components of subsequent evaluation are individualized, depending on the estimated baseline risk, type of cancer and the type of cancer treatment the patient is going to receive.

Clinical History and Examination

The patients with cardiotoxicity are often asymptomatic; hence, the need for a proper clinical history and examination for signs of heart failure like tachycardia, S3 gallop, etc. cannot be overemphasized. High degree of suspicion is warranted while history taking as the usual symptoms of easy fatigue, asthenia, dyspnea, tiredness, etc. which are commonly encountered in cancer patients may indeed be due to cardiac causes.

Electrocardiogram

Electrocardiogram should be done before starting chemotherapy and during the therapy to look for arrhythmias, ST-T changes, QT prolongation, and conduction disturbances. These changes can be transient and nonspecific but still need to be monitored.

Cardiac Biomarkers

Cardiac troponin (cTn) and brain natriuretic peptide (BNP) are the two most commonly used biomarkers for diagnosing cardiac injury in asymptomatic patients receiving chemotherapy. cTn gets released due to injury to cardiomyocytes whereas BNP is a measurement of elevation in LV filling pressure and wall stress. Other biomarker of inflammation (high sensitivity C-reactive protein, interleukin-6, myeloperoxidase, etc.), markers of endothelial dysfunction (plasminogen activator inhibitor, tissue plasminogen activator, etc.), markers of myocardial ischemia (fatty acid binding protein, glycogen phosphorylase binding protein) have also been studied.[10] High sensitivity troponins are good indicator of early cardiac injury in patients treated with trastuzumab and anthracyclines.[11] Both the ASE and the European Society of Cardiology (ESC) recommend measurement of cTn at baseline and during therapy with agents associated with high risk of myocardial dysfunction (e.g. anthracyclines and trastuzumab).[2,4] The exact monitoring protocol varies, as discussed subsequently.

Cardiac Imaging

Cardiac imaging forms the cornerstone of evaluation and management of cardiac complications in patients undergoing treatment for various cancers. The use of LVEF in defining CTRCD makes echocardiography the most integral tool for diagnosis, baseline assessment and serial follow-up of cardiotoxicity. It is also the most preferred tool because of its wider availability, lower cost, noninvasive nature, safety, and repeatability. When needed, other imaging modalities may be used to complement echocardiography. Cardiac magnetic resonance imaging (MRI) is highly accurate for assessment of cardiac structure and function and is therefore used as the reference modality in challenging cases. It is also very useful for evaluation of cardiac masses, pericardial involvement, myocardial fibrosis, and infiltrative conditions.

The role of echocardiography in the evaluation and management of CTRCD is discussed below in greater details.

LV Systolic Function

Cancer therapy-related cardiac dysfunction is diagnosed when there is a decrease in LVEF of >10 percentage points to a value < 53%, confirmed on two examinations at least 2–3 weeks apart.[4] LVEF is determined using the biplane Simpson's method of disks in accordance with the current guidelines from the ASE or other relevant societies.[12] This is done by tracing the LV endocardial border in apical 4-chamber and 2-chamber views at end-diastole and end-systole. If endocardial borders are not well-defined, ultrasonic contrast should be used to improve accuracy and reproducibility. LVEF in the range of >53–73% is considered normal.[4]

Three-dimensional (3D) echocardiography is a more accurate method than two-dimensional (2D) echocardiography for measurement of LVEF. 3D measurement has much lower intraobserver, interobserver, and test-retest variability, and has much better correlation with cardiac MRI.[12,13] For this reason, 3D echocardiography has become the technique of choice for monitoring cardiac effects postchemotherapy.[14] However, it is limited by relative nonavailability, higher cost and the fact that high quality images and expertise are needed to obtain accurate results. For estimation of LVEF by 3D echocardiography, a full-volume dataset of left ventricle is acquired, which can be cropped in any orientation. Processing of this dataset allows estimation of LVEF without any geometric assumptions or mathematical approximations.

Calculation of LVEF should be combined with assessment of wall motion score index. Resting wall motion score index based on 16-segment model of the left ventricle has been shown to be a more sensitive marker of anthracycline-induced CTRCD than LVEF alone.[15]

Vital parameters like heart rate, blood pressure, etc. should be recorded during each echocardiography study to indicate the hydration status of the patient.

LV Diastolic Function

Abnormalities of LV diastolic function occur commonly and may be more sensitive than LVEF for detection of CTRCD. Ganame et al.[16] observed LV diastolic dysfunction just 2 hours after the first dose of anthracycline. More importantly, it was noted that diastolic dysfunction persisted for weeks to months after the therapy even though LVEF was not reduced. Evaluation of mitral inflow pattern and measurement of early diastolic mitral annulus velocity (e') by tissue Doppler provide an indication of LV diastolic function and LV filling pressures.[17] Parameters like mitral inflow E velocity, E/A ratio, lateral mitral e', and lateral mitral S' (i.e. annular systolic velocity) have been shown to represent an early marker of cardiac dysfunction.[18] Left atrial volume estimation, pulmonary artery systolic pressure estimated from tricuspid regurgitation jet, and pulmonary vein flow pattern can also provide additional useful information. In pediatric patients, myocardial performance index [(isovolumic contraction time + isovolumic relaxation time)/ejection time] has been shown to be a predictor of late LV dysfunction post chemotherapy.[19]

Myocardial Strain

Strain is a measure of myocardial deformation and calculates fractional change in the length of the myocardial segment. Strain rate is the rate at which this deformation occurs. Although LV deformation is a complex, multidimensional process, for the sake of simplicity, LV myocardial strain is expressed along three primary coordinates—longitudinal, radial, and circumferential.[20]

Strain imaging has rapidly evolved as an important technique to quantitatively estimate global or regional myocardial mechanical or contractile function and can detect early, subclinical LV dysfunction even before LVEF starts to decrease.[20] Strain imaging can be performed using either tissue Doppler imaging or speckle-tracking; however, tissue Doppler strain is not used routinely because of its angle dependence and poorer signal-noise ratio.

Speckle tracking echocardiography (STE) is the current modality of choice for assessment of myocardial strain.[20] STE overcomes many of the limitations inherent in tissue Doppler imaging. It utilizes computer-based algorithms to bypass technique-based limitations improving accuracy and decreasing inter-/intraobserver variability. It can also measure radial, circumferential, and global strains with 3D analysis of rotational and twist parameters. STE is based on analysis of discrete echo-densities within myocardium, which are referred as "speckles". These speckles form due to interaction of ultrasound beam as it traverses the myocardial tissue. The movement of each speckle is digitally tracked, frame by frame, in all directions of imaging plane and from this data, myocardial velocity, strain, and strain rate are derived. The automated software calculates strain for each myocardial segment, which can be averaged to provide global strain (Figs. 1A to D). Apical 4-chamber, 2-chamber, and 3-chamber views are used for estimating longitudinal strain whereas short-axis views at base, mid and apex of the left ventricle are used for deriving radial and circumferential strain.

Numerous studies have shown that reduction in global longitudinal strain (GLS) is an independent predictor of future development of cardiotoxicity and is able to detect ensuing LV systolic dysfunction even when LVEF is within the normal range (Figs. 1A to D).[11,21-27]

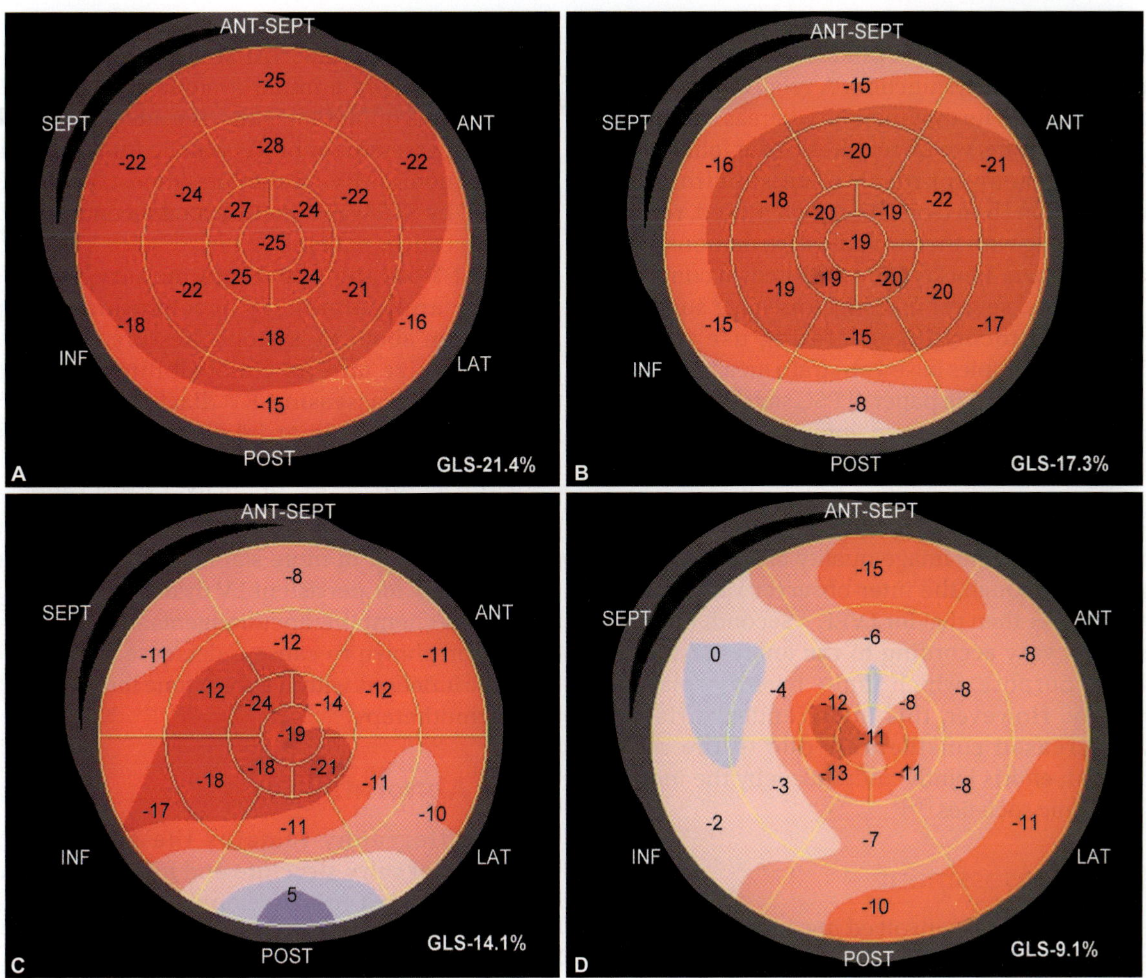

Figs. 1A to D: Different examples of global longitudinal strain (GLS). (A) Normal individual with normal left ventricular ejection fraction (LVEF) and normal GLS. (B, C) patients on chemotherapy with subclinical left ventricular systolic dysfunction (normal LVEF, but reduced GLS), and (D) a patient on chemotherapy with overt LV systolic dysfunction (reduced LVEF 44% with reduced GLS).

In a study by Sawaya et al.[11], 81 women with newly diagnosed HER2-positive breast cancer treated with anthracycline followed by trastuzumab were studied for 15 months using LVEF and peak systolic longitudinal, radial, and circumferential strain. The authors concluded that strain imaging was useful in prediction of subsequent cardiotoxicity and also helped to guide treatment to avoid cardiac side effects.

A systemic review identified six individual studies which had studied the prognostic value of GLS in patients receiving cancer chemotherapy.[28] Subclinical LV dysfunction as defined by GLS had a sensitivity of 65–86% and specificity of 73–95% for predicting subsequent decline in LVEF and/or development of heart failure.

Previous observations and randomized studies have shown that administration of various cardioprotective therapies such as beta-blockers, angiotensin converting enzyme inhibitors, statins, etc. can reduce the risk of developing LV systolic dysfunction, reverse the myocardial dysfunction if it has already set in and improve the overall prognosis.[29-33] However, appropriate timing of institution of these therapies remains unclear. Preliminary observations have suggested that strain imaging, by recognizing early, subclinical LV systolic dysfunction, may be useful for this purpose.[34] However, no randomized study has so far been published to determine the incremental value of strain imaging for guiding management of the patients receiving cancer chemotherapy. SUCCOUR (Strain sUrveillance of Chemotherapy for improving Cardiovascular Outcomes) is the first, international, multicentric randomized study currently underway to address this issue.[35] The study has completed recruitment and the preliminary results should become available soon.

Nonetheless, despite the absence of randomized data, both the ASE and the EACVI recommend measuring GLS in patients who are receiving potentially cardiotoxic drugs for early recognition of cardiotoxicity.[4] A relative percentage reduction in GLS ≥15% is considered to represent subclinical LV systolic dysfunction. A relative decrease of <8% is consistent with no dysfunction, whereas a reduction of 8–15% is a gray zone, which requires closer follow-up.

The management approach once subclinical LV systolic dysfunction (based on GLS) is diagnosed, remains uncertain. Keeping with the available data demonstrating beneficial role of beta-blockers and angiotensin converting enzyme inhibitors, several investigators have suggested management protocols incorporating use of these cardioprotective therapies based on strain measurement.[36] However, the 2016 position paper of ESC states that "cancer treatment should not be stopped, interrupted, or reduced in dose based on a new GLS reduction alone".[2]

At this point, it is imperative to recognize some of the important limitations of strain imaging. First, STE is highly dependent on the image quality and the expertise of the examiner, though the inter-observer variability for GLS is much lower than that for LVEF.[37] Second, the strain measurements vary according to the analysis software used for this purpose, which limits its cross-platform comparability. However, this inter-vendor variability has now decreased considerably due to the recent standardization efforts jointly undertaken by the industry and the academic societies.[38,39]

Right Heart Assessment

The right ventricle can get involved in cancer patients due to preexisting right ventricular (RV) dysfunction, primary or secondary neoplastic involvement or due to cardiotoxic effect of chemotherapy.[40]

Echocardiographic assessment of the right ventricle has remained challenging due to its crescent shape. There is no single 2D echocardiographic plane which allows complete visualization of the RV cavity and as a result, it is not possible to measure RV volume and EF using 2D echocardiography. Hence, M mode, 2D, Doppler, and myocardial strain are all used in combination to evaluate the right heart function.[41] More recently, 3D echocardiography has enabled assessment of RV volumes and EF, but the technique is not yet ready for routine application.[12]

Current guidelines for right heart assessment recommend measuring RV size in parasternal long-axis, short axis, and apical 4-chamber views.[41] RV systolic function is assessed by measuring fractional area change [right ventricular fractional area change (RVFAC)], tricuspid annular plane systolic excursion (TAPSE), tricuspid annular systolic velocity, and RV free wall longitudinal strain. RVFAC is calculated from the RV end-diastolic and end-systolic areas obtained from the RV-focused 4-chamber view. TAPSE and annular systolic velocity track the movement of lateral tricuspid annulus and are measured in the RV-focused apical 4-chamber view. TAPSE is derived using M-mode, whereas tricuspid annular systolic velocity is measured using tissue Doppler imaging. The advent of STE has now simplified assessment of RV systolic function by allowing measurement of RV strain. The importance of RV strain obtained by STE was demonstrated recently in a cohort of 35 breast cancer patients.[42]

Apart from the above, pulmonary artery systolic pressure and pulmonary acceleration time provide information about RV systolic pressure, whereas inferior vena cava size and its collapsibility with respiration are helpful in assessing RV diastolic pressure (which is equivalent to right atrial pressure in the absence of tricuspid inflow obstruction).

Although RV dysfunction is not taken into account in the diagnosis of cardiotoxicity, concomitant RV dysfunction may be a marker of more significant cardiac injury and a potential risk for persistent LV dysfunction during follow-up.[43] Some chemotherapeutic agents such as anthracycline have been shown to cause a decrease in RV systolic and diastolic functions within a short time interval after starting the chemotherapy.[40]

Valve Abnormalities

Echocardiography remains the gold standard for evaluation of valve structure and function.[44,45] The valves can get involved in cancer patients due to neoplastic infiltration or due to the impingement by the tumors. Additionally, nonbacterial thrombotic endocarditis or infective endocarditis can also affect the valves which can lead to impaired valve function, regurgitation, or thromboembolism.[46] Functional regurgitation due to annular dilatation or tethering is seen secondary to ventricular dysfunction. Chemotherapy agents directly do not affect the valves, but pancytopenia caused due to chemotherapy can lead to bacteremia, increasing the risk for endocarditis, especially in patients with predisposing valve lesions like prolapse and bicuspid aortic valves or with indwelling central venous catheters. Concomitant or previous exposure to radiotherapy is known to affect valvular apparatus.[47,48]

Pericardial Involvement

Pericardial involvement can occur due to neoplastic involvement, radiotherapy or certain cancer chemotherapies such as anthracycline, cyclophosphamide, and cytarabine.[49] It can manifest as pericarditis, pericardial effusion, constrictive pericarditis, or cardiac tamponade. Constrictive pericarditis is more often associated with radiotherapy induced cardiotoxicity than with cancer drugs. Echocardiography permits quick recognition of pericardial abnormalities and the assessment of their hemodynamic significance (e.g. tamponade or pericardial constriction). Echocardiography also helps in guiding pericardiocentesis.

Role of Stress Echocardiography

Certain chemotherapeutic agents like 5-fluorouracil, sorafenib, and bevacizumab are known to cause myocardial ischemia. Therefore, in patients undergoing treatment with these agents, stress echocardiography may be required to exclude preexisting coronary artery disease, allow early recognition of CTRCD or to evaluate subclinical LV dysfunction. Additionally, some patients who have a reduced cardiac reserve due to previous exposure to cardiotoxic drugs are advised for stress echocardiography (exercise or pharmacologic) to detect the contractile reserve. Civelli et al. assessed the prognostic value of LV contractile reserve during dobutamine stress echocardiography in 49 female patients undergoing high-dose chemotherapy for poor-prognosis breast cancer.[50] Dobutamine stress echocardiography was performed, before each of the three chemotherapy cycles and at 1, 4, and 7 months after the end of chemotherapy. LV contractile reserve was defined as absolute increase in LVEF from rest to peak dose of dobutamine. It was observed that a 5 unit fall in contractile reserve during serial follow-up of these patients was associated with subsequent reduction in LVEF to <50%. Conversely, in CTRCD, the recovery of LV function during stress echo has been shown to be a predictor of better outcome.[51]

Echocardiographic Monitoring Recommendations

Several different protocols have been recommended for monitoring patients receiving potentially cardiotoxic chemotherapies.[4,36] Figures 2A and B depict the scheme recommended by the ASE.[4] If an agent likely to cause type 1 cardiotoxicity (e.g. anthracyclines) is being used, then evaluation (which includes LVEF, GLS, and cTn) is recommended at baseline, at completion of therapy and 6 months later. If the dose is higher than 240 mg/m^2 of doxorubicin or equivalent, then evaluation is required prior to each additional 50 mg/m^2 dose. In contrast, in patients receiving agents causing type 2 cardiotoxicity (e.g. trastuzumab), evaluation is recommended at baseline and at every 3 months during chemotherapy. Herrmann et al. have proposed a more comprehensive monitoring strategy that takes into account the patient's risk for developing cardiotoxicity.[36] Based on the initial risk assessment, the patients are categorized into very high risk, high risk, intermediate risk, low risk, and very low risk groups (Fig. 3). The subsequent monitoring and management approach are tailored according to the estimated risk.

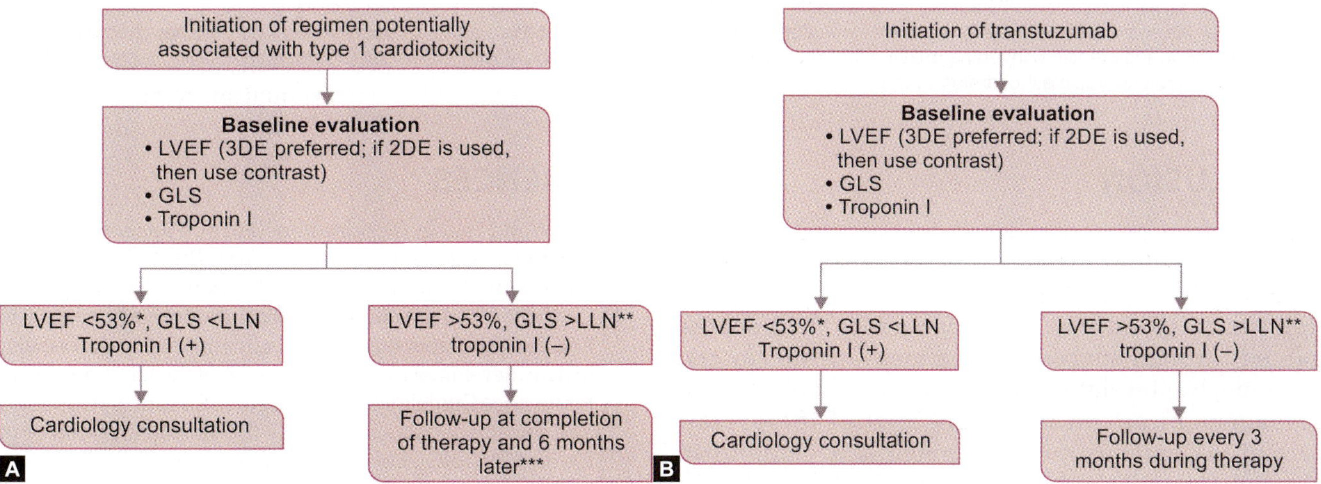

Figs. 2A and B: Monitoring protocol in patients receiving potentially cardiotoxic chemotherapy, as recommended by the American Society of Echocardiography.[4]

* Consider confirmation with cardiac magnetic resonance imaging

** For the reference ranges, please refer the guideline document[4]

*** If the cumulative dose is more than 240 mg/m^2 (or equivalent), recommend measurement of LVEF, GLS and troponin prior to each additional 50 mg/m^2 dose.

(2DE: two-dimensional echocardiography; 3DE: three-dimensional echocardiography; GLS: global longitudinal strain; LLN: lower limit of normal; LVEF: left ventricular ejection fraction)

Step 1: Risk assessment	
Medication-related risk	**Patient-related risk factors**
• **High (risk score 4):** Anthracyclines, Cyclophosphamide, ifosfamide, Clofarabine, Herceptin • **Intermediate (risk score 2):** Docetaxel, Pertuzumab, Sunitinib, Sorafinib • **Low (risk score 1):** Dasatinib, Imatinib, Lapatinib • **Rare (risk score o):** For example, Etoposide, Rituximab, Thalidomide	• Cardiomyopathy or heart failure • Coronary artery disease or equivalent • Hypertension • Diabetes mellitus • Prior or concurrent anthracycline • Prior or concurrent chest radiation • Age <15 or >65 years • Female gender

Step 2: Risk categories	
Categories	**Risk score***
Very high risk	>6
High risk	5–6
Intermediate risk	3–4
Low risk	1–2
Very low risk	0

Step 3: Monitoring and management protocol	
Monitoring protocol	**Management protocol****
• **Routine-** TTE with strain at baseline, before every cycle, at the end of therapy, 3–6 months after completion of therapy and every year thereafter • **Optional-** ECG and cTn with echocardiography during chemotherapy	Initiate ACE-I/ARB, carvedilol, and statins, starting at lowest dose and start chemotherapy in 1 week from initiation to allow steady state, up-titrate as tolerated
• **Routine-** TTE with strain every 3 cycle, end of therapy, 3–6 months and 1 year after chemotherapy; • **Optional-** ECG, cTn with echocardiography during chemotherapy	Initiate ACE-I/ARB, carvedilol, and/or statins
• **Routine-** Echocardiography with strain imaging mid-term, end, and 3–6 months after chemotherapy • **Optional-** ECG, cTn mid-term of chemotherapy	Discuss risk and benefit of medications
• **Optional-** Echocardiography with strain imaging and/or ECG, cTn at the end of chemotherapy	None, monitoring only
• None	None, monitoring only

Fig. 3: Risk assessment. Monitoring and management protocol for patients undergoing cancer chemotherapy, as recommended by Herrmann et al.[36]

* Risk score is calculated by adding drug-related risk score to the number of patient-related risk factors

** Management recommendations are for institution of preventive measures before and with abnormalities during/after chemotherapy. (ACE-I: angiotensin converting enzyme inhibitor; ARB: angiotensin receptor blocker; cTn: cardiac troponin; ECG: electrocardiogram; TTE: transthoracic echocardiography)

CONCLUSION

Cardiotoxicity, primarily CTRCD, is amongst the leading causes of death in patients who have otherwise been successfully treated for their cancers. It is really an unfortunate event that virtually outdoes the benefits gained through successful treatment of the cancer. Accordingly, prevention, early recognition, and effective management are an important goal of the overall care of the patients receiving potentially cardiotoxic chemotherapies. Echocardiography is the most commonly utilized modality for this purpose and is pivotal in the management of these patients. The advent of myocardial strain imaging has rendered echocardiography more sensitive for detection of early CTRCD, though the true incremental value of strain imaging for this purpose is yet to be determined.

REFERENCES

1. The World Health Organization. (2018). Cancer fact sheets. [online] Available from https://www.who.int/news-room/fact-sheets/detail/cancer [Last Accessed November 2019].
2. Zamorano JL, Lancellotti P, Rodriguez Munoz D, et al. 2016 ESC Position Paper on cancer treatments and cardiovascular toxicity developed under the auspices of the ESC Committee for Practice Guidelines: The Task Force for cancer treatments and cardiovascular toxicity of the European Society of Cardiology (ESC). Eur Heart J. 2016;37:2768-801.
3. Seidman A, Hudis C, Pierri MK, et al. Cardiac dysfunction in the trastuzumab clinical trials experience. J Clin Oncol. 2002;20:1215-21.
4. Plana JC, Galderisi M, Barac A, et al. Expert consensus for multimodality imaging evaluation of adult patients during and after cancer therapy: a report from the American Society of Echocardiography and the European Association of

Cardiovascular Imaging. J Am Soc Echocardiogr. 2014;27: 911-39.
5. Pavo N, Raderer M, Hulsmann M, et al. Cardiovascular biomarkers in patients with cancer and their association with all-cause mortality. Heart. 2015;101:1874-80.
6. Baylis RA, Gomez D, Mallat Z, et al. The CANTOS trial: one important step for clinical cardiology but a giant leap for vascular biology. Arterioscler Thromb Vasc Biol. 2017;37:e174-7.
7. Ewer MS, Lippman SM. Type II chemotherapy-related cardiac dysfunction: time to recognize a new entity. J Clin Oncol. 2005;23:2900-2.
8. Cuomo JR, Sharma GK, Conger PD, et al. Novel concepts in radiation-induced cardiovascular disease. World J Cardiol. 2016;8:504-19.
9. Mozdzanowska D, Wozniewski M. Radiotherapy and anthracyclines—cardiovascular toxicity. Contemp Oncol (Pozn). 2015;19:93-7.
10. Tan LL, Lyon AR. Role of biomarkers in prediction of cardiotoxicity during cancer treatment. Curr Treat Options Cardiovasc Med. 2018;20:55.
11. Sawaya H, Sebag IA, Plana JC, et al. Assessment of echocardiography and biomarkers for the extended prediction of cardiotoxicity in patients treated with anthracyclines, taxanes, and trastuzumab. Circ Cardiovasc Imaging. 2012;5:596-603.
12. Lang RM, Badano LP, Mor-Avi V, et al. Recommendations for cardiac chamber quantification by echocardiography in adults: an update from the American Society of Echocardiography and the European Association of Cardiovascular Imaging. J Am Soc Echocardiogr. 2015;28:1-39.
13. Jenkins C, Moir S, Chan J, et al. Left ventricular volume measurement with echocardiography: a comparison of left ventricular opacification, three-dimensional echocardiography, or both with magnetic resonance imaging. Eur Heart J. 2009;30:98-106.
14. Mor-Avi V, Lang RM. Is echocardiography reliable for monitoring the adverse cardiac effects of chemotherapy? J Am Coll Cardiol. 2013;61:85-7.
15. Bountioukos M, Doorduijn JK, Roelandt JR, et al. Repetitive dobutamine stress echocardiography for the prediction of anthracycline cardiotoxicity. Eur J Echocardiogr. 2003;4:300-5.
16. Ganame J, Claus P, Uyttebroeck A, et al. Myocardial dysfunction late after low-dose anthracycline treatment in asymptomatic pediatric patients. J Am Soc Echocardiogr. 2007;20:1351-8.
17. Nagueh SF, Smiseth OA, Appleton CP, et al. Recommendations for the Evaluation of left ventricular diastolic function by echocardiography: An update from the American Society of Echocardiography and the European Association of Cardiovascular Imaging. J Am Soc Echocardiogr. 2016;29: 277-314.
18. Nagiub M, Nixon JV, Kontos MC. Ability of nonstrain diastolic parameters to predict doxorubicin-induced cardiomyopathy: a systematic review with meta-analysis. Cardiol Rev. 2018;26:29-34.
19. Ayhan SS, Ozdemir K, Kayrak M, et al. The evaluation of doxorubicin-induced cardiotoxicity: comparison of Doppler and tissue Doppler-derived myocardial performance index. Cardiology J. 2012;19:363-8.
20. Mor-Avi V, Lang RM, Badano LP, et al. Current and evolving echocardiographic techniques for the quantitative evaluation of cardiac mechanics: ASE/EAE consensus statement on methodology and indications endorsed by the Japanese Society of Echocardiography. J Am Soc Echocardiogr. 2011;24:277-313.
21. Hare JL, Brown JK, Leano R, et al. Use of myocardial deformation imaging to detect preclinical myocardial dysfunction before conventional measures in patients undergoing breast cancer treatment with trastuzumab. Am Heart J. 2009;158:294-301.
22. Stoodley PW, Richards DA, Hui R, et al. Two-dimensional myocardial strain imaging detects changes in left ventricular systolic function immediately after anthracycline chemotherapy. Eur J Echocardiogr. 2011;12:945-52.
23. Poterucha JT, Kutty S, Lindquist RK, et al. Changes in left ventricular longitudinal strain with anthracycline chemotherapy in adolescents precede subsequent decreased left ventricular ejection fraction. J Am Soc Echocardiogr. 2012;25:733-40.
24. Jurcut R, Wildiers H, Ganame J, et al. Strain rate imaging detects early cardiac effects of pegylated liposomal Doxorubicin as adjuvant therapy in elderly patients with breast cancer. J Am Soc Echocardiogr. 2008;21:1283-9.
25. Negishi K, Negishi T, Hare JL, et al. Independent and incremental value of deformation indices for prediction of trastuzumab-induced cardiotoxicity. J Am Soc Echocardiogr. 2013;26:493-8.
26. Sawaya H, Sebag IA, Plana JC, et al. Early detection and prediction of cardiotoxicity in chemotherapy-treated patients. Am J Cardiol. 2011;107:1375-80.
27. Tsai HR, Gjesdal O, Wethal T, et al. Left ventricular function assessed by two-dimensional speckle tracking echocardiography in long-term survivors of Hodgkin's lymphoma treated by mediastinal radiotherapy with or without anthracycline therapy. Am J Cardiol. 2011;107:472-7.
28. Thavendiranathan P, Poulin F, Lim KD, et al. Use of myocardial strain imaging by echocardiography for the early detection of cardiotoxicity in patients during and after cancer chemotherapy: a systematic review. J Am Coll Cardiol. 2014;63:2751-68.
29. Cardinale D, Colombo A, Sandri MT, et al. Prevention of high-dose chemotherapy-induced cardiotoxicity in high-risk patients by angiotensin-converting enzyme inhibition. Circulation. 2006;114:2474-81.
30. Seicean S, Seicean A, Alan N, et al. Cardioprotective effect of beta-adrenoceptor blockade in patients with breast cancer undergoing chemotherapy: follow-up study of heart failure. Circ Heart Fail. 2013;6:420-6.
31. Seicean S, Seicean A, Plana JC, et al. Effect of statin therapy on the risk for incident heart failure in patients with breast cancer receiving anthracycline chemotherapy: an

observational clinical cohort study. J Am Coll Cardiol. 2012;60:2384-90.
32. Bosch X, Rovira M, Sitges M, et al. Enalapril and carvedilol for preventing chemotherapy-induced left ventricular systolic dysfunction in patients with malignant hemopathies: the OVERCOME trial (preventiOn of left Ventricular dysfunction with Enalapril and caRvedilol in patients submitted to intensive ChemOtherapy for the treatment of Malignant hEmopathies). J Am Coll Cardiol. 2013;61:2355-62.
33. Cardinale D, Colombo A, Lamantia G, et al. Anthracycline-induced cardiomyopathy: clinical relevance and response to pharmacologic therapy. J Am Coll Cardiol. 2010;55:213-20.
34. Negishi K, Negishi T, Haluska BA, et al. Use of speckle strain to assess left ventricular responses to cardiotoxic chemotherapy and cardioprotection. Eur Heart J Cardiovasc Imaging. 2014;15:324-31.
35. Negishi T, Thavendiranathan P, Negishi K, et al. Rationale and design of the strain surveillance of chemotherapy for improving cardiovascular outcomes: The SUCCOUR trial. JACC Cardiovasc Imaging. 2018;11:1098-105.
36. Herrmann J, Lerman A, Sandhu NP, et al. Evaluation and management of patients with heart disease and cancer: cardio-oncology. Mayo Clin Proc. 2014;89:1287-306.
37. Farsalinos KE, Daraban AM, Unlu S, et al. Head-to-Head Comparison of Global Longitudinal Strain Measurements among Nine Different Vendors: The EACVI/ASE Inter-Vendor Comparison Study. J Am Soc Echocardiogr. 2015;28:1171-81.
38. Voigt JU, Pedrizzetti G, Lysyansky P, et al. Definitions for a common standard for 2D speckle tracking echocardiography: consensus document of the EACVI/ASE/Industry task force to standardize deformation imaging. J Am Soc Echocardiogr. 2015;28:183-93.
39. Yang H, Marwick TH, Fukuda N, et al. Improvement in Strain Concordance between Two Major Vendors after the Strain Standardization Initiative. J Am Soc Echocardiogr. 2015;28:642-8.
40. Tanindi A, Demirci U, Tacoy G, et al. Assessment of right ventricular functions during cancer chemotherapy. Eur J Echocardiogr. 2011;12:834-40.
41. Rudski LG, Lai WW, Afilalo J, et al. Guidelines for the echocardiographic assessment of the right heart in adults: a report from the American Society of Echocardiography endorsed by the European Association of Echocardiography, a registered branch of the European Society of Cardiology, and the Canadian Society of Echocardiography. J Am Soc Echocardiogr. 2010;23:685-713.
42. Chang WT, Shih JY, Feng YH, et al. The early predictive value of right ventricular strain in epirubicin-induced cardiotoxicity in patients with breast cancer. Acta Cardiol Sin. 2016;32:550-9.
43. Calleja A, Poulin F, Khorolsky C, et al. Right ventricular dysfunction in patients experiencing cardiotoxicity during breast cancer therapy. J Oncol. 2015;2015:609194.
44. Zoghbi WA, Adams D, Bonow RO, et al. Recommendations for noninvasive evaluation of native valvular regurgitation: A Report from the American Society of Echocardiography Developed in Collaboration with the Society for Cardiovascular Magnetic Resonance. J Am Soc Echocardiogr. 2017;30:303-71.
45. Baumgartner H, Hung J, Bermejo J, et al. Echocardiographic assessment of valve stenosis: EAE/ASE recommendations for clinical practice. J Am Soc Echocardiogr. 2009;22:1-23.
46. Edoute Y, Haim N, Rinkevich D, et al. Cardiac valvular vegetations in cancer patients: a prospective echocardiographic study of 200 patients. Am J Med. 1997;102:252-8.
47. Hamza A, Tunick PA, Kronzon I. Echocardiographic manifestations of complications of radiation therapy. Echocardiography. 2009;26:724-8.
48. Lancellotti P, Nkomo VT, Badano LP, et al. Expert consensus for multi-modality imaging evaluation of cardiovascular complications of radiotherapy in adults: a report from the European Association of Cardiovascular Imaging and the American Society of Echocardiography. J Am Soc Echocardiogr. 2013;26:1013-32.
49. Tohda S, Kobayashi H, Suzuki T, et al. [Acute pericarditis caused by daunorubicin in acute myelocytic leukemia]. Rinsho Ketsueki. 1988;29:874-8.
50. Civelli M, Cardinale D, Martinoni A, et al. Early reduction in left ventricular contractile reserve detected by dobutamine stress echo predicts high-dose chemotherapy-induced cardiac toxicity. Int J Cardiol. 2006;111:120-6.
51. Grosu A, Bombardini T, Senni M, et al. End-systolic pressure/volume relationship during dobutamine stress echo: a prognostically useful non-invasive index of left ventricular contractility. Eur Heart J. 2005;26:2404-12.

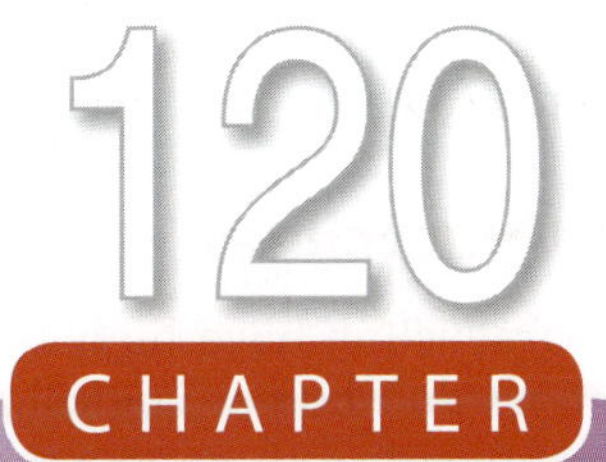

Chemotherapy and Congestive Heart Failure: Role of Multimodality Imaging

Surendra K Chutani, Arun Chutani, Arti Shah, Bharat Kantharia

INTRODUCTION

Advances in treatment have led to improved survival of patients with cancer, but have also increased morbidity and mortality due to treatment side effects. Cardiovascular diseases (CVDs) are one of the most frequent of these side effects, and there is a growing concern that they may lead to premature morbidity and death among cancer survivors. This may be the result of cardiotoxicity, which involves direct effects of the cancer treatment on heart function and structure, or may be due to accelerated development of CVD, especially in the presence of traditional cardiovascular risk factors. The complex issue of CVD because of previous cancer treatment requires the creation of multidisciplinary teams involving specialists in cardiology, oncology, and other related fields. The mutual interest to provide optimal care for patients with cancer and cancer survivors is an important motivation for the development of cardio-oncology teams.

Cardiovascular complications of cancer chemotherapy can be divided into following categories:

- Myocardial dysfunction and heart failure (HF)
- Coronary artery disease (CAD)
- Valvular disease
- Arrhythmias, especially those induced by QT-prolonging drugs
- Arterial hypertension
- Thromboembolic disease
- Peripheral vascular disease and stroke
- Pulmonary hypertension
- Pericardial complications.

CARDIOVASCULAR COMPLICATIONS OF CANCER THERAPY: PATHOPHYSIOLOGY

Myocardial Dysfunction and Heart Failure

Myocardial dysfunction and HF, frequently described as cardiotoxicity, are the most concerning cardiovascular complications of cancer therapies and cause an increase in morbidity and mortality. The time point when cardiotoxicity becomes clinically manifest varies substantially; some cancer treatments induce side effects that appear early after exposure—and therefore may adversely affect oncological therapy—while others generate cardiac injuries resulting in clinical problems only years later. In addition, some cancer drugs, for example, anthracyclines, can induce progressive cardiac remodeling as a late consequence of earlier myocyte damage, resulting in late cardiomyopathy, while others may cause transient cardiac dysfunction without long-term consequences. The prediction of long-term cardiovascular prognosis is frequently challenging because patients with cancer typically receive multiple cancer drugs and sometimes radiation, with the potential for cardiotoxic effects from interactions among the different therapeutic modalities. Left ventricular (LV) dysfunction and HF are relatively common and serious side effects of cancer treatment. Survivors of pediatric cancer, treated with anthracycline and/or mediastinal radiotherapy, have a 15-fold increased lifetime risk for HF compared with matched controls.[1]

Anthracyclines

Anthracycline have high efficacy for treatment of solid tumors and hematological malignancies, and avoiding their use due to concerns about cardiac side effects may negatively affect prognosis. On the other hand, anthracycline may cause irreversible cardiac damage, which in turn affects prognosis. Doxorubicin is associated with a 5% incidence of congestive HF when a cumulative lifetime dose of 400 mg/m^2 is reached, and higher doses lead to an exponential increase in risk, up to 48% at 700 mg/m.

The cardiotoxicity of anthracyclines may be acute, early, or late. Acute toxicity, predominantly supraventricular arrhythmia, transient LV dysfunction, and electrocardiographic (ECG) changes, develops in <1% of patients immediately after infusion and is usually reversible. However, acute cardiac dysfunction may also reflect myocyte injury that eventually can evolve into early or late cardiotoxicity. There are no proven strategies to identify, if cardiac dysfunction is reversible or progressive; however, elevation of cardiac biomarkers may be a way to identify patients at risk for long-term cardiotoxicity. Early effects occur within the first year of treatment, while late effects manifest themselves after several years (median of 7 years after treatment). In patients treated with commonly used anthracycline doses and >65 years of age, the rate of anthracycline-associated HF can be as high as 10%. In addition, if anthracycline-associated cardiac dysfunction is detected early and treated with HF medications, patients frequently have a good functional recovery. Conversely, if patients are identified late after the onset of cardiac dysfunction, HF is typically difficult to treat.

Risk factors for anthracycline-related cardiotoxicity include lifetime cumulative dose, infusion regimen and any condition that increases cardiac susceptibility, including pre-existing cardiac disease, hypertension, concomitant use of other chemotherapies or mediastinal radiation therapy, and older age (>65 years). The developing heart is also particularly vulnerable, and pediatric patients treated with anthracycline are at an exceedingly high risk for anthracycline cardiotoxicity.[2]

Other Conventional Chemotherapies

Other conventional chemotherapies that can induce myocardial dysfunction and HF are cyclophosphamide, cisplatin, ifosfamide, and taxes (paclitaxel and docetaxel). Cyclophosphamide cardiotoxicity is relatively rare and is primarily seen in patients receiving high doses (>140 mg/kg) before bone marrow transplantation. HF typically occurs within days of drug administration, and risk factors include total bolus dose, older age, combination therapy with other cancer drugs, and mediastinal irradiation.

Some alkylating agents similar to cyclophosphamide, such as cisplatin and ifosfamide, infrequently cause HF due to several pathological effects, including myocardial ischemia. Additionally, platinum-containing chemotherapy requires the administration of a high intravenous (IV) volume to avoid platinum-related toxicity. This volume overload in patients with preexisting myocardial impairment, rather than the direct toxicity of these drugs, is often the cause of first or recurrent episodes of HF.

Docetaxel, a drug frequently used in breast cancer, in combination with or after anthracyclines, cyclophosphamide, or trastuzumab, also appears to increase the incidence of HF; however, the contribution of individual agents in multidrug schemes is frequently difficult to assess. Some reports suggest that taxes may be safer in patients with preexisting LV dysfunction, in whom anthracycline should be avoided, but the absolute cardiotoxic risks with taxanes are unknown. However, there is considerable debate with regard to patients with breast cancer for whom the true benefits of using anthracyclines versus taxanes is not as clear as it is for tumors such as lymphomas or sarcomas. The risk-benefit assessment should encompass both the risk factors of the individual patient and the potential efficacy based on the characteristics of the tumor.

IMMUNOTHERAPIES AND TARGETED THERAPIES

More recently, immunotherapies and targeted therapies have led to substantial improvement in the efficacy of cancer drugs. Either inhibition of human epidermal growth factor receptor 2 (HER2) signaling with antibodies [trastuzumab, pertuzumab, trastuzumab-emtansine (T-DM1), or tyrosine kinase inhibitors (TKIs) (lapatinib)] has improved outcomes of patients with HER2-positive breast cancer when used in conjunction with chemotherapies.

When trastuzumab was used concomitantly with antimetabolites and alkylating agents in patients with gastric cancer, the rates of cardiac dysfunction and HF were 5% and <1%, respectively. These data indicate that concomitant or previous use of anthracycline substantially increases the cardiotoxicity of trastuzumab. In a retrospective observational study based on the International Classification of Diseases codes, without access to LVEF data, the cumulative incidence of the composite of cardiac dysfunction or HF in patients treated with anthracycline and trastuzumab was 6.2% and 20.1% after 1 and 5 years, respectively. In contrast to anthracycline, trastuzumab cardiotoxicity typically manifests during treatment. Trastuzumab-induced LV dysfunction and HF are usually reversible with trastuzumab interruption and/or treatment with HF therapies.

The mechanism of anti-HER2 drug-induced cardiotoxicity includes structural and functional changes in contractile proteins and mitochondria, but it rarely leads to cell death, explaining the potential for reversibility. Risk factors for anti-HER2 drug-induced cardiotoxicity include previous exposure to anthracycline, short time, 3 weeks versus 3 months, between anthracycline and anti-HER2 treatment, preexisting arterial hypertension, low LVEF, and older age.

One of the most relevant clinical implications of trastuzumab-induced cardiotoxicity is treatment interruption, which is associated with an increase in cancer recurrence. In patients with HER2-positive breast cancer receiving adjuvant trastuzumab, cardiotoxicity was the most common reason for treatment interruption in 13.5% of patients, 30% for HF and 70% for asymptomatic LVEF decline. In most trastuzumab breast cancer registration trials, treatment was stopped when patients developed HF or (in asymptomatic patients) when LVEF dropped below 45%.

The cardiotoxicity risk of other anti-HER2-targeted therapies (lapatinib, pertuzumab, and T-DM1) appears similar to that of trastuzumab.[3]

INHIBITION OF THE VASCULAR ENDOTHELIAL GROWTH FACTOR SIGNALING PATHWAY

Inhibition of the vascular endothelial growth factor (VEGF) signaling pathway benefits patients diagnosed with one of several different solid cancers, but some of the VEGF inhibitors can cause reversible or irreversible cardiac side effects, particularly when used with or after conventional chemotherapies. In a large trial of patients with breast cancer, where cardiac function was prospectively assessed, the anti-VEGF antibody bevacizumab used after chemotherapy-induced LV dysfunction in 2% of patients and HF [New York Heart Association III or IV (NYHA III or IV)] in 1% of patients. Similarly, cardiotoxicity was found for the TKIs sunitinib, pazopanib, and axitinib. These drugs induce cardiac dysfunction in 3–15% of patients and symptomatic HF in 1–10% of patients. VEGF inhibitors also cause substantial arterial hypertension, potentially affecting cardiac function. Many anti-VEGF cancer drugs inhibit multiple signaling pathways, and identification of the pathophysiological mechanism causing cardiotoxicity.[3]

Inhibition of BCR-ABL Kinase

The inhibition of BCR-ABL kinase by small molecules such as imatinib has profoundly improved the prognosis of patients with several forms of chronic leukemia and some forms of gastrointestinal stromal tumors. Although initial reports suggested a risk for imatinib-induced cardiotoxicity, analysis of large cohorts did not confirm these data. Newer, more potent inhibitors of BCR-ABL, such as nilotinib and ponatinib, have also demonstrated an association with cardiovascular events.

Proteasome Inhibitors

Proteasome inhibitors are a relatively new line of treatment for multiple myeloma. Bortezomib and carfilzomib are the two clinically available drugs potentially causing cardiac dysfunction. Proteasomes, protein complexes responsible for degrading dysfunctional or unneeded proteins, have an important maintenance function in the cardiomyocyte, and cardiac dysfunction and other cardiac issues may be expected if this maintenance function is impaired. The incidence of HF under bortezomib is relatively low (up to 4%) compared with carfilzomib, although it is sometimes aggravated by the concomitant use of steroids. Carfilzomib is a more potent and irreversible proteasomal inhibitor, and preliminary data suggest a substantially higher risk of HF, up to 25%.

Cardiovascular Management of Patients Treated with Anthracyclines

For patients treated with adjuvant anthracycline, baseline cardiac function should be assessed. If systolic dysfunction or significant valvular heart disease (VHD) is found, the patient should be discussed with the oncology team and options for nonanthracycline-containing chemotherapy and/or cardioprotection should be considered. If used, a second assessment of cardiac function should be performed at the end of the treatment, particularly when the patient has an increased risk for cardiotoxicity or consecutive treatment with potentially cardiotoxic targeted therapies will follow. For higher-dose anthracycline-containing regimens and in patients with high baseline risk, earlier assessment of cardiac function after a cumulative total doxorubicin (or equivalent) dose of 240 mg/m^2 should be considered. Measurement of at least one cardiac biomarker—high-sensitivity troponin (I or T) or a natriuretic peptide—may be considered at baseline, and determination of high-sensitivity troponin I has been suggested with each cycle of anthracycline-containing chemotherapy. To date, this suggested strategy has not been validated to prevent or improve longer-term toxicity events, but elevation of cardiac biomarkers identifies patients at greater risk for cardiotoxicity who may benefit from measures to prevent cardiotoxicity.

Patients receiving anti-HER2 therapies frequently, though not always, receive anthracycline before starting the targeted therapy. In such cases, surveillance should begin before anthracycline administration. Standard screening during treatment depends on local protocols and recommendations, but typically, cardiac monitoring is performed every 3 months during and once after completion of anti-HER2 treatment. Some investigators found that the rate of clinically relevant trastuzumab-induced cardiac dysfunction is substantially lower when a confirmatory LV assessment is carried out 3 weeks after an initial asymptomatic LVEF decrease. Several studies have demonstrated an improvement in early detection of LVEF decrease when troponins and speckle tracking echocardiography are used every 3 months during adjuvant trastuzumab treatment. Given the variability in timing of trastuzumab-induced LV dysfunction, measurement of troponin with every cycle may be considered in patients with high baseline risk.[4]

Cardiovascular Management of Patients Treated with VEGF Inhibitors

The optimal timing of surveillance strategies for the various VEGF inhibitors known to cause myocardial dysfunction still needs to be clarified. After baseline assessment, some patients appear to develop LV dysfunction early after treatment onset, whereas in others, this is delayed for several months. If baseline risk is high, it may be appropriate to consider early clinical follow-up in the first 2–4 weeks after starting targeted molecular therapy with, for example, sunitinib, sorafenib, or pazopanib. Thereafter, the drug labels for all of these drugs suggest a periodic reassessment of cardiac function, but do not state specifically when and how. Currently, it is reasonable to consider periodic echocardiography, for example, every 6 months until stability in LVEF values is achieved. However, limited evidence is available to support any specific surveillance strategy. One observational study suggested surveillance every 2–3 months with troponin or N-terminal pro-B-type natriuretic peptide (NT-proBNP), and echocardiography detected myocardial toxicity in 33% of patients taking VEGF inhibitors for renal cell carcinoma.[5]

Diagnostic Tools to Detect Myocardial Toxicity

Electrocardiography

Electrocardiography is recommended in all patients before and during treatment. It is useful to detect any ECG signs of cardiac toxicity, including resting tachycardia, ST-T wave changes, conduction disturbances, QT interval prolongation, or arrhythmias. However, these ECG abnormalities are not specific and can be related to other factors. Of note, these ECG changes can be transitory and are not related to the development of chronic cardiomyopathy.

Echocardiography

Echocardiography is the method of choice for the detection of myocardial dysfunction before, during, and after cancer therapy. Unless three-dimensional (3D) echocardiography is used, which is the best echocardiographic method for measuring LVEF when endocardial definition is clear; the two-dimensional (2D) biplane Simpson method is recommended for estimation of LV volumes and ejection fraction in these patients. Cancer therapeutics-related cardiac dysfunction (CTRCD) is defined as a decrease in the LVEF of >10 percentage points, to a value below the lower limit of normal. This decrease should be confirmed by repeated cardiac imaging done 2–3 weeks after the baseline diagnostic study showing the initial decrease in LVEF. The LVEF decrease may be further categorized as symptomatic or asymptomatic, or with regard to reversibility. Although the exact interval is not established, echocardiographic examination should be repeated during follow-up to confirm recovery, or to detect irreversible LV dysfunction. Echocardiography can also detect other complications of cancer therapy, including valvular and pericardial diseases and findings suggestive of pulmonary hypertension.

The main limitation of 2D echocardiography is its relatively moderate reproducibility, which can be improved by the use of 3D echocardiography. The latter is associated with the best day-to-day reproducibility, but remains dependent on image quality, availability, and operator experience. For serial evaluation of patients with cancer, LVEF measurements should ideally be performed by the same observer with the same equipment to reduce variability. Other useful echocardiographic techniques include contrast echocardiography, indicated in patients with suboptimal echocardiograms to improve delineation of the LV endocardial borders.

Doppler myocardial imaging and deformation imaging is a promising tool and its use should be considered whenever possible. Several recent studies have shown the value of deformation imaging for early detection of LV dysfunction secondary to cancer therapy. Global systolic longitudinal myocardial strain (GLS) has been reported to accurately predict a subsequent decrease in LVEF. A relative percentage reduction of GLS of >15% from baseline is considered abnormal and a marker of early LV subclinical dysfunction. Until standardization of strain imaging through different vendors is fully achieved, the current recommendation is to use the same equipment for the longitudinal follow-up of patients with cancer to facilitate the interpretation of results. These advanced echocardiographic measurements are preferred, when available, to serve as the basis for clinical decisions when performed with adequate expertise at laboratories doing cardiac safety studies. Diastolic dysfunction is common in patients with cancer, both at baseline and during treatment; however, no evidence has shown that treatment should be stopped based on these findings.

Nuclear Cardiac Imaging

Evaluation of LV function using mitigated radionuclide angiography has been used for years to diagnose chemotherapy-induced cardiotoxicity with good accuracy and reproducibility and few technical limitations. However, it is constrained by radiation exposure and provides only limited additional information on cardiac structure and hemodynamics. As echocardiography and mitigated radionuclide angiography have different reference values, the same technique should be performed for baseline and follow-up studies.

Cardiac Magnetic Resonance

Cardiac magnetic resonance (CMR) is a helpful tool for the evaluation of cardiac structure and function. It is useful to determine the cause of LV dysfunction and to clarify left and right ventricular function in challenging cases, i.e. borderline or contradictory results from other imaging modalities. It also serves to evaluate the pericardium, especially in patients with chest irradiation. Late gadolinium imaging may be useful to detect scarring or fibrosis, which may have prognostic implications in the context of impaired LV function. Additionally, CMR is an excellent test for the comprehensive evaluation of cardiac masses and infiltrative conditions. Use of unique tissue characterization capabilities of CMR (e.g. inflammation and edema) will be dependent on acceptance of T2 and T1 mapping and extracellular volume fraction quantification. Diffuse anthracycline fibrosis cannot be evaluated with conventional techniques of late gadolinium enhancement.[6]

Fluoropyrimidines

Fluoropyrimidines such as 5-fluorouracil (5-FU) and its oral form capecitabine are used to treat patients with gastrointestinal and other malignancies. The incidence of myocardial ischemia varies considerably and may be as high as 10%, depending on dose, scheduling, and route of administration. The mechanisms of 5-FU-induced myocardial ischemia are multifactorial and include coronary vasospasm and endothelial injury. Chest pain and ischemic ECG changes typically occur at rest, and less frequently during exercise, within days of drug administration and sometimes persist even after treatment cessation. However, the problem of fluoropyrimidine-induced myocardial ischemia may be clinically underestimated; a recent study found silent ischemia in ~6–7% of 5-FU-treated patients examined using a stress test. 5-FU can also result in acute myocardial infarction.

Cisplatin

Cisplatin may induce arterial thrombosis with subsequent myocardial and cerebrovascular ischemia in ~2 percentage of patients. The pathophysiology is multifactorial, including procoagulant and direct endothelial toxic effects. Cisplatin-treated survivors of testicular cancer have a higher incidence of CAD, with an absolute risk of up to 8% over 20 years.

Immune and Targeted Therapeutics

Among the immune and targeted therapeutics, those inhibiting the VEGF signaling pathway have an increased risk for coronary thrombosis. VEGF signaling is important for endothelial cell survival, and inhibition can induce endothelial injury. The incidence of arterial thrombosis varies depending on the compound and disease studied; for the monoclonal VEGF antibody bevacizumab, it ranges from <1% in the setting of adjuvant breast cancer to 3.8% in metastatic diseases. A recent meta-analysis on the risk of arterial thrombosis induced by anti-VEGF small molecule TKIs found an overall incidence of 1.7% for sorafenib and 1.4% for sunitinib.[123] Sorafenib has also been reported to induce vasospasm.

Valvular Disease: Pathophysiology and Clinical Presentation

Chemotherapeutic agents do not directly affect cardiac valves, but VHD may be observed in patients with cancer for several reasons, including preexisting valve lesions, radiotherapy, infective endocarditis and secondary to LV dysfunction. Radiation-induced VHD has been reported as common, affecting ~10% of treated patients, includes fibrosis and calcification of the aortic root, aortic valve cusps, mitral valve annulus and the base and mid portions of the mitral valve leaflets, sparing the mitral valve tips, and commissures, allowing distinction from rheumatic disease. In patients with Hodgkin lymphoma, radiation dose to the heart valves can increase the risk of clinically significant VHD as the first cardiovascular event after treatment, especially at doses > 30 Gy. However, for patients with mediastinal involvement treated today with 20 or 30 Gy, the 30-year risk would be increased only by ~1.4 percentage.[1]

Diagnostic and Therapeutic Management

Echocardiography is the assessment method of choice, and 3D echocardiography may be useful, particularly for the evaluation of mitral valve commissures. Baseline and repeated echocardiography after radiation therapy involving the heart are recommended in patients with cancer for the diagnosis and follow-up of VHD.

Cardiac magnetic resonance and computed tomography (CT) may be used to assess the severity of VHD, but cardiac CT is mainly useful for detecting extensive calcifications of the ascending aorta, which may lead to a higher operative risk and sometimes prohibit conventional cardiovascular surgery. Cardiac surgery is also frequently challenging in such patients because of mediastinal fibrosis, impaired wound healing and associated coronary artery, myocardial, and pericardial disease. Transcatheter valve implantation (e.g. transcatheter aortic valve implantation) may be a suitable option in this situation.[2]

Arrhythmias: Pathophysiology and Clinical Presentation

Patients with cancer may experience a wide spectrum of cardiac arrhythmias, including sinus tachycardia, bradyarrhythmias or tachyarrhythmias, and conduction defects, some of which may cause severe symptoms, become life threatening, or impose a change in the patient's treatment plan. Arrhythmias can be present at baseline in 16–36% of treated patients with cancer.

QT Prolongation

QT prolongation can be caused by cancer therapies, electrolyte disturbances, predisposing factors, and concomitant medications (e.g. antiemetics, cardiac medications, and antibiotics and psychotropic). QT prolongation can lead to life-threatening arrhythmias such as torsade de pointes. The duration of the QT interval and risk factors for QT prolongation should be controlled before, during and after cancer treatment. The risk of QT prolongation varies with different drugs, with arsenic trioxide being the most relevant. This drug, which is used to treat some leukemias and myelomas, prolongs the QT interval in 26–93% of patients, and life-threatening ventricular tachyarrhythmias have been reported not infrequently. Prolongation of the QTc interval was observed 1–5 weeks after arsenic trioxide infusion and then returned toward baseline by the end of 8 weeks, i.e. before the second course of chemotherapy. Among these, the TKI drug class, and specifically vandetanib, has the second highest incidence of QT prolongation.

Arterial Hypertension—Pathophysiology and Clinical Presentation

Hypertension is a frequent comorbidity in patients with cancer. It can also be a causative factor, such as in renal cancer. VEGF inhibitors have a high risk (11–45%) of inducing new hypertension or destabilizing previously controlled hypertension, including severe hypertension in 2–20% of cases. The incidence and severity depend upon patient age, history of hypertension, and CVD history; type of cancer (i.e. renal vs nonrenal cell cancer), drug type and dose, schedule used and associated cancer therapies. In a meta-analysis of clinical trials, the incidence of hypertension was increased by a factor of 7.5, 6.1, and 3.9, respectively, under bevacizumab, sorafenib, and sunitinib.

Thromboembolic Disease: Pathophysiology and Clinical Presentation

Tumor cells can trigger coagulation through different pathways, including procoagulant, antifibrinolytic, and proaggregating activities; release of proinflammatory and proangiogenic cytokines and interaction with vascular and blood cells through adhesion molecules.

Arterial Thrombosis

Intra-arterial thrombotic events are rare in patients with cancer, with an incidence of ~1%. They occur mostly in metastatic pancreatic, breast, colorectal, and lung cancers, under anthracyclines and taxane- and platinum-based chemotherapies, and affected patients have a poor prognosis. The prothrombotic state may facilitate embolic events secondary to atrial fibrillation. Some cancer therapies, especially VEGF inhibitors, may favor thromboembolic complications. In patients with breast cancer under hormonal therapy, higher rates of arterial thrombotic events are reported under aromatase inhibitors compared with tamoxifen, which are at least partly explained by the more favorable effects of tamoxifen on the lipid profile.

Venous Thrombosis and Thromboembolism

Venous thrombosis and venous thromboembolism (VTE) occur frequently in patients with cancer, may affect up to 20% of hospitalized patients and are frequently under recognized. They can be related to chemotherapy, including its administration route, use of indwelling venous catheters, and to the cancer itself and the patient's previous risk of venous thrombosis. VTE is the most common cause of death after surgery for cancer. Antithrombotic prophylaxis should be given for a minimum of 4 weeks after surgery. VTE is common in ambulatory patients with cancer (bladder, colon, ovary, lung, stomach, and pancreas) during chemotherapy treatment; however, the role of prophylaxis is unclear.

Peripheral Artery Disease

Severe atherosclerotic and nonatherosclerotic peripheral artery disease (PAD) in the lower extremities can occur (in up to 30%) in patients treated with nilotinib, pontine, or BCR-ABL TKIs used for chronic myeloid leukemia, even in the absence of CVD risk factors, although the latter increases the likelihood of PAD. PAD can occur as early as in the first months of therapy or as a late effect several years after treatment. Other cancer therapy-related peripheral arterial toxicity includes Raynaud's phenomenon and ischemic stroke (i.e. with L-asparaginase, cisplatin, methotrexate, 5-FU, and paclitaxel).

Stroke

The risk of stroke is increased—at least doubled—after mediastinal, cervical, or cranial radiotherapy. Endothelial damage and thrombus formation may occur after irradiation of cerebral small vessels. In medium or large vessels, three mechanisms are described: vasa vasorum occlusions with medial necrosis and fibrosis; adventitial fibrosis and accelerated atherosclerosis, leading to increased carotid stiffness and intima-media thickness and advanced. Similar consequences are reported for the aorta and other peripheral arteries, including the subclavian and iliofemoral, with ischemic limb symptoms.[2]

Pulmonary Hypertension—Pathophysiology and Clinical Presentation

Pulmonary hypertension is a rare but serious complication of some cancer agents and stem cell bone marrow transplantation. The TKI imatinib improved hemodynamics in patients with advanced pulmonary arterial hypertension (PAH). However, a drug of the same TKI family—dasatinib, used as second-line treatment for chronic myelogenous leukemia—can induce severe precapillary pulmonary hypertension. This condition appears 8–40 months after exposure to dasatinib, with clinical and hemodynamic presentation suggestive of PAH. Unlike other forms of PAH, this is often reversible after drug discontinuation or replacement with another TKI, such as nilotinib. Recently, cyclophosphamide and other alkylating agents were suggested as contributing to the development of pulmonary veno-occlusive disease, involving predominantly small venules and representing the most severe form of pulmonary hypertension lacking effective pharmacological treatment.

OTHER CARDIOVASCULAR COMPLICATIONS OF CANCER TREATMENT

Pericardial Disease

Acute pericarditis may occur with the use of several chemotherapeutic drugs (predominantly anthracyclines, but also cyclophosphamide, cytarabine, and bleomycin), while it has become uncommon during radiotherapy and is usually associated with pericardiac mediastinal tumors. Acute pericarditis with typical chest pain, fever, ST-T changes, and large effusions, even leading to tamponade, may develop 2–145 months after thoracic radiotherapy, with an absolute cumulative incidence of 2–5%. Transthoracic echocardiography is the method of choice for the evaluation of patients with suspected pericardial disease due to chemotherapy, but CT can be of help, particularly to identify calcification. Treatment of pericardial effusion consists primarily of nonsteroidal anti-inflammatory drugs and colchicine. Pericardiocentesis may be required for large effusions and those causing hemodynamic compromise, eventually followed by surgical pericardial windowing. Delayed pericardial disease may develop 6 months to 15 years after radiation treatment and includes pericarditis and chronic pericardial effusion. Although most cases resolve spontaneously, there are reports of occurrence of chronic and/or constrictive pericarditis after high-dose radiotherapy administration in up to 20% of patients.

Pleural Effusion

Pleural effusion related to the cancer itself, HF, infections, or other causes is common in patients with cancer. Some cancer drugs, e.g. dasatinib and imatinib may induce fluid retention or a reversible pleural effusion through additional unknown mechanisms.

Autonomic Dysfunction

Radiotherapy damage to the cardiac nervous system may lead to sympathetic-vagal imbalance characterized by inappropriate sinus tachycardia, altered heart rate variability, and decreased sensitivity. This may lead to a higher pain threshold or silent ischemia in cancer survivors with manifest CAD. Its management does not differ from that in noncancer patients.[4]

REFERENCES

1. Plana JC, Galderisi M, Barac A, et al. Expert Consensus for multimodality imaging evaluation of adult patients during and after cancer therapy: a report from the American Society of Echocardiography and the European Association of Cardiovascular Imaging. Eur Heart J Cardiovasc Imaging. 2014;15:1063-93.
2. Zamorano JL, Lancellotti P, Rodriguez Munoz D, et al. 2016 ESC Position Paper on cancer treatments and cardiovascular toxicity developed under the auspices of the ESC Committee for Practice Guidelines: The Task Force for cancer treatments and cardiovascular toxicity of the European Society of Cardiology (ESC). Eur Heart J. 2016;37:2768-801.
3. Cardinale D, Colombo A, Bacchiani G, et al. Early detection of anthracycline cardiotoxicity and improvement with heart failure. Circulation. 2015;131:1981-8.
4. Thavendiranathan P, Grant AD, Negishi T, et al. Reproducibility of echocardiographic techniques for sequential assessment of left ventricular ejection fraction and volumes: application to patients undergoing cancer chemotherapy. J Am Coll Cardiol. 2013;61:77-84.
5. Lancellotti P, Nkomo VT, Badano LP, et al. Expert consensus for multi-modality imaging evaluation of cardiovascular complications of radiotherapy in adults: a report from the European Association of Cardiovascular Imaging and the American Society of Echocardiography. Eur Heart J Cardiovasc Imaging. 2013;14:721-40.
6. Plana JC, Thavendiranathan P, Bucciarelli-Ducci C, et al. Multi-modality imaging in the assessment of cardiovascular toxicity in the cancer patient. JACC Cardiovasc Imaging. 2018;11:1173-86.

SECTION 12

Systematics Inflammatory Release Syndrome with Multiorgan Failure and Cardiogenic Shock

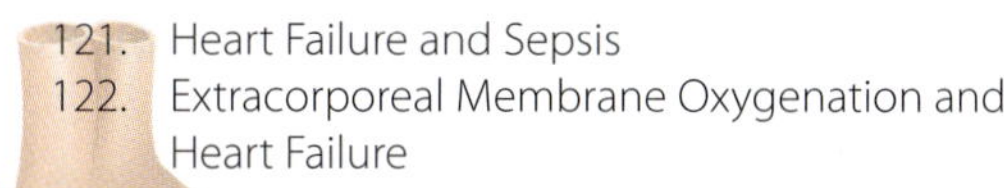

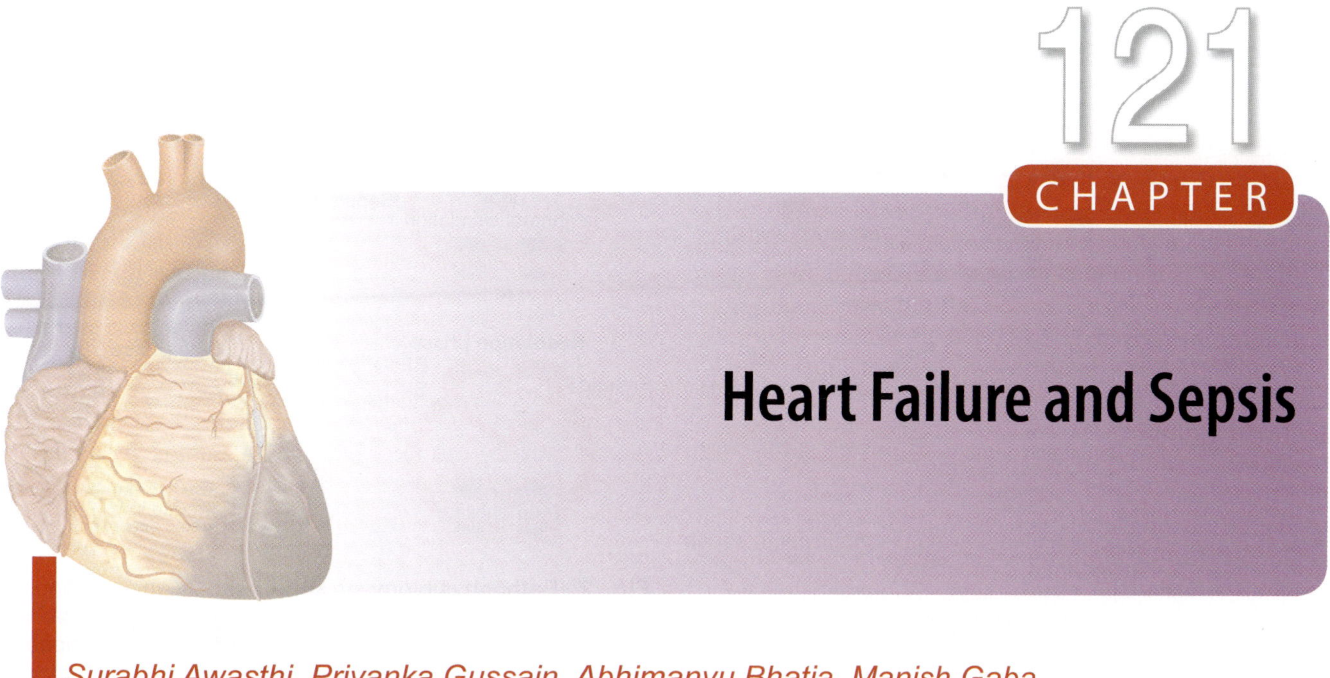

Heart Failure and Sepsis

Surabhi Awasthi, Priyanka Gussain, Abhimanyu Bhatia, Manish Gaba

INTRODUCTION

Sepsis—an "inflam-metabolic" disease—is defined as a systemic inflammatory response. Sepsis is a complex syndrome that has recently been defined as "life-threatening organ dysfunction due to a dysregulated host response to infection". It usually follows bacterial, viral, or fungal infection and can lead to severe sepsis and septic shock characterized by hypotension, ischemia, multiple organ failure, and death. Sepsis is a major health complication causing patient mortality and increased health care cost. Sepsis is responsible for 10% of all intensive care unit (ICU) admissions. The exuberant septic inflammatory response in the organism is complicated by secondary end organ damage. In particular, cardiovascular derangements such as decreased peripheral resistance and increased vascular permeability leading to tissue hypoperfusion are of clinical importance in the therapeutic approach of sepsis. Feared complications in severe sepsis and septic shock are multiorgan failure (MOF) and hemostatic derangements leading to disseminated intravascular coagulation (DIC).

DIAGNOSTIC CRITERIA FOR SEPSIS

Sepsis Definitions Task Force recommended that once infection is suspected, clinicians consider whether it has caused organ dysfunction by determining a sequential organ failure assessment (SOFA) score. The SOFA score ranges from 0 points to 24 points, with up to 4 points accrued across six organ systems (respiratory, cardiovascular, hepatic, coagulation, renal and neurological). With ≥2 new SOFA points, the infected patient is considered septic and may be at ≥10% risk of in-hospital death. Because the SOFA score requires multiple laboratory tests and may be costly to measure repeatedly, the quick SOFA (qSOFA) score was proposed as a clinical prompt to identify patients at high risk of sepsis outside the ICU, whether on the medical ward or in the emergency department. The qSOFA score ranges from 0 points to 3 points, with 1 point each for systolic hypotension (≤100 mm Hg), tachypnea (≥22 breaths/min), or altered mentation. A qSOFA score of ≥2 points has a predictive value for sepsis similar to that of more complicated measures of organ dysfunction.

Criteria for Septic Shock

For clarity, criteria are proposed for septic shock that include:

- Sepsis plus
- The need for vasopressor therapy to elevate mean arterial pressure to ≥65 mm Hg
- A serum lactate concentration >2.0 mmol/L after adequate fluid resuscitation.

MYOCARDIAL DYSFUNCTION IN SEPSIS (FIG. 1)

Sepsis leads to complex intramyocardial inflammatory response that results in sepsis-induced myocardial dysfunction. Several lines of evidence suggest that the ventricular myocardium is depressed during sepsis with features of diastolic dysfunction.

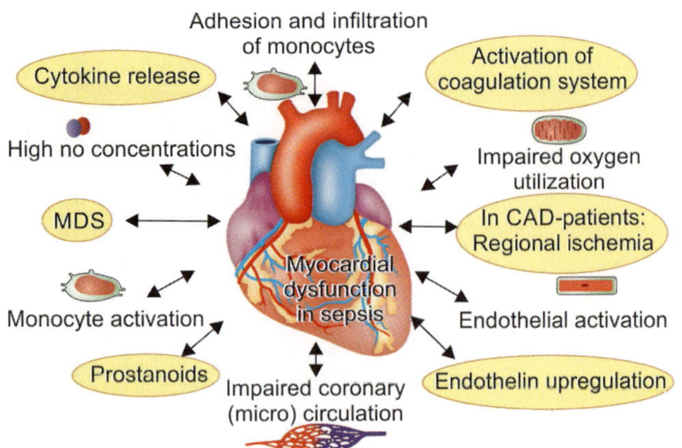

Fig. 1: Synopsis of potential underlying mechanisms in septic myocardial dysfunction.[57]
(CAD: coronary artery disease; MDS: myocardial depressant substance; NO: nitric oxide)

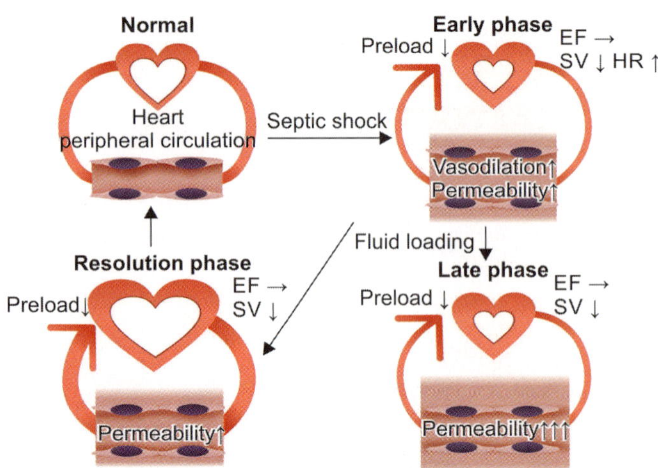

Fig. 2: Pathophysiology of septic shock and secondary myocardial dysfunction.[33] (*A*) In the normal condition, cardiac output is adequate to meet the oxygen demand in peripheral tissues; (*B*) At the very early phase of sepsis, left ventricular ejection fraction (LVEF) is not impaired (typically LVEF >55%), but stroke volume (SV) is low because of insufficient cardiac preload due to a high vascular permeability and vasodilation. The compensatory increase in heart rate (HR) is often insufficient to maintain adequate cardiac output; (*C*) After fluid loading, SV can be recovered especially in the case of survivors while LVEF is temporarily decreased (typically <45%) in part due to high left ventricular end-diastolic volume (LVEDV). This indicates that low LVEF may represent preload optimization and good adaptation. (*D*) During the later phase of sepsis, nonsurvivors are given more fluid than survivors but, nevertheless, have lower LVEDV suggesting a persistent vascular hyperpermeability and preload deficiency. In these cases, LVEF can be retained in part due to low LVEDV and/or ongoing harmful adrenergic overstimulation.
(EF: ejection fraction)

PATHOPHYSIOLOGY OF SEPTIC SHOCK AND SECONDARY MYOCARDIAL DYSFUNCTION (FIG. 2)

Septic distributive shock is a circulatory maldistribution associated with peripheral vasodilation, as well as arterial and capillary shunting. However, the pathophysiology of septic shock comprises both warm (hyperdynamic) and cold (hypodynamic) types. The early phase of septic shock is called hyperdynamic, or warm shock, that is characterized by high cardiac output, low peripheral vascular resistance, and warm extremities. The late phase comprises concomitant hypotension followed by hypodynamic, or cold shock, with low cardiac output, poor peripheral perfusion, cool extremities, and finally, death. Inadequate resuscitation, relative hypovolemia, and an increased afterload were initially thought to be the hemodynamic profile of patients with hypodynamic shock.

Adequate volume resuscitation and the profoundly reduced systemic vascular resistance typically encountered in patients with sepsis lead to a normal or elevated cardiac index. However, despite increased cardiac output and a normal stroke volume, myocardial dysfunction is significant in patients with septic shock. Notably, ejection fraction is lower and end-diastolic volume is higher in survivors, compared to nonsurvivors of shock. This suggests that ventricular dilation might be a compensatory mechanism to maintain adequate cardiac output and protect against myocardial depression.

Importantly, cardiovascular dysfunction in sepsis is associated with a significantly increased mortality rate of 70–90% compared with 20% among patients with sepsis that is not accompanied by cardiovascular impairment. Myocardial edema due to inflammation-induced vascular leakage might also influence cardiac compliance and function.

In addition, ventricular function is influenced by changes in afterload. Pulmonary hypertension will worsen right-heart function, whereas right-heart dilation will impair left-heart function. Endothelial cells producing vasoactive molecules that regulate peripheral vascular resistance are impaired during septic shock, and thus, endothelial dysfunction plays a crucial role in its pathophysiology. This is because impaired endothelium-derived nitric oxide release could alter the physiological regulation of blood flow distribution via coronary vasospasm combined with an increase in peripheral vascular resistance and the associated elevation of cardiac workload and myocardial oxygen demand.

DIRECT MYOCARDIAL DEPRESSION IN SEPSIS AND SEPSIS-INDUCED CARDIOMYOPATHY (FIG. 3)

A major mechanism of direct cardiac depression in sepsis is the attenuation of the adrenergic response at the cardiomyocyte level due to downregulation of β-adrenergic receptors and depression of postreceptor signaling pathways. These changes seem to be mediated by many substances, such as cytokines and nitric oxide. Another mechanism of direct cardiac depression in sepsis is cardiomyocyte injury or death, which can be induced by toxins, complements, damage-associated molecular patterns (DAMPs), and as-yet-unidentified myocardial depressants.

Sepsis also triggers takotsubo cardiomyopathy, also known as stress cardiomyopathy, apical ballooning syndrome, or broken-heart syndrome, which is different from sepsis-induced cardiomyopathy (SIC). Takotsubo cardiomyopathy, typically, occurs when the contractile function of the mid-to-apical segments of the left ventricle (LV) is depressed and there is hyperkinesis of basal walls, producing a balloon-like appearance of the distal ventricle. Several studies have reported that this syndrome is induced by increased catecholamine levels. In takotsubo cardiomyopathy, the left ventricular function usually returns to normal within a few weeks. At a cellular level, changes were shown to be reversible with normalization of the left ventricular ejection fraction, including the cytoskeletal protein derangements, increase in extracellular matrix proteins, and accumulation of intracellular glycogen. Although sepsis and septic shock can trigger takotsubo cardiomyopathy, the etiology and myocardial alterations appear to be different from those of SIC. In SIC, there is global ventricular dysfunction and dilated LV without regional dysfunction. In takotsubo cardiomyopathy, there is typically regional dysfunction, especially characterized by apical ballooning mimicking acute coronary syndrome (ACS). Therefore, the accurate diagnosis of takotsubo cardiomyopathy requires coronary angiography to rule out ACS.

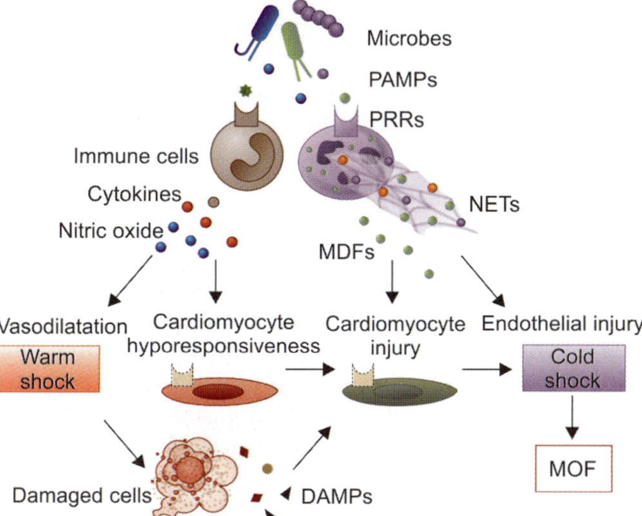

Fig. 3: Direct myocardial depression in sepsis.
(DAMPs: damage-associated molecular patterns; MDF: myocardial depressant factor; MOF: multiple organ failure; NETs: neutrophil extracellular traps; PAMPs: pathogen-associated molecular patterns; PRRs: pattern recognition receptors)

Mechanisms of Sepsis-induced Cardiomyopathy

Diagnosis

Despite the lack of diagnostic criteria for SIC to date, it is known to have three characteristics.

The first is left ventricular dilatation with normal or low filling pressure unlike the "classic" pattern of cardiogenic shock where LV pressures are elevated. Unlike classic cardiomyopathy, it is not associated with high filling pressures for two reasons—increased LV compliance and frequently associated right ventricle dysfunction. It is always reversible.

The second characteristic is depressed ejection fraction. Parker et al. reported that end-diastolic and systolic ventricular volumes were increased but with normal or elevated stroke volume and cardiac index in septic shock survivors.

The third characteristic of SIC is that it should normalize within 7–10 days. Septic cardiomyopathy is acute and reversible, providing the patient recovers. In 90 patients during a 5-year period, Jardin et al. reported that LV ejection fraction is normalized in a few days, as also reported more recently by Bouhemad et al. In SIC diagnosis, the first and second characteristics are particularly important and easy to detect using echocardiography. Thus, echocardiography in sepsis management is the most important thing for diagnosing SIC.

B-type natriuretic peptide (BNP), a diuretic hormone, is released from ventricular myocardium in response to cardiac wall stretch. Recent observational study demonstrated that SIC is associated with BNP rise, although not independently, whereas left ventricular filling pressures do not correlate with the BNP levels.

Troponin is a very sensitive and specific protein of myocardial damage and often used for the diagnosis of ACS. Troponin elevation is common in septic shock patients, and it was estimated that 43–85% of patients with sepsis showed cardiac troponin I elevation. However, the use of troponin to diagnose SIC is limited because there are many causes such as ACS and low renal function that affect troponin levels.

Depression of LV intrinsic contractility is constant in patients with septic shock. Because most parameters of cardiac function are strongly dependent on afterload, especially in this context, cardiac performance evaluated at the bedside reflects intrinsic contractility but also the degree of vasoplegia. Recent advances in echocardiography have allowed better characterization of septic cardiomyopathy. Although it is unclear how septic cardiomyopathy affects outcome, a hyperkinetic state is indicative of profound and persistent vasoplegia associated with a high mortality rate. Preliminary data suggest that the hemodynamic response to dobutamine challenge has a prognostic value, but large studies are required to establish whether inotropic drugs should be used to treat this septic cardiac dysfunction.

Treatment (Fig. 4)

Fluid Resuscitation

It appears to be safe to give patients with severe sepsis or septic shock and a known history of heart failure, at least the recommended 30 mL/kg of fluid resuscitation within the first few hours of sepsis onset. The incidence of adverse clinical events such as intubation rate, continuous positive airway pressure/bilevel positive airway pressure (CPAP/BIPAP) use, cardiovascular complications, acute kidney injury, hospital length of stay, ICU length of stay and mortality are not increased in patients with known heart failure and severe sepsis or septic shock. Volume expansion must always be proposed first to restore central blood volume in the case of absolute or relative hypovolemia. Parker et al. suggested that "massive" fluid infusion maintains a normal cardiac index, despite a significantly impaired LV contractility, through LV preload adaptation. Fluid management in critically-ill patients with sepsis is complex, in part because the clinical endpoints for fluid administration change during the course of the septic episode. Initially, there is a general consensus that fluid administration should be liberal and aggressive. Clinical management during the initial 24 hours of therapy emphasize the use of resuscitation goals that implicate sufficient tissue delivery of oxygen and include not only traditional hemodynamic measurements and urine output but also variables related to oxygen delivery and consumption, such as hemoglobin, lactate levels and mixed venous oxygen saturation. Subsequently, however, patient outcomes are improved in critically-ill septic patients by observing conservative fluid management strategies. The supporting rationale for the application of conservative fluid management strategies during the late stages of sepsis stem from observations of improved patient outcomes from the use of such strategies for the treatment of acute lung injury. Complex patients with both preexisting LVD and sepsis

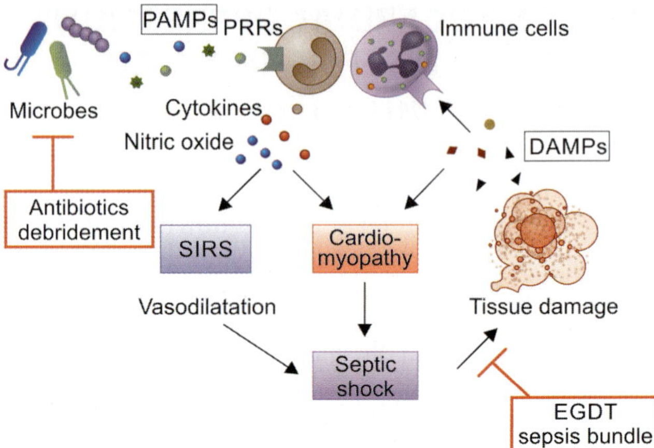

Fig. 4: Management of myocardial dysfunction in septic shock. Prompt and adequate antibiotic therapy, accompanied by surgical removal of the infectious focus, if indicated and feasible, is important to decrease PAMPs arising from invasive microorganisms. Early goal-directed therapy (EGDT), including fluid resuscitation, vasopressor and inotropic therapy, and red blood cell transfusion, is important to reestablish organ perfusion pressure, which helps maintain blood flow to tissues and reduces the release of damage-associated molecular patterns (DAMPs) in patients with septic shock. Sepsis bundle is a selected set of elements of care distilled from Surviving Sepsis Campaign guidelines.
(PAMPs: pathogen-associated molecular patterns; PRRs: pattern recognition receptors; SIRS: systemic inflammatory response syndrome)

might be perceived as being more susceptible than other septic patients to developing respiratory complications from aggressive initial fluid resuscitation because pulmonary edema is a component of the congestive heart failure syndrome. Crystalloids is recommended as the initial fluid in the resuscitation of sepsis; however, a research from septic animal demonstrated that albumin and hypertonic saline were more beneficial on cardiac function com-pared with normal saline.

Noradrenaline

Noradrenaline is recommended as a first-line vasopressor; however, some studies reported that vasopressin also may be effective for septic shock. Current guidance describes that low-dose vasopressin can be added to noradrenaline with the intent of either raising mean arterial pressure or decreasing noradrenaline dosage; however, low-dose vasopressin is not recommended as a single vasopressor.

Dobutamine

Current guidance recommends using dobutamine to increase the cardiac index. However, hemodynamic therapy with dobutamine and dopamine to achieve supranormal values for the cardiac index fails to reduce morbidity or mortality among critically ill patients. It has been shown that use of dobutamine to boost the cardiac index did not improve the outcome of critically ill patients. Furthermore, use of dobutamine was associated with increased 90-day mortality from septic shock, while it has been observed that dobutamine did not improve sublingual microcirculatory, metabolic, hepatosplanchnic, or peripheral perfusion parameters in patients with septic shock.

The ability of inotropic catecholamines to stimulate bacterial proliferation and biofilm formation might be an etiological factor in the development of intravascular catheter colonization and catheter-related infection. This effect of inotropic catecholamines does not seem to be limited to only coagulase-negative *Staphylococcus* but also other Gram-negative bacteria. The growth of these bacteria and production of virulence are associated with inotropic catecholamines. Thus, inotropic catecholamines, such as dobutamine, may have adverse effects in patients with septic shock, and the decrease in β-adrenergic response in patients with SIC may be a protective mechanism to these effects. Thus, β-blockade could be associated with reductions in the heart rate without adverse effects and that this could help to improve survival. For these reasons, despite the beneficial effects of dobutamine, it appears that excessive increases in sympathetic tone during sepsis can create adverse effects.

Levosimendan

Levosimendan can increase contractile myofilament sensitivity to calcium and is a positive inotropic drug. Levosimendan sensitizes troponin C to calcium in a calcium concentration-dependent manner; this increases the effects of calcium on myofilaments during systole. This sensitization is diminished by decreasing calcium concentration level during diastole, and thus, diastolic relaxation remains largely unaffected. In contrast to other inotropic agents, levosimendan does not cause arrhythmias or increase the oxygen consumption. It also opens the ATP-sensitive potassium channels causing smooth muscle membrane hyperpolarization which leads to vasodilation. A meta-analysis evaluated the use of levosimendan in septic shock and reported that it was associated with reduced mortality when compared with standard inotropic therapy. Although levosimendan is also an inotropic agent, it does not stimulate β-adrenergic receptor; but further study is needed to confirm whether it is truly effective in SIC.

Beta-blockers

Beta-blockers can prevent ischemia, decrease oxygen demand (by reducing cardiac output up to 20% without worsening oxygen utilization or increasing lactate levels), and decrease tumor necrosis factor-α (TNF-α) production, allowing for better preservation of cardiac function. Beta-blocking agents could be beneficial because evidence suggests that β-adrenergic stress is a major factor in the pathogenesis of sepsis-induced myocardial dysfunction. The ultra-short-acting β-blocker landiolol is associated with a significant reduction in serum levels of the inflammatory mediator HMGB1 and histological lung damage.

Intra-aortic Balloon Pumping and Extracorporeal Membrane Oxygenation

Intra-aortic balloon pumping (IABP) is expected to increase the cardiac output and reduce the dosage of a vasopressor. In severe septic shock with a low cardiac index, IABP prolongs survival time and lowers vasopressor requirements. There has been successful use of venoarterial extracorporeal membrane oxygenation (ECMO) as a viable rescue therapy to unresponsive severe cardiogenic shock in patients with SIC. This strategy may provide time for antibiotics to work effectively. If both septic and cardiogenic factors contribute to the pathophysiology of shock, venoarterial ECMO may improve the mortality of the most severe group. However, the management of patients who need ECMO is very complex; thus, a well-experienced team should use it in a specialized center. For these reasons, to date, mechanical support with IABP or ECMO seems not to be a standard therapy, although it may be the last option for unresponsive severe cardiogenic shock due to SIC.

Others

Erythropoietin (EPO) is widely used for the treatment of anemia in patients, especially the anemia in patients with chronic kidney disease. The administration of EPO attenuated the impaired systolic contractility in experimental sepsis via activation of the β-common receptor. As the complex and strong interaction between EPO and β common receptor (βcR), selectively activating the tissue-protective βcR–EpoR heterocomplex represents a new therapeutic approach to SIC. MicroRNAs (miRNAs) are a class of small 21–23 nucleotides long RNAs molecules, which have been identified as novel regulators of gene expression at the posttranscriptional level.

Studies involving animal models over 40 years ago demonstrated that serum lactate levels were elevated when tissue oxygenation was decreased by experimental manipulation of the determinants of oxygen delivery. Increased lactate levels have been demonstrated to be associated with poor outcomes in critically-ill patients, patients with circulatory shock, and patients with severe sepsis. Production of lactate appears to be increased both in patients with circulatory shock and sepsis. While there are some data that suggest that lactate clearance may be preserved in circulatory shock, lactate clearance seems to be diminished in some patients with sepsis. It is possible that initial serum lactate levels may be less important a predictor of outcome in septic patients with preexisting left ventricular dysfunction (LVD) than they are in other septic patients.

The relationship between central venous oxygen saturation ($ScVO_2$) and lactate levels in patients with cardiopulmonary disease has been studied, noting that $ScVO_2$ levels were decreased in such patients and associated with increased lactate levels and mortality. The presumed mechanism for this phenomenon is that diminished cardiac output leads to decreased oxygen delivery to tissues, increased oxygen extraction and, therefore, diminished oxygen saturation in blood returning to the heart. Evidence was provided supporting this hypothesis in general, but suggested that short-term decrements in $ScVO_2$ might be associated with adverse clinical outcomes. It has also been shown in a few studies that targets augmenting $ScVO_2$ in septic patients leads to improved clinical outcomes. It has been found that patients with preexisting LVD and sepsis have a lower mean initial $ScVO_2$ than other septic patients. Sepsis is a heterogeneous disorder, and management strategies that target oxygen delivery variables may be particularly appropriate for patients with preexisting LVD.

CONCLUSION

Infections are an important cause of decompensation of existing heart failure or development of SIC which should be early detected and treated using specific protocols and in the presence of sepsis and/or septic shock. Volemic resuscitation, early antibiotic treatment, and referral to cardiac ICUs are considered good clinical practices that can reduce the morbidity and mortality. On the other hand, it has become more and more recognized that sepsis promotes cardiovascular changes with multisystemic involvement that increase the frequency of cardiac and noncardiac events after recovery from sepsis. Heart failure has been an independent predictor of worse clinical outcomes in patients admitted with a primary diagnosis of sepsis. Currently, there are no expert consensus or management guidelines focusing on this critical state. Mortality risk factors for patients with preexisting LVD and sepsis included a low $ScVO_2$, failure to comply with a sepsis bundle of therapies, intubation status, and a source of infection other than the lung, whereas mortality risk factors for septic patients with no previous evidence of cardiac disease included increased lactate levels and a low platelet count. In the near future, levosimendan or mechanical support with venoarterial and venous (VAV) ECMO could be a feasible rescue strategy for a small proportion of patients with combined respiratory and cardiac failure secondary to septic shock with septic cardiomyopathy.

BIBLIOGRAPHY

1. Abou Dagher G, Hajjar K, Khoury C, et al. Outcomes of patients with systolic heart failure presenting with sepsis to the emergency department of a tertiary hospital: a retrospective chart review study from Lebanon. BMJ Open. 2018;8:e022185. oi:10.1136/bmjopen-2018-022185.
2. Agency for Healthcare Research and Quality: HCUP facts and figures: statistics on hospital-based care in the United States, 2008. Rockville (MD): Agency for Healthcare Research and Quality (US); 2010.
3. Alon D, Stein GY, Korenfeld R, et al. Predictors and outcomes of infection-related hospital admissions of heart failure patients. PLoS One. 2013;8(8):e72476.
4. Ammann P, Fehr T, Minder EI, et al. Elevation of troponin I in sepsis and septic shock. Intensive Care Med. 2001;27(6):965-9.
5. Angus DC, Barnato AE, Bell D, et al. A systematic review and meta-analysis of early goal-directed therapy for septic shock: the ARISE, ProCESS and ProMISe Investigators. Intensive Care Med. 2015;41:1549-60.
6. Bouhemad B, Nicolas-Robin A, Arbelot C, et al. Acute left ventricular dilatation and shock-induced myocardial dysfunction. Crit Care Med. 2009;37:441-7.
7. Brines M, Patel NS, Villa P, et al. Nonerythropoietic, tissue-protective peptides derived from the tertiary struc-ture of erythropoietin. Proc Natl Acad Sci U S A. 2008;105(31): 10925-30.
8. Cady LD, Weil MH, Afifi AA, et al. Quantitation of severity of critical illness with special reference to blood lactate. Crit Care Med 1973;1:75-80.
9. Cain SM. Appearance of excess lactate in anesthetized dogs during anemic and hypoxic hypoxia. Am J Physiol. 1965;209:604-10.
10. Centers for Disease Control and Prevention. (2016). Sepsis Data and Reports sheet. [online] Available from https://www.cdc.gov/sepsis/datareports/index.html. [Last accessed November, 2019]
11. Chioléro RL, Revelly JP, Leverve X, et al. Effects of cardiogenic shock on lactate and glucose metabolism after heart surgery. Crit Care Med. 2000;28:3784-91.
12. Christopher W. Seymour CW, Angus DC. Sepsis and Septic Shock. In: Jameson JL, Fauci AS, Kasper DL, Hauser SL, Longo DL, Loscalzo J (Eds). Harrison Principles of Internal Medicine. New York: McGraw-Hill Medical; 2018
13. Combes A, Brodie D, Bartlett R, et al. Position paper for the organization of extracorporeal membrane oxygenation programs for acute respiratory failure in adult patients. Am J Respir Crit Care. 2014;190(5):488-96.
14. Dellinger RP, Levy MM, Rhodes A, et al. Surviving sepsis campaign: international guidelines for management

of severe sepsis and septic shock: 2012. Crit Care Med. 2013;41(2):580-637.
15. Edwards JD. Oxygen transport in cardiogenic and septic shock. Crit Care Med. 1991;19:658-63.
16. Ferro TN, Goslar PW, Romanovsky AA, et al. Smoking in trauma patients: the effects on the incidence of sepsis, respiratory failure, organ failure, and mortality. J Trauma 2010;69:308-12.
17. Finkel MS, Oddis CV, et al. Negative inotropic effects of cytokines on the heart mediated by nitric oxide. Science. 1992;257:387-9.
18. Gattinoni L, Brazzi L, Pelosi P, et al. A trial of goal- oriented hemodynamic therapy in critically ill patients. $ScvO_2$ Collaborative Group. N Eng J Med. 1995;333(16):1025-32.
19. Hagiwara S, Iwasaka H, Maeda H, et al. Landiolol, an ultrashort-acting beta1-adrenoceptor antagonist, has protective effects in an LPS-induced systemic inflammation model. Shock. 2009;31:515-20.
20. Hayes MA, Timmins AC, Yau EH, et al. Elevation of systolic oxygen delivery in the treatment of critically ill patients. N Eng J Med. 1994;330(24):1717-22.
21. Hernandez G, Bruhn A, Luengo C, et al. Effects of dobutamine on systemic, regional and microcirculatory perfusion parameters in septic shock: a randomized, placebo-controlled, double-blind, crossover study. Intensive Care Med. 2013;39(8):1435-43.
22. Hogue B, Chagnon F, Lesur O. Resuscitation fluids and endotoxin-induced myocardial dysfunction: is selection a load-independent differential issue? Shock. 2012;38(3):307-13.
23. Jafri SM, Lavine S, Field BE, et al. Left ventricular diastolic function in sepsis. Crit Care Med. 1990;18:709-14.
24. Jardin F, Brun-Ney D, Auvert B, et al. Sepsis-related cardiogenic shock. Crit Care Med. 1990;18:1055-60.
25. Jardin F, Fourme T, Page B, et al. Persistent preload defect in severe sepsis despite fluid loading: a longitudinal echocardiographic study in patients with septic shock. Chest. 1999;116:1354-9.
26. Jones AE, Trzeciak S, Kline JA. The Sequential Organ Failure Assessment score for predicting outcome in patients with severe sepsis and evidence of hypoperfusion at the time of emergency department presentation. Crit Care Med. 2009;37(5):1649-54.
27. Kakihana Y, Ito T, Nakahara M, et al. Sepsis-induced myocardial dysfunction: pathophysiology and management. J Intensive Care. 2016;4:22.
28. Kakihana Y, Ito T, Nakahara M, et al. Sepsis-induced myocardial dysfunction: pathophysiology and management. J Intensive Care. 2016;4:22.
29. Kakihana Y, Ito T, Nakahara M, et al. Sepsis-induced myocardial dysfunction: pathophysiology and management. J Intensive Care. 2016;4:22.
30. Kasnitz P, Druger GL, Yorra F, et al. Mixed venous oxygen tension and hyperlactatemia: survival in severe cardiopulmonary disease. JAMA. 1976;236:570-4.
31. Kern H, Wittich R, Rohr U, et al. Increased endothelial injury in septic patients with coronary artery disease. Chest. 2001;119:874-83.
32. Khadour FH, Panas D, Ferdinandy P, et al. Enhanced NO and superoxide generation in dysfunctional hearts from endotoxemic rats. Am J Physiol Heart Circ Physiol. 2002;283:H1108-15.
33. Khan AI, Coldewey SM, Patel NS, et al. Erythropoietin attenuates cardiac dysfunction in experimental sepsis in mice via activation of the beta-common receptor. Dis Model Mech. 2013;6(4):1021-30.
34. Krafft P, Steltzer H, Hiesmayr M, et al. Mixed oxygen saturation in critically ill septic shock patients: the role of defined events. Chest. 1993;103:900-6.
35. Kumar A, Haery C, Parrillo JE. Myocardial dysfunction in septic shock. Crit Care Clin. 2000;16(2):251-87.
36. Landesberg G, Jaffe AS, Gilon D, et al. Troponin elevation in severe sepsis and septic shock: the role of left ventricular diastolic dysfunction and right ventricular dilatation. Crit Care Med. 2014;42:790-800.
37. Lemay AC, Anzueto A, Restrepo MI, et al. Predictors of long-term mortality after severe sepsis in the elderly. Am J Med Sci. 2014;347:282-8.
38. Levraut J, Ciebiera JP, Chave S, et al. Mild hyperlactatemia in stable septic patients is due to impaired lactate clearance rather than overproduction. Am J Respir Crit Care Med. 1998;157:1021-6.
39. Lyte M, Freestone PP, Neal CP, et al. Stimulation of *Staphylococcus epidermidis* growth and biofilm formation by catecholamine inotropes. Lancet. 2003;361(9352):130-5.
40. Mehta NJ, Khan IA, Gupta V, et al. Cardiac troponin I predicts myocardial dysfunction and adverse outcome in septic shock. Int J Cardiol. 2004;95(1):13-7.
41. Merx MW, Weber C. Sepsis and the Heart. Circulation. 2007;116(7):793-802.
42. Mikkelsen ME, Miltiades AN, Gaieski DF, et al. Serum lactate is associated with mortality in severe sepsis independent of organ failure and shock. Crit Care Med. 2009;37:1670-7.
43. Mink SN, Jacobs H, et al. N,N',N"-triacetylglucosamine, an inhibitor of lysozyme, prevents myocardial depression in Escherichia coli sepsis in dogs. Crit Care Med. 2004;32: 184-93.
44. Morelli A, Ertmer C, Westphal M, et al. Effect of heart rate control with esmolol on hemodynamic and clinical outcomes in patients with septic shock: a randomized clinical trial. JAMA. 2013;310(16):1683-91.
45. Mozaffarian D, Benjamin EJ, Go AS, et al. Heart Disease and Stroke Statistics—2016 Update. Circulation. 2016;133:e38-360.
46. Munt B, Jue J, Gin K, et al. Diastolic filling in human severe sepsis: an echocardiographic study. Crit Care Med. 1998;26:1829-33.
47. Murphy CV, Schramm GE, Doherty JA, et al. The importance of fluid management in acute lung injury secondary to septic shock. Chest. 2009;136:102-9.
48. Nef HM, Mollmann H, Kostin S, et al. Tako-Tsubo cardiomyopathy: intraindividual structural analysis in the acute phase and after functional recovery. Eur Heart J. 2007;28(20):2456-64.
49. Neill WA, Jensen PE, Rich GB, et al. Effect of decreased O_2 supply to tissue on the lactate: pyruvate ratio in blood. J Clin Invest. 1969;48:1862-9.

50. Ouellette DR, Shah SZ. Comparison of outcomes from sepsis between patients with and without pre-existing left ventricular dysfunction: a case-control analysis. Crit Care. 2014;18:R79.
51. Papanikolaou J, Makris D, Mpaka M, et al. New insights into the mechanisms involved in B-type natriuretic peptide elevation and its prognostic value in septic patients. Crit Care. 2014;18:R94.
52. Parker M, Shelhamer J, Bacharach S, et al. Profound but reversible myocardial depression in patients with septic shock. Ann Intern Med. 1984;100:483-90.
53. Parker MM, Shelhamer JH, Bacharach SL, et al. Profound but reversible myocardial depression in patients with septic shock. Ann Intern Med. 1984;100:483-90.
54. Piper RD, Li FY, Myers ML, et al. Effects of isoproterenol on myocardial structure and function in septic rats. J Appl Physiol (1985). 1999;86:993-1001.
55. Poelaert J, Declerck C, Vogelaers D, et al. Left ventricular systolic and diastolic function in septic shock. Intensive Care Med. 1997;23:553-60.
56. Preiser JC, Zhang H, Vray B, et al. Time course of inducible nitric oxide synthase activity following endotoxin administration in dogs. Nitric Oxide. 2001;5:208-211.
57. Reines HD, Halushka PV, Cook JA, et al. Plasma thromboxane concentrations are raised in patients dying with septic shock. Lancet. 1982;2:174-5.
58. Rivers E, Nguyen B, Havstad S, et al. Earlygoal-directed therapy in the treatment of severe sepsis and septic shock. N Engl J Med. 2001;345:1368-77.
59. Rivers E, Nguyen B, Havstad S, et al. Early goal-directed therapy in the treatment of severe sepsis and septic shock. N Engl J Med. 2001;345:1368-77.
60. Rivers EP. Fluid-management strategies in acute lung injury—liberal, conservative, or both? N Engl J Med. 2006;354:2598-600.
61. Roger VL. Epidemiology of heart failure. Circ Res. 2013;113:646-59.
62. Russell JA, Walley KR, Singer J, et al. Vasopressin versus norepinephrine infusion in patients with septic shock. N Eng J Med. 2008;358(9):877-87.
63. Sato R, Nasu M. A review of sepsis-induced cardiomyopathy. J Intensive Care. 2015;3:48.
64. Schulz R, Nava E, Moncada S. Induction and potential biological relevance of a Ca^{2+}-independent nitric oxide synthase in the myocardium. Br J Pharmacol. 1992;105: 575-80.
65. Schulz R, Rassaf T, Massion PB, et al. Recent advances in the understanding of the role of nitric oxide in cardiovascular homeostasis. Pharmacol Ther. 2005;108:225-56.
66. Shindo T, Kurihara H, Kurihara Y, et al. Upregulation of endothelin-1 and adrenomedullin gene expression in the mouse endotoxin shock model. J Cardiovasc Pharmacol. 1998;31:S541-4.
67. Solomon DB, Minneci PC, Deans KJ, et al. Effects of intra-aortic balloon counterpulsation in a model of septic shock. Crit Care Med. 2009;37(1):7-18.
68. Surviving Sepsis campaign. (2018). [online] Available from http://www.survivingsepsis.org/bundles/Pages/default.aspx. [Last accessed November 2019].
69. Suzuki T, Morisaki H, Serita R, et al. Infusion of beta-adrenergic blocker esmolol attenuates myocardial dysfunction in septic rats. Crit Care Med. 2005;33:2294-301.
70. Tam WS, Fried J, Grotts J, et al. Fluid Resuscitation and Clinical Outcomes in Patients With Known Heart Failure Who Develop Severe Sepsis or Septic Shock. CHEST. 2016;150(4):350A.
71. Ver Elst KM, Spapen HD, Nguyen DN, et al. Cardiac troponins I and T are biological markers of left ventricular dysfunction in septic shock. Clin Chem. 2000;46(5):650-7.
72. Vieillard-Baron A, Schmitt JM, Beauchet A, et al. Early preload adaptation in septic shock? A transesophageal echocardiographic study. Anesthesiology. 2001;94:400-6.
73. Vieillard-Baron A. Septic cardiomyopathy. Ann Intensive Care. 2011;1(1):6.
74. Vincent J-L, Dufaye P, Berré J, et al. Serial lactate determinations during circulatory shock. Crit Care Med. 1983;11:449-51.
75. Walley KR. Sepsis-induced myocardial dysfunction. Curr Opin Crit Care. 2018;24(4):292-9.
76. Wiedemann HP, Wheeler AP, Bernard GR, et al. Comparison of two fluid-management strategies in acute lung injury. N Engl J Med. 2006;354:2564-75.
77. Wilkman E, Kaukonen KM, Pettilä V, et al. Association between inotrope treatment and 90-day mortality in patients with septic shock. Acta Anaesthesiol Scand. 2013;57(4):431-42.
78. Yang LL, Gros R, Kabir MG, et al. Conditional cardiac overexpression of endothelin-1 induces inflammation and dilated cardiomyopathy in mice. Circulation. 2004;109:255-61.
79. Zangrillo A, Putzu A, Monaco F, et al. Levosimendan reduces mortality in patients with severe sepsis and septic shock: a meta-analysis of randomized trials. J Crit Care. 2015;30(5):908-13.

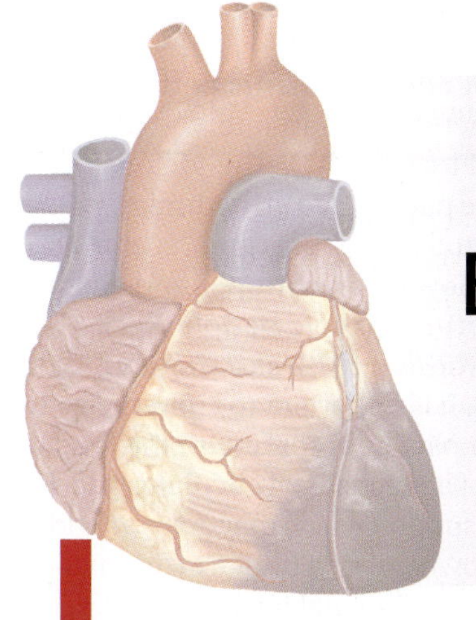

Extracorporeal Membrane Oxygenation and Heart Failure

Poonam Malhotra Kapoor

INTRODUCTION

Heart failure is the pathophysiologic state in which the heart, via an abnormality of cardiac function (detectable or not), fails to pump blood at a rate commensurate with the requirements of the metabolizing tissues or is able to do so only with an elevated diastolic filling pressure. Despite these mechanisms, there is a progressive decline in the ability of the heart to contract and relax, resulting in worsening heart failure and severe diastolic failure (Figs. 1A and B).

EXTRACORPOREAL MEMBRANE OXYGENATION USE IN ADVANCED HEART FAILURE

Acute Heart Failure

Acute heart failure is a rapid onset of symptoms and signs related to abnormal cardiac function. As a result of systolic and diastolic dysfunction, arrhythmias, or preload-after load mismatch, acute heart failure (AHF) leads to higher

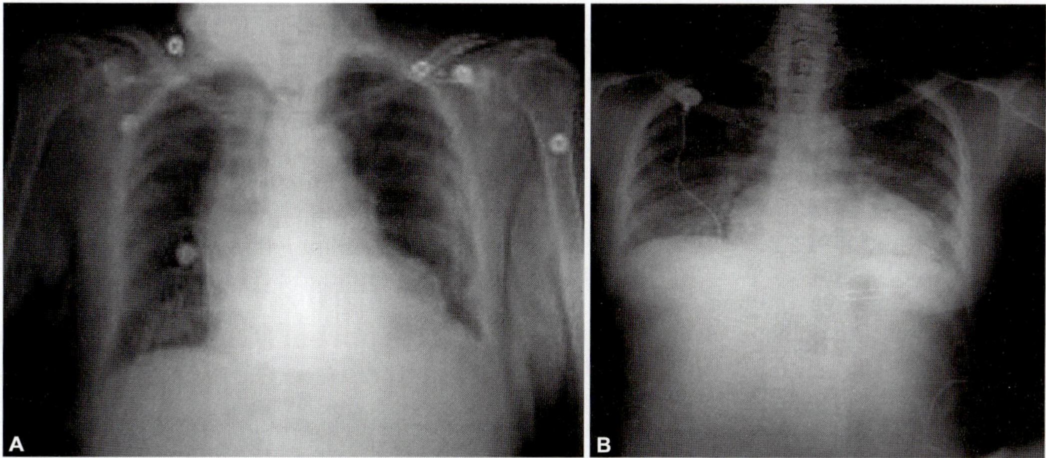

Figs. 1A and B: (A) Chest radiograph shows an enlarge cardiac silhouette and edema at the lung bases, signs of acute heart failure; (B) Acute heart failure secondary to chronic hypertension. The enlarged cardiac silhouette on this anteroposterior (AP) radiograph is caused by acute heart failure due to the effects of chronic high blood pressure on the left ventricle. The heart then becomes enlarged, and fluid accumulates in the lungs (i.e. pulmonary congestion).

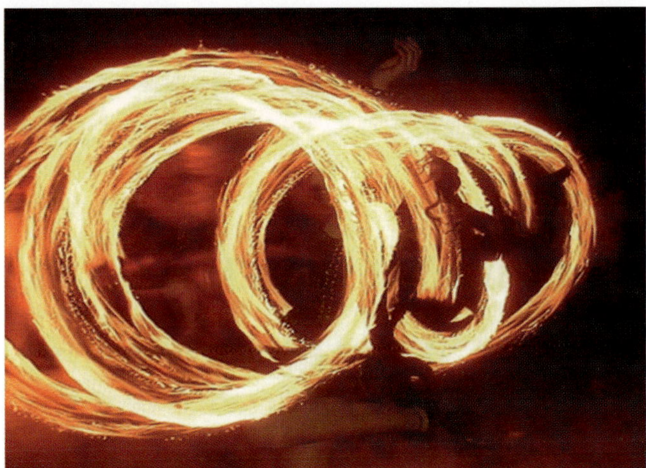

Fig. 2: A vicious circle between systolic and diastolic heart failure → Decompensation → Worsening of the patient → IABP/ECMO/VAD may be needed.
(ECMO: extracorporeal membrane oxygenation; IABP: intra-aortic balloon pump; VAD: ventricular assist devices)

mortality rates used in AHF. A vicious cycle exists between systolic and diastolic heart failure (Fig. 2).

Despite vasopression and inotropes, the patient had arrhythmias, was it sustained hypotension, oligua and all signs of tissue hypoperfusion, the cold peaipheaies.

Typical Case of Heart Failure with Worsening on Inotropes

A typical case presented is as under:

A 59-year-old female with no medical history was referred from a regional hospital with subacute myocardial infarction complicated by cardiogenic shock and a third-degree atrioventricular (AV) block. The left anterior descending artery showed a thrombus which was aspirated and stented (Promus DES 3.0 × 20 mm). Right coronary artery (RCA) was occluded with collateral flow from the left anterior descending artery and stenotic lesion ramus circumflexes were seen. Patient was treated with temporary pacing lead, intra-aortic balloon pump (IABP) and high dose inotropes. Transferred to ward 1 week after weaning the IABP; was put on angiotensin converting enzyme (ACE)-inhibitor, diuretics and epinephrine infusion. The creatine kinase (CK) peak was 5,100 U/I, CK-MB peak 250 µg/L. Inotropes and mechanical ventilation. Echocardiography [Transthoracic echocardiography (TTE)] showed poor LV function and anteroseptal wall new regional wall motion abnormalities with bradycardia.

What would be the Next Step? Is ECMO Needed with the IABP?

In an effort to maintain an adequate tissue perfusion, the body has three defenses: increased heart rate, vascular tone and circulating volume (Flowchart 1). The vicious cycle continues despite above the patient had arrhythmias, was in sustained hypotension (systolic blood pressure <90 mm Hg), despite vasopressures and low dose inotropes and oliguria with signs of tissue hypoperfusion (cold peripheries).

Do we need an ECMO with the IABP as a short bridge to therapy? The answer is YES. It is important to know the goals of treatment and judge the patient according to the level of clinical evidence for need of a mechanical circulatory device (MCS). ECMO is temporary support which may act as a "bridge to recovery" or "bridge to nowhere" or a bridge to destination therapy (DT) or a bridge to decision making (DM).[1]

Does ECMO have a Role in Such a Scenario? Device Selection in AHF

Extracorporeal membrane oxygenation is a modification of the cardiopulmonary bypass circuit which is used routinely in cardiac surgery. It is used as a temporary support, usually awaiting recovery of organs. Today in 2019, in a case of AHF, the utility of IABP–as a destination therapy, remains controversial. The answer is NO! There are a lot of pros and cons for IABP which can be summarized as in Table 1.

In a study done by Sofie Gevaert et al.[2] there is a current trend to use short-term support with ECMO in refractory cardiogenic shock but data from large randomized trials are lacking.

Extracorporeal Membrane Oxygenation

Extracorporeal membrane oxygenation is a rescue therapy used to provide cardiac and/or respiratory support for critically ill patients in whom maximal conventional medical management has failed. ECMO is considered an emergency rescue therapy for patients with:

- Refractory cardiogenic shock
- Their condition is so unstable that they are not eligible for immediate left ventricular assist devices (LVAD) implantation.

Extracorporeal Membrane Oxygenation Brief Historical Background

Extracorporeal life support (ECLS) outside of the operating room was pioneered in the late 1960s. First successful use of ECMO was reported in 1972 by Dr Robert Bartlett with the first baby born with **meconium** aspiration for

Flowchart 1: Pathophysiology and vicious cycle of worsening heart failure.

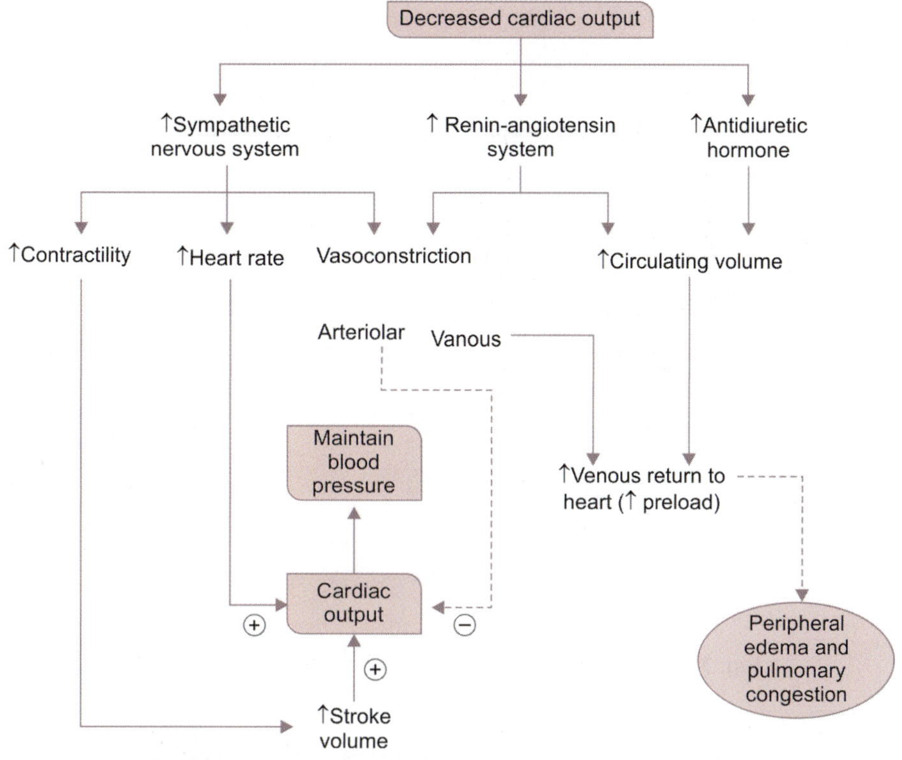

esperanza meaning hope in Figures 3 and 4).[3] ECMO has been best studied as a treatment for respiratory failure in the newborn. An accepted therapy for severe cases of neonatal respiratory distress syndrome and is meconium aspiration, acute respiratory distress syndrome (ARDS), dextro-transposition of the great arteries (dTGA), etc.

So, our patient has a choice of mechanical circulatory support (MCS).

Mechanical circulatory support, either an intra-aortic balloon pump and CentriMag/ventricular assisted devices of percutaneous (Tandem Heart, Impella) or a surgical; LVAD, RVAD, BIVAD (CentriMag, Bio-Medicus, Medos, Heartmate) can also be used or a short ECMO duration, till a definitive device like CentriMag/impella can be made available (definitive therapy) (Fig. 5).

TABLE 1: Pros and cons of intra-aortic balloon pump (IABP) for acute heart failure.

Pros	Cons
• Increases coronary perfusion • Decreases preload and afterload • Modestly increases cardiac output • Mature technology • Easy to transport patients • Patients can be awake • Nurse managed • Relatively inexpensive	• Modestly increases cardiac output • Does not provide a high level of support • Does not unload (rest) the heart • Requires some cardiac function • Requires a stable rhythm • Not without complications • Bleeding, embolism.thrombosis, thrombocytopenia, limb ischemia, aortic dissection, infection/sepsis

CANNULATION FOR EXTRACORPOREAL MEMBRANE OXYGENATION DURING CARDIOMYOPATHY

Figure 6A and B shown cannulation for ECMO during cardiomyopathy.

Extracorporeal Membrane Oxygenation Basics and Importance in Heart Failure

Extracorporeal membrane oxygenation should be considered if the process is severe, acute and potentially reversible. Technique is used to provide life support to the critically ill; temporary support for patients with pulmonary or cardiac failure (or both), when no other form of treatment is likely to be successful. It is an expensive therapy, requiring the weighing of its application, instead of other forms of treatment (Figs. 7 and 8).

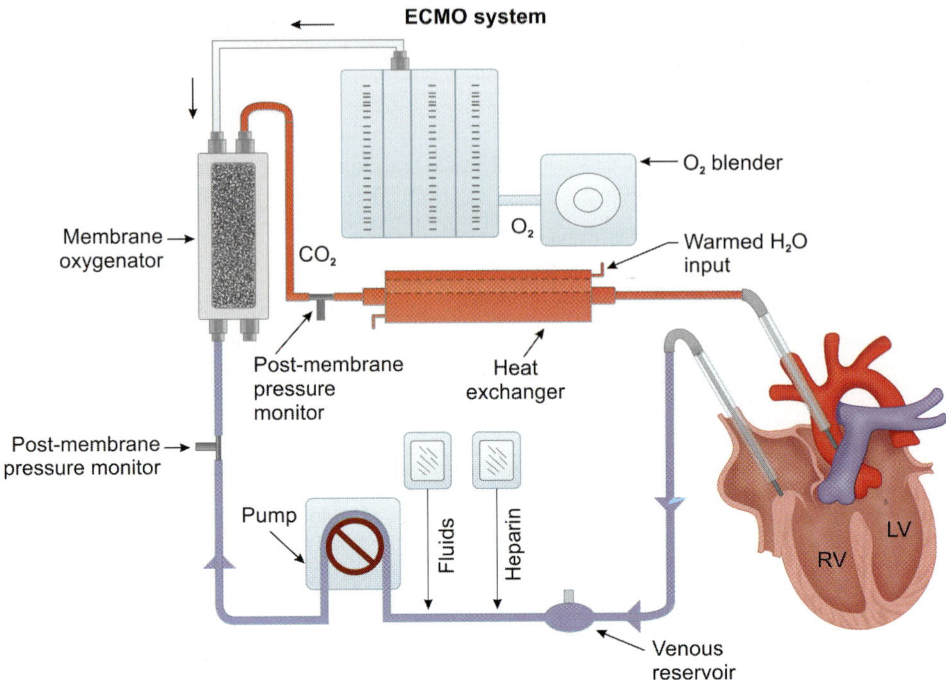

Fig. 3: The extracorporeal membrane oxygenation system.

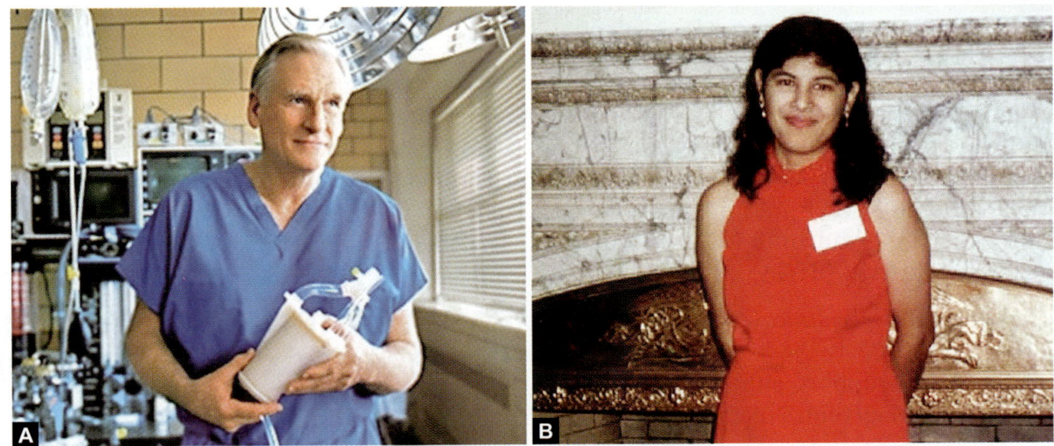

Figs. 4A and B: (A) Dr Robert Bartlett (Father of ECMO) who did the first VA ECMO on a meconium aspiration; (B) ASD baby girl "Esperanza".

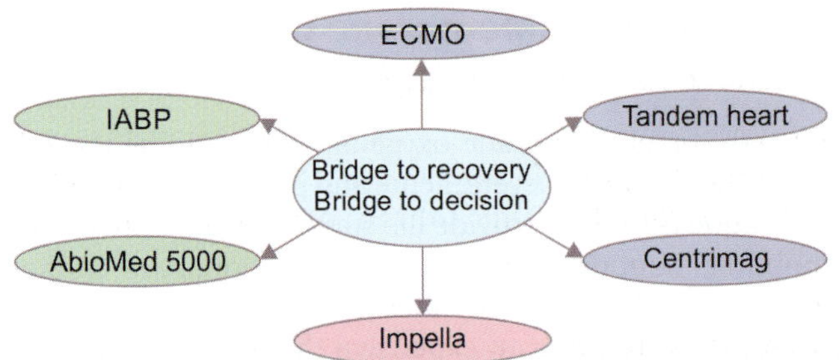

Fig. 5: Short-term device options.
(ECMO: extracorporeal membrane oxygenation; IABP: intra-aortic balloon pump)

Extracorporeal Membrane Oxygenation in India

Extracorporeal membrane oxygenation has grown in India by leaps and bound. Today, robust and active centers are around 50 with Fortis Chennai topping the list.[4,5]

ECMO in Heart Failure can be Used as a Bridge to Bridge

Immediately stabilized circulation improve end-organ perfusion, overall survival comparable between

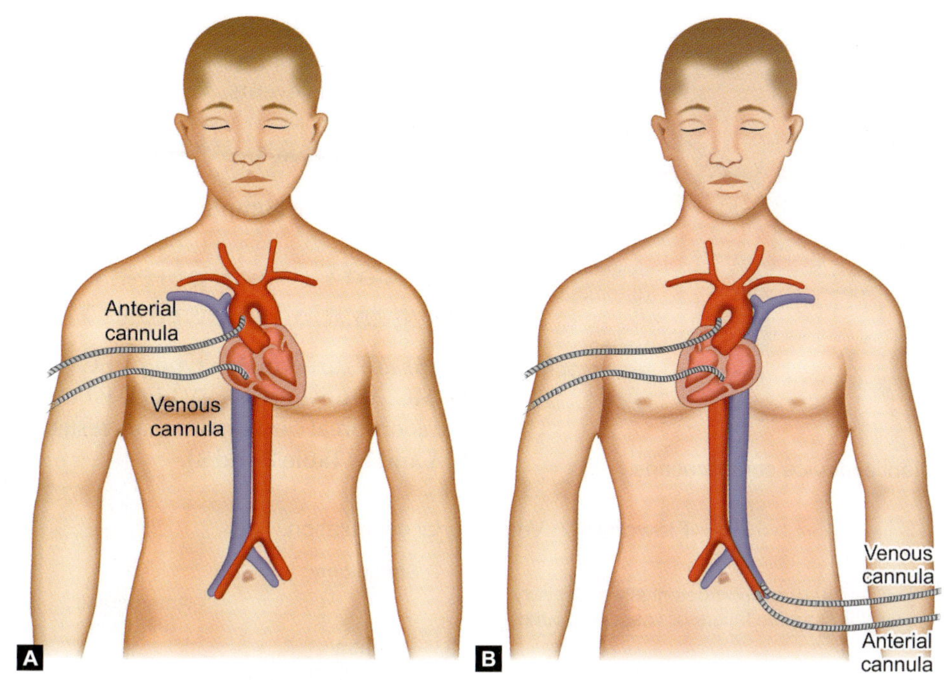

Figs. 6A and B: Cannulation for extracorporeal membrane oxygenation during cardiomyopathy.

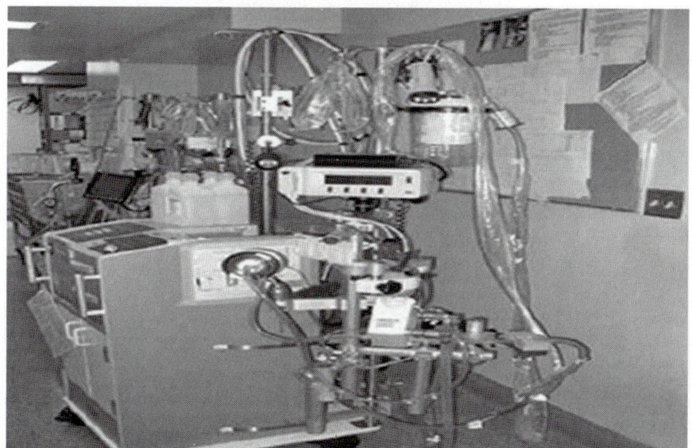

Fig. 7: Extracorporeal membrane oxygenation machine getting miniaturized in 2019.

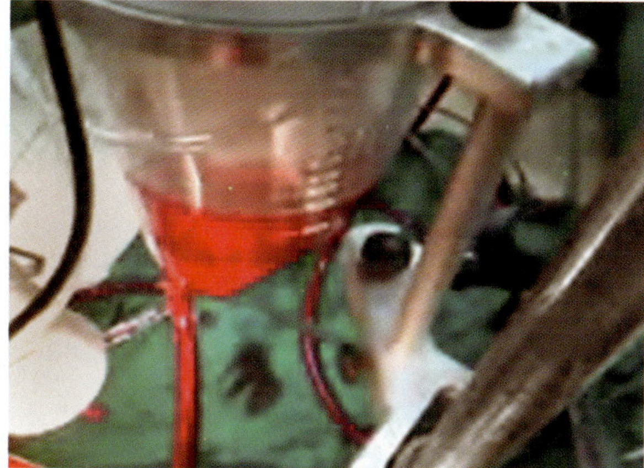

Fig. 8: First extracorporeal membrane oxygenation circuit at All India Institute of Medical Science (AIIMS).

ECMO + LVAD vs LVAD alone. Clinical indicators of poor outcome after ECMO—consider VAD implantation carefully.

Things to Think About? Extracorporeal Membrane Oxygenation Disadvantages

Mechanical ventilation must be continued during ECMO support or ECMO flow can be very volume dependent.

Requires trained team and equipment availability onsite and early in resuscitation or higher risk of infection, bleeding and vascular injury. ECMO with improved survival rates, does have complications and disadvantages as listed in Figure 9.

Complications of Extracorporeal Membrane Oxygenation in Heart Failure

Complications of ECMO falls into three major categories:

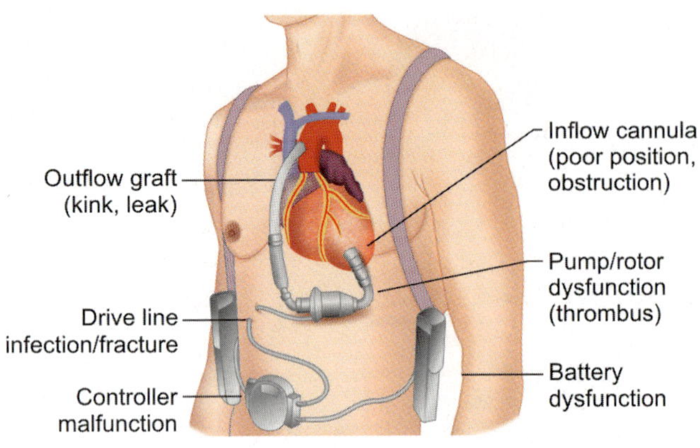

Fig. 9: Potential device complications.

1. Bleeding/hemolysis
2. Mechanical failure
3. Neurologic events.

Potential Device Complications

Potential device complications in Figure 9.

Types of Extracorporeal Membrane Oxygenation (Flowchart 2)

There are three major type of ECMO; venoarterial (VA) ECMO, venovenous (VV) ECMO and rescue ECMO on extracorporeal cardiopulmonary resuscitation (ECPR) (Figs. 10A and B, Table 2 and 3).

Flowchart 2: Venoarterial cannulation.

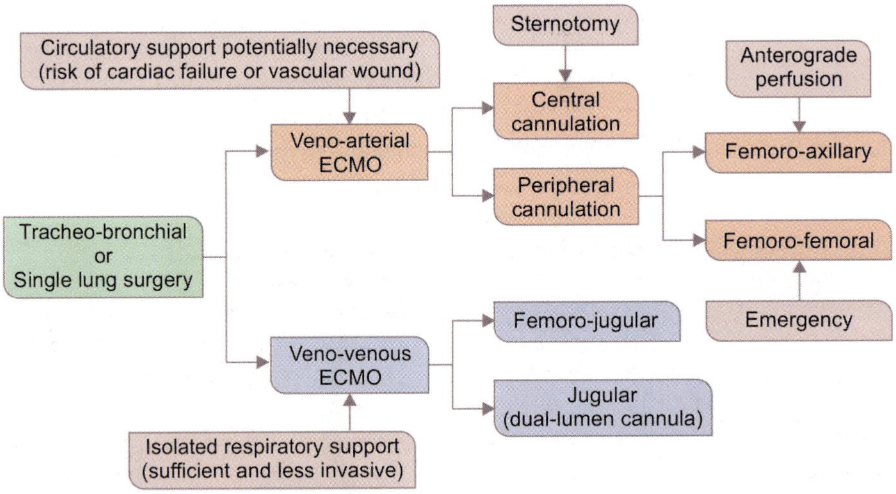

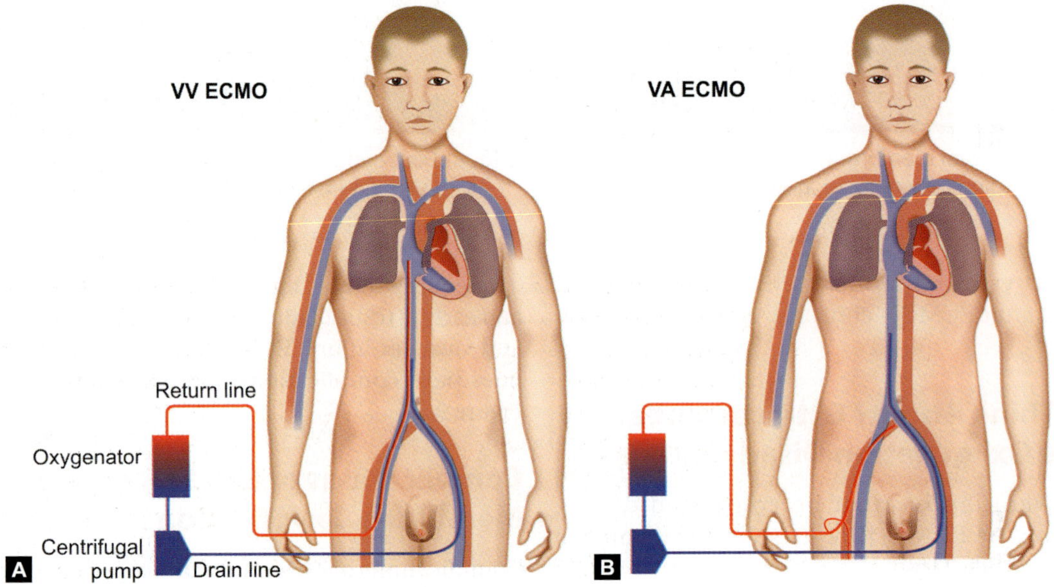

- Tracheo-bronchial or Single lung surgery → Veno-arterial ECMO; Veno-venous ECMO
- Circulatory support potentially necessary (risk of cardiac failure or vascular wound) → Veno-arterial ECMO
- Veno-arterial ECMO → Central cannulation; Peripheral cannulation
- Sternotomy → Central cannulation
- Peripheral cannulation → Femoro-axillary; Femoro-femoral
- Anterograde perfusion → Femoro-axillary
- Emergency → Femoro-femoral
- Isolated respiratory support (sufficient and less invasive) → Veno-venous ECMO
- Veno-venous ECMO → Femoro-jugular; Jugular (dual-lumen cannula)

VV ECMO
VA ECMO
Return line
Oxygenator
Centrifugal pump
Drain line
A
B

Figs. 10 A and B: Venovenous (VV) and venoarterial (VA) extracorporeal membrane oxygenation (ECMO).

TABLE 2: ECMO types and their differences.

Property	*VA ECMO*	*VV ECMO*
Cannulation site	IJV/FV and RCC/Ax/FA/Ao	IJV alone/ IJV-FV/ FV-FV/Saph-saph/RA
PaO_2	60–150 mm Hg	45–80 mm Hg
Indicator of O_2 sufficiency	Mixed ven sat or PaO_2	Combination of SaO_2, PaO_2, cerebral ven sat and pre-membr sat trend
Cardiac effect	↓ preload; ↑ afterload; pulse pr ↓; coronary oxygen by LV blood; `Cardiac stun`	Negligible effects; may improve coronary oxygen; may reduce RV afterload
O_2 delivery capacity	High	Moderate: ↑ cephalad drain
Circulatory support	Partial to complete	Indirect: ↑ delivery of O_2 to coronary and pulmonary circulation

TABLE 3: ECMO types and their grouping.

	Bad lung Good heart	*Good lung Bad heart*	*Bad lung Bad heart*
VV	✓	✗	✗
VA peripheral	✗	✓	✓
VA central	✓ (not required)	✓	✓

(VA: venoarterial, VV: venovenous)

Venovenous/Arterial Extracorporeal Membrane Oxygenation (Flowchart 2, Figs. 11 and 12)

There are the few indications of VV ECMO:
- Cardiogenic shock
- Pulmonary support
- Postcardiotomy
- Postheart/lung transplant.

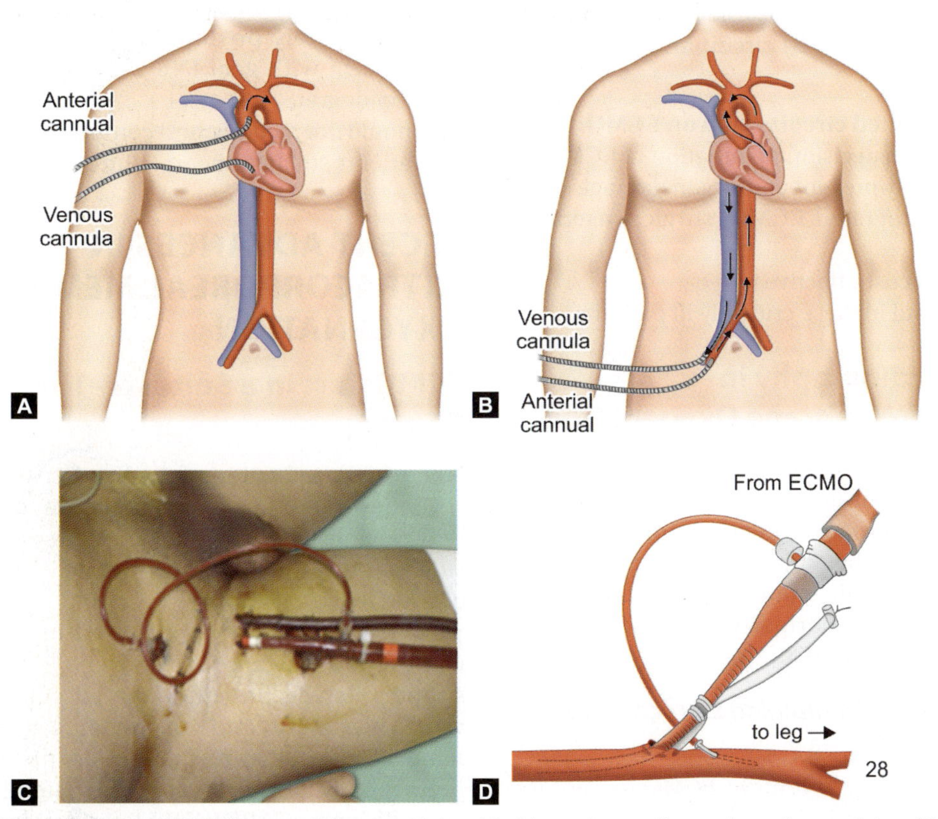

Figs. 11A to D: ECMO cannulation can be guided by echocardiography or image intensifies.

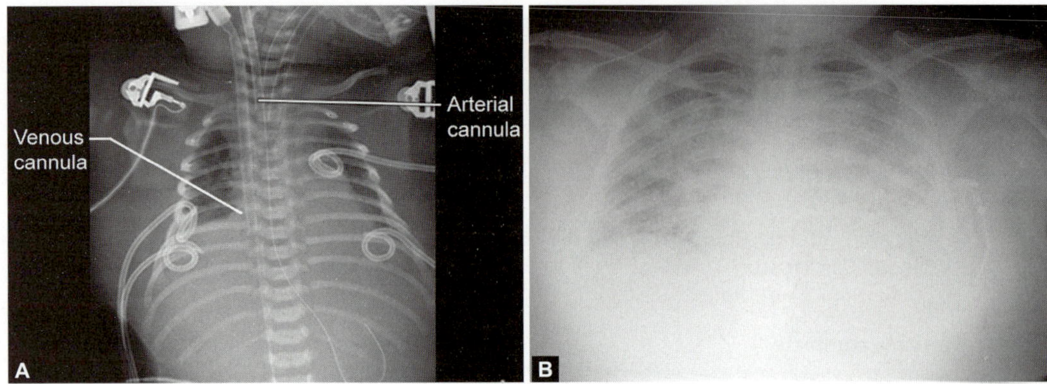

Figs. 12A and B: Chest X-ray of complete whiteout of the patient lung in cardiac heart failure seen on day 1 of venoarterial extracorporeal membrane oxygenation.

The portable VV ECMO machine in heart failure.

- Portable, can be inserted in Cath lab
- 17 to 21 Fr cannulas
- IABP to reduce afterload
- Centrifugal pump at 2 to 4 L/min
- Bridge to surgical VAD, transplant or recovery.

Use of Integrated Extracorporeal Membrane Oxygenator Better Survival Benefit: in neonates undergoing cardiac surgery at AIIMS (Figs. 13 to 15)[6,7]

Integrated ECMO circuitry was established along with cardiopulmonary bypass (CPB) circuit and primed with blood.

Advantages of integrated circuit when on ECMO:

- No time is lost from decision to initiation of ECMO
- Early initiation may prevent end-organ damage
- With a use of integrated ECMO, surgical asepsis is maintained
- The procedure is cost-effective
- Increasing survival in these critically ill patients.

Role of Echocardiography in Extracorporeal Membrane Oxygenation

As ECMO flow depends on right atrial filling, this is monitored by means of echocardiography. During a weaning attempt each partial decrease in ECMO flow should be compensated by an increase in stroke volume without excessive increase in inotropic support. Treatment of acute and critically ill peripartum cardiomyopathy (PPCM) is shown in Flowchart 3.

Echocardiography for Maintaining Extracorporeal Membrane Oxygenation

Echo is useful in the whole process of ECMO as described under: Patient selection for ECMO

Management Considerations in Extracorporeal Membrane Oxygenation for Heart Failure

- *Typically, pulseless*: Use a Doppler or arterial line for blood pressure (BP) assessment [target mean arterial pressure (MAP) 60–80].
- *Afterload sensitive*: An increase against pump propulsion is reflected in decreased pump flow.
- *Anticoagulation status*: Correction of coagulopathy immediately postoperatively and at 24–48 hours, warfarin with goal INR 2–3 ± aspirin, dipyridamole, clopidogrel.
- Should not receive chest compressions during an arrest. Patients still have heart failure.

RECENT ADVANCES IN EXTRACORPOREAL MEMBRANE OXYGENATION

ECMO Cart in a Suitcase–The CARDIOHELP (Fig. 16)

Since the introduction of the first ECMO treatment in the seventies, there has always been the dream of having a fully capable heart and lung assisted system in the size of a suitcase. This dream has come true with the introduction of CARDIOHELP system.

CARDIOHELP system combines a high level of clinical performance for venovenous or venoarterial life support during percutaneous or centrally cannulated ventricular assist, and for providing state-of-the-art CO_2 removal capabilities to enable ideal protective ventilation protocols. All this together with outstanding mobility and cost efficiency. CARDIOHELP system delivers a high level

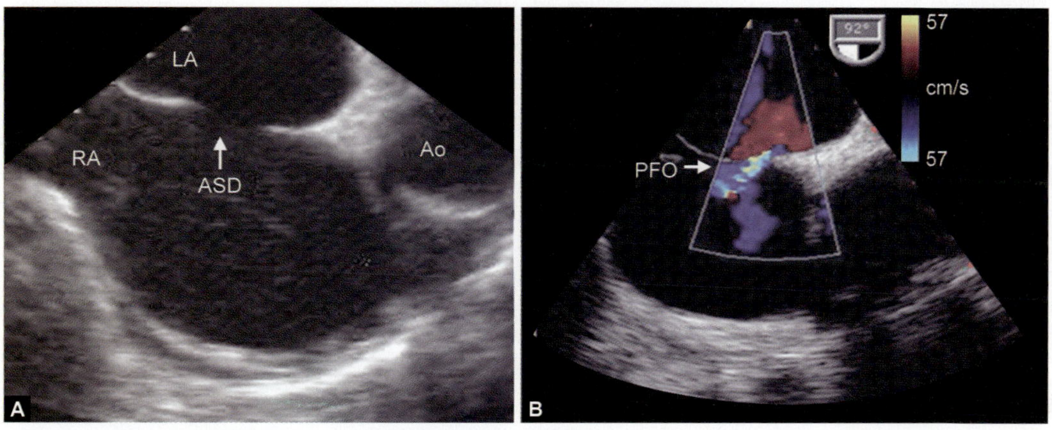

Figs. 13 A and B: (A) Atrial septal defect (ASD); (B) Patent foramen ovale (PFO).

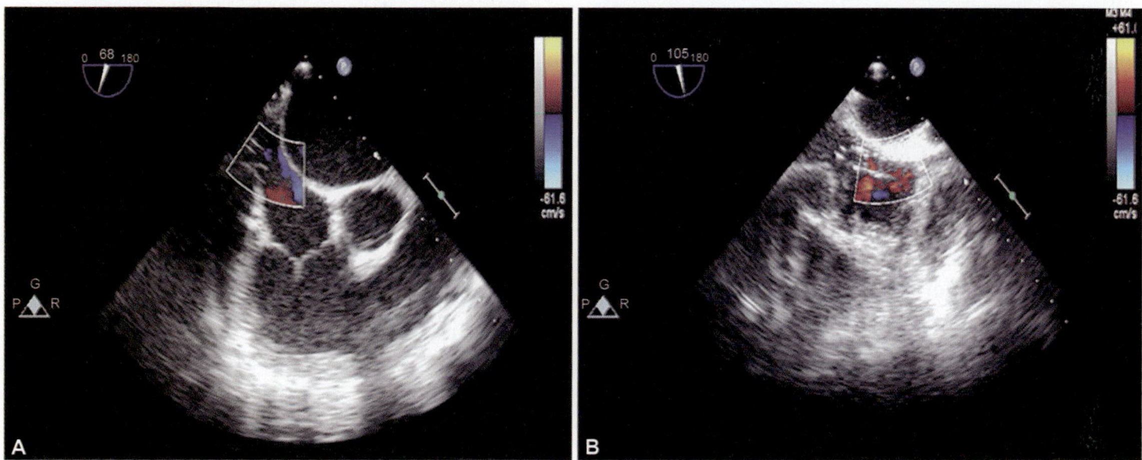

Figs. 14A and B: Insertion and correct placement of cannulas (VA ECMO).

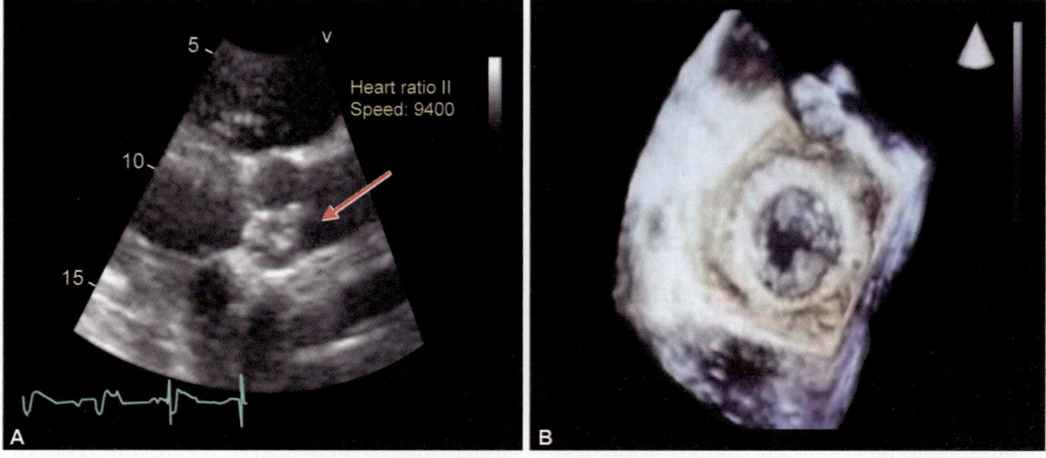

Figs. 15A and B: ECMO complication—thrombosis.

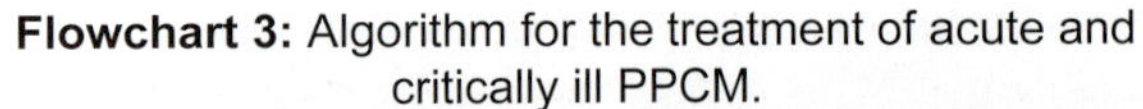

Flowchart 3: Algorithm for the treatment of acute and critically ill PPCM.

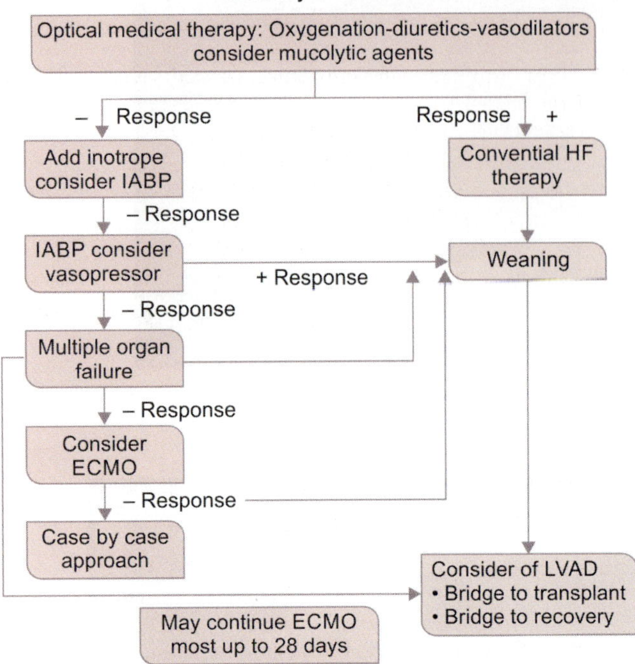

of clinical performance to help clinicians provide the best possible care for their patients.[6,7]

SHORT-TERM MECHANICAL CIRCULATORY SUPPORT

In the past few years, the 4 primary ways by which short-term mechanical circulatory assistance has been most efficiently applied include the following:

1. *Bridge to recovery:* This is for postoperative cardiac or pulmonary failure or both and for transient nonoperative organ failure that has an expectation of meaningful recovery if given enough time to overcome the inciting event.
2. *Bridge to transplant:* This is fairly well established in the area of primary cardiac failure but is becoming a far more important factor in the arena of lung transplantation.
3. *Procedural support:* In this application, various forms of mechanical support are deployed either to improve stability to the patient who requires procedural intervention or prophylactically to the patient who is expected to develop clinical instability during a potential clinically problematic procedure.
4. *Bridge to decision:* Conceptually, this is the most flexible, dynamic, and newest application of short-term mechanical circulatory assistance. This will likely make up the largest portion of short-term mechanical circulatory support in the near future. The rapid advancement of this technology and its increasingly diverse options in terms of actual devices and indications are somewhat juxtaposed to the immediacy of the patient's clinical status and the lack of time to fully assess which type of mid-term and long-term mechanical support, if any, is best applied to that particular clinical indication.

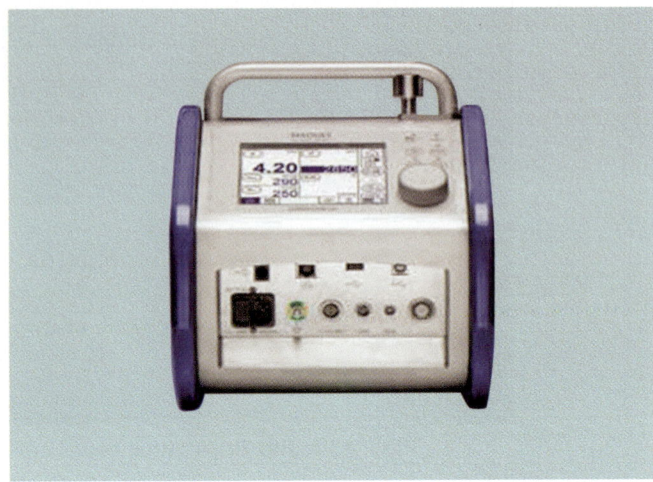

Fig. 16: ECMO cart in a suitcase, with CARDIOHELP, for EC-CPR.

Although medications such as beta-blockers, ACE inhibitors, and angiotensin II receptor blockers can alleviate the symptoms of HF and improve mortality, the gold standard for treating end-stage HF remains heart transplantation. Unfortunately, given the scarcity of available organs, only about 4,500 heart transplantations were performed worldwide in patients of all ages in 2013. The demand for heart transplantations is expected to far exceed the available supply for the foreseeable future.

Mechanical circulatory support devices (MCSDs) replaced some of the mechanical functions of the failing heart to improve cardiac output and organ perfusion. They have the potential to treat many patients with end-stage HF who cannot be transplanted either due to lack of available organs or socioeconomic reasons.

Between June 2006 and December 2014, 15,745 patients were implanted with ventricular assist devices (VADs) and the total artificial heart (TAH) in the United States. These numbers have been rising steadily, from approximately 1,000 devices implanted in 2009 to approximately 2,500 devices implanted in 2014 in the United States.[4] Besides the VAD and the TAH, other types of MCSD exist, including the IABP and ECMO. The IABP, ECMO, and VAD can be utilized as a bridge to recovery (BTR). All four types of MCSD can be utilized as a bridge to transplantation (BTT), whereas only VADs can be utilized as destination therapy (DT).

Successful cardiovascular support requires maintaining perfusion and aggressive volume resuscitation during the first few days on ECMO. Since ECMO promotes release of cytokines and a generalized systemic inflammatory response syndrome, adequate volume resuscitation with crystalloid or colloid is paramount. In addition, inotropic support is often required as the heart recovers.

CONCLUSION

The management of advanced heart failure is a dynamic process that requires frequent reevaluation. Timing of ECMO placement is critical. ECMO for destination therapy has been shown to improve mortality rates and quality of life. There are short-term ECMO (ECPR) options available for emergent situations and ECPR for cardiogenic shock and VA ECMO for heart failure.

REFERENCES

1. Lietz K, Long JW, Kfoury AJ, et al. Outcomes of left ventricular assist device implantation as destination therapy in the post-REMATCH era: implications for patient selection. Circulation. 2007;116(5):497-505.
2. Gevaert S, Belleghem YV, Bouchez S, et al. Acute and critically ill peripartum cardiomyopathy and 'bridge to' therapeutic options: a single center experience with intraaortic balloon pump, extracorporeal membrane oxygenation and continuous-flow left ventricular assist devices. Crit Care. 2011;15(2):R93.
3. Hill JD, O'Brien TJ, Murray JJ, et al. Prolonged Extracorporeal Oxygenation for Acute Post-Traumatic Respiratory Failure (Shock-Lung Syndrome)—Use of the Bramson Membrane Lung. N Engl J Med. 1972;286(12):629-34.
4. Wander GS, Pareek KK, Kapoor PM. A New Therapeutic Modality—Where we are in India. In: Textbook of Medicine Update 2016. New Delhi: Jaypee Brothers Medical Publishers (P) Ltd. 2016. pp. 1634-8.
5. Pooboni S, Goyal V, Oza P, et al. ECMO Challenges and its Future: Indian Scenario. J Card Crit Care. 2017;1(02): 89-94.
6. Singh P, Kapoor PM, Devagourou V, et al. Use of integrated extracorporeal membrane oxygenator in anomalous left coronary artery to pulmonary artery: Better survival benefit. Ann Card Anaesth. 2011;14:240-2.
7. Kapoor PM, Hasija S. Cardio Help: The Future of Extracorporeal Membrane Oxygenation. In: Manual of Extracorporeal Membrane Oxygenation (ECMO) in the ICU. New Delhi: Jaypee Brothers Medical Publishers (P) Ltd. 2013. pp. 243-8.

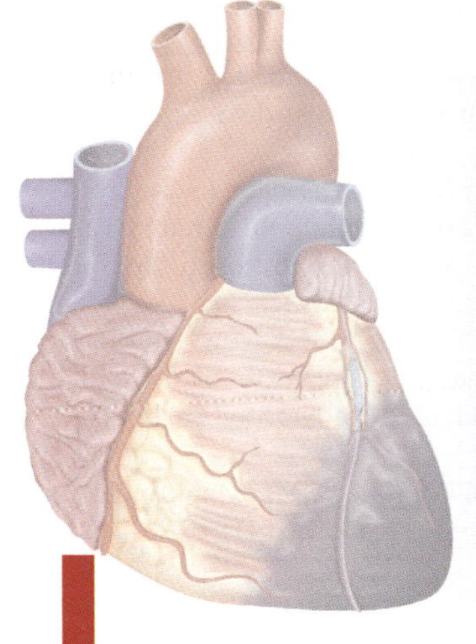

Heart Transplant and Heart Failure

Anuj Sangal, Rajneesh Malhotra

INTRODUCTION

The field of heart transplantation has made undeniable progress since the first human-to-human heart transplant was performed 50 years ago in 1967. It has now entered an era of tremendous growth and innovation. Since 1990, the heart transplant volume has averaged between 2,000 and 2,500 cases/year. Interestingly, over the past 3 years there has been a steady uptrend. In 2016, 3,190 heart transplants were performed. This is an exciting statistic and perhaps reflects increased donor utilization as the number of donors has remained stable. Survival after transplant has steadily improved with recent 1-, 5- and 10-year rates at approximately 90%, 80%, and 65%, respectively.[1] In addition to the technological and pharmaceutical achievements, proper patient selection, superb medical management, meticulous operative care, vigilant surveillance, and responsive long-term follow-up can all be credited for the continuing success in heart transplantation. Further advances in immunosuppression, immune tolerance and personalized medicine hold the key for future gains.

HISTORICAL NOTE

The first human-to-human heart transplant (allograft) was performed in Cape Town, South Africa, by Christiaan Barnard on December 3, 1967.[2] The recipient was Louis Washkansky, a 53-year-old ex-boxer with end-stage ischemic cardiomyopathy. 3 days after the Cape Town operation, Adrian Kantrowitz performed the second human heart transplant in Brooklyn.[3] On January 2, 1968, Barnard performed the third human heart transplant on Philip Blaiberg, a 46-year-old dental surgeon with refractory heart failure, severe coronary artery disease, and a large left ventricular aneurysm. He became the first long-term survivor, living for 18 months. Norman Shumway performed the fourth heart transplant 4 days later, and this patient died 2 weeks later. After this, other heart transplants followed rapidly in a number of institutions. By the end of 1968, cardiac transplantation had been performed in 102 patients in 50 different institutions in 17 countries. The results were generally poor, with 60% mortality by the eighth postoperative day and a mean survival of only 29 days. Since 1980, published data on more than 80,000 cardiac transplantations from over 300 cardiac transplant programs have been reported in the voluntary registry of the International Society for Heart and Lung Transplantation (ISHLT) (Fig. 1).[4]

RISK FACTORS AND CONTRAINDICATIONS FOR CARDIAC TRANSPLANTATION

The risk factors and contraindications for cardiac transplantation are outlined in Boxes 1 and 2.

DONOR EVALUATION AND SELECTION

The donor becomes available when brain death has occurred, and criteria enumerated by the Ad Hoc Committee of the Harvard Medical School are generally used.[5-7] The

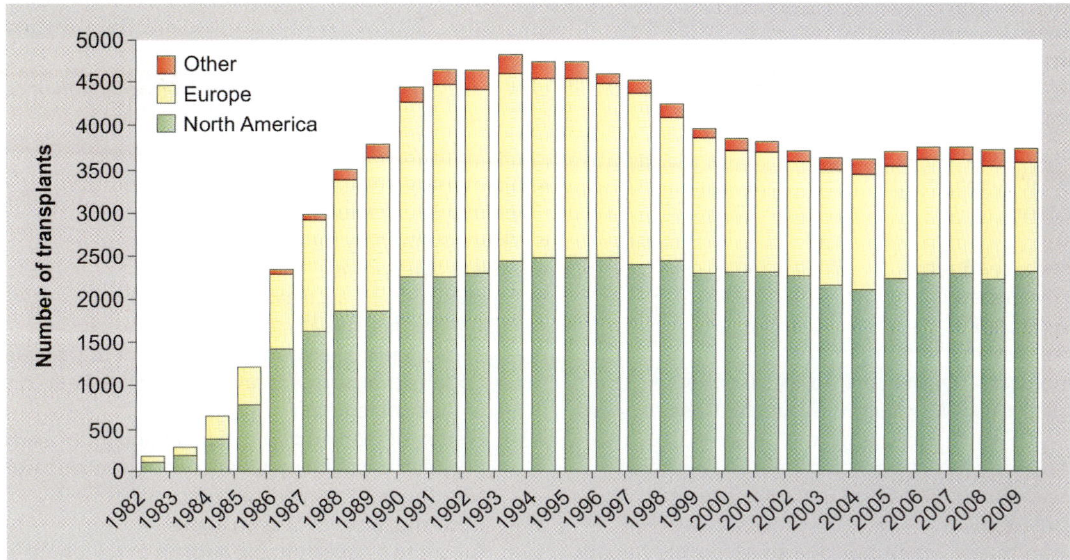

Fig. 1: Number of heart transplants reported by the International Society for Heart and Lung Transplantation (ISHLT).
Source: Adapted from ISHLT. J Heart Lung Transplant. 2011;30(10):1071-132.

BOX 1: Risk factors associated with high morbidity and mortality.

- Pulmonary hypertension (>6 Wood units not responsive to vasodilators or not decreasing to <3 to 4 Wood units, pulmonary artery systolic pressure >70 mm Hg, transpulmonary gradient >15 mm Hg)
- Infection, active, untreated:
  - HIV positive
- End-organ disease, irreversible:
  - Hepatic
  - Renal
  - Pulmonary (FEV_1 <1.5 $L\text{-}sec^{-1}$)
- Pulmonary infarction, recent
- Age >60 years
- Diabetes mellitus with end-organ damage (without end-organ damage also increases risk)
- Peripheral arterial disease or cerebrovascular disease (risk related to severity)
- Gastrointestinal diseases:
  - Chronic active hepatitis
  - Diverticulitis, recent
  - Peptic ulcer disease with active bleeding
- Obesity (> 120% of ideal body weight)
- Malignancy (within 5 years, high risk; remote, less risk)
- Osteoporosis
- Psychiatric disorder:
  - Affective or schizophrenic
  - Personality disorder, including medical noncompliance
- Substance abuse:
  - Tobacco
  - Alcohol
  - Controlled drug
- Lack of social support

donor must be completely unresponsive, without reflexes or movements of breathing. Two flat electroencephalograms obtained 24 hours apart are sometimes required. The donor should be younger than 60 years of age (although occasionally hearts from older donors are used for elderly recipients) and without documented prior myocardial infarction. Coronary angiography is recommended in all potential donors older than age 45 years; the heart is generally not used for transplantation if there is important arteriosclerotic coronary obstruction. A history of smoking also prompts coronary angiography as part of the process of donor selection.

There should have been no prolonged episodes of profound hypotension or cardiac arrest after injury, because poor donor heart function after transplantation is likely to follow such an event. However, echocardiography often allows the heart to be used if ventricular performance is good. Important ventricular arrhythmias usually eliminate a donor.

Immunologic Aspects of Transplant Testing

- ABO compatibility
- HLA typing
- Panel reactive antigens (PRA)
- Crossmatching

Flowchart 1 shows 2017 ACC/AHA/HFSA focused update of the 2013 ACCF/AHA guidelines for the management of heart failure.

BOX 2: Contraindications to heart transplant.

General Contraindications

Presence of any noncardiac condition that would itself shorten life expectancy or increase risk of death from rejection or complications of immunosuppression

Specific Contraindications

- Older age (>about 65 years)
- Active infection
- HIV positive
- Active peptic ulcer disease
- Chronic active hepatitis
- Recent diverticulitis
- Diabetes mellitus with end-organ damage
- Severe peripheral arterial or cerebrovascular disease
- Coexisting active neoplasm (within 5 years, high risk; removed, low risk)
- Morbid obesity (>140% of predicted ideal body weight)
- Creatinine clearance <40 to 50 mL/min, effective renal plasma flow <200 mL/min
- Bilirubin >2.5 mg/dL when not due to reversible hepatic congestion, transaminases >2 × normal
- Severe pulmonary dysfunction with FVC and FEV_1 less than about 40% of predicted, especially with intrinsic lung disease
- Pulmonary artery systolic pressure >60 mm Hg, mean transpulmonary gradient > 15 Wood units
- Acute pulmonary thromboembolism
- Severe osteoporosis
- Smoking within last 6 months
- High risk of life-threatening noncompliance:
  - Inability to make strong commitment to transplantation
  - Cognitive impairment severe enough to limit comprehension of medical regimen
  - History of marked depression or emotional instability
  - Psychiatric instability severe enough to jeopardize incentive for adherence to medical regimen
  - Recurring alcohol or drug abuse
  - Failure to establish stable address or telephone number
  - Previous demonstration of repeated noncompliance with medical therapy or follow-up
  - Lack of independent family or social support system

Flowchart 1: 2017 ACC/AHA/HFSA focused update of the 2013 ACCF/AHA guidelines for the management of heart failure.

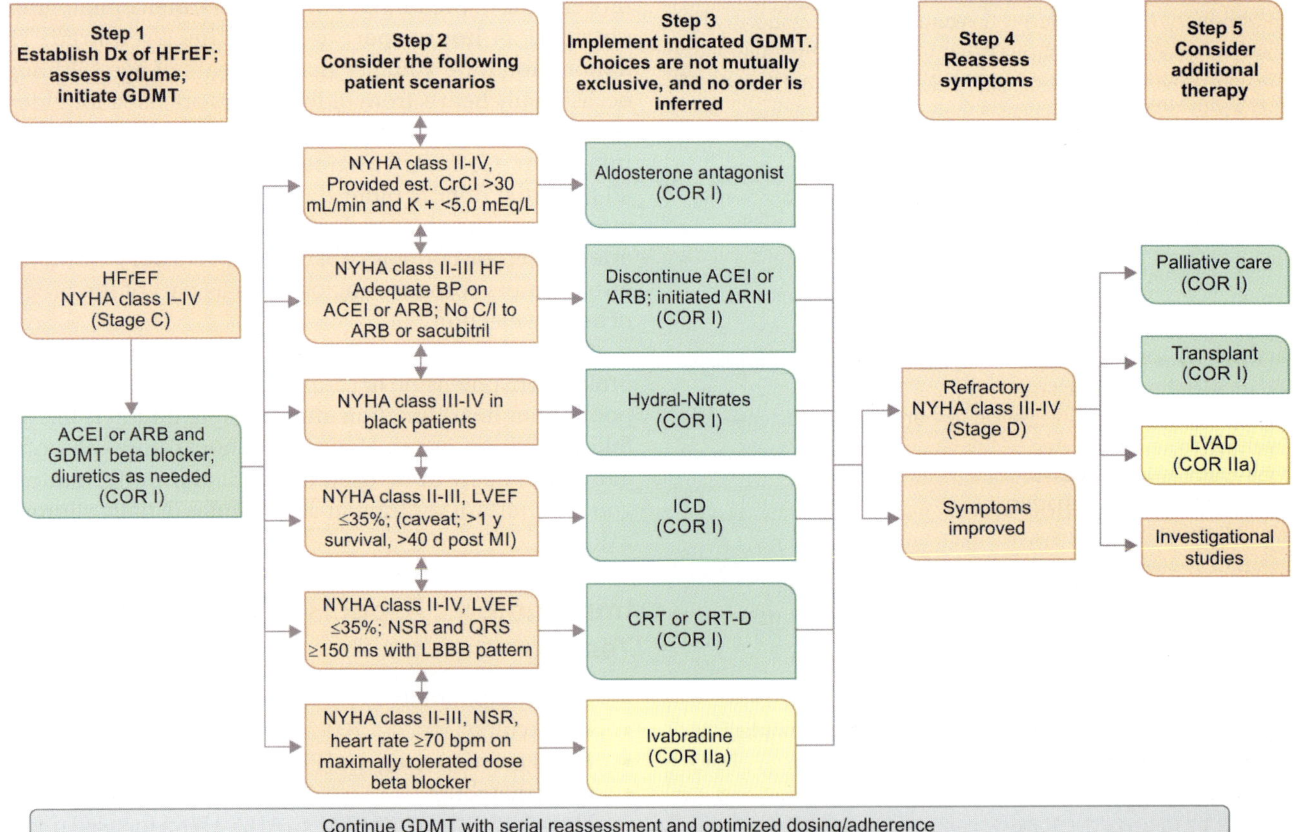

(ACEI: angiotensin-converting enzyme inhibitors; ARB: angiotensin II receptor blockers; ARNI: angiotensin receptor-neprilysin inhibitors; GDMT: guideline-directed medical therapy; HFrEF: heart failure with reduced ejection fraction; LVAD: left ventricular assist device; NYHA: New York Heart Association)

TECHNIQUES OF OPERATION

Donor Heart Procurement

Most donors are donating multiple organs including the heart. Therefore, the donor is prepared from neck to mid-thigh. Preferably, a central venous line and an arterial catheter are placed because marked hypotension may occur while mobilizing the abdominal organs. After median sternotomy, a self-retaining retractor is inserted. While other organ procurement teams proceed, the pericardium is opened and usual stay sutures are applied. The heart is examined for evidence of cardiac injury, congenital anomalies, coronary arteriosclerosis, or other acquired heart disease. The ascending aorta is dissected and mobilized as far as the brachiocephalic takeoff. The superior vena cava (SVC) is completely mobilized, including any pericardial reflection onto it. A purse-string suture is placed on the ascending aorta for cardioplegia infusion. When cardiectomy is ready to begin, 200 units kg^{-1} of heparin are given, and the cardioplegia needle is inserted into the ascending aorta and secured. In this setting, the cardioplegic solution is infused by gravity.

Orthotopic Cardiac Transplantation

Biatrial Technique

Figure 2 shows the biatrial technique for orthotopic cardiac transplantation.

Bicaval Technique

Figure 3 shows the bicaval technique for orthotopic cardiac transplantation.

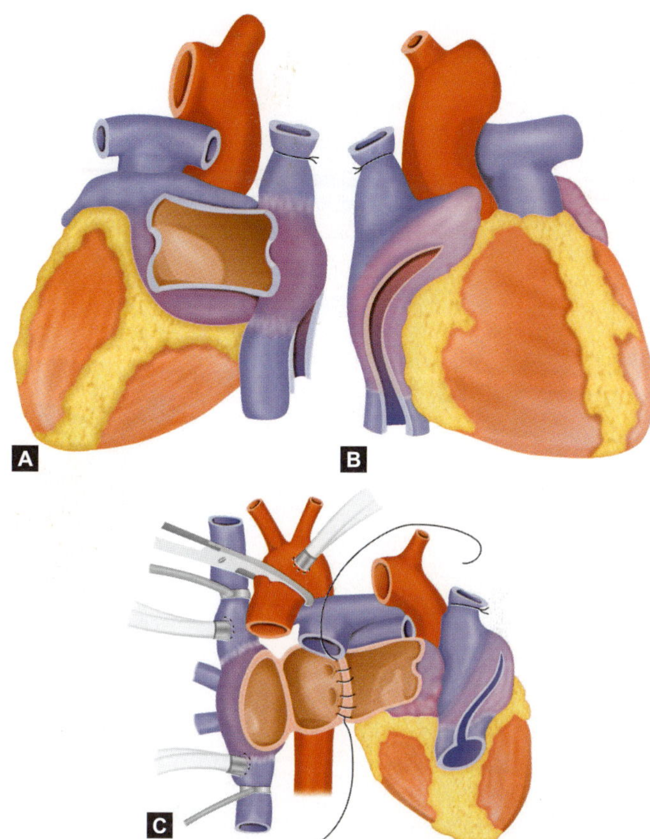

Figs. 2A to C: Orthotopic cardiac transplantation, biatrial technique. (A) Creating donor heart left atrial cuff by incising through pulmonary vein orifices; (B) Creating donor heart right atrial cuff. Incision begins at orifice of inferior vena cava and extends toward right atrial appendage approximately halfway between sulcus terminalis and atrioventricular groove; (C) Left atrial anastomosis is commenced.

SPECIAL FEATURES OF POSTOPERATIVE CARE

Usual care given to patients after cardiac surgery is applied to patients who have received a cardiac transplant.

Cardiac denervation may temporarily lower heart rate; consequently, a chronotropic catecholamine agent may be indicated. Acute distention and failure of the right ventricle resulting from excessive right ventricular afterload is occasionally observed, most commonly in the presence of preexisting recipient pulmonary hypertension or reactive pulmonary vasoconstriction from cardiopulmonary bypass (CPB) or protamine administration. Various agents may dilate pulmonary vasculature, but the most effective combination appears to be milrinone at 0.3–1 μg kg^{-1} min^{-1} and nitric oxide. Rarely, right ventricular mechanical support is required.

Aspirin, 325 mg daily, is given as soon as oral intake is begun and is continued indefinitely to counteract the tendency of the donor heart to develop coronary arteriosclerosis.

Immunosuppressive Modalities

Three situations require specific combinations of immunosuppressive therapies:

1. Initial high-dose immunosuppression to facilitate graft acceptance, minimize the chance of early rejection, and potentially favor induction of tolerance;
2. Maintenance therapy for chronic acceptance of the allograft; and
3. Augmented immunosuppression to reverse episodes of acute rejection.

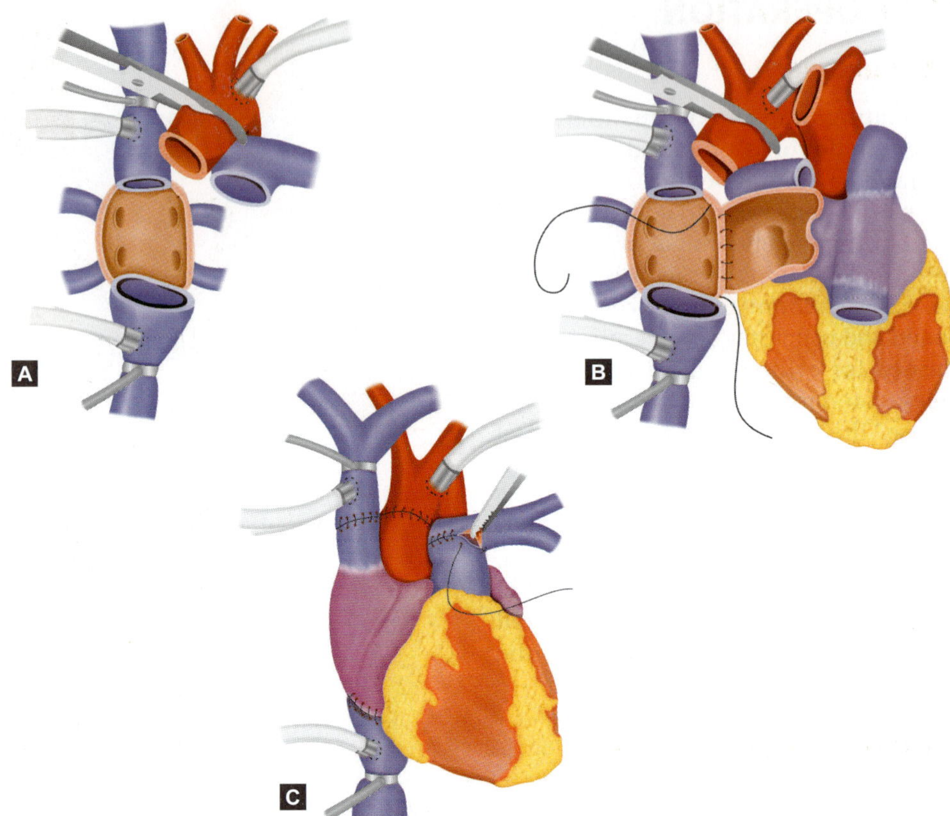

Figs. 3A to C: Orthotopic cardiac transplantation, bicaval technique. (A) Right atrium is divided to create superior and inferior vena caval cuffs. Great vessels are divided as in biatrial method. (B) Commencement of left atrial anastomosis. (C) Completion of bicaval transplant technique, showing inferior vena caval, superior vena caval, aortic, and pulmonary trunk anastomoses.

Although there is considerable variability among institutions, the general strategy involves induction therapy followed by maintenance therapy with initial "triple-drug" immunosuppression followed by gradual tapering or withdrawal of the steroid component.

Induction therapy generally includes monoclonal antibodies like basiliximab/daclizumab or antithymocyte globulin or OKT3. Maintenance immunosuppression generally includes immunosuppressive agents from three general classes, comprising the triple-drug strategy: Calcineurin inhibitors, antiproliferative agents, and steroids.

Plasmapheresis, immunoadsorption, photopheresis, and total lymphoid irradiation are other modalities that may be considered during rejection management.

CONCLUSION

Rejection

Acute cellular rejection (ACR): Major and minor histocompatibility antigens are not expressed equally among all individuals; this increases the potential of such proteins to act as alloantigens and activate alloimmunity by stimulating cytotoxic T cells. T cells respond to these donor antigens either directly or indirectly based on the method of antigen presentation. T cells can either directly recognize donor MHC molecules on allograft or target when presented indirectly by recipient antigen presenting cells (APC). Interleukin-2 (IL-2), tumor necrosis factor-beta (TNF-beta), and interferon-gamma (IFN-gamma), all act as significant mediators during rejection.

Acute humoral/antibody-mediated rejection (AMR): Antibody-mediated humoral rejection is poorly understood. The antibody reacts to donor MHC antigens (HLA-I and II) leading to capillary endothelial changes. Deposition of immunoglobulin and complements within myocardial capillary bed are detectable by immunofluorescence.

Infection

A proactive policy to detect infection is necessary because of the frequent blunting of usual infection signs and symptoms secondary to blunting of the normal inflammatory response by immunosuppressive medications. Infectious complications are closely linked to other post-transplant adverse events, such as malignancy (Epstein-Barr virus), allograft vasculopathy (cytomegalovirus), and acute rejection.

Approximately 40% of recipients suffer one or more infections requiring IV antibiotics, hospitalization, or both during the first year after transplantation.[8-10] In the current era, most infections are successfully treated, with an overall mortality from infection of less than 5% during the first year.[11]

Malignancy

Neoplastic disorders after cardiac transplantation arise from three major causes: Pre-existing malignancies, transmission of malignancy from donor to recipient, and de novo malignancy arising after transplantation. Preexisting malignancy is a relative contraindication to cardiac transplantation unless there is a prolonged malignancy-free interval and strong clinical evidence of cure.

Survival

Survival at 1 year has gradually improved over the past several decades and currently approaches 85%. Risk of death is greatest during the first 3 months after operation. After 1 year, there is a constant mortality of about 4% per year. Survival at 5 years is approximately 70%, at 10 years 50%, and at 15 years 30%. Median survival is 10 years. For patients alive at 1 year, median survival is 13 years.[4]

The most dramatic improvement in survival after heart transplantation over the past 25 years has been during the first 3-6 months. Despite the obvious importance of long-term survival to patients and their families, survival at 1 year has been a benchmark for comparison of institutions as well as eras.

REFERENCES

1. Lund LH, Edwards LB, Dipchand AI, et al. The Registry of the International Society for Heart and Lung Transplantation: thirty-third adult heart transplantation report—2016; focus theme: primary diagnostic indications for transplant. J Heart Lung Transplant. 2016;35(10):1158-69.
2. Barnard CN. The operation. A human cardiac transplant: an interim report of a successful operation performed at Groote Schuur Hospital, Cape Town. S Afr Med J. 1967;41(48): 1271-4.
3. Kantrowitz A, Haller JD, Joos H, et al. Transplantation of the heart in an infant and an adult. Am J Cardiol. 1968;22(6): 782-90.
4. Taylor DO, Edwards LB, Aurora P, et al. Registry of the International Society for Heart and Lung Transplantation: twenty-fifth official adult heart transplant report—2008. J Heart Lung Transplant. 2008;27(9):943-56.
5. A definition of irreversible coma. The Ad Hoc Committee of the Harvard Medical School to Examine the Definition of Brain Death. JAMA. 1968;205(6):337-40.
6. Capron AM. Brain death—well settled yet still unresolved. N Engl J Med. 2001;344(16):1244-6.
7. Smith SH, Kirklin JK, Geer JC, et al. Arteritis in cardiac rejection after transplantation. Am J Cardiol. 1987;59(12):1171-3.
8. Briscoe DM, Alexander SI, Lichtman AH. Interactions between T lymphocytes and endothelial cells in allograft rejection. Curr Opin Immunol. 1998;10(5):525-31.
9. Brasile L, Zerbe T, Rabin B, et al. Identification of the antibody to vascular endothelial cells in patients undergoing cardiac transplantation. Transplantation. 1985;40(6):672-5.
10. Miller LW, Naftel DC, Bourge RC, et al. Infection after heart transplantation: a multi-institutional study. Cardiac Transplant Research Database Group. J Heart Lung Transplant. 1994;13:381-93.
11. Reid KR, Menkis AH, Novick RJ, et al. Reduced incidence of severe infection after heart transplantation with low-intensity immunosuppression. J Heart Lung Transplant. 1991;10(6):894-900.

SECTION 13

Rehabilitation

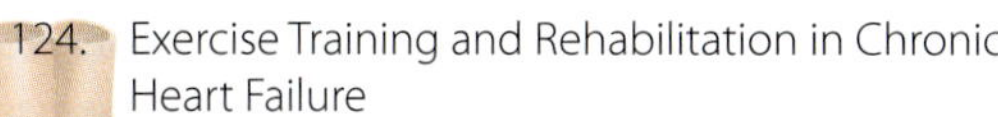

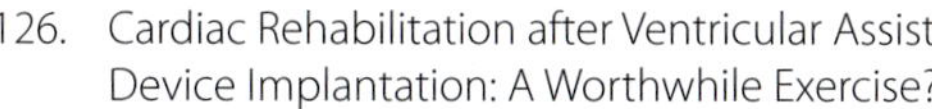

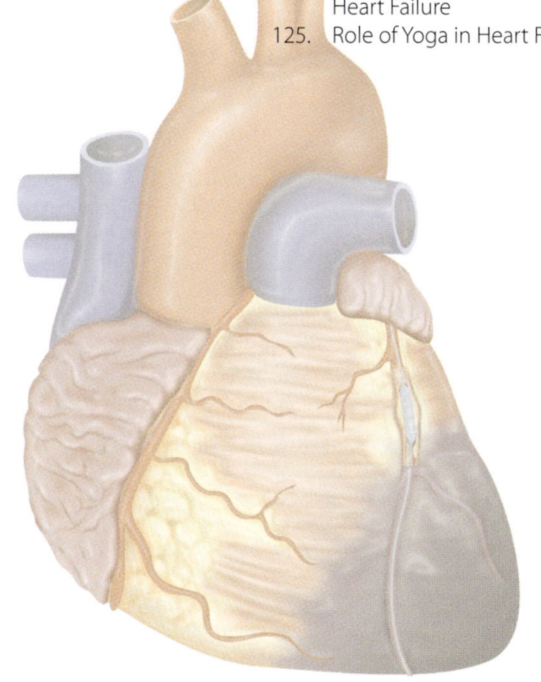

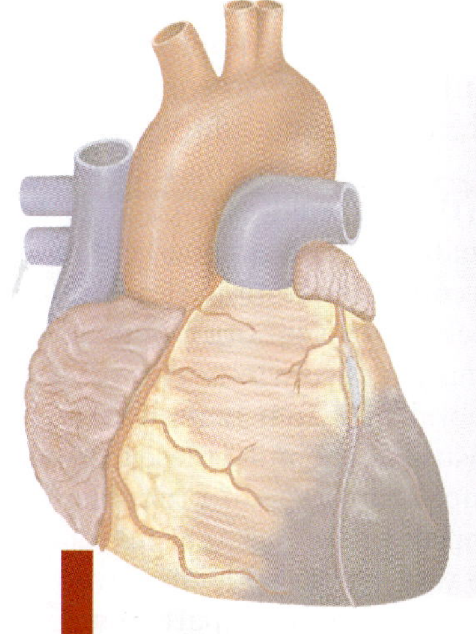

Exercise Training and Rehabilitation in Chronic Heart Failure

JPS Sawhney, Manish Kumar Sharma, Kushal Madan

INTRODUCTION

Heart failure (HF) is one of the serious health problems especially in developing countries. Exercise intolerance, accompanied by significant dyspnea and/or fatigue, is the main symptom of chronic HF and is associated with reduced quality of life (QoL) and increased mortality.

HOW TO DIAGNOSE EXERCISE INTOLERANCE?

New York Heart Association (NYHA) functional classification is a clinically useful, subjective method for stratification of HF patients. Dedicated HF QoL questionnaires, such as the Kansas City Cardiomyopathy, Minnesota Living With HF questionnaires, Duke Activity Status Index, EQ-5D all are easy to perform, cost-free and have prognostic value but have limited insight to define mechanisms of exercise intolerance. 6-minute walk test (6MWT), graded exercise testing with electrocardiography (ECG), and cardiopulmonary exercise testing (CPX) are the objective quantitative methods for the assessment of functional and/or exercise capacity. CPX is the gold standard for the assessment of exercise capacity in cardiac and noncardiac diseases, but this is time consuming and expensive as compared to 6MWT and exercise ECG tests.[1]

Exercise and Primary Prevention in Heart Failure

Several studies have reported that exercise provides protective benefit in preventing HF. In a prospective cohort, cardiorespiratory fitness (CRF) (as measured by maximal oxygen uptake, mL/kg/min) was assessed in 1,873 Finnish males without HF. During a mean follow up of 20.4 years, 152 incident HF events were recorded. This study concluded that men in top-quartile of long-term CRF had 53% lower risk of developing HF. 1 unit higher long-term CRF was associated with a 6% reduced risk of incident HF events, corresponding to a 21% risk reduction of HF per 1-MET increment in CRF.[2] In a pooled analysis of three prospective studies to quantify dose-response association between physical activity and the risk of HF with preserved ejection fraction (HFpEf) and HF with reduced ejection fraction (HfrEF), it was confirmed that there is a dose-dependent association of physical activity with HFpEF but not with HFrEF.[3] These included the Women's Health Initiative (WHI), the Multiethnic Study of Atherosclerosis (MESA), and the Cardiovascular Health Study (CHS).[4-6] In a meta-analysis of 12 prospective studies with 20,203 HF events among 370,460 participants, it was shown that the highest levels of physical activity were associated with significantly reduced risk of HF, suggesting that "more activity is better than some activity for HF prevention".[7]

Exercise Training as Therapy for Heart Failure

Before 1990s, patients with HF were generally confined to bed rest, rather discouraged from exercise. Similar to the exercise-based cardiac rehabilitation programs for myocardial infarction patients, with due course of time, over decades, several studies have demonstrated the safety and efficacy of aerobic exercise training (ET) in patients with

HF. ET is now a well establishes therapy for HF patients and American Heart Association/American College Cardiology (AHA/ACC), European Society of Cardiology (ESC) guidelines recommended individually designed ET for patients with HF as a therapeutic strategy.[8,9]

The HF-ACTION (Heart Failure: A Controlled Trial Investigating Outcomes of Exercise Training), multicenter prospective randomized controlled trial tested the long-term safety and efficacy of aerobic ET in stable HFrEF and NYHA class II to IV patients. Medically, stable 2,331 patients with HFrEF left ventricular ejection fraction (LVEF #35%) randomized to exercise participated in 36 sessions supervised ET with moderate intensity 3 days/week and were followed by up to 2 years of home training. Patients in ET group experienced an 11% reduction in all-cause mortality or hospitalization and a 15% decrease in cardiovascular death or HF hospitalization.[10,11] Following which ESC and AHA have mentioned exercise in stable HF patients as a class I with level of evidence A recommendation in addition to optimal pharmacological therapy in the guidelines.

As compared to HFrEF, there is a limited number of randomized controlled trials to study the effects of ET in HFpEF. In a randomized study of supervised ET, in 53 elderly patients with HFpEF, it was shown that a three days/week exercise program for 16 weeks could increase exercise capacity and physical score (measured on Minnesota Living with HF Questionnaire), while no change was observed in neuroendocrine or LV function.[12] In a recent review of 9 studies on 348 HFpEF patients to analyze the effects of the ET on cardiovascular outcomes, it was reported that peak oxygen uptake, 6MWT distance, ventilator threshold were significantly improved. In the included studies, training consisted of in-hospital and home-based aerobic, endurance and resistance training, walking, treadmill and bicycle ergometer.[13]

There is evidence to show that ET in HF is beneficial not only in addition to medical therapy but also, to device therapy. In a subanalysis of HF-ACTION study in which 1,053 patient with implanted cardioverter defibrillator (ICD) implants were randomized to exercise group vs. control group. It was concluded that ET was not associated with shocks and thus feasible in HFrEF patients with ICDs provided HF has been stable for at least 3 months.[14] In a meta-analysis of 6 clinical trials with ET duration of 12 weeks in HF patients and ICD implantation it was demonstrated that ET was associated with significant improvement in CRF and lower likelihood of ICD shocks.[15]

Exercise Training Modalities

Most of the exercise intervention trials are conducted on chronic, stable HF patients with moderate intensity aerobic training as intervention and are in favor of antiremodeling and improved QoL associated with moderate intensity training. Meta-analyses of HfrEF[16] and HFpEF[17] suggests only modest improvement in peak oxygen consumption (average 3.0 mL/kg/min) during maximal effort exercise.[18] Recently, there has been interest in assessing the role of high intensity interval training (HIIT) in stable HF patients. In a randomized study of 45 patients were assigned either to interval training, moderate continuous training for 30 min/day, 3 days/week for 12 weeks, or to a control group. It was shown that interval training effectively improves oxygen uptake by enhancing cerebral/muscular hemodynamics and QoL in HF patients.[19] Hsu et al. extended these findings by demonstrating that each 1-mL/kg/min increase in VO_{2peak} conferred a 58% improvement in 5-year mortality. The 8-month survival rate was significantly improved in HIIT participants compared to nonexercise participants.[20]

Resistance training is often overlooked for CHF patients but it is supported in guidelines.[21] Systemic reviews and meta-analysis of resistance training in systolic CHF patients have demonstrated improved muscle strength and endurance, increased ability, no deleterious effects on LV function or structure in CHF patients.[22-24]

In one trial of HFpEF, resistance training was included as an adjunct to aerobic ET and it was concluded that benefits from ET (endurance/resistance) are associated with atrial reverse remodeling and improved LV diastolic function.[25] A recent meta-analysis of 10 studies including 240 CHF patients systematically reviewed randomized controlled trials of resistance training as a single intervention on muscle strength, aerobic capacity and QoL. It was concluded that resistance training may be used as primary training modality for those who are unable to participate in aerobic training.[26]

Cardiac Rehabilitation for Chronic Heart Failure

Apart from ET, there is ample evidence to suggest that cardiac rehabilitation program including not only ET but also patient education, improved NYHA status, QOL, 6-minute walk distance, reduced all cause and cardiovascular hospitalizations, and days in the hospital.[27] It has been shown that a multidisciplinary cardiac rehabilitation program extending up to 10 years has shown improvements in exercise capacity, QOL, and HF hospitalizations[28] Rehabilitation Therapy in Older Acute HF Patients REHAB-HF study, suggested the efficacy and safety of multidomain physical rehabilitation intervention to improve physical function and reduce hospitalization in older and frail patients with acute decompensated HF with multiple co-morbidities.[29]

Considering the economic burden of HF management, Dang et al. conducted a comparative study of cost-effectiveness of multidisciplinary management program, ET program and usual care. This study showed that both multidisciplinary management program, ET program were cost-effective compared with usual care from societal perspective.[30] Many published meta-analyses of CR ET with or without counseling have demonstrated symptomatic improvements in CHF along with reduction in cardiac mortality and hospitalizations. There is also evidence to show that CHF related education (counseling) also improves clinical outcomes. In an integrative review of 19 studies representing 3,166 CHF patients it was found that the knowledge and self-care behaviors for HF improved the patient outcomes.[31] In 2013, ACCF/ASHA HF guidelines provided class I recommendation to education for HF patients.[9]

CONCLUSION

Exercise training is nonpharmacological, safe and inexpensive therapeutic strategy for the chronic HF in addition to medial and device therapy. It is not an alternative treatment but a complementary measure in stable HF patients. ET results in improved exercise and functional capacity in both in HFrEF and HFpEF, and appears to reduce HF-related hospitalizations. In spite of class I recommendation from guidelines, only 10% of eligible HF patients are referred to cardiac rehabilitation programs.[32]

REFERENCES

1. Del Buono MG, Arena R, Borlaug BA, et al. Exercise Intolerance in Patients with Heart Failure: JACC State-of-the-Art Review. J Am Coll Cardiol. 2019;73(17):2209-25.
2. Khan H, Kunutsor S, Rauramaa R, et al. Cardio-respiratory fitness and risk of heart failure: a population-based follow-up study. Eur J Heart Fail. 2014;16(2):180-8.
3. Pandey A, LaMonte M, Klein L, et al. Relationship between physical activity, body mass index and risk of heart failure. J Am Coll Cardiol. 2017;69(9):1129-42.
4. Design of the Women's Health Initiative clinical trial and observational study. The Women's Health Initiative Study Group. Control Clin Trials. 1998;19(1):61-109.
5. Bild DE, Bluemke DA, Burke GL, et al. Multi-Ethnic Study of Atherosclerosis: objectives and design. Am J Epidemiol. 2002;156(9):871-81.
6. Fried LP, Borhani NO, Enright P, et al. The Cardiovascular Health Study: design and rationale. Ann Epidemiol. 1991;1(3):263-76.
7. Pandey A, Garg S, Khunger M, et al. Dose–response relationship between physical activity and risk of heart failure. A meta-analysis. Circulation. 2015;132(19):1786-94.
8. Ponikowski P, Voors AA, Anker SD, et al. 2016 ESC guidelines for the diagnosis and treatment of acute and chronic heart failure: the task force for the diagnosis and treatment of acute and chronic heart failure of the European Society of Cardiology (ESC) developed with the special contribution of the Heart Failure Association (HFA) of the ESC. Eur Heart J. 2016;37(27):2129-200.
9. Yancy CW, Jessup M, Bozkurt B, et al. 2013 ACCF/AHA guideline for the management of heart failure: a report of the American College of Cardiology Foundation/American Heart Association Task Force on Practice Guidelines. J Am Coll Cardiol. 2013;62(16):e147-239.
10. O'Connor CM, Whellan DJ, Lee KL, et al. Efficacy and safety of exercise training in patients with chronic heart failure: HF-ACTION randomized controlled trial. JAMA. 2009;301(14):1439-50.
11. Flynn KE, Pina IL, Whellan DJ, et al. Effects of exercise training on health status in patients with chronic heart failure: HF-ACTION randomized controlled trial. JAMA. 2009;301(14):1451-9.
12. Kitzman DW, Brubaker PH, Morgan TM, et al. Exercise training in older patients with heart failure and preserved ejection fraction: a randomized, controlled, single-blind trial. Circ Heart Fail. 2010;3(6):659-67.
13. Leggio M, Fusco A, Loreti C, et al. Effects of exercise training in heart failure with preserved ejection fraction: an updated systematic literature review. Heart Fail Rev. 2019.
14. Piccini JP, Hellkamp AS, Whellan DJ, et al. Exercise training and implantable cardioverter defibrillator shocks in patients with heart failure. JACC Heart Fail. 2013;1(2):142-8.
15. Pandey A, Parashar A, Moore C, et al. Safety and Efficacy of Exercise Training in Patients with an Implantable Cardioverter-Defibrillator: A Meta-Analysis. JACC Clin Electrophysiol. 2017;3(2):117-26.
16. Wisloff U, Stoylen A, Loennechen JP, et al. Superior cardiovascular effect of aerobic interval training versus moderate continuous training in heart failure patients: A randomized study. Circulation. 2007;115(24):3086-94.
17. Taylor RS, Davies EJ, Dalal HM, et al. Effects of exercise training for heart failure with preserved ejection fraction: A systematic review and meta-analysis of comparative studies. Int J Cardiol. 2012;162(1):6-13.
18. Fleg JL, Cooper LS, Borlaug BA, et al. Exercise Training as Therapy for Heart Failure: Current Status and Future Directions. Circ Heart Fail. 2015;8(1):209-20.
19. Fu TC, Wang CH, Lin PS, et al. Aerobic interval training improves oxygen uptake efficiency by enhancing cerebral and muscular hemodynamics in patients with heart failure. Int J Cardiol. 2013;167(1):41-50.
20. Hsu CC, Fu TC, Yuan SS, et al. High-Intensity Interval Training is Associated with Improved Long-Term Survival in Heart Failure Patients. J Clin Med. 2019;8(3):409.
21. Williams MA, Haskell WL, Ades PA, et al. Resistance exercise in individuals with and without cardiovascular disease: 2007 update: A scientific statement from the American Heart Association Council on Clinical Cardiology and Council on

Nutrition, Physical Activity and Metabolism. Circulation. 2007;116(5):572-84.

22. Selig SE, Carey MF, Menzies DG, et al. Moderate-intensity resistance exercise training in patients with chronic heart failure improves strength endurance, heart rate variability, and forearm blood flow. J Card Fail. 2004;10(1):21-30.
23. Savage PA, Shaw AO, Miller MS, et al. Effect of resistance training on physical disability in chronic heart failure. Med Sci Sports Exerc. 2011;43(8):1379-86.
24. Levinger I, Bronks R, Cody DV, et al. The effect of resistance training on left ventricular function and structure of patients with chronic heart failure. Int J Cardiol. 2005;105(2):159-63.
25. Edelmann F, Gelbrich G, Dungen HD, et al. Exercise Training Improves Exercise Capacity and Diastolic Function in Patients with Heart Failure with Preserved Ejection Fraction Results of the Ex-DHF (Exercise training in Diastolic Heart Failure) Pilot Study. J Am Coll Cardiol. 2011;58(17):1780-91.
26. Giuliano C, Karahalios A, Neil C, et al. The effects of resistance training on muscle strength, quality of life and aerobic capacity in patients with chronic heart failure—A meta-analysis. Int J Cardiol. 2017;227:413-23.
27. Davidson PM, Cockburn J, Newton PJ, et al. Can a heart failure-specific cardiac rehabilitation program decrease hospitalizations and improve outcomes in high-risk patients? Eur J Cardiovasc Prev Rehabil. 2010;17(4):393-402.
28. Belardinelli R, Georgiou D, Cianci G, et al. 10-year exercise training in chronic heart failure: a randomized controlled trials. J Am Coll Cardiol. 2012;60(16):1521-8.
29. Reeves GR, Whellan DJ, O'Connor CM. A Novel Rehabilitation Intervention for Older Patients with Acute Decompensated Heart Failure: The REHAB-HF Pilot Study. JACC Heart Fail. 2017;5(5):359-66.
30. Dang W, Yi A, Jhamnani S, et al. Cost-Effectiveness of Multidisciplinary Management Program and Exercise Training Program in Heart Failure. Am J Cardiol. 2017;120(8): 1338-43.
31. Baranson S, Zimmerman L, Young L. An integrative review of interventions promoting self-care of patients with heart failure. J Clin Nurs. 2011;21:448-75.
32. Piepoli MF, Binno S, Corrà U, et al. Committee on Exercise Physiology and Training of the Heart Failure Association of the ESC. ExtraHF survey: the first European survey on implementation of exercise training in heart failure patients. Eur J Heart Fail. 2015;17(6):631-8.

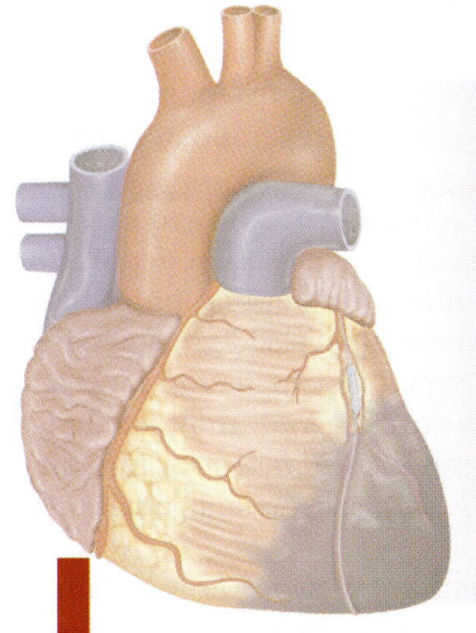

Role of Yoga in Heart Failure

SC Manchanda, Ashish Kumar Jain, Kushal Madan

INTRODUCTION

Heart failure (HF) is one of the serious illnesses with profound clinical and economic impact. A global prevalence has been estimated 62 million people and is expected to continue increasing.[1,2] The survival rates in heart failure are worse than many common cancers. Half of the patients with heart failure die within 5 years of diagnosis. A very large number of patients are readmitted repeatedly due to worsening of heart failure. In India, the prevalence of heart failure is huge although the exact epidemiological data are not available. However, it is estimated that the prevalence is 4.5 million patients approximately and annual incidence is 491,600–1.8 million.[3] Heart failure in India occurs at relatively young age and has a very high mortality rate as compared to western countries.[4] In spite of several advances in the pharmacological and device therapy of heart failure the mortality and morbidity remains very high. Moreover, the compliance of medication is poor especially in developing countries because of the cost and side effects of drugs and a large number of patients do not get guideline based therapy.[5] Hence there is need for additional cost-effective approaches. Yoga and meditation may be one such alternative/adjuvant treatment.

What is Yoga?

Yoga is a profound system of holistic health which originated in India over 5,000 years ago. Yoga is derived from a Sanskrit word "yug" which means to "to join" body with mind or lower human nature to higher.[6] Yoga is not merely a few postures (asanas) but a holistic lifestyle consisting of physical (diet, exercise, avoidance of tobacco), mental (stress management), emotional (control of negative emotions like anger, ego, hostility, jealousy, etc.) and spiritual (faith, moral values) well being. Yoga aims at harmonious development of the body and mind leading to positive thinking, happiness and peace. Although there are many systems of yoga, the commonly practiced is Hatha Yoga which has three components namely physical postures (Asanas), breathing control (Pranayama), and meditation (Dhyan).

Yoga has been shown to be having several beneficial effects on well being, quality of life, stress control, and prevention of lifestyle diseases like hypertension, diabetes, bronchial asthma, cardiovascular diseases, anxiety, depression, etc.[7-9]

RATIONALE FOR USE OF YOGA IN HEART FAILURE

Several studies suggest that heart failure is caused by imbalance of autonomic nervous system, neurohormonal disturbances, inflammation and oxidative stress in which yoga could be helpful (Fig. 1).[10] Yoga is also equivalent to mild exercise, which has been shown to be beneficial in heart failure.

Depression is frequently associated with heart failure and carries a grave prognosis.[11] Yoga has been shown to control depression and thus may be beneficial in heart failure.

Yoga may be especially useful in prevention of heart failure in stage A patients with hypertension, ischemic heart

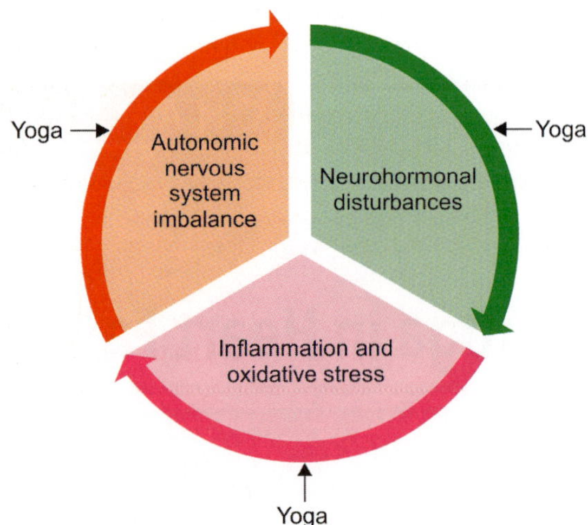

Fig. 1: Yoga can affect the main pathophysiological abnormalities of heart failure.

disease, diabetes, metabolic syndrome, obesity, etc. which can lead to heart failure.[9]

Yoga may also decrease the inflammatory markers and oxidative stress, which also contribute to heart failure.[12]

Scientific studies: There are limited studies available in the literature regarding the role of yoga in heart failure. Krishna et al. in a randomized controlled trial (RCT) of 130 patients of class I-II heart failure reported that ejection fraction (EF) improved from 39% to 53% (38.93 ± 5.1 to 52.96 ± 6.01, $p < 0.01$) in the yoga group after 12 weeks as compared to controls who showed lesser increase of 40–45%. N-terminal pro B-type natriuretic peptide (NT-proBNP) also significantly reduced from 3,965 to 1,395 versus 5,495 to 4,722. There was a correlation between the NT-proBNP decrease and increase in EF. In this study duration of yoga was around 60 minutes per day. Patients did supervised yoga for 2 weeks after which they practiced the same for 3 days under direct supervision and 3 days at their home for total duration of 12 weeks. The yogic practices included asanas, pranayama, and meditation.[13]

Pullen et al. reported improvement in exercise capacity and biomarkers [interleukin-6, C-reactive protein (CRP), and extracellular superoxide dismutase] in a RCT of 40 African American heart failure patients, with yoga for 8 weeks.[14]

Gomes-Neto et al. in a meta-analysis showed improvement in peak oxygen consumption and health-related quality of life in patients with heart failure by yoga.[15] They suggested that it must be considered alternative method of exercise training in patients with heart failure. They used Minnesota Living with Heart Failure Questionnaire (MLHFQ), to assess the improvement in quality of life of heart failure patients post yoga intervention. This questionnaire is validated and reliable for assessment of quality of life in heart failure patients. It is composed of 21 questions which include physical, emotional, socioeconomic aspects of heart failure that adversely affects quality of life of patients. A decrease of five points in total score after a specific intervention is regarded as clinically significant.

Kubo et al. conducted a feasibility study to examine recruitment, retention, adherence, quality of life, depression, and body weight for a multiethnic population of heart failure patients who attended supervised yoga sessions twice a week for 8 weeks. Significant reduction in weight and severity of depression were observed. They concluded that heart failure patients can incorporate yoga into their lives and that it may help with disease management and symptoms.[16]

Recently, a RCT of 3 months of yoga postures, breathing and relaxation has been reported in heart failure patients. Pulmonary function as assessed by forced vital capacity increased by 24% and systolic blood pressure decreased significantly by 11%.[17]

The Support, Education, and Research in Chronic Heart Failure (SEARCH) study utilizing mind fullness meditation therapy demonstrated a significant improvement in the heart failure symptoms as compared to controls at 1 year. The mindfulness group also reported to have significantly lower levels of anxiety and depression.[18] The HEART camp trial assessed the efficacy of a behavioral exercise training program on long-term adherence to exercise in patients with heart failure.[19] Addition of behavior techniques, pedometers and cellphone apps appear worthy of further investigations and may improve the adherence of yoga and exercise activities at home. Some recent publications address novel interventions that may deliver yoga guidance in home settings for example: tele-yoga and exergames.[20,21] Transcendental meditation™ was found to decrease mortality, myocardial infarction, and strokes in African American patients of coronary heart disease with a follow up of 5 years.[22] A very recent multicenter RCT (YOGA CARE) of 4,000 patients after myocardial infarction showed a significant improvement in the quality of life in the yoga group as compared to the standard group.[23] In patients with heart failure and chronic obstructive pulmonary disease (COPD), yoga has also been found to be effective in improving 6-minute walk test, dyspnea on exertion, depression, quality of sleep, and quality of life.[24] Though exercise has been found to be beneficial in patients of heart failure, several patients may not be able to do exercise because of comorbidities. However yoga can be easily incorporated in such patients. Yoga has been shown to produce a significant improvement in exercise capacity, exercise tolerance, flexibility, cardiovascular endurance, and health-related quality of life with no adverse effects in heart failure patients.[14]

Very few studies have been done to assess the safety of yoga in heart failure patients. Esquivel et al. conducted a study on 15 heart failure patients to assess the safety of 8 week yoga program.[25] They have reported that there were no orthopedic injuries or cardiac problems during the yoga sessions. Apart from safety, authors also collected data for physical function (strength, balance, endurance, and flexibility); and psychological functions, quality of life, depression scores, mindfulness before and after 8 weeks of yoga classes.[25] Pullen et al. also reported that there were no adverse events in their study of 8 weeks of yoga in a chronic heart failure group.[26]

Thus, there are studies of yoga in heart failure with encouraging results but have limitations like nonuniform methodology, nonrandomized and short follow up. Hence, large multicentric trials with longer follow up are needed to clarify the exact role of yoga in heart failure.

Possible mechanisms: Exact mechanisms of benefit of yoga are not clear and several mechanisms have been hypothesized.

- *Benefit of yoga as physical activity*: Physical exercise has been consistently shown to be beneficial in patients with heart failure. Meta-analysis of 19 RCTs including 3,647 patients of heart failure showed that heart failure-related hospitalizations were reduced, quality of life improved and mortality was reduced.[27] Yoga has been considered equivalent to mild exercise. Few studies have measured the energy cost of yoga in healthy adults, utilizing a variety of protocols. The first published investigation compared the metabolic equivalents (METs) of a 32-min hatha yoga routine to a 32-min treadmill walk at 4.0 mph.[28] Ten subjects 38–47 years of age, achieved an energy expenditure of 4.1 METs for a yoga routine, compared with 5.4 METs required for treadmill walking. A similar study measured the oxygen requirements of a more dynamic yoga sequence (Ashtanga Vinyasa style) and reported a metabolic demand of 6.7 METs.[29]

  No studies were found that measured the metabolic intensity of yoga on heart failure patients directly, making recommendations unfounded from a scientific perspective. However, it is prudent to recommend that the less vigorous styles of yoga are of reasonable intensity for the heart failure patient who would participate in a yoga therapy (YT) program. Yoga has also been shown to improve VO2 max, anxiety, depression, and quality of life in patients with heart failure with no adverse effects.
- *Improvement in the neurohumoral profile*: Heart failure is associated with increase in several neurohormones like renin angiotensin, cortisol, catecholamines, etc. Yoga has been shown to improve the neurohormonal profile. Regular practice of yoga has been reported to decrease levels of catecholamines, cortisol, nitric oxide, arginine, vasopressin, aldosterone, atrial natriuretic hormone through hypothalamic adrenal pituitary axis.[30] Yoga may also cause behavioral changes which helps the patient to have a better compliance with lifestyle modifications and also reduces stress (Flowchart 1).
- *Improvement in the autonomic nervous system*: Heart failure has been shown to be associated with increased sympathetic activity and yoga has been reported to increase parasympathetic and decrease sympathetic activity thus balancing the autonomic nervous system. This can improve several symptoms in patients with heart failure (Flowchart 1).[30]
- *Inflammation and oxidative stress*: Several studies demonstrate that heart failure is associated with inflammation and oxidative stress as seen by elevated plasma levels of interleukin-6, CRP and TNF-alpha and leptin.[31] Few studies suggest that yoga could reduce the inflammation and oxidative stress.[12] Adiponectin which reduces inflammation and improves endothelial function has also shown to improve with yogic practices.[32]
- *Control of stress and depression*: Depression is prevalent in 20–30% patients in heart failure and has been consistently shown to increase mortality and hospitalization of heart failure patients.[11] Depression may be acting through several mechanisms including neuroendocrinal, autonomic imbalance, and inflammation. Several meta-analysis suggest that yoga could be useful modality to control stress in patients with heart failure[33-36] but no studies are available in heart failure patients.
- *Another mechanism for yoga's physiological effects may be musculoskeletal massage*: There is recent evidence that circulating muscle specific microRNA (miRNA) increase following prolonged exercise in humans and after stretching in animal models. Further evidence suggests that exosomes can act as intercellular communication packets carrying factors such as receptors, transmembrane proteins, kinases, mRNA, miRNA, long noncoding RNA, DNA, and lipids. These metabolic alterations produced by yogic exercises (stretching—asanas) may improve coagulation and inflammatory profiles.[37-39]
- *Yoga may have antiarrhythmic effects* which are beneficial in heart failure. A few studies have suggested that yoga may reduce episodes of atrial fibrillation, ventricular ectopics and significant reduction in device-related ventricular events in patients with implanted cardiovascular-defibrillator (ICD).[40-42]

OTHER BENEFITS OF YOGA

Numerous studies have demonstrated that yoga may be beneficial in controlling several risk factors of heart failure,

Flowchart 1: Psychophysiology of yoga in heart disease—possible mechanisms.

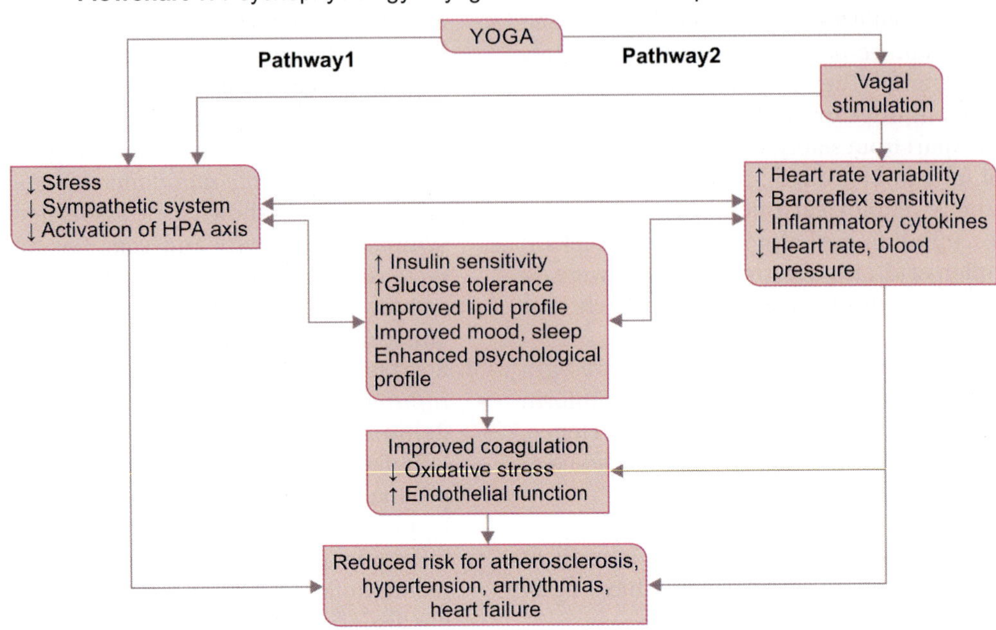

(HPA: hypothalamic–pituitary–adrenal)

Source: Modified from Innes KE, Bourguignon C, Taylor AG. Risk indices associated with the insulin resistance syndrome, cardiovascular disease, and possible protection with yoga: a systematic review. J Am Board Fam Pract. 2005;18:491-519.

e.g. hypertension, diabetes mellitus, obesity, metabolic syndrome, left ventricular hypertrophy, psychosocial stress and may even regress atherosclerosis, and thus, may be useful for prevention of development of heart failure.[9]

CONCLUSION

Heart failure is one of the serious cardiac illnesses, which is associated with very high morbidity and mortality especially in developing countries like India. In spite of tremendous advances in the pharmacological and device-based therapies, the mortality still remains very high. Hence, there is a need for additional therapies. Yoga appears to be one such cost-effective alternative approach. The rationale of using yoga in heart failure appears to be that it can improve the autonomic nervous system imbalance, neurohormonal abnormalities, inflammation, oxidative stress, and depression which are common in heart failure. However, there are very few scientific studies which have utilized yoga as an adjunct therapy in heart failure. Few studies do suggest that yoga is useful in heart failure patients by improving EF, decreasing NT-proBNP levels and improved quality of life. Yoga is also equivalent to mild exercise which has been shown to be beneficial in heart failure. Moreover, exercise may not be feasible in some patients of heart failure but yoga can be easily incorporated. However, larger studies with clinical endpoints are needed.

REFERENCES

1. Mozaffarian D, Benjamin EJ, Go AS, et al. Heart disease and stroke statistics—2015 update: a report from the American Heart Association. Circulation. 2015;131:e29-322.
2. Global, regional, and national disability-adjusted life years (DALYs) for 306 diseases and injuries and healthy life expectancy (HALE) for 188 countries, 1990-2013: quantifying the epidemiological transition. Lancet. 2015;386: 2145-91.
3. Huffman MD, Prabhakaran D. Heart failure: epidemiology and prevention in India. Natl Med J India. 2010;23:283-8.
4. Seth S, Khanal S, Ramakrishnan S, et al. Epidemiology of acute decompensated heart failure in India: The AFAR study (Acute failure registry study). J Pract Cardiovasc Sci. 2015;1:35-8.
5. Sanjay G, Jeemon P, Agarwal A, et al. In-Hospital and Three-Year Outcomes of Heart Failure Patients in South India: The Trivandrum Heart Failure Registry. J Card Fail. 2018;24:842-8.
6. Ananda S. The Complete Book of Yoga: Harmony of Body and Mind, 1st edition. Delhi: Orient Publishing Company; 1981.
7. Raub JA. Psychophysiologic effects of Hatha Yoga on musculoskeletal and cardiopulmonary function: a literature review. J Altern Complement Med. 2002;8:797-812.
8. Ospina MB, Bond K, Karkhaneh M, et al. Meditation practices for health. state of the research. Evid Rep Technol Assess (Full Rep). 2007;(55):1-263.
9. Manchanda SC, Madan K. Yoga and meditation in cardiovascular disease. Clin Res Cardiol. 2014;103:675-80.

10. Mentz RJ, O'Connor CM. Pathophysiology and clinical evaluation of acute heart failure. Nat Rev Cardiol. 2016;13: 28-35.
11. Mbakwem A, Aina F, Amadi C. Expert Opinion—Depression in Patients with Heart Failure: Is Enough Being Done? Card Fail Rev. 2016;2:110-2.
12. Djalilova DM, Schulz PS, Berger AM, et al. Impact of Yoga on Inflammatory Biomarkers: A Systematic Review. Biol Res Nurs. 2019;21:198-209.
13. Krishna BH, Pal P, Pal G, et al. A randomized controlled trial to study the effect of yoga therapy on cardiac function and N terminal Pro BNP in heart failure. Integr Med Insights. 2014;9:1-6.
14. Pullen PR, Nagamia SH, Mehta PK, et al. Effects of yoga on inflammation and exercise capacity in patients with chronic heart failure. J Card Fail. 2008;14:407-13.
15. Gomes-Neto M, Rodrigues-Jr ES, Silva-Jr WM, et al. Effects of Yoga in Patients with Chronic Heart Failure: A Meta-Analysis. Arquivos Brasileiros de Cardiologia. 2014;103:433-9.
16. Kubo A, Hung YY, Ritterman J. Yoga for heart failure patients: A feasibility pilot study with a multiethnic population. Int J Yoga Therap. 2011;21:77-83.
17. Yadav A, Singh S, Singh K, et al. Effect of yoga regimen on lung functions including diffusion capacity in coronary artery disease patients: A randomized controlled study. Int J Yoga. 2015;8:62-7.
18. Sullivan MJ, Wood L, Terry J, et al. The Support, Education, and Research in Chronic Heart Failure Study (SEARCH): a mindfulness-based psychoeducational intervention improves depression and clinical symptoms in patients with chronic heart failure. Am Heart J. 2009;157:84-90.
19. Pozehl BJ, Duncan K, Hertzog M, et al. Study of adherence to exercise in heart failure: the HEART camp trial protocol. BMC Cardiovasc Disord. 2014;14:172.
20. Selman L, McDermott K, Donesky D, et al. Appropriateness and acceptability of a Tele-Yoga intervention for people with heart failure and chronic obstructive pulmonary disease: qualitative findings from a controlled pilot study. BMC Complement Altern Med. 2015;15:21.
21. Seffens WS, Pullen PR. Exergame development study of Kinect for yoga postures. International Association of Yoga Therapy, IYAT Symposium on Yoga Research, 2014. [online] https://www.c.ymcdn.com/sites/www.iayt.org/resource/resmgr/docs_syr2015/syr2014 [Last accessed, 2019].
22. Schneider RH, Grim CE, Rainforth MV, et al. Stress reduction in the secondary prevention of cardiovascular disease: randomized, controlled trial of transcendental meditation and health education in Blacks. Circ Cardiovasc Qual Outcomes. 2012;5:750-8.
23. Prabhakaran D. Effectiveness of a yoga-based cardiac rehabilitation (Yoga-CaRe) program: a multi-centre randomised controlled trial of patients with acute myocardial infarction from India. Chicago, IL: AHA; 2018.
24. Donesky D, Selman L, McDermott K, et al. Evaluation of the Feasibility of a Home-Based TeleYoga Intervention in Participants with Both Chronic Obstructive Pulmonary Disease and Heart Failure. J Altern Complement Med. 2017;23:713-21.
25. Howie-Esquivel J, Lee J, Collier G, et al. Yoga in heart failure: a pilot study. J Card Fail. 2010;16:742-9.
26. Pullen PR, Thompson WR, Benardot D, et al. Benefits of yoga for African American heart failure patients. Med Sci Sports Exerc. 2010;42:651-7.
27. Tucker WJ, Beaudry RI, Liang Y. Exercise training for systolic heart failure: Cochrane systematic review and meta-analysis. Eur J Heart Fail. 2010;12:706-15.
28. DiCarlo LJ, Sparling PB, Hinson BT, et al. Cardiovascular, metabolic, and perceptual responses to hatha yoga standing poses. Med Exerc Nutr Health. 1995;4:107-12.
29. Carroll J, Blansit A, Otto RM, et al. The metabolic requirements of Vinyasa Yoga. Med Sci Sports Exerc. 2003;35:S155.
30. Innes KE, Bourguignon C, Taylor AG. Risk indices associated with the insulin resistance syndrome, cardiovascular disease, and possible protection with yoga: a systematic review. J Am Board Fam Pract. 2005;18:491-519.
31. Djalilova DM, Schulz PS, Berger AM, et al. Impact of Yoga on Inflammatory Biomarkers: A Systematic Review. Biol Res Nurs. 2019;21:198-209.
32. Sarvottam K, Magan D, Yadav RK, et al. Adiponectin, interleukin-6, and cardiovascular disease risk factors are modified by a short-term yoga-based lifestyle intervention in overweight and obese men. J Altern Complement Med. 2013;19:397-402.
33. Mezzacappa ES, Kelsey RM, Katkin ES, et al. Vagal rebound and recovery from psychological stress. Psychosom Med. 2001;63:650-7.
34. Kirkwood G., Rampes H., Tuffrey V., et al. Yoga for anxiety: a systematic review of the research evidence. Br J Sports Med. 2005;39:884-91.
35. Pilkington K, Kirkwood G, Rampes H, et al. Yoga for depression: the research evidence. J Affect Disord. 2005;89:13-24.
36. Shapiro D, Cook IA, Davydov DM, et al. Yoga as a complementary treatment of depression: effects of traits and moods on treatment outcome. Evid Based Complement Alternat Med. 2007;4:493-502.
37. Guescini M, Canonico B, Lucertini F, et al. Muscle releases alpha-sarcoglycan positive extracellular vesicles carrying miRNAs in the bloodstream. PLoS One. 2015;10:e0125094.
38. Corey SM, Vizzard MA, Bouffard NA, et al. Stretching of the back improves gait, mechanical sensitivity and connective tissue inflammation in a rodent model. PLoS One. 2012;7:e29831.
39. Emanueli C, Shearn AI, Angelini GD, et al. Exosomes and exosomal miRNAs in cardiovascular protection and repair. Vascul Pharmacol. 2015;71:24-30.
40. Lakkireddy D, Atkins D, Pillarisetti J, et al. Effect of yoga on arrhythmia burden, anxiety, depression, and quality of life in paroxysmal atrial fibrillation: the YOGA My Heart Study. J Am Coll Cardiol. 2013;61:1177-82.
41. Dabhade AM, Pawar BH, Ghunage MS, et al. Effect of pranayama (breathing exercise) on arrhythmias in the human heart. Explore (NY). 2012;8:12-5.
42. Ravindra PN, Madanmohan, Pavithran P. Effect of pranayam (yoga breathing) and shavasan (relaxation training) on the frequency of benign ventricular ectopics in two patients with palpitations. Int J Cardiol. 2006;108:124-5.

CHAPTER

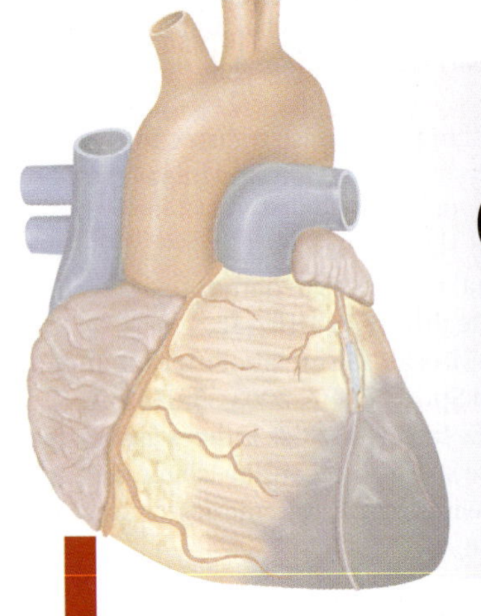

Cardiac Rehabilitation after Ventricular Assist Device Implantation: A Worthwhile Exercise?

Chetan P Shah, Charan Reddy KV

INTRODUCTION

Advanced heart failure (HF) is characterized by a low cardiac output state leading to circulatory insufficiency resulting in life-threatening end-organ hypoperfusion and tissue hypoxia. It is often multifactorial, hemodynamically complex condition associated with high mortality. However, with the advent of newer standardized team-based approach, better mechanical support devices, risk assessment and postoperative care, the outcomes have drastically improved. Although, heart transplantation remains the most important surgical treatment for patients with end-stage HF, it is often limited by donor availability.[1] Ventricular assist devices (VADs) offer good alternative to heart transplantation. They can also be used as bridge to transplant (BTT) or recovery and in destination therapy (DT). Kirklin et al. presented the eighth annual report of the Interagency Registry for Mechanically Assisted Circulatory Support (INTERMACS) in 2017 showing 1-year and 2-year survival rates with continuous-flow mechanical devices to be greater than 80% and greater than 70%, respectively. However, postsurgical recovery and adjustment to a new routine with mechanical equipment is often challenging. As the patient recover, the cardiac insufficiency is relieved, the systemic effects of chronic HF, such as muscle wasting and malnutrition also show improvement. Hence, cardiac rehabilitation (CR) postdevice implantation significantly reduces both morbidity and mortality by treating the frailty associated with end stage HF.[2] With various exciting technologies emerging in the past few years including the development of small portable or permanent pumps and with emergence of DT as an viable alternative to heart transplantation, a growing population of patients with advanced HF are likely to benefit.

INDICATIONS OF MECHANICAL ASSIST DEVICES IN HEART FAILURE

Though there are various guidelines for the use of mechanical assist devices, most agree that it is indicated in advanced HF patients that have symptoms at rest or with minimal exertion and cannot perform most activities of daily living. Other indications include cardiac cachexia, patient refractory or intolerant to conventional HF therapy, inotrope dependent and requiring repeated hospitalization with pulmonary edema. Commonly used objective measurement of functional limitations include a peak VO_2 less than 14 mL/kg/min (or <50% of expected) and a 6-minute walk distance (6MWD) of less than 300 meters. Life expectancy is usually less than 2 years in patients without heart transplantation or mechanical assist device support.[3, 4]

ROLE OF MECHANICAL ASSIST DEVICES IN HEART FAILURE

The field of mechanical support devices maybe new but is a rapidly evolving one, applying expensive technologies to critically ill patient population. In its current state of evolution, the primary role of mechanical support device technology is to prolong and improve the quality of life. Development of mechanical circulatory support (MCS) began in 1953 with the cardiopulmonary bypass to facilitate open heart surgery.[5] As the demand for long-term replacement of diseased heart with transplantation could not be fulfilled due to inadequate supply of donor hearts, there was a clear need for innovative, safe, and durable MCS to treat the growing population of patients with advanced HF. The first-generation VADs were approved by the United States Food and Drug Administration (FDA) for clinical use in 1994. VADs essentially consist of a surgically implanted mechanical pump that increases cardiac output and maintains sufficient blood flow to the peripheral organs.[6]

There are two types of flow characteristics in VADs: Pulsatile-flow and continuous-flow. First generation pulsatile-flow VADs [HeartMate XVE, Novacor left ventricular assist system (LVAS)] were more physiological but only preload dependant, physically large, noisy, less durable with faster depletion of batteries, requiring frequent charging. Second generation nonpulsatile or continuous-flow VADs (HeartMate II, HeartWare, Jarvik 2000 and MicroMed DeBakey) are smaller in profile, quieter, more durable and are both preload and afterload dependent.[7] Currently, third generation devices (HeartMate III, DuraHeart, HeartWare HVAD, Incor and Levacor) have been developed that have better efficiency, smaller size, more durability with lesser incidence of thrombosis than the second generation devices. Other devices extensively studied are biventricular assist device (BiVAD) and total artificial heart (TAH). BiVAD is primarily used for patients with biventricular failure or in right ventricular failure associated with left ventricular disease. TAH (SynCardia TAH) also used in end-stage biventricular failure as a bridge to heart transplantation.

A large-scale randomized controlled trial of VAD implantation therapy showed that VAD implantation dramatically increased the survival rates in end-stage HF with 1-year survival rate of 52% and 25% in people with a VAD vs optimal medical management; respectively.[8] The usage of VAD is not without its complications. The frequency of adverse events in patient with VAD is approximately, twice as high as that in patients with optimal medical management. In particular, the rate of neurological events with VAD is approximately four times higher than that of optimal medical management group. Lazar et al. reported approximately 40% of patients had neurological events after VAD implantation.[9] Other complications seen in VADs include long-term cognitive disorder, coagulopathy, device malfunction and bloodstream infection. Patient on VADs require long-term anticoagulation therapy to prevent potential embolism. However, such therapy also increases the risk of cerebral hemorrhage in the patient.

Though, these mentioned complications have reduced with the use of newer generation VADs, it is imperative that a proper follow-up and subsequent CR is recommended not only to improve the functional capacity of the patient but also to reduce morbidity and mortality.[10]

ROLE OF CARDIAC REHABILITATION IN PATIENT ON VENTRICULAR ASSIST DEVICES

Traditionally, CR was only indicated for patients with ischemic heart disease, HF with reduced ejection fraction (HFrEF) and following heart transplantation. However, with robust clinical data to support, CR in VADs is now set to become a cornerstone in management of advanced HF. CR in patient on VAD is generally considered to be safe and effective.[11] Multidisciplinary approach is needed to achieve optimal clinical outcomes. The various components of CR include: Exercise training, weight management, nutritional counseling, lipid management, diabetes management, blood pressure management, tobacco cessation and psychosocial management. The most commonly followed exercise training protocol in CR include 30–60 minutes of exercise on a treadmill or bicycle ergometer for more than 3 days per week for 6–12 months depending on the training intensity or 50–80% of peak oxygen consumption or subjective fatigue. Resistance training, such as weight training or machine training is also encouraged. A Cochrane meta-analysis found that exercise-based CR was associated with a 25% reduction in mortality and a 39% reduction in hospital readmission rates in patient with advanced HF.[12]

In a systematic review and meta-analysis of six trials with a total of 183 patients was done, and it showed that exercise-based CR was associated with improved peak oxygen uptake (VO_2) in all trials. Similarly, 6MWD also showed significantly improvement.[13] In one of the largest studies conducted by Bachmann et al. to investigate the use of CR among 1,164 medicare beneficiaries who received VAD therapy in 2014, the investigators reported patients characteristics, CR participation rates, and associated risks including subsequent hospitalizations and mortality. Findings are as follows: One-third of VAD-treated patients participated in CR, although on average they completed just two-third of the prescribed regimen, it was found that CR participants had 23% lower adjusted risk for rehospitalization. CR use was also associated with a 47% lower adjusted risk for death at 1 year.

Evidence clearly shows that exercise training improves physical function and emotional status in patients with

HF. Exercise training has been shown to increase maximal oxygen uptake (VO_2 max), improve endothelial function and myocardial flow reserve. It has also been reported that regular exercise training can enhance the fibrinolytic activity in patients with heart disease.[14] Furthermore, in a study, exercise-based CR also lowered the triglycerides levels, increased high-density lipoprotein cholesterol levels in patient with heart disease, thereby, reducing the risk for a neurological stroke.[15]

CONCLUSION

Even though experience remains limited, the results from various trials conducted to-date have been very encouraging. They have clearly shown that CR is associated with significant morbidity and mortality benefits in treating the frailty associated with end-stage HF. However, it is currently being underutilized due to additional expenses it incurs, inadequate home or social support, lack of trained medical professionals and paucity of equipped inpatient rehabilitation centers or nursing facilities. With the emergence of the next generation of fully implantable devices and supportive data to study, one can only hope that in future, important insights into the physiological impact of HF and ways to optimize patients will be made with improved clinical outcomes and fewer adverse events. Appropriate patient selection with a focus on earlier referral and optimization of comorbid conditions is expected to further improve patient outcomes.

REFERENCES

1. American Society of Transplantation and the American Society of Transplant Surgeons. Organ Procurement and Transplantation Network and Scientific Registry of Transplant Recipients 2010 data report. Am J Transplant. 2012;12 (Suppl 1):1-156.
2. Bachmann JM, Duncan MS, Shah AS, et al. Association of cardiac rehabilitation with decreased hospitalizations and mortality after ventricular assist device implantation. JACC Heart Fail. 2018;6(2):130-9.
3. Metra M, Ponikowski P, Dickstein K, et al. Heart Failure Association of the, European Society of Cardiology. Advanced chronic heart failure: position statement from the Study Group on Advanced Heart Failure of the Heart Failure Association of the European Society of Cardiology. Eur J Heart Fail. 2007;9(6-7):684-94.
4. Hunt SA, Abraham WT, Chin MH, et al. ACC/AHA 2005 guideline update for the diagnosis and management of chronic heart failure in the adult: a report of the American College of Cardiology/American Heart Association Task Force on Practice Guidelines (Writing Committee to Update the 2001 Guidelines for the Evaluation and Management of Heart Failure) developed in collaboration with the American College of the Chest Physicians and the International Society for Heart Lung Transplantation: endorsed by the Heart RhythmSociety. Circulation. 2005;112(12):e154-235.
5. Gibbon JH Jr. Application of a mechanical heart and lung apparatus to cardiac surgery. Minn Med. 1954;37(3):171-85.
6. Peura JL, Colvin-Adams M, Francis GS, et al. Recommendations for the use of mechanical circulatory support: device strategies and patient selection: a scientific statement from the American Heart Association. Circulation. 2012;126(22): 2648-67.
7. Slaughter MS, Rogers JG, Milano CA, et al. HeartMate II Investigators. Advanced heart failure treated with continuous-flow left ventricular assist device. N Engl J Med. 2009;361(23):2241-51.
8. Rose EA, Gelijns AC, Moskowitz AJ, et al. Long-term use of a left ventricular assist device for end-stage heart failure. N Engl J Med. 2001;345(20):1435-43.
9. Lazar RM, Shapiro PA, Jaski BE, et al. Neurological events during long term mechanical circulatory support for heart failure: the Randomized Evaluation of Mechanical Assistance for the Treatment of Congestive Heart Failure (REMATCH) experience. Circulation. 2004;109(20):2423-7.
10. Yancy CW, Jessup M, Bozkurt B, et al. 2013 ACCF/AHA Guideline for the Management of Heart Failure: a report of the American College of Cardiology Foundation/American Heart Association Task Force on Practice Guidelines. Circulation. 2013;128(16):e240-327.
11. Alsara O, Perez-Terzic C, Squires RW, et al. Is exercise training safe and beneficial in patients receiving left ventricular assist device therapy? J Cardiopulm Rehabil Prev. 2014;34(4): 233-40.
12. Taylor RS, Sagar VA, Davies EJ, et al. Exercise-based rehabilitation for heart failure. Cochrane Database Syst Rev. 2014;(4):CD003331.
13. Mahfood Haddad T, Saurav A, Smer A. Cardiac Rehabilitation in Patients With Left Ventricular Assist Device: A Systematic Review and Meta-Analysis. J Cardiopulm Rehabil Prev. 2017;37(6):390-6.
14. Womack CJ, Nagelkirk PR, Coughlin AM. Exercise induced changes in coagulation and fibrinolysis in healthy populations and patients with cardiovascular disease. Sports Med. 2003;33(11):795-807.
15. Rankovic G, Djindjic N, Rankovic-Nedin G, et al. The effects of physical training on cardiovascular parameters, lipid disorders and endothelial function. Vojnosanit Pregl. 2012;69(11):956-60.

SECTION 14

Legal and Ethical Issues

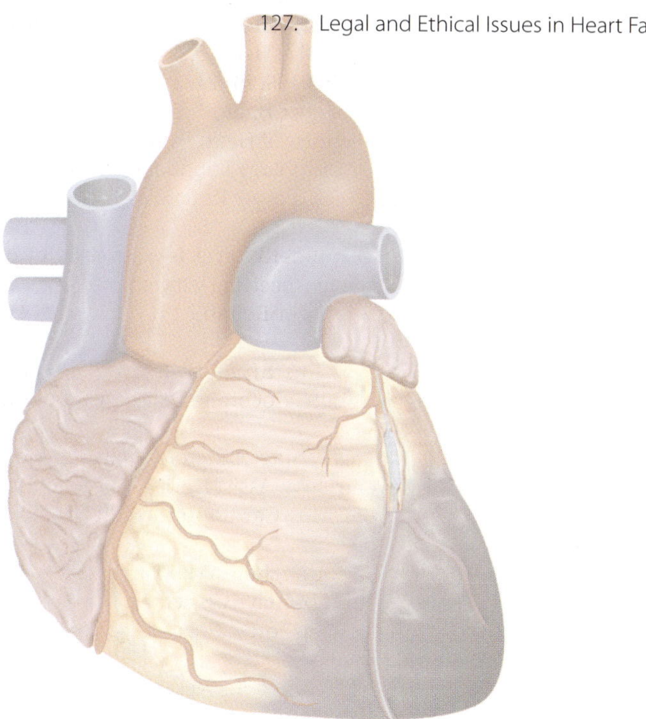

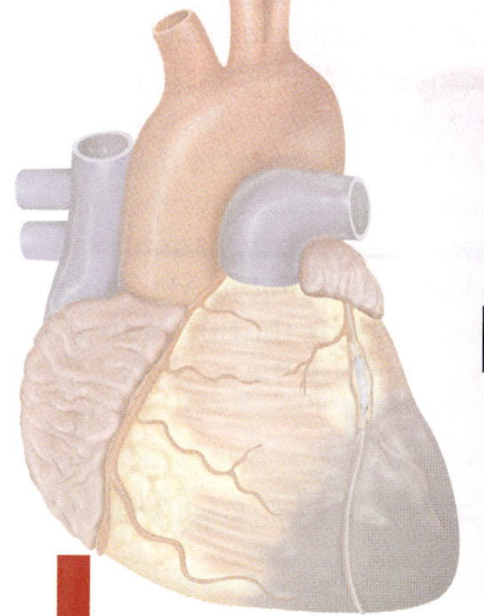

Legal and Ethical Issues in Heart Failure

KK Aggarwal, Sanchita Sharma, Ira Gupta

INTRODUCTION

The prevalence of heart failure is rising globally including in India. This increase can be attributed to the increase in life expectancy and also to the therapeutic advances that have improved survival rate in patients who suffer cardiac events, such as acute myocardial infarction or ventricular arrhythmias.[1] Heart failure is a chronic illness associated with high morbidity and mortality and its treatment is resource intensive.[2] This is especially of concern in our country, where out of pocket spending on health is among the highest in the world. Inequitable distribution of healthcare services, lack of accessibility and affordability further add to the problem. Up till now, heart failure was regarded as just systolic heart failure, but now diastolic heart failure is becoming the new epidemic of the society. There is a new definition of diastolic heart failure. Mixing of definitions can lead to disputes in insurance. There has also been a paradigm shift in the management of heart failure. It has evolved from no management to offering all available management options; this is an ethical conflict the cardiologist faces everyday. Missing the early signs of heart failure can reduce the lifespan of the patient with poor quality of life. Not providing appropriate treatment for systolic and diastolic heart failure including failure to timely use implantable cardioverter-defibrillator (ICD), cardiac resynchronization therapy (CRT) or left ventricular assist device (LVAD) can lead to legal disputes. Other important ethical issues relate to device therapy, end of life care and cardiac transplantation especially in patients with advanced heart failure. Hence there is a need to know the ethical and legal issues in heart failure.

MEDICAL ETHICS

The doctor-patient relationship is a fiduciary relationship and doctors must adhere to the principles of *medical ethics* (autonomy, nonmaleficence, beneficence, and justice), *rules* (fidelity, confidentiality, privacy, and veracity), and *virtues* (compassion, kindness, respect, etc.) in their interactions with the patients which have been laid down by various professional bodies and associations [The Hippocratic Oath, the Declaration of Geneva, the International Code of Medical Ethics, the World Medical Association in its Medical Ethics Manual, United Nations Educational, Scientific and Cultural Organization (UNESCO) Universal Declaration on Bioethics and Human Rights, to name a few] as professional codes of conduct and standards for doctors.

Although the various codes of ethics have been written differently, the common themes running through them all remain unequivocally that of nonmaleficence or "do no harm" and beneficence or "do good" which means doing the right thing for the patient. Patient autonomy has now been thrust to the forefront with the changing character of the doctor-patient relationship; from "*paternalism*" to the current "*patient-centric*". This also forms the basis of "informed consent" which has become especially pertinent as the patient today is more fully informed. Now consent is no longer simply a formality, it is an ethical and legal necessity. Failure to obtain consent is a professional misconduct rendering the doctor liable for disciplinary action and negligence.

Doctors should also respect the principle of justice, where justice means fairness of access to treatment.

INFORMED CONSENT

Consent for the purpose of medical treatment means grant of permission by the patient for an act to be carried out by the doctor, such as a diagnostic, surgical or therapeutic procedure. The relationship between a doctor and his patient is of an implied contract, i.e. a patient enters a doctor's clinic and sits in the examination chair; his consent is implied for examination, diagnosis and consultation.[3]

Any act done without permission is "battery" or physical assault and is liable for punishment.

A signed informed written consent form by itself does not constitute valid consent, though it is an evidence of consent given by the patient or his guardian.

The judgment of the Hon'ble Supreme Court in the case of *Samira Kohli vs Dr Prabha Manchanda & Anr, AIR 2008 SC 1385* is a landmark ruling with regard to informed consent. In this, the Apex Court has elaborated on the components of a valid consent and also defined adequate information to be provided by the doctor: "*... The consent so obtained should be real and valid, which means that: the patient should have the capacity and competence to consent; his consent should be voluntary; and his consent should be on the basis of adequate information concerning the nature of the treatment procedure, so that he knows what is consenting to*".

"Doctor should disclose (a) nature and procedure of the treatment and its purpose, benefits and effect, (b) alternatives if any available, (c) an outline of the substantial risks, and (d) adverse consequences of refusing treatment..."

"...Consent given only for a diagnostic procedure, cannot be considered as consent for therapeutic treatment. Consent given for a specific treatment procedure will not be valid for conducting some other treatment procedure..." which means that blanket consent given at the time of admission may be invalid.

When patient lacks the competence to make a decision about treatment, a substitute decision maker/s must be sought. If doctors do not take substituted consent, they may be subject to claims of having treated the person without informed consent. *Clause 7.16 of the MCI Code of Ethics Regulations, 2002* places the responsibility of obtaining consent from the patient or the guardian, in case of a minor, upon the doctor.

However, consent of a patient is not necessary in case of a medical emergency when the doctor can operate, examine, treat the patient without his/her consent and is protected by the defense of medical necessity of obtaining consent from the patient, if there is no other person available to give consent. *"...This stringent standard of disclosure was subjected to only two exceptions: (i) where there was a genuine emergency, e.g. the patient was unconscious; and (ii) where the information would be harmful to the patient, e.g. where it might cause psychological damage, or where the patient would become so emotionally distraught as to prevent a rational decision."* (Samira Kohli vs Dr Prabha Manchanda, AIR 2008 SC 1385). But, the onus lies on the doctor to prove that the treatment given was life-saving. The facts of the case must be documented.

AUTONOMY AND SHARED DECISION-MAKING

In India, the patient has a legal right to autonomy and self-determination enshrined within *Article 21* of the Constitution of India, 1950, which provides for protection of life and personal liberty by stating *"No person shall be deprived of his life or personal liberty except according to procedure established by law"*.

The patients have the right to information related to their health. In the case of *Aruna Ramchandra Shanbaug versus Union of India, 2011 (15) SCC480*, Hon'ble Supreme Court has observed that *"autonomy means the right to self-determination, where the informed patient has a right to choose the manner of his treatment. To be autonomous the patient should be competent to make decisions and choices."* They also have the right to refuse treatment. Failure to give all the facts to the patients that are necessary for them to take a rational decision about their treatment is a violation of their rights.

Doctors are no longer *"parent figures"* taking decisions on behalf of their patients. Today, the patients are *"equal partners"* in all decisions regarding their care. Doctors and patients collaborate to choose a line of management, out of the many options available, bearing in mind the patient preferences and their goals and values in *"shared decision-making"*.[4]

CONFIDENTIALITY AND PRIVACY

Privacy and confidentiality have often been considered as synonyms. But, the two are not the same.

Privacy is the right of a person (patient) to keep his health information including any other personal information, private and undisclosed. On the other hand, confidentiality is what we, as doctors (or other concerned persons) do with the information that has been entrusted to us. Confidentiality implies the duty of everyone entrusted with any information to keep that information private.

Protecting the privacy of patient information is the ethical duty of the doctor as also mandated in the MCI Code of Ethics Regulations. According to Clause 2.2, "... *Confidences concerning individual or domestic life entrusted by patients to a physician and defects in the disposition or character of patients observed during medical attendance should never be revealed unless their revelation is required by the laws of the State...*"

Clause 7.14: The registered medical practitioner shall not disclose the secrets of a patient that have been learnt in the exercise of his/her profession except:

- In a court of law under orders of the Presiding Judge;
- In circumstances where there is a serious and identified risk to a specific person and/or community; and
- Notifiable diseases.

In case of communicable/notifiable diseases, concerned public health authorities should be informed immediately.

In August 2017, the Hon'ble Supreme Court of India declared the right to privacy as a fundamental right in a historic judgment and said, *"The right to privacy is protected as an intrinsic part of the right to life and personal liberty under Article 21 and as a part of the freedoms guaranteed by Part III of the Constitution".*

DEVICE THERAPY

Cardiovascular implanted electronic devices (CIEDs) are now an integral part of heart failure management. The two main devices used are ICD and CRT which decrease symptoms and hospitalizations and improve survival.[5] Implantable LVADs have emerged as an option for patients with advanced heart failure,[6] where they are either used as bridge to transplant in patients on the waiting list, or as destination therapy in patients who are not eligible for transplant due to a listed contraindication or as bridge-to-decision in patients who are not yet candidates for transplant and in whom LVAD is used as support till a decision is made.[2]

Informed consent, patient autonomy, and shared decision-making are particularly relevant to the use of CIEDs in patients with heart failure.

The informed consent process for devices should take into consideration the estimated risks, patient's expected benefits, whether patient prefers quality of life more than the quantity of life[7] and the later need of device deactivation, including end of life decisions, and the patient preferences.[8] A written consent must also be obtained from the patient, when he/she is alive for removal of device after death.[9]

ADVANCE DIRECTIVES

The Heart Rhythm Society (HRS) Expert Consensus Statement on the management of CIEDs in patients nearing end of life or requesting withdrawal of therapy has recommended that all patients with CIEDs should be encouraged to have advance directives.[10]

Advance medical directives are legal in India as held by the Supreme Court of India in a landmark judgment in the matter of *"Common Cause versus Union of India, 2018 (5) SCC 1"*. Further in the said judgment, the Hon'ble Apex Court has laid down certain guidelines and directions wrt. advance medical directives which shall remain in force till the Parliament makes legislation on this subject. The treating doctor who in *"good faith exercise of professional medical judgment"* abides by an advance directive will not be held liable under criminal law.

DEVICE REUSE

Devices are expensive which makes them inaccessible to many patients. Hence, devices are now being reused, after reprocessing, to lower the cost of treatment.

Informed consent from a patient is mandatory before implanting reused pacemakers/defibrillators. A new device should be used if the patient opts against device reuse.[9] Reusing the device without consent is disrespecting patient autonomy. And, any adverse outcome suffered due to reused device, such as device failure, transmission of infections, may have legal implications with expensive malpractice lawsuits, which could defeat the very purpose of reuse.[11] The liability of the safety and efficacy of the reprocessed devices lies with the hospitals using such devices.[9]

CARDIAC TRANSPLANTATION

Patients with end-stage heart failure refractory to medical treatment can be offered cardiac transplantation as a treatment option.[12] However, many constraints and ethical concerns are attached with organ transplantation.

The shortage of organs is the first and foremost concern with organ transplantation.[13] There is a huge gap between patients who need transplant and the availability of organs. The allocation of resources (organs) brings forth the principle of distributive justice, i.e. fair distribution of resources. Given the shortage of available organs, patient selection for the transplant is an ethical dilemma. Should medical need of the patient be the deciding factor or should the patients who have the best chances of success of transplant be given priority?[14] Organ transplantation is a high-risk procedure and the high costs promote organ trade and trafficking.

MEDICAL RECORDS

Doctors are required to maintain medical records of their inpatients for a period of 3 years as stipulated in *Regulation*

1.3.1 of the MCI Code of Ethics Regulations. All documents must be issued within 72 hours if requested for either by the patients/authorized attendant or legal authorities involved (1.3.2). Failure to comply with the above regulations is professional misconduct liable for disciplinary action.

Regulation 1.3.4 says, "*Efforts shall be made to computerize medical records for quick retrieval*".

Ownership of medical records must be understood very clearly. While hospitals own the physical (or electronic) records, they are only "held in trust by them on behalf of the patient". The information or data "protected health information" contained in the records are owned by the patient.

CONCLUSION

Legal and ethical issues mentioned above should always be considered for prognosticative and therapeutic implications in public interest.

REFERENCES

1. Kirkpatrick JN, Fields AV, Ferrari VA. Medical ethics and the art of cardiovascular medicine. Lancet. 2010;376(9740): 508-9.
2. Guha S, Harikrishnan S, Ray S, et al. CSI position statement on management of heart failure in India. Indian Heart J. 2018;70 Suppl 1:S1-S72.
3. Aggarwal KK. Real consent and not informed consent applicable in India. Ind J Clin Practice. 2014;25(4):392-3.
4. Allen LA, Stevenson LW, Grady KL, et al. Decision making in advanced heart failure: a scientific statement from the American Heart Association. Circulation. 2012;125(15): 1928-52.
5. El-Chami MF, Smith AL, Leon AR. Device Therapy in Heart Failure. In: Baliga R, Haas G. (Eds). Management of Heart Failure. London: Springer; 2015.
6. Gustafsson F, Rogers JG. Left ventricular assist device therapy in advanced heart failure: patient selection and outcomes. Eur J Heart Fail. 2017;19:595-602.
7. Kramer DB, Brock DW, Tedrow UB. Informed consent in cardiac resynchronization therapy: what should be said? Circ Cardiovasc Qual Outcomes. 2011;4(5):573-7.
8. Pitcher D, Soar J, Hogg K, et al. Cardiovascular implanted electronic devices in people towards the end of life, during cardiopulmonary resuscitation and after death: guidance from the Resuscitation Council (UK), British Cardiovascular Society and National Council for Palliative Care. Heart. 2016;102(Suppl 7):A1-A17.
9. Kapoor A, Vora A, Nataraj G, et al. Guidance on reuse of cardiovascular catheters and devices in India: A consensus document. Indian Heart J. 2017;69(3):357-63.
10. Lampert R, Hayes DL, Annas GJ, et al. HRS expert consensus statement on the management of cardiovascular implantable electronic devices (CIEDs) in patients nearing end of life or requesting withdrawal of therapy. Heart Rhythm. 2010;7(7):1008-26.
11. Collier R. The ethics of reusing single-use devices. CMAJ. 2011;183(11):1245.
12. Alraies MC, Eckman P. Adult heart transplant: indications and outcomes. J Thorac Dis. 2014;6(8):1120-8.
13. Ladin K. Organ Donation as a collective action problem: ethical considerations and implications for practice. AMA J Ethics. 2016;18(2):156-62.
14. Nagral S. Ethics of organ transplantation. Indian J Med Ethics. 1995;3(5):19-22.

SECTION 15

Future Directions

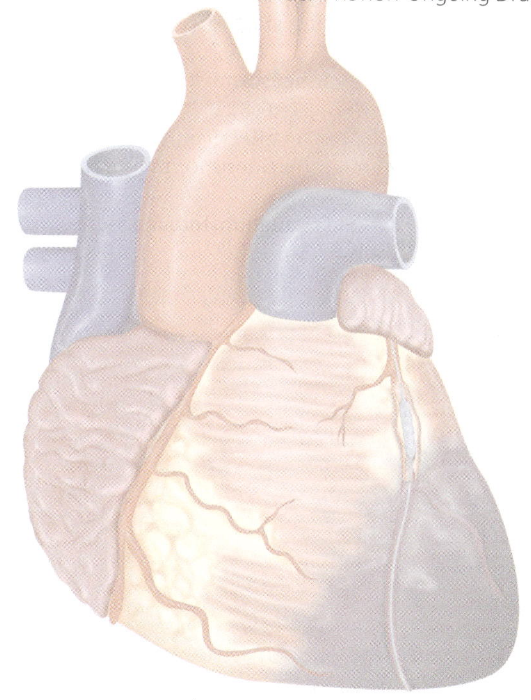

CHAPTER 128

Review Ongoing Drug and Device Trials in HFpEF

Viveka Kumar, Avishek Bagchi, HK Chopra

INTRODUCTION

Heart failure with preserved ejection fraction (HFpEF), also known as diastolic heart failure (DHF), is a clinical entity defined as signs and symptoms of congestive heart failure, in spite of a normal or near normal left ventricular ejection fraction (LVEF ≥50%) and is associated with impaired diastolic function.[1,2] Epidemiologic studies and registries indicate HFpEF accounts for 30–75% of HF cases.[1]

Currently, management of HFpEF is directed toward reducing volume overload, treating coexisting comorbidities, increasing exercise tolerance, educating patients regarding diet and self-care, and managing chronic disease through structured programs.[3] Therapeutic goals include reduction or control of symptoms, prevention of hospitalization and mortality, and improvement in quality of life.[4]

While substantial clinical evidence is available to guide treatment of HFrEF,[4-7] there is minimal evidence-based guidance for the treatment of HFpEF. Clinical trials in HFpEF have been inconclusive, failing to identify therapies that reduce mortality.[8] The neutral outcomes obtained in clinical trials may reflect, at least in part, the phenotypic heterogeneity of HFpEF.

According to the 2013 American College of Cardiology Foundation (ACCF)/American Heart Association (AHA) Guideline for the Management of Heart Failure, Class I recommendations for treating stage C HFpEF include the use of antihypertensive medications to control systolic and diastolic blood pressure and diuretics to relieve symptoms caused by hypervolemia; ClassIIa recommendations include coronary revascularization in patients with coronary artery disease who, despite guideline-directed medical therapy, have symptoms or ischemia; management of atrial fibrillation according to published practice guidelines; and the use of beta-blockers, angiotensin-converting enzyme inhibitors (ACEIs), and angiotensin receptor blockers (ARBs) in patients with hypertension (HTN).[6] In 2017, an update to the 2013 guidelines included a recommendation for a target systolic blood pressure of less than 130 mm Hg for patients with stage C HFpEF and persistent HTN despite management of volume overload.[6] Although limited clinical trial data are available to guide the choice of antihypertensive agent, ACEIs, ARBs, and possibly an angiotensin receptor-neprilysin inhibitor (ARNI), each of which inhibit RAAS, are the preferred choices.[6] While no studies have demonstrated reductions in mortality, use of ARBs may reduce HF hospitalizations.[6,9] The use of aldosterone antagonists may reduce HF hospitalizations in patients with HFpEF with elevated biomarker (i.e. brain natriuretic peptide and N-terminal pro-B-type natriuretic peptide) levels.[1,6,9] A recent meta-analysis that included randomized and non-randomized controlled trials and a pre-post trial suggested exercise training is safe and confers benefits (improved exercise capacity and health-related quality of life) for patients with HFpEF.[10]

EMERGING PHARMACOTHERAPIES FOR HFpEF

Two drug classes with indications for other medical conditions have emerged as potential treatments for HFpEF:

Sodium-glucose cotransporter-2 (SGLT2) inhibitors and combination ARBs/ARNI. Several SGLT2 inhibitors and a first-in-class ARNI are currently under evaluation in late-stage, randomized clinical trials.

Sodium-Glucose Cotransporter-2 Inhibitors

Sodium-glucose cotransporter-2 inhibitors increase urinary glucose excretion by binding to one of two symporters in the kidney nephron, both of which can cotransport glucose and sodium.[11] Four SGLT2 inhibitors—canagliflozin, dapagliflozin, empagliflozin, and ertugliflozin have received approval from the US Food and Drug Administration (FDA) as adjuncts to diet and exercise to improve glycemic control in adults with T2DM.

Evidence for a possible therapeutic role of SGLT2 inhibitors in heart failure prevention or management was provided in RCTs conducted in patients with T2DM. The EMPA-REG OUTCOME (Empagliflozin Cardiovascular Outcomes and Mortality in T2DM),[12] CANVAS (Canagliflozin Cardiovascular Assessment Study),[13] and DECLARE-TIMI 58[14] trial have successfully shown decreased major adverse cardiac events (MACE), the composite of cardiovascular death, nonfatal myocardial infarction, and nonfatal stroke, in diabetics across all risk groups. A meta-analysis of these three trials have demonstrated a moderate reduction (11%) in the risk of MACE that appeared confined to a subset of patients with established atherosclerotic cardiovascular disease and that did not extend to patients with multiple risk factors; in contrast, there were robust reductions in the risk of hospitalization for heart failure (23%) and of progression of renal disease (45%), with these occurring regardless of existing atherosclerotic cardiovascular disease or history of heart failure.[15] The reductions in hospitalization for heart failure that were demonstrated across independent trial programs has led the American Diabetes Association and the European Association for the Study of Diabetes to recommend treatment with SGLT2 inhibitors for patients with T2DM and atherosclerotic disease "in whom HF coexists or is of special concern."[16]

The benefits suggest a class effect that may be applicable across broad populations with T2DM in clinical practice. Interim results from another real-world study [Empagliflozin Comparative Effectiveness and Safety Study (EMPRISE)] indicate empagliflozin was associated with a 44% reduction in relative risk for heart failure hospitalization compared with a glucose-lowering agent in patients with T2DM with and without cardiovascular disease.[17]There are a number of large RCTs which are specifically looking at the effects of SGLT2 inhibition in diabetics with HFpEF. These are summarized in Table 1.

Angiotensin Receptor-Neprilysin Inhibitor

Sacubitril/valsartan represents a first-in-class ARNI combination. As a neprilysin inhibitor, sacubitril augments plasma concentrations of natriuretic peptides [e.g. B-type natriuretic peptide (BNP)] that are involved in the long-term regulation of water and sodium balance and of blood volume and arterial pressure. In addition, sacubitril increases plasma levels of vasodilators such as bradykinin and adrenomedullin but also increases levels of vasoconstrictor peptides, including angiotensin I and II.[18] Coadministration of the ARB valsartan counters vasoconstriction by inhibiting RAAS to reduce blood pressure.[18] The results of a double blind, placebo-controlled RCT (PARADIGM) conducted in patients (N = 8442) with Class II, III, or IV heart failure with ejection fraction ≤40% (i.e., HFrEF) showed sacubitril/valsartan to be superior to enalapril (an ACEI), with significant improvement in the primary endpoint of combined cardiovascular mortality or HF hospitalizations.[19] Following a median follow-up of 27 months, the trial was discontinued, having crossed the threshold for showing overwhelming benefit.[19] Sacubitril/valsartan has received FDA approval and is indicated to reduce the risk of cardiovascular death and hospitalization for heart failure in patients with chronic heart failure [New York Heart Association (NYHA) Class II-IV] and reduced ejection fraction.[6]

For patient with HFpEF, current guidelines recommend sacubitril/valsartan as a possible preferred choice of antihypertensive agent for achieving target systemic blood pressure (<130 mm Hg).[6] This drug decreases sodium and water retention (limiting plasma volume expansion), inhibit the accumulation of inflammatory perivisceral adipose tissue, and has antihypertrophic and antifibrotic effects, which may be of use in treating diastolic dysfunction in HFpEF.[20,21] For patients with HFpEF, the PARAMOUNT study, a phase 2, double-blind, active-controlled proof-of-concept RCT, demonstrated that sacubitril/valsartan treatment was associated with a significantly greater reduction in the level of N-terminal B-type natriuretic peptide (NT-proBNP), a biomarker of left ventricular (LV) wall stress, at 12 weeks than valsartan treatment alone.[22] In addition, significant reduction in left atrial (LA) size and improvement in NYHA HF functional class were noted with sacubitril/valsartan at 36 weeks compared with valsartan alone.[22] Ongoing trials for sacubitril/valsartan in patients with HFpEF are shown in Table 2.

NOVEL DEVICES IN HFpEF (FLOWCHART 1)

All systemic comorbidities involved in HFpEF pathogenesis seem to induce structural cardiac changes (molecular

TABLE 1: SGLT2 inhibitor clinical trials for patients with HFpEF.

Trial/Identifier	*SGLT2 inhibitor*	*Description*
EMPEROR Preserved/ NCT03057951	Empagliflozin	EMPEROR-Preserved, a phase 3 RCT of up to 38 months' duration, is assessing the effect of empagliflozin on long-term morbidity and mortality outcomes in patients (N = 4,126) with chronic HFpEF. The primary outcome measure is the time to first event of composite CV death or HHF. Among secondary endpoints are occurrence of HHF (first and recurrent) and the time to first hospitalization for heart failure. Patients will also be monitored for time of onset of T2DM. The study is expected to be completed in 2020 (2Q).
EMPERIAL Preserved/ NCT03448406	Empagliflozin	EMPERIAL-Preserved, a phase 3 RCT, is evaluating the impact of empagliflozin on exercise ability and HF symptoms in patients (N = 300) with chronic HFpEF, independent of T2DM status. Primary outcomes include the change from baseline to week 12 in exercise capacity, as measured by the distance walked in 6 minutes. Estimated completion date is 2019 (4Q).
EMPA-VISION/ NCT03332212	Empagliflozin	EMPA-Vision is a phase 3 mechanistic RCT of 12 weeks' duration, designed to assess the effect of empagliflozin on cardiac physiology and metabolism; experimental cohorts include patients with HFpEF and patients with HFrEF (N = 86). The primary outcome measure is the change from baseline to week 12 in myocardial creatine phosphate/ adenosine triphosphate ratio in the resting state, as measured using magnetic resonance imaging. The study is expected to be completed in 2019 (4Q).
EMBRACE-HF/ NCT03030222	Empagliflozin	EMBRACE-HF is a phase 4 RCT evaluating the impact of empagliflozin on hemodynamic parameters in patients (N=60) with HF (HFpEF or HFrEF). The primary outcome measure is the change from baseline to end of treatment in pulmonary artery diastolic pressure. The study is scheduled for completion in 2019 (2Q).
PRESERVED-HF/ NCT03030235	Dapagliflozin	PRESERVED-HF is a phase 3 RCT designed to evaluate the effects of dapagliflozin on levels of HF biomarkers (BNP and NT-proBNP), symptoms, health status, quality of life, and echocardiographic parameters in patients with chronic HFpEF (N = 320). The primary outcome measure is the change from baseline in NT-proBNP at weeks 6 and 12; among secondary measures are the changes from baseline to week 12 in the KCCQ summary score and in a 6-minute walk test. The study runs through 2019 (4Q).
DELIVER/ NCT03619213	Dapagliflozin	DELIVER, a phase 3 RCT of up to 33 months' duration, is evaluating whether dapagliflozin, when added to standard of care, reduces CV death or worsening HF in patients with HFpEF (N = 4,700). Primary outcomes include the time to first occurrence of any component of a composite: CV cardiovascular death, HHF, or urgent heart failure visit (outpatient or emergency department). The total number of HHF (first and recurrent) and CV death is a secondary measure. Study completion is expected in 2021 (2Q).
ERADICATE-HF/ NCT03416270	Ertugliflozin	ERADICATE-HF is a phase 2 safety and mechanistic RCT designed to assess how ertugliflozin modifies cardiorenal interactions that regulate fluid volume and neurohormonal activation in patients (N = 36) with T2DM and HF (HFpEF or HFrEF). The primary outcome measure is the difference vs. placebo in proximal sodium reabsorption [acute (week 1) and chronic (week 12)]. The study will be completed in 2021 (1Q).
SOLOIST-WHF/ NCT03521934	Sotagliflozin	SOLOIST-WHF is a phase 3 RCT designed to evaluate mortality and morbidity in hemodynamically stable patients (N = 4,000) (HFrEF and HFpEF) with worsening HF (admitted to a hospital or urgent care visit) with T2DM. Primary measures include the time to first occurrence of either CV death or HHF in patients with HFrEF and in the total population. Study completion is expected in 2021 (1Q).

(BNP: B-type natriuretic peptide; CV: cardiovascular; HF: heart failure; HFpEF: heart failure with preserved ejection fraction; HFrEF: heart failure with reduced ejection fraction; HHF: hospitalization for heart failure; KCCQ: Kansas City Cardiomyopathy Questionnaire; NT-proBNP: N-terminal pro-B type natriuretic peptide; RCT: randomized clinical trial; SGLT2: sodium glucose transporter-2, T2DM: diabetes mellitus)

alteration in cardiomyocytes),[23] myocardial and endothelial inflammation,[24] collagen modification, increased systemic and diastolic ventricular passive stiffness,[25,26] and loss of nitric oxide bioavailability.[24] These molecular and cellular changes translate into biomechanical alterations of cardiac chambers configuration and functioning: Changes

TABLE 2: Sacubitril/valsartan clinical trials for patients with HFpEF.

Trial/identifier	*Description*
PARAGON-HF/ NCT01920711	PARAGON-HF, a multicenter, double-blind, parallel-group, active-controlled phase 3 RCT of up to 57 months' duration, is evaluating the efficacy and safety of sacubitril/valsartan inpatients (N = 4822) with HFpEF. The primary outcome measure is the cumulative number of composite event of CV death and total (first and recurrent) HHF. Secondary outcome measures include the change from baseline to month 8 in: • The clinical summary score of the KCCQ, and • The NYHA functional class. Study completion is expected in 2019 (2Q).
PERSPECTIVE/ NCT02884206	PERSPECTIVE, a multicenter, double-blind, parallel-group, active-controlled phase 3 RCT, is assessing efficacy and safety of sacubitril/valsartan on cognitive function in patients (N = 520) with HFpEF. The primary outcome measure is the change from baseline to week 156 in the CogState Global Cognitive Composite Score. Secondary measures are the change from baseline to week 156 in: • Cortical composite standardized uptake value ratio, • Individual cognitive domains (memory, executive function, and attention), and • Summary score of the instrumental activities of daily living. The study is anticipated to conclude in 2022 (2Q).
PARALLAX/ NCT03066804	PARALLAX, a multicenter, double blind, parallel-group, active-controlled phase 3 RCT, is evaluating the effect of sacubitril/valsartan on NT-proBNP, exercise capacity, symptoms, and safety compared to individualized medical management of comorbidities in patients (N = 2500) with HFpEF. Primary outcome measures are: • The change from baseline to week 12 in NT-proBNP, and • The change from baseline to week 24 in 6-minute walk distance. The trial is expected to be completed in 2019 (4Q).
CNEPi/ NCT03506412	CNEPi, sponsored by the Mayo Clinic in collaboration with the National Institute on Aging, is a proof-of-concept mechanistic phase 4 study for determining efficacy of sacubitril/valsartan in patients (N = 40) with high and low circulating neprilysin levels. The primary outcome measure is the change from baseline to week 5 in biomarkers based on neprilysin levels. Secondary measures are the change from baseline in NT-proANP, NT-proBNP, and NT-proCNP and the change from baseline in plasma cGMP. The study will conclude in 2019 (2Q).

(cGMP: cyclic guanosine monophosphate; CV: cardiovascular; RCT: randomized clinical trial; HFpEF: heart failure with preserved ejection fraction; HHF: hospitalization for heart failure; KCCQ: Kansas City Cardiomyopathy Questionnaire; NT-proANP: N-terminal pro-A type natriuretic peptide: NT-proBNP: N-terminal pro-B type natriuretic peptide; NT-proCNP: N-terminal pro-C type natriuretic peptide; NYHA: New York Heart Association)

in LV geometry and function leading to relaxation and filling impairment, LA remodeling with increase in intra-atrial pressure, inter-atrial dyssynchrony, and changes in systemic and pulmonary vascular compliance.[24] In this context of lack of medical treatment benefits, novel interventional devices and techniques emerged in HFpEF. In each situation, the interventional approach is rather mechanicist, the technique does not target molecular/structural modifications but rather the consequences of those alterations: Increased LA pressure (inter-atrial shunt devices), compromised LV relaxation (LV expanders), or inter-atrial mechanical dyssynchrony (LA pacing).

Inter-atrial Shunt Devices

This concept of creating an iatrogenic inter-atrial shunt was derived from the observation that patients with mitral stenosis and interatrial septal defect (IASD) (Lutembacher syndrome) manifest fewer symptoms compared with patients with mitral stenosis alone.

Currently, there are three devices designed for iatrogenic inter-atrial shunting: V-Wave® (V-Wave Ltd., Or Akiva, Israel), IASD® (DC Devices Inc., Tewksbury, MA, USA), and Atrial flow regulator (Occlutech, Istanbul, Turkey) (AFR).

V-Wave Device

The V-Wave device is an hourglass-shaped nitinol frame covered on the left side with polytetrafluoroethylene polymer and with a trileaflet porcine pericardium valve on the right side to prevent paradoxical embolism and early device closure.[27] This device is implanted through venous femoral access with general anesthesia and transesophageal echocardiography guidance (TEE).

Trials: A first-in-human prospective multicenter single-arm open-label trial assessed the feasibility, safety, and exploratory efficacy of the V-Wave device.[29] The study enrolled eight patients with HF with reduced ejection fraction (HFrEF) and 30 patients with HFpEF, NYHA class III/IV, on guidelines driven maximally tolerated medical and device therapy, with ≥ 1 HF hospitalization in the prior 12 months or elevated NT-proBNP. All patients had the device successfully implanted and 1–2 hospitalization days.

After 1 year, there was significant improvement in the functional status with a decrease in NYHA class in 61% patients ($p < 0.001$), increase in quality of life assessed by KCCQ/MLHFQ (increase with ≥ 5 points) in 74% patients ($p < 0.001$), and an increase in 6-min walk test (6MWT) with 34 min ($p = 0.012$). Also, at 12 months, there was a 2 mm Hg decrease in pulmonary capillary wedge pressure (PCWP) and a minor increase in cardiac index without significant changes in the right-sided cardiac function.[29] Shunt occlusion occurred in 14% of patients (n = 5) after 1 year and 36% of patients had shunt restenosis (n = 13) due to pannus formation in the valve of the device. Patients with permeable shunt were older, had lower glomerular filtration rate, higher PCWP, and had lower exercise tolerance. Also, the patency of the shunt was correlated with a reduced HF hospitalization rate (HR ca. 0.5 vs. 2% $p = 0.008$), a decrease in death, ventricular assist-device implantation, and transplant rate (HR ca. 0.3% vs. 0.6% $p = 0.001$) compared with occluded shunts.[28] Importantly, the primary outcome was device/procedure related major adverse cardiovascular and neurological events (MACNE), defined as death, stroke device embolization, pericardial effusion requiring intervention, reintervention or surgery at 3 and 12 months follow-up. At both 3 and 12 months, the rate of MACNE was 2.6%.[29] At 12 months, the rate of all-cause MACNE was 7.9%, with one patient experiencing nonfatal cardiac tamponade, concluding that the V-Wave system was feasible and safe for HF patients.[29]

Another study enrolled 10 patients with HFrEF NYHA III/IV with LVEF< 40% on optimal medical and device therapy with no evidence of severe right ventricular dysfunction and PCWP > 15 mm Hg.[30] The V-Wave device was successfully implanted in all patients with no procedural complications. At 3 months, NYHA class improved from III to II in 89% of patients and PCWP decreased from 23 to 17 mm Hg with no increase in RAP and mean pulmonary arterial pressure ($p = 0.035$).[30]

A novel trial, RELIEVE-HF, with an estimated enrolment of 500 participants has recently started in September 2018 and is estimated to be completed in 2021 (NCT03499236). It was designed to provide reasonable assurance of safety and effectiveness of the V-Wave device by improving meaningful clinical outcomes in patients with NYHA III/IV irrespective of LVEF, who at baseline are treated with guidelines-directed drug or device therapy[31] (Table 3). To note, all trials designed for V-Wave device were single arm open-label studies.

The Interatrial Septal Defect Device

The IASD device (IASD II, CorviaMedical Inc.) is a bare-metal nitinol frame with an outer diameter of 19 mm which is inserted percutaneously and implanted through atrial transseptal puncture creating an 8 mm shunt. The diameter of the shunt was determined based on predictive hemodynamic modeling which evaluated the relationship between LAP and inter-atrial shunt in humans. The device is flat on the LA side to prevent thrombus formation and curved on the right atrial side to accommodate septal deformations. It is inserted via the femoral vein, with a classic atrial transseptal puncture, under general anesthesia/conscious sedation.[32]

Trials: The first feasibility study of IASD II device was a prospective single-arm single-center study which enrolled 11 patients with HFpEF NYHA III/IV, baseline PCWP ≥ 15 mm Hg at rest, or ≥ 25 mmHg during exercise and ≥ 1 hospitalization for HF within the past 12 months.[22] The device was successfully implanted in all patients with no embolization at echocardiographic evaluation at 1 month. The device was permeable at 1 month in nine patients. The NYHA class improved in seven patients, was worse in one patient and stationary in the remaining. A 50 m increase in 6-MWD (330 vs. 387m, $p = 0.025$) and a better performance in MLWHF score (56 vs. 30, $p = 0.005$) was detected at 1 month. The PCWP decreased significantly (19 vs. 14 mm Hg, baseline vs. 30 days, $p = 0.005$) with no increase in RAP (12 vs. 11 mm Hg, p = NS) and mean pulmonary arterial pressure (30 vs. 27 mm Hg, p = NS).[33]

The Reduce Elevated Left Atrial Pressure in Patients with Heart Failure (REDUCE LAP-HF) study is a multicenter, prospective, nonrandomized, single-arm phase 1 study designed to assess the safety and performance of the IASD in patients with HFpEF with NYHA II-IV despite optimal medical or device therapy.[23] The study enrolled 64 patients with HFpEF, without severe right ventricular dysfunction or pulmonary HTN to receive device insertion after a period of 45 days of screening, and to be reassessed at 6 months. The device was implanted successfully in 97% of patients, in three patients initially being removed because of unsuitable position (n = 2) or a suspected small mobile thrombus in the right atrium (n = 1). However, a second device was deployed in all three patients without incident. No periprocedural or major adverse cardiac or cerebrovascular event, including death, stroke, myocardial infarction, pulmonary or systemic embolism, or need for cardiac surgical intervention for device-related complications were noted during the months of follow-up. At follow-up, all patients with adequate echocardiographic image quality (n = 50) had evidence of left-to-right flow through the device with no right-to-left flow observed.[34]

At 6 months, the quality of life and symptoms of patients improved: Median functional NYHA class decreased by one class in 75% of patients ($p = 0.0001$), mean MLWHF score decreased from 49 to 36 ($p = <0.0001$), mean 6-MWD increased from 313 to 345 m ($p = 0.0023$), and supine

TABLE 3: Future trials of novel interventional devices for HFpEF.

Device	Manufacturer	Condition	Title	Primary outcome	No. of patients	Design
V-Wave	V-Wave Ltd., Or Akiva, Israel	HFpEF, HFrEF	RELIEVE-HF	Safety—percentage of treatment patients experiencing MACNE during the first 30 days Effectiveness—hierarchical composite of death, heart transplant or LVAD, HF hospitalizations, and changes in 6MWDT	500	Prospective, multicenter randomized, patient and observer blinded clinical study
IASD II	Corvia Medical Inc.	HFpEF	REDUCE LAP II	Composite of: • Incidence of and time to cardiovascular mortality or first nonfatal, ischemic stroke in12 months • Total rate per patient year of HF. Changes in baseline KCCQ total summary score	608	Prospective, multicenter, randomized, blinded trial with a nonimplant control group
AFR	Occlutech, Istanbul, Turkey	HFpEF, HFrEF	PRELIEVE	Incidence of SADE: • Device dislocation/ embolization • Damage to the tricuspid or mitral valve • Intractable arrhythmias caused by the device • Any circumstance that requires device removal	30	Prospective, nonrandomized, pilot study
Corolla	CorAssist Cardiovascular Ltd.	HFpEF	CORolla® TAA for heart failure with preserved ejection fraction (HFpEF) and diastolic dysfunction (DD)	• All-cause mortality and SAE after months • Implantation Rating Questionnaire	10	Prospective, single-group, nonrandomized

(6MWDT: 6-min walking distance test; HFpEF: heart failure with preserved ejection fraction; HF: heart failure; HFrEF: heart failure with reduced ejection fraction; KCCQ: Kansas city cardiomyopathy questionnaire score; LVAD: left ventricular assist device; MACCE: major adverse cardiac and cerebrovascular events rate; MACNE: major adverse cardiovascular and neurological events; SADE: serious adverse device effects; SAE: serious adverse event)

exercise duration at the time of right heart catheterization increased from 7.3 to 8.2 min (p = 0.0275). Also, there was a consistent improvement in hemodynamic parameters: Reduction of PCWP at rest in 52% of patients (n = 32) and reduced PCWP measured by right heart catheterization during supine bicycle exercise in 58% of patients (n = 34), and 39% (n = 23) fulfilled both of these criteria, with no significant increase in RAP (9 vs. 11 mm Hg, p = 0.0270), or deterioration of right ventricular function (TAPSE at baseline 20 vs. 6 months 20 mm, p = 0.97). It also noted a consistent reduction of heart failure rehospitalization from 20% (n = 13) to 14% (n =9), with no mean reduction of diuretic dose (mean difference between baseline and 6 months of 0 mg) during the 6 months follow-up. Because there was no difference in the treatment regimen, it was unlikely that medical treatment accounted for the recorded reduction of HF rehospitalization.[34]

In 2016, David M. Kaye et al. published 1-year outcomes after REDUCE LAP-HF study with particular regard to device safety and performance, and the persistence of clinical and hemodynamic effects.[35] The exercise protocol was as previously used, and to account the hemodynamic effect of differences in workload, corrected workload PCWP was calculated as previously described. Echocardiographic evaluation revealed the presence of left-to-right shunting at 12 months postdevice implantation in all patients with adequate image quality (n = 48), with unchanged EF, minor increase in right ventricle ejection fraction (59–65%), modest reduction in LV end-diastolic volume index (69–60 mL/m^2) with concomitant rise in right ventricle end-diastolic index (23–30 mL/m^2). Serial hemodynamic measurements from right side catheterization at 12 months revealed: no improvement in PCWP at rest (16 ± vs. 17 ± 6 mm Hg), and during exercise (33 ± 9 vs. 33 ± 10 mm Hg) with minor increase in right-sided cardiac output at rest (6.3 ± 1.4 L/min vs. 6.7 ± 1.8 L/min), and increase in left-sided cardiac output at rest (4.9 ± 1.5 L/min vs. 5.8 ± 1.5 L/min) compared with the 6 months follow-up. Also at 12 months, there was sustained significant improvement in NYHA class, MLWHF score and 6-MWD test compared with baseline, but no improvement compared with the 6 months follow-up.[35]

Recently, REDUCE LAP-HF I, a phase 2 randomized, parallel-group, blinded multicenter sham-controlled trial evaluated IASD in patients with HFpEF, and published the short-term results.[36] 94 patients with HF NYHA III/IV were enrolled under optimal medical or device treatment with LVEF > 40%, exercise PCWP > 25 mm Hg, and PCWP right atrial pressure gradient > 5 mm Hg to be randomized 1:1 to implantation of IASD device vs. a sham procedure (femoral venous access with intracardiac echocardiography but no IASD placement). The device was successfully implanted in 21 patients of 22 (in one patient, the device could not be placed due to an occluded inferior vena cava filter).[36] No subsequent adverse cardiac, cerebrovascular, and renal events occurred at 1 month. There was no significant decrease in NYHA class or rehospitalization for HF in the IASD group compared with the sham group and baseline after 1 month. There was a significant decrease in exercise PCWP in the IASD group compared with baseline (–3.2 ± 5.2 mm Hg at low workload—20 W and –2.3 ± 4.9 mm Hg at high workload—60 W) and no significant improvement in exercise PCWP in the sham group (0.9 ± 5.1 mm Hg at 20 W and –1.3 ± 4.9 mm Hg at 60 W). There was no significant increase in right atrial pressure at rest and mean pulmonary arterial pressure at rest in the IASD group compared with baseline and control group (p = 0.0673 and p = 0.111). The major limitation of the study is the small period of follow-up and was not powered up to assess clinical endpoints.[36] Three novel trials evaluating IASD device are being planned: Reduce LAP-HF II, Reduce LAP-HF III, and Reduce LAP-HFrEF (Table 3). The first one is a randomized, controlled, blinded trial with a nonimplant control group with 1:1 randomization which will enroll almost 600 patients with HF NYHA III/IV with LVEF over 40% on guideline medical or device therapy.[37] The primary outcome is cardiovascular mortality, ischemic stroke, total rate per patient year of heart failure admissions, and change in baseline KCCQ total summary score at 12 months. The trial is due to be completed in 2024.

Reduce LAP HFrEF is a nonrandomized feasibility trial which will enroll 10 patients with HF with EF <40% with elevated LAP who remain symptomatic despite guideline medical or device therapy.[38] The study will assess the successful device implantation, the permeability of the device at 6 months, and the incidence of major adverse cardiac and cerebrovascular events at 6 months, and is due to be completed in 2024.

Atrial Flow Regulator

The atrial flow regulator (AFR) is a self-expandable double-disk wired mesh with a central penetration that enables inter-atrial shunting. The device is implanted percutaneously via the femoral vein with standard transseptal function and positioned similarly to atrial septal defect occluder devices. It is available in 6, 8, 10-mm fenestration diameters and 1, 24, 30-mm total device diameter.[39,40]

Trials: The first use of AFR was for severe pulmonary HTN based on the fact that atrial septostomy relieves syncope, improves heart filling, cardiac output, and systemic oxygen transport despite hypoxia.[40] Due to the success of the IASD devices in the past decade, the spectrum of indications for AFR extended to HFpEF patients.[39]

Currently, PRELIEVE trial aims to investigate the safety and efficacy of the AFR in patients with HFrEF and HFpEF, with an estimated completion date in 2019.[41]

Left Ventricular Expanders

Left ventricular expanders are devices that aim to improve LV compliance through direct internal or external expansion forces distributed on the LV walls during diastole.[39] Currently, there are two devices made: CORolla® and ImCardia®.

CORolla Assist Device

Interventional procedure CORolla (CorAssist Inc., Haifa, Israel) is an elastic self-expanding device inserted percutaneously (or transfemural) and attached to the endocardium. The device enhances LV diastolic expansion, improves LV filling, and lowers LVEDP and LAP.[42]

Trials: Preclinical studies demonstrated safety and efficacy.[43] The first-in-man procedure was performed in 2013 in a patient with severe aortic stenosis requiring surgery and

Flowchart 1: Physiopathological classification of novel interventional therapies in HFpEF.

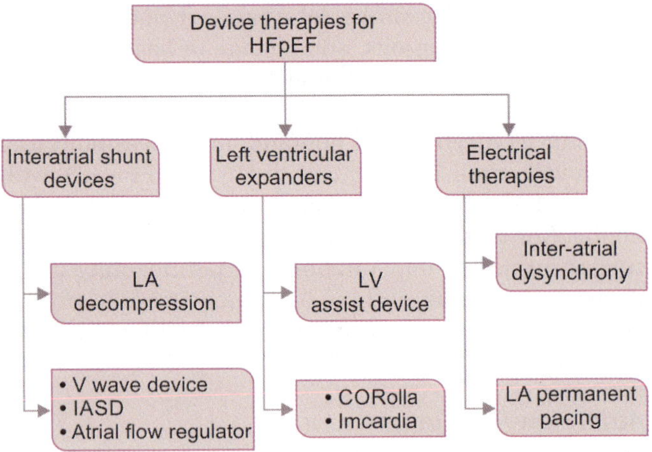

(HFpEF: heart failure with preserved ejection fraction; LA: left atrium; LV: left ventricle)

type IV diastolic dysfunction.[44] The device was surgically implanted. At 6 months follow-up, there was a significant improvement in LV mass, LA indexed volume, and a consistent regression of diastolic dysfunction (from type IV to type I) suggesting a good hemodynamic performance and safety of the device. In 2017, the device was percutaneously inserted (transapical) at RAMBAM Medical Center with the same consistent LV remodeling improvement at 6 months. An ongoing trial (NCT02499601) enrolling 10 patients aims to demonstrate the safety and feasibility of the device during12 months follow-up in patients with HFpEF with NYHA III/IV (Table 3).[45]

ImCardia

ImCardia (CorAssist Inc., Haifa, Israel) is an elastic self-expanding device attached on the epicardial surface of the left ventricle. The device is inserted surgically through an off-pump procedure in patients undergoing surgery for aortic valvular disease.[46]

Trials: Krucoff et al. conducted a study in which 10 patients with severe aortic stenosis underwent surgical treatment concomitant with ImCardia insertion.[46] There were no improvements in NYHA class and 6-MWT at 1 year, but there was a significant LV mass regression (–126 g ± 33 g) and LA area decrease (–2.29 cm^2 ± 3.09 cm^2). The trial was terminated with the conclusion that the device needs further improvement.

Electrical Therapy in HFpEF

Left atrial permanent pacing for atrial dyssynchrony Syndrome

A novel theory suggests that atrial electrical dyssynchrony and LA dysfunction may be the missing key in the physiopathology of HFpEF.[47] Left atrial pacing (coronary sinus pacing) was firstly developed for the management of atrial tachyarrhythmias and it was recently developed for atrial resynchronization in HFpEF patients.[48] The procedure requires a specially designed coronary sinus (CS) lead, with a double 45° angulation at its distal end, ensuring very close contact with the upper wall of the CS.[49] For optimal threshold pacing voltage, the lead can be positioned from the middle to the distal part of CS.

Trials: Recent echocardiographic studies suggest that HFpEF patients present with an increased intra-atrial dyssynchrony and reduced LA diastolic and systolic function compared with normal patients.[50] Furthermore, there is an independent correlation between the severity of the dyssynchrony and reduced LA systolic function with NYHA class >II in patients with HFpEF.[51,52] A study conducted in 2013 by Laurent et al. presented atrial dyssynchrony syndrome as inter-atrial conduction delay (ADS) (P wave duration > 120ms in D II), short left atrioventricular interval (< 70 ms), and increased LA stiffness.[53] The study evaluated the implantation of a lead put inside the coronary sinus for active vs. inactive LA pacing in six patients with HFpEF NYHA III/IV under optimal medical treatment. After 3 months of pacing, there was significant improvement in 6-MWDT (240 ± 25 m vs. 190 ± 15 m, $P < 0.05$), mitral A wave duration was longer (104 ± 8 vs.158 ± 25 ms, $P = 0.002$) and E/A and E/e' ratio was smaller (3.4 ± 1.3 vs. 1.8 ± 0.9, $P = 0.009$, and 22.6 ± 4.6 vs. 15.3 ±4.3, $P = 0.006$, respectively). Importantly, after the inactivation of pacing for 1 week, there was a significant reduction in 6-MWDT with an on/off response. This novel beneficial effect of LA permanent pacing opens a new perspective for the electrical therapy in HfpEF.[53]

Cardiac Contractility Modulation

Cardiac contraction modulation (CCM) is a pacemaker-like therapy that applies nonexcitatory electrical signals (biphasic high-voltage bipolar) to the right ventricular septum during the absolute refractory period. This concept was developed for symptomatic patients with HFrEF with slightly prolonged QRS interval not eligible for CRT therapy.[54] Currently, there are nearly 3,000 devices (Optimizer Smart, Optimizer III, Optimizer IV from Impulse Dynamics) implanted worldwide.[55]

Trials: The benefits of CCM therapy were mostly studied in HFrEF patients.[56] Few studies promise good safety and feasibility with increasing exercise tolerance and symptoms improvement in HFpEF.[57,58] An ongoing trial evaluates the efficacy and safety of CCM therapy in HFpEF patients who have NYHA Class II or III symptoms despite appropriate medication (for potential expansion of the CE Mark indication for use in the HFpEF population).[59]

CONCLUSION

HFpEF is a common and severe condition, with devastating mortality and morbidity rate. Because there are few effective treatments and minimal evidence-based guidance, management of HFpEF is directed toward reducing volume overload, controlling blood pressure, and treating comorbidities. Improving exercise tolerance and managing chronic disease through structured care programs and initiatives promoting health and wellness literacy are also recommended. Reduction or control of symptoms, improvement in quality of life, and prevention of hospitalization and premature death are chief aims of therapy; however, no completed studies to date have demonstrated reductions in mortality.

The failure of medical therapy to improve symptoms in HFpEF gave rise to interventional approaches, based on the subsequent pathophysiology of the disease. Given the recently approached strategies, artificial inter-atrial shunting developed the most, being the only devices tested in a phase 3 trial.[36] Although IASD devices are recently introduced, long-term safety needs to be proven.

The exact duration of antithrombotic therapy needs to be established. Currently, IASD II requires 1-year double antiplatelet therapy, V-Wave requires oral anticoagulation and aspirin for 3 months and AFR requires 6–12 months double antiplatelet therapy. A low dose of aspirin is required in all the devices indefinitely.

Other long-term consideration should be the development of atrial tachyarrhythmias, incidence of cryptogenic stroke, and volume overload of right-sided chambers. LV expanders are a novel approach on HFpEF with positive short-term results but the devices need to be further refined to a standardized technical approach. Two mechanical assist devices were used in HFpEF setting to pump blood from either LA[60] or LV into arterial system. Both studies showed (at least in theory) that these devices could improve hemodynamics in HFpEF patients by increasing the total stroke volume and decompressing LA/LV cavities.

New long-term trials are required in order to prove the benefits, safety, and feasibility of these devices.

REFERENCES

1. Harper AR, Patel HC, Lyon AR. Heart failure with preserved ejection fraction. Clin Med (Lond). 2018;18(Suppl 2): s24 s29.
2. McHugh K, DeVore AD, Wu J, et al. Heart failure with preserved ejection fraction and diabetes: JACC state-of-the-art review. J Am Coll Cardiol. 2019;73(5):602-11.
3. Redfield MM. Heart failure with preserved ejection fraction. New Engl J Med. 2016;375(19):1868-77.
4. Yancy CW, Jessup M, Bozkurt B, et al. 2013 ACCF/AHA guideline for the management of heart failure: executive summary: a report of the American College of Cardiology Foundation/American Heart Association Task Force on Practice Guidelines. Circulation. 2013;128(16):1810-52.
5. Yancy CW, Jessup M, Bozkurt B, et al. 2016 ACC/AHA/HFSA focused update on new pharmacological therapy for heart failure: an update of the 2013 ACCF/AHA Guideline for the Management of Heart Failure: a report of the American College of Cardiology/American Heart Association Task Force on Clinical Practice Guidelines and the Heart Failure Society of America. Circulation. 2016;134(13):e282-e293.
6. Yancy CW, Jessup M, Bozkurt B, et al. 2017 ACC/AHA/HFSA focused update of the 2013 ACCF/AHA guideline for the management of heart failure: a report of the American College of Cardiology/American Heart Association Task Force on Clinical Practice Guidelines and the Heart Failure Society of America. Circulation. 2017;136(6):e137-e161.
7. Yancy CW, Januzzi JL, Allen LA, et al. 2017 ACC expert consensus decision pathway for optimization of heart failure treatment: answers to 10 pivotal issues about heart failure with reduced ejection fraction. J Am Coll Cardiol 2018;71(2):201-30.
8. Martin N, Manoharan K, Thomas J, et al. Beta-blockers and inhibitors of the renin-angiotensin aldosterone system for chronic heart failure with preserved ejection fraction. Cochrane Database Syst Rev. 2018;6:CD012721.
9. Bozkurt B. What is new in heart failure management in 2017? Update on ACC/AHA heart failure guidelines. Curr Cardiol Rep. 2018;20(6):39.
10. Taylor RS, Davies EJ, Dalal HM, et al. Effects of exercise training for heart failure with preserved ejection fraction: a systematic review and meta-analysis of comparative studies. Int J Cardiol. 2012;162(1):6-13.
11. Baar MJB, van Ruiten CC, Muskiet MHA, et al. SGLT2 inhibitors in combination therapy: from mechanisms to clinical considerations in type 2 diabetes management. Diabetes Care. 2018;41(8):1543-56.
12. Zinman B, Wanner C, Lachin JM, et al. Empagliflozin, cardiovascular outcomes, and mortality in type 2 diabetes. N Engl J Med. 2015;373(22):2117-28.
13. Radholm K, Figtree G, Perkovic V, et al. Canagliflozin and heart failure in type 2 diabetes mellitus. Circulation. 2018;138(5):458-68.
14. Wiviott SD, Raz I, Bonaca MP, et al. Dapagliflozin and cardiovascular outcomes in type 2 diabetes. N Engl J Med. 2019;380(4):347-57.
15. Zelniker TA, Wiviott SD, Raz I, et al. SGLT-2 inhibitors for primary and secondary prevention of cardiovascular and renal outcomes in type 2 diabetes: a systematic review and meta-analysis of cardiovascular outcome trials. Lancet. 2019;393(10166):31-9.

16. Davies MJ, D'Alessio DA, Fradkin J, et al. Management of hyperglycemia in type 2 diabetes, 2018. A consensus report by the American Diabetes Association (ADA) and the European Association for the Study of Diabetes (EASD). Diabetes Care. 2018;41(12):2669-701.
17. Boehringer Ingelheim. Initial results from EMPRISE real-world evidence study show Jardiance was associated with reduced risk for hospitalization for heart failure compared with DPP-4 inhibitors in people with type 2 diabetes with and without cardiovascular disease. [online] Available from https://www.boehringer-ingelheim.us/press-release/initial-results-emprise-real-world-evidence-study-showjardiance-was-associated. [Last accessed November, 2019].
18. Gori M, D'Elia E, Senni M. Sacubitril/valsartan therapeutic strategy in HFpEF: Clinical insights and perspectives. Int J Cardiol. 2019;281:158-65.
19. McMurray JJV, Packer M, Desai AS, et al. Angiotensin-neprilysin inhibition versus enalapril in heart failure. N Engl J Med. 2014;371(11):993-1004.
20. Zouein FA, de Castro Bras LE, da Costa DV, et al. Heart failure with preserved ejection fraction: emerging drug strategies. J Cardiovasc Pharmacol. 2013;62(1):13-21.
21. Shah SJ, Kitzman DW, Borlaug BA, et al. Phenotype-specific treatment of heart failure with preserved ejection fraction: a multiorgan roadmap. Circulation. 2016;143(1):73-90.
22. Solomon SD, Zile M, Pieske B, et al. The angiotensin neprilysin inhibitor LCZ696 in heart failure with preserved ejection fraction: a phase 2 double-blind randomised controlled trial. Lancet. 2012;380(9851):1387-95.
23. van Heerebeek L, Borbely A, Niessen HW, et al. Myocardial structure and function differ in systolic and diastolic heart failure. Circulation. 2006;113(16):1966-73.
24. Paulus WJ, Tschope C. A novel paradigm for heart failure with preserved ejection fraction: comorbidities drive myocardial dysfunction and remodeling through coronary microvascular endothelial inflammation. J Am Coll Cardiol. 2013;62(4):263-71.
25. Zile MR, Baicu CF, Gaasch WH. Diastolic heart failure–abnormalities in active relaxation and passive stiffness of the left ventricle. N Engl J Med. 2004;350(19):1953-9.
26. Westermann D, Kasner M, Steendijk P, et al. Role of left ventricular stiffness in heart failure with normal ejection fraction. Circulation. 2008;117(16):2051-60.
27. Amat-Santos IJ, Nombela-Franco L, Garcia B, et al. The V-Wave device for the treatment of heart failure. Initial experience in Europe. Rev Esp Cardiol. 2015;68(9):808-10.
28. Rodes-Cabau J, Bernier M, Amat-Santos IJ, et al. Interatrial shunting for heart failure: early and late results from the first-in-human experience with the V-Wave system. JACC Cardiovasc Interv. 2018;11(22):2300-10.
29. Del Trigo M, Bergeron S, Bernier M, et al. Unidirectional left-to-right interatrial shunting for treatment of patients with heart failure with reduced ejection fraction: a safety and proof-of principle cohort study. Lancet. 2016;387(10025): P1290-1297.
30. ClinicalTrials.gov. Reducing Lung CongestIon Symptoms in Advanced Heart Failure (RELIEVE-HF). [online] Available from https://clinicaltrials.gov/ct2/show/NCT03499236. [Last accessed November, 2019].
31. Kaye D, Shah SJ, Borlaug BA, et al. Effects of an interatrial shunt on rest and exercise hemodynamics: results of a computer simulation in heart failure. J Card Fail. 2014;20(3):212-21.
32. Sondergaard L, Reddy V, Kaye D, et al. Transcatheter treatment of heart failure with preserved or mildly reduced ejection fraction using a novel interatrial implant to lower left atrial pressure. Eur J Heart Fail. 2014;16(7):796-801.
33. Hasenfuss G, Hayward C, Burkhoff D, et al. A transcatheter intracardiac shunt device for heart failure with preserved ejection fraction (REDUCE LAP-HF): a multicentre, open-label, single-arm, phase 1 trial. Lancet. 2016;387(10025): 1298-1304.
34. Kaye DM, Hasenfuß G, Neuzil P, et al. One-year outcomes after transcatheter insertion of an interatrial shunt device for the management of heart failure with preserved ejection fraction. Circ Heart Fail. 2016;9(12).
35. Feldman T, Mauri L, Kahwash R, et al. Transcatheter interatrial shunt device for the treatment of heart failure with preserved ejection fraction [REDUCE LAP-HF I (Reduce Elevated Left Atrial Pressure in patients With Heart Failure)]: a phase 2, randomized, sham controlled trial. Circulation. 2018;137(4):364-75.
36. Clinicaltrials.gov. Reduce Lap-HF Trial II (REDUCELAPHF II). [online] Available from https://clinicaltrials.gov/ct2/show/NCT03088033. [Last accessed November, 2019].
37. ClinicalTrials.gov. REDUCE LAP-HFREF TRIAL. [online] Available from https://clinicaltrials.gov/ct2/show/NCT03093961. [Last accessed November, 2019].
38. Patel MB, Samuel BP, Girgis RE, et al. Implantable atrial flow regulator for severe, irreversible pulmonary arterial hypertension. Eurointervention. 2015;11(6):706-9.
39. Gupta A, Bailey SR. Update on devices for diastolic dysfunction: options for a no option condition? Curr Cardiol Rep. 2018;20(10):85.
40. ClinicalTrials.gov. The Prelieve trial-pilot study to assess safety and efficacy of a novel atrial flow regulator (AFR) in heart failure patients (PRELIEVE). [online] Available from https://clinicaltrials.gov/ct2/show/NCT03030274. [Last accessed November, 2019].
41. Snowden TD. (2010) Reversing heart failure: diastolic recoil in a proposed cardiac support device. [online] Available from http://oaktrust.library.tamu.edu/bitstream/handle/1969.1/154367/Snowden12.pdf?sequence=1&isAllowed=y. [Last accessed November, 2019].
42. M K Heart Failure With Preserved EFx: Corassist. In: TCT 2012, San Francisco (2012)
43. A E (2013) First in man implantation of intra-ventricular device for diastolic heart failure. TCT 2013, San Francisco
44. ClinicalTrials.gov. (2015) CORolla® TAA for heart failure with preserved ejection fraction (HFpEF) and diastolic dysfunction (DD). [online] Available from https://clinicaltrials.gov/ct2/show/NCT02499601. [Last accessed November, 2019].

45. TCT-481: Diastolic heart failure–innovative extra and intraventricular solutions. J Am Coll Cardiol. 2011;58(20 Supplement):B131.
46. Morris DA, Gailani M, Vaz Perez A, et al. Left atrial systolic and diastolic dysfunction in heart failure with normal left ventricular ejection fraction. J Am Soc Echocardiogr. 2011;24(6):651-62.
47. Maass AH, Van Gelder IC. Atrial resynchronization therapy: a new concept for treatment of heart failure with preserved ejection fraction and prevention of atrial fibrillation? Eur J Heart Fail. 2012;14(3):227-9.
48. Daubert C, Leclercq C, Le Breton H, et al. Permanent left atrial pacing with a specifically designed coronary sinus lead. Pacing Clin Electrophysiol. 1997;20(11):2755-64.
49. Sanchis L, Vannini L, Gabrielli L, et al. Interatrial Dyssynchrony may contribute to heart failure symptoms in patients with reserved ejection fraction. Echocardiography. 2015;32(11):1655-61.
50. Liu S, Guan Z, Zheng X, et al. Impaired left atrial systolic function and interatrial dyssynchrony may contribute to symptoms of heart failure with preserved left ventricular ejection fraction: a comprehensive assessment by echocardiography. Int J Cardiol. 2018;257:177-81.
51. Eicher JC, Laurent G, Mathe A, et al. Atrial dyssynchrony syndrome: an overlooked phenomenon and a potential cause of "diastolic" heart failure. Eur J Heart Fail. 2012;14(3):248-58.
52. Laurent G, Eicher JC, Mathe A, et al. Permanent left atrial pacing therapy may improve symptoms in heart failure patients with preserved ejection fraction and atrial dyssynchrony: a pilot study prior to a national clinical research programme. Eur J Heart Fail. 2013;15(1):85-93.
53. Kleemann T. Cardiac contractility modulation. A new form of therapy for patients with heart failure and narrow QRS complex? Herz. 2015;40(7):945-51.
54. Abi-Samra F, Gutterman D. Cardiac contractility modulation: a novel approach for the treatment of heart failure. Heart Fail Rev. 2016;21(6):645-60.
55. Pappone C, Augello G, Rosanio S, et al. First human chronic experience with cardiac contractility modulation by nonexcitatory electrical currents for treating systolic heart failure: mid-term safety and efficacy results from a multicenter study. J Cardiovasc Electrophysiol. 2004;15(4):418-27.
56. Tschope C, Van Linthout S, Spillmann F, et al. Cardiac contractility modulation signals improve exercise intolerance and maladaptive regulation of cardiac key proteins for systolic and diastolic function in HFpEF. Int J Cardiol. 2016;203:1061-6.
57. Borggrefe M, Mann DL. Cardiac contractility modulation in 2018. Circulation. 2018;138(24):2738-40.
58. ClinicalTrials.gov. (2017) CCM in heart failure with preserved ejection fraction (CCM-HFpEF). [online] Available from https://clinicaltrials.gov/ct2/show/NCT03240237?titles=CCM+HFPEF&rank=1. [Last accessed November 2019].
59. Burkhoff D, Maurer MS, Joseph SM, et al. Left atrial decompression pump for severe heart failure with preserved ejection fraction: theoretical and clinical considerations. JACC Heart Fail. 2015;3(4):275-82.
60. Granegger M, Dave H, Knirsch W, et al. A valveless pulsatile pump for the treatment of heart failure with preserved ejection fraction: a simulation study. Cardiovasc Eng Technol. 2018;10:69-79.

Index

Page numbers followed by *b* refer to box, *f* refer to figure, *fc* refer to flow chart, and *t* refer to table.

D

I

L